Wilson and
Gisvold's Textbook of

ORGANIC MEDICINAL AND PHARMACEUTICAL CHEMISTRY

E L E V E N T H   E D I T I O N

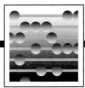

*Wilson and
Gisvold's Textbook of*

ORGANIC MEDICINAL
AND PHARMACEUTICAL
CHEMISTRY

E L E V E N T H   E D I T I O N

Edited by

John H. Block, Ph.D., R.Ph.
Professor of Medicinal Chemistry
Department of Pharmaceutical Sciences
College of Pharmacy
Oregon State University
Corvallis, Oregon

John M. Beale, Jr., Ph.D.
Associate Professor of Medicinal Chemistry and
Director of Pharmaceutical Sciences
St. Louis College of Pharmacy
St. Louis, Missouri

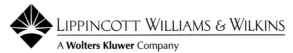

LIPPINCOTT WILLIAMS & WILKINS
A **Wolters Kluwer** Company
Philadelphia · Baltimore · New York · London
Buenos Aires · Hong Kong · Sydney · Tokyo

Editor: David B. Troy
Managing Editor: Matthew J. Hauber
Marketing Manager: Samantha S. Smith
Production Editor: Bill Cady
Designer: Doug Smock
Compositor: Maryland Composition
Printer: Quebecor World

351 West Camden Street
Baltimore, MD 21201

530 Walnut Street
Philadelphia, PA 19106

Printed in the United States of America

First Edition, 1949	Fifth Edition, 1966	Eighth Edition, 1982
Second Edition, 1954	Sixth Edition, 1971	Ninth Edition, 1991
Third Edition, 1956	Seventh Edition, 1977	Tenth Edition, 1998
Fourth Edition, 1962		

Library of Congress Cataloging-in-Publication Data
Wilson and Gisvold's textbook of organic medicinal and pharmaceutical chemistry.—11th
  ed. / edited by John H. Block, John M. Beale Jr.
     p. ; cm.
  Includes bibliographical references and index.
  ISBN 0-7817-3481-9
  1. Pharmaceutical chemistry. 2. Chemistry, Organic. I. Title: Textbook of organic medicinal
and pharmaceutical chemistry. II. Wilson, Charles Owens, 1911–2002 III. Gisvold, Ole,
1904– IV. Block, John H. V. Beale, John Marlowe.
    [DNLM: 1. Chemistry, Pharmaceutical. 2. Chemistry, Organic. QV 744 W754 2004]
  RS403. T43 2004
  615′.19—dc21
                                               2003048849

To purchase additional copies of this book, call our customer service department at **(800) 638-3030** or fax orders to **(301) 824-7390**. International customers should call **(301) 714-2324**.

Visit Lippincott Williams & Wilkins on the Internet: http:// www.LWW.com. Lippincott Williams & Wilkins customer service representatives are available from 8:30 am to 6:00 pm, EST.

03 04 05 06 07
1 2 3 4 5 6 7 8 9 10

The Eleventh Edition of Wilson and Gisvold's Textbook of Organic and Medicinal Pharmaceutical Chemistry *is dedicated to the memory of Jaime N. Delgado and Charles O. Wilson*

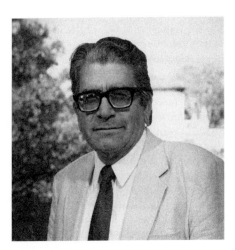

**Jaime N. Delgado
1932–2001**

Professor Jaime N. Delgado served as coeditor for the ninth and tenth editions and was continuing in this role before his death on October 5, 2001. Dr. Delgado studied with Ole Gisvold, one of the two founding editors of this textbook, and he was dedicated to maintaining the standards of excellence established by Gisvold and his coeditor Charles Wilson. He loved teaching medicinal chemistry to students, and this textbook was a powerful aid to him.

A graduate of the University of Texas at Austin and the University of Minnesota, Jaime Delgado began his teaching career as an assistant professor at the University of Texas College of Pharmacy in 1959. He rose through the academic ranks to become professor and head of the Division of Medicinal Chemistry and a leader in research and graduate education. He essentially built both the graduate program and the Division from scratch, and his publication of research and scholarly works brought national recognition to the department.

Although Jaime Delgado became known for his research and scholarship, his first love and his greatest legacy were in teaching and advising undergraduate and graduate students. The University of Texas at Austin awarded him five major teaching awards, and recognized him two times as one of its "best" professors. In 1997, he was elected to the Academy of Distinguished Teachers at the university and was honored as a Distinguished Teaching Professor, a permanent academic title. Former dean James Doluisio described Dr. Delgado's teaching style as "owning the classroom" because of his knowledge, communication skills, and deep conviction that pharmacy is a science-based profession. His enthusiasm and extemporaneous use of the chalkboard were legendary. In addition to his contributions to teaching at the University of Texas, Dr. Delgado traveled extensively in Mexico and South America to present lectures on pharmaceutical education.

Jaime Delgado's first contributions to the *Textbook of Organic Medicinal and Pharmaceutical Chemistry* were made as a chapter author in the seventh and eighth editions. Much of the material he presented came from his lecture notes. Although he was proud of these contributions, which were expanded in the ninth and tenth editions, he considered his role as coeditor in the latter editions one of the highlights of his distinguished career. Jaime was a true gentleman and a pleasure to have as a collaborator. He will be greatly missed by the editors, authors, and professional staff for the *Textbook*.

William A. Remers

Charles O. Wilson
1911–2002

As the chapters for the eleventh edition were being sent to the publisher, I was notified that my colleague and friend, Charles Wilson, had died shortly after Christmas. He was a product of the Pacific Northwest having received all of his degrees from the University of Washington. His first teaching job was at the now discontinued pharmacy school at George Washington University and then he moved to the University of Minnesota. Charles, along with other medicinal chemistry faculty at the University of Minnesota, saw the need for textbooks that presented modern medicinal chemistry. In 1949, he and Professor Ole Gisvold edited *Organic Chemistry in Pharmacy*, which became the first edition of the *Textbook of Medicinal and Pharmaceutical Chemistry*. Continuing in this tradition, Charles and Professor Taito Soine assumed the authorship of *Roger's Inorganic Pharmaceutical Chemistry*, which included eight editions before its discontinuance. Finally, Charles and Professor Tony Jones started the *American Drug Index* series. Charles continued his publishing activities after moving to the University of Texas and then assumed the position of Dean of Oregon State University's School of Pharmacy, where he oversaw a major expansion of its faculty and physical plant.

Although a medicinal chemist, Charles devoted considerable time to his chosen pharmacy profession, students, and community. Charles was an active member of the American Pharmaceutical Association as well as the pharmacy associations in each state where he lived. In addition, he was a registered pharmacist in each state where he taught: Washington, Minnesota, Texas, Oregon, and the District of Columbia. Charles chaired national committees and sections of the American Pharmaceutical Association and the American Association of Colleges of Pharmacy. Related to these, his loyalty to students included organizing student branches of the American Pharmaceutical Association at George Washington University, the University of Minnesota, and the University of Texas. He was actively involved in the local American Red Cross blood program and took the lead in developing the hugely successful student centered blood drives at Oregon State University. In 1960, Charles and his wife, Vaughn, helped launch the AFS (American Field Service) in Corvallis, an international high-school exchange program. He volunteered for Meals on Wheels for over 30 years after his retirement.

We certainly miss this fine gentleman and leader of pharmacy education and the pharmacy profession.

John H. Block

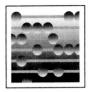

PREFACE

For almost six decades, *Wilson and Gisvold's Textbook of Organic Medicinal and Pharmaceutical Chemistry* has been a standard in the literature of medicinal chemistry. Generations of students and faculty have depended on this textbook not only for undergraduate courses in medicinal chemistry but also as a supplement for graduate studies. Moreover, students in other health sciences have found certain chapters useful at one time or another. The current editors and authors worked on the eleventh edition with the objective of continuing the tradition of a modern textbook for undergraduate students and also for graduate students who need a general review of medicinal chemistry. Because the chapters include a blend of chemical and pharmacological principles necessary for understanding structure–activity relationships and molecular mechanisms of drug action, the book should be useful in supporting courses in medicinal chemistry and in complementing pharmacology courses.

It is our goal that the eleventh edition follow in the footsteps of the tenth edition and reflect the dynamic changes occurring in medicinal chemistry. Recognizing that the search for new drugs involves both synthesis and screening of large numbers of compounds, there is a new chapter on combinatorial chemistry that includes a discussion on how the process is automated. The power of mainframe computing now is on the medicinal chemist's desk. A new chapter describes techniques of molecular modeling and computational chemistry. With a significant percentage of the general population purchasing alternative medicines, there is a new chapter on herbal medicines that describes the chemical content of many of these products.

The previous edition had new chapters on drug latentiation and prodrugs, immunizing biologicals, diagnostic imaging agents, and biotechnology. Expansion of chapters from the tenth edition includes the antiviral chapter that contains the newest drugs that have changed the way HIV is treated. Dramatic progress in the application of molecular biology to the production of pharmaceutical agents has produced such important molecules as modified human insulins, granulocyte colony-stimulating factors, erythro-poietins, and interferons, all products of cloned and, sometimes, modified human genes. The chapter on biotechnology describes these exciting applications. Recent advances in understanding the immune system at the molecular level have led to new agents that suppress or modify the immune response, producing new treatments for autoimmune diseases including rheumatoid arthritis, Crohn's disease, and multiple sclerosis. Techniques of genetic engineering now allow the preparation of pure surface antigens as vaccines while totally eliminating the pathogenic organisms from which they are derived.

The editors welcome the new contributors to the eleventh edition: Doug Henry, Phillip Bowen, Stephen J. Cutler, T. Kent Walsh, Philip Proteau, and Michael J. Deimling. The editors extend thanks to all of the authors who have cooperated in the preparation of the current edition. Collectively, the authors represent many years of teaching and research experience in medicinal chemistry. Their chapters include summaries of current research trends that lead the reader to the original literature. Documentation and references continue to be an important feature of the book.

We continue to be indebted to Professors Charles O. Wilson and Ole Gisvold, the originators of the book and editors of five editions, Professor Robert Doerge, who joined Professors Wilson and Gisvold for the sixth and seventh editions and single-handedly edited the eighth edition, and Professors Jaime Delgado and William Remers who edited the ninth and tenth editions. They and the authors have contributed significantly to the education of countless pharmacists, medicinal chemists, and other pharmaceutical scientists.

John H. Block
John M. Beale, Jr.

1st	1949	Wilson and Gisvold (*Organic Chemistry in Pharmacy*)	6th	1971	Wilson, Gisvold, and Doerge
2nd	1954	Wilson and Gisvold	7th	1977	Wilson, Gisvold, and Doerge
3rd	1956	Wilson	8th	1982	Doerge
4th	1962	Wilson and Gisvold	9th	1991	Delgado and Remers
5th	1966	Wilson	10th	1998	Delgado and Remers

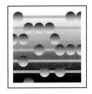

CONTRIBUTORS

JOHN M. BEALE, JR., PH.D.
Associate Professor of Medicinal
  Chemistry and Director of
  Pharmaceutical Sciences
St. Louis College of Pharmacy
St. Louis, Missouri

JOHN H. BLOCK, PH.D., R.PH.
Professor of Medicinal Chemistry
Department of Pharmaceutical
  Sciences
College of Pharmacy
Oregon State University
Corvallis, Oregon

J. PHILLIP BOWEN, PH.D.
Professor of Chemistry and
Director, Center for Biomolecular
  Structure and Dynamics
Computational Chemistry Building
Cedar Street
University of Georgia
Athens, Georgia

C. RANDALL CLARK, PH.D.
Professor of Medicinal Chemistry
Department of Pharmacal Sciences
School of Pharmacy
Auburn University
Auburn, Alabama

GEORGE H. COCOLAS, PH.D.
Professor of Medicinal Chemistry and
  Associate Dean
School of Pharmacy
University of North Carolina at
  Chapel Hill
Chapel Hill, North Carolina

HORACE G. CUTLER, PH.D.
Senior Research Professor
Director of the Natural Products
  Discovery Group
Southern School of Pharmacy
Mercer University
Atlanta, Georgia

STEPHEN J. CUTLER, PH.D.
Professor of Medicinal Chemistry
School of Pharmacy
Mercer University
Atlanta, Georgia

MICHAEL J. DEIMLING, R.PH., PH.D.
Professor of Pharmacology and Chair
Department of Pharmaceutical
  Sciences
School of Pharmacy
Southwestern Oklahoma State
  University
Weatherford, Oklahoma

JACK DERUITER, PH.D.
Professor of Medicinal Chemistry
Department of Pharmacal Sciences
School of Pharmacy
Auburn University
Auburn, Alabama

JACK N. HALL, M.S., R.PH., BCNP
Clinical Lecturer
Department of Radiology/Nuclear
  Medicine
College of Medicine, University of
  Arizona
University of Arizona Health
  Sciences Center
Tucson, Arizona

DOUGLAS R. HENRY
Advisory Scientist
MDL Information Systems, Inc.
San Leandro, California

THOMAS J. HOLMES, JR., PH.D.
Associate Professor
School of Pharmacy
Campbell University
Buies Creek, North Carolina

TIM B. HUNTER, M.D.
Vice-Chairman and Professor
Department of Radiology
University of Arizona
Tucson, Arizona

EUGENE I. ISAACSON, PH.D.
Professor Emeritus of Medicinal
  Chemistry
Department of Pharmaceutical
  Sciences
College of Pharmacy
Idaho State University
Pocatello, Idaho

RODNEY L. JOHNSON, PH.D.
Professor of Medicinal Chemistry
Department of Medicinal
  Chemistry
University of Minnesota
Minneapolis, Minnesota

DANIEL A. KOECHEL, PH.D.
Professor Emeritus—Pharmacology
Department of Pharmacology
Medical College of Ohio
Toledo, Ohio

GUSTAVO R. ORTEGA, R.PH., PH.D.
Professor of Medicinal Chemistry
Department of Pharmaceutical
  Sciences
School of Pharmacy
Southwestern Oklahoma State
  University
Weatherford, Oklahoma

PHILIP J. PROTEAU, PH.D.
Associate Professor of Medicinal
  Chemistry
College of Pharmacy
Oregon State University
Corvallis, Oregon

WILLIAM A. REMERS, PH.D.
Professor Emeritus
Pharmacology and Toxicology
University of Arizona
Tucson, Arizona

THOMAS N. RILEY, PH.D.
Professor of Medicinal Chemistry
Department of Pharmacal Sciences
School of Pharmacy
Auburn University
Auburn, Alabama

FORREST T. SMITH, PH.D.
Associate Professor
Department of Pharmacal Sciences
School of Pharmacy
Auburn University
Auburn, Alabama

GARETH THOMAS, PH.D.
Associate Senior Lecturer
The School of Pharmacy and
    Biomedical Sciences
University of Portsmouth
Portsmouth, England

T. KENT WALSH, D.O.
Director
Nuclear Medicine Program
Southern Arizona V.A. Health Care
    System
Tucson, Arizona

**ROBERT E. WILLETTE,
PH.D.**
President
Duo Research, Inc.
Denver, Colorado

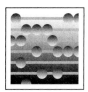

CONTENTS

CHAPTER 1

Introduction

JOHN H. BLOCK AND JOHN M. BEALE, JR.

The discipline of medicinal chemistry is devoted to the discovery and development of new agents for treating diseases. Most of this activity is directed to new natural or synthetic organic compounds. Inorganic compounds continue to be important in therapy, e.g., trace elements in nutritional therapy, antacids, and radiopharmaceuticals, but organic molecules with increasingly specific pharmacological activities are clearly dominant. Development of organic compounds has grown beyond traditional synthetic methods. It now includes the exciting new field of biotechnology using the cell's biochemistry to synthesize new compounds. Techniques ranging from recombinant DNA and site-directed mutagenesis to fusion of cell lines have greatly broadened the possibilities for new entities that treat disease. The pharmacist now dispenses modified human insulins that provide more convenient dosing schedules, cell-stimulating factors that have changed the dosing regimens for chemotherapy, humanized monoclonal antibodies that target specific tissues, and fused receptors that intercept immune cell–generated cytokines.

This book treats many aspects of organic medicinals: how they are discovered, how they act, and how they developed into clinical agents. The process of establishing a new pharmaceutical is exceedingly complex and involves the talents of people from a variety of disciplines, including chemistry, biochemistry, molecular biology, physiology, pharmacology, pharmaceutics, and medicine. Medicinal chemistry, itself, is concerned mainly with the organic, analytical, and biochemical aspects of this process, but the chemist must interact productively with those in other disciplines. Thus, medicinal chemistry occupies a strategic position at the interface of chemistry and biology.

To provide an understanding of the principles of medicinal chemistry, it is necessary to consider the physicochemical properties used to develop new pharmacologically active compounds and their mechanisms of action, the drug's metabolism including possible biological activities of the metabolites, the importance of stereochemistry in drug design, and the methods used to determine what "space" a drug occupies. All of the principles discussed in this book are based on fundamental organic chemistry, physical chemistry, and biochemistry.

The earliest drug discoveries were made by random sampling of higher plants. Some of this sampling, although based on anecdotal evidence, led to the use of such crude plant drugs as opium, belladonna, and ephedrine that have been important for centuries. With the accidental discovery of penicillin came the screening of microorganisms and the large number of antibiotics from bacterial and fungal sources. Many of these antibiotics provided the prototypical structure that the medicinal chemist modified to obtain antibacterial drugs with better therapeutic profiles. With the changes in federal legislation reducing the efficacy requirement for "nutriceutical," the public increasingly is using so-called nontraditional or alternative medicinals that are sold over the counter, many outside of traditional pharmacy distribution channels. It is important for the pharmacist and the public to understand the rigor that is required for prescription-only and FDA-approved nonprescription products to be approved relative to the nontraditional products. It also is important for all people in the health care field and the public to realize that whether these nontraditional products are effective as claimed or not, many of the alternate medicines contain pharmacologically active agents that can potentiate or interfere with physician-prescribed therapy.

Hundreds of thousands of new organic chemicals are prepared annually throughout the world, and many of them are entered into pharmacological screens to determine whether they have useful biological activity. This process of random screening has been considered inefficient, but it has resulted in the identification of new lead compounds whose structures have been optimized to produce clinical agents. Sometimes, a lead develops by careful observation of the pharmacological behavior of an existing drug. The discovery that amantadine protects and treats early influenza A came from a general screen for antiviral agents. The use of amantadine in long-term care facilities showed that it also could be used to treat parkinsonian disorders. More recently, automated high-throughput screening systems utilizing cell culture systems with linked enzyme assays and receptor molecules derived from gene cloning have greatly increased the efficiency of random screening. It is now practical to screen enormous libraries of peptides and nucleic acids obtained from combinatorial chemistry procedures.

Rational design, the opposite approach to high-volume screening, is also flourishing. Significant advances in x-ray crystallography and nuclear magnetic resonance have made it possible to obtain detailed representations of enzymes and other drug receptors. The techniques of molecular graphics and computational chemistry have provided novel chemical structures that have led to new drugs with potent medicinal activities. Development of HIV protease inhibitors and angiotensin-converting enzyme (ACE) inhibitors came from an understanding of the geometry and chemical character of the respective enzyme's active site. Even if the receptor structure is not known in detail, rational approaches based on the physicochemical properties of lead compounds can provide new drugs. For example, the development of cimetidine as an antinuclear drug involved a careful study of the changes in antagonism of H_2-histamine receptors induced by varying the physical properties of structures based on histamine. Statistical methods based on the correlation of physicochemical properties with biological potency are used to explain and optimize biological activity.

As you proceed through the chapters, think of what problem the medicinal chemist is trying to solve. Why were certain structures selected? What modifications were made to produce more focused activity or reduce adverse reactions or produce better pharmaceutical properties? Was the prototypical molecule discovered from random screens, or did the medicinal chemist have a structural concept of the receptor or an understanding of the disease process that must be interrupted?

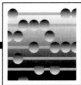

Physicochemical Properties in Relation to Biological Action

JOHN H. BLOCK

Modern drug design, compared with the classical approach—*let's make a change on an existing compound or synthesize a new structure and see what happens*—continues to evolve rapidly as an approach to solving a drug design problem. The combination of increasing power and decreasing cost of desktop computing has had a major impact on solving drug design problems. While drug design increasingly is based on modern computational chemical techniques, it also uses sophisticated knowledge of disease mechanisms and receptor properties. A good understanding of how the drug is transported into the body, distributed throughout the body compartments, metabolically altered by the liver and other organs, and excreted from the patient is required along with the structural characteristics of the receptor. Acid–base chemistry is used to aid in formulation and biodistribution. Structural attributes and substituent patterns responsible for optimum pharmacological activity can often be predicted by statistical techniques such as regression analysis. Computerized conformational analysis permits the medicinal chemist to predict the drug's three-dimensional shape that is *seen* by the receptor. With the isolation and structural determination of specific receptors and the availability of computer software that can estimate the three-dimensional shape of the receptor, it is possible to design molecules that will show an optimum fit to the receptor.

OVERVIEW

A drug is a chemical molecule. Following introduction into the body, a drug must pass through many barriers, survive alternate sites of attachment and storage, and avoid significant metabolic destruction before it reaches the site of action, usually a receptor on or in a cell (Fig. 2-1). At the receptor, the following equilibrium (Rx. 2-1) usually holds:

Drug + Receptor ⇌ Drug-Receptor Complex
↓
Pharmacologic Response

(Rx. 2-1)

The ideal drug molecule will show favorable binding characteristics to the receptor, and the equilibrium will lie to the right. At the same time, the drug will be expected to dissociate from the receptor and reenter the systemic circulation to be excreted. Major exceptions include the alkylating agents used in cancer chemotherapy (see Chapter 12), a few inhibitors of the enzyme acetylcholinesterase (see Chapter 17), suicide inhibitors of monoamine oxidase (see Chapter 14), and the aromatase inhibitors 4-hydroxyandrostenedione and exemestane (see Chapter 23). These pharmacological agents form covalent bonds with the receptor, usually an enzyme's active site. In these cases, the cell must destroy the receptor or enzyme, or, in the case of the alkylating agents, the cell would be replaced, ideally with a normal cell. In other words, the usual use of drugs in medical treatment calls for the drug's effect to last for a finite period of time. Then, if it is to be repeated, the drug will be administered again. If the patient does not tolerate the drug well, it is even more important that the agent dissociate from the receptor and be excreted from the body.

DRUG DISTRIBUTION

Oral Administration

An examination of the *obstacle course* (Fig. 2-1) faced by the drug will give a better understanding of what is involved in developing a commercially feasible product. Assume that the drug is administered orally. The drug must go into solution to pass through the gastrointestinal mucosa. Even drugs administered as true solutions may not remain in solution as they enter the acidic stomach and then pass into the alkaline intestinal tract. (This is explained further in the discussion on acid–base chemistry.) The ability of the drug to dissolve is governed by several factors, including its chemical structure, variation in particle size and particle surface area, nature of the crystal form, type of tablet coating, and type of tablet matrix. By varying the dosage form and physical characteristics of the drug, it is possible to have a drug dissolve quickly or slowly, with the latter being the situation for many of the sustained-action products. An example is orally administered sodium phenytoin, with which variation of both the crystal form and tablet adjuvants can significantly alter the bioavailability of this drug widely used in the treatment of epilepsy.

Chemical modification is also used to a limited extent to facilitate a drug reaching its desired target (see Chapter 5). An example is olsalazine, used in the treatment of ulcerative colitis. This drug is a dimer of the pharmacologically active mesalamine (5-aminosalicylic acid). The latter is not effective orally because it is metabolized to inactive forms

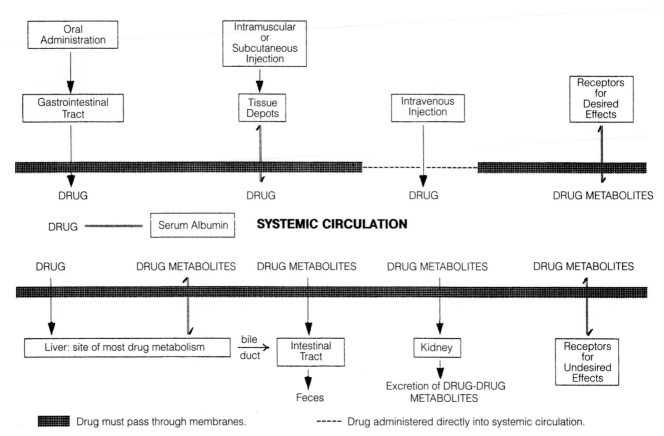

Figure 2-1 ■ Summary of drug distribution.

before reaching the colon. The dimeric form passes through a significant portion of the intestinal tract before being cleaved by the intestinal bacteria to two equivalents of mesalamine.

Olsalazine

Mesalamine

As illustrated by olsalazine, any compound passing through the gastrointestinal tract will encounter a large number and variety of digestive and bacterial enzymes, which, in theory, can degrade the drug molecule. In practice, a new drug entity under investigation will likely be dropped from further consideration if it cannot survive in the intestinal tract or its oral bioavailability is low, necessitating parenteral dosage forms only. An exception would be a drug for which there is no effective alternative or which is more effective than existing products and can be administered by an alternate route, including parenteral, buccal, or transdermal.

In contrast, these same digestive enzymes can be used to advantage. Chloramphenicol is water soluble enough (2.5 mg/mL) to come in contact with the taste receptors on the tongue, producing an unpalatable bitterness. To mask this intense bitter taste, the palmitic acid moiety is added as an ester of chloramphenicol's primary alcohol. This reduces the parent drug's water solubility (1.05 mg/mL) enough so that it can be formulated as a suspension that passes over the bitter taste receptors on the tongue. Once in the intestinal tract, the ester linkage is hydrolyzed by the digestive esterases to the active antibiotic chloramphenicol and the very common dietary fatty acid palmitic acid.

Chloramphenicol: R = H
Chloramphenicol Palmitate: R = CO(CH₂)₁₄CH₃

Olsalazine and chloramphenicol palmitate are examples of *prodrugs*. Most prodrugs are compounds that are inactive in their native form but are easily metabolized to the active agent. Olsalazine and chloramphenicol palmitate are examples of prodrugs that are cleaved to smaller compounds, one of which is the active drug. Others are metabolic precursors to the active form. An example of this type of prodrug is menadione, a simple naphthoquinone that is converted in the liver to phytonadione (vitamin $K_{2(20)}$).

Menadione

Phytonadione (Vitamin $K_{2(20)}$)

Occasionally, the prodrug approach is used to enhance the absorption of a drug that is poorly absorbed from the gastrointestinal tract. Enalapril is the ethyl ester of enalaprilic acid, an active inhibitor of angiotensin-converting enzyme (ACE). The ester prodrug is much more readily absorbed orally than the pharmacologically active carboxylic acid.

Enalapril: R = C_2H_5
Enalaprilic Acid: R = H

Unless the drug is intended to act locally in the gastrointestinal tract, it will have to pass through the gastrointestinal mucosal barrier into venous circulation to reach the site of the receptor. The drug's route involves distribution or partitioning between the aqueous environment of the gastrointestinal tract, the lipid bilayer cell membrane of the mucosal cells, possibly the aqueous interior of the mucosal cells, the lipid bilayer membranes on the venous side of the gastrointestinal tract, and the aqueous environment of venous circulation. Some very lipid-soluble drugs may follow the route of dietary lipids by becoming part of the mixed micelles, incorporating into the chylomicrons in the mucosal cells into the lymph ducts, servicing the intestines, and finally entering venous circulation via the thoracic duct.

The drug's passage through the mucosal cells can be passive or active. As is discussed below in this chapter, the lipid membranes are very complex with a highly ordered structure. Part of this membrane is a series of channels or tunnels that form, disappear, and reform. There are receptors that move compounds into the cell by a process called *pinocytosis*. Drugs that resemble a normal metabolic precursor or intermediate may be actively transported into the cell by the same system that transports the endogenous compound. On the other hand, most drug molecules are too large to enter the cell by an active transport mechanism through the

passages. The latter, many times, pass into the patient's circulatory system by passive diffusion.

Parenteral Administration

Many times there will be therapeutic advantages to bypassing the intestinal barrier by using parenteral (injectable) dosage forms. This is common in patients who, because of illness, cannot tolerate or are incapable of accepting drugs orally. Some drugs are so rapidly and completely metabolized to inactive products in the liver (first-pass effect) that oral administration is precluded. But that does not mean that the drug administered by injection is not confronted by obstacles (Fig. 2-1). Intravenous administration places the drug directly into the circulatory system, where it will be rapidly distributed throughout the body, including tissue depots and the liver, where most biotransformations occur (see below), in addition to the receptors. Subcutaneous and intramuscular injections slow distribution of the drug because it must diffuse from the site of injection into systemic circulation.

It is possible to inject the drug directly into specific organs or areas of the body. Intraspinal and intracerebral routes will place the drug directly into the spinal fluid or brain, respectively. This bypasses a specialized epithelial tissue, the blood–brain barrier, which protects the brain from exposure to a large number of metabolites and chemicals. The blood–brain barrier is composed of membranes of tightly joined epithelial cells lining the cerebral capillaries. The net result is that the brain is not exposed to the same variety of compounds that other organs are. Local anesthetics are examples of administration of a drug directly onto the desired nerve. A spinal block is a form of anesthesia performed by injecting a local anesthetic directly into the spinal cord at a specific location to block transmission along specific neurons.

Most of the injections a patient will experience in a lifetime will be subcutaneous or intramuscular. These parenteral routes produce a depot in the tissues (Fig. 2-1), from which the drug must reach the blood or lymph. Once in systemic circulation, the drug will undergo the same distributive phenomena as orally and intravenously administered agents before reaching the target receptor. In general, the same factors that control the drug's passage through the gastrointestinal mucosa will also determine the rate of movement out of the tissue depot.

The prodrug approach described above also can be used to alter the solubility characteristics, which, in turn, can increase the flexibility in formulating dosage forms. The solubility of methylprednisolone can be altered from essentially water-insoluble methylprednisolone acetate to slightly water-insoluble methylprednisolone to water-soluble methylprednisolone sodium succinate. The water-soluble sodium hemisuccinate salt is used in oral, intravenous, and intramuscular dosage forms. Methylprednisolone itself is normally found in tablets. The acetate ester is found in topical ointments and sterile aqueous suspensions for intramuscular injection. Both the succinate and acetate esters are hydrolyzed to the active methylprednisolone by the patient's own systemic hydrolytic enzymes (esterases).

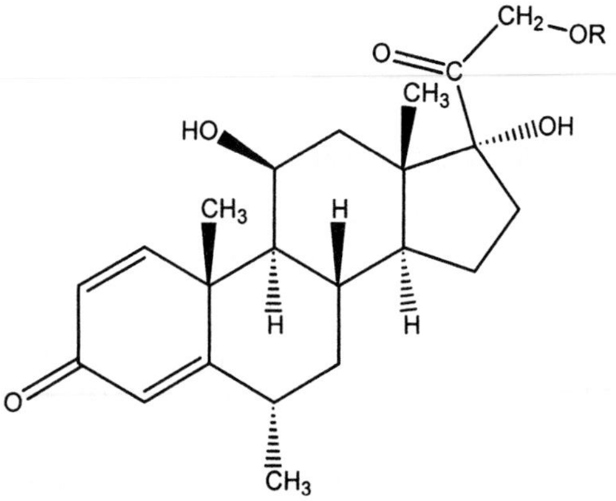

Methylprednisolone: R = H
Methylprednisolone Acetate: R = C(=O)CH₃
Methylprednisolone Sodium Succinate: R = C(=O)CH₂CH₂COO⁻ Na⁺

Another example of how prodrug design can significantly alter biodistribution and biological half-life is illustrated by two drugs based on the retinoic acid structure used systemically to treat psoriasis, a nonmalignant hyperplasia. Etretinate has a 120-day "terminal" half-life after 6 months of therapy. In contrast, the active metabolite, acitretin, has a 33- to 96-hour "terminal" half-life. Both drugs are potentially teratogenic. Female patients of childbearing age must sign statements that they are aware of the risks and usually are administered a pregnancy test before a prescription is issued. Acitretin, with its shorter half-life, is recommended for a female patient who would like to become pregnant, because it can clear her body within a reasonable time frame. When effective, etretinate can keep a patient clear of psoriasis lesions for several months.

Protein Binding

Once the drug enters the systemic circulation (Fig. 2-1), it can undergo several events. It may stay in solution, but many drugs will be bound to the serum proteins, usually albumin (Rx. 2-2). Thus a new equilibrium must be considered. Depending on the equilibrium constant, the drug can remain in systemic circulation bound to albumin for a considerable period and not be available to the sites of biotransformation, the pharmacological receptors, and excretion.

$$\text{Drug } + \text{ Albumin} \rightleftharpoons \text{Drug-Albumin Complex} \qquad \text{(Rx. 2-2)}$$

Protein binding can have a profound effect on the drug's effective solubility, biodistribution, half-life in the body, and interaction with other drugs. A drug with such poor water solubility that therapeutic concentrations of the unbound (active) drug normally cannot be maintained still can be a very effective agent. The albumin–drug complex acts as a reservoir by providing large enough concentrations of free drug to cause a pharmacological response at the receptor.

Protein binding may also limit access to certain body compartments. The placenta is able to block passage of proteins from maternal to fetal circulation. Thus, drugs that normally would be expected to cross the placental barrier and possibly harm the fetus are retained in the maternal circulation, bound to the mother's serum proteins.

Protein binding also can prolong the drug's duration of action. The drug–protein complex is too large to pass through the renal glomerular membranes, preventing rapid excretion of the drug. Protein binding limits the amount of drug available for biotransformation (see below and Chapter 4) and for interaction with specific receptor sites. For example, the large, polar trypanocide suramin remains in the body

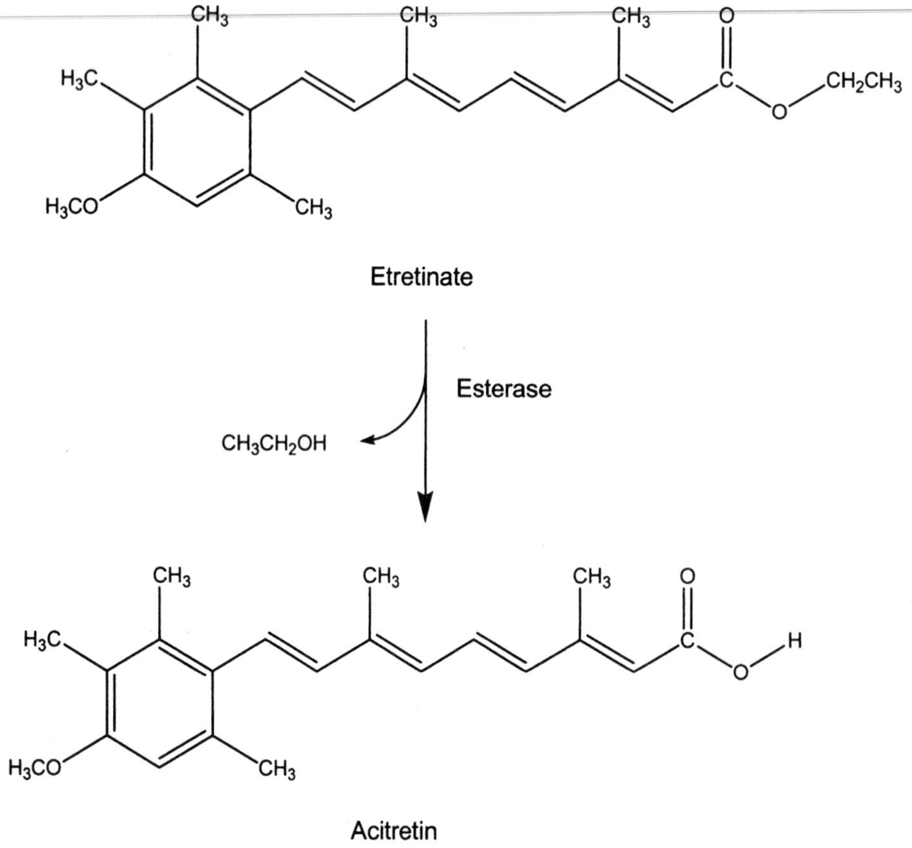

Etretinate

Esterase

CH₃CH₂OH

Acitretin

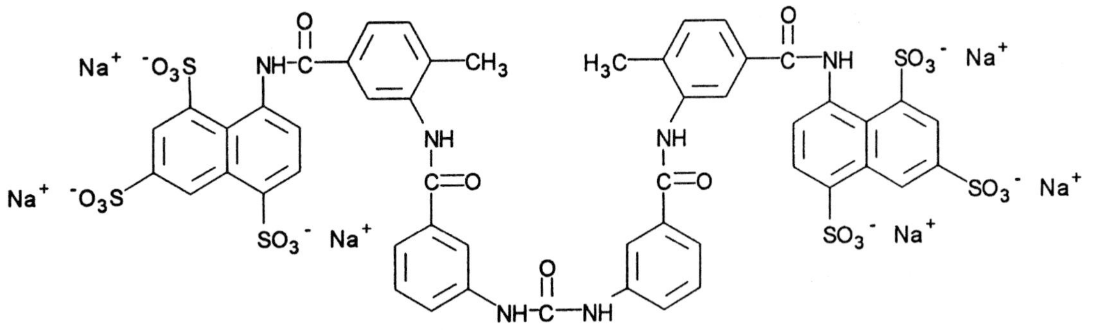

Suramin Sodium

in the protein-bound form for as long as 3 months ($t_{1/2}$ = 50 days). The maintenance dose for this drug is based on weekly administration. At first, this might seem to be an advantage to the patient. It can be, but it also means that, should the patient have serious adverse reactions, a significant length of time will be required before the concentration of drug falls below toxic levels.

The drug–protein binding phenomenon can lead to some clinically significant drug–drug interactions resulting when one drug displaces another from the binding site on albumin. A large number of drugs can displace the anticoagulant warfarin from its albumin-binding sites. This increases the effective concentration of warfarin at the receptor, leading to an increased prothrombin time (increased time for clot formation) and potential hemorrhage.

Tissue Depots

The drug can also be stored in tissue depots. Neutral fat constitutes some 20 to 50% of body weight and constitutes a depot of considerable importance. The more lipophilic the drug, the more likely it will concentrate in these pharmacologically inert depots. The ultra-short-acting, lipophilic barbiturate thiopental's concentration rapidly decreases below its effective concentration following administration. It "disappears" into tissue protein, redistributes into body fat, and then slowly diffuses back out of the tissue depots but in concentrations too low for a pharmacological response. Thus, only the initially administered thiopental is present in high enough concentrations to combine with its receptors. The remaining thiopental diffuses out of the tissue depots into systemic circulation in concentrations too small to be effective (Fig. 2-1), is metabolized in the liver, and is excreted.

In general, structural changes in the barbiturate series (see Chapter 14) that favor partitioning into the lipid tissue stores decrease duration of action but increase central nervous system (CNS) depression. Conversely, the barbiturates with the slowest onset of action and longest duration of action contain the more polar side chains. This latter group of barbiturates both enters and leaves the CNS more slowly than the more lipophilic thiopental.

Drug Metabolism

All substances in the circulatory system, including drugs, metabolites, and nutrients, will pass through the liver. Most molecules absorbed from the gastrointestinal tract enter the portal vein and are initially transported to the liver. A significant proportion of a drug will partition or be transported into the hepatocyte, where it may be metabolized by hepatic enzymes to inactive chemicals during the initial trip through the liver, by what is known as the first-pass effect (see Chapter 4).

Lidocaine is a classic example of the significance of the first-pass effect. Over 60% of this local anesthetic antiarrhythmic agent is metabolized during its initial passage through the liver, resulting in it being impractical to administer orally. When used for cardiac arrhythmias, it is administered intravenously. This rapid metabolism of lidocaine is used to advantage when stabilizing a patient with cardiac arrhythmias. Should too much lidocaine be administered intravenously, toxic responses will tend to decrease because of rapid biotransformation to inactive metabolites. An understanding of the metabolic labile site on lidocaine led to the development of the primary amine analogue tocainide. In contrast to lidocaine's half-life of less than 2 hours, tocainide's half-life is approximately 15 hours, with 40% of the drug excreted unchanged. The development of orally active antiarrhythmic agents is discussed in more detail in Chapter 19.

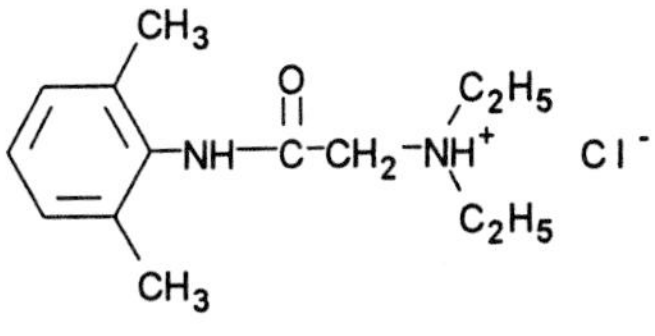

Lidocaine

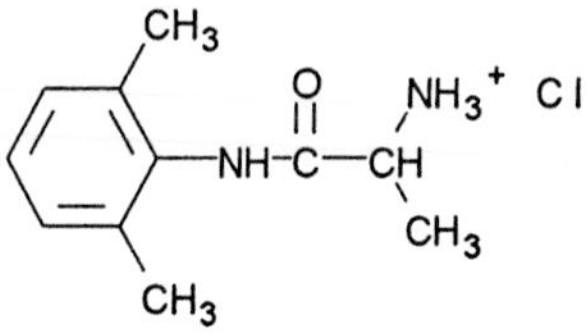

Tocainide

A study of the metabolic fate of a drug is required for all new drug products. Often it is found that the metabolites are also active. Indeed, sometimes the metabolite is the pharmacologically active molecule. These drug metabolites can provide leads for additional investigations of potentially new products. Examples of an inactive parent drug that is converted to an active metabolite include the nonsteroidal anti-inflammatory agent sulindac being reduced to the active sulfide metabolite; the immunosuppressant azathioprine being cleaved to the purine antimetabolite 6-mercaptopurine; and purine and pyrimidine antimetabolites and antiviral agents being conjugated to their nucleotide form (acyclovir phosphorylated to acyclovir triphosphate). Often both the parent drug and its metabolite are active, which has led to additional commercial products, instead of just one being marketed. About 75 to 80% of phenacetin (now withdrawn from the U. S. market) is converted to acetaminophen. In the tricyclic antidepressant series (see Chapter 14), imipramine and amitriptyline are N-demethylated to desipramine and nortriptyline, respectively. All four compounds have been marketed in the United States. Drug metabolism is discussed more fully in Chapter 4.

Sulindac: R = CH₃S(=O)

Active Sulfide Metabolite: R = CH₃S

Azathioprine   6-Mercaptopurine

Acyclovir: R = H

Acyclovir triphosphate: R = O-P-O-P-O-P

Phenacetin: R = OC₂H₅

Acetaminophen: R = OH

Amitriptyline: R = CH₃
Nortriptyline: R = H

Imipramine: R = CH₃
Desipramine: R = H

Although a drug's metabolism can be a source of frustration for the medicinal chemist, pharmacist, and physician and lead to inconvenience and compliance problems with the patient, it is fortunate that the body has the ability to metabolize foreign molecules (xenobiotics). Otherwise, many of these substances could remain in the body for years. This has been the complaint against certain lipophilic chemical pollutants, including the once very popular insecticide DDT. After entering the body, these chemicals reside in body tissues, slowly diffusing out of the depots and potentially harming the individual on a chronic basis for several years. They can also reside in tissues of commercial food animals that have been slaughtered before the drug has "washed out" of the body.

Excretion

The main route of excretion of a drug and its metabolites is through the kidney. For some drugs, enterohepatic circulation (Fig. 2-1), in which the drug reenters the intestinal tract from the liver through the bile duct, can be an important part of the agent's distribution in the body and route of excretion. Either the drug or drug metabolite can reenter systemic circulation by passing once again through the intestinal mucosa. A portion of either also may be excreted in the feces. Nursing mothers must be concerned because drugs and their metabolites can be excreted in human milk and be ingested by the nursing infant.

One should keep a sense of perspective when learning about drug metabolism. As explained in Chapter 4, drug metabolism can be conceptualized as occurring in two stages or phases. Intermediate metabolites that are pharmacologically active usually are produced by phase I reactions. The products from the phase I chemistry are converted into inactive, usually water-soluble end products by phase II reactions. The latter, commonly called *conjugation* reactions, can be thought of as synthetic reactions that involve addition of water-soluble substituents. In human drug metabolism, the main conjugation reactions add glucuronic acid, sulfate, or glutathione. Obviously, drugs that are bound to serum protein or show favorable partitioning into tissue depots are going to be metabolized and excreted more slowly for the reasons discussed above.

This does not mean that drugs that remain in the body for longer periods of time can be administered in lower doses or be taken fewer times per day by the patient. Several variables determine dosing regimens, of which the affinity of the drug for the receptor is crucial. Reexamine Reaction 2-1 and Figure 2-1. If the equilibrium does not favor formation of the drug–receptor complex, higher and usually more frequent doses must be administered. Further, if partitioning into tissue stores or metabolic degradation and/or excretion is favored, it will take more of the drug and usually more frequent administration to maintain therapeutic concentrations at the receptor.

Receptor

With the possible exception of general anesthetics (see Chapter 14), the working model for a pharmacological response consists of a drug binding to a specific receptor. Many drug receptors are the same as those used by endogenously produced ligands. Cholinergic agents interact with the same receptors as the neurotransmitter acetylcholine. Synthetic corticosteroids bind to the same receptors as cortisone and hydrocortisone. Often, receptors for the same ligand are found in a variety of tissues throughout the body. The nonsteroidal anti-inflammatory agents (see Chapter 22) inhibit the prostaglandin-forming enzyme cyclooxygenase, which is found in nearly every tissue. This class of drugs has a long list of side effects with many patient complaints. Note in Figure 2-1 that, depending on which receptors contain bound drug, there may be desired or undesired effects. This is because a variety of receptors with similar structural requirements are found in several organs and tissues. Thus, the nonsteroidal anti-inflammatory drugs combine with the desired cyclooxygenase receptors at the site of the inflammation and the undesired cyclooxygenase receptors in the gastrointestinal mucosa, causing severe discomfort and sometimes ulceration. One of the ''second-generation'' antihistamines, fexofenadine, is claimed to cause less sedation because it does not readily penetrate the blood–brain barrier. The rationale is that less of this antihistamine is available for the receptors in the CNS, which are responsible for the sedation response characteristic of antihistamines. In contrast, some antihistamines are used for their CNS depressant activity because a significant proportion of the administered dose is crossing the blood–brain barrier relative to binding to the histamine H_1 receptors in the periphery.

Although it is normal to think of side effects as undesirable, they sometimes can be beneficial and lead to new products. The successful development of oral hypoglycemic agents used in the treatment of diabetes began when it was found that certain sulfonamides had a hypoglycemic effect. Nevertheless, a real problem in drug therapy is patient compliance in taking the drug as directed. Drugs that cause serious problems and discomfort tend to be avoided by patients.

Summary

One of the goals is to design drugs that will interact with receptors at specific tissues. There are several ways to do this, including *(a)* altering the molecule, which, in turn, can change the biodistribution; *(b)* searching for structures that show increased specificity for the target receptor that will produce the desired pharmacological response while decreasing the affinity for undesired receptors that produce adverse responses; and *(c)* the still experimental approach of attaching the drug to a monoclonal antibody (see Chapter 7) that will bind to a specific tissue antigenic for the antibody. Biodistribution can be altered by changing the drug's solubility, enhancing its ability to resist being metabolized (usually in the liver), altering the formulation or physical characteristics of the drug, and changing the route of administration. If a drug molecule can be designed so that its binding to the desired receptor is enhanced relative to the undesired receptor and biodistribution remains favorable, smaller doses of the drug can be administered. This, in turn, reduces the amount of drug available for binding to those receptors responsible for its adverse effects.

The medicinal chemist is confronted with several challenges in designing a bioactive molecule. A good fit to a specific receptor is desirable, but the drug would normally be expected to dissociate from the receptor eventually. The specificity for the receptor would minimize side effects. The drug would be expected to clear the body within a reasonable time. Its rate of metabolic degradation should allow reasonable dosing schedules and, ideally, oral administration. Many times, the drug chosen for commercial sales has been selected from hundreds of compounds that have been screened. It usually is a compromise product that meets a medical need while demonstrating good patient acceptance.

ACID–BASE PROPERTIES

Most drugs used today can be classified as acids or bases. As is noted shortly, a large number of drugs can behave as either acids or bases as they begin their journey into the patient in different dosage forms and end up in systemic circulation. A drug's acid–base properties can greatly influence its biodistribution and partitioning characteristics.

Over the years, at least four major definitions of acids and bases have been developed. The model commonly used in pharmacy and biochemistry was developed independently by Lowry and Brønsted. In their definition, an *acid* is defined as a proton donor and a *base* is defined as a proton acceptor. Notice that for a base, *there is no mention of the hydroxide ion.*

Acid–Conjugate Base

Representative examples of pharmaceutically important acidic drugs are listed in Table 2-1. Each acid, or proton donor, yields a *conjugate base*. The latter is the product after the proton is lost from the acid. Conjugate bases range from the chloride ion (reaction *a*), which does not accept a proton in aqueous media, to ephedrine (reaction *h*), which is an excellent proton acceptor.

Notice the diversity in structure of these proton donors. They include the classical hydrochloric acid (reaction *a*), the weakly acidic dihydrogen phosphate anion (reaction *b*), the ammonium cation as is found in ammonium chloride (reaction *c*), the carboxylic acetic acid (reaction *d*), the enolic form of phenobarbital (reaction *e*), the carboxylic acid moiety of indomethacin (reaction *f*), the imide of saccharin (reaction *g*), and the protonated amine of ephedrine (reaction *h*). Because all are proton donors, they must be treated as acids when calculating the pH of a solution or percent ionization of the drug. At the same time, as noted below, there are important differences in the pharmaceutical properties of ephedrine hydrochloride (an acid salt of an amine) and those of indomethacin, phenobarbital, or saccharin.

Base–Conjugate Acid

The Brønsted-Lowry theory defines a *base* as a molecule that accepts a proton. The product resulting from the addition of a proton to the base is the *conjugate acid*. Pharmaceutically important bases are listed in Table 2-2. Again, there are a variety of structures, including the easily recognizable base sodium hydroxide (reaction *a*); the basic component of an important physiological buffer, sodium monohydrogen phosphate (reaction *b*), which is also the conjugate base of dihydrogen phosphate (reaction *b* in Table 2-1); ammonia (reaction *c*), which is also the conjugate base of the ammonium cation (reaction *c* in Table 2-1); sodium acetate (reaction *d*), which is also the conjugate base of acetic acid (reaction *d* in Table 2-1); the enolate form of phenobarbital

TABLE 2–1   Examples of Acids

Acid	$\longrightarrow$	H$^+$	+	Conjugate Base
(a) Hydrochloric acid HCl	$\longrightarrow$	H$^+$	+	Cl^{-a}
(b) Sodium dihydrogen phosphate (monobasic sodium phosphate) NaH$_2$PO$_4$ (Na$^+$, H$_2$PO$_4^-$)^a	$\longrightarrow$	H$^+$	+	NaHPO$_4^{2-}$ (Na^{+a}, HPO$_4^{2-}$)
(c) Ammonium chloride NH$_4$Cl (NH$_4^+$, Cl$^-$)^a	$\longrightarrow$	H$^+$	+	NH$_3$ (Cl$^-$)^a
(d) Acetic acid CH$_3$COOH	$\longrightarrow$	H$^+$	+	CH$_3$COO$^-$

(e) Phenobarbital

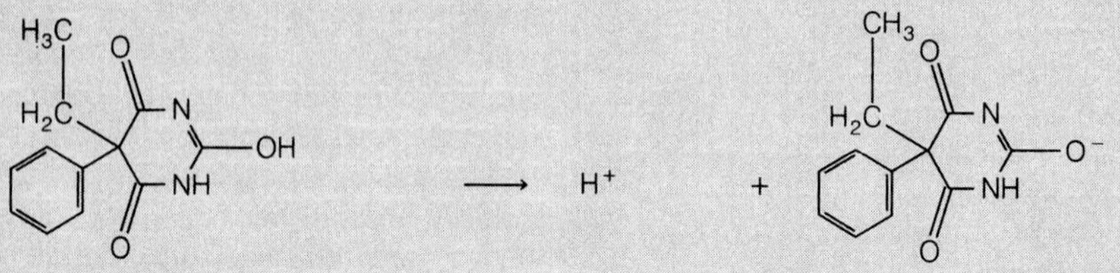

$\longrightarrow$ H$^+$ +

(f) Indomethacin

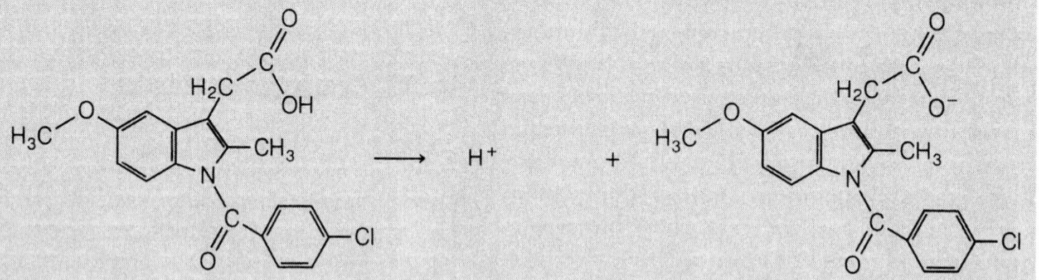

$\longrightarrow$ H$^+$ +

(g) Saccharin

$\longrightarrow$ H$^+$ +

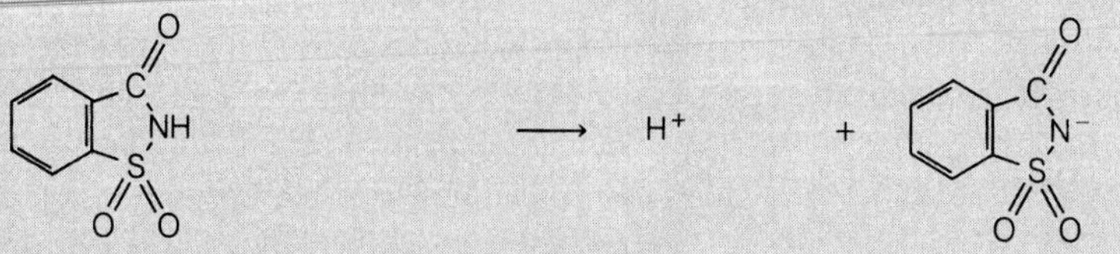

(h) Ephedrine hydrochloride

$\longrightarrow$ H$^+$ (Cl^{-a})   +

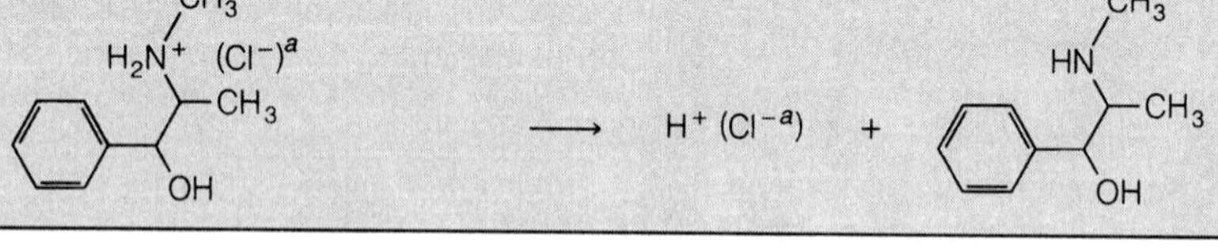

^{a} The sodium cation and chloride anion do not take part in these reactions.

(reaction *e*), which is also the conjugate base of phenobarbital (reaction *e* in Table 2-1); the carboxylate form of indomethacin (reaction *f*), which is also the conjugate base of indomethacin (reaction *f* in Table 2-1); the imidate form of saccharin (reaction *g*), which is also the conjugate base of saccharin (reaction *g* in Table 2-1); and the amine ephedrine (reaction *h*), which is also the conjugate base of ephedrine hydrochloride (reaction *h* in Table 2-1). Notice that the conjugate acid products in Table 2-2 are the reactant acids in Table 2-1. Conversely, most of the conjugate base products in Table 2-1 are the reactant bases in Table 2-2. Also, notice that whereas phenobarbital, indomethacin, and saccharin are un-ionized in the protonated form, the protonated (acidic) forms of ammonia and ephedrine are ionized salts (Table 2-1). The opposite is true for the basic (proton acceptors) forms of these drugs. The basic forms of phenobarbital, indomethacin, and saccharin are anions, whereas ammonia and ephedrine are electronically neutral (Table 2-2). Remember that each of the chemical examples in Tables 2-1 and 2-2 can function as either a proton donor (acid) or proton acceptor

TABLE 2–2 Examples of Bases

Base	+ H⁺ ⟶	Conjugate Acid	

(a) Sodium hydroxide
NaOH (Na^{+a}, OH$^-$)   + H$^+$ ⟶   H$_2$O   + Na^{+a}

(b) Sodium monohydrogen phosphate (dibasic sodium phosphate)
Na$_2$HPO$_4$ (2 Na^{+a}, HPO$_4^{2-}$)   + H$^+$ ⟶   H$_2$PO$_4^-$ + 2 Na^{+a}

(c) Ammonia
NH$_3$ + H$^+$ ⟶   NH$_4^+$

(d) Sodium acetate
CH$_3$COONa (CH$_3$COO$^-$, Na^{+a})   + H$^+$ ⟶   CH$_3$COOH   + Na^{+a}

(e) Phenobarbital sodium

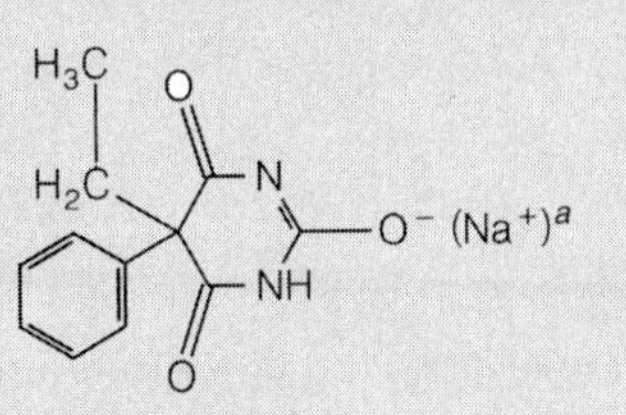

+ H$^+$ ⟶   + Na^{+a}

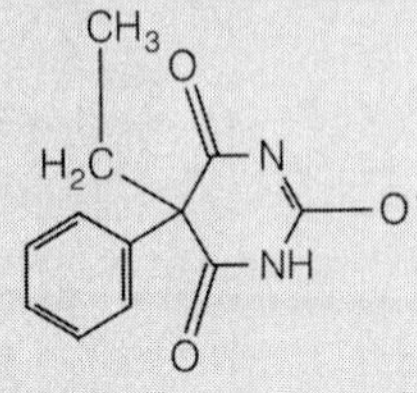

(f) Indomethacin sodium

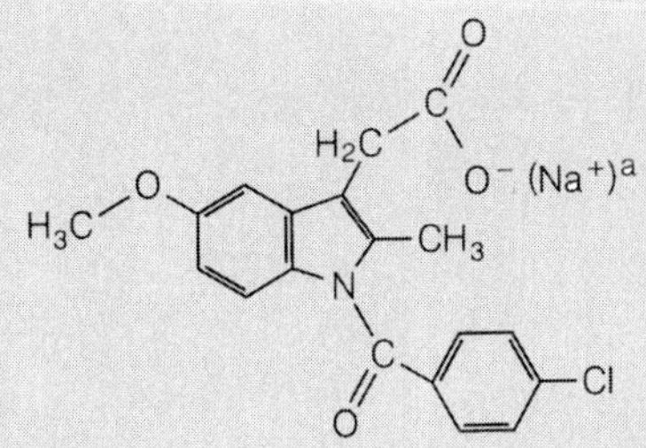

+ H$^+$ ⟶   + Na^{+a}

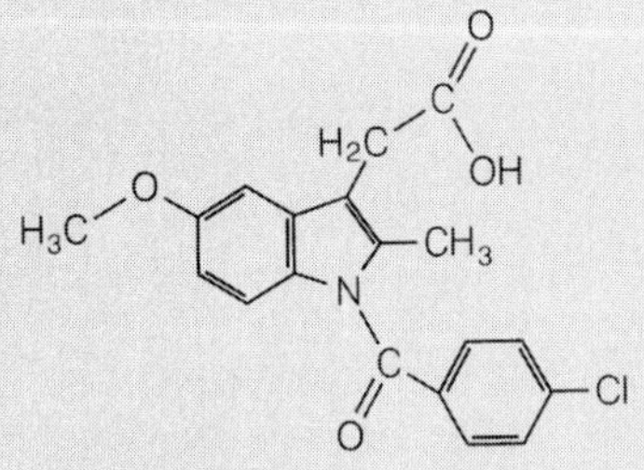

(g) Saccharin sodium

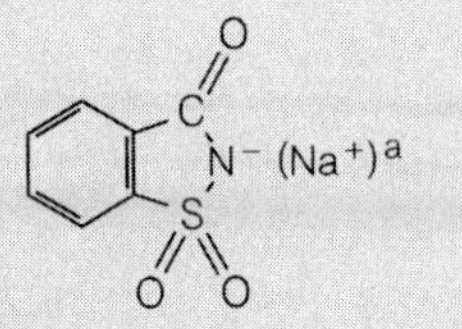

+ H$^+$ ⟶   + Na^{+a}

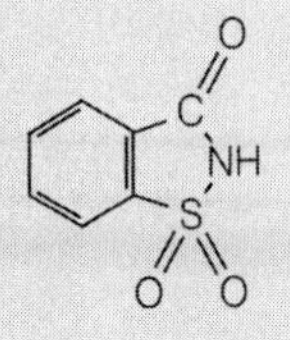

(h) Ephedrine

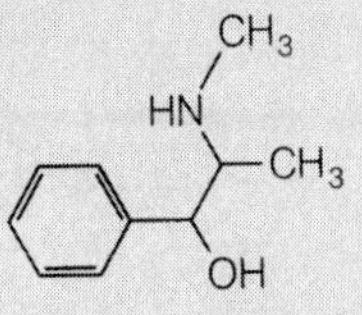

+ H$^+$ ⟶

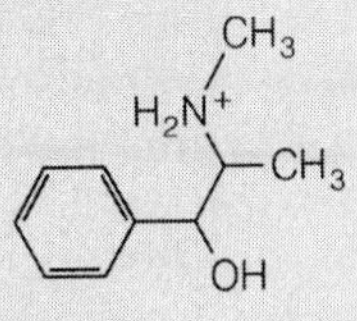

^{a} The sodium cation is present only to maintain charge balance. It plays no direct acid–base role.

(base). This can best be understood by emphasizing the concept of conjugate acid–conjugate base pairing. Complicated as it may seem at first, conjugate acids and conjugate bases are nothing more than the products of an acid–base reaction. In other words, they appear to the right of the reaction arrows. Examples from Tables 2-1 and 2-2 are rewritten in Table 2-3 as complete acid–base reactions.

Careful study of Table 2-3 shows water functioning as a proton acceptor (base) in reactions *a, c, e, g, i, k,* and *m* and a proton donor (base) in reactions *b, d, f, h, j, l,* and *n*. Hence,

water is known as an *amphoteric* substance. Water can be either a weak base accepting a proton to form the strongly acidic hydrated proton or hydronium ion H$_3$O$^+$ (reactions *a, c, e, g, i, k,* and *m*), or a weak acid donating a proton to form the strongly basic (proton accepting) hydroxide anion OH$^-$ (reactions *b, d, f, h, j, l,* and *n*).

Acid Strength

While any acid–base reaction can be written as an equilibrium reaction, an attempt has been made in Table 2-3 to

TABLE 2–3 Examples of Acid–Base Reactions (With the Exception of Hydrochloric Acid, Whose Conjugate Base (Cl⁻) Has No Basic Properties in Water, and Sodium Hydroxide, Which Generates Hydroxide, the Reaction of the Conjugate Base in Water Is Shown for Each Acid)

Acid	+	Base	⇌	Conjugate Acid	+	Conjugate Base
Hydrochloric acid						
(a) HCl	+	H_2O	⟶	H_3O^+	+	Cl^-
Sodium hydroxide						
(b) H_2O	+	$NaOH$	⟶	H_2O	+	$OH^- (Na^+)^a$
Sodium dihydrogen phosphate and its conjugate base, sodium monohydrogen phosphate						
(c) $H_2PO_4^- (Na^+)^a$	+	H_2O	⇌	H_3O^+	+	$HPO_4^{2-} (Na^+)^a$
(d) H_2O	+	$HPO_4^{2-} (2Na^+)^a$	⇌	$H_2PO_4^{2-} (Na^+)^a$	+	$OH^- (Na^+)^a$
Ammonium chloride and its conjugate base, ammonia						
(e) $NH_4^+ (Cl^-)^a$	+	H_2O	⇌	$H_3O^+ (Cl^-)^a$	+	NH_3
(f) H_2O	+	NH_3	⇌	NH_4^+	+	OH^-
Acetic acid and its conjugate base, sodium acetate						
(g) CH_3COOH	+	H_2O	⇌	H_3O^+	+	CH_3COO^-
(h) H_2O	+	$CH_3COO^- (Na^+)^a$	⇌	CH_3COOH	+	$OH^- (Na^+)^a$

Indomethacin and its conjugate base, indomethacin sodium, show the identical acid–base chemistry as acetic acid and sodium acetate, respectively.

Phenobarbital and its conjugate base, phenobarbital sodium

(i) [phenobarbital structure] + H_2O ⇌ H_3O^+ + [phenobarbital anion structure]

(j) H_2O + [phenobarbital sodium structure] $O^- (Na^+)^a$ ⇌ [phenobarbital structure] + $OH^- (Na^+)^a$

Saccharin and its conjugate base, saccharin sodium

(k) [saccharin structure NH] + H_2O ⇌ H_3O^+ + [saccharin anion structure N^-]

(l) H_2O + [saccharin sodium structure $N^- (Na^+)^a$] ⇌ [saccharin structure NH] + $OH^- (Na^+)^a$

Ephedrine HCl and its conjugate base, ephedrine

(m) [ephedrine HCl structure $H_2N^+ (Cl^-)^a$] + H_2O ⇌ $H_3O^+ (Cl^-)^a$ + [ephedrine structure HN]

(n) H_2O + [ephedrine structure HN] ⇌ [ephedrine cation structure H_2N^+] + OH^-

---

[a] The chloride anion and sodium cation are present only to maintain charge balance. These anions play no other acid–base role.

indicate which sequences are unidirectional or show only a small reversal. For hydrochloric acid, the conjugate base, Cl^-, is such a weak base that it essentially does not function as a proton acceptor. That is why the chloride anion was not included as a base in Table 2-2. In a similar manner, water is such a weak conjugate acid that there is little reverse reaction involving water donating a proton to the hydroxide anion of sodium hydroxide.

Two logical questions to ask at this point are how one predicts in which direction an acid–base reaction lies and to what extent the reaction goes to completion. The common physical chemical measurement that contains this information is known as the pK_a. The pK_a is the negative logarithm of the modified equilibrium constant, K_a, for an acid–base reaction written so that water is the base or proton acceptor. It can be derived as follows:

Assume that a weak acid, HA, reacts with water.

$$\begin{array}{cccc} & & \text{Conj.} & \text{Conj.} \\ \text{Acid} & \text{Base} & \text{Acid} & \text{Base} \\ \text{HA} & + \text{ H}_2\text{O} & \rightleftharpoons \text{ H}_3\text{O}^+ & + \text{ A}^- \end{array} \quad \text{(Rx. 2-3)}$$

The equilibrium constant, K_{eq}, for Reaction 2-3 is

$$K_{eq} = \frac{[\text{H}_3\text{O}^-][\text{A}^-]}{[\text{HA}][\text{H}_2\text{O}]} = \frac{[\text{conj. acid}][\text{conj. base}]}{[\text{acid}][\text{base}]}$$

$$\text{(Eq. 2-1)}$$

In a dilute solution of a weak acid, the molar concentration of water can be treated as a constant, 55.5 M. This number is based on the density of water equaling 1. Therefore, 1 L of water weighs 1000 g. With a molecular weight of 18, the molar concentration of water in 1 L of water is

$$[\text{H}_2\text{O}] = \frac{\text{Weight}_{\text{H}_2\text{O}}}{\text{MW}_{\text{H}_2\text{O}}} = \frac{1,000 \text{ g}}{18 \text{ g}} = 55.5 \text{ M}$$

Thus, with $[\text{H}_2\text{O}] = 55.5$, Equation 2-1 can be simplified to

$$K_a = K_{eq}[\text{H}_2\text{O}] = K_{eq}(55.5) = \frac{[\text{H}_3\text{O}^+][\text{A}^-]}{[\text{HA}]}$$

$$= \frac{[\text{conj. acid}][\text{conj. base}]}{[\text{acid}]} \quad \text{(Eq. 2-2)}$$

By definition,

$$pK_a = -\log K_a \quad \text{(Eq. 2-3)}$$

and

$$pH = -\log [\text{H}_3\text{O}^+] \quad \text{(Eq. 2-4)}$$

The modified equilibrium constant, K_a, is customarily converted to pK_a (the negative logarithm) to use on the same scale as pH. Therefore, rewriting Equation 2-2 in logarithmic form produces

$$\log K_a = \log [\text{H}_3\text{O}^+] + \log [\text{A}^-] - \log [\text{HA}] \quad \text{(Eq. 2-5)}$$
$$= \log [\text{H}_3\text{O}^+] + \log [\text{conj. base}] - \log [\text{acid}]$$

Rearranging Equation 2-5 gives

$$-\log [\text{H}_3\text{O}^+] = -\log K_a + \log [\text{A}^-] - \log [\text{HA}] \quad \text{(Eq. 2-6)}$$
$$= -\log K_a + \log [\text{conj. base}] - \log [\text{acid}]$$

Substituting Equations 2-3 and 2-4 into Equation 2-6 produces

$$pH = pK_a + \log \frac{[\text{A}^-]}{[\text{HA}]} = pK_a + \log \frac{[\text{conj. base}]}{[\text{acid}]} \quad \text{(Eq. 2-7)}$$

Equation 2-7 is more commonly called the Henderson-Hasselbalch equation and is the basis for most calculations involving weak acids and bases. It is used to calculate the pH of solutions of weak acids, weak bases, and buffers consisting of weak acids and their conjugate bases or weak bases and their conjugate acids. Because the pK_a is a modified equilibrium constant, it corrects for the fact that weak acids do *not* completely react with water.

A very similar set of equations is obtained from the reaction of a protonated amine, BH^+, in water. The reaction is

$$\begin{array}{cccc} & & \text{Conj.} & \text{Conj.} \\ \text{Acid} & \text{Base} & \text{Acid} & \text{Base} \\ \text{BH}^+ & + \text{ H}_2\text{O} & \rightleftharpoons \text{ H}_3\text{O}^+ & + \text{ B} \end{array} \quad \text{(Rx. 2-4)}$$

The equilibrium constant, K_{eq}, is defined as

$$K_{eq} = \frac{[\text{H}_3\text{O}^+][\text{B}]}{[\text{BH}^+][\text{H}_2\text{O}]} = \frac{[\text{conj. acid}][\text{conj. base}]}{[\text{acid}][\text{base}]} \quad \text{(Eq. 2-8)}$$

Notice that Equation 2-8 is identical to Equation 2-1 when the general [conj. acid][conj. base] representation is used. Therefore, using the same simplifying assumption that water remains at a constant concentration of 55.5 M in dilute solutions, Equation 2-8 can be rewritten as

$$K_a = K_{eq}(55.5) = \frac{[\text{H}_3\text{O}^+][\text{B}]}{[\text{BH}^+]} = \frac{[\text{conj. acid}][\text{conj. base}]}{[\text{acid}]}$$

$$\text{(Eq. 2-9)}$$

Rearranging Equation 2-9 into logarithmic form and substituting the relationships expressed in Equations 2-3 and 2-4 yields the same Henderson-Hasselbalch equation (Eq. 2-10).

$$pH = pK_a + \log \frac{[\text{B}]}{[\text{BH}^+]} = pK_a + \log \frac{[\text{conj. base}]}{[\text{acid}]}$$

$$\text{(Eq. 2-10)}$$

Rather than trying to remember the specific form of the Henderson-Hasselbalch equation for an HA or BH^+ acid, it is simpler to use the general form of the equation (Eq. 2-11) expressed in both Equations 2-7 and 2-10.

$$pH = pK_a + \log \frac{[\text{conj. base}]}{[\text{acid}]} \quad \text{(Eq. 2-11)}$$

With this version of the equation, there is no need to remember whether the species in the numerator/denominator is ionized (A^-/HA) or un-ionized (B/BH^+). The molar concentration of the proton acceptor is the term in the numerator, and the molar concentration of the proton donor is the denominator term.

What about weak bases such as amines? In aqueous solutions, water functions as the proton donor or acid (Rx. 2-5), producing the familiar hydroxide anion (conjugate base).

$$\begin{array}{cccc} & & \text{Conj.} & \text{Conj.} \\ \text{Acid} & \text{Base} & \text{Acid} & \text{Base} \\ \text{H}_2\text{O} & + \text{ B} & \rightleftharpoons \text{ BH}^+ & + \text{ OH}^- \end{array} \quad \text{(Rx. 2-5)}$$

Originally, a modified equilibrium constant, the pK_b, was derived following the same steps that produced Equation 2-2. It is now more common to express the basicity of a chemical in terms of the pK_a, using the relationship in Equation 2-12.

$$pK_a = pK_b - 14 \quad \text{(Eq. 2-12)}$$

TABLE 2–4   Examples of Calculations Requiring the pK_a

1. What is the ratio of ephedrine to ephedrine HCl (pK_a 9.6) in the intestinal tract at pH 8.0? Use Equation 2-11.

$$8.0 = 9.6 + \log \frac{[\text{ephedrine}]}{[\text{ephedrine HCl}]} = -1.6$$

$$\frac{[\text{ephedrine}]}{[\text{ephedrine HCl}]} = 0.025$$

The number whose log is −1.6 is 0.025, meaning that there are 25 parts ephedrine for every 1000 parts ephedrine HCl in the intestinal tract whose environment is pH 8.0.

2. What is the pH of a buffer containing 0.1 M acetic acid (pK_a 4.8) and 0.08 M sodium acetate? Use Equation 2-11.

$$pH = 4.8 + \log \frac{0.08}{0.1} = 4.7$$

3. What is the pH of a 0.1 M acetic acid solution? Use the following equation for calculating the pH of a solution containing either an HA or BH^+ acid.

$$pH = \frac{pK_a - \log [\text{acid}]}{2} = 2.9$$

4. What is the pH of a 0.08 M sodium acetate solution? Remember, even though this is the conjugate base of acetic acid, the pK_a is still used. The pK_w term in the following equation corrects for the fact that a proton acceptor (acetate anion) is present in the solution. The equation for calculating the pH of a solution containing either an A^- or B base is

$$pH = \frac{pK_w + pK_a + \log [\text{base}]}{2} = 8.9$$

5. What is the pH of an ammonium acetate solution? The pK_a of the ammonium (NH_4^+) cation is 9.3. Always bear in mind that the pK_a refers to the ability of the proton donor form to release the proton into water to form H_3O^+. Since this is the salt of a weak acid (NH_4^+) and the conjugate base of a weak acid (acetate anion), the following equation is used. Note that molar concentration is not a variable in this calculation.

$$pH = \frac{pK_{a_1} + pK_{a_2}}{2} = 7.1$$

6. What is the percentage ionization of ephedrine HCl (pK_a 9.6) in an intestinal tract buffered at pH 8.0 (see example 1)? Use Equation 2-14 because this is a BH^+ acid.

$$\% \text{ ionization} = \frac{100}{1 + 10^{(8.0 - 9.6)}} = 97.6\%$$

Only 2.4% of ephedrine is present as the un-ionized conjugate base.

7. What is the percentage ionization of indomethacin (pK_a 4.5) in an intestinal tract buffered at pH 8.0? Use Equation 2-13 because this is an HA acid.

$$\% \text{ ionization} = \frac{100}{1 + 10^{(4.5 - 8.0)}} = 99.97\%$$

For all practical purposes indomethacin is present only as the anionic conjugate base in that region of the intestine buffered at pH 8.0.

Warning! It is *important* to recognize that a pK_a for a base is in reality the pK_a of the conjugate acid (acid donor or protonated form, BH^+) of the base. The pK_a is listed in the Appendix as 9.6 for ephedrine and as 9.3 for ammonia. In reality, this is the pK_a of the protonated form, such as ephedrine hydrochloride (reaction *m* in Table 2-3) and ammonium chloride (reaction *e* in Table 2-3), respectively. This is confusing to students, pharmacists, clinicians, and experienced scientists. It is crucial that the chemistry of the drug be understood when interpreting a pK_a value. When reading tables of pK_a values, such as those found in the Appendix, one must realize that the listed value is for the proton donor form of the molecule, no matter what form is indicated by the name. See Table 2-4 for several worked examples of how the pK_a is used to calculate pHs of solutions, required ratios of [conjugate base]/[acid], and percent ionization at specific pHs.

Just how strong or weak are the acids whose reactions in water are illustrated in Table 2-3? Remember that the K_as or pK_as are modified equilibrium constants that indicate the extent to which the acid (proton donor) reacts with water to form conjugate acid and conjugate base. The equilibrium for a strong acid (low pK_a) in water lies to the right, favoring the formation of products (conjugate acid and conjugate base). The equilibrium for a weak acid (high pK_a) in water lies to the left, meaning that the conjugate acid is a better proton donor than the parent acid is or that the conjugate base is a good proton acceptor.

Refer back to Equation 2-2 and, using the K_a values in Table 2-5, substitute the K_a term for each of the acids. For hydrochloric acid, a K_a of 1.26×10^6 means that the product of the molar concentrations of the conjugate acid, $[H_3O^+]$, and the conjugate base, $[Cl^-]$, is huge relative to the denominator term, $[HCl]$. In other words, there essentially is no unreacted HCl left in an aqueous solution of hydrochloric acid. At the other extreme is ephedrine HCl with a pK_a of 9.6 or a K_a of 2.51×10^{-10}. Here, the denominator representing the concentration of ephedrine HCl greatly predominates over that of the products, which, in this example, is ephedrine (conjugate base) and H_3O^+ (conjugate acid). In other words, the protonated form of ephedrine is a very poor proton donor. It holds onto the proton. Indeed, free ephedrine (the conjugate base in this reaction) is an excellent proton acceptor.

A general rule for determining whether a chemical is strong or weak acid or base is

$pK_a < 2$: strong acid; conjugate base has no meaningful basic properties in water
pK_a 4–6: weak acid; weak conjugate base
pK_a 8–10: very weak acid; conjugate base getting stronger
$pK_a > 12$: essentially no acidic properties in water; strong conjugate base

This delineation is only approximate. Other properties also become important when considering cautions in handling acids and bases. Phenol has a pK_a of 9.9, slightly less than that of ephedrine HCl. Why is phenol considered corrosive to the skin, whereas ephedrine HCl or free ephedrine is considered innocuous when applied to the skin? Phenol has the ability to partition through the normally protective lipid layers of the skin. Because of this property, this extremely weak acid has carried the name carbolic acid. Thus,

TABLE 2–5 Representative K_a and pK$_a$ Values From the Reactions Listed in Table 2-3 (See the Appendix)

Hydrochloric acid	1.26×10^6	−6.1
Dihydrogen phosphate	6.31×10^{-8}	7.2
Ammonia (ammonium)	5.01×10^{-10}	9.3
Acetic acid	1.58×10^{-5}	4.8
Phenobarbital	3.16×10^{-8}	7.5
Saccharin	2.51×10^{-2}	1.6
Indomethacin	3.16×10^{-5}	4.5
Ephedrine (as the HCl salt)	2.51×10^{-10}	9.6

the pK$_a$ simply tells a person the acid properties of the protonated form of the chemical. It does not represent anything else concerning other potential toxicities.

Percent Ionization

Using the drug's pK$_a$, the formulation or compounding pharmacist can adjust the pH to ensure maximum water solubility (ionic form of the drug) or maximum solubility in nonpolar media (nonionic form). This is where understanding the drug's acid–base chemistry becomes important. Note Reactions 2-6 and 2-7:

$$\text{Acid} \quad \underset{\text{Base}}{\text{}} \quad \underset{\text{Acid}}{\overset{\text{Conj.}}{}} \quad \underset{\text{Base}}{\overset{\text{Conj.}}{}}$$

$$HA_{(un\text{-}ionized)} + H_2O \rightleftharpoons H_3O^+ + A^-_{(ionized)} \qquad \text{(Rx. 2-6)}$$

$$\text{Acid} \quad \underset{\text{Base}}{\text{}} \quad \underset{\text{Acid}}{\overset{\text{Conj.}}{}} \quad \underset{\text{Base}}{\overset{\text{Conj.}}{}}$$

$$BH^+_{(ionized)} + H_2O \rightleftharpoons H_3O^+ + B_{(un\text{-}ionized)} \qquad \text{(Rx. 2-7)}$$

Acids can be divided into two types, HA and BH$^+$, on the basis of the ionic form of the acid (or conjugate base). HA acids go from un-ionized acids to ionized conjugate bases (Rx. 2-6). In contrast, BH$^+$ acids go from ionized (polar) acids to un-ionized (nonpolar) conjugate bases (Rx. 2-7). In general, pharmaceutically important HA acids include the inorganic acids (e.g., HCl, H_2SO_4), enols (e.g., barbiturates, hydantoins), carboxylic acids (e.g., low-molecular-weight organic acids, arylacetic acids, *N*-aryl anthranilic acids, salicylic acids), and amides and imides (e.g., sulfonamides and saccharin, respectively). The chemistry is simpler for the pharmaceutically important BH$^+$ acids: They are all protonated amines. A polyfunctional drug can have several pK$_a$s (e.g., amoxicillin). The latter's ionic state is based on amoxicillin's ionic state at physiological pH 7.4 (see the discussion below on percent ionization).

pK$_{a3}$ = 9.6

Amoxicillin

The percent ionization of a drug is calculated by using

Equation 2-13 for HA acids and Equation 2-14 for BH$^+$ acids.

$$\% \text{ ionization} = \frac{100}{1 + 10^{(pK_a - pH)}} \qquad \text{(Eq. 2-13)}$$

$$\% \text{ ionization} = \frac{100}{1 + 10^{(pH - pK_a)}} \qquad \text{(Eq. 2-14)}$$

A plot of percent ionization versus pH illustrates how the degree of ionization can be shifted significantly with small changes in pH. The curves for an HA acid (indomethacin) and BH$^+$ (protonated ephedrine) are shown in Figure 2-2. First, note that when pH = pK$_a$, the compound is 50% ionized (or 50% un-ionized). In other words, when the pK$_a$ is equal to the pH, the molar concentration of the acid equals the molar concentration of its conjugate base. In the Henderson-Hasselbalch equation, pK$_a$ = pH when log [conj. base]/[acid] = 1. An increase of 1 pH unit from the pK$_a$ (increase in alkalinity) causes an HA acid (indomethacin) to become 90.9% in the ionized conjugate base form but results in a BH$^+$ acid (ephedrine HCl) decreasing its percent ionization to only 9.1%. An increase of 2 pH units essentially shifts an HA acid to complete ionization (99%) and a BH$^+$ acid to the nonionic conjugate base form (0.99%).

Just the opposite is seen when the medium is made more acidic relative to the drug's pK$_a$ value. Increasing the hydrogen ion concentration (decreasing the pH) will shift the equilibrium to the left, thereby increasing the concentration of the acid and decreasing the concentration of conjugate base. In the case of indomethacin, a decrease of 1 pH unit below the pK$_a$ will increase the concentration of un-ionized (protonated) indomethacin to 9.1%. Similarly, a decrease of 2 pH units results in only 0.99% of the indomethacin being present in the ionized conjugate base form. The opposite is seen for the BH$^+$ acids. The percentage of ephedrine present as the ionized (protonated) acid is 90.9% at 1 pH unit below the pK$_a$ and is 99.0% at 2 pH units below the pK$_a$. These results are summarized in Table 2-6.

With this knowledge in mind, return to the drawing of amoxicillin. At physiological pH, the carboxylic acid (HA acid; pK$_{a1}$ 2.4) will be in the ionized carboxylate form, the

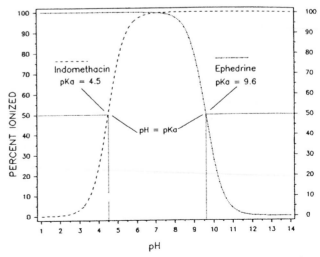

Figure 2–2 ■ Percent ionized versus pH for indomethacin (pK$_a$ 4.5) and ephedrine (pK$_a$ 9.6).

TABLE 2–6 Percentage Ionization Relative to the pK$_a$

	Ionization (%)	
	HA Acids	**BH· Acids**
pK$_a$ − 2 pH units	0.99	99.0
pK$_a$ − 1 pH unit	9.1	90.9
pK$_a$ = pH	50.0	50.0
pK$_a$ + 1 pH unit	90.9	9.1
pK$_a$ + 2 pH units	99.0	0.99

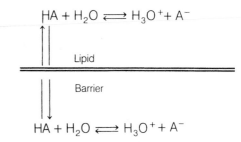

Figure 2–3 ■ Passage of HA acids through lipid barriers.

primary amine (BH$^+$ acid; pK$_{a2}$ 7.4) will be 50% protonated and 50% in the free amine form, and the phenol (HA acid; pK$_{a3}$ 9.6) will be in the un-ionized protonated form. A knowledge of percent ionization makes it easier to explain and predict why the use of some preparations can cause problems and discomfort as a result of pH extremes. Phenytoin (HA acid; pK$_a$ 8.3) injection must be adjusted to pH 12 with sodium hydroxide to ensure complete ionization and maximize water solubility. In theory, a pH of 10.3 will result in 99.0% of the drug being an anionic water-soluble conjugate base. To lower the concentration of phenytoin in the insoluble acid form even further and maintain excess alkalinity, the pH is raised to 12 to obtain 99.98% of the drug in the ionized form. Even then, a cosolvent system of 40% propylene glycol, 10% ethyl alcohol, and 50% water for injection is used to ensure complete solution. This highly alkaline solution is irritating to the patient and generally cannot be administered as an admixture with other intravenous fluids that are buffered more closely at physiological pH 7.4. This decrease in pH would result in the parent un-ionized phenytoin precipitating out of solution.

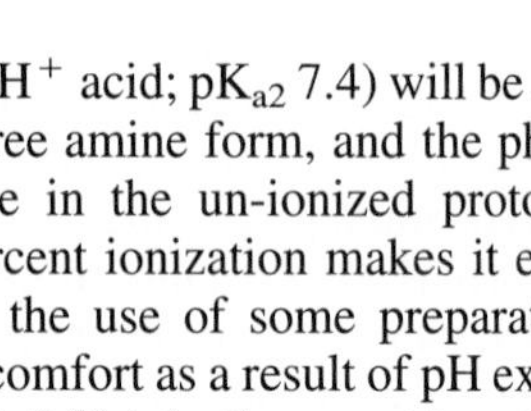

Phenytoin Sodium

Tropicamide is an anticholinergic drug administered as eye drops for its mydriatic response during eye examinations. With a pK$_a$ of 5.2, the drug has to be buffered near pH 4 to obtain more than 90% ionization. The acidic eye drops can sting. Some optometrists and ophthalmologists use local anesthetic eye drops to minimize the patient's discomfort. The only atom with a meaningful pK$_a$ is the pyridine nitrogen. The amide nitrogen has no acid–base properties in aqueous media.

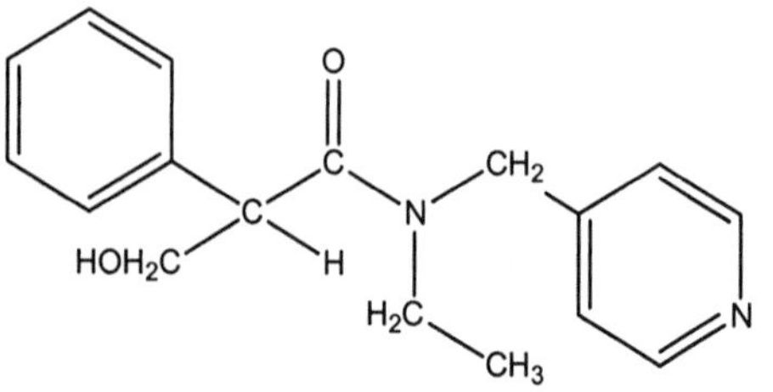

Tropicamide

Adjustments in pH to maintain water solubility can sometimes lead to chemical stability problems. An example is indomethacin (HA acid; pK$_a$ 4.5), which is unstable in alkaline media. Therefore, the preferred oral liquid dosage form is a suspension buffered at pH 4 to 5. Because this is near the drug's pK$_a$, only 50% will be in the water-soluble form. There is a medical indication requiring intravenous administration of indomethacin to premature infants. The intravenous dosage form is the lyophilized (freeze-dried) sodium salt, which is reconstituted just prior to use.

Drug Distribution and pK$_a$

The pK$_a$ can have a pronounced effect on the pharmacokinetics of the drug. As discussed above, drugs are transported in the aqueous environment of the blood. Those drugs in an ionized form will tend to distribute throughout the body more rapidly than will un-ionized (nonpolar) molecules. With few exceptions, the drug must leave the polar environment of the plasma to reach the site of action. In general, drugs pass through the nonpolar membranes of capillary walls, cell membranes, and the blood–brain barrier in the un-ionized (nonpolar) form. For HA acids, it is the parent acid that will readily cross these membranes (Fig. 2-3). The situation is just the opposite for the BH$^+$ acids. The un-ionized conjugate base (free amine) is the species most readily crossing the nonpolar membranes (Fig. 2-4).

Consider the changing pH environment experienced by the drug molecule orally administered. The drug first encounters the acidic stomach, where the pH can range from 2 to 6 depending on the presence of food. HA acids with pK$_a$s of 4 to 5 will tend to be nonionic and be absorbed partially through the gastric mucosa. (The main reason most acidic drugs are absorbed from the intestinal tract rather than the stomach is that the microvilli of the intestinal mucosa provide a huge surface area relative to that found in the gastric mucosa of the stomach.) In contrast, amines (pK$_a$ 9 to 10) will be protonated (BH$^+$ acids) in the acidic stomach

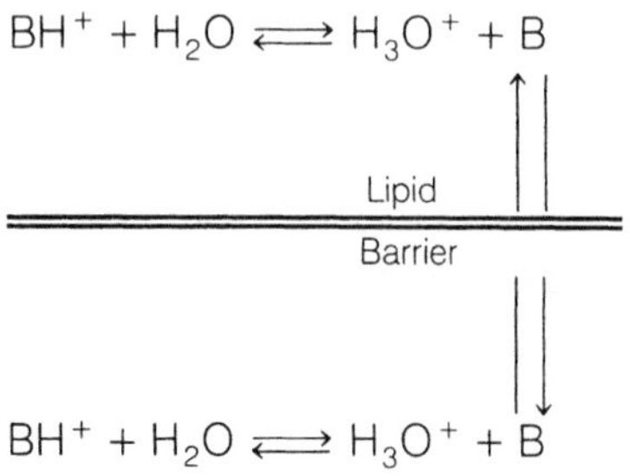

$$BH^+ + H_2O \rightleftharpoons H_3O^+ + B$$

Lipid
Barrier

$$BH^+ + H_2O \rightleftharpoons H_3O^+ + B$$

Figure 2–4 ■ Passage of BH$^+$ acids through lipid barriers.

and usually will not be absorbed until reaching the mildly alkaline intestinal tract (pH ~8). Even here, only a portion of the amine-containing drugs will be in their nonpolar conjugate base form (Fig. 2-4). Remember that the reactions shown in Figures 2-3 and 2-4 are equilibrium reactions with K_a values. Therefore, whenever the nonpolar form of either an HA acid (as the acid) or a B base (the conjugate base of the BH^+ acid) passes the lipid barrier, the ratio of conjugate base to acid (percent ionization) will be maintained. Based on Equations 2-13 and 2-14, this ratio depends on the pK_a (a constant) and the pH of the medium.

For example, once in systemic circulation, the plasma pH of 7.4 will be one of the determinants of whether the drug will tend to remain in the aqueous environment of the blood or partition across lipid membranes into hepatic tissue to be metabolized, into the kidney for excretion, into tissue depots, or to the receptor tissue. A useful exercise is to calculate either the [conj. base]/[acid] ratio using the Henderson-Hasselbalch equation (Eq. 2-11) or percent ionization for ephedrine (pK_a 9.6; Eq. 2-14) and indomethacin (pK_a 4.5; Eq. 2-13) at pH 3.5 (stomach), pH 8.0 (intestine), and pH 7.4 (plasma) (see examples 1, 6, and 7 in Table 2-4). Of course, the effect of protein binding, discussed above, can greatly alter any prediction of biodistribution based solely on pK_a.

STATISTICAL PREDICTION OF PHARMACOLOGICAL ACTIVITY

Just as mathematical modeling is used to explain and model many chemical processes, it has been the goal of medicinal chemists to quantify the effect of a structural change on a defined pharmacological response. This would meet three goals in drug design: *(a)* to predict biological activity in untested compounds, *(b)* to define the structural requirements required for a good fit between the drug molecule and the receptor, and *(c)* to design a test set of compounds to maximize the amount of information concerning structural requirements for activity from a minimum number of compounds tested. This aspect of medicinal chemistry is commonly referred to as quantitative structure–activity relationships (QSAR).

The goals of QSAR studies were first proposed about 1865 to 1870 by Crum-Brown and Fraser, who showed that the gradual chemical modification in the molecular structure of a series of poisons produced some important differences in their action.[1] They postulated that the physiological action, *Φ*, of a molecule is a function of its chemical constitution, *C*. This can be expressed in Equation 2-15:

$$\Phi = f(C) \qquad \text{(Eq. 2-15)}$$

Equation 2-15 states that a defined change in chemical structure results in a predictable change in physiological action. The problem now becomes one of numerically defining chemical structure. It still is a fertile area of research. What has been found is that biological response can be predicted from physical chemical properties such as vapor pressure, water solubility, electronic parameters, steric descriptors, and partition coefficients (Eq. 2-16). Today, the partition coefficient has become the single most important physical chemical measurement for QSAR studies. Note that Equation 2-16 is the equation for a straight line ($Y = mx + b$).

$$\log BR = a(\text{physical chemical property}) + c$$
$$\text{(Eq. 2-16)}$$

where

BR = a defined pharmacological response usually expressed in millimoles such as the inhibitory constant K_i, the effective dose in 50% of the subjects (ED_{50}), the lethal dose in 50% of the subjects (LD_{50}), or the minimum inhibitory concentration (MIC). It is common to express the biological response as a reciprocal, $1/BR$ or $1/C$

a = the regression coefficient or slope of the straight line

c = the intercept term on the *y* axis (when the physical chemical property equals zero)

To understand the concepts in the next few paragraphs, it is necessary to know how to interpret defined pharmacological concepts such as the ED_{50}, which is the amount of the drug needed to obtain the defined pharmacological response. Let's assume that drug A's ED_{50} is 1 mmol and drug B's ED_{50} is 2 mmol. Drug A is twice as potent as drug B. In other words, the smaller the ED_{50} (or ED_{90}, LD_{50}, MIC, etc.), the more potent the substance being tested.

The logarithmic value of the dependent variable (concentration necessary to obtain a defined biological response) is used to linearize the data. As shown below, QSARs are not always linear. Nevertheless, using logarithms is an acceptable statistical technique (taking reciprocals obtained from a Michaelis-Menton study produces the linear Lineweaver-Burke plots found in any biochemistry textbook).

Now, why is the biological response usually expressed as a reciprocal? Sometimes, one obtains a statistically more valid relationship. More importantly, expressing the biological response as a reciprocal usually produces a positive slope (Fig. 2-7). Let us examine the following published example. The BR is the LD_{100} (lethal dose in 100% of the subjects). The mechanism of death is general depression of the CNS. Table 2-7 contains the pertinent data.

The most lethal compound in this assay was chlorpromazine, with a BR (LD_{100}) of only 0.00000631 mmol; and the least active was ethanol, with a BR of 0.087096 mmol. In other words, it takes about 13,800 times as many millimoles of ethanol than of chlorpromazine to kill 100% of the test subjects in this particular assay.

Let's plot BR versus PC (partition coefficient). Figure 2-5 shows the scatter and an attempt at determining a linear fit for the relationship. Note that compounds 1 and 11 lie at a considerable distance from the remaining nine compounds. In addition to the 13,800 times difference in activity, there is a 33,900 times difference in the octanol/water partition coefficient. Also, the regression line whose equation is

$$BR = -0.0000 \, PC + 0.0117 \qquad \text{(Eq. 2-17)}$$

is meaningless statistically. The slope is 0, meaning that the partition coefficient has no effect on biological activity, and yet from the plot and Table 2-7, it is obvious that the higher the octanol/water partition coefficient, the more toxic the compound. The correlation coefficient (r^2) is 0.05, meaning that there is no significant statistical relationship between activity and partition coefficient.

Now, let's see if the data can be linearized by using the logarithms of the biological activity and partition coefficient. Notice that as logarithmic terms, the difference between the LD_{100} of chlorpromazine and ethanol is only 4.14 logarithmic units. Similarly, the difference between chlorproma-

TABLE 2–7   Data Used for a Quantitative Structure–Activity Relationship Study

Compound	Log 1/BR	1/BR	BR	BR × 1000	Log BR	Log PC	PC × 0.01
1. Chlorpromazine	5.20	158489.32	0.000006	0.006310	−5.2000	4.22	165.95869
2. Propoxyphene	5.08	120226.44	0.000008	0.008318	−5.0800	2.36	2.2908677
3. Amitriptyline	4.92	83176.38	0.000012	0.012023	−4.9200	2.50	3.1622777
4. Dothiepin	4.75	56234.13	0.000018	0.017783	−4.7500	2.76	5.7543994
5. Secobarbital	4.19	15488.17	0.000065	0.064565	−4.1900	1.97	0.9332543
6. Phenobarbital	3.71	5128.61	0.000195	0.194984	−3.7100	1.14	0.1380384
7. Chloroform	3.60	3981.07	0.000251	0.251189	−3.6000	1.97	0.9332543
8. Chlormethiazole	3.51	3235.94	0.000309	0.309030	−3.5100	2.12	1.3182567
9. Paraldehyde	2.88	758.58	0.001318	1.318257	−2.8800	0.67	0.0467735
10. Ether	2.17	147.91	0.006761	6.760830	−2.1700	0.89	0.0776247
11. Ethanol	1.06	11.48	0.087096	87.096359	−1.0600	−0.31	0.0048978

From Hansch, C., Björkroth, J. P., and Leo, A.: J. Pharm. Sci. 76:663, 1987.
BR is defined as the LD_{100}, and PC is the octanol–water partition coefficient.

zine's partition coefficient and that of ethanol is 4.53 logarithmic units. Figure 2-6 shows the plot and regression line for log BR versus log PC. Notice that there is an inverse relationship between physicochemical property and biological response. Otherwise, the regression equation is excellent with a correlation coefficient of 0.9191.

$$\log BR = -1.1517 \log PC - 1.4888 \quad \text{(Eq. 2-18)}$$

While there is no statistical advantage to using the log of the reciprocal of the biological response, the positive relationship is consistent with common observation that the biological activity increases as the partition coefficient (or other physicochemical parameter) increases. In interpreting plots like that in Figure 2-7, remember that biological activity is increasing as the amount of compound required to obtain the defined biological response is decreasing. The equation for the line in Figure 2-7 is identical to Equation 2-18, except for the change to positive slope and sign of the intercept. The correlation coefficient also remains the same at 0.9191.

$$\log 1/BR = 1.517 \log PC + 1.4888 \quad \text{(Eq. 2-19)}$$

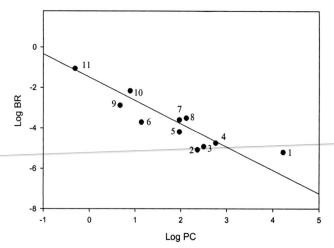

Figure 2–6 ▪ Plot of log BR versus log PC.

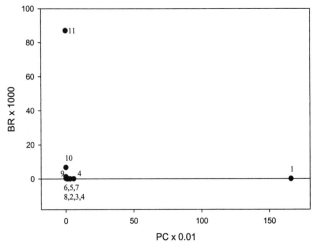

Figure 2–5 ▪ Plot of (BR × 1000) versus (PC × 0.01).

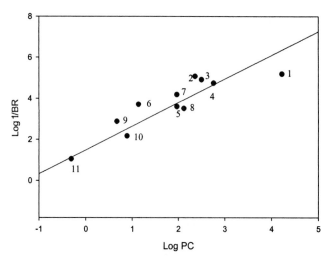

Figure 2–7 ▪ Plot of log 1/BR versus log PC.

As emphasized above, the drug will go through a series of partitioning steps: *(a)* leaving the aqueous extracellular fluids, *(b)* passing through lipid membranes, and *(c)* entering other aqueous environments before reaching the receptor (Fig. 2-1). In this sense, a drug is undergoing the same partitioning phenomenon that happens to any chemical in a separatory funnel containing water and a nonpolar solvent such as hexane, chloroform, or ether. The difference between the separatory funnel model and what actually occurs in the body is that the partitioning in the funnel will reach an equilibrium at which the rate of chemical leaving the aqueous phase and entering the organic phase will equal the rate of the chemical moving from the organic phase to the aqueous phase. This is not the physiological situation. Refer to Figure 2-1 and note that dynamic changes are occurring to the drug, such as it being metabolized, bound to serum albumin, excreted from the body, and bound to receptors. The environment for the drug is not static. Upon administration, the drug will be *pushed* through the membranes because of the high concentration of drug in the extracellular fluids relative to the concentration in the intracellular compartments. In an attempt to maintain equilibrium ratios, the flow of the drug will be from systemic circulation through the membranes onto the receptors. As the drug is metabolized and excreted from the body, it will be *pulled* back across the membranes, and the concentration of drug at the receptors will decrease.

Because much of the time the drug's movement across membranes is a partitioning process, the partition coefficient has become the most common physicochemical property. The question that now must be asked is what immiscible nonpolar solvent system best mimics the water/lipid membrane barriers found in the body? It is now realized that the *n*-octanol/water system is an excellent estimator of drug partitioning in biological systems. Indeed, one could argue that it was fortuitous that *n*-octanol was available in reasonable purity for the early partition coefficient determinations. To appreciate why this is so, one must understand the chemical nature of the lipid membranes.

These membranes are not exclusively anhydrous fatty or oily structures. As a first approximation, they can be considered bilayers composed of lipids consisting of a polar cap and large hydrophobic tail. Phosphoglycerides are major components of lipid bilayers. Other groups of bifunctional lipids include the sphingomyelins, galactocerebrosides, and plasmalogens. The hydrophobic portion is composed largely of unsaturated fatty acids, mostly with *cis* double bonds. In addition, there are considerable amounts of cholesterol esters, protein, and charged mucopolysaccharides in the lipid membranes. The final result is that these membranes are highly organized structures composed of channels for transport of important molecules such as metabolites, chemical regulators (hormones), amino acids, glucose, and fatty acids into the cell and removal of waste products and biochemically produced products out of the cell. The cellular membranes are dynamic, with the channels forming and disappearing depending on the cell's and body's needs (Fig. 2-8).

In addition, the membranes on the surface of nucleated cells have specific antigenic markers, major histocompatibility complex (MHC), by which the immune system monitors the cell's status. There are receptors on the cell surface where hormones such as epinephrine and insulin bind, setting off

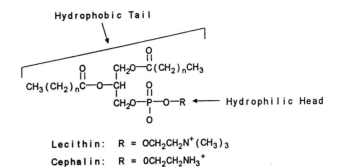

Lecithin: R = $OCH_2CH_2N^+(CH_3)_3$

Cephalin: R = $OCH_2CH_2NH_3^+$

Figure 2–8 ■ General structure of a bifunctional phospholipid. Many of the fatty acid esters will be *cis* unsaturated.

a series of biochemical events within the cell. Some of these receptors are used by viruses to gain entrance into the cells, where the virus reproduces. As newer instrumental techniques are developed, and genetic cloning permits isolation of the genetic material responsible for forming and regulating the structures on the cell surface, the image of a passive lipid membrane has disappeared to be replaced by a very complex, highly organized, dynamically functioning structure.

For purposes of the partitioning phenomenon, picture the cellular membranes as two layers of lipids (Fig. 2-9). The two outer layers, one facing the interior and the other facing the exterior of the cell, consist of the polar ends of the bifunctional lipids. Keep in mind that these surfaces are exposed to an aqueous polar environment. The polar ends of the charged phospholipids and other bifunctional lipids are solvated by the water molecules. There are also considerable amounts of charged proteins and mucopolysaccharides present on the surface. In contrast, the interior of the membrane is populated by the hydrophobic aliphatic chains from the fatty acid esters.

Partition Coefficient

With this representation in mind, a partial explanation can be presented as to why the *n*-octanol/water partitioning system seems to mimic the lipid membranes/water systems found in the body. It turns out that *n*-octanol is not as nonpolar as initially might be predicted. Water-saturated octanol contains 2.3 M water because the small water molecule easily clusters around octanol's hydroxy moiety. *n*-Octanol–saturated water contains little of the organic phase because of the large hydrophobic 8-carbon chain of octanol. The water in the *n*-octanol phase apparently approximates the polar prop-

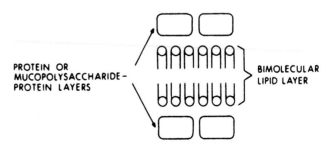

Figure 2–9 ■ Schematic representation of the cell membrane.

erties of the lipid bilayer, whereas the lack of octanol in the water phase mimics the physiological aqueous compartments, which are relatively free of nonpolar components. In contrast, partitioning systems such as hexane/water and chloroform/water contain so little water in the organic phase that they are poor models for the lipid bilayer/water system found in the body. At the same time, remember that the *n*-octanol/water system is only an approximation of the actual environment found in the interface between the cellular membranes and the extracellular/intracellular fluids.

The basic procedure for obtaining a partition coefficient is to shake a weighed amount of chemical in a flask containing a measured amount of water-saturated octanol and octanol-saturated water. Many times, the aqueous phase will be buffered with a phosphate buffer at pH 7.4 to reflect physiological pH. This corrects for the ratio of [conjugate base]/[acid] found in vivo. The amount of chemical in one or both of the phases is determined by an appropriate analytical technique and the partition coefficient calculated from Equation 2-20. The octanol/water partition coefficient has been determined for thousands of compounds, including drugs, agricultural chemicals, biochemical intermediates and metabolites, and common chemicals. Many of these determinations have been obtained in several other organic solvent/water systems, such as ether, chloroform, triolein, and hexane. Equations have been published relating the partition coefficients determined in one solvent/water system to those determined in another.

$$P = \frac{[\text{chemical}]_{\text{oct}}}{[\text{chemical}]_{\text{aq}}} \qquad \text{(Eq. 2-20)}$$

The determination of partition coefficients is tedious and time consuming. Some chemicals are too unstable and either degrade during the procedure, which can take several hours, or cannot be obtained in sufficient purity for an accurate determination. This has led to attempts at approximating the partition coefficient. Perhaps the most popular approach has been high-performance liquid chromatography (HPLC) or thin-layer chromatography (TLC). In each case, the support phase is nonpolar, either by permanent bonding (usually octadecylsilane) or a coating of octanol, mineral oils, or related materials. The mobile phase usually contains some water-miscible organic solvent to hold enough of the chemical whose partition coefficient is being determined in solution. Sometimes the partition coefficient is calculated from the retention data by regression analysis using Equation 2-21. The *a* and *c* terms have the same uses as in Equation 2-16.

$$\log P = a(\log \text{retention}) + c \qquad \text{(Eq. 2-21)}$$

This model has at least two limitations. First, to obtain valid numerical values for *a* and *c* in Equation 2-16, partition coefficients for a group of very closely related compounds must be obtained initially by the classical shake flask method. The retention times for the same group of compounds are then obtained in the identical chromatographic system that will be used for the new compounds. The values for *a* and *c* are obtained using Equation 2-21 using standard linear regression. The second limitation to the chromatographic model is that chromatographic approximations of the partition coefficients usually only work when one is determining the retention times of chemicals of the same chemical class and similar substitution patterns. Because of these limitations, sometimes the medicinal chemist will use the

retention data directly in the prediction of biological response (Eq. 2-22). A chemical's retention on a chromatographic support is the result of a combination of its partitioning, steric, and electronic properties. Because these same physical chemical properties are important variables in determining a drug's biological response, excellent correlations have been obtained between chromatographic retention parameters and biological response. While the model represented by Equation 2-22 is useful in predicting biological response, it is not as definitive as the models presented below (Eqs. 2-23 to 2-25) because the precise physical chemical properties are combined into one chromatographic retention term. In other words, it is not possible to determine the relative importance of lipophilicity, electronic effects, or steric influence on the biological response when using Equation 2-22.

$$\log BR = a(\log \text{retention}) + c \qquad \text{(Eq. 2-22)}$$

Most recently, there has been a concentrated effort to calculate the partition coefficient on the basis of the atomic components of the molecule. Each atom type is assumed to contribute a fixed amount to the chemical's partition coefficient. Because this assumption breaks down quickly, several correction factors are used. Cyclohexene will serve as an example.

$$\log P = 6(\text{carbon atoms}) + 12(\text{hydrogen atoms}) + (n-1)\text{bonds} + \text{double bond correction}$$
$$\log P = 6(0.20) + 12(0.23) + 5(-0.09) + (-0.55)$$
$$= 2.96$$

For purposes of comparison, the observed octanol/water partition coefficient (expressed as a logarithm) is 2.86. Because of the correction factors, these calculations become so complex that they must be done by a computer program that analyzes the structure and identifies those structural attributes requiring correction factors. Convenient as the calculation method may be, its accuracy depends on first determining experimental partition coefficients of chemicals exhibiting very similar chemistry. The values for specific atoms, groups of atoms and bond correction factors are derived from these experimentally determined partition coefficients.

There are several commercial drug design software packages that contain modules that estimate a chemical's partition coefficient. Some use the method described in the previous paragraph. Others use quantum chemical parameters. In all cases, the algorithm must be validated against test sets of diverse chemical structures whose partition coefficients have been determined by the classical shake flask method.

There are simpler methods for estimating lipophilicity that will give reasonably correct results. These are based on the additive effect on the partition coefficient that is seen when varying a series of substituents on the same molecule. Over the years, fairly extensive tables have been developed that contain the contribution (π) of a wide variety of substituents to the partition coefficient. The method can be illustrated for chlorobenzene. The log of P is 2.13 for benzene and 2.84 for chlorobenzene. The π value for the chlorine substituent is obtained by subtracting the log of P values for benzene and chlorobenzene.

$$\pi_{\text{Cl}} = \log P_{\text{chlorobenzene}} - \log P_{\text{benzene}}$$
$$\pi_{\text{Cl}} = 2.84 - 2.13 = 0.71$$

While the π substituent method has its limitations, particularly when there are significant resonance and inductive effects resulting from the presence of multiple substituents, it can work well for a series of compounds that have similar substitution patterns.

Other Physicochemical Parameters

There is a series of other constants that measure the contribution by substituents to the molecule's total physicochemical properties. These include Hammett's Φ constant; Taft's steric parameter, E_s; Charton's steric parameter, ν; Verloop's multidimensional steric parameters, L, B_1, B_5; and molar refractivity, MR. The latter has become the second most useful physicochemical parameter used in classical QSAR modeling. It is a complex term based on the molecule's refractive index, molecular weight, and density and can be considered a measure of the molecule's bulk and electronic character. One reason for its popularity is that it is easy to calculate from tables of atoms, using a minimum of correction factors. Of the listed physicochemical parameters group, it is most easy to locate values for B, Φ, E_s, and MR. A representative list can be found in Table 2-8.

Table 2-8 illustrates several items that must be kept in mind when selecting substituents to be evaluated in terms of the type of factors that influence a biological response. For electronic parameters such as Φ, the location on an aromatic ring is important because of resonance versus inductive effects. Notice the twofold differences seen between Φ_{meta} and Φ_{para} for the three aliphatic substituents and iodo, and severalfold difference for methoxy, amino, fluoro, and phenolic hydroxyl.

Selection of substituents from a certain chemical class may not really test the influence of a parameter on biological activity. There is little numerical difference among the Φ_{meta} or Φ_{para} values for the four aliphatic groups or the four halogens. It is not uncommon to go to the tables and find missing parameters such as the E_s values for acetyl and *N*-acyl.

Nevertheless, medicinal chemists can use information from extensive tables of physicochemical parameters to minimize the number of substituents required to find out if the biological response is sensitive to electronic, steric, and/or partitioning effects.[2] This is done by selecting substituents in each of the numerical ranges for the different parameters. In Table 2-8, there are three ranges of B values (-1.23 to -0.55, -0.28 to 0.56, and 0.71 to 1.55); three ranges of MR values (0.92 to 2.85, 5.02 to 8.88, and 10.30 to 14.96); and two main clusters of Φ values, one for the aliphatic substituents and the other for the halogens. In the ideal situation, substituents are selected from each of the clusters to determine the dependence of the biological response over the largest possible variable space. Depending on the biological responses obtained from testing the new compounds, it is possible to determine if lipophilicity (partitioning), steric bulk (molar refraction), or electron withdrawing/donating properties are important determinants of the desired biological response.

QSAR Models

Currently, there are three models or equations seen in QSAR analysis using physicochemical parameters, represented by Equation 2-23, 2-24, and 2-25. These three equations are illustrated in Figure 2-10, using the logarithm of the partition coefficient (log P) as the physical chemical parameter. First, there is the linear model (Eq. 2-23). When plots of log 1/BR or log BR indicated a nonlinear relationship between biological response and the partition coefficient, a parabolic model was tried (Eq. 2-24). Examination of Figure 2-10 shows an optimum log P (log P_o), where maximum biological activity will be obtained before a decrease in activity is seen. One explanation for this phenomenon is that hydrophilic drugs will tend to stay in the aqueous phase, whereas lipophilic chemicals will prefer the lipid bilayer. In both cases, less drug is being transported to the receptor, resulting in a decrease in the actual concentration of receptor-bound

TABLE 2–8 Sampling of Physicochemical Parameters Used in Quantitative Structure Activity Relationships Investigations

Substituent Group	π	σ_{meta}	σ_{para}	E_s	MR
—H	0.00	0.00	0.00	0.00	1.03
—CH$_3$	0.56	−0.07	−0.17	−1.24	5.65
—CH$_2$CH$_3$	1.02	−0.07	−0.15	−1.31	10.30
—CH$_2$CH$_2$CH$_3$	1.55	−0.07	−0.13	−1.60	14.96
—C(CH$_3$)$_2$	1.53	−0.07	−0.15	−1.71	14.96
—OCH$_3$	−0.02	0.12	−0.27	−0.55	7.87
—NH$_2$	−1.23	−0.16	−0.66	−0.61	5.42
—F	0.14	0.34	0.06	−0.46	0.92
—Cl	0.71	0.37	0.23	−0.97	6.03
—Br	0.86	0.39	0.23	−1.16	8.88
—I	1.12	0.35	0.18	−1.40	13.94
—CF$_3$	0.88	0.43	0.54	−2.40	5.02
—OH	−0.67	0.12	−0.37	−0.55	2.85
—COCH$_3$	−0.55	0.38	0.50		11.18
—NHCOCH$_3$	−0.97	0.21	0.00		14.93
—NO$_2$	−0.8	0.71	0.78	−2.52	7.36
—CN	−0.57	0.56	0.66	−0.51	6.33

From Hansch, C., Leo, A. J.: Substituent Constants for Correlation Analysis in Chemistry and Biology. New York, John Wiley & Sons, 1979.

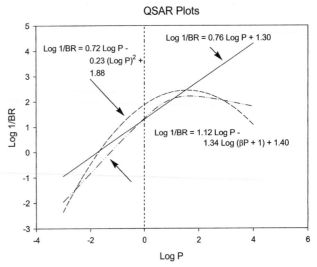

Figure 2–10 ■ Plots of log biological response versus log partition coefficient, using linear, parabolic, and bilinear models.

drug. In other words, the equilibrium seen in Reaction 2-1 shifts to the left. There will be a group of drugs whose log P places them near the top of the parabola; their lipophilic–hydrophilic balance will permit them to penetrate both aqueous and lipid barriers and reach the receptor.

$$\log 1/BR = a (\log P) + c \qquad \text{(Eq. 2-23)}$$
$$\log 1/BR = a (\log P) - b (\log P)^2 + c \qquad \text{(Eq. 2-24)}$$
$$\log 1/BR = a (\log P) - b \log(\beta P + 1) + c \qquad \text{(Eq. 2-25)}$$

The third QSAR equation in current use is the bilinear model (Eq. 2-25). It consists of two straight lines, one ascending and one descending. The β term connects the two lines. There are several interpretations for the β term. One explanation is based on the ratio of the rate constant for diffusion out of the octanol layer into the aqueous environment being different from the rate of diffusion out of the aqueous layer into the octanol layer. In other words, what may be simulated with the bilinear model is recognition that the rate of diffusion from the extracellular fluids into the lipid bilayer differs from the rate of diffusion out of the lipid bilayer into the intracellular environment. Another interpretation is recognition that the kinetics of partitioning through the lipid bilayer differ from the kinetics of binding to the receptor. A third explanation takes into account the different volumes of the aqueous and lipid bilayers in the biological system.

With this background in mind, three examples of QSAR equations taken from the medicinal chemistry literature are presented. One shows a linear relationship (Eq. 2-26), and the others show parabolic (Eq. 2-27) and bilinear (Eq. 2-28) correlations. A study of a group of griseofulvin analogues showed a linear relationship (Eq. 2-26) between the biological response and both lipophilicity (log P) and electronic character (σ).[3] It was suggested that the antibiotic activity may depend on the enone system facilitating the addition of griseofulvin to a nucleophilic group such as the SH moiety in a fungal enzyme.

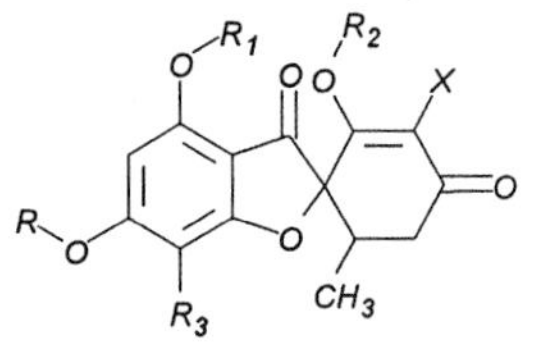

Griseofulvin: $R = R_1 = R_2 = OCH_3$; $R_3 = Cl$; $X = H$

$$\log BR = (0.56)\log P + (2.19)\sigma_x - 1.32 \qquad \text{(Eq. 2-26)}$$

A parabolic relationship (Eq. 2-27) was reported for a series of substituted acetylated salicylates (substituted aspirins) tested for anti-inflammatory activity.[4] A nonlinear relationship exists between the biological response and lipophilicity, and a significant detrimental steric effect is seen with substituents at position 4. The two sterimol parameters used in this equation were L, defined as the length of the substituent along the axis of the bond between the first atom of the substituent and the parent molecule, and B_2, defined as a width parameter. Steric effects were not considered statistically significant at position 3, as shown by the sterimol parameters for substituents at position 3 not being part of Equation 2-27. The optimal partition coefficient (log P_o) for the substituted aspirins in this assay was 2.6. At the same time,

increasing bulk, as measured by the sterimol parameters, decreases activity.

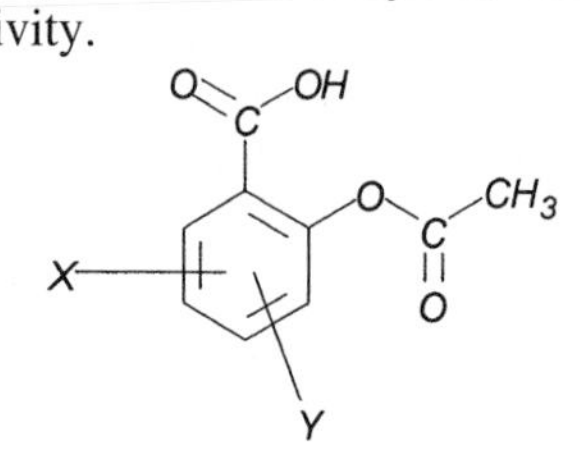

Aspirin: $X = Y = H$

$$\log 1/ED_{50} = 1.03 \log P - 0.20(\log P)^2 - 0.05 L_{(4)} - 0.24 B_{2(4)} + 2.29 \qquad \text{(Eq. 2-27)}$$

In addition to these QSAR models based on biological responses, QSAR is used to analyze pharmacokinetic activity. One example of this (Eq. 2-28) is a simulation of barbiturate absorption, which leads to the bilinear model.[5,6]

$$\log k_{DIFF} =$$
$$0.949 \log P - 1.238 \log(\beta P + 1) - 3.131 \qquad \text{(Eq. 2-28)}$$

where $\beta = -1.271$; log $P_o = 1.79$; and k_{DIFF} = diffusion rate constant.

At this point, it is appropriate to ask the question, are all the determinations of partition coefficients and compilation of physical chemical parameters useful only when a statistically valid QSAR model is obtained? The answer is a firm "no." One of the most useful spinoffs from the field of QSAR has been the application of experimental design to the selection of new compounds to be synthesized and tested. Let's assume that a new series of drug molecules is to be synthesized based on the following structure. The goal is to test the effect of the 16 substituents in Table 2-8 at each of the three positions on our new series. The number of possible analogues is equal to 16^3, or 4096, compounds, assuming that all three positions will always be substituted with one of the substituents from Table 2-7. If hydrogen is included when a position is not substituted, there are 17^3, or 4913, different combinations. The problem is to select a small number of substituents that represent the different ranges or clusters of values for lipophilicity, electronic influence, and bulk. An initial design set could include the methyl and propyl from the aliphatic cluster, fluorine and chlorine from the halogen cluster, N-acetyl and phenol from the substituents showing hydrophilicity, and a range of electronic and bulk values. Including hydrogen, there will be 7^3, or 343, different combinations. Obviously, that is too many for an initial evaluation. Instead, certain rules have been devised to maximize the information obtained from a minimum number of compounds. These include the following:

1. Each substituent must occur more than once at each position on which it is found.
2. The number of times that each substituent at a particular position appears should be approximately equal.
3. No two substituents should be present in a constant combination.
4. When combinations of substituents are a necessity, they should not occur more frequently than any other combination.

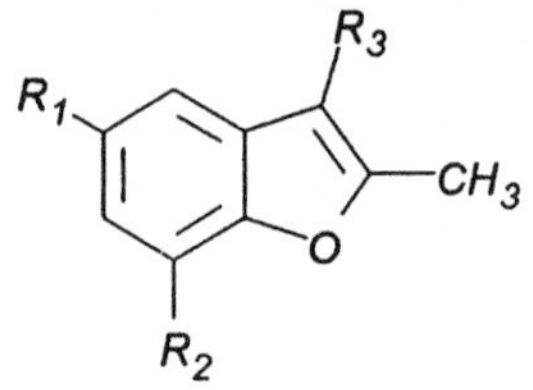

Following these guidelines, the initial test set can be reduced to 24 to 26 compounds. Depending on the precision of the biological tests, it will be possible to see if the data will fit a QSAR model. Even an approximate model usually will indicate the types of substituents to test further and what positions on the molecules are sensitive to substitution and, if sensitive, to what degree variation in lipophilic, electronic, or bulk character is important. Just to ensure that the model is valid, it is a good idea to synthesize a couple of compounds that the model predicts would be inactive. As each group of new compounds is tested, the QSAR model is refined until the investigators have a pretty good idea what substituent patterns are important for the desired activity. These same techniques used to develop potent compounds with desired activity also can be used to evaluate the influence of substituent patterns on undesired toxic effects and pharmacokinetic properties.

In their *pure form,* the rules listed above can be used to select a minimum number of compounds for a test set, using what are known as *identity variables.* No physicochemical parameters are required. In its simplest form, the equation takes the form outlined in Equation 2-29. This approach has been known as a Free-Wilson analysis.[7]

$$\log BR = \Sigma \text{ (substituent contributions)}$$
$$+ \text{ contribution from the base molecule} \quad \text{(Eq. 2-29)}$$

An example is a small set of phosphorus-containing acetylcholinesterase inhibitors that were selected by using the rules for designing a test set and evaluated as possible insecticides.[8] The result is a complex equation that produces a coefficient for each substituent. They are summarized in Table 2-9.

Examination of this table shows that ethyl and ethoxy at R_1, ethoxy and isopropoxy at R_2, and oxo at R_4 have minimal influence on biological activity. In contrast, methyl and isopropoxy at R_1; methoxy, propoxy, and butoxy at R_2; all three nitrophenoxy substituents at R_3; and thio at R_4 significantly influence the biological response. The predicted log 1/BR for the compound, where R_1 = methyl, R_2 = propoxy, R_3 = 4-nitrophenoxy, and R_4 = thio, would be calculated from Equation 2-29:

$$
\begin{aligned}
\log BR &= R_1 + R_2 + R_3 + R_4 + \text{base molecule} \\
&= 0.729 + 0.543 + 0.611 - 1.673 + 5.143 \\
&= 5.353
\end{aligned}
$$

One of the newer QSAR methods combines statistical techniques with molecular modeling and has been referred to as three-dimensional QSAR (3D-QSAR) because the independent variables, usually physicochemical parameters, take into account spatial distances among and between pharmacophores and their location at specific distances from the molecule. Each point has a location on *x, y,* and *z* coordinates. 3D-QSAR depends on the molecular modeling algorithms and is discussed in more detail in Chapter 5. Attempts at including a variety of orientations in space and a variety of biological responses have led to the use of terms such as *four-dimensional* and *five-dimensional QSAR.*[9,10]

Topological Descriptors

An alternate method of describing molecular structure is based on graph theory, in which the bonds connecting the atoms is considered a path that is traversed from one atom to another. Consider Figure 2-11 containing D-phenylalanine and its hydrogen-suppressed graph representation. The numbering is arbitrary and not based on IUPAC or *Chemical Abstracts* nomenclature rules. A connectivity table, Table 2-10, is constructed.

Table 2-10 is a two-dimensional connectivity table for the hydrogen-suppressed phenylalanine molecule. No three-dimensional representation is implied. Further, this type of connectivity table will be the same for molecules with asymmetric atoms (D versus L) or for those that can exist in more than one conformation (i.e., "chair" versus "boat" conformation, *anti* versus *gauche* versus *eclipsed*).

Graph theory is not limited to the paths followed by chemical bonds. In its purest form, the atoms in the phenyl ring of phenylalanine would have paths connecting atom 7 with atoms 9, 10, 11, and 12; atom 8 with atoms 10, 11, and 12; atom 9 with atoms 11 and 12; and atom 10 with atom 12. Also, the graph itself might differentiate neither single, double, and triple bonds nor the type of atom (C, O, and N in the

---

TABLE 2–9 Coefficients for Substituents in a Set of Acetylcholinesterase Inhibitors[a]

$$
\begin{array}{c}
R_2 \\
| \\
R_1\!-\!P\!-\!R_3 \\
\| \\
R_4
\end{array}
$$

R_1 = CH_3, C_2H_5, OCH_3, OC_2H_5, OC_3H_7, $OC(CH_3)_2$

R_2 = OCH_3, OC_2H_5, OC_3H_7, $OC(CH_3)_2$, OC_4H_9

R_3 = $-O(C_6H_4)(2-NO_2)$, $-O(C_6H_4)(3-NO_2)$, $-O(C_6H_4)(4-NO_2)$

R_4 = O, S

R_1		R_2		R_3		R_4	
Methyl	0.729	Methoxy	−0.598	2-Nitrophenoxy	0.856	Oxo	0.052
Ethyl	−0.167	Ethoxy	0.186	3-Nitrophenoxy	−1.134	Thio	−1.673
Ethoxy	−0.168	Propoxy	0.543	4-Nitrophenoxy	0.611		
Propoxy	−0.405	Isopropoxy	−0.164				
Isopropoxy	−1.267	Butoxy	0.786				

From Waisser, K., Macháček, M., and Čeladnik, M.: The use of Free-Wilson model on investigating the relationship between the chemical structure and selectivity of drugs. In Kuchar, M. (ed.). QSAR in Design of Bioactive Molecules. Barcelona, J. R. Prous, 1984.
[a] Contribution from the base molecule = 5.143.

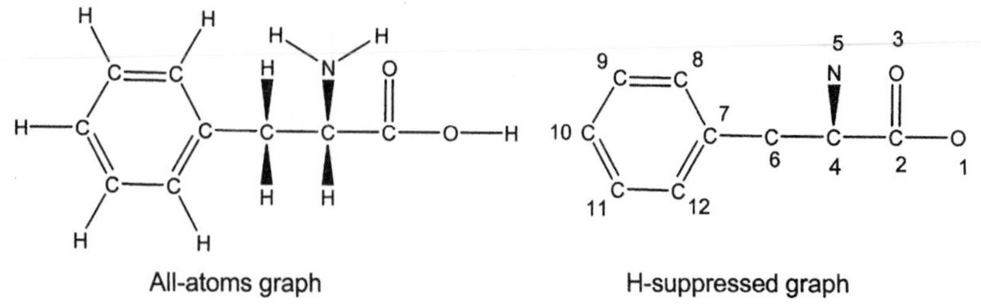

All-atoms graph   H-suppressed graph

D-Phenylalanine

Figure 2–11 ▪ Hydrogen-suppressed graphic representation of phenylalanine.

phenylalanine example). Connectivity tables can be coded to indicate the type of bond.

The most common application of graph theory used by medicinal chemistry is called *molecular connectivity*. It limits the paths to the molecule's actual chemical bonds. Table 2-11 shows several possible paths for phenylalanine, including linear paths and clusters or branching. Numerical values for each path or path-cluster are based on the number of nonhydrogen bonds to each atom. Let's examine oxygen atom 1. There is only one nonhydrogen bond, and it connects oxygen atom 1 to carbon atom 2. The formula is the reciprocal square root of the number of bonds. For oxygen 1, the connectivity value is 1. For carbonyl oxygen 2, it is $2^{-1/2}$, or 0.707. Note that there is no difference between oxygen 1 and nitrogen 5. Both have only one nonhydrogen bond and a connectivity value of 1. Similarly, there is no difference in values for a carbonyl oxygen and a methylene carbon, each having two nonhydrogen bonds. The final connectivity values for a path are the reciprocal square roots of the products of each path. For the second-order path 2C-4C-6C, the reciprocal square root $(3 \times 3 \times 2)^{-1/2}$ is 4.243. The values for each path order are calculated and summed.

As noted above, the method as described so far cannot distinguish between atoms that have the same number of nonhydrogen bonds. A method to distinguish heteroatoms from each other and carbon atoms is based on the difference between the number of valence electrons and possible hydrogen atoms (which are suppressed in the graph). The "va-

lence" connectivity term for an alcohol oxygen would be 6 valence electrons minus 1 hydrogen, or 5. The "valence" connectivity term for a primary amine nitrogen would be 5 valence electrons minus 2 hydrogens, or 3. There are a variety of additional modifications that are done to further differentiate atoms and define their environments within the molecule.

Excellent regression equations using topological indices have been obtained. A problem is interpreting what they mean. Is it lipophilicity, steric bulk, or electronic terms that define activity? The topological indices can be correlated with all of these common physicochemical descriptors. Another problem is that it is difficult to use the equation to decide what molecular modifications can be made to enhance activity further, again because of ambiguities in physicochemical interpretation. Should the medicinal chemist increase or decrease lipophilicity at a particular location on the molecule? Should specific substituents be increased or decreased? On the other hand, topological indices can be very valuable in classification schemes that are described below. They do describe the structure in terms of rings, branching, flexibility, etc.

Classification Methods

Besides regression analysis, there are other statistical techniques used in drug design. These fit under the classification of multivariate statistics and include discriminant analysis,

TABLE 2–10   Connectivity Table for Hydrogen-Suppressed Phenylalanine

Atom	O-1	C-2	O-3	C-4	N-5	C-6	C-7	C-8	C-9	C-10	C-11	C-12
O-1		X										
C-2	X		X	X								
O-3		X										
C-4		X			X	X						
N-5				X								
C-6				X			X					
C-7						X		X				X
C-8							X		X			
C-9								X		X		
C-10									X		X	
C-11										X		X
C-12							X				X	

TABLE 2–11 Examples of Paths Found in the Phenylalanine Molecule

1st Order Path	2nd Order Path	3rd Order Path	4th Order Path	5th Order Path	Path-Cluster
1O-2C	1O-2C-3O	1O-2C-4C-6C	1O-2C-4C-6C-7C	1O-2C-4C-6C-7C-8C	1O-2C-3O-4C
2C-3O	1O-2C-4C	3O-2C-4C-5N	3O-2C-4C-6C-7C	1O-2C-4O-6C-7C-12C	2C-4C-5N-6C
2C-4C	3O-2C-4C	3O-2C-4C-6C	2C-4C-6C-7C-8C	2C-4C-6C-7C-8C-9C	6C-7C-8C-12C
4C-5N	2C-4C-5N	1O-2C-4C-5N	2C-4C-6C-7C-12C	2C-4C-6C-7C-12C-11C	
4C-6C	2C-4C-6C	2C-4C-6C-7C	4C-6C-7C-8C-9C	3O-2C-4C-6C-7C-8C	
6C-7C	5N-4C-6C	5N-4C-6C-7C	4C-6C-7C-12C-11C	3O-2C-4C-6C-7C-12C	
7C-8C	4C-6C-7C	4C-6C-7C-8C	5N-4C-6C-7C-8C	4C-6C-7C-8C-9C-10C	
8C-9C	6C-7C-8C	4C-6C-7C-12C	5N-4C-6C-7C-12C	4C-6C-7C-12C-11C-10C	
7C-12C	6C-7C-12C	6C-7C-8C-9C	6C-7C-8C-9C-10C	5N-4C-6C-7C-8C-9C	
9C-10C	7C-8C-9C	6C-7C-12C-11C	6C-7C-12C-11C-10C	5N-4C-6C-7C-12C-11C	
10C-11C	7C-12C-11C	7C-8C-9C-10C	7C-8C-9C-10C-11C	6C-7C-8C-9C-10C-11C	
11C-12C	8C-9C-10C	7C-12C-11C-10C	7C-12C-11C-10C-9C	6C-7C-12C-11C-10C	
	9C-10C-11C	8C-9C-10C-11C	8C-9C-10C-11C-12C	7C-8C-9C-10C-11C-12C	
	10C-11C-12C	9C-10C-11C-12C		7C-12C-11C-10C-9C-8C	

principal component analysis, and pattern recognition. The latter can consist of a mixture of statistical and nonstatistical methodologies. The goal usually is to try to ascertain what physicochemical parameters and structural attributes contribute to a class or type of biological activity. Then the chemicals are classified into groupings such as carcinogenic/noncarcinogenic, sweet/bitter, active/inactive, and depressant/stimulant.

The term *multivariate* is used because of the wide variety and number of independent or descriptor variables that may be used. The same physicochemical parameters seen in QSAR analyses are used, but in addition, the software in the computer programs "breaks" the molecule down into substructures. These structural fragments also become variables. Examples of the typical substructures used include carbonyls, enones, conjugation, rings of different sizes and types, N-substitution patterns, and aliphatic substitution patterns such as 1,3- or 1,2-disubstituted. The end result is that for even a moderate-size molecule typical of most drugs, there can be 50 to 100 variables.

The technique is to develop a large set of chemicals well characterized in terms of the biological activity that is going to be predicted. This is known as the *training set*. Ideally, it should contain hundreds, if not thousands, of compounds, divided into active and inactive types. In reality, sets smaller than 100 are studied. Most of these investigations are retrospective ones in which the investigator locates large data sets from several sources. This means that the biological testing likely followed different protocols. That is why classification techniques tend to avoid using continuous variables such as ED_{50}, LD_{50}, and MIC. Instead, arbitrary endpoints such as active or inactive, stimulant or depressant, sweet or sour, are used.

Once the training set is established, the multivariate technique is carried out. The algorithms are designed to group the underlying commonalities and select the variables that have the greatest influence on biological activity. The predictive ability is then tested with a test set of compounds that have been put through the same biological tests used for the training set. For the classification model to be valid, the investigator must select data sets whose results are not intuitively obvious and could not be classified by a trained medicinal chemist. Properly done, classification methods can identify structural and physicochemical descriptors that can be powerful predictors and determinants of biological activity.

There are several examples of successful applications of this technique.[11] One study consisted of a diverse group of 140 tranquilizers and 79 sedatives subjected to a two-way classification study (tranquilizers versus sedatives). The ring types included phenothiazines, indoles, benzodiazepines, barbiturates, diphenylmethanes, and a variety of heterocyclics. Sixty-nine descriptors were used initially to characterize the molecules. Eleven of these descriptors were crucial to the classification, 54 had intermediate use and depended on the composition of the training set, and 4 were of little use. The overall range of prediction accuracy was 88 to 92%. The results with the 54 descriptors indicate an important limitation when large numbers of descriptors are used. The inclusion or exclusion of descriptors and parameters can depend on the composition of the training set. The training set must be representative of the population of chemicals that are going to be evaluated. Indeed, repeating the study on different randomly selected training sets is important.

Classification techniques lend themselves to studies lacking quantitative data. An interesting classification problem involved olfactory stimulants, in which the goal was to select chemicals that had a musk odor. A group of 300 unique compounds was selected from a group of odorants that included 60 musk odorants plus 49 camphor, 44 floral, 32 ethereal, 41 mint, 51 pungent, and 23 putrid odorants. Initially, 68 descriptors were evaluated. Depending on the approach, the number of descriptors was reduced to 11 to 16, consisting mostly of bond types. Using this small number, the 60 musk odorants could be selected from the remaining 240 compounds, with an accuracy of 95 to 97%.

The use of classification techniques in medicinal chemistry has matured over years of general use. The types of descriptors have expanded to spatial measurements in three-dimensional space similar to those used in 3D-QSAR (see below). Increasingly, databases of existing compounds are scanned for molecules that possess what appear to be the desired parameters. If the scan is successful, compounds that are predicted to be active provide the starting point for synthesizing new compounds for testing. One can see parallels between the search of chemical databases and screening plant, animal, and microbial sources for new compounds. Although the statistical and pattern recognition methodologies have been in use for a very long time, there still needs to be considerable research into their proper use, and further testing of their predictive power is needed. The goal of scanning databases of already-synthesized compounds to select compounds for pharmacological evaluation will require considerable additional development of the various multivariate techniques.

COMBINATORIAL CHEMISTRY

Elegant as the statistical techniques described above are, the goal remains to synthesize large numbers of compounds so promising marketable products are not missed. At the same time, traditional synthetic and biological testing are very costly. This has led to the technique called *combinatorial chemistry*. The latter uses libraries of chemical moieties that react with a parent or base molecule in a small number of defined synthetic steps. Return to the two examples presented with the discussion of the Free-Wilson analysis above. As the number of different substituents is considered, literally more than 10,000 compounds are possible. Remember that the medicinal chemist can select subsets of substituents that vary in lipophilicity, steric bulk, induction, and resonance effects and use the four rules for placing and use of the substituents. If this process is properly done, a relatively small number of compounds will be obtained that show the dual importance of each of the physicochemical parameters being evaluated at each position on the molecule and the effect of specific moieties at each position. This "rational" approach to drug design assumes that there is some understanding of the target receptor and that there is a lead molecule, commonly called the *prototype molecule*. A classic example is the dihydrofolate reductase inhibitor methotrexate, which has been one of the prototypes that laboratories have used to synthesize and test new inhibitors. Another example is benzodiazepine, which has a defined structure whose activity varies with the substituents.

What about the situation in which little is known about the mechanisms causing the disease process? Until recently, this has been the normal situation when searching for new molecules with the desired pharmacological response. With the discovery of penicillin came the realization that microbial organisms produced "antibiotics." This started screenings of microbial products, looking for new antibiotics. In a similar manner, thousands of synthetic compounds and plant extracts have been screened for anticancer activity. Some have called this "irrational" drug design, but it has produced most of the drugs currently prescribed. This approach also is very expensive, particularly when one realizes the cost to synthesize, isolate, and test each new compound plus the time and expense necessary to take an active compound through efficacy and safety testing before its release to the general public is approved by government regulatory agencies.

Combinatorial chemistry is one method of reducing the cost of drug discovery in which the goal is to find new leads or prototype compounds or to optimize and refine the structure–activity relationships.[12,13] Libraries of "reactive" chemical moieties provide the chemical diversity of products that will be screened for activity. The chemistry is elegant but relatively simple, in that the same few reactions are required to make thousands of compounds in a particular series. The reactions must be clean and reproducible and have high yields. Often, solid-state synthetic methods are used in which compounds are "grown" onto polymer support. Robotics can be used to reduce further the cost of synthesis. Biological testing can also be automated in a process called *high-throughput screening,* which can test tens to hundreds of structures at a time. Many times it is possible to take advantage of gene cloning techniques, clone the desired receptor, and measure the binding of the newly synthesized compounds to the cloned receptor.

To maintain some focus on the needed structures, information theory has been used to construct the libraries of substituents. These libraries tend to maximize chemical diversity in terms of physicochemical parameters. Many of these libraries are sold commercially by firms specializing in this technique. The synthetic methodologies cover the spectrum from producing thousands of relatively pure compounds to producing mixtures of compounds that are tested as mixtures. Of course, mixtures can be difficult to classify, and it can be difficult to determine which products in the mixture are active and which are inactive. Elegant methods have been developed that chemically "tag" each compound with a small peptide, nucleotide, or other small molecule that is pharmacologically inert. When mixtures of products are obtained, they are screened for activity. Only those mixtures that are biologically active are retained. In a process called *deconvolution,* the synthesis is repeated in an iterative manner, producing smaller and sometimes overlapping mixtures. The screening is repeated until the active compounds are identified. Examine Table 2-12. This simplified outline shows how four steps will identify the three active components in a 20-compound investigation. (Keep in mind that the actual combinatorial process will produce hundreds or thousands of compounds for testing.)

Assume that the project calls for synthesizing 20 compounds, A to T. Rather than carry out 20 distinct syntheses followed by 20 separate screening experiments, all of which can take weeks, four combinatorial syntheses are carried out such that four mixtures containing five compounds each are obtained. Only the three mixtures that test positive in the screening assay are retained. The synthesis is repeated producing five mixtures of three components each, and the testing is repeated. Six more syntheses are carried out this time, producing overlapping two-component mixtures, and the assays are repeated. It is now possible to determine that compounds B, H, and N are active. Instead of 20 syntheses and 20 assays, only 15 were required. Further, time-consuming purification of each mixture was not required. This process is very similar to that carried out by natural-product chemists. The microbial, plant, or animal tissue is extracted with a variety of solvents, beginning with nonpolar hydrocarbons

TABLE 2-12 Simplified Deconvolution Scheme for a 20-Compound Combinatorial Chemistry Screen

A	B[a]	C	D	E	F	G	H[a]	I	J	K	L	M	N[a]	O	P	Q	R	S	T
Carry out the synthesis producing four five-component mixtures. Screen the mixtures.																			
AB[a]CDE					FGH[a]IJ					KLM[a]NO					PQRST				
Retain only the three mixtures containing active components. Repeat the synthesis producing three-component mixtures and repeat the screening.																			
AB[a]C				DEF			GH[a]I			JKL				MN[a]O					
Discard the inactive mixtures. Repeat the synthesis producing overlapping two-component products and repeat the screening.																			
AB[a]			B[a]C			GH[a]			H[a]I			MN[a]			N[a]O				
Only compounds B, H, and N need to be chemically characterized.																			

[a] Indicates an active compound.

and ending with an alcohol or water, and the fractions are screened for activity. Only the active fractions are retained. The latter are more carefully fractionated, using biological assays to follow the purification. In either combinatorial synthesis or natural product isolation, once active compounds are identified, larger-scale, more focused syntheses can be done, using QSAR-derived experimental design and/or molecular modeling (see below) to yield compounds different from those produced from the combinatorial library of chemical fragments.

Other methods that are used commonly in combinatorial chemistry include attaching structures of known composition to polystyrene beads (one compound per bead) or synthesizing structures onto a microchip-sized matrix where a compound's location gives its identity. The latter is called *spatially addressable synthesis*. This topic is covered in more detail in Chapter 3.

MOLECULAR MODELING (COMPUTER-AIDED DRUG DESIGN)

The low cost of powerful desktop computers gives the medicinal chemist the ability to "design" the molecule on the basis of an estimated fit onto a receptor or have similar spatial characteristics found in the prototypical lead compound. Of course, this assumes that the molecular structure of the receptor is known in enough detail for a reasonable estimation of its three-dimensional shape. When a good understanding of the geometry of the active site is known, databases containing the three-dimensional coordinates of the chemicals in the database can be searched rapidly by computer programs that select candidates likely to fit in the active site. As shown below, there have been some dramatic successes with use of this approach, but first one must have an understanding of ligand (drug)–receptor interactions and conformational analysis.

Drug–Receptor Interactions

At this point, let us assume that the drug has entered the systemic circulation (Fig. 2-1), passed through the lipid bar-

riers, and is now going to make contact with the receptor. As illustrated in Reaction 2-1, this is an equilibrium process. A good ability to fit the receptor favors binding and the desired pharmacological response. In contrast, a poor fit favors the reverse reaction. With only a small amount of drug bound to the receptor, there will be a much smaller pharmacological effect. Indeed, if the amount of drug bound to the receptor is too small, there may be no discernible response. Many variables contribute to a drug's binding to the receptor. These include the structural class, the three-dimensional shape of the molecule, and the types of chemical bonding involved in the binding of the drug to the receptor.

Most drugs that belong to the same pharmacological class have certain structural features in common. The barbiturates act on specific CNS receptors, causing depressant effects; hydantoins act on CNS receptors, producing an anticonvulsant response; benzodiazepines combine with the γ-aminobutyric acid (GABA) receptors, with resulting anxiolytic activity; steroids can be divided into such classes as corticosteroids, anabolic steroids, progestogens, and estrogens, each acting on specific receptors; nonsteroidal anti-inflammatory agents inhibit enzymes required for the prostaglandin cascade; penicillins and cephalosporins inhibit enzymes required to construct the bacterial cell wall; and tetracyclines act on bacterial ribosomes.

Receptor

With the isolation and characterization of receptors becoming a common occurrence, it is hard to realize that the concept of receptors began as a postulate. It had been realized early that molecules with certain structural features would elucidate a specific biological response. Very slight changes in structure could cause significant changes in biological activity. These structural variations could increase or decrease activity or change an agonist into an antagonist. This early and fundamentally correct interpretation called for the drug (ligand) to fit onto some surface (the receptor) that had fairly strict structural requirements for proper binding of the drug. The initial receptor model was based on a rigid lock-and-key concept, with the drug (key) fitting into a receptor (lock). It has been used to explain why certain structural attributes produce a predictable pharmacological action. This model still is useful, although one must realize that both the drug and the receptor can have considerable flexibility. Molecular graphics, using programs that calculate the preferred conformations of drug and receptor, show that the receptor can undergo an adjustment in three-dimensional structure when the drug makes contact. Using space-age language, the drug "docks" with the receptor.

More complex receptors now are being isolated, characterized, and cloned. The first receptors to be isolated and characterized were the reactive and regulatory sites on enzymes. Acetylcholinesterase, dihydrofolate reductase, angiotensin, and HIV protease-converting enzyme are examples of enzymes whose active sites (the receptors) have been modeled. Most drug receptors probably are receptors for natural ligands used to regulate cellular biochemistry and function and to communicate between cells. Receptors include a relatively small region of a macromolecule, which may be an isolatable enzyme, a structural and functional component of a cell membrane, or a specific intracellular substance such as a protein or nucleic acid. Specific regions of these macromolecules are visualized as being oriented in space in a manner that permits their functional groups to interact with the complementary functional groups of the drug. This interaction initiates changes in structure and function of the macromolecule, which lead ultimately to the observable biological response. The concept of spatially oriented functional areas forming a receptor leads directly to specific structural requirements for functional groups of a drug, which must complement the receptor.

It now is possible to isolate membrane-bound receptors, although it still is difficult to elucidate their structural chemistry, because once separated from the cell membranes, these receptors may lose their native shape. This is because the membrane is required to hold the receptor in its correct tertiary structure. One method of receptor isolation is affinity chromatography. In this technique, a ligand, often an altered drug molecule known to combine with the receptor, is attached to a chromatographic support phase. A solution containing the desired receptor is passed over this column. The receptor will combine with the ligand. It is common to add a chemically reactive grouping to the drug, resulting in the receptor and drug covalently binding with each other. The drug–receptor complex is washed from the column and then characterized further.

A more recent technique uses recombinant DNA. The gene for the receptor is located and cloned. It is transferred into a bacterium, yeast, or animal, which then produces the receptor in large enough quantities to permit further study. Sometimes it is possible to determine the DNA sequence of the cloned gene. By using the genetic code for amino acids, the amino acid sequence of the protein component of the receptor can be determined, and the receptor then modeled, producing an estimated three-dimensional shape. The model for the receptor becomes the template for designing new ligands. Genome mapping has greatly increased the information on receptors. Besides the human genome, the genetic composition of viruses, bacteria, fungi, and parasites has increased the possible sites for drugs to act. The new field of proteomics studies the proteins produced by structural genes.

The discussion above in this chapter emphasizes that the cell membrane is a highly organized, dynamic structure that interacts with small molecules in specific ways; its focus is on the lipid bilayer component of this complex structure. The receptor components of the membranes appear to be mainly protein. They constitute a highly organized region of the cell membrane. The same type of molecular specificity seen in such proteins as enzymes and antibodies is also a property of drug receptors. The nature of the amide link in proteins provides a unique opportunity for the formation of multiple internal hydrogen bonds, as well as internal formation of hydrophobic, van der Waals', and ionic bonds by side chain groups, leading to such organized structures as the α helix, which contains about four amino acid residues for each turn of the helix. An organized protein structure would hold the amino acid side chains at relatively fixed positions in space and available for specific interactions with a small molecule.

Proteins can potentially adopt many different conformations in space without breaking their covalent amide linkages. They may shift from highly coiled structures to partially disorganized structures, with parts of the molecule existing in "random chain" or "folded sheet" structures, contingent on the environment. In the monolayer of a cell membrane, the interaction of a small foreign molecule with an organized protein may lead to a significant change in the structural and physical properties of the membrane. Such changes could well be the initiating events in the tissue or organ response to a drug, such as the ion-translocating effects produced by interaction of acetylcholine and the cholinergic receptor.

The large body of information now available on relationships between chemical structure and biological activity strongly supports the concept of flexible receptors. The fit of drugs onto or into macromolecules is rarely an all-or-none process as pictured by the earlier lock-and-key concept of a receptor. Rather, the binding or partial insertion of groups of moderate size onto or into a macromolecular pouch appears to be a continuous process, at least over a limited range, as indicated by the frequently occurring regular increase and decrease in biological activity as one ascends a homologous series of drugs. A range of productive associations between drug and receptor may be pictured, which leads to agonist responses, such as those produced by cholinergic and adrenergic drugs. Similarly, strong associations may lead to unproductive changes in the configuration of the macromolecule, leading to an antagonistic or blocking response, such as that produced by anticholinergic agents and HIV protease inhibitors. Although the fundamental structural unit of the drug receptor is generally considered to be protein, it may be supplemented by its associations with other units, such as mucopolysaccharides and nucleic acids.

Humans (and mammals in general) are very complex organisms that have developed specialized organ systems. It is not surprising that receptors are not distributed equally throughout the body. It now is realized that, depending on the organ in which it is located, the same receptor class may behave differently. This can be advantageous by focusing drug therapy on a specific organ system, but it can also cause adverse drug responses because the drug is exerting two different responses based on the location of the receptors. An example is the selective estrogen receptor modulators

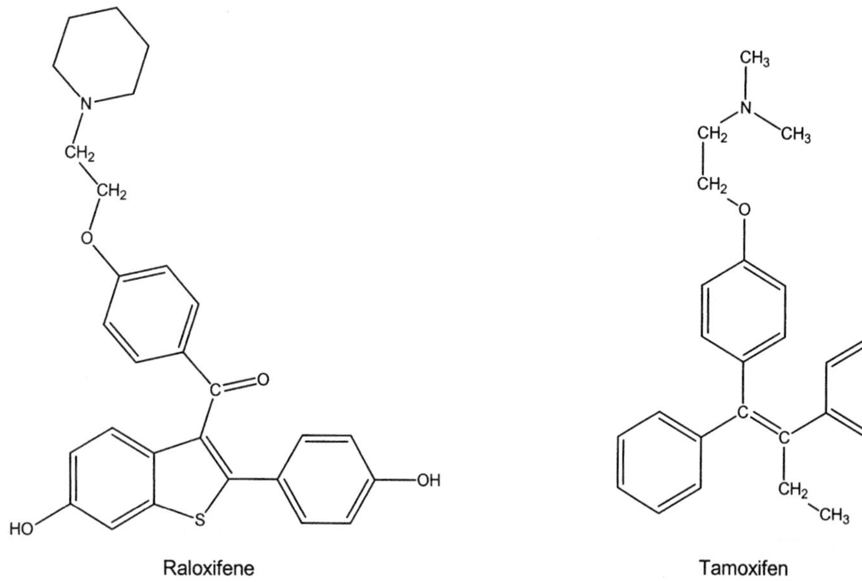

Figure 2–12 ■ Selective SERMs.

Raloxifene

Tamoxifen

(SERMs). They cannot be classified simply as agonists or antagonists. Rather they can be considered variable agonists and antagonists. Their selectivity is very complex because it depends on the organ in which the receptor is located.

This complexity can be illustrated with tamoxifen and raloxifene (Fig. 2-12). Tamoxifen is used for estrogen-sensitive breast cancer and for reducing bone loss from osteoporosis. Unfortunately, prolonged treatment increases the risk of endometrial cancer because of the response from the uterine estrogen receptors. Thus, tamoxifen is an estrogen antagonist in the mammary gland and an agonist in the uterus and bone. In contrast, raloxifene does not appear to have much agonist property in the uterus but, like tamoxifen, is an antagonist in the breast and agonist in the bone.

There are a wide variety of phosphodiesterases throughout the body. These enzymes hydrolyze the cyclic phosphate esters of adenosine monophosphate (cAMP) and guanosine monophosphate (cGMP). Although the substrates for this family of enzymes are cAMP and cGMP, there are differences in the active sites. Figure 2-13 illustrates three drugs used to treat erectile dysfunction (sildenafil, tadalafil, and vardenafil). These three take advantage of the differences in active site structural requirements between phosphodiesterase type 5 and the other phosphodiesterases. They have an important role in maintaining a desired lifestyle: treatment of erectile dysfunction caused by a variety of medical conditions. The drugs approved for this indication were discovered by accident. The goal was to develop a newer treatment of angina. The approach was to develop phosphodiesterase inhibitors that would prolong the activity of cGMP. The end result was drugs that were not effective inhibitors of the phosphodiesterase that would treat angina, but were effective inhibitors of the one found in the corpus cavernosum. The vasodilation in this organ results in penile erection.

Drug–Receptor Interaction: Forces Involved

A biological response is produced by the interaction of a drug with a functional or organized group of molecules, which may be called the *biological receptor site*. This interaction would be expected to take place by using the same bonding forces as are involved when simple molecules interact. These, together with typical examples, are collected in Table 2-13.

Most drugs do not possess functional groups of a type that would lead to ready formation of strong and essentially irreversible covalent bonds between drug and biological receptors. In most cases, it is desirable to have the drug leave the receptor site when the concentration decreases in the extracellular fluids. Therefore, most useful drugs are held to their receptors by ionic or weaker bonds. When relatively long-lasting or irreversible effects are desired (e.g., antibacterial, anticancer), drugs that form covalent bonds with the receptor are effective and useful. The alkylating agents, such as the nitrogen mustards used in cancer chemotherapy, furnish an example of drugs that act by formation of covalent bonds (see Chapter 12).

Covalent bond formation between drug and receptor is the basis of Baker's concept of *active-site-directed irreversible inhibition*.[14] Considerable experimental evidence on the nature of enzyme inhibitors supports this concept. Compounds studied possess appropriate structural features for reversible and highly selective association with an enzyme. If, in addition, the compounds carry reactive groups capable of forming covalent bonds, the substrate may be irreversibly bound to the drug–receptor complex by covalent bond formation with reactive groups adjacent to the active site. The diuretic drug ethacrynic acid (see Chapter 18) is an α,β-unsaturated ketone, thought to act by covalent bond formation with sulfhydryl groups of ion transport systems in the renal tubules. Another example of a drug that covalently binds to the receptor is selegiline (see Chapter 14), an inhibitor of monoamine oxidase-B. Other examples of covalent bond formation between drug and biological receptor site include the reaction of arsenicals and mercurials with cysteine sulfhydryl groups, the acylation of bacterial cell wall constituents by penicillin, and the phosphorylation of the serine hydroxyl moiety at the active site of cholinesterase by organic phosphates.

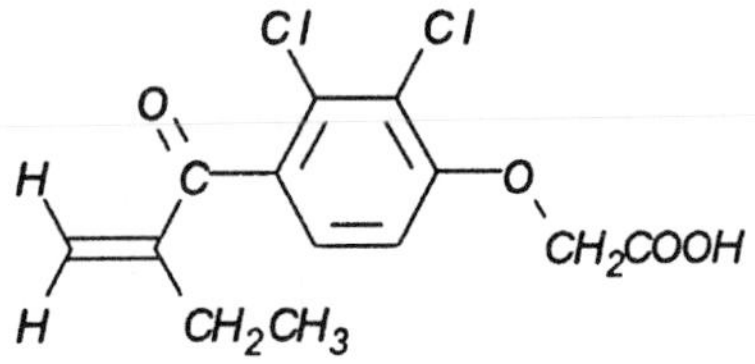

Ethacrynic Acid

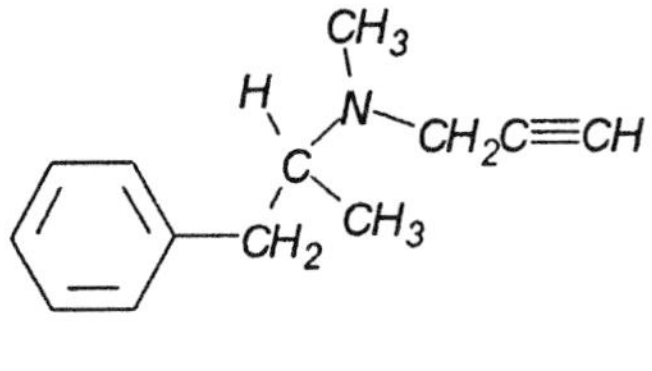

Selegiline

Keep in mind that it is desirable to have most drug effects reversible. For this to occur, relatively weak forces must be involved in the drug–receptor complex yet be strong enough that other binding sites will not competitively deplete the site of action. Compounds with high structural specificity may orient several weakly binding groups so that the summation of their interactions with specifically oriented complementary groups on the receptor provides a total bond strength

sufficient for a stable combination. Consequently, drugs acting by virtue of their structural specificity will bind to the receptor site by hydrogen bonds, ionic bonds, ion–dipole and dipole–dipole interactions, and van der Waals' and hydrophobic forces.

Considering the wide variety of functional groups found on a drug molecule and receptor, there will be a variety of secondary bonding forces. Ionization at physiological pH would normally occur with the carboxyl, sulfonamido, and aliphatic amino groups, as well as the quaternary ammonium group at any pH. These sources of potential ionic bonds are frequently found in active drugs. Differences in electronegativity between carbon and other atoms, such as oxygen and nitrogen, lead to an asymmetric distribution of electrons (dipoles) that are also capable of forming weak bonds with regions of high or low electron density, such as ions or other dipoles. Carbonyl, ester, amide, ether, nitrile, and related groups that contain such dipolar functions are frequently found in equivalent locations in structurally specific drugs.

The relative importance of the *hydrogen bond* in the formation of a drug–receptor complex is difficult to assess. Many drugs possess groups such as carbonyl, hydroxyl, amino, and imino, with the structural capabilities of acting as acceptors or donors in the formation of hydrogen bonds. However, such groups would usually be solvated by water,

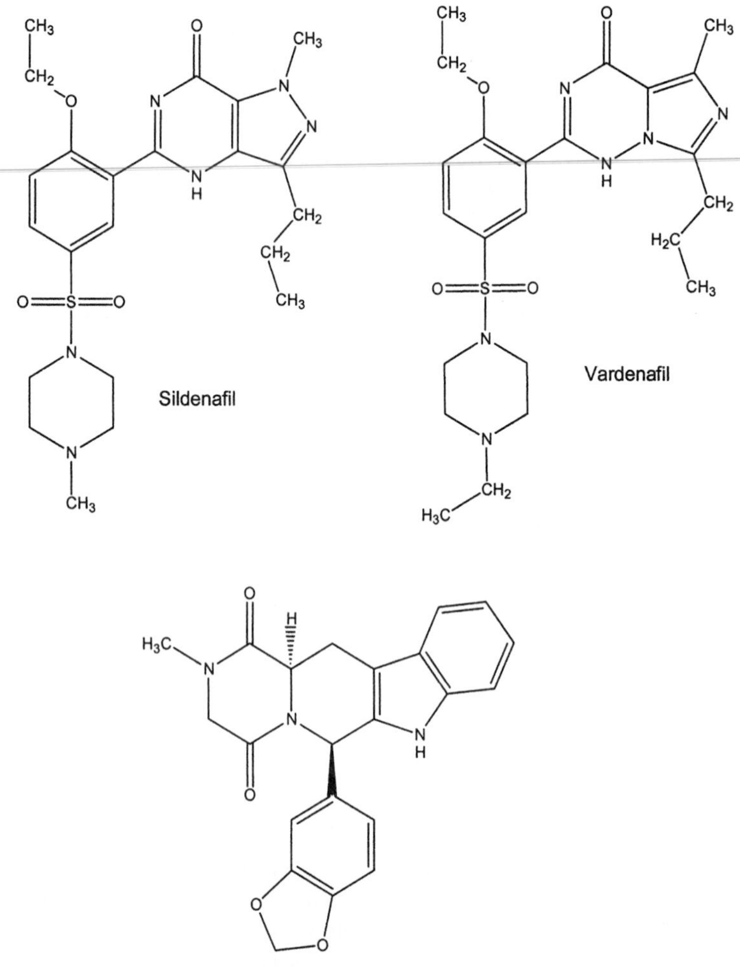

Sildenafil

Vardenafil

Tadalafil

Figure 2–13 ■ Examples of phosphodiesterase type 5 inhibitors.

TABLE 2–13 Types of Chemical Bonds

Bond Type	Bond Strength (kcal/mol)	Example
Covalent	40–140	$CH_3—OH$
Reinforced ionic	10	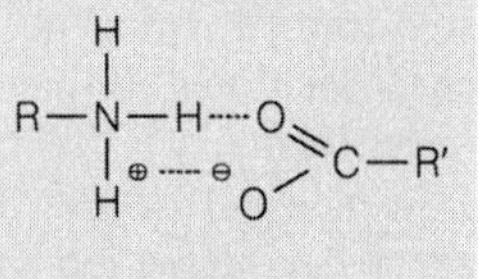 *(structure shown)*
Ionic	5	$R_4N^{\oplus} \cdots {}^{\ominus}I$
Hydrogen	1–7	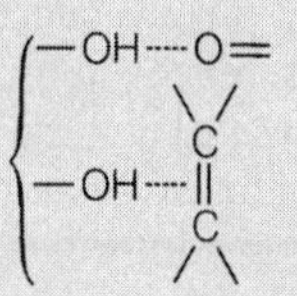 *(structure shown)*
Ion-dipole	1–7	$R_4N^{\oplus} \cdots :NR_3$
Dipole-dipole	1–7	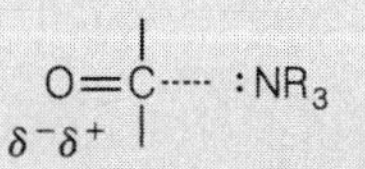 *(structure shown)*
van der Waals'	0.5–1	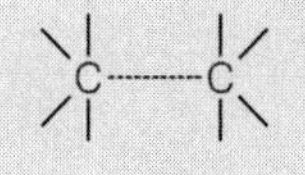 *(structure shown)*
Hydrophobic	1	See text

Adapted from a table in Albert, A: Selective Toxicity. New York, John Wiley & Sons, 1986; 183.

as would the corresponding groups on a biological receptor. Relatively little net change in free energy would be expected in exchanging a hydrogen bond with a water molecule for one between drug and receptor. However, in a drug–receptor combination, several forces could be involved, including the hydrogen bond, which would contribute to the stability of the interaction. Where multiple hydrogen bonds may be formed, the total effect may be sizable, such as that demonstrated by the stability of the protein α helix and by the stabilizing influence of hydrogen bonds between specific base pairs in the double-helical structure of DNA.

Van der Waals' forces are attractive forces created by the polarizability of molecules and are exerted when any two uncharged atoms approach each other very closely. Their strength is inversely proportional to the seventh power of the distance. Although individually weak, the summation of their forces provides a significant bonding factor in higher-molecular-weight compounds. For example, it is not possible to distill normal alkanes with more than 80 carbon atoms, because the energy of ~80 kcal/mol required to separate the molecules is approximately equal to the energy required to break a carbon–carbon covalent bond. Flat structures, such as aromatic rings, permit close approach of atoms. With van der Waals' forces of ~0.5 to 1.0 kcal/mol for each atom, about six carbons (a benzene ring) would be necessary to match the strength of a hydrogen bond. The aromatic ring

is frequently found in active drugs, and a reasonable explanation for its requirement for many types of biological activity may be derived from the contributions of this flat surface to van der Waals' binding to a correspondingly flat receptor area.

The *hydrophobic bond* is a concept used to explain attractive interactions between nonpolar regions of the receptor and the drug. Explanations such as the ''isopropyl moiety of the drug fits into a hydrophobic cleft on the receptor composed of the hydrocarbon side chains of the amino acids valine, isoleucine, and leucine'' are commonly used to explain why a nonpolar substituent at a particular position on the drug molecule is important for activity. Over the years, the concept of hydrophobic bonds has developed. There has been considerable controversy over whether the bond actually exists. Thermodynamic arguments on the gain in entropy (decrease in ordered state) when hydrophobic groups cause a partial collapse of the ordered water structure on the surface of the receptor have been proposed to validate a hydrophobic bonding model. There are two problems with this concept. First, the term *hydrophobic* implies repulsion. The term for attraction is *hydrophilicity*. Second, and perhaps more important, there is no truly water-free region on the receptor. This is true even in the areas populated by the nonpolar amino acid side chains. An alternate approach is to consider only the concept of hydrophilicity and lipophilicity. The predominating water molecules solvate polar moieties, effectively squeezing the nonpolar residues toward each other.

Steric Features of Drugs

Regardless of the ultimate mechanism by which the drug and the receptor interact, the drug must approach the receptor and fit closely to its surface. Steric factors determined by the stereochemistry of the receptor site surface and that of the drug molecules are, therefore, of primary importance in determining the nature and the efficiency of the drug–receptor interaction. With the possible exception of the general anesthetics, such drugs must possess a high structural specificity to initiate a response at a particular receptor.

Some structural features contribute a high structural rigidity to the molecule. For example, aromatic rings are planar, and the atoms attached directly to these rings are held in the plane of the aromatic ring. Hence, the quaternary nitrogen and carbamate oxygen attached directly to the benzene ring in the cholinesterase inhibitor neostigmine are restricted to the plane of the ring, and consequently, the spatial arrangement of at least these atoms is established.

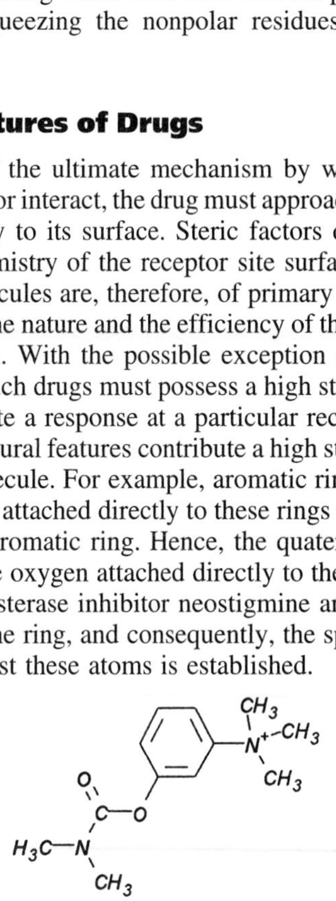

Neostigmine

The relative positions of atoms attached directly to multiple bonds are also fixed. For the double bond, *cis* and *trans* isomers result. For example, diethylstilbestrol exists in two fixed stereoisomeric forms: *trans*-diethylstilbestrol is estrogenic, whereas the *cis* isomer is only 7% as active. In *trans*-diethylstilbestrol, resonance interactions and minimal steric interference tend to hold the two aromatic rings and connecting ethylene carbon atoms in the same plane.

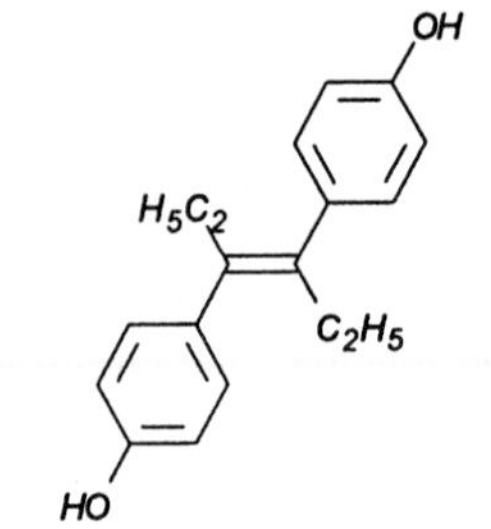

trans-Diethylstilbestrol

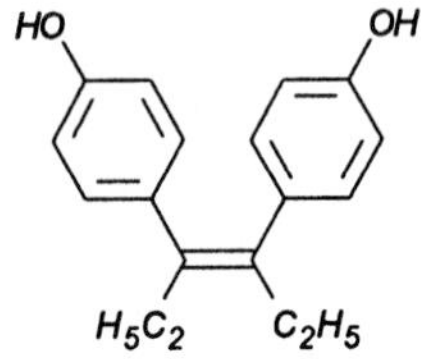

cis-Diethylstilbestrol

Geometric isomers, such as the *cis* and the *trans* isomers, hold structural features at different relative positions in space. These isomers also have significantly different physical and chemical properties. Therefore, their distributions in the biological medium are different, as are their capabilities

for interacting with a biological receptor in a structurally specific manner. The United States Pharmacopeia recognizes that there are drugs with vinyl groups whose commercial form contains both their *E* and *Z* isomers. Figure 2-14 provides four examples of these mixtures.

More subtle differences exist for *conformational* isomers. Like geometric isomers, these exist as different arrangements in space for the atoms or groups in a single classic structure. Rotation about bonds allows interconversion of conformational isomers. However, an energy barrier between isomers is often high enough for their independent existence and reaction. Differences in reactivity of functional groups or interaction with biological receptors may be due to differences in steric requirements of the receptors. In certain semirigid ring systems, conformational isomers show significant differences in biological activities. Methods for calculating these energy barriers are discussed in Chapter 28.

Open chains of atoms, which form an important part of many drug molecules, are not equally free to assume all possible conformations; some are sterically preferred. Energy barriers to free rotation of the chains are present, because of interactions of nonbonded atoms. For example, the atoms tend to position themselves in space so that they occupy staggered positions, with no two atoms directly facing each other (eclipsed). Nonbonded interactions in polymethylene chains tend to favor the most extended *anti* conformations, although some of the partially extended *gauche* conformations also exist. Intramolecular bonding between

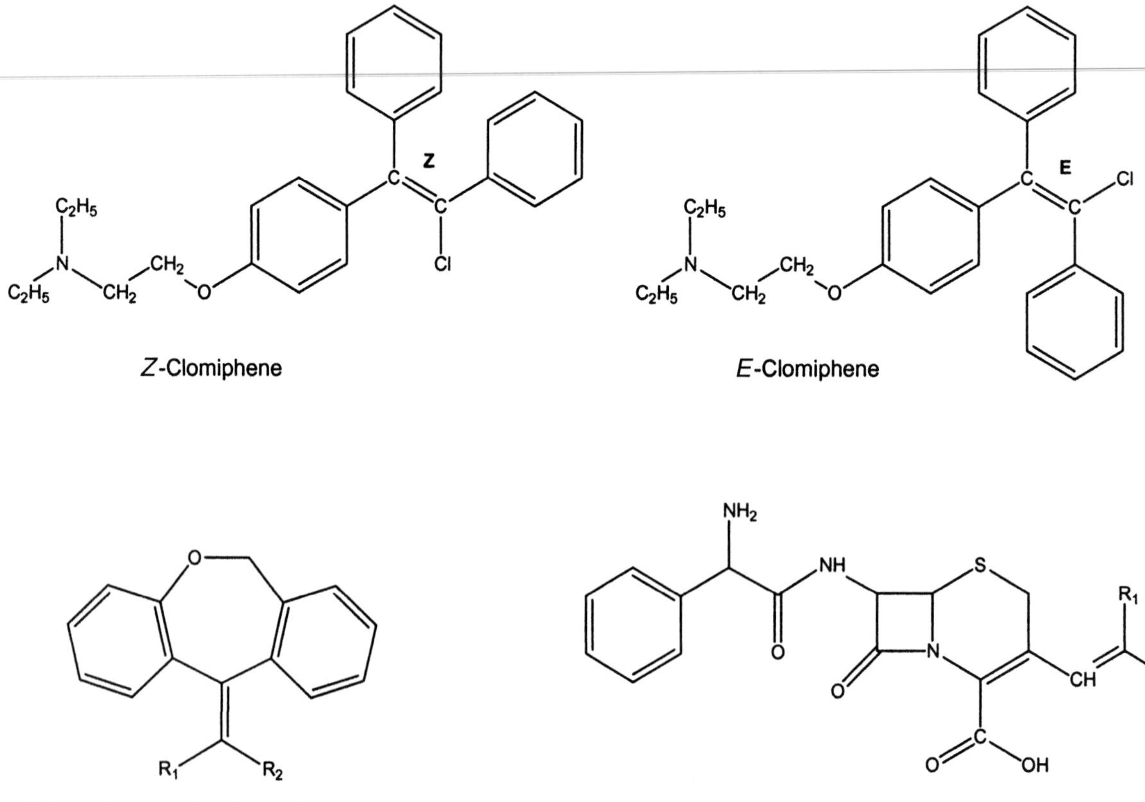

Z-Clomiphene

E-Clomiphene

Z-Doxepin: R₁ = CH₂CH₂N(CH₃)₂; R₂ = H
E-Doxepin: R₁ = H; R₂ = CH₂CH₂N(CH₃)₂

Z-Cefprozil: R₁ = H; R₂ = CH₃
E-Cefprozil: R₁ = CH₃; R₂ = H

Figure 2–14 ■ Examples of *E* and *Z* isomers.

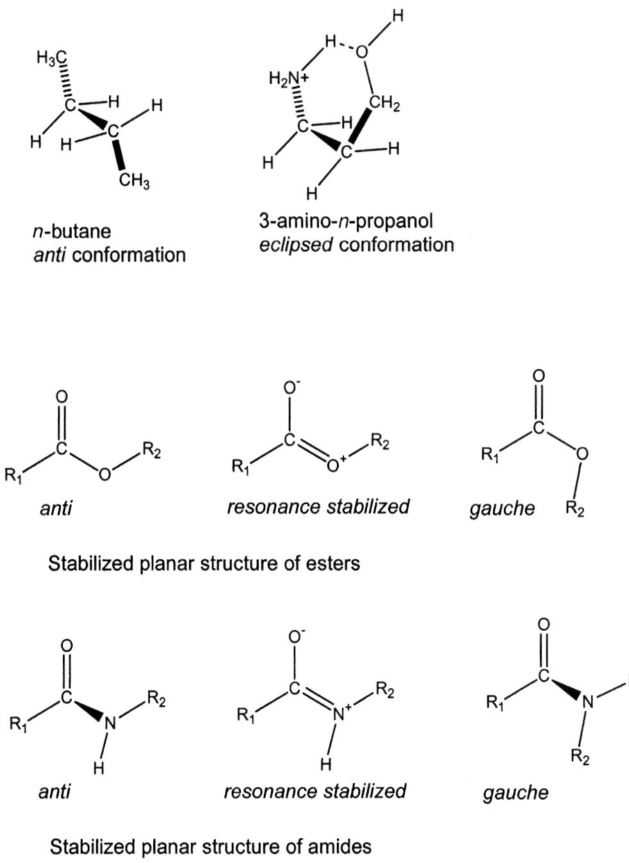

n-butane
anti conformation

3-amino-*n*-propanol
eclipsed conformation

anti   *resonance stabilized*   *gauche*

Stabilized planar structure of esters

anti   *resonance stabilized*   *gauche*

Stabilized planar structure of amides

Figure 2–15 ■ Effect of noncarbon atoms on a molecule's configuration.

substituent groups can make what might first appear to be an unfavorable conformation favorable.

The introduction of atoms other than carbon into a chain strongly influences the conformation of the chain (Fig. 2-15). Because of resonance contributions of forms in which a double bond occupies the central bonds of esters and amides, a planar configuration is favored in which minimal steric interference of bulky substituents occurs. Hence, an ester may exist mainly in the *anti*, rather than the *gauche*, form. For the same reason, the amide linkage is essentially planar, with the more bulky substituents occupying the *anti* position. Therefore, ester and amide linkages in a chain tend to hold bulky groups in a plane and to separate them as far as possible. As components of the side chains of drugs, ester and amide groups favor fully extended chains and also add polar character to that segment of the chain.

In some cases, *dipole–dipole interactions* appear to influence structure in solution. Methadone may exist partially in a cyclic form in solution because of dipolar attractive forces between the basic nitrogen and carbonyl group or because of hydrogen bonding between the hydrogen on the nitrogen and the carbonyl oxygen (Fig. 2-16). In either conformation, methadone may resemble the conformationally more rigid potent analgesics including morphine, meperidine, and their analogues (see Chapter 23), and it may be this form that interacts with the analgesic receptor. Once the interaction between the drug and its receptor begins, a flexible drug molecule may assume a different conformation than that predicted from solution chemistry.

An intramolecular *hydrogen bond,* usually formed between donor hydroxy and amino groups and acceptor oxygen and nitrogen atoms, might be expected to add stability to a particular conformation of a drug in solution. However, in aqueous solution, donor and acceptor groups tend to be

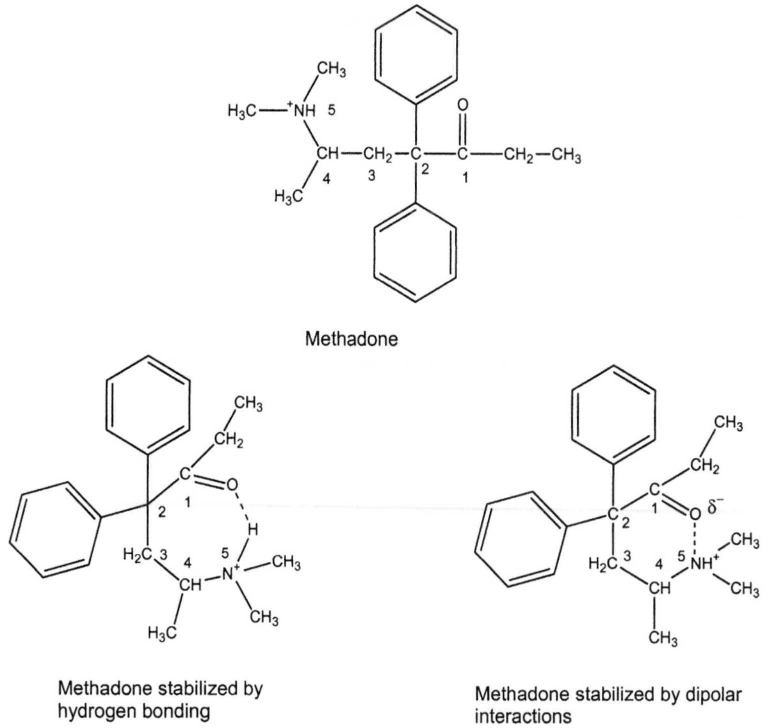

Methadone

Methadone stabilized by hydrogen bonding

Methadone stabilized by dipolar interactions

Figure 2–16 ■ Stabilization of conformations by secondary bonding forces.

bonded to water, and little gain in free energy would be achieved by the formation of an intramolecular hydrogen bond, particularly if unfavorable steric factors involving nonbonded interactions were introduced in the process. Therefore, internal hydrogen bonds likely play only a secondary role to steric factors in determining the conformational distribution of flexible drug molecules.

Hydrogen-bonding donor groups

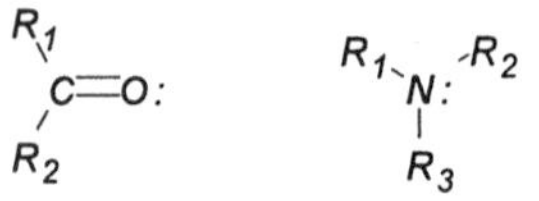

Hydrogen-bonding acceptor groups

Conformational Flexibility and Multiple Modes of Action

It has been proposed that the conformational flexibility of most open-chain neurohormones, such as acetylcholine, epinephrine, serotonin, histamine, and related physiologically active biomolecules, permits multiple biological effects to be produced by each molecule, by virtue of their ability to interact in a different and unique conformation with different biological receptors. Thus, it has been suggested that acetylcholine may interact with the muscarinic receptor of postganglionic parasympathetic nerves and with acetylcholinesterase in the fully extended conformation and, in a different, more folded structure, with the nicotinic receptors at ganglia and at neuromuscular junctions (Fig. 2-17).

Conformationally rigid acetylcholine-like molecules have been used to study the relationships between these various possible conformations of acetylcholine and their biological effects (Fig. 2-17). (+)-*trans*-2-Acetoxycyclopropyl trimethylammonium iodide, in which the quaternary nitrogen atom and acetoxyl groups are held apart in a conformation approximating that of the extended conformation of acetylcholine, was about 5 times more active than acetylcholine in its muscarinic effect on dog blood pressure and was as active as acetylcholine in its muscarinic effect on the guinea pig ileum.[15] The (+)-*trans* isomer was hydrolyzed by acetylcholinesterase at a rate equal to the rate of hydrolysis of acetylcholine. It was inactive as a nicotinic agonist. In contrast, the (−)-*trans* isomer and the mixed (±)-*cis* isomers were, respectively, 1/500 and 1/10,000 as active as acetylcholine in muscarinic tests on guinea pig ileum and were inactive as nicotinic agonists. Similarly, the *trans* diaxial relationship between the quaternary nitrogen and acetoxyl group led to maximal muscarinic response and rate of hydrolysis by true acetylcholinesterase in a series of isomeric

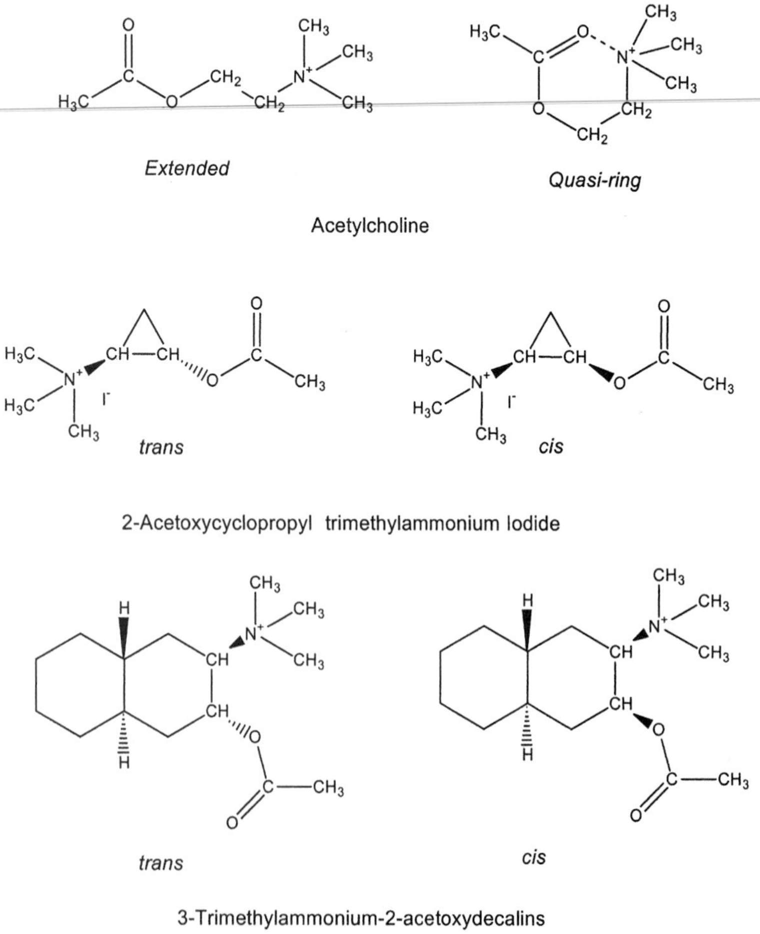

Extended

Quasi-ring

Acetylcholine

2-Acetoxycyclopropyl trimethylammonium Iodide

trans

cis

3-Trimethylammonium-2-acetoxydecalins

Figure 2–17 ■ Acetylcholine conformations (only one each of the two possible *trans* and *cis* isomers is represented).

3-trimethylammonium-2-acetoxydecalins.[16] These results could be interpreted as either that acetylcholine was acting in a *trans* conformation at the muscarinic receptor and not acting in a *cisoid* conformation at the nicotinic receptor or that the nicotinic response is highly sensitive to steric effects of substituents being used to orient the molecule. This approach in studying the cholinergic receptor is covered in more detail in Chapter 17.

Optical Isomerism and Biological Activity

The widespread occurrence of differences in biological activities for *optical activities* has been of particular importance in the development of theories on the nature of drug–receptor interactions. Most commercial drugs are asymmetric, meaning that they cannot be divided into symmetrical halves. While D and L isomers have the same physical properties, a large number of drugs are *diastereomeric*, meaning that they have two or more asymmetric centers. Diastereomers have different physical properties. Examples are the diastereomers ephedrine and pseudoephedrine. The former has a melting point of 79° and is soluble in water, whereas pseudoephedrine's melting point is 118°, and it is only sparingly soluble in water. Keep in mind that receptors will be asymmetric because they are mostly protein, meaning that they are constructed from L-amino acids. A ligand fitting the hypothetical receptor shown in Figure 2-18 will have to have a positively charged moiety in the upper left corner and a hydrophobic region in the upper right. Therefore, one would predict that optical isomers will also have different biological properties. Well-known examples of this phenomenon include (–)-hyoscyamine, which exhibits 15 to 20 times more mydriatic activity than (+)-hyoscyamine, and (–)-ephedrine, which shows 3 times more pressor activity than (+)-ephedrine, 5 times more pressor activity than (+)-pseudoephedrine, and 36 times more pressor activity than (–)-pseudoephedrine. All of ascorbic acid's antiscorbutic properties reside in the (+) isomer. A postulated fit to epinephrine's receptor can explain why (–)-epinephrine ex-

hibits 12 to 15 times more vasoconstrictor activity than (+)-epinephrine. This is the classical three-point attachment model. For epinephrine, the benzene ring, benzylic hydroxyl, and protonated amine must have the stereochemistry seen with the (–) isomer to match up with the hydrophobic or aromatic region, anionic site, and a hydrogen-bonding center on the receptor. The (+) isomer (the mirror image) will not align properly on the receptor.

Frequently, the generic name indicates a specific stereoisomer. Examples include levodopa, dextroamphetamine, dextromethorphan, levamisole, dexmethylphenidate, and levothyroxine. Sometimes the difference in pharmacological activity between stereoisomers is dramatic. The dextrorotatory isomers in the morphine series are cough suppressants with less risk of substance abuse, whereas the levorotatory isomers (Fig. 2-19) contain the analgesic activity and significant risk of substance abuse. While the direction of optical rotation is opposite to that of the morphine series, dextropropoxyphene contains the analgesic activity, and the *levo* isomer contains antitussive activity.

Figure 2-19 contains examples of drugs with asymmetric carbons. Some were originally approved as racemic mixtures, and later a specific isomer was marketed with claims of having fewer adverse reactions in patients. An example of the latter is the local anesthetic levobupivacaine, which is the *S* isomer of bupivacaine. Both the *R* and *S* isomers have good local anesthetic activity, but the *R* isomer may cause depression of the myocardium leading to decreased cardiac output, heart block hypotension, bradycardia, and ventricular arrhythmias. In contrast, the *S* isomer shows less cardiotoxic responses but still good local anesthetic activity. Escitalopram is the *S* isomer of the antidepressant citalopram. There is some evidence that the *R* isomer, which contains little of the desired selective serotonin reuptake inhibition, contributes more to the adverse reactions than does the *S* isomer.

As dramatic as the above examples of stereoselectivity may be, sometimes it may not be cost-effective to resolve the drug into its stereoisomers. An example is the calcium

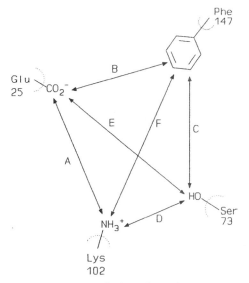

Figure 2–18 ■ Diagram of a hypothetical receptor site, showing distances between functional groups.

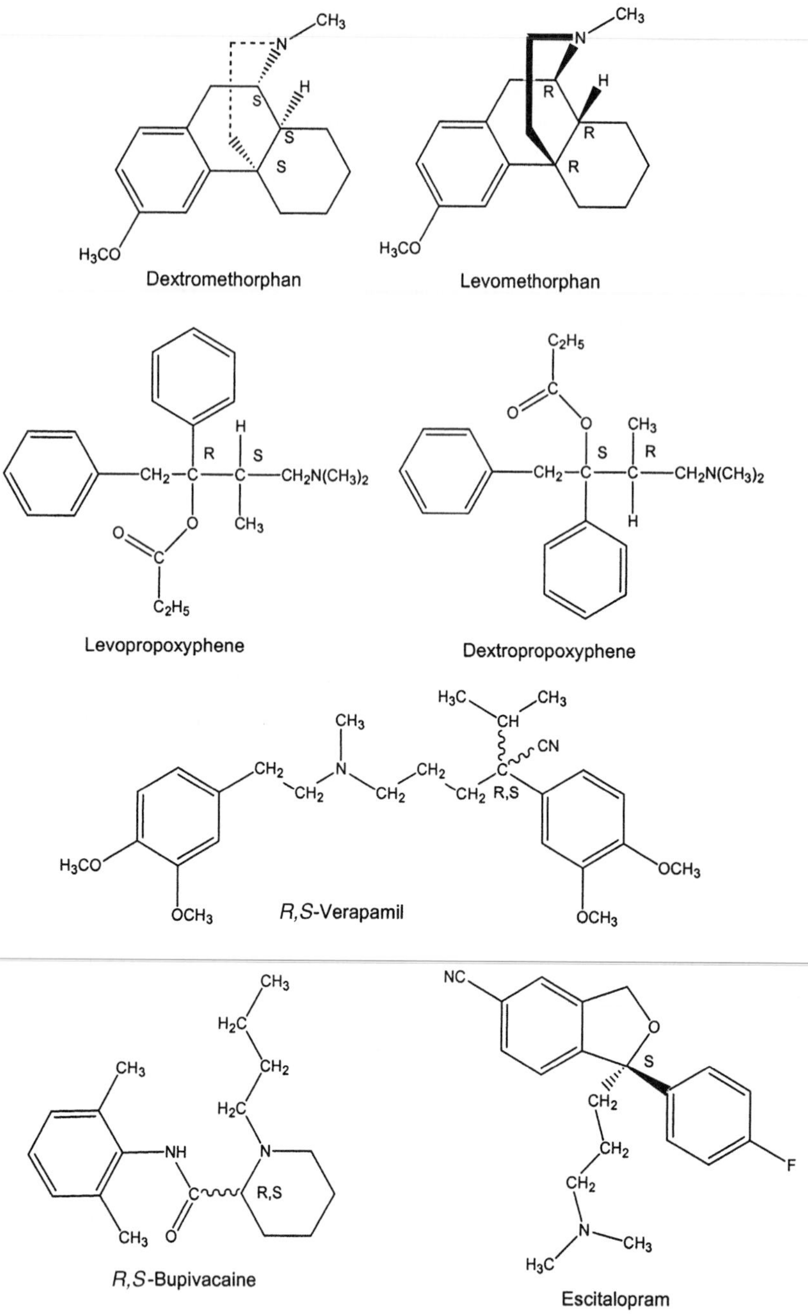

Figure 2-19 ■ Examples of drug stereoisomers.

channel antagonist verapamil, which illustrates why it is difficult to conclude that one isomer is superior to the other. *S*-Verapamil is a more active pharmacological stereoisomer than *R*-verapamil, but the former is more rapidly metabolized by the first-pass effect. (First-pass refers to orally administered drugs that are extensively metabolized as they pass through the liver. See Chapter 4.) *S*- and *R*-warfarin are metabolized by two different cytochrome P-450 isozymes. Drugs that either inhibit or induce these enzymes can significantly affect warfarin's anticoagulation activity.

Because of biotransformations after the drug is administered, it sometimes makes little difference whether a racemic mixture or one isomer is administered. The popular nonsteroidal anti-inflammatory drug (NSAID) ibuprofen is sold as the racemic mixture. The *S* enantiomer contains the anti-inflammatory activity by inhibiting cyclooxygenase. The *R* isomer does have centrally acting analgesic activity, but it is converted to the *S* form in vivo (Fig. 2-20).

In addition to the fact that most receptors are asymmetric, there are other reasons why stereoisomers show different biological responses. Active transport mechanisms involve asymmetric carrier molecules, which means that there will be preferential binding of one stereoisomer over others. When differences in physical properties exist, the distribution of isomers between body fluids and tissues where the receptors are located will differ. The enzymes responsible for drug metabolism are asymmetric, which means that biological half-lives will differ among possible stereoisomers

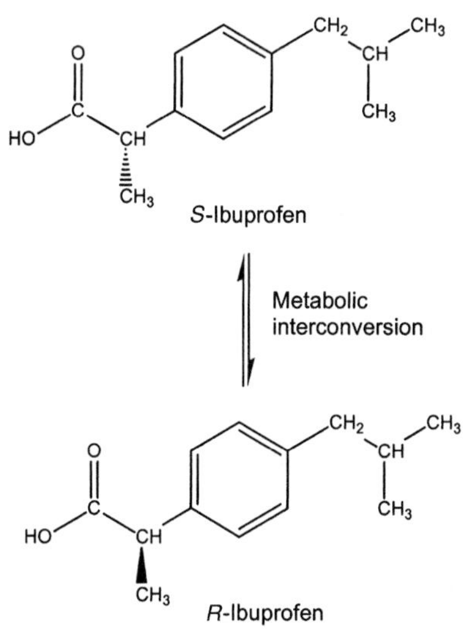

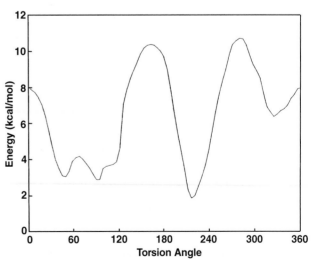

Figure 2–20 ■ Metabolic interconversion of *R*- and *S*-ibuprofen.

of the same molecule. The latter may be a very important variable because the metabolite may actually be the active molecule.

Calculated Conformations

It should now be obvious that medicinal chemists must obtain an accurate understanding of the active conformation of the drug molecule. Originally, molecular models were constructed from kits containing a variety of atoms of different valence and oxidation states. Thus, there would be carbons suitable for carbon–carbon single, double, and triple bonds; carbon–oxygen bonds for alcohols or ethers and the carbonyl moiety; carbon–nitrogen bonds for amines, amides, imines, and nitrites; and carbons for three-, four-, five-, and larger-member rings. More complete sets include a variety of heteroatoms including nitrogen, oxygen, and sulfur in various oxidation states. These kits might be ball and stick, stick or wire only, or space filling. The latter contained attempts at realistically visualizing the effect of a larger atom such as sulfur relative to the smaller oxygen. The diameters of the atoms in these kits are proportional to the van der Waals' radii, usually corrected for overlap effects. In contrast, the wire models usually depict accurate intraatomic distances between atoms. A skilled chemist using these kits usually can obtain a reasonably accurate three-dimensional representation. This is particularly true if it is a moderately simple molecule with considerable rigidity. An extreme example is a steroid with the relatively inflexible fused-ring system. In contrast, molecules with chains consisting of several atoms can assume many shapes. Yet, only one shape or conformation can be expected to fit onto the receptor. The number of conformers can be estimated from Equation 2-30. Calculating the *global minimum*, the lowest energy conformation, can be a difficult computational problem. Assume that there are three carbon–carbon freely rotatable single bonds that are rotated in 10° increments. Equation 2-30 states that there are 46,656 different conformations. A typical en-

ergy diagram is shown in Figure 2-21. Notice that some of the minima are nearly equivalent, and it is easy to move from one minimum to another. From energy diagrams, it is difficult to answer the question, which of the ligand's low or moderately low conformations fits onto the receptor? This question can be answered partially by assuming that lower energy conformations are more highly populated and thus more likely to interact with the receptor. Nevertheless, specific interactions like hydrogen bond formation and dipole–dipole interactions can affect the energy levels of different conformations. Therefore, the bound conformation of a drug is seldom its lowest energy conformation.

$$\text{Number of conformers} = \left(\frac{360}{\text{angle increment}}\right)^{\text{No. rotatable bonds}}$$

(Eq. 2-30)

There are three common quantitative ways to obtain estimations of preferred molecular shapes required for a good fit at the receptor. The first, which is the oldest and considered the most accurate, is x-ray crystallography. When properly done, resolution down to a few angstrom units can be obtained. This permits an accurate mathematical description of the molecule, providing atomic coordinates in three-dimensional space that can be drawn by using a chemical graphics program. A serious limitation of this technique is the requirement for a carefully grown crystal. Some chemicals will not form crystals. Others form crystals with mixed symmetries. Nevertheless, with the newer computational techniques, including high-speed computers, large databases of x-ray crystallographic data are now available. These databases can be searched for structures, including substructures, similar to the molecule of interest. Depending on how close is the match, it is possible to obtain a pretty good idea of the low-energy conformation of the drug molecule. This is a common procedure for proteins and nucleic acids after obtaining the amino acid and nucleotide sequences, respectively. Obtaining these sequences is now largely an automated process.

There also is the "debate" that asks if the conformation

Figure 2–21 ■ Diagram showing the energy maxima and minima as two substituted carbons connected by a single bond are rotated 360° relative to each other.

found in the crystal represents the conformation ''seen'' by the receptor. For rigid molecules, it probably is. The question is very difficult to answer for flexible molecules. A common technique is to determine the crystal structure of a protein accurately and then *soak* the crystal in a nonaqueous solution of the drug. This allows the drug molecules to diffuse into the active site. The resulting crystal is reanalyzed using different techniques, and the bound conformation of the drug can be determined rapidly without redoing the entire protein. Often, the structure of a bound drug can be determined in a day or less.

Because of the drawbacks to x-ray crystallography, two purely computational methods that require only a knowledge of the molecular structure are used. The two approaches are known as *quantum mechanics* and *molecular mechanics*. Both are based on assumptions that (*a*) a molecule's three-dimensional geometry is a function of the forces acting on the molecule and (*b*) these forces can be expressed by a set of equations that pertain to all molecules. For the most part, both computational techniques assume that the molecule is in an isolated system. Solvation effects from water, which are common to any biological system, tend to be ignored, although this is changing with increased computational power. Calculations now can include limited numbers of water molecules, where the number depends on the amount of available computer time. Interestingly, many crystals grown for x-ray analysis can contain water in the crystal lattice. High-resolution nuclear magnetic resonance (NMR) provides another means of obtaining the structures of macromolecules and drugs in solution.

There are fundamental differences between the quantum and molecular mechanics approaches. They illustrate the dilemma that can confront the medicinal chemist. Quantum mechanics is derived from basic theoretical principles at the atomic level. The model itself is exact, but the equations used in the technique are only approximate. The molecular properties are derived from the electronic structure of the molecule. The assumption is made that the distribution of electrons within a molecule can be described by a linear sum of functions that represent an atomic orbital. (For carbon, this would be s, p_x, p_y, etc.) Quantum mechanics is computation intensive, with the calculation time for obtaining an approximate solution increasing by approximately N^4 times, where N is the number of such functions. Until the advent of the high-speed supercomputers, quantum mechanics in its *pure* form was restricted to small molecules. In other words, it was not practical to conduct a quantum mechanical analysis of a drug molecule.

To make this technique more practical, simplifying techniques have been developed. While the computing time is decreased, the accuracy of the outcome is also lessened. In general, use of calculations of the quantum mechanics type in medicinal chemistry is a method that is *still waiting to happen*. It is being used by laboratories with access to large-scale computing, but there is considerable debate about its utility because so many simplifying approximations must be made for larger molecules.

In contrast, medicinal chemists are embracing molecular mechanics. This approach is derived from empirical observations. In contrast to quantum mechanics, the equations in molecular mechanics have exact solutions. At the same time, the parameters that are used in these equations are adjusted to ensure that the outcome fits experimental observations. In place of the fundamental electronic structure used in quantum mechanics, molecular mechanics uses a model consisting of balls (the atoms) connected by springs (the bonds). The total energy of a molecule consists of the sum of the following energy terms:

E_c: stretching and compressing of the bonds (springs)
E_b: bending about a central atom
E_t: rotation about bonds
E_v: van der Waals' interactions
E_u: electrostatic interactions

Each atom is defined (parameterized) in terms of these energy terms. What this means is that the validity of molecular mechanics depends on the accuracy of the parameterization process. Historically, saturated hydrocarbons have proved easy to parameterize, followed by selective heteroatoms such as ether oxygens and amines. Unsaturated systems, including aromaticity, caused problems because of the delocalization of the electrons, but this seems to have been solved. Charged atoms such as the carboxylate anion and protonated amine can prove to be a real problem, particularly if the charge is delocalized. Nevertheless, molecular mechanics is being used increasingly by medicinal chemists to gain a better understanding of the preferred conformation of drug molecules and the macromolecules that compose a receptor. The computer programs are readily available and run on relatively inexpensive, but powerful, desktop computers.

In summary, quantum mechanics attempts to model the position or distribution of the electrons or bonds, while molecular mechanics attempts to model the positions of the nuclei or atoms. Quantum mechanics calculations are used commonly to generate or verify molecular mechanics parameters. Larger structures can be studied by use of molecular mechanics, and with simulation techniques such as molecular dynamics, the behavior of drugs in solution or even in passage through bilayer membranes can be studied.

The only way to test the validity of the outcome from either quantum or molecular mechanics calculations is to compare the calculated structure or property with actual experimental data. Obviously, crystallographic data provide a reliable measure of the accuracy of at least one of the low-energy conformers. Since that is not always feasible, other physical chemical measurements are used for comparison. These include comparing calculated vibrational energies, heats of formation, dipole moments, and relative conformational energies with measured values. When results are inconsistent, the parameter values are adjusted. This readjustment of the parameters is analogous to the fragment approach for calculating octanol/water partition coefficients. The values for the fragments and the accompanying correction factors are determined by comparing calculated partition coefficients with a large population of experimentally determined partition coefficients.

Three-Dimensional Quantitative Structure–Activity Relationships

With molecular modeling becoming more common, the QSAR paradigm that traditionally used physicochemical descriptors on a two-dimensional molecule can be adapted to three-dimensional space. Essentially, the method requires knowledge of the three-dimensional shape of the molecule. Indeed, accurate modeling of the molecule is crucial. A reference (possibly the prototype molecule) or shape is selected against which all other molecules are compared. The original method called for overlapping the test molecules with the reference molecule and minimizing the differences in overlap. Then distances were calculated between arbitrary locations on the molecule. These distances were used as variables in QSAR regression equations. While overlapping rigid ring systems such as tetracyclines, steroids, and penicillins are relatively easy, flexible molecules can prove challenging. Examine the following hypothetical molecule. Depending on the size of the various *R* groups and the type of atom represented by *X*, a family of compounds represented by this molecule could have a variety of conformations. Even when the conformations might be known with reasonable certainty, the reference points crucial for activity must be identified. Is the overlap involving the tetrahedral carbon important for activity? Or should the five-membered ring provide the reference points? And which way should it be rotated? Assuming that R_b is an important part of the pharmacophore, should the five-membered ring be rotated so that R_b is pointed down or up? These are not trivial questions, and successful 3D-QSAR studies have depended on just how the investigator positions the molecules relative to each other. There are several instances in which apparently very similar structures have been shown to bind to a given receptor in different orientations.

There are a variety of algorithms for measuring the degree of conformational and shape similarities, including molecular shape analysis (MSA),[17] distance geometry,[18] and molecular similarity matrices.[19,20] Many of the algorithms use graph theory, in which the bonds that connect the atoms of a molecule can be thought of as paths between specific points on the molecule. Molecular connectivity is a commonly used application of graph theory.[21-23]

Besides comparing how well a family of molecules overlaps with a reference molecule, there are sophisticated software packages that determine the physicochemical parameters located at specific distances from the surface of the molecule. An example of this approach is comparative molecular field analysis (CoMFA). This technique is described in more detail in Chapter 3.

Database Searching and Mining

As pointed out above, receptors are being isolated and cloned. This means that it is possible to determine their structures. Most are proteins, which means determining their amino acid sequence. This can be done either by degrading the protein or by obtaining the nucleotide sequence of the structural gene coding for the receptor and using the triplet genetic code to determine the amino acid sequence. The parts of the receptor that bind the drug (ligand) can be determined by site-directed mutagenesis. This alters the nucleotide sequence at specific points on the gene and, therefore, changes specific amino acids. Also, keep in mind that many enzymes become receptors when the goal is to alter their activity. Examples of the latter include acetylcholinesterase, monoamine oxidase, HIV protease, rennin, ACE, and tetrahydrofolate reductase.

The starting point is a database of chemical structures. They may belong to large pharmaceutical or agrochemical firms that literally have synthesized the compounds in the database and have them ''sitting on the shelf.'' Alternatively, the database may be constructed so that several different chemical classes and substituent patterns are represented. (See discussion of isosterism in the next section.) The first step is to convert the traditional or historical two-dimensional molecules into three-dimensional structures whose intramolecular distances are known. Keeping in mind the problems of finding the ''correct'' conformation for flexible molecule, false hits and misses might result from the search. Next, the dimensions of the active site must be determined. Ideally, the receptor has been crystallized, and from the coordinates, the intramolecular distances between what are assumed to be key locations are obtained. If the receptor cannot be crystallized, there are methods for estimating the three-dimensional shape based on searching crystallographic databases and matching amino acid sequences of proteins whose tertiary structure has been determined.

Fortunately, the crystal structures of literally thousands of proteins have been determined, and their structures have been stored in the Brookhaven Protein Databank. It is now known that proteins with similar functions have similar amino acid sequences in various regions of the protein. These sequences tend to show the same shapes in terms of α helix, parallel and antiparallel β-pleated forms, turns in the chain, etc. Using this information plus molecular mechanics parameters, the shape of the protein and the dimensions of the active site can be estimated. Figure 2-18 contains the significant components of a hypothetical active site. Notice that four amino acid residues at positions 25, 73, 102, and 147 have been identified as important either for binding the ligand to the site or for the receptor's intrinsic activity. Keep in mind that Figure 2-18 is a two-dimensional representation of a three-dimensional image. Therefore, the distances between amino acid residues must take into account the fact that each residue is above or below the planes of the other three residues. For an artificial ligand to ''dock,'' or fit into the site, six distances must be considered: *A*, Lys–Glu; *B*, Glu–Phe; *C*, Phe–Ser; *D*, Ser–Lys; *E*, Glu–Phe; and *F*, Lys–Phe. In reality, not all six distances may be important. In selecting potential ligands, candidates might include a positively charged residue (protonated amine), aromatic ring, hydrogen bond donor or acceptor (hydroxy, phenol, amine, nitro), and hydrogen bond acceptor or a negatively charged residue (carboxylate) that will interact with the aspartate, phenylalanine, serine, and lysine residues, respectively. A template is constructed containing the appropriate residues at the proper distances with correct geometries, and the chemical database is searched for molecules that fit the template. A degree of fit or match is obtained for each ''hit.'' Their biological responses are obtained, and the model for the receptor is further refined. New, better-defined ligands may be synthesized.

In addition to the interatomic distances, the chemical databases will contain important physicochemical values including partition coefficients, electronic terms, molar refractivity, pKₐs, solubilities, and steric values. Arrangements of atoms may be coded by molecular connectivity or other topological descriptors. The result is a "flood of data" that requires interpretation, large amounts of data storage, and rapid means of analysis. Compounds usually must fit within defined limits that estimate absorption, distribution, metabolism, and excretion (ADME).

Chemical databases can contain hundreds of thousands of molecules that could be suitable ligands for a receptor. But, no matter how good the fit is to the receptor, the candidate molecule is of no use if the absorption is poor or if the drug is excreted too slowly from the body. An analysis of 2,245 drugs has led to a set of "rules" called the *Lipinski Rule of Five*.[24,25] A candidate molecule is more likely to have poor absorption or permeability if

1. The molecular weight exceeds 500
2. The calculated octanol/water partition coefficient exceeds 5
3. There are more than 5 H-bond donors expressed as the sum of O–H and N–H groups
4. There are more than 10 H-bond acceptors expressed as the sum of N and O atoms

The rapid evaluation of large numbers of molecules is sometimes called *high-throughput screening* (Fig. 2-22). The screening can be in vitro, often measuring how well the tested molecules bind to cloned receptors or enzyme active sites. Robotic devices are available for this testing. Based on the results, the search for viable structures is narrowed, and new compounds are synthesized. The criteria for activity will be based on structure and physicochemical values. QSAR models can be developed to aid in designing new active ligands.

Alternatively, the search may be virtual. Again starting with the same type of database and the dimensions of the active site, the ability of the compounds in the database to fit or bind is estimated. The virtual receptor will include both its dimensions and physicochemical characteristic. Keeping in mind that the receptor is a protein, there will be hydrogen bond acceptors and donors (serine, threonine, tyrosine), positively and negatively charged side chains (lysine, histidine, glutamic acid, aspartic acid), nonpolar or hydrophobic side chains (leucine, isoleucine, valine, alanine), and induced dipoles (phenylalanine, tyrosine). The type of groups that will be attracted or repulsed by the type of amino acid side chain is coded into the chemical database. The virtual screening will lead to development of a refined model for good binding, and the search is repeated. When the model is considered valid, it must be tested by actual screening in biological test systems and by synthesizing new compounds to test its validity.

Isosterism

The term *isosterism* has been used widely to describe the selection of structural components—the steric, electronic, and solubility characteristics that make them interchangeable in drugs of the same pharmacological class. The concept

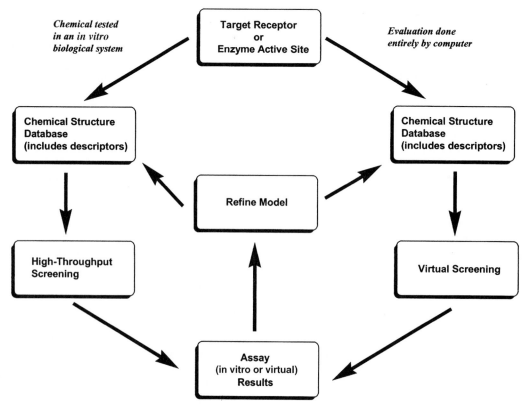

Figure 2–22 ■ High-throughput screening.

of isosterism has evolved and changed significantly in the years since its introduction by Langmuir in 1919.[26] Langmuir, while seeking a correlation that would explain similarities in physical properties for nonisomeric molecules, defined *isosteres* as compounds or groups of atoms having the same number and arrangement of electrons. Isosteres that were isoelectric (i.e., with the same total charge as well as the same number of electrons) would possess similar physical properties. For example, the molecules N_2 and CO both possess 14 total electrons and no charge and show similar physical properties. Related examples described by Langmuir were CO_2, N_2O, N_3^-, and NCO^- (Table 2-14).

With increased understanding of the structures of molecules, less emphasis has been placed on the number of electrons involved, because variations in hybridization during bond formation may lead to considerable differences in the angles, lengths, and polarities of bonds formed by atoms with the same number of peripheral electrons. Even the same atom may vary widely in its structural and electronic characteristics when it forms part of a different functional group. Thus, nitrogen is part of a planar structure in the nitro group but forms the apex of a pyramidal structure in ammonia and amines.

Groups of atoms that impart similar physical or chemical properties to a molecule because of similarities in size, electronegativity, or stereochemistry are now frequently referred to by the general term of *isostere*. The early recognition that benzene and thiophene were alike in many of their properties led to the term *ring equivalents* for the vinylene group (—CH＝CH—) and divalent sulfur (—S—). This concept has led to replacement of the sulfur atom in the phenothiazine ring system of tranquilizing agents with the vinylene group to produce the dibenzodiazepine class of antidepressant drugs (see Chapter 14). The vinylene group in an aromatic ring system may be replaced by other atoms isosteric to sulfur, such as oxygen (furan) or NH (pyrrole); however, in such cases, aromatic character is significantly decreased.

Examples of isosteric pairs that possess similar steric and electronic configurations are the carboxylate (COO^-) and sulfonamide (SO_2NR^-) ions, ketone ($C＝O$) and sulfone ($O＝S＝O$) groups, chloride (Cl^-) and trifluoromethyl (CF_3) groups. Divalent ether (—O—), sulfide (—S—), amine (—NH—), and methylene (—CH_2—) groups, although dis-

similar electronically, are sufficiently alike in their steric nature to be frequently interchangeable in designing new drugs.

Compounds may be altered by isosteric replacements of atoms or groups, to develop analogues with select biological effects or to act as antagonists to normal metabolites. Each series of compounds showing a specific biological effect must be considered separately, for there are no general rules that predict whether biological activity will be increased or decreased. Some examples of this type follow.

When a group is present in a part of a molecule in which it may be involved in an essential interaction or may influence the reactions of neighboring groups, isosteric replacement sometimes produces analogues that act as antagonists. The 6-NH_2 and 6-OH groups appear to play essential roles in the hydrogen-bonding interactions of base pairs during nucleic acid replication in cells. The substitution of the significantly weaker hydrogen-bonding isosteric sulfhydryl groups results in a partial blockage of this interaction and a decrease in the rate of cellular synthesis.

Similarly, replacement of the hydroxyl group of pteroylglutamic acid (folic acid) by the amino group leads to aminopterin, a folate antimetabolite. Addition of the methyl group to the *p*-aminobenzoate nitrogen produced methotrexate, which is used in cancer chemotherapy, for psoriasis, and as an immunosuppressant in rheumatoid arthritis.

As a better understanding of the nature of the interactions between drug-metabolizing enzymes and biological receptors develops, selection of isosteric groups with particular electronic, solubility, and steric properties should permit the rational preparation of drugs that act more selectively. At the same time, results obtained by the systematic application of the principles of isosteric replacement are aiding in the understanding of the nature of these receptors.

SELECTED WEB PAGES

The field of drug design, particularly those aspects that are computer intensive, is increasingly being featured on Web pages. Faculty and students might find it instructive to search the Web at regular intervals. Many university chemistry departments have organized Web pages that provide excellent linkages. Listed below are a small number of representative sites that feature drug design linkages. Some have excellent illustrations. These listings should not be considered any type of endorsement by the author, editors, or publisher. Indeed, some of these sites may disappear.

http://www.nih.gov/
(Search terms: QSAR; molecular modeling)
http://www.pharma.ethz.ch/qsar/
http://www.scamag.com/links/default.html
http://www.imb-jena.de/IMAGE.html
http://www.cooper.edu/engineering/chemechem/monte.html
http://triton.ps.toyaku.ac.jp/~dobashi/database/indexe.html
http://www.clunet.edu/BioDev/omm/gallery.htm
http://www.netsci.org/Science/Compchem/feature19.html
http://clogp.pomona.edu/medchem/chem/qsar-db/index.html
http://qcpe.chem.indiana.edu/
http://www.umass.edu/microbio/rasmol/index2.htm
http://www.webmo.net/

TABLE 2–14 Commonly Used Alicyclic Chemical Isosteres

A. Univalent atoms and groups
   (1) —CH_3 —NH_2 —OH   —F   —Cl
   (2) —Cl   —SH
   (3) —Br   —*i*—Pr

B. Bivalent atoms and groups
   (1) —CH_2—   —NH—   —O—   —S—
   (2) —$COCH_2R$ —CONHR
   (3) —CO_2R —COSR

C. Trivalent atoms and groups
   (1) —CH＝   —N＝

From Silverman, R. B.: The Organic Chemistry of Drug Design and Drug Action. New York, Academic Press, 1992.

REFERENCES

1. Crum-Brown, A., and Fraser, T.: R. Soc. Edinburgh 25:151, 1868–1869.
2. Hansch, C., Leo, A., and Hoekman, D.: Exploring QSAR: Hydrophobic, Electronic, and Steric Constants. Washington, DC, American Chemical Society, 1995.
3. Hansch, C., and Lien, E. J.: J. Med. Chem. 14:653, 1971.
4. Dearden, J. C., and George, E.: J. Pharm. Pharmacol. 31:S45P, 1979.
5. Kubinyi, H.: The bilinear model. In Kuchar, M. (ed.). QSAR in Design of Bioactive Molecules. Barcelona, J. R. Prous, 1984.
6. Kubinyi, H.: J. Med. Chem. 20:625, 1971.
7. Free, S. M., and Wilson, J. W.: J. Med. Chem. 7:395, 1964.
8. Waisser, K., Macháček, M., and Čeladník, M.: The use of Free-Wilson model on investigating the relationship between the chemical structure and selectivity of drugs. In Kuchar, M. (ed.). QSAR in Design of Bioactive Molecules. Barcelona, J. R. Prous, 1984.
9. Krasowski, M.D., Hong, X., Hopfinger, A. J., and Harrison, N. L.: J. Med. Chem. 45:3210, 2002.
10. Vedani, A., and Dobler, M.: J. Med. Chem. 45:2139, 2002.
11. Stuper, A. J., Brügger, W. E., and Jurs, P. C.: Computer Assisted Studies of Chemical Structure and Biological Function. New York, John Wiley & Sons, 1979.
12. Baum, R., and Borman, S.: Chem. Eng. News 74:28, 1996.
13. Gordon, E. M., Barrett, R. W., Dower, W. J., et al.: J. Med. Chem. 37:1385, 1994.
14. Baker, B. R.: J. Pharm. Sci. 53:347, 1964.
15. Chiou, C. Y., Long, J. P., Cannon, J. G., and Armstrong, P. D.: J. Pharmacol. Exp. Ther. 166:243, 1969.
16. Smissman, E., Nelson, W., Day, J., and LaPidus, J.: J. Med. Chem. 9:458, 1966.
17. Hopfinger, A. J., and Burke, B. J.: Molecular shape analysis: a formalism to quantitatively establish spatial molecular similarity. In Johnson, M. A., Maggiora, G. M. (eds.). Concepts and Applications of Molecular Similarity. New York, John Wiley & Sons, 1990.
18. Srivastava, S., Richardson, W. W., Bradely, M. P., and Crippen, G. M.: Three-dimensional receptor modeling using distance geometry and Voronoi polyhydra. In Kubinyi, H. (ed.). 3D-QSAR in Drug Design: Theory, Methods and Applications. Leiden, The Netherlands, ESCOM, 1993.
19. Good, A. C., Peterson, S. J., and Richards, W. G.: J. Med. Chem. 36:2929, 1993.
20. Good, A. C., and Richards, W. G.: Drug Inf. J. 30:371, 1996.
21. Kier, L. B., and Hall, L. H.: Molecular Connectivity in Chemistry and Drug Research. New York, Academic Press, 1976.
22. Kier, L. B., and Hall, L. H.: Molecular Connectivity in Structure-Activity Analysis. New York, Research Studies Press (Wiley), 1986.
23. Bonchev, D.: Information Theoretic Indices for Characterization of Chemical Structures. New York, Research Studies Press (Wiley), 1983.
24. Lipinski, C. A.: J. Pharmacol. Toxicol. Methods 44:235, 2000.
25. Lipinski, C. A., Lombardo, F., Dominy, B. W., and Feeney, P. J.: Adv. Drug Deliv. Rev. 46:3, 2001.
26. Langmuir, I.: J. Am. Chem. Soc. 41:1543, 1919.

SELECTED READING

Abraham, D. (ed.): Burger's Medicinal Chemistry and Drug Discovery, 6th ed. New York, Wiley-Interscience, 2003.
Albert, A.: Selective Toxicity, 7th ed. New York, Chapman & Hall, 1985.
Dean, P. M. (ed.): Molecular Similarity in Drug Design. New York, Chapman & Hall, 1995.
Devillers, J. and Balaban, A. T., (eds.): Topological Indices and Related Descriptors in QSAR and QSPR. Amsterdam, Gordon and Breach, 1999.
Franke, R.: Theoretical drug design methods. In Nauta, W. T., and Rekker, R. F. (eds.). Pharmacochemistry Library, vol. 7. New York, Elsevier, 1984.
Güner, O. F. (ed.): Pharmacophore Perception, Development, and Use in Drug Design. La Jolla, CA, International University Line, 2000.
Hansch, C., and Leo, A.: Exploring QSAR, vol. 1. Fundamentals and Applications in Chemistry and Biology. Washington, DC, American Chemical Society, 1995.
Keverling Buisman, J. A.: Biological activity and chemical structure. In Nauta, W. T., Rekker, R. F. (eds.). Pharmacochemistry Library, vol. 2. New York, Elsevier, 1977.
Kier, L. B., and Hall, L. H.: Molecular Structure Description, the Electrotopological State. New York, Academic Press, 1999.
Leach, A. R.: Molecular Modeling Principles and Applications. Essex, England, Longman 1996.
Leo, A., Hansch, C., and Hoekman, D.: Exploring QSAR, vol. 2. Hydrophobic, Electronic, and Steric Constants. Washington, DC, American Chemical Society, 1995.
Martin, Y. C.: Quantitative drug design. In Grunewald, G. (ed.). Medicinal Research, vol. 8. New York, Dekker, 1978.
Mutschler, E., and Windterfeldt, E. (eds.). Trends in Medicinal Chemistry. Berlin, VCH Publishers, 1987.
Olson, E. C., and Christoffersen, R. E.: Computer assisted drug design. In Comstock, M. J. (ed.). ACS Symposium Series, vol. 112. Washington, DC, American Chemical Society, 1979.
Rappé, A. K., and Casewit, C. J.: Molecular Mechanics Across Chemistry. Sausalito, CA, 1997.
Silverman, R. B.: The Organic Chemistry of Drug Design and Drug Action. New York, Academic Press, 1992.
Topliss, J. G.: Quantitative Structure-Activity Relationships of Drugs. Medicinal Chemistry, A Series of Monographs, vol. 19. New York, Academic Press, 1983.
Young, D.: Computational Chemistry, A Practical Guide for Applying Techniques to Real World Problems. New York, Wiley-Interscience, 2001.

Combinatorial Chemistry

DOUGLAS R. HENRY

The term *paradigm shift* is an overused one, but in the mid-1980s a true paradigm shift occurred in the way new drugs are synthesized and screened for activity. Prior to then, most drug compounds were synthesized in milligram quantities in a *serial* one-at-a-time fashion. After synthesis, the compound was sent to a biologist, who tested it in several in vitro assays and returned the results to the chemist. Based on the assay results, the chemist would apply some structure–activity relationship (SAR) or use chemical intuition to decide what changes to make in future versions of the molecule to improve activity. Using this iterative process, a chemist would be able to synthesize only a handful of structures per week. Since the yield of marketable drugs from compounds synthesized and tested is only about 1 in 10,000, the road to success has been a long and expensive one, taking 6 to 12 years and costing $500 to $800 million per drug.

In the mid-1980s, this approach to drug synthesis changed dramatically with the introduction of combinatorial chemistry. The drug discovery process became a highly *parallel* one, in which hundreds or even thousands of structures could be synthesized at one time. Interestingly, biologists had for some time been using high-throughput screening (HTS) to perform their in vitro assays, running assays in 96-well microtiter plates and even using laboratory robotics for pipetting and analysis. The bottleneck had become the synthesis of the compounds to test. Chemists realized that syntheses could also be conducted by using a parallel approach. The term *combinatorial chemistry* was coined to refer to the parallel generation of all possible *combinations* of substituents or components in a synthetic experiment. Whereas the yield from a serial synthesis is a single compound, the yield from a combinatorial synthesis is a chemical *library*. Figure 3-1 shows two common types of chemical libraries—a *generic* library, based on a single parent or scaffold structure and multiple substituents or residues, and a *mixture* library, containing a variety of structure types. The total number of structures in a library is either the product of the various numbers of substituents (for a generic library) or the total number of structures in a mixture. The goal of combinatorial chemistry is to be able to synthesize, purify, chemically analyze, and biologically test all the structures in the library, using as few synthetic experiments as possible. This chapter describes how combinatorial chemistry and HTS are being used in drug design and discovery to find new lead structures in a shorter time.

HOW IT BEGAN: PEPTIDES AND OTHER LINEAR STRUCTURES

Combinatorial chemistry was first applied to the synthesis of peptides, since a convenient method for the automated synthesis of these compounds was already in widespread use. In 1963, Merrifield introduced the efficient synthesis of peptides on a solid support or resin (Fig. 3-2).[1] This made the rapid, automated synthesis of peptides possible, and earned Merrifield a Nobel Prize in 1984. A key feature of his approach is the attachment of a growing peptide chain to an inert polymer bead, usually about 100 μm in diameter, composed of polystyrene cross-linked with divinyl benzene. Such beads were originally designed for size exclusion chromatography. The beads can be immersed in solvents, washed, heated, etc., and when the synthesis is complete, the beads can be filtered from solution, and the reaction products can be cleaved from the polymer, yielding pure products. A Hungarian chemist, Arpad Furka, realized that Merrifield's approach could be extended to allow the synthesis of all possible combinations of a given set of amino acids in a limited number of steps. He accomplished this by splitting and remixing portions of the peptide-bound resin at each step in the synthesis (Fig. 3-3). His description of the use of combinatorial chemistry to synthesize polypeptides appeared in the Hungarian patent literature in 1982. Apparently, it is the first literature reference to a combinatorial chemistry experiment.[2]

As seen in Figure 3-3, the advantage of split-and-mix synthesis is that all 27 tripeptides can be synthesized in just three steps, instead of 27 steps. The disadvantage of this approach is that in the end, one obtains three *mixtures* of beads with tripeptides attached, rather than the pure compounds themselves. If activity is detected in one of the mixtures, it becomes necessary to go back and resynthesize some or all of the structures in that mixture, to see which tripeptide is responsible for the activity. As we shall see, various methods for *tagging* and *deconvoluting* combinatorial libraries have been devised that reduce or eliminate the need for resynthesis.

The first combinatorial chemistry experiments were applied to the study of *epitopes*—the short sequences of amino acids responsible for antibody recognition and binding to proteins.[3] Early researchers used solid-phase resin beads in vials, microtiter plates, columns, and porous plastic mesh "tea bags." They also used brush-like arrays of plastic pins, at the ends of which compounds could be synthesized. Other media that have been used include paper and polymer sheets and glass chips—basically anything that can immobilize a structure for the purpose of exposing it to reagents and solvents (Fig. 3-4).

Peptides, of course, make poor oral drug molecules because they hydrolyze in the acidity of the stomach. As combinatorial methods were applied to the synthesis of drugs, a need developed for methods of generating small (molecular weight, <500) nonpeptide molecules as potential drug leads. Among the first alternatives that were studied were Chiron's "peptoids"—molecules in which the variation occurs in

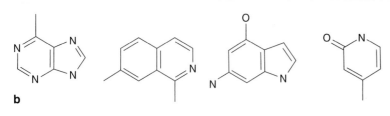

a

b

Figure 3–1 ■ Generic **(a)** and mixture **(b)** combinatorial libraries. The size of the generic library is the product of the various numbers of substituents (here, 2 × 2 × 4 × 5, or 80). The size of the mixture library is simply the total number of structures.

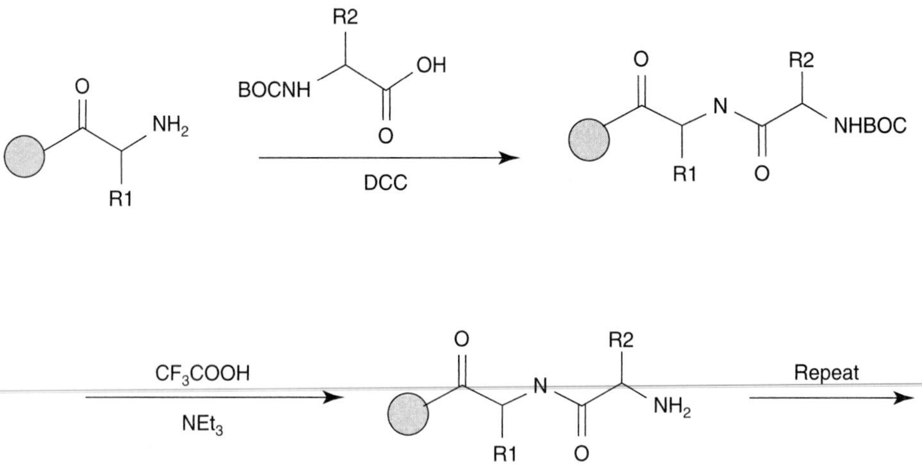

R_1 = H, 4′-OH

R_2 = 5-Cl, 4-COOH+5Cl

R_3 = CH3, CH(CH3)2, CH2Ph(4-OH), CH2Ph,

R_4 = H, CH3, CH2CH3, CH2CH=CH2, CH2Ph

Figure 3–2 ■ Merrifield synthesis on a polymer bead support. The growing peptide chain is attached to a polymer support, usually in the form of small beads. The next amino acid (bearing R2) is attached, and its protecting group (BOC) is removed with acid/base treatment. *BOC*, butyloxycarbonyl; *DCC*, dicyclohexylcarbodiimide.

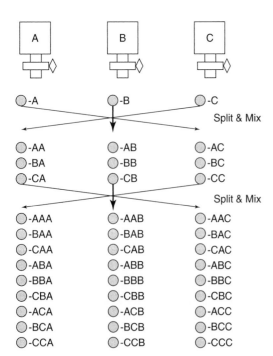

Split & Mix

Split & Mix

Figure 3–3 ■ Split-and-mix synthesis of tripeptides. In the first step, all the beads in a given container have a single monopeptide. These are all mixed together, then split into three aliquots and re-treated, attaching a second peptide. After just one more step, all 27 possible combinations exist, spread among the three containers.

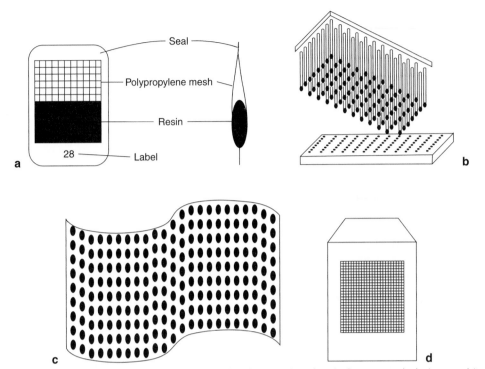

Figure 3–4 ▪ Various approaches to immobilizing and separating chemical compounds during combinatorial synthesis have been devised. **a.** Tea bag synthesis. **b.** Pins and "lollypops." **c.** Dots on cellulose. **d.** Spatial arrays on microchips.

(molecular weight, <500) the attachment to the amide nitrogen (Fig. 3-5).[4] Although these structures could potentially place side chain functional groups in positions similar to those on the corresponding peptides, they differ significantly in that they lack peptide hydrogen bonds and chiral centers. They also show more rotational flexibility than the corresponding peptides, since the peptoid amide bonds show less double-bond character than those in peptides. Miller demonstrated the stability of peptoids to a number of enzymes, including chymotrypsin, papain, pepsin, and carboxypeptidase A.[5] Zuckerman et al.[6] demonstrated in 1994 that biologically active peptoids could be obtained by using combinatorial chemistry. He used 24 monomers to generate tripeptoids, each of which had one hydroxylic, one aromatic, and one diverse side chain. Limiting the composition of the peptoids

in this way limited the total number of compounds to just 204. Nevertheless, several potent ligands were found, including a nanomolar α-adrenergic inhibitor (Fig. 3-6a) and a similarly active μ-opiate receptor ligand (Fig. 3-6b).[6] Because of the ease of synthesis, other classes of linear chain

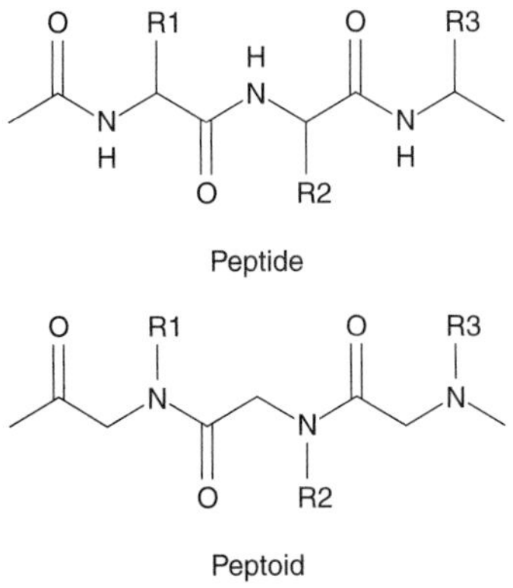

Figure 3–5 ▪ Comparison of peptide and peptoid.

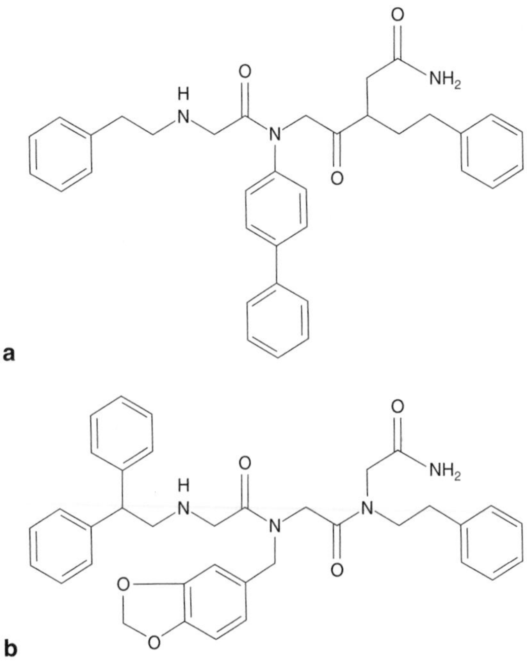

Figure 3–6 ▪ Biologically active peptoids. Compound **a** is an α-adrenergic inhibitor, while compound **b** is a μ-opiate receptor ligand.

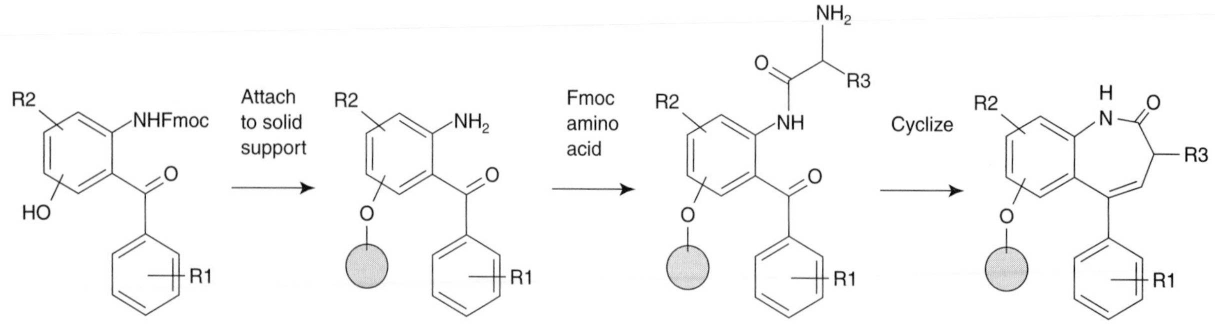

Figure 3–7 ■ Synthesis of 1,4-benzodiazepines on a solid support. *Fmoc*, 9-fluorenylmethoxycarbonyl, a common organic protecting group.

molecules have been investigated. These include oligonucleotides (DNA and RNA), oligoureas, and carbohydrates.

DRUG-LIKE MOLECULES

The real advance in combinatorial chemistry for drug discovery purposes was the introduction of synthetic methodology to yield true drug-like structures. Bunin and Ellman[7] in 1992 demonstrated the synthesis of 1,4-benzodiazepine compounds, using three components: a 2-aminobenzophenone, a protected amino acid, and an alkyl halide (Fig. 3-7). Although we normally think of benzodiazepines as muscle relaxants and tranquilizers, a search for drug structures containing the benzodiazepine scaffold returns antiviral,

alcohol-deterrent, uterine-relaxant, antineoplastic, anticonvulsant, antiulcerative, analgesic, antiarthritic, and sedative structures, among many others. For this reason, the demonstration of the solid-phase synthesis of these structures virtually opened the door to the use of combinatorial chemistry in drug discovery.

In the decade since the first drug molecules were generated by using combinatorial chemistry, solid-phase syntheses have been discovered for most common classes of drug structure. Some examples of these are shown in Figure 3-8. Of necessity, the reactions that can be performed in combinatorial chemistry are simpler than many reactions that a chemist using standard synthetic procedures can perform. Extremes of temperature and pressure, the use of highly caustic reagents, inert atmospheres, and multistep reactions are gen-

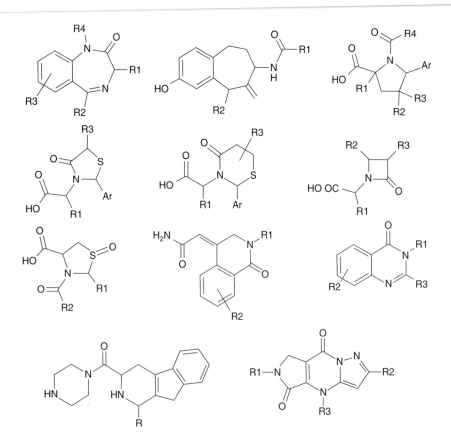

Figure 3–8 ■ Examples of drug-like structures that can be generated by solid-phase synthesis. (Structures drawn from Balkenhohl, F., et al.: Combinatorial synthesis of small organic molecules. Angew. Chem. Int. Ed. Engl. 35:2288–2337, 1996.)

erally avoided in combinatorial chemistry. Also, the reactions should not yield alternative products. The yield of reactions in combinatorial chemistry should be high (80% or more), but this can often be achieved by using an excess of reagent and then washing the beads afterward to remove the excess. An important recent advance in combinatorial chemistry is the use of microwave heating in place of standard heating methods.[8]

Other classes of therapeutically important compounds that have been synthesized successfully by using solid-phase combinatorial chemistry include carbohydrates and natural products.[9] Polysaccharides are important for various carbohydrate–protein interactions. Carbohydrate antibiotics, including vancomycin and aminoglycosides, have been the targets of combinatorial chemistry, as well as complex oligosaccharides like the one shown in Figure 3-9.[10] A vari-

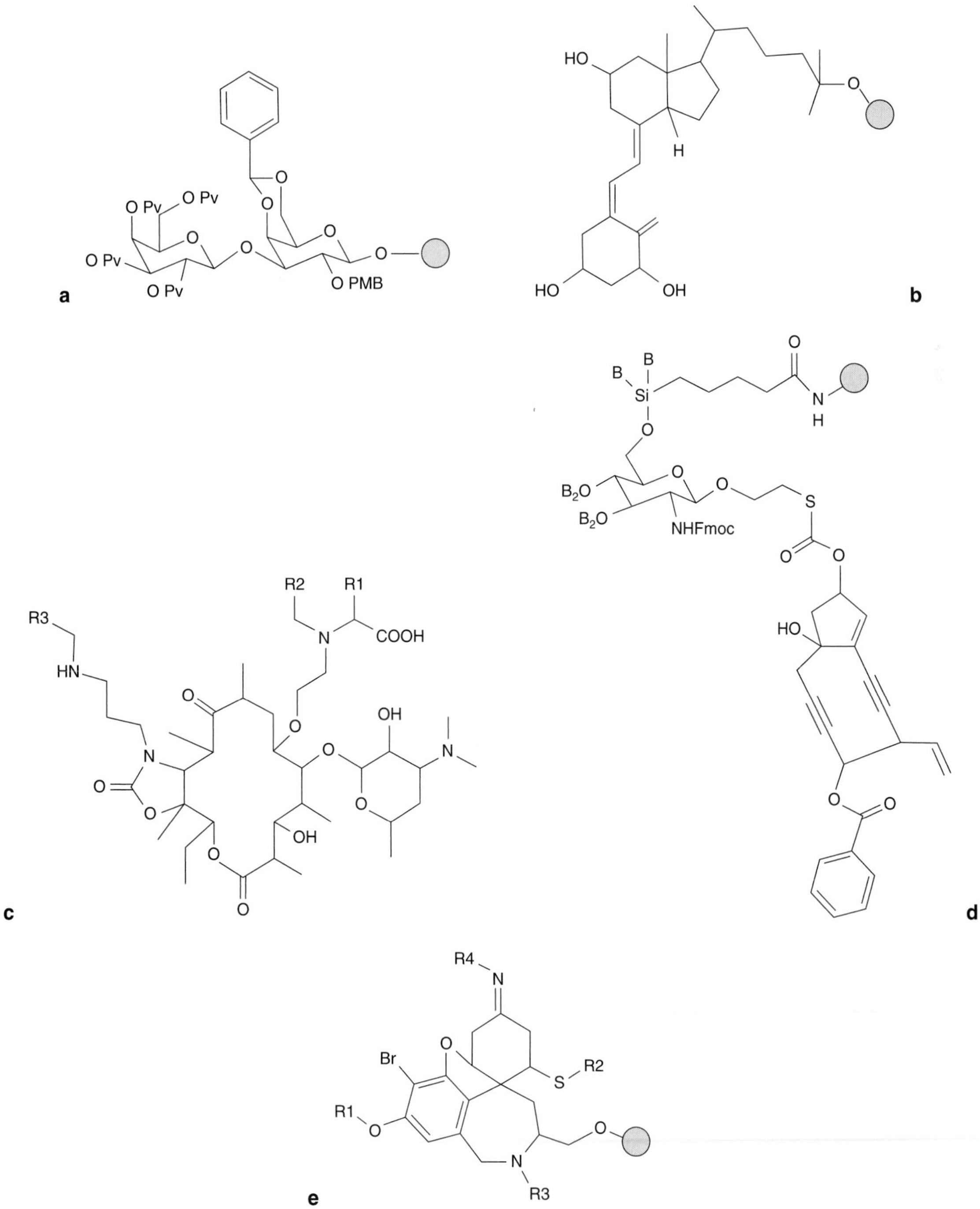

Figure 3–9 ■ Carbohydrate and natural product synthetic targets. **a.** *Bauhinia purpurea* lectin ligand analogues. **b.** Vitamin D₃ analogues. **c.** Erythromycin analogues. **d.** Neocarzinostatin anticancer agents. **e.** Galanthamine cholinesterase inhibitors. In most cases, the molecules are assembled by connecting large subfragments in a small number of synthetic steps rather than by attempting total synthesis. *Fmoc*, 9-fluorenylmethoxycarbonyl, a common organic protecting group.

ety of natural products are being studied, mainly in the areas of infectious disease and cancer but also as scaffolds for many other therapeutic categories. Figure 3-9 shows examples of natural products that have been studied, including vitamin D analogues, erythromycin-like antibiotics, anticancer neocarzinostatins, and galanthamine, a cholinesterase inhibitor.[11]

SUPPORTS AND LINKERS

Most solid-state combinatorial chemistry is conducted by using polymer beads 10 to 750 μm in diameter. These beads swell in organic solvents, allowing the free diffusion of solvent and reagent into the interior of the bead and greatly expanding the available area for the attachment of product. The polymers are inert, except for the functional groups to which the molecules are attached. In general, the compounds to be synthesized are not attached directly to the polymer molecules. They are usually attached using a ''linker'' moiety that *(a)* enables attachment in a way that can be easily reversed without destroying the molecule that is being synthesized and *(b)* allows some room for rotational freedom of the molecules attached to the polymer. Sometimes, the molecules attached to the polymer are used directly as substrates in in vitro assays without removing them from the

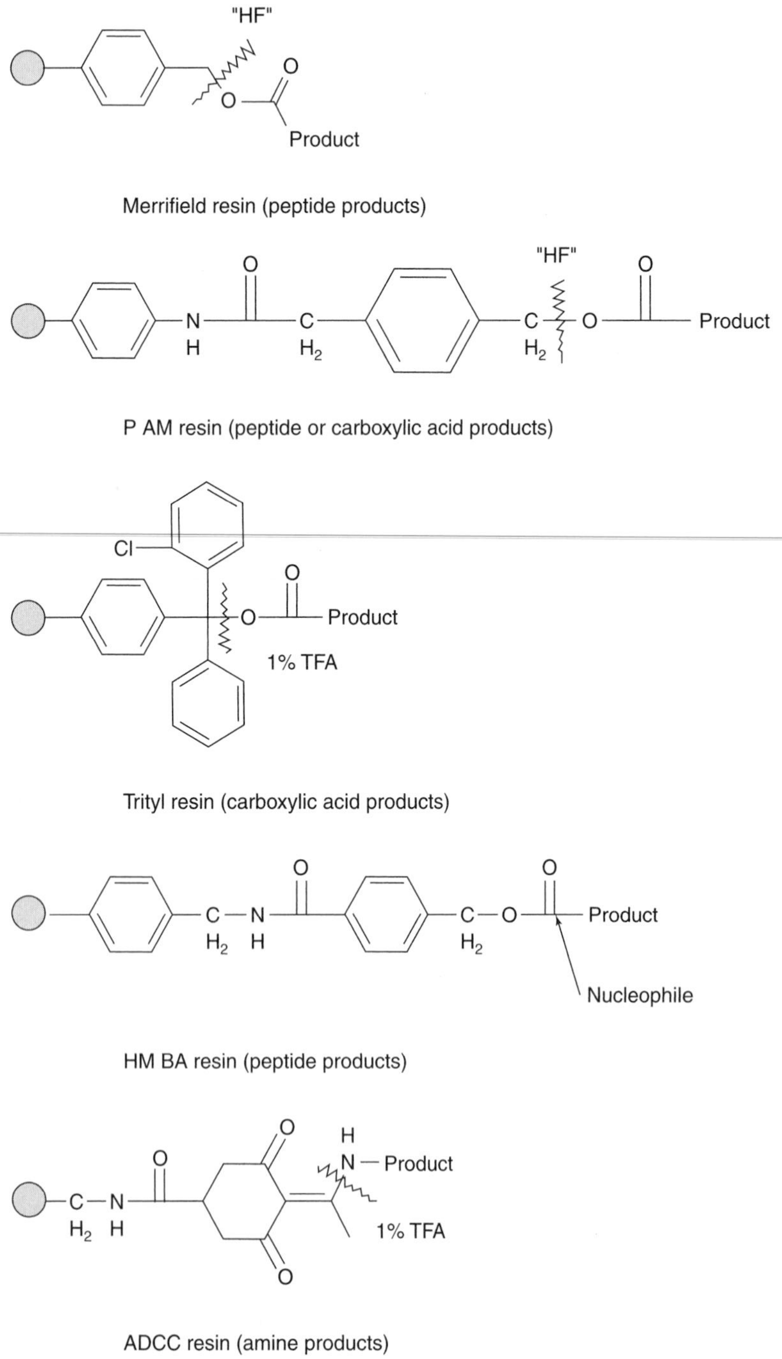
"HF"
Product
Merrifield resin (peptide products)
"HF"
Product
P AM resin (peptide or carboxylic acid products)
Cl
Product
1% TFA
Trityl resin (carboxylic acid products)
Product
Nucleophile
HM BA resin (peptide products)
N — Product
1% TFA
ADCC resin (amine products)

Figure 3–10 ■ Common linker functional groups and the reagents that cleave the product. Note that different linkers provide different spacing and steric freedom between the product and the support. *HF*, hydrofluoric acid; *TFA*, trifluoroacetic acid.

polymer. In such cases, if the molecules are too tightly packed on the polymer, the enzyme molecules cannot gain access to the substrates. A similar situation exists for access by some of the reagents and catalysts used to synthesize the molecules. In general, about 1 mmol of linker is attached per gram of solid support. The types of solid supports that are used include

- **Polystyrene resins.** Polystyrene cross-linked with divinyl benzene (about 1% cross-linking). These are common resins used in size exclusion chromatography.
- **TentaGel resins.** Polystyrene in which some of the phenyl groups have polyethylene glycol (PEG) groups attached in the *para* position. The free OH groups of the PEG allow the attachment of compounds to be synthesized.
- **Polyacrylamide resins.** Like "super glue," these resins swell better in polar solvents and, since they contain amide bonds, more closely resemble biological materials.
- **Glass and ceramic beads.** Not a type of organic resin but sometimes used when high-temperature or high-pressure reactions are needed.

To support the attachment of a synthetic target, the polymer is usually modified by equipping it with a linker or anchor group. Such groups must be stable under the reaction conditions, but they must be susceptible to a "cleavage" reaction that allows removal of the product. Some common linkers are shown in Figure 3-10, along with the reagents that cleave the product from the resin.

Some specialized linkers have been developed to meet particular reaction or product conditions. So-called traceless linkers can be cleaved from the resin with no residual functionality left. This allows the attachment of aryl and alkyl products that do not have OH or NH functionality. These linkers usually include a silyl group ($-Si(CH_3)_2-$) that is sensitive to acids and can be cleaved to give unsubstituted phenyl or alkyl products. A class of linkers known as "safety-catch" linkers are inert to the synthesis conditions but have to be chemically transformed to allow final liberation of the product from the resin. Typically, two reactions are required to break the linker (hence the name). A rather elegant approach to linker chemistry is to use linkers that are sensitive to ultraviolet (UV) light. The Affymax group has used these in the synthesis of carboxylic acid and carboxamide products.[12] Finally, some groups have used linkers that can only be cleaved by enzymes.[13]

SOLUTION-PHASE COMBINATORIAL CHEMISTRY

Most ordinary synthetic chemistry takes place in solution. When a reaction must be modified to accommodate a solid support, it takes time and resources to develop and optimize the reaction conditions. Indeed, a combinatorial chemist may spend months designing a solid-phase reaction and gathering the necessary materials but then conduct the entire synthesis in a matter of hours or days! Many reactions cannot ever be run on solid supports because of poor yields or failed reactions. For these reasons, there has been much interest in using solution-phase chemistry for the preparation of combinatorial libraries. Unlike one-bead one-compound synthesis described above, solution-phase combinatorial chemistry often leads to a mixture of products. Imagine reacting a set of 10 amines with 10 acid chlorides, all in one flask, and with the reactants and conditions chosen so that no reaction of amines with amines or chlorides with chlorides occurs, only reactions between amines and chlorides. The result would be a mixture of 100 amides, one for each possible combination of amine and acid chloride. The resulting mixture could then be tested for activity, under the assumption that the inactive amides did not interfere with binding of active molecules (not always a valid assumption). If activity is found, smaller subsets of amines and chlorides can be tested to eventually find the structure(s) responsible for activity.

Researchers have gone one step further by reacting multiple kinds of reactants together to produce some rather amazing mixtures. Figure 3-11 shows an example of a four-component Ugi reaction that yields, after appropriate further transformation of the intermediate product, a mixture of carboxylic acids, esters and thioesters, pyrroles, 1,4-benzodiazepine-2,5-diones, and even a monosaccharide.[14] Despite the diversity of the chemistry, the yields of products in such mixture-based experiments are often found to be about 90% or better. Although this is an extreme example of a multicomponent reaction, it illustrates the utility of solution-phase chemistry for generating great diversity in chemical libraries.

An approach that is intermediate between solid-phase chemistry and solution-phase chemistry is to use soluble polymers as a support for the product. PEG is a common vehicle in many pharmaceutical preparations. Depending on the degree of polymerization, PEG can be liquid or solid at room temperature and show varying degrees of solubility in aqueous and organic solvents. Each molecule of PEG has an OH group at either end:

$$HOCH_2CH_2O-[CH_2CH_2O]_n-CH_2CH_2OH$$

By converting one OH group to a methyl ether (MeO–PEG–OH), it is possible to attach a carboxylic acid functionality to the free OH and use solution-phase combinatorial chemistry to synthesize, for example, *N*-aryl-sulfonamide structures.[15] The resulting mixture of PEG-bound sulfonamides can be separated by use of chromatography. Another type of soluble support is dendrimers. These are large, highly branched molecules with terminal amino groups that can be used like the OH groups of PEG for the attachment of products. Finally, a class of molecules known as fluorous phases are a form of "liquid Teflon," consisting mainly of long chains of ($—CF_2-$) groups attached to a silicon atom. When these phases are used as a soluble support for synthesis, the resulting product can be readily separated from any organic solvents and reaction by-products by extracting the reaction mixture with fluorocarbon solvents.[16] A unique application using complementary DNA as a "support" has been reported by Harvard researchers.[17] To "encourage" pairs of molecules in solution to react under mild conditions, they attach short strands of complementary DNA or RNA to the structures to "zip" the structures together and promote reaction. The DNA is then removed, yielding product that would not otherwise be synthesized. Using this method makes it possible to prevent reaction of certain pairs of structures as well.

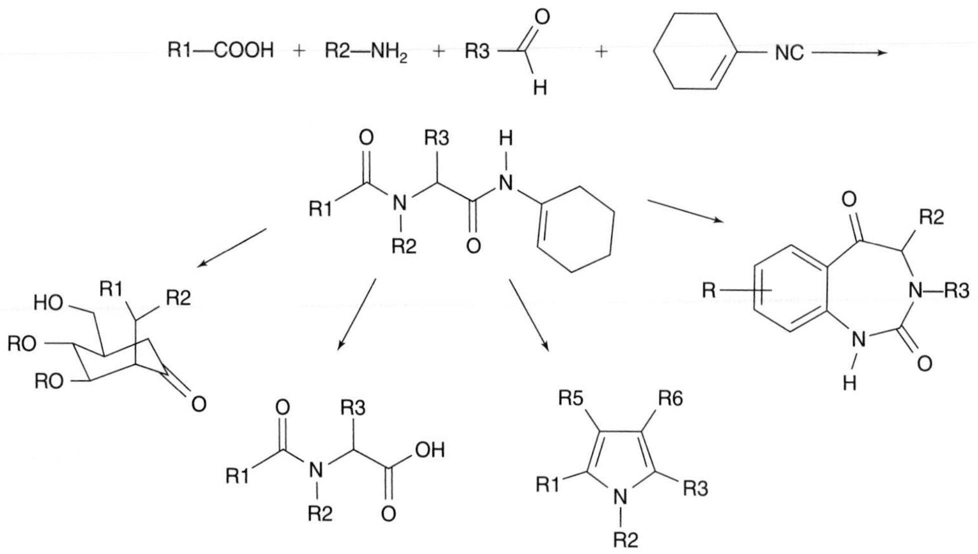

Figure 3–11 ■ Four-component Ugi reaction reported by Keating and Armstrong.[14] A combinatorial mixture of the intermediate cyclohexenyl amide can be split into several portions, and each can be further reacted to give a variety of products, all of which will be combinatorial. (Reaction redrawn from description from Keating, T. A., and Armstrong, R. W.: Molecular diversity via a convertible isocyanide in the Ugi four-component condensation. J. Am. Chem. Soc. 117:7842–7843, 1995.)

POOLING STRATEGIES

Although some solid-phase combinatorial chemistry is conducted by use of the one-bead one-compound strategy, chemists have devised numerous other approaches to pooling reactants and intermediates to generate libraries. The goal is generally to achieve a balance between the simplicity of mixing everything together in one step but then having to "deconvolute" the resulting mixture and working with more, but smaller, mixtures. It has been likened to someone giving you a rake and a magnet and telling you to go find and describe a needle in a field of hay. You can make one big haystack you know contains the needle, then have to deal with ever-smaller "subhaystacks," or you can use more clever approaches, such as dividing the field into regions, using overlapping regions, etc. The major approaches that have been used include the following:

- **One-bead one-compound strategy.** With this strategy, a specific quantity of beads is allocated for each possible structure in the library; those beads contain only molecules of the given library member. The beads may be tagged in various ways (see the next section) to help identify the synthetic compound. The advantage of one-bead one-compound strategy is the simplicity of analysis and screening. The disadvantage is keeping the beads separate and having to deal with a large number of syntheses in parallel. As advances were made in robotics and automation, the problems were reduced, and today, probably most combinatorial experiments involve a one-bead one-compound strategy.
- **Iterative deconvolution.** This is the strategy first described 20 years ago when combinatorial chemistry was started. Reexamine Figure 3-3 and imagine starting at the bottom of the figure with three groups of beads. Each group has beads bearing a variety of compounds, but a given structure only appears in one of the groups. Suppose the active structure is ABC (we pretend here there is only one—in reality there will probably

be several) in the third group. Since it is in the third group, we know a C in position 3 is needed for activity. We synthesize a smaller library of the structures, in three groups: AAC + BAC + CAC, ABC + BBC + CBC, and ACC + BCC + CCC. We do this by skipping the last set of pooling shown in Figure 3-3. Now when we screen these mixtures, we find activity in the middle group of beads. This tells us that a B in position 2 is required for activity. The final step is to synthesize ABC, BBC, and CBC, keeping them separate, and screen each, to find ABC as the active structure.

- **Subtractive deconvolution.** This is similar to iterative deconvolution but uses negative logic, namely, leave out a functional group, and if activity is absent, the functional group that is missing must be needed for activity. This is particularly useful for quantitative structure–activity relationship (QSAR)-type studies in which, say, a —Cl group is placed at several positions on a phenyl ring. The entire library is screened as a mixture to get the baseline activity level. If activity is detected, a set of sublibraries is prepared, with each missing one building block (subtraction of a functional group). Sublibraries that are missing functional groups from the active compound(s) will be less active than the parent library. The least active sublibraries identify the most important functional groups. A reduced library containing only these functional groups is then prepared, and the most active compounds are identified by either one-compound synthesis or iterative deconvolution.
- **Bogus-coin detection.** This begins with generating and screening the entire library as a single mixture. If activity is detected, the building blocks are divided into three groups (α, β, and γ), and additional sublibraries are prepared. In these subsets, the number of building blocks from the α group is decreased, the number from the β group is increased, and the number from the γ group is unchanged. The resulting effect on activity (up, down, unchanged) suggests which group of building blocks was contributing most to activity. This approach is applied iteratively to zoom in on the groups that are most active.
- **Orthogonal pooling.** The term *orthogonal* means perpendicular or uncorrelated. In this type of pooling, we distribute the

functional groups to be considered into sets of libraries, A, B, C, etc., which can contain mixtures of the same compounds. However, the functional groups are distributed such that any subset in A and B shares only one functional group. For example, if we have a very small library of structures—aa, ab, and ac—we might put aa and ab into group A, aa and ac into group B, and ab and ac into group C. If ab is the active structure, screening A, B, and C would show activity in A and C, but not in B, telling us that ab (the only structure in common) is the active one.

- **Positional scanning.** This is a noniterative screening strategy in which a subset library is created with a single building block fixed at one position and all building blocks in the other positions. In principle, by selecting the functional group from the most active subset at each position, the most active compound overall is discovered. This ignores interactions between building blocks, which may complicate the results.

Certain problems with mixtures must be considered when pooling. Complex mixtures with only one or a few active structures can have solubility problems, especially if the compounds are poorly soluble. The inactive compounds contribute to the total ionic concentration but not to the activity. Sometimes, compounds that have a common scaffold will have many active species, arising from the scaffold and not the substituents. Thus, many poorly active structures may show additivity of activity, leading us to think the mixture contains a single active structure (false-positive results). Finally, partial binding of inactive structures can sometimes prevent an active structure from showing full activity (false-negative results).

DETECTION, PURIFICATION, AND ANALYSIS

Detection, analysis, and purification of combinatorial libraries places high demands on existing analytical techniques because *(a)* the quantities to be analyzed are very small, sometimes picomoles of material, *(b)* the analysis should be nondestructive, to allow recovery of the compound if possible, and *(c)* the methods must be suitable for rapid, parallel analysis—analysis cannot be the rate-limiting step in the procedure. No single analytical technique can fit all the requirements, so usually some "hyphenated" analytical techniques are used, for example, high-performance liquid chromatography with a mass spectrometer detection system (HPLC-MS). We describe this and other techniques in this section.

Chromatography is usually the first step in the analysis of a combinatorial mixture. If we start with solid-phase chemistry, we chemically cleave the compounds from the support and filter off the beads, giving a solution containing the compounds we synthesized. If the solution contains just a single compound, we might use a spectrophotometer, to measure infrared (IR) and ultraviolet (UV) absorbance or fluorescence directly, or even nuclear magnetic resonance (NMR) spectroscopy, to determine the structure of the compound in solution. If the solution contains a mixture of compounds, one must separate them before determining their structures. HPLC is a standard approach. A sample of the mixture is injected into the flow of solvent entering a chromatographic column. The components in the mixture travel down the column at different rates, depending on their affin-

ity for the stationary phase in the column, and they exit or *elute* from the column at different times. They are detected by some optical method (UV absorption, fluorescence, refractive index, etc.) that gives rise to peaks on a graphical readout. Sometimes, the output from the column is passed into a spectrophotometer or mass spectrometer to generate a spectrum for each fraction of the output. These spectra can be interpreted to determine the structure of the compound that caused a given peak. It is also possible to use much larger chromatographic columns and run *preparative* HPLC to separate up to several milligrams of material for further analysis or biological assay.

Chromatographic separations and analyses can be fully automated. Thus, a chemist can place all the reaction vessels, microtiter plates, etc. from a combinatorial experiment into racks and use a robotic system to draw samples, inject them into the HPLC, and collect the data output into computer files or databases—all without further intervention from the chemist (except to wash the dishes!). For this reason, speed and solvent handling are special concerns with combinatorial experiments. One approach that has been adopted to speed up analyses and reduce the amount of solvent that must be consumed is *supercritical fluid chromatography* (SFC). Here, the solvent is not a common organic solvent such as acetone or ethanol. Instead, it is a pressurized gas like CO_2 that evaporates from the output, leaving pure compound behind. Another advantage of SFC is speed; since the solvent molecules are small, diffusion is rapid, and separations take place in about half the time of ordinary HPLC separations or less. Finally, the amount of "solvent" that is consumed is significantly lower with SFC. A disadvantage is that certain compounds may not separate as well under SFC as under HPLC.[18]

IR spectroscopy is often applied in combinatorial chemistry. Since IR light can be reflected from materials, one can analyze resin beads directly, without cleaving the products from them. Since the loading of product on any given bead is very small, usually computer-enhanced methods like Fourier transform IR (FTIR) are needed to enhance the very small spectral signal from one or a few beads. Interestingly, the shape of the beads has been found to affect the IR spectra results, and flattened rather than spherical beads give stronger IR signals.[19] NMR spectroscopy gives more structural information than IR or UV spectroscopy, but it has traditionally not been nearly as sensitive. Compounds are normally cleaved from solid support before analysis by NMR, since NMR on solid resin or on resin swollen by solvent gives broadened peaks and low resolution. A type of NMR called *magic angle spinning* NMR, in which the sample is inserted into the magnetic field at an angle of about 55°, reduces the peak broadening and has been used to analyze swollen polymer beads directly. Recent improvements and the use of "nanoprobes" have allowed NMR analysis of 100-mμ beads bearing less than 800 pmol of compound. Other NMR techniques that have been used to analyze combinatorial mixtures include various "two-dimensional" (2D) NMR techniques that use multiple magnetic fields, HPLC-NMR, capillary electrophoresis coupled to NMR (CE-NMR), and even NMR to detect the binding of drugs to receptors to identify active agents. This latter technique has been termed *SAR with NMR*.[20]

Mass spectrometry (MS) is the technique most widely

used for combinatorial library analysis. The measurements can be made on resin beads directly, a wide range of compounds can be analyzed, and MS analyses can be highly automated. Included among a number of MS techniques in use are

- **Electrospray ionization.** A solution containing the compounds to be analyzed is passed into a mass spectrometer through an electrically charged capillary. The droplets that emerge from the capillary bear strong electric charges themselves, and they literally ''explode'' into smaller and smaller droplets and eventually into singly charged ions that are detected by the mass spectrometer.
- **Matrix-assisted laser desorption/ionization time-of-flight (MALDI-TOF).** Quite a mouthful, it simply means the sample is embedded in some solid matrix (e.g., 2,5-dihydroxybenzoic acid) and then bombarded with a laser. Sample molecules are vaporized and ionized in a ''gentle'' fashion that allows whole-molecule ions of the sample to be analyzed. The analysis is done with use of a time-of-flight analyzer, in which ions of different mass travel different distances in a given amount of time.
- **Other less-used MS techniques.** These include secondary-ion MS (SIMS) in which the sample is hit by a metal ion rather than the electron beam itself, and Fourier transform MS.

A very important use of MS in combinatorial chemistry is in quality control of combinatorial libraries. As much as possible, we would like to have pure compounds generated in high yield, with no side reactions or by-products. We also need to verify that every component actually exists in a library (i.e., that no reactions failed). Only MS provides the sensitivity and versatility to perform this checking with both solid-phase and solution-phase libraries

ENCODING COMBINATORIAL LIBRARIES

Once we have found a mixture or sublibrary that shows biological activity, how do we determine exactly which structure or structures are responsible for the activity? We can purify and analyze as described in the previous section, but if no direct analysis is available, we need to *encode* or *tag* the support or the molecules themselves, using physical or molecular ''barcodes.'' An obvious approach that can be used only with small libraries is to physically label each vial of one-bead one-compound resin. This may be practical for a few tens of compounds, but what if we have a library of 32,000 compounds, or even 1,000,000 compounds, in a mixture? Clearly, there is a need for a more automated means of identifying the structures that are in the library.

The most common approach to encoding solid-phase libraries is to attach a chemical tag to the resin beads as the target molecule gets synthesized. Typically, at each step in the reaction, a tag is attached that is unique for the given step. For example, if we are creating a tripeptide and we have 10 possible amino acids at each position, we need to attach either a single tag that says ''the tripeptide on this bead has amino acid Ala at position 1, Phe at position 2, and Gly at position 3,'' or we need to attach three different tags, one for each position.

One of the earliest types of chemical encoding was the attachment of oligonucleotides (usually single-strand DNA)

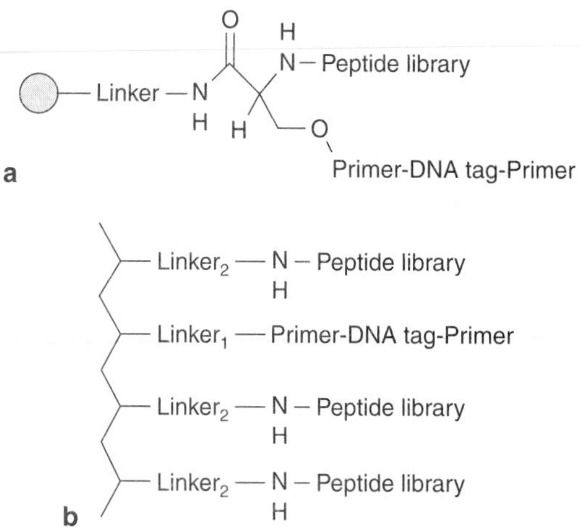

Figure 3–12 ■ Two ways of attaching DNA tags to solid supports. **a.** A DNA tag is attached with each peptide molecule via a bifunctional serine residue. **b.** The DNA and peptide groups have separate linkers.

to beads on which peptides or peptoids were being built.[21] Since there are 20 possible amino acids and only four nucleotide bases, enough bases must be attached at each amino acid addition step to identify properly the amino acid being attached. Although three bases are used in the DNA genetic code, it is customary to use up to six bases for library tagging. For decoding, the DNA tag is amplified by use of the *polymerase chain reaction* (PCR), the same reaction that is used in forensic DNA analysis. For this reason, the chemical tag must also bear PCR primer sequences.

Two types of anchors have been used to connect the DNA tags to the solid support (Fig. 3-12). In one type, the growing DNA chain is attached to the α carbon of a serine group that is anchored to the solid support by a linker molecule. The growing peptide chain is attached to the serine amino group, possibly through a spacer. In the second type of anchor, the DNA chain has its own anchor to the solid support. In this case, fewer DNA tags are attached than the number of polypeptide molecules.[22]

If DNA tags cannot be used, one can label beads by using a ''binary'' approach. Suppose we are building a tripeptide with four possible amino acids at each position. We can use binary digits to encode which amino acid is at a given position as follows (each binary ''number'' is read from the right) (Table 3-1): Thus, using 18 different tags (3×6) we can encode for any of the ($4^3 = 64$) members of the library. For example, if the product is Ala-Gly-Lys, the encoding

TABLE 3–1 Binary Encoding of a Tripeptide, Using 18 Possible Tags

Amino Acid	Position 1	Position 2	Position 3
Ala	00 00 00	00 00 00	00 00 00
Phe	00 00 01	00 01 00	01 00 00
Gly	00 00 10	00 10 00	10 00 00
Lys	00 00 11	00 11 00	11 00 00

would be 00 00 00 00 10 00 11 00 00, and 3 of the 18 possible tags would be attached to the support, along with the tripeptide. It is common to use polyhalogenated aromatic compounds as tags, such as

where X represents some combination of halogen atoms. The halogens make the tags show up clearly in MS analysis of the mixture, and by varying the chain length n, the tag can be made flexible enough not to interfere with attachment of the product. Other chemical tags that have been used include isotopically labeled peptides and dyes.

When it is not possible to use chemical tags, one must physically label the solid or liquid support itself. One alternative is to use radiofrequency encoding, in which tiny microchips are added to the resin or to the solution phase. As various reactions are conducted to generate the products, at each step a radiofrequency signal is stored in the microchip. This signal can be recalled to identify the sequence of reactions that generated the product (a similar principle is used when your dog or cat gets a small identification (ID) pellet implanted under the skin of the neck). Laser optical encoding is yet another approach, in which the solid support consists of a ceramic chip covered with a polypropylene–polystyrene polymer solid phase. The barcode pattern is actually burned into the ceramic at each step in the reaction and is decoded visually with use of a microscope. Finally, one can embed semiconductor particles into the solid phase that fluoresce at different wavelengths. These are called "quantum dots" by their manufacturer.[23]

HIGH-THROUGHPUT SCREENING (HTS)

Without the ability to screen libraries rapidly for activity, there would be no combinatorial chemistry. Fortunately, the biologists are just as adept at developing rapid high-throughput assays as the chemists are at generating structures. HTS is an extremely broad topic, encompassing enzymes, organelles, cells, various tissues, whole organs, and even whole-animal testing, via cassette dosing. This section briefly discusses only a part of the role of HTS in drug discovery, with emphasis on a few recent developments.[24]

Successful HTS programs integrate several activities, including target identification (genomics and molecular biology groups), reagent preparation (protein expression and purification groups), compound management (information management group), assay development (biologist and pharmacologist), and high-throughput library screening (biologists and chemists). Formerly, these activities were handled separately, and multiple handoffs of samples were involved. It is becoming more common to integrate the activities and share expertise. This increases efficiency of the screening process. Another route to increasing efficiency is a move to

higher-density screening platforms. The standard layout for HTS has been a 96-well microtiter plate (12×8). Denser formats, up to 1,536 wells per plate, are increasingly being used. This requires advances in liquid handling, precision of detection, and laboratory automation.

One of the first activities in developing a HTS assay is selecting the target. About 500 targets are currently being used by drug companies. Of these, cell membrane receptors, mostly G-protein–coupled receptors, make up the largest group (about 45% of the total). Enzymes make up the next largest group (28%), followed by hormones (11%), unknowns (7%), ion channels (5%), nuclear receptors (2%), and finally DNA (2%).[25] It is expected that the annotation of the human genome will add additional targets, although the rate of this addition is not known. New targets must be part of some regulatory pathway in the cell and should be sensitive to some disease state, not be expressed all the time and everywhere in the cell.

The next concern in HTS is the library to be screened. Throughout our discussion, we have perhaps offered the impression that a given library for a particular project was the only set of compounds that were ever screened for activity. In fact, much HTS involves screening compounds that are part of the corporate storehouse of compounds synthesized in the past, or they may be a library purchased from a vendor. Such libraries usually consist of microtiter plates containing frozen or dried samples of compound—perhaps only micrograms per well. The size of such libraries may range from a few thousand compounds to nearly a million. The cost of completely screening such a library against just a single assay may amount to over $300,000, so such large-scale screens are conducted rather infrequently, compared with routine day-to-day screens. It has been estimated that one must screen at least 120,000 "quality" compounds (i.e., diverse drug-like structures) to discover a single-lead series for a therapeutically sound target.[26]

As discussed above in the section on pooling strategies, one can reduce the screening effort by pooling groups of structures and running assays on mixtures of compounds. This also conserves reagents and biological material, has smaller storage requirements, and requires fewer personnel. There are potential problems with pooling. A number of factors limit the number of different compounds we can test in a given well, including ionization, reactivity, and solubility. Compounds can enter a screening program in a nonrandom order, such that a given assay plate may have compounds that are highly similar structurally. This may give rise to false-positive hits. False-negative hits are less likely to arise from pooling. Another concern is the use of replicates—compounds from the same series—in a given assay. If only one representative of a given series is present, the chance of missing that series as a possible lead series is greater than if multiple members are present. Therefore, it is common to include several members of each series in a given assay when possible.

To be effective, a given compound must dissolve completely in the assay medium. It is common to add a small amount (1%) of dimethyl sulfoxide (DMSO) to the assay to assist solvation. The best concentration of compound to use is somewhat debatable. High concentrations (10 μM and above) often lead to more false positives than screening at a low concentration (3 μM). The reason for this may be nonspecific binding at the higher concentration.

Just as there are several ways to detect and identify members of a combinatorial library, there are many ways to measure activity in HTS assays. Any such method must be accurate, reproducible, and have a high signal-to-noise ratio (S/N). Typically, the result of HTS is a qualitative (yes/no) or semiquantitative one (high-medium-low), rather than a precise value (e.g., KI_{50} or LD_{50}). The methods for detection in HTS fall into the categories of *nonradiometric* and *radiometric*.

Nonradiometric methods include absorbance, fluorescence, and luminescence spectroscopy. Enzyme assays are a common example. The assay is usually run at or below the K_m value of the substrate, with only about 5% of the substrate consumed during the assay, and multiple enzyme turnovers occur during the assay. Sometimes enzyme reactions are coupled, especially if the target reaction does not produce a product that can be detected directly in the assay. An example is carboxypeptidase, which is coupled to the reduction of NADP to NADPH, giving rise to absorbance at 340 nm.

Radiometric methods include filtration and scintillation proximity assay (SPA). These assays use radioisotopes, so safe storage and handling are of concern. In filtration assay, a radioactive substrate bound to a capture group is cleaved by its enzyme, removing the radioactivity from the capture group. The mixture is filtered through special filter paper that the capture group sticks to, but everything else passes through. A scintillation fluid is added, and the radioactivity of the filter is measured. The degree to which the radioactivity is retained measures the strength of the inhibition (Fig. 3-13a).

SPA is a newer, simpler method (Fig. 3-13b). We start with the same radioactive substrate, which may not necessarily need a capture group. The enzyme and potential drug are added, causing the cleavage of the substrate to some degree. Now, instead of filtering, a special resin bead coated with a

scintillant—a compound that fluoresces in the near presence of the radioactive substrate (near being about 20 μm)—is added to the mixture. The lysed and unlysed substrate binds to the beads, and if the radioactive part of the substrate is still attached, the bead will fluoresce. If not, the radioactive parts of the substrate floating in the solution will be too far from the beads to cause any fluorescence. The presence of fluorescence implies that the test compound inhibited the enzyme. The advantage of SPA over filtration is that no filtering of the solution is needed, so beads can be added directly to the assay mixture in wells or test tubes. Also, special scintillation fluid is not needed. The beads for SPA can be engineered to attach a variety of substrate types.

Other HTS assay advances include the use of microorganisms such as bacteria and yeast, the cloning and expression of mammalian receptors in microorganisms, probing protein–protein interactions, and very importantly, DNA and protein arrays. These are too involved to discuss here, but excellent reviews exist.[24, 27] The increasing use of HTS to screen for a molecule's absorption, distribution, metabolism, excretion, and toxicity (ADMET) properties has been covered as well.[28]

VIRTUAL (IN SILICO) SCREENING

Virtual, or in silico, screening refers to the use of computers to predict whether a compound will show desired properties or activity on the basis of its two-dimensional (2D) or three-dimensional (3D) chemical structure or its physicochemical properties. The motivation for using virtual screening arises from the flood of new structures coming from combinatorial chemistry, the expense and time required to run conventional HTS, the ethical concerns about using animal tissue instead of predictive models, and an increasing failure rate for structures coming out of combinatorial programs. In general, a virtual screening program attempts to answer one or both of these questions:

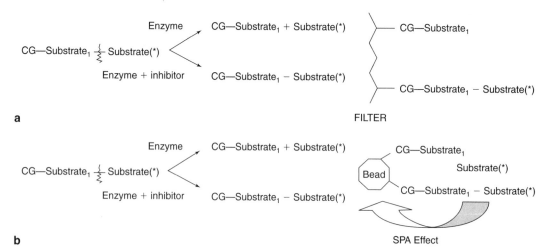

a

b

Figure 3–13 ■ Comparison of filtration and scintillation proximity assays. **a.** In filtration assay, the enzyme, substrate, and inhibitor are mixed; the uninhibited enzyme splits the radioactive portion (*) off the substrate, and filtering the mixture, followed by measuring the radioactivity of the filter, tells how much inhibition has occurred. **b.** In SPA, the same mixture is treated with resin beads containing a scintillant that fluoresces only in close proximity to the radioactive source. Any radioactivity that was split off by the enzyme does not need to be filtered in SPA.

1. Will a particular compound show sufficient binding to a known receptor?
2. Will a particular compound possess any undesirable ADMET properties?

To answer these questions, we must build computer models of the interaction of drugs with receptors (docking, molecular modeling, quantum mechanics) and models for predicting ADMET properties on the basis of chemical structure (QSAR models). Like much of drug discovery, the virtual screening process is a cyclic one. We start with a collection of structures and run predictive models on them, generating some subset of "best" structures. We then test these structures in real assays or screens to see if the predictions were accurate. Finally, we incorporate information learned from the real assays back into our predictive models to improve them for future use.[29]

Models for the prediction of binding arise from the field of molecular modeling. This includes molecular mechanics (predicting the 3D structure of molecules from the standpoint of the atomic nuclei) and quantum mechanics (predicting the 3D structure of molecules from the standpoint of their electrons). We can generate fairly accurate 3D structures of stand-alone molecules with either of these approaches. We can also model the interaction of two molecules and predict whether they will show hydrogen bonding or electrostatic or lipophilic interactions. If we know the 3D structure of a receptor, we can predict whether a given compound will "fit" into the receptor with sufficiently tight binding to prevent normal substrates from binding, i.e., an enzyme inhibitor (or drug). Typically, this does not consider any effects of transport, metabolism, interaction with solvent, etc. Consequently, the existing models for the binding of drugs to receptors are rather crude, with errors of 50% or more. Nevertheless, for the purpose of screening, this is often adequate. If a structure is predicted to show tight binding, it will probably be synthesized and tested in a real HTS assay, to obtain a more accurate estimate of its activity.[30] An interesting application of high-throughput docking is the United Devices screensaver.[31] This is a PC program that can be downloaded to run in the background and participate in worldwide projects to screen large databases of structures against such targets as cancer and anthrax.

We can combine the prediction of binding to a receptor with the design of molecules. If we start with a set of building blocks and a known receptor, we can align complementary building blocks with pockets in the receptor, in conformations that maximize hydrogen bonding and other interactions. When the fragments are aligned, we can then connect the fragments with appropriately sized spacer fragments to "build" a drug molecule within the confines of the receptor. This approach is sometimes called *de novo* or *structure-based* drug design. As our models for binding to receptors improve, this approach is becoming more popular.[32]

In 1997, researchers at Pfizer looked at the previous 10 years' worth of drug design, including all of their combinatorial chemistry efforts.[33] They found that since the introduction of combinatorial chemistry, chemists had tended to design larger, more complex, and more lipophilic structures than in the past. Since the structures were supposed to be designed as lead structures rather than optimized drug molecules, it was becoming more difficult to optimize them into

drugs. This led Lipinski to enumerate some rules for the rejection of structures. He proposed rejecting any structures that fail two or more of the following criteria:

- Molecular weight should be <500.
- Number of hydrogen bond donors (NH, OH) should be fewer than 5.
- Number of hydrogen bond acceptors (—N—, —O—, —S—) should be fewer than 10.
- Calculated log P value should be less than 5.

Since the number 5 shows up in many of these criteria, they have become known as the "rule of five." These and similar rules have become widely adopted by drug companies in their discovery programs. They fall under the general category of "business rules"—guidelines for the proper conduct of business and research. One should be cautious though and use them as guidelines and not strict rules, to avoid missing important drug structures that happen to fail the rules but still show high activity and acceptable ADMET properties.[34] The "rule of five" is designed to be a yes/no filter for the rejection of structures. More quantitative models designed to predict some value or level of property have also been developed. Examples include predicting Caco-2 cell permeability (Caco-2 cells are human intestinal epithelial cells that can be layered and studied in vitro)[35] and predicting binding to cytochrome P-450 (a major liver enzyme involved in metabolism).[36]

CHEMICAL DIVERSITY AND LIBRARY DESIGN

The universe of drug-molecule–sized compounds that could be synthesized is enormous. For example, a polypeptide with 100 residues could regenerate 100^{20} or 10^{40} possible structures. If just 1 g of each were synthesized, it would be a mass comparable to the mass of the known universe (about 10^{50} kg!) (Peterson, J.: Universe in the Balance. *New Scientist* 168:26, 2000). Clearly, a combinatorial chemist needs to select carefully the scaffolds and building blocks that will make up the library to be synthesized. Since the 1980s, chemists have adopted many computational techniques to aid in the design and selection of library structures. These techniques have been borrowed largely from the fields of QSAR and molecular modeling. This section describes some of the most common computational approaches to library design.

Typically in drug design there are four possible scenarios for the amount of information we are starting with[37]

1. We do not know the structure of the receptor, and we do not have any known ligands or inhibitors. This is mainly a case for high-throughput in vitro screening of existing drug databases and libraries, in the hope that some structure may bind to the receptor and serve as a starting point for lead development. Often it is straightforward to find existing structures with micromolar potency. The problem then becomes one of deciding how to modify the structures to yield ones that are novel from a patent standpoint and show suitable biopharmaceutical properties.
2. We do not know the structure of the receptor, but we do have known ligands or inhibitors. This was once the most common

situation in drug design. The usual approach to selecting structures for further testing is to find structures in chemical databases that are similar in structure and properties to the known inhibitors. A common approach is to develop a pharmacophore model for the receptor, based on superimposing structures with known activity. This can then be used as a *search query* in a chemical structure database to find structures that have the same functional groups in the same relative positions.

3. We do know the structure of the receptor and we have known ligands or inhibitors. This is increasingly becoming the state of affairs for known receptors. There are about 100 known receptor–ligand complexes published in the Protein Data Bank that have relevance to existing human illness. Pharmaceutical companies have many more examples. As soon as one drug company patents a drug with activity for a known receptor, other companies are quick to use this information to try to develop novel structures with greater potency, longer-lasting activity, fewer side effects, etc. This is especially true if the market for the agent is a large one. The techniques for finding new drugs in this situation combine *(a)* pharmacophore discovery using known ligands with *(b)* docking and molecular modeling of new structures to see how well they fit into the receptor. This is known as *virtual screening,* and it is becoming more important all the time. The quality of virtual screening results depends on the quality of the protein and drug molecule structures we start with and the accuracy of the mathematical functions that predict the degree of binding from such factors as steric, electrostatic, hydrogen bonding, and lipophilic interactions between the drug and the receptor.

4. In the final scenario, we know the structure of the receptor, but we do not have known ligands or inhibitors. This is a less likely case than scenario 3, but the decoding of the human genome may change that. Of the 30,000 or more genes that are being annotated from the genome, it is estimated that perhaps 10% may have some relevance to human disease. This would represent 3,000 new enzyme targets for drug designers to work with. Researchers expect 10 or more new targets to be elucidated each year, so this promises to be a long-term project. In many cases, the enzyme or structural protein that a gene encodes may be difficult to crystallize for x-ray analysis or to study in solution using NMR. In such cases, protein molecular modeling may be used to predict the structure of the enzyme. A common approach is *homology* modeling, in which sequences of the unknown protein are assigned secondary and tertiary structures based on those of known proteins with similar sequences. IBM has embarked on a project known as ''Blue Gene,'' to try to predict the structures and receptor sites of all the protein products of the human genome, over a period of a few years, using supercomputers. Once the enzyme structures are known or predicted, virtual screening can be used to find drug molecules that might fit into the receptor.

Assuming that one of the above scenarios holds for a given drug discovery project, one commonly proceeds through a sequence of chemical libraries on the way to lead discovery and optimization. This process has several phases, and the libraries that are designed at any given phase show varying levels of diversity, size, and specificity for the given receptor. The goal of library design is to select a subset of molecules from some larger collection such that we are taking samples from various regions of chemical space. If the library is an initial or *exploratory* library, we want to sample as much chemical space as possible, so we seek structures with high diversity. If the library is a more *focused* library, we want to sample a smaller region of chemical space in the neighborhood of the most active structure discovered in the exploratory library. If the library is an *optimization* li-

brary, we want to look for small changes in the basic structure, to find the best combination of substituents that will yield the highest activity.

The first task is to define and quantify chemical *diversity*. This requires a definition of chemical *similarity*, since diversity is essentially the opposite of similarity. There are several ways to quantify molecular similarity. Two common approaches in combinatorial chemistry are *(a)* to define similarity as the closeness of structures to each other in the space of some physicochemical or topological descriptors (e.g., log *P*, solubility, or polar molecular surface area) and *(b)* to define similarity as the number of simple structural features the compounds have in common (e.g., carbonyl groups, phenyl rings, etc.).

Consider the molecules in Table 3-2. If the first molecule, diethylstilbestrol, is used as a similarity probe in a database of drug structures, several other structures can be found (some of which are estrogens, but many of which have other activities). The most similar structures do have estrogenic activity, and they have values similar to those of some of the other descriptors in the table. Some descriptors by themselves would be poor predictors of molecular similarity. For example, one can find many structures with similar log *P* values but with different structural characteristics. For this reason, there has been some controversy about what the ''best'' approach to similarity and diversity is.[38] In the design of exploratory libraries, the goal is to sample a wide variety of chemical structures, so it is reasonable to use diversity measures that focus on structural differences, such as 2D molecular similarity. We select molecules that are dissimilar to each other. In the design of optimization libraries, the goal is often twofold: to increase potency and to optimize ADMET properties. Minor changes in the structure are usually made at this point, so all the structures show high 2D similarity to each other. But minor changes in substituents can change physicochemical properties and modify the interaction of the drug with the receptor, so the other descriptors in Table 3-2 are often more useful in the lead optimization stage of a project. An example of a simple change that causes a large decrease in binding affinity is seen in Figure 3-14, where the replacement of a H atom by a methyl group reduces activity 80-fold.[39]

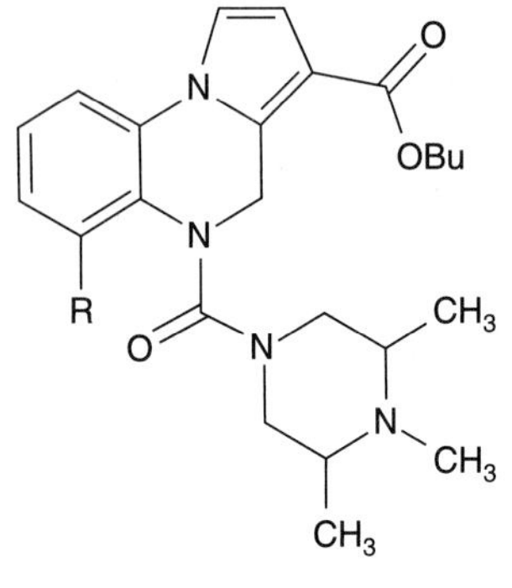

R = H (6.7 nM)
R = Me (470 nM)

Figure 3–14 ■ Changing a H atom to a methyl group has a large effect on binding to the α-aminobutyric acid ($GABA_A$) receptor.

TABLE 3–2 Similarity of Structures to Diethylstilbestrol (DES), Using Various Descriptors

Molecule	Log P	Polar Surface Area	No. of H-Bond Acceptors	No. of H-Bond Donors	No. of Rotatable Bonds	2D Molecular Similarity to DES
	5.64	40.5	2	2	2	100
	7.91	29.5	1	2	5	76
	6.78	52.6	0	4	8	56
	5.68	40.5	2	2	5	40
	5.34	20.2	1	1	0	36
	5.58	40.5	2	2	4	33

Having decided on some measure(s) of diversity, the next step is to actually select structures from the starting collection. Typically, we select either whole compounds for HTS or reagents to be used in a particular synthetic step. The selection process consists of using similarity/diversity measures to pick compounds that sample chemical space in a manner appropriate for the library being generated. Thus, for an exploratory library, we would pick diverse structures with as much structural variation as possible, perhaps subject to some rules about size, lipophilicity, etc. For an optimization library, we would pick substituents for a given scaffold that span traditional QSAR space, which includes steric, electronic, and lipophilic properties of the substituents.

The methods of selecting structures come mainly from statistics and QSAR.[40] They include the following:

- **Random selection.** Here we let the computer pick structures at random from the initial collection. We may "bias" the random selection by filtering the structures as they are picked and rejecting ones that we know we do not want or that are too similar to structures already picked.
- **Visual selection.** If we have selected, for example, 10 descriptors for our chemical space, it is difficult to find display methods that can display data in high dimensions. There are *projection* methods in statistics that can make a "shadow" of the points in high-dimensional space onto two or three dimensions, at which point a standard two-dimensional (2D) or three-dimensional (3D) scatterplot can be used to see how the points are distributed and to select compounds. A standard method for this projection is *principal components analysis* (PCA). In this approach, we generate a couple of new descriptors, the principal components, that are linear combinations of the original descriptors ($pc_1 = w_1x_1 + w_2x_2 + \cdots$) with each descriptor ($x$) weighted ($w$) according to how much it contributes to the overall variation of the data.
- **Binning.** If we partition chemical space into regions, like squares on a checkerboard, we can pick molecules from each region to build our library. Probably some regions will have many structures in them, and we may pick several from such areas. Some regions will be empty. These are termed *holes* in our collection, and we may want to design structures with property values that would help fill these holes.
- **Cluster analysis.** This method involves using statistical procedures that try to discover natural groupings of compounds on the basis of similarity or distance between them. Cluster methods function either by partitioning space on the basis of the density of the compounds (e.g., K-means clustering) or by linking the compounds in a tree-like structure (hierarchical clustering). The result is to assign each compound to a group or cluster. Compounds within a cluster are more similar or closer to each other, on average, than to compounds in other clusters.
- **Experimental design.** If we have selected a subset of structures from our collection, we can use any of several statistical measures to quantify the diversity of our subset. Further, there are statistical selection procedures that, if followed, will make it more likely (but not guarantee) that we pick more and more diverse subsets. These are *optimization* procedures, and they are widely used in the design of experiments, statistical surveys, etc. An example of a common procedure is one called *D-optimal selection*, which is designed to pick a subset of points that are as widely separated from each other as possible.
- **Genetic algorithms.** This optimization procedure is inspired by the way genetics and natural selection work. To use a genetic algorithm, we pretend that our collection is an artificial "genome." Each structure in the collection is a base or string of bases in the genome (instead of A, T, G, and C, the base designation is just 1 or 0). We start by generating random strings of 1s and 0s to represent the genome. Each string is measured for the diversity the structures in the string represent. This is called the *fitness* of the string. Then, we apply the genetic operations of mutation, crossover, and recombination, to generate new populations of 1s and 0s. Some of these will have higher fitness values (more diversity) than others. Over time, as we repeat the genetic operations, the overall genome will tend to improve toward more diverse collections of structures.

Most of these methods, including calculating descriptors and measuring molecular similarity are part of combinatorial chemistry software systems. These systems are provided by molecular modeling and by chemical information companies such as Accelrys, Daylight, MDL, and Tripos. They usually function in the context of a chemical structure database. Such databases can store 2D structures, 3D models, reactions, generic structures, building blocks, and all the physicochemical and inventory data in a single repository, sometimes called a *data warehouse*. Chemical data are indexed and accessed by structure or structure ID. Biological data are typically indexed and accessed by assay or test ID. For this reason, most drug companies have traditionally stored chemical and biological data separately and used different systems for access. In the past few years, it has become common to store both chemical structures and biology data in relational databases such as Oracle. This trend toward integration of the two types of data is motivated in large part by the flood of information that combinatorial chemistry and HTS are generating. Most large pharmaceutical companies are synthesizing and testing 1000 times as many structures today as they were 15 to 20 years ago, with a similar increase in the amount of information that must be collected, organized, stored, and interpreted. The drug companies are taking a cue from large retailers and financial vendors and adopting "data mining" techniques to search for hidden associations, clusters, and predictive relationships in the mountains of data they are collecting in their databases.[41]

REPORT CARD ON COMBINATORIAL CHEMISTRY: HAS IT WORKED?

A report published in 1998 showed that virtually all of the major pharmaceutical firms had adopted combinatorial chemistry to some extent in their drug discovery process.[42] The degree of adoption ranged from 16 to 100% of new drug synthesis, with an average of 66%. Clearly, the pharmaceutical firms have a big stake in combinatorial chemistry, but has it really worked out? As of this writing, the pharmaceutical firms are suffering large increases in research and development expenses, but with a decline in the number of new drugs in the pipeline. Many firms have a large fraction of their blockbuster drugs (>$1 billion in sales per year) going off patent in the next few years. Part of the problem has been the pursuit of only a few, highly profitable, therapeutic targets. For example, there are at least seven statin anti-cholesterol drugs on the market; the most profitable one, Lipitor, currently collects about $7 billion in sales per year for its developer. Another problem has been the marketing of drugs that appeared to be safe, even throughout clinical trials, but were later found to cause serious and even fatal side effects (e.g., Seldane and Baycol).

There is little question that combinatorial chemistry has been effective in generating large numbers of lead structures. Many pharmaceutical companies began using combinatorial chemistry to build up their in-house libraries of structures that could be "mined" for activity against newly discovered receptors. A typical pharmaceutical firm has access to information on 10 to 20 million structures from commercial sources (various chemical software vendors and the Ameri-

---

TABLE 3–3   Examples of Lead Structures Obtained by Combinatorial Chemistry

Structure	Source	Target	Mechanism
	Merck	HIV-1 integrase	Block viral integration
	SmithKline Beecham	Human 5-HT$_6$ serotonin receptor	Antagonist; cognitive disorders
	Abbott	Interleukin-2	Cytokine inhibition
	Pfizer	Farnesyl transferase a	Inhibition
	Parke Davis	KDO-8-P synthetase	Inhibition; antibacterial

can Chemical Society Chemical Abstracts Service). In addition, large companies have their own multimillion-compound databases. Golebiowski et al.[43] describe how lead structures with a wide variety of activity have been obtained with use of combinatorial chemistry. Some examples are shown in Table 3-3, demonstrating the variety of structural types that have been generated. An industry perspective published in 2001 reported 46 compounds in human clinical trials that originated from HTS of libraries that were identified between 1992 and 1998.[44]

What can be argued is whether the goal of generating lead structures is sufficient, in light of an increasing rejection rate of candidate drugs in clinical trials, caused by side effects and other ADMET-related failures. Most researchers would agree that we need to predict the "drugability" of a lead better before much testing, if any, is done. As mentioned in the section on virtual screening, much work is being devoted to the development of better in vitro and computational methods for predicting ADMET properties. Alternatives to combinatorial chemistry are appearing in the literature. An example is the "non-combinatorial" approach of Everett et al.[45] These authors argue that the goal of combinatorial chemistry should be the quality, not the quantity, of leads.

Some trends that are appearing in the literature include *(a)* smaller libraries, a few thousand carefully selected structures rather than 250,000 hastily designed ones; *(b)* more attention to ADMET properties in the early phases of drug discovery; *(c)* miniaturization of syntheses and assays, using *microfluidics* and *nanotechnology,* both for speed and to conserve resources; and *(d)* an integration of genomic and combinatorial chemistry technology for better use human genome information in the design of new drugs.[46] Most chemists agree that combinatorial chemistry, after 20 years of evaluation, is a vital, but not the only, implement in the drug discovery toolkit that should be used. Like other tools, it can be applied intelligently to great benefit, or it can be misused.

RESOURCES FOR COMBINATORIAL CHEMISTRY

Books

Beck-Sicklinger, A., and Weber, P.: Combinatorial Strategies in Biology and Chemistry. New York, John Wiley & Sons, 2002. (The finest short introduction available)

Bunin, B. A.: The Combinatorial Index. New York, Academic Press, 1998 (a comprehensive, chemistry-oriented reference).

Czarnik, A. W., and DeWitt, S. H. (eds.): A Practical Guide to Combinatorial Chemistry. Washington, DC, American Chemical Society, 1997.

Fenniri, H., Combinatorial Chemistry—A Practical Approach. Oxford, UK, Oxford University Press, 2000. (Laboratory experiments)

Ghose, A. K., and Viswanadhan, V. N.: Combinatorial Library Design and Evaluation. Principles, Software Tools, and Applications in Drug Discovery. New York, Marcel Dekker, 2001.

Gordon, E. M., and Kerwin, J. J. F. (eds.): Combinatorial Chemistry and Molecular Diversity in Drug Discovery. New York, Wiley-Liss, 1998.

Terrett, N.: Combinatorial chemistry. In Compton, R. G., Davies, S. G., and Evans, J. (eds.). Oxford Chemistry Masters. Oxford, UK, Oxford University Press, 1998. (A brief, highly readable introduction)

Journals

Combinatorial Chemistry and High-Throughput Screening—Bentham Publishers
Drug Discovery Today—Reed Elsevier
Journal of Chemical Information and Computer Sciences—American Chemical Society
Journal of Combinatorial Chemistry—American Chemical Society
Modern Drug Discovery—American Chemical Society
Molecular Diversity—Kluwer
Nature Reviews Drug Discovery—Nature Publishing Group
Trends in Biotechnology (TIBTECH)—Elsevier

Videos

Chemical Diversity: Applications of Computational Approaches. Washington, DC, American Chemical Society, 1995.
Chemical Diversity: Synthetic Techniques of Combinatorial Chemistry. Washington, DC, American Chemical Society, 1995.

Web Sites

http://www.combi-web.com—Corporate-sponsored web portal. Accessed Dec. 3, 2002.
http://www.combichem.net/home/login.asp—Recent developments. Accessed Dec. 3, 2002.
http://www.combinatorial.com—Web site for The Combinatorial Index text. Accessed Dec. 3, 2002.
http://www.geocities.com/ResearchTriangle/Lab/4688/ combinatorial chemistry.htm—Unofficial Combinatorial Chemistry Web site. Updated Mar. 5, 2002.
http://www.microarrays.org—University of California at San Francisco site. Accessed Dec. 3, 2002.

COMBINATORIAL CHEMISTRY TERMINOLOGY

The following terms are some of the most common used in combinatorial chemistry and HTS. More complete glossaries can be found in Beck-Sicklinger, A., and Weber, P.: Combinatorial Strategies in Biology and Chemistry. New York, John Wiley & Sons, 2002, and in MacLean, D., et al.: Glossary of terms used in combinatorial chemistry. J. Comb. Chem. 2:562–578, 2000.

ADMET (also ADME, ADMET-PK): The collection of a molecule's properties related to *a*bsorption, *d*istribution, *m*etabolism, *e*xcretion, *t*oxicity, and *p*harmaco*k*inetics. These factors are being increasingly considered in combinatorial library design, to yield molecules that will be more suitable as drugs.

Aptamer: RNA molecule that displays specific binding to a target, usually a protein. Aptamers are often used in microarrays in place of antibodies, to bind peptide ligands.

Array synthesis: The form of parallel synthesis in which the reaction vessels are maintained in a particular spatial arrangement, such as a grid in a microtiter plate. Such arrays generated on a microscopic basis are termed a *spatially addressable library.*

Backbone: A linear scaffold to which substituents are attached. Common backbones include the α carbon backbones of peptides and peptoids.

Bead: A spherical particle of solid support. Typically 50 to 100

μm in diameter, they swell in solvent, allowing access by synthetic reagents for reaction, washing, etc. The *loading* on a bead is the amount of synthetic target that can be attached to a single bead, which is in the nanomolar range.

Binary encoding: Encoding technique of a library based on the presence or absence of tags on a bead. Thus, the sequence 011001 would encode the presence of three of six possible tags. The number of combinations that can be encoded is 2^n, where n is the number of positions in the string.

Binning: A computational procedure to allow selecting chemical structures across a wide range of diversity. The structures are grouped into bins on the basis of common physical or chemical structures.

Building block: One of a set of interchangeable reagents that can be used in the synthesis of a generic library.

Capacity: Theoretical amount of material that could be attached to a bead. Because of steric hindrance of the synthetic target, it may be greater than the actual amount.

Capillary electrophoresis: Method of separating components of a mixture by placing the mixture at one end of a capillary filled with gel. A continuous gradient of electronic charge across the capillary causes the components to separate, much like a chromatographic separation but based on charge, size, and shape of the molecules.

Cleavage: The process of releasing a compound from a solid support, allowing assay or analysis in solution. Special reagents or even enzymes may be used to release the compound without reacting with or altering it.

Cluster analysis: Statistical or pattern recognition technique to group a set of structures into ''natural'' groupings or clusters on the basis of physicochemical or structural properties. It is similar to binning in its result, and both methods are commonly used to select a representative sample of structures, either for screening or as building blocks for combinatorial synthesis.

Combinatorial: Relating to combinations of objects.

Combinatorial chemistry: Using a combinatorial process to prepare sets of compounds from building blocks.

Combinatorial library: A set of compounds prepared by combinatorial chemistry.

Cross-linking: The property of a polymer used in a solid support such that long strands of polymer are interconnected at various points by relatively short sequences—much like rungs on a flexible ladder. Cross-linking affects the properties of the polymer, including its ability to swell in different solvents.

Decode: To ''read'' a chemical or electronic tag attached to a bead or other solid support, for the purpose of determining the sequence of reaction steps that were applied to the given bead. This allows determining the composition of the synthetic target on the bead.

Deconvolute: To make the results of a combinatorial experiment less complex, usually by backtracking and reanalyzing or resynthesizing a subset of the structures in the library. The goal of deconvolution is to determine which of a mixture of compounds is actually responsible for activity.

Dendrimer: A polymer having a very highly branched structure. Dendrimers can be used in place of solid supports for attachment of synthetic targets, and then they can be separated by using size exclusion chromatography.

Descriptor: A numerical representation of a molecular property, either a bulk property (like log P) or a two-dimensional (2D) or three-dimensional (3D) structural property. When descriptors encode the presence or absence of a property, they are usually represented by 1s and 0s, and the collection of descriptors is called a *fingerprint* of the molecule.

Directed (focused) library: A library that uses a limited number of building blocks chosen on the basis of information or some hypothesis that defines the functionalities needed for activity.

A directed library lies midway between an initial *exploration* library and a final *optimization* library in its size and overall diversity.

Diversity: The ''unrelatedness'' of a set of, for example, building blocks or members of a combinatorial library. Measured using physicochemical or structural descriptors, a set with high diversity spans a larger fraction of ''chemical space.'' Cluster analysis is one technique used to quantify diversity.

Dynamic library: A mixture of compounds in a dynamic equilibrium with, for example, a synthetic process. If a receptor is introduced into the system, the equilibrium will shift to produce more of the compounds that bind tightly with the receptor.

Encoding: The process of adding a chemical or electronic tag to a bead for the purpose of ''recording'' the sequence of reaction steps to which the bead has been exposed. By *decoding* the resulting tag, perhaps by treating a DNA tag with polymerase chain reaction and analyzing the oligonucleotide, the exact nature of the synthetic target on the bead can be determined.

Enumeration: The process of explicitly describing all of the specific structures that a generic structure or library contains.

Epitope: The region of a protein strand that is recognized by an antibody.

Fingerprint: An array of numbers (n_1, n_2, . . .) that numerically represents a given structure as values of physicochemical or structural descriptors. Commonly, the numbers are binary (0 or 1), but they may also be counts (whole numbers) or values.

Flow cytometry: Technique for characterizing or separating particles such as beads or cells, often on the basis of their fluorescence. Used to separate beads that have biologically active molecules attached.

Fluorous synthesis: An approach to solution-phase synthesis that uses highly fluorinated compounds as soluble supports for combinatorial chemistry. The addition of water or organic solvents causes a phase separation of the fluorinated support for subsequent cleavage of the synthetic target structure.

Generic structure: General structural formula of a library, consisting of a *scaffold* (parent structure) plus *residues* (R groups). A simple example is R_1-$CH_2C(=O)NH$-R_2.

Genetic algorithm: Method of library design by selecting substituents for a library in a stepwise fashion, based on the fitness of the resulting library for some purpose (e.g., biological activity). At each step, the substituents are modified by use of the genetic principles of recombination, crossover, mutation, etc. Selection of the ''fittest'' combinations of substituents yields a library that is locally optimal for the given purpose.

Green fluorescent protein (GFP): A protein isolated from jellyfish that has its own fluorescence. It can be modified at various positions to generate molecules that fluoresce at different wavelengths. The DNA for this protein can be inserted into the genomes of cells to give them a fluorescent label.

High-throughput screening (HTS): The process for rapidly assessing the activity of samples from a combinatorial library or other compound collection, usually done by running parallel assays in plates of 96 or more wells. A screening rate of 100,000 assays per day is termed *ultrahigh-throughput screening*.

Hit: A compound that has some required level of activity.

HPLC: High-performance liquid chromatography. Solvent is pumped under high pressure through a chromatographic column containing a very finely divided support. The compounds in the mixture separate according to their affinity for the support and *elute* from the column at different times, to be detected by use of some optical or even mass spectrometric detector (HPLC-MS).

In silico screening: See *virtual screening*.

Lead compound: First compound in the development of a drug that has the desired biological and physicochemical properties. It typically has micromolar potency, and by optimizing various positions of the molecule, the potency can be increased to nanomolar, at which point it would be considered for drug candidacy.

Library: A collection of structures, either a *generic* library (based on some scaffold plus multiple residues) or a *mixture* library (containing diverse scaffolds). The number of specific structures in a library is either the product of the numbers of residues possible at each variable position (for a generic library) or simply the sum of the number of structures (for a mixture library).

Linker: A chemical chain that connects the solid or soluble support to the synthetic target in a combinatorial experiment. The linker is decomposed when the desired compound is cleaved from the support.

Lipinski "rule of five": A set of criteria for predicting the oral bioavailability of a compound on the basis of simple molecular properties (molecular weight, <500; log P, <5; number of hydrogen-bond donors, <5; and number of hydrogen-bond acceptors, <10). Typically, the criteria are applied to a library to filter structures from the library before any synthesis takes place. Any structure exceeding two or more criteria is rejected.

Liquid-phase chemistry: The process of using a large, soluble molecule as the support for a combinatorial chemistry experiment.

Loading: Characteristic property of a solid support that describes the amount of a specific chemical species that can be attached synthetically to a unit mass of support.

Mapping: Analyzing the sequence of a protein with regard to a desired property to identify the residues involved in binding or activity. Typically, this involves generating short, overlapping sequences of the protein, perhaps on a microarray, and testing for activity.

Markush structure: A type of structure representation in which very general terms, such as *alkyl* or *alcohol*, can be used to describe the substituents in a generic structure. Used in the patent literature and adapted for combinatorial chemistry publications.

Member: Either *(a)* a particular substituent at a given position in a generic structure (an R-group member) or *(b)* an enumerated structure of a generic library, which corresponds to a given selection of substituents (a member of a library).

Mesh size: The density of wires in a sieve; also, a term to describe the size of particles. A 100- to 200-mesh particle will pass through a 100-mesh filter but be trapped by a 200-mesh filter and consist of particles 75 to 150 μm in diameter.

Microarray: Masks can be used in the same way that stencils are used to make printed circuit boards, to either allow or block UV light from causing chemical reactions in a small defined area. In this way, a library of hundreds or thousands of compounds can be synthesized in a grid layout, over a very small area, perhaps a fraction of a square inch. The resulting microarray can be exposed to a given receptor, and examining the chip under UV light can reveal which structures have bound to the receptor.

Mimetics: Compounds that share the desired properties of other molecules (e.g., the affinity for a given receptor) but do not share the undesirable properties, such as susceptibility to proteases. An important class of mimetics is peptide mimetics.

Mimotope: A compound that imitates an epitope; typically, a nonpeptide sequence that can bind to a particular antibody. Mimotopes were an important class of compounds studied in early combinatorial chemistry experiments.

Monomer: A member of a set of building blocks that can be repeatedly incorporated into a library (e.g., amino acids in a peptide library).

Neural network: Computational procedure to generate a predictive model for some property or response. The model consists of input "nodes" (the input data), a set of "hidden" nodes, and one or more output nodes (the predictions). Each node behaves like a neuron, with a threshold value of input below which it will not "fire" any output. The interconnection of nodes allows the network to deal with complex nonlinear relationships. The network is trained by iteratively adjusting the weights at the nodes on the basis of the difference between the observed and the predicted output.

Omission library: Strategy for identifying active library members by the systematic omission of building blocks from mixtures. Observation of reduced activity in a certain pool suggests that the building block that was omitted in that pool contributes to activity.

One-bead one-compound strategy: The earliest strategy for solid-phase combinatorial chemistry, in which each bead has molecules of only a single structure attached rather than a mixture of structures.

Orthogonal design: *(a)* Using protecting groups or linkers in a combinatorial experiment that do not interfere with each other chemically; or *(b)* a pooling strategy in which a given library member appears in more than one pool, mixed with other members. Pools have only one structure in common, so a hit in several pools implies that a given member is responsible for the activity.

Peptoid: Oligomer of repeating N-substituted glycines that can emulate a peptide, without being susceptible to acid degradation in the gastrointestinal tract.

Phage display: Use of bacteriophage viruses as vessels for presenting short peptide segments of their native surface proteins. By varying the gene sequences of the phages in a combinatorial manner, libraries of peptides can be generated and tested.

Pharmacophore: The ensemble of steric, electronic, and lipophilic factors needed to ensure interaction of a drug molecule with a given receptor. Pharmacophores are most useful in searching a three-dimensional (3D) structure database and in filtering structures for virtual screening.

Photolithography: The process by which successive masking generates light patterns that direct chemical transformations in certain areas of a photosensitive surface. Coupling different building blocks to discrete sites on the surface gives rise to spatially addressable microarrays of compounds.

Pin: An elongated device in which the tip acts as a solid support. An array of pins, fitting into wells of a microtiter plate, can be used for parallel synthesis of a combinatorial library.

Polyethylene glycol (PEG): Polymer widely used in pharmacy as an ointment base. It has been used as a soluble support and as a linker in combinatorial synthesis. Its structure is

$$HOCH_2CH_2O[CH_2CH_2O]_nCH_2CH_2OH$$

Polymerase chain reaction(PCR): Technique for amplification of small amounts of DNA, starting with a few molecules and yielding sufficient material to analyze the sequence. Also widely used in forensic DNA analysis.

Pool: *(a)* A subset of a given combinatorial library; or *(b)* the process of combining and mixing library components.

Pool/split (split and mix, split and pool): Strategy for assembling a combinatorial library. The solid support is divided into portions, each of which is subjected to a given reaction with a single building block. Pooling the portions gives a single batch with a mixture of components. Repeating the split, react, and mix sequence results in a library in which each discrete bead of solid support carries a single library member (one-bead one-compound strategy). The number of members equals the product of the number of building blocks incorporated at each step (i.e., fully combinatorial).

Positional scan: Strategy for identifying individual compounds of interest in a library. A collection of sublibraries is prepared, equal in number to the total number of building blocks in the whole library. In each pool, one substituent position is held constant by incorporating a single building block while the other positions use all possible building blocks. Activity in a given pool implies that the given substituent at the given position is essential for activity.

Principal components analysis: Computational approach to reduce the dimensionality (i.e., the number of variables) in a data analysis, by weighting variables according to their contribution to the overall variation. A plot of points in the first two principal components is like a two-dimensional (2D) "shadow" of the multidimensional data that can be used to find clusters and relationships among the points (i.e., compounds).

Property space: Multidimensional representation of a set of compounds as points in space. Each axis of the space represents some descriptor, either whole property or computed from the two-dimensional (2D) or three-dimensional (3D) chemical structure. Compounds that are similar to each other chemically will cluster together in property space. A further assumption used in library design is that structurally similar compounds will share similar biological activity.

Protecting group: Chemical group that reversibly blocks functional groups on a synthetic target, to prevent them from entering into undesired side reactions. For example, an OH group might be protected by converting it to an ester, then hydrolyzing the ester back to an alcohol when the synthesis is complete.

Radiofrequency encoding: The process of embedding into solid supports the minute electronic devices that emit radiofrequency signals upon stimulation with an electromagnetic source. The signals can be used to track the reaction history of the given bead and thus the makeup of the compounds attached.

Ratio encoding: Strategy in which the quantities of tags on a bead give information about the compound identity rather than the nature of the tags.

Residue: The portion of a chemical structure that can be identified as coming from a particular building block, such as the alanine residue in a polypeptide. In a generic structure, the residues are the substituents that correspond to the R-groups in the structure.

Resin: Insoluble polymeric material to which linkers, synthetic targets, and tags are attached. Sometimes, resins are simply used to scavenge side products of a reaction. In chromatography, resin beads are used to separate compounds by size or by the charge on a molecule.

Resynthesis: Preparation of individual members or subsets of a combinatorial library, to follow up on some property of interest.

Reverse transcriptase: An enzyme that can reverse transcribe RNA into its corresponding DNA.

Ribozyme: RNA molecule with enzyme catalytic activity.

Robotic system: An automated system, usually controlled by a computer, to transfer materials by physical movement of a delivery device or by movement of the reaction vessels. Robotic systems can be general purpose, and capable of being reprogrammed to do a variety of different tasks, or may be specialized, as part of a *turnkey* system.

Safety-catch linker: A linker that is cleaved by performing two reactions instead of the customary one. This provides greater control over the timing of the release of the synthetic target.

Scaffold: The core portion of a generic structure, common to all the members of the library. Note that in the case of Ph-R_1-$CH_2CH_2COOR_2$, the scaffold consists of two disconnected fragments, separated by the R_1 substituent.

Scavenger resin: A resin introduced into a combinatorial experiment to react with undesired materials (excess reagent or side products) and remove them from the experiment.

Selectivity: Measure of a compound's tendency to bind only to a certain target receptor. Drug molecules should have high selectivity as well as potency.

Solid support: Insoluble, functionalized polymeric material to which library members or reagents may be attached, often via a linker, allowing them to be readily separated from solvent, excess reagent, etc. Typically, the solid support swells in solvent, allowing reactions to occur in the interior of the bead or other form. This greatly increases the available surface area for reaction.

Soluble support: Typically, a large molecule that is soluble in some solvents and, upon the addition of other solvents, separates into phases. The molecule can serve as a support for attaching members of a combinatorial library. The advantage over solid supports is that reactions are more complete in liquid phase. Sometimes termed liquid-phase chemistry. An example of a soluble support is PEG, which is soluble in polar solvents but separates from organic ones.

Spacer: Same as a linker.

Spatially addressable: Having the ability to identify part or all of the structure of a library component or pool from its physical location in a grid or array.

Spot synthesis: Solid-phase synthesis at certain points (spots) on a two-dimensional (2D) surface (e.g., a cellulose membrane). Recently, the techniques of ink-jet printing have been applied to spot synthesis, yielding very dense arrays of compounds.

Sublibrary: A subset of a combinatorial library in which, for example, the substituent at one position is held constant while other positions are varied. Also called a *pool*.

Supercritical fluid chromatography (SFC): HPLC using a "solvent" such as liquid CO_2 under high pressure. The advantage is that the carrier evaporates, simplifying the detection of the compounds as they elute from the chromatographic column.

Tag: A nonreactive chemical functionality attached to a solid support that carries information about the reaction history of the given support and thus can at least partially identify the attached synthetic target. An example is attaching various DNA bases to the bead at each synthetic step. The resulting oligonucleotide can be multiplied by using PCR and identified analytically.

Tea bag: A type of reaction vessel consisting of a porous mesh bag that encloses the resin but allows passage of reagents and solvents. Several tea bags can be immersed in a given reagent and then manipulated from one reagent to the next to generate combinatorial libraries.

Virtual library: A combinatorial library that has no physical existence; rather, it exists in a computer or on paper. Such libraries can be generated automatically and screened against physiochemical filters like the "rule of five" or be docked into receptors by use of molecular modeling.

Virtual screening: The selection of compounds by evaluating their fitness by use of computational model. Also called *in silico screening*.

REFERENCES

1. Merrifield, R. B.: Solid phase peptide synthesis. I. The synthesis of a tetrapeptide. J. Am. Chem. Soc. 85:2149–2154, 1963.
2. Furka, A.: Combinatorial chemistry: 20 years . . . . Drug Discovery Today 7:1–4, 2002.
3. Houghten, R. A.: General method for the rapid solid-phase synthesis of large numbers of peptides: specificity of antigen-antibody interaction at the level of individual amino acids. Proc. Natl. Acad. Sci. U. S. A. 82:5131–5135, 1985.
4. Simon, R. J., Kania, R. S., Zuckermann, R. N., et al.: Peptoids: a modular approach to drug discovery. Proc. Natl. Acad. Sci. U. S. A. 89:9367–9371, 1992.
5. Miller, S. M., et al.: Proteolytic studies of homologous peptide and N-

substituted glycine peptoid oligomers. Bioorg. Med. Chem. Lett. 4: 2657–2662, 1994.

6. Zuckerman, R. N., et al.: Discovery of nanomolar ligands for 7-trans-membrane G-protein-coupled receptors from a diverse N-(substituted)-glycine peptoid library. J. Med. Chem. 37:2678–2685, 1994.

7. Bunin, B. A., and Ellman, J. A.: A general and expedient method for the solid-phase synthesis of 1,4-benzodiazepine derivatives. J. Am. Chem. Soc. 114:10997–10998, 1992.

8. Larhed, M., and Hallberg, A.: Microwave-assisted high-speed chemistry: a new technique in drug discovery. Drug Discovery Today 6: 406–416, 2001.

9. Balkenhohl, F., et al.: Combinatorial synthesis of small organic molecules. Angew. Chem. Int. Ed. Engl. 35:2288–2337, 1996.

10. Marcaurelle, L. A., and Seeberger, P. H.: Combinatorial carbohydrate chemistry. Curr. Opin. Chem. Biol. 6:289–296, 2002.

11. Nielsen, J.: Combinatorial synthesis of natural products. Curr. Opin. Chem. Biol. 6:297–305, 2002.

12. Holmes, C. P.: Model studies for new o-nitrobenzyl photolabile linkers: substituent effects on the rates of photochemical cleavage. J. Org. Chem. 62:2370–2380, 1997.

13. Reents, R., Jeyaraj, D. A., and Waldman, H.: Enzymatically cleavable linker groups in polymer-supported synthesis. Drug Discovery Today 7:71–75, 2002.

14. Keating, T. A., and Armstrong, R. W.: Molecular diversity via a convertible isocyanide in the Ugi four-component condensation. J. Am. Chem. Soc. 117:7842–7843, 1995.

15. Han, H., et al.: Liquid-phase combinatorial synthesis. Proc. Natl. Acad. Sci. U. S. A. 92:6419–6423, 1995.

16. Studer, A., et al.: Fluorous synthesis: a fluorous-phase strategy for improving separation efficiency in organic synthesis. Science 275: 823–826, 1997.

17. Calderone, C. T., et al.: Directing otherwise incompatible reactions in a single solution using DNA-templated organic synthesis. Angew. Chem. Int. Ed. Engl. 41:4104–4108, 2002.

18. Hughes, I., and Hunter, D.: Techniques for analysis and purification in high-throughput chemistry. Curr. Opin. Chem. Biol. 5:243–247, 2001.

19. Yan, B., and Kumaravel, G.: Probing solid-phase reactions by monitoring the IR bands of compounds on a single 'flattened' resin bead. Tetrahedron 52:843–848, 1996.

20. Shuker, S. B., et al.: Discovering high-affinity ligands for proteins: SAR by NMR. Science 274:1531–1534, 1996.

21. Brenner, S., and Lerner, R. A.: Encoded combinatorial chemistry. Proc. Natl. Acad. Sci. U. S. A. 89:5381–5383, 1992.

22. Nielsen, J., Brenner, S., and Janda, K. D.: Synthetic methods for the implementation of encoded combinatorial chemistry. J. Am. Chem. Soc. 115:9812–9813, 1993.

23. http://www.qdots.com, Quantum dots. 2002.

24. Landro, J. A., et al.: HTS in the new millennium—the role of pharmacology and flexibility. J. Pharmacol. Toxicol. Methods 44:273–289, 2000.

25. Drews, J.: Drug discovery: a historical perspective. Science 287: 1960–1964, 2000.

26. Spencer, R. W.: High-throughput screening of historic collections: observations on file size, biological targets, and file diversity. Biotechnol. Bioeng. 61:61–67, 1998.

27. Venton, D. L., and Woodbury, C. P.: Screening combinatorial libraries. Chemometr. Intell. Lab. Syst. 48:131–150, 1999.

28. Tarbit, M. H., and Berman, J.: High-throughput approaches for evaluating absorption, distribution, metabolism and excretion properties of lead compounds. Curr. Opin. Chem. Biol. 2:411–416, 1998.

29. Walters, W. P., Stahl, M. T., and Murcko, M. A.: Virtual screening—an overview. Drug Discovery Today 3:160–178. 1998.

30. Shoichet, B. K., et al.: Lead discovery using molecular docking. Curr. Opin. Chem. Biol. 6:439–446, 2002.

31. http://www.grid.org/projects/patriot.htm, United Devices agent software download. 2002.

32. Böhm, J.-J., and Stahl, M.: Structure-based library design: molecular modelling merges with combinatorial chemistry. Curr. Opin. Chem. Biol. 4:283–286, 2000.

33. Lipinski, C. A., et al.: Experimental and computational approaches to estimate solubility and permeability in drug discovery and development settings. Adv. Drug Deliv. Rev. 23:3–25, 1997.

34. Oprea, T. I.: Virtual screening in lead discovery: a viewpoint. Molecules 7:51–62, 2002.

35. Oprea, T. I., and Gottfries, J.: Toward minimalistic modeling of oral drug absorption. J. Mol. Model. Graph. 17:261–274, 1999.

36. Zuegge, J., et al.: A fast virtual screening filter for cytochrome P450 3A4 inhibition liability of compound libraries. QSAR 21:249–256, 2002.

37. Adang, E. P., and Hermkens, P. H. H.: The contribution of combinatorial chemistry to lead generation: an interim analysis. Curr. Med. Chem. 8:985–998, 2001.

38. Spellmeyer, D. C., and Grootenhuis, P. D. J.: Recent developments in molecular diversity: computational approaches to combinatorial chemistry. Ann. Rep. Med. Chem. 34:287–296, 1999.

39. Jacobsen, E. J., et al.: Piperazine imidazo[1,5-a]quinoxaline ureas as high affinity GABA—a ligand of dual functionality. J. Med. Chem. 42:1123, 1999.

40. Martin, E. J., and Critchlow, R. E.: Beyond mere diversity: tailoring combinatorial libraries for drug discovery. J. Comb. Chem. 1:32–45, 1999.

41. Oprea, T. I., et al.: Chemical information management in drug discovery: optimizing the computational and combinatorial chemistry interfaces. J. Mol. Model. Graph. 18:512–524, 2000.

42. Merritt, A. T.: Uptake of new technology in lead optimization for drug discovery. Drug Discovery Today 3:505–510, 1998.

43. Golebiowski, A., Klopfenstein, S. R., and Portlock, D. E.: Lead compounds discovered from libraries. Curr. Opin. Chem. Biol. 5:273–284, 2001.

44. Owens, J., et al.: News in brief/miscellaneous—first HTS drug candidates reach clinical trials. Drug Discovery Today 6:230, 2001.

45. Everett, J., et al.: The application of non-combinatorial chemistry to lead discovery. Drug Discovery Today 6:779–785, 2001.

46. Lenz, G. R., Nash, H. M., and Jindal, S.: Chemical ligands, genomics, and drug discovery. Drug Discovery Today 5:145–156, 2000.

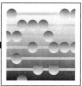

Metabolic Changes of Drugs and Related Organic Compounds

STEPHEN J. CUTLER AND JOHN H. BLOCK

Metabolism plays a central role in the elimination of drugs and other foreign compounds *(xenobiotics)* from the body. A solid understanding of drug metabolic pathways is an essential tool for pharmacists in their role of selecting and monitoring appropriate drug therapy for their patients. Most organic compounds entering the body are relatively lipid soluble *(lipophilic)*. To be absorbed, they must traverse the lipoprotein membranes of the lumen walls of the gastrointestinal (GI) tract. Then, once in the bloodstream, these molecules can diffuse passively through other membranes and be distributed effectively to reach various target organs to exert their pharmacological actions. Because of reabsorption in the renal tubules, lipophilic compounds are not excreted to any substantial extent in the urine. Xenobiotics then meet their metabolic fate through various enzyme systems that change the parent compound to render it more water soluble *(hydrophilic)*. Once the metabolite is sufficiently water soluble, it may be excreted from the body. The statements above show that a working knowledge of the ADME (absorption, distribution, metabolism, and excretion) principles is vital for successful determination of drug regimens.

If lipophilic drugs, or xenobiotics, were not metabolized to polar, readily excretable water-soluble products, they would remain indefinitely in the body, eliciting their biological effects. Thus, the formation of water-soluble metabolites not only enhances drug elimination, but also leads to compounds that are generally pharmacologically inactive and relatively nontoxic. Consequently, drug metabolism reactions have traditionally been regarded as *detoxication* (or *detoxification*) processes.[1] Unfortunately, it is incorrect to assume that drug metabolism reactions are always detoxifying. Many drugs are biotransformed to pharmacologically active metabolites. These metabolites may have significant activity that contributes substantially to the pharmacological or toxicological effect(s) ascribed to the parent drug. Occasionally, the parent compound is inactive when administered and must be metabolically converted to a biologically active drug (metabolite).[2, 3] These types of compounds are referred to as *prodrugs*. In addition, it is becoming increasingly clear that not all metabolites are nontoxic. Indeed, many adverse effects (e.g., tissue necrosis, carcinogenicity, teratogenicity) of drugs and environmental contaminants can be attributed directly to the formation of chemically reactive metabolites that are highly detrimental to the body.[4–6] This concept is more important when the patient has a disease state that inhibits or expedites xenobiotic metabolism. Also, more and more drug metabolites are being found in our sewage systems. These compounds may be nontoxic to humans but harmful to other animals or the environment.

GENERAL PATHWAYS OF DRUG METABOLISM

Drug metabolism reactions have been divided into two categories: *phase I (functionalization)* and *phase II (conjugation)* reactions.[1, 7] Phase I, or functionalization reactions, include oxidative, reductive, and hydrolytic biotransformations (Table 4-1).[8] The purpose of these reactions is to introduce a functional polar group(s) (e.g., OH, COOH, NH_2, SH) into the xenobiotic molecule to produce a more water soluble compound. This can be achieved by direct introduction of the functional group (e.g., aromatic and aliphatic hydroxylation) or by modifying or "unmasking" existing functionalities (e.g., reduction of ketones and aldehydes to alcohols; oxidation of alcohols to acids; hydrolysis of ester and amides

TABLE 4–1 General Summary of Phase I and Phase II Metabolic Pathways

Phase I or Functionalization Reactions
Oxidative reactions
Oxidation of aromatic moieties
Oxidation of olefins
Oxidation at benzylic, allylic carbon atoms, and carbon atoms α to carbonyl and imines
Oxidation at aliphatic and alicyclic carbon atoms
Oxidation involving carbon–heteroatom systems:
Carbon–nitrogen systems (aliphatic and aromatic amines; includes N-dealkylation, oxidative deamination, N-oxide formation, N-hydroxylation)
Carbon–oxygen systems (O-dealkylation)
Carbon–sulfur systems (S-dealkylation, S-oxidation, and desulfuration)
Oxidation of alcohols and aldehydes
Other miscellaneous oxidative reactions
Reductive Reactions
Reduction of aldehydes and ketones
Reduction of nitro and azo compounds
Miscellaneous reductive reactions
Hydrolytic Reactions
Hydrolysis of esters and amides
Hydration of epoxides and arene oxides by epoxide hydrase

Phase II or Conjugation Reactions
Glucuronic acid conjugation
Sulfate conjugation
Conjugation with glycine, glutamine, and other amino acids
Glutathione or mercapturic acid conjugation
Acetylation
Methylation

to yield COOH, NH$_2$, and OH groups; reduction of azo and nitro compounds to give NH$_2$ moieties; oxidative N-, O-, and S-dealkylation to give NH$_2$, OH, and SH groups). Although phase I reactions may not produce sufficiently hydrophilic or inactive metabolites, they generally tend to provide a functional group or "handle" on the molecule that can undergo subsequent phase II reactions.

The purpose of phase II reactions is to attach small, polar, and ionizable endogenous compounds such as glucuronic acid, sulfate, glycine, and other amino acids to the functional "handles" of phase I metabolites or parent compounds that already have suitable existing functional groups to form water-soluble conjugated products. Conjugated metabolites are readily excreted in the urine and are generally devoid of pharmacological activity and toxicity in humans. Other phase II pathways, such as methylation and acetylation, terminate or attenuate biological activity, whereas glutathione (GSH) conjugation protects the body against chemically reactive compounds or metabolites. Thus, phase I and phase II reactions complement one another in detoxifying, and facilitating the elimination of, drugs and xenobiotics.

To illustrate, consider the principal psychoactive constituent of marijuana, Δ^9-tetrahydrocannabinol (Δ^9-THC, also known as Δ^1-THC, depending on the numbering system being used). This lipophilic molecule (octanol/water partition coefficient ~6,000)[9] undergoes allylic hydroxylation to give 11-hydroxy-Δ^9-THC in humans.[10, 11] More polar than its parent compound, the 11-hydroxy metabolite is further oxidized to the corresponding carboxylic acid derivative Δ^9-THC-11-oic acid, which is ionized (pK$_a$ COOH ~5) at physiological pH. Subsequent conjugation of this metabolite (either at the COOH or phenolic OH) with glucuronic acid leads to water-soluble products that are readily eliminated in the urine.[12]

In the above series of biotransformations, the parent Δ^9-THC molecule is made increasingly polar, ionizable, and hydrophilic. The attachment of the glucuronyl moiety (with its ionized carboxylate group and three polar hydroxyl groups; see structure) to the Δ^9-THC metabolites notably favors partitioning of the conjugated metabolites into an aqueous medium. This is an important point in using urinalysis to identify illegal drugs.

The purpose of this chapter is to provide the student with a broad overview of drug metabolism. Various phase I and phase II biotransformation pathways (see Table 4-1) are outlined, and representative drug examples for each pathway are presented. Drug metabolism examples in humans are emphasized, although discussion of metabolism in other mammalian systems is necessary. The central role of the cytochrome P-450 monooxygenase system in oxidative drug biotransformation is elaborated. Discussion of other enzyme systems involved in phase I and phase II reactions is presented in their respective sections. In addition to stereochemical factors that may affect drug metabolism, biological factors such as age, sex, heredity, disease state, and species variation are considered. The effects of enzyme induction and inhibition on drug metabolism and a section on pharmacologically active metabolites are included.

SITES OF DRUG BIOTRANSFORMATION

Although biotransformation reactions may occur in many tissues, the liver is, by far, the most important organ in drug metabolism and detoxification of endogenous and exogenous compounds.[13] Another important site, especially for orally administered drugs, is the intestinal mucosa. The latter contains the cytochrome P-450 (CYP) 3A4 isozyme (see discussion on cytochrome nomenclature below) and P-glycoprotein that can capture the drug and secrete it back into the intestinal tract. In contrast, the liver, a well-perfused organ, is particularly rich in almost all of the drug-metabolizing enzymes discussed in this chapter. Orally administered

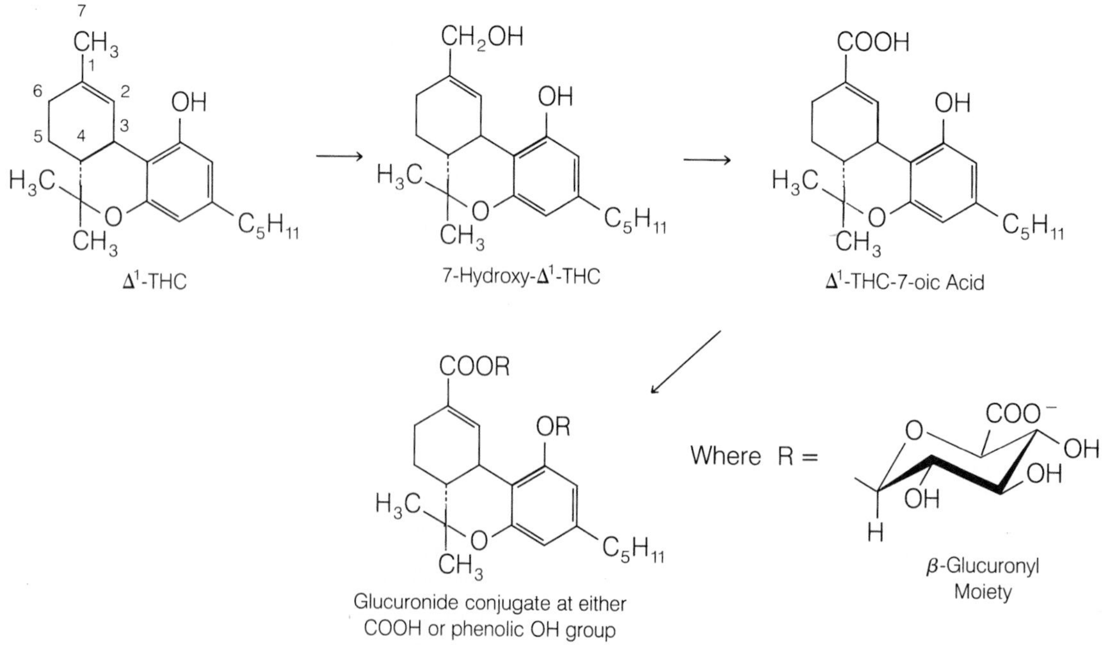

Δ^1-THC

7-Hydroxy-Δ^1-THC

Δ^1-THC-7-oic Acid

Glucuronide conjugate at either COOH or phenolic OH group

Where R =

β-Glucuronyl Moiety

drugs that are absorbed into the bloodstream through the GI tract must pass through the liver before being further distributed into body compartments. Therefore, they are susceptible to hepatic metabolism known as the *first-pass effect* before reaching the systemic circulation. Depending on the drug, this metabolism can sometimes be quite significant and result in decreased oral bioavailability. For example, in humans, several drugs are metabolized extensively by the first-pass effect.[14] The following list includes some of those drugs:

Isoproterenol	Morphine	Propoxyphene
Lidocaine	Nitroglycerin	Propranolol
Meperidine	Pentazocine	Salicylamide

Some drugs (e.g., lidocaine) are removed so effectively by first-pass metabolism that they are ineffective when given orally.[15] Nitroglycerin is administered buccally to bypass the liver.

Because most drugs are administered orally, the intestine appears to play an important role in the extrahepatic metabolism of xenobiotics. For example, in humans, orally administered isoproterenol undergoes considerable sulfate conjugation in the intestinal wall.[16] Several other drugs (e.g., levodopa, chlorpromazine, and diethylstilbestrol)[17] are also reportedly metabolized in the GI tract. Esterases and lipases present in the intestine may be particularly[18] important in carrying out hydrolysis of many ester prodrugs (see "Hydrolytic Reactions," below). Bacterial flora present in the intestine and colon appear to play an important role in the reduction of many aromatic azo and nitro drugs (e.g., sulfasalazine).[19, 20] Intestinal β-glucuronidase enzymes can hydrolyze glucuronide conjugates excreted in the bile, thereby liberating the free drug or its metabolite for possible reabsorption (enterohepatic circulation or recycling).[21]

Although other tissues, such as kidney, lungs, adrenal glands, placenta, brain, and skin, have some drug-metabolizing capability, the biotransformations that they carry out often are more substrate selective and more limited to particular types of reaction (e.g., oxidation, glucuronidation).[22] In many instances, the full metabolic capabilities of these tissues have not been explored fully.

ROLE OF CYTOCHROME P-450 MONOOXYGENASES IN OXIDATIVE BIOTRANSFORMATIONS

Of the various phase I reactions that are considered in this chapter, oxidative biotransformation processes are, by far, the most common and important in drug metabolism. The general stoichiometry that describes the oxidation of many xenobiotics (R-H) to their corresponding oxidized metabolites (R-OH) is given by the following equation:[23]

$$RH + NADPH + O_2 + H^+ \rightarrow ROH + NADP^+ + H_2O$$

The enzyme systems carrying out this biotransformation are referred to as *mixed-function oxidases* or *monooxygenases*.[24, 25] There is a large family that carry out the same basic chemical reactions. Their nomenclature is based on

TABLE 4–2 Cytochrome P-450 Enzymes Nomenclature

CYP-Arabic Number-Capital Letter-Arabic Number
1. CYP: cytochrome P-450 enzymes
2. Arabic number: Family (CYP 1, CYP 2, CYP 3, etc.)
   Must have more than 40% identical amino acid sequence
3. Capital letter: Subfamily (CYP 1A, CYP 2C, CYP 3A, etc.)
   Must have more than 55% identical amino acid sequence
4. Arabic number: Individual enzyme in a subfamily (CYP 1A2, CYP 2C9, CYP 2D6, CYP 2E1, CYP 3A4, etc.)
   Identity of amino acid sequences can exceed 90%

amino acid homology and is summarized in Table 4-2. There are four components to the name. CYP refers to the cytochrome system. This is followed by the arabic number that specifies the cytochrome family (CYP1, CYP2, CYP 3, etc.). Next is a capital letter that represents the subfamily (CYP 1A, CYP 1B, CYP 2A, CYP 2B, CYP 3A, CYP 3B, etc.). Finally the cytochrome name ends with another arabic number that specifies the specific enzyme responsible for a particular reaction (CYP 1A2, CYP 2C9, CYP 2C19, CYP 3A4, etc.).

The reaction requires both molecular oxygen and the reducing agent NADPH (reduced form of nicotinamide adenosine dinucleotide phosphate). During this oxidative process, one atom of molecular oxygen (O_2) is introduced into the substrate R-H to form R-OH and the other oxygen atom is incorporated into water. The mixed-function oxidase system[26] is actually made up of several components, the most important being the superfamily of cytochrome P-450 enzymes (currently at 57 genes) [http://drnelson.utmem.edu/CytochromeP450.html], which are responsible for transferring *an oxygen atom* to the substrate R-H. Other important components of this system include the NADPH-dependent cytochrome P-450 reductase and the NADH-linked cytochrome b_5. The latter two components, along with the cofactors NADPH and NADH, supply the reducing equivalents (electrons) needed in the overall metabolic oxidation of foreign compounds. The proposed mechanistic scheme by which the cytochrome P-450 monooxygenase system catalyzes the conversion of molecular oxygen to an "activated oxygen" species is elaborated below.

The cytochrome P-450 enzymes are heme proteins.[27] The heme portion is an iron-containing porphyrin called *protoporphyrin IX*, and the protein portion is called the *apoprotein*. Cytochrome P-450 is found in high concentrations in the liver, the major organ involved in the metabolism of xenobiotics. The presence of this enzyme in many other tissues (e.g., lung, kidney, intestine, skin, placenta, adrenal cortex) shows that these tissues have drug-oxidizing capability too. The name *cytochrome P-450* is derived from the fact that the reduced (Fe^{2+}) form of this enzyme binds with carbon monoxide to form a complex that has a distinguishing spectroscopic absorption maximum at 450 nm.[28]

One important feature of the hepatic cytochrome P-450 mixed-function oxidase system is its ability to metabolize an almost unlimited number of diverse substrates by a variety of oxidative transformations.[29] This versatility is believed to be due to the substrate nonspecificity of cytochrome P-450 as well as to the presence of multiple forms of the enzyme.[30] Some of these P-450 enzymes are selectively inducible by various chemicals (e.g., phenobarbital, benzo[*a*]pyrene, 3-methylcholanthrene).[31] One of these inducible forms of the enzyme (cytochrome P-448)[32] is of particular interest and is discussed below.

The cytochrome P-450 monooxygenases are located in the endoplasmic reticulum, a highly organized and complex network of intracellular membranes that is particularly abundant in tissues such as the liver.[33] When these tissues are disrupted by homogenization, the endoplasmic reticulum loses its structure and is converted into small vesicular bodies known as *microsomes*. Mitochondria house many of the cytochrome enzymes that are responsible for the biosynthesis of steroidal hormones and metabolism of certain vitamins.

Microsomes isolated from hepatic tissue appear to retain all of the mixed-function oxidase capabilities of intact hepatocytes; because of this, microsomal preparations (with the necessary cofactors, e.g., NADPH, Mg^{2+}) are used frequently for in vitro drug metabolism studies. Because of its membrane-bound nature, the cytochrome P-450 monooxygenase system appears to be housed in a lipoidal environment. This may explain, in part, why lipophilic xenobiotics are generally good substrates for the monooxygenase system.[34]

The catalytic role that the cytochrome P-450 monooxygenase system plays in the oxidation of xenobiotics is summarized in the cycle shown in Figure 4-1.[35-37] The initial step of this catalytic reaction cycle starts with the binding of the substrate to the oxidized (Fe^{3+}) resting state of cytochrome P-450 to form a P-450-substrate complex. The next step involves the transfer of one electron from NADPH-dependent cytochrome P-450 reductase to the P-450-substrate complex. This one-electron transfer reduces Fe^{3+} to Fe^{2+}. It is this reduced (Fe^{2+}) P-450-substrate complex that is capable of binding dioxygen (O_2). The dioxygen–P-450-substrate complex that is formed then undergoes another one-electron reduction (by cytochrome P-450 reductase-NADPH and/or cytochrome b_5 reductase-NADH) to yield what is believed to be a peroxide dianion–P-450 (Fe^{3+})-substrate complex. Water (containing one of the oxygen atoms from the original dioxygen molecule) is released from the latter intermediate to form an activated oxygen–P-450-substrate complex (Fig. 4-2). The activated oxygen [FeO]$^{3+}$ in this complex is highly electron deficient and a potent oxidizing agent. The activated oxygen is transferred to the substrate (RH), and the oxidized substrate product (ROH) is released from the enzyme complex to regenerate the oxidized form of cytochrome P-450.

The key sequence of events appears to center around the alteration of a dioxygen–P-450-substrate complex to an activated oxygen–P-450-substrate complex, which can then effect the critical transfer of oxygen from P-450 to the substrate.[37, 38] In view of the potent oxidizing nature of the activated oxygen being transferred, it is not surprising cytochrome P-450 can oxidize numerous substrates. The mechanistic details of oxygen activation and transfer in cytochrome P-450-catalyzed reactions continue to be an active area of

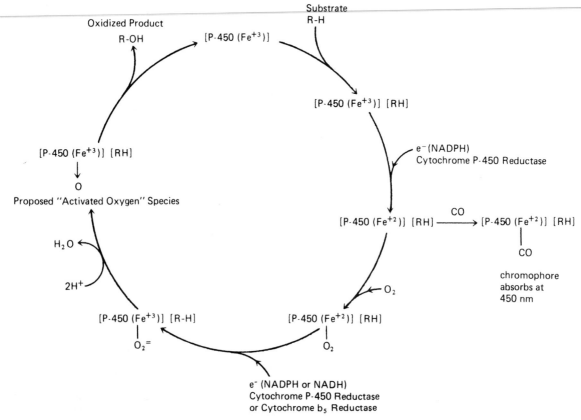

Figure 4–1 ■ Proposed catalytic reaction cycle involving cytochrome P-450 in the oxidation of xenobiotics.

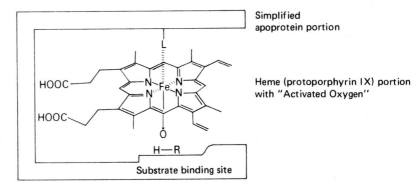

Figure 4–2 ■ Simplified depiction of the proposed activated oxygen–cytochrome P-450-substrate complex. Note the simplified apoprotein portion and the heme (protoporphyrin IX) portion or cytochrome P-450 and the close proximity of the substrate R-H undergoing oxidation.

research in drug metabolism.[34] The many types of oxidative reaction carried out by cytochrome P-450 are enumerated in the sections below. Many of these oxidative pathways are summarized schematically in Figure 4-3 (see also Table 4-1).[37]

The versatility of cytochrome P-450 in carrying out a variety of oxidation reactions on a multitude of substrates may be attributable to the multiple forms of the enzyme. Consequently, the student must realize that the biotransformation of a parent xenobiotic to several oxidized metabolites is carried out not just by one form of P-450 but, more likely, by several different forms. Extensive studies indicate that the apoprotein portions of various cytochrome P-450s differ from one another in their tertiary structure (because of differences in amino acid sequence or the makeup of the polypeptide chain).[27, 30, 39–41] Because the apoprotein portion is important in substrate binding and catalytic transfer of activated oxygen, these structural differences may account for some substrates being preferentially or more efficiently oxidized

by one particular form of cytochrome P-450. Finally, because of the enormous number of uncommon reactions that are catalyzed by P-450, the reader is directed to other articles of interest.[42]

OXIDATIVE REACTIONS

Oxidation of Aromatic Moieties

Aromatic hydroxylation refers to the mixed-function oxidation of aromatic compounds *(arenes)* to their corresponding phenolic metabolites *(arenols)*.[43] Almost all aromatic hydroxylation reactions are believed to proceed initially through an epoxide intermediate called an ''arene oxide,'' which rearranges rapidly and spontaneously to the arenol product in most instances. The importance of arene oxides in the formation of arenols and in other metabolic and toxico-

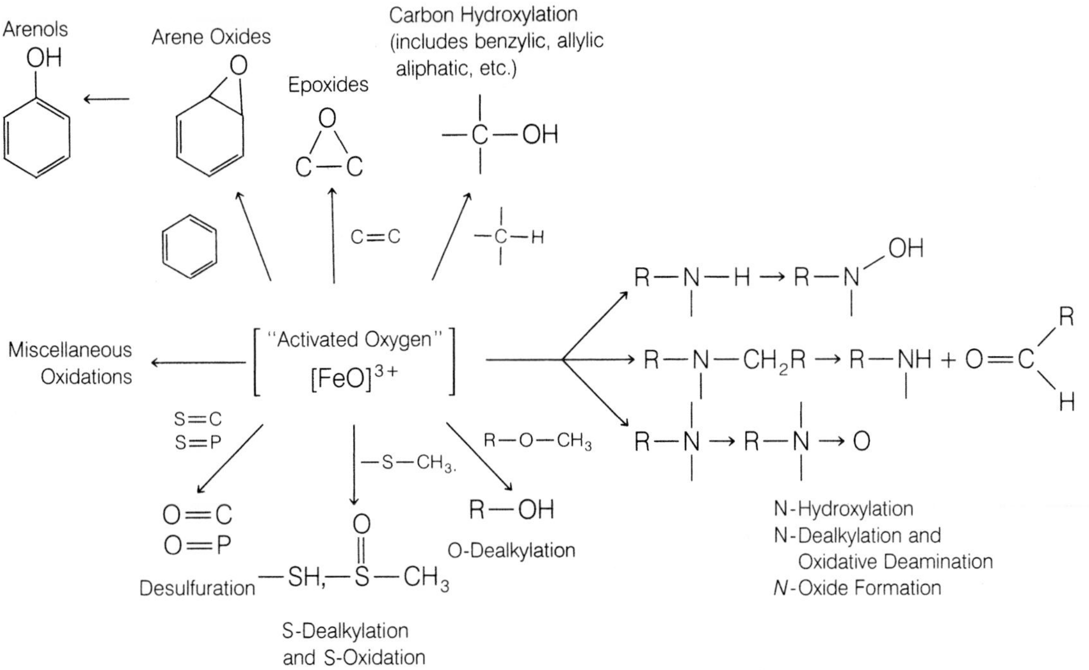

Figure 4–3 ■ Schematic summary of cytochrome P-450-catalyzed oxidation reactions. (Adapted from Ullrich, V.: Top. Curr. Chem. 83:68, 1979.)

logic reactions is discussed below.[44, 45] Our attention now focuses on the aromatic hydroxylation of several drugs and xenobiotics.

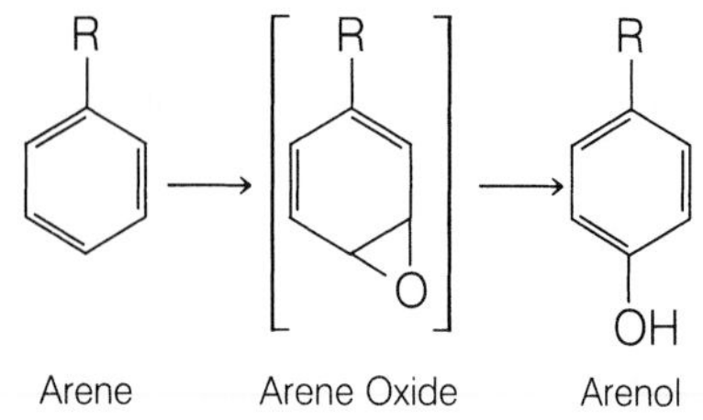

Arene — Arene Oxide — Arenol

Most foreign compounds containing aromatic moieties are susceptible to aromatic oxidation. In humans, aromatic hydroxylation is a major route of metabolism for many drugs containing phenyl groups. Important therapeutic agents such as propranolol,[46, 47] phenobarbital,[48] phenytoin,[49, 50] phenylbutazone,[51, 52] atorvastatin,[53] 17α-ethinylestradiol,[54, 55] and (S)(−)-warfarin,[56] among others, undergo extensive aromatic oxidation (Fig. 4-4 shows structure and site of hydroxylation). In most of the drugs just mentioned, hydroxylation occurs at the *para* position.[57] Most phenolic metabolites formed from aromatic oxidation undergo further conversion to polar and water-soluble glucuronide or sulfate conjugates,

which are readily excreted in the urine. For example, the major urinary metabolite of phenytoin found in humans is the *O*-glucuronide conjugate of *p*-hydroxyphenytoin.[49, 50] Interestingly, the *para*-hydroxylated metabolite of phenylbutazone, oxyphenbutazone, is pharmacologically active and has been marketed itself as an anti-inflammatory agent (Tandearil, Oxalid).[51, 52] Of the two enantiomeric forms of the oral anticoagulant warfarin (Coumadin), only the more active S(−) enantiomer has been shown to undergo substantial aromatic hydroxylation to 7-hydroxywarfarin in humans.[56] In contrast, the (R)(+) enantiomer is metabolized by keto reduction[56] (see "Stereochemical Aspects of Drug Metabolism," below).

Often, the substituents attached to the aromatic ring may influence the ease of hydroxylation.[57] As a general rule, microsomal aromatic hydroxylation reactions appear to proceed most readily in activated (electron-rich) rings, whereas deactivated aromatic rings (e.g., those containing electron-withdrawing groups Cl, $-N^+R_3$, COOH, SO_2NHR) are generally slow or resistant to hydroxylation. The deactivating groups (Cl, $-N^+H=C$) present in the antihypertensive clonidine (Catapres) may explain why this drug undergoes little aromatic hydroxylation in humans.[58, 59] The uricosuric agent probenecid (Benemid), with its electron-withdrawing car-

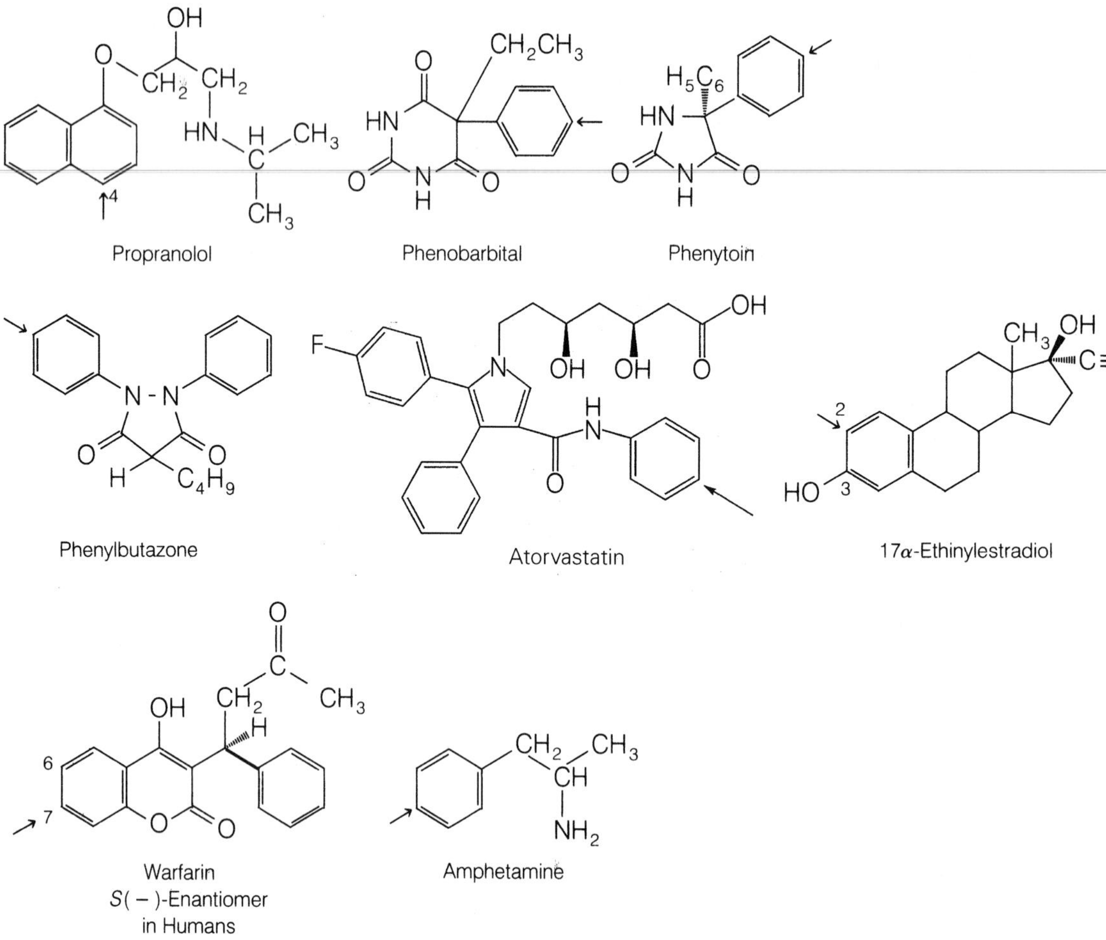

Figure 4–4 ■ Examples of drugs and xenobiotics that undergo aromatic hydroxylation in humans. *Arrow* indicates site of aromatic hydroxylation.

boxy and sulfamido groups, has not been reported to undergo any aromatic hydroxylation.[60]

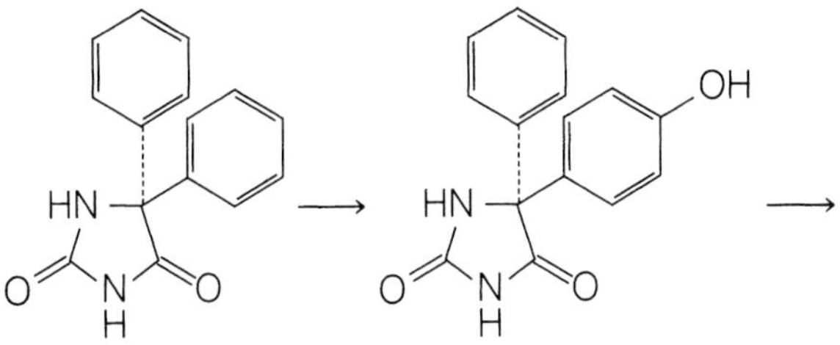

Phenytoin

p-Hydroxyphenytoin

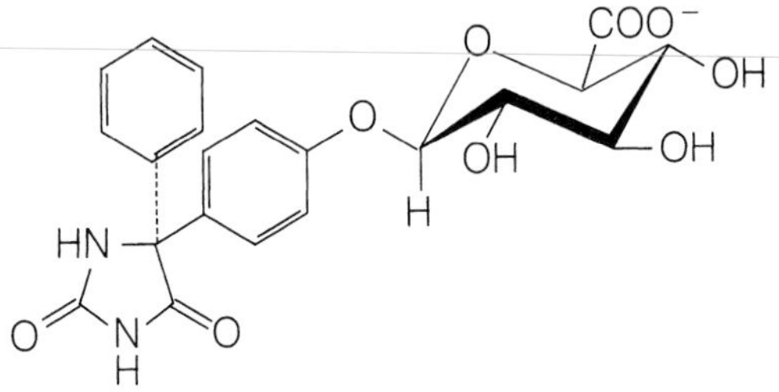

O-Glucuronide Conjugate

In compounds with two aromatic rings, hydroxylation occurs preferentially in the more electron-rich ring. For example, aromatic hydroxylation of diazepam (Valium) occurs primarily in the more activated ring to yield 4'-hydroxydiazepam.[61] A similar situation is seen in the 7-hydroxylation of the antipsychotic agent chlorpromazine (Thorazine)[62] and in the *para*-hydroxylation of p-chlorobiphenyl to p-chloro-p'-hydroxybiphenyl.[63]

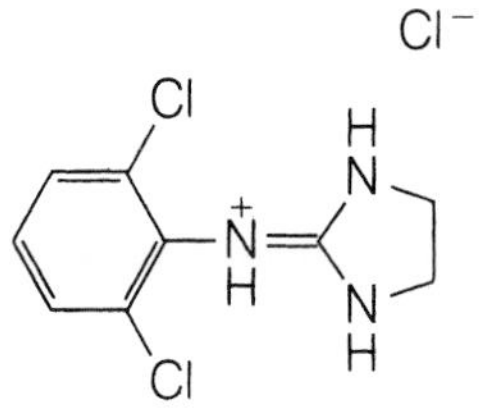

Clonidine Hydrochloride

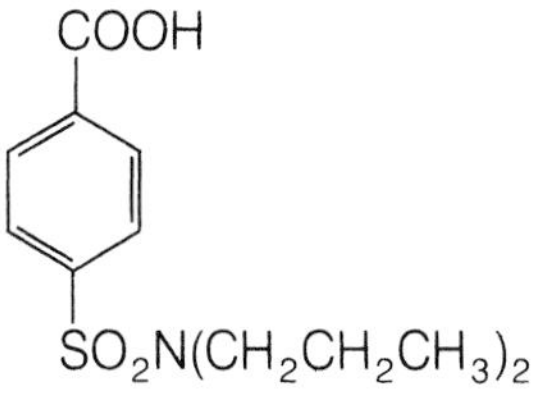

Probenecid

Recent environmental pollutants, such as polychlorinated biphenyls (PCBs) and 2,3,7,8-tetrachlorodibenzo-p-dioxin (TCDD), have attracted considerable public concern over their toxicity and health hazards. These compounds appear to be resistant to aromatic oxidation because of the numerous electronegative chlorine atoms in their aromatic rings. The metabolic stability coupled to the lipophilicity of these environmental contaminants probably explains their long persistence in the body once absorbed.[64–66]

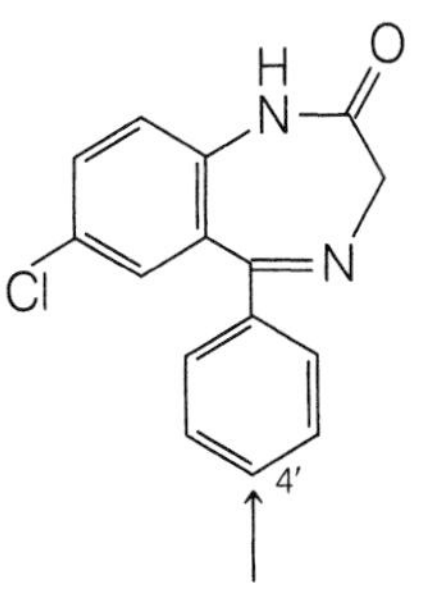

Diazepam

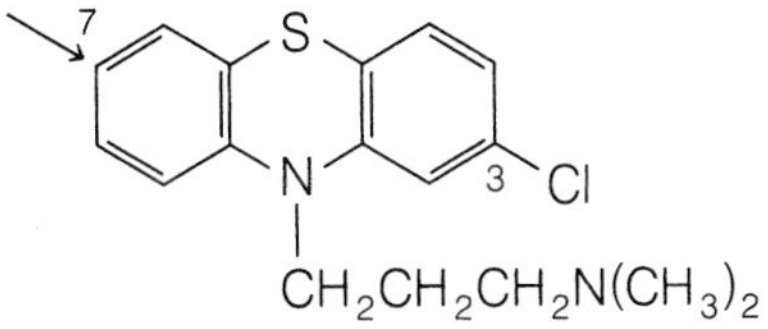

Chlorpromazine

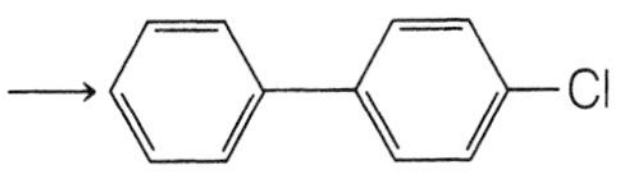

p-Chlorobiphenyl

Arene oxide intermediates are formed when a double bond in aromatic moieties is epoxidized. Arene oxides are of significant toxicologic concern because these intermediates are electrophilic and chemically reactive (because of the strained three-membered epoxide ring). Arene oxides are mainly detoxified by spontaneous rearrangement to arenols, but enzymatic hydration to *trans*-dihydrodiols and enzymatic conjugation with GSH also play very important roles (Fig. 4-5).[43, 44] If not effectively detoxified by the first three pathways in Figure 4-5, arene oxides will bind covalently with nucleophilic groups present on proteins, DNA, and RNA, thereby leading to serious cellular damage.[5, 43] This, in part, helps explain why benzene can be so toxic to mammalian systems.

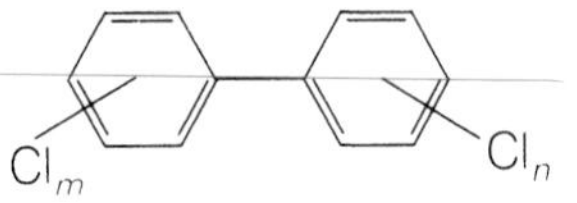

Polychlorinated Biphenyl Mixtures

The number of chlorine atoms (m, n) present in two aromatic rings varies considerably

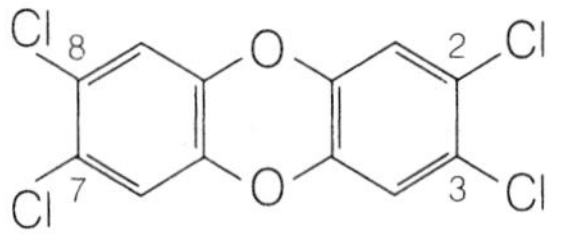

2,3,7,8-Tetrachlorodibenzo-p-dioxin (TCDD)

Quantitatively, the most important detoxification reaction for arene oxides is the spontaneous rearrangement to corresponding arenols. Often, this rearrangement is accompanied by a novel intramolecular hydride (deuteride) migration called the "NIH shift."[67] It was named after the National Institutes of Health (NIH) laboratory in Bethesda, Maryland, where this process was discovered. The general features of the NIH shift are illustrated with the mixed-function aromatic oxidation of 4-deuterioanisole to 3-deuterio-4-hydroxyanisole in Figure 4-6.[68]

After its metabolic formation, the arene oxide ring opens in the direction that generates the most resonance-stabilized carbocation (positive charge on C-3 carbon is resonance stabilized by the OCH_3 group). The zwitterionic species (positive charge on the C-3 carbon atom and negative charge on the oxygen atom) then undergoes a 1,2-deuteride shift (NIH shift) to form the dienone. Final transformation of the dienone to 3-deuterio-4-hydroxyanisole occurs with the preferential loss of a proton because of the weaker bond energy of the C-H bond (compared with the C-D bond). Thus, the deuterium is retained in the molecule by undergoing this intramolecular NIH shift. The experimental observation of an NIH shift for aromatic hydroxylation of a drug or xenobiotic is taken as indirect evidence for the involvement of an arene oxide.

In addition to the NIH shift, the zwitterionic species may undergo direct loss of D^+ to generate 4-hydroxyanisole, in which there is no retention of deuterium (Fig. 4-6). The alternative pathway (direct loss of D^+) may be more favorable than the NIH shift in some aromatic oxidation reactions. Therefore, depending on the substituent group on the arene, some aromatic hydroxylation reactions do not display any NIH shift.

Two extremely important enzymatic reactions also aid in neutralizing the reactivity of arene oxides. The first of these involves the hydration (i.e., nucleophilic attack of water on the epoxide) of arene oxides to yield inactive *trans*-dihydrodiol metabolites (Fig. 4-5). This reaction is catalyzed by

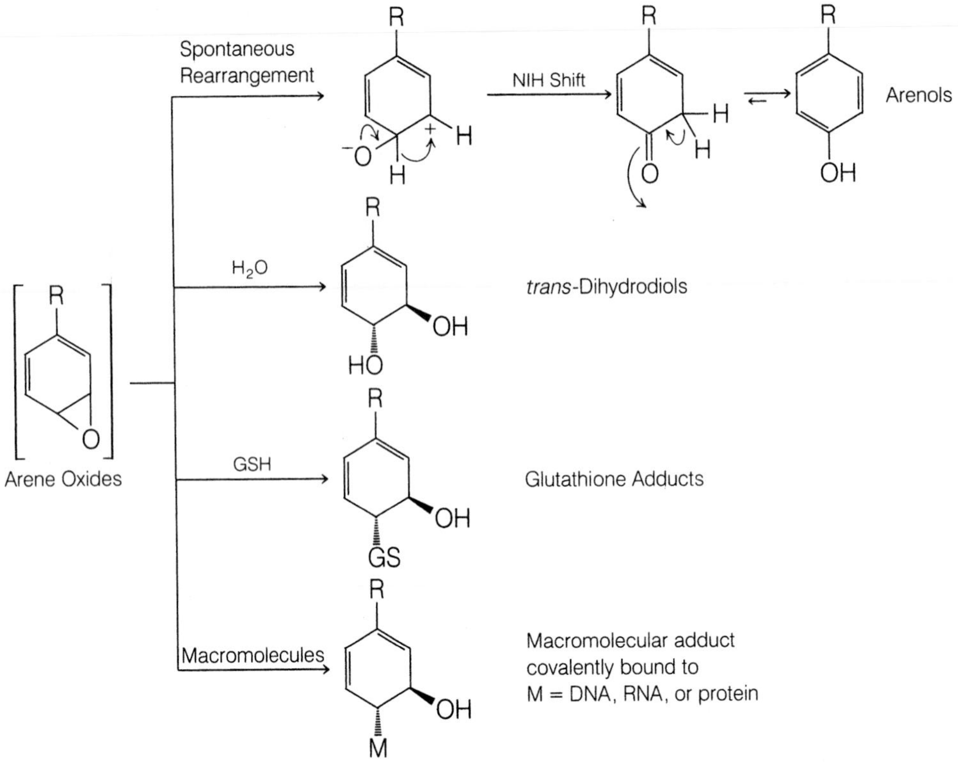

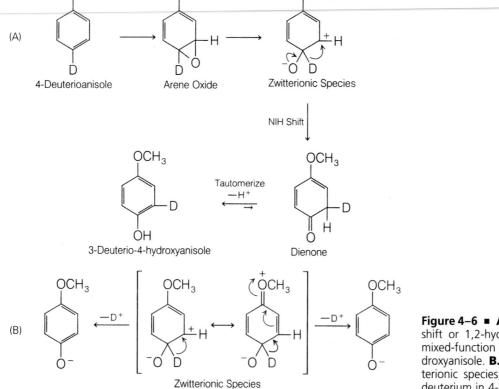

Figure 4–5 ■ Possible reaction pathways for arene oxides. (Data are from Daly, J. W., et al.: Experientia 28:1129, 1972; Jerina, D. M., and Daly, J. W.: Science 185:573, 1974; and Kaminsky, L. S.: In Anders, M. W. (ed.). Bioactivation of Foreign Compounds. New York, Academic Press, 1985, p. 157.)

Figure 4–6 ■ **A.** General features of the NIH shift or 1,2-hydride (deuteride) shift in the mixed-function oxidation of 4-deuterio-4-hydroxyanisole. **B.** Direct loss of D+ from zwitterionic species, leading to no retention of deuterium in 4-hydroxyanisole.

microsomal enzymes called *epoxide hydrases*.[69, 70] Often, epoxide hydrase inhibitors, such as cyclohexene oxide and 1,1,1-trichloropropene-2,3-oxide, have been used to demonstrate the detoxification role of these enzymes. Addition of these inhibitors is accompanied frequently by increased toxicity of the arene oxide being tested, because formation of nontoxic dihydrodiols is blocked. For example, the mutagenicity of benzo[α]pyrene-4,5-oxide, as measured by the Ames *Salmonella typhimurium* test system, is potentiated when cyclohexene oxide is added.[71] Dihydrodiol metabolites have been reported in the metabolism of several aromatic hydrocarbons (e.g., naphthalene, benzo[α]pyrene, and other related polycyclic aromatic hydrocarbons).[43] A few drugs (e.g., phenytoin,[72] phenobarbital,[73] glutethimide[74]) also yield dihydrodiol products as minor metabolites in humans. Dihydrodiol products are susceptible to conjugation with glucuronic acid, as well as enzymatic dehydrogenation to the corresponding catechol metabolite, as exemplified by the metabolism of phenytoin.[72]

A second enzymatic reaction involves nucleophilic ring opening of the arene oxide by the sulfhydryl group present in GSH to yield the corresponding *trans*-1,2-dihydro-1-*S*-glutathionyl-2-hydroxy adduct, or GSH adduct (Fig. 4-5).[44] The reaction is catalyzed by various GSH S-transferases.[75] Because GSH is found in practically all mammalian tissues, it plays an important role in the detoxification not only of arene oxides but also of a variety of other chemically reactive and potentially toxic intermediates. Initially, GSH adducts formed from arene oxides are modified in a series of reactions to yield "premercapturic acid" or mercapturic acid metabolites.[76] Since it is classified as a phase II pathway, GSH conjugation is covered in greater detail below.

Because of their electrophilic and reactive nature, arene oxides also may undergo spontaneous reactions with nucleophilic functionalities present on biomacromolecules.[44, 45] Such reactions lead to modified protein, DNA, and RNA structures and often cause dramatic alterations in how these macromolecules function. Much of the cytotoxicity and irreversible lesions caused by arene oxides are presumed to result from their covalent binding to cellular components. Several well-established examples of reactive arene oxides that cause serious toxicity are presented below.

Administration of bromobenzene to rats causes severe liver necrosis.[77] Extensive in vivo and in vitro studies indicate that the liver damage results from the interaction of a chemically reactive metabolite, 4-bromobenzene oxide, with hepatocytes.[78] Extensive covalent binding to hepatic tissue

| Cyclohexane oxide | 1,1,1-Trichloropropene 2,3-oxide | Benzo[a]pyrene 4,5-oxide |

Phenytoin   Arene Oxide   *trans*-Dihydrodiol Metabolite (conjugated)

p-Hydroxyphenytoin (conjugated as glucuronide)   Catechol Metabolite

Arene Oxide   Glutathione Adduct   "Premercapturic Acid" Derivative   Mercapturic Acid Derivative

was confirmed by use of radiolabeled bromobenzene. The severity of necrosis correlated well with the amount of covalent binding to hepatic tissue. Use of diethyl maleate or large doses of bromobenzene in rats showed that the depletion of hepatic GSH led to more severe liver necrosis.

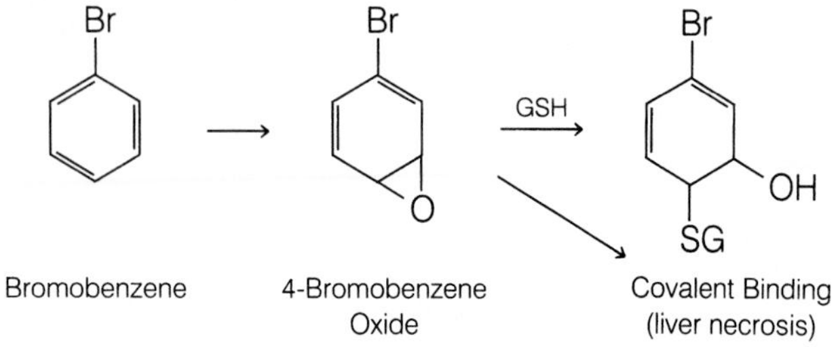

Bromobenzene   4-Bromobenzene   Covalent Binding
Oxide   (liver necrosis)

Polycyclic aromatic hydrocarbons are ubiquitous environmental contaminants that are formed from auto emission, refuse burning, industrial processes, cigarette smoke, and other combustion processes. Benzo[α]pyrene, a potent carcinogenic agent, is perhaps the most extensively studied of the polycyclic aromatic hydrocarbons.[79] Inspection of its structure reveals that aromatic hydroxylation of benzo[α]pyrene can occur at a number of positions. The identification of several dihydrodiol metabolites is viewed as indirect evidence for the formation and involvement of arene oxides in the metabolism of benzo[α]pyrene. Although certain arene oxides of benzo[α]pyrene (e.g., 4,5-oxide, 7,8-oxide, 9,10-oxide) appear to display some mutagenic and tumorigenic activity, it does not appear that they represent the ultimate reactive species responsible for benzo[α]pyrene's carcinogenicity. In recent years, extensive studies have led to the characterization of a specific sequence of metabolic reactions (Fig. 4-7) that generate a highly reactive intermediate that covalently binds to DNA. Metabolic activation of benzo[α]pyrene to the ultimate carcinogenic species involves an initial epoxidation reaction to form the 7,8-oxide, which is then

converted by epoxide hydrase to (−)-7(R),8(R)-dihydroxy-7,8-dihydrobenzo[α]pyrene.[80] The two-step enzymatic formation of this *trans*-dihydrodiol is stereospecific. Subsequent epoxidation at the 9,10-double bond of the latter metabolite generates predominantly (+)-7(R),8(S)-dihydroxy-9(R),10(R)-oxy-7,8,9,10-tetrahydrobenzo[α]pyrene or (+)7,8-diol-9,10-epoxide. It is this key electrophilic diol epoxide metabolite that readily reacts with DNA to form many covalently bound adducts.[81–83] Careful degradation studies have shown that the principal adduct involves attack of the C-2 amino group of deoxyguanosine at C-10 of the diol epoxide. Clearly, these reactions are responsible for genetic code alterations that ultimately lead to the malignant transformations. Covalent binding of the diol epoxide metabolite to deoxyadenosine and to deoxycytidine also has been established.[84]

Another carcinogenic polycyclic aromatic hydrocarbon, 7,12-dimethylbenz[α]anthracene, also forms covalent adducts with nucleic acids (RNA).[85] The ultimate carcinogenic reactive species apparently is the 5,6-oxide that results from epoxidation of the 5,6-double bond in this aromatic hydrocarbon. The arene oxide intermediate binds covalently to guanosine residues of RNA to yield the two adducts.

Oxidation of Olefins

The metabolic oxidation of olefinic carbon–carbon double bonds leads to the corresponding epoxide (or oxirane). Epoxides derived from olefins generally tend to be somewhat more stable than the arene oxides formed from aromatic compounds. A few epoxides are stable enough to be directly measurable in biological fluids (e.g., plasma, urine). Like their arene oxide counterparts, epoxides are susceptible to enzymatic hydration by epoxide hydrase to form *trans*-1,2-dihydrodiols (also called *1,2-diols* or *1,2-dihydroxy com-*

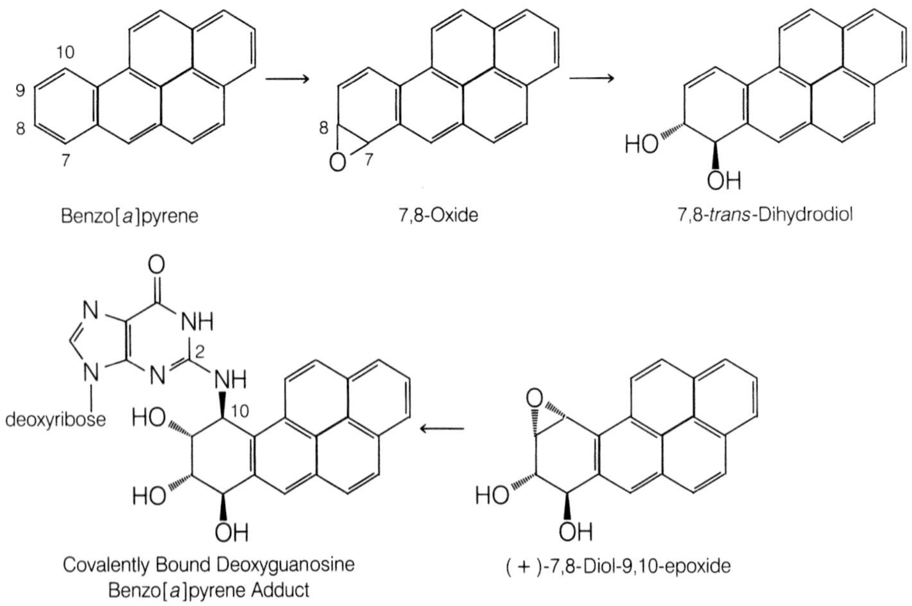

Benzo[a]pyrene   7,8-Oxide   7,8-*trans*-Dihydrodiol

Covalently Bound Deoxyguanosine
Benzo[a]pyrene Adduct

(+)-7,8-Diol-9,10-epoxide

Figure 4–7 ■ Metabolic sequence leading to the formation of the ultimate carcinogenic species of benzo[a]pyrene: (+)-7*R*,8*S*-dihydroxy-9*R*,10-oxy-7,8,9,10-tetrahydrobenzo[a]pyrene or (+)-7,8-diol-9,10-epoxide.

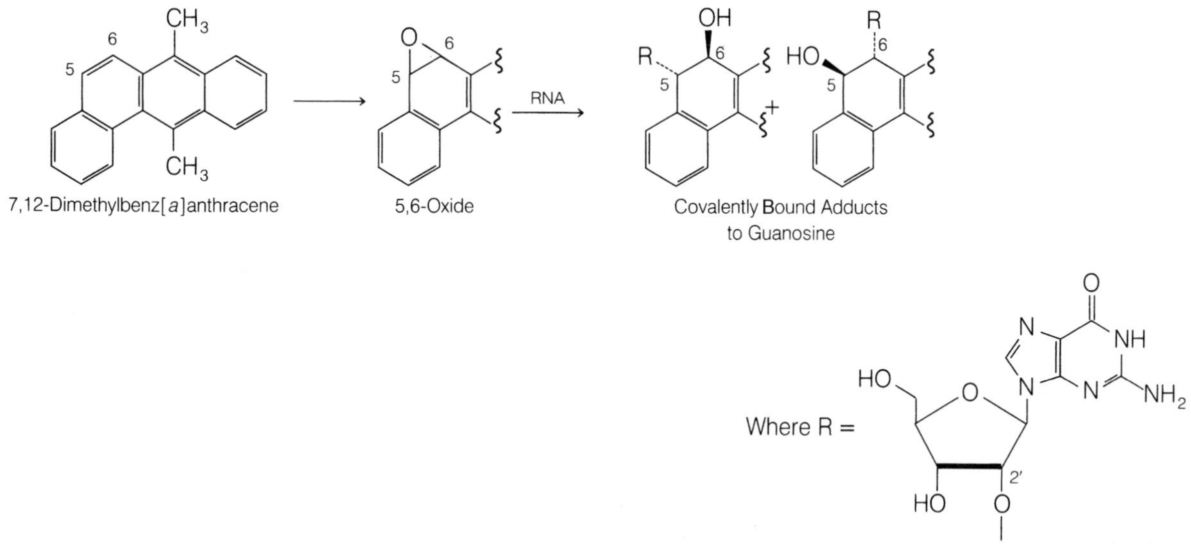

7,12-Dimethylbenz[*a*]anthracene　　5,6-Oxide　　Covalently Bound Adducts to Guanosine

Where R =

pounds).[69, 70] In addition, several epoxides undergo GSH conjugation.[86]

A well-known example of olefinic epoxidation is the metabolism, in humans, of the anticonvulsant drug carbamazepine (Tegretol) to carbamazepine-10,11-epoxide.[87] The epoxide is reasonably stable and can be measured quantitatively

in the plasma of patients receiving the parent drug. The epoxide metabolite may have marked anticonvulsant activity and, therefore, may contribute substantially to the therapeutic effect of the parent drug.[88] Subsequent hydration of the epoxide produces 10,11-dihydroxycarbamazepine, an important urinary metabolite (10 to 30%) in humans.[87]

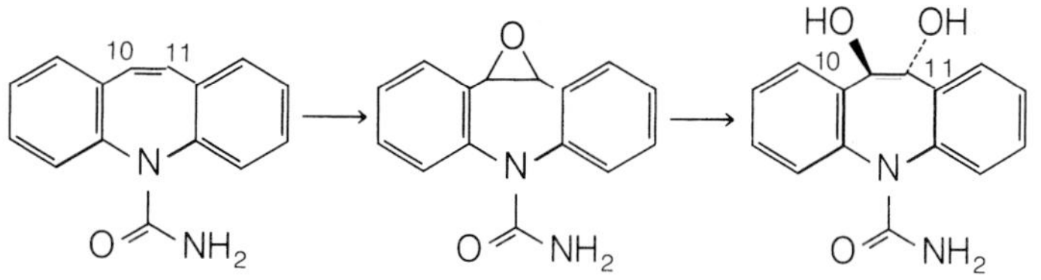

Carbamazepine　　Carbamazepine-10,11-epoxide　　*trans*-10,11-Dihydroxy-carbamazepine

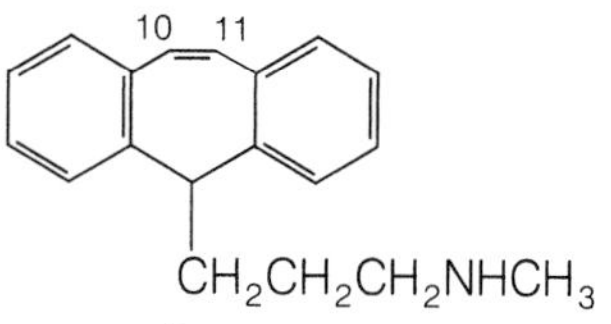

Protriptyline

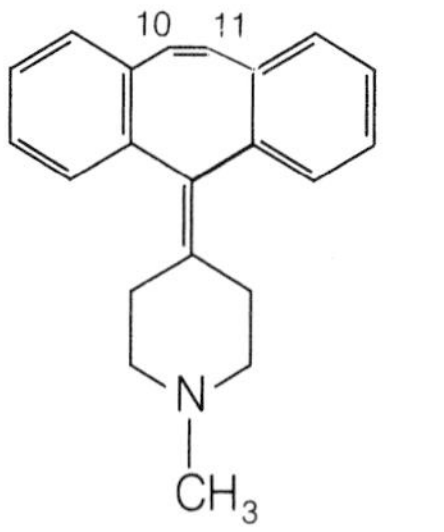

Cyproheptadine

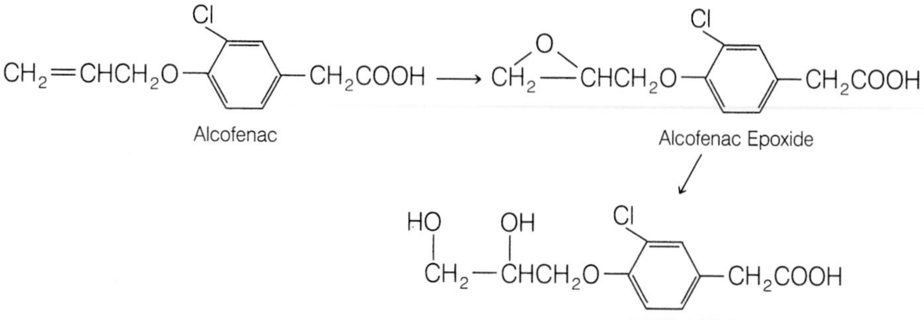

Alcofenac　　Alcofenac Epoxide

Dihydroxyalcofenac

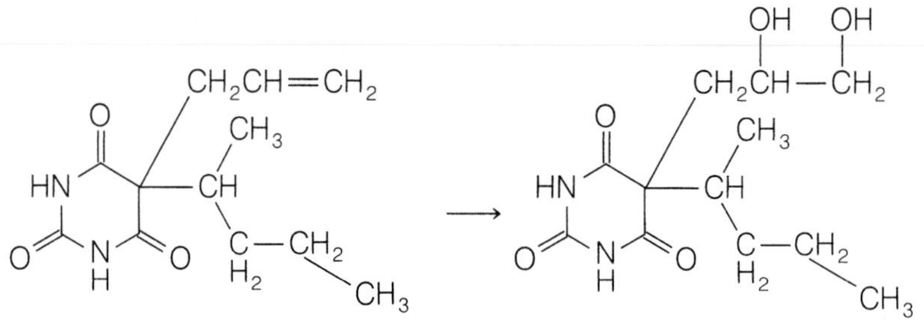

Secobarbital

Secodiol
5-(2,3-Dihydroxypropyl)-5-
(1-methylbutyl)-barbituric Acid

Epoxidation of the olefinic 10,11-double bond in the antipsychotic agent protriptyline (Vivactil)[89] and in the H_1-histamine antagonist cyproheptadine (Periactin)[90] also occurs. Frequently, the epoxides formed from the biotransformation of an olefinic compound are minor products, because of their further conversion to the corresponding 1,2-diols. For instance, dihydroxyalcofenac is a major human urinary metabolite of the once clinically useful anti-inflammatory agent alclofenac.[91] The epoxide metabolite from which it is derived, however, is present in minute amounts. The presence of the dihydroxy metabolite (secodiol) of secobarbital, but not the epoxide product, has been reported in humans.[92]

Indirect evidence for the formation of epoxides comes also from the isolation of GSH or mercapturic acid metabolites. After administration of styrene to rats, two urinary metabolites were identified as the isomeric mercapturic acid derivatives resulting from nucleophilic attack of GSH on the intermediate epoxide.[93] In addition, styrene oxide covalently

binds to rat liver microsomal proteins and nucleic acids.[94] These results indicate that styrene oxide is relatively reactive toward nucleophiles (e.g., GSH and nucleophilic groups on protein and nucleic acids).

There are, apparently, diverse metabolically generated epoxides that display similar chemical reactivity toward nucleophilic functionalities. Accordingly, the toxicity of some olefinic compounds may result from their metabolic conversion to chemically reactive epoxides.[95] One example that clearly links metabolic epoxidation as a biotoxication pathway involves aflatoxin B_1. This naturally occurring carcinogenic agent contains an olefinic (C2–C3) double bond adjacent to a cyclic ether oxygen. The hepatocarcinogenicity of aflatoxin B_1 has been clearly linked to its metabolic oxidation to the corresponding 2,3-oxide, which is extremely reactive.[96, 97] Extensive in vitro and in vivo metabolic studies indicate that this 2,3-oxide binds covalently to DNA, RNA, and proteins. A major DNA adduct has been isolated and

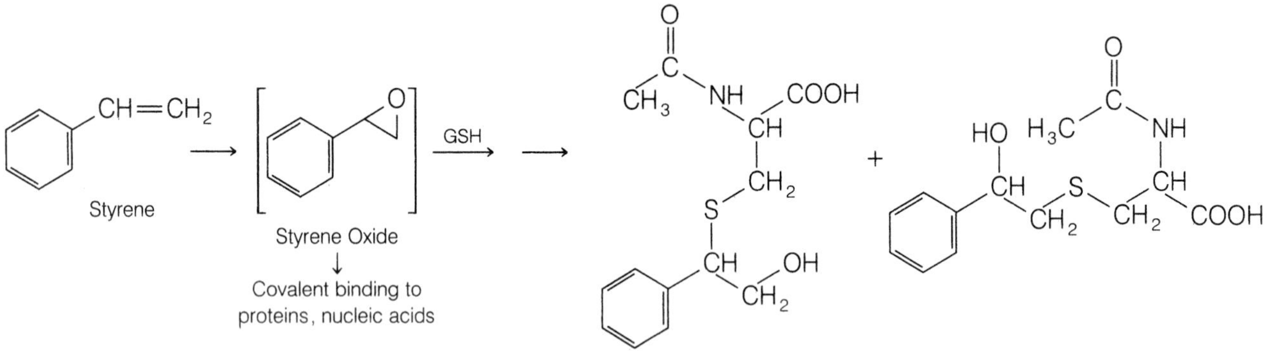

Styrene

Styrene Oxide
↓
Covalent binding to
proteins, nucleic acids

Mercapturic Acid
Derivative (major)

Mercapturic Acid
Derivative (minor)

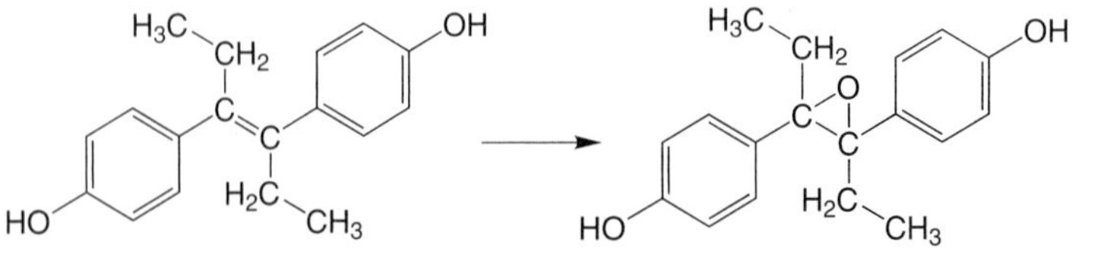

Diethylstilbestrol

Diethylstilbestrol Epoxide
↓
Possible covalent binding to
proteins and/or nucleic acids

characterized as 2,3-dihydro-2-(N^7-guanyl)-3-hydroxyafla-toxin B_1.[98, 99]

Other olefinic compounds, such as vinyl chloride,[100] stilbene,[101] and the carcinogenic estrogenic agent diethylstilbestrol (DES),[102, 103] undergo metabolic epoxidation. The corresponding epoxide metabolites may be the reactive species responsible for the cellular toxicity seen with these compounds.

An interesting group of olefin-containing compounds causes the destruction of cytochrome P-450.[104, 105] Compounds belonging to this group include allylisopropylacetamide,[106, 107] secobarbital,[108, 109] and the volatile anesthetic agent fluroxene.[110] It is believed that the olefinic moiety present in these compounds is activated metabolically by cytochrome P-450 to form a very reactive intermediate that covalently binds to the heme portion of cytochrome P-450.[111–113] The abnormal heme derivatives, or "green pigments," that result from this covalent interaction have been characterized as N-alkylated protoporphyrins in which the N-alkyl moiety is derived directly from the olefin administered.[104, 105, 111–113] Long-term administration of the above-mentioned three agents is expected to lead to inhibition of oxidative drug metabolism, potential drug interactions, and prolonged pharmacological effects.

Oxidation at Benzylic Carbon Atoms

Carbon atoms attached to aromatic rings (benzylic position) are susceptible to oxidation, thereby forming the corresponding alcohol (or carbinol) metabolite.[114, 115] Primary alcohol metabolites are often oxidized further to aldehydes and carboxylic acids ($CH_2OH \rightarrow CHO \rightarrow COOH$), and secondary alcohols are converted to ketones by soluble alcohol and aldehyde dehydrogenases.[116] Alternatively, the alcohol may be conjugated directly with glucuronic acid.[117] The benzylic carbon atom present in the oral hypoglycemic agent tolbuta-mide (Orinase) is oxidized extensively to the corresponding alcohol and carboxylic acid. Both metabolites have been isolated from human urine.[118] Similarly, the "benzylic" methyl group in the anti-inflammatory agent tolmetin (Tolectin) undergoes oxidation to yield the dicarboxylic acid product as the major metabolite in humans.[119, 120] The selective COX-2 anti-inflammatory agent celecoxib undergoes benzylic oxidation at its C-5 methyl group to give hydroxy-celecoxib as a major metabolite.[121] Significant benzylic hydroxylation occurs in the metabolism of the β-adrenergic blocker metoprolol (Lopressor) to yield α-hydroxymetoprolol.[122, 123] Additional examples of drugs and xenobiotics undergoing benzylic oxidation are shown in Figure 4-8.

Oxidation at Allylic Carbon Atoms

Microsomal hydroxylation at allylic carbon atoms is commonly observed in drug metabolism. An illustrative example of allylic oxidation is given by the psychoactive component of marijuana, Δ^1-tetrahydrocannabinol Δ^1-THC. This molecule contains three allylic carbon centers (C-7, C-6, and C-3). Allylic hydroxylation occurs extensively at C-7 to yield 7-hydroxy- Δ^1-THC as the major plasma metabolite in humans.[10, 11] Pharmacological studies show that this 7-hydroxy metabolite is as active as, or even more active than, Δ^1-THC per se and may contribute significantly to the overall central nervous system (CNS) psychotomimetic effects of the parent compound.[124, 125] Hydroxylation also occurs to a minor extent at the allylic C-6 position to give both the epimeric 6α- and 6β-hydroxy metabolites.[10, 11] Metabolism does not occur at C-3, presumably because of steric hindrance.

The antiarrhythmic agent quinidine is metabolized by allylic hydroxylation to 3-hydroxyquinidine, the principal plasma metabolite found in humans.[126, 127] This metabolite shows significant antiarrhythmic activity in animals and possibly in humans.[128]

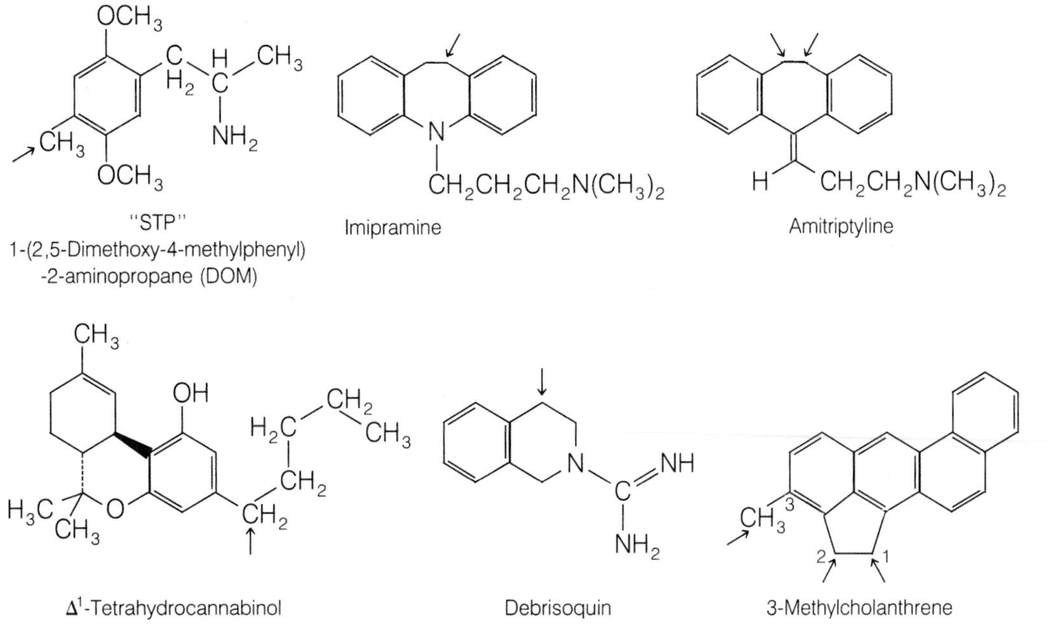

Figure 4–8 ■ Examples of drugs and xenobiotics undergoing benzylic hydroxylation. *Arrow* indicates site of hydroxylation.

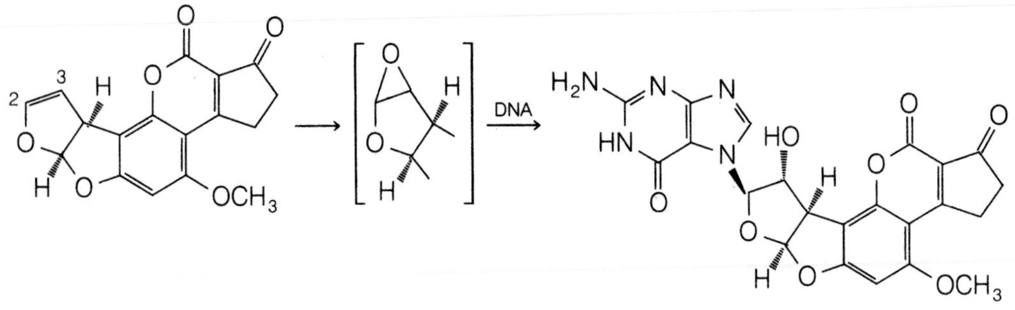

Aflatoxin B$_1$ 2,3-Expoxide   2,3-Dihydro-2-(N^7-guanyl)-3-hydroxyaflatoxin B$_1$

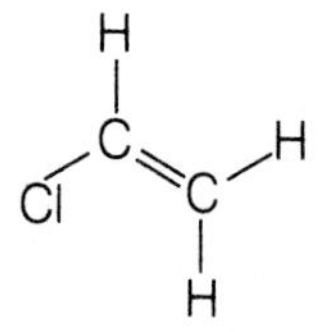

Vinyl Chloride

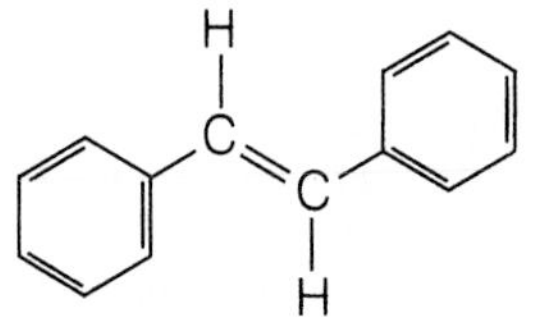

Stilbene

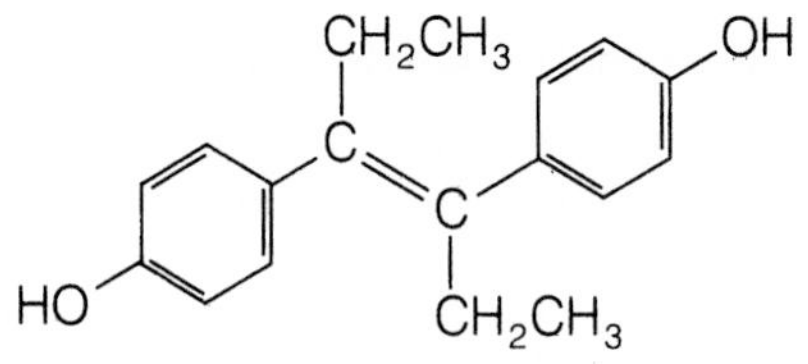

Diethylstilbestrol
(DES)

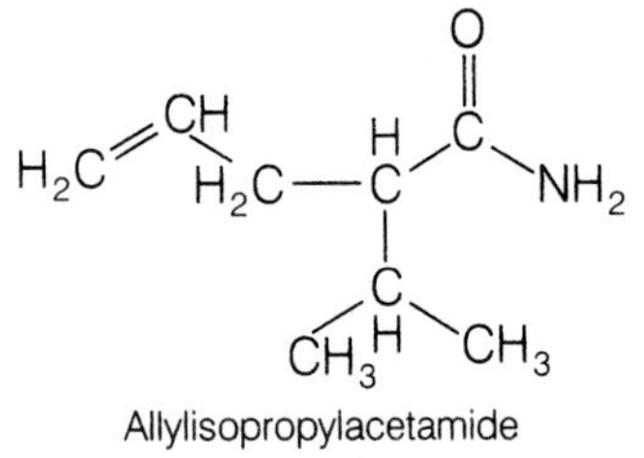

Allylisopropylacetamide 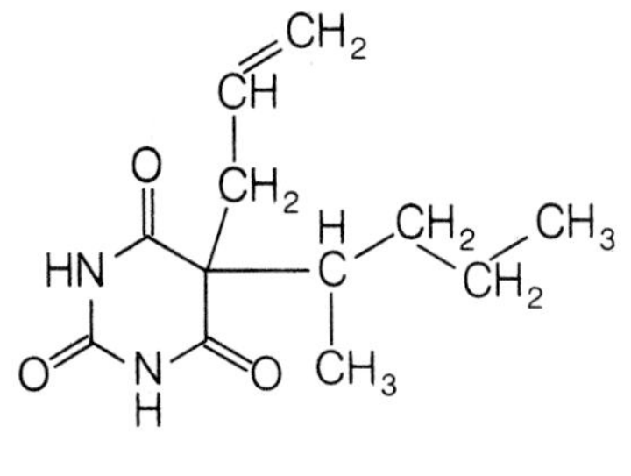   Secobarbital

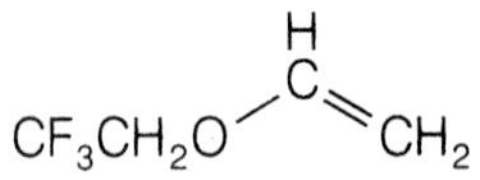

Fluroxene

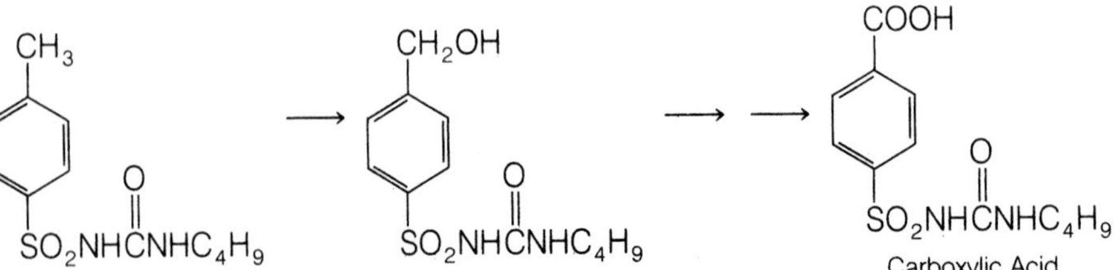

Tolbutamide   Alcohol Metabolite   Carboxylic Acid Metabolite

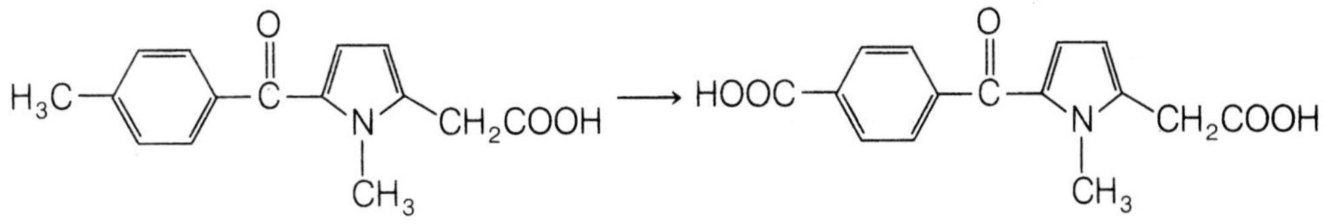

Tolmetin → Dicarboxylic Acid Metabolite

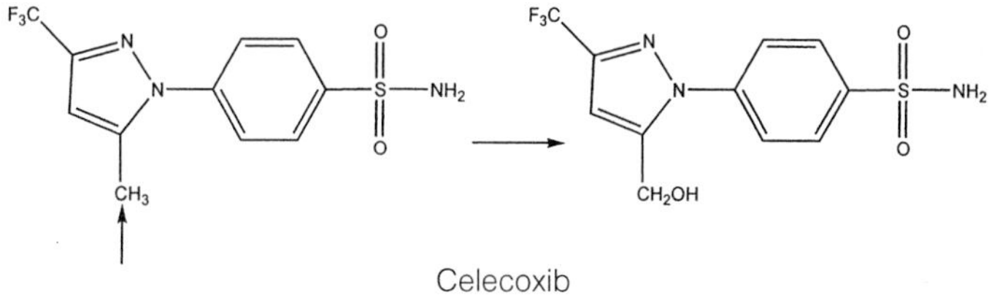

Celecoxib
4-(5-Methyl-3-trifluoromethyl-pyrazol-1-yl)-benzenesulfonamide

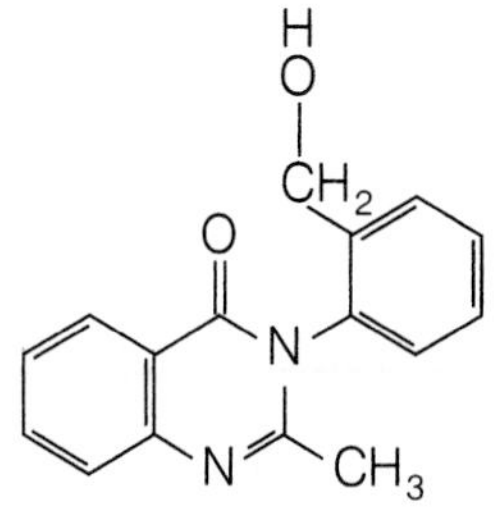

2′-Hydroxymethylmethaqualone

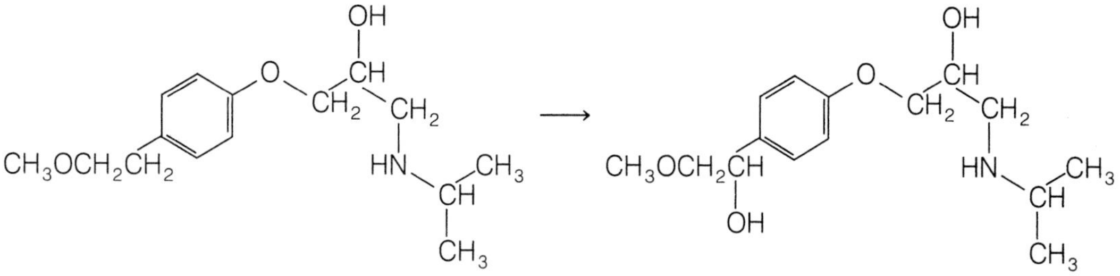

Metroprolol → α-Hydroxymetroprolol

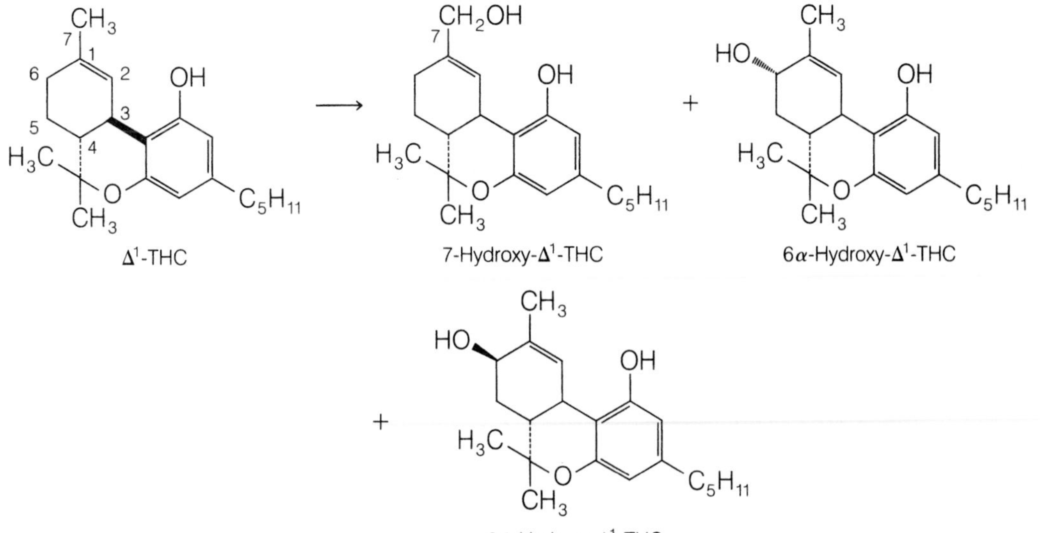

Δ¹-THC → 7-Hydroxy-Δ¹-THC + 6α-Hydroxy-Δ¹-THC

+ 6β-Hydroxy-Δ¹-THC

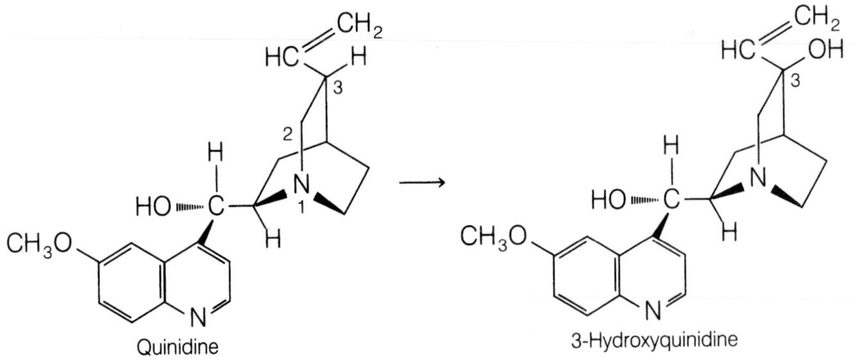

Quinidine → 3-Hydroxyquinidine

Other examples of allylic oxidation include the sedative hypnotic hexobarbital (Sombulex) and the analgesic pentazocine (Talwin). The 3′-hydroxylated metabolite formed from hexobarbital is susceptible to glucuronide conjugation as well as further oxidation to the 3′-oxo compound.[129, 130] Hexobarbital is a chiral barbiturate derivative that exists in two enantiomeric forms. Studies in humans indicate that the pharmacologically less active $(R)(-)$ enantiomer is metabolized more rapidly than its $(S)(+)$ isomer.[131] Pentazocine undergoes allylic hydroxylation at the two terminal methyl groups of its *N*-butenyl side chain to yield either the *cis* or *trans* alcohol metabolites shown in the diagrams. In humans, more of the *trans* alcohol is formed.[132, 133]

For the hepatocarcinogenic agent safrole, allylic hydroxylation is involved in a bioactivation pathway leading to the formation of chemically reactive metabolites.[134] This process involves initial hydroxylation at the C-1′ carbon of safrole, which is both allylic and benzylic. The hydroxylated metabolite then undergoes further conjugation to form a sulfate ester. This chemically reactive ester intermediate presumably undergoes nucleophilic displacement reactions with DNA or RNA in vitro to form covalently bound adducts.[135] As shown in the scheme, nucleophilic attack by DNA, RNA, or other nucleophiles is facilitated by a good leaving group (e.g., SO_4^{2-}) at the C-1′ position. The leaving group tendency of the alcohol OH group itself is not enough

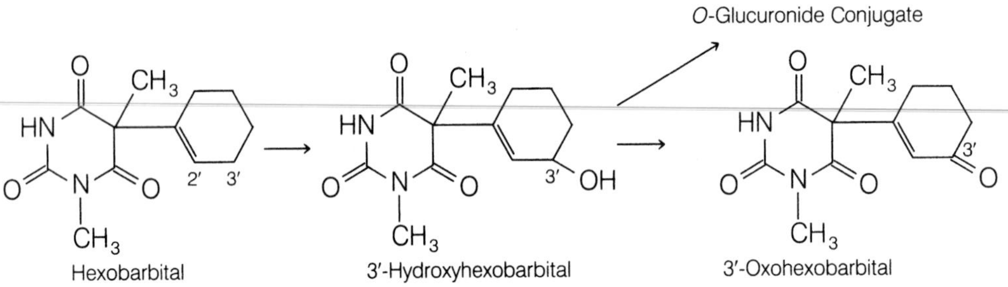

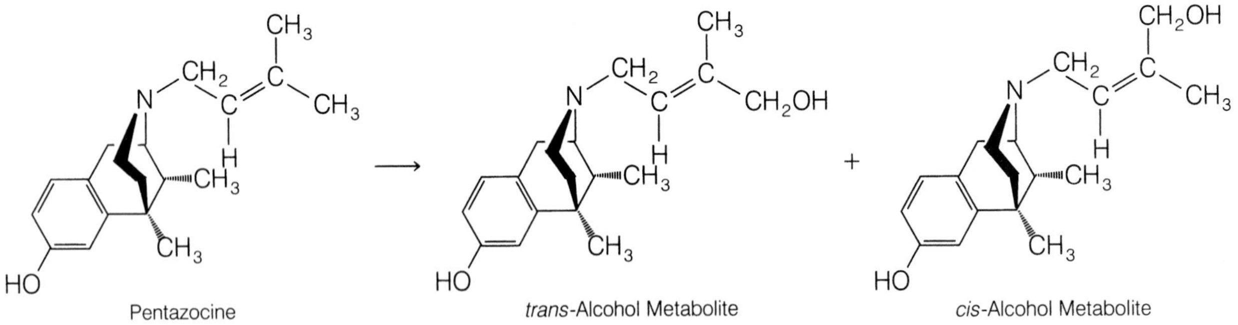

Hexobarbital → 3′-Hydroxyhexobarbital → *O*-Glucuronide Conjugate; 3′-Oxohexobarbital

Pentazocine → *trans*-Alcohol Metabolite + *cis*-Alcohol Metabolite

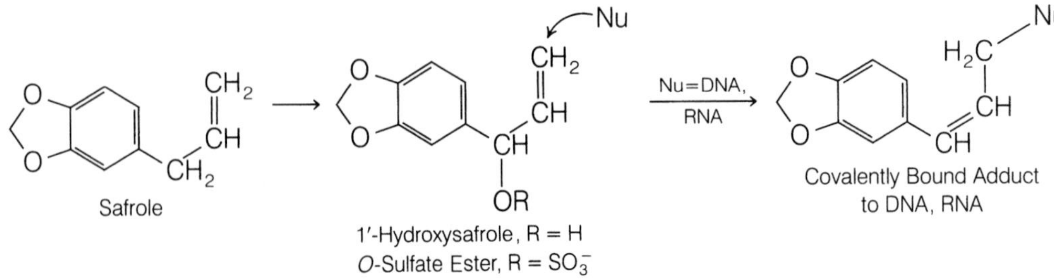

Safrole → 1′-Hydroxysafrole, R = H / *O*-Sulfate Ester, R = SO_3^- → Covalently Bound Adduct to DNA, RNA

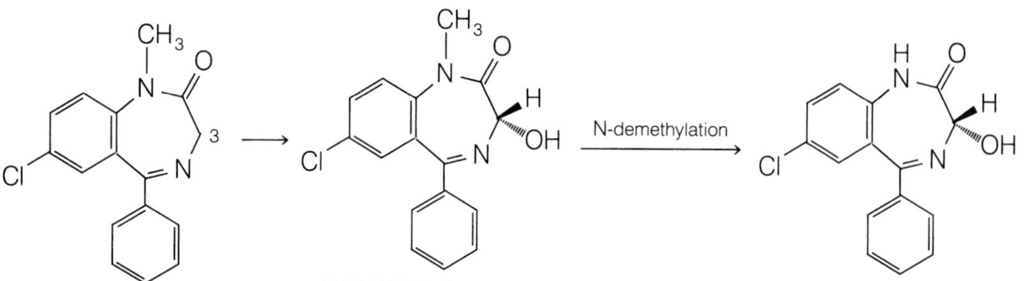

Diazepam → (3S) N-Methyloxazepam or 3-Hydroxydiazepam → N-demethylation → Oxazepam

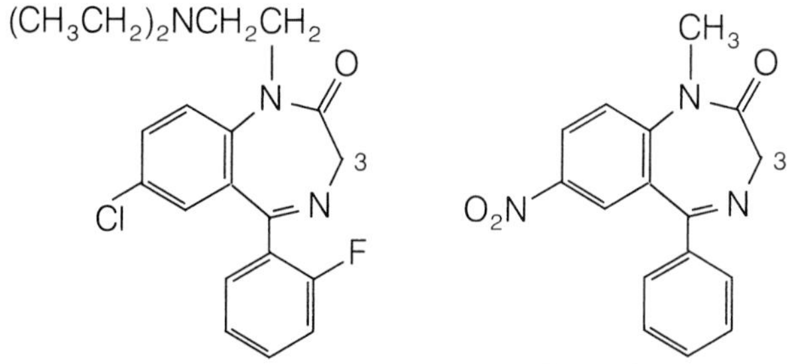

Flurazepam Nimetazepam

to facilitate displacement reactions. Importantly, allylic hydroxylation generally does not lead to the generation of reactive intermediates. Its involvement in the biotoxification of safrole appears to be an exception.

Oxidation at Carbon Atoms α to Carbonyls and Imines

The mixed-function oxidase system also oxidizes carbon atoms adjacent (i.e., α) to carbonyl and imino (C=N) functionalities. An important class of drugs undergoing this type of oxidation is the benzodiazepines. For example, diazepam (Valium), flurazepam (Dalmane), and nimetazepam are oxidized to their corresponding 3-hydroxy metabolites.[136–138] The C-3 carbon atom undergoing hydroxylation is α to both a lactam carbonyl and an imino functionality.

For diazepam, the hydroxylation reaction proceeds with remarkable stereoselectivity to form primarily (90%) 3-hydroxydiazepam (also called *N*-methyloxazepam), with the (S) absolute configuration at C-3.[139] Further N-demethylation of the latter metabolite gives rise to the pharmacologically active 3(S)(+)-oxazepam.

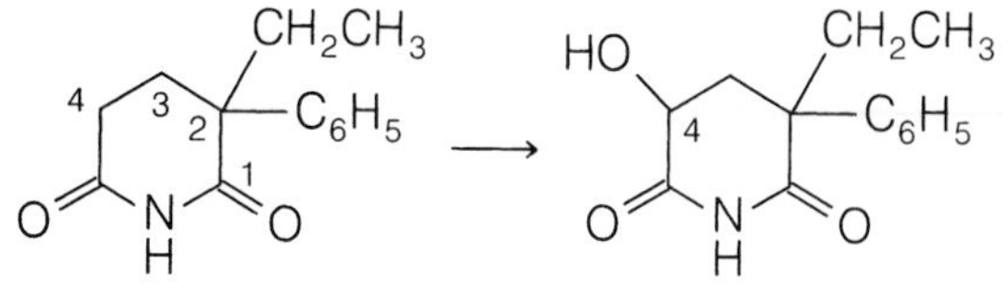

Glutethimide → 4-Hydroxyglutethimide

ω Oxidation

$\omega - 1$ Oxidation

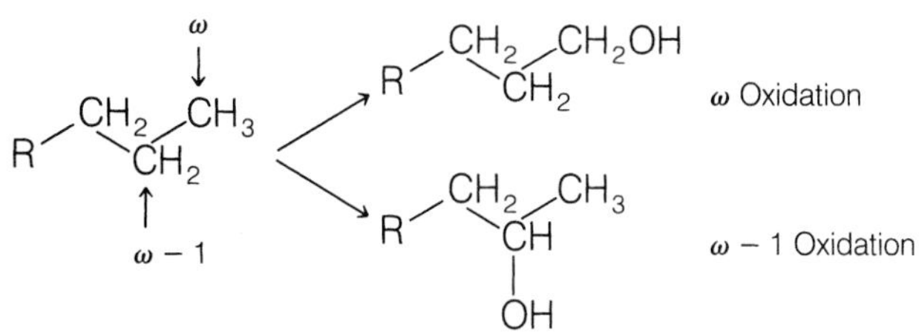

Hydroxylation of the carbon atom α to carbonyl functionalities generally occurs only to a limited extent in drug metabolism. An illustrative example involves the hydroxylation of the sedative hypnotic glutethimide (Doriden) to 4-hydroxyglutethimide.[140, 141]

Oxidation at Aliphatic and Alicyclic Carbon Atoms

Alkyl or aliphatic carbon centers are subject to mixed-function oxidation. Metabolic oxidation at the terminal methyl group often is referred to as ω *oxidation*, and oxidation of the penultimate carbon atom (i.e., next-to-the-last carbon) is called $\omega - 1$ *oxidation*.[114, 115] The initial alcohol metabolites formed from these enzymatic ω and $\omega - 1$ oxidations are susceptible to further oxidation to yield aldehyde, ketones, or carboxylic acids. Alternatively, the alcohol metabolites may undergo glucuronide conjugation.

Aliphatic ω and $\omega - 1$ hydroxylations commonly take place in drug molecules with straight or branched alkyl chains. Thus, the antiepileptic agent valproic acid (Depakene) undergoes both ω and $\omega - 1$ oxidation to the 5-hydroxy and 4-hydroxy metabolites, respectively.[142, 143] Further oxidation of the 5-hydroxy metabolite yields 2-*n*-propylglutaric acid.

Numerous barbiturates and oral hypoglycemic sulfonylureas also have aliphatic side chains that are susceptible to oxidation. Note that the sedative hypnotic amobarbital (Amytal) undergoes extensive $\omega - 1$ oxidation to the corresponding 3′-hydroxylated metabolite.[144] Other barbiturates, such as pentobarbital,[145, 146] thiamylal,[147] and secobarbital,[92] reportedly are metabolized by way of ω and $\omega - 1$ oxidation. The *n*-propyl side chain attached to the oral hypoglycemic agent chlorpropamide (Diabinese) undergoes extensive $\omega - 1$ hydroxylation to yield the secondary alcohol 2′-hydroxychlorpropamide as a major urinary metabolite in humans.[148]

Omega and $\omega - 1$ oxidation of the isobutyl moiety present in the anti-inflammatory agent ibuprofen (Motrin) yields the

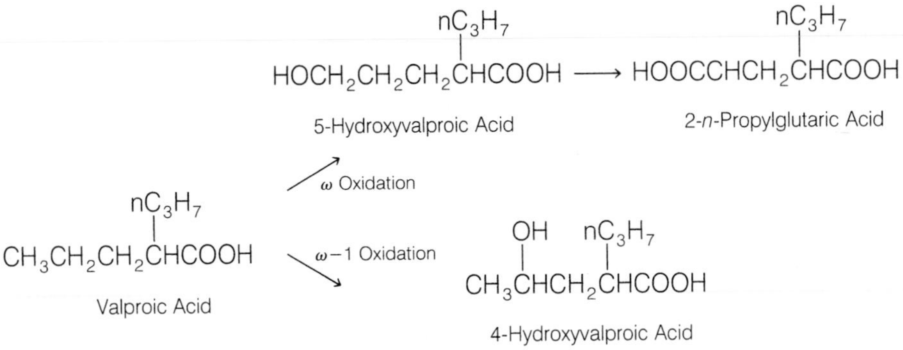

$$HOCH_2CH_2CH_2\overset{\overset{\displaystyle nC_3H_7}{|}}{CH}COOH \longrightarrow HOOCCHCH_2\overset{\overset{\displaystyle nC_3H_7}{|}}{CH}COOH$$

5-Hydroxyvalproic Acid   2-*n*-Propylglutaric Acid

ω Oxidation

$$CH_3CH_2CH_2\overset{\overset{\displaystyle nC_3H_7}{|}}{CH}COOH$$

Valproic Acid

ω−1 Oxidation

$$CH_3\overset{\overset{\displaystyle OH}{|}}{CH}CH_2\overset{\overset{\displaystyle nC_3H_7}{|}}{CH}COOH$$

4-Hydroxyvalproic Acid

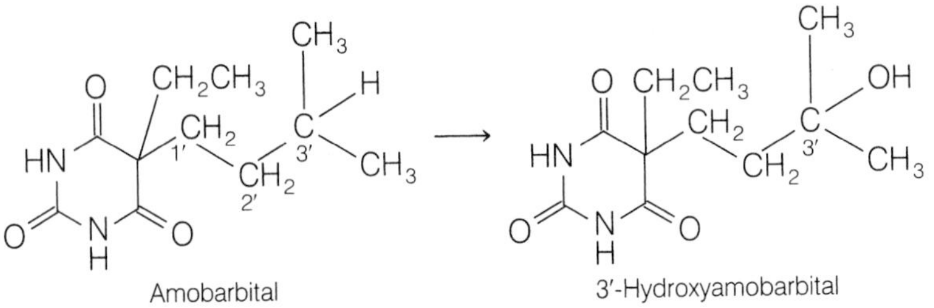

Amobarbital   3'-Hydroxyamobarbital

corresponding carboxylic acid and tertiary alcohol metabolites.[149] Additional examples of drugs reported to undergo aliphatic hydroxylation include meprobamate,[150] glutethimide,[140, 141] ethosuximide,[151] and phenylbutazone.[152]

The cyclohexyl group is commonly found in many medicinal agents, and is also susceptible to mixed-function oxidation (alicyclic hydroxylation).[114, 115] Enzymatic introduction of a hydroxyl group into a monosubstituted cyclohexane ring generally occurs at C-3 or C-4 and can lead to *cis* and *trans* conformational stereoisomers, as shown in the diagrammed scheme.

An example of this hydroxylation pathway is seen in the metabolism of the oral hypoglycemic agent acetohexamide

(Dymelor). In humans, the *trans*-4-hydroxycyclohexyl product is reportedly a major metabolite.[153] Small amounts of the other possible stereoisomers (namely, the *cis*-4-, *cis*-3-, and *trans*-3-hydroxycyclohexyl derivatives) also have been detected. Another related oral hypoglycemic agent, glipizide, is oxidized in humans to the *trans*-4- and *cis*-3-hydroxylcyclohexyl metabolites in about a 6:1 ratio.[154]

Two human urinary metabolites of phencyclidine (PCP) have been identified as the 4-hydroxypiperidyl and 4-hydroxycyclohexyl derivatives of the parent compound.[155, 156] Thus, from these results, it appears that "alicyclic" hydroxylation of the six-membered piperidyl moiety may parallel closely the hydroxylation pattern of the cyclohexyl moiety.

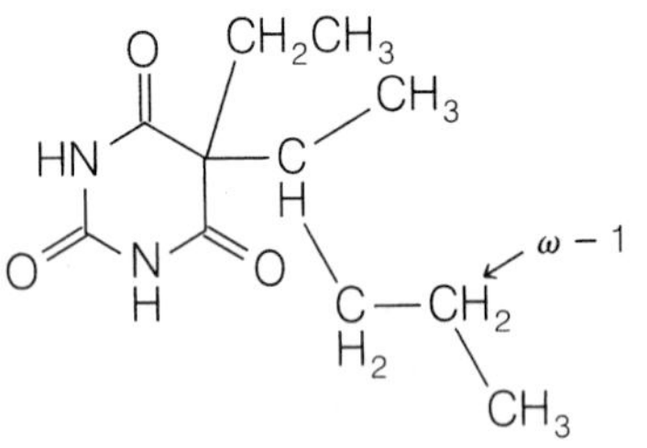

Pentobarbital

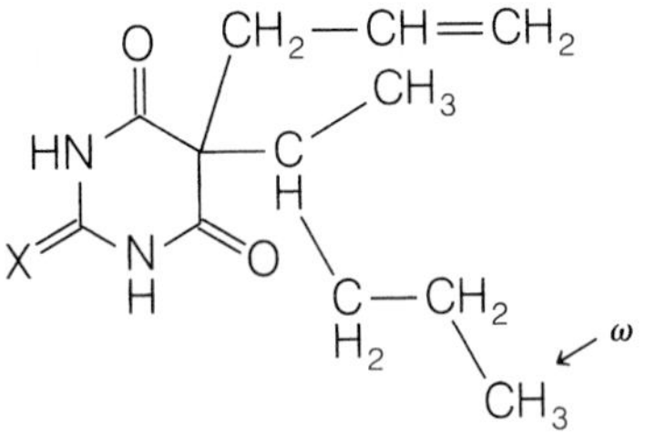

Thiamylal X = S
Secobarbital X = O

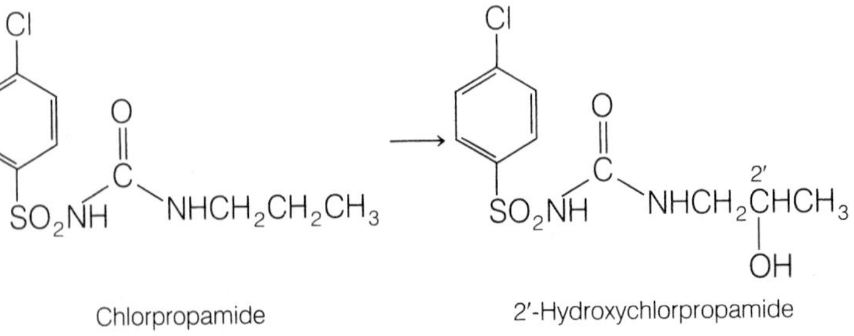

Chlorpropamide   2'-Hydroxychlorpropamide

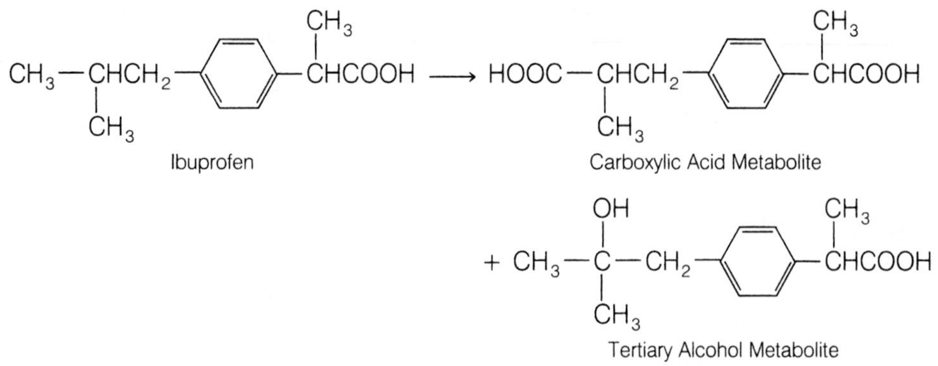

Ibuprofen → Carboxylic Acid Metabolite

+ Tertiary Alcohol Metabolite

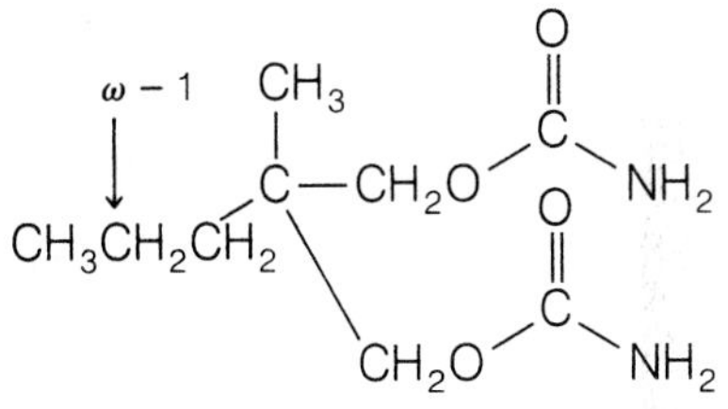

Meprobamate 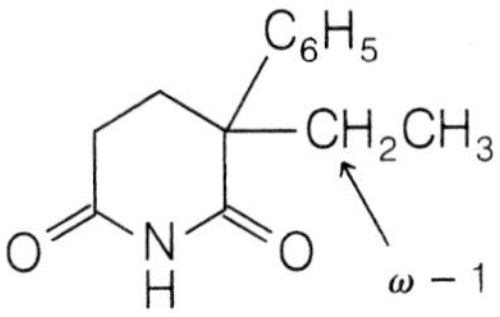   Glutethimide 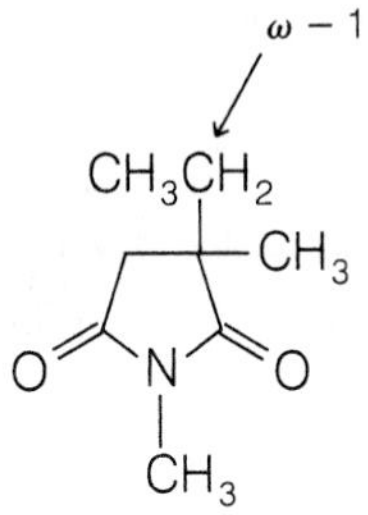   Ethosuximide 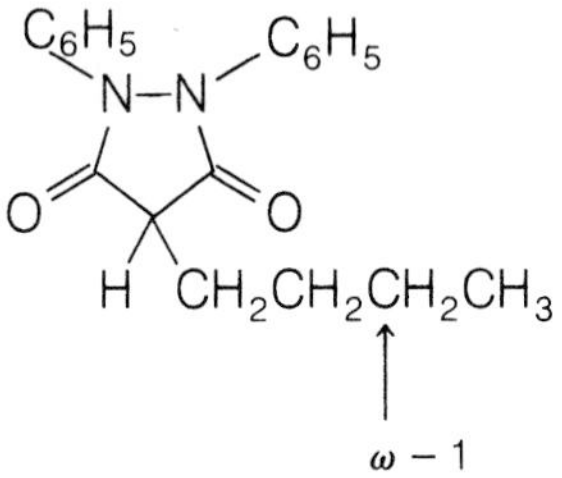   Phenylbutazone

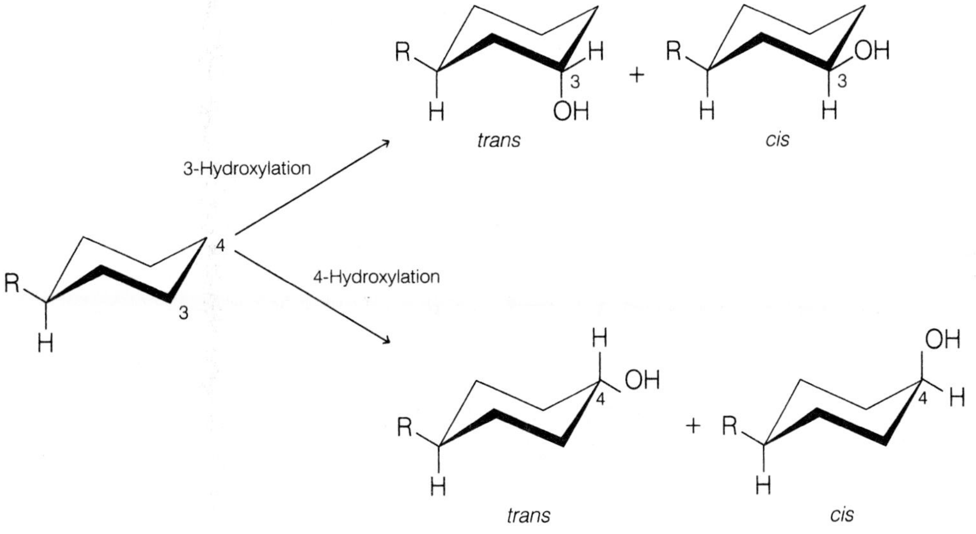

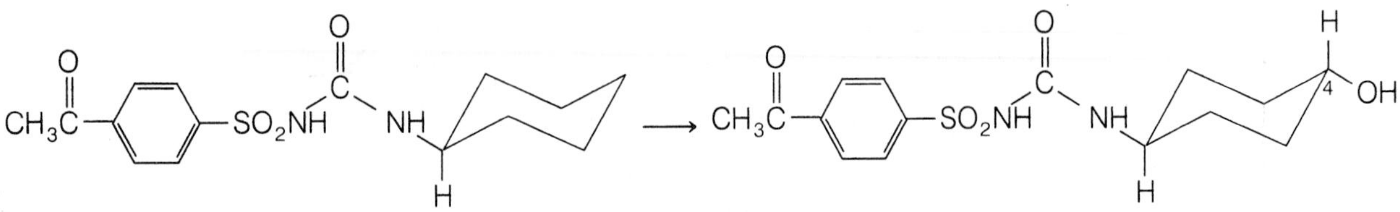

3-Hydroxylation

trans + *cis*

4-Hydroxylation

trans + *cis*

Acetohexamide → *trans*-4-Hydroxyacetohexamide

The stereochemistry of the hydroxylated centers in the two metabolites has not been clearly established. Biotransformation of the antihypertensive agent minoxidil (Loniten) yields the 4'-hydroxypiperidyl metabolite. In the dog, this product is a major urinary metabolite (29 to 47%), whereas in humans it is detected in small amounts (~3%).[157, 158]

Oxidation Involving Carbon–Heteroatom Systems

Nitrogen and oxygen functionalities are commonly found in most drugs and foreign compounds; sulfur functionalities occur only occasionally. Metabolic oxidation of carbon–nitrogen, carbon–oxygen, and carbon–sulfur systems principally involves two basic types of biotransformation processes:

1. Hydroxylation of the α-carbon atom attached directly to the heteroatom (N, O, S). The resulting intermediate is often unstable and decomposes with the cleavage of the carbon–heteroatom bond:

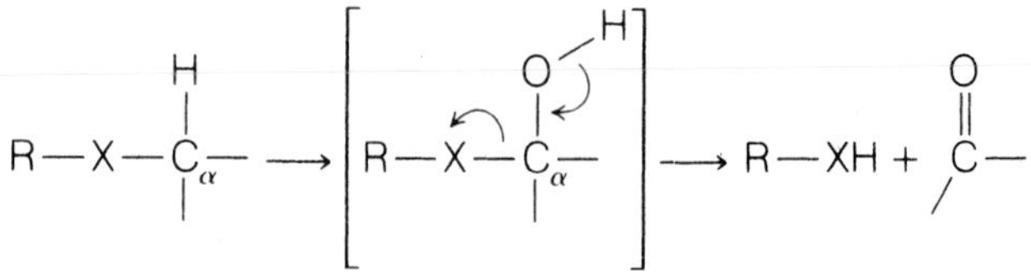

Where X = N,O,S   Usually Unstable

Oxidative N-, O-, and S-dealkylation as well as oxidative deamination reactions fall under this mechanistic pathway.

2. Hydroxylation or oxidation of the heteroatom (N, S only, e.g., N-hydroxylation, *N*-oxide formation, sulfoxide, and sulfone formation).

Several structural features frequently determine which pathway will predominate, especially in carbon–nitrogen systems. Metabolism of some nitrogen-containing compounds is complicated by the fact that carbon- or nitrogen-

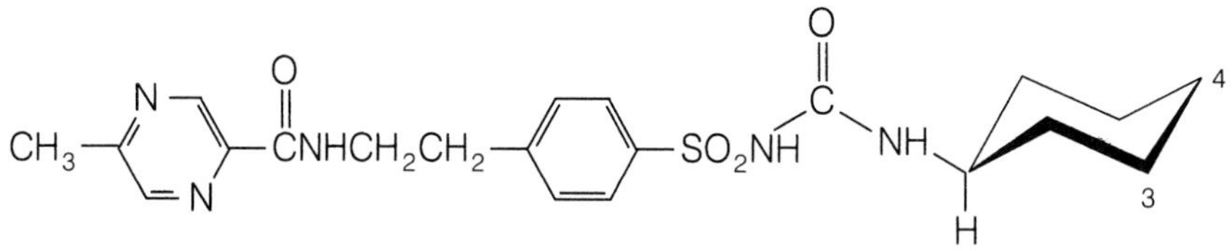

Glipizide

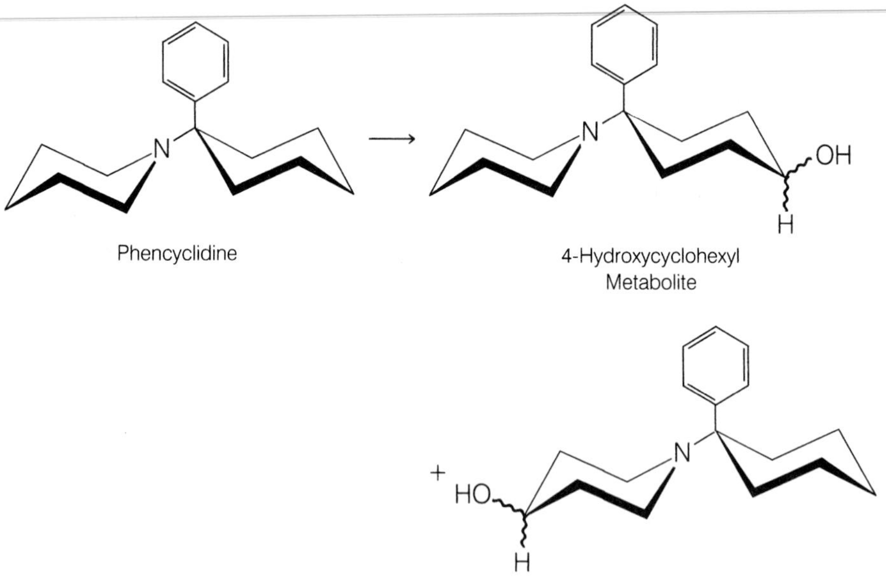

Phencyclidine

4-Hydroxycyclohexyl Metabolite

4-Hydroxypiperidyl Metabolite

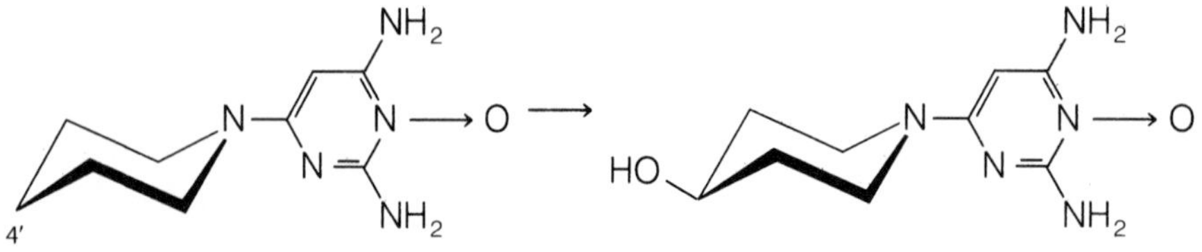

Minoxidil

4'-Hydroxyminoxidil

hydroxylated products may undergo secondary reactions to form other, more complex metabolic products (e.g., oxime, nitrone, nitroso, imino). Other oxidative processes that do not fall under these two basic categories are discussed individually in the appropriate carbon–heteroatom section. The metabolism of carbon–nitrogen systems will be discussed first, followed by the metabolism of carbon–oxygen and carbon–sulfur systems.

OXIDATION INVOLVING CARBON–NITROGEN SYSTEMS

Metabolism of nitrogen functionalities (e.g., amines, amides) is important because such functional groups are found in many natural products (e.g., morphine, cocaine, nicotine) and in numerous important drugs (e.g., phenothiazines, antihistamines, tricyclic antidepressants, β-adrenergic agents, sympathomimetic phenylethylamines, benzodiazepines).[159] The following discussion divides nitrogen-containing compounds into three basic classes:

1. Aliphatic (primary, secondary, and tertiary) and alicyclic (secondary and tertiary) amines
2. Aromatic and heterocyclic nitrogen compounds
3. Amides

The susceptibility of each class of these nitrogen compounds to either α-carbon hydroxylation or N-oxidation and the metabolic products that are formed are discussed.

The hepatic enzymes responsible for carrying out α-carbon hydroxylation reactions are the cytochrome P-450 mixed-function oxidases. The N-hydroxylation or N-oxidation reactions, however, appear to be catalyzed not only by cytochrome P-450 but also by a second class of hepatic mixed-function oxidases called *amine oxidases* (sometimes called *N-oxidases*).[160] These enzymes are NADPH-dependent flavoproteins and do not contain cytochrome P-450.[161, 162] They require NADPH and molecular oxygen to carry out N-oxidation.

Tertiary Aliphatic and Alicyclic Amines.

The oxidative removal of alkyl groups (particularly methyl groups) from tertiary aliphatic and alicyclic amines is carried out by hepatic cytochrome P-450 mixed-function oxidase enzymes. This reaction is commonly referred to as *oxidative N-dealkylation*.[163] The initial step involves α-carbon hydroxylation to form a carbinolamine intermediate, which is unstable and undergoes spontaneous heterolytic cleavage of the C–N bond to give a secondary amine and a carbonyl moiety (alde-

hyde or ketone).[164, 165] In general, small alkyl groups, such as methyl, ethyl, and isopropyl, are removed rapidly.[163] N-dealkylation of the *t*-butyl group is not possible by the carbinolamine pathway because α-carbon hydroxylation cannot occur. The first alkyl group from a tertiary amine is removed more rapidly than the second alkyl group. In some instances, bisdealkylation of the tertiary aliphatic amine to the corresponding primary aliphatic amine occurs very slowly.[163] For example, the tertiary amine imipramine (Tofranil) is monodemethylated to desmethylimipramine (desipramine).[166, 167] This major plasma metabolite is pharmacologically active in humans and contributes substantially to the antidepressant activity of the parent drug.[168] Very little of the bisdemethylated metabolite of imipramine is detected. In contrast, the local anesthetic and antiarrhythmic agent lidocaine is metabolized extensively by N-deethylation to both monoethylglycylxylidine and glycyl-2,6-xylidine in humans.[169, 170]

Numerous other tertiary aliphatic amine drugs are metabolized principally by oxidative N-dealkylation. Some of these include the antiarrhythmic disopyramide (Norpace),[171, 172] the antiestrogenic agent tamoxifen (Nolvadex),[173] diphenhydramine (Benadryl),[174, 175] chlorpromazine (Thorazine),[176, 177] and (+)-α-propoxyphene (Darvon).[178] When the tertiary amine contains several different substituents capable of undergoing dealkylation, the smaller alkyl group is removed preferentially and more rapidly. For example, in benzphetamine (Didrex), the methyl group is removed much more rapidly than the benzyl moiety.[179]

An interesting cyclization reaction occurs with methadone on N-demethylation. The demethylated metabolite normethadone undergoes spontaneous cyclization to form the enamine metabolite 2-ethylidene-1,5-dimethyl-3,3-diphenylpyrrolidine (EDDP).[180] Subsequent N-demethylation of EDDP and isomerization of the double bond leads to 2-ethyl-5-methyl-3,3-diphenyl-1-pyrroline (EMDP).

Many times, bisdealkylation of a tertiary amine leads to the corresponding primary aliphatic amine metabolite, which is susceptible to further oxidation. For example, the bisdesmethyl metabolite of the H_1-histamine antagonist brompheniramine (Dimetane) undergoes oxidative deamination and further oxidation to the corresponding propionic acid metabolite.[181] Oxidative deamination is discussed in greater detail when we examine the metabolic reactions of secondary and primary amines.

Like their aliphatic counterparts, alicyclic tertiary amines are susceptible to oxidative N-dealkylation reactions. For example, the analgesic meperidine (Demerol) is metabolized

| Tertiary Amine | Carbinolamine | Secondary Amine | Carbonyl Moiety (aldehyde or ketone) |

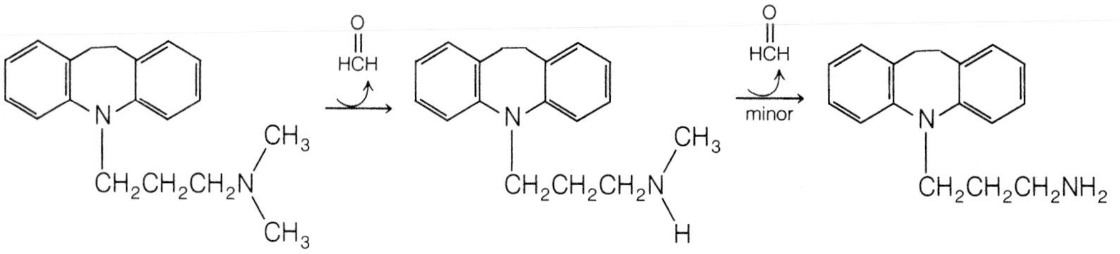

Imipramine → Desmethylimipramine (desipramine) → Bisdesmethylimipramine

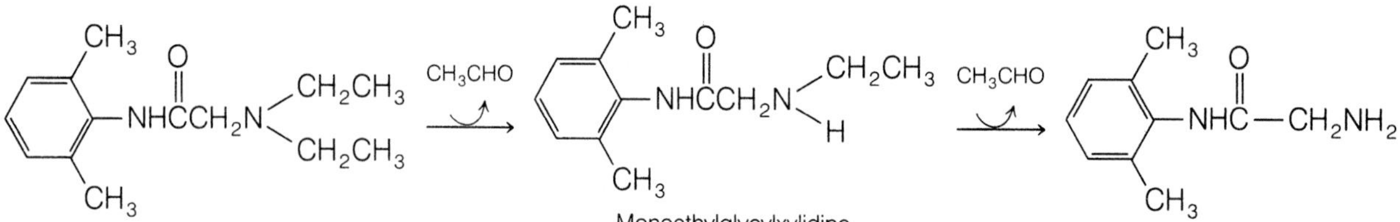

Lidocaine → Monoethylglycylxylidine (MEGX) → Glycyl-2,6-xylidine

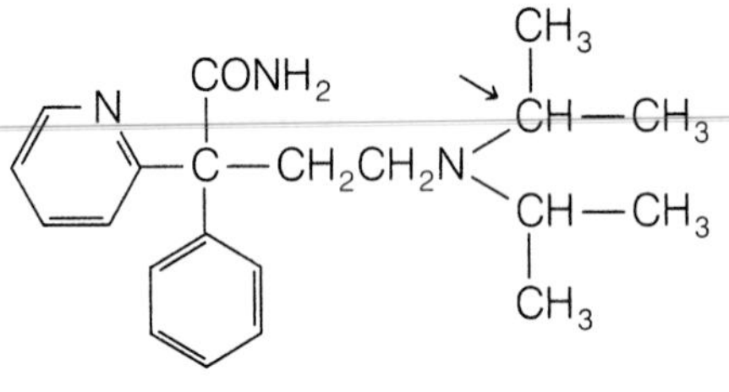

Disopyramide

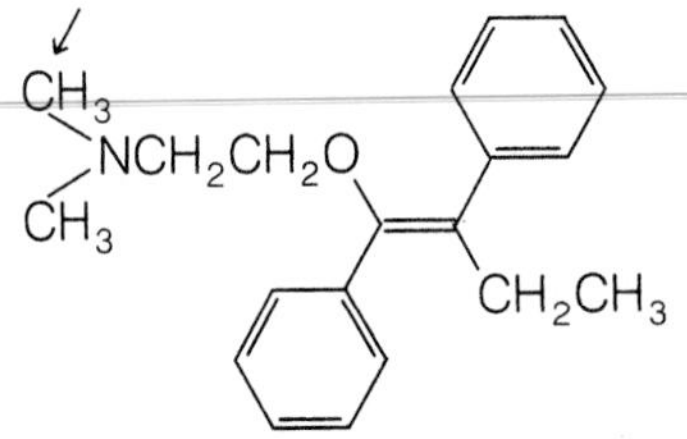

Tamoxifen

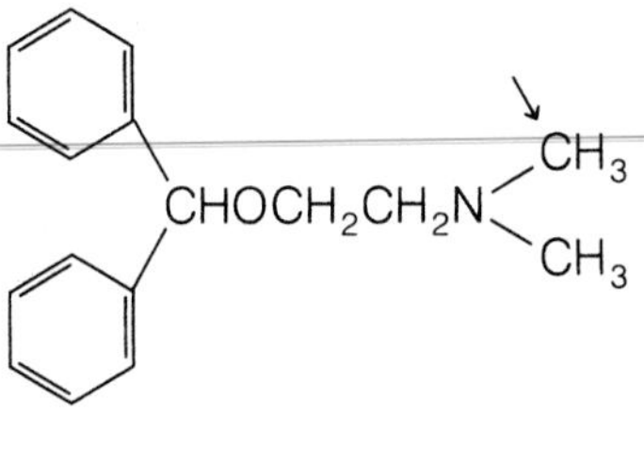

Diphenhydramine

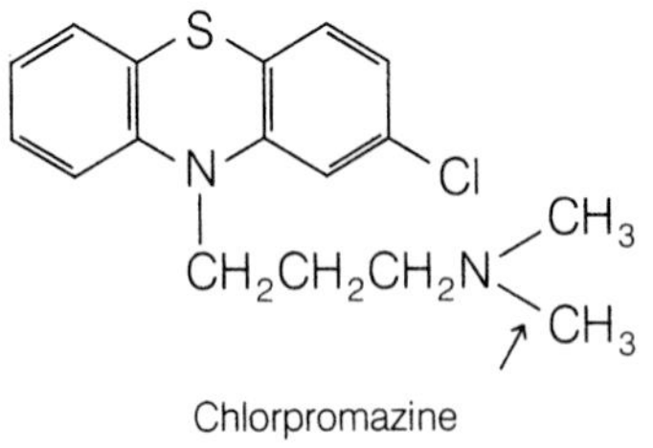

Chlorpromazine

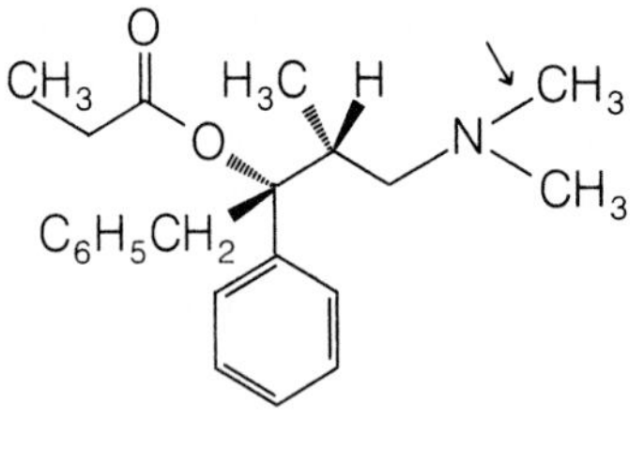

(+)-α-Propoxyphene

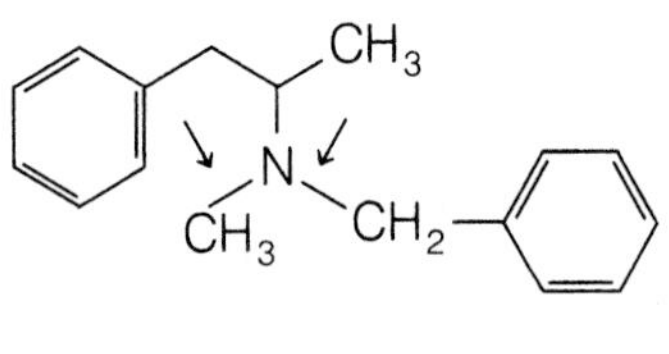

Benzphetamine (N-demethylation and N-debenzylation)

principally by this pathway to yield normeperidine as a major plasma metabolite in humans.[182] Morphine, *N*-ethylnormorphine, and dextromethorphan also undergo some N-dealkylation.[183]

Direct N-dealkylation of *t*-butyl groups, as discussed above, is not possible by the α-carbon hydroxylation pathway. In vitro studies indicate, however, that *N-t*-butylnor-

chlorocyclizine is, indeed, metabolized to significant amounts of norchlorocyclizine, whereby the *t*-butyl group is lost.[184] Careful studies showed that the *t*-butyl group is removed by initial hydroxylation of one of the methyl groups of the *t*-butyl moiety to the carbinol or alcohol product.[185] Further oxidation generates the corresponding carboxylic acid that, on decarboxylation, forms the *N*-isopropyl deriva-

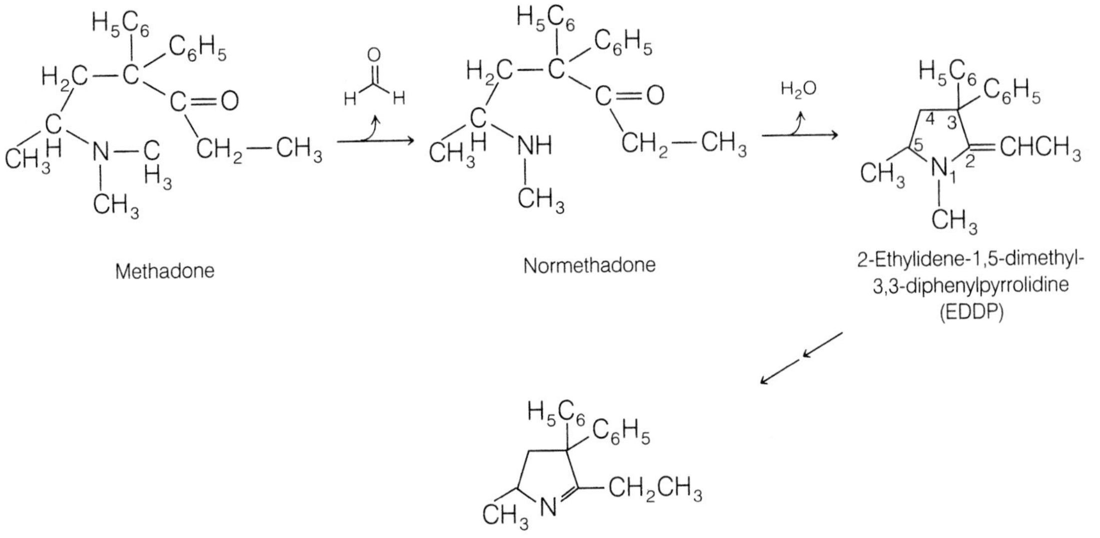

Methadone → Normethadone → 2-Ethylidene-1,5-dimethyl-3,3-diphenylpyrrolidine (EDDP)

2-Ethyl-5-methyl-3,3-diphenyl-1-pyrroline (EMDP)

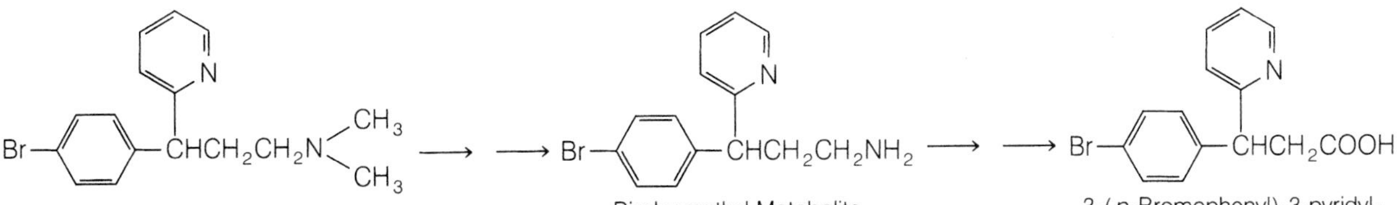

Brompheniramine → Bisdesmethyl Metabolite → 3-(*p*-Bromophenyl)-3-pyridyl-propionic acid

tive. The *N*-isopropyl intermediate is dealkylated by the normal α-carbon hydroxylation (i.e., carbinolamine) pathway to give norchlorocyclizine and acetone. Whether this is a general method for the loss of *t*-butyl groups from amines is still unclear. Indirect N-dealkylation of *t*-butyl groups is not observed significantly. The *N*-*t*-butyl group present in many β-adrenergic antagonists, such as terbutaline and salbutamol, remains intact and does not appear to undergo any significant metabolism.[186]

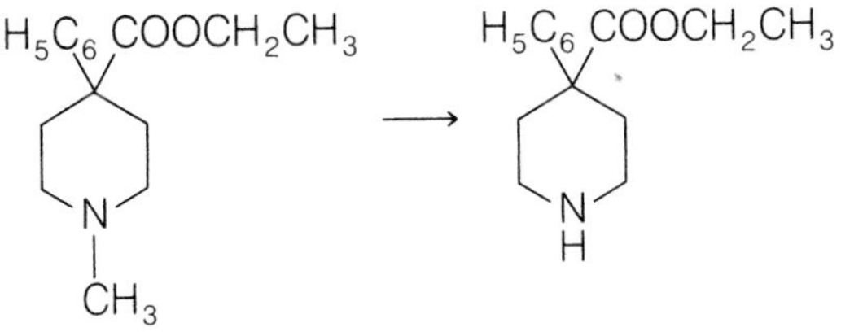

Meperidine → Normeperidine

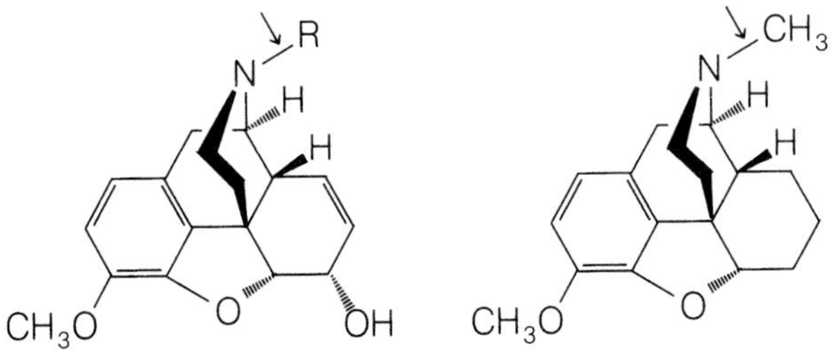

Morphine   R = CH₃
N-Ethylnormorphine   R = CH₂CH₃

Dextromethorphan

Alicyclic tertiary amines often generate lactam metabolites by α-carbon hydroxylation reactions. For example, the tobacco alkaloid nicotine is hydroxylated initially at the ring carbon atom α to the nitrogen to yield a carbinolamine intermediate. Furthermore, enzymatic oxidation of this cyclic carbinolamine generates the lactam metabolite cotinine.[187, 188]

Formation of lactam metabolites also has been reported to occur to a minor extent for the antihistamine cyproheptadine (Periactin)[189, 190] and the antiemetic diphenidol (Vontrol).[191]

N-oxidation of tertiary amines occurs with several drugs.[192] The true extent of *N*-oxide formation often is complicated by the susceptibility of *N*-oxides to undergo in vivo reduction back to the parent tertiary amine. Tertiary amines such as H₁-histamine antagonists (e.g., orphenadrine, tripelenamine), phenothiazines (e.g., chlorpromazine), tricyclic antidepressants (e.g., imipramine), and narcotic analgesics (e.g., morphine, codeine, and meperidine) reportedly form *N*-oxide products. In some instances, *N*-oxides possess pharmacological activity.[193] A comparison of imipramine *N*-oxide with imipramine indicates that the *N*-oxide itself possesses antidepressant and cardiovascular activity similar to that of the parent drug.[194, 195]

Secondary and Primary Amines.

Secondary amines (either parent compounds or metabolites) are susceptible to oxidative N-dealkylation, oxidative deamination, and N-oxidation reactions.[163, 196] As in tertiary amines, N-dealkylation of secondary amines proceeds by the carbinolamine path-

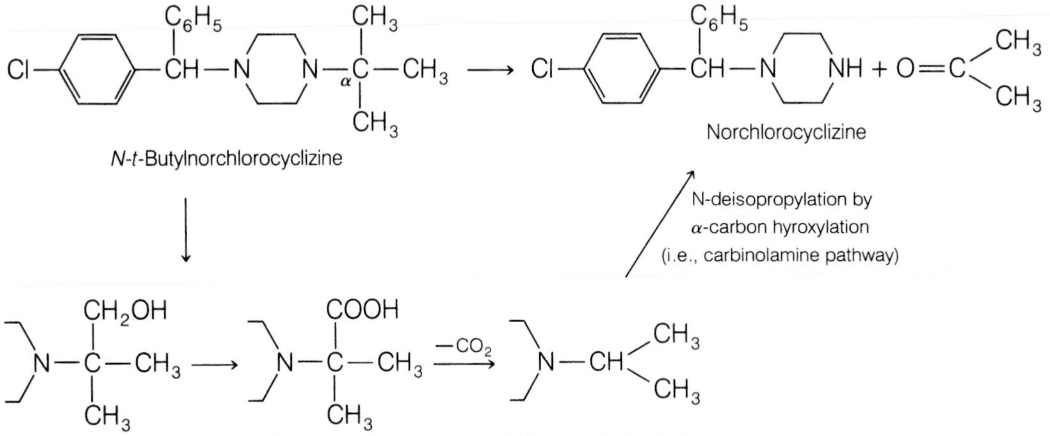

N-t-Butylnorchlorocyclizine

Norchlorocyclizine

N-deisopropylation by
α-carbon hyroxylation
(i.e., carbinolamine pathway)

Alcohol or Carbinol

Carboxylic Acid

N-Isopropyl Metabolite

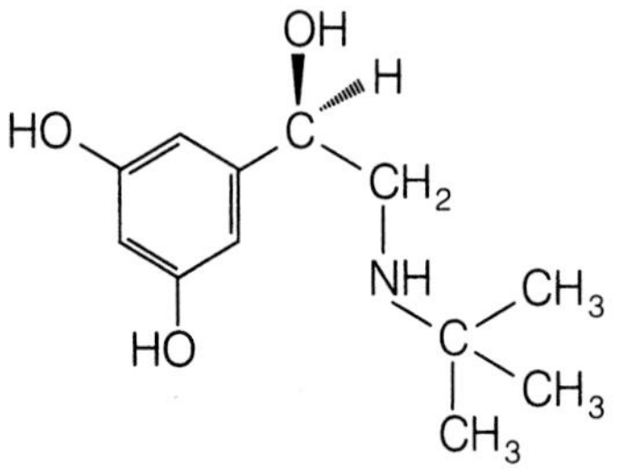

Terbutaline

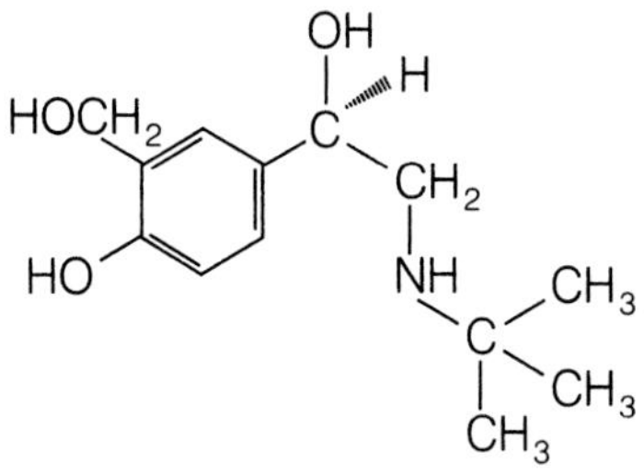

Salbutamol

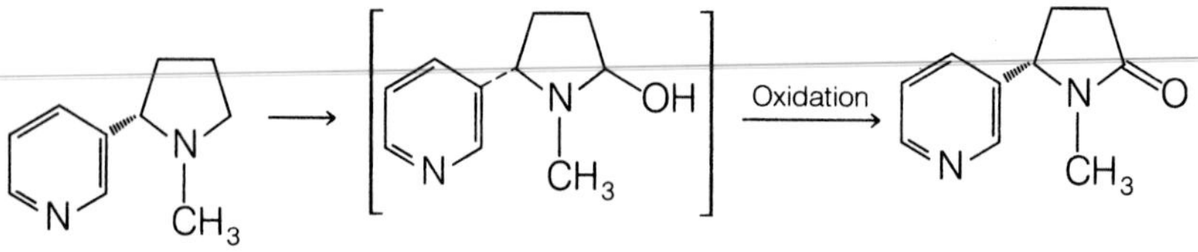

Nicotine

Carbinolamine

Cotinine

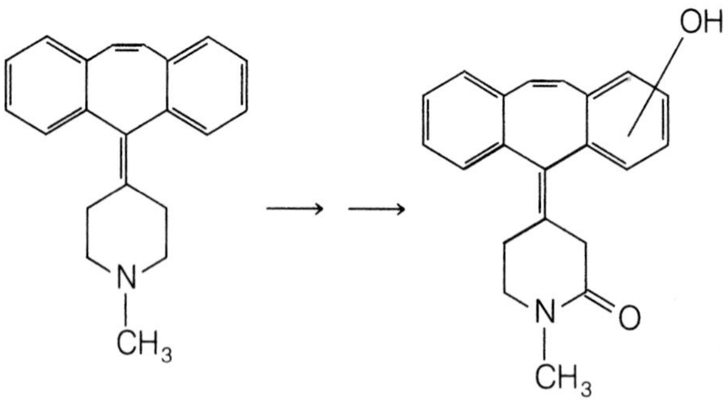

Cyproheptadine

Lactam Metabolite

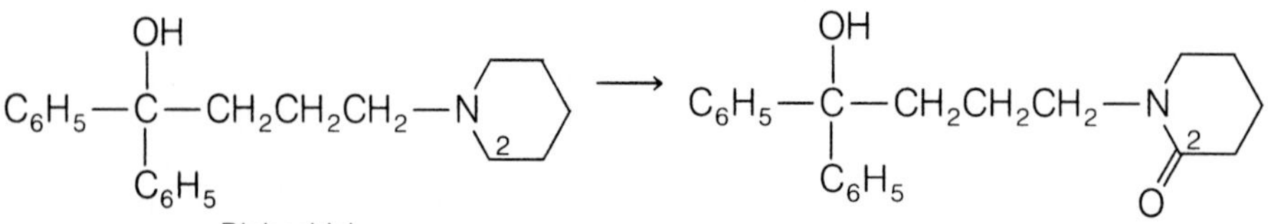

Diphenidol

2-Oxodiphenidol

way. Dealkylation of secondary amines gives rise to the corresponding primary amine metabolite. For example, the α-adrenergic blockers propranolol[46, 47] and oxprenolol[197] undergo N-deisopropylation to the corresponding primary amines. N-dealkylation appears to be a significant biotransformation pathway for the secondary amine drugs methamphetamine[198, 199] and ketamine,[200, 201] yielding amphetamine and norketamine, respectively.

The primary amine metabolites formed from oxidative dealkylation are susceptible to *oxidative deamination*. This process is similar to N-dealkylation, in that it involves an initial α-carbon hydroxylation reaction to form a carbinolamine intermediate, which then undergoes subsequent carbon–nitrogen cleavage to the carbonyl metabolite and ammonia. If α-carbon hydroxylation cannot occur, then oxidative deamination is not possible. For example, deamination does not occur for norketamine because α-carbon hydroxylation cannot take place.[200, 201] With methamphetamine, oxidative deamination of primary amine metabolite amphetamine produces phenylacetone.[198, 199]

In general, dealkylation of secondary amines is believed to occur before oxidative deamination. Some evidence indicates, however, that this may not always be true. Direct deamination of the secondary amine also has occurred. For example, in addition to undergoing deamination through its desisopropyl primary amine metabolite, propranolol can undergo a direct oxidative deamination reaction (also by α-carbon hydroxylation) to yield the aldehyde metabolite and isopropylamine (Fig. 4-9).[202] How much direct oxidative deamination contributes to the metabolism of secondary amines remains unclear.

Primary Amine   Carbinolamine   Carbonyl   Ammonia

Some secondary alicyclic amines, like their tertiary amine analogues, are metabolized to their corresponding lactam derivatives. For example, the anorectic agent phenmetrazine (Preludin) is metabolized principally to the lactam product 3-oxophenmetrazine.[203] In humans, this lactam metabolite is a major urinary product. Methylphenidate (Ritalin) also reportedly yields a lactam metabolite, 6-oxoritalinic acid, by oxidation of its hydrolyzed metabolite, ritalinic acid, in humans.[204]

Metabolic N-oxidation of secondary aliphatic and alicyclic amines leads to several N-oxygenated products.[196] N-hydroxylation of secondary amines generates the corresponding *N*-hydroxylamine metabolites. Often, these hydroxylamine products are susceptible to further oxidation (either spontaneous or enzymatic) to the corresponding nitrone derivatives. *N*-benzylamphetamine undergoes metabolism to both the corresponding *N*-hydroxylamine and the nitrone metabolites.[205] In humans, the nitrone metabolite of phenmetrazine (Preludin), found in the urine, is believed to be formed by further oxidation of the *N*-hydroxylamine intermediate *N*-hydroxyphenmetrazine.[203] Importantly,

Propranolol   Oxprenolol

Methamphetamine   Amphetamine   Phenylacetone

Ketamine   Norketamine

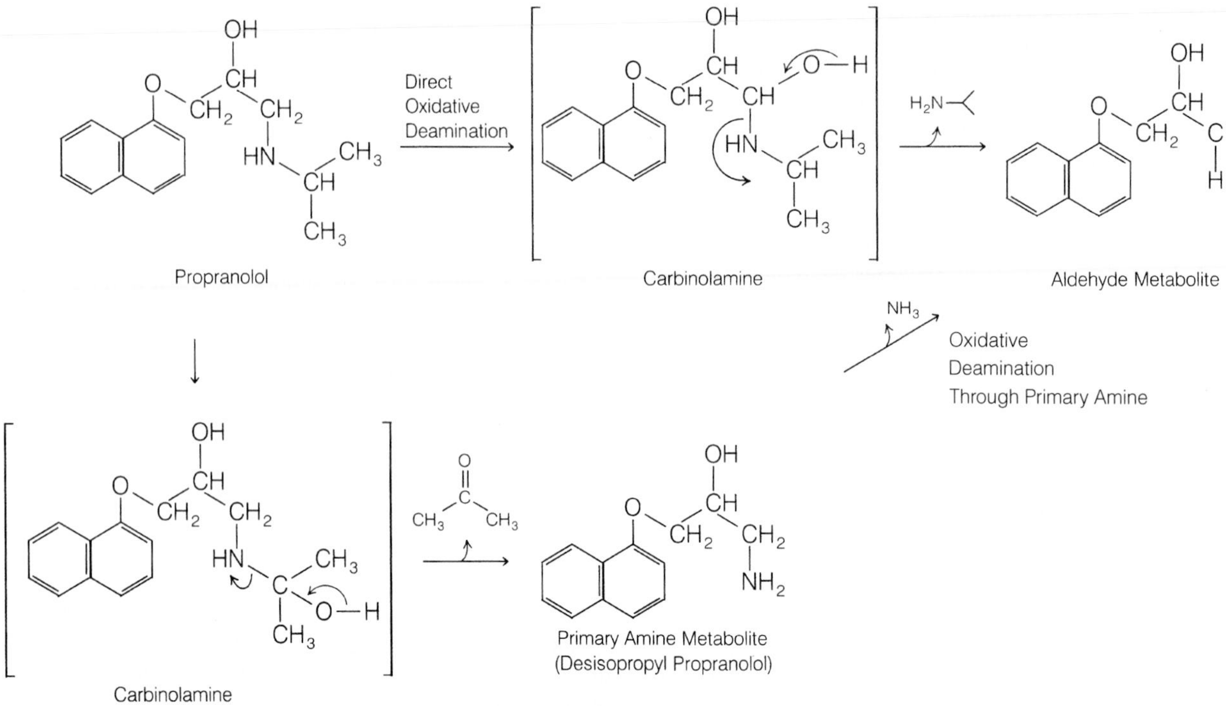

Figure 4–9 ■ Metabolism of propranolol to its aldehyde metabolite by direct deamination of the parent compound and by deamination of its primary amine metabolite, desisopropyl propranolol.

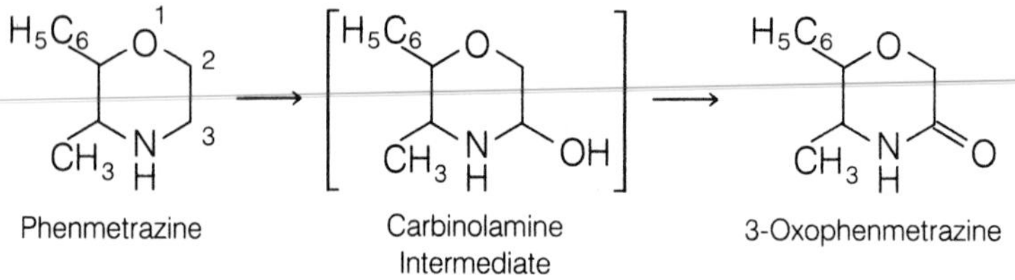

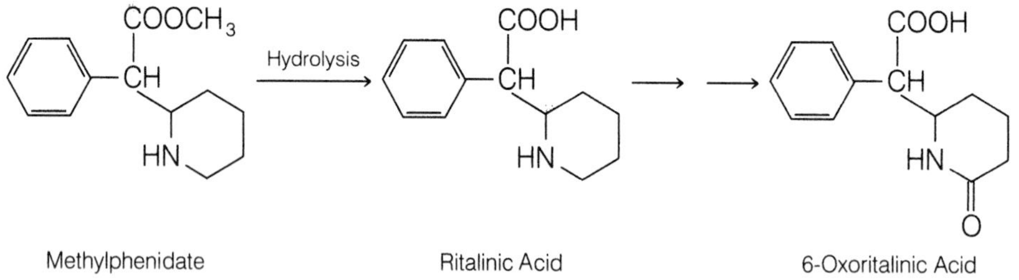

much less N-oxidation occurs for secondary amines than oxidative dealkylation and deamination.

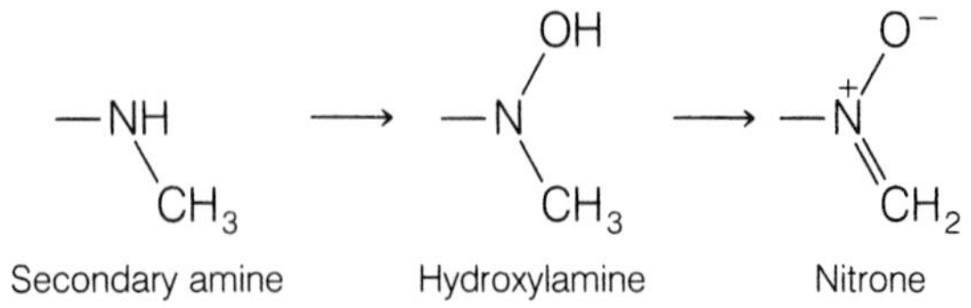

Primary aliphatic amines (whether parent drugs or metab-olites) are biotransformed by oxidative deamination (through the carbinolamine pathway) or by N-oxidation. In general, oxidative deamination of most exogenous primary amines is carried out by the mixed-function oxidases discussed above. Endogenous primary amines (e.g., dopamine, norepinephrine, tryptamine, and serotonin) and xenobiotics based on the structures of these endogenous neurotransmitters are metabolized, however, via oxidative deamination by a specialized family of enzymes called *monoamine oxidases* (MAOs).[206]

MAO is a flavin (FAD)-dependent enzyme found in two isozyme forms, MAO-A and MAO-B, and widely distributed in both the CNS and peripheral organs. In contrast, cytochrome P-450 exists in a wide variety of isozyme forms and is an NADP-dependent system. Also the greatest variety of CYP isozymes, at least the ones associated with the metabolism of xenobiotics, are found mostly in the liver and intestinal mucosa. MAO-A and MAO-B are coded by two genes, both on the X-chromosome and have about 70% amino acid sequence homology. Another difference between the CYP and MAO families is cellular location. CYP enzymes are found on the endoplasmic reticulum of the cell's cytosol, whereas the MAO enzymes are on the outer mitochondrial membrane. In addition to the xenobiotics illustrated in the reaction schemes, other drugs metabolized by the MAO system include phenylephrine, propranolol, timolol and other β-adrenergic agonists and antagonists and a variety of phenylethylamines.[206]

Structural features, especially the α substituents of the primary amine, often determine whether carbon or nitrogen oxidation will occur. For example, compare amphetamine with its α-methyl homologue phentermine. In amphetamine, α-carbon hydroxylation can occur to form the carbinolamine intermediate, which is converted to the oxidatively deaminated product phenylacetone.[67] With phentermine, α-carbon hydroxylation is not possible and precludes oxidative deamination for this drug. Consequently, phentermine would be expected to undergo N-oxidation readily. In humans, p-hydroxylation and N-oxidation are the main pathways for biotransformation of phentermine.[207]

Indeed, N-hydroxyphentermine is an important (5%) urinary metabolite in humans.[207] As discussed below, N-hydroxylamine metabolites are susceptible to further oxidation to yield other N-oxygenated products.

Xenobiotics, such as the hallucinogenic agents mescaline[208, 209] and 1-(2,5-dimethoxy-4-methylphenyl)-2-aminopropane (DOM or "STP"),[210, 211] are oxidatively deaminated. Primary amine metabolites arising from N-

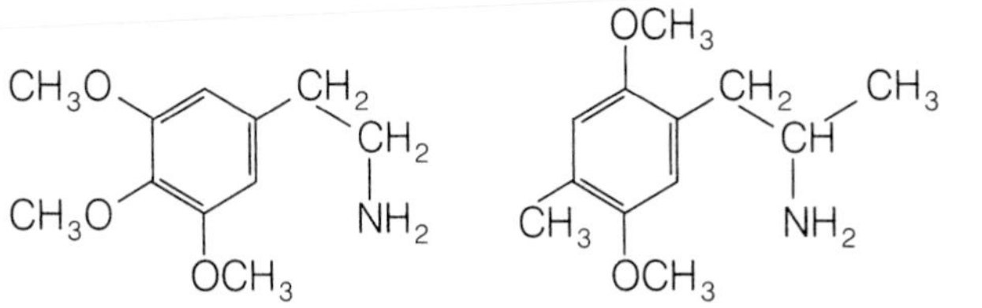

Mescaline

1-(2,5-Dimethoxy-4-methylphenyl)-
2-aminopropane
DOM or "STP"

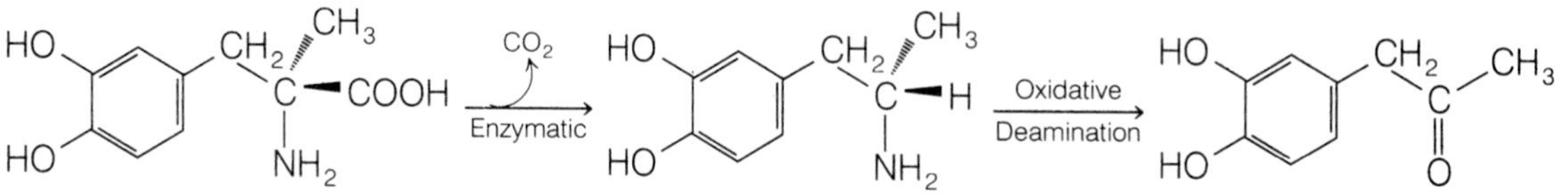

$S(-)$-α-Methyldopa $S(+)$-α-Methyldopamine   3,4-Dihydroxyphenylacetone

dealkylation or decarboxylation reactions also undergo deamination. The example of the bisdesmethyl primary amine metabolite derived from bromopheniramine is discussed above (see section on tertiary aliphatic and alicyclic amines).[181] In addition, many tertiary aliphatic amines (e.g., antihistamines) and secondary aliphatic amines (e.g., propranolol) are dealkylated to their corresponding primary amine metabolites, which are amenable to oxidative deamination. $(S)(+)$-α-Methyldopamine resulting from decarboxylation of the antihypertensive agent $(S)(-)$-α-methyldopa (Aldomet) is deaminated to the corresponding ketone metabolite 3,4-dihydroxyphenylacetone.[212] In humans, this ketone is a major urinary metabolite.

The N-hydroxylation reaction is not restricted to α-substituted primary amines such as phentermine. Amphetamine has been observed to undergo some N-hydroxylation in vitro to *N*-hydroxyamphetamine.[213, 214] *N*-Hydroxyamphetamine is, however, susceptible to further conversion to the imine or oxidation to the oxime intermediate. Note that the oxime intermediate arising from this N-oxidation pathway can undergo hydrolytic cleavage to yield phenylacetone, the same product obtained by the α-carbon hydroxylation (carbi-

nolamine) pathway.[215, 216] Thus, amphetamine may be converted to phenylacetone through either the α-carbon hydroxylation or the N-oxidation pathway. The debate concerning the relative importance of the two pathways is ongoing.[217-219] The consensus, however, is that both metabolic pathways (carbon and nitrogen oxidation) are probably operative. Whether α-carbon or nitrogen oxidation predominates in the metabolism of amphetamine appears to be species dependent.

In primary aliphatic amines, such as phentermine,[207] chlorphentermine (*p*-chlorphentermine),[219] and amantadine,[220] N-oxidation appears to be the major biotransformation pathway because α-carbon hydroxylation cannot occur. In humans, chlorphentermine is N-hydroxylated extensively. About 30% of a dose of chlorphentermine is found in the urine (48 hours) as *N*-hydroxychlorphentermine (free and conjugated) and an additional 18% as other products of N-oxidation (presumably the nitroso and nitro metabolites).[219] In general, *N*-hydroxylamines are chemically unstable and susceptible to spontaneous or enzymatic oxidation to the nitroso and nitro derivatives. For example, the *N*-hydroxylamine metabolite of phentermine undergoes further oxida-

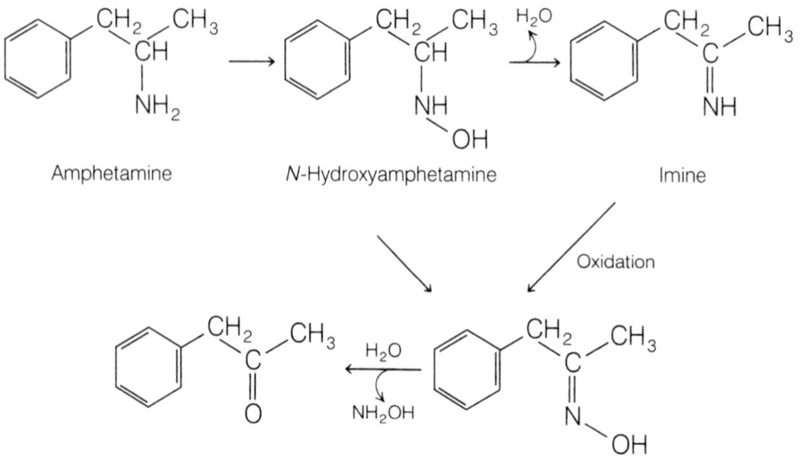

Amphetamine   *N*-Hydroxyamphetamine   Imine

Oxidation

Phenylacetone   Oxime

tion to the nitroso and nitro products.[207] The antiviral and antiparkinsonian agent amantadine (Symmetrel) reportedly undergoes N-oxidation to yield the corresponding *N*-hydroxy and nitroso metabolites in vitro.[220]

Aromatic Amines and Heterocyclic Nitrogen Compounds. The biotransformation of aromatic amines parallels the carbon and nitrogen oxidation reactions seen for aliphatic amines.[221–223] For tertiary aromatic amines, such as *N,N*-dimethylaniline, oxidative N-dealkylation as well as *N*-oxide formation take place.[224] Secondary aromatic amines may undergo N-dealkylation or N-hydroxylation to give the corresponding *N*-hydroxylamines. Further oxidation of the *N*-hydroxylamine leads to nitrone products, which in turn may be hydrolyzed to primary hydroxylamines.[225] Tertiary and secondary aromatic amines are encountered rarely in medicinal agents. In contrast, primary aromatic amines are found in many drugs and are often generated from enzymatic reduction of aromatic nitro compounds, reductive cleavage of azo compounds, and hydrolysis of aromatic amides.

N-oxidation of primary aromatic amines generates the *N*-hydroxylamine metabolite. One such case is aniline, which is metabolized to the corresponding *N*-hydroxy product.[223] Oxidation of the hydroxylamine derivative to the nitroso derivative also can occur. When one considers primary aromatic amine drugs or metabolites, N-oxidation constitutes only a minor pathway in comparison with other biotransformation pathways, such as N-acetylation and aromatic hydroxylation, in humans. Some N-oxygenated metabolites have been reported, however. For example, the antileprotic agent dapsone and its N-acetylated metabolite are metabolized significantly to their corresponding *N*-hydroxylamine derivatives.[226] The *N*-hydroxy metabolites are further conjugated with glucuronic acid.

Methemoglobinemia toxicity is caused by several aromatic amines, including aniline and dapsone, and is a result of the bioconversion of the aromatic amine to its *N*-hydroxy derivative. Apparently, the *N*-hydroxylamine oxidizes the Fe^{2+} form of hemoglobin to its Fe^{3+} form. This oxidized (Fe^{3+}) state of hemoglobin (called *methemoglobin* or *ferrihemoglobin*) can no longer transport oxygen, which leads to serious hypoxia or anemia, a unique type of chemical suffocation.[227]

Diverse aromatic amines (especially azoamino dyes) are known to be carcinogenic. N-oxidation plays an important role in bioactivating these aromatic amines to potentially reactive electrophilic species that covalently bind to cellular protein, DNA, or RNA. A well-studied example is the carcinogenic agent *N*-methyl-4-aminoazobenzene.[228, 229] N-oxidation of this compound leads to the corresponding hydroxylamine, which undergoes sulfate conjugation. Because of the good leaving-group ability of the sulfate (SO_4^{2-}) anion, this conjugate can ionize spontaneously to form a highly reactive, resonance-stabilized nitrenium species. Covalent adducts between this species and DNA, RNA, and proteins have been characterized.[230, 231] The sulfate ester is believed to be the ultimate carcinogenic species. Thus, the example indicates that certain aromatic amines can be bioactivated to reactive intermediates by N-hydroxylation and *O*-sulfate conjugation. Whether primary hydroxylamines can be bioactivated similarly is unclear. In addition, it is not known if this biotoxification pathway plays any substantial role in the toxicity of aromatic amine drugs.

N-oxidation of the nitrogen atoms present in aromatic heterocyclic moieties of many drugs occurs to a minor extent. Clearly, in humans, N-oxidation of the folic acid antagonist trimethoprim (Proloprim, Trimpex) has yielded approximately equal amounts of the isomeric 1-*N*-oxide and 3-*N*-oxide as minor metabolites.[232] The pyridinyl nitrogen atom present in nicotinine (the major metabolite of nicotine) undergoes oxidation to yield the corresponding *N*-oxide metabolite.[233] Another therapeutic agent that has been observed to undergo formation of an *N*-oxide metabolite is metronidazole.[234]

Phentermine   Chlorphentermine   Amantadine

Chlorphentermine → *N*-Hydroxychlorphentermine → Nitroso Metabolite → Nitro Metabolite

$$RCH_2NHOH \longrightarrow RCH_2-N{=}O \longrightarrow RCH_2-\overset{+}{N}\underset{O^-}{\overset{O}{\diagdown}}$$

Hydroxylamine   Nitroso   Nitro

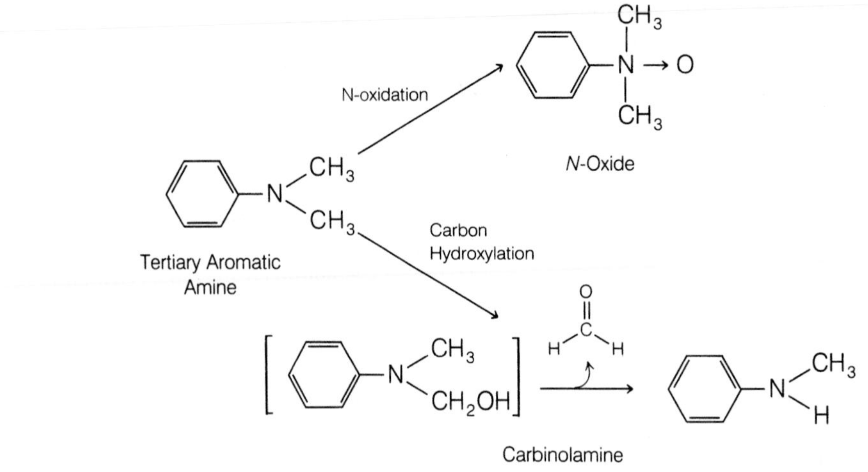

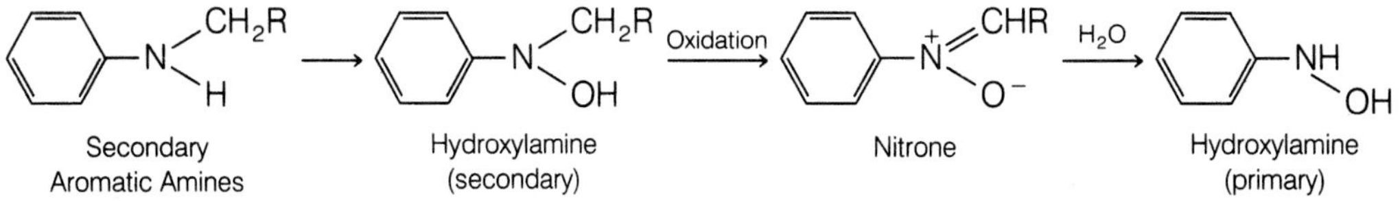

N-Oxide

Tertiary Aromatic Amine

Carbinolamine

Secondary Aromatic Amines

Hydroxylamine (secondary)

Nitrone

Hydroxylamine (primary)

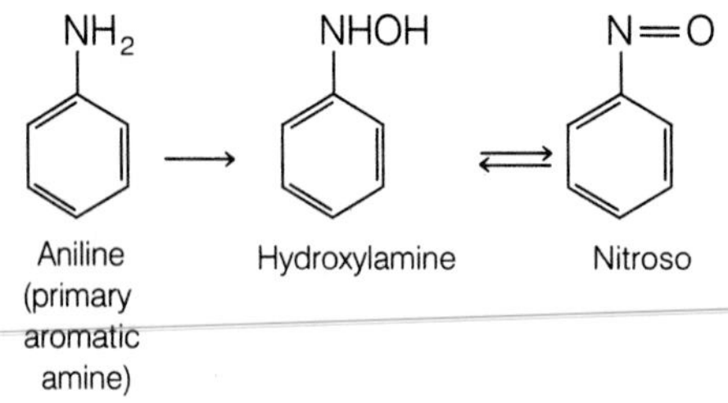

Aniline (primary aromatic amine)

Hydroxylamine

Nitroso

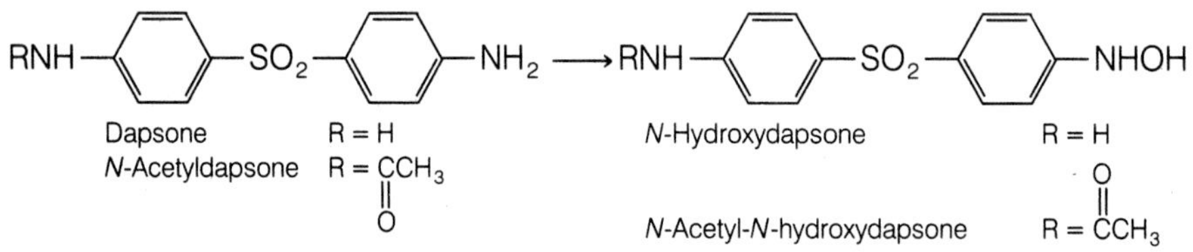

Dapsone	R = H
N-Acetyldapsone	R = CCH₃

N-Hydroxydapsone R = H

N-Acetyl-*N*-hydroxydapsone R = CCH₃

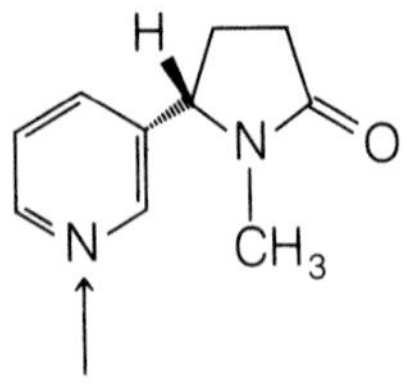

Cotinine

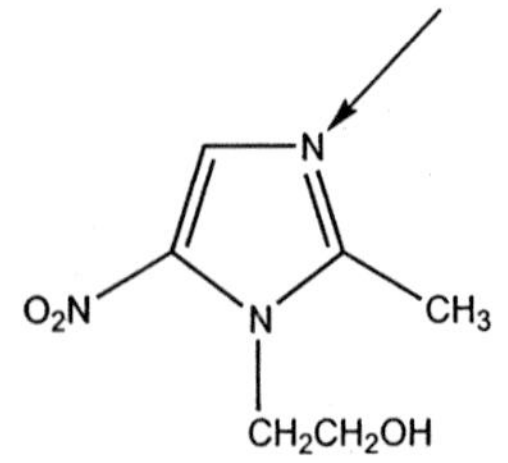

Metronidazole
2-(2-Methyl-5-nitro-imidazol-1-yl)-ethanol

Amides. Amide functionalities are susceptible to oxidative carbon–nitrogen bond cleavage (via α-carbon hydroxylation) and N-hydroxylation reactions. Oxidative dealkylation of many N-substituted amide drugs and xenobiotics has been reported. Mechanistically, oxidative dealkylation proceeds via an initially formed carbinolamide, which is unstable and fragments to form the N-dealkylated product. For example, diazepam undergoes extensive N-demethylation to the pharmacologically active metabolite desmethyldiazepam.[235]

Various other *N*-alkyl substituents present in benzodiazepines (e.g., flurazepam)[136–138] and in barbiturates (e.g., hexobarbital and mephobarbital)[128] are similarly oxidatively N-dealkylated. Alkyl groups attached to the amide moiety of some sulfonylureas, such as the oral hypoglycemic chlorpropamide,[236] also are subject to dealkylation to a minor extent.

In the cyclic amides or lactams, hydroxylation of the alicy-

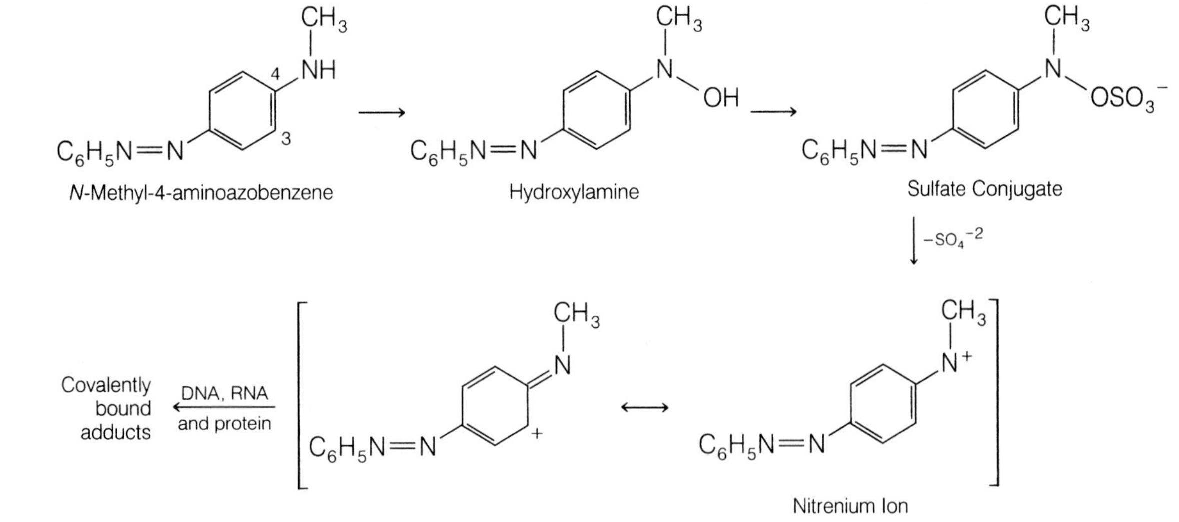

N-Methyl-4-aminoazobenzene → Hydroxylamine → Sulfate Conjugate

Covalently bound adducts ← DNA, RNA and protein ← Nitrenium Ion

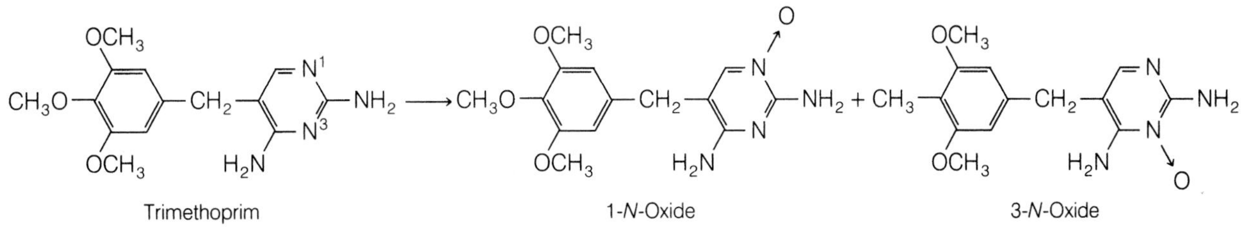

Trimethoprim → 1-N-Oxide + 3-N-Oxide

clic carbon α to the nitrogen atom also leads to carbinolamides. An example of this pathway is the conversion of cotinine to 5-hydroxycotinine. Interestingly, the latter carbinolamide intermediate is in tautomeric equilibrium with the ring-opened metabolite γ-(3-pyridyl)-γ-oxo-N-methylbutyramide.[237]

Metabolism of the important cancer chemotherapeutic agent cyclophosphamide (Cytoxan) follows a hydroxylation pathway similar to that just described for cyclic amides. This drug is a cyclic phosphoramide derivative and, for the most part, is the phosphorous counterpart of a cyclic amide. Because cyclophosphamide itself is pharmacologically inac-

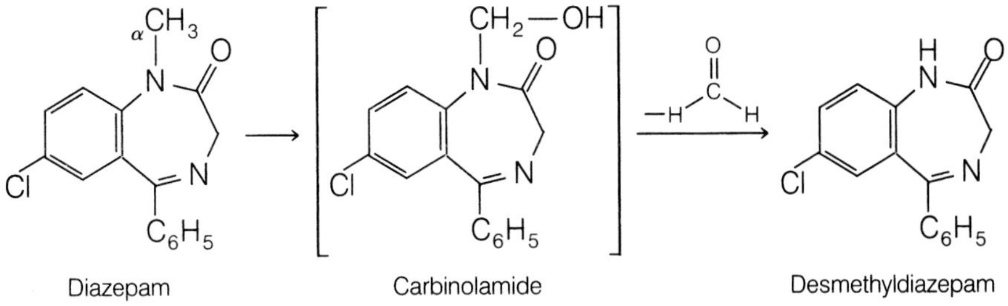

Diazepam → Carbinolamide → Desmethyldiazepam

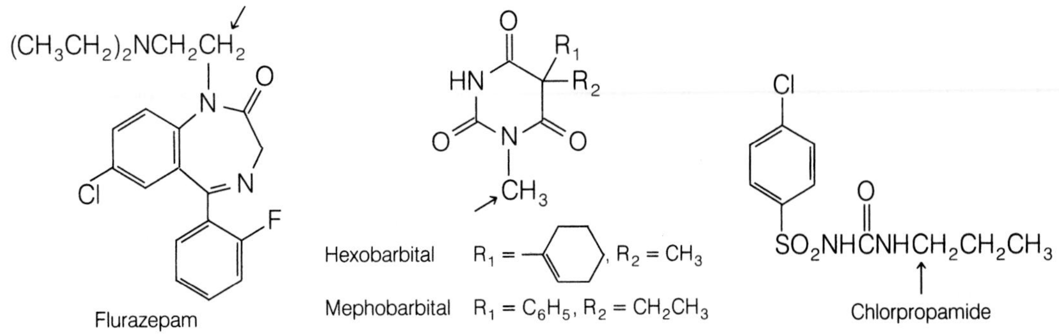

Flurazepam

Hexobarbital $R_1 =$ ⬡ , $R_2 = CH_3$

Mephobarbital $R_1 = C_6H_5$, $R_2 = CH_2CH_3$

Chlorpropamide

Cotinine · 5-Hydroxycotinine · γ-(3-Pyridyl)-γ-oxo-*N*-methylbutyramide

tive,[238] metabolic bioactivation is required for the drug to mediate its antitumorigenic or cytotoxic effects. The key biotransformation pathway leading to the active metabolite involves an initial carbon hydroxylation reaction at C-4 to form the carbinolamide 4-hydroxycyclophosphamide.[239, 240] 4-Hydroxycyclophosphamide is in equilibrium with the ring-opened dealkylated metabolite aldophosphamide. Although it has potent cytotoxic properties, aldophosphamide undergoes a further elimination reaction (reverse Michael reaction) to generate acrolein and the phosphoramide mustard *N,N*-bis(2-chloro-ethyl)phosphorodiamidic acid. The latter is the principal species responsible for cyclophosphamide's antitumorigenic properties and chemotherapeutic effect. Enzymatic oxidation of 4-hydroxycyclophosphamide and aldophosphamide leads to the relatively nontoxic metabolites 4-ketocyclophosphamide and carboxycyclophosphamide, respectively.

N-hydroxylation of aromatic amides, which occurs to a minor extent, is of some toxicological interest, since this biotransformation pathway may lead to the formation of chemically reactive intermediates. Several examples of cytotoxicity or carcinogenicity associated with metabolic N-hydroxylation of the parent aromatic amide have been reported. For example, the well-known hepatocarcinogenic 2-acetylaminofluorene (AAF) undergoes an N-hydroxylation reaction catalyzed by cytochrome P-450 to form the corresponding N-hydroxy metabolite (also called a hydroxamic

acid).[241] Further conjugation of this hydroxamic acid produces the corresponding *O*-sulfate ester, which ionizes to generate the electrophilic nitrenium species. Covalent binding of this reactive intermediate to DNA is known to occur and is likely to be the initial event that ultimately leads to malignant tumor formation.[242] Sulfate conjugation plays an important role in this biotoxification pathway (see "Sulfate Conjugation," for further discussion).

Acetaminophen is a relatively safe and nontoxic analgesic agent if used at therapeutic doses. Its metabolism illustrates the fact that a xenobiotic commonly produces more than one metabolite. Its metabolism also illustrates the effect of age, since infants and young children carry out sulfation rather than glucuronidation (see discussion at the end of this chapter). New pharmacists must realize that at one time acetanilide and phenacetin were more widely used than acetaminophen, even though both are considered more toxic because they produce aniline derivatives. Besides producing toxic aniline and *p*-phenetidin, these two analgesics also produce acetaminophen. When large doses of the latter drug are ingested, extensive liver necrosis is produced in humans and animals.[243, 244] Considerable evidence argues that this hepatotoxicity depends on the formation of a metabolically generated reactive intermediate.[245] Until recently,[246, 247] the accepted bioactivation pathway was believed to involve an initial N-hydroxylation reaction to form *N*-hydroxyacetaminophen.[248] Spontaneous dehydration of this *N*-hydrox-

Cyclophosphamide · 4-Hydroxycyclophosphamide · 4-Ketocyclophosphamide · Phosphoramide Mustard *N,N*-bis(2-Chloroethyl)-phosphorodiamidic Acid · Acrolein · Aldophosphamide · Carboxyphosphamide

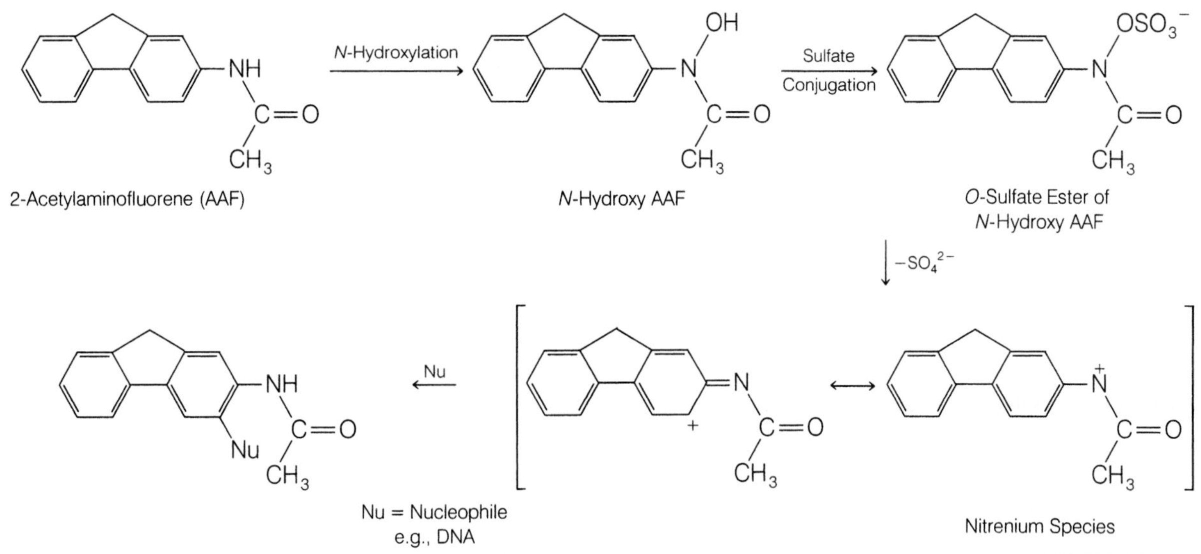

2-Acetylaminofluorene (AAF)

N-Hydroxy AAF

O-Sulfate Ester of
N-Hydroxy AAF

Nu = Nucleophile
e.g., DNA

Nitrenium Species

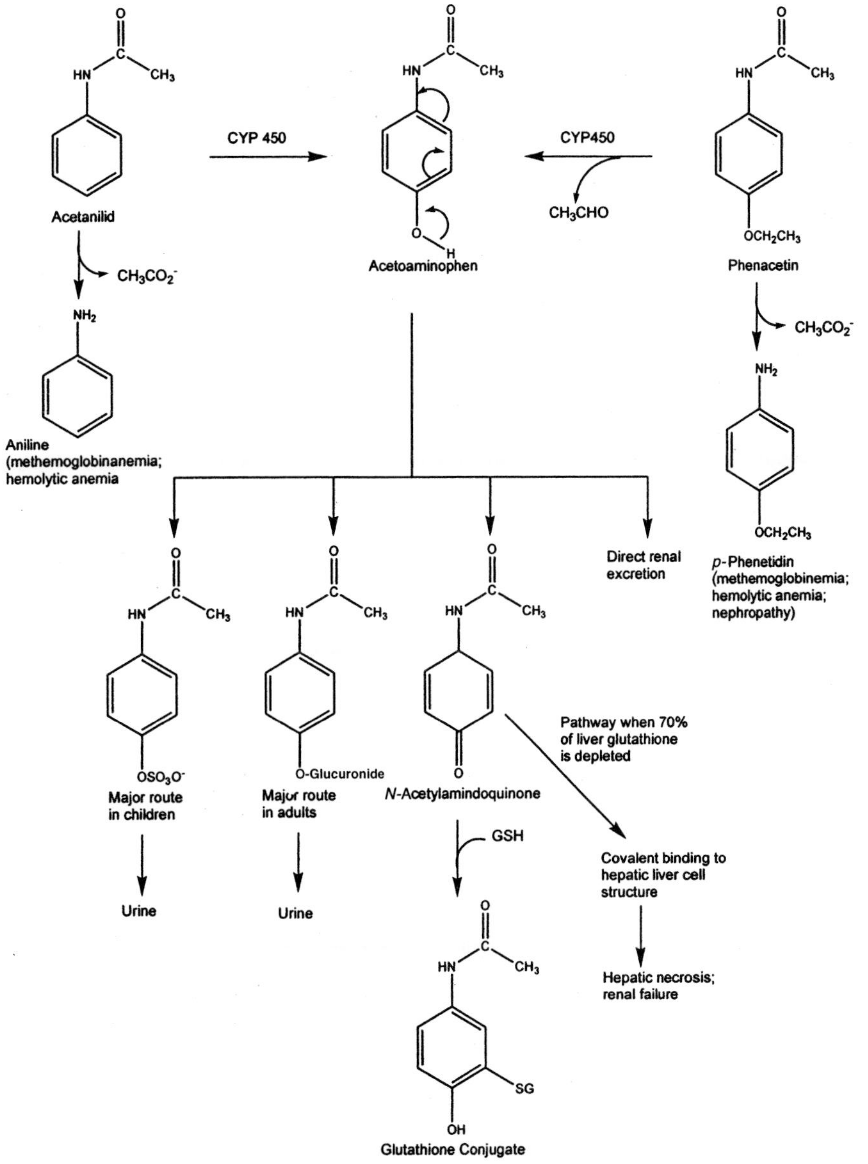

Acetanilid

CYP 450

Acetoaminophen

CYP450

CH₃CHO

Phenacetin

Aniline
(methemoglobinanemia;
hemolytic anemia

p-Phenetidin
(methemoglobinemia;
hemolytic anemia;
nephropathy)

Direct renal
excretion

OSO₃⁻
Major route
in children

O-Glucuronide
Major route
in adults

N-Acetylamindoquinone

Pathway when 70%
of liver glutathione
is depleted

Urine

Urine

GSH

Covalent binding to
hepatic liver cell
structure

Hepatic necrosis;
renal failure

Glutathione Conjugate

yamide produces *N*-acetylimidoquinone, the proposed reactive metabolite. Usually, the GSH present in the liver combines with this reactive metabolite to form the corresponding GSH conjugate. If GSH levels are sufficiently depleted by large doses of acetaminophen, covalent binding of the reactive intermediate occurs with macromolecules present in the liver, thereby leading to cellular necrosis. Studies indicate, however, that the reactive *N*-acetylimidoquinone intermediate is not formed from *N*-hydroxyacetaminophen.[245–247] It probably arises through some other oxidative process. Therefore, the mechanistic formation of the reactive metabolite of acetaminophen remains unclear.

OXIDATION INVOLVING CARBON–OXYGEN SYSTEMS

Oxidative O-dealkylation of carbon–oxygen systems (principally ethers) is catalyzed by microsomal mixed function oxidases.[163] Mechanistically, the biotransformation involves an initial α-carbon hydroxylation to form either a hemiacetal or a hemiketal, which undergoes spontaneous carbon–oxygen bond cleavage to yield the dealkylated oxygen species (phenol or alcohol) and a carbon moiety (aldehyde or ketone). Small alkyl groups (e.g., methyl or ethyl) attached to oxygen are O-dealkylated rapidly. For example, morphine is the metabolic product of O-demethylation of codeine.[249] The antipyretic and analgesic activities of phenacetin (see drawing of acetaminophen metabolism) in humans appear to be a consequence of O-deethylation to the active metabolite acetaminophen.[250] Several other drugs containing ether groups, such as indomethacin (Indocin),[251, 252] prazosin (Minipress),[253, 254] and metoprolol (Lopressor),[122, 123] have reportedly undergone significant O-demethylation to their corresponding phenolic or alcoholic metabolites, which are further conjugated. In many drugs that have several nonequivalent methoxy groups, one particular methoxy group often appears to be O-demethylated selectively or preferentially. For example, the 3,4,5-trimethoxyphenyl moiety in both mescaline[255] and trimethoprim[232] undergoes O-demethylation to yield predominantly the corresponding 3-O-demethylated metabolites. 4-O-demethylation also occurs to a minor extent for both drugs. The phenolic and alcoholic metabolites formed from oxidative O-demethylation are susceptible to conjugation, particularly glucuronidation.

OXIDATION INVOLVING CARBON–SULFUR SYSTEMS

Carbon–sulfur functional groups are susceptible to metabolic S-dealkylation, desulfuration, and S-oxidation reactions. The first two processes involve oxidative carbon–sulfur bond cleavage. S-dealkylation is analogous to O- and N-dealkylation mechanistically (i.e., it involves α-carbon hydroxylation) and has been observed for various sulfur xenobiotics.[163, 256] For example, 6-(methylthio)purine is demethylated oxidatively in rats to 6-mercaptopurine.[257, 258] S-demethylation of methitural[259] and S-debenzylation of 2-benzylthio-5-trifluoromethylbenzoic acid also have been reported. In contrast to O- and N-dealkylation, examples of drugs undergoing S-dealkylation in humans are

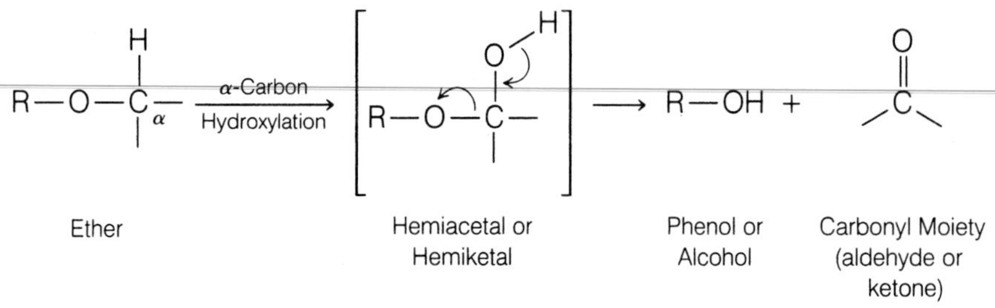

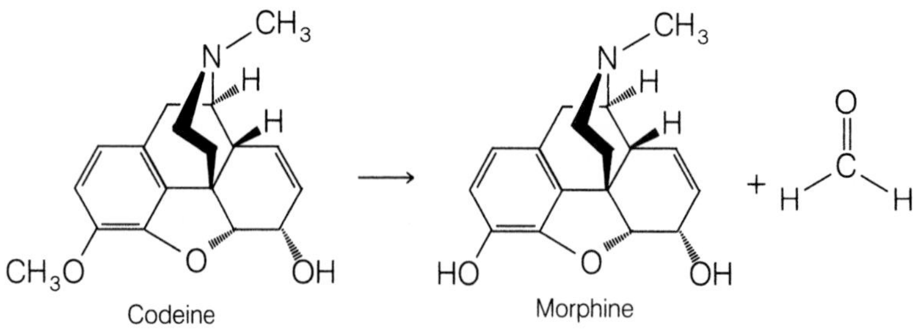

Ether → Hemiacetal or Hemiketal → Phenol or Alcohol + Carbonyl Moiety (aldehyde or ketone)

Codeine → Morphine +

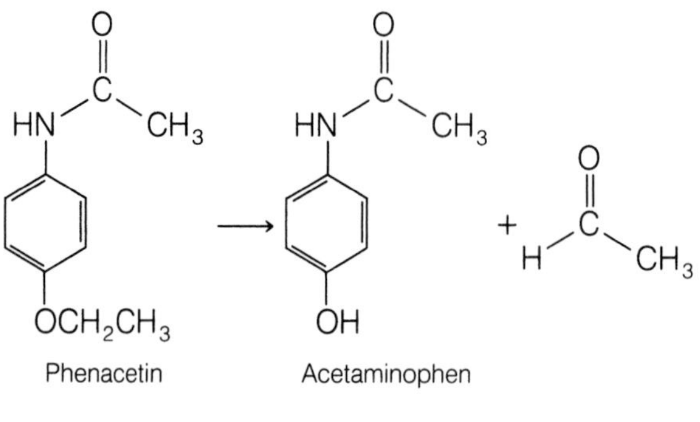

Phenacetin → Acetaminophen +

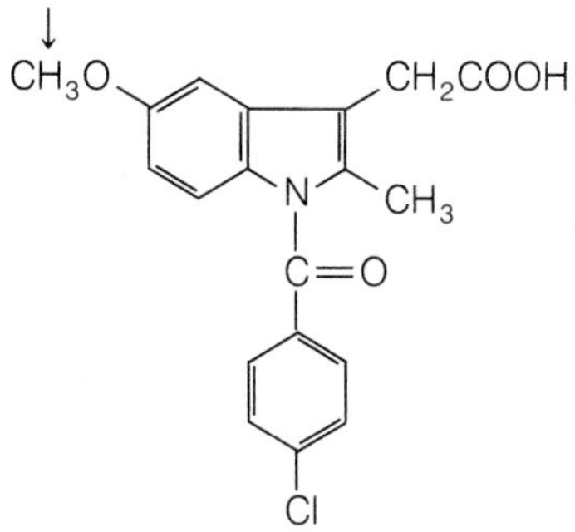

Indomethacin

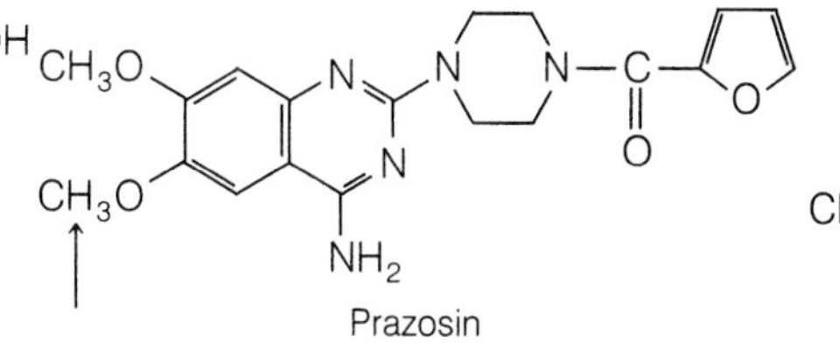

Prazosin

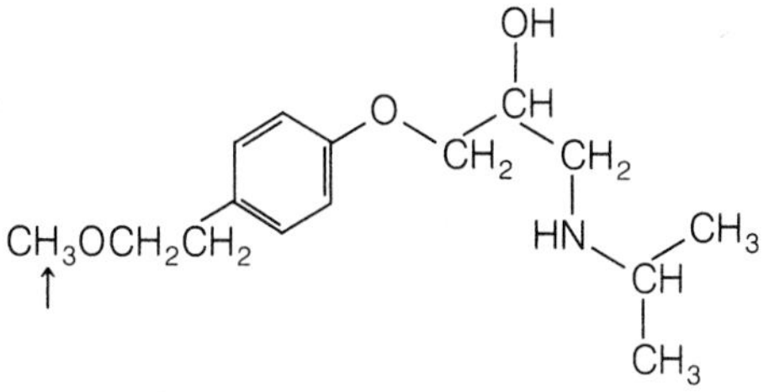

Metoprolol

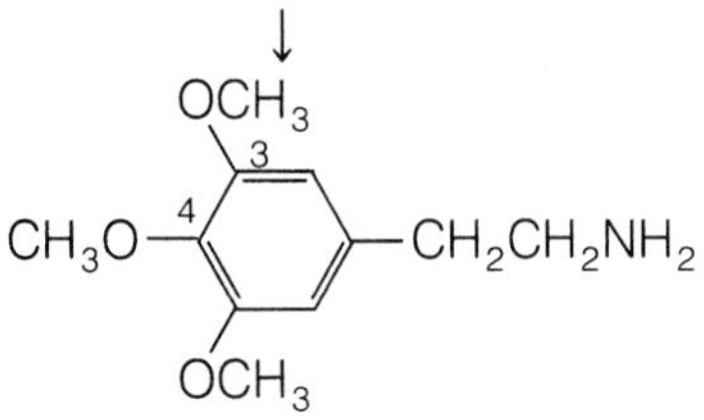

Mescaline

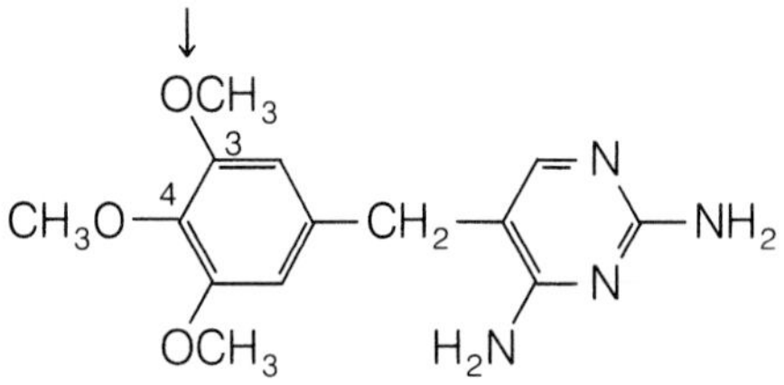

Trimethoprim

limited because of the small number of sulfur-containing medicinals and the competing metabolic S-oxidation processes (see diagram).

Oxidative conversion of carbon–sulfur double bonds (C = S) (thiono) to the corresponding carbon–oxygen double bond (C = O) is called *desulfuration*. A well-known drug example of this metabolic process is the biotransformation of thiopental to its corresponding oxygen analogue pentobarbital.[260, 261] An analogous desulfuration reaction also occurs with the P = S moiety present in a number of organophosphate insecticides, such as parathion.[262, 263] Desulfuration of parathion leads to the formation of paraoxon, which is the active metabolite responsible for the anticholinesterase activity of the parent drug. The mechanistic details of desulfuration are poorly understood, but it appears to involve microsomal oxidation of the C = S or P = S double bond.[264]

Organosulfur xenobiotics commonly undergo S-oxidation to yield sulfoxide derivatives. Several phenothiazine derivatives are metabolized by this pathway. For example, both sulfur atoms present in thioridazine (Mellaril)[265, 266] are susceptible to S-oxidation. Oxidation of the 2-methylthio group yields the active sulfoxide metabolite mesoridazine. Interestingly, mesoridazine is twice as potent an antipsychotic agent as thioridazine in humans and has been introduced into clinical use as Serentil.[267]

S-oxidation constitutes an important pathway in the metabolism of the H_2-histamine antagonists cimetidine (Tagamet)[268] and metiamide.[269] The corresponding sulfoxide derivatives are the major human urinary metabolites.

Sulfoxide drugs and metabolites may be further oxidized to sulfones (-SO_2-). The sulfoxide group present in the immunosuppressive agent oxisuran is metabolized to a sulfone moiety.[270] In humans, dimethylsulfoxide (DMSO) is found primarily in the urine as the oxidized product dimethylsulfone. Sulfoxide metabolites, such as those of thioridazine, reportedly undergo further oxidation to their sulfone -SO_2- derivatives.[265, 266]

Oxidation of Alcohols and Aldehydes

Many oxidative processes (e.g., benzylic, allylic, alicyclic, or aliphatic hydroxylation) generate alcohol or carbinol metabolites as intermediate products. If not conjugated, these alcohol products are further oxidized to aldehydes (if primary alcohols) or to ketones (if secondary alcohols). Aldehyde metabolites resulting from oxidation of primary alcohols or from oxidative deamination of primary aliphatic amines often undergo facile oxidation to generate polar carboxylic acid derivatives.[116] As a general rule, primary alcoholic groups and aldehyde functionalities are quite vulnera-

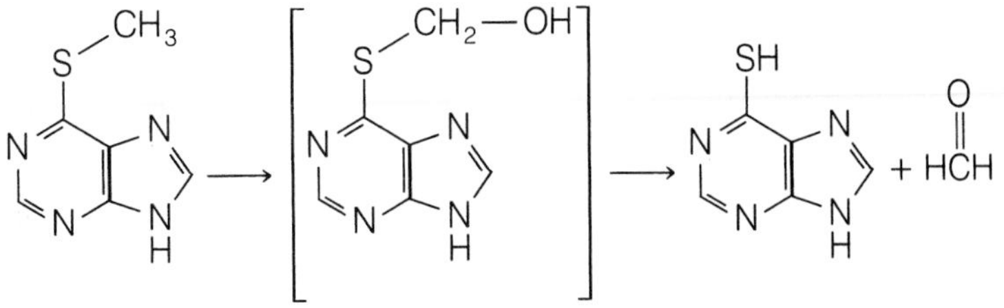

6-(Methylthio)-purine

6-Mercaptopurine

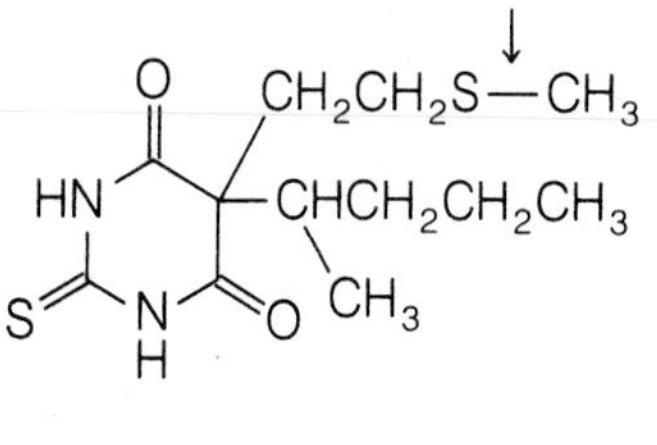

Methitural

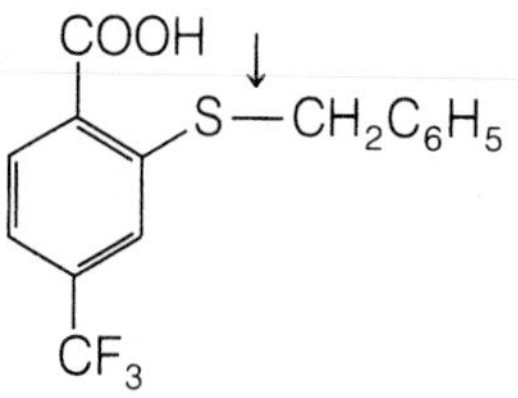

2-Benzylthio-5-
trifluoromethylbenzoic Acid

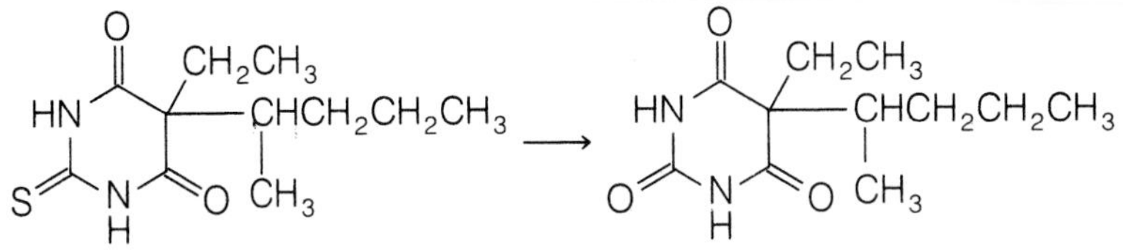

Thiopental → Pentobarbital

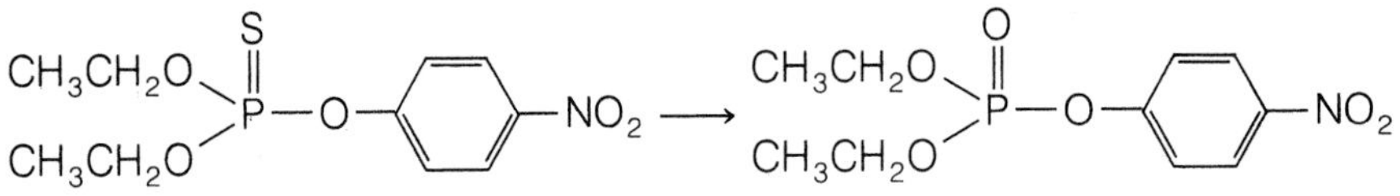

Parathion → Paraoxon

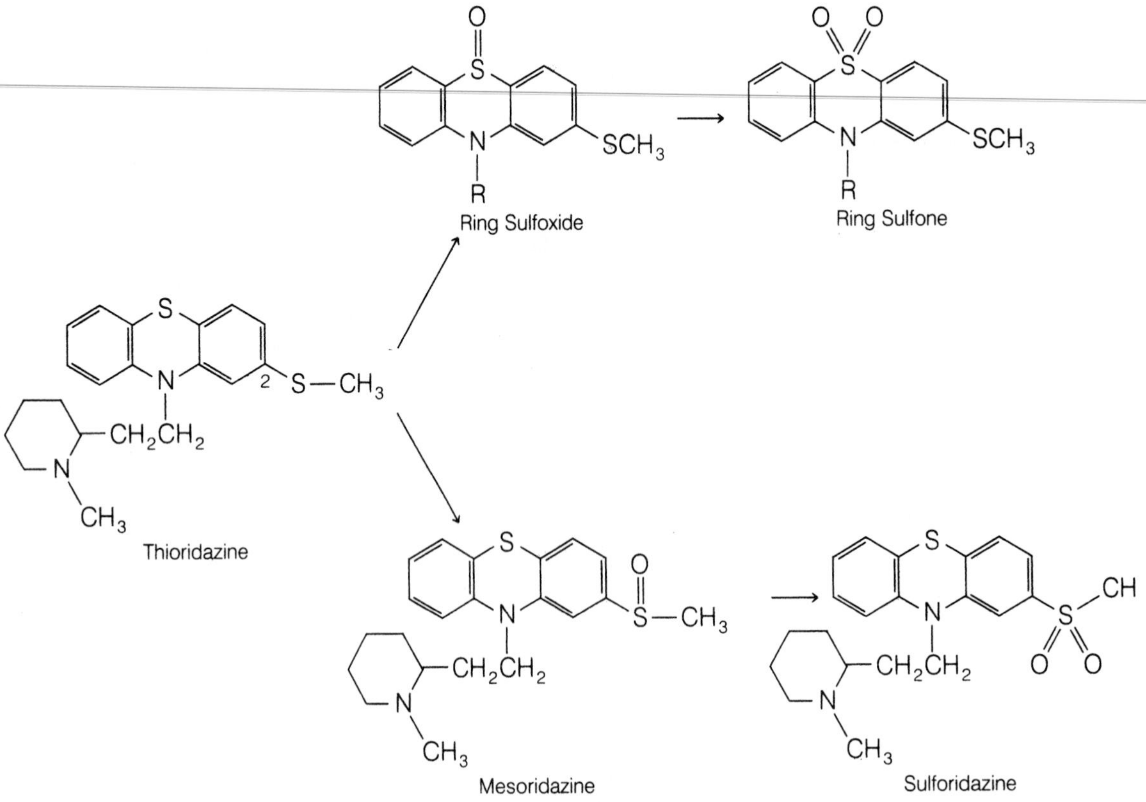

Ring Sulfoxide → Ring Sulfone

Thioridazine

Mesoridazine

Sulforidazine

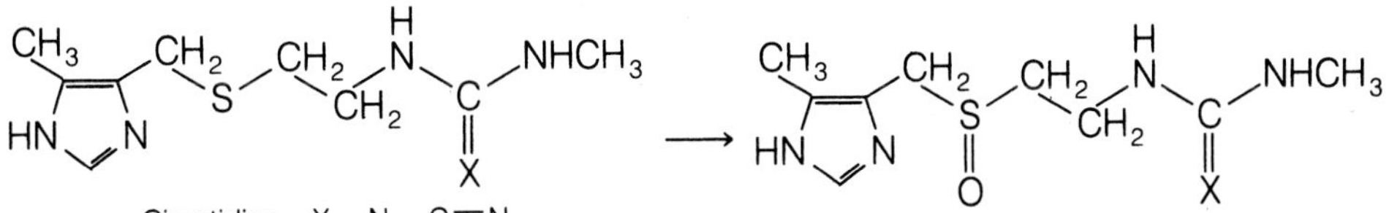

Cimetidine X = N—C≡N
Metiamide X = S

Sulfoxide Metabolite

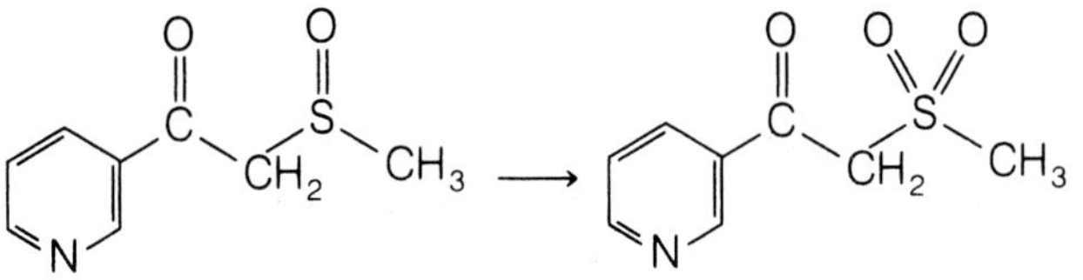

Oxisuran

Sulfone Metabolite

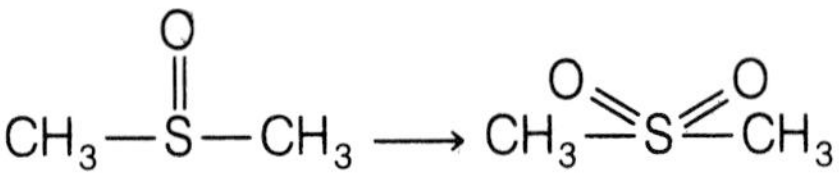

Dimethyl Sulfoxide → Dimethyl Sulfone

ble to oxidation. Several drug examples in which primary alcohol metabolites and aldehyde metabolites are oxidized to carboxylic acid products are cited in sections above.

Although secondary alcohols are susceptible to oxidation, this reaction is not often important because the reverse reaction, namely, reduction of the ketone back to the secondary alcohol, occurs quite readily. In addition, the secondary alcohol group, being polar and functionalized, is more likely to be conjugated than the ketone moiety.

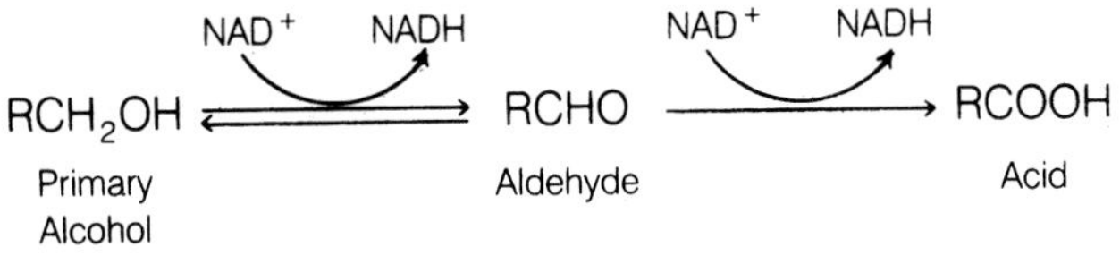

$$RCH_2OH \underset{NADH}{\overset{NAD^+}{\rightleftarrows}} RCHO \underset{NADH}{\overset{NAD^+}{\longrightarrow}} RCOOH$$

Primary   Aldehyde   Acid
Alcohol

The bioconversion of alcohols to aldehydes and ketones is catalyzed by soluble alcohol dehydrogenases present in the liver and other tissues. NAD$^+$ is required as a coenzyme, although NADP$^+$ also may serve as a coenzyme. The reaction catalyzed by alcohol dehydrogenase is reversible but often proceeds to the right because the aldehyde formed is further oxidized to the acid. Several aldehyde dehydrogenases, including aldehyde oxidase and xanthine oxidase, carry out the oxidation of aldehydes to their corresponding acids.[116, 271–273]

Metabolism of cyclic amines to their lactam metabolites has been observed for various drugs (e.g., nicotine, phenmetrazine, and methylphenidate). It appears that soluble or microsomal dehydrogenase and oxidases are involved in oxidizing the carbinol group of the intermediate carbinolamine to a carbonyl moiety.[273] For example, in the metabolism of medazepam to diazepam, the intermediate carbinolamine (2-hydroxymedazepam) undergoes oxidation of its 2-hydroxy group to a carbonyl moiety. A microsomal dehydrogenase carries out this oxidation.[274]

Other Oxidative Biotransformation Pathways

In addition to the many oxidative biotransformations discussed above, oxidative aromatization or dehydrogenation and oxidative dehalogenation reactions also occur. Metabolic aromatization has been reported for norgestrel. Aromatization or dehydrogenation of the A ring present in this steroid leads to the corresponding phenolic product 17α-ethinyl-18-homoestradiol as a minor metabolite in women.[275] In mice, the terpene ring of Δ^1-THC or $\Delta^{1,6}$-THC undergoes aromatization to give cannabinol.[276, 277]

Many halogen-containing drugs and xenobiotics are metabolized by oxidative dehalogenation. For example, the volatile anesthetic agent halothane is metabolized principally to trifluoroacetic acid in humans.[278, 279] It has been postulated that this metabolite arises from cytochrome P-450-mediated hydroxylation of halothane to form an initial carbinol intermediate that spontaneously eliminates hydrogen bromide (dehalogenation) to yield trifluoroacetyl chloride. The latter acyl chloride is chemically reactive and reacts rapidly with water to form trifluoroacetic acid. Alternatively, it can acylate tissue nucleophiles. Indeed, in vitro studies indicate that halothane is metabolized to a reactive intermediate (presumably trifluoroacetyl chloride), which covalently binds to liver microsomal proteins.[280, 281] Chloroform also appears to be metabolized oxidatively by a similar dehalogenation pathway to yield the chemically reactive species phosgene. Phosgene may be responsible for the hepato- and nephrotoxicity associated with chloroform.[282]

A final example of oxidative dehalogenation concerns the antibiotic chloramphenicol. In vitro studies have shown that the dichloroacetamide portion of the molecule undergoes oxidative dechlorination to yield a chemically reactive oxamyl chloride intermediate that can react with water to form

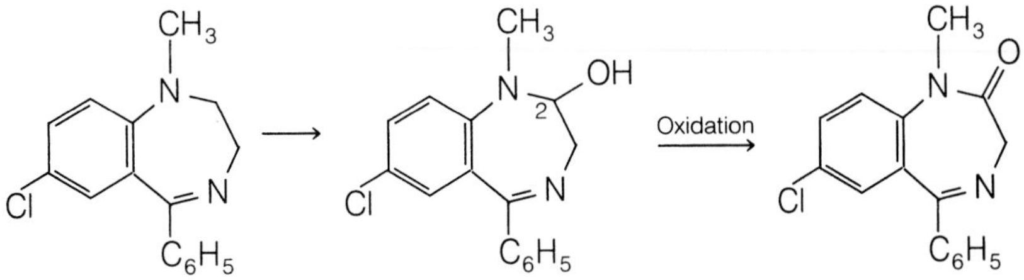

Medazepam → 2-Hydroxymedazepam —Oxidation→ Diazepam

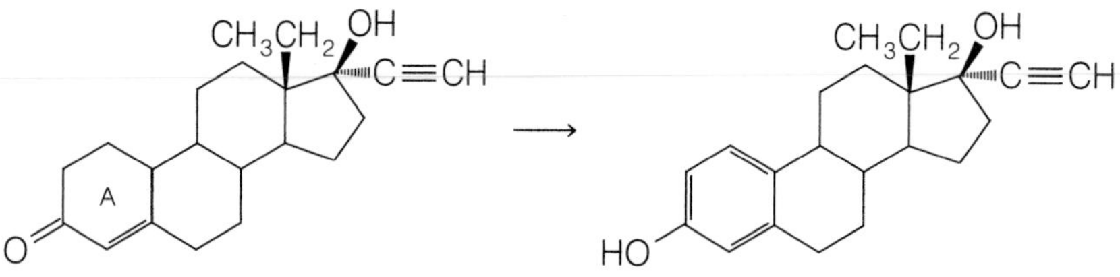

Norgestrel → 17α-Ethinyl-18-homoestradiol

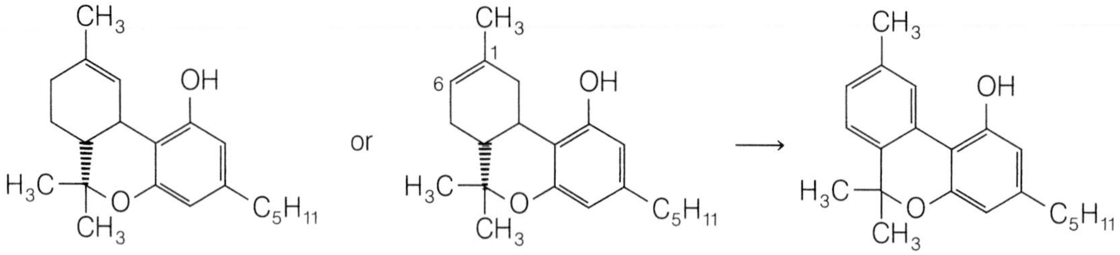

Δ^1-THC or $\Delta^{1,6}$-THC → Cannabinol

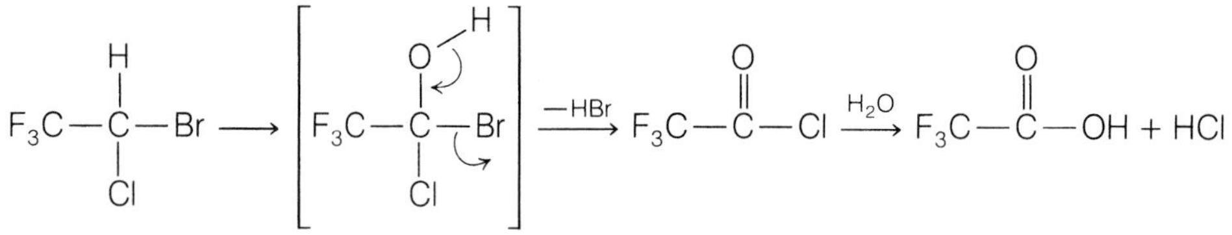

Halothane → Carbinol Intermediate → Trifluoroacetyl Chloride → Trifluoroacetic Acid

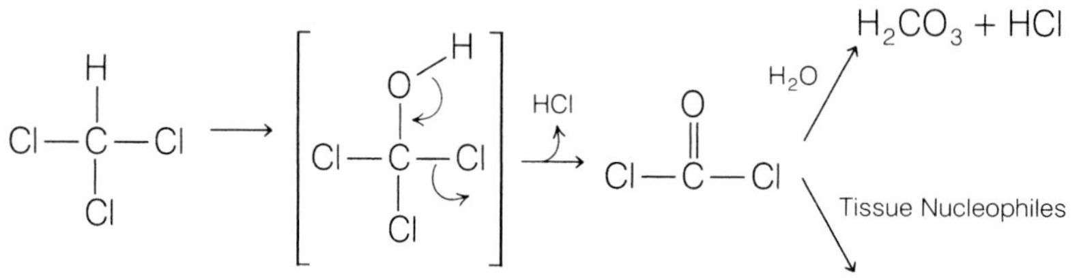
H_2CO_3 + HCl
H_2O
HCl
Tissue Nucleophiles

Chloroform → Phosgene → Covalent Binding

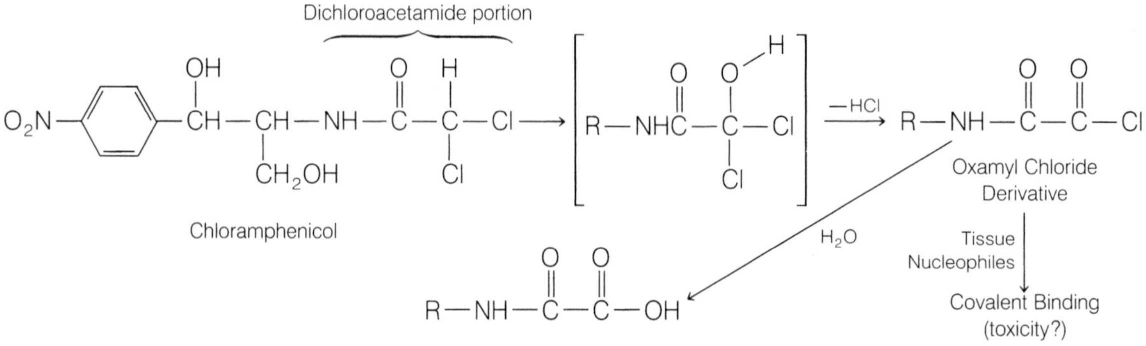
Dichloroacetamide portion
−HCl
Oxamyl Chloride Derivative
H_2O
Tissue Nucleophiles
Covalent Binding (toxicity?)

Chloramphenicol

Oxamic Acid Derivative

the corresponding oxamic acid metabolite or can acylate microsomal proteins.[283, 284] Thus, it appears that in several instances, oxidative dehalogenation can lead to the formation of toxic and reactive acyl halide intermediates.

REDUCTIVE REACTIONS

Reductive processes play an important role in the metabolism of many compounds containing carbonyl, nitro, and azo groups. Bioreduction of carbonyl compounds generates alcohol derivatives,[116, 285] whereas nitro and azo reductions lead to amino derivatives.[286] The hydroxyl and amino moieties of the metabolites are much more susceptible to conjugation than the functional groups of the parent compounds. Hence, reductive processes, as such, facilitate drug elimination.

Reductive pathways that are encountered less frequently in drug metabolism include reduction of *N*-oxides to their corresponding tertiary amines and reduction of sulfoxides to sulfides. Reductive cleavage of disulfide linkages and reduction of carbon–carbon double bonds also occur, but constitute only minor pathways in drug metabolism.

Reduction of Aldehyde and Ketone Carbonyls

The carbonyl moiety, particularly the ketone group, is encountered frequently in many drugs. In addition, metabolites containing ketone and aldehyde functionalities often arise from oxidative deamination of xenobiotics (e.g., propranolol, chlorpheniramine, amphetamine). Because of their ease of oxidation, aldehydes are metabolized mainly to carboxylic acids. Occasionally, aldehydes are reduced to primary alcohols. Ketones, however, are generally resistant to oxidation and are reduced mainly to secondary alcohols. Alcohol metabolites arising from reduction of carbonyl compounds generally undergo further conjugation (e.g., glucuronidation).

Diverse soluble enzymes, called *aldo-keto reductases,* carry out bioreduction of aldehydes and ketones.[116, 287] They are found in the liver and other tissues (e.g., kidney). As a general class, these soluble enzymes have similar physiochemical properties and broad substrate specificities and require NADPH as a cofactor. Oxidoreductase enzymes that carry out both oxidation and reduction reactions also can reduce aldehydes and ketones.[287] For example, the important liver alcohol dehydrogenase is an NAD$^+$-dependent oxidoreductase that oxidizes ethanol and other aliphatic alcohols to aldehydes and ketones. In the presence of NADH or

NADPH, however, the same enzyme system can reduce carbonyl derivatives to their corresponding alcohols.[116]

Few aldehydes undergo bioreduction because of the relative ease of oxidation of aldehydes to carboxylic acids. One frequently cited example of a parent aldehyde drug undergoing extensive enzymatic reduction, however, is the sedative–hypnotic chloral hydrate. Bioreduction of this hydrated aldehyde yields trichloroethanol as the major metabolite in humans.[288] Interestingly, this alcohol metabolite is pharmacologically active. Further glucuronidation of the alcohol leads to an inactive conjugated product that is readily excreted in the urine.

Chloral Hydrate   Chloral   Trichloroethanol

Aldehyde metabolites resulting from oxidative deamination of drugs also undergo reduction to a minor extent. For example, in humans the β-adrenergic blocker propranolol is converted to an intermediate aldehyde by N-dealkylation and oxidative deamination. Although the aldehyde is oxidized primarily to the corresponding carboxylic acid (naphthoxylactic acid), a small fraction also is reduced to the alcohol derivative (propranolol glycol).[289]

Two major polar urinary metabolites of the histamine H$_1$ antagonist chlorpheniramine have been identified in dogs as the alcohol and carboxylic acid products (conjugated) derived, respectively, by reduction and oxidation of an aldehyde metabolite. The aldehyde precursor arises from bis-N-demethylation and oxidative deamination of chlorpheniramine.[290]

Bioreduction of ketones often leads to the creation of an asymmetric center and, thereby, two possible stereoisomeric alcohols.[116, 291] For example, reduction of acetophenone by a soluble rabbit kidney reductase leads to the enantiomeric alcohols (S)(−)- and (R)(+)-methylphenylcarbinol, with the (S)(−) isomer predominating (3:1 ratio).[292] The preferential formation of one stereoisomer over the other is termed *product stereoselectivity* in drug metabolism.[291] Mechanistically, ketone reduction involves a ''hydride'' transfer from the reduced nicotinamide moiety of the cofactor NADPH or NADH to the carbonyl carbon atom of the ketone. It is generally agreed that this step proceeds with considerable *stereoselectivity.*[116, 291] Consequently, it is not surprising to find many reports of xenobiotic ketones that are reduced preferentially to a predominant stereoisomer. Often, ketone reduction yields alcohol metabolites that are pharmacologically active.

Although many ketone-containing drugs undergo significant reduction, only a few selected examples are presented in detail here. The xenobiotics that are not discussed in the text have been structurally tabulated in Figure 4-10. The keto group undergoing reduction is designated with an arrow.

Ketones lacking asymmetric centers in their molecules, such as acetophenone or the oral hypoglycemic acetohexamide, usually give rise to predominantly one enantiomer on reduction. In humans, acetohexamide is metabolized rapidly in the liver to give principally (S)(−)-hydroxyhexamide.[293, 294] This metabolite is as active a hypoglycemic agent as its parent compound and is eliminated through the

Propranolol → N-dealkylation → N-Desisopropyl Propranolol → Oxidative Deamination → Aldehyde Intermediate → Oxidation → Naphthoxylactic Acid

Reduction → Propranolol Glycol (conjugated)

Chlorpheniramine → 1) bis-N-demethylation 2) Oxidative Deamination → Aldehyde Metabolite

Reduction → 3-(*p*-Chlorobenzyl)-3-(2-pyridyl)-propan-1-ol

Oxidation → 3-(*p*-Chlorobenzyl)-3-(2-pyridyl)-propanoic Acid

Acetophenone → *S*(−)-Methyl Phenyl Carbinol (75%) + *R*(+)-Methyl Phenyl Carbinol (25%)

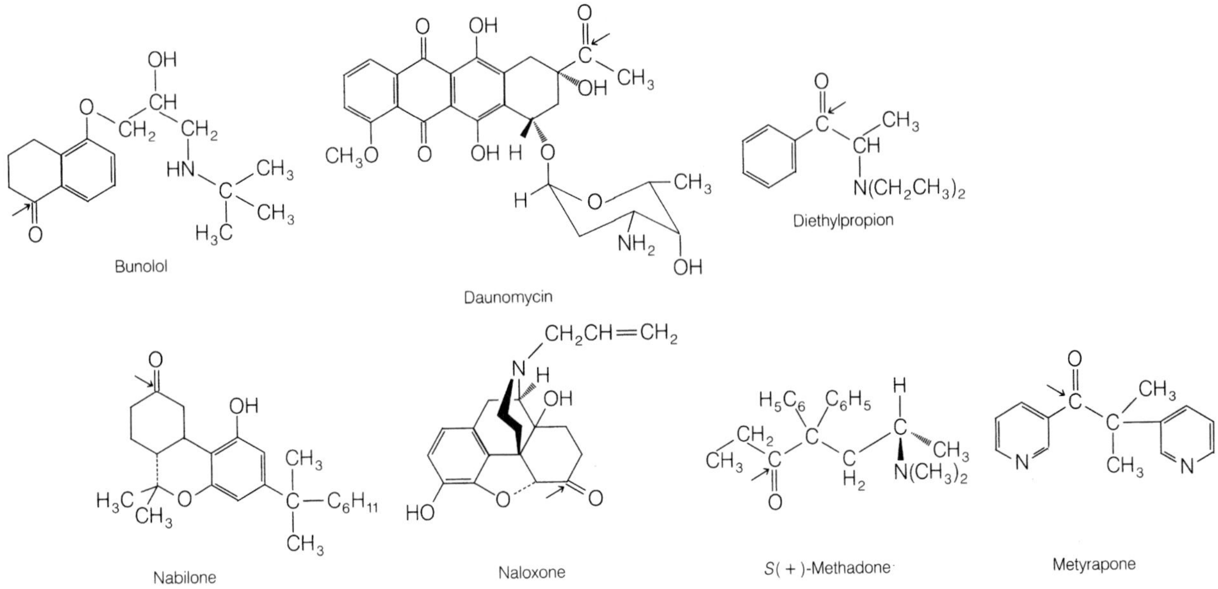

Figure 4–10 ■ Additional examples of xenobiotics that undergo extensive ketone reduction, not covered in the text. *Arrow* indicates the keto group undergoing reduction.

kidneys.[295] Acetohexamide usually is not recommended in diabetic patients with renal failure, because of the possible accumulation of its active metabolite, hydroxyhexamide.

When chiral ketones are reduced, they yield two possible diastereomeric or epimeric alcohols. For example, the $(R)(+)$ enantiomer of the oral anticoagulant warfarin undergoes extensive reduction of its side chain keto group to generate the $(R,S)(+)$ alcohol as the major plasma metabolite in humans.[56, 296] Small amounts of the $(R,R)(+)$ diastereomer also are formed. In contrast, the $(S)(-)$ enantiomer undergoes little ketone reduction and is primarily 7-hydroxylated (i.e., aromatic hydroxylation) in humans.

Reduction of the 6-keto functionality in the narcotic antagonist naltrexone can lead to either the epimeric 6α- or 6β-hydroxy metabolites, depending on the animal species.[297, 298] In humans and rabbits, bioreduction of naltrexone is highly stereoselective and generates only

6β-naltrexol, whereas in chickens, reduction yields only 6α-naltrexol.[297–299] In monkeys and guinea pigs, however, both epimeric alcohols are formed (predominantly 6β-naltrexol).[300, 301] Apparently, in the latter two species, reduction of naltrexone to the epimeric 6α- and 6β-alcohols is carried out by two distinctly different reductases found in the liver.[299–301]

Reduction of oxisuran appears not to be an important pathway by which the parent drug mediates its immunosuppressive effects. Studies indicate that oxisuran has its greatest immunosuppressive effects in those species that form alcohols as their major metabolic products (e.g., human, rat).[302–306] In species in which reduction is a minor pathway (e.g., dog), oxisuran shows little immunosuppressive activity.[304–306] These findings indicate that the oxisuran alcohols (oxisuranols) are pharmacologically active and contribute substantially to the overall immunosuppressive effect of the

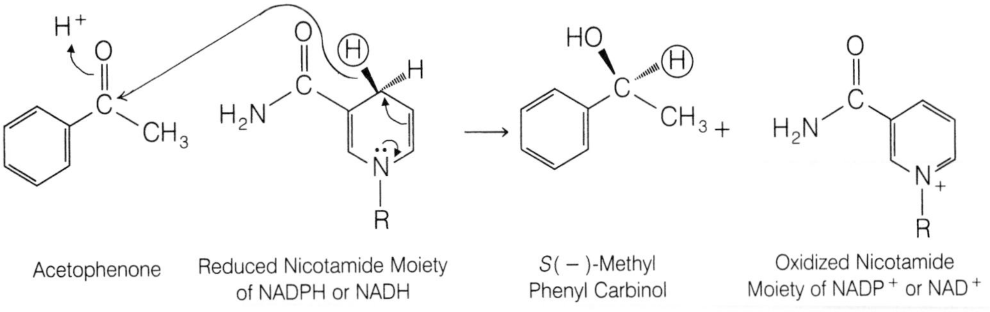

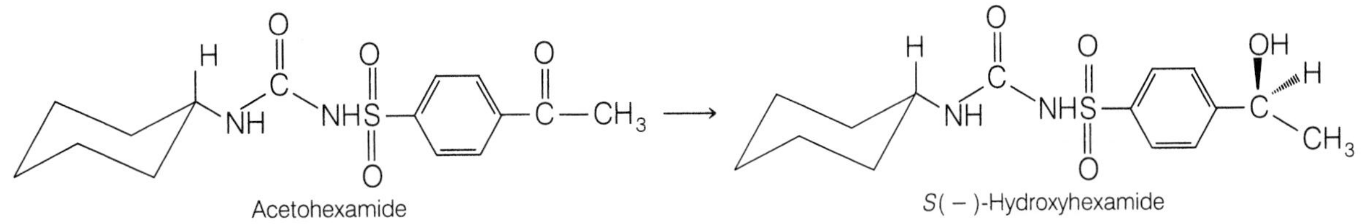

R(+)-Warfarin → R,S-(+)-Alcohol Major Diastereomer + R,R-(+)-Alcohol Minor Diastereomer

Naltrexone → 6β-Naltrexol and/or 6α-Naltrexol

parent drug. The sulfoxide group in oxisuran is chiral, by virtue of the lone pair of electrons on sulfur. Therefore, reduction of oxisuran leads to diastereomeric alcohols.

Oxisuran → Oxisuranols (diastereomeric mixture)

Reduction of α,β-unsaturated ketones results in reduction not only of the ketone group but of the carbon–carbon double bond as well. Steroidal drugs often fall into this class, including norethindrone, a synthetic progestin found in many oral contraceptive drug combinations. In women, the major plasma and urinary metabolite of norethindrone is the $3\beta,5\beta$-tetrahydro derivative.[307]

Ketones resulting from metabolic oxidative deamination processes are also susceptible to reduction. For instance, rabbit liver microsomal preparations metabolize amphetamine to phenylacetone, which is reduced subsequently to 1-

Norethindrone → 3β,5β-Tetrahydronorethindrone

Amphetamine → Phenylacetone → (Reduction) → 1-Phenyl-2-propanol

(−)-Ephedrine → (N-demethylation and Oxidative Deamination) → 1-Hydroxy-1-phenyl-propan-2-one → (Reduction) → 1-Phenyl-1,2-propanediol (as glucuronide conjugate)

phenyl-2-propanol.[308] In humans, a minor urinary metabolite of (-)-ephedrine has been identified as the diol derivative formed from keto reduction of the oxidatively deaminated product 1-hydroxy-1-phenylpropan-2-one.[309]

Reduction of Nitro and Azo Compounds

The reduction of aromatic nitro and azo xenobiotics leads to aromatic primary amine metabolites.[286] Aromatic nitro compounds are reduced initially to the nitroso and hydroxylamine intermediates, as shown in the following metabolic sequence:

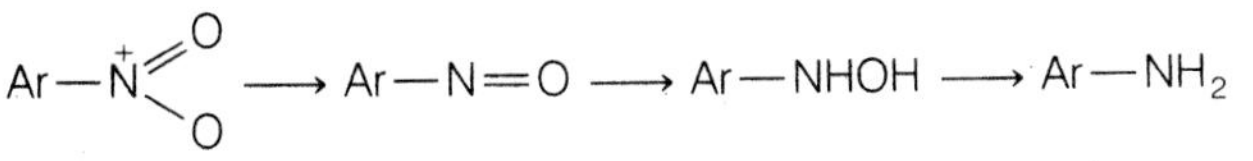

$$Ar-\overset{+}{N}\overset{O}{\underset{O}{=}} \longrightarrow Ar-N=O \longrightarrow Ar-NHOH \longrightarrow Ar-NH_2$$

Nitro Nitroso Hydroxylamine Amine

Azo reduction, however, is believed to proceed via a hydrazo intermediate (-NH-NH-) that subsequently is cleaved reductively to yield the corresponding aromatic amines:

$$Ar-N=N-Ar' \longrightarrow Ar-NH-NH-Ar' \longrightarrow$$

Azo Hydrazo

$$Ar-NH_2 + H_2N-Ar'$$

Amines

Bioreduction of nitro compounds is carried out by NADPH-dependent microsomal and soluble nitro reductases present in the liver. A multicomponent hepatic microsomal reductase system requiring NADPH appears to be responsible for azo reduction.[310–312] In addition, bacterial reductases present in the intestine can reduce nitro and azo compounds, especially those that are absorbed poorly or excreted mainly in the bile.[313, 314]

Various aromatic nitro drugs undergo enzymatic reduction to the corresponding aromatic amines. For example, the 7-nitro benzodiazepine derivatives clonazepam and nitrazepam are metabolized extensively to their respective 7-amino metabolites in humans.[315, 316] The skeletal muscle relaxant dantrolene (Dantrium) also reportedly undergoes reduction to aminodantrolene in humans.[317, 318]

For some nitro xenobiotics, bioreduction appears to be a minor metabolic pathway in vivo, because of competing oxidative and conjugative reactions. Under artificial anaerobic in vitro incubation conditions, however, these same nitro xenobiotics are enzymatically reduced rapidly. For example, most of the urinary metabolites of metronidazole found in humans are either oxidation or conjugation products. Reduced metabolites of metronidazole have not been detected.[319] When incubated anaerobically with guinea pig liver preparations, however, metronidazole undergoes considerable nitro reduction.[320]

Bacterial reductase present in the intestine also tends to complicate in vivo interpretations of nitro reduction. For example, in rats, the antibiotic chloramphenicol is not reduced in vivo by the liver but is excreted in the bile and, subsequently, reduced by intestinal flora to form the amino metabolite.[321, 322]

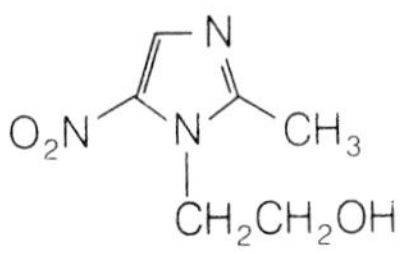

Metronidazole

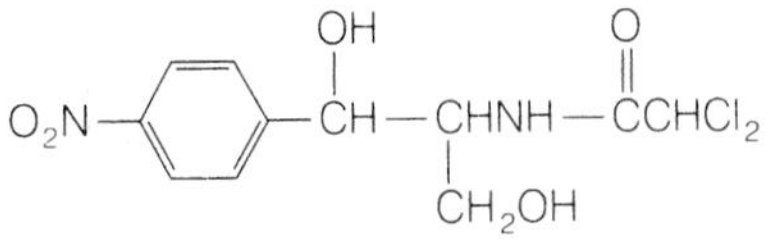

Chloramphenicol

The enzymatic reduction of azo compounds is best exemplified by the conversion of sulfamidochrysoidine (Prontosil) to the active sulfanilamide metabolite in the liver.[323] This reaction has historical significance, for it led to the discovery of sulfanilamide as an antibiotic and eventually to the development of many of the therapeutic sulfonamide drugs. Bacterial reductases present in the intestine play a significant role in reducing azo xenobiotics, particularly those that are absorbed poorly.[313, 314] Accordingly, the two azo dyes tartrazine[324, 325] and amaranth[326] have poor oral absorption because of the many polar and ionized sulfonic acid groups present in their structures. Therefore, these two azo compounds are metabolized primarily by bacterial reductases present in the intestine. The importance of intestinal reduction is further revealed in the metabolism of sulfasalazine (formerly salicylazosulfapyridine, Azulfidine), a drug used in the treatment of ulcerative colitis. The drug is ab-

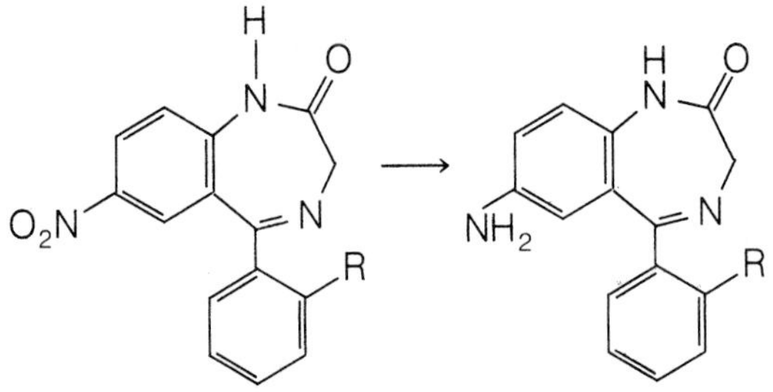

Clonazepam, R = Cl
Nitrazepam, R = H

7-Amino Metabolite

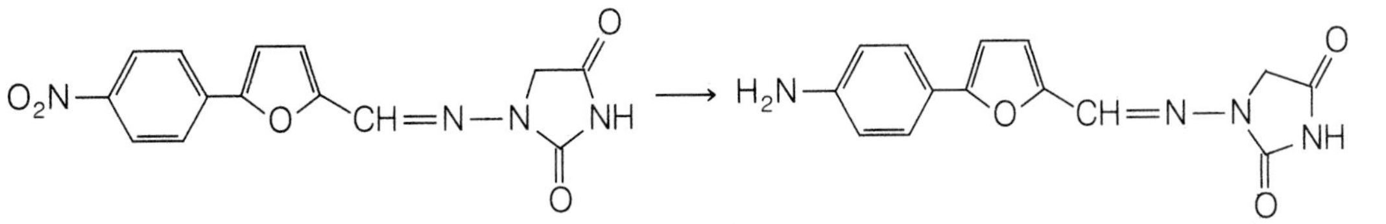

Dantrolene

Aminodantrolene

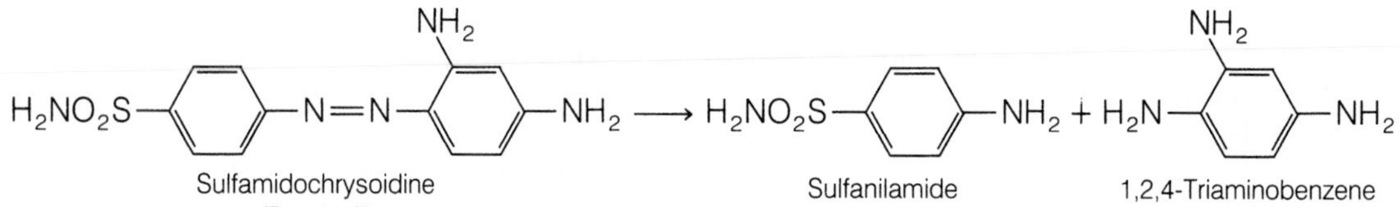

Sulfamidochrysoidine
(Prontosil)

Sulfanilamide

1,2,4-Triaminobenzene

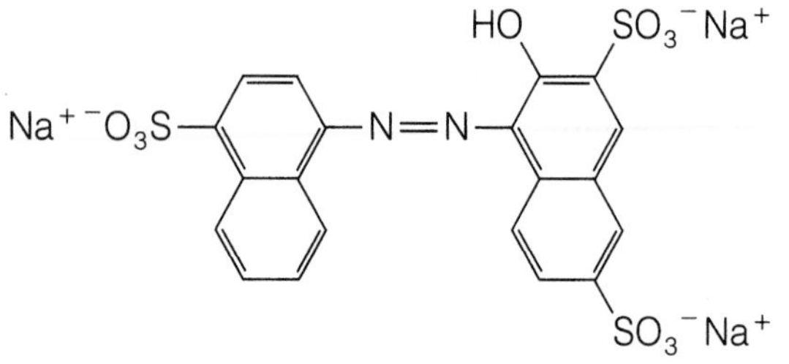

Tartrazine

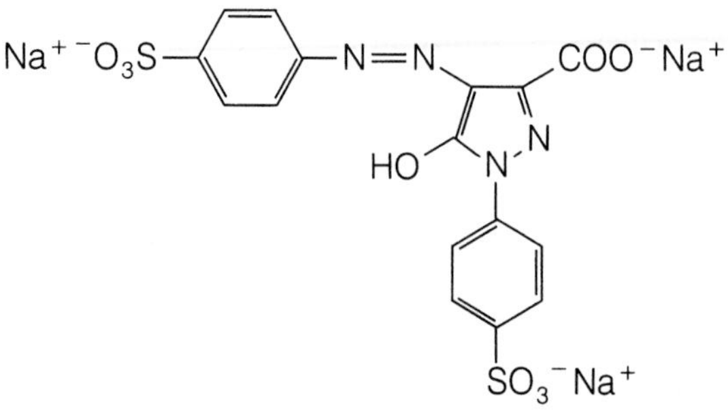

Amaranth

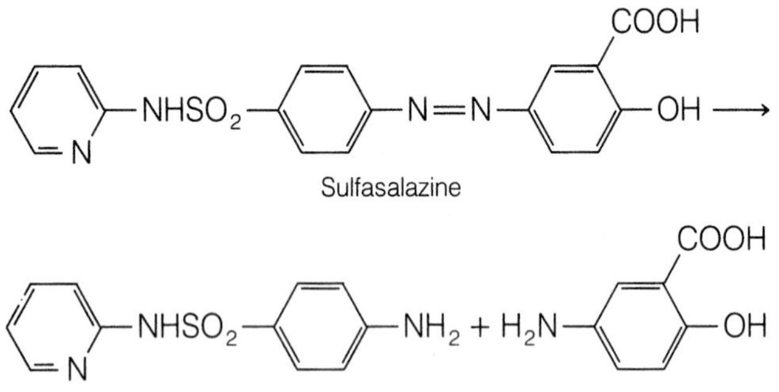

Sulfasalazine

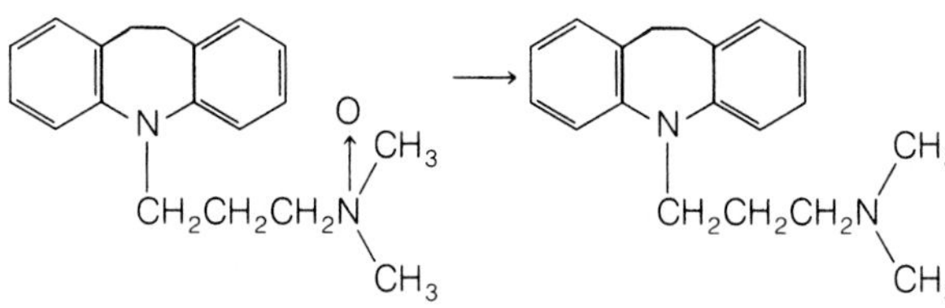

Imipramine *N*-Oxide

Imipramine

Sulfapyridine

5-Aminosalicylic Acid

sorbed poorly and undergoes reductive cleavage of the azo linkage to yield sulfapyridine and 5-aminosalicylic acid.[327, 328] The reaction occurs primarily in the colon and is carried out principally by intestinal bacteria. Studies in germ-free rats, lacking intestinal flora, have demonstrated that sulfasalazine is not reduced to any appreciable extent.[329]

Miscellaneous Reductions

Several minor reductive reactions also occur. Reduction of *N*-oxides to the corresponding tertiary amine occurs to some extent. This reductive pathway is of interest because several tertiary amines are oxidized to form polar and water-soluble *N*-oxide metabolites. If reduction of *N*-oxide metabolites occurs to a significant extent, drug elimination of the parent tertiary amine is impeded. *N*-Oxide reduction often is assessed by administering the pure synthetic *N*-oxide in vitro

or in vivo and then attempting to detect the formation of the tertiary amine. For example, imipramine *N*-oxide undergoes reduction in rat liver preparations.[330]

Reduction of sulfur-containing functional groups, such as the disulfide and sulfoxide moieties, also constitutes a minor reductive pathway. Reductive cleavage of the disulfide bond in disulfiram (Antabuse) yields *N,N*-diethyldithiocarbamic acid (free or glucuronidated) as a major metabolite in humans.[331, 332] Although sulfoxide functionalities are oxidized mainly to sulfones ($-SO_2-$), they sometimes undergo reduction to sulfides. The importance of this reductive pathway is seen in the metabolism of the anti-inflammatory agent sulindac (Clinoril). Studies in humans show that sulindac undergoes reduction to an active sulfide that is responsible for the overall anti-inflammatory effect of the parent drug.[333, 334] Sulindac or its sulfone metabolite exhibits little anti-inflammatory activity. Another example of sulfide for-

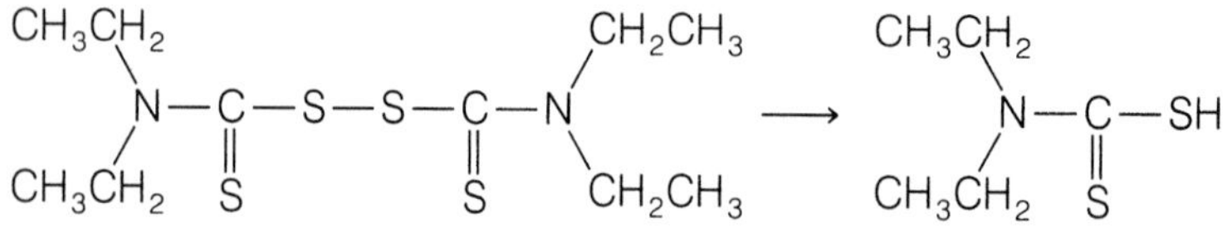

Disulfiram

N,N-Diethylthiocarbamic
Acid

Sulindac → Sulindac Sulfide Metabolite

mation involves the reduction of DMSO to dimethyl sulfide. In humans, DMSO is metabolized to a minor extent by this pathway. The characteristic unpleasant odor of dimethyl sulfide is evident on the breath of patients who use this agent.[335]

CH$_3$—S—CH$_3$ ⟶ CH$_3$SCH$_3$

Dimethyl Sulfoxide   Dimethyl Sulfide

HYDROLYTIC REACTIONS

Hydrolysis of Esters and Amides

The metabolism of ester and amide linkages in many drugs is catalyzed by hydrolytic enzymes present in various tissues and in plasma. The metabolic products formed (carboxylic acids, alcohols, phenols, and amines) generally are polar and functionally more susceptible to conjugation and excretion than the parent ester or amide drugs. The enzymes carrying out ester hydrolysis include several nonspecific esterases found in the liver, kidney, and intestine as well as the pseudo-cholinesterases present in plasma.[336, 337] Amide hydrolysis appears to be mediated by liver microsomal amidases, esterases, and deacylases.[337]

Hydrolysis is a major biotransformation pathway for drugs containing an ester functionality. This is because of the relative ease of hydrolyzing the ester linkage. A classic example of ester hydrolysis is the metabolic conversion of aspirin (acetylsalicylic acid) to salicylic acid.[338] Of the two ester moieties present in cocaine, it appears that, in general, the methyl group is hydrolyzed preferentially to yield benzoylecgonine as the major human urinary metabolite.[339] The

hydrolysis of cocaine to methyl ecgonine, however, also occurs in plasma and, to a minor extent, blood.[340, 341] Methylphenidate (Ritalin) is biotransformed rapidly by hydrolysis to yield ritalinic acid as the major urinary metabolite in humans.[342] Often, ester hydrolysis of the parent drug leads to pharmacologically active metabolites. For example, hydrolysis of diphenoxylate in humans leads to diphenoxylic acid (difenoxin), which is, apparently, 5 times more potent an antidiarrheal agent than the parent ester.[343] The rapid metabolism of clofibrate (Atromid-S) yields p-chlorophenoxyisobutyric acid (CPIB) as the major plasma metabolite in humans.[344] Studies in rats indicate that the free acid CPIB is responsible for clofibrate's hypolipidemic effect.[345]

Aspirin (Acetylsalicylic acid) → Salicylic Acid + Acetic Acid

Many parent drugs have been chemically modified or derivatized to generate so-called prodrugs to overcome some undesirable property (e.g., bitter taste, poor absorption, poor solubility, irritation at site of injection). The rationale behind the prodrug concept was to develop an agent that, once inside the biological system, would be biotransformed to the active parent drug.[18] The presence of esterases in many tissues and plasma makes ester derivatives logical prodrug candidates because hydrolysis would cause the ester prodrug to revert to the parent compound. Accordingly, antibiotics such as chloramphenicol and clindamycin have been derivatized as their palmitate esters to minimize their bitter taste and to improve their palatability in pediatric liquid suspensions.[346, 347] After oral administration, intestinal esterases

Cocaine → Benzoylecgonine + Methylecgonine

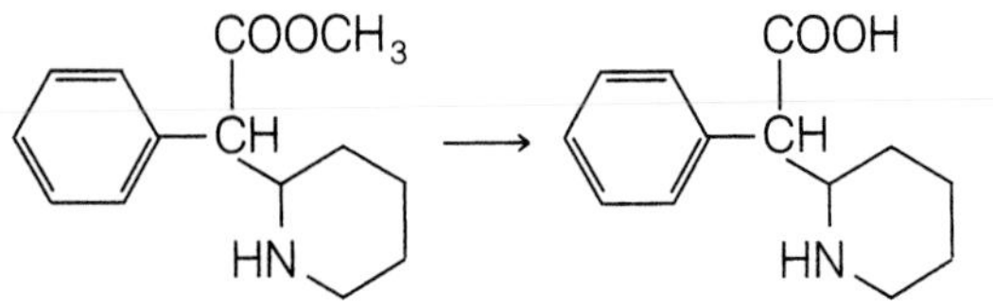

Methylphenidate → Ritalinic Acid

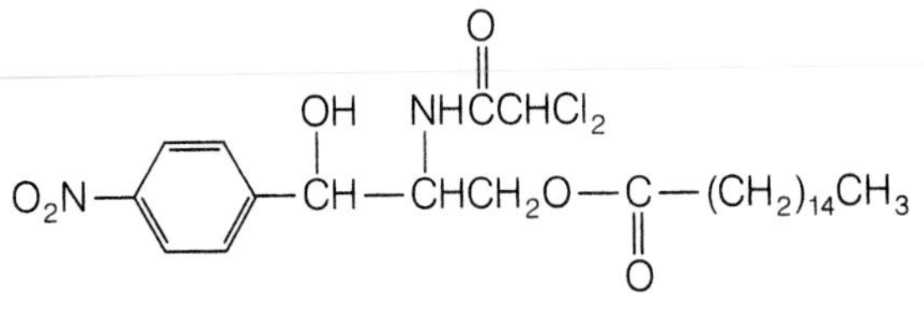

Chloramphenicol Palmitate

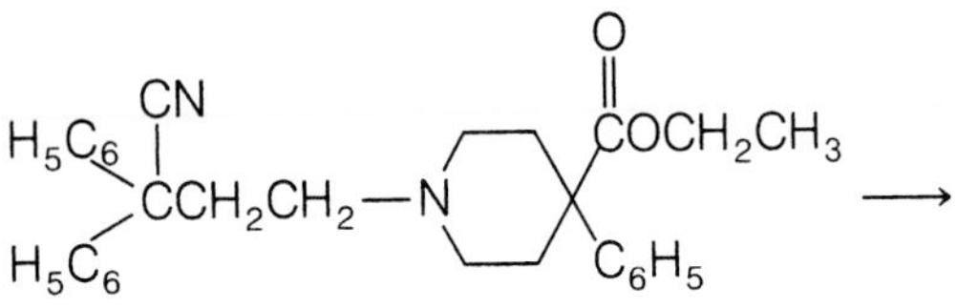

Diphenoxylate →

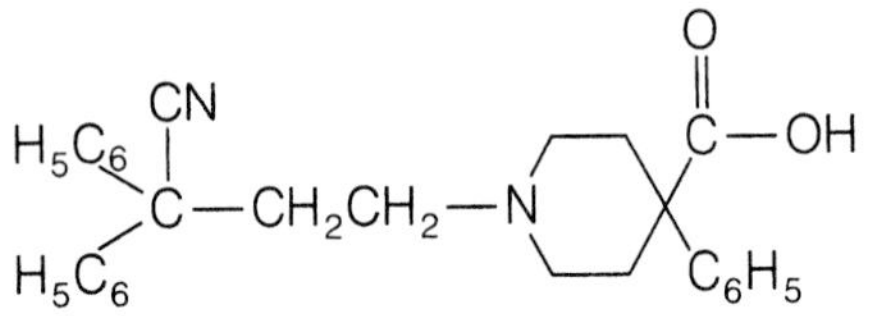

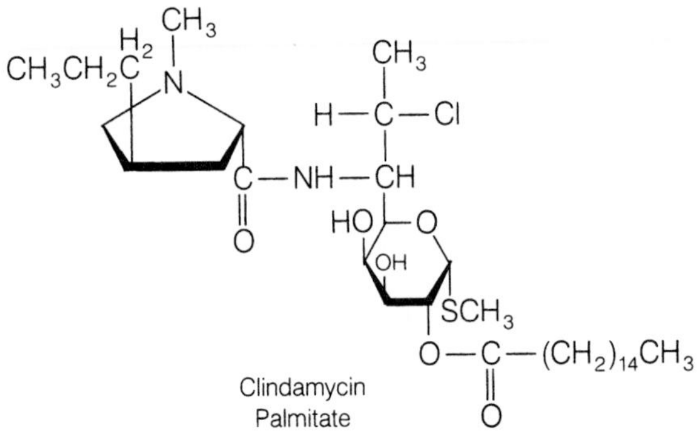

Clindamycin Palmitate

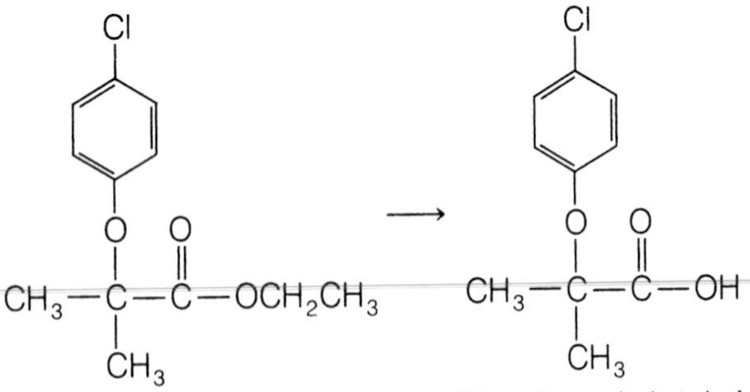

Diphenoxylic Acid (Difenoxin)

Clofibrate → p-Chlorophenoxyisobutyric Acid

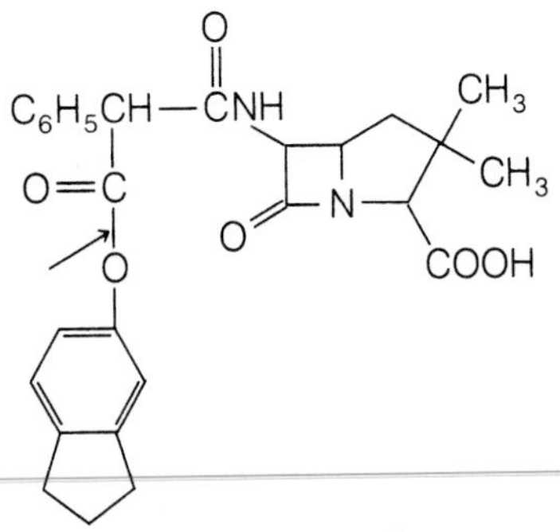

Carbenicillin Indanyl Ester

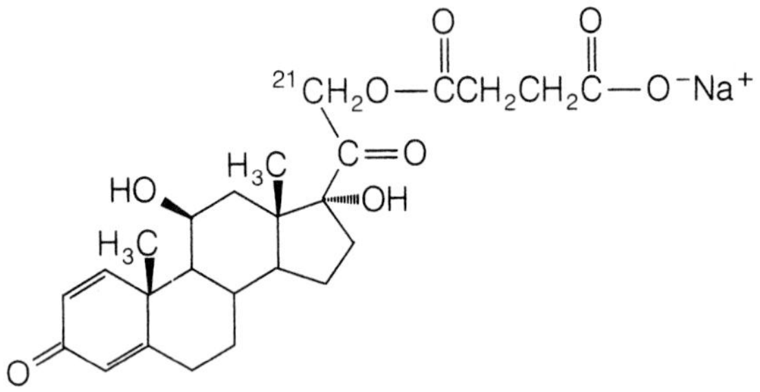

and lipases hydrolyze the palmitate esters to the free antibiotics. To improve the poor oral absorption of carbenicillin, a lipophilic indanyl ester has been formulated (Geocillin).[348] Once orally absorbed, the ester is hydrolyzed rapidly to the parent drug. A final example involves derivatization of prednisolone to its C-21 hemisuccinate sodium salt. This water-soluble derivative is extremely useful for parenteral administration and is metabolized to the parent steroid drug by plasma and tissue esterases.[349]

Amides are hydrolyzed slowly in comparison to esters.[337] Consequently, hydrolysis of the amide bond of procainamide is relatively slow compared with hydrolysis of the ester linkage in procaine.[336, 350] Drugs in which amide cleavage has been reported to occur, to some extent, include lidocaine,[351] carbamazepine,[87] indomethacin,[251, 252] and prazosin (Minipress).[253, 254] Amide linkages present in barbiturates (e.g., hexobarbital)[352, 353] as well as in hydantoins (e.g., 5-phenylhydantoin)[354, 355] and succinimides (phensuximide)[354, 355] are also susceptible to hydrolysis.

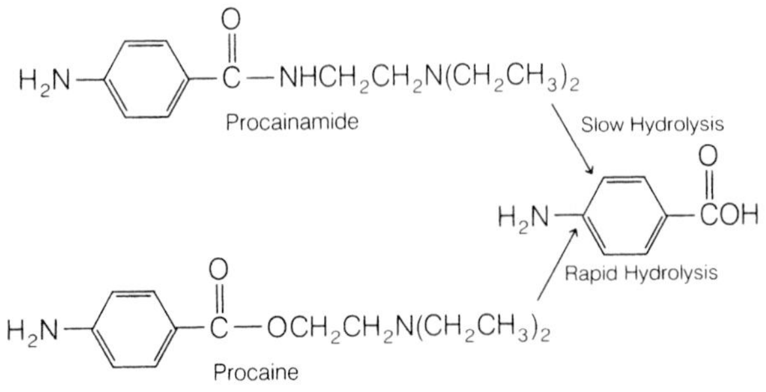

Miscellaneous Hydrolytic Reactions

Hydrolysis of recombinant human peptide drugs and hormones at the N- or C-terminal amino acids by carboxy- and

Prednisolone Hemisuccinate Sodium Salt

Procainamide

Slow Hydrolysis / Rapid Hydrolysis

Procaine

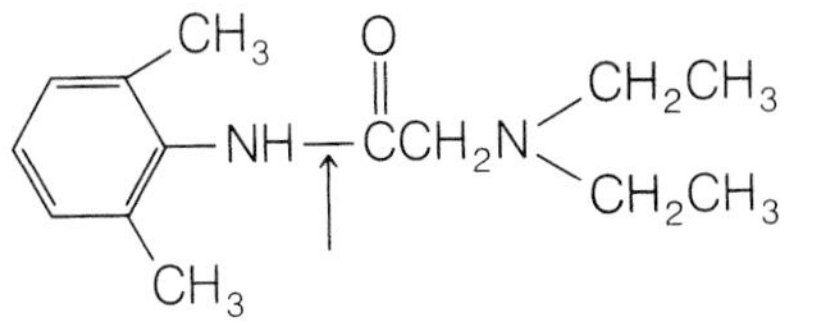

Lidocaine

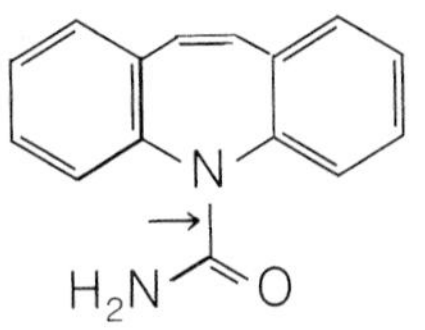

Carbamazepine

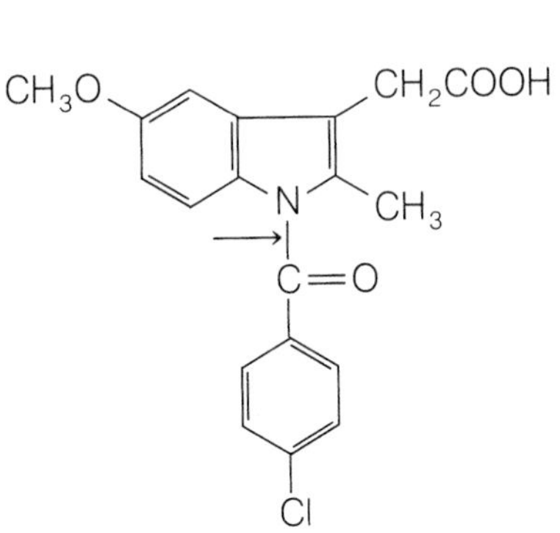

Indomethacin

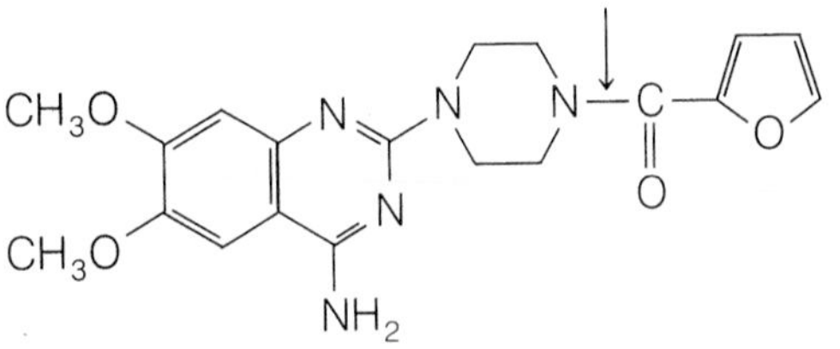

Prazosin

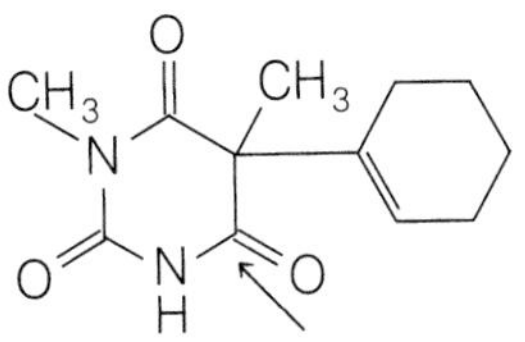

Hexobarbital

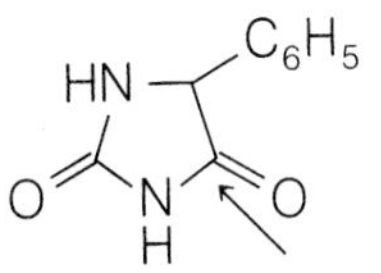

5-Phenylhydantoin

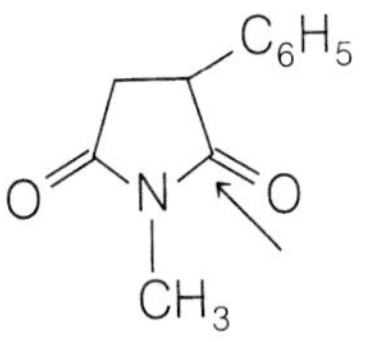

Phensuximide

aminopeptidases and proteases in blood and other tissues is a well-recognized hydrolytic reaction.[356, 357] Examples of peptides or protein hormones undergoing hydrolysis include human insulin, growth hormone (GH), prolactin, parathyroid hormone (PTH), and atrial natriuretic factor (ANF).[358]

In addition to hydrolysis of amides and esters, hydrolytic cleavage of other moieties occurs to a minor extent in drug metabolism,[8] including the hydrolysis of phosphate esters (e.g., diethylstilbestrol diphosphate), sulfonylureas, cardiac glycosides, carbamate esters, and organophosphate compounds. Glucuronide and sulfate conjugates also can undergo hydrolytic cleavage by β-glucuronidase and sulfatase enzymes. These hydrolytic reactions are discussed in the following section. Finally, the hydration or hydrolytic cleavage of epoxides and arene oxides by epoxide hydrase is considered a hydrolytic reaction.

PHASE II OR CONJUGATION REACTIONS

Phase I or functionalization reactions do not always produce hydrophilic or pharmacologically inactive metabolites. Various phase II or conjugation reactions, however, can convert these metabolites to more polar and water-soluble products. Many conjugative enzymes accomplish this objective by at-

taching small, polar, and ionizable endogenous molecules, such as glucuronic acid, sulfate, glycine, and glutamine, to the phase I metabolite or parent xenobiotic. The resulting conjugated products are relatively water soluble and readily excretable. In addition, they generally are biologically inactive and nontoxic. Other phase II reactions, such as methylation and acetylation, do not generally increase water solubility but mainly serve to terminate or attenuate pharmacological activity. The role of GSH is to combine with chemically reactive compounds to prevent damage to important biomacromolecules, such as DNA, RNA, and proteins. Thus, phase II reactions can be regarded as truly detoxifying pathways in drug metabolism, with a few exceptions.

A distinguishing feature of most phase II reactions is that the conjugating group (glucuronic acid, sulfate, methyl, and acetyl) is activated initially in the form of a coenzyme before transfer or attachment of the group to the accepting substrate by the appropriate transferase enzyme. In other cases, such as glycine and glutamine conjugation, the substrate is activated initially. Many endogenous compounds, such as bilirubin, steroids, catecholamines, and histamine, also undergo conjugation reactions and use the same coenzymes, although they appear to be mediated by more specific transferase enzymes. The phase II conjugative pathways discussed include those listed above in this chapter. Although other conjugative pathways exist (e.g., conjugation with glycosides, phosphate, and other amino acids and conversion of cyanide to thiocyanate), they are of minor importance in drug metabolism and are not covered in this chapter.

Glucuronic Acid Conjugation

Glucuronidation is the most common conjugative pathway in drug metabolism for several reasons: (a) a readily available supply of D-glucuronic acid (derived from D-glucose), (b) numerous functional groups that can combine enzymatically with glucuronic acid, and (c) the glucuronyl moiety (with its ionized carboxylate [pK$_a$ 3.2] and polar hydroxyl groups), which, when attached to xenobiotic substrates, greatly increases the water solubility of the conjugated product.[117, 359-361] Formation of β-glucuronides involves two steps: synthesis of an activated coenzyme, uridine-5'-diphospho-α-D-glucuronic acid (UDPGA), and subsequent transfer of the glucuronyl group from UDPGA to an appropriate substrate.[117, 360, 361] The transfer step is catalyzed by microsomal enzymes called *UDP-glucuronyltransferases*. They are found primarily in the liver but also occur in many other tissues, including kidney, intestine, skin, lung, and brain.[360, 361] The sequence of events involved in glucuronidation is summarized in Figure 4-11.[117, 360, 361] The synthesis of the coenzyme UDPGA uses α-D-glucose-1-phosphate as its initial precursor. Note that all glucuronide conjugates have the β configuration or β linkage at C-1 (hence, the term *β-glucuronides*). In contrast, the coenzyme UDPGA has an α linkage. In the enzymatic transfer step, it appears that nucleophilic displacement of the α-linked UDP moiety from UDPGA by the substrate RXH proceeds with complete inversion of configuration at C-1 to give the β-glucuronide. Glucuronidation of one functional group usually suffices to effect excretion of the conjugated metabolite; diglucuronide conjugates do not usually occur.

The diversity of functional groups undergoing glucuronidation is illustrated in Table 4-3 and Figure 4-12. Metabolic products are classified as oxygen–, nitrogen–, sulfur–, or carbon–glucuronide, according to the heteroatom attached to the C-1 atom of the glucuronyl group. Two important functionalities, the hydroxy and carboxy, form *O*-glucuron-

TABLE 4–3 Types of Compounds Forming Oxygen, Nitrogen, Sulfur, and Carbon Glucuronides[a]

Oxygen Glucuronides
Hydroxyl compounds
Phenols: morphine, acetaminophen, *p*-hydroxyphenytoin
Alcohols: tricholoroethanol, chloramphenicol, propranolol
Enols: 4-hydroxycoumarin
N-Hydroxyamines: *N*-hydroxydapsone
N-Hydroxyamides: *N*-hydroxy-2-acetylaminofluorene
Carboxyl compounds
Aryl acids: benzoic acid, salicylic acid
Arylalkyl acids: naproxen, fenoprofen
Nitrogen Glucuronides
Arylamines: 7-amino-5-nitroindazole
Alkylamines: desipramine
Amides: meprobamate
Sulfonamides: sulfisoxazole
Tertiary amines: cyproheptadine, tripelennamine
Sulfur Glucuronides
Sulfhydryl groups: methimazole, propylthiouracil, diethylthiocarbamic acid
Carbon Glucuronides
3,5-Pyrazolidinedione: phenylbutazone, sulfinpyrazone

[a] For structures and site of β-glucuronide attachment, see Figure 4-12).

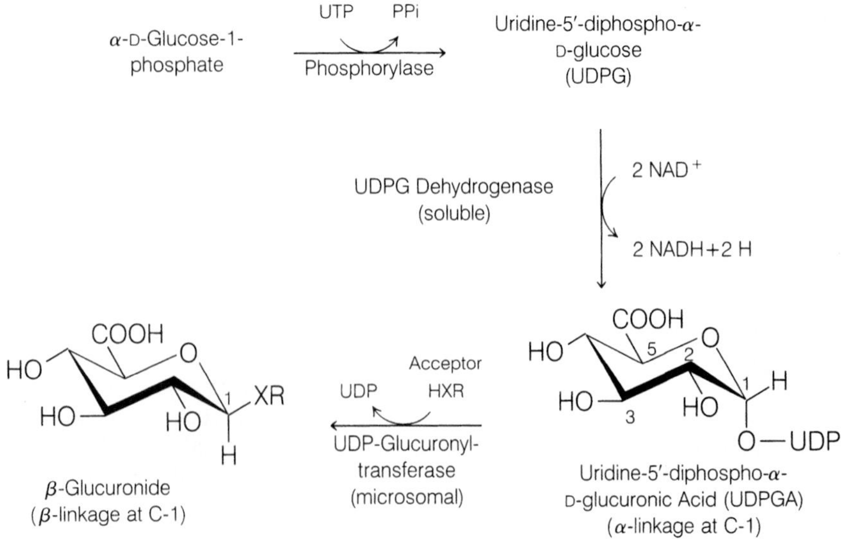

ides. Phenolic and alcoholic hydroxyls are the most common functional groups undergoing glucuronidation in drug metabolism. As we have seen, phenolic and alcoholic hydroxyl groups are present in many parent compounds and arise through various phase I metabolic pathways. Morphine,[362, 363] acetaminophen,[364] and *p*-hydroxyphenytoin (the major metabolite of phenytoin)[49, 50] are a few examples of phenolic compounds that undergo considerable glucuronidation. Alcoholic hydroxyls, such as those present in trichloroethanol (major metabolite of chloral hydrate),[288] chloramphenicol,[365] and propranolol,[366, 367] are also com-

Figure 4–11 ■ Formation of UDPGA and β-glucuronide conjugates.

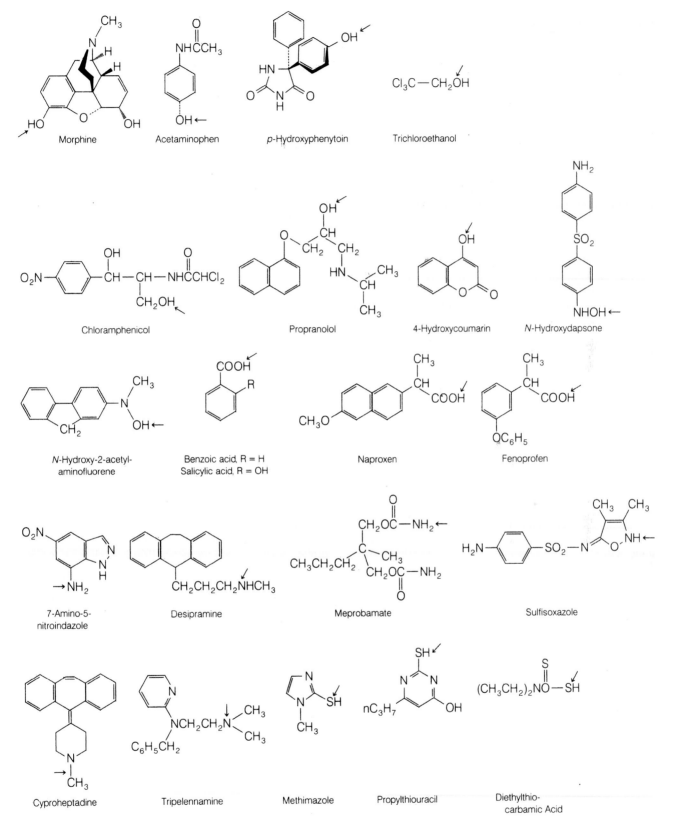

Figure 4–12 ■ Structure of compounds that undergo glucuronidation. *Arrows* indicate sites of β-glucuronide attachment.

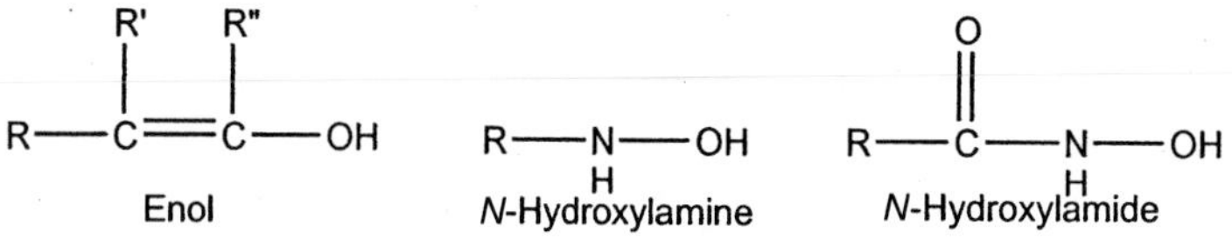

monly glucuronidated. Less frequent is glucuronidation of other hydroxyl groups, such as enols,[368] *N*-hydroxylamines,[226] and *N*-hydroxylamides.[241] For examples, refer to the list of glucuronides in Table 4-3.

The carboxy group is also subject to conjugation with glucuronic acid. For example, arylaliphatic acids, such as the anti-inflammatory agents naproxen[369] and fenoprofen,[370, 371] are excreted primarily as their *O*-glucuronide derivatives in humans. Carboxylic acid metabolites such as those arising from chlorpheniramine[290] and propranolol[289] (see "Reduction of Aldehyde and Ketone Carbonyls," above) form *O*-glucuronide conjugates. Aryl acids (e.g., benzoic acid,[372] salicylic acid[373, 374]) also undergo conjugation with glucuronic acid, but conjugation with glycine appears to be a more important pathway for these compounds.

Occasionally, *N*-glucuronides are formed with aromatic amines, aliphatic amines, amides, and sulfonamides. Representative examples are found in the list of glucuronides in Table 4-3. Glucuronidation of aromatic and aliphatic amines is generally a minor pathway in comparison with *N*-acetylation or oxidative processes (e.g., oxidative deamination). Tertiary amines, such as the antihistaminic agents cyproheptadine (Periactin)[375] and tripelennamine,[376] form interesting quaternary ammonium glucuronide metabolites.

Because the thiol group (SH) does not commonly occur in xenobiotics, *S*-glucuronide products have been reported for only a few drugs. For instance, the thiol groups present in methimazole (Tapazole),[377] propylthiouracil,[378, 379] and *N,N*-diethyldithiocarbamic acid (major reduced metabolite of disulfiram, Antabuse)[380] undergo conjugation with glucuronic acid.

The formation of glucuronides attached directly to a carbon atom is relatively novel in drug metabolism. Studies in humans have shown that conjugation of phenylbutazone (Butazolidin)[381, 382] and sulfinpyrazone (Anturane)[383] yield the corresponding *C*-glucuronide metabolites:

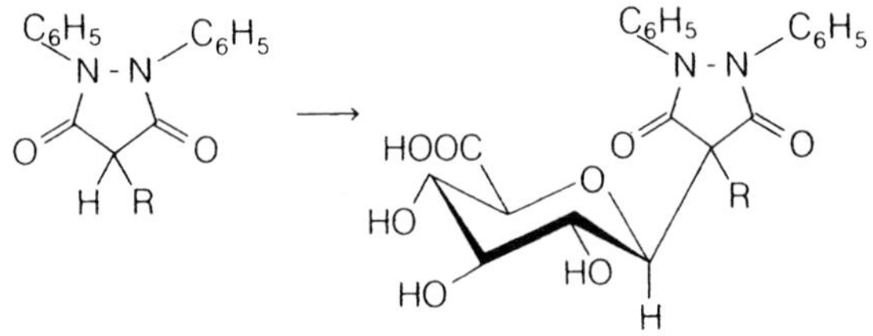

C-Glucuronide Metabolite

Phenylbutazone, R $= CH_2CH_2CH_2CH_3$
Sulfinpyrazone, R $= CH_2CH_2SC_6H_5$ $\overset{\parallel}{O}$

Besides xenobiotics, a number of endogenous substrates, notably bilirubin[384] and steroids,[385] are eliminated as glucuronide conjugates, which are excreted primarily in the urine. As the relative molecular mass of the conjugate exceeds 300 Da, however, biliary excretion may become an important route of elimination.[386] Glucuronides that are excreted in the bile are susceptible to hydrolysis by β-glucuronidase enzymes present in the intestine. The hydrolyzed product may be reabsorbed in the intestine, thus leading to enterohepatic recycling.[22] β-Glucuronidases are also present in many other tissues, including the liver, the endocrine system, and the reproductive organs. Although the function of these hydrolytic enzymes in drug metabolism is unclear, it appears that, in terms of hormonal and endocrine regulation, β-gluc-

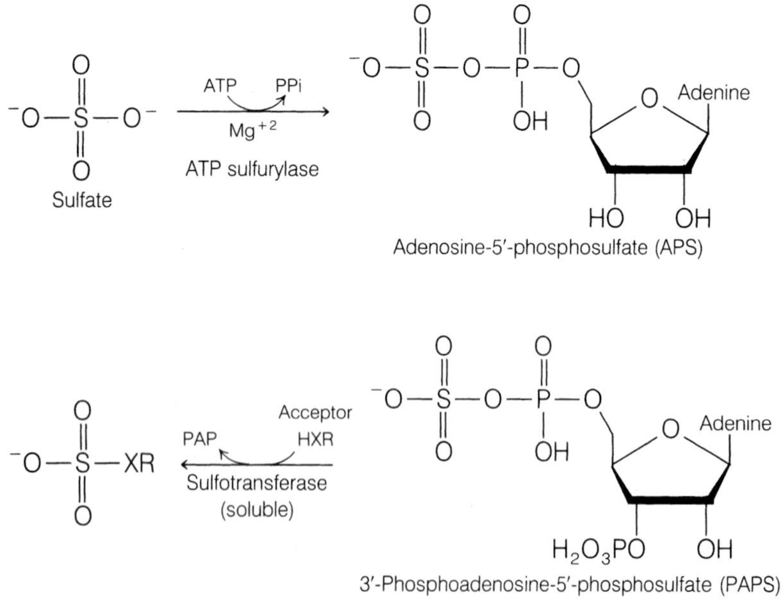

Figure 4–13 ■ Formation of PAPS and sulfate conjugates.

uronidases may liberate active hormones (e.g., steroids) from their inactive glucuronide conjugates.[22]

In neonates and children, glucuronidating processes are often not developed fully. In such subjects, drugs and endogenous compounds (e.g., bilirubin) that are metabolized normally by glucuronidation may accumulate and cause serious toxicity. For example, neonatal hyperbilirubinemia may be attributable to the inability of newborns to conjugate bilirubin with glucuronic acid.[387] Similarly, the inability of infants to glucuronidate chloramphenicol has been suggested to be responsible for the gray baby syndrome, which results from accumulation of toxic levels of the free antibiotic.[388]

Sulfate Conjugation

Conjugation of xenobiotics with sulfate occurs primarily with phenols and, occasionally, with alcohols, aromatic amines, and *N*-hydroxy compounds.[389–391] In contrast to glucuronic acid, the amount of available sulfate is rather limited. The body uses a significant portion of the sulfate pool to conjugate numerous endogenous compounds such as steroids, heparin, chondroitin, catecholamines, and thyroxine. The sulfate conjugation process involves activation of inorganic sulfate to the coenzyme 3′-phosphoadenosine-5′-phosphosulfate (PAPS). Subsequent transfer of the sulfate group from PAPS to the accepting substrate is catalyzed by various soluble sulfotransferases present in the liver and other tissues (e.g., kidney, intestine).[392] The sequence of events involved in sulfoconjugation is depicted in Figure 4-13. Sulfate conjugation generally leads to water-soluble and inactive metabolites. It appears, however, that the *O*-sulfate conjugates of some *N*-hydroxy compounds give rise to chemically reactive intermediates that are toxic.[241]

Phenols compose the main group of substrates undergoing sulfate conjugation. Thus, drugs containing phenolic moieties are often susceptible to sulfate formation. For example, the antihypertensive agent α-methyldopa (Aldomet) is metabolized extensively to its 3-*O*-sulfate ester in humans.[393, 394] The β-adrenergic bronchodilators salbutamol (albut-erol)[395] and terbutaline (Brethine, Bricanyl)[396] also undergo sulfate conjugation as their principal route of metabolism in humans. For many phenols, however, sulfoconjugation may represent only a minor pathway. Glucuronidation of phenols is frequently a competing reaction and may predominate as the conjugative route for some phenolic drugs. In adults, the major urinary metabolite of the analgesic acetaminophen is the *O*-glucuronide conjugate, with the concomitant *O*-sulfate conjugate being formed in small amounts.[364] Interestingly, infants and young children (ages 3 to 9 years) exhibit a different urinary excretion pattern: the *O*-sulfate conjugate is the main urinary product.[397, 398] The explanation for this reversal stems from the fact that neonates and young children have a decreased glucuronidating capacity because of undeveloped glucuronyltransferases or low levels of these enzymes. Sulfate conjugation, however, is well developed and becomes the main route of acetaminophen conjugation in this pediatric group.

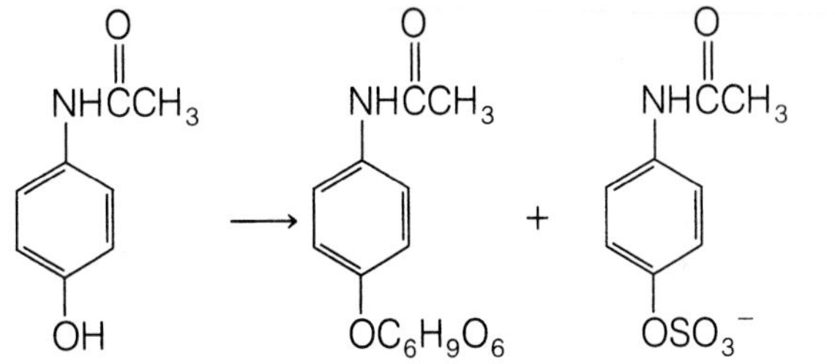

Acetaminophen   *O*-Glucuronide Conjugate   *O*-Sulfate Conjugate

Other functionalities, such as alcohols (e.g., aliphatic C_1 to C_5 alcohols, diethylene glycol)[399, 400] and aromatic amines (e.g., aniline, 2-naphthylamine),[401, 402] can also form sulfate conjugates. These reactions, however, have only minor importance in drug metabolism. The sulfate conjugation of *N*-hydroxylamines and *N*-hydroxylamides takes place as well, occasionally. *O*-Sulfate ester conjugates of *N*-hydroxy compounds are of considerable toxicological concern because they can lead to reactive intermediates that are responsible

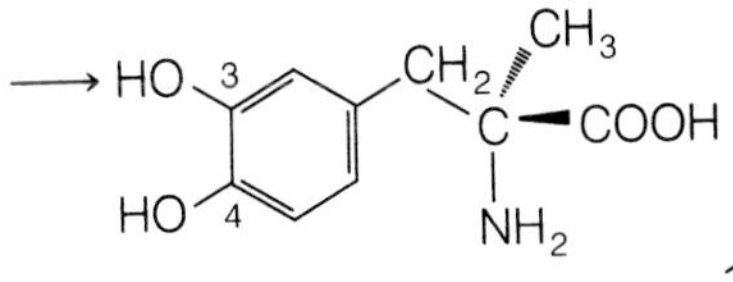

α-Methyldopa

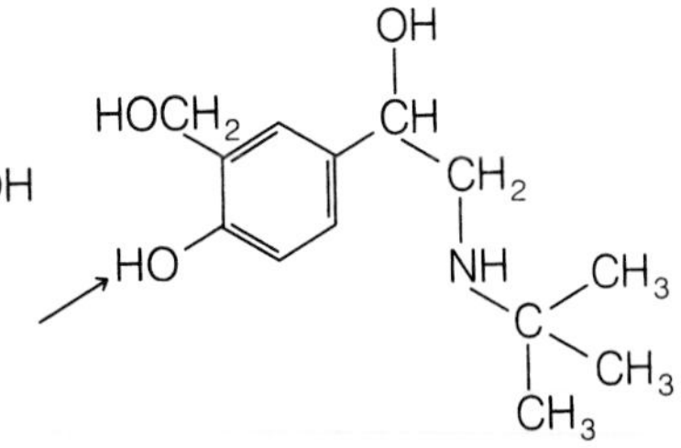

Salbutamol
(Albuterol)

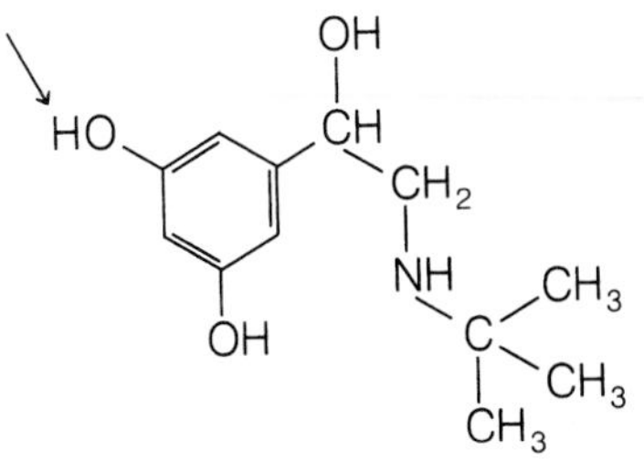

Terbutaline

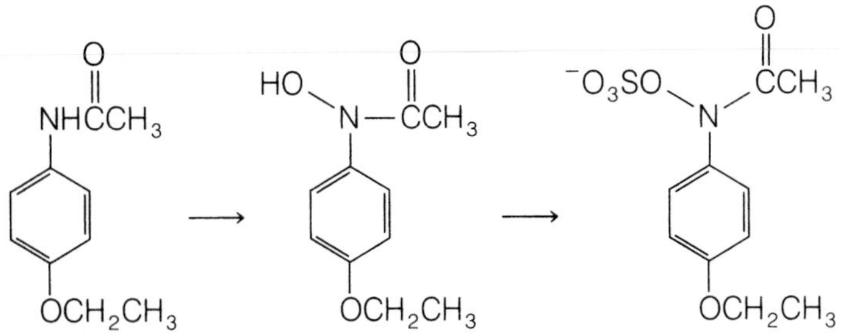

for cellular toxicity. The carcinogenic agents *N*-methyl-4-aminoazobenzene and 2-acetylaminofluorene are believed to mediate their toxicity through N-hydroxylation to the corresponding *N*-hydroxy compounds (see earlier section on N-hydroxylation of amines and amides). Sulfoconjugation of the *N*-hydroxy metabolites yields *O*-sulfate esters, which presumably are the ultimate carcinogenic species. Loss of SO_4^{2-} from the foregoing sulfate conjugates generates electrophilic nitrenium species, which may react with nucleophilic groups (e.g., NH_2, OH, SH) present in proteins, DNA, and RNA to form covalent linkages that lead to structural and functional alteration of these crucial biomacromolecules.[403] The consequences of this are cellular toxicity (tissue necrosis) or alteration of the genetic code, eventually leading to cancer. Some evidence supporting the role of sulfate conjugation in the metabolic activation of *N*-hydroxy compounds to reactive intermediates comes from the observation that the degree of hepatotoxicity and hepatocarcinogenicity of *N*-hydroxy-2-acetyl-aminofluorene depends markedly on the level of sulfotransferase activity in the liver.[404, 405]

The discontinued analgesic phenacetin is metabolized to *N*-hydroxyphenacetin and subsequently conjugated with sulfate.[406] The *O*-sulfate conjugate of *N*-hydroxyphenacetin binds covalently to microsomal proteins.[407] This pathway may represent one route leading to reactive intermediates that are responsible for the hepatotoxicity and nephrotoxicity associated with phenacetin. Other pathways (e.g., arene oxides) leading to reactive electrophilic intermediates are also possible.[6]

Conjugation With Glycine, Glutamine, and Other Amino Acids

The amino acids glycine and glutamine are used by mammalian systems to conjugate carboxylic acids, particularly aromatic acids and arylalkyl acids.[408, 409] Glycine conjugation is common to most mammals, whereas glutamine conjugation appears to be confined mainly to humans and other primates. The quantity of amino acid conjugates formed from xenobiotics is minute because of the limited availability of amino acids in the body and competition with glucuronidation for carboxylic acid substrates. In contrast with glucuronic acid and sulfate, glycine and glutamine are not converted to activated coenzymes. Instead, the carboxylic acid substrate is activated with adenosine triphosphate (ATP) and coenzyme A (CoA) to form an acyl-CoA complex. The latter intermediate, in turn, acylates glycine or glutamine under the influence of specific glycine or glutamine N-acyltransferase enzymes. The activation and acylation steps take place in the mitochondria of liver and kidney cells. The sequence of metabolic events associated with glycine and glutamine conjuga-

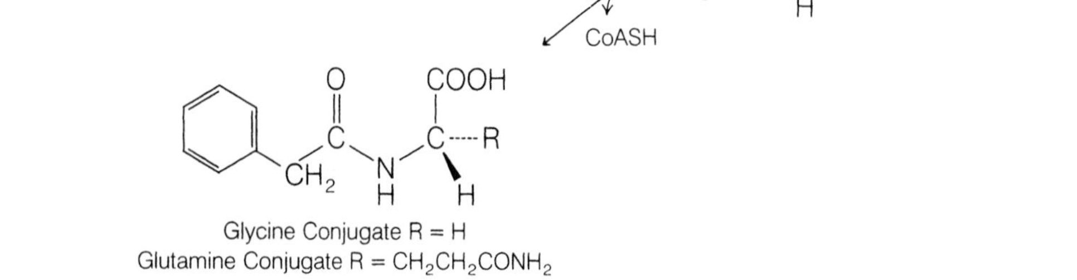

Figure 4–14 ▪ Formation of glycine and glutamine conjugates of phenylacetic acid.

tion of phenylacetic acid is summarized in Figure 4-14. Amino acid conjugates, being polar and water soluble, are excreted mainly renally and sometimes in the bile.

Benzoic Acid, R = H
Salicylic Acid, R = OH

Hippuric Acid, R = H
Salicyluric Acid, R = OH

Aromatic acids and arylalkyl acids are the major substrates undergoing glycine conjugation. The conversion of benzoic acid to its glycine conjugate, hippuric acid, is a well-known metabolic reaction in many mammalian systems.[410] The extensive metabolism of salicylic acid (75% of dose) to salicyluric acid in humans is another illustrative example.[411, 412] Carboxylic acid metabolites resulting from oxidation or hydrolysis of many drugs are also susceptible to glycine conjugation. For example, the H$_1$-histamine antagonist brompheniramine is oxidized to a propionic acid metabolite that is conjugated with glycine in both human and dog.[181] Similarly, *p*-fluorophenylacetic acid, derived from the metabolism of the antipsychotic agent haloperidol (Haldol), is found as the glycine conjugate in the urine of rats.[413] Phenylacetic acid and isonicotinic acid, resulting from the hydrolysis of, respectively, the anticonvulsant phenacemide (Phenurone)[414] and the antituberculosis agent isoniazid,[415] also are conjugated with glycine to some extent.

Glutamine conjugation occurs mainly with arylacetic acids, including endogenous phenylacetic[416] and 3-indolylacetic acid.[417] A few glutamine conjugates of drug metabolites have been reported. For example, in humans, the 3,4-dihydroxy-5-methoxyphenylacetic acid metabolite of mescaline is found as a conjugate of glutamine.[418] Diphenylmethoxyacetic acid, a metabolite of the antihistamine diphenhydramine (Benadryl), is biotransformed further to the corresponding glutamine derivative in the rhesus monkey.[419]

Several other amino acids are involved in the conjugation of carboxylic acids, but these reactions occur only occasionally and appear to be highly substrate and species dependent.[409, 420] Ornithine (in birds), aspartic acid and serine (in rats), alanine (in mouse and hamster), taurine (H$_2$NCH$_2$CH$_2$SO$_3$H) (in mammals and pigeons), and histidine (in African bats) are among these amino acids.[420]

GSH or Mercapturic Acid Conjugates

GSH conjugation is an important pathway for detoxifying chemically reactive electrophilic compounds.[421–428] It is now generally accepted that reactive electrophilic species manifest their toxicity (e.g., tissue necrosis, carcinogenicity, mutagenicity, teratogenicity) by combining covalently with nucleophilic groups present in vital cellular proteins and nucleic acids.[4, 429] Many serious drug toxicities may be explained also in terms of covalent interaction of metabolically generated electrophilic intermediates with cellular nucleophiles.[5, 6] GSH protects vital cellular constituents against chemically reactive species by virtue of its nucleophilic sulfhydryl (SH) group. The SH group reacts with electron-deficient compounds to form S-substituted GSH adducts (Fig. 4-15).[421–428]

GSH is a tripeptide (γ-glutamyl-cysteinylglycine) found in most tissues. Xenobiotics conjugated with GSH usually are not excreted as such, but undergo further biotransformation to give S-substituted N-acetylcysteine products called mercapturic acids.[76, 86, 424–428] This process involves enzymatic cleavage of two amino acids (namely, glutamic acid and glycine) from the initially formed GSH adduct and subsequent N-acetylation of the remaining S-substituted cysteine residue. The formation of GSH conjugates and their conversion to mercapturic acid derivatives are outlined in Figure 4-15.

Conjugation of a wide spectrum of substrates with GSH is catalyzed by a family of cytoplasmic enzymes known as glutathione S-transferases.[75] These enzymes are found in most tissues, particularly the liver and kidney. Degradation of GSH conjugates to mercapturic acids is carried out principally by renal and hepatic microsomal enzymes (Fig. 4-15).[76] Unlike other conjugative phase II reactions, GSH conjugation does not require the initial formation of an activated coenzyme or substrate. The inherent reactivity of the nucleophilic GSH toward an electrophilic substrate usually provides sufficient driving force. The substrates susceptible to GSH conjugation are quite varied and encompass many chemically different classes of compounds. A major prerequisite is that the substrate be sufficiently electrophilic. Compounds that react with GSH do so by two general mechanisms: (a) nucleophilic displacement at an electron-deficient carbon or heteroatom or (b) nucleophilic addition to an electron-deficient double bond.[421–423]

Many aliphatic and arylalkyl halides (Cl, Br, I), sulfates (OSO$_3^-$), sulfonates (OSO$_2$R), nitrates (NO$_2$), and organo-

Brompheniramine

3-(*p*-Bromophenyl)-3-(2-pyridyl)-propionic Acid

Glycine Conjugate

Haloperidol → p-Fluorophenylacetic Acid → Glycine Conjugate

Phenacemide →(Hydrolysis)→ Phenylacetic Acid → Glycine Conjugate

Isoniazid (R = H) or N-Acetylisoniazid (R = COH₃) →(Hydrolysis)→ Isonicotinic Acid → Glycine Conjugate

Mescaline → 3,4-Dihydroxy-5-methoxyphenylacetic Acid → Glutamine Conjugate

Diphenhydramine → Diphenylmethoxyacetic Acid → Glutamine Conjugate

phosphates (O-P[OR]₂) possess electron-deficient carbon atoms that react with GSH (by aliphatic nucleophilic displacement) to form GSH conjugates, as shown:

$$GSH \overset{+\delta}{\curvearrowright} \overset{}{C}H_2 \overset{-\delta}{-} X \longrightarrow GS-CH_2 + HX$$

R = Alkyl, Aryl, Benzylic, Allylic
X = Br, Cl, I, OSO₃⁻, OSO₂R, OPO(OR)₂

The carbon center is rendered electrophilic as a result of the electron-withdrawing group (e.g., halide, sulfate, phosphate) attached to it. Nucleophilic displacement often is facilitated when the carbon atom is benzylic or allylic or when X is a good leaving group (e.g., halide, sulfate). Many industrial chemicals, such as benzyl chloride ($C_6H_5CH_2Cl$), allyl chloride ($CH_2=CHCH_2Cl$), and methyl iodide, are known to be toxic and carcinogenic. The reactivity of these three halides toward GSH conjugation in mammalian systems is

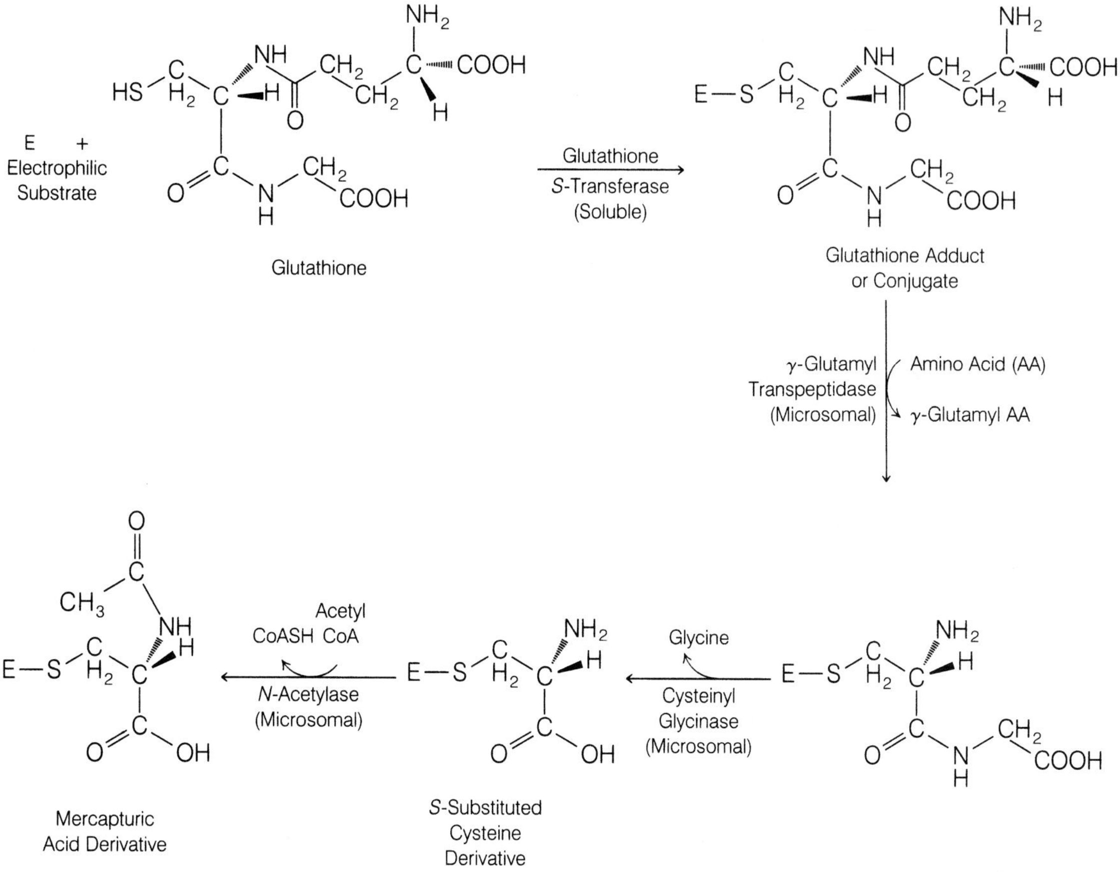

Figure 4–15 ■ Formation of GSH conjugates of electrophilic xenobiotics or metabolites (E) and their conversion to mercapturic acids.

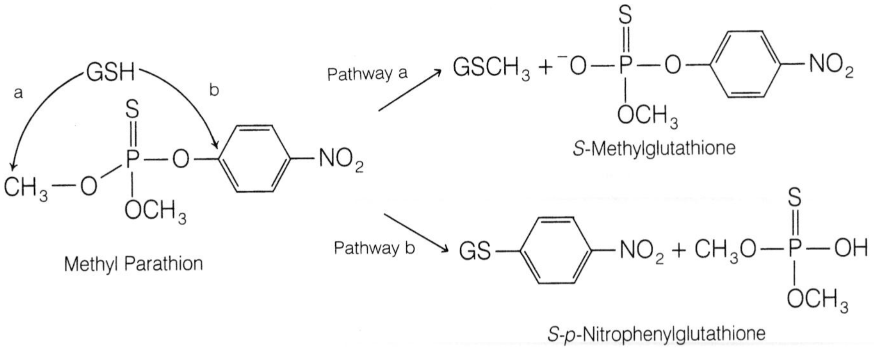

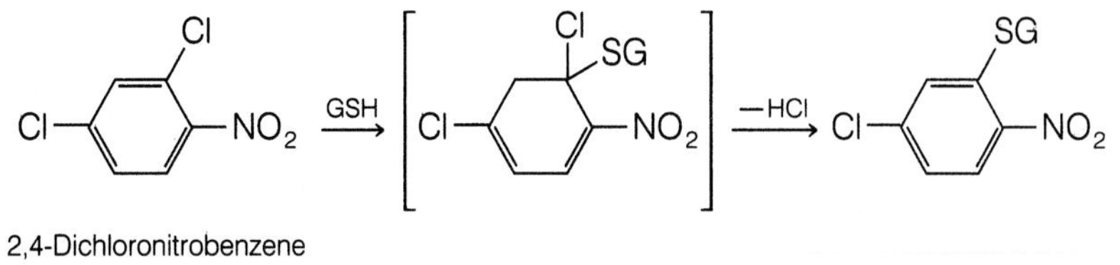

demonstrated by the formation of the corresponding mercapturic acid derivatives.[424–428] Organophosphate insecticides, such as methyl parathion, are detoxified by two different GSH pathways.[430, 431] Pathway ''a'' involves aliphatic nucleophilic substitution and yields *S*-methylglutathione. Pathway ''b'' involves aromatic nucleophilic substitution and produces *S*-*p*-nitrophenylglutathione. Aromatic or heteroaromatic nucleophilic substitution reactions with GSH occur only when the ring is rendered sufficiently electron-deficient by the presence of one or more strongly electron-withdrawing substituents (e.g., NO$_2$, Cl). For example, 2,4-dichloronitrobenzene is susceptible to nucleophilic substitution by GSH, whereas chlorobenzene is not.[432]

The metabolism of the immunosuppressive drug azathioprine (Imuran) to 1-methyl-4-nitro-5-(S-glutathionyl)imidazole and 6-mercaptopurine is an example of heteroaromatic nucleophilic substitution involving GSH.[433-435] Interestingly, 6-mercaptopurine formed in this reaction appears to be responsible for azathioprine's immunosuppressive activity.[436]

Azathioprine

1-Methyl-4-nitro-5-(S-glutathionyl)imidazole

6-Mercaptopurine

Arene oxides and aliphatic epoxides (or oxiranes) represent a very important class of substrates that are conjugated and detoxified by GSH.[437] The three-membered oxygen-containing ring in these compounds is highly strained and, therefore, reactive toward ring cleavage by nucleophiles (e.g., GSH, H$_2$O, or nucleophilic groups present on cellular macromolecules). As discussed above, arene oxides and epoxides are intermediary products formed from cytochrome P-450 oxidation of aromatic compounds (arenes) and olefins, respectively. If reactive arene oxides (e.g., benzo[α]pyrene-4,5-oxide, 4-bromobenzene oxide) and aliphatic epoxides (e.g., styrene oxide) are not "neutralized" or detoxified by glutathione S-transferase, epoxide hydrase, or other pathways, they ultimately covalently bind to cellular macromolecules and cause serious cytotoxicity and carcinogenicity. The isolation of GSH or mercapturic acid adducts from benzo[α]pyrene, bromobenzene, and styrene clearly demonstrates the importance of GSH in reacting with the reactive epoxide metabolites generated from these compounds.

GSH conjugation involving substitution at heteroatoms, such as oxygen, is seen often with organic nitrates. For example, nitroglycerin (Nitrostat) and isosorbide dinitrate (Isordil) are metabolized by a pathway involving an initial

GSH conjugation reaction. The GSH conjugate products, however, are not metabolized to mercapturic acids but instead are converted enzymatically to the corresponding alcohol derivatives and glutathione disulfide (GSSG).[438]

The nucleophilic addition of GSH to electron-deficient carbon–carbon double bonds occurs mainly in compounds with α,β-unsaturated double bonds. In most instances, the double bond is rendered electron deficient by resonance or conjugation with a carbonyl group (ketone or aldehyde), ester, nitrile, or other. Such α,β-unsaturated systems undergo so-called Michael addition reactions with GSH to yield the corresponding GSH adduct.[421-428] For example, in rats and dogs, the diuretic agent ethacrynic acid (Edecrin) reacts with GSH to form the corresponding GSH or mercapturic acid derivatives.[439] Not all α,β-unsaturated compounds are conjugated with GSH. Many steroidal agents with α,β-unsaturated carbonyl moieties, such as prednisone and digitoxigenin, have evinced no significant conjugation with GSH. Steric factors, decreased reactivity of the double bond, and other factors (e.g., susceptibility to metabolic reduction of the ketone or the C=C double bond) may account for these observations.

Occasionally, metabolic oxidative biotransformation reactions may generate chemically reactive α,β-unsaturated systems that react with GSH. For example, metabolic oxidation of acetaminophen presumably generates the chemically reactive intermediate *N*-acetylimidoquinone. Michael addition of GSH to the imidoquinone leads to the corresponding mercapturic acid derivative in both animals and humans.[245, 248] 2-Hydroxyestrogens, such as 2-hydroxy-17β-estradiol, undergo conjugation with GSH to yield the two isomeric mercapturic acid or GSH derivatives. Although the exact mechanism is unclear, it appears that 2-hydroxyestrogen is oxidized to a chemically reactive orthoquinone or semiquinone intermediate that reacts with GSH at either the electrophilic C-1 or C-4 position.[440, 441]

In most instances, GSH conjugation is regarded as a detoxifying pathway that protects cellular macromolecules such as protein and DNA against harmful electrophiles. In a few cases, GSH conjugation has been implicated in causing toxicity. Often, this is because the GSH conjugates are themselves electrophilic (e.g., vicinal dihaloethanes) or give rise to metabolic intermediates (e.g., cysteine metabolites of ha-

Nitroglycerin

Isosorbide

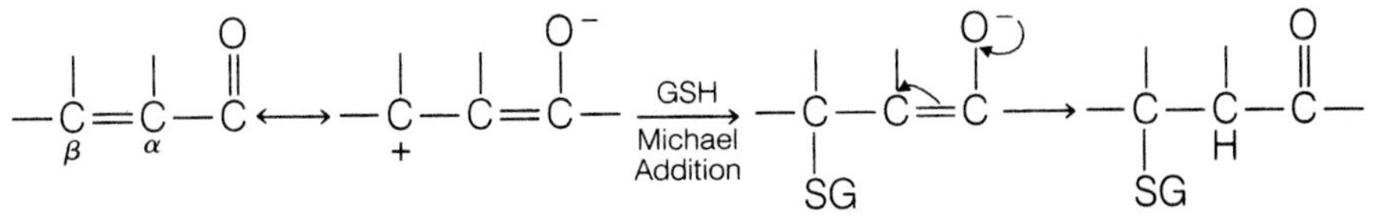

α-β-Unsaturated
System

Glutathione
Adduct

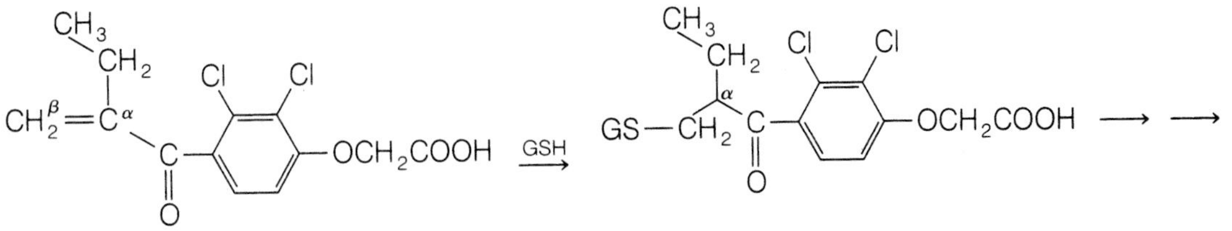

Ethacrynic Acid
(note α,β-unsaturated
ketone moiety)

GSH

Glutathione adduct
of Ethacrynic Acid

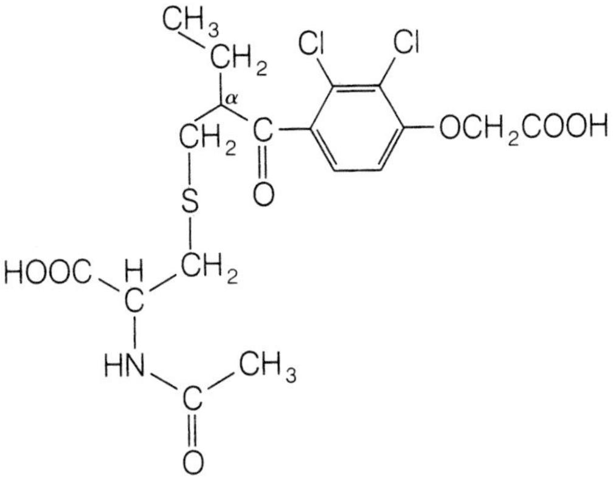

Mercapturic Acid Derivative

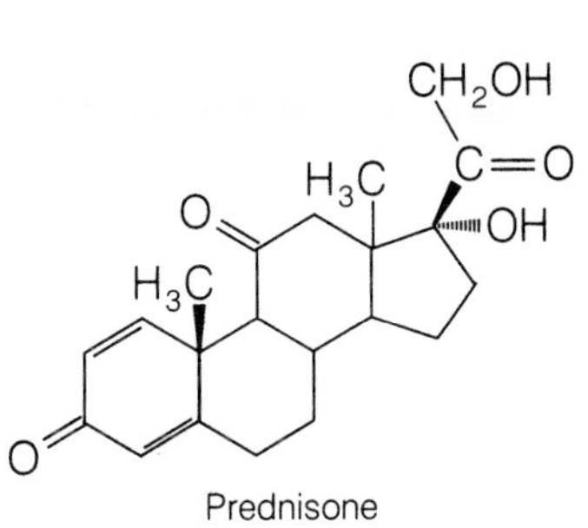

Prednisone

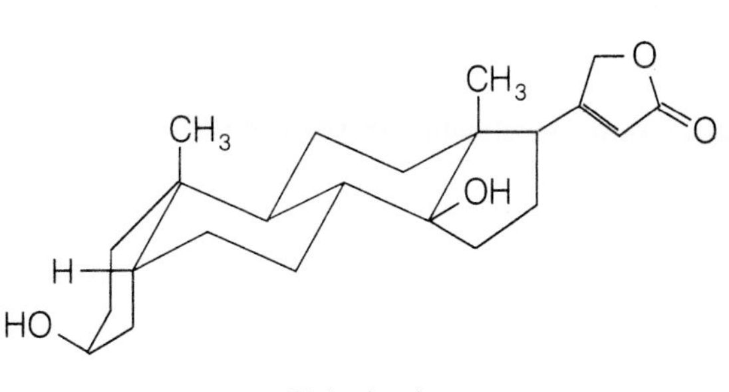

Digitoxigenin

loalkenes) that are electrophilic.[424–428] 1,2-Dichloroethane, for example, reacts with GSH to produce S-(2-chloroethyl)glutathione; the nucleophilic sulfur group in this conjugate can internally displace the chlorine group to give rise to an electrophilic three-membered ring episulfonium ion. The covalent interaction of the episulfonium intermediate with the guanosine moiety of DNA may contribute to the mutagenic and carcinogenic effects observed for 1,2-dichloroethane.[425–427] The metabolic conversion of GSH conjugates to reactive cysteine metabolites is responsible for the nephrotoxicity associated with some halogenated alkanes and alkenes.[428] The activation pathway appears to involve γ-glutamyl transpeptidase and cysteine conjugate β-lyase,

two enzymes that apparently target the conjugates to the kidney.

Acetylation

Acetylation constitutes an important metabolic route for drugs containing primary amino groups.[408, 442, 443] This encompasses primary aromatic amines ($ArNH_2$), sulfonamides ($H_2NC_6H_4SO_2NHR$), hydrazines (—$NHNH_2$), hydrazides (—$CONHNH_2$), and primary aliphatic amines. The amide derivatives formed from acetylation of these amino functionalities are generally inactive and nontoxic. Because water solubility is not enhanced greatly by N-acetylation, it ap-

Acetaminophen   N-Acetylimidoquinone   Mercapturic Acid Derivative

2-Hydroxy-17β-estradiol   Orthoquinone   Semiquinone

pears that the primary function of acetylation is to terminate pharmacological activity and detoxification. A few reports indicate, however, that acetylated metabolites may be as active as (e.g., *N*-acetylprocainamide),[444, 445] or more toxic than (e.g., *N*-acetylisoniazid),[446, 447] their corresponding parent compounds.

The acetyl group used in N-acetylation of xenobiotics is supplied by acetyl-CoA.[408] Transfer of the acetyl group from this cofactor to the accepting amino substrate is carried out by soluble N-acetyltransferases present in hepatic reticuloendothelial cells. Other extrahepatic tissues, such as the lung, spleen, gastric mucosa, red blood cells, and lymphocytes, also show acetylation capability. N-Acetyltransferase enzymes display broad substrate specificity and catalyze the acetylation of several drugs and xenobiotics (Fig. 4-16).[442, 443] Aromatic compounds with a primary amino group, such as aniline,[408] *p*-aminobenzoic acid,[448, 449] *p*-aminosalicylic acid,[418] procainamide (Pronestyl),[444, 445, 448, 449] and dapsone (Avlosulfon),[450] are especially susceptible to N-acetylation. Aromatic amine metabolites resulting from the reduction of aryl nitro compounds also are N-acetylated. For example, the anticonvulsant clonazepam (Klonopin) undergoes nitro reduction to its 7-amino metabolite, which in turn is N-acetylated.[315] Another related benzodiazepam analogue, nitrazepam, follows a similar pathway.[316]

The metabolism of a number of sulfonamides, such as sulfanilamide,[451] sulfamethoxazole (Gantanol),[452] sulfisoxazole (Gantrisin),[452] sulfapyridine[453] (major metabolite from azo reduction of sulfasalazine, Azulfidine), and sulfamethazine,[408] occurs mainly by acetylation at the N-4 position. With sulfanilamide, acetylation also takes place at the sulfamido N-1 position.[451] N-Acetylated metabolites of sulfon-

amides tend to be less water soluble than their parent compounds and have the potential of crystallizing out in renal tubules *(crystalluria),* thereby causing kidney damage. The frequency of crystalluria and renal toxicity is especially high with older sulfonamide derivatives, such as sulfathiazole.[1, 420] Newer sulfonamides, such as sulfisoxazole and sulfamethoxazole, however, are metabolized to relatively water-soluble acetylated derivatives, which are less likely to precipitate out.

The biotransformation of hydrazine and hydrazide derivatives also proceeds by acetylation. The antihypertensive hydralazine (Apresoline)[454, 455] and the MAO inhibitor phenelzine (Nardil)[456] are two representative hydrazine compounds that are metabolized by this pathway. The initially formed *N*-acetyl derivative of hydralazine is unstable and cyclizes intramolecularly to form 3-methyl-*s*-triazolo[3,4-*α*]phthalazine as the major isolable hydralazine metabolite in humans.[454, 455] The antituberculosis drug isoniazid or isonicotinic acid hydrazide (INH) is metabolized extensively to *N*-acetylisoniazid.[446, 447]

The acetylation of some primary aliphatic amines such as histamine,[457] mescaline,[208, 209] and the bis-N-demethylated metabolite of *α*(−)-methadol[458–460] also has been reported. In comparison with oxidative deamination processes, N-acetylation is only a minor pathway in the metabolism of this class of compounds.

The acetylation pattern of several drugs (e.g., isoniazid, hydralazine, procainamide) in the human population displays a bimodal character in which the drug is conjugated either rapidly or slowly with acetyl-CoA.[461, 462] This phenomenon is termed *acetylation polymorphism.* Individuals are classified as having either slow or rapid acetylator pheno-

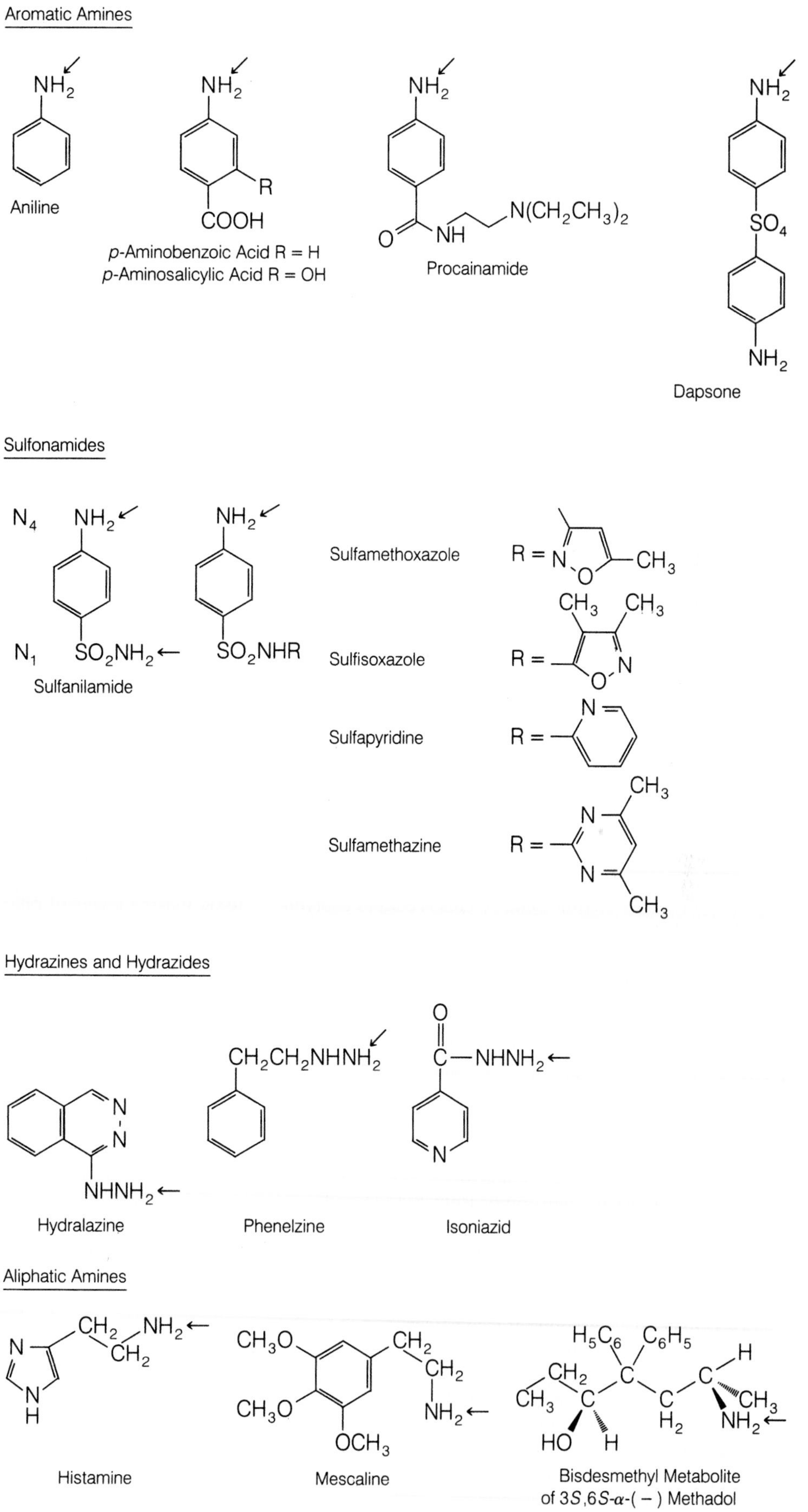

Aromatic Amines

Aniline

p-Aminobenzoic Acid R = H
p-Aminosalicylic Acid R = OH

Procainamide

Dapsone

Sulfonamides

Sulfanilamide

Sulfamethoxazole   R =

Sulfisoxazole   R =

Sulfapyridine   R =

Sulfamethazine   R =

Hydrazines and Hydrazides

Hydralazine   Phenelzine   Isoniazid

Aliphatic Amines

Figure 4–16 ■ Examples of different types of compound undergoing N-acetylation. *Arrows* indicate sites of N-acetylation.

Histamine   Mescaline   Bisdesmethyl Metabolite
of 3*S*,6*S*-α-(–) Methadol

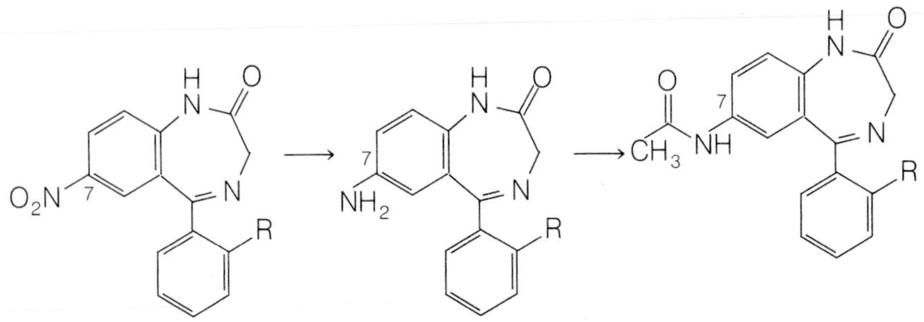

Clonazepam, R = Cl
Nitrazepam, R = H

7-Amino Metabolite

7-Acetamido Metabolite
or
N-Acetylated Metabolite

Sulfanilamide R = H

Sulfamethoxazole R =

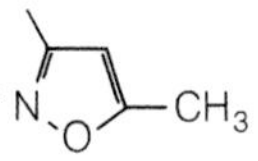

Sulfisoxazole R =

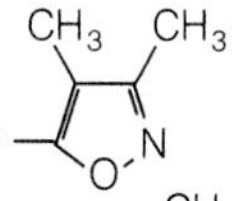

Sulfamethazine R =

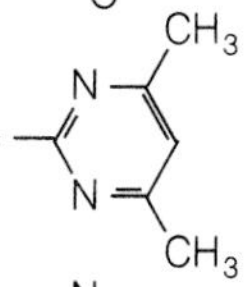

Sulfapyridine R =

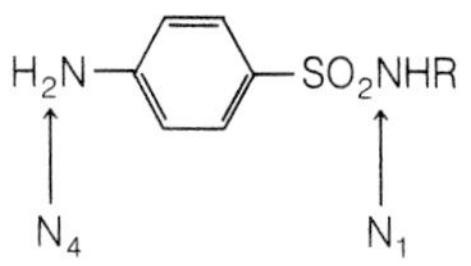

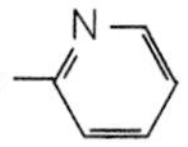

Sulfonamide Nomenclature

types. This variation in acetylating ability is genetic and is caused mainly by differences in N-acetyltransferase activity. The proportion of rapid and slow acetylators varies widely among different ethnic groups throughout the world. Oddly, a high proportion of Eskimos and Asians are rapid acetylators, whereas Egyptians and some Western European groups are mainly slow acetylators.[462] Other populations are intermediate between these two extremes. Because of the bimodal distribution of the human population into rapid and slow acetylators, there appears to be significant individual variation in therapeutic and toxicological responses to drugs displaying acetylation polymorphism.[408, 461, 462] Slow acetylators seem more likely to develop adverse reactions, whereas rapid acetylators are more likely to show an inadequate therapeutic response to standard drug doses.

The antituberculosis drug isoniazid illustrates many of these points. The plasma half-life of isoniazid in rapid acetylators ranges from 45 to 80 minutes; in slow acetylators the half-life is about 140 to 200 minutes.[463] Thus, for a given fixed-dosing regimen, slow acetylators tend to accumulate higher plasma concentrations of isoniazid than do rapid acetylators. Higher concentrations of isoniazid may explain the greater therapeutic response (i.e., higher cure rate) among slow acetylators, but they probably also account for the greater incidence of adverse effects (e.g., peripheral neuritis and drug-induced systemic lupus erythematosus syndrome) observed among slow acetylators.[462] Slow acetylators of isoniazid apparently are also more susceptible to certain drug interactions involving drug metabolism. For example, phenytoin toxicity associated with concomitant use with isoniazid appears to be more prevalent in slow acetylators than in rapid acetylators.[464] Isoniazid inhibits the metabolism of phenytoin, thereby leading to an accumulation of high and toxic plasma levels of phenytoin.

Interestingly, patients who are rapid acetylators appear to be more likely to develop isoniazid-associated hepatitis.[446, 447] This liver toxicity presumably arises from initial hydrolysis of the N-acetylated metabolite *N*-acetylisoniazid to acetylhydrazine. The latter metabolite is further converted (by cytochrome P-450 enzyme systems) to chemically reactive acylating intermediates that covalently bind to hepatic tissue, causing necrosis. Pathological and biochemical studies in experimental animals appear to support this hypothesis. Therefore, rapid acetylators run a greater risk of incurring liver injury by virtue of producing more acetylhydrazine.

The tendency of drugs such as hydralazine and procainamide to cause lupus erythematosus syndrome and to elicit formation of antinuclear antibodies (ANAs) appears related to acetylator phenotype, with greater prevalence in slow acetylators.[465, 466] Rapid acetylation may prevent the immunological triggering of ANA formation and the lupus syndrome. Interestingly, the N-acetylated metabolite of procainamide is as active an antiarrhythmic agent as the parent drug[444, 445] and has a half-life twice as long in humans.[467] These findings indicate that *N*-acetylprocainamide may be a promising alternative to procainamide as an antiarrhythmic agent with less lupus-inducing potential.

Hydralazine → *N*-Acetylhydralazine → [−H₂O] → 3-Methyl-*s*-triazolo-[3,4-*a*]phthalazine

Isoniazid → N-acetylation → *N*-Acetylisoniazid → Hydrolysis → $CH_3\overset{O}{\overset{\|}{C}}NHNH_2$ + Acetylhydrazine + Isonicotinic Acid

N-oxidation Cytochrome P-450 Mediated

Reactive intermediates possibly, $CH_3\overset{O}{\overset{\|}{C}}+,CH_3\overset{O}{\overset{\|}{C}}\cdot$ → Covalent Binding → Liver Damage

Methylation

Methylation reactions play an important role in the biosynthesis of many endogenous compounds (e.g., epinephrine and melatonin) and in the inactivation of numerous physiologically active biogenic amines (e.g., norepinephrine, dopamine, serotonin, and histamine).[468] Methylation, however, constitutes only a minor pathway for conjugating drugs and xenobiotics. Methylation generally does not lead to polar or water-soluble metabolites, except when it creates a quaternary ammonium derivative. Most methylated products tend to be pharmacologically inactive, although there are a few exceptions.

Norepinephrine, R = OH
Dopamine, R = H
→ COMT →
Normetanephrine, R = OH
3-Methoxytyramine, R = H

The coenzyme involved in methylation reactions is *S*-adenosylmethionine (SAM). The transfer of the activated methyl group from this coenzyme to the acceptor substrate is catalyzed by various cytoplasmic and microsomal methyltransferases (Fig. 4-17).[468, 469] Methyltransferases of particular importance in the metabolism of foreign compounds include catechol-*O*-methyltransferase (COMT), phenol-*O*-

methyltransferase, and nonspecific N-methyltransferases and S-methyltransferases.[358] One of these enzymes, COMT, should be familiar because it carries out O-methylation of such important neurotransmitters as norepinephrine and dopamine and thus terminates their activity. Besides being present in the central and peripheral nerves, COMT is distributed widely in other mammalian tissues, particularly the liver and kidney. The other methyltransferases mentioned are located primarily in the liver, kidney, or lungs. Transferases that specifically methylate histamine, serotonin, and epinephrine are not usually involved in the metabolism of xenobiotics.[468]

Foreign compounds that undergo methylation include catechols, phenols, amines, and *N*-heterocyclic and thiol compounds. Catechol and catecholamine-like drugs are metabolized by COMT to inactive monomethylated catechol products. Examples of drugs that undergo significant O-methylation by COMT in humans include the antihypertensive (S)(−)α-methyldopa (Aldomet),[470, 471] the antiparkinsonism agent (S)(−)-dopa (levodopa),[472] isoproterenol (Isuprel),[473] and dobutamine (Dobutrex).[474] The student should note the marked structural similarities between these drugs and the endogenous catecholamines such as norepinephrine and dopamine. In the foregoing four drugs, COMT selectively O-methylates only the phenolic OH at C-3. Bismethylation does not occur. Catechol metabolites arising from aromatic hydroxylation of phenols (e.g., 2-hydroxylation of 17α-ethinylestradiol)[54, 55] and from the arene oxide dihy-

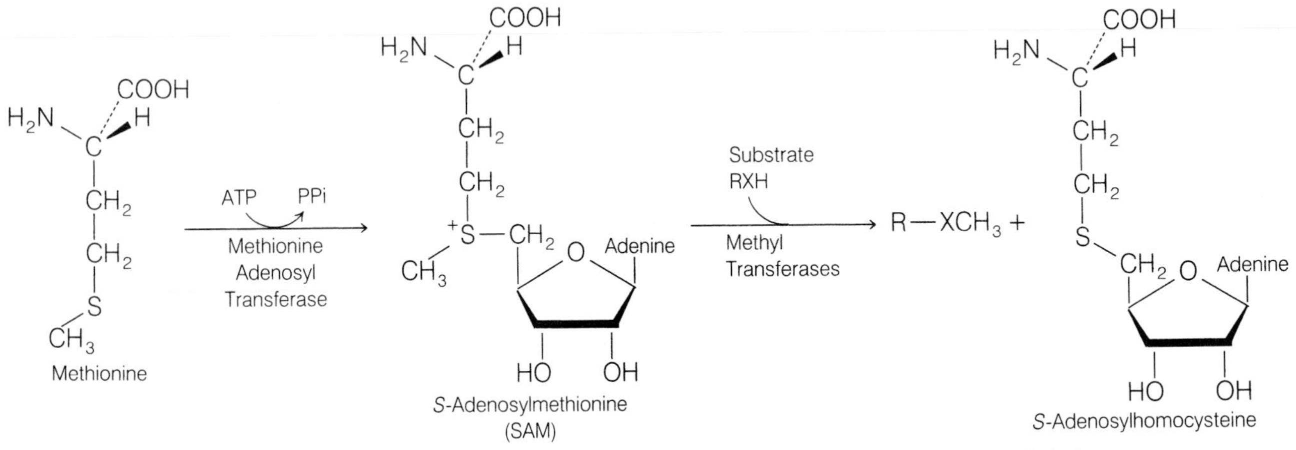

Figure 4–17 ■ Conjugation of exogenous and endogenous substrates *(RXH)* by methylation.

drodiol–catechol pathway (see section above on oxidation of aromatic moieties, e.g., the catechol metabolite of phenytoin)[475] also undergo O-methylation. Substrates undergoing O-methylation by COMT must contain an aromatic 1,2-dihydroxy group (i.e., catechol group). Resorcinol (1,3-dihydroxybenzene) or *p*-hydroquinone (1,4-dihydroxybenzene) derivatives are not substrates for COMT. This explains why isoproterenol undergoes extensive O-methylation[473] but terbutaline (which contains a resorcinol moiety) does not.[396]

Occasionally, phenols have been reported to undergo O-methylation but only to a minor extent.[468] One interesting example involves the conversion of morphine to its O-methylated derivative, codeine, in humans. This metabolite is formed in significant amounts in tolerant subjects and may account for up to 10% of the morphine dose.[476]

Although N-methylation of endogenous amines (e.g., histamine, norepinephrine) occurs commonly, biotransformation of nitrogen-containing xenobiotics to N-methylated metabolites occurs to only a limited extent. Some examples reported include the N-methylation of the antiviral and antiparkinsonism agent amantadine (Symmetrel) in dogs[477] and the in vitro N-methylation of norephedrine in rabbit lung preparations.[468] N-methylation of nitrogen atoms present in heterocyclic compounds (e.g., pyridine derivatives) also takes place. For example, the pyridinyl nitrogens of nicotine[187, 188] and nicotinic acid[478] are N-methylated to yield quaternary ammonium products.

Thiol-containing drugs, such as propylthiouracil,[479] 2,3-dimercapto-1-propanol (BAL),[480] and 6-mercaptopurine,[481, 482] also have been reported to undergo S-methylation.

FACTORS AFFECTING DRUG METABOLISM

Drugs and xenobiotics often are metabolized by several different phase I and phase II pathways to give a number of metabolites. The relative amount of any particular metabolite is determined by the concentration and activity of the enzyme(s) responsible for the biotransformation. The rate of metabolism of a drug is particularly important for its pharmacological action as well as its toxicity. For example, if the rate of metabolism of a drug is decreased, this generally increases the intensity and duration of the drug action. In addition, decreased metabolic elimination may lead to accumulation of toxic levels of the drug. Conversely, an increased rate of metabolism decreases the intensity and duration of action as well as the drug's efficacy. Many factors may affect drug metabolism, and they are discussed in the following sections. These include age, species and strain, genetic or hereditary factors, sex, enzyme induction, and enzyme inhibition.[32, 483–486]

Age Differences

Age-related differences in drug metabolism are generally quite apparent in the newborn.[487, 488] In most fetal and newborn animals, undeveloped or deficient oxidative and conjugative enzymes are chiefly responsible for the reduced metabolic capability seen. In general, the ability to carry out metabolic reactions increases rapidly after birth and approaches adult levels in about 1 to 2 months. An illustration of the influence of age on drug metabolism is seen in the duration of action (sleep time) of hexobarbital in newborn and adult mice.[489] When given a dose of 10 mg/kg of body weight, the newborn mouse sleeps more than 6 hours. In contrast, the adult mouse sleeps for fewer than 5 minutes when given the same dose.

In humans, oxidative and conjugative (e.g., glucuronidation) capabilities of newborns are also low compared with those of adults. For example, the oxidative (cytochrome P-450) metabolism of tolbutamide appears to be markedly lower in newborns.[490] Compared with the half-life of 8 hours in adults, the plasma half-life of tolbutamide in infants is more than 40 hours. As discussed above, infants possess poor glucuronidating ability because of a deficiency in glucuronyltransferase activity. The inability of infants to conjugate chloramphenicol with glucuronic acid appears to be responsible for the accumulation of toxic levels of this antibiotic, resulting in the so-called gray baby syndrome.[388] Similarly, neonatal hyperbilirubinemia (or kernicterus) results from the inability of newborn babies to glucuronidate bilirubin.[387]

The effect of old age on drug metabolism has not been as well studied. There is some evidence in animals and humans that drug metabolism diminishes with old age.[491, 492]

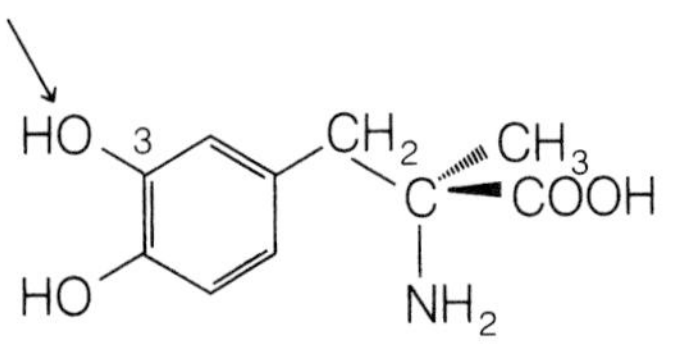

S(−)-α-Methyldopa

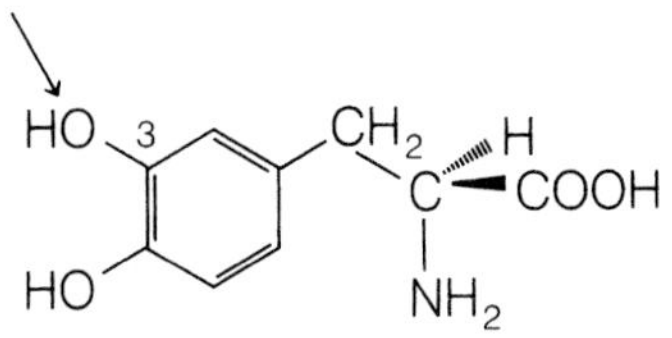

S(−)-Dopa

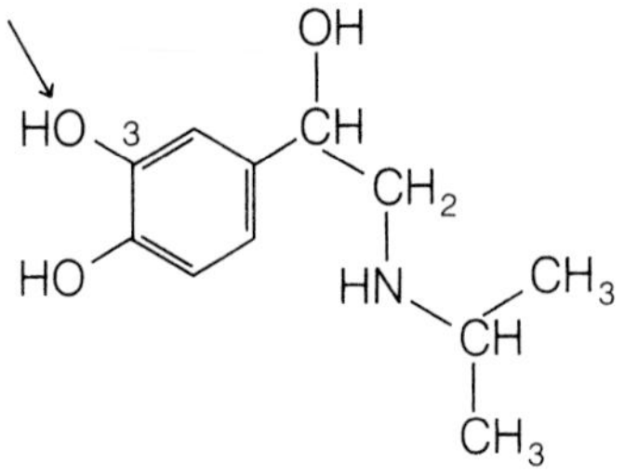

Isoproterenol

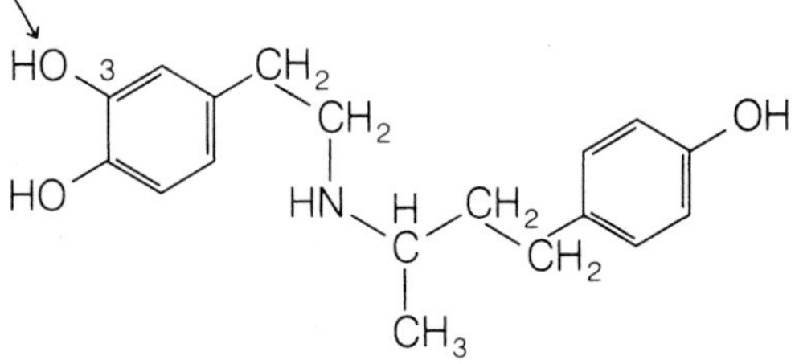

Dobutamine

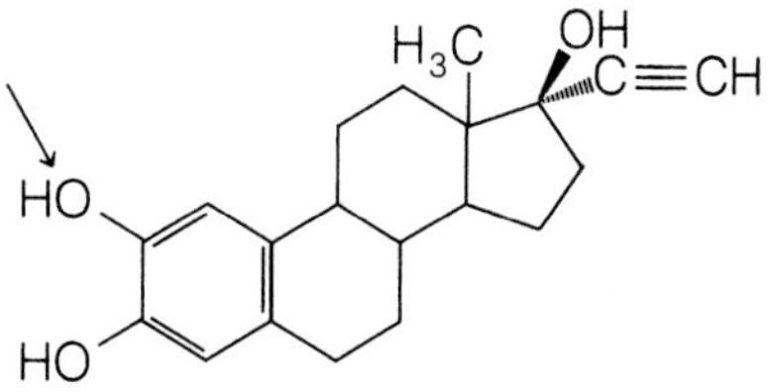

2-Hydroxy-17α-ethinylestradiol

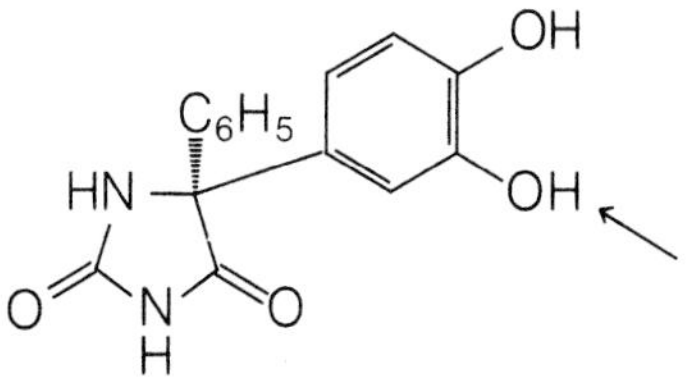

Catechol Metabolite
of Phenytoin

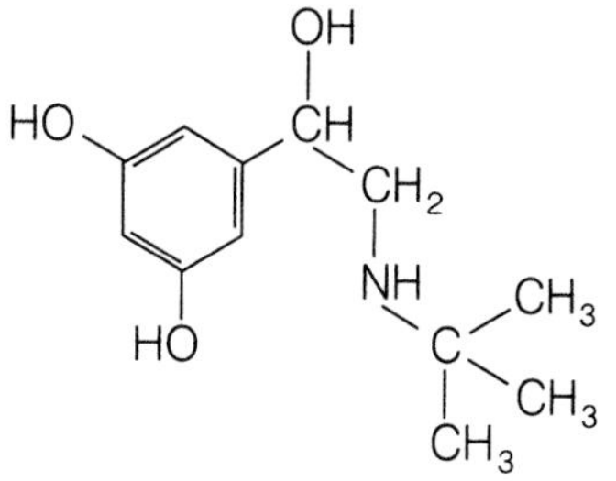

Terbutaline
(not a substrate for COMT)

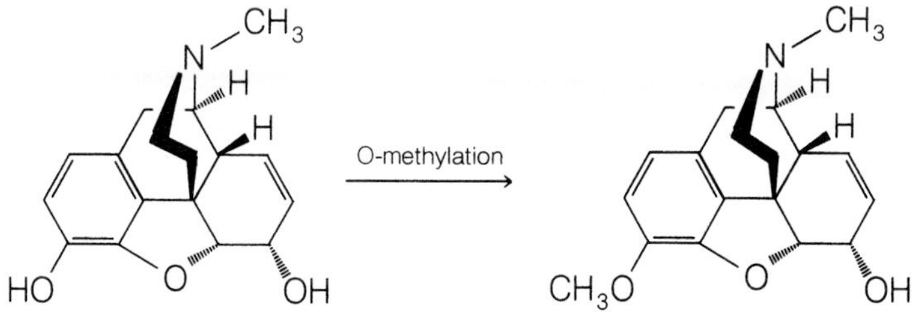

Morphine

O-methylation

Codeine

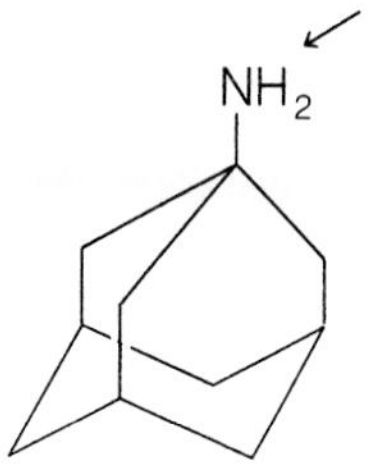

Amantadine

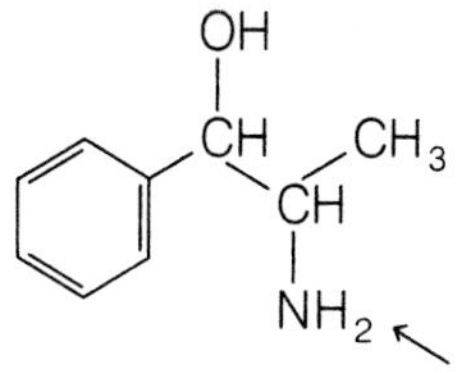

Norephedrine

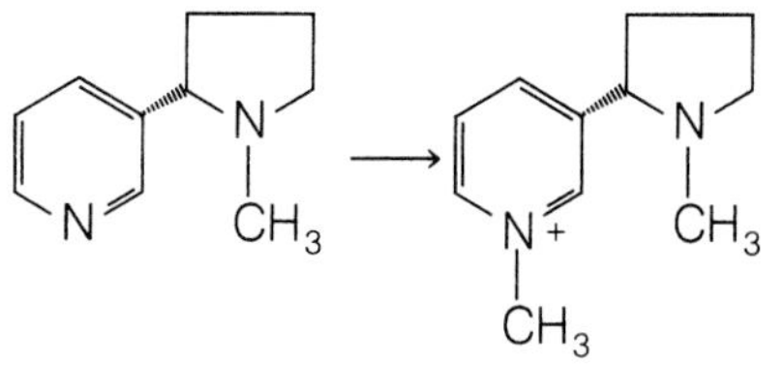

Nicotine

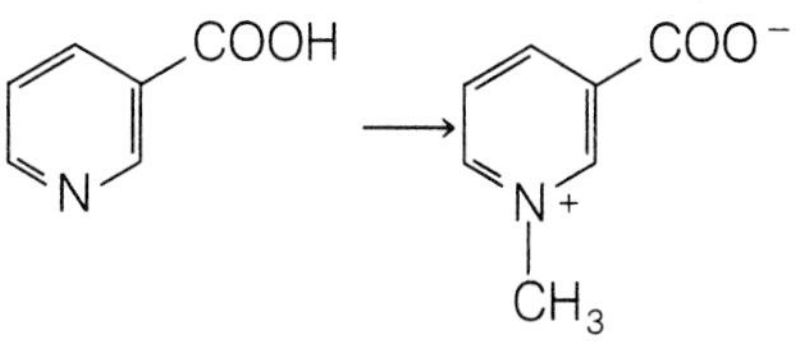

Nicotinic Acid

Trigonelline

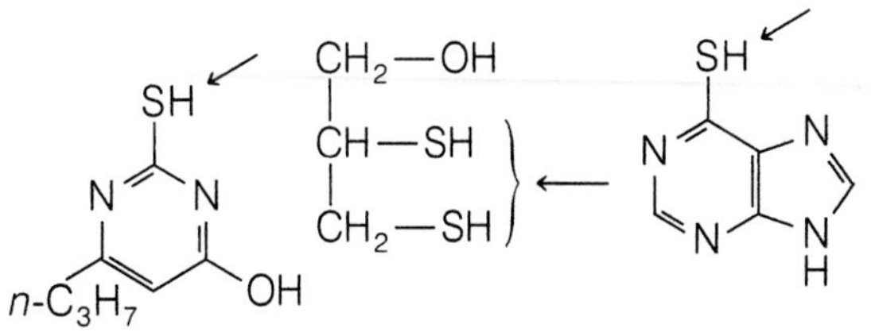

Propylthiouracil

2,3-Dimercapto-1-
propanol (BAL)

6-Mercaptopurine

Much of the evidence, however, is based on prolonged plasma half-lives of drugs that are metabolized totally or mainly by hepatic microsomal enzymes (e.g., antipyrine, phenobarbital, acetaminophen). In evaluating the effect of age on drug metabolism, one must differentiate between "normal" loss of enzymatic activity with aging and the effect of a diseased liver from hepatitis, cirrhosis, etc., plus decreased renal function, because much of the water-soluble conjugation products are excreted in the liver.

Species and Strain Differences

The metabolism of many drugs and foreign compounds is often species dependent. Different animal species may biotransform a particular xenobiotic by similar or markedly different metabolic pathways. Even within the same species, individual variations (strain differences) may result in significant differences in a specific metabolic pathway.[493, 494] This is a problem when a new drug is under development. A new drug application requires the developer to account for the product as it moves from the site of administration to final elimination from the body. It is difficult enough to find appropriate animal models for a disease. It is even harder to find animal models that mimic human drug metabolism.

Species variation has been observed in many oxidative biotransformation reactions. For example, metabolism of amphetamine occurs by two main pathways: oxidative deamination or aromatic hydroxylation. In the human, rabbit, and guinea pig, oxidative deamination appears to be the predominant pathway; in the rat, aromatic hydroxylation appears to be the more important route.[495] Phenytoin is another drug that shows marked species differences in metabolism. In the human, phenytoin undergoes aromatic oxidation to yield primarily $(S)(-)$-p-hydroxyphenytoin; in the dog, oxidation occurs to give mainly $(R)(+)$-m-hydroxyphenytoin.[496] There is a dramatic difference not only in the position (i.e., *meta* or *para*) of aromatic hydroxylation but also in which of the two phenyl rings (at C-5 of phenytoin) undergoes aromatic oxidation.

Species differences in many conjugation reactions also have been observed. Often, these differences are caused by the presence or absence of transferase enzymes involved in the conjugative process. For example, cats lack glucuronyltransferase enzymes and, therefore, tend to conjugate phenolic xenobiotics by sulfation instead.[497] In pigs, the situation is reversed: pigs are not able to conjugate phenols with sulfate (because of lack of sulfotransferase enzymes) but appear to have good glucuronidation capability.[497] The conjugation of

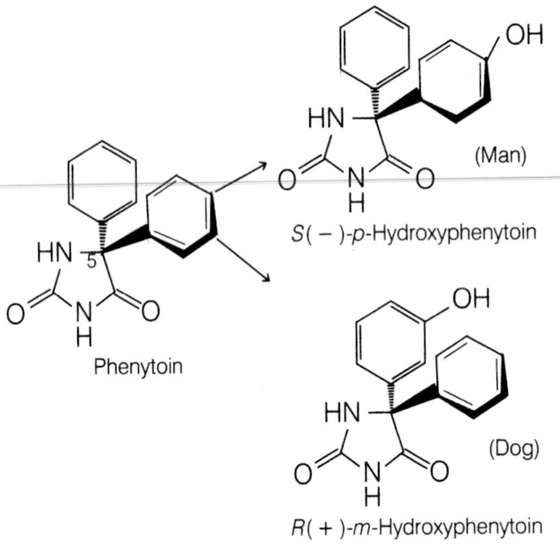

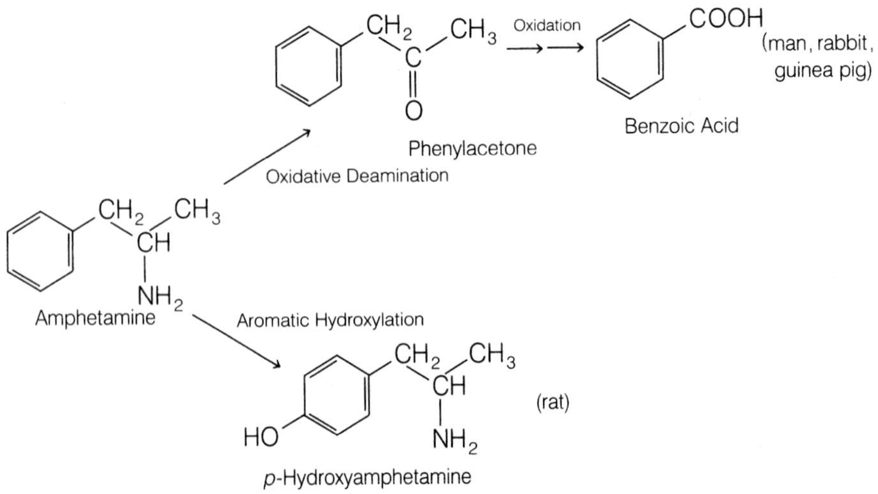

Phenytoin

$S(-)$-p-Hydroxyphenytoin (Man)

$R(+)$-m-Hydroxyphenytoin (Dog)

Phenylacetone

Benzoic Acid (man, rabbit, guinea pig)

Oxidative Deamination

Amphetamine

Aromatic Hydroxylation

p-Hydroxyamphetamine (rat)

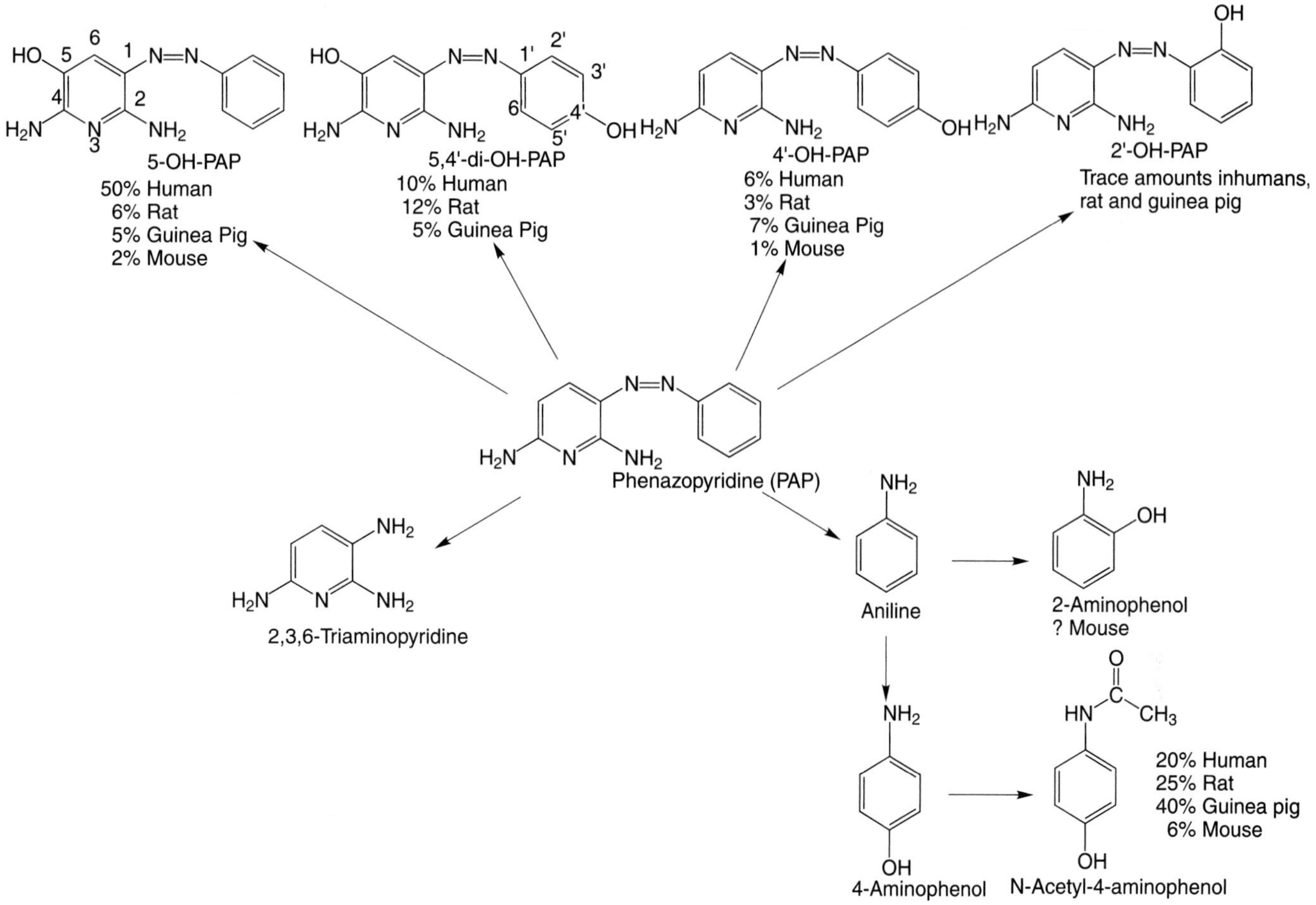

Figure 4–18 ■ Phenazopyridine metabolism in humans, guinea pigs, rats and mice.

aromatic acids with amino acids (e.g., glycine, glutamine) depends on the animal species as well as on the substrate. For example, glycine conjugation is a common conjugation pathway for benzoic acid in many animals. In certain birds (e.g., duck, goose, turkey), however, glycine is replaced by the amino acid ornithine.[498] Phenylacetic acid is a substrate for both glycine and glutamine conjugation in humans and other primates. Nonprimates, such as the rabbit and rat, excrete phenylacetic acid only as the glycine conjugate, however.[499] The metabolism of the urinary antiseptic, phenazopyridine (Pyridium) depends strongly on the animal. The diazo linkage remains intact in over half of the metabolites in humans, whereas 40% of the metabolites in the guinea pig result from its cleavage. The metabolic product pattern in human or guinea pig does not correlate with that of either rat or mouse (Fig. 4-18).[500]

Strain differences in drug metabolism exist, particularly in inbred mice and rabbits. These differences apparently are caused by genetic variations in the amount of metabolizing enzyme present among the different strains. For example, in vitro studies indicate that cottontail rabbit liver microsomes metabolize hexobarbital about 10 times faster than New Zealand rabbit liver microsomes.[501] Interindividual differences in drug metabolism in humans are considered below.

Hereditary or Genetic Factors

Marked individual differences in the metabolism of several drugs exist in humans.[463] Many of these genetic or hered-

itary factors are responsible for the large differences seen in the rate of metabolism of these drugs. The frequently cited example of the biotransformation of the antituberculosis agent isoniazid is discussed above under acylation. Genetic factors also appear to influence the rate of oxidation of drugs like phenytoin, phenylbutazone, dicumarol, and nortriptyline.[502, 503] The rate of oxidation of these drugs varies widely among different individuals; these differences, however, do not appear to be distributed bimodally, as in acetylation. In general, individuals who tend to oxidize one drug rapidly are also likely to oxidize other drugs rapidly. Numerous studies in twins (identical and fraternal) and in families indicate that oxidation of these drugs is under genetic control.[503]

Many patients state that they do not respond to codeine and codeine analogues. It now is realized that their CYP 2D6 isozyme does not readily O-demethylate codeine to form morphine. This genetic polymorphism is seen in about 8% of Caucasians, 4% of African Americans, and less than 1% of Asians.[504] Genetic polymorphism with CYP isozymes is well documented as evidenced by the many examples in this chapter. There is limited evidence of polymorphism involving MAO-A and MAO-B. The chemical imbalances seen with some mental diseases may be the cause.[206]

Sex Differences

The rate of metabolism of xenobiotics also varies according to gender in some animal species. A marked difference is observed between female and male rats. Adult male rats metabolize several foreign compounds at a much faster rate than female rats (e.g., N-demethylation of aminopyrine, hexobarbital oxidation, glucuronidation of *o*-aminophenol). Apparently, this sex difference also depends on the substrate, because some xenobiotics are metabolized at the same rate in both female and male rats. Differences in microsomal oxidation are under the control of sex hormones, particularly androgens; the anabolic action of androgens seems to increase metabolism.[505]

Sex differences in drug metabolism appear to be species

dependent. Rabbits and mice, for example, do not show a significant sex difference in drug metabolism.[505] In humans, there have been a few reports of sex differences in metabolism. For instance, nicotine and aspirin seem to be metabolized differently in women and men.[506, 507] On the other hand, gender differences can become significant in terms of drug–drug interactions based on the drug's metabolism. For women, the focus is on drugs used for contraception. Note in Table 4-4 that the antibiotic rifampin, a CYP 3A4 inducer, can shorten the half-life of oral contraceptives.

TABLE 4–4 Clinically Significant Cytochrome P-450-Based Drug–Drug Interactions

Agent	Substrates	Inhibitors	Inducers	Agent	Substrates	Inhibitors	Inducers
CYP 1A2	Amitriptyline	Cimetidine	Carbamazepine		Imipramine		
	Clomipramine	Ciprofloxacin	Phenobarbital		Meperidine		
	Clozapine	Clarithromycin	Phenytoin		Methadone		
	Desipramine	Enoxacin	Primidone		Mexiletine		
	Fluvoxamine	Erythromycin	Rifampin		Nortriptyline		
	Haloperidol	Fluvoxamine	Ritonavir		Oxycodone		
	Imipramine	Isoniazid	Smoking		Propafenone		
	Ropinirole	Nalidixic acid	St. John's wort		Propoxyphene		
	Tacrine	Norfloxacin			Thioridazine		
	Theophylline	Troleandomycin			Tramadol		
	(*R*)-Warfarin	Zileuton			Trazodone		
CYP 2C9	Diazepam	Amiodarone	Carbamazepine	CYP 3A4	Alfentanil	Amiodarone	Carbamazepine
	Phenytoin	Chloramphenicol	Phenobarbital		Alprazolam	Cimetidine	Efavirenz
	(*S*)-Warfarin	Cimetidine	Phenytoin		Amlodipine	Ciprofloxacin	Ethosuximide
		Fluconazole	Primidone		Atorvastatin	Clarithromycin	Garlic supplements
		Fluoxetine	Rifampin				
		Fluvoxamine	Rifapentine		Busulfan	Cyclosporine	Modafinil
		Isoniazid			Carbamazepine	Delavirdine	Nevirapine
		Metronidazole			Cisapride	Diltiazem	Oxcarbazepine
		Voriconazole			Clarithromycin	Efavirenz	Phenobarbital
		Zafirlukast			Cyclosporine	Erythromycin	Phenytoin
CYP 2C19	Phenytoin	Fluoxetine	Carbamazepine		Dihydroergotamine	Fluconazole	Primidone
	Thioridazine	Fluvoxamine	Phenobarbital		Disopyramide	Fluoxetine	Rifabutin
		Modafinil	Phenytoin		Doxorubicin	Fluvoxamine	Rifampin
		Omeprazole			Dronabinol	Grapefruit	Rifapentine
		Topiramate			Ergotamine	Indinavir	St. John's wort
CYP 2D6	Amitriptyline	Amiodarone	St. John's wort		Erythromycin	Isoniazid	
	Atomoxetine	Cimetidine			Estrogens, oral contraceptives	Itraconazole	
	Codeine	Fluoxetine				Ketoconazole	
	Desipramine	Paroxetine			Ethinyl estradiol	Metronidazole	
	Dextromethorphan	Quinidine			Ethosuximide	Miconazole	
	Donepezil	Ritonavir			Etoposide	Nefazodone	
	Doxepin	Sertraline			Felodipine	Nelfinavir	
	Fentanyl				Fentanyl	Nifedipine	
	Flecainide				Indinavir	Norfloxacin	
	Haloperidol				Isradipine	Quinine	
	Hydrocodone				Itraconazole	Ritonavir	

Abstracted from Levien, T. L., and Baker, D. E.: Pharmacist's Letter, December 2002, Detail-Document #150400 (Pharmacist's Letter used as sources: Hansten, P. D., and Horn, J. R.: Drug Interactions Analysis and Management. Vancouver, WA, Applied Therapeutics, 2002; and Tatro, D. S. (ed.): Drug Interaction Facts. St. Louis, Facts & Comparisons, 2002.)

Enzyme Induction

The activity of hepatic microsomal enzymes, such as the cytochrome P-450 mixed-function oxidase system, can be increased markedly by exposure to diverse drugs, pesticides, polycyclic aromatic hydrocarbons, and environmental xenobiotics. The process by which the activity of these drug-metabolizing enzymes is increased is termed *enzyme induction*.[508–511] The increased activity is apparently caused by an increased amount of newly synthesized enzyme. Enzyme induction often increases the rate of drug metabolism and decreases the duration of drug action. (See Table 4-4 for a list of clinically significant drug–drug interactions based on one drug inducing the metabolism of a second drug.)

Inducing agents may increase the rate of their own metabolism as well as those of other unrelated drugs or foreign compounds (Table 4-4).[32] Concomitant administration of two or more drugs often may lead to serious drug interactions as a result of enzyme induction. For instance, a clinically critical drug interaction occurs with phenobarbital and warfarin.[512] Induction of microsomal enzymes by phenobarbital increases the metabolism of warfarin and, consequently, markedly decreases the anticoagulant effect. Therefore, if a patient is receiving warfarin anticoagulant therapy and begins taking phenobarbital, careful attention must be paid to readjustment of the warfarin dose. Dosage readjustment is also needed if a patient receiving both warfarin and phenobarbital therapy suddenly stops taking the barbiturate. The ineffectiveness of oral contraceptives in women on concurrent phenobarbital or rifampin therapy has been attributed to the enhanced metabolism of estrogens (e.g., 17α-ethynylestradiol) caused by phenobarbital[513] and rifampin[514] induction.

Inducers of microsomal enzymes also may enhance the metabolism of endogenous compounds, such as steroidal hormones and bilirubin. For instance, phenobarbital can increase the metabolism of cortisol, testosterone, vitamin D, and bilirubin in humans.[508, 509] The enhanced metabolism of vitamin D_3 induced by phenobarbital and phenytoin appears to be responsible for the osteomalacia seen in patients on long-term therapy with these two anticonvulsant drugs.[515] Interestingly, phenobarbital induces glucuronyltransferase enzymes, thereby enhancing the conjugation of bilirubin with glucuronic acid. Phenobarbital has been used occasionally to treat hyperbilirubinemia in neonates.[516]

In addition to drugs, other chemicals, such as polycyclic aromatic hydrocarbons (e.g., benzo[α]pyrene, 3-methylcholanthrene) and environmental pollutants (e.g., pesticides, polychlorinated biphenyls, TCDD), may induce certain oxidative pathways and, thereby, alter drug response.[508, 509, 511] Cigarette smoke contains minute amounts of polycyclic aromatic hydrocarbons, such as benzo[α]pyrene, which are potent inducers of microsomal cytochrome P-450 enzymes. This induction increases the oxidation of some drugs in smokers. For example, theophylline is metabolized more rapidly in smokers than in nonsmokers. This difference is reflected in the marked difference in the plasma half-life of theophylline between smokers ($t\frac{1}{2}$ 4.1 hours) and nonsmokers ($t\frac{1}{2}$ 7.2 hours).[517] Other drugs, such as phenacetin, pentazocine, and propoxyphene, also reportedly undergo more rapid metabolism in smokers than in nonsmokers.[518–520] Occupational and accidental exposure to chlorinated pesticides and insecticides can also stimulate drug metabolism. For instance, the half-life of antipyrine in workers occupationally exposed to the insecticides lindane and DDT is reportedly significantly shorter (7.7 vs. 11.7 hours) than in control subjects.[521] A case was reported in which a worker exposed to chlorinated insecticides failed to respond (i.e., decreased anticoagulant effect) to a therapeutic dose of warfarin.[522]

As discussed above, multiple forms (isozymes) of cytochrome P-450 have been demonstrated.[31, 40–42] Many chemicals selectively induce one or more distinct forms of cytochrome P-450.[31] (See Table 4-4.) Enzyme induction also may affect toxicity of some drugs by enhancing the metabolic formation of chemically reactive metabolites. Particularly important is the induction of cytochrome P-450 enzymes involved in the oxidation of drugs to reactive intermediates. For example, the oxidation of acetaminophen to a reactive imidoquinone metabolite appears to be carried out by a phenobarbital-inducible form of cytochrome P-450 in rats and mice. Numerous studies in these two animals indicate that phenobarbital pretreatment increases in vivo hepatotoxicity and covalent binding as well as increases formation of reactive metabolite in microsomal incubation mixtures.[243–245, 248] Induction of cytochrome P-448 is of toxicological concern because this particular enzyme is involved in the metabolism of polycyclic aromatic hydrocarbons to reactive and carcinogenic intermediates.[80, 523] Consequently, the metabolic bioactivation of benzo[α]pyrene to its ultimate carcinogenic diol epoxide intermediate is carried out by cytochrome P-448 (see section above on aromatic oxidation for the bioactivation pathway of benzo[α]pyrene to its diol epoxide).[523] Thus, it is becoming increasingly apparent that enzyme induction may enhance the toxicity of some xenobiotics by increasing the rate of formation of reactive metabolites.

Enzyme Inhibition

Several drugs, other xenobiotics including grapefruit, and possibly other foods can inhibit drug metabolism (Table 4-5).[32, 483–486] With decreased metabolism, a drug often accumulates, leading to prolonged drug action and serious ad-

TABLE 4–5 Potential Drug—Grapefruit Interactions Based on Grapefruit Inhibition of CYP 3A4

Drug	Result
Amiodarone	Increased bioavailability
Diazepam	Increased AUC
Carbamazepine	Increased AUC, peak and trough plasma concentrations
Cisapride	Increased AUC
Cyclosporine, tacrolimus	Increased AUC and serum concentrations
Atorvastatin, simvastatin	Increased absorption and plasma concentrations
Saquinavir	Increased absorption and plasma concentrations

Abstracted from Kehoe, W. A.: Pharmacist's Letter, 18, September 2002, Detail Document #180905.

AUC, area under the curve.

verse effects. Enzyme inhibition can occur by diverse mechanisms, including substrate competition, interference with protein synthesis, inactivation of drug-metabolizing enzymes, and hepatotoxicity leading to impairment of enzyme activity. Some drug interactions resulting from enzyme inhibition have been reported in humans.[524, 525] For example, phenylbutazone (limited to veterinary use) stereoselectively inhibits the metabolism of the more potent (S)(−) enantiomer of warfarin. This inhibition may explain the excessive hypoprothrombinemia (increased anticoagulant effect) and many instances of hemorrhaging seen in patients on both warfarin and phenylbutazone therapy.[56] The metabolism of phenytoin is inhibited by drugs such as chloramphenicol, disulfiram, and isoniazid.[512] Interestingly, phenytoin toxicity as a result of enzyme inhibition by isoniazid appears to occur primarily in slow acetylators.[464] Several drugs, such as dicumarol, chloramphenicol, and phenylbutazone,[512] inhibit the biotransformation of tolbutamide, which may lead to a hypoglycemic response.

The grapefruit–drug interaction is complex. It may be caused by the bioflavonoids or the furanocoumarins. Grapefruit's main bioflavonoid, naringin, is a weak CYP inhibitor, but the product of the intestinal flora, naringenin, does inhibit CYP 3A4. The literature is very confusing because many of the studies were done in vitro, and they cannot always be substantiated under in vivo conditions. In addition, components in grapefruit also activate P-glycoprotein, which would activate the efflux pump in the gastric mucosa and thus interfere with oral absorption of the certain drugs. The combination of CYP enzyme inhibition and P-glycoprotein activation can lead to inconclusive results.[526] The general recommendation when a drug interaction is suspected is that the patient avoid grapefruit and its juice.

Miscellaneous Factors Affecting Drug Metabolism[32, 483–486]

Other factors also may influence drug metabolism. Dietary factors, such as the protein-to-carbohydrate ratio, affect the metabolism of a few drugs. Indoles present in vegetables such as Brussels sprouts, cabbage, and cauliflower, and polycyclic aromatic hydrocarbons present in charcoal-broiled beef induce enzymes and stimulate the metabolism of some drugs. Vitamins, minerals, starvation, and malnutrition also apparently influence drug metabolism. Finally, physiological factors, such as the pathological state of the liver (e.g., hepatic cancer, cirrhosis, hepatitis), pregnancy, hormonal disturbances (e.g., thyroxine, steroids), and circadian rhythm, may markedly affect drug metabolism.

Stereochemical Aspects of Drug Metabolism

Many drugs (e.g., warfarin, propranolol, hexobarbital, glutethimide, cyclophosphamide, ketamine, and ibuprofen) often are administered as racemic mixtures in humans. The two enantiomers present in a racemic mixture may differ in pharmacological activity. Usually, one enantiomer tends to be much more active than the other. For example, the (S)(−) enantiomer of warfarin is 5 times more potent as an oral anticoagulant than the (R)(+) enantiomer.[527] In some instances, the two enantiomers may have totally different pharmacological activities. For example, (+)-α-propoxyphene (Darvon) is an analgesic, whereas (−)-α-propoxyphene (Novrad) is an antitussive.[528] Such differences in activity between stereoisomers should not be surprising, since Chapter 2 explains that stereochemical factors generally have a dramatic influence on how the drug molecule interacts with the target receptors to elicit its pharmacological response. By the same token, the preferential interaction of one stereoisomer with drug-metabolizing enzymes may lead one to anticipate differences in metabolism for the two enantiomers of a racemic mixture. Indeed, individual enantiomers of a racemic drug often are metabolized at different rates. For instance, studies in humans indicate that the less active (+) enantiomer of propranolol undergoes more rapid metabolism than the corresponding (−) enantiomer.[529] Allylic hydroxylation of hexobarbital occurs more rapidly with the R(−) enantiomer in humans.[530] The term *substrate stereoselectivity* is used frequently to denote a preference for one stereoisomer as a substrate for a metabolizing enzyme or metabolic process.[291]

Individual enantiomers of a racemic mixture also may be metabolized by different pathways. For instance, in dogs, the (+) enantiomer of the sedative–hypnotic glutethimide (Doriden) is hydroxylated primarily α to the carbonyl to yield 4-hydroxyglutethimide, whereas the (−) enantiomer undergoes aliphatic ω − 1 hydroxylation of its C-2 ethyl group.[140, 141] Dramatic differences in the metabolic profile of two enantiomers of warfarin also have been noted. In humans, the more active (S)(−) isomer is 7-hydroxylated (aromatic hydroxylation), whereas the (R)(+) isomer undergoes keto reduction to yield primarily the (R,S) warfarin alcohol as the major plasma metabolite.[56, 296] Although numerous other examples of substrate stereoselectivity or enantioselectivity in drug metabolism exist, the examples presented should suffice to emphasize the point.[291, 531]

Drug biotransformation processes often lead to the creation of a new asymmetric center in the metabolite (i.e., stereoisomeric or enantiomeric products). The preferential metabolic formation of a stereoisomeric product is called *product stereoselectivity*.[291] Thus, bioreduction of ketone xenobiotics, as a general rule, produces predominantly one stereoisomeric alcohol (see ''Reduction of Ketone Carbonyls,'' above).[116, 291] The preferential formation of (S)(−)-hydroxyhexamide from the hypoglycemic agent acetohexamide[293, 294] and the exclusive generation of 6β-naltrexol from naltrexone[297, 298] (see "Reduction of Ketone Carbonyls" for structure) are two examples of highly stereoselective bioreduction processes in humans.

Oxidative biotransformations display product stereoselectivity, too. For example, phenytoin contains two phenyl rings in its structure, both of which a priori should be susceptible to aromatic hydroxylation. In humans, however, *p*-hydroxylation occurs preferentially (approximately 90%) at the pro-(*S*)-phenyl ring to give primarily (*S*)(−)-5-(4-hydroxyphenyl)-5-phenylhydantoin. Although the other phenyl ring also is *p*-hydroxylated, it occurs only to a minor extent (10%).[496] Microsomal hydroxylation of the C-3 carbon of diazepam and desmethyldiazepam (using mouse liver preparations) has been reported to proceed with remarkable stereoselectivity to yield optically active metabolites with the 3(*S*) absolute configuration.[139] Interestingly, these two metabolites are pharmacologically active and one of them, oxazepam, is marketed as a drug (Serax). The allylic hydroxylation of the *N*-butenyl side group of the analgesic pentazocine (Talwin) leads to two possible alcohols (*cis* and *trans* alcohols). In human, mouse, and monkey, pentazocine is metabolized predominantly to the *trans* alcohol metabolite, whereas the rat primarily tends to form the *cis* alcohol.[129, 130] The product stereoselectivity observed in this biotransformation involves *cis* and *trans* geometric stereoisomers.

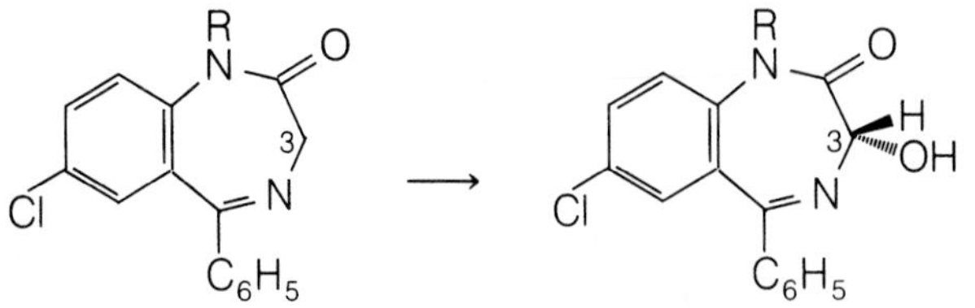

Diazepam, R = CH₃
Desmethyldiazepam, R = H

(3*S*) *N*-Methyloxazepam, R = CH₃
S(+)-Oxazepam, R = H

The term *regioselectivity*[532] has been introduced in drug metabolism to denote the selective metabolism of two or more similar functional groups (e.g., OCH_3, OH, NO_2) or two or more similar atoms that are positioned in different regions of a molecule. For example, of the four methoxy groups present in papaverine, the 4-OCH_3 group is regioselectively O-demethylated in several species (e.g., rat, guinea pig, rabbit, and dog).[533] Trimethoprim (Trimpex, Proloprim) has two heterocyclic sp^2 nitrogen atoms (N^1 and N^3) in its structure. In dogs, it appears that oxidation occurs regioselectively at N^3 to give the corresponding 3-*N*-oxide.[232] Nitroreduction of the 7-nitro group in 5,7-dinitroindazole to yield the 7-amino derivative in the mouse and rat occurs with high regioselectivity.[534] Substrates amenable to O-methylation by COMT appear to proceed with remarkable regioselectivity, as typified by the cardiotonic agent dobutamine (Dobutrex).

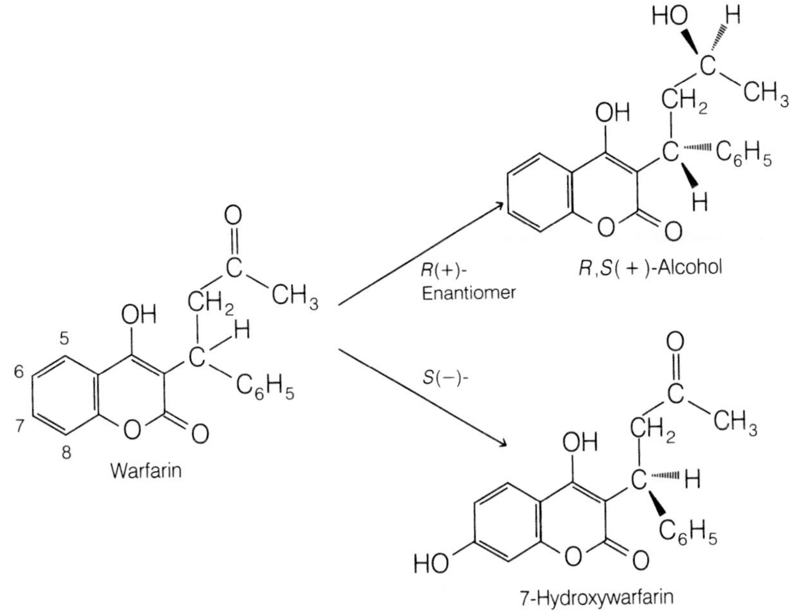

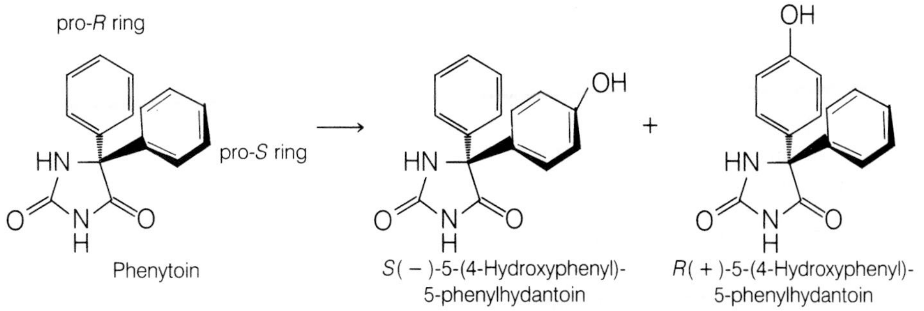

Warfarin

R(+)-Enantiomer

R,*S*(+)-Alcohol

S(−)-

7-Hydroxywarfarin

pro-*R* ring

pro-*S* ring

Phenytoin

S(−)-5-(4-Hydroxyphenyl)-
5-phenylhydantoin

R(+)-5-(4-Hydroxyphenyl)-
5-phenylhydantoin

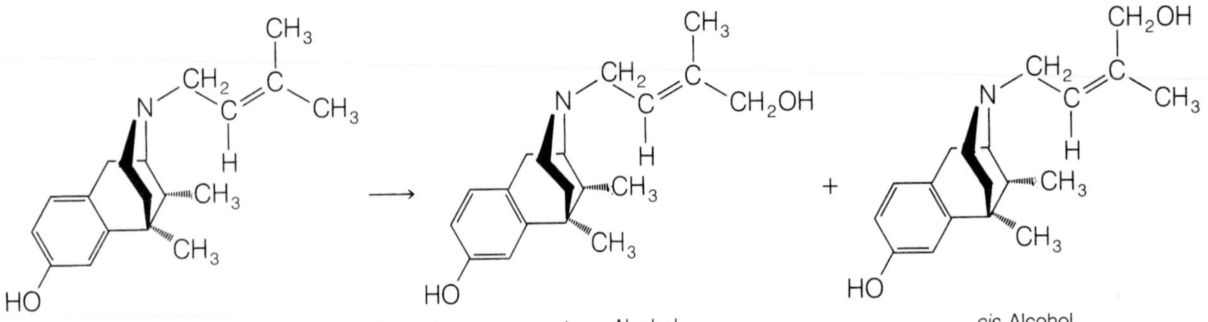

Pentazocine → *trans*-Alcohol + *cis*-Alcohol

O-methylation occurs exclusively with the phenolic hydroxy group at C-3.[474]

Pharmacologically Active Metabolites

The traditional notion that drug metabolites are inactive and insignificant in drug therapy has changed dramatically in recent years. Increasing evidence indicates that many drugs are biotransformed to pharmacologically active metabolites that contribute to the therapeutic as well as toxic effects of the parent compound. Metabolites shown to have significant therapeutic activity in humans are listed in Table 4-4.[2, 535] The parent drug from which the metabolite is derived and the biotransformation process involved also are given.

How significantly an active metabolite contributes to the therapeutic or toxic effects ascribed to the parent drug depends on its relative activity and quantitative importance (e.g., plasma concentration). In addition, whether the metabolite accumulates after repeated administration (e.g., desmethyldiazepam in geriatric patients) or in patients with renal failure is determinant.

From a clinical standpoint, active metabolites are especially important in patients with decreased renal function. If renal excretion is the major pathway for elimination of the active metabolite, then accumulation is likely to occur in patients with renal failure. Especially with drugs such as procainamide, clofibrate, and digitoxin, caution should be exercised in treating patients with renal failure.[2, 413] Many of the toxic effects seen for these drugs have been attributed to high plasma levels of their active metabolites. For example, the combination of severe muscle weakness and tenderness (myopathy) seen with clofibrate in renal failure patients is believed to be caused by high levels of the active metabolite chlorophenoxyisobutyric acid.[536, 537] Cardiovascular toxicity owing to digitoxin and procainamide in anephric subjects has been attributed to high plasma levels of digoxin and *N*-acetylprocainamide, respectively. In such situations, appropriate reduction in dosage and careful monitoring of plasma levels of the parent drug and its active metabolite often are recommended.

The pharmacological activity of some metabolites has led many manufacturers to synthesize these metabolites and to market them as separate drug entities (Table 4-6). For example, oxyphenbutazone (Tandearil, Oxalid) is the *p*-hydroxylated metabolite of the anti-inflammatory agent phenylbutazone (Butazolidin, Azolid), nortriptyline (Aventyl) is the N-demethylated metabolite of the tricyclic antidepressant amitriptyline (Elavil), oxazepam (Serax) is the N-demethylated

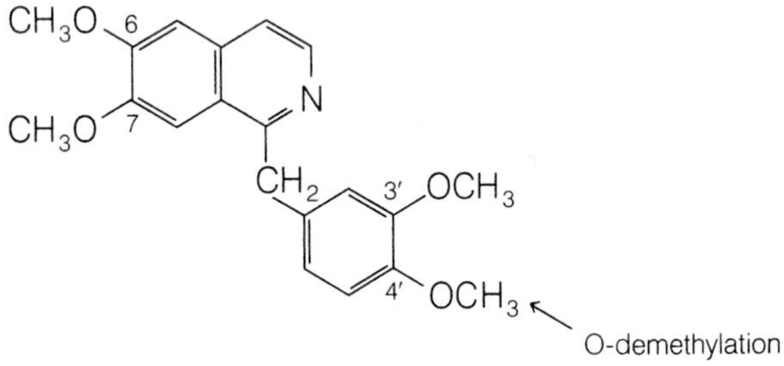

Papaverine

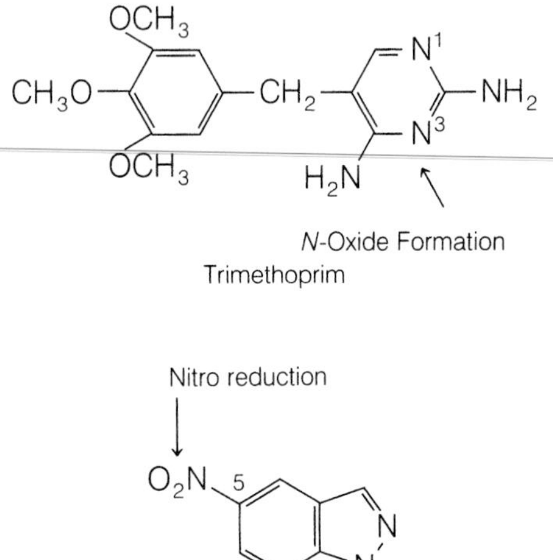

Trimethoprim

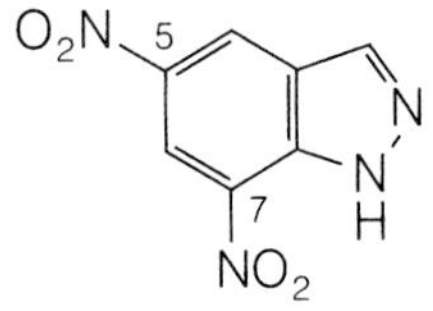

N-Oxide Formation

Nitro reduction

5,7-Dinitroindazole

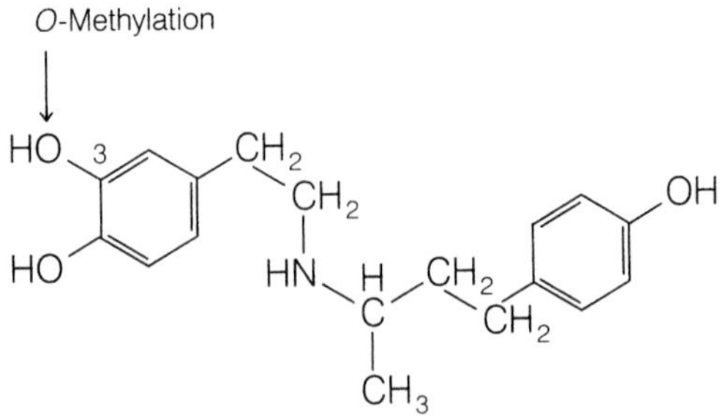

O-Methylation

Dobutamine

TABLE 4–6 Pharmacologically Active Metabolites in Humans

Parent Drug	Metabolite	Biotransformation Process
Acetohexamide	Hydroxyhexamide	Ketone reduction
Acetylmethadol	Noracetylmethadol	N-Demethylation
Amitriptyline	Nortriptyline	N-Demethylation
Azathioprine	6-Mercaptopurine	Glutathione conjugation
Carbamazepine	Carbamazepine-9,10-epoxide	Epoxidation
Chloral hydrate	Trichloroethanol	Aldehyde reduction
Chlorpromazine	7-Hydroxychlorpromazine	Aromatic hydroxylation
Clofibrate	Chlorophenoxyisobutyric acid	Ester hydrolysis
Cortisone	Hydrocortisone	Ketone reduction
Diazepam	Desmethyldiazepam and oxazepam	N-Demethylation and 3-hydroxylation
Digitoxin	Digoxin	Alicyclic hydroxylation
Diphenoxylate	Diphenoxylic acid	Ester hydrolysis
Imipramine	Desipramine	N-Demethylation
Mephobarbital	Phenobarbital	N-Demethylation
Metoprolol	α-Hydroxymethylmetoprolol	Benzylic hydroxylation
Phenacetin	Acetaminophen	O-Deethylation
Phenylbutazone	Oxybutazone	Aromatic hydroxylation
Prednisone	Prednisolone	Ketone reduction
Primidone	Phenobarbital	Hydroxylation and oxidation to ketone
Procainamide	N-Acetylprocainamide	N-Acetylation
Propranolol	4-Hydroxypropranolol	Aromatic hydroxylation
Quinidine	3-Hydroxyquinidine	Allylic hydroxylation
Sulindac	Sulfide metabolite of sulindac	Sulfoxide reduction
Thioridazine	Mesoridazine	S-oxidation
Warfarin	Warfarin alcohols	Ketone reduction

and 3-hydroxylated metabolite of diazepam (Valium), and mesoridazine (Serentil) is the sulfoxide metabolite of the antipsychotic agent thioridazine (Mellaril).

Antivirals that are used in treating herpes simplex virus, varicella-zoster virus, and/or human cytomegalovirus must be bioactivated.[538] These include acyclovir, valacyclovir, penciclovir, famciclovir, and ganciclovir, which must be phosphorylated on the pentose-like side chain to the triphosphate derivative to be effective in inhibiting the enzyme DNA polymerase. The antiviral cidovir is dispensed as a monophosphate and only needs to be diphosphylated for conversion to the active triphosphate metabolite. The nucleoside antivirals that are used in treating AIDS/HIV must also undergo a similar metabolic conversion to the triphosphate metabolite.[539] The triphosphate derivative acts as a competitive inhibitor of the enzyme, reverse transcriptase, which normally uses the triphosphorylated form of nucleic acids. Examples include zidovudine, stavudine, zalcitabine, lamivudine, and didanosine.

One of the more recent uses of drug metabolism in the development of a novel agent includes the example of oseltamivir, a neuraminidase inhibitor used in treating influenza. Ro-64-0802, the lead drug, showed promise against both influenza A and B viruses in vitro but was not very effective when used in vivo. To improve the oral bioavailability, the ethyl ester, oseltamivir, was developed as a prodrug. Administration of the more lipophilic oseltamivir allowed good penetration of the active metabolite in various tissues, especially in the lower respiratory tract. The metabolism proceeds via a simple ester hydrolysis to yield the active free carboxylic acid.[540]

REFERENCES

1. Williams, R. T.: Detoxication Mechanisms, 2nd ed. New York, John Wiley & Sons, 1959.
2. Drayer, D. E.: Clin. Pharmacokinet. 1:426, 1976.
3. Drayer, D. E.: Drugs 24:519, 1982.
4. Jollow, D. J., et al.: Biological Reactive Intermediates. New York, Plenum Press, 1977.
5. Gillette, J. R., et al.: Annu. Rev. Pharmacol. 14:271, 1974.
6. Nelson, S. D., et al.: In Jerina, D. M. (ed.). Drug Metabolism Concepts. Washington, DC, American Chemical Society, 1977, p. 155.
7. Testa, B., and Jenner, P.: Drug Metab. Rev. 7:325, 1978.
8. Low, L. K., and Castagnoli, N., Jr.: In Wolff, M. E. (ed.). Burger's Medicinal Chemistry, Part 1, 4th ed. New York, Wiley-Interscience, 1980, p. 107.
9. Gill, E. W., et al.: Biochem. Pharmacol. 22:175, 1973.
10. Wall, M. E., et al.: J. Am. Chem. Soc. 94:8579, 1972.
11. Lemberger, L.: Drug Metab. Dispos. 1:641, 1973.
12. Green, D. E., et al.: In Vinson, J. A. (ed.). Cannabinoid Analysis in Physiological Fluids. Washington, DC, American Chemical Society, 1979, p. 93.
13. Williams, R. T.: In Brodie, B. B., and Gillette, J. R. (eds.). Concepts in Biochemical Pharmacology, Part 2. Berlin, Springer-Verlag, 1971, p. 226.
14. Rowland, M.: In Melmon, K. L., and Morelli, H. F. (eds.). Clinical Pharmacology: Basic Principles in Therapeutics, 2nd ed. New York, Macmillan, 1978, p. 25.
15. Benowitz, N. L., and Meister, W.: Clin. Pharmacokinet. 3:177, 1978.
16. Connolly, M. E., et al.: Br. J. Pharmacol. 46:458, 1972.
17. Gibaldi, M., and Perrier, D.: Drug Metab. Rev. 3:185, 1974.
18. Sinkula, A. A., Yalkowsky, S. H.: J. Pharm. Sci. 64:181, 1975.
19. Scheline, R. R.: Pharmacol. Rev. 25:451, 1973.
20. Peppercorn, M. A., and Goldman, P.: J. Pharmacol. Exp. Ther. 181: 555, 1972.
21. Levy, G. A., and Conchie, J.: In Dutton, G. J. (ed.). Glucuronic Acid, Free and Combined. New York, Academic Press, 1966, p. 301.
22. Testa, B., and Jenner, P.: Drug Metabolism: Chemical and Biochemical Aspects. New York, Marcel Dekker, 1976, p. 419.

23. Powis, G., and Jansson, I.: Pharmacol. Ther. 7:297, 1979.
24. Mason, H. S.: Annu. Rev. Biochem. 34:595, 1965.
25. Hayaishi, O.: In Hayaishi, O. (ed.). Oxygenases. New York, Academic Press, 1962, p. 1.
26. Mannering, G. J.: In LaDu, B. N., et al. (eds.). Fundamentals of Drug Metabolism and Disposition. Baltimore, Williams & Wilkins, 1971, p. 206.
27. Sato, R., and Omura, T. (eds.): Cytochrome P-450. New York, Academic Press, 1978.
28. Omura, T., and Sato, R.: J. Biol. Chem. 239:2370, 1964.
29. Gillette, J. R.: Adv. Pharmacol. 4:219, 1966.
30. Nelson, D. R., Koymans, L., Kamataki, T., et al.: Pharmacogenetics 6:1, 1996.
31. Schuetz, E.G.: Curr. Drug Metab. 2:139, 2001.
32. Claude, A.: In Gillette, J. R., et al. (eds.). Microsomes and Drug Oxidations. New York, Academic Press, 1969, p. 3.
33. Hansch, D.: Drug Metab. Rev. 1:1, 1972.
34. Ortiz de Montellano, P. R.: Cytochrome P-450. New York, Plenum Press, 1986, p. 217.
35. Estabrook, R. W., and Werringloer, J.: In Jerina, D. M. (ed.). Drug Metabolism Concepts. Washington, DC, American Chemical Society, 1977, p. 1.
36. Trager, W. F.: In Jenner, P., and Testa, B. (eds.). Concepts in Drug Metabolism, Part A. New York, Marcel Dekker, 1980, p. 177.
37. Ullrich, V.: Top. Curr. Chem. 83:68, 1979.
38. White, R. E., and Coon, M. J.: Annu. Rev. Biochem. 49:315, 1980.
39. Guengerich, F. P. (ed.): Mammalian Cytochromes P-450, vols. 1 and 2. Boca Raton, FL, CRC Press, 1987.
40. Schenkman, J. B., and Kupfer, D. (eds.): Hepatic Cytochrome P-450 Monooxygenase System. New York, Pergamon Press, 1982.
41. Ioannides, C. (ed.): Cytochromes P450: Metabolic and Toxicological Aspects. Boca Raton, FL, CRC Press, 1996.
42. Guengerich, F. P.: Curr. Drug Metab. 2:93, 2001.
43. Daly, J. W., et al.: Experientia 28:1129, 1972.
44. Jerina, D. M., and Daly, J. W.: Science 185:573, 1974.
45. Kaminsky, L. S.: In Anders, M. W. (ed.). Bioactivation of Foreign Compounds. New York, Academic Press, 1985, p. 157.
46. Walle, T., and Gaffney, T. E.: J. Pharmacol. Exp. Ther. 182:83, 1972.
47. Bond, P.: Nature 213:721, 1967.
48. Whyte, M. P., and Dekaban, A. S.: Drug Metab. Dispos. 5:63, 1977.
49. Witkin, K. M., et al.: Ther. Drug Monit. 1:11, 1979.
50. Richens, A.: Clin. Pharmacokinet. 4:153, 1979.
51. Burns, J. J., et al.: J. Pharmacol. Exp. Ther. 113:481, 1955.
52. Yü, T. F., et al.: J. Pharmacol. Exp. Ther. 123:63, 1958.
53. Black A. E., Hayes R. N., Roth B. D., et al.: Drug Metab. Dispos. 27(8):916, 1999.
54. Williams, M. C., et al.: Steroids 25:229, 1975.
55. Ranney, R. E.: J. Toxicol. Environ. Health 3:139, 1977.
56. Lewis, R. J., et al.: J. Clin. Invest. 53:1697, 1974.
57. Daly, J.: In Brodie, B. B., and Gillette, J. R. (eds.). Concepts in Biochemical Pharmacology, Part 2. Berlin, Springer-Verlag, 1971, p. 285.
58. Lowenthal, D. T.: J. Cardiovasc. Pharmacol. 2(Suppl.):S29, 1980.
59. Davies, D. S., et al.: Adv. Pharmacol. Ther. 7:215, 1979.
60. Dayton, P. G., et al.: Drug Metab. Dispos. 1:742, 1973.
61. Schreiber, E. E.: Annu. Rev. Pharmacol. 10:77, 1970.
62. Hollister, L. E., et al.: Res. Commun. Chem. Pathol. Pharmacol. 2:330, 1971.
63. Safe, S., et al.: J. Agric. Food Chem. 23:851, 1975.
64. Allen, J. R., et al.: Food Cosmet. Toxicol. 13:501, 1975.
65. Vinopal, J. H., et al.: Arch. Environ. Contamin. Toxicol. 1:122, 1973.
66. Hathway, D. E. (Sr. Reporter): Foreign Compound Metabolism in Mammals, vol. 4. London, Chemical Society, 1977, p. 234.
67. Guroff, G., et al.: Science 157:1524, 1967.
68. Daly, J., et al.: Arch. Biochem. Biophys. 128:517, 1968.
69. Oesch, F.: Prog. Drug Metab. 3:253, 1978.
70. Lu, A. A. H., and Miwa, G. T.: Annu. Rev. Pharmacol. Toxicol. 20:513, 1980.
71. Ames, B. N., et al.: Science 176:47, 1972.
72. Maguire, J. H., et al.: Ther. Drug Monit. 1:359, 1979.
73. Harvey, D. G., et al.: Res. Commun. Chem. Pathol. Pharmacol. 3:557, 1972.
74. Stillwell, W. G.: Res. Commun. Chem. Pathol. Pharmacol. 12:25, 1975.
75. Jakoby, W. B., et al.: In Arias, I. M., and Jakoby, W. B. (eds.). Gluta-thione, Metabolism and Function. New York, Raven Press, 1976, p. 189.
76. Boyland, E.: In Brodie, B. B., and Gillette, J. R. (eds.). Concepts in Biochemical Pharmacology, Part 2. Berlin, Springer-Verlag, 1971, p. 584.
77. Brodie, B. B., et al.: Proc. Natl. Acad. Sci. U. S. A. 68:160, 1971.
78. Jollow, D. J., et al.: Pharmacology 11:151, 1974.
79. Gelboin, H. V., et al.: In Jollow, D. J., et al. (eds.). Biological Reactive Intermediates. New York, Plenum Press, 1977, p. 98.
80. Thakker, D. R., et al.: Chem. Biol. Interact. 16:281, 1977.
81. Weinstein, I. B., et al.: Science 193:592, 1976.
82. Jeffrey A. M., et al.: J. Am. Chem. Soc. 98:5714, 1976.
83. Koreeda, M., et al.: J. Am. Chem. Soc. 98:6720, 1976.
84. Straub, K. M., et al.: Proc. Natl. Acad. Sci. U. S. A. 74:5285, 1977.
85. Kasai, H., et al.: J. Am. Chem. Soc. 99:8500, 1977.
86. Chausseaud, L. F.: Drug Metab. Rev. 2:185, 1973.
87. Pynnönen, S.: Ther. Drug Monit. 1:409, 1979.
88. Eadie, M. J., and Tyrer, J. H.: Anticonvulsant Therapy, 2nd ed. Edinburgh, Churchill-Livingstone, 1980, p. 142.
89. Hucker, H. B., et al.: Drug Metab. Dispos. 3:80, 1975.
90. Hintze, K. L., et al.: Drug Metab. Dispos. 3:1, 1975.
91. Slack, J. A., and Ford-Hutchinson, A. W.: Drug Metab. Dispos. 8:84, 1980.
92. Waddell, W. J.: J. Pharmacol. Exp. Ther. 149:23, 1965.
93. Seutter-Berlage, F., et al.: Xenobiotica 8:413, 1978.
94. Marniemi, J., et al.: In Ullrich, V., et al. (eds.). Microsomes and Drug Oxidations. Oxford, Pergamon Press, 1977, p. 698.
95. Garner, R. C.: Prog. Drug Metab. 1:77, 1976.
96. Swenson, D. H., et al.: Biochem. Biophys. Res. Commun. 60:1036, 1974.
97. Swenson, D. H., et al.: Biochem. Biophys. Res. Commun. 53:1260, 1973.
98. Essigman, J. M., et al.: Proc. Natl. Acad. Sci. U. S. A. 74:1870, 1977.
99. Croy, R. G., et al.: Proc. Natl. Acad. Sci. U. S. A. 75:1745, 1978.
100. Henschler, D., and Bonser, G.: Adv. Pharmacol. Ther. 9:123, 1979.
101. Watabe, T., and Akamatsu, K.: Biochem. Pharmacol. 24:442, 1975.
102. Metzler, M.: J. Toxicol. Environ. Health 1(Suppl.):21, 1976.
103. Neuman, H. G., and Metzler, M.: Adv. Pharmacol. Ther. 9:113, 1979.
104. Ortiz de Montellano, P. R., and Correia, M. A.: Annu. Rev. Pharmacol. Toxicol. 23:481, 1983.
105. Ortiz de Montellano, P. R.: In Anders, M. W. (ed.). Bioactivation of Foreign Compounds. New York, Academic Press, 1985, p. 121.
106. DeMatteis, F.: Biochem. J. 124:767, 1971.
107. Levin, W., et al.: Arch. Biochem. Biophys. 148:262, 1972.
108. Levin, W., et al.: Science 176:1341, 1972.
109. Levin, W., et al.: Drug Metab. Dispos. 1:275, 1973.
110. Ivanetich, K. M., et al.: In Ullrich, V., et al.: (eds.). Microsomes and Drug Oxidations. Oxford, Pergamon Press, 1977, p. 76.
111. Ortiz de Montellano, P. R., et al.: Biochem. Biophys. Res. Commun. 83:132, 1978.
112. Ortiz de Montellano, P. R., et al.: Arch. Biochem. Biophys. 197:524, 1979.
113. Ortiz de Montellano, P. R., et al.: Biochemistry 21:1331, 1982.
114. Beckett, A. H., and Rowland, M.: J. Pharm. Pharmacol. 17:628, 1965.
115. Dring, L. G., et al.: Biochem. J. 116:425, 1970.
116. McMahon, R. E.: In Brodie, B. B., and Gillette, J. R. (eds.). Concepts in Biochemical Pharmacology, Part 2. Berlin, Springer-Verlag, 1971, p. 500.
117. Dutton, G.: In Brodie, B. B., and Gillette, J. R. (eds.). Concepts in Biochemical Pharmacology, Part 2. Berlin, Springer-Verlag, 1971, p. 378.
118. Thomas, R. C., and Ikeda, G. J.: J. Med. Chem. 9:507, 1966.
119. Selley, M. L., et al.: Clin. Pharmacol. Ther. 17:599, 1975.
120. Sumner, D. D., et al.: Drug Metab. Dispos. 3:283, 1975.
121. Tang C., Shou M., Mei Q., et al.: J. Pharmacol. Exp. Ther. 293(2):453, 2000.
122. Borg, K. O., et al.: Acta Pharmacol. Toxicol. 36(Suppl. 5):125, 1975.
123. Hoffmann, K. J.: Clin. Pharmacokinet. 5:181, 1980.
124. Lemberger, L., et al.: Science 173:72, 1971.
125. Lemberger, L., et al.: Science 177:62, 1972.
126. Carroll, F. I., et al.: J. Med. Chem. 17:985, 1974.
127. Drayer, D. E., et al.: Clin. Pharmacol. Ther. 27:72, 1980.
128. Drayer, D. E., et al.: Clin. Pharmacol. Ther. 24:31, 1978.
129. Bush, M. T., and Weller, W. L.: Drug Metab. Rev. 1:249, 1972.
130. Thompson, R. M., et al.: Drug Metab. Dispos. 1:489, 1973.

131. Breimer, D. D., and Van Rossum, J. M.: J. Pharm. Pharmacol. 25: 762, 1973.
132. Pittman, K. A., et al.: Biochem. Pharmacol. 18:1673, 1969.
133. Pittman, K. A., et al.: Biochem. Pharmacol. 19:1833, 1970.
134. Miller, J. A., and Miller, E. C.: In Jollow, D. J., et al. (eds.). Biological Reactive Intermediates. New York, Plenum Press, 1977, p. 14.
135. Wislocki, P. G., et al.: Cancer Res. 36:1686, 1976.
136. Garattini, S., et al.: In Usdin, E., Forrest, I. (eds.). Psychotherapeutic Drugs, Part 2. New York, Marcel Dekker, 1977, p. 1039.
137. Greenblatt, D. J., et al.: Clin. Pharmacol. Ther. 17:1, 1975.
138. Yanagi, Y., et al.: Xenobiotica 5:245, 1975.
139. Corbella, A., et al.: J. Chem. Soc. Chem. Commun. 721, 1973.
140. Keberle, H., et al.: Arch. Int. Pharmacodyn. 142:117, 1963.
141. Keberle, H., et al.: Experientia 18:105, 1962.
142. Ferrandes, B., and Eymark, P.: Epilepsia, 18:169, 1977.
143. Kuhara, T., and Matsumoto, J.: Biomed. Mass Spectrom. 1:291, 1974.
144. Maynert, E. W.: J. Pharmacol. Exp. Ther. 150:117, 1965.
145. Palmer, K. H., et al.: J. Pharmacol. Exp. Ther. 175:38, 1970.
146. Holtzmann, J. L., and Thompson, J. A.: Drug Metab. Dispos. 3:113, 1975.
147. Carroll, F. J., et al.: Drug Metab. Dispos. 5:343, 1977.
148. Thomas, R. C., and Judy, R. W.: J. Med. Chem. 15:964, 1972.
149. Adams, S. S., and Buckler, J. W.: Clin. Rheum. Dis. 5:359, 1979.
150. Ludwig, B. J., et al.: J. Med. Pharm. Chem. 3:53, 1961.
151. Horning, M. G., et al.: Drug Metab. Dispos. 1:569, 1973.
152. Dieterle, W., et al.: Arzneimittelforschung 26:572, 1976.
153. McMahon, R. E., et al.: J. Pharmacol. Exp. Ther. 149:272, 1965.
154. Fuccella, L. M., et al.: J. Clin. Pharmacol. 13:68, 1973.
155. Lin, D. C. K., et al.: Biomed. Mass Spectrom. 2:206, 1975.
156. Wong, L. K., and Biemann, K.: Clin. Toxicol. 9:583, 1976.
157. Thomas, R. C., et al.: J. Pharm. Sci. 64:1360, 1366, 1975.
158. Gottlieb, T. B., et al.: Clin. Pharmacol. Ther. 13:436, 1972.
159. Gorrod, J. W. (ed.): Biological Oxidation of Nitrogen. Amsterdam, Elsevier-North Holland, 1978.
160. Gorrod, J. W.: Chem. Biol. Interact. 7:289, 1973.
161. Ziegler, D. M., et al.: Drug Metab. Dispos. 1:314, 1973.
162. Ziegler, D. M., et al.: Arch. Biochem. Biophys. 150:116, 1972.
163. Gram, T. E.: In Brodie, B. B., and Gillette, J. R. (eds.). Concepts in Biochemical Pharmacology, Part 2. Berlin, Springer-Verlag, 1971, p. 334.
164. Brodie, B. B., et al.: Annu. Rev. Biochem. 27:427, 1958.
165. McMahon, R. E.: J. Pharm. Sci. 55:457, 1966.
166. Crammer, J. L., and Scott, B.: Psychopharmacologia 8:461, 1966.
167. Nagy, A., and Johansson, R.: Arch. Pharm. (Weinheim) 290:145, 1975.
168. Gram, L. F., et al.: Psychopharmacologia 54:255, 1977.
169. Collinsworth, K. A., et al.: Circulation 50:1217, 1974.
170. Narang, P. K., et al.: Clin. Pharmacol. Ther. 24:654, 1978.
171. Hutsell, T. C., and Kraychy, S. J.: J. Chromatogr. 106:151, 1975.
172. Heel, R. C., et al.: Drugs 15:331, 1978.
173. Adam, H. K., et al.: Biochem. Pharmacol. 27:145, 1979.
174. Chang, T. K., et al.: Res. Commun. Chem. Pathol. Pharmacol. 9:391, 1974.
175. Glazko, A. J., et al.: Clin. Pharmacol. Ther. 16:1066, 1974.
176. Hammar, C. G., et al.: Anal. Biochem. 25:532, 1968.
177. Beckett, A. H., et al.: J. Pharm. Pharmacol. 25:188, 1973.
178. Due, S. L., et al.: Biomed. Mass Spectrom. 3:217, 1976.
179. Beckett, A. H., et al.: J. Pharm. Pharmacol. 23:812, 1971.
180. Pohland, A., et al.: J. Med. Chem. 14:194, 1971.
181. Bruce, R. B., et al.: J. Med. Chem. 11:1031, 1968.
182. Szeto, H. H., and Inturri, C. E.: J. Chromatogr. 125:503, 1976.
183. Misra, A. L.: In Adler, M. L., et al. (eds.). Factors Affecting the Action of Narcotics. New York, Raven Press, 1978, p. 297.
184. Kamm, J. J., et al.: J. Pharmacol. Exp. Ther. 182:507, 1972.
185. Kamm, J. J., et al.: J. Pharmacol. Exp. Ther. 184:729, 1973.
186. Goldberg, M. E. (ed.): Pharmacological and Biochemical Properties of Drug Substances, vol. 1. Washington, DC, American Pharmaceutical Association, 1977, pp. 257, 311.
187. Gorrod, J. W., and Jenner, P.: Essays Toxicol. 6:35, 1975.
188. Beckett, A. H., and Triggs, E. J.: Nature 211:1415, 1966.
189. Hucker, H. B., et al.: Drug Metab. Dispos. 2:406, 1974.
190. Wold, J. S., and Fischer, L. J.: J. Pharmacol. Exp. Ther. 183:188, 1972.
191. Kaiser, C., et al.: J. Med. Chem. 15:1146, 1972.
192. Bickel, M. H.: Pharmacol. Rev. 21:325, 1969.
193. Jenner, P.: In Gorrod, J. W. (ed.). Biological Oxidation of Nitrogen. Amsterdam, Elsevier-North Holland, 1978, p. 383.
194. Faurbye, A., et al.: Am. J. Psychiatry 120:277, 1963.
195. Theobald, W., et al.: Med. Pharmacol. Exp. 15:187, 1966.
196. Coutts, R., and Beckett, A. H.: Drug Metab. Rev. 6:51, 1977.
197. Leinweber, F.-J., et al.: J. Pharm. Sci. 66:1570, 1977.
198. Beckett, A. H., and Rowland, M.: J. Pharm. Pharmacol. 17:109S, 1965.
199. Caldwell, J., et al.: Biochem. J. 129:11, 1972.
200. Wieber, J., et al.: Anesthesiology 24:260, 1975.
201. Chang, T., and Glazko, A. J.: Anesthesiology 21:401, 1972.
202. Tindell, G. L., et al.: Life Sci. 11:1029, 1972.
203. Franklin, R. B., et al.: Drug Metab. Dispos. 5:223, 1977.
204. Barlett, M. F., and Egger, H. P.: Fed. Proc. 31:537, 1972.
205. Beckett, A. H., and Gibson, G. G.: Xenobiotica 8:73, 1978.
206. Benedetti, M. S.: Fundam. Clin. Pharmacol. 15:75, 2001.
207. Beckett, A. H., and Brookes, L. G.: J. Pharm. Pharmacol. 23:288, 1971.
208. Charalampous, K. D., et al.: J. Pharmacol. Exp. Ther. 145:242, 1964.
209. Charalampous, K. D., et al.: Psychopharmacologia 9:48, 1966.
210. Ho, B. T., et al.: J. Med. Chem. 14:158, 1971.
211. Matin, S., et al.: J. Med. Chem. 17:877, 1974.
212. Au, W. Y. W., et al.: Biochem. J. 129:110, 1972.
213. Parli, C. J., et al.: Biochem. Biophys. Res. Commun. 43:1204, 1971.
214. Lindeke, B., et al.: Acta Pharm. Suecica 10:493, 1973.
215. Hucker, H. B.: Drug Metab. Dispos. 1:332, 1973.
216. Parli, C. H., et al.: Drug Metab. Dispos. 3:337, 1973.
217. Wright, J., et al.: Xenobiotica 7:257, 1977.
218. Gal, J., et al.: Res. Commun. Chem. Pathol. Pharmacol. 15:525, 1976.
219. Beckett, A. H., and Bélanger, P. M.: J. Pharm. Pharmacol. 26:205, 1974.
220. Bélanger, P. M., and Grech-Bélanger, O.: Can. J. Pharm. Sci. 12:99, 1977.
221. Weisburger, J. H., and Weisburger, E. K.: Pharmacol. Rev. 25:1, 1973.
222. Miller, E. C., and Miller, J. A.: Pharmacol. Rev. 18:805, 1966.
223. Weisburger, J. H., and Weisburger, E. K.: In Brodie, B. B., and Gillette, J. R. (eds.). Concepts in Biochemical Pharmacology, Part 2. Berlin, Springer-Verlag, 1971, p. 312.
224. Uehleke, H.: Xenobiotica 1:327, 1971.
225. Beckett, A. H., and Bélanger, P. M.: Biochem. Pharmacol. 25:211, 1976.
226. Israili, Z. H., et al.: J. Pharmacol. Exp. Ther. 187:138, 1973.
227. Kiese, M.: Pharmacol. Rev. 18:1091, 1966.
228. Lin, J.-K., et al.: Cancer Res. 35:844, 1975.
229. Poirer, L. A., et al.: Cancer Res. 27:1600, 1967.
230. Lin, J.-K., et al.: Biochemistry 7:1889, 1968.
231. Lin, J.-K., et al.: Biochemistry 8:1573, 1969.
232. Schwartz, D. E., et al.: Arzneimittelforschung 20:1867, 1970.
233. Dagne, E., and Castagnoli, N., Jr.: J. Med. Chem. 15:840, 1972.
234. Essien E. E., Ogonor, J. I., Coker H. A., Bamisile M. M: J. Pharm. Pharmacol. 39(10):843, 1987.
235. Garrattini, S., et al.: Drug Metab. Rev. 1:291, 1972.
236. Brotherton, P. M., et al.: Clin. Pharmacol. Ther. 10:505, 1969.
237. Langone, J. J., et al.: Biochemistry 12:5025, 1973.
238. Grochow, L. B., and Colvin, M.: Clin. Pharmacokinet. 4:380, 1979.
239. Colvin, M., et al.: Cancer Res. 33:915, 1973.
240. Connors, T. A., et al.: Biochem. Pharmacol. 23:115, 1974.
241. Irving, C. C.: In Fishman, W. H. (ed.). Metabolic Conjugation and Metabolic Hydrolysis, vol. 1. New York, Academic Press, 1970, p. 53.
242. Miller, J., and Miller, E. C.: In Jollow, D. J., et al. (eds.). Biological Reactive Intermediates. New York, Plenum Press, 1970, p. 6.
243. Jollow, D. J., et al.: J. Pharmacol. Exp. Ther. 187:195, 1973.
244. Prescott, L. F., et al.: Lancet 1:519, 1971.
245. Hinson, J. A.: Rev. Biochem. Toxicol. 2:103, 1980.
246. Hinson, J. A., et al.: Life Sci. 24:2133, 1979.
247. Nelson, S. D., et al.: Biochem. Pharmacol. 29:1617, 1980.
248. Potter, W. Z., et al.: J. Pharmacol. Exp. Ther. 187:203, 1973.
249. Adler, T. K., et al.: J. Pharmacol. Exp. Ther. 114:251, 1955.
250. Brodie, B. B., and Axelrod, J.: J. Pharmacol. Exp. Ther. 97:58, 1949.
251. Duggan, D. E., et al.: J. Pharmacol. Exp. Ther. 181:563, 1972.
252. Kwan, K. C., et al.: J. Pharmacokinet. Biopharm. 4:255, 1976.
253. Brogden, R. N., et al.: Drugs 14:163, 1977.
254. Taylor, J. A., et al.: Xenobiotica 7:357, 1977.
255. Daly, J., et al.: Ann. N. Y. Acad. Sci. 96:37, 1962.

256. Mazel, P., et al.: J. Pharmacol. Exp. Ther. 143:1, 1964.
257. Sarcione, E. J., and Stutzman, L.: Cancer Res. 20:387, 1960.
258. Elion, G. B., et al.: Proc. Am. Assoc. Cancer Res. 3:316, 1962.
259. Taylor, J. A.: Xenobiotica 3:151, 1973.
260. Brodie, B. B., et al.: J. Pharmacol. Exp. Ther. 98:85, 1950.
261. Spector, E., and Shideman, F. E.: Biochem. Pharmacol. 2:182, 1959.
262. Neal, R. A.: Arch. Intern. Med. 128:118, 1971.
263. Neal, R. A.: Biochem. J. 103:183, 1967.
264. Neal, R. A.: Rev. Biochem. Toxicol. 2:131, 1980.
265. Gruenke, L., et al.: Res. Commun. Chem. Pathol. Pharmacol. 10:221, 1975.
266. Zehnder, K., et al.: Biochem. Pharmacol. 11:535, 1962.
267. Aguilar, S. J.: Dis. Nerv. Syst. 36:484, 1975.
268. Taylor, D. C., et al.: Drug Metab. Dispos. 6:21, 1978.
269. Taylor, D. C.: In Wood, C. J., and Simkins, M. A. (eds.). International Symposium on Histamine H₂-Receptor Antagonists. Welwyn Garden City, UK, Smith, Kline & French, 1973, p. 45.
270. Crew, M. C., et al.: Xenobiotica 2:431, 1972.
271. Hucker, H. B., et al.: J. Pharmacol. Exp. Ther. 154:176, 1966.
272. Hucker, H. B., et al.: J. Pharmacol. Exp. Ther. 155:309, 1967.
273. Hathway, D. E. (Sr. Reporter): Foreign Compound Metabolism in Mammals, vol. 3. London, Chemical Society, 1975, p. 512.
274. Schwartz, M. A., and Kolis, S. J.: Drug Metab. Dispos. 1:322, 1973.
275. Sisenwine, S. F., et al.: Drug Metab. Dispos. 3:180, 1975.
276. McCallum, N. K.: Experientia 31:957, 1975.
277. McCallum, N. K.: Experientia 31:520, 1975.
278. Cohen, E. N., and Van Dyke, R. A.: Metabolism of Volatile Anesthetics. Reading, MA, Addison-Wesley, 1977.
279. Cohen, E. N., et al.: Anesthesiology 43:392, 1975.
280. Van Dyke, R. A., et al.: Drug Metab. Dispos. 3:51, 1975
281. Van Dyke, R. A., et al.: Drug Metab. Dispos. 4:40, 1976.
282. Pohl, L.: Rev. Biochem. Toxicol. 1:79, 1979.
283. Pohl, L., et al.: Biochem. Pharmacol. 27:335, 1978.
284. Pohl, L., et al.: Biochem. Pharmacol. 27:491, 1978.
285. Parke, D. V.: The Biochemistry of Foreign Compounds. Oxford, Pergamon Press, 1968, p. 218.
286. Gillette, J. R.: In Brodie, B. B., and Gillette, J. R. (eds.). Concepts in Biochemical Pharmacology, Part 2. Berlin, Springer-Verlag, 1971, p. 349.
287. Bachur, N. R.: Science 193:595, 1976.
288. Sellers, E. M., et al.: Clin. Pharmacol. Ther. 13:37, 1972.
289. Pritchard, J. F., et al.: J. Chromatogr. 162:47, 1979.
290. Osterloh, J. D., et al.: Drug Metab. Dispos. 8:12, 1980.
291. Jenner, P., and Testa, B.: Drug Metab. Rev. 2:117, 1973.
292. Culp, H. W., and McMahon, R. E.: J. Biol. Chem. 243:848, 1968.
293. McMahon, R. E., et al.: J. Pharmacol. Exp. Ther. 149:272, 1965.
294. Galloway, J. A., et al.: Diabetes 16:118, 1967.
295. Yü, T. F., et al.: Metabolism 17:309, 1968.
296. Chan, K. K., et al.: J. Med. Chem. 15:1265, 1972.
297. Pollock, S. H., and Blum, K.: In Blum, K., et al. (eds.). Alcohol and Opiates. New York, Academic Press, 1977, p. 359.
298. Chatterjie, N., et al.: Drug Metab. Dispos. 2:401, 1974.
299. Dayton, H., and Inturrisi, C. E.: Drug Metab. Dispos. 4:474, 1974.
300. Roerig, S., et al.: Drug Metab. Dispos. 4:53, 1976.
301. Malspeis, L., et al.: Res. Commun. Chem. Pathol. Pharmacol. 14:393, 1976.
302. Bachur, N. R., and Felsted, R. L.: Drug Metab. Dispos. 4:239, 1976.
303. Crew, M. C., et al.: Clin. Pharmacol. Ther. 14:1013, 1973.
304. DiCarlo, F. J., et al.: Xenobiotica 2:159, 1972.
305. Crew, M. C., et al.: Xenobiotica 2:431, 1972.
306. DiCarlo, F. J., et al.: J. Reticuloendothel. Soc. 14:387, 1973.
307. Gerhards, E., et al.: Acta Endocrinol. 68:219, 1971.
308. Wright, J., et al.: Xenobiotica 7:257, 1977.
309. Kawai, K., and Baba, S.: Chem. Pharm. Bull. (Tokyo) 24:2728, 1976.
310. Gillette, J. R., et al.: Mol. Pharmacol. 4:541, 1968.
311. Fouts, J. R., and Brodie, B. B.: J. Pharmacol. Exp. Ther. 119:197, 1957.
312. Hernandez, P. H., et al.: Biochem. Pharmacol. 16:1877, 1967.
313. Scheline, R. R.: Pharmacol. Rev. 25:451, 1973.
314. Walker, R.: Food Cosmet. Toxicol. 8:659, 1970.
315. Min, B. H., and Garland, W. A.: J. Chromatogr. 139:121, 1977.
316. Rieder, J., and Wendt, G.: In Garattini, S., et al. (eds.). The Benzodiazepines. New York, Raven Press, 1973, p. 99.
317. Conklin, J. D., et al.: J. Pharm. Sci. 62:1024, 1973.
318. Cox, P. L., et al.: J. Pharm. Sci. 58:987, 1969.
319. Stambaugh, J. E., et al.: J. Pharmacol. Exp. Ther. 161:373, 1968.
320. Mitchard, M.: Xenobiotica 1:469, 1971.
321. Glazko, A. J., et al.: J. Pharmacol. Exp. Ther. 96:445, 1949.
322. Smith, G. N., and Worrel, G. S.: Arch. Biochem. Biophys. 24:216, 1949.
323. Tréfouël, J., et al.: C. R. Seances Soc. Biol. Paris 190:756, 1935.
324. Jones, R., et al.: Food Cosmet. Toxicol. 2:447, 1966.
325. Jones, R., et al.: Food Cosmet. Toxicol. 4:419, 1966.
326. Ikeda, M., and Uesugi, T.: Biochem. Pharmacol. 22:2743, 1973.
327. Peppercorn, M. A., and Goldman, P.: J. Pharmacol. Exp. Ther. 181:555, 1972.
328. Das, E. M.: Scand. J. Gastroenterol. 9:137, 1974.
329. Schröder, H., and Gustafsson, B. E.: Xenobiotica 3:225, 1973.
330. Bickel, M. H., and Gigon, P. L.: Xenobiotica 1:631, 1971.
331. Eldjarn, L.: Scand. J. Clin. Lab. Invest. 2:202, 1950.
332. Staub, H.: Helv. Physiol. Acta 13:141, 1955.
333. Duggan, D. E., et al.: Clin. Pharmacol. Ther. 21:326, 1977.
334. Duggan, D. E., et al.: J. Pharmacol. Exp. Ther. 20:8, 1977.
335. Kolb, H. K., et al.: Arzneimittelforschung 15:1292, 1965.
336. LaDu, B. N., and Snady, H.: In Brodie, B. B., and Gillette, J. R. (eds.). Concepts in Biochemical Pharmacology, Part 2. Berlin, Springer-Verlag, 1971, p. 477.
337. Junge, W., and Krisch, K.: CRC Crit. Rev. Toxicol. 3:371, 1975.
338. Davison, C.: Ann. N. Y. Acad. Sci. 179:249, 1971.
339. Kogan, M. J., et al.: Anal. Chem. 49:1965, 1977.
340. Inaba, T., et al.: Clin. Pharmacol. Ther. 23:547, 1978.
341. Stewart, D. J., et al.: Life Sci. 1557, 1977.
342. Wells, R., et al.: Clin. Chem. 20:440, 1974.
343. Rubens, R., et al.: Arzneimittelforschung 22:256, 1972.
344. Gugler, L., and Jensen, C.: J. Chromatogr. 117:175, 1976.
345. Houin, G., et al.: Eur. J. Clin. Pharmacol. 8:433, 1975.
346. Sinkula, A. A., et al.: J. Pharm. Sci. 62:1106, 1973.
347. Martin, A. R.: In Wilson, C. O., et al. (eds.). Textbook of Organic Medicinal and Pharmaceutical Chemistry, 7th ed. Philadelphia, J. B. Lippincott, 1977, p. 304.
348. Knirsch, A. K., et al.: J. Infect. Dis. 127:S105, 1973.
349. Stella, V.: In Higuchi, T., and Stella, V. (eds.): Prodrugs as Novel Drug Delivery Systems. Washington, DC, American Chemical Society, 1975, p. 1.
350. Mark, L. C., et al.: J. Pharmacol. Exp. Ther. 102:5, 1951.
351. Nelson, S. D., et al.: J. Pharm. Sci. 66:1180, 1977.
352. Tsukamoto, H., et al.: Chem. Pharm. Bull. (Tokyo) 3:459, 1955.
353. Tsukamoto, H., et al.: Chem. Pharm. Bull. (Tokyo) 3:397, 1955.
354. Dudley, K. H., et al.: Drug Metab. Dispos. 6:133, 1978.
355. Dudley, K. H., et al.: Drug Metab. Dispos. 2:103, 1974.
356. Humphrey, M. J., and Ringrose, P. S.: Drug Metab. Rev. 17:283, 1986.
357. Kompella, U. B., and Lee, V. H. L.: Adv. Parenteral Sci. 4:391, 1992.
358. Moore, J. A., and Wroblewski, V. J.: In Ferraiolo, B. L., et al. (eds.). Protein Pharmacokinetics and Metabolism. New York, Plenum Press, 1992, p. 93.
359. Dutton, G. J., et al.: In Parke, D. V., and Smith, R. L. (eds.). Drug Metabolism: From Microbe to Man. London, Taylor & Francis, 1977, p. 71.
360. Dutton, G. J.: In Dutton, G. J. (ed.). Glucuronic Acid, Free and Combined. New York, Academic Press, 1966, p. 186.
361. Dutton, G. D., et al.: Prog. Drug Metab. 1:2, 1977.
362. Brunk, S. F., and Delle, M.: Clin. Pharmacol. Exp. Ther. 16:51, 1974.
363. Berkowitz, B. A., et al.: Clin. Pharmacol. Exp. Ther. 17:629, 1975.
364. Andrews, R. S., et al.: J. Int. Med. Res. 4(Suppl. 4):34, 1976.
365. Thies, R. L., and Fischer, L. J.: Clin. Chem. 24:778, 1978.
366. Walle, T., et al.: Fed. Proc. 35:665, 1976.
367. Walle, T., et al.: Clin. Pharmacol. Ther. 26:167, 1979.
368. Roseman, S., et al.: J. Am. Chem. Soc. 76:1650, 1954.
369. Segre, E. J.: J. Clin. Pharmacol. 15:316, 1975.
370. Rubin, A., et al.: J. Pharm. Sci. 61:739, 1972.
371. Rubin, A., et al.: J. Pharmacol. Exp. Ther. 183:449, 1972.
372. Bridges, J. W., et al.: Biochem. J. 118:47, 1970.
373. Gibson, T., et al.: Br. J. Clin. Pharmacol. 2:233, 1975.
374. Tsuichiya, T., and Levy, G.: J. Pharm. Sci. 61:800, 1972.
375. Porter, C. C., et al.: Drug Metab. Dispos. 3:189, 1975.
376. Chaundhuri, N. K., et al.: Drug Metab. Dispos. 4:372, 1976.
377. Sitar, D. S., and Thornhill, D. P.: J. Pharmacol. Exp. Ther. 184:432, 1973.
378. Lindsay, R. H., et al.: Pharmacologist 18:113, 1976.

379. Sitar, D. S., and Thornhill, D. P.: J. Pharmacol. Exp. Ther. 183:440, 1972.
380. Dutton, G. J., and Illing, H. P. A.: Biochem. J. 129:539, 1972.
381. Dieterle, W., et al.: Arzneimittelforschung 26:572, 1976.
382. Richter, J. W., et al.: Helv. Chim. Acta 58:2512, 1975.
383. Dieterle, W., et al.: Eur. J. Clin. Pharmacol. 9:135, 1975.
384. Schmid, R., and Lester, R.: In Dutton, G. J. (ed.). Glucuronic Acid, Free and Combined. New York, Academic Press, 1966, p. 493.
385. Hadd, H. E., and Blickenstaff, R. T.: Conjugates of Steroid Hormones. New York, Academic Press, 1969.
386. Smith, R. L.: The Excretory Function of Bile: The Elimination of Drugs and Toxic Substance in Bile. London, Chapman & Hall, 1973.
387. Stern, L., et al.: Am. J. Dis. Child. 120:26, 1970.
388. Weiss, C. F., et al.: N. Engl. J. Med. 262:787, 1960.
389. Dodgson, K. S.: In Parke, D. V., and Smith, R. L. (eds.). Drug Metabolism: From Microbe to Man. London, Taylor & Francis, 1977, p. 91.
390. Roy, A. B.: In Brodie, B. B., and Gillette, J. R. (eds.). Concepts in Biochemical Pharmacology, Part 2. Berlin, Springer-Verlag, 1971, p. 536.
391. Williams, R. T.: In Bernfeld, P. (ed.). Biogenesis of Natural Products, 2nd ed. Oxford, Pergamon Press, 1967, p. 611.
392. Roy, A. B.: Adv. Enzymol. 22:205, 1960.
393. Kwan, K. C., et al.: J. Pharmacol. Exp. Ther. 198:264, 1976.
394. Stenback, O., et al.: Eur. J. Clin. Pharmacol. 12:117, 1977.
395. Lin, C., et al.: Drug Metab. Dispos. 5:234, 1977.
396. Nilsson, H. T., et al.: Xenobiotica 2:363, 1972.
397. Miller, R. P., et al.: Clin. Pharmacol. Ther. 19:284, 1976.
398. Levy, G., et al.: Pediatrics 55:818, 1975.
399. James, S. P., and Waring, R. H.: Xenobiotica 1:572, 1971.
400. Bostrum, H., and Vestermark, A.: Acta Physiol. Scand. 48:88, 1960.
401. Boyland, E., et al.: Biochem. J. 65:417, 1957.
402. Roy, A. B.: Biochem. J. 74:49, 1960.
403. Irving, C. C.: In Gorrod, J. W. (ed.). Biological Oxidation of Nitrogen. Amsterdam, Elsevier-North Holland, 1978, p. 325.
404. Irving, C. C.: Cancer Res. 35:2959, 1975.
405. Jackson, C. D., and Irving, C. C.: Cancer Res. 32:1590, 1972.
406. Hinson, J. A., and Mitchell, J. R.: Drug Metab. Dispos. 4:430, 1975.
407. Mulder, G. J., et al.: Biochem. Pharmacol. 26:189, 1977.
408. Weber, W.: In Brodie, B. B., and Gillette, J. R. (eds.). Concepts in Biochemical Pharmacology, Part 2. Berlin, Springer-Verlag, 1971, p. 564.
409. Williams, R. T., and Millburn, P.: In Blaschko, H. K. F. (ed.). MTP International Review of Science, Biochemistry Series One, vol. 12, Physiological and Pharmacological Biochemistry. Baltimore, University Park Press, 1975, p. 211.
410. Bridges, J. W., et al.: Biochem. J. 118:47, 1970.
411. Wan, S. H., and Riegelman, S.: J. Pharm. Sci. 61:1284, 1972.
412. Von Lehmann, B., et al.: J. Pharm. Sci. 62:1483, 1973.
413. Braun, G. A., et al.: Eur. J. Pharmacol. 1:58, 1967.
414. Tatsumi, K., et al.: Biochem. Pharmacol. 16:1941, 1967.
415. Weber, W. W., and Hein, D. W.: Clin. Pharmacokinet. 4:401, 1979.
416. James, M. O., et al.: Proc. R. Soc. Lond. B. Biol. Sci. 182:25, 1972.
417. Smith, R. L., and Caldwell, J.: In Parke, D. V., and Smith, R. L. (eds.). Drug Metabolism: From Microbe to Man. London, Taylor & Francis, 1977, p. 331.
418. Williams, R. T.: Clin. Pharmacol. Ther. 4:234, 1963.
419. Drach, J. C., et al.: Proc. Soc. Exp. Biol. Med. 135:849, 1970.
420. Caldwell, J.: In Jenner, P., and Testa, B. (eds.). Concepts in Drug Metabolism, Part A. New York, Marcel Dekker, 1980, p. 211.
421. Jerina, D. M., and Bend, J. R.: In Jollow, D. J., et al. (eds.). Biological Reactive Intermediates. New York, Plenum Press, 1977, p. 207.
422. Chasseaud, L. F.: In Arias, I. M., and Jakoby, W. B. (eds.). Glutathione: Metabolism and Function. New York, Raven Press, 1976, p. 77.
423. Ketterer, B.: Mutat. Res. 202:343, 1988.
424. Mantle, T. J., Pickett, C. B., and Hayes, J. D. (eds.): Glutathione S-Transferases and Carcinogenesis. London, Taylor & Francis, 1987.
425. Foureman, G. L., and Reed, D. J.: Biochemistry 26:2028, 1987.
426. Rannung, U., et al.: Chem. Biol. Interact. 20:1, 1978.
427. Olson, W. A., et al.: J. Natl. Cancer Inst. 51:1993, 1973.
428. Monks, T. J., and Lau, S. S.: Toxicology 52:1, 1988.
429. Weisburger, E. K.: Annu. Rev. Pharmacol. Toxicol. 18:395, 1978.
430. Hollingworth, R. M., et al.: Life Sci. 13:191, 1973.
431. Benke, G. M., and Murphy, S. D.: Toxicol. Appl. Pharmacol. 31:254, 1975.
432. Bray, H. G., et al.: Biochem. J. 67:607, 1957.
433. Chalmers, A. H.: Biochem. Pharmacol. 23:1891, 1974.
434. de Miranda, P., et al.: J. Pharmacol. Exp. Ther. 187:588, 1973.
435. de Miranda, P., et al.: J. Pharmacol. Exp. Ther. 195:50, 1975.
436. Elion, G. B.: Fed. Proc. 26:898, 1967.
437. Jerina, D. M.: In Arias, I. M., and Jakoby, W. B. (eds.). Glutathione: Metabolism and Function. New York, Raven Press, 1976, p. 267.
438. Needleman, P.: In Needleman, P. (ed.). Organic Nitrates. Berlin, Springer-Verlag, 1975, p. 57.
439. Klaasen, C. D., and Fitzgerald, T. J.: J. Pharmacol. Exp. Ther. 191:548, 1974.
440. Kuss, E., et al.: Hoppe Seyler Z. Physiol. Chem. 352:817, 1971.
441. Nelson, S. D., et al.: Biochem. Biophys. Res. Commun. 70:1157, 1976.
442. Weber, W.: In Fishman, W. H. (ed.). Metabolic Conjugation and Metabolic Hydrolysis, vol. 3. New York, Academic Press, 1973, p. 250.
443. Williams, R. T.: Fed. Proc. 26:1029, 1967.
444. Elson, J., et al.: Clin. Pharmacol. Ther. 17:134, 1975.
445. Drayer, D. E., et al.: Proc. Soc. Exp. Biol. Med. 146:358, 1974.
446. Mitchell, J. R., et al.: Ann. Intern. Med. 84:181, 1976.
447. Nelson, S. D., et al.: Science 193:193, 1976.
448. Giardina, E. G., et al.: Clin. Pharmacol. Ther. 19:339, 1976.
449. Giardina, E. G., et al.: Clin. Pharmacol. Ther. 17:722, 1975.
450. Peters, J. H., and Levy, L.: Ann. N. Y. Acad. Sci. 179:660, 1971.
451. Reimerdes, E., and Thumim, J. H.: Arzneimittelforschung 20:1171, 1970.
452. Vree, T. B., et al.: In Merkus, F. W. H. M. (ed.). The Serum Concentration of Drugs. Amsterdam, Excerpta Medica, 1980, p. 205.
453. Garrett, E. R.: Int. J. Clin. Pharmacol. 16:155, 1978.
454. Reidenberg, M. W., et al.: Clin. Pharmacol. Ther. 14:970, 1973.
455. Israili, Z. H., et al.: Drug Metab. Rev. 6:283, 1977.
456. Evans, D. A. P., et al.: Clin. Pharmacol. Ther. 6:430, 1965.
457. Tabor, H., et al.: J. Biol. Chem. 204:127, 1953.
458. Sullivan, H. R., and Due, S. L.: J. Med. Chem. 16:909, 1973.
459. Sullivan, H. R., et al.: J. Am. Chem. Soc. 94:4050, 1972.
460. Sullivan, H. R., et al.: Life Sci. 11:1093, 1972.
461. Drayer, D. E., and Reidenberg, M. M.: Clin. Pharmacol. Ther. 22:251, 1977.
462. Lunde, P. K. M., et al.: Clin. Pharmacokinet. 2:182, 1977.
463. Kalow, W.: Pharmacogenetics: Heredity and the Response to Drugs. Philadelphia, W. B. Saunders, 1962.
464. Kutt, H., et al.: Am. Rev. Respir. Dis. 101:377, 1970.
465. Alarcon-Segovia, D.: Drugs 12:69, 1976.
466. Reidenberg, M. M., and Martin, J. H.: Drug Metab. Dispos. 2:71, 1974.
467. Strong, J. M., et al.: J. Pharmacokinet. Biopharm. 3:233, 1975.
468. Axelrod, J.: In Brodie, B. B., and Gillette, J. R. (eds.). Concepts in Biochemical Pharmacology, Part 2. Berlin, Springer-Verlag, 1971, p. 609.
469. Mudd, S. H.: In Fishman, W. H. (ed.). Metabolic Conjugation and Metabolic Hydrolysis, vol. 3. New York, Academic Press, p. 297.
470. Young, J. A., and Edwards, K. D. G.: Med. Res. 1:53, 1962.
471. Young, J. A., and Edwards, K. D. G.: J. Pharmacol. Exp. Ther. 145:102, 1964.
472. Shindo, H., et al.: Chem. Pharm. Bull. (Tokyo) 21:826, 1973.
473. Morgan, C. D., et al.: Biochem. J. 114:8P, 1969.
474. Weber, R., and Tuttle, R. R.: In Goldberg, M. E. (ed.). Pharmacological and Biochemical Properties of Drug Substances, vol. 1. Washington, DC, American Pharmaceutical Association, 1977, p. 109.
475. Glazko, A. J.: Drug Metab. Dispos. 1:711, 1973.
476. Börner, U., and Abbott, S.: Experientia 29:180, 1973.
477. Bleidner, W. E., et al.: J. Pharmacol. Exp. Ther. 150:484, 1965.
478. Komori, Y., and Sendju, Y.: J. Biochem. 6:163, 1926.
479. Lindsay, R. H., et al.: Biochem. Pharmacol. 24:463, 1975.
480. Bremer, J., and Greenberg, D. M.: Biochim. Biophys. Acta 46:217, 1961.
481. Allan, P. W., et al.: Biochim. Biophys. Acta 114:647, 1966.
482. Elion, G. B.: Fed. Proc. 26:898, 1967.
483. Testa, B., and Jenner, P.: Drug Metabolism: Chemical and Biochemical Aspects. New York, Marcel Dekker, 1976, pp. 329–418.
484. Testa, B., and Jenner, P: Drug Metab. Rev. 12:1, 1981.
485. Murray, M., and Reidy, G. F.: Pharmacol. Ther. 42:85, 1990.
486. Murray, M.: Clin. Pharmacokinet. 23:132, 1992.
487. Ward, R. M., et al.: In Avery, G. S. (ed.). Drug Treatment, 2nd ed. Sydney, ADIS Press, 1980, p. 76.

488. Morselli, P. L.: Drug Disposition During Development. New York, Spectrum, 1977.
489. Jondorf, W. R., et al.: Biochem. Pharmacol. 1:352, 1958.
490. Nitowsky, H. M., et al.: J. Pediatr. 69:1139, 1966.
491. Crooks, J., et al.: Clin. Pharmacokinet. 1:280, 1976.
492. Crooks, J., and Stevenson, I. H. (eds.): Drugs and the Elderly. London, Macmillan, 1979.
493. Williams, R. T.: Ann. N. Y. Acad. Sci. 179:141, 1971.
494. Williams, R. T.: In LaDu, B. N., et al. (eds.). Fundamentals of Drug Metabolism and Disposition. Baltimore, Williams & Wilkins, 1971, p. 187.
495. Williams, R. T., et al.: In Snyder, S. H., and Usdin, E. (eds.). Frontiers in Catecholamine Research. New York, Pergamon Press, 1973 p. 927.
496. Butler, T. C., et al.: J. Pharmacol. Exp. Ther. 199:82, 1976.
497. Williams, R. T.: Biochem. Soc. Trans. 2:359, 1974.
498. Bridges, J. W., et al.: Biochem. J. 118:47, 1970.
499. Williams, R. T.: Fed. Proc. 26:1029, 1967.
500. Thomas, B. H. et al, J. Pharm. Sci., 79:321, 1990.
501. Cram, R. L., et al.: Proc. Soc. Exp. Biol. Med. 118:872, 1965.
502. Kutt, H., et al.: Neurology 14:542, 1962.
503. Vesell, E. S.: Prog. Med. Genet. 9:291, 1973.
504. Pelkonen, O., et al.: In Pacifici, G. M., and Pelkonen, O. (eds.). Interindividual Variability in Human Drug Metabolism. New York, Taylor & Francis, 2001, p. 269.
505. Kato, R.: Drug Metab. Rev. 3:1, 1974.
506. Beckett, A. H., et al.: J. Pharm. Pharmacol. 23:62S, 1971.
507. Menguy, R., et al.: Nature 239:102, 1972.
508. Conney, A. H.: Pharmacol. Rev. 19:317, 1967.
509. Snyder, R., and Remmer, H.: Pharmacol. Ther. 7:203, 1979.
510. Parke, D. V.: In Parke, D. V. (ed.). Enzyme Induction. London, Plenum Press, 1975, p. 207.
511. Estabrook, R. W., and Lindenlaub, E. (eds.): The Induction of Drug Metabolism. Stuttgart, Schattauer Verlag, 1979.
512. Hansten, P. D.: Drug Interactions, 4th ed. Philadelphia, Lea & Febiger, 1979, p. 38.
513. Laenger, H., and Detering, K.: Lancet 600, 1974.
514. Skolnick, J. L., et al.: JAMA 236:1382, 1976.
515. Dent, C. E., et al.: Br. Med. J. 4:69, 1970.
516. Yeung, C. Y., and Field, C. E.: Lancet 135, 1969.
517. Jenne, J., et al.: Life Sci. 17:195, 1975.
518. Pantuck, E. J., et al.: Science 175:1248, 1972.
519. Pantuck, E. J., et al.: Clin. Pharmacol. Ther. 14:259, 1973.
520. Vaughan, D. P., et al.: Br. J. Clin. Pharmacol. 3:279, 1976.
521. Kolmodin, B., et al.: Clin. Pharmacol. Ther. 10:638, 1969.
522. Jeffrey, W. H., et al.: JAMA 236:2881, 1976.
523. Gelboin, H. V., and Ts'o, P. O. P. (eds.): Polycyclic Hydrocarbons and Cancer: Environment, Chemistry, Molecular and Cell Biology. New York, Academic Press, 1978.
524. Vesell, E. S., and Passananti, G. T.: Drug Metab. Dispos. 1:402, 1973.
525. Anders, M. W.: Annu. Rev. Pharmacol. 11:37, 1971.
526. Kehoe, W. A.: Pharmacist's Letter, 18:#180905, September 2002.
527. Hewick, D., and McEwen, J.: J. Pharm. Pharmacol. 25:458, 1973.
528. Casy, A. F.: In Burger, A. (ed.). Medicinal Chemistry, Part 1, 3rd ed. New York, Wiley-Interscience, 1970, p. 81.
529. George, C. F., et al.: Eur. J. Clin. Pharmacol. 4:74, 1972.
530. Breimer, D. D., and Van Rossum, J. M.: J. Pharm. Pharmacol. 25: 762, 1973.
531. Low, L. K., and Castagnoli, N., Jr.: Annu. Rep. Med. Chem. 13:304, 1978.
532. Testa, B., and Jenner, P.: J. Pharm. Pharmacol. 28:731, 1976.
533. Belpaire, F. M., et al.: Xenobiotica 5:413, 1975.
534. Woolhouse, N. M., et al.: Xenobiotica 3:511, 1973.
535. Drayer, D. E.: US Pharm. (Hosp. Ed.) 5:H15, 1980.
536. Pierides, A. M., et al.: Lancet 2:1279, 1975.
537. Gabriel, R., and Pearce, J. M. S.: Lancet 2:906, 1976.
538. Gallois-Montbrun, S., Schneider, B., Chen, Y., et al.: J. Biol. Chem. 277(42):39953, 2002.
539. Stein, D. S., and Moore, K. H.: Pharmacotherapy 21(1), 11, 2001.
540. Sweeny, D. J., Lynch, G., Bidgood, et al.: Drug Metab. Dispos. 28(7): 737, 2000.

SELECTED READING

Aitio, A. (ed.): Conjugation Reactions in Drug Biotransformation. Amsterdam, Elsevier, 1978.

Anders, M. W. (ed.): Bioactivation of Foreign Compounds. New York, Academic Press, 1985.
Baselt, R. C., and Cravey, R. H.: Disposition of Toxic Drugs and Chemicals in Man. Foster City, CA, Chemical Toxicology Institute, 1995.
Benford, D. J., Bridges, J. W., and Gibson, G. G. (eds.): Drug Metabolism—From Molecules to Man. London, Taylor & Francis, 1987.
Brodie, B. B., and Gillette, J. R. (eds.): Concepts in Biochemical Pharmacology, Part 2. Berlin, Springer-Verlag, 1971.
Caldwell, J.: Conjugation reactions in foreign compound metabolism. Drug Metab. Rev. 13:745, 1982.
Caldwell, J., and Jakoby, W. B. (eds.): Biological Basis of Detoxification. New York, Academic Press, 1983.
Caldwell, J., and Paulson, G. D. (eds.): Foreign Compound Metabolism. London, Taylor & Francis, 1984.
Creasey, W. A.: Drug Disposition in Humans. New York, Oxford University Press, 1979.
DeMatteis, F., and Lock, E. A. (eds.): Selectivity and Molecular Mechanisms of Toxicity. London, Macmillan, 1987.
Dipple, A., Micheijda, C. J., and Weisburger, E. K.: Metabolism of chemical carcinogens. Pharmacol. Ther. 27:265, 1985.
Drayer, D. E.: Pharmacologically active metabolites of drugs and other foreign compounds. Drugs 24:519, 1982.
Dutton, G. J.: Glucuronidation of Drugs and Other Compounds. Boca Raton, FL, CRC Press, 1980.
Estabrook, R. W., and Lindenlaub, E. (eds.): Induction of Drug Metabolism. Stuttgart, Schattauer Verlag, 1979.
Ferraiolo, B. L., Mohler, M. A., and Gloff, C. A. (eds.): Protein Pharmacokinetics and Metabolism. New York, Plenum Press, 1992.
Gibson, G. G., and Skett, P.: Introduction to Drug Metabolism. London, Chapman & Hall, 1986.
Gorrod, J. W. (ed.): Drug Toxicity. London, Taylor & Francis, 1979.
Gorrod, J. W., and Damani, L. A. (eds.): Biological Oxidation of Nitrogen in Organic Molecules. Chichester, UK, Ellis Horwood, 1985.
Gorrod, J. W., Oelschlager, H., and Caldwell, J. (eds.): Metabolism of Xenobiotics. London, Taylor & Francis, 1988.
Gram, T. E. (ed.): Extrahepatic Metabolism of Drugs and Other Foreign Compounds. New York, SP Medical and Scientific, 1980.
Guengerich, F. P.: Analysis and characterization of drug metabolizing enzymes. In Hayes, A. W. (ed.). Principles and Methods of Toxicology, 3rd ed. New York, Raven Press, 1994.
Guengerich, F. P. (ed.): Mammalian Cytochromes P-450, vols. 1 and 2. Boca Raton, FL, CRC Press, 1987.
Hathway, D. E.: Mechanisms of Chemical Carcinogenesis. London, Butterworths, 1986.
Hodgson, E., and Levi, P. E. (eds.): A Textbook of Modern Toxicology. New York, Elsevier, 1987.
Humphrey, M. I., and Ringrose, P. S.: Peptides and related drugs: a review of their absorption, metabolism and excretion. Drug Metab. Rev. 17: 283, 1986.
Jakoby, W. B. (ed.): Detoxification and drug metabolism. Methods Enzymol. 77: 1981.
Jakoby, W. B. (ed.): Enzymatic Basis of Detoxification, vols. 1 and 2. New York, Academic Press, 1980.
Jakoby, W. B., Bend, J. R., and Caldwell, J. (eds.): Metabolic Basis of Detoxification: Metabolism of Functional Groups. New York, Academic Press, 1982.
Jeffrery, E. H.: Human Drug Metabolism. From Molecular Biology to Man. Boca Raton, FL, CRC Press, 1993.
Jenner, P., and Testa, B.: The influence of stereochemical factors on drug disposition. Drug Metab. Rev. 2:117, 1973.
Jenner, P., and Testa, B. (eds.): Concepts in Drug Metabolism, Parts A and B. New York, Marcel Dekker, 1980, 1981.
Jerina, D. M. (ed.): Drug Metabolism Concepts. Washington, DC, American Chemical Society, 1977.
Jollow, D. J., et al. (eds.): Biological Reactive Intermediates: Formation, Toxicity and Inactivation. New York, Plenum Press, 1977.
Kauffman, F. C. (ed.): Conjugation–Deconjugation Reactions in Drug Metabolism and Toxicity. Berlin, Springer-Verlag, 1994.
Klaasen, C. D. (ed.): Casarett & Doull's Toxicology, 5th ed. New York, McGraw-Hill, 1996.
La Du, B. N., Mandel, H. G., and Way, E. L. (eds.): Fundamentals of Drug Metabolism and Drug Disposition. Baltimore, Williams & Wilkins, 1971.
Low, L. K., and Castagnoli, N.: Drug biotransformations. In Wolff, M. E.

(ed.). Burger's Medicinal Chemistry, Part 1, 4th ed. New York, Wiley-Interscience, 1980, p. 107.

Mitchell, J. R., and Horning, M. G. (eds.): Drug Metabolism and Drug Toxicity. New York, Raven Press, 1984.

Monks, T. J., and Lau, S. S.: Reactive intermediates and their toxicological significance. Toxicology 52:1, 1988.

Mulder, G. J. (ed.): Sulfate Metabolism and Sulfate Conjugation. London, Taylor & Francis, 1985.

Nelson, S. D.: Chemical and biological factors influencing drug biotransformation. In Wolff, M. E. (ed.). Burger's Medicinal Chemistry, Part 1, 4th ed. New York, Wiley-Interscience, 1980, p. 227.

Nelson, S. D.: Metabolic activation and drug toxicity. J. Med. Chem. 25: 753, 1982.

Ortiz de Montellano, P. R. (ed.): Cytochrome P-450: Structure, Mechanism, and Biochemistry. New York, Plenum Press, 1986.

Pacifici, G. M., and Pelkonen O. (eds.): Interindividual Variability in Human Drug Metabolism, New York, Taylor & Francis, 2001.

Parke, D. V.: The Biochemistry of Foreign Compounds. New York, Pergamon Press, 1968.

Parke, D. V., and Smith, R. L. (eds.): Drug Metabolism: From Microbe to Man. London, Taylor & Francis, 1977.

Paulson, G. D., et al. (eds.): Xenobiotic Conjugation Chemistry. Washington, DC, American Chemical Society, 1986.

Reid, E., and Leppard, J. P. (eds.): Drug Metabolite Isolation and Detection. New York, Plenum Press, 1983.

Sato, R., and Omura, T. (eds.): Cytochrome P-450. New York, Academic Press, 1978.

Schenkman, J. B., and Greim, H. (eds.): Cytochrome P450. Berlin, Springer-Verlag, 1993.

Schenkman, J. B., and Kupfer, D. (eds.): Hepatic Cytochrome P-450 Monooxygenase System. New York, Pergamon Press, 1982.

Siest, G. (ed.): Drug Metabolism: Molecular Approaches and Pharmacological Implications. New York, Academic Press, 1985.

Singer, B., and Grunberger, D.: Molecular Biology of Mutagens and Carcinogens. New York, Plenum Press, 1983.

Snyder, R., et al. (eds.): Biological Reactive Intermediates II, Parts A and B. New York, Plenum Press, 1982.

Snyder, R., et al. (eds.): Biological Reactive Intermediates III: Animal Models and Human Disease, Parts A and B. New York, Plenum Press, 1986.

Tagashira, Y., and Omura, T. (eds.): P-450 and Chemical Carcinogenesis. New York, Plenum Press, 1985.

Testa, B., and Caldwell, J. (eds.): The Metabolism of Drugs and Other Xenobiotics. London, Academic Press, 1995.

Testa, B., and Jenner, P.: Drug Metabolism: Chemical and Biochemical Aspects. New York, Marcel Dekker, 1976.

Timbrell, J. A.: Principles of Biochemical Toxicology. London, Taylor & Francis, 1982.

Williams, R. T.: Detoxification Mechanisms, 2nd ed. New York, Wiley, 1959.

CHAPTER 5

Prodrugs and Drug Latentiation

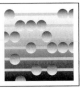

FORREST T. SMITH AND C. RANDALL CLARK

HISTORY

In 1958, Albert initially coined the term *prodrug* and used it to refer to a pharmacologically inactive compound that is transformed by the mammalian system into an active substance by either chemical or metabolic means.[1] This included both compounds that are designed to undergo a transformation to yield an active substance and those that were discovered by serendipity to do so. These two situations were distinguished by Harper, who in 1959 introduced the term *drug latentiation* to refer to drugs that were specifically designed to require bioactivation.[2]

These ideas led to the development of a number of currently used drugs that have advantages over their nonprodrug counterparts. The type of prodrug to be produced depends on the specific aspect of the drug's action that requires improvement and the type of functionality that is present in the active drug. Generally, prodrug approaches are undertaken to improve patient acceptability of the agent (i.e., reduce pain associated with administration), alter absorption, alter distribution, alter metabolism, or alter elimination. The chemical nature of the prodrugs that can be prepared is somewhat limited, however, by the chemical nature of the active species.

Recently, the terms *hard drugs* and *soft drugs* were introduced.[3, 4] Hard drugs are compounds that are designed to contain the structural characteristics necessary for pharmacological activity but in a form that is not susceptible to metabolic or chemical transformation. In this way, the production of any toxic metabolite is avoided, and there is increased efficiency of action. Since the drug is not inactivated by metabolism, it may be less readily eliminated. On the other hand, soft drugs are active compounds that after exerting their desired pharmacological effect are designed to undergo metabolic inactivation to give a nontoxic product. Thus soft drugs are considered to be the opposite of prodrugs.

BASIC CONCEPTS

A prodrug by definition is inactive and must be converted into an active species within the biological system. There are a variety of mechanisms by which this conversion may be accomplished. Generally, the conversion to an active form is most often carried out by metabolizing enzymes within the body. Conversion to an active form may be accomplished by chemical means (e.g., hydrolysis or decarboxylation), although this is less common. Chemical transformation does not depend on the presence or relative amounts of metaboliz-

ing enzymes, and therefore, less interpatient variability in activation is seen; since such compounds are chemically unstable, however, storage of these compounds may present a problem.

Prodrugs can be conveniently grouped into carrier-linked prodrugs and bioprecursor prodrugs.[5] Carrier-linked prodrugs are drugs that have been attached through a metabolically labile linkage to another molecule, the so-called promoiety, which is not necessary for activity but may impart some desirable property to the drug, such as increased lipid or water solubility or site-directed delivery. Several advantages may be gained by generating a prodrug: increased absorption, alleviation of pain at the site of injection if the agent is given parenterally, elimination of an unpleasant taste associated with the drug, decreased toxicity, decreased metabolic inactivation, increased chemical stability, and prolonged or shortened action, whichever is desired in a particular agent. An example of such a prodrug form of chloramphenicol is provided below (Scheme 5-1).[6]

Administration of a drug parenterally may cause pain at the site of injection, especially if the drug begins to precipitate out of solution and damage the surrounding tissue. This situation can be remedied by preparing a drug with increased solubility in the administered solvent. Since chloramphenicol has low water solubility, the succinate ester was prepared to increase the water solubility of the agent and facilitate parenteral administration. The succinate ester itself is inactive as an antibacterial agent, so it must be converted to chloramphenicol for this agent to be effective. This occurs in the plasma to give the active drug and succinate. The ester hydrolysis reaction can be catalyzed by esterases present in large amounts in the plasma. The ability to prepare ester-type prodrugs depends, of course, on the presence of either a hydroxyl group or a carboxyl moiety in the drug molecule. The promoiety should be easily and completely removed after it has served its function and should be nontoxic, as is indeed the case with succinate. The selection of the appropriate promoiety depends on which properties are sought for the agent. If it is desirable to increase water solubility, then a promoiety containing an ionizable function or numerous polar functional groups is used. If, on the other hand, the goal is to increase lipid solubility or decrease water solubility, a nonpolar promoiety is appropriate.

A slight variation on the *carrier-linked prodrug* approach is seen with *mutual prodrugs* in which the carrier also has activity. The antineoplastic agent estramustine, which is used in the treatment of prostatic cancer, provides an example of such an approach (Scheme 5-2).[7] Estramustine is composed of a phosphorylated steroid (17α-estradiol) linked to a normustard [$HN(CH_2CH_2Cl)_2$] through a carbamate linkage. The steroid portion of the molecule helps to concentrate the

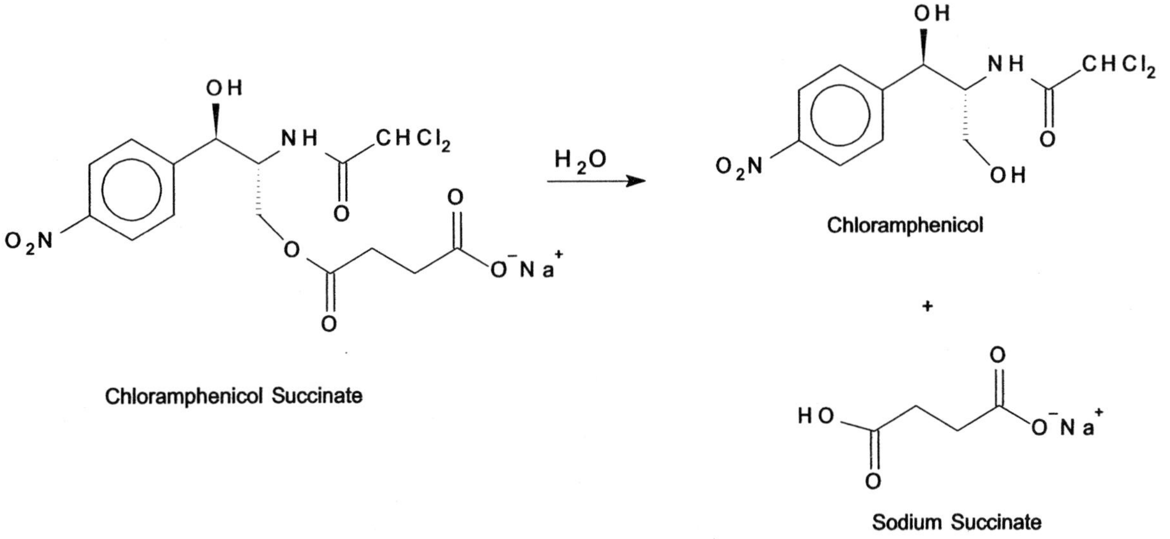

Scheme 5-1 ■ Hydrolysis of chloramphenicol succinate.

drug in the prostate, where hydrolysis occurs to give the normustard and CO_2. The normustard then acts as an alkylating agent and exerts a cytotoxic effect. The 17α-estradiol also has an antiandrogenic effect on the prostate and, thereby, slows the growth of the cancer cells. Since both the steroid and the mustard possess activity, estramustine is termed a *mutual prodrug*. Note that phosphorylation of the estradiol can be used to increase the water solubility, which also constitutes a prodrug modification. Both types of esters (carbamates and phosphates) are hydrolyzed by chemical or enzymatic means.

In contrast to carrier-linked prodrugs, bioprecursor prodrugs contain no promoiety but rather rely on metabolism to introduce the functionality necessary to create an active species. For example, the nonsteroidal anti-inflammatory drug (NSAID) sulindac is inactive as the sulfoxide and must be reduced metabolically to the active sulfide (Scheme 5-3).[8] Sulindac is administered orally, absorbed in the small intestine, and subsequently reduced to the active species. Administration of the inactive form has the benefit of reducing the gastrointestinal (GI) irritation associated with the sulfide. This example also illustrates one of the problems associated with this approach, namely, participation of alternate metabolic paths that may inactivate the compound. In this case, after absorption of sulindac, irreversible metabolic oxidation of the sulfoxide to the sulfone can also occur to give an inactive compound.

Although seen less frequently, some prodrugs rely on chemical mechanisms for conversion of the prodrug to its active form. For example, hetacillin is a prodrug form of ampicillin in which the amide nitrogen and α-amino functionalities have been allowed to react with acetone to give an imidazolidinone ring system (Scheme 5-4).[9–14] This decreases the basicity of the α-amino group and reduces pro-

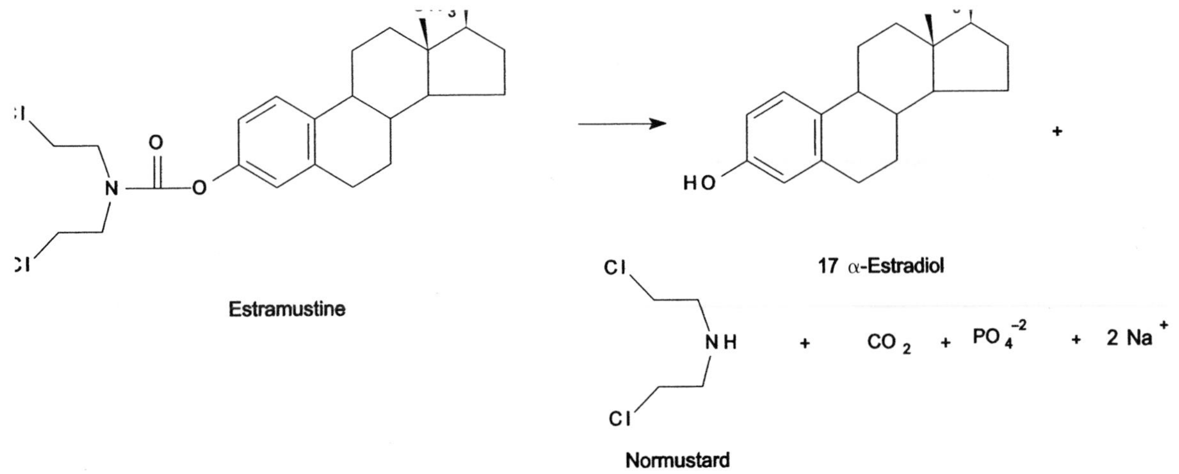

Scheme 5-2 ■ Activation of estramustine.

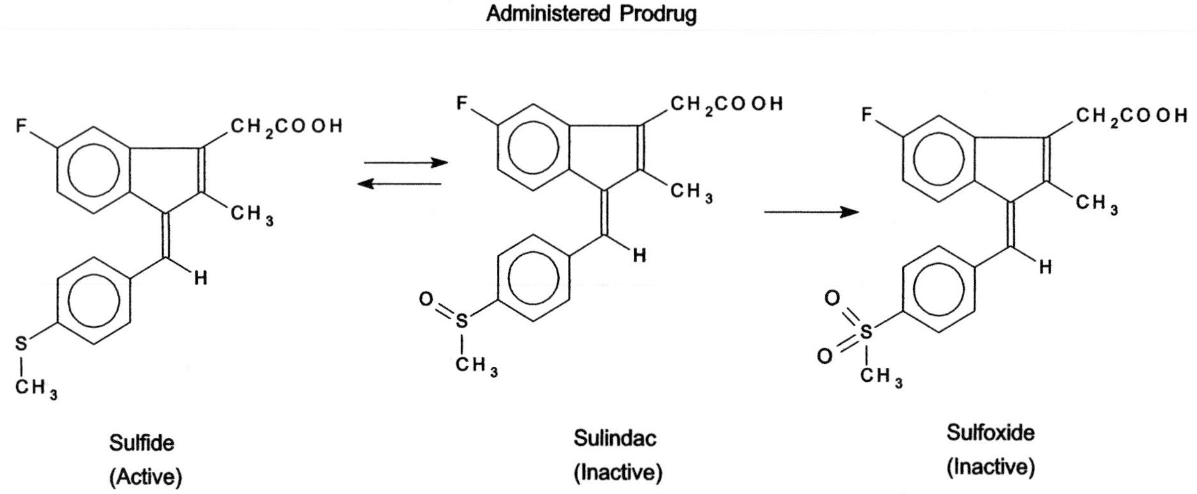

Administered Prodrug

Scheme 5-3 ▪ Metabolism of sulindac.

tonation in the small intestine so that the agent is more lipophilic. In this manner, the absorption of the drug from the small intestine is increased after oral dosing, and chemical hydrolysis after absorption regenerates ampicillin. In such an approach, the added moiety, or promoiety, in this case acetone, must be nontoxic and easily removed after it has performed its function.

PRODRUGS OF FUNCTIONAL GROUPS

As mentioned above, there are a variety of different types of prodrugs, and a comprehensive discussion of each individual agent is beyond the scope of this chapter. The major types of prodrugs (grouped according to functional group) and bioprecursor drugs (grouped according to type of metabolic activation), however, are discussed briefly below.

Carboxylic Acids and Alcohols

Prodrugs of agents that contain carboxylic acid or alcohol functionalities can often be prepared by conversion to an ester. This is the most common type of prodrug because of the ease with which the ester can be hydrolyzed to give the active drug. Hydrolysis is normally accomplished by esterase enzymes present in plasma and other tissues that are capable of hydrolyzing a wide variety of ester linkages (Scheme 5-5).[15] Included below are a number of the different types of esterases that prodrugs may use:

Ester hydrolase
Lipase
Cholesterol esterase
Acetylcholinesterase
Carboxypeptidase
Cholinesterase

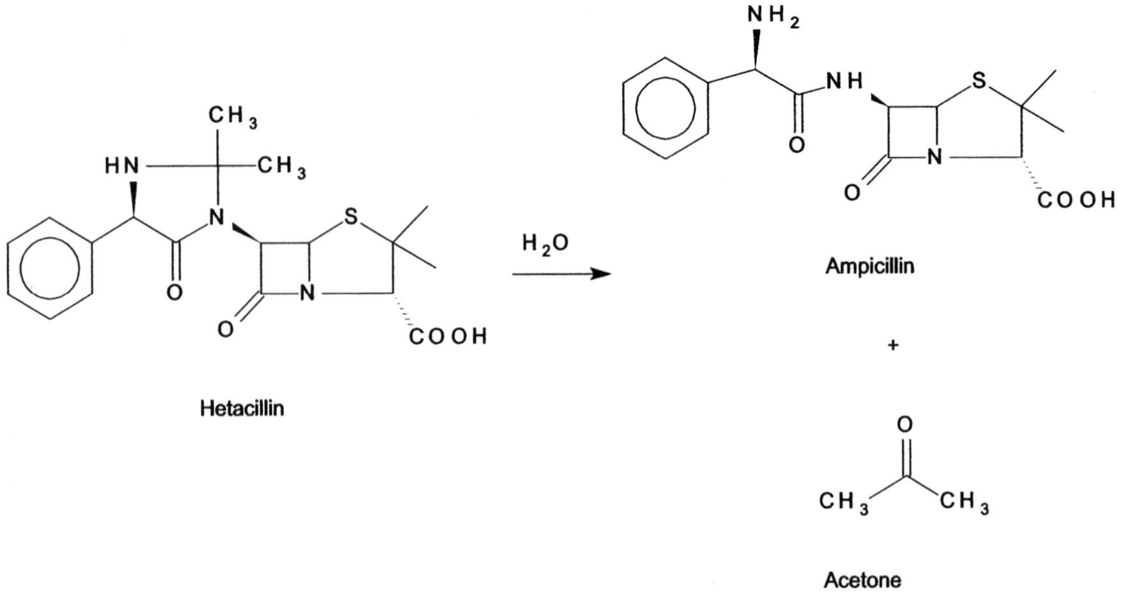

Scheme 5-4 ▪ Hydrolysis of hetacillin.

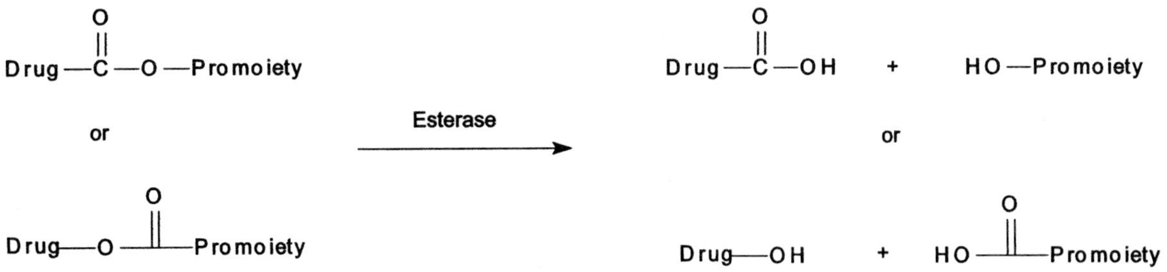

Scheme 5–5 ■ Activation of ester prodrugs.

In addition to these agents, microflora present within the gut produce a wide variety of enzymes that can hydrolyze esters. Chemical hydrolysis of the ester function may also occur to some extent. An additional factor that has contributed to the popularity of esters as prodrugs is the ease with which they can be formed. If the drug molecule contains either an alcohol or carboxylic acid functionality, an ester prodrug may be synthesized easily. The carboxylic or alcohol promoiety can be chosen to provide a wide range of lipophilic or hydrophilic properties to the drug, depending on what is desired. Manipulation of the steric and electronic properties of the promoiety allows control of the rate and extent of hydrolysis. This can be an important consideration when the active drug must be revealed at the correct point in its movement through the biological system.

When it is desired to decrease water solubility, a nonpolar alcohol or carboxylic acid is chosen as the prodrug moiety. Decreasing the hydrophilicity of the compound may yield a number of benefits, including increased absorption, decreased dissolution in the aqueous environment of the stomach, and a longer duration of action. An example of increased absorption by the addition of a nonpolar carboxylic acid is seen with dipivefrin HCl (Scheme 5-6). This is a prodrug form of epinephrine in which the catechol hydroxyl groups have been used in the formation of an ester linkage with pivalic acid.[16] The agent is used in the treatment of open-angle glaucoma. The increased lipophilicity relative to epi-nephrine allows the agent, when applied, to move across the membrane of the eye easily and achieve higher intraocular concentrations. Hydrolysis of the ester functions then occurs in the cornea, conjunctiva, and aqueous humor to generate the active form, epinephrine. Using pivalic acid as the promoiety increases the steric bulk around the scissile ester bond, which slows the ester hydrolysis relative to less bulky groups, yet still allows this reaction to proceed after the drug has crossed the membrane barriers of the eye. In addition to this benefit, the catechol system is somewhat susceptible to oxidation, and protecting the catechol as the diester prevents this oxidation and the resulting drug inactivation.

Decreasing the water solubility of a drug by the formation of a prodrug may have additional benefits beyond simply increasing absorption. A number of agents have an unpleasant taste when given orally. This results when the drug begins to dissolve in the mouth and then is capable of interacting with taste receptors. This can present a significant problem, especially in pediatric patients, and may lead to low compliance. A prodrug with reduced water solubility does not dissolve to any appreciable extent in the mouth and, therefore, does not interact with taste receptors. This approach has been used in the case of the antibacterial chloramphenicol, which produces a bitter taste when given as the parent drug (Scheme 5-7). The hydrophobic palmitate ester does not dissolve to any appreciable extent in the mouth, so there is little chance for interaction with taste receptors.[17]

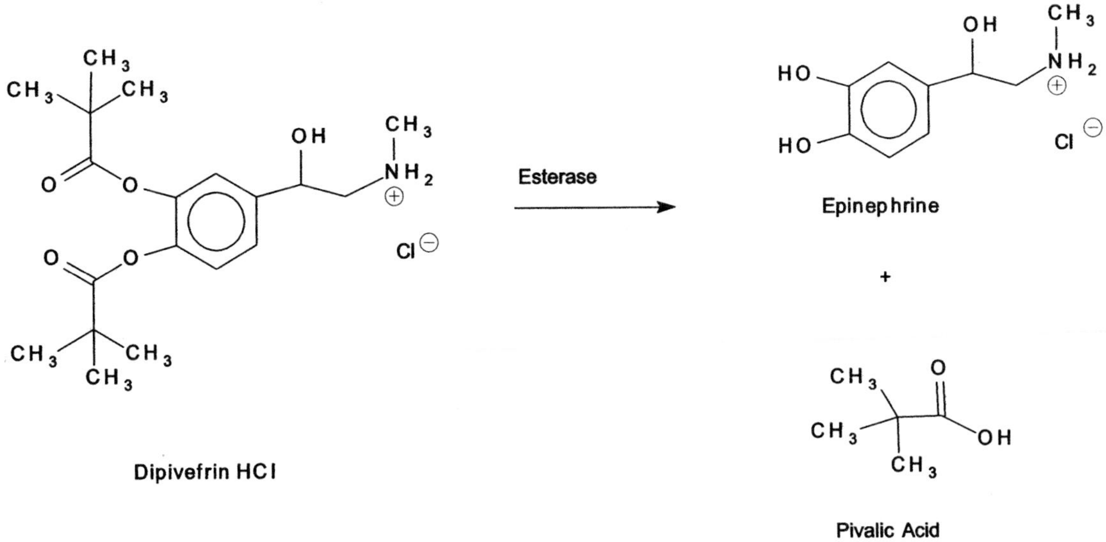

Scheme 5–6 ■ Hydrolysis of dipivefrin HCl.

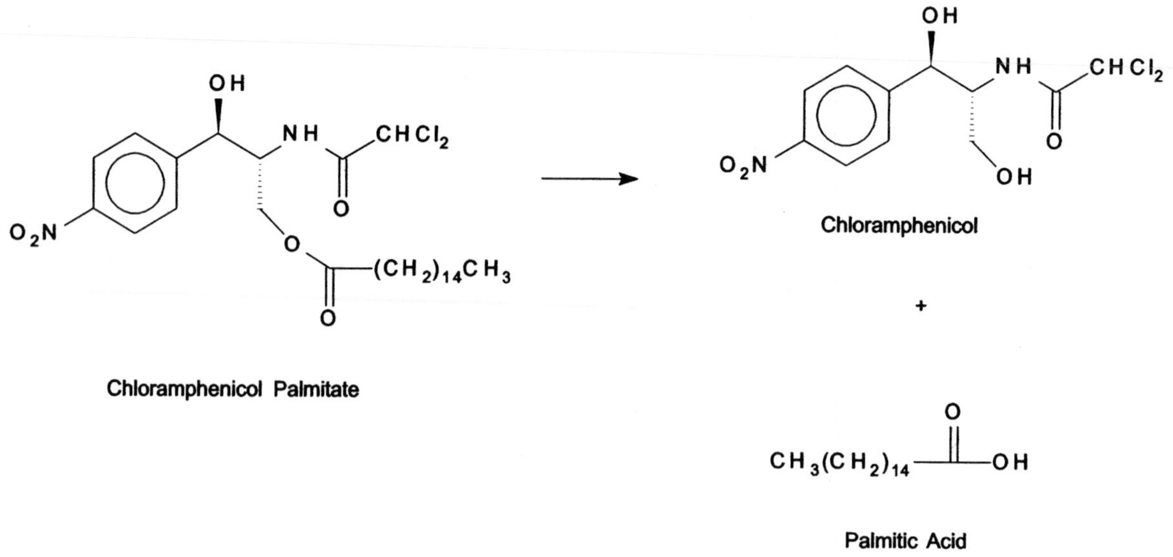

Scheme 5-7 ■ Hydrolysis of chloramphenicol palmitate.

The ester moiety is subsequently hydrolyzed in the GI tract, and the agent is absorbed as chloramphenicol.

Listed below are a number of other agents that have been converted into ester prodrugs and other types of prodrugs to overcome an unpleasant taste:

Chloramphenicol palmitate
N-Acetyl sulfisoxazole
N-Acetyl sulfamethoxypyridazine
Erythromycin estolate
Clindamycin palmitate
Troleandomycin

Not all carboxylic esters are easily hydrolyzed in vivo. Steric inhibition around the ester in some cases prevents the prodrug from being hydrolyzed. This is seen in the β-lactams, in which it is often desirable to increase the hydrophobicity of the agent to improve absorption or prevent dissolution in the stomach where acid-catalyzed decomposition may occur. Simple esters of the carboxylic acid moiety, however, are not hydrolyzed in vivo to the active carboxylate (Scheme 5-8).

A solution to this problem was to use the so-called double-ester approach, in which an additional ester or carbonate

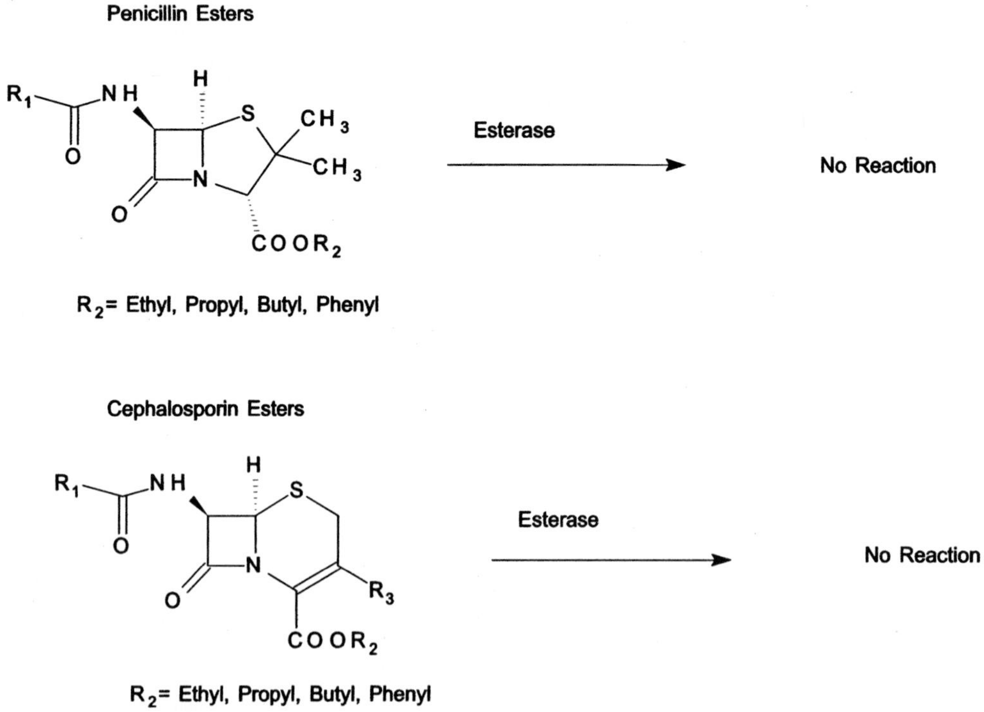

Scheme 5-8 ■ Simple esters of β-lactams with resistance to enzymatic hydrolysis.

function is incorporated into the R_2 substituent further removed from the heterocyclic nucleus.[18, 19] Hydrolysis of such a function occurred readily, and the moiety was selected so that chemical hydrolysis of the second ester occurred quickly. This is seen in the cephalosporin cefpodoxime proxetil, where a carbonate function was used (Scheme 5-9).[20] The carbonate is also susceptible to the action of esterase enzymes, and the unstable product undergoes further reaction to give the active carboxylate. This approach is frequently used to improve absorption or prevent dissolution in the stomach and the subsequent acid-catalyzed decomposition of aminopenicillins and second- and third-generation

cephalosporins (cefpodoxime proxetil has been classified as both a second- and a third-generation agent) so that these agents can be administered orally (see Scheme 5-10 for several examples).

To increase the hydrophilicity of an agent, several different types of ester prodrugs have been used, including succinates, phosphates, and sulfonates. All are ionized at physiological pH and, therefore, increase the water solubility of the agents, making them more suitable for parenteral or oral administration when high water solubility is desirable (Scheme 5-11).

Succinate esters containing an ionizable carboxylate are

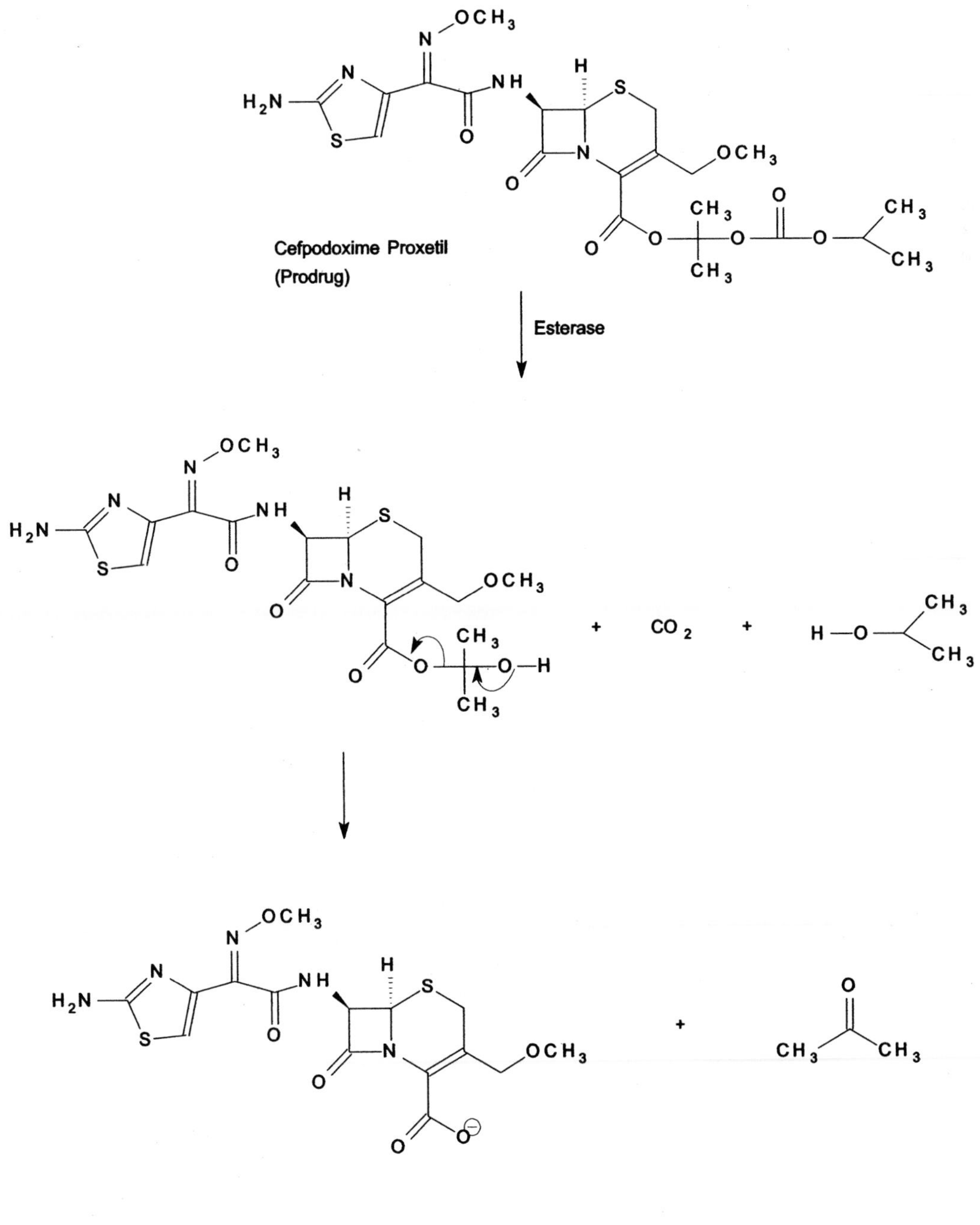

Scheme 5–9 ■ Hydrolysis mechanism of cefpodoxime proxetil.

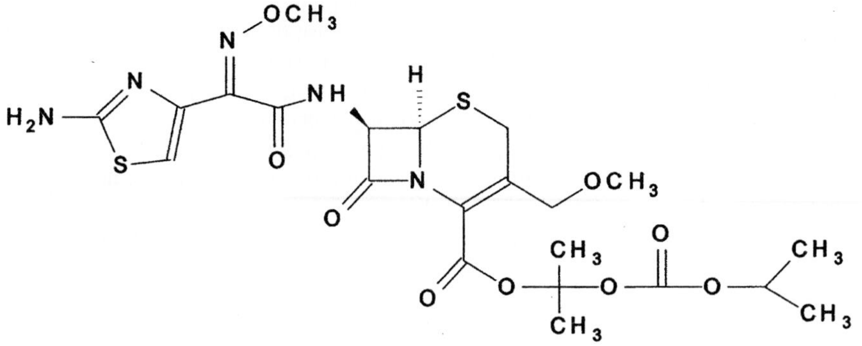

Cefpodoxime Proxetil

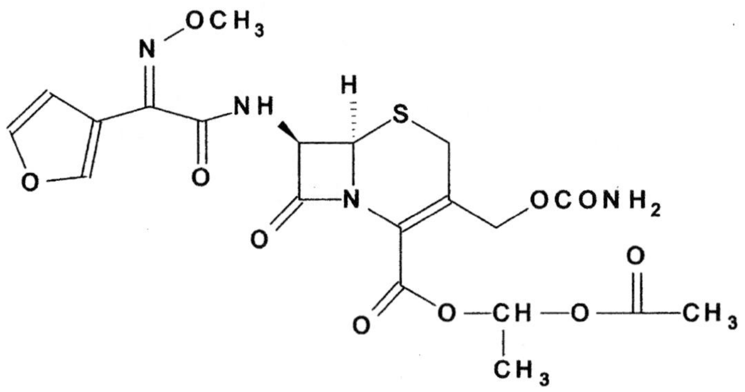

Cefuroxime Axetil

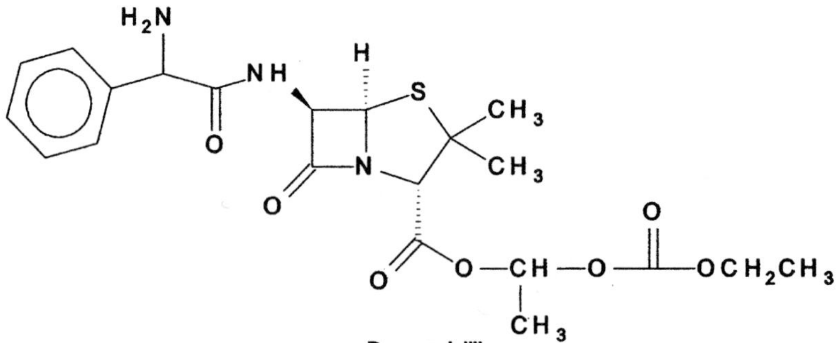

Bacampicillin

Scheme 5–10 ■ Some examples of double esters of β-lactams.

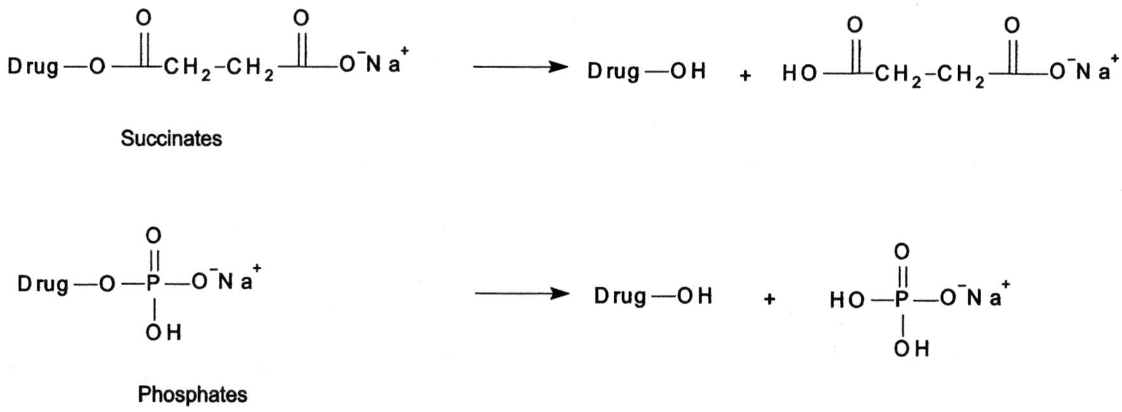

Succinates

Phosphates

Scheme 5–11 ▪ Succinate and phosphate esters.

useful when rapid in vivo hydrolysis of the ester functionality is required. The rapid hydrolysis is related to the intramolecular attack of the carboxylate on the ester linkage, which does not require the participation of enzymes (Scheme 5-12). As a result, these agents may be somewhat unstable in solution and should be dissolved immediately prior to administration.

Phosphate esters of alcohols offer another method of increasing the water solubility of an agent. The phosphates are completely ionized at physiological pH and generally hydrolyzed rapidly in vivo by phosphatase enzymes. Ionization of the phosphate function imparts high stability to these derivatives in solution, and solutions for administration can be stored for long periods of time without hydrolysis of the phosphate. Such an approach has been used to produce clindamycin phosphate, which produces less pain at the injection site than clindamycin itself (Scheme 5-13). Pain after parenteral administration is associated with local irritation caused by low aqueous solubility or highly acidic or basic solutions. With clindamycin phosphate, the reduction in pain is attributed to the increased water solubility of the agent.

Amines

Derivatization of amines to give amides has not been widely used as a prodrug strategy because of the high chemical stability of the amide linkage and the lack of amidase enzymes necessary for hydrolysis. There have been efforts at incorporating amines into peptide linkages in which the peptide serves to increase cellular uptake by use of an amino acid transporter. The amino acids are then cleaved by specific peptidase enzymes. A more common approach has been to use Mannich bases as a prodrug form of the amines. Mannich bases result from the reaction of two amines with an aldehyde or ketone. As seen with hetacillin (see Scheme 5-4), the effect of forming the Mannich base is to lower the basicity of the amine and, thereby, increase lipophilicity and absorption.

When nitrogen is present in an amide linkage, it is sometimes desirable to use the amide nitrogen as one of the amines necessary to form a Mannich base. This approach was used with the antibiotic tetracycline—the amide nitrogen was allowed to react with formaldehyde and pyrrolidine to give the Mannich base rolitetracycline (Scheme 5-14).[21] In this case, addition of the basic pyrrolidine nitrogen introduces an additional ionizable functionality and increases the water solubility of the parent drug. The Mannich base hydrolyzes completely and rapidly in aqueous media to give the active tetracycline.

Azo Linkage

Amines have occasionally been incorporated into an azo linkage to produce a prodrug. In fact, it was an azo dye, prontosil, that led to the discovery of the sulfonamides as the first antibacterials to be used to treat systemic infections.[22] Although prontosil itself was inactive in vitro, it was active

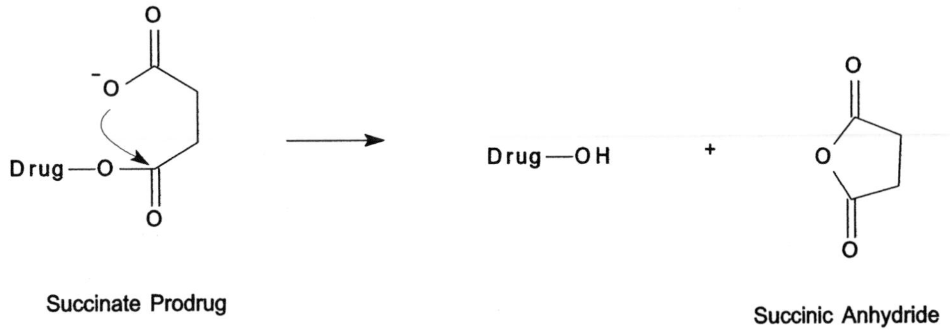

Succinate Prodrug

Succinic Anhydride

Scheme 5–12 ▪ Intramolecular cleavage of succinate esters.

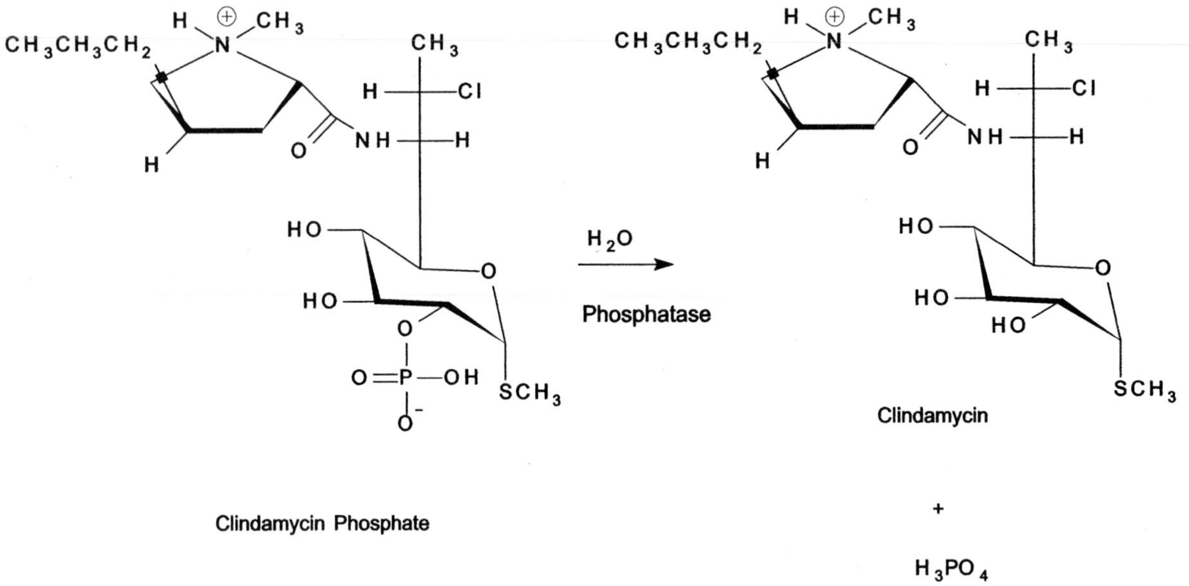

Scheme 5–13 ■ Clindamycin activation by phosphate hydrolysis.

in vivo and was converted by azo reductase enzymes in the gut to sulfanilamide, the active species (Scheme 5-15).

Although prontosil is no longer used as an antibacterial, this type of linkage appears in sulfasalazine, which is used in the treatment of ulcerative colitis. The azo linkage is broken in the gut by the action of azo reductases produced by microflora. This releases the active agent, aminosalicylic acid, which has an anti-inflammatory effect on the colon, and sulfapyridine (Scheme 5-16). The advantage of this prodrug approach is that the combination of cleavage of the azo link-

age and generation of aminosalicylic acid prior to absorption prevents the systemic absorption of the agent and helps concentrate the active agent at the site of action.

Carbonyl Compounds

A number of different functionalities have been evaluated as prodrug derivatives of carbonyls (e.g., aldehydes and ketones), although this approach has not found wide clinical use. These have generally involved derivatives in which the

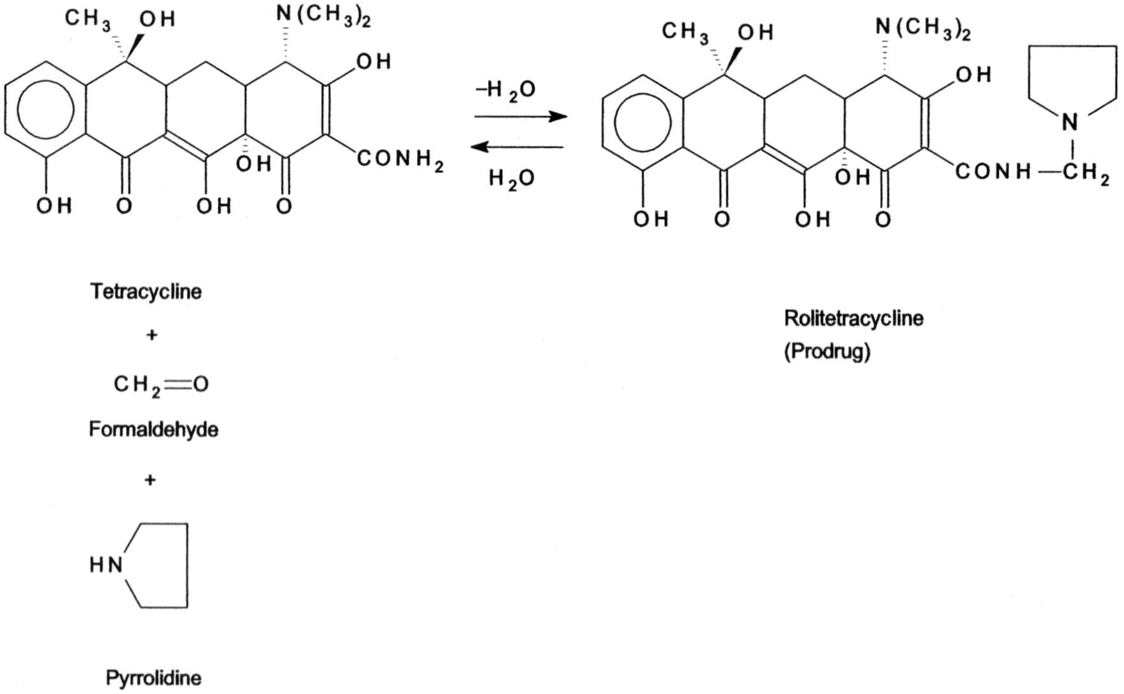

Scheme 5–14 ■ Rolitetracycline synthesis and activation.

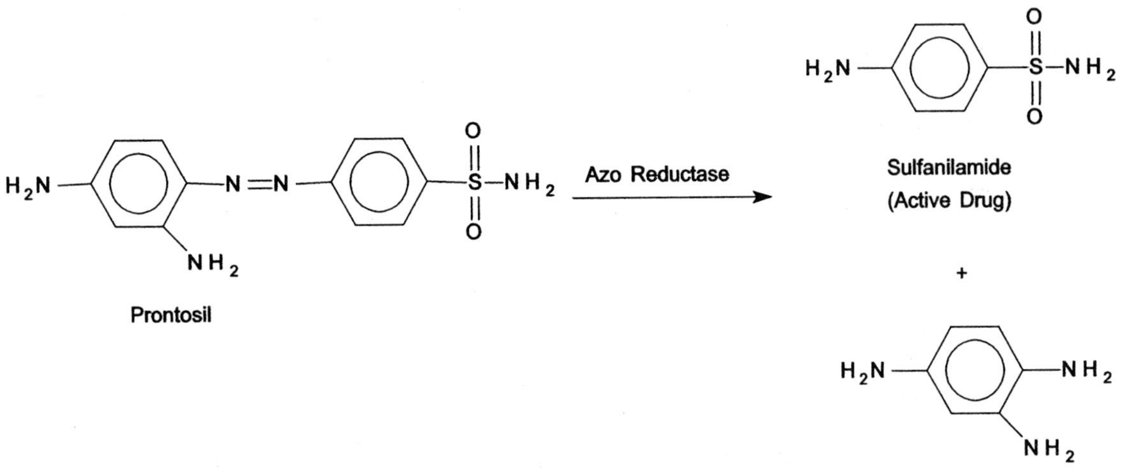

Scheme 5–15 ■ Azo cleavage of prontosil.

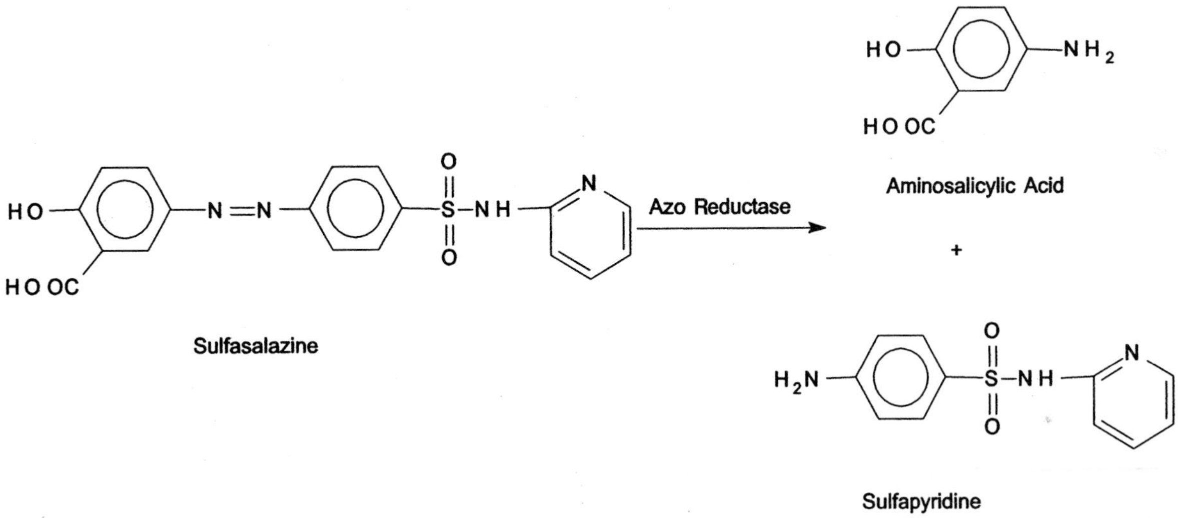

Scheme 5–16 ■ Action of azo reductase on sulfasalazine.

sp² hybridized carbonyl carbon is converted to an sp³ hybridized carbon attached to two heteroatoms, such as oxygen, nitrogen, or sulfur. Under hydrolysis conditions, these functionalities are reconverted to the carbonyl compounds. An example of this approach is methenamine, shown below (Scheme 5-17).[23] Methenamine releases formaldehyde in the urine, which acts as an antibacterial agent by reacting with nucleophiles present in bacteria. The agent is administered in enteric-coated capsules to protect it from premature hydrolysis in the acidic environment of the stomach. After dissolution of the enteric-coated capsules in the intestine, the agent is absorbed and moves into the bloodstream, eventually ending up in the urine, where the acidic pH catalyzes the chemical hydrolysis to give formaldehyde. Use of this

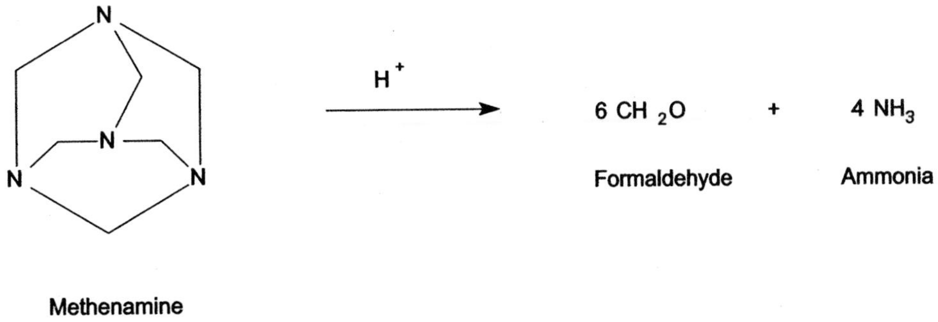

Scheme 5–17 ■ Methenamine hydrolysis.

prodrug approach prevents the systemic release of formaldehyde and reduces toxicity.

Other prodrug approaches have involved the use of oximes, imines, and enol esters, although these types of compounds have not been used clinically. A number of agents contain imine and oxime linkages, such as many of the third-generation cephalosporins (e.g., cefotaxime, ceftizoxime), but these are not prodrugs.

BIOPRECURSOR PRODRUGS

As indicated above, bioprecursor prodrugs do not contain a carrier or promoiety but rather contain a latent functionality that is metabolically or chemically transformed to the active drug molecule. The types of activation often involve oxidative activation, reductive activation, phosphorylation, and in some cases chemical activation. Of these, oxidation is commonly seen, since a number of endogenous enzymes can carry out these transformations. Phosphorylation has been widely exploited in the development of antiviral agents, and many currently available agents depend on this type of activation.

The abundance of oxidizing enzymes in the body has made this type of bioactivation a popular route. Isozymes of cytochrome P-450 can oxidize a wide variety of functionalities, generally to produce more polar compounds that can be excreted directly or undergo phase 2 conjugation reactions and subsequently undergo elimination. This occurs in a fairly predictable manner and, therefore, has been successfully exploited in prodrug approaches.

A good example of a prodrug that requires oxidative activation is the NSAID nabumetone (Relafen) (Scheme 5-18).[24] NSAIDs produce stomach irritation, which in patients with preexisting conditions or patients taking large amounts of NSAIDs for extended periods may be severe. This irritation is associated in part with the presence of an acidic functionality in these agents. The carboxylic acid functionality commonly found in these agents is un-ionized in the highly acidic environment of the stomach. As a result, these agents are more lipophilic in nature and may pass into the cells of the gastric mucosa. The intracellular pH of these cells is more basic than that of the stomach lumen, and the NSAID becomes ionized. This results in backflow of H^+ from the lumen into these cells, with concomitant cellular damage. This type of damage could be prevented if the carboxylic acid function could be eliminated from these agents; this functional group is required for activity, however.

Nabumetone contains no acidic functionality and passes through the stomach without producing the irritation normally associated with this class of agents. Subsequent absorption occurs in the intestine, and metabolism in the liver produces the active compound as shown in Scheme 5-18. This approach, however, did not completely eliminate the gastric irritation associated with nabumetone, since it is due only in part to a direct effect on the stomach. Inhibition of the target enzyme, cyclooxygenase, while having an anti-inflammatory effect, also results in the increased release of gastric acid, which irritates the stomach. So, while nabumetone induces less gastric irritation than other NSAIDs, this undesirable effect was not completely eliminated by a prodrug approach. Such an effect was also seen above with the NSAID sulindac (see Scheme 5-3), whose GI irritation was reduced but not completely eliminated.

Reductive activation is occasionally seen as a method of prodrug activation but, because there are fewer reducing enzymes, is generally less common than oxidative activation. One of the best known examples of reductive activation is for the antineoplastic agent mitomycin C, which is used in the treatment of bladder and lung cancer (Scheme 5-19).[25–28] Mitomycin C contains a quinone functionality that undergoes reduction to give a hydroquinone. This is important because of the differential effect of the quinone and hydroquinone on the electron pair of the nitrogen. Whereas the quinone has an electron-withdrawing effect on this electron pair, the hydroquinone has an electron-releasing effect, which allows these electrons to participate in the expulsion of methoxide and the subsequent loss of the carbamate to generate a reactive species that can alkylate DNA.

The cascade of events that leads to an alkylating active drug species is initiated by the reduction of the quinone functionality in mitomycin C. The selectivity of mitomycin for hypoxic cells is minimal, however. The selectivity is determined in part by the reduction potential of the quinone, which can be influenced by the substituents attached to the ring. In an effort to modify the reduction potential of mitomycin C, various analogues have been prepared and tested for antineoplastic activity. It was hoped that the reduction potential could be altered so that the analogues would only be activated in hypoxic conditions, such as those found in slow-growing solid tumors that are poorly vascularized. In these tissues with a low oxygen content it was thought that reductive metabolism might be more prevalent than in nor-

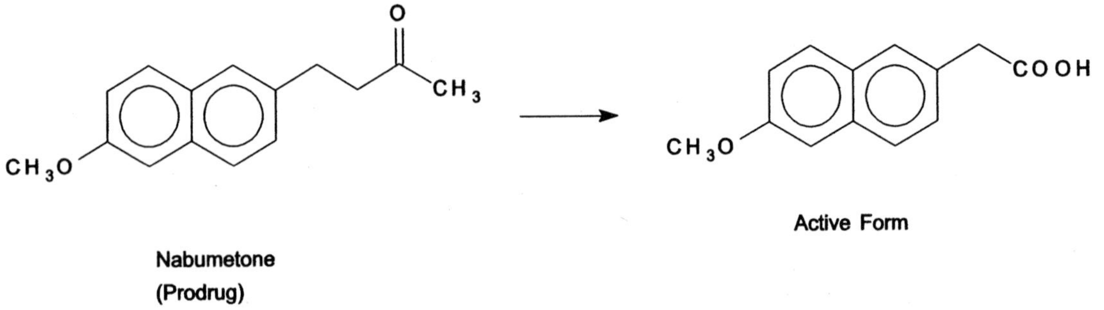

Nabumetone

(Prodrug)

Active Form

Scheme 5–18 ■ Oxidative activation of nabumetone.

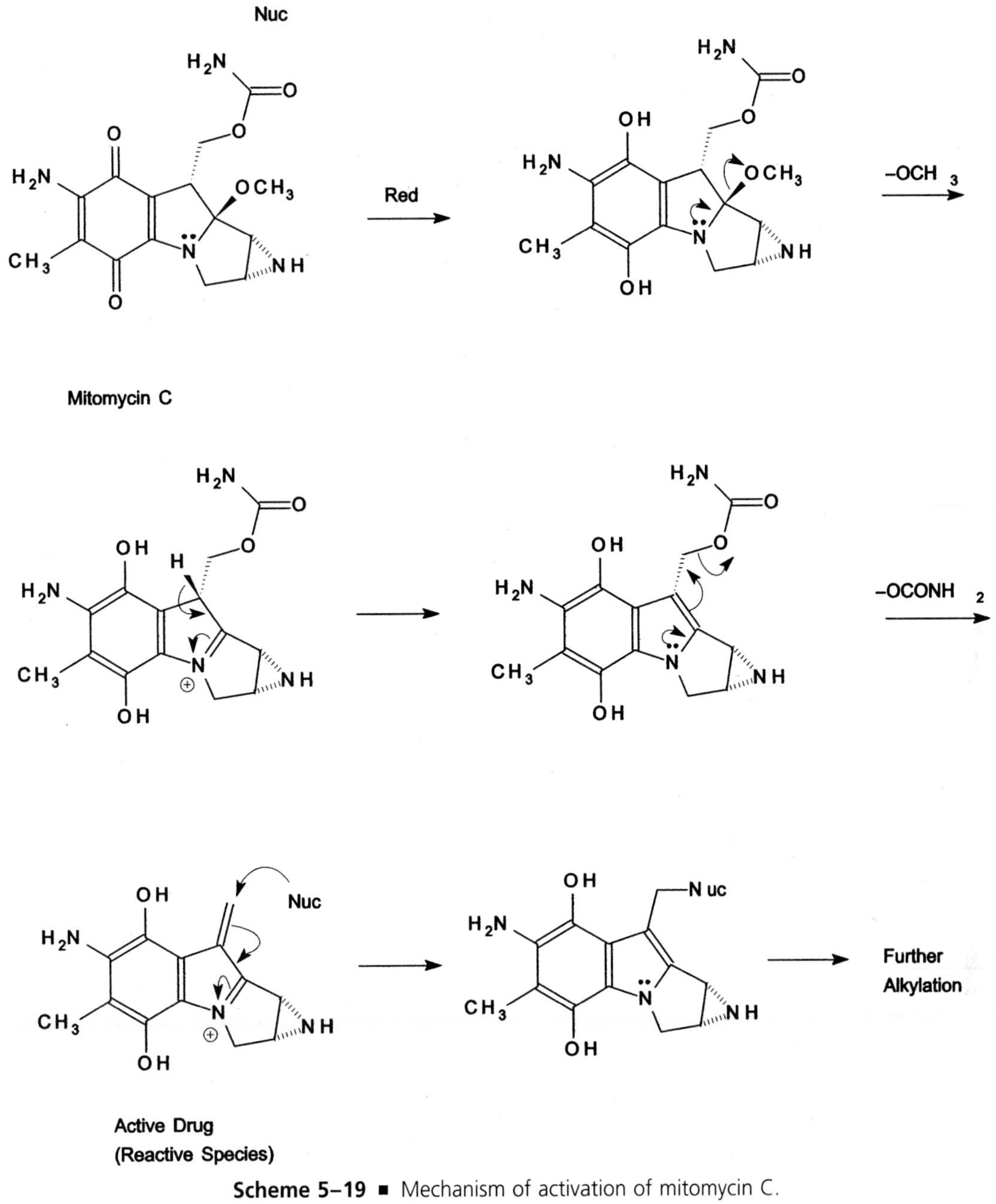

Scheme 5-19 ■ Mechanism of activation of mitomycin C.

mal tissues, so the agents would be selectively activated and, therefore, selectively toxic.

Although mitomycin was the first agent used clinically to be recognized as requiring reductive activation, it is only modestly selective for hypoxic cells. A much more selective agent, tirapazamine, is currently undergoing phase III clinical trials.[29] Tirapazamine is reported to be 100 to 200 times more selective for hypoxic cells than for normal cells. The mechanism of activation involves a one-electron reduction that is catalyzed by a number of enzymes, including cytochrome P-450 and cytochrome P-450 reductase to give a radical species (Scheme 5-20). This species, which is shown as a carbon-centered radical, can initiate breaks in the DNA chain under hypoxic conditions. Under aerobic conditions, hydroxide radical is formed, which can initiate chain breaks.

Phosphorylation is a common metabolic function of the body, which is used to produce high-energy phosphodiester bonds such as those present in ATP and GTP. The body then typically uses these molecules to phosphorylate other molecules and, in the process of doing so, activates these molecules. The type of activation achieved depends on the molecule phosphorylated, but in many cases, phosphorylation introduces a leaving group, which can be displaced by an incoming nucleophile. This is seen, for example, in the synthesis of DNA and RNA, in which nucleotides are added to the 3′ end of a growing chain of DNA or RNA (Scheme 5-21).

Phosphorylation is commonly required for the bioactivation of antiviral agents. These agents are commonly nucleosides, which must be converted to the nucleotides to have

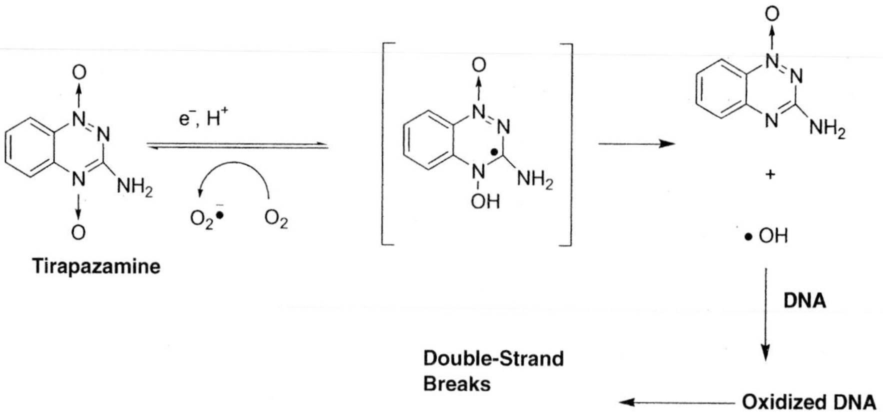

Scheme 5–20 ■ Reductive activation of tirapazamine.

activity. Most often, antiviral agents disrupt the synthesis or function of DNA or RNA, which is generally accomplished by conversion to the triphosphate. Since normal cells are also involved in the synthesis of DNA and RNA, compounds have been sought that would be converted to the triphosphates, the active form, in greater amounts in infected cells than in normal cells. Therefore, nucleosides that have higher affinity for the viral kinase enzymes than the mammalian kinases are desirable and have greater selective toxicity.

This can be seen in the prodrug idoxuridine, which was the first agent to show clinical effectiveness against viruses (Scheme 5-22).[30] The nucleoside enters the cell, where it is phosphorylated. In virally infected cells, this phosphorylation is accomplished preferentially by viral thymidine ki-

nase, because the idoxuridine is a better substrate for the viral enzyme than for the corresponding mammalian enzyme. Therefore, the drug is activated to a greater extent in the virally infected cells and achieves some selective toxicity, although this selectivity is rather low, and there is significant toxicity to normal cells. Once the drug has been phosphorylated to the triphosphate stage, it can inhibit DNA synthesis in a number of ways, including inhibition of viral DNA polymerase and incorporation into DNA, which results in incorrect base pairing that disrupts the ability of DNA to function as a template for DNA and RNA synthesis.

In addition to the selective toxicity mentioned, the prodrug approach offers the additional advantage of increased cell penetration. The prodrug can easily enter the cell via active

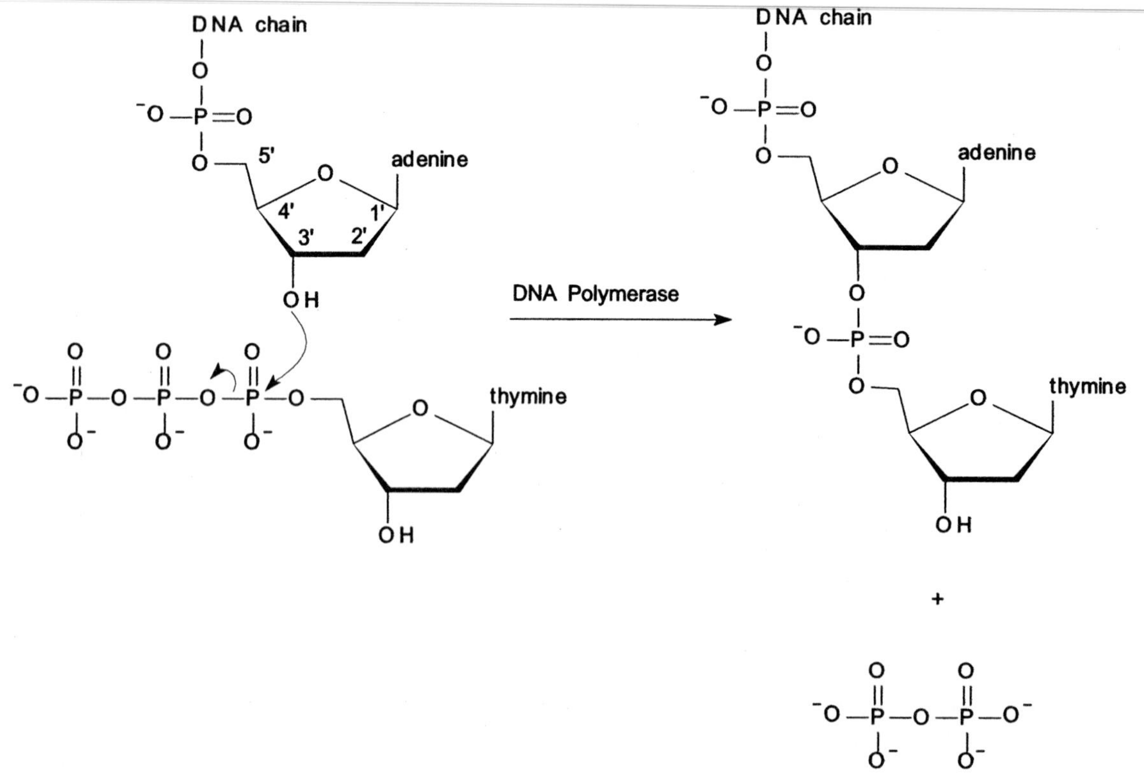

Scheme 5–21 ■ DNA synthesis.

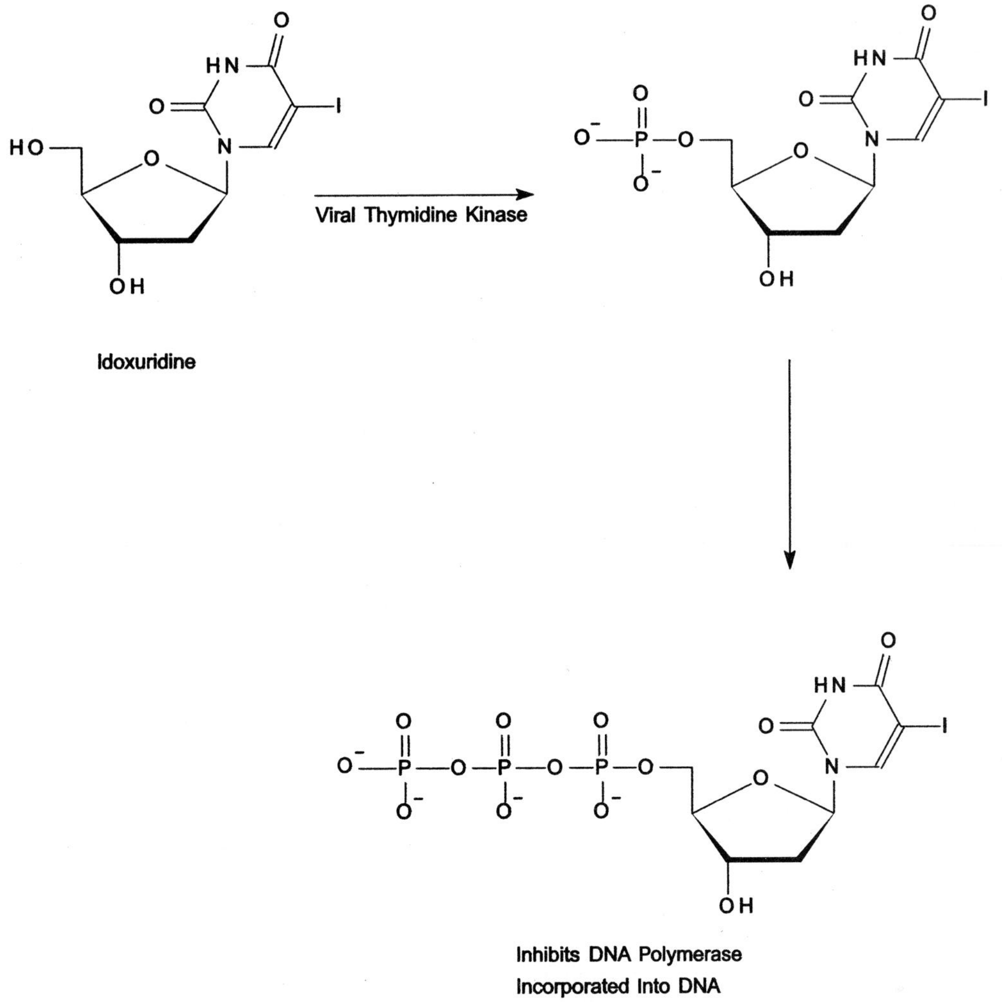

Scheme 5–22 ■ Idoxuridine activation.

transport mechanisms, whereas the active nucleotides are unable to use this process and are too polar to cross the membrane via passive diffusion.

A good example of chemical activation is seen with the proton pump inhibitors such as omeprazole. In this case, chemical activation is provided by the highly acidic environment in and around the parietal cell of the stomach (Scheme 5-23). This allows protonation of nitrogen on the benzimidazole ring followed by attachment of the pyridine nitrogen. Ring opening then gives the sulfenic acid that subsequently cyclizes with the loss of water. Attachment by a sulfhydryl group present on the proton pump of the parietal cell then occurs and inactivates this enzyme, preventing further release of H^+ into the GI tract, which is useful in treating gastric ulceration.

CHEMICAL DELIVERY SYSTEMS

The knowledge gained from drug metabolism and prodrug studies may be used to target a drug to its site of action. Site-specific chemical delivery systems take advantage of

higher levels of activity in a metabolic or chemical pathway at the target site. A prodrug form of the active drug is designed to serve as a substrate in that specific pathway, thus yielding a high concentration of active drug at the target site. Site-specific chemical delivery requires that the prodrug reaches the target site and that the enzymatic or chemical process exists at the target site for conversion of the prodrug to the active drug. Many factors are involved in the relative success of site-specific drug delivery, including extent of target organ perfusion, rate of conversion of prodrug to active drug in both target and nontarget sites, and input/output rates of prodrug and drug from the target sites.

Site-specific chemical delivery systems represent but one approach to the selective delivery of drug molecules to their site of action for increased therapeutic effectiveness and limited side effects. Other than chemical drug delivery, many carrier systems have been evaluated for drug delivery, including proteins, polysaccharides, liposomes, emulsions, cellular carriers (erythrocytes and leukocytes), magnetic control targeting, and implanted mechanical pumps.[31] As the fate of drugs in the human body has become more clearly understood, research activity to improve the delivery of active drug to the target site has increased. The basic goal

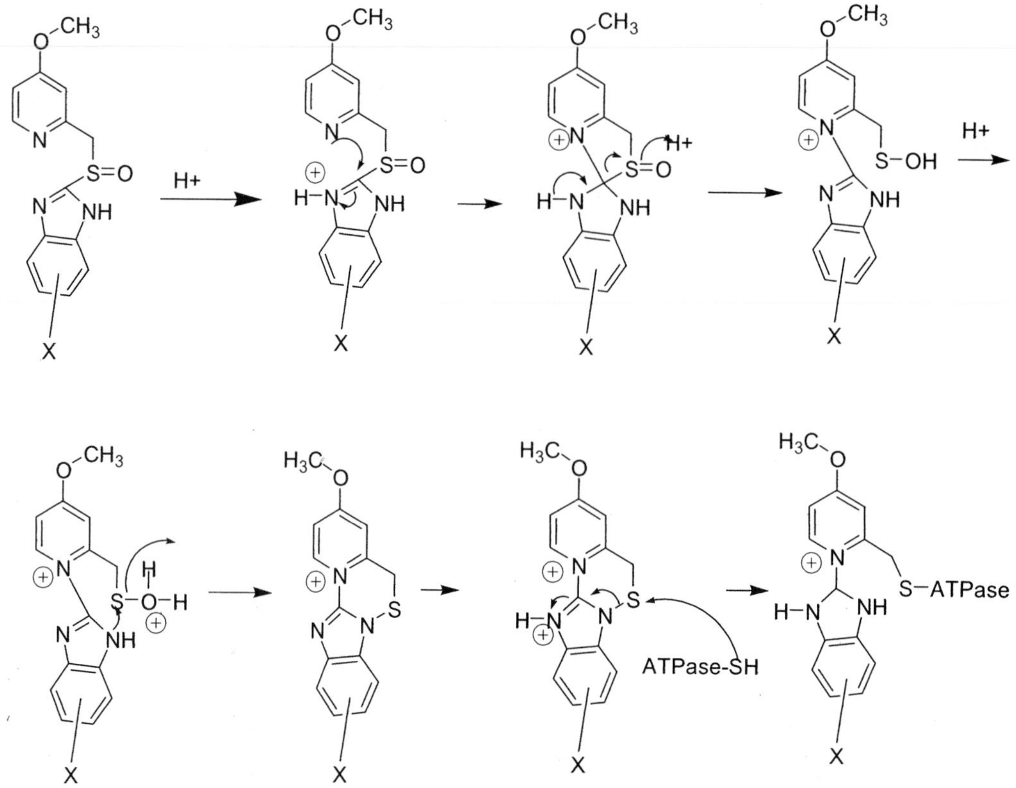

Scheme 5–23 ■ Mechanism of activation of proton pump inhibitors.

of these efforts is to protect the drug from the nonspecific biological environment and to protect the nonspecific bio-environment from the drug to achieve some site-specific drug delivery. Site-specific drug delivery has been evaluated extensively for drugs with narrow therapeutic windows, such as many of the anticancer drugs.

The site-specific delivery of the active drug via its prodrug counterpart requires that the prodrug be readily transported to the site of action and rapidly absorbed at the site. On arrival at the target site, the prodrug should be selectively converted to drug relative to its rate of conversion at nontarget sites. Since high metabolic activity occurs in highly perfused tissues such as liver and kidney, delivery to these organs has a natural advantage. Unfortunately, prodrug delivery of active drug to other organs or tissues is disadvantaged for the same reasons.

Furthermore, it is highly desirable to have the active drug, once formed, migrate from the target site at a slow rate. On the basis of all these requirements, clearly site-specific delivery of drug to the target by a prodrug chemical delivery system is a far more complex undertaking than designing a prodrug to improve one aspect of its overall properties. Yet there are several excellent examples of site-specific chemical delivery systems in use in modern drug therapy. The target sites include cancer cells, GI tract, kidney and urinary tract, bacterial cells, viral material, ocular tissue, and the blood–brain barrier.

The prodrug methenamine, described above in this chapter (Scheme 5-17), can be considered a site-specific chemical delivery system for the urinary tract antiseptic agent formaldehyde.[31] The low pH of the urine promotes the hydrolysis

of methenamine to formaldehyde, the active antibacterial agent. The rate of hydrolysis increases with increased acidity (decreased pH), and this can be promoted by administration of urinary pH-lowering agents or by diet. The pH of the plasma is buffered to about 7.4, and the rate of hydrolysis is low, preventing systemic toxicity from formaldehyde. As mentioned above, this compound is administered in enteric-coated tablets that prevent dissolution and, therefore, premature hydrolysis in the highly acidic environment of the stomach.

A number of prodrugs for cancer chemotherapy have been designed for selective delivery of active drug to tumor tissue, based on higher levels of activating enzyme in the tumor cell than in normal tissue.[32] Many enzymatic systems show higher activity in tumor cells than in normal tissue because of the higher growth rates associated with tumor tissue. Peptidases and proteolytic enzymes are among those systems showing higher activity in and near tumor cells. Thus, one means of attempting to produce higher rates of drug incorporation into tumors than in surrounding normal tissue involves deriving a drug molecule with an amino acid or peptide fragment.

Capecitabine is an example of a prodrug chemical delivery system that requires a series of enzymatic steps for conversion to the active antitumor drug species, 5-fluorouracil (Scheme 5-24).[33] Tumors located in tissues with high levels of the required enzymes should respond best to treatment with capecitabine. Esterase activity occurs primarily in the liver, allowing the intact ester capecitabine to be the absorbed species following oral administration. The ester hydrolysis product itself shows some specific toxicity toward

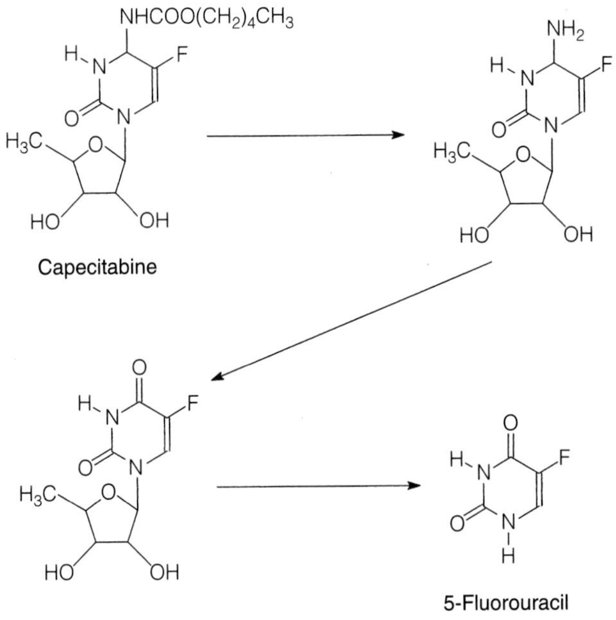

Scheme 5–24 ▪ Metabolic conversion of capecitabine.

GI tract tissue, which prevents this molecule from serving as an effective prodrug delivery form of 5-fluorouracil. The other two enzymes involved in the formation of 5-fluorouracil occur in high concentrations in target tissues such as cervix, breast, kidney, and colon.

There is considerable current interest in the general concept of tumor-activated prodrugs, and a number of strategies have been proposed for drug targeting in tumor cells.[34] One of the more interesting approaches is linking an exogenous (nonhuman) enzyme to a tumor-specific antibody. Based on an immunological response, the antibody would carry the exogenous enzyme to the tumor surface, where it would be available for prodrug activation. Prodrugs activated by this exogenous enzyme would be converted to the active species only at the tumor site. Since the activating exogenous enzyme is not normally found in human tissue, maximum accuracy in drug targeting should be achieved in this antibody-directed enzyme prodrug therapy.

The antiviral drugs, such as idoxuridine (Scheme 5-22), are an interesting example of site-specific chemical delivery.[26] These drugs serve as substrates for phosphorylating enzymes found in viruses, and the phosphorylated species is the active antiviral agent. The active phosphorylated species is incorporated into viral DNA, disrupting viral replication and, thus, producing the antiviral effect. These drugs do not undergo phosphorylation by mammalian cells, so the prodrug is specific for those sites where it serves as a substrate for phosphorylation enzymes. One of the requirements for site-specific chemical delivery discussed above was the proper input/output ratios for prodrug and active drug species at the target. The relative physicochemical properties of prodrug and its phosphorylated derivative suggest an appropriate input/output ratio for site specificity. The prodrug can readily penetrate the virus, and the increased polarity of the phosphorylated derivative would serve to retain that active species inside the virus. The combination of increased polarity and viral retention of the active phosphorylated species likely reduces any human toxicity that might be associated with this active species.

The amino acid drug L-dopa can be considered a site-specific chemical delivery system that delivers the drug dopamine to the brain. The brain has an active transport system that operates to incorporate L amino acids into the central nervous system (CNS), and L-dopa is transported into the brain in this manner. Once across the blood–brain barrier, L-dopa undergoes decarboxylation, as shown in Scheme 5-25, to yield the active metabolite, dopamine. Direct systemic administration of dopamine does not produce significant levels of the drug in the brain because of its high polarity and poor membrane permeability as well as its facile metabolic degradation by oxidative deamination. Dopamine formed on the inside of the blood–brain barrier is held there, however, because of the poor membrane permeability of this drug. Although some specificity for brain tissue is achieved by this delivery method, peripheral side effects of L-dopa are the direct result of decarboxylation to dopamine in other organ systems. In this case, the enzyme activating system is not localized at the target site, and its presence in other tissues and organs leads to undesirable side effects.

Another example of the chemical delivery of a drug to the brain and CNS is the prodrug form of 2-PAM (pro-2-PAM), an important antidote for the phosphate and carbamate acetylcholinesterase inhibitors used in insecticides and nerve gases.[35] The polar properties of 2-PAM, a permanent cationic species, prevent this drug from being absorbed following oral administration and restrict the drug from access to the brain, even after IV administration. Pro-2-PAM is a dihydropyridine derivative that undergoes metabolic and chemical oxidation to yield the active drug 2-PAM (Scheme 5-26). The nonionic pro-2-PAM can easily cross the blood–brain barrier, and oxidation to 2-PAM within the brain essentially traps the active cationic drug species inside the brain. Oxidation of the dihydropyridine ring of pro-2-PAM occurs throughout the mammalian system, not just in the brain, and the levels of the resulting 2-PAM are approximately the same in peripheral tissue as in the brain. IV ad-

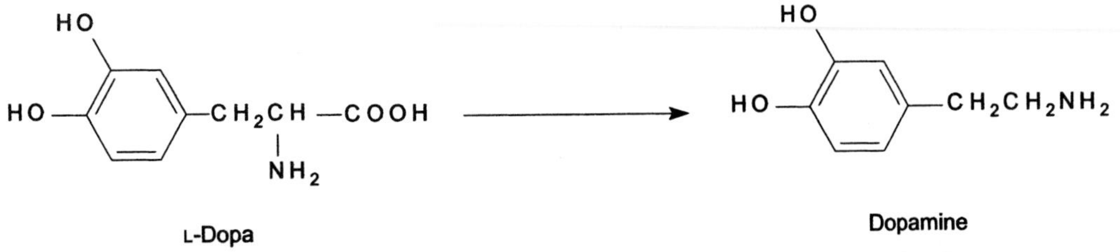

Scheme 5–25 ▪ Decarboxylation of L-dopa in the CNS to yield the active drug dopamine.

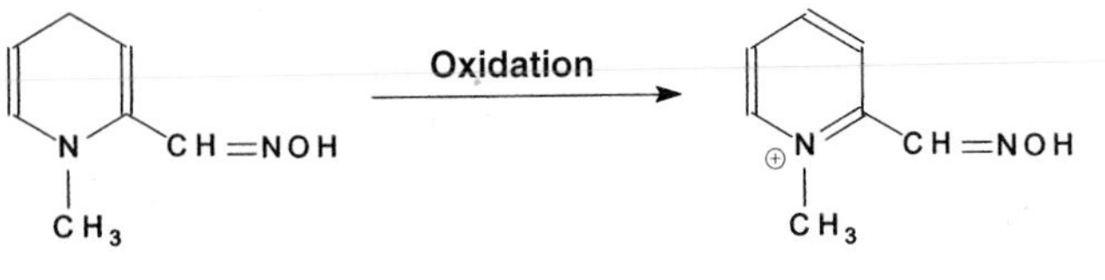

Scheme 5–26 ■ Oxidation of pro-2-PAM.

ministration of pro-2-PAM, however, yields brain levels of 2-PAM that are approximately 10 times higher than those achieved by IV administration of the parent drug.

The delivery of drugs across the blood–brain barrier has been a significant issue in the design of many therapeutic compounds. Only very lipophilic drugs can cross into the brain without the aid of some active uptake process, such as the one that operates to incorporate essential amino acids into the CNS. The facile oxidation of the dihydropyridine ring system has been extensively investigated as a general process for chemical delivery of a number of drugs to the CNS. The approach has been described as a chemical delivery system, not just a prodrug designed to penetrate the blood–brain barrier.[36] This process is a multistep procedure involving delivery of the drug–dihydropyridine derivative to the brain via facile diffusion across the blood–brain barrier, followed by oxidation to the quaternary pyridine cation, which is trapped in the brain. The drug is then released from the pyridine cation by a second metabolic/chemical event. A number of functional groups can be added to the dihydropyridine to facilitate the derivatization of various functional groups found in CNS drugs. Since many CNS drugs are amines, amides of dihydropyridine carboxylic acids are often prepared and used to deliver the drugs across the blood–brain barrier into the brain. Additionally, these amide derivatives often serve to protect the amines from metabolic degradation before they reach the target site. Primary amines such as dopamine and norepinephrine and many others are readily metabolized and degraded by oxidative deamination before reaching the CNS. The dihydropyridine derivative of a dopamine ester, shown in Scheme 5-27, has access to the

CNS via passive absorption of the tertiary amine, which on oxidation restricts the resulting pyridinium amide to the brain. Amide hydrolysis then delivers the active form of the drug at or near its site of action. The amide hydrolysis step may be slower than the dihydropyridine oxidation step, and thus a reservoir of pyridinium amide precursor may be available for conversion to the active drug species.

The use of prodrug concepts has been very successful in the delivery of active drug species to the human eye following local application. Lipophilic esters of epinephrine, such as the dipivaloyl ester described above (see Scheme 5-6), show better corneal penetration following direct application to the eye than the more polar parent drug epinephrine.[35] The esterases necessary for the hydrolysis of the prodrug are readily available in the eye and skin. The more polar drug species, epinephrine, is then localized within the lipophilic membrane barriers of the eye, and the drug remains available at the target site to produce its antiglaucoma effects. The local application of the prodrug species to the skin or eye allows metabolic processes to activate the drug without concern for competitive reactions at other tissues or sites of loss.

The delivery of drugs to the colon and lower GI tract has taken advantage of the unique enzymatic processes found in colon bacteria. The glucosidase activity of these bacteria allows hydrolysis of glucoside derivatives of drugs in the colon and provides higher concentrations of active drug.[32] A number of steroid drugs (Scheme 5-28) demonstrate increased effectiveness in the lower GI tract following administration as their glucoside derivatives. The polar glucoside derivatives of the steroids are not well absorbed into the bloodstream from the GI tract and remain available to serve as substrates for the bacteria that are found primarily in the human colon.

The prodrug approach for the delivery of anticancer drugs to the site of action has been used in a number of cases in an effort to increase effectiveness and lower side effects. Several enzyme systems that show higher activity in and near the cancer cells have been evaluated for their ability to activate the prodrug species. In most cases, the enzyme activity level is simply higher near the faster growing cancer cells,

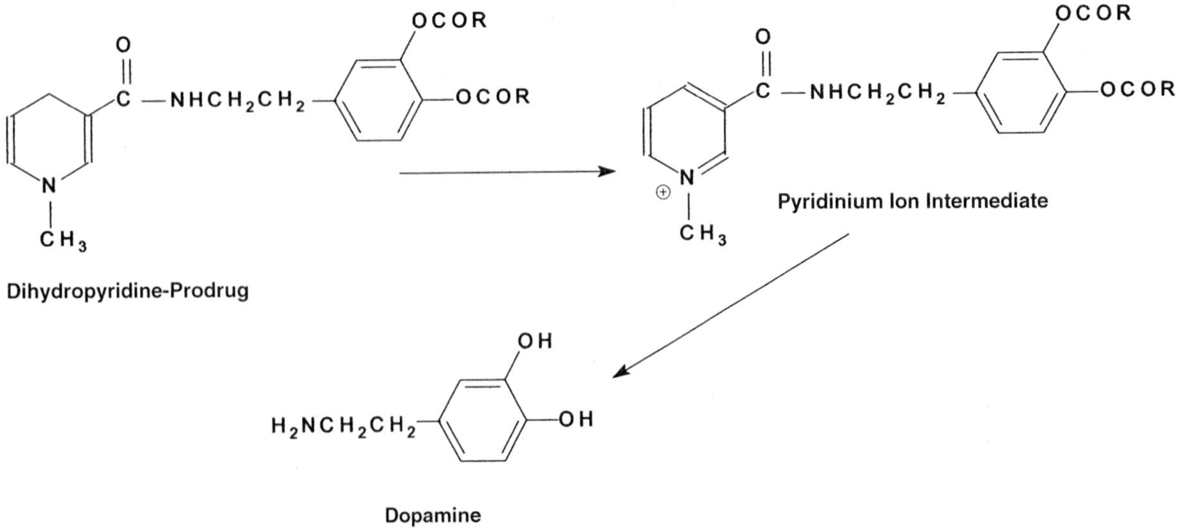

Scheme 5–27 ■ Dihydropyridine-based drug delivery system for dopamine.

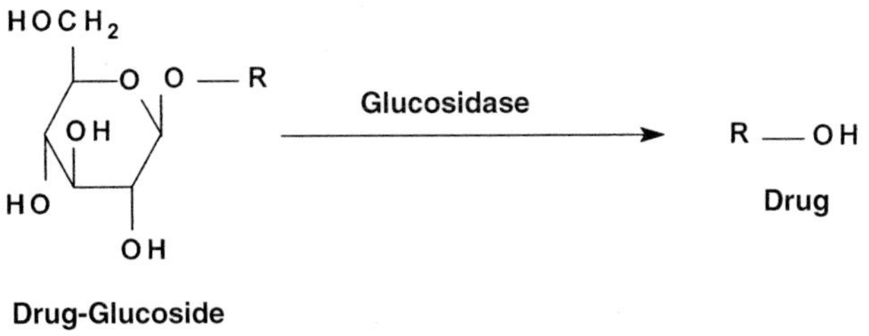

Drug-Glucoside

Scheme 5–28 ■ Activation of drug-glucoside by bacterial glucosidase.

but the presence of the enzymes in normal tissue prevents the possibility of complete site specificity for these agents.

This brief discussion of site-specific drug delivery shows that in some cases the prodrug was in use before its mechanism of delivery and specificity was discovered. Thus, some compounds were discovered to represent site-specific drug delivery well after they were placed into therapeutic use. An evaluation of the properties of these agents has produced the framework for the design of other prodrugs with target sites in specific tissues. This process is really no different from the general drug discovery process in which a unique substance is observed to have desirable pharmacological effects, and studies of its properties lead to the design of better drugs.

REFERENCES

1. Albert, A.: Nature 182:421, 1958.
2. Harper, N. J.: J. Med. Pharm. Chem. 1:467, 1959.
3. Ariens, E. J., and Simonis, A. M.: Optimization of pharmacokinetics—an essential aspect of drug development by metabolic stabilization. In Deverling Busiman, J. A. (ed.). Strategy in Drug Research. Amsterdam, Elsevier, 1982, pp. 165–178.
4. Bodor, N.: Med. Res. Rev. 4:449, 1984.
5. Silverman, R.: Prodrugs and drug delivery systems. In The Organic Chemistry of Drug Design and Drug Action. New York, Academic Press, 1992, Chap. 8, pp. 352–401.
6. Glazko, A. J., Carnes, H. E., Kazenko, A., et al.: Antibiot. Annu. 792: 752–802, 1957.
7. Riley, T. N.: J. Chem. Educ. 65:947–953, 1988.
8. Duggan, D. E.: Drug Metab. Rev. 12:325–337, 1981.
9. Hardcastle, G. A., Johnson, D. A., Panetta, C. A., et al.: J. Org. Chem. 31:897–899, 1966.
10. Tsuji, A., and Yamana, T.: Chem. Pharm. Bull. 22:2434–2443, 1974.
11. Jusko, W. J., and Lewis, G. P.: J. Pharm. Sci. 62:69–76, 1973.
12. Jusko, W. J., Lewis, G. P., and Schmitt, G. W.: Clin. Pharm. Ther. 14: 90–99, 1973.
13. Schwartz, M. A., and Hayton, W. L.: J. Pharm. Sci. 61:906–909, 1972.
14. Bungarrd, H.: Acta Pharm. Suec. 13:9–26, 1976.
15. Sinkula, A. A., and Yalkowsky, S. H.: J. Pharm. Sci. 64:181, 1975.
16. Wei, C. P., Anderson, J. A., and Leopold, I.: Invest. Ophthalmol. Vis. Sci. 17:315–321, 1978.
17. Sinkula, A. A., Morozowich, W., and Rowe, E. L.: J. Pharm. Sci. 62: 1106–1111, 1973.
18. Jansen, A. B. A., and Russell, T. J.: J. Chem. Soc., 1965, 2127.
19. Bodin, N. D., Ekström, B., Forsgren, U., et al.: Antimicrob. Agents Chemother. 8:518, 1975.
20. Hughes, G. S., Heald, D. L., Barker, K. B., et al.: Clin. Pharmacol. Ther. 46:1989, 1989.
21. Vej-Hansen, B., and Bundgaard, H.: Arch. Pharm. Chem. Sci. Educ. 7:65, 1979.
22. Tréfouël, J., Tréfouël, M. J., Nitti, F., and Bovet, D.: C. R. Soc. Biol. 120:756, 1935.
23. Notari, R. E.: J. Pharm. Sci. 62:865–881, 1973.
24. Mangan, F. R., Flack, J. D., and Jackson, D.: Am. J. Med. 83(4B):6, 1987.
25. Moore, H. W., and Czerniak, R.: Med. Res. Rev. 1:249, 1981.
26. Moore, H. W.: Science 197:527, 1977.
27. Iyer, V. N., and Szybalski, W.: Science 145:55, 1964.
28. Remers, W. A.: Mitomycin and porfiromycin. In The Chemistry of Antitumor Antibiotics. New York, Wiley, 1979, pp. 221–276.
29. Brown, J. M.: Br. J. Cancer 67:1163, 1993.
30. Kaufman, H. E.: Proc. Soc. Exp. Biol. Med. 109:251, 1962.
31. Friend, D. R.: Med. Res. Rev. 7:53, 1987.
32. Jungheim, L. N., and Shepherd, T. A.: Chem. Rev. 94:1553, 1994.
33. Miwa, M., Nishida, U. M., Sawada, N., et al.: Eur. J. Cancer 34:1274, 1998.
34. Denny, W. A.: Eur. J. Med. Chem. 36:577, 2001.
35. Stella, V. J.: J. Med. Chem. 23:1275, 1980.
36. Bodor, N.: Adv. Drug Res. 13:255, 1984.

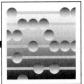

C H A P T E R **6**

Biotechnology and Drug Discovery

JOHN M. BEALE, JR.

BIOTECHNOLOGY: AN OVERVIEW

Developments in biotechnology in recent times have been quite dramatic. The years between 1999 and 2001 witnessed a tremendous increase in the number of biotechnology-related pharmaceutical products in development, and a number of important new drugs progressed through trials and into the clinic. A good reflection of the impact of biotechnology is the GenBank database. GenBank is an electronic repository of gene sequence information, specifically the nucleotide sequences of complementary DNA (cDNA), representing the messenger RNA (mRNA), and genomic clones that have been isolated and sequenced by scientists worldwide.[1, 2] The growth of the GenBank database has been rapid, and it has been increasing steadily since about 1992.[3] Figures 6-1 and 6-2 graphically depict these growth rates.

In October 2002, the Pharmaceutical Research and Manufacturers Association (PhRMA) reported that 371 biotechnology-derived medicines were in testing at various stages and that nearly 200 diseases are being targeted by research conducted by 144 companies and the National Cancer Institute. Of these—all of which are in human trials or awaiting Food and Drug Administration (FDA) approval—178 are new drugs for cancer, 47 are new drugs for infectious diseases, 26 are new drugs for autoimmune diseases, 22 are new drugs for neurological disorders, and 21 are new drugs for human immunodeficiency virus (HIV) and acquired immunodeficiency syndrome (AIDS) and related conditions.[4] PhRMA also reported 194 new medicines targeted for pediatric use.[5] Approved drugs derived from biotechnology also treat or help prevent myocardial infarction, stroke, multiple sclerosis, leukemia, hepatitis, rheumatoid arthritis, breast cancer, diabetes, congestive heart failure, lymphoma, renal cancer, cystic fibrosis, and other diseases. The number of approvals of biotechnology drugs per year has been increasing steadily. These data are shown in Figure 6-3.

The Human Genome Project, an international effort to obtain complete genetic maps, including nucleotide sequences, of each of the 24 human chromosomes, has spawned much new knowledge and technology. It is awesome to consider that in the mere 30 years since 1972, the science has reached the stage of attempting genetic cures for some diseases, such as cystic fibrosis and immune deficiency disorders.

BIOTECHNOLOGY AND PHARMACEUTICAL CARE

As it affects medicine and pharmaceutical care, biotechnology has forever altered the drug discovery process and the thinking about patient care. Extensive screening programs once drove drug discovery on natural or synthetic compounds. Now, the recombinant DNA (rDNA)-driven drug discovery process is beginning to yield new avenues for the preparation of some old drugs. For example, insulin, once prepared by isolation from pancreatic tissue of bovine or porcine species, can now be prepared in a pure form identical with human insulin. Likewise, human growth hormone, once isolated from the pituitary glands of the deceased, can now be prepared in pure form. Recombinant systems such as these provide high-yielding, reproducible batches of the drug and uniform dosing for patients.

LITERATURE OF BIOTECHNOLOGY

Many good literature sources on biotechnology exist for the pharmacist and medicinal chemist. These cover topics such as management issues in biotechnology,[6–14] implementation of instruction on biotechnology in education,[15–22] costs of biotechnology drugs,[23–26] implementation in a practice setting,[27–42] regulatory issues,[43–46] product evaluation and formulation,[47, 48] patient compliance,[49, 50] and finding information.[51–53] Additionally, there are a number of general texts,[54–60] review articles,[61–65] and a general resource reference catalogue.[66] Any good biochemistry textbook is also a useful resource.

BIOTECHNOLOGY AND NEW DRUG DEVELOPMENT

The tools of biotechnology are also being brought to bear in the search for new biological targets for presently available drugs as well as for the discovery of new biological molecules with therapeutic utility. Molecular cloning of novel receptors can provide access to tremendous tools for the testing of drugs (e.g., the adrenergic receptors), while cloning of a novel growth factor might potentially provide a new therapeutic agent. Biotechnology is also being used to screen compounds for biological activity. By using cloned and expressed genes, it is possible to generate receptor proteins to facilitate high-throughput screening of drugs in vitro or in cell culture systems rather than in animals or tissues. Biotechnology is being investigated in completely novel approaches to the battle against human disease, including the use of antisense oligonucleotides and gene replacement therapies for the treatment of diseases such as cystic fibrosis

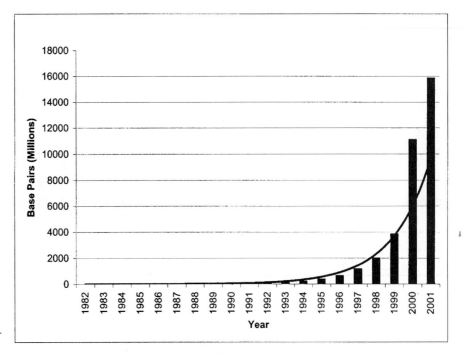

Figure 6–1 ■ Yearly growth of Gen-Bank in base pairs.

and the use of monoclonal antibodies for the treatment of cancer.

Biotechnology encompasses many subdisciplines including genomics, proteomics, gene therapy, made-to-order molecules, computer-assisted drug design, and pharmacogenomics. A goal of biotechnology in the early 21st century is to eliminate the "one drug fits all" paradigm for pharmaceutical care.[58]

The drugs that are elaborated by biotechnological methods are proteins and, hence, require special handling. There are some basic requirements of pharmaceutical care for the pharmacist working with biotechnologically derived products:[41]

- An understanding of how the handling and stability of biopharmaceuticals differs from other drugs that pharmacists dispense
- Knowledge of preparation of the product for patient use, including reconstitution or compounding if required
- Patient education on the disease, benefits of the prescribed biopharmaceutical, potential side effects or drug interactions to be aware of, and the techniques of self-administration
- Patient counseling on reimbursement issues involving an expensive product
- Monitoring of the patient for compliance

The pharmacist must maintain an adequate knowledge of agents produced through the methods of biotechnology and

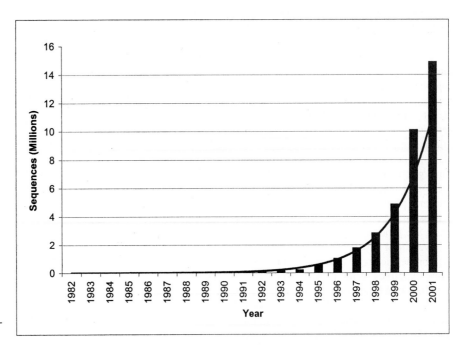

Figure 6–2 ■ Yearly growth of Gen-Bank in terms of gene sequences.

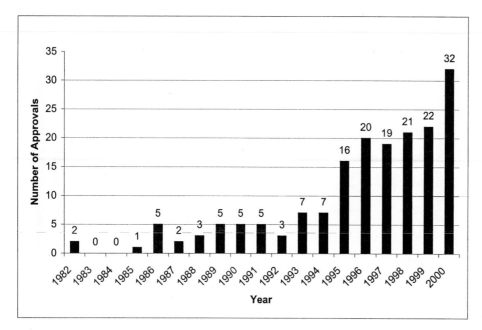

Figure 6–3 ■ Yearly approvals of biotechnology-derived drugs and vaccines.

remain "in the loop" for new developments. The language of biotechnology encompasses organic chemistry, biochemistry, physiology, pharmacology, medicinal chemistry, immunology, molecular biology, and microbiology. A pharmacist has studied in all of these areas and is uniquely poised to use these skills to provide pharmaceutical care with biotechnological agents when needed.

The key techniques that unlocked the door to the biotechnology arena are those of rDNA, also known as *genetic engineering*. rDNA techniques allow scientists to manipulate genetic programming, create new genomes, and extract genetic material (genes) from one organism and insert it into another to produce proteins.

THE BIOTECHNOLOGY OF RECOMBINANT DNA (rDNA)

Since its inception in the mid-1970s, rDNA[67–74] (genetic engineering) technology has driven much of the fundamental research and practical development of novel drug molecules and proteins. rDNA technology provides the ability to isolate genetic material from any source and insert it into cells (plant, fungal, bacterial, animal) and even live animals and plants, where it is expressed as part of the receiving organism's genome. Before discussing techniques of genetic engineering, a review of some of the basics of cellular nucleic acid and protein chemistry is relevant.[75–77]

Most of the components that contribute to cellular homeostasis are proteins—so much so that more than half of the dry weight of a cell is protein. Histones, cellular enzymes, membrane transport systems, and immunoglobulins are just a few examples of the proteins that carry out the biological functions of a living human cell. Proteins are hydrated three-dimensional structures, but at their most basic level, they are composed of linear sequences of amino acids that fold to create the spatial characteristics of the protein. These linear

sequences are called the *primary structure* of the protein, and they are encoded from DNA through RNA. The information flow sequence DNA → RNA → protein has for many years been called the biological "Central Dogma."[78, 79] The specific sequence of amino acids is encoded in genes. Genes are discrete segments of linear DNA that compose the chromosomes in the nucleus of a cell. The Human Genome Project has revealed that there are between 30,000 and 35,000 functional genes in a human, encompassing about 3,400,000,000 base pairs (bp).[80]

As depicted in Figure 6-4, in the nucleus of the cell, double-stranded DNA undergoes a process of transcription (catalyzed by RNA polymerase) to yield a single-stranded molecule of pre-mRNA. Endonucleases then excise nonfunctional RNA sequences called *introns* from the pre-mRNA to yield functional mRNA. In the cytoplasm, mRNA complexes with the ribosomes, and the codons are read and translated into proteins. The process of protein synthesis in *Escherichia coli* begins with the activation of amino acids as aminoacyl-transfer RNA (tRNA) derivatives. All 20 of the amino acids undergo this activation, an ATP-dependent step catalyzed by aminoacyl-tRNA synthetase. Initiation involves the mRNA template, *N*-formylmethionyl tRNA, the initiation codon (AUG), initiation factors, and the ribosomal subunits. Elongation occurs (using several elongation factors) with the aminoacyl-tRNAs being selected by recognition of their specific codons and forming new peptide bonds with neighboring amino acids. When biosynthesis of the specific protein is finished, a termination codon in the mRNA is recognized, and release factors disengage the protein from the elongation complex. Finally, the protein is folded and posttranslational processing occurs.[81, 82] Processes that might be used in this step include removal of initiating residues and signaling sequences, proteolysis, modification of terminal residues, and attachment of phosphate, methyl, carboxyl, sulfate, carbohydrate, or prosthetic groups that help the protein achieve its final three-dimensional shape. Spe-

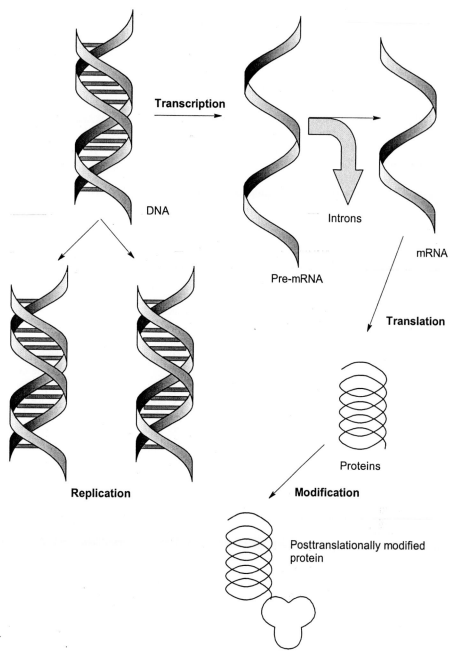

Transcription

DNA

Introns

mRNA

Pre-mRNA

Translation

Proteins

Replication

Modification

Posttranslationally modified protein

Figure 6–4 ■ Path from DNA to protein.

cialized chaperone proteins can also direct the three-dimensional formation. Posttranslational modifications occur in mammalian cells in the endoplasmic reticulum or the Golgi apparatus before the protein is transported out of the cell. Most posttranslational modifications occur only in higher organisms, not in bacteria. The three-base genetic codon system is well known and has been conserved among all organisms. This allows rDNA procedures to work and facilitates the development of a model for the amino acid sequence of a protein by correlation with the codon sequence of the genome.

Recombinant DNA (rDNA) Technology

The fundamental techniques involved in working with rDNA involve isolating or copying a gene; inserting the precise gene into a transmissible vector that can be transcribed, amplified, and propagated by a host cell's biochemical machinery; transferring it to that host cell; and facilitating the transcription into mRNA and translation into proteins. Cloned DNA can also be removed or altered by using an appropriate restriction endonuclease. Since genes encode the language of proteins, in theory it is possible to create any protein if one can obtain a copy of the corresponding gene. rDNA methods require:[83]

- An efficient method for cleaving and rejoining phosphodiester bonds on fragments of DNA (genes) derived from an array of different sources
- Suitable vectors or carriers capable of replicating both themselves and the foreign DNA linked to them
- A means of introducing the rDNA into a bacterial, yeast, plant, or mammalian cell

- Procedures for screening and selecting a clone of cells that has acquired the rDNA molecule from a large population of cells

There are two primary methods for cloning DNA[84] using genomic and cDNA libraries as the primary sources of DNA fragments, which, respectively, represent either the chromosomal DNA of a particular organism or the cDNA prepared from mRNA present in a given cell, tissue, or organ. In the first method, a library of DNA fragments is created from a cell's genome, which represents all of the genes present. The library is then screened against special DNA probes. Lysing the genomic contents to generate fragments of different sizes and compositions, some of which should contain the genetic sequences that encode the specific activity that one is seeking, creates the library. With knowledge of the protein sequence that the gene specifies, DNA probes can be synthesized that should hybridize with corresponding fragments in the library. By labeling the probes with fluorescent or radioactive tags, probe molecules that hybridize and form double-helical DNA can be identified and isolated electrophoretically. The DNA from the library can then be amplified by a technique such as the polymerase chain reaction (PCR), inserted into a vector, and transferred into a host cell. A comparison of these methods is given in Table 6-1.

The second major method for cloning DNA represents only genes that are being expressed[84] at a given time and involves first the isolation of the mRNA that encodes the amino acid sequence of the protein of interest. Treating the mRNA with the viral enzyme reverse transcriptase in the presence of nucleoside triphosphates (NTPs) causes a strand of DNA to be synthesized complementary to the mRNA matrix, affording a RNA–DNA hybrid. The RNA strand is broken down in alkaline conditions, yielding a single-stranded molecule of DNA. The DNA polymerase reaction affords a complementary or copy strand of DNA (cDNA), which on fusion of a promotor sequence can be attached to a transport vector. Figure 6-5 depicts these reactions.

If the amino acid sequence of a protein (and, hence, the codon sequence) is known, automated synthesis of DNA through chemical or enzymatic means represents a third way that genes can be engineered. This method is useful only for

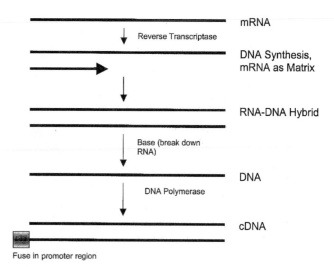

Figure 6–5 ■ Method for preparation of cDNA from a mRNA transcript.

relatively small proteins. In principle, for the preparation of a genomic library the cellular origin of the DNA is not an issue, whereas the cellular origin of mRNA is central to the preparation of a cDNA library. Therefore, genomic libraries vary from species to species but not from tissue to tissue within that species. cDNA varies with tissue and the developmental stages of cells, tissues, or species. Another important distinction is that the fragment of DNA from eukaryotic chromosomes will contain exons (protein coding segments) and introns (noncoding segments between exons), whereas in cDNA the introns are spliced out.

Restriction Endonucleases[84, 85]

The restriction endonuclease (or restriction enzyme) is probably best described as a set of ''molecular scissors'' in nature. Restriction endonucleases are bacterial enzymes that, as the name implies, cleave internal phosphodiester bonds of a DNA molecule. The cleavage site on a segment of DNA lies within a specific nucleotide sequence of about six to eight base pairs. More than 500 restriction endonucleases have been discovered, and these react with more than 100 different cleavage sites. The chemical reaction of the restriction endonuclease releases the 3′ end of one base as an alcohol and the 5′ end as a monophosphate. The general reaction is shown in Figure 6-6.

The recognition sites for restriction endonucleases are specific palindromic sequences of DNA[85] not more than 8 bp long. A number of these palindromes are listed in Table 6-2. A palindrome is a sequence of letters that reads the same way forward and backward, for instance: ''A man, a plan, a canal: Panama!,'' ''DNA-land,'' ''Did Hannah see bees? Hannah did.'' Restriction endonucleases cleave DNA at palindromic sites to yield several types of cuts:

$$\begin{array}{ccc} \downarrow & & \\ 5'\ CCTAGG\ 3' & \rightarrow & 5'\ CCTAG\ 3' \\ 3'\ GGATCC\ 5' & & 3'\ GATCC\ 5' \\ \uparrow & & \end{array}$$

The above cut yields an overhanging C/C ''sticky'' end that

TABLE 6–1 Characteristics of Genomic Versus cDNA Libraries

Characteristic	Genomic	cDNA
Source of genetic material	Genomic DNA	Cell or tissue mRNA
Complexity (independent recombinants)	>100,000	5,000–20,000
Size range of recombinants (bp[a])	1,000–50,000	30–10,000
Presence of introns	Yes	No
Presence of regulatory elements	Yes	Maybe
Suitable for heterologous expression	Maybe	Yes

[a]bp, base pairs.

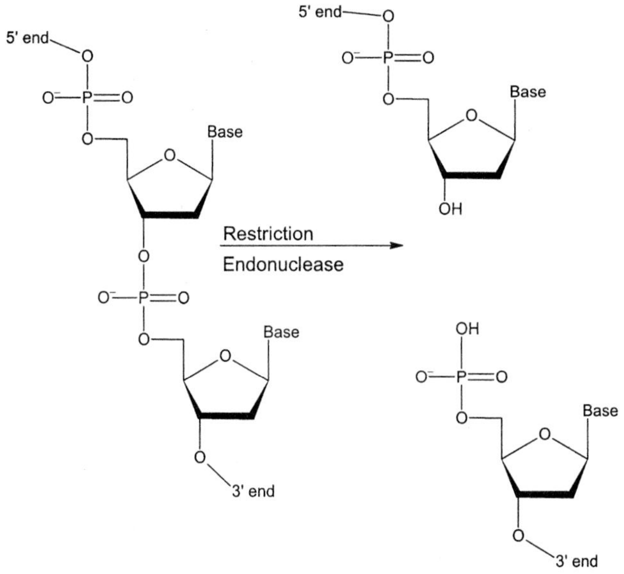

Figure 6–6 ■ Mechanism of a restriction endonuclease reaction.

is relatively easy to ligate with complementary ends of other DNA molecules. A cut from an endonuclease like *Hae*III:

5′ CC↓GG 3′   →   5′ CC GG 3′
3′ GG↑CC 5′   3′ GG CC 5′

requires more complicated methods to ligate into vector DNA. Palindromic cleavage sites for some selected restriction enzymes are given in Table 6-2. The *arrow* shows the cleavage site. The restriction endonucleases are a robust group of enzymes that form a toolbox for investigators working in the field of genetic engineering. About the only caveat to their use is an obvious one: they must be chosen to not make their cut inside the gene of interest.

DNA Ligases[86]

When the gene of interest has been excised from its flanking DNA by the appropriate restriction endonucleases and the vector DNA has been opened (using the same restriction endonuclease to break phosphodiester bonds), the two different DNA molecules are brought together by annealing. In the first step of this process, heating unwinds the double-stranded DNA of the vector. The insert or passenger DNA is added to the heated mixture, and subsequent cooling facilitates pairing of complementary strands. Then, phosphodiester bonds are regenerated, linking the two DNA molecules,

vector and insert. A total of four such bonds must be reformed, two on each strand at the 5′ and 3′ sites. This process is termed *ligation,* and the enzymes that catalyze the reaction are named *DNA ligases.* Typically, ATP or another energy source is required to drive the ligation reaction, and linker fragments of DNA are used to facilitate coupling. There are several different types of ligation reactions that are used, depending on the type of restriction endonuclease product that was formed. The sticky-ended DNA, using complementary vector and insert ends that easily base pair at the cuts, is probably the easiest to accomplish, although methods exist to ligate the blunt-ended varieties, using DNA ligase.

The Vector[84]

There are several methods available for introducing DNA into host cells. DNA molecules that can maintain themselves by replication are called *replicons*. Vectors are subsets of replicons. In genetic engineering, the vector (carrier) is the most widely used method for the insertion of foreign, or passenger, genetic material into a cell. Vectors are genetic elements such as plasmids or viruses that can be propagated and that have been engineered so that they can accept fragments of foreign DNA. Depending on the vector, they may have many other features, including multiple cloning sites (a region containing multiple restriction enzyme sites into which an insert can be installed or removed), selection markers, and transcriptional promoters. The passenger DNA must integrate into the host cell's DNA or be carried into the cell as part of a biologically active molecule that can replicate independently. If this result is not achieved, the inserted gene will not be successfully transcribed. The most commonly used biological agent for transporting genes into bacterial and yeast cells is the plasmid, such as the *E. coli* bacterial plasmid pBR322. A plasmid is a small, double-stranded, closed circular extrachromosomal DNA molecule. This plasmid contains 4,361 bp and can transport relatively small amounts of DNA. Plasmids occur in many species of bacteria and yeasts. Sometimes, plasmids carry their own genes, e.g., the highly transmissible genes for antibiotic resistance in some bacterial species. An important feature of a plasmid is that it has an origin of replication *(ori)* site that allows it to multiply independently of a host cell's DNA. Although there can be more than one copy of a plasmid in a cell, the copy number is controlled by the plasmid itself.

Another type of cloning vector is the bacteriophage (Fig. 6-7). Bacteriophage λ (lambda) possesses a genome of approximately 4.9×10^5 bp and can package large amounts of genetic material without affecting the infectivity of the phage. A large DNA library can be created, packaged in

TABLE 6–2   Palindromic Cleavage Sites

*Alu*I	*Asu*II	*Bal*I	*Bam*H1	*Bgl*II	*Cla*I	*Eco*RI
AG↓CT	**TT↓CGAA**	**TGG↓CCA**	**G↓GATCC**	**A↓GATCT**	**AT↓CGAT**	**G↓AATTC**
*Eco*RV	*Hae*III	*Hha*I	*Hind*II	*Hind*III	*Hpa*II	*Kpn*I
GAT↓ATC	GG↓CC	GCG↓C	GTPy↓PuAC	A↓AGCTT	C↓CGG	GGTAC↓C
*Mbo*I	*Pst*I	*Pvu*I	*Sal*I	*Sma*I	*Xma*I	*Not*I
↓GATC	CTGCA↓G	CGAT↓CG	G↓TCGAC	CCC↓GGG	C↓CCGGG	GC↓GGCCGC

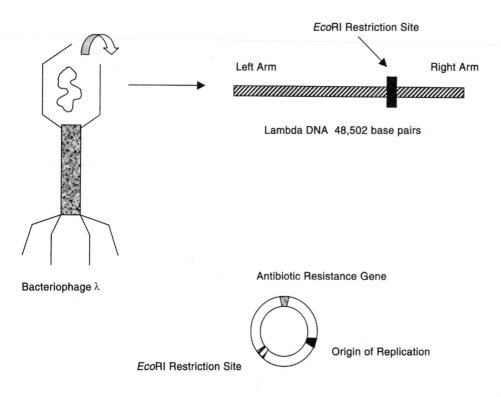

EcoRI Restriction Site

Left Arm   Right Arm

Lambda DNA 48,502 base pairs

Bacteriophage λ

Antibiotic Resistance Gene

EcoRI Restriction Site

Origin of Replication

E. coli plasmid pBR322   4,361 base pairs

Figure 6–7 ▪ Types of cloning vectors: a bacteriophage and a plasmid.

bacteriophage *λ*, and when the virus infects, inserted into cells. Hybridization is then detected by screening with DNA probes.[87] In addition, there are special vectors called phagemids, vaccinia and adenovirus for cloning into mammalian cells, and yeast artificial chromosomes (YACs) that facilitate cloning in yeasts.[88] Differences among these vectors concern the size of the insert that they will accept, the methods used in the selection of the clones, and the procedures for propagation.

Once the passenger DNA has been created and the plasmid vector cut (both with the same restriction enzyme), the insert is ligated into the plasmid along with a promoter (a short DNA sequence that enhances the transcription of the adjacent gene). Often, a gene imparting antibiotic resistance linked to the desired gene is inserted as a selection tool. The idea behind this is that if the gene is inserted in the proper location, the bacterial cell will grow on a medium containing the antibiotic. Bacteria that do not contain the resistance gene and, hence, lack the required gene will not grow. This makes the task of screening for integration of the desired gene easier. After the molecule is ligated, the vector is finally a rDNA molecule that can be inserted into a host cell.

Host cells can be bacteria (e.g., *E. coli*), eukaryotic yeast (*Saccharomyces cerevisiae*), or mammalian cell lines including Chinese hamster ovary (CHO), African green monkey kidney (VERO), and baby hamster kidney (BHK). It is easy to grow high concentrations of bacteria and yeast cells in fermenters to yield high protein concentrations. Mammalian cell culture systems typically give poorer protein yields, but sometimes this is acceptable, especially when the product demands the key posttranslational modifications that do not occur in bacteria. Host cells containing the vector are grown

in small-scale cultures and screened for the desired gene.[89] When the clone providing the best protein yield is located, the organism is grown under carefully controlled conditions and used to inoculate pilot-scale fermentations. Parameters such as production medium composition, pH, aeration, agitation, and temperature are investigated at this stage to optimize the fermentation. The host cells divide and the plasmids in them replicate, producing the desired ''new'' protein. The fermentation is scaled up into larger bioreactors for large-scale isolation of the recombinant protein. Obviously, the cultures secrete their own natural proteins along with the cloned protein. Purification steps are required before the recombinant protein is suitable for testing as a new, genetically engineered pharmaceutical agent. Once the host cell line expressing the recombinant gene is isolated, it is essential to maintain selection pressure on it so that it does not spontaneously lose the plasmid. Typically, this pressure is applied by maintaining the cells on medium containing an antibiotic to which they bear a resistance gene.

SOME TYPES OF CLONING

A listing of some types of cloning is given in Table 6-3.

Functional Expression Cloning[90]

Functional expression cloning focuses on obtaining a specific cDNA of known function. There are many variations on this approach, but they all rely on the ability to search for and isolate cDNAs based on some functional activity

TABLE 6–3   Cloning Strategies

Strategy	Advantages	Disadvantages	Example
Positional	Provides information underlying the genetic basis of known diseases	3.3×10^9 bp, difficult to use with diseases caused by multiple interacting alleles	Cystic fibrosis gene product
Protein purification	Yields genetic information encoding proteins of known structure and function	Protein purification, especially for low-abundance proteins, is exacting; availability of appropriate libraries, incomplete coding sequences	β_2-Adrenergic receptor
Antibody based	Yields genetic information encoding proteins of known structure and function	Involves protein purification, unrecognized cross-reactivity, incomplete coding sequences	Vitamin D receptor
Functional expression	Yields genetic information encoding a functionally active protein; does not require protein purification	Function must be compatible with existing library-screening technology	Substance K receptor
Homology based	Identification of related genes or gene families; relatively simple	Depends on preexisting gene sequence; can yield incomplete genes or genes of unknown function	Muscarinic receptor
Expressed sequence tagging	High throughput; identification of novel cDNAs	Incomplete coding sequences or genes of unknown function	
Total genomic sequencing	Knowledge of total genome; identification of all potential gene products	3.3×10^9 bp, labor intensive; genes of unknown function	*Haemophilus influenzae*

that can be measured, e.g., the electrophysiological measurement of ion conductances following expression of cDNAs in frog oocytes. By incrementally subdividing the cDNAs into pools and following the activity, it is possible to obtain a single cDNA clone that encodes the functionality. The advantage of functional expression cloning is that it does not rely on knowledge of the primary amino acid sequence. This is a definite advantage when attempting to clone proteins of low abundance.

Positional Cloning[90]

Positional cloning can be used to localize fragments of DNA representing genes prior to isolating the DNA. An example of the use of positional cloning is the cloning of the gene responsible for cystic fibrosis (CF). By studying the patterns of inheritance of the disease and then comparing these with known chromosomal markers (linkage analysis), it was possible, without knowing the function of the gene, to locate the gene on human chromosome 7. Then, by using a technique known as *chromosome walking,* the gene was localized to a DNA sequence that encodes a protein now known as the cystic fibrosis transmembrane conductance regulator (CFTR). This protein, previously unknown, was shown to be defective in CF patients and could account for many of the symptoms of the disease. Like functional cloning, positional cloning has the advantage that specific knowledge of the protein is not required. It is also directly relevant to the understanding of human disease, and it can provide important new biological targets for drug development and the treatment of disease.

Homology-Based Cloning

Another cloning strategy involves the use of previously cloned genes to guide identification and cloning of evolutionarily related genes. This approach, referred to as *homol-ogy-based cloning,* takes advantage of the fact that nucleotide sequences encoding important functional domains of proteins tend to be conserved during the process of evolution. Thus, nucleotide sequences encoding regions involved with ligand binding or enzymatic activity can be used as probes that will hybridize to complementary nucleotide sequences that may be present on other genes that bind similar ligands or have similar enzymatic activity. This approach can be combined with PCR[91, 92] to amplify the DNA sequences. The use of homology-based cloning has the advantages that it can be used to identify families of related genes, does not rely on the purification or functional activity of a given protein, and can provide novel targets for drug discovery. Its usefulness is offset by the possibility that the isolated fragment may not encode a complete or functional protein or that in spite of knowledge of the shared sequence, the actual function of the clone may be difficult to identify.

EXPRESSION OF CLONED DNA

Once cloned, there are many different possibilities for the expression and manipulation of DNA sequences. As it concerns the use of cloned genes in the process of drug discovery and development, there are many obvious ways in which the expression of DNA sequences can be applied. One of the most obvious is in replacement of older technologies that involve the purification of proteins for human use from either animal sources or human by-products, such as blood. An example of this is factor VIII, a clotting cascade protein used for the treatment of the genetically linked bleeding disorder hemophilia. Until recently, the only source of purified factor VIII was human blood, and tragically, before the impact of AIDS was fully appreciated, stocks of factor VIII had become contaminated with HIV-1, resulting in the infection of as many as 75% of the patients receiving this product. The gene encoding factor VIII has since been cloned, and recombinant factor VIII is now available as a product purified from cultured mammalian cells. Other recombinant clotting factors, including factors VIIa and IX, are under development and, together with recombinant factor VIII, will eliminate the risk of exposure to human pathogens.

Other examples in which the expression of cloned human genes offers alternatives to previously existing products include human insulin, which is now a viable replacement for purified bovine and porcine insulin for the treatment of diabetes, and human growth hormone, which is used for the treatment of growth hormone deficiency in children (dwarfism). Unlike insulin, growth hormones from other animal species are ineffective in humans; thus until human recombinant growth hormone became available, the only source of human growth hormone was the pituitary glands of cadavers. This obviously limited the supply of human growth hormone and, like factor VIII, exposed patients to potential contamination by human pathogens. Recombinant human growth hormone can now be produced by expression in bacterial cells.

The expression of cloned genes can be integrated into rational drug design by providing detailed information about the structure and function of the sites of drug action. With the cloning of a gene comes knowledge of the primary amino acid sequence of an encoded receptor protein. This information can be used to model its secondary structure and in an initial attempt to define the protein's functional domains, such as its ligand-binding site. Such a model can then serve as a basis for the design of experiments that can be used to test the model and facilitate further refinement. Of particular use are mutagenesis experiments that use rDNA techniques to change a primary amino acid sequence so that the consequences can be studied. In addition, expression of a cloned target protein can be used to generate samples for various biophysical determinations, such as x-ray crystallography. This technique, which can provide detailed information about the three-dimensional molecular structure of a protein, frequently requires large amounts of protein, which in some cases is only available with the use of recombinant expression systems.

Like the many strategies used to clone genes, there are many strategies for their expression, involving the use of either bacterial or eukaryotic cells and specialized vectors compatible with expression in host cells. Since these cells do not normally express the protein of interest, this methodology is often referred to as *heterologous expression*. It is also possible to prepare cRNA from rDNA, which can then be used for either in vitro expression or injection directly into cells. In the former situation, purified ribosomes are used in the test tube to convert cRNA into protein; for the latter situation, the endogenous cellular ribosomes make the protein. A relatively new development for the expression of cloned genes is the use of animals that have the cloned gene stably integrated into their genome. Such transgenic animals can potentially make very large amounts of recombinant protein, which can be harvested from the milk, blood, and ascites fluid.

The choice of a particular expression system depends on a number of factors. Protein yield, requirements for biological activity, and compatibility of the expressed protein with the host organism are a few. An example of the compatibility issue is that bacteria do not process proteins in exactly the same ways as do mammalian cells, so that the expression of human proteins in bacteria will not always yield an active product or any product at all. Cases like these may require expression in mammalian cell cultures. The choice of an expression system also reflects the available vectors and corresponding host organisms. A basic requirement for the heterologous expression of a cloned gene is the presence of a promoter that can function in the host organism and a mechanism for introducing the cloned gene into the organism. The promoter is the specific site at which DNA polymerase binds to initiate transcription and is usually specific for the host organism. As in gene cloning, the vectors are either plasmids or viruses that have been engineered to accept rDNA and that contain promoters that direct the expression of the rDNA. The techniques for introducing the vector into the organism vary widely and depend on whether one is interested in transient expression of the cloned gene or in stable expression. In the latter case, integration into the host genome is usually required; transient expression simply requires getting the vector into the host cell.

MANIPULATION OF DNA SEQUENCE INFORMATION

Perhaps the greatest impact of rDNA technology lies in its ability to alter a DNA sequence and create entirely new molecules that, if reintroduced into the genome, can be inherited and propagated in perpetuity. The ability to alter a DNA sequence, literally in a test tube, at the discretion of an individual, corporation, or nation, brings with it important questions about ownership, ethics, and social responsibility. There is no question, however, that potential benefits to the treatment of human disease are great.

There are three principal reasons for using rDNA technology to alter DNA sequences. The first is simply to clone the DNA to facilitate subsequent manipulation. The second is to intentionally introduce mutations so that the site-specific effect on protein structure and function can be studied.[93, 94] The third reason is to add or remove sequences to obtain some desired attribute in the recombinant protein. For example, recent studies with factor VIII show that the protein contains a small region of amino acids that are the major determinant for the generation of anti–factor VIII antibodies in a human immune system. This autoimmune response of the patient inhibits the activity of factor VIII, which is obviously a serious therapeutic complication for patients who are using factor VIII for the treatment of hemophilia. By altering the DNA sequence encoding this determinant, however, the amino acid sequence can be changed both to reduce the antigenicity of the factor VIII molecule and to make it transparent to any existing anti–factor VIII antibodies (i.e., changing the epitope eliminates the existing antibody recognition sites).

It is possible to combine elements of two proteins into one new recombinant protein. The resulting protein, referred to as a *chimeric* or *fusion protein,* may then have some of the functional properties of both of the original proteins.

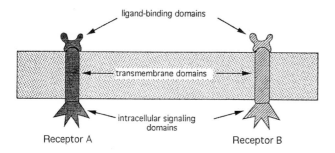

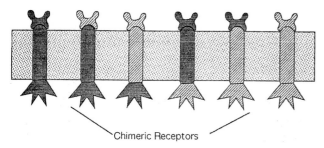

Figure 6–8 ■ Chimeric receptors.

This is illustrated in Figure 6-8 for two receptors labeled *A* and *B*. Each receptor has functional domains that are responsible for ligand binding, integration into the plasma membrane, and activation of intracellular signaling pathways. Using rDNA techniques, one can exchange these functional domains to create chimeric receptors that, for example, contain the ligand-binding domain of receptor B but the transmembrane and intracellular signaling domains of receptor A. The application of the fusion protein strategy is discussed further in connection with the human growth hormone receptor (under the heading, Novel Drug-Screening Strategies) and with denileukin diftitox.

Another reason for combining elements of two proteins into one recombinant protein is to facilitate its expression and purification. For example, recombinant glutathione S-transferase (GST), cloned from the parasitic worm *Schistosoma japonicum*, is strongly expressed in *E. coli* and has a binding site for glutathione. Heterologous sequences encoding the functional domains from other proteins can be fused, in frame, to the carboxy terminus of GST, and the resulting fusion protein is often expressed at the same levels as GST itself. In addition, the resulting fusion protein still retains the ability to bind glutathione, which means that affinity chromatography, using glutathione that has been covalently bonded to agarose, can be used for a single-step purification of the fusion protein. The functional activity of the heterologous domains that have been fused to GST can then be studied either as part of the fusion protein or separately following treatment of the fusion protein with specific proteases that cleave at the junction between GST and the heterologous domain. Purified fusion proteins can also be used to generate antibodies to the heterologous domains and for other biochemical studies. Sometimes, fusion proteins are made to provide a recombinant protein that can be easily identified. An example of this is a technique called *epitope tagging,* in which well-characterized antibody recognition sites are fused with recombinant proteins. The resulting recombinant

protein can then be identified by immunofluorescence or can be purified with antibodies that recognize the epitope.

NEW BIOLOGICAL TARGETS FOR DRUG DEVELOPMENT

One of the outcomes of the progress that has been made in the identification and cloning of genes is that many proteins encoded by these genes represent entirely new targets for drug development. In some cases, the genes themselves may represent the ultimate target for the treatment of a disease in the form of gene therapy. The cloning of the cystic fibrosis gene is an example of both a new drug target and a gene that could potentially be used to treat the disease. The protein encoded by this gene, CFTR, is a previously unknown integral membrane protein that functions as a channel for chloride ions. Mutations in *CFTR* underlie the pathophysiology of cystic fibrosis, and in principle, replacement or coexpression of the defective gene with the healthy, nonmutated gene would cure the disease. It is also possible, however, that by understanding the structure and function of the healthy CFTR, drugs could be designed to interact with the mutated CFTR and improve its function.

An important outgrowth of the study of new drug targets is the recognition that many traditional targets, such as enzymes and receptors, are considerably more heterogeneous than previously thought. Thus, instead of one enzyme or receptor, there may be several closely related subtypes, or isoforms, each with the potential of representing a separate drug target. This can be illustrated with the enzyme cyclooxygenase (COX), which is pivotal to the formation of prostaglandins and which is the target of aspirin and the nonsteroidal anti-inflammatory agents (NSAIDs). Until recently, COX was considered to be a single enzyme, but pharmacological and gene cloning studies have revealed that there are at least three enzyme forms, named COX-1, COX-2, and COX-3. Interestingly, they are differentially regulated. COX-1 is expressed constitutively in many tissues, whereas the expression of COX-2 is induced by inflammatory processes. Thus, the development of COX-2 selective agents can yield NSAIDs with the same efficacy as existing (nonselective) agents but with fewer side effects, such as those on the gastric mucosa.

The elucidation of the family of adrenergic receptors is another example in which molecular cloning studies have revealed previously unknown heterogeneity, with the consequence of providing new targets for drug development. The adrenergic receptors mediate the physiological effects of the catecholamines epinephrine and norepinephrine. They are also the targets for many drugs used in the treatment of such conditions as congestive heart failure, asthma, hypertension, glaucoma, and benign prostatic hypertrophy. Prior to the molecular cloning and purification of adrenergic receptors, the pharmacological classification of this family of receptors consisted of four subtypes: α_1, α_2, β_1, and β_2. The initial cloning of the α-adrenergic receptor in 1986 and subsequent gene cloning studies revealed at least nine subtypes: β_1, β_2, β_3, α_{1A}, α_{1B}, α_{1D}, α_{2A}, α_{2B}, and α_{2C} (Chapter 16).

The evidence that there are nine subtypes of adrenergic receptors is very important in terms of understanding the

TABLE 6–4 Selected Examples of Receptor Subtype Heterogeneity

Receptor Superfamily	Original Subtypes	Present Subtypes
G-protein-coupled		
Adrenergic	β_1, β_2, α_1, α_2	β_1, β_2, β_3, α_{1A}, α_{1B}, α_{1D}, α_2A, α_2B, α_2C,
Dopamine	D_1, D_2	D_1, $D_2{}^a$, D_3, D_4, D_5
Prostaglandin E_2	EP_1, EP_2, EP_3	EP_1, EP_2, $EP_3{}^a$, EP_4
Receptor tyrosine kinase neurotrophins	Nerve growth factor receptor	TrkA,[a] TrkB, TrkC[a]
DNA binding		
Estrogen	Estrogen receptor	ERR1, ERR2
Thyroid hormone	Thyroid hormone receptor	$TR\alpha$, $TR\beta$
Retinoic acid	Retinoic acid receptor	$RAR\alpha$, $RAR\beta$
Ligand-activated channels		
Glycine	Glycine and/or strychnine receptor	α_1, α_2, α_3 (multisubunit)[b]
$GABA_A$	GABA and/or benzodiazepine receptor	α_1, α_2, α_3, α_4, α_5, α_6 (multisubunit)[b]

[a] Alternative mRNA splicing creates additional receptor heterogeneity.

[b] Only the heterogeneity of the ligand-binding subunit is listed; a multisubunit structure combined with the heterogeneity of the other subunits creates a very large number of potential subtypes.

physiology of the adrenergic receptors and of developing drugs that can selectively interact with these subtypes. For example, in the case of the α_2-agonist *p*-aminoclonidine, an agent used to lower intraocular pressure (IOP) in the treatment of glaucoma, it may now be possible to explain some of the drug's pharmacological side effects (e.g., bradycardia and sedation) by invoking interactions with the additional α_2-adrenergic receptor subtypes. Of considerable interest is the possibility that these pharmacological effects (i.e., lowering of IOP, bradycardia, and sedation) are each mediated by one of the three different α_2-receptor subtypes. If this is true, it might be possible to develop a subtype-selective α_2-agonist that lowers IOP but does not cause bradycardia or sedation. Likewise, it might even be possible to take advantage of the pharmacology and develop α_2-adrenergic agents that selectively lower heart rate or produce sedation.

The discovery of subtypes of receptors and enzymes by molecular cloning studies seems to be the rule rather than the exception and is offering a plethora of potential new drug targets (Table 6-4). To note just a few: 5 dopamine receptor subtypes have been cloned, replacing 2 defined pharmacologically (Chapter 15); 7 serotonin receptor subtypes have been cloned, replacing 3; 4 genes encoding receptors for prostaglandin E_2 have been isolated, including 12 additional alternative mRNA splice variants; and 3 receptors for nerve growth factor have been cloned, replacing 1.

NOVEL DRUG-SCREENING STRATEGIES

The combination of the heterologous expression of cloned DNA, the molecular cloning of new biological targets, and the ability to manipulate gene sequences has created powerful new tools that can be applied to the process of drug discovery and development. In its most straightforward application, the ability to simply express newly identified receptor protein targets offers a novel means of obtaining information that may be difficult, or even impossible, to obtain

from more complex native biological systems. There is a reason for this. A newly identified protein can be expressed in isolation. Even for closely related enzyme or receptor subtypes, heterologous expression of the individual subtype can potentially provide data that are specific for the subtype being expressed, whereas the data from native biological systems will reflect the summation of the individual subtypes that may be present.

The potential advantage of heterologous expression is illustrated in Figure 6-9 for the interaction of a drug with multiple binding sites. In *panel A,* which can represent the data obtained from a native biological system, the data are complex, and the curve reflects interactions of the drug with two populations of receptors: one with high affinity, representing 50% of the total receptor population, and one with low affinity, representing the remaining 50%. The individual contributions of these two populations of receptors are indicated in *panel B,* which could also reflect the data obtained if rDNA encoding these two receptors were expressed individually in a heterologous expression system. Although in some cases the data, as in *panel A,* can be analyzed with success, frequently they cannot, especially if more than two subtypes are present or if any one subtype makes up less than 10% of the total receptor population or if the affinities of the drug for the two receptor populations differ by less than 10-fold.

Another important reason for integrating heterologous expression into drug-screening strategies is that data can usually be obtained for the human target protein rather than an animal substitute. This does not mean that organ preparations or animal models will be totally replaced. For the purposes of the identification of lead compounds and the optimization of selectivity, affinity, etc., however, the use of recombinant expression systems provides some obvious advantages.

By combining heterologous expression with novel functional assays, it is possible to increase both specificity and throughput (the number of compounds that can be screened

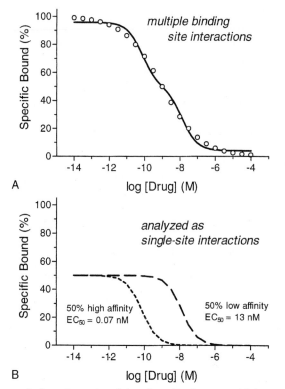

A

B

Figure 6–9 ■ Convoluted data from binding to multiple receptor subtypes versus classic mass action.

per unit time). For example, reporter genes have been developed that respond to a variety of intracellular second messengers, such as the activation of guanine nucleotide-binding proteins (G proteins), and levels of cAMP, or calcium. One approach to the development of novel functional assays involves the use of promoter regions in DNA that control the transcription of genes. This approach is exemplified by the cAMP *r*esponse *e*lement (CRE). This is a specifically defined sequence of DNA that is a binding site for the *c*AMP *r*esponse *e*lement-*b*inding (CREB) protein. In the unstimulated condition, the binding of CREB to the CRE prevents the transcription and expression of genes that follow it (Fig. 6-10). When CREB is phosphorylated by cAMP-dependent protein kinase (PKA), however, its conformation changes, permitting the transcription and expression of the downstream gene. Thus, increases in intracellular cAMP, such as those caused by receptors that activate adenylyl cyclase (e.g., β-adrenergic, vasopressin, and many others), will stimulate the activity of PKA, which, in turn, results in the phosphorylation of CREB and the activation of gene transcription.

In nature, there are a limited number of genes whose activity is regulated by a CRE. Biologically, however, the expression of almost any gene can be regulated in a cAMP-dependent fashion if it is placed downstream of a CRE, using rDNA techniques. If the products of the expression of the downstream gene can be easily detected, they can serve as reporters for any receptor or enzyme that can modulate the formation of cAMP in the cell. The genes encoding chloramphenicol acetyl transferase (CAT), luciferase, and β-galactosidase are three examples of potential "reporter genes" whose products can be easily detected. Sensitive enzymatic assays have been developed for all of these enzymes; thus any changes in their transcription will be quickly reflected by changes in enzyme activity. By coexpressing the reporter gene along with the genes encoding receptors and enzymes that modulate cAMP formation, it is possible to obtain very sensitive functional measures of the activation of the coexpressed enzyme or receptor.

Another example of the use of a reporter gene for high-throughput drug screening is the *r*eceptor *s*election and *a*mplification *t*echnology (r-SAT) assay. This assay takes advantage of the fact that the activation of several different classes of receptors can cause cellular proliferation. If genes for such receptors are linked with a reporter gene, such as

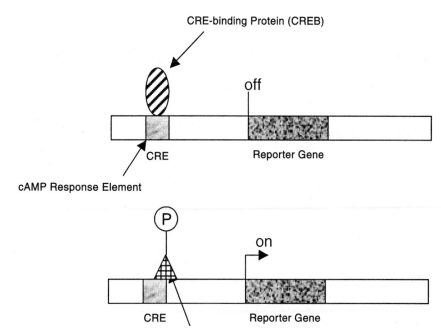

Figure 6–10 ■ Activation of transcription by a cAMP response element (CRE). CREB is phosphorylated by cAMP-dependent protein kinase.

β-galactosidase, the activity of the reporter will be increased as the number of cells increase as a consequence of receptor activation. Initially, a limitation of this assay was that it only worked with receptors that normally coupled to cellular proliferation; by making a mutation in one of the second-messenger proteins involved with the proliferative response, however, it was possible to get additional receptors to work in this assay. This second-messenger protein, G_q, was cloned, and a recombinant chimera was made that included part of another second messenger known as G_i. In native cells, receptors that activate G_i are not known for their stimulation of cell proliferation, but when such receptors are coexpressed in the r-SAT assay with the chimeric G_q, their activity can be measured.

A similar strategy involving chimeric proteins has been used for receptors whose second-messenger signaling pathways are not clearly understood. For example, the development of potential therapeutic agents acting on the human growth hormone receptor has been difficult because of a lack of a good signaling assay. The functional activity of other receptors that are structurally and functionally related to the growth hormone receptor can be measured, however, in a cell proliferation assay. One such receptor that has been cloned is the murine receptor for granulocyte colony-stimulating factor (G-CSF). By making a recombinant chimeric receptor containing the ligand-binding domain of the human growth hormone receptor with the second-messenger–coupling domain of the murein G-CSF receptor, it was possible to stimulate cellular proliferation with human growth hormone.

In addition to providing a useful pharmacological screen for human growth hormone analogues, the construction of this chimeric receptor provides considerable insight into the mechanism of agonist-induced growth hormone receptor activation. The growth hormone–binding domain is clearly localized to the extracellular amino terminus of the receptor, while the transmembrane and intracellular domains are implicated in the signal transduction process. It was also determined that successful signal transduction required receptor dimerization by the agonist (i.e., simultaneous interaction of two receptor molecules with one molecule of growth hormone). On the basis of this information, a mechanism-based strategy was used for the design of potential antagonists. Thus, human growth hormone analogues were prepared that were incapable of producing receptor dimerization and were found to be potent antagonists.

PROCESSING OF THE RECOMBINANT PROTEIN

Processing the fermentation contents to isolate a recombinant protein is often a difficult operation, requiring as much art as science. In the fermentation broth are whole bacterial cells, lysed cells, cellular fragments, nucleotides, normal bacterial proteins, the recombinant protein, and particulate medium components. If a Gram-negative bacterium such as *E. coli* has been used, lipopolysaccharide endotoxins (pyrogens) may be present. When animal cell cultures are used, it is commonly assumed that virus particles may be present. Viruses can also be introduced by the culture nutrients, gen-

erated by an infected cell line, or introduced by animal serum. Purification of a rDNA protein while maintaining the factors that keep it in its active three-dimensional conformation from this mixture may be difficult because each step must be designed to ensure that the protein remains intact and pharmacologically active. Assays must be designed that allow the activity of the protein to be assessed at each purification step. Consequently, the structure and activity of the recombinant protein must be considered at all stages of purification, and assays must be conducted to measure the amount of purified, intact protein.

A general scheme for purification of a rDNA protein is as follows:[95]

- *Particulate removal.* Particulates may be removed by centrifugation, filtration, ultrafiltration, and tangential flow filtration. Virus particles may be inactivated by heating if the rDNA peptide can tolerate the procedure.
- *Concentration.* The volume of the mixture is reduced, which increases the concentration of the contents. Often, concentration is achievable by the filtration step, especially if ultrafiltration is used.
- *Initial purification.* The initial purification of the mixture is sometimes accomplished by precipitation of the proteins, using a slow, stepwise increase of the ionic strength of the solution (salting out). Ammonium sulfate is a typical salt that can be used in cold, aqueous solutions. Water-miscible organic solvents such as trichloroacetic acid and polyethylene glycol change the dielectric constant of the solution and also effect precipitation of proteins.
- *Intermediate purification.* In this stage, the proteins may be dialyzed against water to remove salts that were used in the precipitation step. Ion exchange chromatography is used to effect a somewhat crude separation of the proteins based on their behavior in a pH or salt gradient on the resin. Another step that may be taken is size exclusion (gel filtration) chromatography. Gels of appropriate molecular weight cutoffs can yield a somewhat low-resolution separation of proteins of a desired molecular weight. If a native bacterial protein that has been carried this far is nearly the same molecular weight as the rDNA protein, no separation will occur.
- *Final purification.* Final purification usually involves the use of high-resolution chromatography, typically high-performance liquid chromatography. An abundance of commercial stationary phases allows various types of adsorption chromatography (normal and reversed phase), ion exchange chromatography, immunoaffinity chromatography, hydrophobic interaction chromatography, and size exclusion chromatography. The protein fractions are simply collected when they elute from the column and are concentrated and assayed for activity.
- *Sterilization and formulation.* This step can be accomplished by ultrafiltration to remove pyrogens or by heating if the protein can withstand this. Formulation might involve reconstitution into stable solutions for administration or determining the optimum conditions for stability when submitting for clinical trials.

Complicating factors include *(a)* proteins unfolding into an inactive conformation during processing (it may not be possible to refold the protein correctly) and *(b)* proteases that are commonly produced by bacterial, yeast, and mammalian cells, which may partially degrade the protein.

PHARMACEUTICS OF RECOMBINANT DNA (rDNA)-PRODUCED AGENTS

rDNA methods have facilitated the production of very pure, therapeutically useful proteins. The physicochemical and pharmaceutical properties of these agents are those of proteins, which means that pharmacists must understand the chemistry (and the chemistry of instability) of proteins to store, handle, dispense, reconstitute, and administer these protein drugs. Instabilities among proteins may be physical or chemical. In the former case, the protein might stick to glass vessels or flocculate, altering the dose that the patient will receive. In the latter case, chemical reactions taking place on the protein may alter the type or stereochemistry of the amino acids, change the position of disulfide bonds, cleave the peptide chains themselves, and alter the charge distribution of the protein. Any of these can cause unfolding (denaturation) of the protein and loss of activity, rendering the molecule useless as a drug. Chemical instability can be a problem during the purification stages of a protein, when the molecule might be subjected to acids or bases, but instability could occur at the point of administration when, for example, a lyophilized protein is reconstituted. The pharmacist must understand a few concepts of the chemical and physical instability of proteins to predict and handle potential problems.

Chemical Instability of Proteins[67]

See Figure 6-11.

- *Hydrolysis*. Hydrolytic reactions of the peptide bonds can break the polymer chain. Aspartate residues hydrolyze 100 times faster in dilute acids than do other amino acids under the same conditions. As a general rule of peptide hydrolysis, Asp-Pro > Asp-X or X-Asp bonds. This property of Asp is probably due to an autocatalytic function of the Asp side chain carboxyl group. Asn, Asp, Gln, and Glu hydrolyze exceptionally easily if they occur next to Gly, Ser, Ala, and Pro. Within these groupings, Asn and Gln accelerate hydrolysis more at low pH, while Asp and Glu hydrolyze most readily at high pH, when the side chain carboxyl groups are ionized.
- *Deamidation*. Gln and Asn undergo hydrolytic reactions that deamidate their side chains. These reactions convert neutral amino acid residues into charged ones. Gln is converted to Glu and Asn to Asp. The amino acid type is changed, but the chain is not cleaved. This process is, effectively, primary sequence isomerization, and it may influence biological activity. The deamidation reaction of Asn residues is accelerated under neutral or alkaline pH conditions. A five-membered cyclic imide intermediate formed by intramolecular attack of the nitrogen atom on the carbonyl carbon of the Asn side chain is the accelerant. The cyclic imide spontaneously hydrolyzes to give a mixture of residues—the aspartyl peptide and an iso form.
- *Racemization*. Base-catalyzed racemization reactions can occur in any of the amino acids except glycine, which is achiral. Racemizations yield proteins with mixtures of L- and D-amino acid configurations. The reaction occurs following the abstraction of the α-hydrogen from the amino acid to form a carbanion. As should be expected, the stability of the carbanion controls the rate of the reaction. Asp, which undergoes racemization via a cyclic imide intermediate, racemizes 105 times faster than free Asn. By comparison, other amino acids

in a protein racemize about 2 to 4 times faster than their free counterparts.
- *β-Elimination*. Proteins containing Cys, Ser, Thr, Phe, and Lys undergo facile β-elimination in alkaline conditions that facilitate formation of an α carbanion.
- *Oxidation*. Oxidation can occur at the sulfur-containing amino acids Met and Cys and at the aromatic amino acids His, Trp, and Tyr. These reactions can occur during protein processing as well as in storage. Methionine (CH_3-S-R) is oxidizable at low pH by hydrogen peroxide or molecular oxygen to yield a sulfoxide (R-SO-CH_3) and a sulfone (R-SO_2-CH_3). The thiol group of Cys (R-SH) can undergo successive oxidation to the corresponding sulfenic acid (R-SOH), disulfide (R-S-S-R), sulfinic acid (R-SO_2H), and sulfonic acid (R-SO_3H). A number of factors, including pH, influence these reactions. Free –SH groups can be converted into disulfide bonds (-S-S-) and vice versa. In the phenomenon of disulfide exchange, disulfide bonds break and reform in different positions, causing incorrect folding of the protein. Major changes in the three-dimensional structure of the peptide can abolish activity. Oxidation of the aromatic rings of His, Trp, and Tyr residues is believed to occur with a variety of oxidizing enzymes.

Physical Instability of Proteins[96]

Chemical alterations are not the only source of protein instability. A protein is a large, globular polymer that exists in some specific forms of secondary, tertiary, and quaternary structure. A protein is not a fixed, rigid structure. The molecule is in dynamic motion, and the structure samples an array of three-dimensional space. During this motion, noncovalent intramolecular bonds can break, reform, and break again, but the overall shape remains centered around an energy minimum that represents the most likely (and pharmacologically active) conformer of the molecule. Any major change in the conformation can abolish the activity of the protein. Small drug molecules do not demonstrate this problem. A globular protein normally folds so that the hydrophobic groups are directed to the inside and the hydrophilic groups are directed to the outside. This arrangement facilitates the water solubility of the protein. If the normal protein unfolds, it can refold to yield changes in hydrogen bonding, charge, and hydrophobic effects. The protein loses its globular structure, and the hydrophobic groups can be repositioned to the outside. The unfolded protein can subsequently undergo further physical interactions. The loss of the globular structure of a protein is referred to as *denaturation*.

Denaturation is, by far, the most widely studied aspect of protein instability. In the process, the three-dimensional folding of the native molecule is disrupted at the tertiary and, possibly, the secondary structure level. When a protein denatures, physical structure rather than chemical composition changes. The normally globular protein unfolds, exposing hydrophobic residues and abolishing the native three-dimensional structure. Factors that affect the denaturation of proteins are temperature, pH, ionic strength of the medium, inclusion of organic solutes (urea, guanidine salts, acetamide, and formamide), and the presence of organic solvents such as alcohols or acetone. Denaturation can be reversible or irreversible. If the denatured protein can regain its native form when the denaturant is removed by dialysis, reversible denaturation will occur. Denatured proteins are generally insoluble in water, lack biological activity, and become sus-

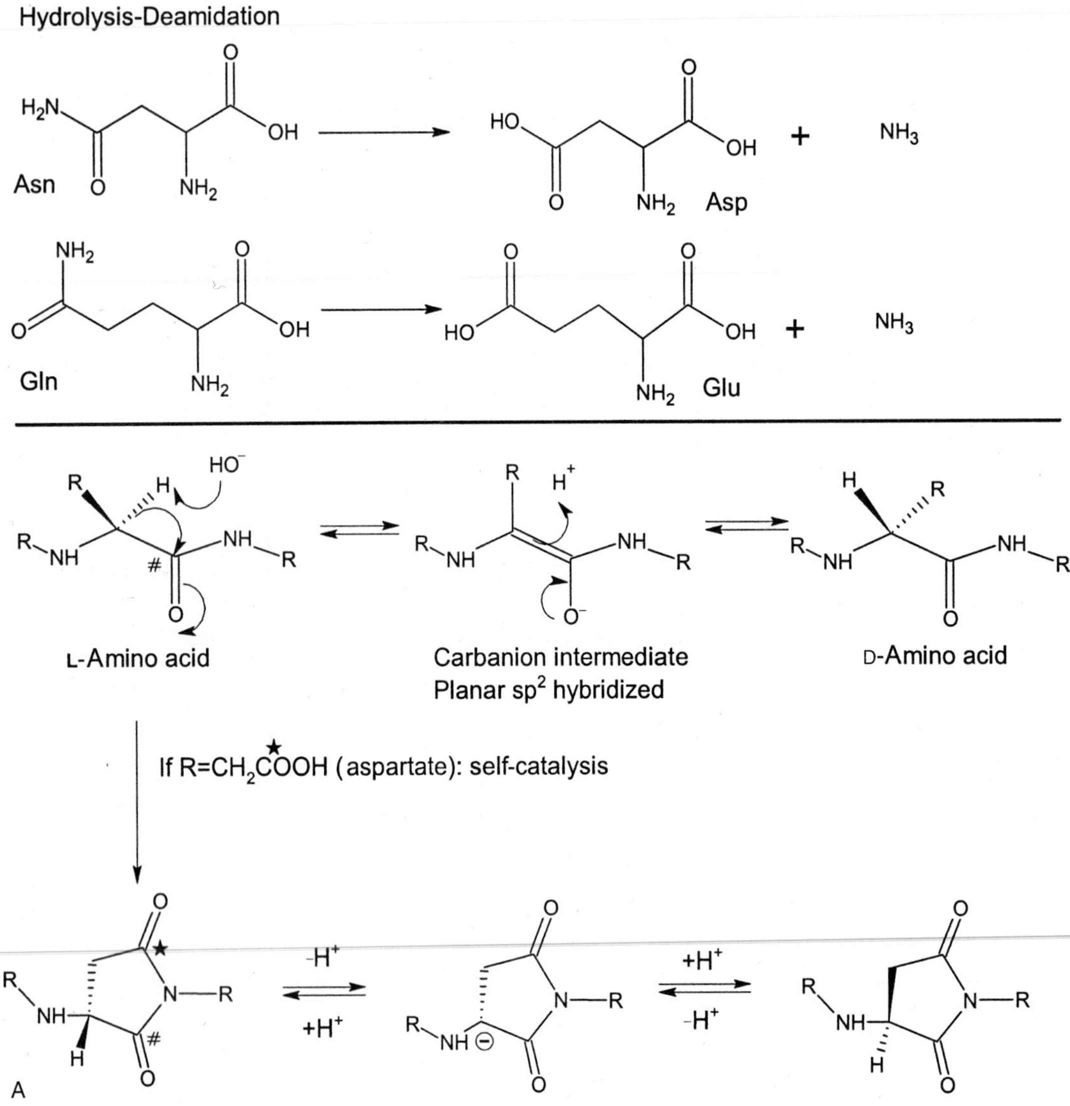
Hydrolysis-Deamidation
Asn
Asp
NH3
Gln
Glu
NH3
L-Amino acid
Carbanion intermediate
Planar sp2 hybridized
D-Amino acid
If R=CH2COOH (aspartate): self-catalysis
-H+
+H+
+H+
-H+
A

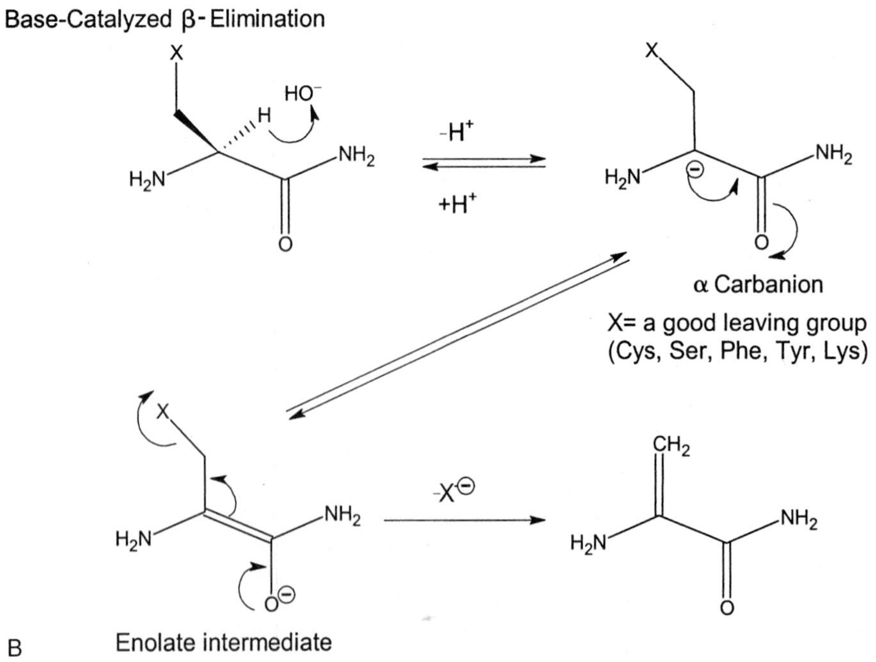
Base-Catalyzed β-Elimination
-H+
+H+
α Carbanion
X= a good leaving group
(Cys, Ser, Phe, Tyr, Lys)
-X⊖
Enolate intermediate
B

Figure 6–11 ▪ **A.** Protein decomposition reactions. **B.** β-Elimination.

ceptible to enzymatic hydrolysis. The air–water interface presents a hydrophobic surface that can facilitate protein denaturation. Interfaces like these are commonly encountered in drug delivery devices and intravenous (IV) bags.

Surface adsorption of proteins is characterized by adhesion of the protein to surfaces, such as the walls of the containers of the dosage form and drug delivery devices, ampuls, and IV tubing. Proteins can adhere to glass, plastics, rubber, polyethylene, and polyvinylchloride. This phenomenon is referred to as *flocculation*. The internal surfaces of intravenous delivery pumps and IV delivery bags pose particular problems of this kind. Flocculated proteins cannot be dosed properly.

Aggregation results when protein molecules, in aqueous solution, self-associate to form dimers, trimers, tetramers, hexamers, and large macromolecular aggregates. Self-association depends on the pH of the medium as well as solvent composition, ionic strength, and dielectric properties. Moderate amounts of denaturants (below the concentration that would cause denaturation) may also cause protein aggregation. Partially unfolded intermediates have a tendency to aggregate. Concentrated protein solutions, such as an immunoglobulin for injection, may aggregate with storage time on the shelf. The presence of particulates in the preparation is the pharmacist's clue that the antibody solution is defective.

Precipitation usually occurs along with denaturation. Detailed investigations have been conducted with insulin, which forms a finely divided precipitate on the walls of an infusion device or its dosage form container. It is believed that insulin undergoes denaturation at the air–water interface, facilitating the precipitation process. The concentration of zinc ion, pH, and the presence of adjuvants such as protamine also affect the precipitation reaction of insulin.

Immunogenicity of Biotechnologically Produced Drugs[97, 98]

Proteins by their very nature are antigens. A human protein, innocuous at its typical physiological concentration, may exhibit completely different immunogenic properties when administered in the higher concentration that would be used as a drug. Unless a biotechnology-derived protein is engineered to be 100% complementary to the human form, it will differ among several major epitopes. The protein may have modifications of its amino acid sequence (substitutions of one amino acid for another). There may be additions or deletions of amino acids, N-terminal methionyl groups, incorrect or abnormal folding patterns, or oxidation of a sulfur-containing side chain of a methionine or a cysteine. Additionally, when a protein has been produced by using a bacterial vector, a finite amount of immunoreactive material may pass into the final product. All of these listed items contribute to the antigenicity of a biotechnologically produced protein. When it is administered to a human patient, the host's immune system will react to the protein just as it would to a microbial attack and neutralize it. This is why research has been undertaken to create 100% human protein drugs, such as insulin, which patients will need to take for a long time. In addition, some of the most promising biotechnology products, the monoclonal antibodies, are produced in mice by use of *humanized* genes to avoid human reaction to the mouse antibody.

DELIVERY AND PHARMACOKINETICS OF BIOTECHNOLOGY PRODUCTS[99]

As with any drug class, the medicinal chemist and pharmacist must be concerned with the absorption, distribution, metabolism, and excretion (ADME) parameters of protein drugs. Biotechnology-produced drugs add complexities that are not encountered with "traditional" low-molecular-weight drug molecules. ADME parameters are necessary to compute pharmacokinetic and pharmacodynamic parameters for a given protein. As for any drug, these parameters are essential in calculating the optimum dose for a given response, determining how often to administer the drug to obtain a steady state, and adjusting the dose to obtain the best possible residence time at the receptor (pharmacodynamic parameters).

Delivery of drugs with the molecular weights and properties of proteins into the human body is a complex task. The oral route cannot be used with a protein because the acidity of the stomach will catalyze its hydrolysis unless the drug is enteric coated. Peptide bonds are chemically labile, and proteolytic enzymes that are present throughout the body can attack and destroy protein drugs. Hydrolysis and peptidase decomposition also occur during membrane transport through the vascular endothelium, at the site of administration, and at sites of reaction in the liver, blood, kidneys, and most tissues and fluids of the body. It is possible to circumvent these enzymes by saturating them with high concentrations of drug or by coadministering peptidase inhibitors. Oxidative metabolism of aromatic rings and sulfur oxidation can also occur. Proteins typically decompose into small fragments that are readily hydrolyzed, and the individual amino acids are assimilated into new peptides. A potentially serious hindrance to a pharmacokinetic profile is the tendency of proteins administered as drugs to bind to plasma proteins such as serum albumin. If this happens, they enter a new biodistribution compartment from which they may slowly exit. Presently, the routes of administration that are available for protein drugs are largely subcutaneous and intramuscular. Much ongoing research is targeted at making peptide drugs more bioavailable. An example of this is conjugation of interleukin-2 with polyethylene glycol (PEG). These so-called pegylated proteins tend to have a slower elimination clearance and a longer $t_{1/2}$ than interleukin-2 alone. Another strategy being used is the installation of a prosthetic sugar moiety onto the peptide. The sugar moiety will adjust the partition coefficient of the drug, probably making it more water soluble.

RECOMBINANT DRUG PRODUCTS

Hormones

Human Insulin, Recombinant.[100–102]   Human insulin was the first pharmacologically active biological macromolecule to be produced through genetic engineering. The FDA approved the drug in 1982 for the treatment of type I (insulin-dependent) diabetes (see Chapter 25). The insulin protein is a two-chain polypeptide containing 51 amino acid residues. Chain A is composed of 21 amino acids, and chain B con-

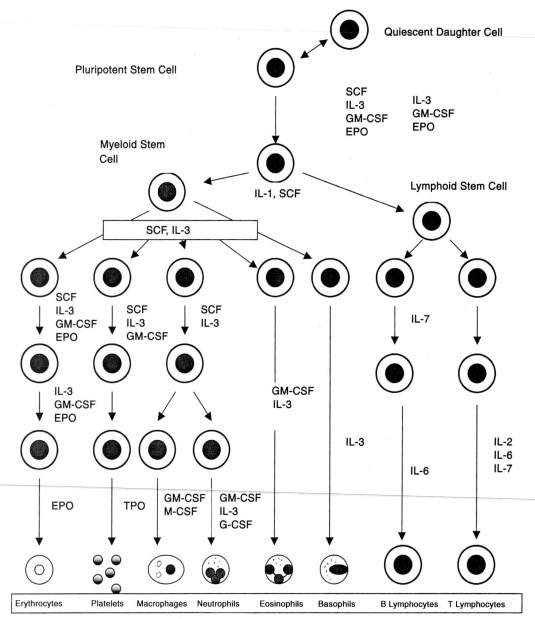

Figure 6–12 ■ Cytokine-mediated cascade leading to different blood cell types. *EPO,* erythropoietin; *G-CSF,* granulocyte colony-stimulating factor; *GM-CSF,* granulocyte-macrophage colony-stimulating factor; *IL-X,* interleukins; *M-CSF,* macrophage colony-stimulating factor; *SCF,* stem cell factor; *TPO,* thrombopoietin.

the kidney, and it activates the proliferation and differentiation of specially committed erythroid progenitors in the bone marrow. Epoetin alfa (Epogen) is a 165-amino acid glycoprotein that is manufactured in mammalian cells by rDNA technology. The protein is heavily glycosylated and has a molecular mass of approximately 30,400 Da. Erythropoietin is composed of four antiparallel α helices. The rDNA protein has the same amino acid sequence as natural erythropoietin.

Epoetin is indicated to treat anemia of chronic renal failure patients, anemia in zidovudine-treated HIV-infected patients, and in cancer patients taking chemotherapy. The results in these cases have been dramatic; most patients respond with a clinically significant increase in hematocrit.

Filgrastim.[114, 115] Filgrastim, granulocyte colony-stimulating factor (G-CSF), Neupogen, stimulates the proliferation of granulocytes (especially neutrophils) by mobilizing hematopoietic stem cells in the bone marrow. Endogenous G-CSF is a glycoprotein produced by monocytes, fibroblasts, and endothelial cells. G-CSF is a protein of 174 amino acids, with a molecular mass of approximately 18,800 Da. The native protein is glycosylated.

Filgrastim selectively stimulates proliferation and differentiation of neutrophil precursors in the bone marrow. This leads to the release of mature neutrophils into the circulation from the bone marrow. Filgrastim also affects mature neutrophils by enhancing phagocytic activity, priming the cellular metabolic pathways associated with the respiratory burst, enhancing antibody-dependent killing, and increasing the expression of some functions associated with cell surface antigens.

In patients receiving chemotherapy with drugs such as cyclophosphamide, doxorubicin, and etoposide, the incidence of neutropenia accompanied by fever is rather high. Administration of G-CSF reduces the time of neutrophil recovery and duration of fever in adults with acute myelogenous leukemia. The number of infections, days that antibiotics are required, and duration of hospitalization are also reduced.

Filgastrim[116] is identical with G-CSF in its amino acid sequence, except that it contains an N-terminal methionine that is necessary for expression of the vector in *E. coli*. The protein is not glycosylated. Filgrastim is supplied in a 0.01 M sodium acetate buffer containing 5% sorbitol and 0.004% polysorbate 80. It should be stored at 2 to 8°C without freezing. Under these conditions, the shelf life is 24 months. Avoid shaking when reconstituting; although the foaming will not harm the product, it may alter the amount of drug that is drawn into a syringe.

Sargramostim.[117, 118]

Sargramostim, granulocyte-macrophage colony-stimulating factor (GM-CSF), Leukine, is a glycoprotein of 127 amino acids, consisting of three molecular subunits of 19,500, 16,800, and 15,500 Da. The endogenous form of GM-CSF is produced by T lymphocytes, endothelial fibroblasts, and macrophages. Recombinant GM-CSF, produced in *S. cerevisiae*, differs from native human GM-CSF only by substitution of a leucine for an arginine at position 23. This substitution facilitates expression of the gene in the yeast. The site of glycosylation in the recombinant molecule may possibly differ from that of the native protein.

Sargramostim binds to specific receptors on target cells and induces proliferation, activation, and maturation. Administration to patients causes a dose-related increase in the peripheral white blood cell count. Unlike G-CSF, GM-CSF is a multilineage hematopoietic growth factor that induces partially committed progenitor cells to proliferate and differentiate along the granulocyte and the macrophage pathways. It also enhances the function of mature granulocytes and macrophages/monocytes. GM-CSF increases the chemotactic, antifungal, and antiparasitic activities of granulocytes and monocytes. It also increases the cytotoxicity of monocytes toward neoplastic cell lines and activates polymorphonuclear leukocytes to inhibit the growth of tumor cells.

Sargramostim is used to reconstitute the myeloid tissue after autologous bone marrow transplant and following chemotherapy in acute myelogenous leukemia. The preparation decreases the incidence of infection, decreases the number of days that antibiotics are required, and decreases the duration of hospital stays.

Sargramostim is supplied as a solution or powder (for solution). Both forms should be stored at 2 to 8°C without freezing. The liquid and powder have expiration dates of 24 months. The reconstituted powder and the aqueous solution should not be shaken.

Becaplermin.[119]

Becaplermin, Regranex Gel, an endogenous polypeptide that is released from cells that are involved in the healing process, is a recombinant human platelet-derived growth factor (r-hPDGF-BB). The "BB" signifies that becaplermin is the homodimer of the B chain.

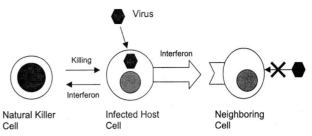

Figure 6–13 ■ Antiviral mechanism of action of the interferons.

Becaplermin is produced by a recombinant strain of *S. cerevisiae* containing the gene for the B chain of PDGF. The protein has a molecular mass of approximately 25 kDa and is a homodimer composed of two identical polypeptide chains that are linked by disulfide bonds. It is a growth factor that activates cell proliferation, differentiation, and function, and it is released from cells involved in the healing process.

Becaplermin is formulated as a gel recommended for topical use in the treatment of ulcerations of the skin secondary to diabetes.

Interferons

The interferons are a family of small proteins or glycoproteins of molecular masses ranging from 15,000 to 25,000 Da and 145 to 166 amino acids long. Eukaryotic cells secrete interferons in response to viral infection. Their mechanism of action is bimodal. The immediate effect is the recruitment of natural killer (NK) cells to kill the host cell harboring the virus (Fig. 6-13). Interferons then induce a state of viral resistance in cells in the immediate vicinity, preventing spread of the virus. Additionally, interferons induce a cascade of antiviral proteins from the target cell, one of which is 2′,5′-oligoadenylate synthetase. This enzyme catalyzes the conversion of ATP into 2′,5′-oligoadenylate, which activates ribonuclease R, hydrolyzing viral RNA. Interferons can be defined as cytokines that mediate antiviral, antiproliferative, and immunomodulatory activities.

Three classes of interferon (IFN) have been characterized: α (alpha), β (beta), and γ (gamma) (see Table 6-6). α-Interferons are glycoproteins derived from human leukocytes. β-Interferons are glycoproteins derived from fibroblasts and macrophages. They share a receptor with α-interferons. γ-Interferons are glycoproteins derived from human T lympho-

TABLE 6–6 Interferons Used Therapeutically

Interferon Type	Endogenous Source	Available Drug Products
Alpha	Leukocytes	Interferon alfa-2a
		Interferon alfa-2b
		Interferon alfa-2c
Beta	Fibroblasts, macrophages	Beta-1a
		Beta-1b
Gamma	T Lymphocytes, natural killer cells	Gamma-1b

TABLE 6–7   Summary of the α-Interferons

	Interferon Alfa-2a	Interferon Alfa-2b	Interferon Alfa-n1	Interferon Alfa-n3	Interferon Alfacon-1
Trade name	Roferon A	Intron A	Wellferon	Alferon N	Infergen
Dosage form	Solution, powder	Solution, powder	Solution	Solution	Solution
Solvent	Sodium chloride, excipients	Buffered saline	Buffered saline	Buffered saline	Phosphate-buffered saline
Indications	Hairy cell leukemia, AIDS-related Kaposi's sarcoma, chronic hepatitis C	Hairy cell leukemia, AIDS-related Kaposi's sarcoma, condylomata acuminata, chronic hepatitis B, chronic hepatitis C	Chronic hepatitis C	Condylomata acuminata	Chronic hepatitis C
Routes[a]	SC, IM, IV, infusion or intralesional	SC, IM, IV, infusion or intralesional	SC or IM	Intralesional	SC
Source	*E. coli*	*E. coli*	Human lymphoblastoid cell line	Human leukocytes	*E. coli*

[a] SC, subcutaneously; IM, intramuscularly; IV, intravenously.

cytes and NK cells. These interferons are acid labile and used to be called "type 2 interferon." The receptor for IFN-γ is smaller than that for IFN-α and IFN-β, 90 to 95 kDa versus 95 to 110 kDa, respectively. The three classes are not homogeneous, and each may contain several different molecular species. For example, at least 18 genetically and molecularly distinct human α-interferons have been identified, each differing in the amino acid substitution at positions 23 and 34. Interferons alfa-2a, alfa-2b, and alfa-2c have been purified and are either in clinical use or in development. A listing of commercially available α-interferons is given in Table 6-7.

As a class, the interferons possess some common side effects. These are flu-like symptoms, headache, fever, muscle aches, back pain, chills, nausea and vomiting, and diarrhea. At the injection site, pain, edema, hemorrhage, and inflammation are common. Dizziness is also commonly reported.

For the pharmacist, when predicting drug interactions with the interferons, cytochrome P-450 metabolism should always be a key consideration. Most of the interferons inhibit cytochrome P-450, causing drugs that are metabolized by this route to reach higher-than-normal and, possibly, toxic concentrations in the blood and tissues.

PRODUCTS: α-INTERFERONS

Interferon Alfa-2a (Recombinant).[120]

Interferon alfa-2a (recombinant), Roferon A, is expressed in an *E. coli* system and purified by using high-affinity mouse monoclonal antibody chromatography. The protein consists of 165 amino acids with a molecular mass of approximately 19,000 Da. and contains lysine at position 23 and histidine at position 34.

Interferon alfa-2a is used in the treatment of hairy cell leukemia and AIDS-related Kaposi's sarcoma in selected patients over 18 years of age. It is also used to treat chronic hepatitis C, and in patients with this disease, interferon alfa-2a can normalize serum alanine aminotransferase (ALT) levels, improve liver histology, and decrease viral load. The drug has a direct antiproliferative activity against tumor

cells. Modulation of the host immune response probably plays a role in the antitumor activity of interferon alfa-2a.

The interferon is supplied as a solution or as a powder for solution. The solution contains 0.72% NaCl. The powder contains 0.9% NaCl, 0.17% human serum albumin, and 0.33% phenol. The interferon vials, if properly stored at 2 to 8°C without freezing, expire in 30 months. Prefilled syringes expire in 24 months. The solutions should not be shaken because the albumin will cause frothing.

Pegylated Interferon Alfa-2a.[121]

Pegylated interferon alfa-2a, Pegasys, is a covalent conjugate of recombinant interferon alfa-2a (approximate molecular mass, 20 kDa) with a singly-branched bis-monomethoxypolyethylene glycol (PEG) chain (approximate molecular mass, 40 kDa). The PEG moiety is linked at a single site to the interferon alfa moiety by a stable amide bond to lysine. Peginterferon alfa-2a has an approximate molecular mass of 60 kDa. Pegasys provides sustained therapeutic serum levels for up to a full week (168 hours). The drug is approved for the treatment of adults with chronic hepatitis C who have compensated liver disease and who have not been previously treated with interferon alfa. Efficacy has also been demonstrated in patients with compensated cirrhosis.

Interferon Alfa-2b (Recombinant).[122]

Interferon alfa-2b, Intron A, a water-soluble protein of 165 amino acids and an approximate molecular mass of 19,200 Da, is expressed from a recombinant strain of *E. coli*. This interferon molecule possesses an arginine at position 23 and a histidine at position 34.

Interferon alfa-2b is a broad-spectrum agent. It is indicated for hairy cell leukemia, condyloma acuminata (genital or venereal warts), AIDS-related Kaposi's sarcoma, and chronic hepatitis B and C infections.

Intron A can be administered by the SC, IM, or IV routes, by infusion or by intralesional routes. The dose is 1 to 35 million IU/day, depending on the application. The drug is supplied as a solution or as a powder for solution, and both forms contain albumin, glycine, and sodium phosphate buffer. Hence, they should not be shaken. Vials of solution should be stored at 2 to 8°C without freezing. The powder is stable for 18 months at room temperature or 7 days at 45°C.

Interferon Alfa-n1.[123]

Interferon alfa-n1, Wellferon, is a mixture of α-interferons isolated from a human lymphoblastoid cell line after induction with mouse parainfluenza virus type 1 (Sendai strain). Each of the subtypes of IFN-α in this product consists of 165 or 166 amino acids with an average molecular mass of 26,000 Da. The product is a mixture of each of the nine predominant subtypes of IFN-α.

Interferon alfa-n1 is indicated to treat chronic hepatitis C in patients 18 years of age or older who have no decompensated liver disease. The exact mechanism of action for interferon alfa-n1 in the treatment of this disease has not been elucidated.

This drug may be administered SC or IM, with a usual dose of 3 million IU 3 times per week. Interferon alfa-n1 is supplied as a solution containing tromethamine and buffered saline with human albumin as a stabilizer. Hence, the solution should not be shaken. The solution should be stored at 2 to 8°C without freezing, and should be discarded if freezing occurs. Properly stored solution expires in 24 months.

Interferon Alfa-n3.[124]

Interferon alfa-n3, Alferon N, is an α-interferon expressed from human leukocytes that are antigen-stimulated with avian Sendai virus. The Sendai virus is propagated in chicken eggs. The protein consists of at least 14 molecular subtypes. The average chain length is 166 amino acids, and the molecular mass range is 16,000 to 27,000 Da. The polydisperse interferon alfa-n3 is extremely pure because it is processed by affinity chromatography over a bed of mouse monoclonal antibodies specifically raised for the protein.

Interferon alfa-n3 is indicated for intralesional treatment of refractory or recurrent condyloma acuminata (genital warts) in patients 18 years of age or older. These warts are associated with human papilloma virus (HPV). Interferon alfa-n3 is especially useful in patients who haven't responded well to other modalities (podophyllin resin, surgery, laser, or cryotherapy). Interferon alfa-n3 is also being investigated for the treatment of non-Hodgkin's lymphoma, herpes simplex, rhinovirus, vaccinia, and varicella zoster. A usual dose in condyloma acuminata is 250,000 IU/wart, injected with a 30-gauge needle around the base of the lesion.

Interferon alfa-n3 is contraindicated in persons sensitive to mouse immunoglobulin G, egg protein, and neomycin.

Interferon alfa-n3 is supplied as a solution with the protein in phosphate-buffered saline with phenol as a preservative. The solution should be stored at 2 to 8°C without freezing. Properly stored solution expires at 18 months.

Interferon Alfacon-1 (Recombinant).

Interferon alfacon-1 (recombinant), Infergen,[125] is a "consensus" interferon that shares structural elements of IFN-α and several subtypes. The range of activity is about the same as the other alpha species, but the specific activity is greater.

The 166-amino acid sequence of alfacon-1 is synthetic. It was developed by comparing several natural IFN-α subtypes and assigning the *most common* amino acid to each variable position. Additionally, four amino acid changes were made to facilitate synthesis. The DNA sequence is also constructed by chemical synthesis. Interferon alfacon-1 differs from interferon alfa-n2 at 20/166 amino acids, yielding 88% homology. The protein has a molecular mass of approximately 19,400 Da.

Interferon alfacon-1 is used in the treatment of chronic hepatitis C virus infection in patients 18 years of age or older with compensated liver disease and who have anti-HCV serum antibodies or HCV RNA.

The drug is administered by the subcutaneous route in a dose of 9 μg 3 times per week. Interferon alfacon-1 is supplied as a solution in phosphate-buffered saline. It should be stored at 2 to 8°C without freezing. Avoid shaking the solution.

PRODUCTS: β-INTERFERONS

A listing of two commercially available IFN-βs is given in Table 6-8.

Interferon Beta-1a (Recombinant).[126]

Interferon beta-1a (recombinant), Avonex, is a glycoprotein with 166 amino acids. It has a molecular mass of approximately 22,000 Da. The site of glycosylation is at the asparagine residue at position 80. Interferon beta-1a possesses a cysteine residue at position 17, as does the native molecule. Natural IFN-β and interferon beta-1a are glycosylated, with each containing a single carbohydrate moiety. The overall complex has 89% protein and 11% carbohydrate by weight. Recombinant interferon beta-1a is expressed in CHO cells containing the recombinant gene for human IFN-β and is equivalent to the human form secreted by fibroblasts.

Interferon beta-1a is indicated for the treatment of relapsing forms of multiple sclerosis. Patients treated with interferon beta-1a demonstrate a slower progression to disability and a less noticeable breakdown of the blood–brain barrier

TABLE 6–8 *β*-Interferons

	Interferon Beta-1a (Avonex)	Interferon Beta-1b (Betaseron)
Recombinant system	CHO cells	*Escherichia coli*
Type	Asn$_{80}$ complex carbohydrate	Not glycosylated
Concentration	30 μg or 6 million IU/mL	250 μg or 8 million IU/mL
Supplied form	Powder for reconstitution	Powder for reconstitution
Diluent	Sterile water–no preservatives	NaCl 0.54% without preservatives
Storage	2–8°C; do not freeze	2–8°C; do not freeze
Dosage	30 μg once a week	250 μg every other day
Route	Intramuscular	Subcutaneous
Notable side effects	Injection site reactions, 3%; no necrosis	Injection site reactions, 85%; necrosis, 5%

as observed in gadolinium-enhanced magnetic resonance imaging (MRI).

Although the exact mechanism of action of interferon beta-1a in multiple sclerosis has not been elucidated, it is known that the drug exerts its biological effects by binding to specific receptors on the surface of human cells. This binding initiates a cascade of intracellular events that lead to the expression of interferon-induced gene products. These include 2′,5′-oligoadenylate synthetase and β_2 microglobulin. These products have been measured in the serum and in cellular fractions of blood collected from patients treated with interferon beta-1a. The functionally specific interferon-induced proteins have not been defined for multiple sclerosis.

Adverse effects include a flu-like syndrome at the start of therapy that decreases in severity as treatment progresses. Interferon beta-1a is a potential abortifacient and an inhibitor of cytochrome P-450.

The dosage form is a powder for solution that is reconstituted in sterile water. Excipients are human albumin, sodium chloride, and phosphate buffer. The solution can be stored at 2 to 8°C and should be discarded if it freezes. The lyophilized powder expires in 15 months. After reconstitution, the solution should be used within 6 hours. The solution should not be shaken because of the albumin content.

Interferon Beta-1b (Recombinant).[127]

Interferon beta-1b, Betaseron, is a protein that is expressed in a recombinant *E. coli*. It is equivalent in type to the interferon that is expressed by human fibroblasts. Interferon beta-1b possesses 165 amino acids and has an approximate molecular mass of 18.5 kDa. The native form has 166 amino acids and weighs 23 kDa. Interferon beta-1b contains a serine residue at position 17 rather than the cysteine in native IFN-β and does not contain the complex carbohydrate side chains found in the natural molecule. In addition to its antiviral activity, interferon beta-1b possesses immunomodulating activity.

Interferon beta-1b is administered SC to decrease the frequency of clinical exacerbation in ambulatory patients with relapsing–remitting multiple sclerosis (RRMS). RRMS is characterized by unpredictable attacks resulting in neurological deficits, separated by variable periods of remission.

Although it is not possible to delineate the mechanisms by which interferon beta-1b exerts its activity in MS, it is known that the interferon binds to specific receptors on cell surfaces and induces the expression of a number of interferon-induced gene products, such as 2′,5′-oligoadenylate synthetase and protein kinase. Additionally, interferon beta-1b blocks the synthesis of INF-γ, which is believed to be involved in MS attacks.

Interferon beta-1b is supplied as powder for solution with albumin and/or dextrose as excipients. It should be stored at 2 to 8°C without freezing. After reconstitution the solution can be stored in the refrigerator for 3 hours. The solution should not be shaken.

A major difference between interferon beta-1a and beta-1b is that beta-1b causes more hemorrhage and necrosis at the injection site than does interferon beta-1a.

PRODUCTS: γ-INTERFERON

Interferon Gamma-1b (Recombinant).[128]

Interferon gamma-1b, Actimmune, is a recombinant protein expressed in *E. coli*. IFN-γ is the cytokine that is secreted by human T lymphocytes and NK cells. It is a single-chain glycoprotein composed of 140 amino acids. The crystal structure of the protein reveals several helical segments arranged to approximate a toric shape.

Interferon gamma-1b is indicated for reducing the frequency and severity of serious infections associated with chronic granulomatous disease, an inherited disorder characterized by deficient phagocyte oxidase activity. In this disease, macrophages try to respond to invading organisms but lack the key oxidative enzymes to dispose of them. To compensate, additional macrophages are recruited into the infected region and form a granulomatous structure around the site. IFN-γ can stimulate the oxidative burst in macrophages and may reverse the situation.

Interferon gamma-1b is supplied as a solution in sterile water for injection. The solution must be stored at 2 to 8°C, without freezing. The product cannot tolerate more than 12 hours at room temperature.

THE INTERLEUKINS

Aldesleukin.[129]

Aldesleukin, T-cell growth factor, thymocyte-stimulating factor, Proleukin, is recombinant interleukin-2 (IL-2) expressed in an engineered strain of *E. coli* containing an analogue of the human IL-2 gene. The recombinant product is a highly purified protein of 133 amino acids with an approximate molecular mass of 15,300 Da. Unlike native IL-2, aldesleukin is not glycosylated, has no N-terminal alanine, and has serine substituted for Cys at site 125. Aldesleukin exists in solution as biologically active, non-covalently bound microaggregates with an average size of 27 IL-2 molecules. This contrasts with traditional solution aggregates of proteins, which often form irreversibly bound structures that are biologically inactive.

Aldesleukin enhances lymphocyte mitogenesis and stimulates long-term growth of human IL-2-dependent cell lines. IL-2 also enhances the cytotoxicity of lymphocytes. Induction of NK cell and lymphocyte-activated killer (LAK) cell activity occurs, as does induction of production. In mouse and human tumor cell lines, aldesleukin activates cellular immunity in patients with profound lymphocytosis, eosinophilia, and thrombocytopenia. Aldesleukin also activates the production of cytokines, including tumor necrosis factor (TNF), IL-1, and IFN-γ. In vivo experiments in mouse tumor models have shown inhibition of tumor growth. The mechanism of the antitumor effect of aldesleukin is unknown.

Aldesleukin is indicated for the treatment of metastatic renal cell carcinoma in adults. It is also indicated for the treatment of metastatic melanoma in adults. Research is under way on the use of aldesleukin for the treatment of various cancers (including head and neck cancers), treatment of acute myelogenous leukemia, and adjunct therapy in the treatment of Kaposi's sarcoma. Renal and hepatic function is typically impaired during therapy with aldesleukin, so interaction with other drugs that undergo elimination by these organs is possible.

Aldesleukin is supplied as a powder for solution. After reconstitution, the solution should not be shaken. The preparation is solubilized with sodium dodecyl sulfate in a phosphate buffer. Aldesleukin should be stored as nonreconstituted powder at 2 to 8°C and never frozen. Reconstituted vials can be frozen and thawed once in 7 days without loss of activity. It expires over a period of 18 months.

Denileukin Diftitox (Recombinant).[130]

Denileukin diftitox, recombinant, Ontak, is an example of a drug that acts like a Trojan horse. One part of the molecule is involved in recognition and binds selectively with the diseased cell, and a highly toxic second part of the molecule effects a kill. Denileukin diftitox is a fusion protein expressed by a recombinant strain of *E. coli*. It is a rDNA-derived cytotoxic protein composed of the amino acid sequences for diphtheria toxin fragments A and B (Met$_1$-Thr$_{387}$)-His, followed by the sequences for IL-2 (Ala$_1$-Thr$_{133}$). The fusion protein has a molecular mass of 58,000 Da. We can think of this large protein as a molecule of diphtheria toxin in which the receptor-binding domain has been replaced by IL-2 sequences, thereby changing its binding specificity. Cells that express the high-affinity (α,β,γ) IL-2 receptor bind the protein tightly. The IL-2 component is used as a director to bring the cytotoxic species in contact with tumor cells. The diphtheria toxin inhibits cellular protein synthesis and the cells die. Malignant cells in certain leukemias and lymphomas, including cutaneous T-cell lymphoma, express the high-affinity IL-2 receptor on their cell surfaces. It is these cells that denileukin diftitox targets.

Denileukin diftitox is indicated for the treatment of persistent or recurrent cutaneous T-cell lymphoma whose malignant cells express the CD25 component of the IL-2 receptor.

Denileukin diftitox is supplied as a frozen solution in water for injection. It should be stored at −10°C or colder. It is suggested that the vials be thawed in a refrigerator at 2 to 8°C for less than 24 hours or at room temperature for 1 to 2 hours. Prepared solutions should be used within 6 hours. The drug is administered by IV infusion from a bag or through a syringe pump.

Oprelvekin (Recombinant).[131, 132]

Oprelvekin, Neumega, is recombinant human IL-11 that is expressed in a recombinant strain of *E. coli* as a thioredoxin and/or rhIL-11 fusion protein. The fusion protein is cleaved and purified to obtain the rhIL-11 protein. The protein is 177 amino acids in length and has a mass of approximately 19,000 Da. Oprelvekin differs from the natural 178-amino acid IL-11 by lacking an N-terminal proline. This alteration has not resulted in differences in bioactivity either in vitro or in vivo.

IL-11 is a thrombopoietic growth factor. It directly stimulates the proliferation of hematopoietic stem cells as well as megakaryocyte progenitor cells. This process induces megakaryocyte maturation and increased production of platelets. The primary hematopoietic activity of oprelvekin is stimulation of megakaryocytopoiesis and thrombopoiesis. Primary osteoblasts and mature osteoclasts express mRNAs for both IL-11 and its receptor, IL-11R alpha. Hence, both bone-forming and bone-resorbing cells are possible targets for IL-11.

Oprelvekin is indicated for the prevention of severe thrombocytopenia. It reduces the need for platelet transfusions after myelosuppressive chemotherapy in patients with nonmyeloid malignancies who are at high risk for severe thrombocytopenia. Efficacy has been demonstrated in persons who have experienced severe thrombocytopenia following a previous chemotherapy cycle.

Oprelvekin causes many adverse reactions. Among these are edema, neutropenic fever, headache, nausea and/or vomiting, dyspnea, and tachycardia. Patients must be monitored closely.

Oprelvekin is supplied as a lyophilized powder for reconstitution. Excipients include glycine and phosphate buffer components. The powder has a shelf life of 24 months. It should be stored at 2 to 8°C. If it is frozen, thaw it before reconstitution.

Tumor Necrosis Factor (Recombinant).[133–135]

The TNFs (Etanercept, Enbrel) are members of a family of cytokines that are produced primarily in the innate immune system by activated mononuclear phagocytes. Along with IL-1, TNF is typically the first cytokine to be produced upon infection, and its reactions can be both positive and negative. On the one hand, TNF can cause cytotoxicity and inflammation, and on the other hand, it serves as a signal to the adaptive immune response. The TNFs are all endogenous pyrogens, and they cause chills, fever, and flu-like symptoms. There are two forms of TNF: TNF-α (cachectin) and TNF-β (lymphotoxin). Both bind to the same receptor and cause similar effects.

Etanercept is a dimeric fusion protein consisting of the extracellular ligand-binding portion of the human 75-kDa (p75) TNF receptor (TNFR) linked to the Fc portion of human isotype IgG$_1$. The Fc component of etanercept contains the CH$_2$ domain, the CH$_3$ domain, and the hinge region, but not the CH$_1$ domain of IgG$_1$. These regions are responsible for the biological effects of immunoglobulins. Etanercept is produced in recombinant CHO cultures. It consists of a peptide chain of 934 amino acids and has a molecular mass of approximately 150 kDa. It binds specifically to TNF and blocks its interaction with cell surface TNFRs. Each etanercept molecule binds specifically to two TNF molecules in the synovial fluid of rheumatoid arthritis patients. It is equally efficacious at blocking TNF-α and TNF-β. The drug is indicated for reducing signs and symptoms and inhibiting the progression of structural damage in patients with moderately to severely active rheumatoid arthritis. Etanercept is also indicated for reducing signs and symptoms of moderately to severely active polyarticular-course juvenile rheumatoid arthritis in patients 4 years of age and older who have had an inadequate response to one or more disease-modifying antirheumatic drugs (DMARDS). Etanercept is also indicated for reducing signs and symptoms of active arthritis in patients with psoriatic arthritis.

ENZYMES

Blood-Clotting Factors

The blood clotting system of the human body is typically in a carefully balanced homeostatic state. If damage occurs to a blood vessel wall, a clot will form to wall off the damage so that the process of regeneration can begin. Normally this process is highly localized to the damaged region, so that the hemostatic response does not cause thrombi to migrate to distant sites or persist longer than it is needed. Lysis of blood clots occurs through the conversion of plasminogen to plasmin, which causes fibrinolysis, converting insoluble fibrin to soluble fibrinopeptides. The plasminogen–plasmin conversion is catalyzed by several blood and tissue activators, among them urokinase, kallikrein, plasminogen activators, and some undefined inhibitors. More specifically, the conversion of plasminogen to plasmin is catalyzed by two extremely specific serine proteases: a urokinase plasminogen activator (uPA) and a tissue plasminogen activator (tPA). This section focuses on tPA.

Human tPA is a serine protease that is synthesized in the vascular endothelial cells. It is a single-chain peptide composed of 527 amino acids and has a molecular mass of approximately 64,000 Da. About 7% of the mass of the molecule consists of carbohydrate. The molecule contains 35 Cys residues. These are fully paired, giving the tPA molecule 17 disulfide bonds. There are four N-linked glycosylation sites recognized by consensus sequences Asn-X-Ser/Thr at residues 117, 184, 218, and 448. It is suspected that Thr_{61} bears an O-fucose residue. There are two forms of tPA that differ by the presence or absence of a carbohydrate group at Asp_{184}. Type I tPA is glycosylated at Asn_{117}, Asn_{184}, and Asn_{448}, while type II tPA lacks a glycosyl group at Asn_{184}. Asn_{218} is typically unsubstituted in both forms. Asn_{117} contains a high-mannose oligosaccharide, while Asn substituents 184 and 448 are complex carbohydrate substituted. During the process of fibrinolysis the single-chain protein is cleaved between Arg_{275} and Ile_{276} by plasmin to yield 2-chain tPA. Two-chain tPA consists of a heavy chain (the A chain, derived from the N terminus) and a light chain (B chain), linked by a single disulfide bond between Cys_{264} and Cys_{395}. The A chain bears some unique structural features: the finger region (residues 6 to 36), the growth factor region (approximate residues 44 to 80), and two kringle domains. These domains are disulfide-closed loops, mostly β sheet in structure. The finger and kringle 2 are responsible for tPA binding to fibrin and for the activation of plasminogen. The function of kringle 1 is not known. The B chain contains the serine protease domain that contains the His-Asp-Ser unit that cleaves plasminogen.

Tissue Plasminogen Activator, Recombinant.[136, 137]

tPA (recombinant), alteplase (Activase), is identical with endogenous tPA. rtPA lacks a glycosyl residue at Asn_{184}. At one time, rtPA was produced in two-chain form in CHO cultures. Now, large-scale cultures of recombinant human melanoma cells in fermenters are used to produce a product that is about 80% single-chain rtPA.

Alteplase is used to improve ventricular function following an acute myocardial infarction, including reducing the incidence of congestive heart failure and decreasing mortality. The drug is also used to treat acute ischemic stroke after computed tomography (CT) or other diagnostic imaging has ruled out intracranial hemorrhage. rtPA is also used in cases of acute pulmonary thromboembolism and is being investigated for unstable angina pectoris.

Alteplase is supplied as powder for injection, and in reconstituted form (normal saline or 5% dextrose in water) is intended for IV infusion only. The solution expires in 8 hours at room temperature and must be prepared just before use.

Reteplase.

Reteplase (Retavase) is a deletion mutant variant of tPA that is produced in recombinant *E. coli*. The deletions are in domains responsible for half-life, fibrin affinity, and thrombolytic potency. It consists of the kringle-2 domain and protease domain of tPA but lacks the kringle-1 domain and the growth factor domain. It is considered a third-generation thrombolytic agent and has a mechanism of action similar to that of alteplase. Reteplase acts directly by catalyzing the cleavage of plasminogen and initiating thrombolysis. It has high thrombolytic potency. A comparison of alteplase and reteplase is given in Table 6-9.

Tenecteplase.[137]

Tenecteplase is a tPA produced by recombinant CHO cells. The molecule is a 527-amino acid glycoprotein developed by introducing the following modifications to the cDNA construct: Thr_{103} to Asp, Asp_{117} to Gln, both within the kringle-1 domain, and a tetraalanine substitution at amino acids 296 to 299 in the protease domain. The drug is a sterile, lyophilized powder recommended for single intravenous bolus administration after reconstitution with sterile water. Tenecteplase should be administered immediately after reconstitution.

Factor VIII.[138]

Antihemophilic factor VIII (recombinant), Recombinate, Kogenate, Bioclate, Helixate, is a plasma protein that functions in the normal blood-clotting cascade by increasing the V_{max} for the activation of clotting factor X by factor IXa in the presence of calcium ions and negatively charged phospholipids. Factor VIII is used in the treatment of hemophilia A. Hemophilia A is a congenital disorder characterized by bleeding. The introduction of factor VIII as a drug has improved the quality of life and the life expectancy of individuals with this disorder. Unfortunately, it has been necessary to rely on an unsure source (human plasma) for the factor. Exposure of patients to alloantigens and viruses has been a concern. Factor VIII derived from a recombinant source will potentially eliminate many of these problems and provide an essentially unlimited supply of the drug.

Factor VIII is biosynthesized as a single-chain polypeptide of 2,332 amino acids. The protein is very heavily glycosylated. Shortly after biosynthesis, peptide cleavage occurs and plasma factor VIII circulates as an 80-kDa light chain associated with a series of heavy chains of approximately 210 kDa in a metal ion-stabilized complex. Factor VIII possesses 25 potential N-linked glycosylation sites and 22 Cys residues. The 210-kDa heavy chain is further cleaved by proteases to yield a series of proteins of molecular mass 90

TABLE 6–9 Comparison of the Pharmacokinetic Parameters of Alteplase and Reteplase

Pharmacokinetic Parameter	Alteplase	Reteplase
Effective $t_{1/2}$ (minutes)	5	13–16
Volume of distribution (L)	8.1	6
Plasma clearance (mL/min)	360–620	250–450

to 188 kDa. The 90- to 188-kDa protein molecules form a metal ion-stabilized complex with the light chain.

Recombinant factor VIII is produced in two recombinant systems: in batch culture of transfected CHO cells or in continuous culture of baby hamster kidney (BHK) cells. There are four types of recombinant factor VIII available. All four are produced by inserting a cDNA construct encoding the entire peptide sequence into the CHO cell or BHK cell line. The CHO cell product contains a $Gal\alpha[1\rightarrow3]Gal$ unit, whereas the BHK enzyme does not. Recombinant factor VIII is polydisperse, containing multiple peptide homologues including an 80-kDa protein and various modifications of an approximately 90-kDa subunit protein. The product contains no blood products and is free of microbes and pyrogens.

Recombinant factor VIII is indicated for the treatment of classical hemophilia (hemophilia A) and for the prevention and treatment of hemorrhagic episodes and perioperative management of patients with hemophilia A. The drug is also indicated for the treatment of hemophilia A in persons who possess inhibitors to factor VIII.

Recombinant factor VIII is supplied in sterile, single-dose vials. The product is stabilized with human albumin and lyophilized. The product must be stored at 2 to 8°C, without freezing. In some instances the powder may be stored at room temperature for up to 3 months without loss of biological activity. Shaking of the reconstituted product should be avoided because of the presence of the albumin. The drug must be administered by intravenous bolus or drip infusion within 3 hours of reconstitution.

Since trace amounts of mouse or hamster protein may copurify with recombinant factor VIII, one should be cautious when administering the drug to individuals with known hypersensitivity to plasma-derived antihemophilic factor or with hypersensitivity to biological preparations with trace amounts of mouse or hamster proteins.

Clotting Factor IX (Recombinant).[139, 140]

When a person is deficient in clotting factor IX (Christmas factor), hemophilia B results. Hemophilia B affects primarily males and accounts for about 15% of all cases of hemophilia. Treatment involves replacement of factor IX so that the blood will clot. Recombinant coagulation factor IX (BeneFix) is a highly purified protein produced in recombinant CHO cells, free of blood products. The product is a glycoprotein of molecular mass approximately 55,000 Da. It consists of 415 amino acids in a single chain. The primary amino acid sequence of BeneFix is identical with the Ala_{148} allelic form of plasma-derived factor IX, and it has structural and functional characteristics similar to those of the endogenous protein. The recombinant protein is purified by chromatography, followed by membrane filtration. SDS-polyacrylamide gel electrophoresis shows that the product exists primarily as a single component.

Clotting factor IX, recombinant, is indicated for the control and prevention of hemorrhagic episodes in persons with hemophilia B (Christmas' disease), including the control and prevention of bleeding in surgical procedures.

BeneFix is supplied as a sterile lyophilized powder. It should be stored at 2 to 8°C. The product will tolerate storage at room temperature not above 25°C for 6 months. The drug becomes unstable following reconstitution and must be used within 3 hours.

Drotrecogin Alfa.[141]

About 750,000 people are diagnosed with sepsis in the United States each year, and of these, an estimated 30% will die from it, despite treatment with intravenous antibiotics and supportive care. Patients with severe sepsis often experience failures of various systems in the body, including the circulatory system, the kidneys, and clotting. Drotrecogin alfa (activated), rotrecogin alfa (activated) (Xigris), is a recombinant form of human activated protein C. Activated protein C exerts an antithrombotic effect by inhibiting factors Va and VIIIa. In vitro data indicate that activated protein C has indirect profibrinolytic activity through its ability to inhibit plasminogen activator inhibitor-1 (PAI-1) and to limit generation of activated thrombin-activatable fibrinolysis inhibitor. Additionally, in vitro data indicate that activated protein C may exert an anti-inflammatory effect by inhibiting TNF production by monocytes, by blocking leukocyte adhesion to selectins, and by limiting the thrombin-induced inflammatory responses within the microvascular epithelium.

Vials of drotrecogin alfa should be stored at 2 to 8°C without freezing. The reconstituted solution is stable for 14 hours at 25°C.

Anticoagulant

Lepirudin, Recombinant.[142]

Leeches (*Hirudo medicinalis*) have been used medicinally for centuries to treat injuries in which blood engorges the tissues. The logic behind this is solid: leeches produce an agent known as *hirudin* that is a potent, specific thrombin inhibitor. Leeches have been used to prevent thrombosis in the microvasculature of reattached digits. Lepirudin (Refludan) is a rDNA-derived protein produced in yeast. It has a molecular mass of approximately 7,000 Da. Lepirudin differs from the natural polypeptide, in that it has an N-terminal leucine instead of isoleucine and is missing a sulfate function at Tyr_{63}.

Other Enzymes

Recombinant Human Deoxyribonuclease I (DNAse).[143]

DNAse is a human endonuclease, normally present in saliva, urine, pancreatic secretions, and blood. The enzyme catalyzes the hydrolysis of extracellular DNA into oligonucleotides. Aerosolized recombinant human DNAse (rhDNAse), dornase alfa, Pulmozyme, has been formulated into an inhalation agent for the treatment of pulmonary disease in patients with cystic fibrosis (CF).

Among the clinical manifestations of CF are obstruction of the airways by viscous, dehydrated mucus. Pulmonary function is diminished, and microbes can become entrapped in the viscid matrix. A cycle of pulmonary obstruction and infection leads to progressive lung destruction and eventual death before the age of 30 for most CF patients. The immune system responds by sending in neutrophils, and these accumulate and eventually degenerate, releasing large amounts of DNA. The high levels of extracellular DNA released and the mucous glycoproteins are responsible for the degenerating lung function. The DNA-rich secretions also bind to aminoglycoside antibiotics typically used to treat the infections. In vitro studies showed that the viscosity of the secretions could be reduced by application of DNAse I.

Before DNAse was purified and sequenced from human

sources, a partial DNA sequence from bovine DNAse (263 amino acids) was used to create a library that could be used to screen a human pancreatic DNA library. This facilitated the development of the human recombinant protein. The endogenous human and recombinant protein sequences are identical.

Recombinant human deoxyribonuclease I (rhDNAse) was cloned, sequenced, and expressed to examine the potential of DNAse I as a drug for use in CF. It has been shown that cleavage of high-molecular-weight DNA into smaller fragments by treatment with aerosolized rhDNAse improves the clearance of mucus from the lungs and reduces the exacerbations of respiratory symptoms requiring parenteral antibiotics.

rhDNAse I is a monomeric glycoprotein consisting of 260 amino acids produced in CHO cell culture. The molecule possesses four Cys residues and two sites that probably contain N-linked glycosides. The molecular mass of the molecule is about 29 kDa. DNAse I is an endonuclease that cleaves double-stranded DNA (and to some extent single-stranded DNA) into 5'-phosphate-terminated polynucleotides. Activity depends on the presence of calcium and magnesium ions.

Pulmozyme is approved for use in the treatment of CF patients, in conjunction with standard therapies, to reduce the frequency of respiratory infections requiring parenteral antibiotics and to improve pulmonary function. The dose is delivered at a level of 2.5 mg daily with a nebulizer. Pulmozyme is not a replacement for antibiotics, bronchodilators, and daily physical therapy.

Cerezyme. Type 1 Gaucher's disease is a hereditary condition occurring in about 1:40,000 individuals. It is characterized by a functional deficiency in β-glucocerebrosidase enzyme activity and the resulting accumulation of lipid glucocerebroside in tissue macrophages, which become engorged and are termed *Gaucher's cells*. Gaucher's cells typically accumulate in the liver, spleen, and bone marrow and, occasionally, in lung, kidney, and intestine. Secondary hematological sequelae include severe anemia and thrombocytopenia in addition to characteristic progressive hepatosplenomegaly. Skeletal complications are common and are frequently the most debilitating and disabling feature of Gaucher's disease. Possible skeletal complications are osteonecrosis, osteopenia with secondary pathological fractures, remodeling failure, osteosclerosis, and bone crises.

Cerezyme (Imiglucerase)[144] is a recombinant, macrophage-targeted variant of human β-glucocerebrosidase, purified from CHO cells. It catalyzes the hydrolysis of the glycolipid glucocerebroside to glucose and ceramide following the normal degradation pathway for membrane lipids.

Cerezyme is supplied as a lyophilized powder for reconstitution. The powder should be stored at 2 to 8°C until used. The reconstituted product for IV infusion is stable for 12 hours at room temperature.

VACCINES

Vaccines and immunizing biologicals are covered thoroughly in Chapter 7 of this text, so no lengthy discussion is given here. Vaccine production is a natural application of rDNA technology, aimed at achieving highly pure and efficacious products. Currently, there are four rDNA vaccines approved for human use. A number of others are in clinical trials for some rather exotic uses. It would appear that biotechnological approaches to vaccines will bring about some very useful drugs.

PRODUCTS

Recombivax and Engerix-B.[145] Recombivax and Engerix-B are interchangeable for immunization against hepatitis B virus (HBV, serum hepatitis). Both contain a 226-amino acid polypeptide composing 22-nm-diameter particles that possess the antigenic epitopes of the HBV surface coat (S) protein. The products from two manufacturers are expressed from recombinant *S. cerevisiae*. It is recommended that patients receive 3 doses, with the second dose 1 month after the first and the third dose 6 months after the first. The route and site of injection are IM in deltoid muscle or, for infants and young children, in the anterolateral thigh. The vaccines achieve 94 to 98% immunogenicity among adults 20 to 39 years of age 1 to 2 months after the third dose. Adults over 40 years of age reach 89% immunogenicity. Infants, young children, and adolescents achieve 96 to 99% immunogenicity.

The vaccine is supplied as a suspension adsorbed to aluminum hydroxide. The shelf life is 36 months. The vaccine should be stored at 2 to 8°C and should be discarded if frozen. Freezing destroys potency.

LYMErix.[146] Lyme disease is caused by the spirochete *Borrelia burgdorferi*. The microorganism is transmitted primarily by ticks and is endemic in heavily wooded areas and forests. The disease produces arthritis-like symptoms. A vaccine against Lyme disease was created by developing a recombinant *E. coli* that contains the gene for the bacterial outer surface protein. This protein (OspA) is a single polypeptide chain of 257 amino acids with covalently bound lipids at the N terminus. The vaccine is formulated as a suspension with aluminum hydroxide as an adsorption adjuvant. In testing, subjects between 15 and 70 years immunized with 3 doses of LYMErix at 0, 1, and 12 months demonstrated a 78% decrease in the likelihood of infection.

LYMErix has a shelf life of 24 months. It should be stored at 2 to 8°C and must be discarded if frozen. If necessary, the vaccine can tolerate 4 days at room temperature.

Comvax. Comvax is a combination of *Haemophilus influenzae* type b conjugate and hepatitis B (recombinant). It was recently approved by the Advisory Committee on Immunization Practices (ACIP). Each 0.5-mL dose contains 7.5 μg of *H. influenzae* type b polyribosylribitol phosphate (PRP), 125 μg of *Neisseria meningitidis* outer membrane protein complex (OMPC), and 5 μg of hepatitis B surface antigen (HbsAg) on an aluminum hydroxide adjuvant. The Committee on Infectious Diseases, the American Academy of Pediatrics, and the Advisory Academy of Family Physicians recommend that all infants receive the vaccine. Three doses should be administered at ages 2, 4, and 12 to 15 months. The vaccine should not be administered to infants younger than 6 weeks because of potential suppression of

TABLE 6–10 Vaccines Developed Using Biotechnology

Vaccine	Type	Use	Phase of Development
MAGE-12 : 170–178	Vaccine	Breast, colorectal, lung cancers; melanoma; sarcoma	II
MART-1 melanoma vaccine	Vaccine	Metastatic melanoma	II
Mylovenge	Vaccine	Multiple myeloma	II
Myeloma-derived idiotypic Ag vaccine	Vaccine	Multiple myeloma	I
Melacine melanoma theraccine, therapeutic vaccine	Therapeutic vaccine	Stage 4 malignant melanoma	III
NBI-6024	Peptide therapeutic vaccine	Type I diabetes	II
Anti-Gastrin therapeutic vaccine	Vaccine	Gastroesophageal reflux disease	III
Helivax *Helicobacter pylori* vaccine	Cellular vaccine	*Helicobacter pylori* infection	II
Hepatitis E vaccine	Recombinant subunit vaccine	Hepatitis E prophylaxis	II
StreptAvax	Vaccine	Group A streptococci, including necrotizing fasciitis, strep throat, and rheumatic fever	II

the immune response to PRP-OMPC with subsequent doses of Comvax TM. The series should be completed by 12 to 15 months.

Vaccines in Development

Quite a number of biotechnology-generated vaccines are in development (Table 6-10). Some of them are in the category of "therapeutic vaccines." These vaccines are designed to bind to cellular receptors, endogenous molecules, and so on, producing specific pharmacological effects. For example, if a cell has a particular receptor that binds a ligand to activate the cell, binding an antibody raised by a specific vaccine to the receptor will prevent activation. If a tumor has a requirement for such a receptor–ligand binding, using a vaccine to develop antibody to the receptor or the ligand should prevent or slow cellular proliferation.

PREPARATION OF ANTIBODIES[147–149]

Hybridoma (Monoclonal Antibody [Mab]) Techniques

In a humoral immune response, B-lymphocyte-derived plasma cells produce antibodies with variations in chemical structure. Biologically, these variations extend the utility of the secreted antibody. These variations are caused by affinity maturation, the tendency for the affinity of antibody for antigen to increase with each challenge, and mutation at the time of somatic recombination. These phenomena produce antibodies with slightly different specificities. Because the clones of antibody-producing cells provide more than one structural type of antibody, they are called *polyclonal antibodies*. Another type of antibody consists of highly homogeneous populations of hybrid proteins produced by one clone of specially prepared B lymphocytes. These antibodies, lacking structural variations, are highly "focused" on their antigenic counterparts' determinants or epitopes, and are called *monoclonal*.

A problem with creating MAbs is that one cannot simply prepare an antibody-producing B lymphocyte and propagate it. Such cells live only briefly in the laboratory environment. Instead, antibody-producing cells are fused with an immortal (tumor) cell line to create *hybridomas*—long-lived, antibody-secreting cells. The trick is to select the monoclonal cells that produce the desired antibody. The hybridoma technique has opened the door to new therapeutic antibodies, imaging agents, radiological diagnostic test kits, targeted radionuclide delivery agents, and home test kits.

In the hybridoma method (Fig. 6-14), a mouse or other small animal is sensitized with an antigen. When a high enough titer of antibody against the selected antigen has been attained, the animal is sacrificed and its spleen cells are collected. The spleen cells contain a large number of B lymphocytes, and it is certain that some will be able to produce antigen-specific antibodies. Because the spleen cells are normal B lymphocytes, they have a very short lifetime in cell cultures. Therefore, a method must be used to extend their lifetime.

To produce MAbs, B cells are fused with immortal myeloma cells in the presence of fusogens such as polyethylene glycol. This procedure produces genetically half-normal and half-myeloma cells. Since the myeloma cells are immortal, the longevity problem is solved. The selection process depends on two different myeloma cell lines: one lacking the enzyme hypoxanthine-guanine phosphoribosyl transferase (HGPRT), a key enzyme in the nucleotide salvage pathways, and the other lacking the *Tk* gene, a key gene in the pyrimidine biosynthetic pathways. The spleen B cells are HGPRT and *Tk* (+), while the myeloma cells are HGPRT and *Tk* (−). This myeloma cell line cannot survive in a medium containing aminopterin, a thymidylate synthetase inhibitor, because it cannot synthesize pyrimidines. The HGPRT (−) cell line cannot use the purine salvage pathways to make nucleotides, forcing it to use thymidylate synthetase. With thymidylate synthetase inhibited, the cell dies. After fusion, cells are maintained on a medium containing hypoxanthine, aminopterin, and thymidine (HAT). Only cells that are "cor-

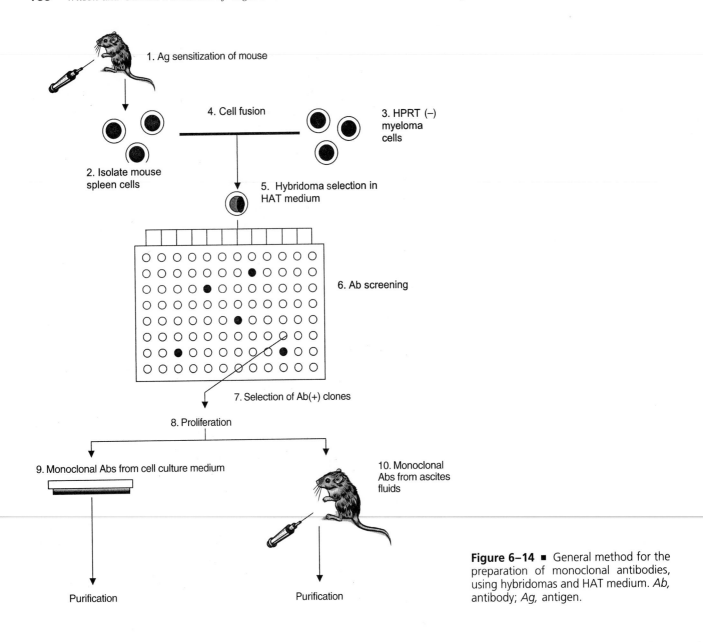

Figure 6–14 ■ General method for the preparation of monoclonal antibodies, using hybridomas and HAT medium. *Ab*, antibody; *Ag*, antigen.

rectly'' fused between one spleen cell (HGPRT [+]) and one myeloma cell (immortal), i.e., a hybridoma, can survive in HAT medium. Fused myeloma cells (myeloma–myeloma) lack the correct genes and cannot survive. Fused spleen cells (spleen–spleen) cannot grow in culture. Thus, only the fused hybridoma (myeloma–spleen) survives. Hypoxanthine and thymidine furnish precursors for the growth of HGPRT (+) cells. Aminopterin suppresses cells that failed to fuse. Hybridomas can be isolated in a 96-well plate and transferred into larger cultures for proliferation. The culture medium will eventually contain a high concentration of MAb against the original antigen. This antibody can be purified to homogeneity.

Monoclonal antibodies, being proteins, tend to be highly immunogenic in humans. This is especially true of the MAbs produced in mouse culture. Humans begin to develop antibodies to mouse MAbs after a single dose. This is natural. The human host is mounting an antibody response to a foreign antigen. The human antimouse antibody response

(known as *HAMA*) has tended to limit the use of monoclonals in human therapy.

In developing a method for making MAbs useful in humans, it is necessary to remove the mouse immunogenic characteristics from the MAb. The antigen-recognition region (Fab) of the MAb must retain its ability to bind to the antigen, however. If this feature is altered, the antibody will likely be useless. Within the light and heavy chains of the Fab portions of antibody molecules are regions that are called *complementarity-determining regions* or CDRs. Each chain possesses three of these. One of the CDRs, CDR3, is located at the juncture of the variable and common domains. CDR3 is also referred to as the *hypervariable region* because most of the variability of the antibody molecule is concentrated there. These must be intact for specific antigen–antibody binding. Immune responses against murine MAb are directed against not only the variable regions, but also the constant regions. Hence, to decrease the immunogenicity of an MAb one must create antibodies that have been ''humanized.'' In MAb production, usually the V_H and V_L domains of a human antibody are replaced by the corresponding regions from the mouse antibody, leaving the specificity intact, but using human constant regions that should not be immunogenic. Antibodies like these are called *chimeric,* and they are less immunogenic and have a longer half-life in human patients. Examples of chimeric MAbs are abciximab, rituximab, infliximab, and basiliximab.

Methods are available for the development of MAbs with 95 to 100% human sequence. By using transgenic mice, all of the essential human antibody genes can be expressed.

Monoclonal Antibody Drugs

Rituximab.[150, 151]   Rituximab (Rituxan, Chimeric) is an MAb directed against the CD20 antigen expressed on the surfaces of normal and malignant B lymphocytes. The MAb is produced in mammalian (CHO) suspension culture and is a chimeric (murine/human) MAb of the IgG_1 κ type. The protein is composed of murine light and heavy chain variable regions and human constant regions. Rituximab is indicated for the treatment of patients with relapsed or refractory, low-grade or follicular, CD20(+) B cell non-Hodgkin's lymphoma. Rituximab binds specifically to antigen CD20 (human B-lymphocyte-restricted differentiation antigen, a hydrophobic transmembrane protein expressed on pre- and mature-B lymphocytes). CD20 is a protein of 35 to 37 kDa, and it may play a role in B cell activation and regulation and may be a calcium ion channel. The antigen is also expressed on more than 90% of non-Hodgkin's lymphoma B cells but is not found on hematopoietic stem cells, pro-B cells, normal plasma cells, or other normal tissues. CD20 regulates the early steps in the activation process for cell-cycle initiation and differentiation.

Gemtuzumab Ozogamicin.[152, 153]   Gemtuzumab ozogamicin (Mylotarg, fusion molecule) is an MAb derived from the CD33 antigen, a sialic acid-dependent adhesion protein expressed on the surface of leukemia blasts and immature normal cells of myelomonocytic origin but not on normal hematopoietic stem cells. CD33 binds sialic acid and appears to regulate signaling in myeloid cells. The antibody is recombinant, humanized IgG_4 κ, linked with the cytotoxic antitumor antibiotic ozogamicin (from the calicheamicin family). More than 98.3% of the amino acids of gemtuzumab are of human origin. The constant region of the MAb contains human sequences, while the CDRs derive from a murine antibody that binds CD33. The antibody is linked to N-acetyl-γ-calicheamicin via a bifunctional linker.

Gemtuzumab ozogamicin is indicated for the treatment of patients with CD33-positive acute myeloid leukemia in first relapse among adults 60 years of age or older who are not considered candidates for cytotoxic chemotherapy.

Gemtuzumab ozogamicin binds to the CD33 antigen expressed by hematopoietic cells. This antigen is expressed on the surface of leukemic blasts in more than 80% of patients with acute myeloid leukemia. CD33 is also expressed on normal and leukemic myeloid colony-forming cells, including leukemic clonogenic precursors, but it is not expressed on pluripotent hematopoietic stem cells or nonhematopoietic cells. Binding of the anti-CD33 antibody results in a complex that is internalized. On internalization the calicheamicin de-

rivative is released inside the lysosomes of the myeloid cells. The released calicheamicin derivative binds to the minor groove of DNA and causes double-strand breaks and cell death.

Alemtuzumab.[154, 155]   Alemtuzumab (Campath) is humanized MAb (Campath-1H) that is directed against the 21- to 28-kDa cell surface glycoprotein CD52. CD52 is expressed on the surface of normal and malignant B and T lymphocytes, NK cells, monocytes, macrophages, and tissues of the male reproductive system. The Campath-1H antibody is an IgG_1 κ form with humanized variable and constant regions and CDRs from a rat MAb, Campath-1G.

Alemtuzumab is indicated for the treatment of B-cell chronic lymphocytic leukemia in patients who have been treated with alkylating agents and who have failed on this therapy. Alemtuzumab binds to CD52, a nonmodulating antigen that is present on the surface of essentially all B and T lymphocytes; most monocytes, macrophages, and NK cells; and a subpopulation of granulocytes. The proposed mechanism of action is antibody-dependent lysis of leukemic cells following cell surface binding.

Basiliximab.[156–158]   Baliximab (Simulect, Chimeric) is an MAb produced by a mouse monoclonal cell line that has been engineered to produce the basiliximab IgG_1 κ antibody glycoprotein. The product is chimeric (murine/human). Basiliximab is indicated for prophylaxis of acute organ rejection in patients receiving renal transplantation when used as part of a regimen of immunosuppressants and corticosteroids. Basiliximab is also indicated in pediatric renal transplantation.

Basiliximab specifically binds to the IL-2 receptor α chain (the CD25 antigen, part of the three-component IL-2 receptor site). These sites are expressed on the surfaces of activated T lymphocytes. Once bound it blocks the IL-2α receptor with extremely high affinity. This specific, high-affinity binding to IL-2α competitively inhibits IL-2-mediated activation of lymphocytes, a critical event in the cellular immune response in allograft rejection.

Daclizumab.[159, 160]   Molecularly, daclizumab (Zenapax, Chimeric) is an immunoglobulin G (IgG_1) MAb that binds specifically to the α subunit of the IL-2 receptor (the complete, high-affinity activated IL-2 receptor consists of interacting α, β, and γ subunits). IL-2 receptors are expressed on the surfaces of activated lymphocytes, where they mediate lymphocyte clonal expansion and differentiation. Daclizumab is a chimeric protein (90% human and 10% mouse) IgG_1. The MAb targets only recently activated T cells that have interacted with antigen and have developed from their naïve form into their activated form. It is at this time that the IL-2 receptors are expressed. The human amino acid sequences of daclizumab derive from constant domains of human IgG, and the variable domains are derived from the fused Eu myeloma antibody. The murine sequences derive from CDRs of a mouse anti-IL2α antibody.

The indications for daclizumab are prophylaxis of acute organ rejection in patients receiving renal transplants, as part of an immunosuppressant regimen including cyclosporine and corticosteroids. The mechanism of action is the same as that of basiliximab.

Muromonab-CD3. [161–163] Muromonab-CD3 (murine, Orthoclone-OKT3) is an unmodified mouse immunoglobulin, an IgG_{2a}, monoclonal. It binds a glycoprotein on the surface of mature T lymphocytes. Mature T cells have, as part of the signal transduction machinery of the T-cell receptor complex, a set of three glycoproteins that are collectively called CD3. Together with the protein zeta, the CD3 molecules become phosphorylated when the T-cell receptor is bound to a peptide fragment and the major histocompatibility complex. The phosphorylated CD3 and zeta molecules transmit information into the cell, ultimately producing transcription factors that enter the nucleus and direct the T-cell activity. By binding to CD3, muromonab-CD3 prevents signal transduction into T cells.

Muromonab-CD3 blocks the function of T cells that are involved in acute renal rejection. Hence, it is indicated for the treatment of acute allograft rejection in heart and liver transplant recipients resistant to standard steroid therapies.

Abciximab. [164, 165] Abciximab (ReoPro, chimeric) is an MAb engineered from the glycoprotein IIb/IIIa receptor of human platelets. The preparation is fragmented, containing only the Fab portion of the antibody molecule. This MAb is a chimeric human–mouse immunoglobulin. The Fab fragments may contain mouse variable heavy- and light-chain regions and human constant heavy- and light-chain regions.

Abciximab is indicated as an adjunct to percutaneous transluminal coronary angioplasty or atherectomy for the prevention of acute cardiac ischemic complications in patients at high risk for abrupt closure of a treated coronary vessel. Abciximab appears to decrease the incidence of myocardial infarction.

Abciximab binds to the intact GPIIb/GPIIIa receptor, which is a member of the integrin family of adhesion receptors and the major platelet-specific receptors involved in aggregation. The antibody prevents platelet aggregation by preventing the binding of fibrinogen, the von Willebrand factor, and other adhesion molecules on activated platelets. The inhibition of binding to the surface receptors may be due to steric hindrance or conformational effects preventing large molecules from approaching the receptor.

Trastuzumab. [166, 167] Trastuzumab (Herceptin, humanized) is an MAb engineered from the human epidermal growth factor receptor type 2 (HER2) protein. This MAb is a human–murine immunoglobulin. It contains human structural domains (framework) and the CDR of a murine antibody (4D5) that binds specifically to HER2. $IgG_1 \kappa$ is the type structure, and the antibody is monoclonal. The protein inhibits the proliferation of human tumor cells that overexpress HER2.

Trastuzumab is indicated for use as a single agent for the treatment of patients with metastatic breast cancer whose tumors overexpress the HER2 protein and who have not received chemotherapy for their metastatic disease.

The HER2 proto-oncogene encodes a transmembrane receptor protein of 185 kDa that is structurally related to the epidermal growth factor receptor HER2. Overexpression of this protein is observed in 25 to 30% of primary breast cancers. Trastuzumab binds with high affinity to the extracellular domain of HER2. It inhibits the proliferation of human tumor cells that overexpress HER2. Trastuzumab also mediates the process of antibody-mediated cellular cytotoxicity (ADCC). This process, leading to cell death, is preferentially exerted on HER2-overexpressing cancer cells over those that do not overexpress HER2.

Infliximab. [168, 169] The MAb infliximab (Remicade, chimeric) is produced from cells that have been sensitized with human TNF-α. The MAb is a chimeric human–mouse immunoglobulin. The constant regions are of human peptide sequence and the variable regions are murine. The MAb is of type $IgG_1 \kappa$.

Infliximab is indicated for the treatment of moderately to severely active Crohn's disease to decrease signs and symptoms in patients who had an inadequate response to conventional treatments. Infliximab binds specifically to TNFα. It neutralizes the biological activity of TNFα by binding with high affinity to soluble and transmembrane forms of the TNF. Infliximab destroys TNFα-producing cells. An additional mechanism by which infliximab could work is as follows: by inhibiting TNFα, pathways leading to IL-1 and IL-6 are inhibited. These interleukins are inflammatory cytokines. Inhibiting their production blocks some of the inflammation common to Crohn's disease.

Monoclonal Antibody Radionuclide Test Kits

Arcitumomab. [170] Arcitumomab (CEA-Scan) is a murine monoclonal Fab$'$ fragment of IMMU-4, an MAb generated in murine ascites fluid. Both IMMU-4 and arcitumomab react with carcinoembryonic antigen (CEA), a tumor-associated antigen whose expression is increased in a variety of carcinomas, especially those of the GI tract. The preparation is a protein, murine Ig Fab fragment from IgG_1, for chemical labeling with Tc-99m.

Arcitumomab/Tc-99m is for use with standard diagnostic evaluations for detecting the presence, location, and extent of recurrent or metastatic colorectal carcinoma involving the liver, extrahepatic abdomen, and pelvis, with a histologically confirmed diagnosis. IMMU-4 (and the Fab$'$ fragments of arcitumomab) bind to carcinoembryonic antigen (CEA), whose expression is increased in carcinoma. Arcitumomab/Tc-99m is injected, and the radionuclide scan is read 2 to 5 hours later.

Nofetumomab Merpentan. [171] Nofetumomab merpentan (Verluma Kit) is the Fab fragment derived from the murine MAb NR-LU-10. The product is a protein, IgG_{2b}, monoclonal that has been fragmented from NR-LU-10. Nofetumomab possesses only the Fab portion. NR-LU-10 and nofetumomab are directed against a 40-kDa protein antigen that is expressed in a variety of cancers and some normal tissues.

Nofetumomab is indicated for the detection and evaluation of extensive-stage disease in patients with biopsy-confirmed, previously untreated small cell lung cancer by bone scan, CT scan (head, chest, abdomen) or chest x-ray.

Nofetumomab merpentan possesses a linker and a chelator that binds the technetium to the peptide. This is a phenthioate ligand, 2,3,5,6-tetrafluorophenyl-4,5-bis-*S*-[1-ethoxyethyl]-thioacetoamidopentanoate, hence the name *merpentan*.

Satumomab Pendetide.[172] Satumomab pendetide (OncoScint, murine) is a kit for In-111. Satumomab is prepared from a murine antibody raised to a membrane-enriched extract of human breast carcinoma hepatic metastasis. It is a protein, IgG_1 κ antibody, and monoclonal. The MAb recognizes tumor-associated glycoprotein (TAG) 72, a mucin-like molecule with a mass greater than 100,000 Da.

Satumomab is indicated as a diagnostic aid in determining the extent and location of extrahepatic malignant disease in patients with known colorectal and ovarian cancer. This agent is used after standard diagnostic tests are completed and when additional information is needed. The cancer must be recurrent or previously diagnosed by other methods.

Satumomab localizes to TAG 72. The antibody is chemically modified so that it links to radioactive indium-111, which is mixed with the antibody just prior to injection. Imaging techniques will reveal the localization of the satumomab as "hot spots." To link the indium-111 to the satumomab protein, a linker-chelator is used. This is glycyltyrosyl-(N,ϵ-diethylenetriaminepentaacetic acid)-lysine hydrochloride.

Imciromab Pentetate.[173] Imciromab pentetate (murine; Myoscint Kit for the preparation of indium-111 imciromab pentetate) is a murine immunoglobulin fragment raised to the heavy chain of human myosin. The drug is a protein of the IgG_2 κ class. It is monoclonal, consisting of the Fab-binding fragments only, and it is bound to the linker-chelator diethylenetriamine pentaacetic acid for labeling with indium-111. Imciromab binds to the heavy chain of human myosin, the intracellular protein found in cardiac and skeletal muscle cells.

Imciromab pentetate is indicated for detecting the presence and location of myocardial injury in patients after a suspected myocardial infarction. In normal myocardium, intracellular proteins such as myosin are isolated from the extravascular space by the cell membrane and are inaccessible to antibody binding. After myocyte injury the cell membrane loses integrity and becomes permeable to macromolecules, which allows Imciromab-In-111 to enter the cells, where it binds to intracellular myosin. The drug localizes in infarcted tissues, where radionuclide scanning can visualize it.

Capromab Pendetide.[174] Capromab (ProstaScint Kit for the preparation of In-111 capromab pendetide, murine) is an MAb (murine IgG_1 κ) that derives from an initial sensitization with a glycoprotein expressed by prostate epithelium known as *prostate surface membrane antigen* (PSMA). The MAb recognizes PSMA specifically and thus is specific for prostate adenocarcinomas. The drug is used in newly diagnosed patients with proven prostate cancer who are at high risk for pelvic lymph metastasis. PSMA has been found in many primary and metastatic prostate cancer lesions. The cytoplasmic domain marker 7E11-C5.3 reacts with more than 95% of adenocarcinomas evaluated.

To join the indium-111 to the antibody, a linker-chelator is used. This moiety is glycyltyrosyl-(N-ethylenetriamine-pentaacetic acid)-lysine HCl.

A Therapeutic Radionuclide Monoclonal Antibody[175]

Ibritumomab Tiuxetan. Ibritumomab (Zevalin kits to prepare In-111 Zevalin and Y-90 Zevalin, murine) is an MAb derived from an initial sensitization with CD20 antigen, expressed on the surface of normal and malignant B cells. The antibody is a murine IgG_1 κ subtype, directed against CD20 antigen. It is produced in a CHO cell line. Ibritumomab is indicated for use as a multistage regimen to treat patients with relapsed or refractory low-grade, follicular, or transformed B-cell non-Hodgkin's lymphoma, including patients with rituximab-refractory follicular non-Hodgkin's lymphoma.

Ibritumomab tiuxetan binds specifically to CD20 antigen (human B-lymphocyte-restricted differentiation antigen). CD20 is expressed on pre-B and mature-B lymphocytes and on more than 90% of B-cell non-Hodgkin's lymphoma. When the CDR of ibritumomab tiutuxan binds to the CD20 antigen, apoptosis is initiated. The tiutuxan chelate binds indium-111 and yttrium-90 tightly. Beta emission induces cellular damage by forming free radicals in the target cells and neighboring cells. Tiutuxan is [N-[2-bis(carboxymethyl)amino]-3-(p-isothiocyanatophenyl)propyl]-[N-[2-bis(carboxymethyl)amino]2-(methyl)-ethyl]glycine.

In-Home Test Kits[176]

There are a variety of MAb-based in-home test kits that are designed to detect pregnancy and ovulation. For example, a pregnancy test kit targets the antigen human chorionic gonadotropin and displays a certain sign if the test is positive. The other type of test kit predicts ovulation by targeting luteinizing hormone in the urine. Just before ovulation, luteinizing hormone surges. The test kit is designed to detect and signal the time of ovulation. These test kits, based on the complex techniques of MAbs, are designed to be as simple and error-free as possible for patients.

GENOMICS

Genomics[177] is a term that means "a study of genes and their functions." Currently, genomics is probably the central driving force for new drug discovery and for novel treatments for disease. Gene therapy is a concept that is often discussed. The human genome project, which was largely completed in the year 2000, provided over 4 billion base pairs of data that have been deposited in public databases. Sequencing the genome itself was an enormous task, but the correlation of genomic data with disease states, sites of microbial attachment, and drug receptor sites is still in its infancy. Once these problems are solved, genomic data will be used to diagnose and treat disease and to develop new drugs specifically for disease states (and possibly specific for a patient). Studying the genetics of biochemical pathways will provide an entry into enzyme-based therapies. There will undoubtedly be a host of new targets for drug therapy. Because deciphering the information that the genomic sequence provides is a complex undertaking, these benefits are probably going to occur years in the future.

Unraveling the Genomic Code to Determine Structure–Function Relationships: Bioinformatics

When considering the topic of bioinformatics, one must recognize that this is a broad term covering many different research areas. The roots of bioinformatics lie in the decades-old field of computational biology. Advances in computer technology that yielded faster computations fueled the expansion of this field into many different scientific areas, as did the development of new mathematical algorithms that allowed highly sophisticated problems to be solved quickly. For instance, with the computer technology available in 2003, it is relatively straightforward to determine a three-dimensional structure of a protein by x-ray crystallography, by nuclear magnetic resonance–distance geometry–molecular dynamics approaches, or to compare a large set of genes structurally. Out of bioinformatics have grown some new scientific disciplines: functional genomics, structural genomics, and evolutionary genomics. The term *bioinformatics* is routinely applied to experiments in genomics that rely on sophisticated computations.

One reason why computational methods are so critical is that biological macromolecules must be simulated in a three-dimensional environment for realistic comparisons and visualizations to be made. A typical molecule is represented in a computer by a set of three Cartesian coordinates per atom that specify the position of each atom in space. There are sets of 3-atom and dihedral angles to specify interatomic connectivity, and designations for the start and end points of chains, where needed. Fortunately it is a relatively simple matter to build or download molecules from databases. Although the Cartesian coordinate system provides the relative positions of the atoms in space, the computer offers the opportunity to let the molecule evolve in the fourth dimension, time. This is where energy minimization routines and molecular dynamics simulations are used.

Functional Genomics

Functional genomics seeks to make an *inference* about the function of a gene (Fig. 6-15). Given a novel gene sequence to be tested, the functional genomics method starts by comparing the new gene with genetic sequences in a database. In some cases, the name of the gene, a function, or a close analogy to previously identified genes can be made. The test

gene is then used as a template to construct, in a computer, a three-dimensional model of the protein. The three-dimensional model is refined by searching databases for possible folded structures of the protein product. Lastly, the likely folded structure of the protein from the new gene is *inferred* by comparison with folding patterns of proteins of known structure and function.

The above method is not without difficulty. There is a lot of genetic overlap between organisms of different types. Usually, as a first step, the genomic sequences of prokaryotes and *Archaebacteria* are subtracted out, but there can still be overlap with organisms such as yeasts. In addition, the human genome possesses introns and exons, and the genetic components that encode one protein may lie on parts of one chromosome that are separated by a large number of nucleotides, or the gene may even be distributed over more than one chromosome.

DNA Microarrays[178, 179]

Each cell in the human body contains a full set of chromosomes and an identical complement of genes. At any given time in a given cell, only a fraction of these genes may be expressed. It is the expressed genes that give each cell its uniqueness. We use the term *gene expression* to describe the transcription of the information contained in the DNA code into mRNA molecules that are translated into the proteins that perform the major functions of the cell. The amount and type of mRNA that is produced by a cell provides information on which genes are being expressed and how the cell responds dynamically to changing conditions (e.g., disease). Gene expression can act as an "on/off" switch to control which genes are expressed, and a level regulator, somewhat like a volume control, that increases or decreases the level of expression as necessary. Thus, genes can be on or off, and low or high.

Historically, scientists wishing to study gene expression could analyze mRNA from cell lines, but the complexity of the task meant that only a few genes could be studied at once. The advent of DNA microarray technology allows scientists to analyze expression of thousands of genes in a single experiment, quickly and efficiently. DNA microarray technology facilitates the identification and classification of DNA sequence information and takes steps toward assigning functions to the new genes. The fundamental precept of microarray technology is that any mRNA molecule can hybridize to the DNA template from which it originated.

In a typical microarray experiment, an array is constructed of many DNA samples. Automation that was developed for the silicon chip industry helps in this procedure, spotting thousands of different DNA samples on glass plates, silicon chips, or nylon wafers. mRNA isolated from probe cells is treated with a mixture of fluorescent-tagged (usually red, green, and yellow) nucleotides in the presence of reverse transcriptase. This process generates fluorescent-tagged cDNA. The fluors will emit light when excited with a laser. The labeled nucleic acids are considered *mobile probes* that, when incubated with the stationary DNA, hybridize or bind to the complementary molecules (sequences that can base pair with each other). After hybridization, bound cDNA is detected by use of a laser scanner. Data on the presence or absence of fluorescence, the color, and the intensity at the

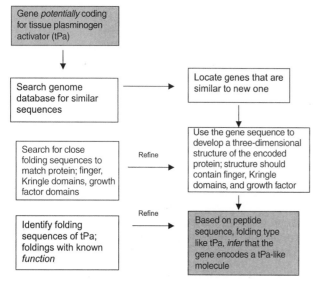

Figure 6–15 ■ Functional genomics.

various points in the array are acquired in a computer for analysis.

As an example, we can consider two cells: cell type 1, a healthy cell, and cell type 2, a diseased cell. Both cell types contain an identical set of four genes: A, B, C, and D. mRNA is isolated from each cell type and used to create fluorescent-tagged cDNA. In this case, red and green are used. Labeled samples are mixed and incubated with a microarray that contains the immobilized genes A, B, C, and D. The tagged molecules bind to the sites on the array corresponding to the genes being expressed in each cell. A robotic scanner, also a product of silicon chip technology, excites the fluorescent labels, and images are stored in a computer. The computer can compute the red-to-green fluorescence ratio, subtract out background noise, and so on. The computer creates a table of the intensity of red to green fluorescence for every point in the matrix. Perhaps both cells express the same levels of gene A, cell 1 expresses more of gene B, cell 2 (the diseased cell) expresses more of gene C, and neither cell expresses gene D. This is a simplistic explanation; experiments have been reported in which as many as 30,000 spots have been placed in the microarray.

DNA microarrays can detect changes in gene expression levels, expression patterns (e.g., the cell cycle), genomic gains and losses (e.g., lost or broken parts of chromosomes in cancer cells), and mutations in DNA (single nucleotide polymorphism [SNPs]). SNPs are also of interest because they may provide clues about how different people respond to a single drug in different ways.

Proteomics[180, 181]

The word *proteome* describes *prot*ein expressed by a gen*ome*. Proteomics is a scientific endeavor that attempts to study the sum total of all of the proteins in a cell from the point of view of their individual functions and how the interaction of specific proteins with other cellular components affects the function of these proteins. Not surprisingly, this is a very complex task. There are many more proteins than there are genes, and in biochemical pathways, a protein rarely acts by itself. At present, we know that the expression of multiple genes is involved for any given disease process. "Simply" knowing the gene sequence rarely unmasks the function of the encoded protein or its relevance to a disease. Consequently, the science of proteomics is not developed to the point at which drug discovery can be driven by gene sequence information. There have been, however, some significant technology-driven approaches to the field. High-throughput high-resolution mass spectroscopy allows the amino acid sequences of proteins to be determined very quickly. The technique of two-dimensional gel electrophoresis has likewise advanced the science of proteomics. Proteomics will, undoubtedly, eventually provide targets for drug discovery and the detection of disease states.

Pharmacogenomics[182]

When pharmaceutical companies develop new drugs for any given disease state, they are limited by a lack of knowledge about how individual patients will respond to the agent. No simple algorithms exist that facilitate prediction of whether a patient will respond negatively (an adverse drug reaction), positively (the desired outcome), or not at all. Consequently, drugs are developed for an "average" patient. The manufacturer relies on clinical studies to expose potential adverse reactions and publishes them in statistical format to guide the physician. Nevertheless, when a physician prescribes a drug to a patient he or she has no way of knowing the outcome. Statistics show clearly that a single drug does not provide a positive outcome in all patients. This "one drug does not fit all" concept has its basis in the genetics of a patient, and the science of studying these phenomena is called *pharmacogenomics*.

A patient's response to a drug, positive or negative, is a highly complex trait that may be influenced by the activities of many different genes. Absorption, distribution, metabolism, and excretion, as well as the receptor-binding relationship, are all under the control of proteins, lipids, and carbohydrates, which are in turn under the control of the patient's genes. When the fact that a person's genes display small variations in their DNA base content was recognized, genetic prediction of response to drugs or infectious microbes became possible. Pharmacogenomics is the science that looks at the inherited variations in genes that dictate drug response and tries to define the ways in which these variations can be used to predict if a patient will have a positive response to a drug, an adverse one, or none at all.

Cataloging the genetic variations is an important phase of present research activity. Scientists look for SNPs in a person's gene sequences. SNPs are viewed as markers for slight genomic variation. Unfortunately, traditional gene sequencing is slow and expensive, preventing for now the general use of SNPs as diagnostic tools. DNA microarrays may make it possible to identify SNPs quickly in a patient's cells. SNP screening may help to determine a response to a drug before it is prescribed. Obviously, this would be a tremendous tool for the physician.

ANTISENSE TECHNOLOGY

During the process of transcription, double-stranded DNA is separated into two strands by polymerases. These strands are named the *sense* (coding or [+] strand) and the *antisense* (template or [−] strand). The antisense DNA strand serves as the template for mRNA synthesis in the cell. Hence, the code for ribosomal protein synthesis is normally transmitted through the antisense strand. Sometimes, the sense DNA strand will code for a molecule of RNA. In this case, the resulting RNA molecule is called *antisense RNA*. Antisense RNA sequences were first reported to be naturally occurring molecules in which endogenous strands formed complementarily to cellular mRNA, resulting in the repression of gene expression. Hence, they may be natural control molecules. Rationally designed antisense oligonucleotide interactions occur when the base pairs of a synthetic, specifically designed antisense molecule align precisely with a series of bases in a target mRNA molecule.

Antisense oligonucleotides may inhibit gene expression transiently by masking the ribosome-binding site on mRNA, blocking translation and thus preventing protein synthesis, or permanently by cross-linkage between the oligonucleotide and the mRNA. Most importantly, ribonuclease H

(RNase H) can recognize the DNA–RNA duplex (antisense DNA binding to mRNA), or a RNA–RNA duplex (antisense RNA interacting with mRNA), disrupting the base pairing interactions and digesting the RNA portion of the double helix. Inhibition of gene expression occurs because the digested mRNA is no longer competent for translation and resulting protein synthesis.

Antisense technology is beginning to be used to develop drugs that might be able to control disease by blocking the genetic code, interfering with damaged or malfunctioning genes. Among the possible therapeutic antisense agents under investigation are agents for chronic myelogenous leukemia, HIV infection and AIDS, cytomegalovirus retinitis in AIDS patients, and some inflammatory diseases.

GENE THERAPY

Gene therapy arguably represents the ultimate application of rDNA technology to the treatment of disease. There are two ways to envision gene therapy: *(a)* the replacement of a defective gene with a normal gene or *(b)* the addition of a gene whose product can help fight a disease such as a viral infection or cancer. In the former case, replacement of a defective gene, an actual cure can be effected instead of just treating the symptoms. For example, in cystic fibrosis, a defective gene has been clearly identified as the cause of the disease. It is possible that replacement of the defective gene with a corrected one could produce a cure. Similar possibilities exist for other inherited genetic disorders such as insulin-dependent diabetes, growth hormone deficiency, hemophilia, and sickle cell anemia.

The ability to transfer genes into other organisms has other important applications, including the heterologous production of recombinant proteins (discussed above) and the development of animal models for the study of human diseases. Another area of exploration is the introduction of recombinant genes as biological response modifiers, for example, in preventing rejection following organ transplantation. If genes encoding host major histocompatibility complexes could be introduced into transplanted cells, the transplanted tissue might be recognized as "self." It might also be possible to introduce genes for substances such as transforming growth factor-β that would decrease local cell-mediated immune responses. An opposite strategy might be considered for the treatment of cancer, whereby transplanted cells could be used to target cancer cells, increasing local cell-mediated immune responses.

The transfer of genes from one organism to another is termed *transgenics,* and an animal that has received such a transgene is referred to as a *transgenic animal*. If the transgene is incorporated into the *germ cells* (eggs and sperm), it will be inherited and passed on to successive generations. If the transgene is incorporated into other cells of the body *(somatic cells)*, it will be expressed only as long as the newly created transgenic cells are alive. Hence, if a terminally differentiated, postmitotic cell receives a transgene it will not undergo further cell division, whereas if a transgene is created in an undifferentiated stem cell, the product will continuously be expressed in new cells.

AFTERWORD

Clearly, biotechnology has become an integral part of pharmaceutical care. Pharmacists need to become comfortable with biotechnology and its language to deliver this kind of care to their patients. This chapter has tried to present an overview of the major biotechnological arenas present in the year 2003. The field is advancing rapidly, and every pharmacist must stay current with the literature on biotechnology.

Acknowledgments

Portions of this chapter included material from the tenth edition chapter by John W. Regan. The author is grateful for the use of this content.

REFERENCES

1. NCBI, NLM, NIH, Bethesda, MD 20894. e-mail info@ncbi.nlm.nih.gov.
2. Benson, D. A.: Nucl. Acids Res. 30(1):17–20, 2002.
3. GenBank, NCBI. https://www.ncbi.nlm.nih.gov/GenBank/genbankstats.html.
4. Pharmaceutical Research and Manufacturers Association: New Medicines in Biotechnology Survey. Washington, DC, Pharmaceutical Research and Manufacturers Association, 2002.
5. Pharmaceutical Research and Manufacturers Association: New Medicines in Development for Pediatrics Survey. Washington, DC, Pharmaceutical Research and Manufacturers Association, 2002.
6. Akinwande, K., et al.: Hosp. Formul. 28(9):773–780, 1993.
7. Mahoney, C. D.: Hosp. Formul. 27(Suppl. 2):2–3, 1992.
8. Wordell, C. J.: Hosp. Pharm. 27(6):521–528, 1992.
9. Seltzer, J. L., et al.: Hosp. Formul. 27(4):379–392, 1992.
10. Schneider, P. J.: Pharm. Pract. Manage. Q. 18(2):32–36, 1998.
11. Huber, S. L.: Am. J. Hosp. Pharm. 50(7 Suppl. 3):531–533, 1993.
12. Bleeker, G. C.: Am. J. Hosp. Pharm. 50(7 Suppl. 3):527–530, 1993.
13. Herfindal, E. T.: Am. J. Hosp. Pharm. 46(12):2516–2520, 1989.
14. Dasher, T.: Am. Pharm. NS35(2):9–10, 1995.
15. Vizirianakis, I. S.: Eur. J. Pharm. Sci. 15(3):243–250, 2002.
16. Baumgartner, R. P.: Hosp. Pharm. 26(11):939–946, 1991.
17. Rospond, R. M., and Do, T. T.: Hosp. Pharm. 26(9):823–827, 1991.
18. Brodie, D. C., and Smith, W. E.: Am. J. Hosp. Pharm. 42(1):81–95, 1985.
19. Slavkin, H. C. Technol. Health Care 4(3):249–253, 1996.
20. Stewart, C. F., and Fleming, R. A.: Am. J. Hosp. Pharm. 46(11 Suppl. 2):54–58, 1989.
21. Tami, J., and Evens, R. P.: Pharmacotherapy 16(4):527–536, 1996.
22. Koeller, J.M.: Am. J. Hosp. Pharm. 46(Suppl. 2):511–515, 1989.
23. Wagner, M.: Mod. Healthcare 22(2):24–29, 1992.
24. Dana, W. J., and Farthing, K.: Pharm. Pract. Manage. Q. 18(2):23–31, 1988.
25. Santell, J. P.: Am. J. Health Syst. Pharm. 53(2):139–155, 1996.
26. Reid, B.: Nat. Biotechnol. 20(4):322, 2002.
27. Piascik, P.: Pharm. Pract. Manage. Q. 18(2):1–12, 1998.
28. Piascik, P.: Am. Pharm. NS35(6):9–10, 1995.
29. Roth, R.: Am. Pharm. NS34(4):31–33, 1994.
30. Taylor, K. S.: Hosp. Health Network 67(17):36–38, 1993.
31. Wade, D. A., and Levy, R. A.: Am. Pharm. NS32(9):33–37, 1992.
32. Lumisdon, K.: Hospitals 65(23):32–35, 1991.
33. Crane, V. S., Gilliland, M., and Trussell, R. G.: Top. Hosp. Pharm. Manage. 10(4):23–30, 1991.
34. Zilz, D. A.: Am. J. Hosp. Pharm. 47(8):1759–1765, 1990.
35. Zarus, S. A.: Curr. Concepts Hosp. Pharm. Manage. 11(4):12–19, 1989.
36. Schneider, P. J.: Pharm. Pract. Manage. Q. 18(2):32–36, 1998.
37. Manuel, S. M.: Am. Pharm. NS34(11):14–15, 1994.
38. Gillouzo, A.: Cell Mol. Biol. 47(8):1307–1308, 2001.
39. Sindelar, R. D.: Drug Top. 137:66–78, 1993.

40. McKinnon, B.: Drug Benefit Trends 9(12):30–34, 1997.
41. Wolf, B. A.: Ther. Drug Monit. 18(4):402–404, 1996.
42. Vermeij, P., and Blok, D.: Pharm. World Sci. 18(3):87–93, 1996.
43. Lambert, K.: Curr. Opin. Biotechnol. 8(3):347–349, 1997.
44. Beatrice, M.: Curr. Opin. Biotechnol. 8(3):370–378, 1997.
45. Romac, D. R., et al.: Formulary 30(9):520–531, 1995.
46. McGarity, T. O.: Issues Sci. Technol. 1(3):40–56, 1985.
47. Columbo P., et al.: Eur. J. Drug Metab. Pharmacokinet. 21(2):87–91, 1996.
48. Berthold, W., and Walter, J.: Biologicals 22(2):135–150, 1994.
49. Roth, R., and Constantine, L. M.: Am. Pharm. NS35(7):19–21, 1995.
50. Santell, J. P.: Am. J. Hosp. Pharm. 51(2):177–187, 1994.
51. Piascek, P.: Am. Pharm. NS33(4):18–19, 1993.
52. Piascek, M. M.: Am. J. Hosp. Pharm. 48(10 Suppl. 11):14–18, 1992.
53. Piascek, P., and Alexander, S.: Am. Pharm. NS35(11):8–9, 1995.
54. Glick, B. R., and Pasternak, J. J. (eds.): Molecular Biotechnology: Principles and Applications of Recombinant DNA, 2nd ed. Washington, DC, ASM Press, 1998.
55. Franks, F. (ed.): Protein Biotechnology. Totowa, NJ, Humana Press, 1993.
56. Bains, W.: Biotechnology from A to Z, 2nd ed. Oxford, England, : Oxford University Press, 1998.
57. Alberts, B., Bray, D., Lewis, J., et al. (eds.): Molecular Biology of the Cell, 3rd ed. New York, NY, Garland Publishing, 1994.
58. Wolfe, S. L.: An Introduction to Cell and Molecular Biology. Belmont, CA, Wadsworth Publishing, 1995.
59. Williams, D. A., and Lemke, T. L. (eds.): Foye's Principles of Medicinal Chemistry, 5th ed. New York, Lippincott Williams & Wilkins, 2001, pp. 981–1015.
60. Sindelar, R. D.: Drug Top. Suppl:3–13, 2001.
61. Fields, S.: Am. Pharm. NS33:4:28–29, 1993.
62. Roth, R.: Am. Pharm. NS34(4):31–34, 1997.
63. Allen, L. V.: Am. Pharm. NS34:31–33, 1994.
64. Evens, R., Louie, S. G., Sindelar, R., et al.: Biotech. Rx: Biotechnology in Pharmacy Practice: Science, Clinical Applications, and Pharmaceutical Care—Opportunities in Therapy Management. Washington, DC, American Pharmaceutical Association, 1997.
65. Zito, S. W. (ed.): Pharmaceutical Biotechnology: A Programmed Text. Lancaster, PA: 1992, Technomic Publishing, 1992.
66. Biotechnology Resource Catalog. Philadelphia: Philadelphia College of Pharmacy and Science, 1993.
67. Watson, J. D., Hopkins, N. H., Roberts, J. W., et al.: Molecular Biology of the Gene, 4th ed. Menlo Park, CA, Benjamin Cummings, 1987.
68. Davis, L. G., Dibner, M. D., and Battey, J. F.: Basic Methods in Molecular Biology. New York, Elsevier, 1986.
69. Wu–Pong, S., and Rojanaskul, Y. (eds.): Biopharmaceutical Drug Design and Development. Totowa, NJ, Humana Press, 1999.
70. Ausubel, F. M., Brent, R., et al.: Current Protocols in Molecular Biology. New York, Greene, Wiley-Interscience, 1988.
71. Davis, L. G.: Background to Recombinant DNA Technology. In Pezzuto, J. M., Johnson, M. E., and Manasse, H. R. (eds.). Biotechnology and Pharmacy. New York, Chapman & Hall, 1993, pp. 1–38.
72. Watson, J. D., et al.: Recombinant DNA, 2nd ed. New York, Scientific American Books, 1992, pp. 13–32.
73. Greene, J. J., and Rao, V. B. (eds.): Recombinant DNA: Principles and Methodologies. New York, Marcel Dekker, 1998.
74. Kreuzer, H., and Massey, A.: Recombinant DNA and Biotechnology. Washington, DC, ASM Press, 1996.
75. Nelson, D. L., and Cox, M. M. (eds.): Lehninger: Principles of Biochemistry. New York, Worth Publishers, 2000, pp. 905–1119.
76. Devlin, T. M. (ed.): Textbook of Biochemistry with Clinical Correlations, 3rd ed. New York, John Wiley & Sons, 1992, pp. 607–766.
77. Horton, H. R., Moran, L. A., Ochs, R. S., et al. (eds.): Principles of Biochemistry, 2nd ed. Upper Saddle River, NJ, Prentice-Hall, 1996, pp. 561–692.
78. Crick, F. H. C.: Symp. Soc. Exp. Biol. 12:128–163, 1958.
79. Watson, J. D.: Molecular Biology of the Gene. New York, W. A. Benjamin, 1970.
80. Jordan, E.: Am. J. Hum. Genet. 51:1–6, 1992.
81. Voet, D., and Voet, J. G.: Biochemistry, 2nd ed. New York, John Wiley & Sons, 1995, pp. 944–945.
82. Johnson, M. E., and Kahn, M.: In Pezzuto, J. M., Johnson, M. E., and Manasse, H. R. (eds.). Biotechnology and Pharmacy. New York, 1993, pp. 369–371.
83. Paolella, P.: Introduction to Molecular Biology. Boston, WCB McGraw–Hill, 1988, p. 176.
84. Davis, L. G.: In Pezzuto, J. M., Johnson, M. E., and Manasse, H. R. (eds.). Biotechnology and Pharmacy. New York, 1993, pp. 10–11.
85. Rojanaskul, Y., and Dokka, S.: In Wu-Pong, S., and Rojanaskul, Y. (eds.). Biopharmaceutical Drug Design and Development. Totowa, NJ, Humana Press, 1999, pp. 39–40.
86. Paolella, P.: Introduction to Molecular Biology. Boston, WCB McGraw–Hill, 1988, pp. 177–178.
87. Rojanaskul, Y., Dokka, S.: In Wu-Pong, S., Rojanaskul, Y. (eds.). Biopharmaceutical Drug Design and Development. Totowa, NJ, Humana Press, 1999, pp. 38–39.
88. Green, E. D., and Olson, M. V.: Proc. Natl. Acad. Sci. U. S. A. 87: 1213–1217, 1990.
89. Kadir, F.: Production of Biotech Compounds—Cultivation and Downstream Processing. In Crommelin, D. J. A., and Sindelar, R. D. (eds.). Pharmaceutical Biotechnology: An Introduction for Pharmacists and Pharmaceutical Scientists, Amsterdam, The Netherlands: Harwood Academic Publishers, 1997, pp. 53–70.
90. Riordan, J. R, et al.: Science 245:1066–1073, 1989.
91. Rommens, J. M., et al.: Science 245:1059–1065, 1989.
92. Heldebrand, G. E., et al.: In Pezzuto, J. M., Johnson, M. E., and Manasse, H. R. (eds.). Biotechnology and Pharmacy. New York, 1993, pp. 198–199.
93. Rojanaskul, Y., and Dokka, S. In Wu-Pong, S., and Rojanaskul, Y. (eds.). Biopharmaceutical Drug Design and Development. Totowa, NJ, Humana Press, 1999, pp. 43–45.
94. Katz, E. D., and Dong, M. W.: BioTechniques 8:628–632, 1990.
95. Kadir, F.: Production of Biotech Compounds—Cultivation and Downstream Processing. In Crommelin, D. J. A., and Sindelar, R. D. (eds.). Pharmaceutical Biotechnology: An Introduction for Pharmacists and Pharmaceutical Scientists, Amsterdam, The Netherlands, Harwood Academic Publishers, 1997, pp. 61–65.
96. Burgess, D. J.: In Pezzuto, J. M., Johnson, M. E., and Manasse, H. R. (eds.). Biotechnology and Pharmacy. New York, 1993, pp. 118–122.
97. Dillman, R. O.: Antibody Immunoconj. Radiopharm. 1990:1–15.
98. Wettendorff, M., et al.: Proc. Natl. Acad. Sci. U. S. A. 86:3787–3791, 1989.
99. Burgess, D. J. In Pezzuto, J. M., Johnson, M. E., and Manasse, H. R. (eds.). Biotechnology and Pharmacy. New York, 1993, pp. 124–143.
100. Facts and Comparisons. St. Louis, MO, Facts and Comparisons, 2000, pp. 287–290.
101. American Hospital Formulary Service Drug Information, 1989. Bethesda, MD, ASHP, 1989, pp. 2714–2728.
102. Beals, J. M, and Kovach, P. M.: In Crommelin, D. J. A., and Sindelar, R. D. (eds.). Pharmaceutical Biotechnology: An Introduction for Pharmacists and Pharmaceutical Scientists. Amsterdam, The Netherlands, Harwood Academic Publishers, 1997, p. 220.
103. Riley, T. N., and DeRuiter, J.: US Pharmacist 25(10):56–64, 2000.
104. Facts and Comparisons. St. Louis, MO, Facts and Comparisons, 2000, pp. 313–314.
105. Facts and Comparisons. St. Louis, MO, Facts and Comparisons, 2000, pp. 344–346.
106. Marian, M.: In Crommelin, D. J. A., and Sindelar, R. D. (eds.). Pharmaceutical Biotechnology: An Introduction for Pharmacists and Pharmaceutical Scientists. Amsterdam, The Netherlands, Harwood Academic Publishers, 1997, pp. 241–253.
107. Facts and Comparisons. St. Louis, MO, Facts and Comparisons, 2000, pp. 247–250.
108. Sam T, DeBoer W.: Follicle Stimulating Hormone. In Crommelin, D. J. A., and Sindelar, R. D. (eds.). Pharmaceutical Biotechnology: An Introduction for Pharmacists and Pharmaceutical Scientists. Amsterdam, The Netherlands, Harwood Academic Publishers, 1997, pp. 315–320.
109. Buckland, P. R., et al.: Biochem. J. 235:879–882, 1986.
110. Pharmaceutical Research and Manufacturers Association: Biotechnology Medicines in Development. PhRMA 2002 Annual Survey. Washington, DC, Pharmaceutical Research and Manufacturers Association, 2002.
111. Graber, S. E., and Krantz, S. B.: Annu. Rev. Med. 29:51–66, 1978.
112. Egric, J. C., Strickland, T. W., Lane J., et al.: Immunobiology 72: 213–224, 1986.
113. Eschenbach, J. W., et al.: Ann. Intern. Med. 111:992–1000, 1989.
114. Zsebo, K. M, Cohen, A. M., et al.: Immunobiology 72:175–184, 1986.
115. Souza, L. M., Boone, T. C., et al.: Science 232:61–65, 1986.

116. Heil, G., Hoelzer, D., et al.: Blood 90:4710–4718, 1997.
117. Metcalf, D.: Blood 67(2):257–267, 1986.
118. Vadhan-Raj, S., Keating, M., et al.: N. Engl. J. Med. 317:1545–1552, 1987.
119. Facts and Comparisons. St. Louis, MO, Facts and Comparisons, 2000, pp. 192–194.
120. Grabenstein, J. D. (ed.): Immunofacts: Vaccines and Immunologic Drugs. St. Louis, MO, Facts and Comparisons, 2002, pp. 695–704.
121. Pegasys. Roche Pharmaceuticals Company Stat/Gram. Nutley, NJ, Hoffman-LaRoche, 2003.
122. Grabenstein, J. D. (ed.): Immunofacts: Vaccines and Immunologic Drugs, St. Louis, MO, Facts and Comparisons, 2002, pp. 705–717.
123. Grabenstein, J. D. (ed.): Immunofacts: Vaccines and Immunologic Drugs, St. Louis, MO, Facts and Comparisons, 2002, pp. 737–740 and references therein.
124. Grabenstein, J. D. (ed.): Immunofacts: Vaccines and Immunologic Drugs, St. Louis, MO, Facts and Comparisons, 2002, pp. 741–745 and references therein.
125. Grabenstein, J. D. (ed.): Immunofacts: Vaccines and Immunologic Drugs, St. Louis, MO, Facts and Comparisons, 2002, pp. 746–752 and references therein.
126. Grabenstein, J. D. (ed.): Immunofacts: Vaccines and Immunologic Drugs, St. Louis, MO, Facts and Comparisons, 2002, pp. 756–764 and references therein.
127. Grabenstein, J. D. (ed.): Immunofacts: Vaccines and Immunologic Drugs, St. Louis, MO, Facts and Comparisons, 2002, pp. 765–770 and references therein.
128. Grabenstein, J. D. (ed.): Immunofacts: Vaccines and Immunologic Drugs, St. Louis, MO, Facts and Comparisons, 2002, pp. 771–775 and references therein.
129. Grabenstein, J. D. (ed.): Immunofacts: Vaccines and Immunologic Drugs, St. Louis, MO, Facts and Comparisons, 2002, pp. 776–787 and references therein.
130. Grabenstein, J. D. (ed.): Immunofacts: Vaccines and Immunologic Drugs, St. Louis, MO, Facts and Comparisons, 2002, pp. 788–794 and references therein.
131. Grabenstein, J. D. (ed.): Immunofacts: Vaccines and Immunologic Drugs, St. Louis, MO, Facts and Comparisons, 2002, pp. 795–802 and references therein.
132. Murray, K. M., and Dahl, S. L.: Ann. Pharmacother. 31(11):1335–1338, 1997.
133. Weinblatt, M., et al.: Arthritis Rheum. 40(Suppl):S126, 1997.
134. Moreland, L. W., et al.: N. Engl. J. Med. 337:141–147, 1997.
135. Verstraate, M., Lijnen, H., and Cullen, D.: Drugs 50(1):29–42, 1995.
136. Facts and Comparisons. St. Louis, MO, Facts and Comparisons, 2000, pp. 183–189.
137. Cannon, C. P, Gibson, C. M., et al.: Circulation 98:2805–2814, 1998.
138. Facts and Comparisons. St. Louis, MO, Facts and Comparisons, 2000, p. 193.
139. Shapiro, A. D., Ragni, M. V., Lusher, J. M., et al.: Thromb. Haemost. 75(1):30–35, 1996.
140. Facts and Comparisons. St. Louis, MO, Facts and Comparisons, 2000, p. 195.
141. Bernard, G. R., et al.: N. Engl. J. Med. 344:699–709, 2001.
142. Fabrizio, M.: J. Am. Soc. Extra Corporeal Tech. 331:117–125, 2001.
143. Facts and Comparisons. St. Louis, MO, Facts and Comparisons, 2000, pp. 679–680.
144. Facts and Comparisons. St. Louis, MO, Facts and Comparisons, 2000, pp. 355.
145. Facts and Comparisons. St. Louis, MO, Facts and Comparisons, 2000, pp. 1529–1531.
146. Facts and Comparisons. St. Louis, MO, Facts and Comparisons, 2000, pp. 1505–1508.
147. Reichmann, L., et al.: Nature 332:323–327, 1983.
148. Cobbold, S. P., and Waldmann, H. Nature 334:460–462, 1984.
149. Adair, J. R., et al.: In Crommelin, D. J. A., and Sindelar, R. D. (eds.). Pharmaceutical Biotechnology: An Introduction for Pharmacists and Pharmaceutical Scientists. Amsterdam, The Netherlands, Harwood Academic Publishers, 1997, pp. 279–287.
150. Coiffier, B., et al.: N. Engl. J. Med. 346(4):280–282, 2002.
151. Maloney, D. G., et al.: Blood 90:2188–2195, 1997.
152. Grabenstein, J. D. (ed.): Immunofacts: Vaccines and Immunologic Drugs, St. Louis, MO, Facts and Comparisons, 2002, pp. 406–413 and references therein.
153. Voliotis, D., et al.: Ann. Oncol. 11(4):95–100, 2000.
154. Grabenstein, J. D. (ed.): Immunofacts: Vaccines and Immunologic Drugs, St. Louis, MO, Facts and Comparisons, 2002, pp. 414–422 and references therein.
155. McConnell, H.: Blood 100:768–773, 2002.
156. Billaud, E. M.: Therapie 55(1):177–183, 2000.
157. Ponticelli, C., et al.: Drugs 1(1):55–60, 1999.
158. Kirkman, R. L.: Transplant. Proc. 31(1–2):1234–1235, 1999.
159. Vincenti, F.: N. Engl. J. Med. 338:161–165, 1998.
160. Oberholzer, J., et al.: Transplant. Int. 14(2):169–171, 2000.
161. Chan, G. L. C., Gruber, S. A., et al.: Crit. Care Clin. 6:841–892, 1990.
162. Hooks, M. A., Wade, C. S., and Milliken, W. J.: Pharmacotherapy 11:26–37, 1991.
163. Todd, P. A., and Brogden, R. N.: Drugs 37:871–899, 1989.
164. Topol, E. J., and Serruys, P. W.: Circulation 98:1802–1820, 1998.
165. Grabenstein, J. D. (ed.): Immunofacts: Vaccines and Immunologic Drugs, St. Louis, MO, Facts and Comparisons, 2002, pp. 455–462 and references therein.
166. Gelmon, K., Arnold, A., et al.: Proc. Am. Soc. Clin. Oncol. 20(69a): Abstr. 271, 2001.
167. Slamon, D. J., Leyland–Jones, B., et al.: N. Engl. J. Med. 344(11): 783–792, 2000.
168. Grabenstein, J. D. (ed.): Immunofacts: Vaccines and Immunologic Drugs, St. Louis, MO, Facts and Comparisons, 2002, pp. 473–482 and references therein.
169. Hanauer, S. B.: N. Engl. J. Med. 334:841, 1996.
170. Bogard, W. C., Jr., et al.: Semin. Nucl. Med. 19(3):202–220, 1989.
171. Kassis, A. I.: J. Nucl. Med. 32(9):1751–1753, 1991.
172. Reilly, R. M.: Clin. Pharmacol. Ther. 10(5):359–375, 1991.
173. Reilly, R. M., et al.: Clin. Pharmacokinet. 28:126–142, 1995.
174. Grabenstein, J. D. (ed.): Immunofacts: Vaccines and Immunologic Drugs, St. Louis, MO, Facts and Comparisons, 2002, pp. 535–543 and references therein.
175. Grabenstein, J. D. (ed.): Immunofacts: Vaccines and Immunologic Drugs, St. Louis, MO, Facts and Comparisons, 2002, pp. 544–554 and references therein.
176. Quattrocchi, E., and Hove, I. US Pharm. 23(4):54–63, 1998.
177. Rios, M.: Pharm. Tech. 25(1):34–40, 2000.
178. Ramsey, G.: Nat. Biotech. 16:40–44, 1998.
179. Khan, J., et al.: Biochim. Biophys. Acta 1423:17–28, 1999.
180. Persidis, A.: Nat. Biotech. 16:393–394, 1998.
181. Borman, S.: Chem. Eng. News 78:31–37, 2000.
182. Lau, K. F., and Sakul, H.: Annu. Rep. Med. Chem. 36:261–269, 2000.

Immunobiologicals

JOHN M. BEALE, JR.

The immune system constitutes the body's defense against infectious agents. It protects the host by identifying and eliminating or neutralizing agents that are recognized as nonself. The entire range of immunological responses affects essentially every organ, tissue, and cell of the body. Immune responses include, in part, antibody (Ab) production, allergy, inflammation, phagocytosis, cytotoxicity, transplant and tumor rejection, and the many signals that regulate these responses.[1] At its most basic, the human immune system can be described in terms of the cells that compose it. Every aspect of the immune system, whether innate and nonspecific or adaptive and specific, is controlled by a set of specialized cells. Thus, this discussion of some of the fundamentals of immunology begins with the cells of the immune system.

CELLS OF THE IMMUNE SYSTEM

All immune cells derive from *pluripotent* stem cells in the bone marrow. These are cells that can differentiate into any other cell type, given the right kind of stimulus (Scheme 7-1). A variety of modes of differentiation beyond the stem cell give rise to unique cellular types, each with a specific function in the immune system. The first stage of differentiation gives rise to two intermediate types of stem cells and creates a branch point.[2] These cells are the myeloid cells (myeloid lineage) and the lymphoid cells (lymphoid lineage). Carrying the lineage further leads to additional branching. The myeloid cells differentiate into erythrocytes and platelets and also monocytes and granulocytes. The lymphoid cell differentiates into B cells and T cells, the cells that are at the center of adaptive immunity. The switching system for each pathway and cell type is governed by a number of colony-stimulating factors, stem cell factors, and interleukins. These control proliferation, differentiation, and maturation of the cells.

Major Histocompatibility Antigens—Self Versus Nonself

The development of most immune responses depends on the recognition of what is *self* and what is *not self*. This determination must be clear and must be done in a very general way. This recognition is achieved by the expression of specialized surface markers on human cells. The major group of markers involved in this recognition consists of surface proteins. These are referred to as the *major histocompatibility complex*[3] (MHC) or *major histocompatibility antigens*. Proteins expressed on the cell surfaces are class I MHCs and class II MHCs. Both classes are highly polymorphic and so are highly specific to each individual. Class I

MHCs can be found on virtually all nucleated cells in the human body, while class II MHC molecules are associated only with B lymphocytes and macrophages. Class I MHCs are markers that are recognized by natural killer cells and cytotoxic T lymphocytes. When a class I MHC is coexpressed with viral antigens on virus-infected cells, cytotoxic target cells are signaled. Class II MHC molecules are markers indicating that a cooperative immune state exists between immunocompetent cells, such as between an antigen-presenting cell and a T-helper cell during the induction of Ab formation.

Granulocytes[4]

If one views a granulocyte under a microscope, one can observe dense intracytoplasmic granules. The granules contain inflammatory mediators and digestive enzymes that destroy invading pathogens, control the rate and pathway of migration of chemotactic cells, and cause dilation of blood vessels at the infected site. The increased blood flow ensures that an ample supply of granulocytes and inflammatory mediators reaches the site of infection. There is a family of granulocytic cells, each member with its own specialized function. Under microscopic examination, some granulocytes are seen to be multinuclear and some mononuclear. The configuration of the nuclear region and the staining behavior provide ways of classifying granulocytes. The group is discussed below.

Neutrophils[4]

Neutrophils are the primary innate defense against pathogenic bacteria. They make up most (50 to 75%) of the leukocyte fraction in the blood. Microscopically, neutrophils have multilobed nuclei. They respond to chemical motility factors such as complement mediators released from infected or inflamed tissues and migrate to a site of infection by the process of chemotaxis. There, they recognize, adhere to, and phagocytose invading microbes.

Phagocytes

The phagocytic process is initiated by contact and adhesion of an invading cell with a phagocyte cell membrane. Adhesion triggers a process whereby the phagocytic cell extrudes pseudopodia that surround the adhering microbe. As this process progresses, the microbe is actually surrounded by the phagocyte cell membrane. Then, invagination of the membrane fully engulfs the particle, and the membrane is resealed, with the particle encased inside an intracellular vacuolar body called a *phagosome*. Lysosomes in the cytoplasm then fuse with the phagosome to form *phagolyso-*

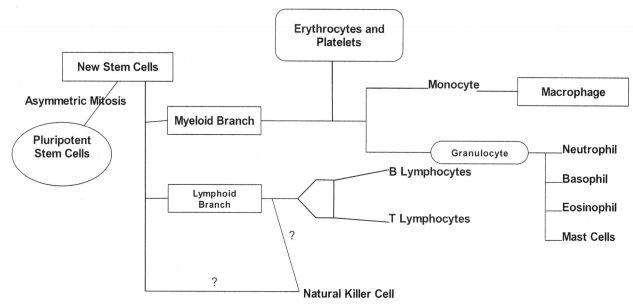

Scheme 7–1 ■ Lineages of blood cells. All blood cells derive from a pluripotent stem cell. A variety of cytokines direct the cells into their specific populations.

somes. The antimicrobial compounds in the phagosomes and lysosomes kill the engulfed pathogen and enzymatically cleave its remains into smaller pieces.

Eosinophils[5]

Eosinophils are granulocytes that can function as phagocytes, but much less efficiently than neutrophils can. They are present as 2 to 4% of blood leukocytes. Their name derives from the intense staining reaction of their intracellular granules with the dye eosin. Eosinophil granules contain inflammatory mediators such as histamine and leukotrienes, so it makes sense that these cells are associated with the allergic response. Clues to the functions of eosinophils come from their behavior in certain disease states. Eosinophil counts are elevated above normal in the tissues in many different diseases, but they are recognized primarily for their diagnostic role in parasitic infections and in allergies. Eosinophils have a unique mode of action that lends to their extreme importance. Unlike neutrophils, eosinophils need not phagocytose a parasite to kill it. Indeed, some parasites are too large to allow phagocytosis. Eosinophils can physically surround a large parasite, forming a cell coat around the invader. Eosinophil granules release oxidative substances capable of destroying even large, multicellular parasites. Hence, even when phagocytosis fails, a mechanism exists to destroy large parasites.

Mast Cells and Basophils

Mast cells and basophils also release the inflammatory mediators commonly associated with allergy. Mast cells are especially prevalent in the skin, lungs, and nasal mucosa; their granules contain histamine. Basophils, present at only 0.2% of the leukocyte fraction in the blood, also contain histamine granules, but the basophiles found circulating in the blood and not isolated in connective tissue. Both mast cells and basophils have high-affinity immunoglobulin E

(IgE) receptors. Complexes of antigen molecules with IgE receptors on the cell surface lead to cross-linking of IgE and distortion of the cell membrane. The distortion causes the mast cell to degranulate, releasing mediators of the allergic response. Because of its association with hypersensitivity, IgE has been called ''reagin'' in the allergy literature. Diagnostically, IgE levels are elevated in allergy, systemic lupus erythematosus, and rheumatoid arthritis. Cromolyn sodium is a drug that prevents mast cell degranulation and thus blocks the allergic response. Cromolyn is used in asthma.

Macrophages and Monocytes[4, 5]

Macrophages and monocytes are mononuclear cells that are capable of phagocytosis. In addition to their phagocytic capabilities, they biosynthesize and release soluble factors (complement, monokines) that govern the acquired immune response. The half-life of monocytes in the bloodstream is about 10 hours, during which time they migrate into tissues and differentiate into macrophages. A macrophage is a terminally differentiated monocyte. Macrophages possess a true anatomical distribution because they develop in the tissues to have specialized functions. Special macrophages are found in tissues such as the liver, lungs, spleen, gastrointestinal (GI) tract, lymph nodes, and brain. These specific macrophages are called either *histiocytes* (generic term) or by certain specialized names (*Kupffer cells* in liver, *Langerhans cells* in skin, *alveolar macrophages* in lung) (Table 7-1). The entire macrophage network is called the *reticuloendothelial system*. Other macrophages exist free in the tissues, where they carry out more nonspecific functions. Macrophages kill more slowly than neutrophils but have a much broader spectrum. It has been estimated that more than 100 soluble inflammatory substances are produced by macrophages. These substances account for macrophages' prolific abilities to direct, modulate, stimulate, and retard the immune response.

Macrophages possess a very specialized function; they

TABLE 7–1 Reticuloendothelial System

Tissue	Cell
Liver	Kupffer cells
Lung	Alveolar macrophages (dust cells)
Peritoneum	Peritoneal macrophages
Spleen	Dendritic cells
Skin	Langerhans cells
Brain	Microglial cells

act as *antigen-presenting cells* (APCs) (Fig. 7-1). APCs are responsible for the preprocessing of antigens, amplifying the numbers of antigenic determinant units and presenting these determinant structures to the programming cells of the immune system. APCs internalize an organism or particle and digest it into small fragments still recognizable as antigen. The fragments are conjugated with molecules of the major histocompatibility complex 2 (MHC-II). These complexes are responsible for self or nonself cell recognition and ascertain that cells being processed are not self. MHCs also direct the binding of the antigenic determinant with immunoreactive cells. Once the antigen–MHC-II complex forms, it undergoes transcytosis to the macrophage's cell surface, where B lymphocytes and helper T cells recognize the anti-

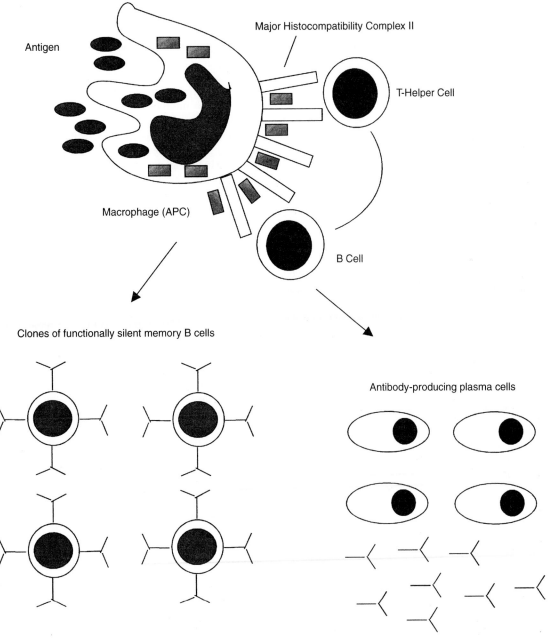

Figure 7–1 ■ Antigen capture and presentation by a macrophage lead to clones of Ab-producing plasma cells and memory B cells.

gen via the B surface Ab and T-cell receptors. It is this step that transfers specificity and memory information from the determinant into the immune system through the modulation of B-cell differentiation. Under the regulatory influence of the helper T cells, B cells are stimulated to differentiate into plasma cells that produce Ab. The helper T cells accelerate and retard the process as necessary. Thus, unlike the granulocytes, which have only destructive functions, monocytes and macrophages regulate and program the immune response.

The Lymphoid Cell Line: B and T Cells[2]

The lymphoid cell line differentiates into two types of lymphocytes, the B lymphocytes and the T lymphocytes. These cells constitute only about 20 to 45% of blood leukocytes. They are small cells, only slightly larger than an erythrocyte, but B and T cells can be identified microscopically by large nuclei that occupy most of the cytoplasmic volume. The nuclei are large to contain enough DNA to enable the T and B cells to biosynthesize massive amounts of protein needed to carry out their immune functions. T lymphocytes are involved in cell-mediated immunity; B lymphocytes differentiate into Ab-producing plasma cells. B lymphocytes express antibodies on their surfaces that bind antigens. T lymphocytes express specialized T-cell receptors on their surfaces that bind major histocompatibility complex 1 (MHC-1) and 2 (MHC-2) complexed with antigenic peptide fragments.

IMMUNITY

Immunity in humans can be conceptualized in a number of different ways. If just the type and specificity of the immune response are considered, the ideas of *innate* and *acquired* immunity are used. If only the components that are involved in the immune response are considered, the processes can be divided into *humoral* and *cellular* immunity. If the location of the immune response is considered, we find that the immune system consists of *serosal* (in the serum) immunity and *mucosal* (on mucosal epithelium surfaces) immunity.

Innate Immunity

Innate immunity is the most basic form of immunity and includes immune systems that are present in a human from birth. A clear distinction must be made between innate immunity and acquired (adaptive) immunity, which develops after birth, and then only after an antigenic challenge (Table 7-2). Innate immunity is the first line of defense against

invasion by microbes and can be characterized as fast in response, nonspecific, and lacking in memory of the challenge. Acquired immunity develops through a complex system of reactions that are triggered by invasion with an infectious agent. It is slow in response to an infection, is *highly specific*, and has memory of previous infections. The memory, or anamnestic response, is responsible for the extremely rapid development of the immune response with subsequent challenges and is a hallmark of acquired immunity.

There are three separate components of innate immunity that work in concert to provide the whole response. There are physical barriers, cellular barriers, and soluble factors. The physical barriers include the largest, most exposed organ of the body (the skin), the mucosa, and its associated mucus. The keratinized layer of protein and lipid in the stratum corneum of the skin protects physically against a variety of environmental, biological, and chemical assaults. The protection afforded by mucosal surfaces, such as are found in the throat, mouth, nose, and GI tract, is due to a surface epithelium. The epithelium consists of single or multiple layers of epithelial cells with tight gap junctions between them. This type of structure provides an impermeable physical barrier to microorganisms. Most of the time, epithelium is further protected by the secretion of mucus, such as from goblet cells in the GI mucosa. Mucus is a viscous layer consisting of glycopeptide and an acidic glycoprotein called mucin. Mucus can prevent penetration of microbial cells into the epithelium, significantly decreasing the possibility of infection by the mucosal route. Other components of the physical barriers in innate immunity are the tears (containing lysozyme), the acidic pH of the stomach, the low pH and flow of the urine, and the cilia in the lungs that constantly beat upward to remove inspired particulates and microbes.

Two components of the cellular innate immune response have already been discussed, granulocytes in the blood and tissue macrophages. When an infection occurs in the tissues, chemotactic factors liberated at the site migrate down a concentration gradient to the surrounding area. These agents make the capillary beds porous. Neutrophils follow the concentration gradient across the endothelium to the site of infection. There are three types of chemotactic factors: *(a)* formylmethionyl (f-Met) peptides released from the invading bacteria, *(b)* leukotrienes secreted by phagocytes, and *(c)* peptide fragments released from activated complement proteins such as C_{3a} and C_{5a}. Neutrophils and macrophages engulf and destroy microorganisms by phagocytosis. Nonphagocytic cells are also involved in the innate immune response, providing soluble chemical factors that enhance the innate response.

Soluble factors of innate immunity include *(a)* bactericidal factors, *(b)* complement, and *(c)* interferon. A bactericidal factor (Table 7-3) is an agent that kills bacteria. Perhaps the most fundamental bactericidal factor is the acid in the stomach. Secreted by goblet cells in the mucosal epithelial lining, stomach acid is responsible for disposing of most of the microbes that are consumed orally. Phagocytes or hepatocytes produce the other bactericidal factors. Most of these are directed toward the phagosome, where the predigested, phagocytically encapsulated bacterial cell is enclosed. The antimicrobial factors kill the immobilized microbes.

There are two types of antimicrobial factors, those that

TABLE 7–2 Characteristics of Innate Versus Acquired Immunity

Innate Immunity	Acquired Immunity
Present from birth	Develops later
Rapid	Slow
Nonspecific	Specific
No memory	Memory

TABLE 7–3 Bactericidal Factors

Factor	Formation	Site of Action
Oxygen ions and radicals	Induced	Phagosomes
Acid hydrolases	Preformed	Lysosomes
Cationic proteins	Preformed	Phagosomes
Defensins	Preformed	Phagosomes or extracellular
Lactoferrin	Preformed	Phagosomes

are preformed inside the phagocyte and one that is *induced* in response to the phagocytic process. The most important of the antimicrobial mechanisms is the respiratory burst, which generates oxygen radicals—superoxide, hydroxyl radicals, and hydrogen peroxide. The respiratory burst is the only induced mechanism. All of the active oxygen species are highly destructive to bacterial as well as host cells, so they are not produced until they are needed. The defensins are arginine- or cysteine-rich bactericidal peptides that exhibit an extremely broad spectrum of antimicrobial activity. The defensins will kill bacteria (Gram positive and Gram negative), fungi, and even some viruses. The mechanism of action of the defensins is unknown, but since the peptides are highly charged in an opposite sense to bacterial cell membranes, an electrostatic, membrane-disruptive interaction might be involved. Bacteria have an absolute requirement for iron, and to compete with the host for this element, they secrete high-affinity siderophore factors that scavenge iron from the host's stores. Lactoferrin is a substance produced by the host that binds iron more tightly than the bacterial chelator, preventing the invading organism's access to a critical nutrient. Lysozyme is an important component of the antimicrobial system. This enzyme hydrolyzes [1-4]-glycosidic bonds, as in the peptidoglycan of bacterial cell walls. Lysozyme is present in almost all body fluids, including tears and saliva.

Hepatocytes produce an array of *acute phase proteins* (Table 7-4) that are released into the serum during inflammation or infection. These proteins do not act directly on bacteria, but they augment the bactericidal activity of other antimicrobial factors.

COMPLEMENT[5]

Complement is a system of at least 20 separate proteins and cofactors that continuously circulate in the bloodstream.

TABLE 7–4 Acute Phase Factors

Acute Phase Factor	Function/Activity
C-reactive protein	Chemotaxis and enhancement of phagocytosis
α_1-Antitrypsin	Inhibition of proteases
Complement factors	Control of the complement cascade
Fibrinogen	Blood coagulation

Complement acts to kill bacterial cells that are missed by the neutrophils and the macrophages. There are actually two separate complement pathways. One, the *classical pathway,* operates in the adaptive or acquired immune response. The classical pathway has an absolute requirement for an Ab–antigen complex as a trigger. The other, the *alternative pathway,* requires no Ab or antigen to initiate and is operative in innate immunity. Both pathways operate in a tightly regulated cascade fashion. The proteins normally circulate as inactive proenzymes. When the pathways are activated, the product of each step activates the subsequent step.

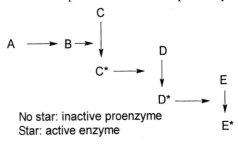

No star: inactive proenzyme
Star: active enzyme

THE ALTERNATIVE PATHWAY

In the alternative pathway, C3 is the initiating peptide (Fig.7-2). In the serum, C3 is somewhat unstable (it is sensitive to proteases) and spontaneously decomposes into a large, active C3b fragment and a smaller, catalytically inactive C3a fragment. C3b now becomes bound to a surface, and it has two fates. We can define two types of surfaces. One, the nonactivating surface, is a surface that contains sialic acid or other acidic polysaccharides. The other, an activating surface, contains none of the acidic polysaccharides or sialic acid. This type conforms to a bacterial cell surface. Under normal circumstances, C3b will bind to a nonactivating surface. On binding, the C3b fragment becomes associated with factor H, a β-globulin that associates with an α chain on C3b. Sialic acid increases the affinity for factor H 100-fold. Factor H alters the shape of C3b in such a way that it becomes susceptible to attack by factor I, a serine esterase that cleaves the α chain of C3b, producing inactive iC3b. Attack by another protease produces a fragment designated C3c. In this pathway, factor H accelerates the decay of C3b. When factors H and I work together they destroy C3b as fast as it is produced and shut down the pathway.

If C3b binds to an activating surface, the ability to bind to factor H is reduced, and C3b binds to a protein called factor B, forming C3bB. Bound factor B is cleaved by factor D into a fragment called Bb. The complex C3bBb has high C3-convertase activity and stimulates the pathway further. Factor P (properdin) binds to the complex, extending the half-life of C3bBbP. This fragment binds to the terminal complement components (C5 to C9), creating a membrane attack complex and thus lysing the cell.

INTERFERONS

An important antiviral system is provided by the interferons (Table 7-5 and Fig. 7-3). The interferons are peptides that, when viral infection occurs, carry out three distinct functions. First, they send a signal to a natural killer cell that essentially leads to the self-destruction of the infected cell. Second, they induce an antiviral state in neighboring cells,

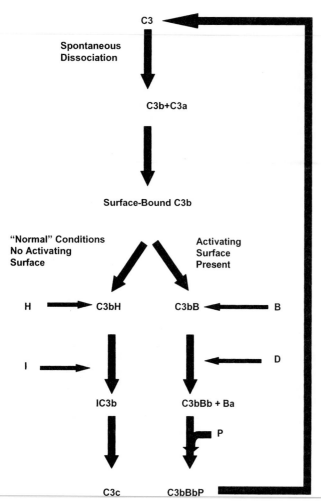

Figure 7–2 ■ Control of the alternative complement pathway by activating surfaces. When complement component C3b binds to a surface, there exist two possible outcomes. Under normal conditions, when no activating surface is present (e.g., if C3b has contacted normal tissue), sequential addition of blood cofactors H and I converts C3b into C3c, inactivating the complement protein. If an activating surface such as a microbe or damaged tissue is encountered, sequential addition of factors B and D drives the alternative pathway to the normal properdin (P) intermediate, and the complement cascade is triggered. The properdin-containing component (C3bBbP) feeds back to the beginning of the pathway, generating more C3.

limiting the viral infection. Third, when interferon receptors are bound on a target cell, the induction of the formation of antiviral proteins occurs. One such protein is the enzyme, 2′,5′- oligoadenylate synthetase. This enzyme catalyzes the reaction that converts ATP into 2′,5′-oligoadenylate. This compound activates ribonuclease R, which possesses the specificity to hydrolyze viral RNA and thus can stop propagation of the virus inside the cell.

Acquired (Adaptive) Immunity

When the host is exposed to an antigen or organism that has been contacted previously, the *adaptive immune response* ensues. The adaptive immune response works through the B and T lymphocytes, which possess surface receptors specific for each invading organism. To account for all possible permutations of antigenic structure, natural and synthetic, that the host might encounter, the adaptive immune system uses genetic recombination of DNA and RNA splicing as a way of encoding its antibodies. Lymphocytes can recognize an estimated 10^7 different types of antigens through this genetic recombination mechanism, far more than a person is likely to encounter during a lifetime. Adaptive immunity is Ab-mediated immunity, based on circulating pools of antibodies that react with, and inactivate, antigens. These antibodies are found in the globulin fraction of the serum. Consequently, antibodies are also referred to as *immunoglobulins* (Ig). The adaptive immune response has the property of *memory*. The sensitivity, specificity, and memory for a particular antigen are retained, and subsequent exposures stimulate an enhanced response. Hence, the adaptive immune response differs from the innate in two respects: *specificity* and *memory*.

The adaptive immune response, like the innate, can be divided into two branches: humoral immunity and cell-mediated immunity (CMI). Humoral immunity is circulating immunity and is mediated by B lymphocytes and differentiated B lymphocytes known as plasma cells. Cell-mediated immunity is controlled by the T lymphocytes. The immune function of T lymphocytes cannot be transferred by serum alone; the T cells must be present, whereas the immunity of the humoral system can be isolated from the serum and transferred. T cells are specially tailored to deal with intracellular infections (such as virus-infected cells), whereas B cells secrete soluble antibodies that can neutralize pathogens before their entry into host cells. Both B and T cells possess specific receptors on their surfaces to recognize unique stimulatory antigens. When B cells are stimulated, they express specific immunoglobulins or surface antibodies that are capable of binding to the antigen. A fraction of the B-cell

TABLE 7–5 Interferons

Interferon	Producing Cells	Producing Mechanism	Isotypes	Molecular Mass	Receptor
Type 1					
IFN-α	Leukocytes		17	16–27 kDa	95–110 kDa
IFN-β	Fibroblasts	Viral infection	1	20 kDa	95–110 kDa
Type 2					
IFN-γ	T lymphocytes	Mitogen stimulation	1	20–24 kDa	90–95 kDa

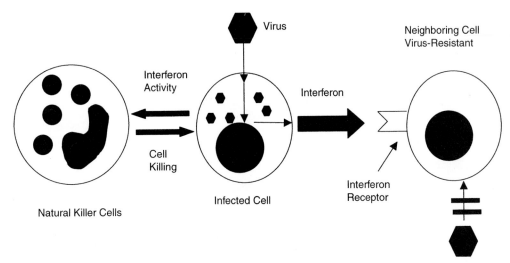

Figure 7–3 ■ The function of interferon. When a virus infects a host cell, the cell expresses interferon. Interferon activates natural killer cells, causing killing of the infected host cells and elimination of the reservoir of infection. At the same time, interferon induces an antiviral state in neighboring cells, effectively breaking the cycle of infection.

population does not differentiate into Ab-producing cells but forms a pool of cells that retain the immunological memory. T cells express a specific antigen receptor, the T-cell receptor, similar in structure to the surface immunoglobulin receptor of B cells. This receptor is activated by a piece of processed antigen (presented with MHC-II). Activated T cells release soluble factors such as interleukins, cytokines, interferons, lymphokines, and colony-stimulating factors, all of which regulate the immune response. Interactions with some of these help to regulate the B-cell activity, directing the innate immune response.

THE CLASSICAL COMPLEMENT PATHWAY

The classical complement pathway differs from the alternative pathway in that it requires a trigger in the form of an antigen–Ab complex. Only two antibodies can fix complement, IgG and IgM. The classical pathway is shown in Figure 7-4. The small fragments that are cleaved from the proenzymes have activities such as chemotactic stimulation and anaphylaxis. The *bar* over the names of some components of the pathway denotes an active complex. Note that the classical pathway does not operate with C1 to C9 in sequence. Rather, the sequence is C1, C4, C2, C3, C5, C6, C7, C8, and C9.

IMMUNOGLOBULIN STRUCTURE AND FUNCTION

An Ab or Ig is composed of peptide chains with carbohydrate pendant groups. A schematic of the Ab IgG is shown in Figure 7-5. The peptide chains form the quaternary structure of the immunoglobulin, while the carbohydrate moieties serve as antigen-recognition groups and probably as conformation-stabilizing units. The general structure of the Ig looks something like a Y, with the antigen-binding regions at the bifurcated end. In this area are peptide sequences that are ''programmable'' by the immune system to allow the Ig to recognize a large number of antigens.

Treatment with either of two enzymes, papain or pepsin,

digests an Ab into fragments that are useful in understanding its molecular structure. Papain clips the Ab into two fragments that contain the antigen-binding regions. These fragments have been termed the Fab, or antigen-binding, fragment. The remaining part of the Ab after papain digestion contains two peptide chains linked by a disulfide bond.

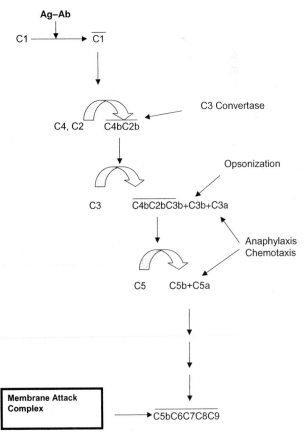

Figure 7–4 ■ Classical complement pathway.

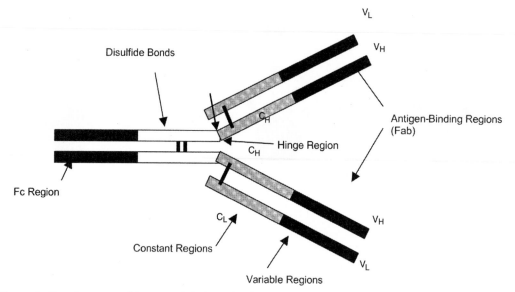

Figure 7–5 ■ Structure of immunoglobulin G (IgG), showing antigen-binding regions and key elements of the molecule.

Treatment of the same Ab with pepsin yields the two Fab units joined by the disulfide bond, plus two of the distal peptide chains. These distal units have been crystallized and, hence, are termed the Fc fragment (for "crystallizable"). The disulfide bond, therefore, provides a demarcation between the two molecular regions. The nomenclature of an Ab includes a high-molecular-weight, or heavy, chain on the inside and a low-molecular-weight, or light, chain on the outside.

IMPORTANT FEATURES OF ANTIBODY MOLECULAR STRUCTURE[4, 6]

As stated above, the tip end of the Fab region binds antigen. There are two of these regions, so we say that the Ab is *bivalent* and can bind two antigen molecules. The overall amino acid sequence of the Ab dictates its conformation. The peptide sequence for most antibodies is similar, except for the hypervariable regions. The amino acid sequence at the end of the heavy chain (Fc) determines the class of the Ig (i.e., IgG, IgM, etc.). All antibodies resemble each other in basic shape, but each has a unique amino acid sequence that is complementary to the antigen in a "lock and key" interaction (antigen–Ab specificity). Some, such as IgM, are pentamers of IgG (Fig.7-6). In reality, the lock-and-key model is too simplistic, and an induced fit model is preferred.

ANTIBODY PRODUCTION AND PROGRAMMING OF THE IMMUNE SYSTEM

The main element of the programming portion of the immune system is the macrophage. A common property of macrophages is *phagocytosis,* the capacity to engulf a particle or cell through invagination and sealing off of the cell membrane. The macrophages involved in the immune response set in motion a unique amplification process, so that a large response is obtained relative to the amount of antigen processed. The macrophages engulf antigenic particles and

incorporate them into their cytoplasm, where the antigens are fragmented. The fragments are then combined with MHC-II, displayed on the cell membrane of the macrophage, and presented to the immune system. The presented antigens interact with B cells, causing differentiation to plasma cells and Ab secretion. T-helper cells also interact with the presented antigen and are stimulated to cause the B cells to proliferate and mature. Plasma cells are monoclonal (genetically identical) and produce monoclonal Ab. The process,

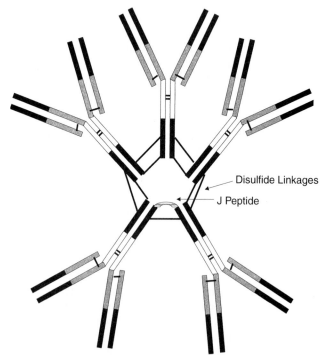

Figure 7–6 ■ Pentameric structure of immunoglobulin M (IgM).

from the pluripotent stem cell, to the B and T cells, to the plasma cells is shown in Figure 7-1.

ANTIBODY FORMATION[5]

Figure 7-1 also indicates the actual Ab-producing steps. Plasma cells are clones of Ab-producing cells, which amplify the Ab response by their sheer numbers. The plasma cells can easily be regenerated if called on to do so by the memory functions. A population of plasma cells is shown at the bottom of the diagram. These are identical and amplify and produce large quantities of Ab, proportionally much greater than the amount of antigen that was initially processed.

ANAMNESTIC RESPONSE[5]

Because the programmed immune system has the property of memory, subsequent exposures to the same antigen are immediately countered. The actual memory response is referred to as the *anamnestic response,* a secondary response of high Ab titer to a particular antigen. This is due to "memory cell" formation as a result of the initial antigen stimulus (sensitization or immunization). The anamnestic response is demonstrated in Figure 7-7.

ANTIGEN–ANTIBODY REACTIONS[4]

An Ab is bivalent, and an antigen is multivalent, so lattice formation can occur (Fig. 7-8). The complex may be fibrous, particulate, matrix-like, soluble, or insoluble. These characteristics dictate the means of its disposal. Four fundamental reactions describe these processes: neutralization, precipitation, agglutination, and bacteriolysis.

Neutralization. Neutralization is an immunological disposal reaction for bacteria and for toxins (which are small and soluble). Once they bind the Ab, they are no longer toxic because their active site structures are covered and they cannot bind their targets. Examples of toxins are tetanospasmin (tetanus toxin; *Clostridium tetani*) and diphtheria toxin. Both react with specific receptors in the inhibitory interneurons of the nervous system, causing spastic paralysis or flac-

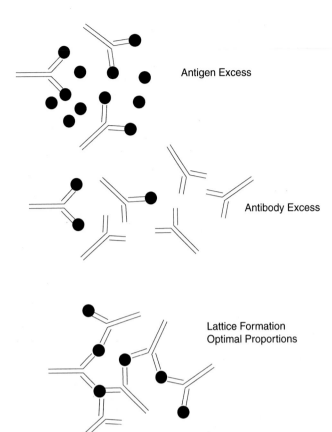

Figure 7–8 ▪ Combining ratios of Ab and antigen. Because the Ab is bivalent, there exist a set of conditions under which optimal proportions yield a stable lattice structure, neutralizing the antigen. If antigen or Ab is in excess, the lattice will not form.

cid paralysis, respectively. When an Ab blocks the toxin's receptor-binding region, it can no longer bind to the neural receptors and is rendered harmless. The toxin–Ab complex is soluble and requires no further processing. The complex can then be eliminated by the kidneys. Bacteria are immobilized by neutralization.

Precipitation. When a soluble antigen reacts with an Ab, it may form an insoluble particulate precipitate. Such a complex cannot remain in the bloodstream in its insoluble state. These species must be removed by the spleen or through the reticuloendothelial system by phagocytosis.

Agglutination. Bacterial cells may be aggregated by binding to antibodies that mask negative ionic surface charges and cross-link cellular structures (Fig. 7-8). The bacteria are thus immediately immobilized. This limits their ability to maintain an infection, but it forms a particulate matrix. This type of complex must also undergo elimination through the reticuloendothelial system.

Bacteriolysis. Bacteriolysis is a complement-mediated reaction. The last five proteins in the cascade self-assemble to produce a membrane attack complex that disrupts the cell membranes of bacteria, acting like bacitracin or amphotericin B. The cell membranes lose integrity, cell contents leak

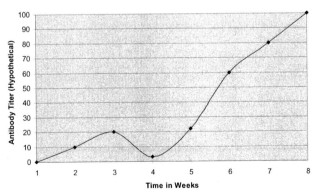

Figure 7–7 ▪ Diagram of the time course of the anamnestic (memory) response. After the first immunization (week 1), the titer of Ab increases slowly to a low level and wanes. A challenge with the same antigen (shown in the diagram at week 4) elicits rapid development of a high titer of Ab in the blood.

out, membrane transport systems fail, and the cell dies. This type of reaction yields products that require no special treatment.

ANTIBODY TYPES AND REACTIONS

Ab types and reactions are classified on the basis of variations in a common section of the Fc fragment that governs biological activity in a general way.

IgG. IgG (Fc = γ) (Fig. 7-5) participates in precipitation reactions, toxin neutralizations, and complement fixation. IgG is the major (70%) human Ig. The Fab tip fixes antigen, and the Fc fragment can fix complement to yield agglutination or lysis. IgG is the only immunoglobulin that crosses the transplacental barrier and the neonatal stomach, so it provides maternal protection. IgG constitutes about 75% of the total Ab in the circulation. It is present at a concentration of about 15 mg/mL and has a half-life of 3 weeks, the longest of any of the Ab types. The light chains of IgG can possess either κ or λ variants. These slight differences in structure are called *isotypes,* and the phenomenon is termed *isotypic variation.*

IgM. IgM (Fc = μ) (Fig. 7-6) is present at a concentration of about 1.5 mg/mL and has a half-life of less than 1 week. This Ab participates in opsonization, agglutination reactions, and complement fixation. Opsonization, as stated above, is a "protein coating" or tagging of a bacterium that renders it more susceptible to phagocytosis. A complex of the Fc portion of IgM plus C3b of complement is that protein. IgM is the first immunoglobulin formed during immunization, but it wanes and gives way to IgG. IgM is a pentamer, and its agglutination potency is about 1,000 times that of IgG. IgM is also responsible for the A, B, and O blood groups. The fundamental monomeric IgM structure is much like that of IgG. The pentamer is held together by disulfide bonds and a single J (joining) peptide. The affinity of an IgM monomer for antigen is less than that of IgG, but the multimeric structure raises the *avidity* of the molecule for an antigen.

IgA. IgA (Fc = α) (Fig. 7-9) is found in exocrine gland secretions (milk, saliva, tears), where it protects mucous membranes (e.g., in the respiratory tract). It is present in the serum as a monomer at a concentration of 1 to 2 mg/mL, but humans secrete about 1 g of the dimer per day in the mucosal fluids. Secretory IgA consists of two IgG-like units linked together at the Fc regions by a peptide known as the secretory fragment and a J fragment. The secretory fragment

is actually part of the membrane receptor for IgA. The IgA molecule on the mucosal side of the membrane binds antigen, then binds to the receptor. By a process of transcytosis, the IgA–antigen complex is moved from the mucosa to the bloodstream, where IgG and IgM can react. Because it is distributed on the mucosa, IgA has an anatomically specific distribution, unlike the other antibodies. IgA is the mediator of oral polio vaccination (the mucosal reaction gives way to systemic protection).

IgD. IgD (Fc = δ) is present on the surface of B cells and, along with monomeric surface IgM, is an antigen receptor that activates immunoglobulin production. There is less than 0.1 mg/mL in the bloodstream, and the half-life is only 3 days.

IgE. IgE (Fc = ϵ) is the Ab responsible for hypersensitivity reactions. IgE complexes have a high affinity for host cell surfaces and can damage the host. High levels of IgE are found in persons with allergies of various types, as well as in autoimmune diseases. The Fc fragment is responsible for the Ig–cell reactivity. An Ab-plus-antigen reaction yields the typical Ab–antigen complex. The Fc portion of the Ab is actually part of the mast cell. When antigen binds to the Fab portion of the Ab, the IgE molecules become cross-linked. This probably distorts the membrane of the mast cells and stimulates them to release histamine, which causes bronchial constriction, itching, redness, and anaphylaxis.

ACQUISITION OF IMMUNITY

Several types of immunity must be considered when describing vaccines and other immunobiologicals. Some are artificial and some are natural. *Natural immunity* is endowed by phagocytic white blood cells, lysozyme in tears, the skin, and so on. *Acquired immunity* is acquired after birth (or by passage from mother to fetus). Thus, immunity may be classified as

- *Active acquired immunity*: The host produces his or her own Ab.
- *Naturally acquired active immunity*: Occurs on recovery from a disease (or from antigen exposure).
- *Artificially acquired active immunity*: Occurs as a response to sensitization by a vaccine or toxoid.
- *Passive acquired immunity*: The subject receives Ab from an outside source, such as a γ-globulin injection, or by transplacental transfer.
- *Naturally acquired passive immunity*: Temporary neonatal protection from maternal IgG passes to the fetus in utero; this type of immunity is not long-lasting.
- *Artificially acquired passive immunity*: An Ab is given by injection, e.g., by an antitoxin or a γ-globulin injection.

Definitions of Immunobiologicals

Immunobiologicals include antigenic substances, such as vaccines and toxoids, or Ab-containing preparations, such as globulins and antitoxins, from human or animal donors. These products are used for active or passive immunization or therapy. All of the following are examples of immunobiologicals:

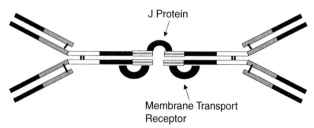

J Protein

Membrane Transport Receptor

Figure 7–9 ■ Structure of immunoglobulin A (IgA), the mucosal Ab that protects the GI tract and the respiratory mucosa.

- *Vaccine*: A suspension of live (usually attenuated) or inactivated microorganisms (e.g., bacteria, viruses, or rickettsiae) or fractions thereof, administered to induce immunity and prevent infectious disease or its sequelae. Some vaccines contain highly defined antigens, e.g., the polysaccharide of *Haemophilus influenzae* type b (Hib) or the surface antigen of hepatitis B; others have antigens that are complex or incompletely defined, e.g., killed *Bordetella pertussis* or live attenuated viruses.
- *Toxoid*: A modified bacterial toxin that has been made nontoxic but retains the ability to stimulate the formation of antitoxin.
- *Immune globulin (IG)*: A sterile solution containing antibodies from human blood. It is obtained by cold ethanol fractionation of large pools of blood plasma and contains 15 to 18% protein. Intended for intramuscular administration, IG is primarily intended for routine maintenance of immunity in certain immunodeficient persons and for passive immunization against measles and hepatitis A. IG does not transmit hepatitis B virus, human immunodeficiency virus (HIV), or other infectious diseases.
- *Intravenous immune globulin (IGIV)*: A product derived from blood plasma from a donor pool similar to the IG pool but prepared so it is suitable for intravenous use. IGIV does not transmit infectious diseases. It is primarily used for replacement therapy in primary Ab deficiency disorders and for the treatment of Kawasaki's disease, immune thrombocytopenia purpura, hypogammaglobulinemia in chronic lymphocytic leukemia, and some cases of HIV infection.
- *Specific immune globulin*: Special preparations obtained from blood plasma from donor pools preselected for a high Ab content against a specific antigen (e.g., hepatitis B immune globulin, varicella-zoster immune globulin, rabies immune globulin, tetanus immune globulin, vaccinia immune globulin, and cytomegalovirus immune globulin). Like IG and IGIV, these preparations do not transmit infectious disease.
- *Antitoxin*: A solution of antibodies (e.g., diphtheria antitoxin and botulinum antitoxin) derived from the serum of animals immunized with specific antigens. Antitoxins are used to confer passive immunity and for treatment.

Vaccination denotes the physical act of administering a vaccine or toxoid. *Immunization* is a more inclusive term denoting the process of inducing or providing immunity artificially by administering an immunobiological. Immunization may be active or passive.

Immunobiologicals (Vaccines and Toxoids)[6–10]

A *vaccine* may be defined as a solution or suspension of killed or live/attenuated virus, killed rickettsia, killed or live/attenuated bacteria, or antigens derived from these sources, which are used to confer active, artificially acquired immunity against that organism or related organisms. When administered, the vaccine represents the initial exposure, resulting in the acquisition of immunity. A subsequent exposure or challenge (a disease) results in the anamnestic, or memory, response.

METHODS OF VACCINE PRODUCTION

Vaccine production methods have varied greatly over the years and are best discussed according to a parallel chronological and sophistication approach.

Killed (Inactivated) Pathogen.
In this method, the normal pathogen is treated with a strong, denaturing disinfectant like formaldehyde or phenol. The process denatures the proteins and carbohydrates that are essential for the organism to live and infect a host, but if treated properly, the surface antigens are left intact. The process must be done carefully to control the unwinding of proteins or carbohydrates by denaturation, since the preparation must be recognized as the original antigen. The main problems with killed pathogen vaccines are: *(a)* if the vaccine is not inactivated totally, disease can result; *(b)* if the preparation is overtreated, vaccine failure usually results because of denaturation; *(c)* the production laboratory must grow the pathogen in large quantities to be commercially useful, putting laboratory technicians at risk; and *(d)* the patient may experience abnormal and harmful responses, such as fever, convulsions, and death. These vaccines typically are viewed as "dirty" vaccines, and some, like the pertussis vaccine, have been associated with problems serious enough to warrant their temporary removal from the market.

Live/Attenuated Pathogens.
The word *attenuated* for our purposes simply means "low virulence." The true pathogen is altered phenotypically so that it cannot invade the human host and cannot get ahead of the host's immune system. Low-pathogenicity strains such as these were originally obtained by passage of the microbes through many generations of host animals. The idea was that the animal and the pathogen, if both were to survive, needed to adapt to live with each other without either partner being killed. Poliovirus is attenuated in this fashion in monkey kidney tissue. In a live/attenuated vaccine, antigenicity is still required, as is infectivity (polio vaccine yields an infection), but the host's immune system must be able to stay ahead of the infection. The key problems are: *(a)* the vaccine cannot be used if the patient is immunocompromised, has fever or malignancy, or is taking immunosuppressive drugs; *(b)* these vaccines should not be used during pregnancy; and *(c)* the attenuated organism commonly reverts to the virulent strain, which was the reason for the failure of some early polio vaccines. Today, biological quality control is very stringent, and these problems have been eliminated.

Live/Attenuated Related Strain.
The live/attenuated related strain is antigenically related so that it can provide cross-immunity to the pathogen. For example, cowpox virus can be used in place of smallpox virus. The strains are antigenically similar enough so that the host's immune system reacts to the related strain to provide protection against the normal pathogen. The main advantage is that a true pathogen is not being used so that the chance of contracting the actual disease is zero. The problem with such vaccines is that they cause an infection. Cowpox is known to spread to the central nervous system in 1 in 10^5 cases, causing a potentially fatal form of meningitis.

Cellular Antigen From a Pathogen.
The surface antigen (i.e., what is recognized as foreign) is harvested from the pathogen, purified, and reconstituted into a vaccine preparation. These antigens can take a number of forms, including the carbohydrate capsule, as in *Neisseria meningitidis*; pili, as in *N. gonorrhoeae*; flagella from motile bacteria (the basis for an experimental cholera vaccine); or the viral

protein coat, as in the vaccine for hepatitis B. Advantages of the method are that there is virtually no chance of disease, contamination, or reversion and there are no storage problems. This method is currently as close to a ''perfect approach'' as we have. A problem is that the pathogen must be grown under careful control or an unsure source must be relied on. For example, hepatitis B vaccine was originally prepared from the serum of a controlled population of human carriers. Imagine the impact if one of the carriers developed another blood-borne disease. Additionally, these are strain-specific antigens (e.g., *N. gonorrhoeae* may require 1,500 different pilar antigens). Acellular vaccines may exhibit lower antigenicity in the very young and may require several injections for full immunological competence. To be safe and consistent, the antigenic component must be identified. Given the complex nature of biological materials, this is not always easy or even possible.

Genetically Engineered Pathogens.[5]

The techniques of genetic engineering have allowed the pharmaceutical industry to prepare absolutely pure surface antigens while totally eliminating the pathogenic organism from the equation. As shown in Figure 7-10, the virus contains surface antigens (designated by *filled circles*). Inside the viral capsule is a circular piece of DNA containing genes for the various biological molecules of the virus. The diagram shows, at about 3 o'clock, a small piece of DNA that codes for the surface antigen. The strategy is to isolate this piece of DNA and insert it into a rapidly growing expression vector for production of the surface protein. In this case, *Escherichia coli* serves as an excellent vector. It contains a plasmid that can be removed, clipped open, and used as a cassette to carry the viral DNA. Additionally, *E. coli* can be grown in batch to produce the viral surface antigen. To begin, the DNA is removed from the virus and the plasmid is removed from the vector. Viral and bacterial nucleic acid is treated with a restriction endonuclease, which cleaves the DNA and plasmid at designated restriction sites. The viral DNA is cleaved into a number of fragments, each of which is ligated into the *E. coli* plasmid with a ligase enzyme. Plasmids are inserted into *E. coli,* and the organism is grown in batch fermentation. The organisms containing the gene for the viral surface protein can be separated by screening and purified to serve as the ultimate antigen producer—free of contamination or pathogenic viral particles. The pure antigen may then be constituted into a vaccine and used in human hosts.

USE OF VACCINES IN COMBINATION: DOSING[5, 11]

Types of Vaccines.

There are three basic types of vaccine preparations that are used clinically:

1. A *simple* vaccine contains one strain of a disease-causing organism (e.g., plague vaccine, *Pasteurella pestis,* and smallpox vaccine).
2. A *multivalent* vaccine is prepared from two or more strains of an organism that cause the same disease (e.g., polio is trivalent). Administration of the multiple strains is required for full protection because their antigens are not cross-immunizing. The immune system must mount a separate immune response to each strain.
3. A *polyvalent* vaccine is prepared from two or more organisms that cause different diseases. Polyvalent vaccines are given for convenience, primarily so that a child can be given one shot rather than several. The measles–mumps–rubella (MMR) vaccine is of the polyvalent type.

Types of Dosing.

Vaccines can be administered according to a variety of dosing regimens, depending on the vaccine type and the purpose of the injection:

1. A *single-dose vaccine* is usually assumed to confer, with one shot, ''lifetime immunity.'' The smallpox vaccine was a single-dose vaccine.
2. In a *multiple-dosing* regimen, several doses are given, spaced weeks or months apart, to get maximum immunogenicity. Multiple dosing is usually done with inactivated vaccines, which are less antigenic. Multiple dosing is not the same as a booster dose.
3. A *booster dose* is administered years after the initial immunization schedule (regardless of single or multiple first dose). As a patient ages, Ab levels may wane. A booster is used to bolster immunity. Also, boosters are used if a patient is known or suspected to have been exposed to a pathogen (e.g., tetanus).
4. A *coadministered vaccine* is possible only if one vaccine does not interfere with another.
5. There are two physical forms of vaccines: A *fluid vaccine* is a solution or a suspension of the vaccine in saline of an aqueous buffer; the solution or suspension in an *adsorbed vaccine* is adsorbed on a matrix of aluminum or calcium phosphate. Like a sustained-release dosage form, in theory there is longer exposure via a depot injection. The higher surface area of the matrix will be exposed to the immune system. Generally, adsorbed vaccines are preferred.

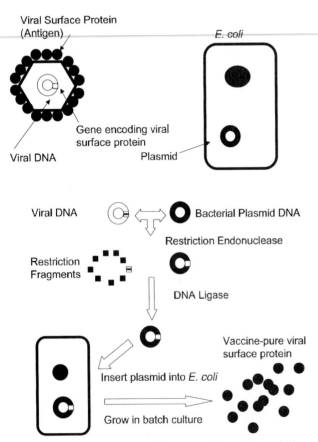

Figure 7–10 ■ Preparation of a genetically engineered Ab.

Pharmaceutical Principles of Vaccines.

As expected for a live biological preparation, heat destroys live viral and bacterial vaccines. If the agent is not killed, the antigen may be altered. Like many biologicals, lyophilized vaccines are unstable after reconstitution. Ice crystals formed inside the protein structure during freeze-drying expand during thawing and disrupt the structure of the vaccine. Live vaccines can be inactivated by minute amounts of detergent. Detergent residue adhering to glassware is concentrated enough to act as a disinfectant. It is safe to use only plastic implements specified for the vaccine. The suspending medium may be sterile water, saline, or more complex systems containing protein or other constituents derived from the medium in which the vaccine is produced (e.g., serum proteins, egg antigens, and cell culture-derived antigens). Concentrated Ab suspensions (γ-globulins) are typical amphiphilic proteins and aggregate on storage. If injected, the particulates may cause anaphylaxis. Preservatives may be components of vaccines, antitoxins, and globulins. These components are present to inhibit or prevent bacterial growth in viral cultures or the final product or to stabilize the antigens or antibodies. Allergic reactions can occur if the recipient is sensitive to one of these additives (e.g., mercurial compounds [thimerosal], phenols, albumin, glycine, or neomycin).

Storage and Handling of Immunobiologicals.

Failure to follow the exact recommendations for storage and handling of immunobiologicals can lead to an impotent preparation. During reconstituting, storing, and handling of immunobiologicals, the most important recommendation is to follow the package insert exactly. Vaccines should always be stored at their recommended temperature. Certain vaccines, such as polio vaccine, are sensitive to increased temperature. Other vaccines, such as oral polio vaccine, diphtheria and tetanus toxoids, and acellular pertussis vaccine, hepatitis B vaccine, influenza vaccine, and Hib conjugate vaccine (Hib-CV) (among others), are sensitive to freezing.

Viral Vaccines[12]

SMALLPOX VACCINE (DRYVAX)

Smallpox vaccine is live *vaccinia* (cowpox) virus grown on the skin of a bovine calf. Smallpox is a highly lethal and disfiguring disease that was common throughout history. Smallpox vaccine was used routinely in the United States but today is no longer recommended. (There have been no reported cases of smallpox since the 1940s.) In 1982, smallpox was declared eradicated worldwide. With smallpox, the risks of the vaccine outweigh the benefits; the vaccine penetrates the central nervous system and potentially fatal encephalitis occurs in 1 in 10^5 patients. After exposure to smallpox, the vaccine can be injected to lessen the severity of the disease.

INFLUENZA VACCINE[13, 14, 15, 16, 17]

Influenza vaccine is a multivalent inactivated influenza virus or viral subunits (split vaccine). The virus is grown on chick embryo and inactivated by exposure to ultraviolet (UV) light or formaldehyde. The antigen type is protein. The vaccine in the United States contains thimerosal, a mercurial, as a preservative. *Influenza* is a respiratory tract infection with a 2-day incubation period. The disease may be devastating and can lead to pneumonia. Without the vaccine, influenza is common in epidemics and pandemics. To clarify, the *flu* is a GI infection with diarrhea and vomiting. Influenza requires weeks of incubation. Influenza is caused by two main genetic strains each year (A and B): type A is most common in humans; type B is less common. The virus mutates very rapidly, and vaccines must be tailored yearly. The World Health Organization (WHO) and the Centers for Disease Control and Prevention (CDC) monitor the migration of the disease from Southeast Asia, type the strains causing the occurrences, and order a vaccine to counter the organisms most likely to enter the United States. Influenza A viruses are categorized according to two cell surface protein antigens: hemagglutinin (H) and neuraminidase (N). Each of these is divided further into subtypes (H1, H2; N1, N2). Individual strains within a subtype are named for the location, isolation sequence number, and year of isolation (e.g., A/Beijing/2/90 [H1N1]). For example, the WHO-recommended formula for 2001 to 2002 included the following antigens: A/New Caledonia/20/99 (H1N1), A/Moscow/10/99 (H3N2), B/Sichuan/379/99, 15 μg each per 0.5 mL. A typical vaccine will be a mixture of three strains. Strains are selected each year in the spring on the basis of the disease trends observed and are released in the autumn. In general, those patients who are at high risk for complications from influenza are

- Persons 65 years of age or older
- Residents of nursing homes and other chronic-care facilities that house persons of any age who have chronic medical conditions
- Adults and children who have chronic disorders of the pulmonary or cardiovascular systems, including asthma
- Adults and children who have required medical follow-up or hospitalization during the preceding year because of chronic metabolic diseases (including diabetes mellitus), renal dysfunction, hemoglobinopathies, or immunosuppression (including immunosuppression caused by medications or HIV infection)
- Children and teenagers (aged 6 months to 18 years) who are receiving long-term aspirin therapy and, therefore, might be at risk for developing Reye's syndrome after influenza infection
- Women who will be in the second or third trimester of pregnancy during the influenza season
- Health care workers and those in close contact with persons at high risk, including household members
- Household members (including children) of persons in groups at high risk, including persons with pulmonary disorders, such as asthma, and health care workers who are at higher risk because of close contact

It is impossible to contract influenza from the vaccine. The only side effects may be local pain and tenderness at the injection site, with low-grade fever in 3 to 5% of patients. Aspirin and acetaminophen are effective in combating these symptoms. Allergic reactions are rare but may be seen in persons allergic to eggs. Immunity to influenza vaccine takes 2 weeks to develop. Some people fear the vaccine because of reports of a strange paralysis and lack of nerve sensation associated with the 1976 swine flu vaccine. This problem, Guillain-Barré syndrome, was associated only with this 1976 vaccine and has not been associated with vaccines since.[17]

POLIO VACCINES[18–20]

Polio is a dangerous viral infection that affects both muscle mass and the spinal cord. Some children and adults who contract polio become paralyzed, and some may die due to respiratory paralysis. Polio was the cause of the "infantile paralysis" epidemic of 1950 to 1953, which led to many paralyzed children and the specter of patients spending their lives in an iron lung. Serious cases of polio cause muscle pain and may make movement of the legs and/or arms difficult or impossible and, as stated above, may make breathing difficult. Milder cases last a few days and may cause fever, sore throat, headache, and nausea. Interest in polio has increased because of recent local outbreaks; large numbers of people are unimmunized. There are no drugs or special therapies to cure polio; treatment is only supportive. The symptoms of polio may reappear 40 to 50 years after a severe infection. This phenomenon is known as postpolio muscle atrophy (PPMA). PPMA is not a reinfection or reactivation of the virus but is probably a form of rapid aging in polio survivors. There are two types of polio vaccines.

Inactivated Polio Vaccine (IPV).

There are several synonyms for the IPV vaccine: IPV, e-IPV, ep-IPV, and the Salk vaccine (1954 [IPOL, Aventis-Pasteur]). e-IPV is an enhanced potency poliovirus, more potent and immunogenic than any of the previous IPV formulations. e-IPV is recommended for all four infant doses because of the incidence of rare cases of oral polio vaccine (OPV)–associated paralytic poliomyelitis. e-IPV is also preferred for adults for the same reason. IPV is a trivalent (strains 1, 2, 3) vaccine grown in monkey kidney culture and subjected to elaborate precautions to ensure inactivation (typically, formaldehyde is used). The antigen form is whole virus. The antigen type is protein. The vaccine is injected to cause induction of active systemic immunity from polio but does not stop polio carriers, who shed the virus from the oral and nasal cavities.

Trivalent Oral Polio Vaccine (TOPV).

TOPV (Sabin vaccine, 1960) is a live attenuated whole virus vaccine (antigen type, protein) containing polio strains 1, 2, and 3. The virus culture is grown on monkey kidney tissue with use of an elaborate attenuation protocol. Oral administration of the vaccine yields a local GI infection, and the initial immune response is via IgA (mucosal, local to the GI tract). The IgA–antigen complex undergoes transcytosis across the mucosal membrane, and systemic immunity is induced as IgM and IgG form. A major caution with TOPV is that it is a live vaccine and must never be injected. Indications are

- Mass vaccination campaigns to control outbreaks of paralytic polio.
- Unvaccinated children who will travel in less than 4 weeks to areas where polio is endemic.
- Children of parents who do not accept the recommended number of vaccine injections. These children may receive OPV only for the third or fourth dose or both. In such cases, the health care provider should administer OPV only after discussing the risk of OPV–associated paralytic poliomyelitis with parents or caregivers.
- e-IPV is recommended for routine use in all four immunizing doses in infants and children.

- The WHO has advocated giving children e-IPV instead of TOPV to prevent exposure of others to virus shed through the nose and mouth.[29, 30]

RUBELLA VACCINE[21]

German measles is a disease that was once called the "3-day measles" and was considered a normal childhood illness. It is a mild disease with few consequences, except in the first trimester of pregnancy. In these mothers, rubella causes birth defects in 50% of cases. Defects may include heart disease, deafness, blindness, learning disorders, and spontaneous abortion of the fetus. Symptoms of rubella are a low-grade fever, swollen neck glands, and a rash that lasts for about 3 days. About 1 of every 10 women of childbearing age in the United States is not protected against rubella. Also, 20% of all adults escaped this normal childhood disease or are not vaccinated.

Rubella vaccine (German measles vaccine, live, Meruvax II, Merck) is a live, attenuated rubella virus produced in human diploid cell culture. The antigen form of the vaccine is whole virus. The antigen type is protein. The vaccine is administered as part of the normal immunization schedule at 15 months. Side effects are minimal, but there may be some soreness and pain at the site of injection and stiffness of the joints.

A problem with the vaccine is that administration of a live virus is contraindicated in pregnancy. Indications are

- Persons aged 12 months to puberty should be immunized routinely.
- Previously unimmunized children of susceptible pregnant women should receive the MMR vaccine. The trivalent vaccine is preferred for persons likely to be susceptible to mumps and rubella.
- Immunization of susceptible nonpregnant adolescent or adult women of childbearing potential is called for if precautions to avoid pregnancy are observed.
- Almost all children and some adults require more than one dose of MMR vaccine.
- On the first routine visit to the obstetrician-gynecologist, the immune status should be checked. If the woman is not immunized against rubella, the physician should administer the vaccine and stress avoiding pregnancy for 3 months.
- If the patient is already pregnant, the physician should not administer the vaccine.
- If exposure is suspected, the cord blood should be monitored for the presence of rubella antibodies.
- All unimmunized women should be vaccinated immediately after delivery of the baby.

MEASLES VACCINE (ATTENUVAX, MERCK)[21]

Measles is a very serious, highly contagious disease. It causes a high fever, rash, and a cough lasting 1 to 2 weeks. Some patients experience extreme sensitivity to light. The rash may occur inside the eyelids, producing a very painful condition. In the United States, between 3,000 and 28,000 cases occur each year, depending on factors such as weather and localized outbreaks. Outbreaks are very common in neighborhoods and schools. One of 10 children contracting measles will develop an ear infection or pneumonia. Measles may infect the brain (encephalitis) and lead to convulsions, hearing loss, and mental disability. In the United States, 1 of every 500 to 10,000 children contracting measles dies from it. Severe sickness and death are more common in babies and adults than in elementary schoolchildren or teenagers. Measles has been linked to multiple sclerosis. In 1977, a severe epidemic occurred in the United States, and 50,000 cases were reported. Only 60% of the population was vaccinated.

Measles vaccine is composed of live/attenuated measles virus that is grown on chick embryo culture with an attenuation protocol. Indications are

- Selective induction of active immunity against measles virus.
- Trivalent MMR vaccine is the preferred immunizing form for most children and many adults.
- Almost all children and many adults require more than one dose of MMR.
- Prior to international travel, persons susceptible to any of the three viruses should receive the single-antigen vaccine or the trivalent vaccine, as appropriate.
- Most persons born before 1956 are likely to have contracted the disease naturally and are not considered susceptible.
- Persons born after 1956 or those who lack adequate documentation of having had the disease should be vaccinated.

The vaccine is required by law at 15 months and again at 11 to 12 years of age. The vaccine can be administered after exposure to measles to lessen the disease severity. This is because Ab to the vaccine develops in 7 days, while the incubation period for the disease is 11 days. The vaccine should not be administered in pregnancy and should always be administered with great care to women of childbearing age. Because measles vaccine is cultivated in egg medium, care must be used in patients who are allergic to eggs and egg products. For this reason, a test dose regimen is used. The administration protocol is shown below in Table 7-6.

MUMPS VACCINE[22, 23]

Mumps virus causes fever, headache, and a painful swelling of the parotid glands under the jaw. Mumps can be serious and is highly contagious. Prior to the vaccine, the disease was passed from child to child with ease. The disease runs its course over several days. Between 4,500 and 13,000 cases of mumps occur as outbreaks in the United States every year. In severe cases, mumps may cause inflammation of the coverings of the brain and spinal cord (meningitis); this occurs in about 10% of infected persons. Swelling of the brain itself occurs in 1 of 200 patients. Men may experience a painful swelling of the testicles (orchitis), which may presage sterility. Women may experience a corresponding infection of the ovaries. Male teens are often sicker than other groups of either sex. Mumps early in childhood has been linked to the development of juvenile diabetes.

The mumps vaccine (Mumpsvax, Merck) is a live, attenuated virus grown on chick embryo culture with attenuation protocols. The antigen form is whole virus. The antigen type is protein. Indications are

- Induction of artificially acquired active immunity against mumps.
- Before international travel, immunize any susceptible individuals with the single-antigen vaccine or the trivalent MMR vaccine, as appropriate.
- Most children and some adults need more than one dose of MMR vaccine.
- Persons born prior to 1956 are generally considered immune.

Caution. Mumps vaccine is supplied with a diluent. Use only this diluent for reconstitution. Addition of a diluent with an antimicrobial preservative can render the vaccine inactive. The vaccine is normally administered to children at 15 months of age and again at 11 to 12 years. Because mumps vaccine is cultivated in egg medium, care used to be advised in patients allergic to eggs and egg products. Recent data show that persons who are allergic to egg and egg products fail to react to the mumps vaccine.

COMBINATION PRODUCTS (POLYVALENT VIRAL VACCINES)

If two or more vaccines are free of interference with each other, they can be administered as a mixture (polyvalent) for convenience. Examples of polyvalent viral vaccines are measles–rubella (MR), rubella–mumps (RM), and measles–mumps–rubella (MMR). MMR is indicated for routine immunization at 15 months (not given at less than 1 year unless the child has been exposed or lacks immunocompetence). This is because maternal Abs interfere with development of vaccine immunity in small children. If the MMR is given at less than 1 year, revaccination is needed at 15 months of age.

CHICKENPOX VACCINE[24–29]

Chickenpox is caused by varicella-zoster virus. Every year, about 3.5 million people in the United States, mostly children, contract chickenpox. The incidence peaks between 3 and 9 years of age. Chickenpox causes a generalized rash, with 300 to 500 blister-like lesions occurring on the scalp, face, and trunk. Symptoms include loss of appetite, malaise, and headache. The disease is usually benign but can lead to bacterial superinfection, pneumonia, encephalitis, and Reye's syndrome. About 50 to 100 previously healthy children die of the disease. About 2% of all cases occur in adults, who have more serious symptoms than children have.

Varicella vaccine (Varivax, Merck) is derived from live virus from a child with natural varicella. The virus has been attenuated by passage through a series of guinea pig and human cell cultures. The final preparation is a lyophilized live, attenuated virus. The antigen form is whole virus. The antigen type is protein. The vaccine is well tolerated, with pain and redness at the injection site as the only side effects. The vaccine has shown tremendous success in reducing infections. Indications are

- The vaccine is recommended for children 12 months to 12 years old as a single dose.
- Adults who are exposed to chickenpox should continue to receive varicella-zoster immune globulin (VZIG).
- In elderly persons, varicella vaccine can boost immunity to varicella-zoster virus and may prevent or attenuate herpes zoster (shingles) attacks.

HEPATITIS VACCINES[30–40]

Hepatitis is a complex of diseases that causes fever, nausea, abdominal pain, jaundice, liver failure, and death. There are five clinically recognized types (A, B, C, D, and E).

Hepatitis A Vaccine.   Hepatitis A virus (HAV; infectious hepatitis) causes an acute disease with an abrupt onset.

TABLE 7–6 Recommended Childhood Immunization Schedule—United States January to December 2000

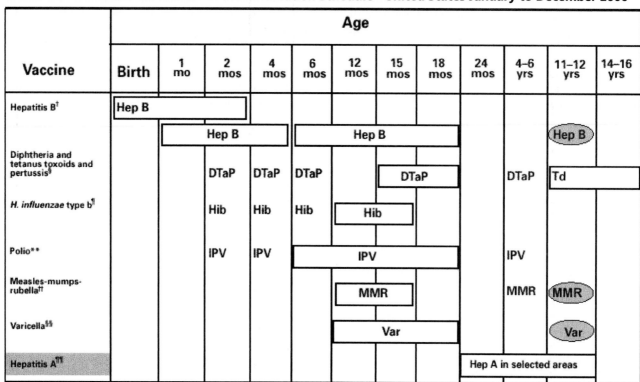

Vaccine	Birth	1 mo	2 mos	4 mos	6 mos	12 mos	15 mos	18 mos	24 mos	4–6 yrs	11–12 yrs	14–16 yrs
Hepatitis B[†]	Hep B											
			Hep B			Hep B					Hep B	
Diphtheria and tetanus toxoids and pertussis[§]			DTaP	DTaP	DTaP		DTaP			DTaP	Td	
***H. influenzae* type b**[¶]			Hib	Hib	Hib	Hib						
Polio[**]			IPV	IPV		IPV				IPV		
Measles-mumps-rubella[††]						MMR				MMR	MMR	
Varicella[§§]						Var					Var	
Hepatitis A[¶¶]									Hep A in selected areas			

▭ Range of recommended ages for vaccination

⬭ Vaccines to be given if previously recommended doses were missed or were given earlier than the recommended minimum age

▓ Recommended in selected states and/or regions.

On October 22, 1999, the Advisory Committee on Immunization Practices (ACIP) recommanded that Rotashield [rhesus rotavirus vaccine-tetravalent (RRV-TV)] the only U.S.-licensed rotavirus vaccine, no longer be used in the United States (*MMWR*, Vol. 48, No. 43. November 6, 1999) Parents should be reassured that children who received rotavirus vaccine before July 1999 are not now at increased risk for intussusception

*This schedule indicates the recommended ages for routine administration of licensed childhood vaccines as of November 1, 1999. Any dose not given at the recommended age should be given as a "catch-up" vaccination at any subsequent visit when indicated and feasible. Additional vaccines may be licensed and recommended during the year. Licensed combination vaccines may be used whenever any components of the combination are indicated and the vaccine's other components are not contraindicated. Providers should consult the manufacturers' package inserts for detailed recommendations.

[†]**Infants born to hepatitis B surface antigen (HBsAg)-negative mothers** should receive the first dose of hepatitis B vaccine (Hep B) by age 2 months. The second dose should be administered at least 1 month after the first dose. The third dose should be administered at least 4 months after the first dose and at least 2 months after the second dose, but not before age 6 months. **Infants born to HBsAg-positive mothers** should receive Hep B and 0.5 mL hepatitis B immune globulin (HBIG) within 12 hours of birth at separate sites. The second dose is recommended at age 1–2 months, and the third dose at age 6 months. **Infants born to mothers whose HBsAg status is unknown** should receive Hep B within 12 hours of birth. Maternal blood should be drawn at delivery to determine the mother's HBsAg status; if the HBsAg test is positive, the infant should receive HBIG as soon as possible (no later than age 1 week). **All children and adolescents (through age 18 years)** who have not been vaccinated against hepatitis B may begin the series during any visit. Providers should make special efforts to vaccinate children who were born in or whose parents were born in areas of the world where hepatitis B virus infection is moderately or highly endemic.

[§]The fourth dose of diphtheria and tetanus toxoids and acellular pertussis vaccine (DTaP) can be administered as early as age 12 months, provided 6 months have elapsed since the third dose and the child is unlikely to return at age 15–18 months. Tetanus and diphtheria toxoids (Td) are recommended at age 11–12 years if at least 5 years have elapsed since the last dose of diphtheria and tetanus toxoids and pertussis vaccine (DTP), DTaP, or diphtheria and tetanus toxoids (DT). Subsequent routine Td boosters are recommended every 10 years.

[¶]Three *Haemophilus influenzae* type b (Hib) conjugate vaccines are licensed for infant use. If Hib conjugate vaccine (PRP-OMP) (PedvaxHIB or ComVax [Merck]) is administered at ages 2 months and 4 months, a dose at age 6 months is not required. Because clinical studies in infants have demonstrated that using some combination products may induce a lower immune response to the Hib vaccine component, Dta/Hib combination products should not be used for primary vaccination in infants at ages 2, 4, or 6 months unless approved by the Food and Drug Administration for these ages.

[**]To eliminate the risk for vaccine-associated paralytic poliomyelitis (VAPP), an all-inactivated poliovirus vaccine (IPV) schedule is now recommended for routine childhood polio vaccination in the United States. All children should receive four doses of IPV; at age 2 months, age 4 months, between ages 6 and 18 months, and between ages 4 and 6 years. Oral poliovirus vaccine (OPV) (if available) may be used only for the following special circumstances: 1) mass vaccination campaigns to control outbreaks of paralytic polio; 2) unvaccinated children who will be traveling in <4 weeks to areas where polio is undemic or epidemic; and 3) children of parents who do not accept the recommended number of vaccine injections. Children of parents who do not accept the recommended number of vaccine injections may receive OPV only for the third or fourth dose or both; in this situation, health-care providers should administer OPV only after discussing the risk for VAPP with parents or caregivers. During the transition to an all-IPV schedule, recommendations for the use of remaining OPV supplies in physicians' offices and clinics have been issued by the American Academy of Pediatrics (*Pediatrics*, Vol. 104, No. 6 December 1999).

[‡‡]The second dose of measles, mumps, and rubella vaccine (MMR) is recommended routinely at age 4–6 years but may be administered during any visit, provided at least 4 weeks have elapsed since receipt of the first dose and that both doses are administered beginning at or after age 12 months. Those who previously have not received the second dose should complete the schedule no later than the routine visit to a health-care provider at age 11–12 years.

[§§]Varicella (Var) vaccine is recommended at any visit on or after the first birthday for susceptible children, i.e., those who lack a reliable history of chickenpox (as judged by a health-care provider) and who have not been vaccinated. Susceptible persons aged ≥ 13 years should receive two doses given at least 4 weeks apart.

[¶¶]Hepatitis A vaccine (Hep A) is recommended for use in selected states and regions. Information is available from local public health authorities and *MMWR*, Vol. 48, No. RR. 12, October 1, 1999.

Use of trade names and commercial sources is for identification only and does not constitute or imply endorsement by CDC or the U.S. Department of Health and Human Services.

Source: Advisory Committee on Immunization Practices (ACIP), American Academy of Family Physicians (AAFP), and American Academy of Pediatrics (AAP).

About 15 to 50 days of incubation are required before the disease becomes clinically noticeable. The primary sign is jaundice. The disease lasts several weeks and is followed by complete recovery. Hepatitis A is transmitted when the virus is taken in by mouth. The fecal-oral route and close contact, unwashed food, and contaminated water account for most of the routes of transmission. The sexual anal-oral route is also a route of spread. Children under the age of 3 frequently have no symptoms but can transmit the disease to adults in child care centers. An injection of hepatitis A immune globulin is one way of preventing the disease but is only effective for about 30 days.

The hepatitis A vaccine (Havrix) is an inactivated preparation that is produced by propagation of the virus in cultured human diploid cells and then is inactivated with formalin. The antigen form is lysed whole viruses. The antigen type is protein. The course of immunization involves two injections over a 4-week period and a booster 12 months after the first injection. Indications are

- Persons traveling outside the United States, except to Australia, Canada, Japan, New Zealand, and Western Europe
- Persons with chronic liver disease
- Persons living in an outbreak zone
- Persons who inject medications
- Persons engaging in high-risk sexual activity
- Child care workers caring for children less than 2 years of age
- Developing countries with poor sanitation

Side effects are minor and usually limited to soreness at the injection site and fever.

Hepatitis B Vaccine. Hepatitis B virus (HBV), the cause of serum hepatitis, is a much more insidious, chronic disease, transmitted by needles, mucosal contact, blood, or high-risk sexual activity. The highest risk for contraction of hepatitis B is among intravenous drug abusers. The disease is linked to cirrhosis and liver cancer. There are about 200,000 new cases reported per year in the United States; of these, 10% become carriers, one fifth die from cirrhosis, and 1,000 die from liver cancer. The hepatitis B vaccine was first introduced in 1981. Initially, it was prepared as an inactivated vaccine from the plasma of carefully screened human, high-titer carriers and/or donors. In 1986, the recombinant DNA (rDNA) vaccine (Engerix B, Recombivax) was introduced to the market. The rDNA vaccine contains only viral subunits and may be used with hepatitis B immune globulin in a postexposure setting to boost the ability of the host to resist the infection. In adults, three doses should be given, at 0, 1, and 6 months. In children, the vaccine is given at birth, 1 month, and 9 months. Administration may be delayed in premature infants whose immune systems are not fully developed. If not immunized at birth, a child should receive three doses by 18 months. If the mother tests positive for hepatitis B, the vaccine plus the immune globulin must be given at or shortly after birth. The vaccine is 95% effective and is typically without side effects. A number of high-risk groups have been identified: health care workers, student health care workers, people living in high-risk environments, and dentists. They should receive a three-dose course of the vaccine. In most other cases, a physician can judge whether a patient is at high risk or not. Side effects of the vaccine are minor.

Hepatitis C Vaccine. Hepatitis C virus (HCV) was once called hepatitis non-A, non-B but has been recognized as a separate entity. HCV infection is spread primarily by the parenteral route (transfusions), and unlike HBV, maternal-fetal and sexual transmission are uncommon. Acute infection may show few symptoms; fewer than 25% of patients develop full-blown hepatitis. Administration of interferon alpha (IFN-α) during the early acute phase can cure most patients. Unfortunately, 50 to 60% of those with HCV infection develop chronic hepatitis. This is often manifested by periodic increases in hepatic enzyme levels. Cirrhosis develops in 20% of chronic infectees; this usually requires 15 to 20 years to develop. Patients with HCV are at risk for hepatocellular carcinoma. Estimates are that 150,000 to 170,000 new cases occur in the United States per year. Intravenous drug users, transfusion patients, and health care workers are at highest risk.

Development of a HCV vaccine proved difficult but was accomplished in 1998. There are 15 genotypes, and the virus can modulate its antigens within the host's body. A new approach using genetic material from the virus, analogous to the approach to the influenza vaccine, is said to be promising.[44]

Hepatitis E. Hepatitis E virus (HEV) causes disease clinically indistinguishable from hepatitis A. Symptoms include malaise, anorexia, abdominal pain, arthritis-like symptoms, and fever. Distinguishing HEV from HAV must be done genetically. The incubation period is 2 to 9 weeks. The disease is usually mild and resolves in 2 weeks, with no sequelae. The fatality rate is 0.1 to 1%, except in pregnant women where the rate soars to 20%. No outbreaks have been reported in the United States as of 1996. There is currently no vaccine against HEV.

ROTAVIRUS VACCINE

There will soon be a new rotavirus vaccine included in the Recommended Childhood Immunization schedule. This vaccine is used to provide immunity against rotavirus, the most common cause of severe diarrhea in children in the United States. All children have at least one rotavirus infection in the first 5 years of life, and there are about 20 deaths per year in this country. Children between the ages of 3 and 24 months of age have the highest rates of severe disease and hospitalization. The rotavirus vaccine is an oral vaccine, given as a series of three doses. It is recommended that the vaccine be administered at 2, 4, and 6 months of age. The most common side effect seems to be fever.

Bacterial Vaccines[41–44]

PERTUSSIS VACCINE

Pertussis, also known as whooping cough, is a highly communicable infection caused by *Bordetella pertussis*. *B. pertussis* produces an endotoxin that causes a spectrum of symptoms in a host. Pertussis occurs mainly in children, and there is no effective treatment once the disease becomes manifest.

Bordetella endotoxin attacks the tracheal mucosa and causes extreme irritation. The inflammatory responses produce the characteristic "whooping inspiration" associated with pertussis. The swollen and irritated tissues may lead to choking in children. The cough may last for months and is often called the "hundred-day cough." About 4,200 cases of pertussis occur yearly in the United States. Pertussis is most dangerous to babies (less than 1 year old). Even with the best supportive medical care, complications occur. At least 50% of pertussis patients must be hospitalized, 16% get pneumonia, 2% develop convulsions, and 1 in 200 babies dies or has lifelong complications.

Pertussis vaccine has been highly controversial in recent years. The original vaccine consisted of killed pertussis bacilli (*B. pertussis*) and was considered somewhat "dirty." Side effects such as fever and convulsions were common, and health authorities in the United States, Japan, and the United Kingdom decided that the risk of the vaccine outweighed the risk of contracting the disease. In all three of these countries, pertussis vaccine was removed from the routine immunization schedules. Almost immediately, pertussis, which had been held in check, began to occur in epidemics. In 1992, a new vaccine was developed that consists of bacterial fractions, combined with tetanus and diphtheria toxoids. This vaccine, called Acell-Immune, or DTaP, is safe and highly effective and has been added to the routine immunization schedule. The vaccine is adsorbed and is used for routine immunization as the polyvalent preparation diphtheria–tetanus–pertussis (DTP) (at 2, 4, 6, and 15 months and at 4 to 6 years). Pertussis vaccination is recommended for most children. There is also a diphtheria–tetanus–pertussis whole-cell pertussis vaccine (DTwP) on the market, but it is considered to be higher in side effects than DTaP. Lastly, a DTaP/Hib vaccine preparation is on the market and is recommended for use only as the fourth dose of the series. At present, the only indication is

- Induction of active immunity against diphtheria and tetanus toxins and pertussis from age 6 weeks up to the seventh birthday

HAEMOPHILUS INFLUENZAE TYPE B CONJUGATE VACCINE (Hib-CV)

H. influenzae type B (Hib) causes the most common type of bacterial meningitis and is a major cause of systemic disease in children less than 6 years old. The chances of contracting the disease are about 1 in 200. Of these contractees, 60% of all patients develop meningitis, while 40% display systemic signs. Hib is a tremendous problem in daycare centers, where the risk of contracting the disease is 400 times greater than in the general population. Hib has approximately a 10% mortality rate, and one third of all survivors have some sort of permanent damage, such as hearing loss, blindness, or impaired vision. Hib can also cause a throat inflammation that results in fatal choking or ear, joint, and skin infections.

Hib-CV is a sterile, lyophilized capsular polysaccharide from Hib vaccine, conjugated to various protein fragments. The antigen type is polysaccharide (phosphoribosyl ribitol phosphate) conjugated to protein. The conjugation produces a stronger, longer-lasting response through the adjuvant effect. Hib-CV is safe and almost completely effective and is a mandatory part of the childhood immunization schedule. The various forms of Hib-CV on the market are not generically equivalent. Indications are

- Induction of artificially acquired active immunity against invasive disease caused by encapsulated Hib
- Routine immunization of all infants beginning at 2 months of age, recommended in the United States
- Immunization of risk groups including children attending daycare centers, persons of low socioeconomic status, and household contacts of Hib cases

TUBERCULOSIS VACCINE

Tuberculosis (TB) is a serious disease caused by *Mycobacterium tuberculosis*. The organism becomes established in the lungs and forms walled-off abscesses that shield the bacterium from the immune system. The disease is diagnosed by a chest x-ray. Until the 1940s, persons with TB were sent to sanatoria, special hospitals to isolate TB patients. The vaccine is referred to as the bacillus Calmette-Guérin (BCG) vaccine and is a live/attenuated strain of *Mycobacterium bovis*. The antigenic form is the whole bacterium, and the antigen type is protein. The vaccine is of questionable efficacy and has been judged only 50 to 77% effective. The duration of protection is highly questionable. The incidence of TB in the United States is so low that the vaccine is not indicated in most cases. Indications are

- Induction of artificially acquired active immunity against *M. tuberculosis* var. *hominis* to lower the risk of serious complications from tuberculosis
- Recommended for PPD skin test–negative infants and children at high risk of intimate and prolonged exposure to persistently treated or ineffectively treated patients with infectious pulmonary tuberculosis
- Persons who are continuously exposed to tuberculosis patients who have mycobacteria resistant to isoniazid and rifampin and who cannot be removed from the source of exposure
- Health care workers in an environment where a high proportion of *M. tuberculosis* isolates are resistant to both isoniazid (INH) and rifampin, where there is a strong possibility of transmission of infection, and where infection control procedures have failed

An adverse effect of the BCG vaccine includes a positive TB skin test. A red blister forms within 7 to 10 days, then ulcerates and scars within 6 months. BCG is a live vaccine, so it cannot be administered to immunosuppressed patients, burn patients, or pregnant women unless exposed (and even then not in the first trimester).

CHOLERA VACCINE

Cholera is a disease caused by *Vibrio cholerae* that presents as severe, watery diarrhea caused by an enterotoxin secreted by the 01-serotype of *V. cholerae*. The disease occurs in pandemics in India, Bangladesh, Peru, and Latin America. The organisms never invade the enteric epithelium; instead, they remain in the lumen and secrete their enterotoxin. There are about 17 known virulence-associated genes necessary for colonization and toxin secretion. Secretory diarrhea is caused by release of an enterotoxin called *cholera toxin,* which is nearly identical with *E. coli* enterotoxin. It is composed of five binding peptides B and a catalytic peptide A. The peptides B bind to ganglioside GM_1 on the surface of the epithelial cells, setting in motion a series of events that causes diarrhea. The vaccine consists of whole cells of *V. cholerae* 01 that have been inactivated. The antigen form of the vaccine is whole bacterium, and the antigen type is protein toxin and lipopolysaccharide. Indications are

- Induction of active immunity against cholera, such as in individuals traveling to or residing in epidemic or endemic areas
- Individuals residing in areas where cholera is endemic

MENINGOCOCCAL POLYSACCHARIDE VACCINE

Meningococcal vaccine is an inactivated vaccine composed of capsular polysaccharide fragments of *Neisseria meningitidis*. There are four polysaccharide serotypes represented in the vaccine: A, C, Y, and W-135. The type A polysaccharide consists of a polymer of *N*-acetyl-*O*-mannosamine phosphate; the group C polysaccharide is mostly *N*-acetyl-*O*-acetylneuraminic acid. Indications are

- Induction of active immunity against selected strains of *N. meningitidis*
- Military recruits during basic training
- College freshmen and those living in dormitories
- Travelers to countries with epidemic meningococcal disease
- Household or institutional contacts of those with meningococcal disease
- Immunosuppressed persons (HIV, *S. pneumoniae*)
- To stop certain meningococcal group C outbreaks

PNEUMOCOCCAL VACCINE

Pneumococcus is also known as *Streptococcus pneumoniae* or diplococcus. The microorganism protects itself from the immune system by producing a capsular polysaccharide that is highly antigenic. This polysaccharide is used to prepare the vaccine. The antigen form of pneumococcal vaccine is capsular polysaccharide fragments, and the antigen type is a polysaccharide mixture. The antigen is 23-valent. Indications are

- Induction of active immunity against pneumococcal disease caused by the pneumococcal antigen types included in the vaccine (the vaccine protects against pneumococcal pneumonia, pneumococcal bacteremia, and other pneumococcal infections)
- All adults at least 65 years old
- All immunocompetent individuals who are at increased risk of the disease because of pathological conditions
- Children at least 2 years old with chronic illness associated with increased risk of pneumococcal disease or its complications

Toxoids

Toxoids are detoxified toxins used to initiate active immunity (i.e., create an antitoxin). They are typically produced by formaldehyde treatment of the toxin. They are safe and unquestionably efficacious.

DISEASE STATES

All of these diseases are produced not by a bacterium but by an exotoxin produced by that organism. For example,

powerful exotoxins are produced by *Corynebacterium diphtheriae* and *Clostridium tetani*. The exotoxins are the most serious part of the disease. In both of the above disease states, survival does not confer immunity to subsequent infections, so lifelong vaccine boosters are needed.

In diphtheria, the exotoxin causes production of a pseudomembrane in the throat; the membrane then adheres to the tonsils. The organism releases a potent exotoxin that causes headache, weakness, fever, and adenitis. Severe diphtheria carries a 10% fatality rate. Only a few cases per year are reported in the United States.

Tetanus is caused by a skin wound with anaerobic conditions at the wound site. A potent exotoxin (tetanospasmin) is produced that attacks the nervous system. The first sign of disease is jaw stiffness; eventually the jaw becomes fixed (lockjaw). The disease is essentially a persistent tonic spasm of the voluntary muscles. Fatality from tetanus is usually through asphyxia. Even with supportive treatment, tetanus is about 30% fatal in the United States. Recovery requires prolonged hospitalization. There have been 50 to 90 reported cases per year in the United States since 1975. There is no natural immunity to the exotoxin. The general rule of thumb is to follow the childhood immunization schedule carefully and immunize all persons of questionable immunization status. Adults require a booster every 10 years; patients who cannot remember their last one are due for another.

CLINICALLY USED TOXOIDS

Adsorbed Tetanus Toxoid. Tetanus is a disease that is also known as lockjaw. The causative organism is the anaerobic spore-forming bacterium *Clostridium tetani*. The organism in the toxoid, adsorbed tetanus toxoid (T, adsorbed), is designated inactivated. The antigen form is toxoid, and the antigen type is protein. This toxoid lasts approximately 10 years. A booster is recommended if injured or every 5 years. Reactions other than pain at the site of injection are rare. Fluid tetanus toxoid is recommended only for the rare individual who is hypersensitive to the aluminum adjuvant.

Adsorbed Diphtheria and Tetanus Toxoid. This is recommended for children less than 7 years old who should not get pertussis vaccine (designated DT).

Adsorbed Tetanus and Diphtheria Toxoid for Adults. Adsorbed tetanus and diphtheria toxoid for adults (designated Td) is for children older than 7 years and for adults. It has a lower level of diphtheria toxoid (1/15) because older children are much more sensitive to "D." It is used for immunization of schoolchildren.

DTP. DTP is D and T toxoids with pertussis vaccine.

DTP Adsorbed. DTP adsorbed is used for early vaccination of infants in repeated doses, starting at 2 to 3 months.

Routine Childhood Immunization Schedule

Table 7-6 shows the Routine Childhood Immunization Schedule formulated by the Advisory Committee on Immunization Practices (2000). This schedule should be followed for all children and young adults regardless of economic circumstances.

REFERENCES

1. Grabenstein, J. D.: Immunofacts. St. Louis, MO, Facts and Comparisons, 2002, pp. 3–8.
2. Shen, W.-G., and Louie, S. G.: Immunology for Pharmacy Students. Newark, NJ, Harwood Academic Publishers, 2000, p. 2.
3. Shen, W.-G., and Louie, S. G.: Immunology for Pharmacy Students. Newark, NJ, Harwood Academic Publishers, 2000, pp. 10-11.
4. Hall, P. D., and Tami, J. A.: Function and evaluation of the immune system. In Di Piro, J. T., et al. (eds.). Pharmacotherapy, a Pathophysiologic Approach, 3rd ed. Norwalk, CT, Appleton & Lange, 1997, pp. 1647–1660 (and references therein).
5. Cremers, N.: Antigens, antibodies, and complement: Their nature and interaction. In Burrows, W. (ed.). Textbook of Microbiology, 20th ed. Philadelphia, W. B. Saunders, 1973, pp. 303–347.
6. Leder, P.: Sci. Am. 247:72–83, 1982.
7. Gilbert, P.: Fundamentals of immunology. In Hugo, W. B., and Russell, A. D. (eds.). Pharmaceutical Microbiology, 4th ed. London, Blackwell, 1987.
8. Bussert, P. D.: Sci. Am. 246:82–95, 1981.
9. Hood, L.: The immune system. In Alberts, B., et al. (eds.). The Molecular Biology of the Cell. New York, Garland, 1983, pp. 95–1012.
10. Sprent, J.: Cell 76:315–322, 1994.
11. Plotkin, S. L., and Plotkin, S. A.: A short history of vaccination. In Plotkin, S. A., and Mortimer, E. A., Jr. (eds.). Vaccines. Philadelphia, W. B. Saunders, 1988.
12. Hopkins, D. R.: Princes and Peasants: Smallpox in History. Chicago, University of Chicago Press, 1983, p. 1.
13. CDC: MMWR 43:1–3, 1994.
14. CDC: MMWR 44:937–943, 1996.
15. CDC: MMWR 41:103–107, 1992.
16. Barker, W. H., and Mullolly, J. P.: JAMA 244:2547–2549, 1980.
17. CDC: MMWR 40:700–708; 709–711, 1991.
18. CDC: Immunization Information. Polio, March 9, 1995.
19. CDC: MMWR 40:1–94, 1991.
20. CDC:. MMWR 43:3–12, 1994.
21. CDC: MMWR 45:304–307, 1996.
22. CDC: MMWR 31:617–625, 1982.
23. CDC: MMWR 39:11–15, 1991.
24. Varivax varicella virus vaccine live (OKA/Merck) prescribing information. Darmstadt, Germany, Merck & Co., 1995.
25. Varivax (recombinant OKA varicella zoster) vaccine ready for prescribing. Merck & Co. Recommendations and Procedures. Merck & Co. House Organ, 1996.
26. White, C. J.: Pediatr. Infect. Dis. 11:19–23, 1992.
27. Lieu, T. A., et al.: JAMA 271: 375–381, 1980.
28. Halloran, M. E.: Am. J. Epidemiol. 140:81–104, 1994.
29. Hadler, S. C.: Ann. Intern. Med. 108:457–458, 1988.
30. Revelle, A.: FDA Electronic Bull. Board, March 17, 1995, p. 95.
31. Grabenstein, J. D.: Immunofacts. St. Louis, MO, Facts and Comparisons, 2002, pp. 152–169.
32. Innis, B. L.: JAMA 271:1328–1334, 1994.
33. Revelle, M.: FDA Electronic Bull. Board, Feb. 22, 1995. FDA Reports, Feb. 27, 1995, pp. 5–6.
34. Alter, M. J., et al.: JAMA 263:1218–1222, 1990.
35. Interferon treatment for hepatitis B and C. American Liver Foundation. http://www.gastro.com.
36. Hepatitis C virus. Bug Bytes Newsletter 1, Dec. 27, 1994.
37. Mast, E. E., and Alter, M. J.: Semin. Virol. 4:273–283, 1993.
38. Hodder, S. L., and Mortimer, E. A.: Epidemiol. Rev. 14:243–267, 1992.
39. Rappuoli, R., et al.: Vaccine 10:1027–1032, 1992.
40. Englund, J., et al.: Pediatrics 93:37–43, 1994.
41. Fine, P., and Chen, R.: Am. J. Epidemiol. 136:121–135, 1992.
42. American Academy of Pediatrics Committee on Infectious Diseases: Pediatrics 92:480–488,1993.
43. Rietschel, E. T., and Brade, H.: Sci. Am. 257:54–61, 1992.
44. CDC: MMWR CDC Surveill. Summ. 41:1–9, 1992.

Anti-infective Agents

JOHN M. BEALE, JR.

The history of work on the prevention of bacterial infection can be traced back to the 19th century when Joseph Lister (in 1867) introduced antiseptic principles for use in surgery and posttraumatic injury.[1] He used phenol (carbolic acid) as a wash for the hands, as a spray on an incision site, and on bandages applied to wounds. Lister's principles caused a dramatic decrease in the incidence of postsurgical infections.

Around 1881 and continuing to 1900, microbiologist Paul Ehrlich, a disciple of Robert Koch, began work with a set of antibacterial dyes and antiparasitic organic arsenicals. His goal was to develop compounds that retained antimicrobial activity at the expense of toxicity to the human host; he called the agents that he sought ''magic bullets.'' At the time that Ehrlich began his experiments, there were only a few compounds that could be used in treating infectious diseases, and none was very useful in the treatment of severe Gram-positive and Gram-negative infections. Ehrlich discovered that the dyes and arsenicals could stain target cells *selectively* and that the antimicrobial properties of the dyes paralleled the staining activity. This discovery was the first demonstration of *selective toxicity,* the property of certain chemicals to kill one type of organism while not harming another. Selective toxicity is the main tenet of modern antimicrobial chemotherapy, and Ehrlich's seminal discovery paved the way for the development of the sulfonamides and penicillins and the elucidation of the mechanisms of *their* selective toxicity. Prior to Ehrlich's studies, the *local* antimicrobial properties of phenol and iodine were well known, but the only useful *systemic* agents were the herbal remedies cinchona for malaria and ipecac for amebic dysentery. Ehrlich's discovery of compound 606, the effective antisyphilitic drug Salvarsan,[2, 3] was a breakthrough in the treatment of a serious, previously untreatable disease.

Salvarsan

Until the 1920s, most successful anti-infective agents were based on the group IIB element mercury and the group VA elements arsenic and antimony. Atoxyl (sodium arsanilate, arsphenamine) was used for sleeping sickness.[4] Certain dyes, such as gentian violet and methylene blue, were also found to be somewhat effective, as were a few chemical congeners of the quinine molecule. Some of these agents represented significant achievements in anti-infective therapy, but they also possessed some important limitations. Heavy metal toxicity after treatment with mercury, arsenic, and antimony severely limited the usefulness of agents containing these elements.

Arsphenamine

Just prior to 1950, great strides were made in anti-infective therapy. The sulfonamides and sulfones (this chapter), more effective phenolic compounds such as hexachlorophene, synthetic antimalarial compounds (Chapter 9), and a number of antibiotics (Chapter 10) were introduced to the therapeutic armamentarium.

Anti-infective agents may be classified according to a variety of schemes. The chemical type of the compound, the biological property, and the therapeutic indication may be used singly or in combination to describe the agents. In this textbook, a combination of these classification schemes is used to organize the anti-infective agents. When several chemically divergent compounds are indicated for a specific disease or group of diseases, the therapeutic classification is used, and the drugs are subclassified according to chemical type. When the information is best unified and presented in a chemical or biological classification system, as for the sulfonamides or antibacterial antibiotics, then one of these classification systems is used.

This chapter addresses an extremely broad base of anti-infective agents, including the local compounds (alcohols, phenols, oxidizing agents, halogen-containing compounds, cationic surfactants, dyes, and mercurials), preservatives, antifungal agents, synthetic antibacterial drugs, antitubercular and antiprotozoal agents, and anthelmintics. Other chapters in this text are devoted to antibacterial antibiotics (Chapter 10), antiviral agents (Chapter 11), and antineoplastic antibiotics (Chapter 12).

Anti-infective agents that are used locally are called *germicides,* and within this classification there are two primary subtypes (see Table 8-1) and a number of other definitions of sanitization. Antiseptics are compounds that kill (*-cidal*) or prevent the growth of (*-static*) microorganisms when applied to *living tissue*. This caveat of use on living tissue points to the properties that the useful antiseptic must have. The ideal antiseptic must have low enough toxicity that it can be used directly on skin or wounds; it will exert a rapid and sustained lethal action against microorganisms (the

TABLE 8–1 Definitions and Standards for Removing Microorganisms

Antisepsis	Application of an agent to living tissue for the purpose of preventing infection
Decontamination	Destruction or marked reduction in the number or activity of microorganisms
Disinfection	Chemical or physical treatment that destroys most vegetative microbes or viruses, but not spores, in or on inanimate surfaces
Sanitization	Reduction of microbial load on an inanimate surface to a level considered acceptable for public health purposes
Sterilization	A process intended to kill or remove all types of microorganisms, including spores, and usually including viruses with an acceptably low probability of survival
Pasteurization	A process that kills nonsporulating microorganisms by hot water or steam at 65–100°C

spectrum may be narrow or broad depending on the use). The agent should have a low surface tension so that it will spread into the wound; it should retain activity in the presence of body fluids (including pus), be nonirritating to tissues, be nonallergenic, lack systemic toxicity when applied to skin or mucous membranes, and not interfere with healing. No antiseptic available today meets all of these criteria. A few antibiotics, such as bacitracin, polymyxin, silver sulfadiazine, and neomycin, are poorly absorbed through the skin and mucous membranes and are used topically for the treatment of local infections; they have been found very effective against infections such as these. In general, however, the

topical use of antibiotics has been restricted by concern about the development of resistant microbial strains and possible allergic reactions. These problems can reduce the usefulness of these antibiotics for more serious infections.

A *disinfectant* is an agent that prevents transmission of infection by the destruction of pathogenic microorganisms when applied to *inanimate objects*. The ideal disinfectant exerts a rapidly lethal action against all potentially pathogenic microorganisms and spores, has good penetrating properties into organic matter, shares compatibility with organic compounds (particularly soaps), is not inactivated by living tissue, is noncorrosive, and is esthetically pleasing (nonstaining and odorless). Locally acting anti-infective drugs are widely used by the lay public and are prescribed by members of the medical profession (even though the effectiveness of many of the agents has not been established completely). The germicide may be harmful in certain cases (i.e., it may retard healing). Standardized methods for evaluating and comparing the efficacy of germicides have only recently been developed.

Numerous classes of chemically divergent compounds possess local anti-infective properties. Some of these are outlined in Table 8-2.

The most important means of preventing transmission of infectious agents from person to person or from regions of high microbial load, such as the mouth, nose, or gut, to potential sites of infection is simply *washing the hands*. In fact, one of the breakthroughs in surgical technique in the 1800s was the finding that the incidence of postsurgical infection decreased dramatically if surgeons washed their hands before operating. Regular hand washing is properly done without disinfection to minimize drying, irritation, and sensitization of the skin. Simple soap and warm water remove bacteria efficiently. Skin disinfectants along with soap and

TABLE 8–2 Common Sterilants and Their Range of Use

	Bacteria			Viruses			Other		
	Gram-positive	Gram-negative	Acid-fast	Spores	Lipophilic	Hydrophilic	Fungi	Amebic Cysts	Prions
Alcohols (isopropanol, ethanol)	+++	+++	+	−	+	±	N/A	N/A	−
Aldehydes (glutaraldehyde, formaldehyde)	+++	+++	++	+	+	++	+	N/A	−
Chlorhexidine gluconate	+++	++	−	−	±	−	N/A	N/A	−
Sodium hypochlorite, chlorine dioxide	+++	+++	++	+ (pH 7.6)	+	+ (high conc.)	++	+	++ (high conc.)
Hexachlorophene	+	−	−	−	−	−	−	−	−
Povidone–Iodine	+++	+++	+	+ (high conc.)	+	−	+	+	−
Phenols, quaternary ammonium	+++	+++	±	−	+	−	N/A	N/A	−
Strong oxidizing agents, cresols	+++	++/−	−	−	+	−	−	−	−

water are usually used as preoperative surgical scrubs and sterilants for surgical incisions.

EVALUATION OF THE EFFECTIVENESS OF A STERILANT

Evaluation of the effectiveness of antiseptics, disinfectants, and other sterilants (Table 8-1), although seemingly simple in principle, is an extremely complex task. One must consider the intrinsic resistance of the microbe, the microbial load, the mixture of the population of microorganisms present, the amount and nature of organic material present (e.g., blood, feces, tissue), the concentration and stability of the disinfectant or sterilant, the time and temperature of exposure, the pH, and the hydration and binding of the agent to surfaces. In summary, a host of parameters must be considered for each sterilant, and experimental assays may be difficult. Specific, standardized assays of activity are defined for each use. Toxicity for human subjects must also be evaluated. The Environmental Protection Agency (EPA) regulates disinfectants and sterilants and the Food and Drug Administration (FDA) regulates antiseptics.

There are some problems with improper use of these agents. Antiseptics and disinfectants may become contaminated by resistant microorganisms (e.g., spores), *Pseudomonas aeruginosa*, or *Serratia marcescens* and may actually transmit infection. Most topical antiseptics interfere with wound healing to some degree, so they should be used according to the proper directions and for a limited length of time.

ALCOHOLS AND RELATED COMPOUNDS

Alcohols and aldehydes have been used as antiseptics and disinfectants for many years.[5] Two of the most commonly used antiseptics and disinfectants are ethyl and isopropyl alcohol.

The antibacterial potencies of the primary alcohols (against test cultures of *Staphylococcus aureus*) increase with molecular weight until the 8-carbon atom octanol is reached. In general, one oxygen atom is capable of solubilizing seven or eight carbon atoms in water. As the primary alcohol chain length increases, van der Waals' interactions increase, and the ability to penetrate microbial membranes increases. As water solubility decreases, the apparent antimicrobial potency diminishes with molecular weight. Branching of the alcohol chain decreases antibacterial potency; weaker van der Waals' forces brought about by branching do not penetrate bacterial cell membranes as efficiently. The isomeric alcohols' potencies decrease in the order primary > secondary > tertiary. Despite this fact, 2-propanol (isopropyl alcohol) is used commercially instead of *n*-propyl alcohol, because it is less expensive. Isopropyl alcohol is slightly more active than ethyl alcohol against vegetative bacterial growth, but both alcohols are largely ineffective against spores. The activity of alcohols against microorganisms is due to the ability of alcohols to denature important proteins and carbohydrates.

Alcohol, USP. Ethanol (ethyl alcohol, wine spirit) is a clear, colorless, volatile liquid with a burning taste and a characteristic pleasant odor. It is flammable, miscible with water in all proportions, and soluble in most organic solvents. Commercial ethanol contains ~95% ethanol by volume. This concentration forms an azeotrope with water that distills at 78.2°C. Alcohol has been known for centuries as a product of fermentation from grain and many other carbohydrates. Ethanol can also be prepared synthetically by the sulfuric acid–catalyzed hydration of ethylene

The commerce in, and use of, alcohol in the United States is strictly controlled by the Treasury Department, which has provided the following definition for "alcohol": "The term *alcohol* means that substance known as ethyl alcohol, hydrated oxide of ethyl, or spirit of wine, from whatever source or whatever process produced, having a proof of 160 or more and not including the substances commonly known as whiskey, brandy, rum, or gin."

Denatured alcohol is ethanol that has been rendered unfit for use in intoxicating beverages by the addition of other substances. *Completely denatured alcohol* contains added wood alcohol (methanol) and benzene and is unsuitable for either internal or external use. *Specially denatured alcohol* is ethanol treated with one or more substances so that its use may be permitted for a specialized purpose. Examples are iodine in alcohol for tincture of iodine, methanol, and other substances in mouthwashes and aftershave lotions, and methanol in alcohol for preparing plant extracts.

The primary medicinal use of alcohol is external, as an antiseptic, preservative, mild counterirritant, or solvent. Rubbing alcohol is used as an astringent, rubefacient, and a mild local anesthetic. The anesthetic effect is due to the evaporative refrigerant action of alcohol when applied to the skin. Ethanol has even been injected near nerves and ganglia to alleviate pain. It has a low narcotic potency and has been used internally in diluted form as a mild sedative, a weak vasodilator, and a carminative.

Alcohol is metabolized in the human body by a series of oxidations:

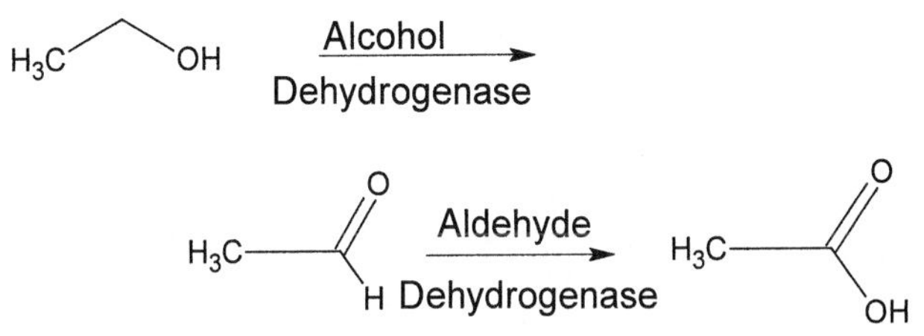

Acetaldehyde causes nausea, vomiting, and vasodilatory flushing. This fact has been used in aversion therapy with the drug disulfiram, which blocks aldehyde dehydrogenase, allowing acetaldehyde to accumulate.

Alcohol is used in the practice of pharmacy for the preparation of spirits, tinctures, and fluidextracts. *Spirits* are preparations containing ethanol as the sole solvent, whereas *tinctures* are hydroalcoholic mixtures. Many fluidextracts contain alcohol as a cosolvent.

The accepted bactericidal concentration of 70% alcohol is not supported by a study that discovered that the kill rates of microorganisms suspended in alcohol concentrations between 60 and 95% were not significantly different.[6] Concentrations below 60% are also effective, but longer contact times are necessary. Concentrations above 70% can be used safely for preoperative sterilization of the skin.[7] Alcohols are flammable and must be stored in cool, well-ventilated areas.

Dehydrated Ethanol, USP.

Dehydrated ethanol, or *absolute ethanol,* contains not less than 99% w/w of C_2H_5OH. It is prepared commercially by azeotropic distillation of an ethanol:benzene mixture, with provisions made for efficient removal of water. Absolute ethanol has a very high affinity for water and must be stored in tightly sealed containers. This form of ethanol is used primarily as a chemical reagent or solvent but has been injected for the local relief of pain in carcinomas and neuralgias. Absolute alcohol cannot be ingested because there is always some benzene remaining from the azeotropic distillation that cannot be removed.

Isopropyl Alcohol, USP.

Isopropanol (2-propanol) is a colorless, volatile liquid with a characteristic odor and a slightly bitter taste. It is considered a suitable substitute for ethanol in most cases but must not be ingested. Isopropyl alcohol is prepared commercially by the sulfuric acid–catalyzed hydration of propylene:

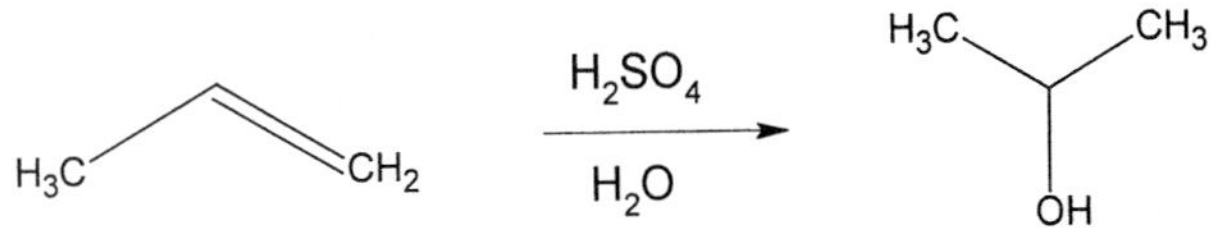

The alcohol forms a constant-boiling mixture with water that contains 91% v/v of 2-propanol. Isopropyl alcohol is used primarily as a disinfectant for the skin and for surgical instruments. The alcohol is rapidly *bactericidal* in the concentration range of 50 to 95%. A 40% concentration is considered equal in antiseptic efficacy to a 60% ethanol in water solution. *Azeotropic isopropyl alcohol, USP,* is used on gauze pads for sterilization of the skin prior to hypodermic injections. Isopropyl alcohol is also used in pharmaceuticals and toiletries as a solvent and preservative.

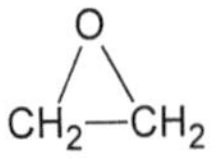

Ethylene Oxide.

Ethylene oxide, C_2H_4O, is a colorless flammable gas that liquefies at 12°C. It has been used to sterilize temperature-sensitive medical equipment and certain pharmaceuticals that cannot be heat sterilized in an autoclave. Ethylene oxide diffuses readily through porous materials and very effectively destroys all forms of microorganisms at ambient temperatures.[8]

Ethylene oxide forms explosive mixtures in air at concentrations ranging from 3 to 80% by volume. The explosion hazard is eliminated when the gas is mixed with sufficient concentrations of carbon dioxide. *Carboxide* is a commercial sterilant containing 10% ethylene oxide and 90% carbon dioxide by volume that can be handled and released in air without danger of explosion. Sterilization is accomplished in a sealed, autoclave-like chamber or in gas-impermeable bags.

The mechanism of the germicidal action of ethylene oxide probably involves the alkylation of functional groups in nucleic acids and proteins by nucleophilic opening of the oxide ring. Ethylene oxide is a nonselective alkylating agent and as such is extremely toxic and potentially carcinogenic. Exposure to skin and mucous membranes should be avoided, and inhalation of the gas should be prevented by use of an appropriate respiratory mask during handling and sterilization procedures.

Aldehydes

Formaldehyde Solution, USP.

Formalin is a colorless aqueous solution that officially contains not less than 37% w/v of formaldehyde (HCHO), with methanol added to retard polymerization. Formalin is miscible with water and alcohol and has a characteristic pungent aroma. Formaldehyde readily undergoes oxidation and polymerization, leading to formic acid and paraformaldehyde, respectively, so the preparation should be stored in tightly closed, light-resistant containers. Formalin must be stored at temperatures above 15°C to prevent cloudiness, which develops at lower temperatures.

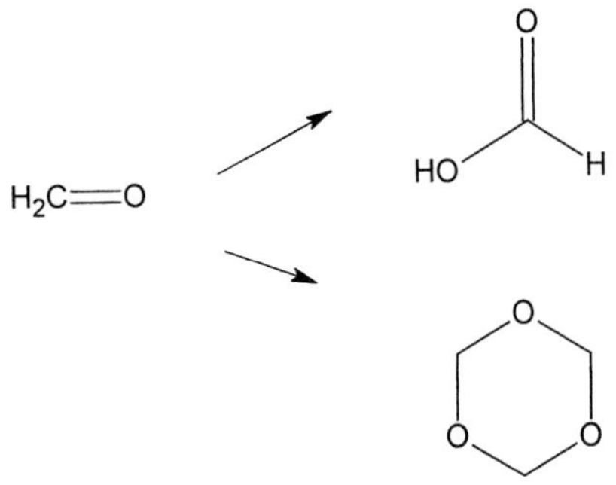

The germicidal action of formaldehyde is slow but powerful. The mechanism of action is believed to involve direct, nonspecific alkylation of nucleophilic functional groups (amino, hydroxyl, and sulfhydryl) in proteins and nucleic acids to form carbinol derivatives. The action of formaldehyde is not confined to microorganisms. The compound is irritating to mucous membranes and causes hardening of the skin. Oral ingestion of the solution leads to severe gastrointestinal distress. Contact dermatitis is common with formalin, and pure formaldehyde is suspected to be a carcinogen.

Glutaraldehyde Disinfectant Solution, USP.

Glutaraldehyde (Cidex, a 5-carbon dialdehyde) is used as a dilute solution for sterilization of equipment and instruments that cannot be autoclaved. Commercial glutaraldehyde is stabilized in alkaline solution. The preparation actually consists of two components, glutaraldehyde and buffer, which are mixed together immediately before use. The activated solution contains 2% glutaraldehyde buffered at pH 7.5 to 8.0. Stabilized glutaraldehyde solutions retain over 80% of their original activity 30 days after preparation,[9] whereas the nonstabilized alkaline solutions lose about 44% of their activity after 15 days. At higher pH (>8.5), glutaraldehyde rapidly polymerizes. Nonbuffered solutions of glutaraldehyde are acidic, possibly because of an acidic proton on the cyclic hemiacetal form. The acidic solutions are stable but lack sporicidal activity.

Glutaraldehyde   Glutaraldehyde Hemiacetal

PHENOLS AND THEIR DERIVATIVES

Phenol, USP, remains the standard to which the activity of most germicidal substances is compared. The *phenol coefficient* is defined as the ratio of a dilution of a given test disinfectant to the dilution of phenol that is required to kill (to the same extent) a strain of *Salmonella typhi* under carefully controlled time and temperature conditions. As an example, if the dilution of a test disinfectant is 10-fold greater than the dilution of phenol, the phenol coefficient is 10. Obviously, the phenol coefficient of phenol itself is 1.0. The phenol coefficient test has many drawbacks. Phenols and other germicides do not kill microorganisms uniformly, so variations in the phenol coefficient will occur. Moreover, the conditions used to conduct the test are difficult to reproduce exactly, so high variability between different measurements and laboratories is expected. Hence, the phenol coefficient may be unreliable.

A number of phenols are actually more bactericidal than phenol itself. Substitution with alkyl, aryl, and halogen (especially in the *para* position) groups increases bactericidal activity. Straight-chain alkyl groups enhance bactericidal activity more than branched groups. Alkylated phenols and resorcinols are less toxic than the parent compounds while retaining bactericidal properties. Phenols denature bacterial proteins at low concentrations, while lysis of bacterial cell membranes occurs at higher concentrations.

Phenol, USP.   Phenol (carbolic acid) is a colorless to pale pink crystalline material with a characteristic "medicinal odor." It is soluble to the extent of 1 part to 15 parts water, very soluble in alcohol, and soluble in methanol and salol (phenyl salicylate).

Phenol

Phenol exhibits germicidal activity (general protoplasmic poison), is caustic to skin, exerts local anesthetic effects, and must be diluted to avoid tissue destruction and dermatitis.

Sir Joseph Lister introduced phenol as a surgical antiseptic in 1867, and it is still used occasionally as an antipruritic in phenolated calamine lotion (0.1 to 1.0% concentrations). A 4% solution of phenol in glycerin has been used to cauterize small wounds. Phenol is almost obsolete as an antiseptic and disinfectant.

Liquified Phenol, USP.   Liquified phenol is simply phenol containing 10% water. The liquid form is convenient for adding phenol to a variety of pharmaceutical preparations because it can be measured and transferred easily. The water content, however, precludes its use in fixed oils or liquid petrolatum because the solution is not miscible with lipophilic ointment bases.

p-Chlorophenol.   *p*-Chlorophenol is used in combination with camphor in liquid petrolatum as an external antiseptic and anti-irritant. The compound has a phenol coefficient of about 4.

p-Chlorophenol

p-Chloro-m-xylenol.   *p*-Chloro-*m*-xylenol (PC-MX; Metasep) is a nonirritating antiseptic agent with broad-spectrum antibacterial and antifungal properties. It is marketed in a 2% concentration as a shampoo. It has also been used topically for the treatment of tinea (ringworm) infections such as athlete's foot (tinea pedis) and jock itch (tinea cruris).

p-Chloro-*m*-xylenol

Hexachlorophene, USP.   Hexachlorophene, 2,2'-methylenebis(3,4,6-trichlorophenol); 2,2'-dihydroxy-3,5,6,3',5', 6'-hexachlorodiphenylmethane (Gamophen, Surgicon, pHisoHex) is a white to light tan crystalline powder that is insoluble in water but is soluble in alcohol and most other organic solvents. A biphenol such as hexachlorophene will, in general, possess greater potency than a monophenol. In addition, as expected, the increased degree of chlorination of hexachlorophene increases its antiseptic potency further.

Hexachlorophene

Hexachlorophene is easily adsorbed onto the skin and enters the sebaceous glands. Because of this, topical application elicits a prolonged antiseptic effect, even in low concentrations. Hexachlorophene is used in concentrations of 2 to 3% in soaps, detergent creams, lotions, and shampoos for a variety of antiseptic uses. It is, in general, effective against Gram-positive bacteria, but many Gram-negative bacteria are resistant.

The systemic toxicity of hexachlorophene in animals after oral and parenteral administration had been known for some time, but in the late 1960s and early 1970s, reports of neurotoxicity in infants bathed in hexachlorophene and in burn patients cleansed with the agent prompted the FDA to ban its use in over-the-counter (OTC) antiseptic and cosmetic preparations.[10] Hexachlorophene is still available by prescription.

Cresol, NF. "Cresol" is actually a mixture of three isomeric methylphenols:

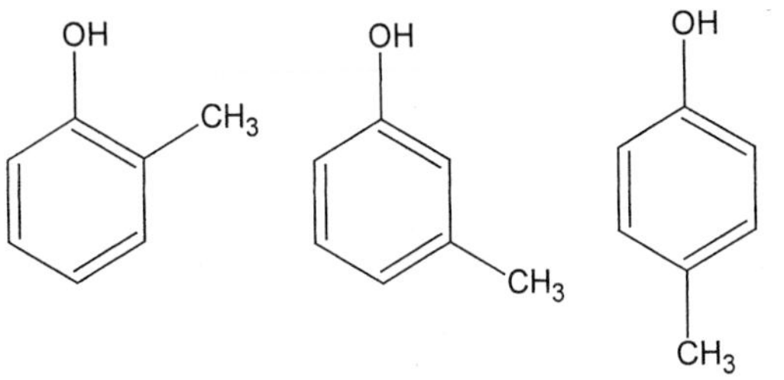

Cresols

The mixture occurs as a yellow to brownish-yellow liquid that has a characteristic odor of creosote. Cresol is obtained from coal tar or petroleum by alkaline extraction into aqueous medium, acidification, and fractional distillation. The mixture is an inexpensive antiseptic and disinfectant. It possesses a phenol coefficient of 2.5. Cresol is sparingly soluble in water, although alcohols and other organic solvents will solubilize it. The drawback to its use as an antiseptic is its unpleasant odor.

Chlorocresol, NF. 4-Chloro-3-methylphenol occurs as colorless crystals. Chlorocresol is only slightly soluble in water. At the low concentration that can be achieved in aqueous media the compound is only useful as a preservative.

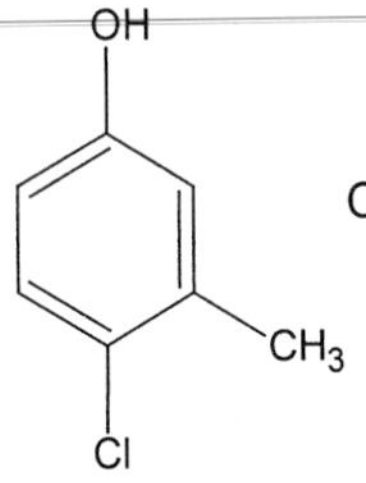

Chlorocresol

Thymol, NF. Isopropyl *m*-cresol is extracted from oil of *Thymus vulgaris* (thyme, of the mint family) by partitioning into alkaline aqueous medium followed by acidification. The crystals obtained from the mother liquor are large and colorless, with a thyme-like odor. Thymol is only slightly soluble in water, but it is extremely soluble in alcohols and other organic solvents. Thymol has mild fungicidal properties and is used in alcohol solutions and in dusting powders for the treatment of tinea (ringworm) infections.

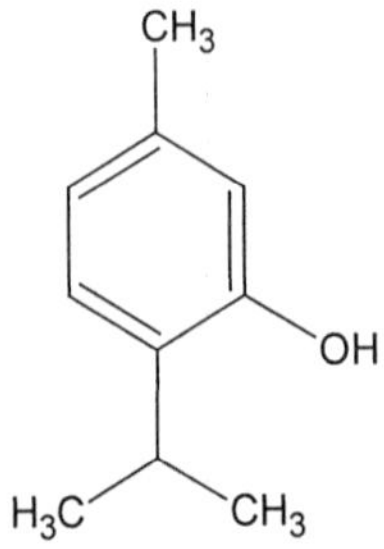

Thymol

Eugenol, USP. 4-Allyl-2-methoxyphenol is obtained primarily from clove oil. It is a pale yellow liquid with a strong aroma of cloves and a pungent taste. Eugenol is only slightly soluble in water but is miscible with alcohol and other organic solvents. Eugenol possesses both local anesthetic and antiseptic activity and can be directly applied on a piece of cotton to relieve toothaches. Eugenol is also used in mouthwashes because of its antiseptic property and pleasant taste. The phenol coefficient of eugenol is 14.4.

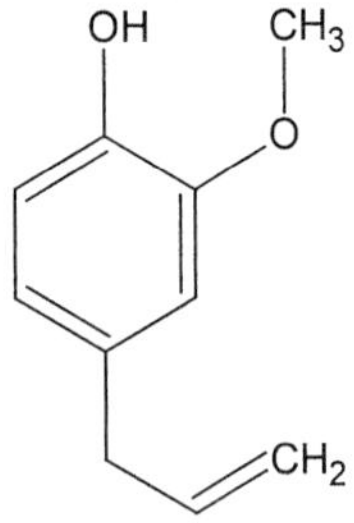

Eugenol

Resorcinol, USP. *m*-Dihydroxybenzene (resorcin), or resorcinol, is prepared synthetically. It crystallizes as white needles or as an amorphous powder that is soluble in water and alcohol. Resorcinol is light sensitive and oxidizes readily, so it must be stored in tight, light-resistant containers. It is much less stable in solution, especially at alkaline pH. Resorcinol is only a weak antiseptic (phenol coefficient 0.4). Nevertheless, it is used in 1 to 3% solutions and in ointments and pastes in concentrations of 10 to 20% for the treatment of skin conditions such as ringworm, eczema, psoriasis, and seborrheic dermatitis. In addition to its antiseptic action, resorcinol is a *keratolytic* agent. This property causes the stratum corneum of the skin to slough, opening the barrier to penetration for antifungal agents.

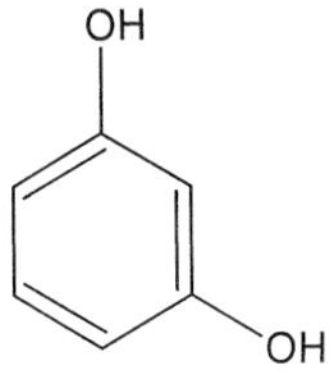

Resorcinol

Hexylresorcinol, USP. 4-Hexylresorcinol, or "hexylresorcinol," is a white crystalline substance with a faint phenolic odor. When applied to the tongue it produces a sensation of numbness. It is freely soluble in alcohol but only slightly soluble in water (1 part to 20,000 parts). Hexylresorcinol is an effective antiseptic, possessing both bactericidal and fungicidal properties. The phenol coefficient of hexylresorcinol against *S. aureus* is 98. As is typical for alkylated phenols, hexylresorcinol possesses surfactant properties. The compound also has local anesthetic activity. Hexylresorcinol is formulated into throat lozenges because of its local anesthetic and antiseptic properties. These preparations are probably of little value. Hexylresorcinol (in the concentration in the lozenge) is probably not antiseptic, and the local anesthetic property can anesthetize the larynx, causing temporary laryngitis.

HO

Hexylresorcinol

CH₃

OXIDIZING AGENTS

In general, the oxidizing agents that are of any value as germicidal agents depend on their ability to liberate oxygen in the tissues. Many of these agents are inorganic compounds, including hydrogen peroxide, a number of metal peroxides, and sodium perborate. All of these react in the tissues to generate oxygen and oxygen radicals. Other oxidizing agents, such as $KMnO_4$, denature proteins in microorganisms through a direct oxidation reaction. Oxidizing agents are especially effective against anaerobic bacteria and can be used in cleansing contaminated wounds. The bubbles that form during the liberation of oxygen help to dislodge debris. The effectiveness of the oxidizing agents is somewhat limited by their generally poor penetrability into infected tissues and organic matter. Additionally, the action of the oxidizers is typically transient.

Carbamide Peroxide Topical Solution, USP. Carbamide peroxide (Gly-Oxide) is a stable complex of urea and hydrogen peroxide. It has the molecular formula $H_2NCONH_2 \cdot H_2O_2$. The commercial preparation is a solution of 12.6% carbamide peroxide in anhydrous glycerin. When mixed with water, hydrogen peroxide is liberated. Carbamide peroxide is used as both an antiseptic and disinfectant. The preparation is especially effective in the treatment of oral ulcerations or in dental care. The oxygen bubbles that are liberated remove debris.

Hydrous Benzoyl Peroxide, USP. Hydrous benzoyl peroxide (Oxy-5, Oxy-10, Vanoxide) is a white granular powder. In its pure powder form it is explosive. The compound is formulated with 30% water to make it safer to handle.

Benzoyl Peroxide

Compounded at 5 and 10% concentrations, benzoyl peroxide is both keratolytic and keratogenic. It is used in the treatment of acne. Benzoyl peroxide induces proliferation of epithelial cells, leading to sloughing and repair.[11]

HALOGEN-CONTAINING COMPOUNDS

IODOPHORS

Elemental iodine (I_2) is probably the oldest germicide still in use today. It was listed in 1830 in USP-II as a tincture and a liniment. Iodine tincture (2% iodine in 50% alcohol with sodium iodide), strong iodine solution (Lugol's solution, 5% iodine in water with potassium iodide), and iodine solution (2% iodine in water with sodium iodide) are currently official preparations in the USP. The iodide salt is admixed to increase the solubility of the iodine and to reduce its volatility. Iodine is one of the most effective and useful of the germicides. It probably acts to inactivate proteins by iodination of aromatic residues (phenylalanyl and tyrosyl) and oxidation (sulfhydryl groups). Mixing with a number of nonionic and cationic surfactants can solubilize iodine. Complexes form that retain the germicidal properties of the iodine while reducing its volatility and removing its irritant properties.[12] In some of the more active, nonionic surfactant complexes, it is estimated that approximately 80% of the dissolved iodine remains available in bacteriologically active form. These active complexes, called *iodophors*, are both bactericidal and fungicidal.

Povidone-Iodine USP. Povidone-iodine (Betadine, Isodine, PVP-iodine) is a charge-transfer complex of iodine with the nonionic surfactant polymer polyvinylpyrrolidone (PVP). The complex is extremely water soluble and releases iodine very slowly. Hence, the preparation provides a nontoxic, nonvolatile, and nonstaining form of iodine that is not irritating to the skin or to wounds. Approximately 10% of the iodine in the complex is bioavailable. Povidone-iodine is used as an aqueous solution for presurgical disinfection of the incision site. It can also be used to treat infected wounds and damage to the skin, and it is effective for local bacterial and fungal infections. A number of other forms of PVP-iodine are available, including aerosols, foams, ointments, surgical scrubs, antiseptic gauze pads, sponges, mouthwashes, and a preparation that disinfects whirlpool baths and hot tubs.

Povidone-Iodine

CHLORINE-CONTAINING COMPOUNDS

Chlorine and chlorine-releasing compounds have been used in the disinfection of water supplies for more than a century. The discovery that hypochlorous acid (HClO) is the active germicidal species that is formed when chlorine is dissolved in water led to the development and use of the first inorganic hypochlorite salts such as NaOCl and Ca(OCl)₂. Later, organic N-chloro compounds were developed as disinfectants. These compounds release hypochlorous acid when dissolved in water, especially in the presence of acid. Two equally plausible mechanisms have been proposed for the germicidal action of hypochlorous acid: the chlorination of amide nitrogen atoms and the oxidation of sulfhydryl groups in proteins. Organic compounds that form stable *N*-chloro derivatives include amides, imides, and amidines. *N*-Chloro compounds slowly release HOCl in water. The antiseptic effect of these agents is optimal at around pH 7.

Halazone, USP. *p*-Dichlorosulfamoylbenzoic acid is a white, crystalline, photosensitive compound with a faint chlorine odor. Halazone is only slightly soluble in water at pH 7 but becomes very soluble in alkaline solutions. The sodium salt of halazone is used to disinfect drinking water.

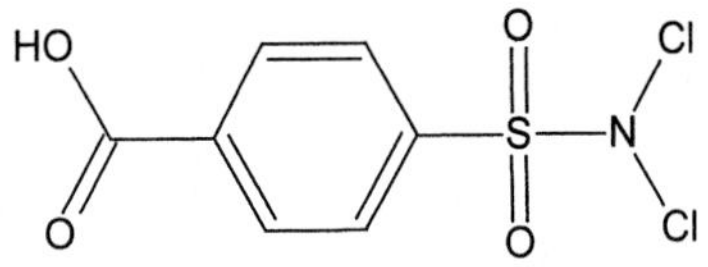

Halazone

Chloroazodin. *N,N*-Dichlorodicarbonamidine (Azochloramid) is a bright yellow crystalline solid with a faint odor of chlorine. It is mostly insoluble in water and organic solvents and is unstable to light or heat. Chloroazodin will explode if heated above 155°C. The compound is soluble enough in water to be used in very dilute solution to disinfect wounds, as packing for dental caries, and for lavage and irrigation. A glyceryltriacetate solution is used as a wound dressing. The antiseptic action of chloroazodin is long lasting because of its extremely slow reaction with water.

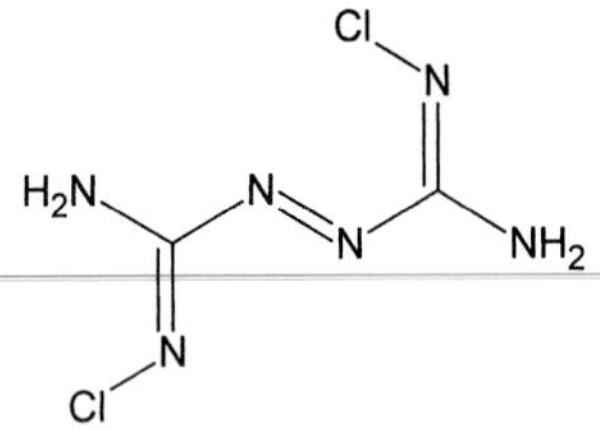

Chloroazodin

Oxychlorosene Sodium. Oxychlorosene (Clorpactin) is a complex of the sodium salt of dodecylbenzenesulfonic acid and hypochlorous acid. The complex slowly releases hypochlorous acid in solution.

Oxychlorosene occurs as an amorphous white powder that has a faint odor of chlorine. It combines the germicidal properties of HOCl with the emulsifying, wetting, and keratolytic actions of an anionic detergent. The agent has a marked and rapid *-cidal* action against most microorganisms, including both Gram-positive and Gram-negative bacteria, molds, yeasts, viruses, and spores. Oxychlorosene is used to treat localized infections (especially when resistant organisms are present), to remove necrotic tissue from massive infections or radiation necrosis, to counteract odorous discharges, to act as an irritant, and to disinfect cysts and fistulas. Oxychlorosene is marketed as a powder for reconstitution into a solution. A typical application uses a 0.1 to 0.5% concentration in water. Dilutions of 0.1 to 0.2% are used in urology and ophthalmology.

CATIONIC SURFACTANTS

All of the cationic surfactants are quaternary ammonium compounds (Table 8-3). As such, they are always ionized in water and exhibit surface-active properties. The compounds, with a polar head group and nonpolar hydrocarbon chain, form micelles by concentrating at the interface of immiscible solvents. The surface activity of these compounds, exemplified by lauryl triethylammonium sulfate, results from two structural moieties: *(a)* a cationic head group, which has a high affinity for water, and *(b)* a long hydrocarbon tail, which has an affinity for lipids and nonpolar solvents.

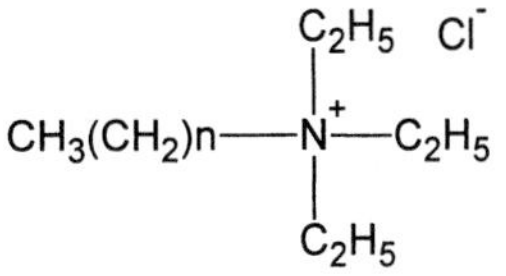

At the right concentration (the critical micelle concentration), the molecules concentrate at the interface between immiscible solvents, such as water and lipid, and water-in-oil or oil-in-water emulsions may be formed with the ammonium head group in the water layer and the nonpolar hydrocarbon chain associated with the oil phase. The synthesis and antimicrobial actions of the members of this class of compounds were first reported in 1908, but it was not until the pioneering work of Gerhard Domagk in 1935[13] that attention was directed to their usefulness as antiseptics, disinfectants, and preservatives.

The cationic surfactants exert a bactericidal action against a broad spectrum of Gram-positive and Gram-negative bacteria. They are also active against several pathogenic species of fungi and protozoa. All spores resist these agents. The mechanism of action probably involves dissolution of the surfactant into the microbial cell membrane, destabilization, and subsequent lysis. The surfactants may also interfere with enzymes associated with the cell membrane.

The cationic surfactants possess several other properties. In addition to their broad-spectrum antimicrobial activity,

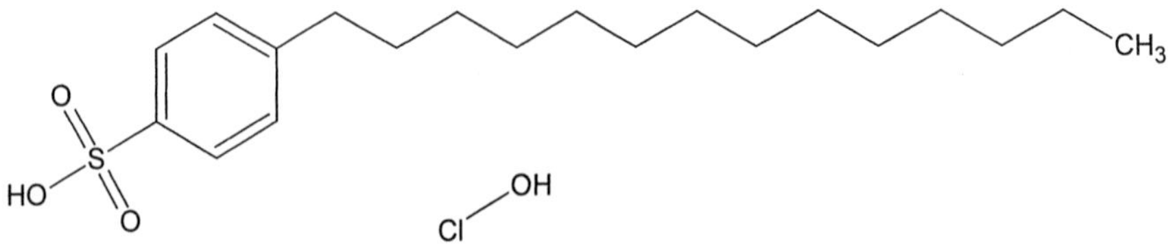

Oxychlorosene

TABLE 8–3 Analogues of Dimethylbenzylammonium Chloride

Compound	R
Benzalkonium Chloride	R = nC$_8$H$_{17}$ to C$_{16}$H$_{33}$
Benzethonium Chloride	R =
Methylbenzethonium Chloride	R =

they are useful as germicides. They are highly water soluble, relatively nontoxic, stable in solution, nonstaining, and noncorrosive. The surface activity causes a keratolytic action in the stratum corneum and, hence, provides good tissue penetration. In spite of these advantages, the cationic surfactants present several difficulties. Soaps and other anionic detergents inactivate them. All traces of soap must be removed from skin and other surfaces before they are applied. Tissue debris, blood, serum, and pus reduce the effectiveness of the surfactants. Cationic surfactants are also adsorbed on glass, talc, and kaolin to reduce or prevent their action. The bactericidal action of cationic surfactants is slower than that of iodine. Solutions of cationic surfactants intended for disinfecting surgical instruments, gloves, etc. should never be reused because they can harbor infectious microorganisms, especially *Pseudomonas* and *Enterobacter* spp.

Benzalkonium Chloride. Alkylbenzyldimethylammonium chloride (Zephiran) is a *mixture* of alkylbenzyldimethylammonium chlorides of the general formula [C$_6$H$_5$CH$_2$N(CH$_3$)$_2$R]$^+$Cl$^-$, where R represents a mixture of alkyl chains beginning with C$_8$H$_{17}$ and extending to higher

homologues with C$_{12}$H$_{25}$, C$_{14}$H$_{29}$, and C$_{16}$H$_{33}$. The higher-molecular-weight homologues compose the major fractions. Although variations in the physical and antimicrobial properties exist between individual members of the mixture, they are of little importance in the chemistry of the overall product. Benzalkonium chloride occurs as a white gel that is soluble in water, alcohol, and organic solvents. Aqueous solutions are colorless, slightly alkaline, and very foamy.

Benzalkonium chloride is a detergent, an emulsifier, and a wetting agent. It is used as an antiseptic for skin and mucous membranes in concentrations of 1:750 to 1:20,000. For irrigation, 1:20,000 to 1:40,000 concentrations are used. For storage of surgical instruments, 1:750 to 1:5,000 concentrations are used, with 0.5% NaNO$_3$ added as a preservative.

Methylbenzethonium Chloride, USP. Benzyldimethyl[2-[2-[[4-(1,1,3,3-tetramethylbutyl)tolyl]oxy]ethoxy]ethyl]ammonium chloride (Diaparene) is a mixture of methylated derivatives of methylbenzethonium chloride. It is used specifically for the treatment of diaper rash in infants, caused by the yeast *Candida albicans*, which produces ammonia. The agent is also used as a general antiseptic. Its properties are virtually identical to those of benzethonium chloride.

Benzethonium Chloride, USP. Benzyldimethyl[2-[2-[*p*-(1,1,3,3-tetramethylbutyl)phenoxy]ethoxy]ethyl]ammonium chloride (Phemerol chloride) is a colorless crystalline powder that is soluble in water, alcohol, and most organic solvents. The actions and uses of this agent are similar to those of benzalkonium chloride. It is used at a 1:750 concentration for skin antisepsis. For the irrigation of mucous membranes, a 1:5,000 solution is used. A 1:500 tincture is also available.

Cetylpyridinium Chloride, USP. 1-Hexadecylpyridinium chloride is a white powder that is very soluble in water and alcohol. In this compound, the quaternary nitrogen atom is a member of an aromatic pyridine ring.

The cetyl derivative is the most active of a series of alkylpyridinium compounds. It is used as a general antiseptic in concentrations of 1:100 to 1:1,000 for intact skin, 1:1,000 for minor lacerations, and 1:2,000 to 1:10,000 for the irrigation of mucous membranes. Cetylpyridinium chloride is also available in the form of throat lozenges and a mouthwash at a 1:20,000 dilution.

Chlorhexidine Gluconate, USP. 1,6-Di(4'-chlorophenyldiguanido)hexane gluconate (Hibiclens) is the most effective of a series of antibacterial biguanides originally developed in Great Britain.[14]

The antimicrobial properties of the biguanides were discovered as a result of earlier testing of these compounds as possible antimalarial agents (Chapter 9). Although the biguanides are technically not bisquaternary ammonium compounds and, therefore, should probably be classified separately, they share many physical, chemical, and antimicrobial properties with the cationic surfactants. The biguanides are strongly basic, and they exist as dications at physiological pH. In chlorhexidine, the positive charges are counterbalanced by gluconate anions (not shown). Like cationic surfactants, these undergo inactivation when mixed with anionic detergents and complex anions such as phosphate, carbonate, and silicate.

Chlorhexidine has broad-spectrum antibacterial activity but is not active against acid-fast bacteria, spores, or viruses. It has been used for such topical uses as preoperative skin disinfection, wound irrigation, mouthwashes, and general sanitization. Chlorhexidine is not absorbed through skin or mucous membranes and does not cause systemic toxicity.

DYES

Organic dyes were used very extensively as anti-infective agents before the discovery of the sulfonamides and the antibiotics. A few cationic dyes still find limited use as anti-infectives. These include the triphenylmethane dyes gentian violet and basic fuchsin and the thiazine dye methylene blue. The dyes form colorless *leucobase* forms under alkaline conditions. Cationic dyes are active against Gram-positive bacteria and many fungi; Gram-negative bacteria are generally resistant. The difference in susceptibility is probably related to the cellular characteristics that underlie the Gram stain.

Gentian Violet, USP. Gentian violet is variously known as hexamethyl-*p*-rosaniline chloride, crystal violet, methyl violet, and methylrosaniline chloride. It occurs as a green powder or green flakes with a metallic sheen. The compound is soluble in water (1:35) and alcohol (1:10) but insoluble in nonpolar organic solvents. Gentian violet is available in vaginal suppositories for the treatment of yeast infections. It is also used as a 1 to 3% solution for the treatment of ringworm and yeast infections. Gentian violet has also been used orally as an anthelmintic for strongyloidiasis (threadworm) and oxyuriasis.

Basic Fuchsin, USP. Basic fuchsin is a mixture of the chlorides of rosaniline and *p*-rosaniline. It exists as a green

crystalline powder with a metallic appearance. The compound is soluble in water and in alcohol but insoluble in ether. Basic fuchsin is a component of carbol–fuchsin solution (Castellani's paint), which is used topically in the treatment of fungal infections, notably ringworm and athlete's foot.

Methylene Blue, USP. Methylene blue is 3,7-bis(dimethylamino)-phenazathionium chloride (Urised). The compound occurs as a dark green crystalline powder with a metallic appearance that is soluble in water (1:25) and alcohol (1:65).

Hexamethyl-*p*-Rosaniline Cloride

Leucobase

TABLE 8–5   Clinical Types of Fungal Infection

Type	Disease State	Causative Organism
Superficial infections	Tinea versicolor	*Pityrosporum orbiculare*
	Piedra	*Trichosporon cutaneum* (white)
		Piedraia hortae (black)
Cutaneous infections	Ringworm of scalp, HAIRLESS skin, nails	Dermatophytes, *Microsporum, Trichophyton, Epidermophyton*
	Candidosis of skin, mucous membranes, nails; sometimes generalized	*Candida albicans* and related forms
Subcutaneous infections	Chromomycosis	*Fonsecaea pedrosoi* and related forms
	Mycotic mycetoma	*Allescheria boydii, Madurella mycetomi*, et al.
	Entomophthoromycosis	*Basidiobolus haptosporus*
		Conidiobolus coronatus
Systemic infections	Histoplasmosis	*Histoplasma capsulatum*
	Blastomycosis	*Blastomyces dermatitidis*
	Paracoccidioidomycosis	*Paracoccidioides brasiliensis*
	Coccidioidomycosis	*Coccidioides immitis*
	Cryptococcosis	*Cryptococcus neoformans*
	Sporotrichosis	*Sporothrix schenckii*
	Aspergillosis	*Aspergillus fumigatus*
	Mucormycosis	*Mucor* spp., *Absidia* spp., *Rhizopus* spp.
	Histoplasmosis duboisii	*Histoplasma capsulatum* var. *duboisii*

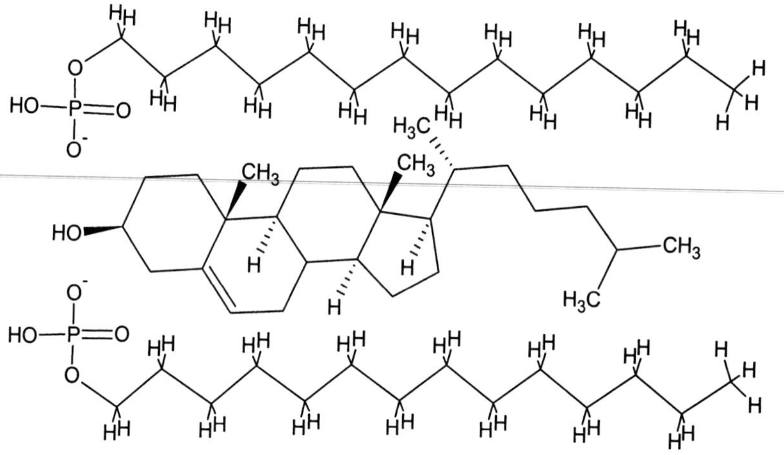

Figure 8–1 ■ Cholesterol embedded in a lipid bilayer.

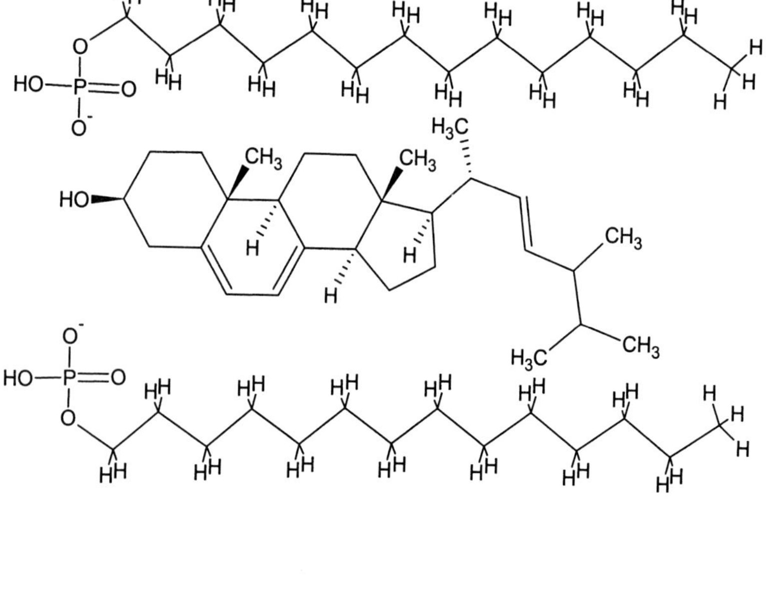

Figure 8–2 ■ Ergesterol embedded in a lipid bilayer.

to a variety of chronic disease outcomes. Granuloma with caseation and fibrocaseous pulmonary granuloma are potential outcomes of infection with *Histoplasma capsulatum,* and thrombotic arteritis, a thrombosis characterized by a purulent coagulative necrosis and invasion of blood vessels, may be caused during aspergillosis and mucormycosis. The large numbers of fungal species of many morphotypes, their disease etiology, and the diversity of outcomes make medical mycology a complex field.

Topical Agents for Dermatophytoses

Collectively, the dermatophytoses are called *tinea,* or *ringworm.* Since these infections tend to be topical, their treatment has been directed to surface areas of the skin. The skin is a formidable barrier to drug penetration, and many of the topical agents work best if an adjuvant is added that opens the barrier function of the skin. Keratolytic agents such as salicylic acid or other *α*-hydroxy compounds perform this function reasonably well.

FATTY ACIDS

Adults have an acidic, fatty substance in and on the skin called *sebum.* Sebum functions as a natural antifungal agent, part of the innate immune system. Fatty acids have been used for years with the idea that if a substance similar to sebum could be applied to the infected area, the effect of the sebum would be augmented and fungi could be eradicated. The application of fatty acids or their salts does in fact have an antifungal effect, albeit a feeble one.

The higher-molecular-weight fatty acids have the advantage of having lower volatility. Salts of fatty acids are also fungicidal and provide nonvolatile forms for topical application.

Propionic Acid.   Propionic acid is an antifungal agent that is nonirritating and nontoxic. After application, it is present in perspiration in low concentration (~0.01%). Salt forms with sodium, potassium, calcium, and ammonium are also fungicidal. Propionic acid is a clear, corrosive liquid with a characteristic odor. It is soluble in water and alcohol. The salts are usually used because they are nonvolatile and odorless.

Zinc Propionate.   Zinc propionate occurs as an anhydrous form and as a monohydrate. It is very soluble in water but only sparingly soluble in alcohol. The salt is unstable to moisture, forming zinc hydroxide and propionic acid. Zinc propionate is used as a fungicide, particularly on adhesive tape.

Sodium Caprylate.   Sodium caprylate is prepared from caprylic acid, which is a component of coconut and palm oils. The salt precipitates as cream-colored granules that are soluble in water and sparingly soluble in alcohol.

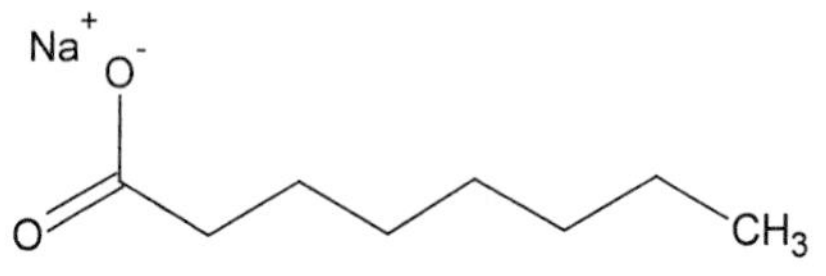

Sodium caprylate is used topically to treat superficial dermatomycoses caused by *C. albicans* and *Trichophyton, Microsporum,* and *Epidermophyton* spp. The sodium salt can be purchased in solution, powder, and ointment forms.

Zinc Caprylate.   Zinc caprylate is a fine white powder that is insoluble in water or alcohol. The compound is used as a topical fungicide. The salt is highly unstable to moisture.

Undecylenic Acid, USP.   10-Undecenoic acid (Desenex, Cruex) has the following molecular formula:

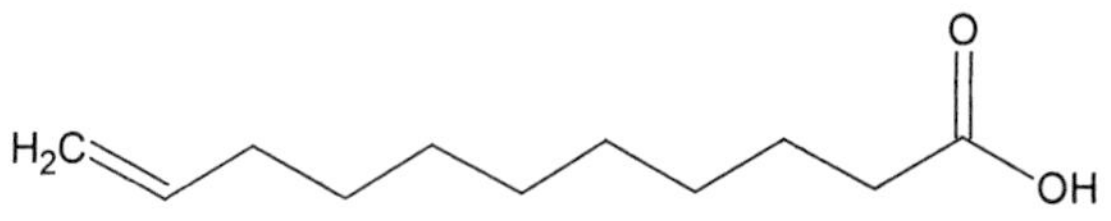

The acid is obtained from the destructive distillation of castor oil. Undecylenic acid is a viscous yellow liquid. It is almost completely insoluble in water but is soluble in alcohol and most organic solvents.

Undecylenic acid is one of the better fatty acids for use as a fungicide, although cure rates are low. It can be used in concentrations up to 10% in solutions, ointments, powders, and emulsions for topical administration. The preparation should never be applied to mucous membranes because it is a severe irritant. Undecylenic acid has been one of the agents traditionally used for athlete's foot *(tinea pedis).* Cure rates are low, however.

Triacetin, USP.   Glyceryl triacetate (Enzactin, Fungacetin) is a colorless, oily liquid with a slight odor and a bitter taste. The compound is soluble in water and miscible with alcohol and most organic solvents.

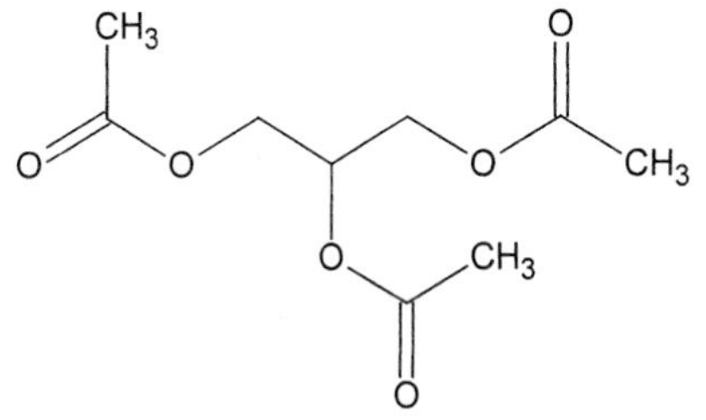

The activity of triacetin is due to the acetic acid released by hydrolysis of the compound by esterases present in the skin. Acid release is a self-limiting process because the esterases are inhibited below pH 4.

Salicylic Acid and Resorcinol.   Salicylic acid is a strong aromatic acid (pK_a 2.5) with both antiseptic and keratolytic properties. It occurs as white, needle-like crystals or a fluffy crystalline powder, depending on how the compound was brought out of solution. Salicylic acid is only slightly soluble in water but is soluble in most organic solvents. The greater acidity of salicylic acid and its lower solubility in water compared with *p*-hydroxybenzoic acid are the consequence of intramolecular hydrogen bonding.

Salicylic acid is used externally in ointments and solutions for its antifungal and keratolytic properties. By itself, salicylic acid is a poor antifungal agent.

m-Hydroxyphenol (resorcinol) possesses antiseptic and keratolytic activity. It occurs as white, needle-like crystals and has a slightly sweet taste. Resorcinol is soluble in water, alcohols, and organic solvents.

Benzoic Acid. Benzoic acid possesses appreciable antifungal effects, but it cannot penetrate the outer layer of the skin in infected areas. Therefore, benzoic acid when used as an antifungal agent must be admixed with a keratolytic agent. Suitable mixtures are benzoic acid and salicylic acid and benzoic acid and resorcinol. An old preparation that is still in use is Whitfield's Ointment, USP. This ointment contains benzoic acid, 6%, and salicylic acid, 6%, in a petrolatum base. The cure rates from preparations like these are low.

PHENOLS AND THEIR DERIVATIVES

Several phenols and their derivatives possess topical antifungal properties. Some of these, such as hexylresorcinols and parachlorometaxylenol (below) have been used for the treatment of tinea infections. Two phenolic compounds, clioquinol and haloprogin, are still official in the USP. A third agent, ciclopirox olamine, is not a phenol but has properties like those of phenols. All of these agents appear to interfere with cell membrane integrity and function in susceptible fungi.

Haloprogin, USP. 3-Iodo-2-propynyl-2,4,5-trichlorophenyl ether (Halotex) crystallizes as white to pale yellow forms that are sparingly soluble in water and very soluble in ethanol. It is an ethereal derivative of a phenol. Haloprogin is used as a 1% cream for the treatment of superficial tinea infections. Formulations of haloprogin should be protected

from light because the compound is photosensitive. Haloprogin is available as a solution and a cream, both in a 1% concentration. Haloprogin is probably not the first topical agent that should be recommended. While the cure rates for topical fungal infections are relatively high, they come at a high price. The lesion typically worsens before it improves. Inflammation and painful irritation are common.

Clioquinol, USP. 5-Chloro-7-iodo-8-quinolinol, 5-chloro-8-hydroxy-7-iodoquinoline, or iodochlorhydroxyquin (Vioform) occurs as a spongy, light-sensitive, yellowish white powder that is insoluble in water. Vioform was initially used as a substitute for iodoform in the belief that it released iodine in the tissues. It has been used as a powder for many skin conditions, such as atopic dermatitis, eczema, psoriasis, and impetigo. A 3% ointment or cream has been used vaginally as a treatment for *Trichomonas vaginalis* vaginitis. The best use for Vioform is in the topical treatment of fungal infections such as athlete's foot and jock itch. A combination with hydrocortisone (Vioform HC) is also available.

Ciclopirox Olamine, USP.[25] 6-Cyclohexyl-1-hydroxyl-4-methyl-2(1*H*)-pyridinone ethanolamine salt (Loprox) is a broad-spectrum antifungal agent intended only for topical use. It is active against dermatophytes as well as pathogenic yeasts (*C. albicans*) that are causative agents for superficial fungal infections.

Ciclopirox is considered an agent of choice in the treatment of cutaneous candidiasis, tinea corporis, tinea cruris, tinea pedis, and tinea versicolor. It is a second-line agent for the treatment of onychomycosis (ringworm of the nails). Loprox is formulated as a cream and a lotion, each containing 1% of the water-soluble ethanolamine salt. Ciclopirox is believed to act on cell membranes of susceptible fungi at low concentrations to block the transport of amino acids into the cells. At higher concentrations, membrane integrity is lost, and cellular constituents leak out.

Nucleoside Antifungals

Flucytosine, USP.[26]   5-Fluorocytosine, 5-FC, 4-amino-5-fluoro-2(1*H*)-pyrimidinone, 2-hydroxy-4-amino-5-fluoro-pyrimidine (Ancobon). 5-Fluorocytosine is an orally active antifungal agent with a very narrow spectrum of activity. It is indicated only for the treatment of serious systemic infections caused by susceptible strains of *Candida* and *Cryptococcus* spp.

The mechanism of action of 5-fluorocytosine has been studied in detail and is presented in Figure 8-3. The drug enters the fungal cell by active transport on ATPases that normally transport pyrimidines. Once inside the cell, 5-fluorocytosine is deaminated in a reaction catalyzed by cytosine deaminase to yield 5-fluorouracil (5-FU). 5-Fluorouracil is the active metabolite of the drug. 5-Fluorouracil enters into pathways of both ribonucleotide and deoxyribonucleotide synthesis. The fluororibonucleotide triphosphates are incorporated into RNA, causing faulty RNA synthesis. This pathway causes cell death. In the deoxyribonucleotide series, 5-fluorodeoxyuridine monophosphate (F-dUMP) binds to 5,10-methylenetetrahydrofolic acid, interrupting the one-carbon pool substrate that feeds thymidylate synthesis. Hence, DNA synthesis is blocked.

Resistance to 5-FC is very common, and it occurs at a number of levels. A main one is at the step in which the drug is transported into the fungal cell. The transport system simply becomes impermeable to 5-FC. The cytosine deaminase step is another point at which resistance occurs, and the UMP pyrophosphorylase reaction is a third point at which fungal cells can become resistant. Regardless of which of these mechanisms operates, fungal resistance develops rapidly and completely when 5-FC is administered. After a few dosing intervals the drug is essentially useless. One strategy used to decrease resistance and to prolong the effect of 5-FC is to administer it with the polyene antibiotic amphotericin B. The antibiotic creates holes in the fungal cell membrane, bypassing the transport step and allowing 5-FC to enter. Additionally, a lower dose of 5-FC can be used, preventing resistance by other mechanisms for a longer period.

Antifungal Antibiotics[27, 28]

The antifungal antibiotics make up an important group of antifungal agents. All of the antibiotics are marked by their complexity. There are two classes: the polyenes, which contain a large number of agents with only a few being useful, and griseofulvin (one member of the class).

POLYENES

A number of structurally complex antifungal antibiotics have been isolated from soil bacteria of the genus *Streptomyces*. The compounds are similar, in that they contain a system of conjugated double bonds in macrocyclic lactone rings. They differ from the erythromycin-type structures (macrolides; see Chapter 10), in that they are larger and contain the conjugated *-ene* system of double bonds. Hence, they are called the *polyene antibiotics*. The clinically useful polyenes fall into two groupings on the basis of the size of the macrolide ring. The 26-membered-ring polyenes, such as natamycin (pimaricin), form one group, while the 38-membered macrocycles, such as amphotericin B and nystatin, form the other group. Also common to the polyenes are (*a*) a series

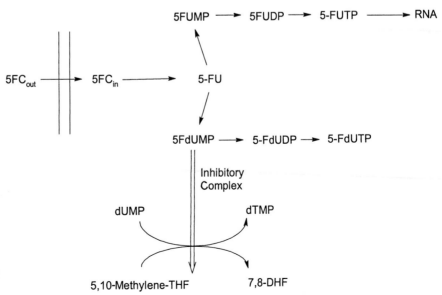

Figure 8–3 ■ Mechanism of action of 5-fluorocytosine.

of hydroxyl groups on the acid-derived portion of the ring and *(b)* a glycosidically linked deoxyaminohexose called *mycosamine*. The number of double bonds in the macrocyclic ring differs also. Natamycin, the smallest macrocycle, is a pentaene; nystatin is a hexaene; and amphotericin B is a heptaene.

The polyenes have no activity against bacteria, rickettsia, or viruses, but they are highly potent, broad-spectrum antifungal agents. They do have activity against certain protozoa, such as *Leishmania* spp. They are effective against pathogenic yeasts, molds, and dermatophytes. Low concentrations of the polyenes in vitro will inhibit *Candida* spp., *Coccidioides immitis*, *Cryptococcus neoformans*, *Histoplasma capsulatum*, *Blastomyces dermatitidis*, *Mucor mucedo*, *Aspergillus fumigatus*, *Cephalosporium* spp., and *Fusarium* spp.

The use of the polyenes for the treatment of systemic infections is limited by the toxicities of the drugs, their low water solubilities, and their poor chemical stabilities. Amphotericin B, the only polyene useful for the treatment of serious systemic infections, must be solubilized with a detergent. The other polyenes are indicated only as topical agents for superficial fungal infections.

The mechanism of action of the polyenes has been studied in some detail. Because of their three-dimensional shape, a barrel-like nonpolar structure capped by a polar group (the sugar), they penetrate the fungal cell membrane, acting as ''false membrane components,'' and bind closely with ergosterol, causing membrane disruption, cessation of membrane enzyme activity, and loss of cellular constituents, especially potassium ions. In fact, the first observable in vitro reaction upon treating a fungal culture with amphotericin B is the loss of potassium ions. The drug is fungistatic at low concentrations and fungicidal at high concentrations. This suggests that at low concentrations the polyenes bind to a membrane-bound enzyme component, such as an ATPase.

Amphotericin B, USP.

The isolation of amphotericin B (Fungizone) was reported in 1956 by Gold et al.[29] The compound was purified from the fermentation beer of a soil culture of the actinomycete *Streptomyces nodosus*, which was isolated in Venezuela. The first isolate from the streptomycete was a separable mixture of two compounds, designated amphotericins A and B. In test cultures, compound B proved to be more active, and this is the one used clinically.[30] The structure and absolute stereochemistry are as shown.

Amphotericin B is believed to interact with membrane sterols (ergosterol in fungi) to produce an aggregate that forms a transmembrane channel. Intermolecular hydrogen bonding interactions among hydroxyl, carboxyl, and amino groups stabilize the channel in its open form, destroying symport activity and allowing the cytoplasmic contents to leak out. The effect is similar with cholesterol. This explains the toxicity in human patients. As the name implies, amphotericin B is an amphoteric substance, with a primary amino group attached to the mycosamine ring and a carboxyl group on the macrocycle. The compound forms deep yellow crystals that are sparingly soluble in organic solvents but insoluble in water. Although amphotericin B forms salts with both acids and bases, the salts are only slightly soluble in water (~0.1 mg/mL) and, hence, cannot be used systemically. To create a parenteral dosage form, amphotericin B is stabilized as a buffered colloidal dispersion in micelles with sodium deoxycholate.[31] The barrel-like structure of the antibiotic develops interactive forces with the micellar components, creating a soluble dispersion. The preparation is light, heat, salt, and detergent sensitive.

Parenteral amphotericin B is indicated for the treatment of severe, potentially life-threatening fungal infections, including disseminated forms of coccidioidomycosis and histoplasmosis, sporotrichosis, North American blastomycosis, cryptococcosis, mucormycosis, and aspergillosis.

The usefulness of amphotericin B is limited by a high prevalence of adverse reactions. Nearly 80% of patients treated with amphotericin B develop nephrotoxicity. Fever, headache, anorexia, gastrointestinal distress, malaise, and muscle and joint pain are common. Pain at the site of injection and thrombophlebitis are frequent complications of intravenous administration. The drug must never be administered intramuscularly. The hemolytic activity of amphotericin B may be a consequence of its ability to leach cholesterol from erythrocyte cell membranes.

For fungal infections of the central nervous system (CNS) (e.g., cryptococcosis), amphotericin B is mixed with cerebrospinal fluid (CSF) that is obtained from a spinal tap. The solution of amphotericin B is then reinjected through the tap. For severe infections, this procedure may need to be repeated many times.

Amphotericin B for injection is supplied as a sterile lyophilized cake or powder containing 50 mg of antibiotic with

41 mg of sodium deoxycholate to be dispersed in 10 mL of water. The infusion, providing 0.1 mg/mL, is prepared by further dilution (1:50) with 5% dextrose for injection. Normal saline cannot be used because it will break the micelles. The suspension should be freshly prepared and used within 24 hours. Even the powder should be refrigerated and protected from light.

A number of sterile dosage forms[32] with amphotericin B admixed with a lipid carrier have been developed with the goal of counteracting the dose-limiting toxicity of the drug following parenteral administration. These include amphotericin B colloidal dispersion (Amphocil, Amphocyte), which contains nearly equal parts of the drug and cholesterol sulfate in a suspension of disk-like particles; Abelcet, a 1:1 combination of amphotericin B with L-*α*-dimyristoylphosphatidylcholine (7 parts) and L-*α*-dimyristoylphosphatidylglycerol (3 parts) to create a suspension of ribbon-like sheets; and liposomal amphotericin B (AmBisome), a small laminar vesicular preparation consisting of an approximately 1:10 molar ratio of amphotericin B and lipid (hydrogenated soy phosphatidyl choline, cholesterol, and distearoylphosphatidylcholine in a 10:5:4 ratio) for an aqueous suspension.

The rationale behind these lipid preparations is simple: amphotericin B should have a greater avidity for the lipid vehicle than for cholesterol in cell membranes. Hence, toxicity should be reduced. Lipid-associated amphotericin B should be drawn into the reticuloendothelial system, concentrating in the lymphatic tissues, spleen, liver, and lungs, where infectious fungi tend to locate. Lipases elaborated by the fungi and the host should release the drug from the lipid carrier, making it available to bind ergosterol in fungal cell membranes to exert its fungistatic and fungicidal activities.

Clinical use of each of the approved lipid preparations has shown reduced renal toxicity. Liposomal amphotericin B has been approved specifically for the treatment of pulmonary aspergillosis because of its demonstrated superiority to the sodium deoxycholate–stabilized suspension.

Amphotericin B is also used topically to treat cutaneous and mucocutaneous mycoses caused by *C. albicans*. The drug is supplied in a variety of topical forms, including a 3% cream, a 3% lotion, a 3% ointment, and a 100-mg/mL oral suspension. The oral suspension is intended for the treatment of oral and pharyngeal candidiasis. The patient should swish the suspension in his or her mouth and swallow it. The suspension has a very bad taste, so compliance may be a problem. A slowly developing resistance to amphotericin B has been described. This is believed to relate to alterations in the fungal cell membrane.

Nystatin, USP. Nystatin (Mycostatin) is a polyene antibiotic that was first isolated in 1951 from a strain of the actinomycete *Streptomyces noursei* by Hazen and Brown.[33] It occurs as a yellow to light tan powder. Nystatin is very slightly soluble in water and sparingly soluble in organic solvents. The compound is unstable to moisture, heat, and light.

The aglycone portion of nystatin is called *nystatinolide*. It consists of a 38-membered macrolide lactone ring containing single tetraene and diene moieties separated by two methylene groups.[34] The aglycone also contains eight hydroxyl groups, one carboxyl group, and the lactone ester functionality. The entire compound is constructed by linking the aglycone to mycosamine. The complete structure of nystatin has been determined by chemical degradation and x-ray crystallography.[35]

Nystatin is not absorbed systemically when administered by the oral route. It is nearly insoluble under all conditions. It is also too toxic to be administered parenterally. Hence, it is used only as a topical agent. Nystatin is a valuable agent for the treatment of local and gastrointestinal monilial infections caused by *C. albicans* and other *Candida* species. For the treatment of cutaneous and mucocutaneous candidiasis, it is supplied as a cream, an ointment, and a powder. Vaginal tablets are available for the control of vaginal candidiasis. Oral tablets and troches are used in the treatment of gastrointestinal and oral candidiasis. Combinations of nystatin with tetracycline can be used to prevent monilial overgrowth caused by the destruction of bacterial microflora of the intestine during tetracycline therapy.

Although nystatin is a pure compound of known structure, its dosage is still expressed in terms of units. One milligram of nystatin contains not less than 2,000 USP units.

Natamycin, USP.[36, 37] Natamycin (pimaricin; Natacyn) is a polyene antibiotic obtained from cultures of *Streptomyces natalensis*.

The natamycin structure consists of a 26-membered lactone ring containing a tetraene chromophore, an α,β-unsaturated lactone carbonyl group, three hydroxyl groups, a carboxyl group, a *trans* epoxide, and a glycosidically joined mycosamine. Like the other polyene antibiotics, natamycin is amphoteric.

The mechanism action of the smaller polyenes differs from that of amphotericin B and nystatin. The 26-membered-ring polyenes cause both potassium ion leakage and cell lysis at the same concentration, whereas the 38-membered-ring polyenes cause potassium leakage at low, fungistatic concentrations and cell lysis at high, fungicidal concentrations. The smaller polyenes are fungistatic and fungicidal within the same concentration range.

Natamycin possesses in vitro activity against a number of yeasts and filamentous fungi, including *Candida, Aspergillus, Cephalosporium, Penicillium,* and *Fusarium* spp. The drug is supplied as a 5% ophthalmic suspension intended for the treatment of fungal conjunctivitis, blepharitis, and keratitis.

Other Antifungal Antibiotics

Griseofulvin, USP. Griseofulvin (Grisactin, Gris-PEG, Grifulvin) was first reported in 1939 by Oxford et al.[38] as an antibiotic obtained from the fungus *Penicillium griseofulvum*. It was isolated originally as a "curling factor" in plants. Application of extracts containing the antibiotic to fungus-infected leaf parts caused the leaf to curl up. The drug has been used for many years for its antifungal action in plants and animals. In 1959, griseofulvin was introduced into human medicine for the treatment of tinea infections by the systemic route.

Griseofulvin is an example of a rare structure in nature, a spiro compound. The structure of griseofulvin was determined by Grove et al.[39] to be 7-chloro-2',4,6-trimethoxy-6',β-methylspiro[benzofuran-2(3H)-1'-[2]cyclohexene]-3,4'-dione. The compound is a white, bitter, heat-stable powder or crystalline solid that is sparingly soluble in water but soluble in alcohol and other nonpolar solvents. It is very stable when dry.

Griseofulvin has been used for a long time for the systemically delivered treatment of refractory ringworm infections of the body, hair, nails, and feet caused by species of dermatophytic fungi including *Trichophyton, Microsporum,* and *Epidermophyton*. After systemic absorption, griseofulvin is carried by the systemic circulation and capillary beds to the skin, nails, and hair follicles, where it concentrates in keratin precursor cells, which are gradually exfoliated and replaced by healthy tissue. Griseofulvin is a fungistatic agent, and as the new, healthy tissue develops, the drug prevents reinfection. Treatment must be continued until all of the infected tissue has been exfoliated, because old tissues will still support and harbor fungal growth. Therapy in slow-growing tissues, such as the nails, must be continued for several months. Compliance with the drug regimen is mandatory. In some cases, such as with the nails, it is possible to observe new, healthy tissue growing in to replace the infected tissue. Griseofulvin neither possesses antibacterial activity nor is effective against *Pityrosporum obiculare,* the organism that causes tinea versicolor.

Few adverse effects have been reported for griseofulvin. The most common ones are allergic reactions such as rash and urticaria, gastrointestinal upset, headache, dizziness, and insomnia.

The oral bioavailability of griseofulvin is very poor. The compound is highly lipophilic with low water solubility. The most successful attempts at improving absorption have centered on creating micronized (ultramicrosized, microsized) griseofulvin. Reducing the particle size, in theory, should improve dissolution in the stomach and absorption. The efficiency of gastric absorption of griseofulvin ultramicrosized versus the microsized form is about 1.5, allowing a dosage reduction of one third. Several structural derivatives have been synthesized, but they have failed to improve absorption. Perhaps the best advice that the pharmacist can give a patient who is about to use griseofulvin is to take the drug with a fatty meal, as with salad dressing.

Griseofulvin is a mitotic spindle poison.[39, 40] In vitro, it rapidly arrests cell division in metaphase. It causes a rapid, reversible dissolution of the mitotic spindle apparatus, probably by binding with the tubulin dimer that is required for microtubule assembly. The selective toxicity to fungi is probably due to the propensity of the drug to concentrate in tissues rich in keratin, where dermatophytes typically establish infections.

Allylamines and Related Compounds

The allylamine class of antifungal agents was discovered as a result of random screening of a chemical inventory for compounds with antifungal activity. Structure–activity studies in the series subsequently led to the discovery of compounds with enhanced potency and potential oral activity, such as terbinafine.[41, 42] Investigation of the mechanism of action of the allylamines demonstrated that the compounds interfere with an early step in ergosterol biosynthesis, namely, the epoxidation of squalene catalyzed by squalene epoxidase. Squalene epoxidase[43] forms an epoxide at the C2–C3 position of squalene (Fig. 8-4). Opening of the epox-

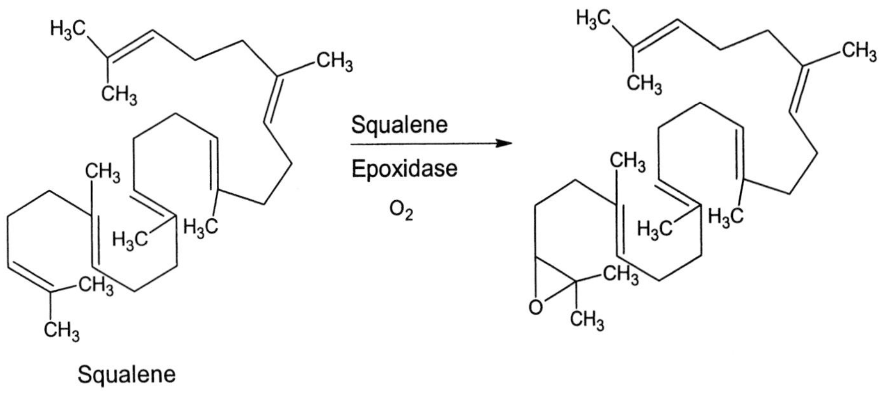

Figure 8–4 ■ Squalene epoxidase reaction.

Squalene

ide under acid catalysis yields a carbocation that initiates the "squalene zipper" reaction that forms the steroid nucleus. Inhibition of squalene epoxidase shuts down the biosynthesis of ergosterol and causes an accumulation of squalene, which destabilizes the fungal cell membrane. The allylamines exert a fungicidal action against dermatophytes and other filamentous fungi, but their action against pathogenic yeasts, such as *Candida* spp., is largely fungistatic. Although mammalian squalene epoxidase is weakly inhibited by the allylamines, cholesterol biosynthesis does not appear to be altered.

Two allylamines, naftifine and terbinafine, have been approved as topical agents for the treatment of tinea pedis, tinea cruris, and tinea corporis caused by *Trichophyton rubrum, Trichophyton mentagrophytes,* or *Epidermophyton floccosum,* respectively. The topical agent tolnaftate, while not an allylamine, inhibits squalene epoxidase and has a spectrum of activity similar to that of the allylamines. Hence, tolnaftate is classified with the allylamines. The allylamines are weak bases that form hydrochloride salts that are slightly soluble in water.

Naftifine Hydrochloride, USP. *N*-Methyl-*N*-(3-phenyl-2-propenyl)-1-naphthalenemethanamine hydrochloride (Naftin) is a white crystalline powder that is soluble in polar solvents such as ethanol and methylene chloride. It is supplied in a 1% concentration in a cream and in a gel for the topical treatment of ringworm, athlete's foot, and jock itch. Although unapproved for these uses, naftifine has shown efficacy for treatment of ringworm of the beard, ringworm of the scalp, and tinea versicolor.

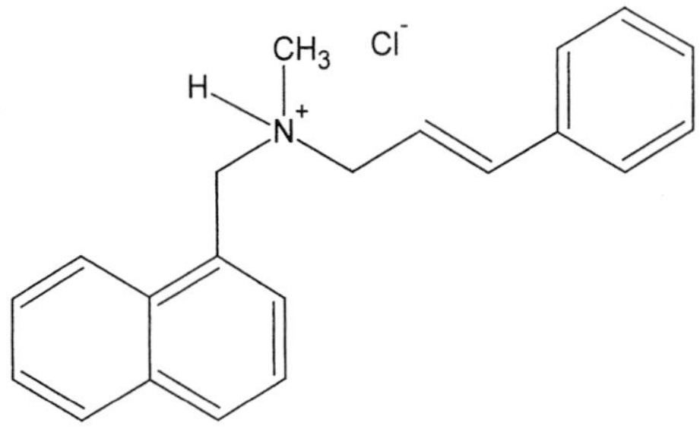

Terbinafine Hydrochloride, USP. (*E*)-*N*-(6,6-dimethyl-2-hepten-4-ynyl)-*N*-methyl-1-naphthalene-methanamine hydrochloride (Lamisil) is an off-white crystalline material that is soluble in polar organic solvents such as metha-

nol, ethanol, and methylene chloride but is only slightly soluble in water. The highly lipophilic free base is insoluble in water. Terbinafine hydrochloride is available in a 1% cream for topical administration for the treatment of tinea pedis, tinea corporis, and tinea cruris. Terbinafine is more potent than naftifine and has also demonstrated oral activity against onychomycosis (ringworm of the nails). It has not been approved in the United States for oral administration.

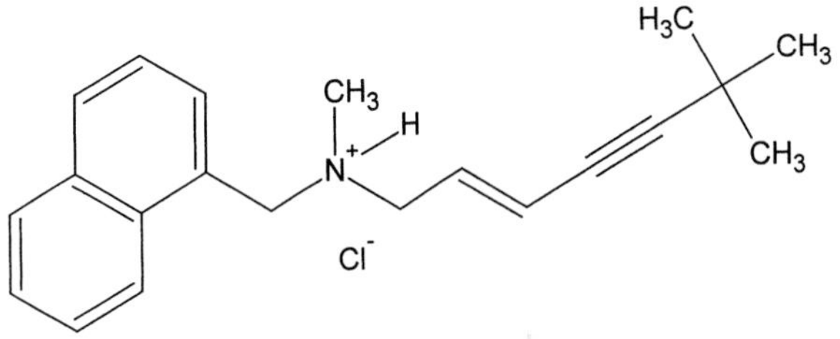

Tolnaftate, USP. *O*,2-Naphthyl *m,N*-dimethylthiocarbanilate (Tinactin, Aftate, NP-27) is a white crystalline solid that is insoluble in water, sparingly soluble in alcohol, and soluble in most organic solvents. The compound, a thioester of β-naphthol, is fungicidal against dermatophytes, such as *Trichophyton, Microsporum,* and *Epidermophyton* spp., that cause superficial tinea infections. Tolnaftate is available in a concentration of 1% in creams, powders, aerosols, gels, and solutions for the treatment of ringworm, jock itch, and athlete's foot. Tolnaftate has been shown to act as an inhibitor of squalene epoxidase[44] in susceptible fungi, so it is classified with the allylamine antimycotics. Tolnaftate is formulated into preparations intended to be used with artificial fingernails to counteract the increased chance of ringworm of the nail beds.

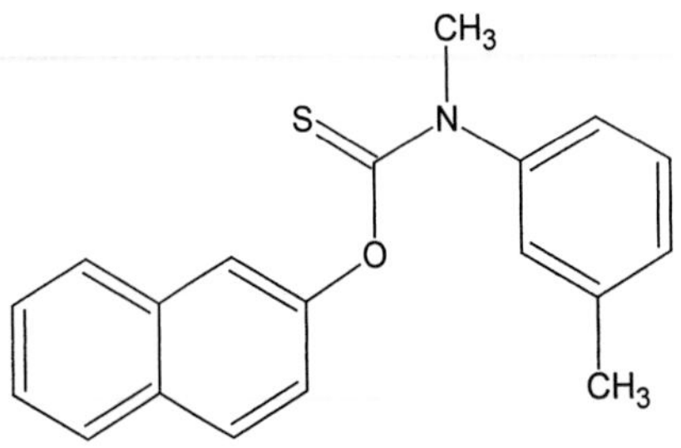

Azole Antifungal Agents

The azoles represent a class of synthetic antifungal agents that possess a unique mechanism of action. With these drugs, one can achieve selectivity for the infecting fungus over the host. Depending on the azole drug used, one can treat infections ranging from simple dermatophytoses to life-threatening, deep systemic fungal infections. Research currently under way in the United States is aimed at developing more potent azoles and compounds that penetrate the blood–brain barrier more effectively. The first members of the class were highly substituted imidazoles, such as clotrimazole and miconazole. Structure–activity studies revealed that the imidazole ring could be replaced with a bioisosteric 1,2,4-triazole ring without adversely affecting the antifungal properties of the molecule. Hence, the more generic term *azoles* refers to this class of antifungal agents.

ANTIFUNGAL SPECTRUM

The azoles tend to be effective against most fungi that cause superficial infections of the skin and mucous membranes, including the dermatophytes such as *Trichophyton, Epidermophyton,* and *Microsporum* spp. and yeasts such as *C. albicans.* On the other hand, they also exhibit activity against yeasts that cause systemic infections, including *Coccidioides immitis, Cryptococcus neoformans, Paracoccidioides brasiliensis, Petriellidium boydii, Blastomyces dermatitidis,* and *Histoplasma capsulatum.*

MECHANISM OF ACTION

The effects of the azoles on fungal biochemistry have been studied extensively, but there is still much to be learned.[45] At high in vitro concentrations (micromolar), the azoles are fungicidal; at low in vitro concentrations (nanomolar), they are fungistatic. The fungicidal effect is clearly associated with damage to the cell membrane, with the loss of essential cellular components such as potassium ions and amino acids. The fungistatic effect of the azoles at low concentration has been associated with inhibition of membrane-bound enzymes. A cytochrome P-450–class enzyme, lanosterol 14α-demethylase, is the likely target for the azoles.[46] P-450 possesses a heme moiety as part of its structure (Fig. 8-5), and the basic electron pairs of the azole rings can occupy a binding site on P-450, preventing the enzyme from turning over. The function of lanosterol 14α-demethylase is to oxidatively remove a methyl group from lanosterol during ergosterol biosynthesis.

When demethylation is inhibited, the 14α-sterol accumulates in the membrane, causing destabilization. As this happens, repair mechanisms, such as chitin synthesis, are initiated to patch the damage. This degrades membrane function further. Lanosterol 14α-demethylase is also required for mammalian biosynthesis of cholesterol, and the azoles are known to inhibit cholesterol biosynthesis.[47] In general, higher concentrations of the azoles are needed to inhibit the mammalian enzyme. This provides selectivity for antifungal action. The 1,2,4-triazoles appear to cause a lower incidence of endocrine effects and hepatotoxicity than the corresponding imidazoles, possibly because of a lower affinity for the mammalian cytochrome P-450 enzymes involved.[48] The primary mode of resistance to the triazoles and imidazoles in

C. albicans is the development of mutations in *ERG 11,* the gene coding for C14-α-sterol demethylase. These mutations appear to protect heme in the enzyme pocket from binding to azole but allow access of the natural substrate of the enzyme, lanosterol. Cross-resistance is conferred to all azoles. Increased azole efflux by the ATP-binding cassette (ABC-1, which normally transports cholesterol) and major facilitator superfamily transporters can add to fluconazole resistance in *C. albicans* and *C. glabrata.* Increased production of C14-α-sterol demethylase could be another cause of resistance.

STRUCTURE–ACTIVITY RELATIONSHIPS

The basic structural requirement for members of the azole class is a weakly basic imidazole or 1,2,4-triazole ring (pK$_a$ of 6.5 to 6.8) bonded by a nitrogen–carbon linkage to the rest of the structure. At the molecular level, the amidine nitrogen atom (N-3 in the imidazoles, N-4 in the triazoles) is believed to bind to the heme iron of enzyme-bound cytochrome P-450 to inhibit activation of molecular oxygen and prevent oxidation of steroidal substrates by the enzyme. The most potent antifungal azoles possess two or three aromatic rings, at least one of which is halogen substituted (e.g., 2,4-dichlorophenyl, 4-chlorophenyl, or 2,4-difluorophenyl), and other nonpolar functional groups. Only 2, and/or 2,4 substitution yields effective azole compounds. The halogen atom that yields the most potent compounds is fluorine, although functional groups such as sulfonic acids have been shown to do the same. Substitution at other positions of the ring yields inactive compounds. Presumably, the large nonpolar portion of these molecules mimics the nonpolar steroidal part of the substrate for lanosterol 14α-demethylase, lanosterol, in shape and size.

The nonpolar functionality confers high lipophilicity to the antifungal azoles. The free bases are typically insoluble in water but are soluble in most organic solvents, such as ethanol. Fluconazole, which possesses two polar triazole moieties, is an exception, in that it is sufficiently water soluble to be injected intravenously as a solution of the free base.

Clotrimazole, USP. 1-(o-Chloro-α,α-diphenylbenzyl)-imidazole (Lotrimin, Gyne-Lotrimin, Mycelex) is a broad-spectrum antifungal drug that is used topically for the treatment of tinea infections and candidiasis. It occurs as a white crystalline solid that is sparingly soluble in water but soluble in alcohol and most organic solvents. It is a weak base that can be solubilized by dilute mineral acids.

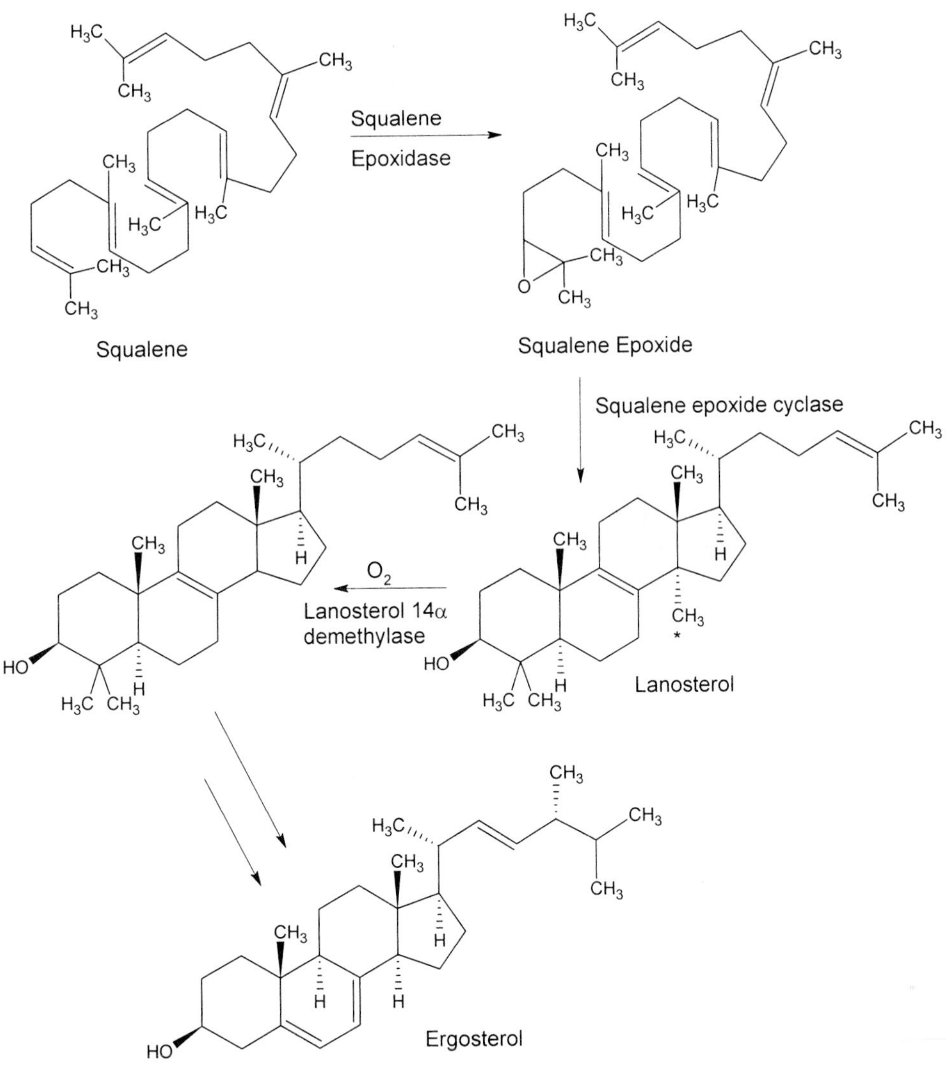

Figure 8–5 ▪ The inhibitory action of azole antifungal agents on the lanosterol 14-α-demethylase reaction.

Clotrimazole is available as a solution in polyethylene glycol 400, a lotion, and a cream in a concentration of 1%. These are all indicated for the treatment of tinea pedis, tinea cruris, tinea capitis, tinea versicolor, or cutaneous candidiasis. A 1% vaginal cream and tablets of 100 mg and 500 mg are available for vulvovaginal candidiasis. Clotrimazole is extremely stable, with a shelf life of more than 5 years.

Although clotrimazole is effective against a variety of pathogenic yeasts and is reasonably well absorbed orally, it causes severe gastrointestinal disturbances. It is also extensively protein bound and, hence, is not considered optimally bioavailable. Clotrimazole is not considered suitable for the treatment of systemic infections.

Econazole Nitrate, USP. 1-[2-[(4-Chlorophenyl)methoxy]-2-(2,4-dichlorophenyl)ethyl]-1*H*-imidazole (Spectazole) is a white crystalline nitric acid salt of econazole. It is only slightly soluble in water and most organic solvents.

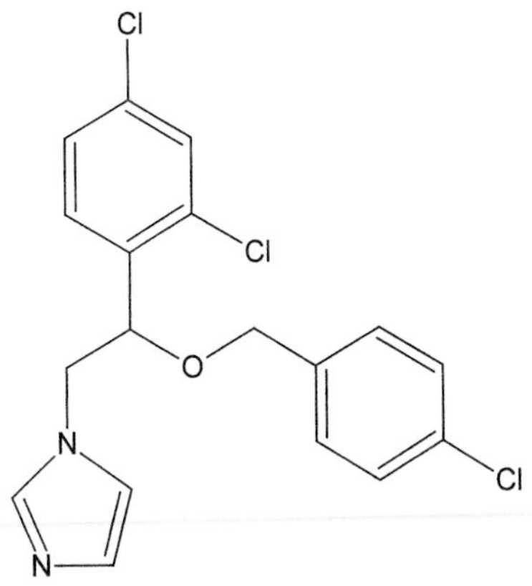

Econazole is used as a 1% cream for the topical treatment of local tinea infections and cutaneous candidiasis.

Butoconazole Nitrate, USP. 1-[4-(4-Chlorophenyl)-2-[(2,6-dichlorophenyl)-thio]butyl]-1*H*-imidazole (Femstat) is an extremely broad-spectrum antifungal drug that is specifically effective against *C. albicans*. It is supplied as a vaginal cream containing 2% of the salt. It is intended for the treatment of vaginal candidiasis.

Sulconazole Nitrate, USP. 1-[2,4-Dichloro-β-[*p*-chlorobenzyl)thio]phenethyl]imidazole mononitrate (Exelderm) is the white crystalline nitric acid salt of sulconazole. It is sparingly soluble in water but soluble in ethanol. The salt is used in a solution and a cream in 1% concentration for the treatment of local tinea infections, such as jock itch, athlete's foot, and ringworm.

Oxiconazole Nitrate, USP. (Z)-1-(2,4-dichlorophenyl)-2-(1*H*-imidazol-1-yl)ethanone-*O*-[2,4-dichlorophenyl) methyl]oxime mononitrate (Oxistat) is a white crystalline nitric acid salt. It is used in cream and lotion dosage forms in 1% concentration for the treatment of tinea pedis, tinea corporis, and tinea capitis.

Tioconazole, USP. 1-[2-[(2-chloro-3-thienyl)methoxy]-2-(2,4-dichlorophenyl)ethyl]-1*H*-imidazole (Vagistat) is

used for the treatment of vulvovaginal candidiasis. A vaginal ointment containing 6.5% of the free base is available. Tioconazole is more effective against *Torulopsis glabrata* than are other azoles.

Miconazole Nitrate, USP. 1-[2-(2,4-Dichlorophenyl)-2-[2,4-dichlorophenyl]methoxy]ethyl]-1*H*-imidazole mononitrate (Monistat, Micatin) is a weak base with a pK_a of 6.65. The nitric acid salt occurs as white crystals that are sparingly soluble in water and most organic solvents.

The free base is available in an injectable form, solubilized with polyethylene glycol and castor oil, and intended for the treatment of serious systemic fungal infections, such as candidiasis, coccidioidomycosis, cryptococcosis, petriellidiosis, and paracoccidioidomycosis. It may also be used for the treatment of chronic mucocutaneous candidiasis. Although serious toxic effects from the systemic administration of miconazole are comparatively rare, thrombophlebitis, pruritus, fever, and gastrointestinal upset are relatively common.

Miconazole nitrate is supplied in a variety of dosage forms (cream, lotion, powder, and spray) for the treatment of tinea infections and cutaneous candidiasis. Vaginal creams and suppositories are also available for the treatment of vaginal candidiasis. A concentration of 2% of the salt is used in most topical preparations.

Ketoconazole, USP. 1-Acetyl-4-[4-[[2-(2,4-dichlorophenyl)-2(1*H*-imidazole-1-ylmethyl)-1,3-dioxolan-4-yl]methoxy]phenyl]piperazine (Nizoral) is a broad-spectrum imidazole antifungal agent that is administered orally for the treatment of systemic fungal infections. It is a weakly basic compound that occurs as a white crystalline solid that is very slightly soluble in water.

The oral bioavailability of ketoconazole depends on an acidic pH for dissolution and absorption. Antacids and drugs such as H_2-histamine antagonists and anticholinergics that inhibit gastric secretion interfere with its oral absorption.

Ketoconazole is extensively metabolized to inactive metabolites, and the primary route of excretion is enterohepatic. It is estimated to be 95 to 99% bound to protein in the plasma.

Hepatotoxicity, primarily of the hepatocellular type, is the most serious adverse effect of ketoconazole. Ketoconazole is known to inhibit cholesterol biosynthesis,[47] suggesting that lanosterol 14α-demethylase is inhibited in mammals as well as in fungi. High doses have also been reported to lower testosterone and corticosterone levels, reflecting the inhibition of cytochrome P-450–requiring enzymes involved in human steroid hormone biosynthesis.[48] Cytochrome P-450 oxidases responsible for the metabolism of various drugs may also be inhibited by ketoconazole to cause enhanced effects. Thus, ketoconazole causes clinically significant increases in plasma concentrations of cyclosporine, phenytoin, and terfenadine. It may also enhance responses to sulfonylurea hypoglycemic and coumarin anticoagulant drugs.

Ketoconazole is a racemic compound, consisting of the *cis-2S,4R* and *cis-2R,4S* isomers. An investigation of the relative potencies of the four possible diastereomers of ketoconazole against rat lanosterol 14α-demethylase[49] indicated that the 2*S*,4*R* isomer was 2.5 times more active than its 2*R*,4*S* enantiomer. The *trans* isomers, 2*S*,4*S* and 2*R*,4*R*, are much less active.[49]

Ketoconazole is recommended for the treatment of the following systemic fungal infections: candidiasis (including oral thrush and the chronic mucocutaneous form), coccidioidomycosis, blastomycosis, histoplasmosis, chromomycosis, and paracoccidioidomycosis. It is also used orally to treat severe refractory cutaneous dermatophytic infections not responsive to topical therapy or oral griseofulvin. The antifungal actions of ketoconazole and the polyene antibiotic amphotericin B are reported to antagonize each other.

Ketoconazole is also used topically in a 2% concentration in a cream and in a shampoo for the management of cutaneous candidiasis and tinea infections.

Terconazole, USP. *cis*-1-[4-[[2-(2,4-Dichlorophenyl)-2-(1*H*-1,2,4-triazol-1-ylmethyl)-1,3-dioxolan-4-yl)methoxy]phenyl]-4-(1 methylethyl)piperazine (Terazol), or terconazole, is a triazole derivative that is used exclusively for the control of vulvovaginal moniliasis caused by *C. albicans* and other *Candida* species. It is available in creams containing 0.4 and 0.8% of the free base intended for 7-day and 3-day treatment periods, respectively. Suppositories containing 80 mg of the free base are also available.

Itraconazole, USP. 4-[4-[4-[4-[[2-(2,4-Dichlorophenyl)-2-1*H*-1,2,4-triazol-1-ylmethyl)-1,3-dioxolan-4-yl]methoxy]phenyl]-1-piperazinyl]phenyl]-2,4-dihydro-2-(1-methylpropyl)-3*H*-1,2,4-triazol-3-one (Sporanox) is a unique member of the azole class that contains two triazole moieties in its structure, a weakly basic 1,2,4-triazole and a nonbasic 1,2,4-triazol-3-one.

Itraconazole is an orally active, broad-spectrum antifungal agent that has become an important alternative to ketoconazole. An acidic environment is required for optimum solubilization and oral absorption of itraconazole. Drugs such as H_2-histamine antagonists and antacids, which reduce stomach acidity, reduce its gastrointestinal absorption. Food greatly enhances the absorption of itraconazole, nearly doubling its oral bioavailability. The drug is avidly bound to plasma proteins (nearly 99% at clinically effective concentrations) and extensively metabolized in the liver. Only one of the numerous metabolites, namely 1-hydroxyitraconazole, has significant antifungal activity. Virtually none of the unchanged drug is excreted in the urine. Thus, the dosage need not be adjusted in patients with renal impairment. The terminal elimination half-life of itraconazole ranges from 24 to 40 hours.

The primary indications for itraconazole are for the treatment of systemic fungal infections including blastomycosis, histoplasmosis (including patients infected with human immunodeficiency virus [HIV]), nonmeningeal coccidioidomycosis, paracoccidioidomycosis, and sporotrichosis. It may also be effective in the treatment of pergellosis, disseminated and deep organ candidiasis, coccidioidal meningitis, and cryptococcosis.

In general, itraconazole is more effective and better tolerated than is ketoconazole. Unlike ketoconazole, it is not hepatotoxic and does not cause adrenal or testicular suppression in recommended therapeutic doses.[14] Nonetheless, itraconazole can inhibit cytochrome P-450 oxidases involved in drug and xenobiotic metabolism and is known to increase plasma levels of the antihistaminic drugs terfenadine and astemizole.

Fluconazole, USP. α-(2,4-Difluorophenyl)-α-(1*H*-1,2, 4-triazol-1-ylmethyl)-1*H*-1,2,4-triazole-1-ethanol or 2,4-difluoro-α,α-bis(1*H*-1, 2,4-triazol-1-ylmethyl)benzyl alcohol (Diflucan) is a water-soluble bis-triazole with broad-spectrum antifungal properties that is suitable for both oral and intravenous administration as the free base. Intravenous solutions of fluconazole contain 2 mg of the free base in 1 mL of isotonic sodium chloride or 5% dextrose vehicle.

The oral bioavailability of fluconazole, following administration of either tablet or oral suspension dosage forms, is excellent. Apparently, the presence of two weakly basic triazole rings in the molecule confers sufficient aqueous solubility to balance the lipophilicity of the 2,4-difluorophenyl group. The oral absorption of fluconazole, in contrast to the oral absorption of ketoconazole or itraconazole, is not affected by alteration in gastrointestinal acidity or the presence of food.

Fluconazole has a relatively long elimination half-life, ranging from 27 to 34 hours. It penetrates well into all body cavities, including the CSF. Plasma protein binding of fluconazole is less than 10%; the drug is efficiently removed from the blood by hemodialysis. Fluconazole experiences little or

no hepatic metabolism and is excreted substantially unchanged in the urine. A small amount of unchanged fluconazole (~10%) is excreted in the feces. Side effects of fluconazole are largely confined to minor gastrointestinal symptoms. Inhibition of cytochrome P-450 oxidases by fluconazole can give rise to clinically significant interactions involving increased plasma levels of cyclosporine, phenytoin, and the oral hypoglycemic drugs (tolbutamide, glipizide, and glyburide). Fluconazole does not appear to interfere with corticosteroid or androgen biosynthesis in dosages used to treat systemic fungal infections.

Fluconazole is recommended for the treatment and prophylaxis of disseminated and deep organ candidiasis. It is also used to control esophageal and oropharyngeal candidiasis. Because of its efficient penetration into CSF, fluconazole is an agent of choice for the treatment of cryptococcal meningitis and for prophylaxis against cryptococcosis in AIDS patients. Although fluconazole is generally less effective than either ketoconazole or itraconazole against nonmeningeal coccidioidomycosis, it is preferred therapy for coccidioidal meningitis. Fluconazole lends itself to one-dose therapies for vaginal candidiasis.

NEWER ANTIFUNGAL STRATEGIES

A new azole, voriconazole,[50] is presently in clinical trials in the United States.

Unlike fluconazole, voriconazole has potent activity against a broad variety of fungi, including the clinically important pathogens. Several publications have substantiated the use of voriconazole against some of the newer and rarer fungal pathogens. Voriconazole is more potent than itraconazole against *Aspergillus* spp. and is comparable to posaconazole,[50] another azole that is in clinical trials, in its activity against *C. albicans*. In general, *Candida* spp. that are less susceptible to fluconazole possess higher MICs to voriconazole. The in vitro activity of posaconazole appears to be similar to that of voriconazole. Posaconazole is now in phase III clinical trials, and evidence of the efficacy of posaconazole against a variety of fungal models, especially the rarer ones, continues to accumulate. Posaconazole exhibits high oral bioavailability, but its low water solubility makes its formulation into an intravenous solution impossible.

A search for potential prodrug forms of posaconazole has yielded a possible candidate, SCH 59884. The compound is inactive in vitro but is dephosphorylated in vivo to yield the active 4-hydroxybutyrate ester. This compound is hydrolyzed to the parent compound in the serum. Posaconazole undergoes extensive enterohepatic recycling, and most of the dose is eliminated in the bile and feces.

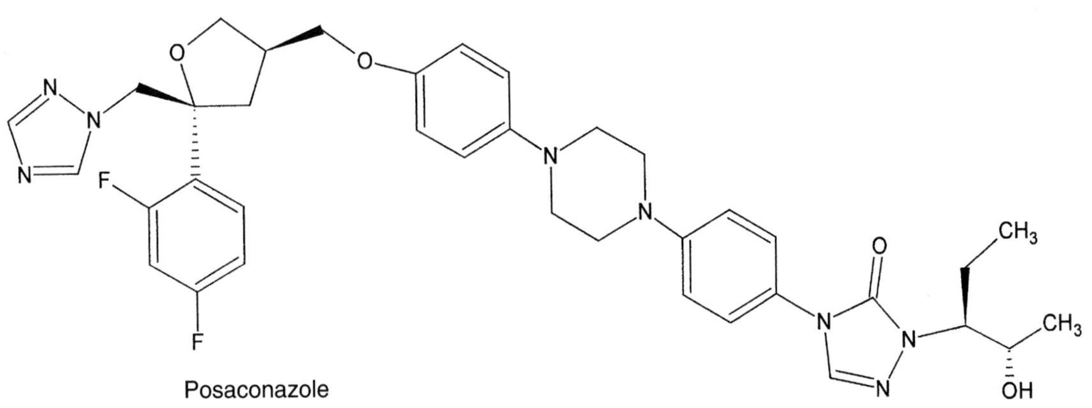

Posaconazole

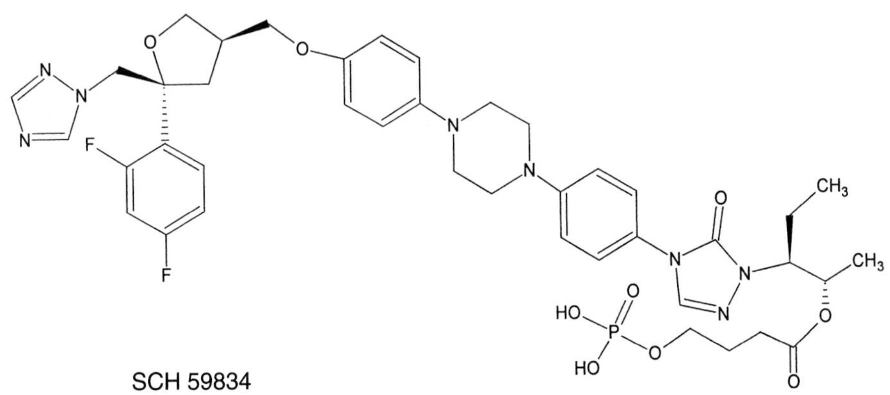

SCH 59834

Syn2869 is a novel broad-spectrum compound that contains the piperazine-phenyl-triazolone side chain common to itraconazole and posaconazole, and it displays potency and an antifungal spectrum similar to those of the latter. Syn2869 demonstrates better activity than itraconazole in animal models of *C. albicans, C. glabrata, and Cryptococ-*

cus neoformans. The oral bioavailability (F) is 60%, and higher tissue-to-serum ratios than those found for itraconazole were claimed to contribute to the greater efficacy of the compound in a model of invasive pulmonary aspergillosis. Syn2869 also demonstrates considerable activity against the common mold pathogens.

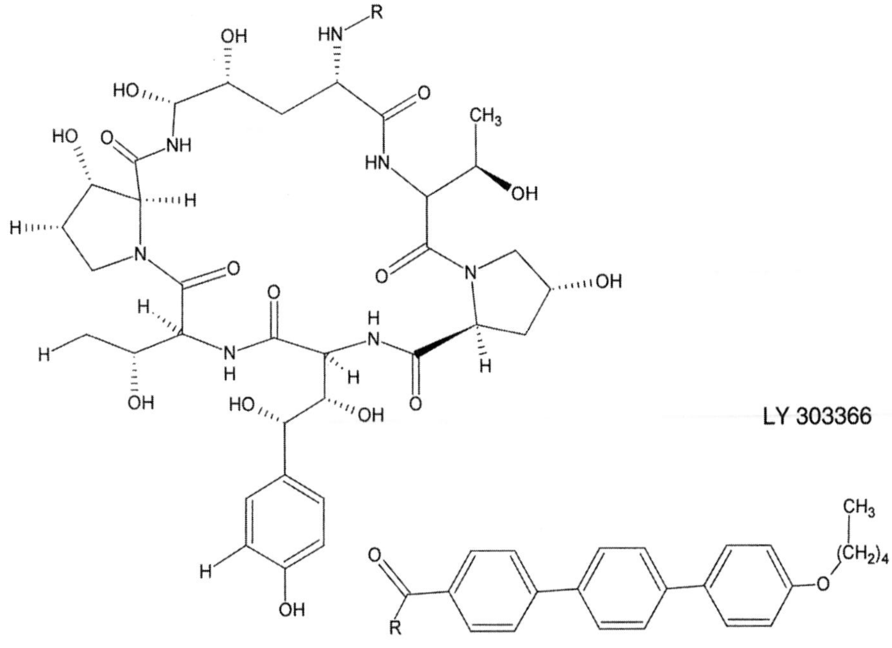

LY 303366

ECHINOCANADINS AND PNEUMOCANADINS

Echinocanadins[51] and the closely related pneumocanadins[52] are natural products that were discovered in the 1970s. They act as noncompetitive inhibitors of (1,3)-β-d-glucan synthase,[53] an enzyme complex that forms stabilizing glucan polymers in the fungal cell wall. Three water-soluble derivatives of the echinocanadins and pneumocanadins are in end-stage clinical development but have not yet been marketed.

LY 303366 is a pentyloxyterphenyl side chain derivative of echinocanadin B that was discovered at Eli Lilly. It was licensed for parenteral use in 2000. Studies have shown that the MICs of LY 303366 against *Candida* spp. range from 0.08 to 5.12 μg/mL, and similar activity was obtained against *Aspergillus* spp. Studies show highly potent activity of the compound in animal models of disseminated candidiasis, pulmonary aspergillosis, and esophageal candidiasis.

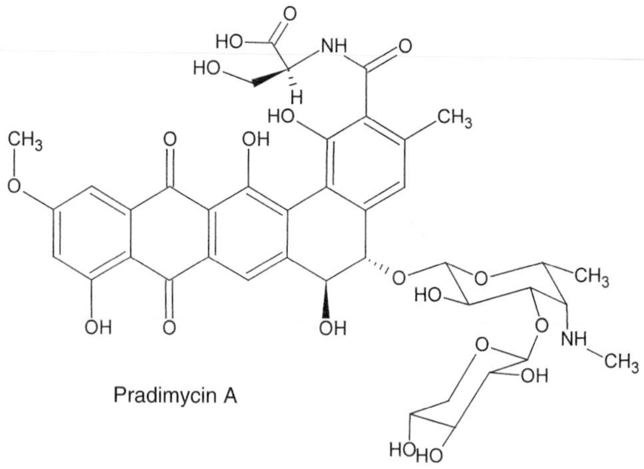

AUREOBASIDINS[54]

Aureobasidin A is a cyclic depsipeptide that is produced by fermentation in cultures of *Aureobasidium pullulan*. Aureobasidin A acts as a tight-binding noncompetitive inhibitor of the enzyme inositol phosphorylceramide synthase (IPC synthase[55]), which is an essential enzyme for fungal sphingolipid biosynthesis. A unique structural feature of the aureobasidins is the N-methylation of four of seven amide nitrogen atoms. The lack of tautomerism dictated by N-methylation may contribute to forming a stable solution conformer that is shaped somewhat like an arrowhead, the presumed biologically active conformation of aureobasidin-A.

The pradimycins and benanomycins are naphthacenequinones that bind mannan in the presence of Ca^{2+} to disrupt the cell membrane in pathogenic fungi. Both demonstrate good in vitro and in vivo activity against *Candida* spp. and *Cryptococcus neoformans* clinical isolates.

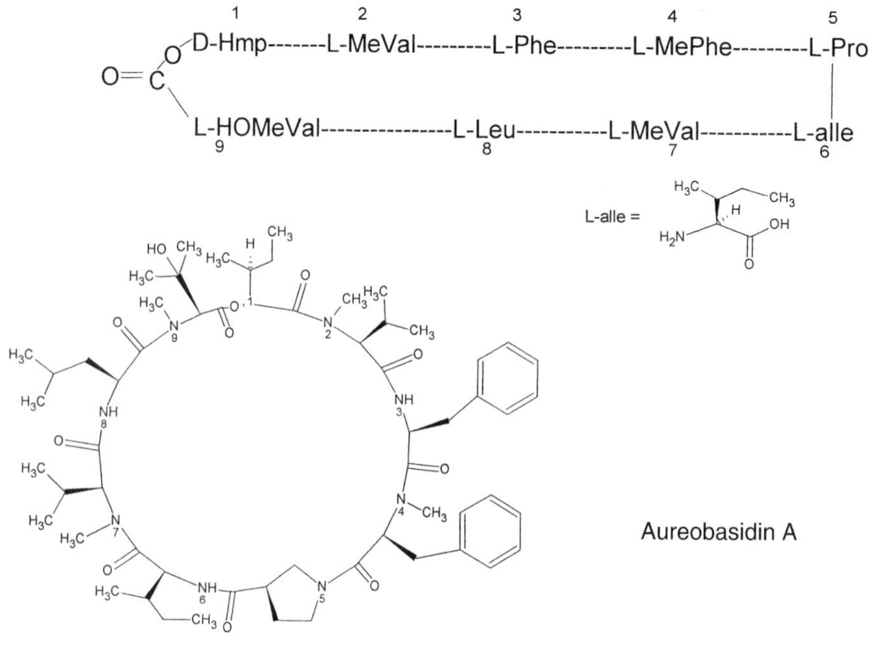

Pradimycin A

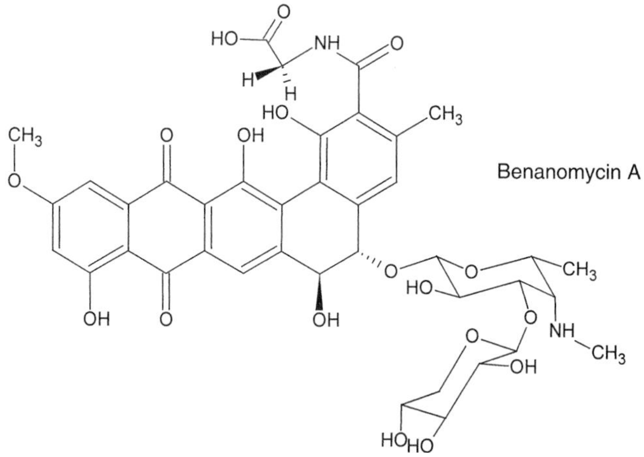

Benanomycin A

Aureobasidin A

SYNTHETIC ANTIBACTERIAL AGENTS

A number of organic compounds obtained by chemical synthesis on the basis of model compounds have useful antibacterial activity for the treatment of local, systemic, and/or urinary tract infections. Some chemical classes of synthetic antibacterial agents include the sulfonamides, certain nitroheterocyclic compounds (e.g., the nitrofurans and metronidazole), and the quinolones. Some antibacterial agents that fail to achieve adequate concentrations in the plasma or tissues for the treatment of systemic infections following oral or parenteral administration are concentrated in the urine, where they can be effective for eradicating urinary tract infections. Nitrofurantoin (a nitrofuran), nalidixic acid (a quinolone), and methenamine are examples of such urinary tract anti-infectives.

Quinolones

The quinolones comprise a series of synthetic antibacterial agents patterned after nalidixic acid, a naphthyridine derivative introduced for the treatment of urinary tract infections in 1963. Isosteric heterocyclic groupings in this class include the quinolones (e.g., norfloxacin, ciprofloxacin, and lomefloxacin), the naphthyridines (e.g., nalidixic acid and enoxacin), and the cinnolines (e.g., cinoxacin). Up to the present time, the clinical usefulness of the quinolones has been largely confined to the treatment of urinary tract infections. For urinary tract infections, good oral absorption, activity against common Gram-negative urinary pathogens, and comparatively higher urinary (compared with plasma and tissue) concentrations are the key useful properties. As a result of extensive structure–activity investigations leading to compounds with enhanced potency, extended spectrum of activity, and improved absorption and distribution properties, the class has evolved to the point that certain newer members are useful for the treatment of a variety of serious systemic infections. In fact, these more potent analogues are sometimes classified separately (from the urinary tract–specific agents) as the fluoroquinolones, because all members of the group have a 6-fluoro substituent in common.

Structure–activity studies have shown that the 1,4-dihydro-4-oxo-3-pyridinecarboxylic acid moiety is essential for antibacterial activity. The pyridone system must be annulated with an aromatic ring. Isosteric replacements of nitrogen for carbon atoms at positions 2 (cinnolines), 5 (1,5-naphthyridines), 6 (1,6-naphthyridines), and 8 (1,8-naphthyridines) are consistent with retention of antibacterial activity. Although the introduction of substituents at position 2 greatly reduces or abolishes activity, positions 5, 6, 7 (especially), and 8 of the annulated ring may be substituted with good effects. For example, piperazinyl and 3-aminopyrrolidinyl substitutions at position 7 have been shown to convey enhanced activity on members of the quinolone class against *P. aeruginosa.* Fluorine atom substitution at position 6 is also associated with significantly enhanced antibacterial activity. Alkyl substitution at the 1 position is essential for activity, with lower alkyl (methyl, ethyl, cyclopropyl) compounds generally having progressively greater potency. Aryl substitution at the 1 position is also consistent with antibacterial activity, with a 2,4-difluorophenyl group providing optimal potency. Ring condensations at the 1,8, 5,6, 6,7, and 7,8 positions also lead to active compounds.

The effective antibacterial spectrum of nalidixic acid and the earliest members of the quinolone class (e.g., oxolinic acid and cinoxacin) are largely confined to Gram-negative bacteria, including common urinary pathogens such as *Escherichia coli, Klebsiella, Enterobacter, Citrobacter,* and *Proteus* spp. *Shigella, Salmonella,* and *Providencia* are also susceptible. Strains of *P. aeruginosa, Neisseria gonorrhoeae,* and *Haemophilus influenzae* are resistant, as are the Gram-positive cocci and anaerobes. Newer members of the class possessing 6-fluoro and 7-piperazinyl substituents exhibit an extended spectrum of activity that includes effectiveness against additional Gram-negative pathogens (e.g., *P. aeruginosa, H. influenzae,* and *N. gonorrhoeae*), Gram-positive cocci (e.g., *S. aureus*), and some streptococci. The quinolones generally exhibit poor activity against most anaerobic bacteria, including most *Bacteroides* and *Clostridium* species. In many cases, bacterial strains that have developed resistance to the antibacterial antibiotics, such as penicillin-resistant gonococci, methicillin-resistant *S. aureus,* and aminoglycoside-resistant *P. aeruginosa* are susceptible to the quinolones.

The bactericidal action of nalidixic acid and its congeners is known to result from the inhibition of DNA synthesis. This effect is believed to be due to the inhibition of bacterial DNA gyrase (topoisomerase II), an enzyme responsible for introducing negative supercoils into circular duplex DNA.[56] Negative supercoiling relieves the torsional stress of helical DNA, facilitates unwinding, and, thereby, allows transcription and replication to occur. Although nalidixic acid inhibits gyrase activity, it binds only to single-stranded DNA and not to either the enzyme or double-helical DNA.[56] Bacterial DNA gyrase is a tetrameric enzyme consisting of two A and two B subunits, encoded by the *gyrA* and *gyrB* genes. Bacterial strains resistant to the quinolones have been identified, with decreased binding affinity to the enzyme because of amino acid substitution in either A or B subunits resulting from mutations in either *gyrA*[57] or *gyrB*[58] genes.

The highly polar quinolones are believed to enter bacterial cells through densely charged porin channels in the outer bacterial membrane. Mutations leading to altered porin proteins can lead to decreased uptake of quinolones and cause resistance.[59] Also, there is evidence for energy-dependent efflux of quinolones by some bacterial species. A quantitative structure–activity relationship (QSAR) study of bacterial cellular uptake of a series of quinolones[60] revealed an inverse relationship of uptake versus log P (a measure of lipophilicity) for Gram-negative bacteria, on the one hand, but a positive correlation of quinolone uptake to log P in Gram-positive bacteria, on the other. This result probably reflects the observed differences in outer envelope structures of Gram-negative and Gram-positive bacteria.[61]

The incidence (relatively low, <1%) of CNS effects associated with the quinolones (e.g., irritability, tremor, sleep disorders, vertigo, anxiety, agitation, convulsions) has been attributed to antagonism of γ-aminobutyric acid (GABA) receptors in the brain by the quinolones. Only fluoroquinolones having a 1-piperidino, a 3-amino-1-pyrrolidino, or similar basic moiety at the 7 position appear to have this property.[61] The low incidence of CNS effects for most quinolones is apparently due to their inability to penetrate the blood–brain barrier

Another property of the quinolone class is phototoxicity, extreme sensitivity to sunlight. Quinolones possessing a halogen atom at the 8 position (e.g., lomefloxacin) have the highest incidence of phototoxicity, while those having an amino (e.g., sparfloxacin) or methoxy group at either the 5 or the 8 position have the lowest incidence.[61]

The antibacterial quinolones can be divided into two classes on the basis of their dissociation properties in physiologically relevant conditions. The first class, represented by nalidixic acid, oxolinic acid (no longer marketed in the United States), and cinoxacin, possesses only the 3-carboxylic acid group as an ionizable functionality. The pK_a values for the 3-carboxyl group in nalidixic acid and other quinolone antibacterial drugs fall in the range of 5.6 to 6.4 (Table 8-6).[62] These comparatively high pK_a values relative to the pK_a of 4.2 for benzoic acid are attributed to the acid-weakening effect of hydrogen bonding of the 3-carboxyl group to the adjacent 4-carbonyl group.[62]

The second class of antibacterial quinolones embraces the broad-spectrum fluoroquinolones (namely, norfloxacin, enoxacin, ciprofloxacin, ofloxacin, lomefloxacin, and sparfloxacin), all of which possess, in addition to the 3-carboxylic acid group, a basic piperazino functionality at the 7 position and a 6-fluoro substituent. The pK_a values for the more basic nitrogen atom of the piperazino group fall in the range of 8.1 to 9.3 (Table 8-6).[62] At most physiologically relevant pH values, significant dissociation of both the 3-carboxylic acid and the basic 7-(1-piperazino) groups occurs, leading to significant fractions of zwitterionic species. As an example, the dissociation equilibria for norfloxacin are illustrated in Figure 8-6.[62, 63]

The tendency for certain fluoroquinolones (e.g., norfloxacin and ciprofloxacin) in high doses to cause crystalluria in alkaline urine is, in part, due to the predominance of the comparatively less soluble zwitterionic form. Solubility data presented for ofloxacin in the 15th edition of the *United States Pharmacopoeia* dramatically illustrate the effect of pH on water solubility of compounds of the fluoroquinolone class. Thus, the solubility of ofloxacin in water is 60 mg/mL at pH values ranging from 2 to 5, falls to 4 mg/mL at pH 7 (near the isoelectric point, pI), and rises to 303 mg/mL at pH 9.8.

The excellent chelating properties of the quinolones provide the basis for their incompatibility with antacids, hematinics, and mineral supplements containing divalent or trivalent metals. The quinolones may form 1:1, 2:1, or 3:1 chelates with metal ions such as Ca^{+2}, Mg^{+2}, Zn^{+2}, Fe^{+2}, Fe^{+3}, and Bi^{+3}. The stoichiometry of the chelate formed depends on a variety of factors, such as the relative concentrations of chelating agent (quinolone) and metal ion present, the valence (or charge) on the metal ion, and the pH. Since such chelates are often insoluble in water, coincidental oral administration of a quinolone with an antacid, a hematinic, or a mineral supplement can significantly reduce the oral bioavailability of the quinolone. As an example, the insoluble 2:1 chelate formed between ciprofloxacin and magnesium ion is shown in Figure 8-7. The presence of divalent ions (such as Mg^{+2}) in the urine may also contribute to the comparatively lower solubility of certain fluoroquinolones in urine than in plasma.

Nalidixic Acid, USP. 1-Ethyl-1,4-dihydro-7-methyl-4-oxo-1,8-naphthyridine-3-carboxylic acid (NegGram) occurs as a pale buff crystalline powder that is sparingly soluble in water and ether but soluble in most polar organic solvents.

Nalidixic acid is useful in the treatment of urinary tract infections in which Gram-negative bacteria predominate. The activity against indole-positive *Proteus* spp. is particularly noteworthy, and nalidixic acid and its congeners represent important alternatives for the treatment of urinary tract infections caused by strains of these bacteria resistant to other agents. Nalidixic acid is rapidly absorbed, extensively metabolized, and rapidly excreted after oral administration. The 7-hydroxymethyl metabolite is significantly more active than the parent compound. Further metabolism of the active metabolite to inactive glucuronide and 7-carboxylic acid metabolites also occurs. Nalidixic acid possesses a $t_{\frac{1}{2}elim}$ of 6 to 7 hours. It is eliminated, in part, unchanged in the urine and 80% as metabolites.

Cinoxacin, USP. 1-Ethyl-1,4-dihydro-4-oxo[1,3]dioxolo[4,5g]cinnoline-3-carboxylic acid (Cinobac) is a close congener (isostere) of oxolinic acid (no longer marketed in the United States) and has antibacterial properties similar to those of nalidixic and oxolinic acids.

TABLE 8–6 Dissociation and Isoelectric Constants for Antibacterial Quinolones

Quinolone	$pK_1{}^a$	$pK_2{}^a$	pI^a	$QH^{\pm}/QH^{\circ}$
Nalidixic acid	6.03	—	—	—
Norfloxacin	6.39	8.56	7.47	118
Enoxacin	6.15	8.54	7.35	238
Ciprofloxacin	6.08	8.73	7.42	444
Ofloxacin	5.88	8.06	6.97	146
Lomefloxacin	5.65	9.04	7.35	3,018

Data are taken from Ross, D. L., and Riley, C. M.: J. Pharm. Biomed. Anal. 12:1325, 1994.
[a]Each value represents an average of literature values.

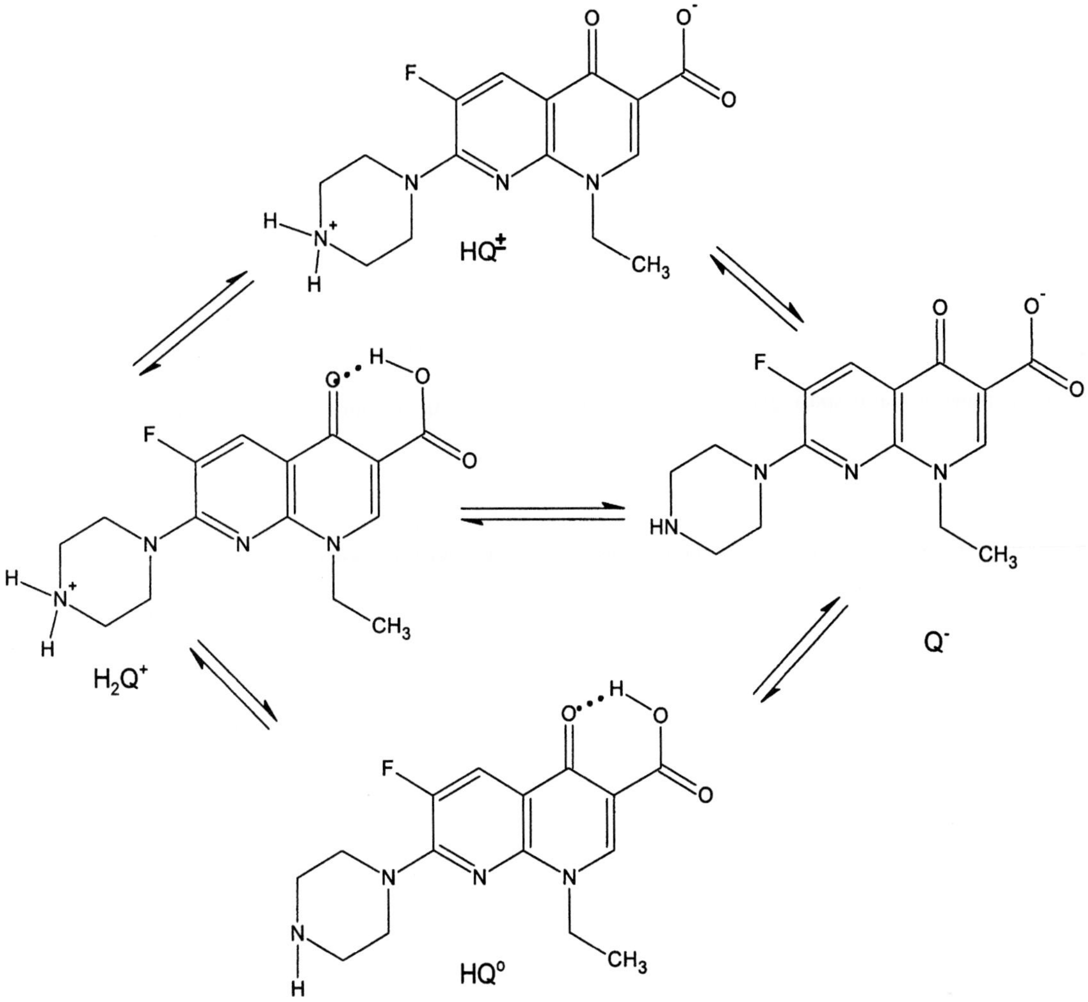

Figure 8–6 ■ Ionization equilibria in the quinolone antibacterial drugs.

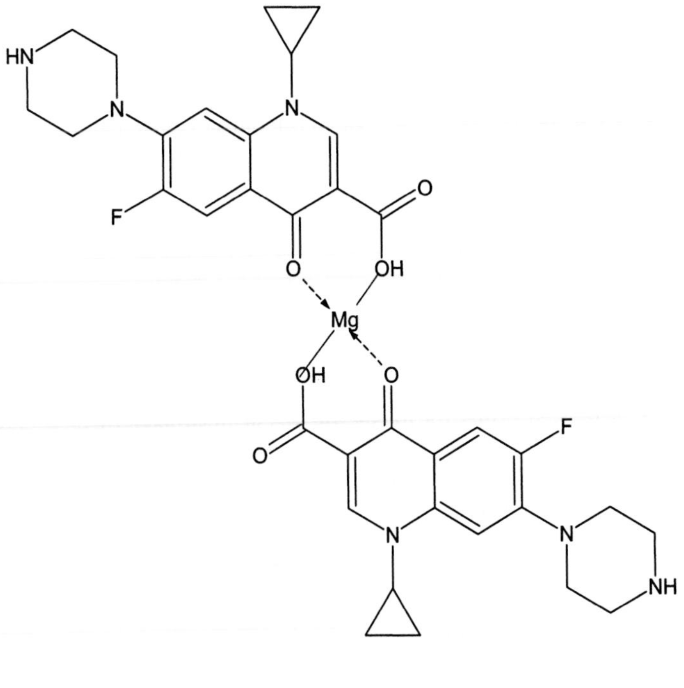

Figure 8–7 ■ A 2:1 chelate of a Mg²⁺ ion by ciprofloxacin.

It is recommended for the treatment of urinary tract infections caused by strains of Gram-negative bacteria susceptible to these agents. Early clinical studies indicate that the drug possesses pharmacokinetic properties superior to those of either of its predecessors. Thus, following oral administration, higher urinary concentrations of cinoxacin than of nalidixic acid or oxolinic acid are achieved. Cinoxacin appears to be more completely absorbed and less protein bound than nalidixic acid.

Norfloxacin. 1-Ethyl-6-fluoro-1,4-dihydro-4-oxo-7-(1-piperazinyl)-3-quinolinecarboxylic acid (Noroxin) is a pale yellow crystalline powder that is sparingly soluble in water. This quinoline has broad-spectrum activity against Gram-negative and Gram-positive aerobic bacteria. The fluorine atom provides increased potency against Gram-positive organisms, whereas the piperazine moiety improves antipseudomonal activity. Norfloxacin is indicated for the treatment of urinary tract infections caused by *E. coli, K. pneumoniae, Enterobacter cloacae, Proteus mirabilis,* indole-positive *Proteus* spp. including *P. vulgaris, Providencia rettgeri, Morganella morganii, P. aeruginosa, S. aureus,* and *S. epidermidis,* and group D streptococci. It is generally not effective against obligate anaerobic bacteria. Norfloxacin in a single 800-mg oral dose has also been approved for the treatment of uncomplicated gonorrhea. The oral absorption of norfloxacin is about 40%. The drug is 15% protein bound and is metabolized in the liver. The $t_{\frac{1}{2}elim}$ is 4 to 8 hours. Approximately 30% of a dose is eliminated in the urine and feces.

The oral absorption of norfloxacin is rapid and reasonably efficient. Approximately 30% of an oral dose is excreted in the urine in 24 hours, along with 5 to 8% consisting of less active metabolites. There is significant biliary excretion, with about 30% of the original drug appearing in the feces.

Enoxacin, USP. 1-Ethyl-6-fluoro-1,4-dihydro-4-oxo-7-(1-piperazinyl)-1,8-naphthyridine-3-carboxylic acid (Penetrex) is a quinolone with broad-spectrum antibacterial activity that is used primarily for the treatment of urinary tract infections and sexually transmitted diseases. Enoxacin has been approved for the treatment of uncomplicated gonococcal urethritis and has also been shown to be effective in chancroid caused by *Haemophilus ducreyi.* A single 400-mg dose is used for these indications. Enoxacin is also approved for the treatment of acute (uncomplicated) and chronic (complicated) urinary tract infections.

Enoxacin is well absorbed following oral administration. Oral bioavailability approaches 98%. Concentrations of the drug in the kidneys, prostate, cervix, fallopian tubes, and myometrium typically exceed those in the plasma. More than 50% of the unchanged drug is excreted in the urine. Metabolism, largely catalyzed by cytochrome P-450 enzymes in the liver, accounts for 15 to 20% of the orally administered dose of enoxacin. The relatively short elimination half-life of enoxacin dictates twice-a-day dosing for the treatment of urinary tract infections.

Some cytochrome P-450 isozymes, such as CYP1A2, are inhibited by enoxacin, resulting in potentially important interactions with other drugs. For example, enoxacin has been reported to decrease theophylline clearance, causing increased plasma levels and increased toxicity. Enoxacin forms insoluble chelates with divalent metal ions present in antacids and hematinics, which reduce its oral bioavailability.

Ciprofloxacin, USP. 1-Cyclopropyl-6-fluoro-1,4-dihydro-4-oxo-7-(1-piperazinyl)-3-quinolinecarboxylic acid (Cipro, Cipro IV) is supplied in both oral and parenteral dosage forms. The hydrochloride salt is available in 250-, 500-, and 750-mg tablets for oral administration. Intravenous solutions containing 200 mg and 400 mg are provided in concentrations of 0.2% in normal saline and 1% in 5% dextrose solutions.

The bioavailability of ciprofloxacin following oral administration is good, with 70 to 80% of an oral dose being absorbed. Food delays, but does not prevent, absorption. Significant amounts (20 to 35%) of orally administered ciprofloxacin are excreted in the feces, in part because of biliary excretion. Biotransformation to less active metabolites accounts for about 15% of the administered drug. Approximately 40 to 50% of unchanged ciprofloxacin is excreted in the urine following oral administration. This value increases to 50 to 70% when the drug is injected intravenously. Somewhat paradoxically, the elimination half-life of ciprofloxacin is shorter following oral administration ($t_{\frac{1}{2}}$, 4 hours) than it is following intravenous administration ($t_{\frac{1}{2}}$, 5 to 6 hours). Ciprofloxacin inhibits the P-450 species CYP1A2.

The oral dose of this quinolone is typically 25% higher than the parenteral dose for a given indication. Probenecid significantly reduces the renal clearance of ciprofloxacin, presumably by inhibiting its active tubular secretion. Ciprofloxacin is widely distributed to virtually all parts of the body, including the CSF, and is generally considered to provide the best distribution of the currently marketed quinolones. This property, together with the potency and broad antibacterial spectrum of ciprofloxacin, accounts for the numerous therapeutic indications for the drug. Ciprofloxacin also exhibits higher potency against most Gram-negative bacterial species, including *P. aeruginosa,* than other quinolones.

Ciprofloxacin is an agent of choice for the treatment of bacterial gastroenteritis caused by Gram-negative bacilli such as enteropathogenic *E. coli,* salmonella (including *S. typhi*), *Shigella* spp., *Vibrio* spp., and *Aeromonas hydrophilia.* It is widely used for the treatment of respiratory tract infections and is particularly effective for controlling bronchitis and pneumonia caused by Gram-negative bacteria. Ciprofloxacin is also used for combating infections of the skin, soft tissues, bones, and joints. Both uncomplicated and complicated urinary tract infections caused by Gram-negative bacteria can be treated effectively with ciprofloxacin. It is particularly useful for the control of chronic infections characterized by renal tissue involvement. The drug also has important applications in controlling venereal diseases. A combination of ciprofloxacin with the cephalosporin antibiotic ceftriaxone is recommended as the treatment of choice for disseminated gonorrhea, while a single-dose treatment with ciprofloxacin plus doxycycline, a tetracycline antibiotic (Chapter 10), can usually eradicate gonococcal urethritis. Ciprofloxacin has also been used for chancroid. The drug has been approved for postexposure treatment of inhalational anthrax.

Injectable forms of ciprofloxacin are incompatible with drug solutions that are alkaline because of the reduced solubility of the drug at pH 7. Thus, intravenous solutions should not be mixed with solutions of ticarcillin sodium, mezlocillin sodium, or aminophylline. Ciprofloxacin may also induce crystalluria under the unusual circumstance that urinary pH rises above 7 (e.g., with the use of systemic alkalinizers or a carbonic anhydrase inhibitor or through the action of urease elaborated by certain species of Gram-negative bacilli).

Ofloxacin, USP. 9-Fluoro-2,3-dihydro-3-methyl-10-(4-methyl-1-piperazin-yl)-7-oxo-7*H*-pyrido[1,2,3-de]-1,4,-benzoxazine-6-carboxylic acid (Floxin, Floxin IV) is a member of the quinolone class of antibacterial drugs wherein the 1 and 8 positions are joined in the form of a 1,4-oxazine ring. The ring system is numbered beginning with the oxazine oxygen atom as shown below.

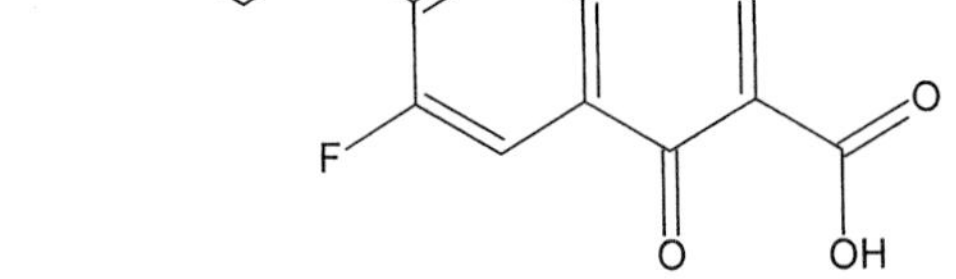

Ofloxacin resembles ciprofloxacin in its antibacterial spectrum and potency. Like ciprofloxacin, this quinolone is

also widely distributed into most body fluids and tissues. In fact, higher concentrations of ofloxacin are achieved in CSF than can be obtained with ciprofloxacin. The oral bioavailability of ofloxacin is superior (95 to 100%) to that of ciprofloxacin, and metabolism is negligible (~3%). The amount of an administered dose of ofloxacin excreted in the urine in a 24- to 48-hour period ranges from 70 to 90%. There is relatively little biliary excretion of this quinolone. Although food can slow the oral absorption of ofloxacin, blood levels following oral or intravenous administration are comparable. The elimination half-life of ofloxacin ranges from 4.5 to 7 hours.

Ofloxacin has been approved for the treatment of infections of the lower respiratory tract, including chronic bronchitis and pneumonia, caused by Gram-negative bacilli. It is also used for the treatment of pelvic inflammatory disease (PID) and is highly active against both gonococci and chlamydia. In common with other fluoroquinolones, ofloxacin is not effective in the treatment of syphilis. A single 400-mg oral dose of ofloxacin in combination with the tetracycline antibiotic doxycycline is recommended by the Centers for Disease Control and Prevention (CDC) for the outpatient treatment of acute gonococcal urethritis. Ofloxacin is also used for the treatment of urinary tract infections caused by Gram-negative bacilli and for prostatitis caused by *E. coli.* Infections of the skin and soft tissues caused by staphylococci, streptococci, and Gram-negative bacilli may also be treated with ofloxacin.

Because ofloxacin has an asymmetric carbon atom in its structure, it is obtained and supplied commercially as a racemate. The racemic mixture has been resolved, and the enantiomers independently synthesized and evaluated for antibacterial activity.[64] The 3*S*(−) isomer is substantially more active (8 to 125 times, depending on the bacterial species) than the 3*R*(+) isomer and has recently been marketed as levofloxacin (Levaquin) for the same indications as the racemate.

Lomefloxacin, USP. 1-Ethyl-6,8-difluoro-1,4-dihydro-7-(3-methyl-1-piperazinyl)-4-oxo-3-quinolinecarboxylic acid (Maxaquin) is a difluorinated quinolone with a longer elimination half-life (7 to 8 hours) than other members of its class. It is the only quinolone for which once-daily oral dosing suffices. The oral bioavailability of lomefloxacin is estimated to be 95 to 98%. Food slows, but does not prevent, its oral absorption. The extent of biotransformation of lomefloxacin is only about 5%, and high concentrations of unchanged drug, ranging from 60 to 80%, are excreted in the urine. The comparatively long half-life of lomefloxacin is apparently due to its excellent tissue distribution and renal reabsorption and not due to plasma protein binding (only ~10%) or enterohepatic recycling (biliary excretion is estimated to be ~10%).

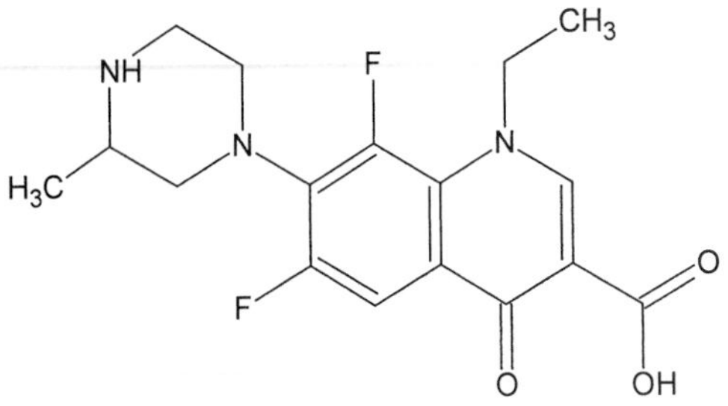

Lomefloxacin has been approved for two primary indications. First, it is indicated for acute bacterial exacerbations of chronic bronchitis caused by *H. influenzae* or *Moraxella (Branhamella) catarrhalis,* but not if *Streptococcus pneumoniae* is the causative organism. Second, it is used for prophylaxis of infection following transurethral surgery. Lomefloxacin also finds application in the treatment of acute cystitis and chronic urinary tract infections caused by Gram-negative bacilli.

Lomefloxacin reportedly causes the highest incidence of phototoxicity (photosensitivity) of the currently available quinolones. The presence of a halogen atom (fluorine, in this case) at the 8 position has been correlated with an increased chance of phototoxicity in the quinolones.[40]

Sparfloxacin. Sparfloxacin, (*cis*)-5-amino-1-cyclopropyl-7-(3,5-dimethyl)-1-piperazinyl)-6,8-difluoro-1,4-dihydro-4-oxo-3-quinolinecarboxylic acid, is a newer fluoroquinolone.

This compound exhibits higher potency against Gram-positive bacteria, especially staphylococci and streptococci, than the fluoroquinolones currently marketed. It is also more active against chlamydia and the anaerobe *Bacteroides fragilis.* The activity of sparfloxacin against Gram-negative bacteria is also very impressive, and it compares favorably with ciprofloxacin and ofloxacin in potency against *Mycoplasma* spp., *Legionella* spp., mycobacteria, and *Listeria monocytogenes.* Sparfloxacin has a long elimination half-life of 18 hours, which permits once-a-day dosing for most indications. The drug is widely distributed into most fluids and tissues. Effective concentrations of sparfloxacin are achieved for the treatment of skin and soft tissue infections, lower respiratory infections (including bronchitis and bacterial pneumonias), and pelvic inflammatory disease caused by gonorrhea and chlamydia. Sparfloxacin has also been recommended for the treatment of bacterial gastroenteritis and cholecystitis. The oral bioavailability of sparfloxacin is claimed to be good, and sufficient unchanged drug is excreted to be effective for the treatment of urinary tract infections. Nearly 20% of an orally administered dose is excreted as an inactive glucuronide.

The incidence of phototoxicity of sparfloxacin is the lowest of the fluoroquinolones, because of the presence of the 5-amino group, which counteracts the effect of the 8-fluorosubstituent.

Nitrofurans

The first nitroheterocyclic compounds to be introduced into chemotherapy were the nitrofurans. Three of these compounds—nitrofurazone, furazolidone, and nitrofurantoin—have been used for the treatment of bacterial infections of various kinds for nearly 50 years. A fourth nitrofuran, nifurtimox, is used as an antiprotozoal agent to treat trypanosomiasis and leishmaniasis. Another nitroheterocyclic of considerable importance is metronidazole, which is an amebicide (a trichomonicide) and is used for the treatment of systemic infections caused by anaerobic bacteria. This important drug is discussed below in this chapter.

The nitrofurans are derivatives of 5-nitro-2-furaldehyde, formed on reaction with the appropriate hydrazine or amine derivative. Antimicrobial activity is present only when the nitro group is in the 5 position.

The mechanism of antimicrobial action of the nitrofurans has been extensively studied, but it still is not fully understood. In addition to their antimicrobial actions, the nitrofurans are known to be mutagenic and carcinogenic under certain conditions. It is thought that DNA damage caused by metabolic reaction products may be involved in these cellular effects.

Nitrofurazone. 5-Nitro-2-furaldehyde semicarbazone (Furacin) occurs as a lemon-yellow crystalline solid that is sparingly soluble in water and practically insoluble in organic solvents. Nitrofurazone is chemically stable, but moderately light sensitive.

It is used topically in the treatment of burns, especially when bacterial resistance to other agents may be a concern. It may also be used to prevent bacterial infection associated with skin grafts. Nitrofurazone has a broad spectrum of activity against Gram-positive and Gram-negative bacteria, but it is not active against fungi. It is bactericidal against most bacteria commonly causing surface infections, including *S. aureus, Streptococcus* spp., *E. coli, Clostridium perfringens, Enterobacter (Aerobacter) aerogenes,* and *Proteus* spp.; however, *P. aeruginosa* strains are resistant.

Nitrofurazone is marketed in solutions, ointments, and suppositories in a usual concentration of 0.2%.

Furazolidone, USP. 3-[(5-Nitrofurylidene)amino]-2-oxazolidinone (Furoxone) occurs as a yellow crystalline powder with a bitter aftertaste. It is insoluble in water or alcohol. Furazolidone has bactericidal activity against a relatively broad range of intestinal pathogens, including *S. aureus*, *E. coli*, *Salmonella*, *Shigella*, *Proteus* spp., *Enterobacter*, and *Vibrio cholerae*. It is also active against the protozoan *Giardia lamblia*. It is recommended for the oral treatment of bacterial or protozoal diarrhea caused by susceptible organisms. The usual adult dosage is 100 mg 4 times daily.

Only a small fraction of an orally administered dose of furazolidone is absorbed. Approximately 5% of the oral dose is detectable in the urine in the form of several metabolites. Some gastrointestinal distress has been reported with its use. Alcohol should be avoided when furazolidone is being used because the drug can inhibit aldehyde dehydrogenase.

Nitrofurantoin, USP. Nitrofurantoin, 1-(5-nitro-2-furfurylidene)-1-aminohydantoin (Furadantin, Macrodantin), is a nitrofuran derivative that is suitable for oral use. It is recommended for the treatment of urinary tract infections caused by susceptible strains of *E. coli*, enterococci, *S. aureus*, and *Klebsiella, Enterobacter,* and *Proteus* spp. The most common side effects are gastrointestinal (anorexia, nausea, and vomiting); however, hypersensitivity reactions (pneumonitis, rashes, hepatitis, and hemolytic anemia) have occasionally been observed. A macrocrystalline form (Macrodantin) is claimed to improve gastrointestinal tolerance without interfering with oral absorption.

Methenamine and Its Salts

Methenamine, USP. The activity of hexamethylenetetramine (Urotropin, Uritone) depends on the liberation of formaldehyde. The compound is prepared by evaporating a solution of formaldehyde and strong ammonia water to dryness.

The free base exists as an odorless white crystalline powder that sublimes at about 260°C. It dissolves in water to form an alkaline solution and liberates formaldehyde when warmed with mineral acids. Methenamine is a weak base with a pK_a of 4.9.

Methenamine is used internally as a urinary antiseptic for the treatment of chronic urinary tract infections. The free base has practically no bacteriostatic power; formaldehyde release at the lower pH of the kidney is required. To optimize the antibacterial effect, an acidifying agent such as sodium biphosphate or ammonium chloride generally accompanies the administration of methenamine.

Certain bacterial strains are resistant to the action of methenamine because they elaborate urease, an enzyme that hydrolyzes urea to form ammonia. The resultant high urinary pH prevents the activation of methenamine, rendering it ineffective. This problem can be overcome by the coadministration of the urease inhibitor acetohydroxamic acid (Lithostat).

Methenamine Mandelate, USP. Hexamethylenetetramine mandelate (Mandelamine) is a white crystalline powder with a sour taste and practically no odor. It is very soluble in water and has the advantage of providing its own acidity, although in its use the custom is to carry out a preliminary acidification of the urine for 24 to 36 hours before administration.

Methenamine Hippurate, USP. Methenamine hippurate (Hiprex) is the hippuric acid salt of methenamine. It is readily absorbed after oral administration and is concentrated in the urinary bladder, where it exerts its antibacterial activity. Its activity is increased in acid urine.

Urinary Analgesics

Pain and discomfort frequently accompany bacterial infections of the urinary tract. For this reason, certain analgesic agents, such as the salicylates or phenazopyridine, which concentrate in the urine because of their solubility properties, are combined with a urinary anti-infective agent.

Phenazopyridine Hydrochloride, USP. Phenazopyridine hydrochloride, 2,6-diamino-3-(phenylazopyridine hydrochloride (Pyridium), is a brick-red fine crystalline powder. It is slightly soluble in alcohol, in chloroform, and in water.

Phenazopyridine Hydrochloride

Phenazopyridine hydrochloride was formerly used as a urinary antiseptic. Although it is active in vitro against staphylococci, streptococci, gonococci, and *E. coli*, it has no useful antibacterial activity in the urine. Thus, its present utility lies in its local analgesic effect on the mucosa of the urinary tract.

Usually, phenazopyridine is given in combination with urinary antiseptics. For example, it is available as Azo-Gantrisin, a fixed-dose combination with the sulfonamide antibacterial sulfisoxazole, and as Urobiotic, a combination with the antibiotic oxytetracycline and the sulfonamide sulfamethizole (Chapter 10). The drug is rapidly excreted in the urine, to which it gives an orange-red color. Stains in fabrics may be removed by soaking in a 0.25% solution of sodium dithionite.

Antitubercular Agents

Ever since Koch identified the tubercle bacillus, *Mycobacterium tuberculosis,* there has been keen interest in the development of antitubercular drugs. The first breakthrough in antitubercular chemotherapy occurred in 1938 with the observation that sulfanilamide had weak bacteriostatic properties. Later, the sulfone derivative dapsone (4,4'-diaminodiphenylsulfone) was investigated clinically. Unfortunately, this drug, which is still considered one of the most effective drugs for the treatment of leprosy and which also has useful antimalarial properties, was considered too toxic because of the high dosages used. The discovery of the antitubercular activity of the aminoglycoside antibiotic streptomycin by Waksman et al. in 1944 ushered in the modern era of tuberculosis treatment. This development was quickly followed by discoveries of the antitubercular properties of *p*-aminosalicylic acid (PAS) first and then, in 1952, of isoniazid. Later, the usefulness of the synthetic drug ethambutol and, eventually, of the semisynthetic antibiotic rifampin was discovered.

Combination therapy, with the use of two or more antitubercular drugs, has been well documented to reduce the emergence of strains of *Mycobacterium tuberculosis* resistant to individual agents and has become standard medical practice. The choice of antitubercular combination depends on a variety of factors, including the location of the disease (pulmonary, urogenital, gastrointestinal, or neural), the results of susceptibility tests and the pattern of resistance in the locality, the physical condition and age of the patient, and the toxicities of the individual agents. For some time, a combination of isoniazid and ethambutol, with or without streptomycin, was the preferred choice of treatment among clinicians in this country. However, the discovery of the tuberculocidal properties of rifampin resulted in its replacement of the more toxic antibiotic streptomycin in most regimens. The synthetic drug pyrazinamide, because of its sterilizing ability, is also considered a first-line agent and is frequently used in place of ethambutol in combination therapy. Second-line agents for tuberculosis include the antibiotics cycloserine, kanamycin, and capreomycin and the synthetic compounds ethionamide and *p*-aminosalicylic acid (PAS).

A major advance in the treatment of tuberculosis was signaled by the introduction of the antibiotic rifampin into therapy. Clinical studies indicated that when rifampin is included in the regimen, particularly in combination with isoniazid and ethambutol (or pyrazinamide), the period required for successful therapy is shortened significantly. Previous treatment schedules without rifampin required maintenance therapy for at least 2 years, whereas those based on the isoniazid–rifampin combination achieved equal or better results in 6 to 9 months.

Once considered to be on the verge of worldwide eradication, as a result of aggressive public health measures and effective chemotherapy, tuberculosis has made a comeback of alarming proportions in recent years.[65] A combination of factors has contributed to the observed increase in tuberculosis cases, including the worldwide AIDS epidemic, the general relaxation of public health policies in many countries, the increased overcrowding and homelessness in major cities, and the increased emergence of multidrug-resistant strains of *M. tuberculosis.*

The development of drugs useful for the treatment of leprosy has long been hampered, in part, by the failure of the causative organism, *Mycobacterium leprae,* to grow in cell culture. However, the recent availability of animal models, such as the infected mouse footpad, now permits in vivo drug evaluations. The increasing emergence of strains of *M. leprae* resistant to dapsone, long considered the mainstay for leprosy treatment, has caused public health officials to advocate combination therapy.

Mycobacteria other than *M. tuberculosis* and *M. leprae,* commonly known as "atypical" mycobacteria, were first established as etiological agents of diseases in the 1950s. Atypical mycobacteria are primarily saprophytic species that are widely distributed in soil and water. Such organisms are not normally considered particularly virulent or infectious. Diseases attributed to atypical mycobacteria are on the increase, however, in large part because of the increased numbers of immunocompromised individuals in the population resulting from the AIDS epidemic and the widespread use of immunosuppressive agents with organ transplantation.

The most common disease-causing species are *Mycobacterium avium* and *Mycobacterium intracellulare,* which have similar geographical distributions, are difficult to distinguish microbiologically and diagnostically, and are thus considered a single complex (MAC). The initial disease attributed to MAC resembles tuberculosis, but skin and musculoskeletal tissues may also become involved. The association of MAC and HIV infection is dramatic. An overwhelming disseminated form of the disease occurs in severely immunocompromised patients, leading to high morbidity and mortality. Another relatively common atypical mycobacterium, *Mycobacterium kansasii,* also causes pulmonary disease and can become disseminated in immunocompromised patients. Patients infected with *M. kansasii* can usually be treated effectively with combinations of antitubercular drugs. MAC infections, in contrast, are resistant to currently available chemotherapeutic agents.

Isoniazid, USP. Isonicotinic acid hydrazide, isonicotinyl hydrazide, or INH (Nydrazid) occurs as a nearly colorless crystalline solid that is very soluble in water. It is prepared by reacting the methyl ester of isonicotinic acid with hydrazine.

Isoniazid

Isoniazid is a remarkably effective agent and continues to be one of the primary drugs (along with rifampin, pyrazinamide, and ethambutol) for the treatment of tuberculosis. It is not, however, uniformly effective against all forms of the disease. The frequent emergence of strains of the tubercle bacillus resistant to isoniazid during therapy was seen as the major shortcoming of the drug. This problem has been largely, but not entirely, overcome with the use of combinations.

The activity of isoniazid is manifested on the growing tubercle bacilli and not on resting forms. Its action, which is considered bactericidal, is to cause the bacilli to lose lipid content by a mechanism that has not been fully elucidated. The most generally accepted theory suggests that the principal effect of isoniazid is to inhibit the synthesis of mycolic acids,[66, 67] high-molecular-weight, branched β-hydroxy fatty acids that constitute important components of the cell walls of mycobacteria.

A mycobacterial catalase–peroxidase enzyme complex is required for the bioactivation of isoniazid.[68] A reactive species, generated through the action of these enzymes on the drug, is believed to attack a critical enzyme required for mycolic acid synthesis in mycobacteria.[69] Resistance to INH, estimated to range from 25 to 50% of clinical isolates of INH-resistant strains, is associated with loss of catalase and peroxidase activities, both of which are encoded by a single gene, *katG*.[70] The target for the action of INH has recently been identified as an enzyme that catalyzes the NADH-specific reduction of 2-*trans*-enoylacyl carrier protein, an essential step in fatty acid elongation.[71] This enzyme is encoded by a specific gene, *inhA*, in *M. tuberculosis*.[72] Approximately 20 to 25% of INH-resistant clinical isolates display mutations in the *inhA* gene, leading to altered proteins with apparently reduced affinity for the active form of the drug. Interestingly, such INH-resistant strains also display resistance to ethionamide, a structurally similar antitubercular drug.[72] On the other hand, mycobacterial strains deficient in catalase/peroxidase activity are frequently susceptible to ethionamide.

Although treatment regimens generally require long-term administration of isoniazid, the incidence of toxic effects is remarkably low. The principal toxic reactions are peripheral neuritis, gastrointestinal disturbances (e.g., constipation, loss of appetite), and hepatotoxicity. Coadministration of pyridoxine is reported to prevent the symptoms of peripheral neuritis, suggesting that this adverse effect may result from antagonism of a coenzyme action of pyridoxal phosphate. Pyridoxine does not appear to interfere with the antitubercular effect of isoniazid. Severe hepatotoxicity rarely occurs with isoniazid alone; the incidence is much higher, however, when it is used in combination with rifampin.

Isoniazid is rapidly and almost completely absorbed following oral administration. It is widely distributed to all tissues and fluids within the body, including the CSF. Ap-

proximately 60% of an oral dose is excreted in the urine within 24 hours in the form of numerous metabolites as well as the unchanged drug. Although the metabolism of isoniazid is very complex, the principal path of inactivation involves acetylation of the primary hydrazine nitrogen. In addition to acetylisoniazid, the isonicotinyl hydrazones of pyruvic and α-ketoglutaric acids, isonicotinic acid, and isonicotinuric acid have been isolated as metabolites in humans.[73] The capacity to inactivate isoniazid by acetylation is an inherited characteristic in humans. Approximately half of persons in the population are fast acetylators (plasma half-life, 45 to 80 minutes), and the remainder slow acetylators (plasma half-life, 140 to 200 minutes).

Ethionamide, USP. 2-Ethylthioisonicotinamide (Trecator SC) occurs as a yellow crystalline material that is sparingly soluble in water. This nicotinamide has weak bacteriostatic activity in vitro but, because of its lipid solubility, is effective in vivo. In contrast to the isoniazid series, 2-substitution enhances activity in the thioisonicotinamide series.

Ethionamide

Ethionamide is rapidly and completely absorbed following oral administration. It is widely distributed throughout the body and extensively metabolized to predominantly inactive forms that are excreted in the urine. Less than 1% of the parent drug appears in the urine.

Ethionamide is considered a secondary drug for the treatment of tuberculosis. It is used in the treatment of isoniazid-resistant tuberculosis or when the patient is intolerant to isoniazid and other drugs. Because of its low potency, the highest tolerated dose of ethionamide is usually recommended. Gastrointestinal intolerance is the most common side effect associated with its use. Visual disturbances and hepatotoxicity have also been reported.

Pyrazinamide, USP. Pyrazinecarboxamide (PZA) occurs as a white crystalline powder that is sparingly soluble in water and slightly soluble in polar organic solvents. Its antitubercular properties were discovered as a result of an investigation of heterocyclic analogues of nicotinic acid, with which it is isosteric. Pyrazinamide has recently been elevated to first-line status in short-term tuberculosis treatment regimens because of its tuberculocidal activity and comparatively low short-term toxicity. Since pyrazinamide is not active against metabolically inactive tubercle bacilli, it is not considered suitable for long-term therapy. Potential hepatotoxicity also obviates long-term use of the drug. Pyrazinamide is maximally effective in the low pH environment that exists in macrophages (monocytes). Evidence suggests bioactivation of pyrazinamide to pyrazinoic acid by an amidase present in mycobacteria.[74]

Pyrazinamide

Because bacterial resistance to pyrazinamide develops rapidly, it should always be used in combination with other drugs. Cross-resistance between pyrazinamide and either isoniazid or ethionamide is relatively rare. The mechanism of action of pyrazinamide is not known. Despite its structural similarities to isoniazid and ethionamide, pyrazinamide apparently does not inhibit mycolic acid biosynthesis in mycobacteria.

Pyrazinamide is well absorbed orally and widely distributed throughout the body. The drug penetrates inflamed meninges and, therefore, is recommended for the treatment of tuberculous meningitis. Unchanged pyrazinamide, the corresponding carboxylic acid (pyrazinoic acid), and the 5-hydroxy metabolite are excreted in the urine. The elimination half-life ranges from 12 to 24 hours, which allows the drug to be administered on either once-daily or even twice-weekly dosing schedules. Pyrazinamide and its metabolites are reported to interfere with uric acid excretion. Therefore, the drug should be used with great caution in patients with hyperuricemia or gout.

Ethambutol, USP.   Ethambutol, (+)-2,2′-(ethylenediimino)-di-1-butanol dihydrochloride, or EMB (Myambutol), is a white crystalline powder freely soluble in water and slightly soluble in alcohol.

Ethambutol Dihydrochloride

Ethambutol is active only against dividing mycobacteria. It has no effect on encapsulated or other nonproliferating forms. The in vitro effect may be bacteriostatic or bactericidal, depending on the conditions. Its selective toxicity toward mycobacteria appears to be related to the inhibition of the incorporation of mycolic acids into the cell walls of these organisms.

This compound is remarkably stereospecific. Tests have shown that, although the toxicities of the *dextro, levo,* and *meso* isomers are about equal, their activities vary considerably. The *dextro* isomer is 16 times as active as the *meso* isomer. In addition, the length of the alkylene chain, the nature of the branching of the alkyl substituents on the nitrogens, and the extent of N-alkylation all have a pronounced effect on the activity.

Ethambutol is rapidly absorbed after oral administration, and peak serum levels occur in about 2 hours. It is rapidly excreted, mainly in the urine. Up to 80% is excreted unchanged, with the balance being metabolized and excreted as 2,2′-(ethylenediimino)dibutyric acid and the corresponding dialdehyde.

Ethambutol is not recommended for use alone, but in combinations with other antitubercular drugs in the chemotherapy of pulmonary tuberculosis.

Aminosalicylic Acid.   4-Aminosalicylic acid (PAS) occurs as a white to yellowish-white crystalline solid that darkens on exposure to light or air. It is slightly soluble in water but more soluble in alcohol. Alkali metal salts and the nitric acid salt are soluble in water, but the salts of hydrochloric acid and sulfuric acid are not. The acid undergoes decarboxylation when heated. An aqueous solution has a pH of ~3.2.

p-Aminosalicylic Acid

PAS is administered orally in the form of the sodium salt, usually in tablet or capsule form. Symptoms of gastrointestinal irritation are common with both the acid and the sodium salt. A variety of enteric-coated dosage forms have been used in an attempt to overcome this disadvantage. Other forms that are claimed to improve gastrointestinal tolerance include the calcium salt, the phenyl ester, and a combination with an anion exchange resin (Rezi-PAS). An antacid such as aluminum hydroxide is frequently prescribed.

The oral absorption of PAS is rapid and nearly complete, and it is widely distributed into most of the body fluids and tissues, with the exception of the CSF, in which levels are significantly lower. It is excreted primarily in the urine as both unchanged drug and metabolites. The *N*-acetyl derivative is the principal metabolite, with significant amounts of the glycine conjugate also being formed. When administered with isoniazid (which also undergoes *N*-acetylation), PAS increases the level of free isoniazid. The biological half-life of PAS is about 2 hours.

The mechanism of antibacterial action of PAS is similar to that of the sulfonamides. Thus, it is believed to prevent the incorporation of *p*-aminobenzoic acid (PABA) into the dihydrofolic acid molecule catalyzed by the enzyme dihydrofolate synthetase. Structure–activity studies have shown that the amino and carboxyl groups must be *para* to each other and free; thus, esters and amides must readily undergo hydrolysis in vivo to be effective. The hydroxyl group may be *ortho* or *meta* to the carboxyl group, but optimal activity is seen in the former.

For many years, PAS was considered a first-line drug for the chemotherapy of tuberculosis and was generally included in combination regimens with isoniazid and streptomycin. However, the introduction of the more effective and generally better tolerated agents, ethambutol and rifampin, has relegated it to alternative drug status.

Aminosalicylate Sodium, USP.   Sodium 4-aminosalicylate (sodium PAS), a salt, occurs in the dihydrate form as a yellow-white powder or crystalline solid. It is very soluble in water in the pH range of 7.0 to 7.5, at which it is the most stable. Aqueous solutions decompose readily and darken. Two pH-dependent types of reactions occur: decarboxylation (more rapid at low pH) and oxidation (more rapid at high pH). Therefore, solutions should be prepared within 24 hours of administration.

Clofazimine. Clofazimine (Lamprene) is a basic red dye that exerts a slow bactericidal effect on *M. leprae*, the bacterium that causes leprosy. It occurs as a dark red crystalline solid that is insoluble in water.

Clofazimine

Clofazimine is used in the treatment of lepromatous leprosy, including dapsone-resistant forms of the disease. In addition to its antibacterial action, the drug appears to possess anti-inflammatory and immune-modulating effects that are of value in controlling neuritic complications and in suppressing erythema nodosum leprosum reactions associated with lepromatous leprosy. It is frequently used in combination with other drugs, such as dapsone or rifampin.

The mechanisms of antibacterial and anti-inflammatory actions of clofazimine are not known. The drug is known to bind to nucleic acids and concentrate in reticuloendothelial tissue. It can also act as an electron acceptor and may interfere with electron transport processes.

The oral absorption of clofazimine is estimated to be about 50%. It is a highly lipid-soluble drug that is distributed into lipoidal tissue and the reticuloendothelial system. Urinary excretion of unchanged drug and metabolites is negligible. Its half-life after repeated dosage is estimated to be about 70 days. Severe gastrointestinal intolerance to clofazimine is relatively common. Skin pigmentation, ichthyosis and dryness, rash, and pruritus also occur frequently.

Clofazimine has also been used to treat skin lesions caused by *M. ulcerans*.

Antitubercular Antibiotics

RIFAMYCINS

The rifamycins are a group of chemically related antibiotics obtained by fermentation from cultures of *Streptomyces mediterranei*. They belong to a class of antibiotics called the *ansamycins* that contain a macrocyclic ring bridged across two nonadjacent positions of an aromatic nucleus. The term *ansa* means "handle," describing well the topography of the structure. The rifamycins and many of their semisynthetic derivatives have a broad spectrum of antimicrobial activity. They are most notably active against Gram-positive bacteria and *M. tuberculosis*. However, they are also active against some Gram-negative bacteria and many viruses. Rifampin, a semisynthetic derivative of rifamycin B, was released as an antitubercular agent in the United States in 1971. A second semisynthetic derivative, rifabutin, was approved in 1992 for the treatment of atypical mycobacterial infections.

The chemistry of rifamycins and other ansamycins has been reviewed.[75] All of the rifamycins (A, B, C, D, and E) are biologically active. Some of the semisynthetic derivatives of rifamycin B are the most potent known inhibitors of DNA-directed RNA polymerase in bacteria,[76] and their action is bactericidal. They have no activity against the mammalian enzyme. The mechanism of action of rifamycins as inhibitors of viral replication appears to differ from that for their bactericidal action. Their net effect is to inhibit the formation of the virus particle, apparently by preventing a specific polypeptide conversion.[77] Rifamycins bind to the β subunit of bacterial DNA-dependent RNA polymerases to prevent chain initiation.[78] Bacterial resistance to rifampin has been associated with mutations leading to amino acid substitution in the β subunit.[78] A high level of cross-resistance between various rifamycins has been observed.

Rifampin, USP. Rifampin (Rifadin, Rimactane, Rifampicin) is the most active agent in clinical use for the treatment of tuberculosis. A dosage of as little as 5 μg/mL is effective against sensitive strains of *M. tuberculosis*. Rifampin is also highly active against staphylococci and *Neisseria, Haemophilus, Legionella,* and *Chlamydia* spp. Gram-negative bacilli are much less sensitive to rifampin. However, resistance to rifampin develops rapidly in most species of bacteria, including the tubercle bacillus. Consequently, rifampin is used only in combination with other antitubercular drugs, and it is ordinarily not recommended for the treatment of other bacterial infections when alternative antibacterial agents are available.

Rifampin

Toxic effects associated with rifampin are relatively infrequent. It may, however, interfere with liver function in some patients and should neither be combined with other potentially hepatotoxic drugs nor used in patients with impaired hepatic function (e.g., chronic alcoholics). The incidence of hepatotoxicity was significantly higher when rifampin was combined with isoniazid than when either agent was combined with ethambutol. Allergic and sensitivity reactions to rifampin have been reported, but they are infrequent and usually not serious. Rifampin is a powerful inducer of hepatic cytochrome P-450 oxygenases. It can markedly potentiate the actions of drugs that are inactivated by these enzymes. Examples include oral anticoagulants, barbiturates, benzodiazepines, oral hypoglycemic agents, phenytoin, and theophylline.

Rifampin is also used to eradicate the carrier state in asymptomatic carriers of *Neisseria meningitidis* to prevent outbreaks of meningitis in high-risk areas such as military facilities. Serotyping and sensitivity tests should be performed before its use because resistance develops rapidly. However, a daily dose of 600 mg of rifampin for 4 days suffices to eradicate sensitive strains of *N. meningitidis*. Rifampin has also been very effective against *M. leprae* in experimental animals and in humans. When it is used in the treatment of leprosy, rifampin should be combined with dapsone or some other leprostatic agent to minimize the emergence of resistant strains of *M. leprae*.

Other, nonlabeled uses of rifampin include the treatment of serious infections such as endocarditis and osteomyelitis caused by methicillin-resistant *S. aureus* or *S. epidermidis*, Legionnaires' disease when resistant to erythromycin, and prophylaxis of *H. influenzae*-induced meningitis.

Rifampin occurs as an orange to reddish brown crystalline powder that is soluble in alcohol but only sparingly soluble in water. It is unstable to moisture, and a desiccant (silica gel) should be included with rifampin capsule containers. The expiration date for capsules stored in this way is 2 years. Rifampin is well absorbed after oral administration to provide effective blood levels for about 8 hours. Food, however, markedly reduces its oral absorption, and rifampin should be administered on an empty stomach. The drug is distributed in effective concentrations to all body fluids and tissues except the brain, despite the fact that it is 70 to 80% protein bound in the plasma. The principal excretory route is through the bile and feces, and high concentrations of rifampin and its primary metabolite, deacetylrifampin, are found in the liver and biliary system. Deacetylrifampin is also biologically active. Equally high concentrations of rifampin are found in the kidneys, and although substantial amounts of the drug are passively reabsorbed in the renal tubules, its urinary excretion is significant. Patients should be made aware that rifampin causes a reddish orange discoloration of the urine, stool, saliva, tears, and skin. It can also permanently discolor soft contact lenses.

Rifampin is also available in a parenteral dosage form consisting of a lyophilized sterile powder that, when reconstituted in 5% dextrose or normal saline, provides 600 mg of active drug in 10 mL for slow intravenous infusion. The parenteral form may be used for initial treatment of serious cases and for retreatment of patients who cannot take the drug by the oral route. Parenteral solutions of rifampin are stable for 24 hours at room temperature. Although rifampin is stable in the solid state, in solution it undergoes a variety of chemical changes whose rates and nature are pH and temperature dependent.[79] At alkaline pH, it oxidizes to a quinone in the presence of oxygen; in acidic solutions, it hydrolyzes to 3-formyl rifamycin SV. Slow hydrolysis of the ester functions also occurs, even at neutral pH.

Rifabutin, USP.

Rifabutin, the spiroimidazopiperidyl derivative of rifamycin B was approved in the United States for the prophylaxis of disseminated MAC in AIDS patients on the strength of clinical trials establishing its effectiveness. The activity of rifabutin against MAC organisms greatly ex-

Rifamycin

ceeds that of rifamycin. This rifamycin derivative is not effective, however, as monotherapy for existing disseminated MAC disease.

Rifabutin is a very lipophilic compound with a high affinity for tissues. Its elimination is distribution limited, with a half-life averaging 45 hours (range, 16 to 69 hours). Approximately 50% of an orally administered dose of rifabutin is absorbed, but the absolute oral bioavailability is only about 20%. Extensive first-pass metabolism and significant biliary excretion of the drug occur, with about 30 and 53% of the orally administered dose excreted, largely as metabolites, in the feces and urine, respectively. The 25-*O*-desacetyl and 31-hydroxy metabolites of rifabutin have been identified. The parent drug is 85% bound to plasma proteins in a concentration-independent manner. Despite its greater potency against *M. tuberculosis* in vitro, rifabutin is considered inferior to rifampin for the short-term therapy of tuberculosis because of its significantly lower plasma concentrations.

Although rifabutin is believed to cause less hepatotoxicity and induction of cytochrome P-450 enzymes than rifampin, these properties should be borne in mind when the drug is used prophylactically. Rifabutin and its metabolites are highly colored compounds that can discolor skin, urine, tears, feces, etc.

Rifabutin

Cycloserine, USP. D-(+)-4-Amino-3-isoxazolidinone (Seromycin) is an antibiotic that has been isolated from the fermentation beer of three different *Streptomyces* species: *S. orchidaceus, S. garyphalus,* and *S. lavendulus.* It occurs as a white to pale yellow crystalline material that is very soluble in water. It is stable in alkaline, but unstable in acidic, solutions. The compound slowly dimerizes to 2,5-bis(aminoxymethyl)-3,6-diketopiperazine in solution or standing.

The structure of cycloserine was reported simultaneously by Kuehl et al.[80] and Hidy et al.[81] to be D-(+)-4-amino-3-isoxazolidinone. It has been synthesized by Stammer et al.[82] and by Smart et al.[83] Cycloserine is stereochemically related to D-serine. However, the L-form has similar antibiotic activity.

Cycloserine is presumed to exert its antibacterial action by preventing the synthesis of cross-linking peptide in the formation of bacterial cell walls.[84] Rando[85] has recently suggested that it is an antimetabolite for alanine, which acts as a suicide substrate for the pyridoxal phosphate–requiring enzyme alanine racemase. Irreversible inactivation of the enzyme thereby deprives the cell of the D-alanine required for the synthesis of the cross-linking peptide.

Although cycloserine exhibits antibiotic activity in vitro against a wide spectrum of both Gram-negative and Gram-positive organisms, its relatively weak potency and frequent toxic reactions limit its use to the treatment of tuberculosis. It is recommended for patients who fail to respond to other tuberculostatic drugs or who are known to be infected with organisms resistant to other agents. It is usually administered orally in combination with other drugs, commonly isoniazid.

Sterile Capreomycin Sulfate, USP. Capastat sulfate, or capreomycin, is a strongly basic cyclic peptide isolated from *S. capreolus* in 1960 by Herr et al.[86] It was released in the United States in 1971 exclusively as a tuberculostatic drug. Capreomycin, which resembles viomycin (no longer marketed in the United States) chemically and pharmacologically, is a second-line agent used in combination with other antitubercular drugs. In particular, it may be used in place of streptomycin when either the patient is sensitive to, or the strain of *M. tuberculosis* is resistant to, streptomycin. Similar to viomycin, capreomycin is a potentially toxic drug. Damage to the eighth cranial nerve and renal damage, as with viomycin, are the more serious toxic effects associated with capreomycin therapy. There are, as yet, insufficient clinical data for a reliable comparison of the relative toxic potentials of capreomycin and streptomycin. Cross-resistance among strains of tubercle bacilli is rare between capreomycin and streptomycin.

Four capreomycins, designated IA, IB, IIA, and IIB, have been isolated from cultures of *S. capreolus.* The clinical agent contains primarily IA and IB. The close chemical relationship between capreomycins IA and IB and viomycin was established,[87] and the total synthesis and proof of structure of the capreomycins were later accomplished.[88] The structures of capreomycins IIA and IIB correspond to those of IA and IB but lack the β-lysyl residue. The sulfate salts are freely soluble in water.

ANTIPROTOZOAL AGENTS

In the United States and other countries of the temperate zone, protozoal diseases are of minor importance, whereas bacterial and viral diseases are widespread and are the cause of considerable concern. On the other hand, protozoal diseases are highly prevalent in tropical Third World countries, where they infect both human and animal populations, causing suffering, death, and enormous economic hardship. Protozoal diseases that are found in the United States are malaria, amebiasis, giardiasis, trichomoniasis, toxoplasmosis, and, as a direct consequence of the AIDS epidemic, *Pneumocystis carinii* pneumonia (PCP).

Although amebiasis is generally thought of as a tropical disease, it actually has a worldwide distribution. In some areas with temperate climates in which sanitation is poor, the prevalence of amebiasis has been estimated to be as high as 20% of the population. The causative organism, *Enta-*

moeba histolytica, can invade the wall of the colon or other parts of the body (e.g., liver, lungs, or skin). An ideal chemotherapeutic agent would be effective against both the intestinal and extraintestinal forms of the parasite.

Amebicides that are effective against both intestinal and extraintestinal forms of the disease are limited to the somewhat toxic alkaloids emetine and dehydroemetine, the nitroimidazole derivative metronidazole, and the antimalarial agent chloroquine (Chapter 9). A second group of amebicides that are effective only against intestinal forms of the disease includes the aminoglycoside antibiotic paromomycin, the 8-hydroxyquinoline derivative iodoquinol, the arsenical compound carbarsone, and diloxanide.

Other protozoal species that colonize the intestinal tract and cause enteritis and diarrhea are *Balantidium coli* and the flagellates *Giardia lamblia* and *Cryptosporidium* spp. Balantidiasis responds best to tetracycline. Metronidazole and iodoquinol may also be effective. Giardiasis may be treated effectively with furazolidone, metronidazole, or the antimalarial drug quinacrine (Chapter 9). Cryptosporidiosis is normally self-limiting in immunocompetent patients and is not normally treated. The illness can be a serious problem in AIDS patients because no effective therapy is currently available.

Trichomoniasis, a venereal disease caused by the flagellated protozoan *Trichomonas vaginalis*, is common in the United States and throughout the world. Although it is not generally considered serious, this affliction can cause serious physical discomfort. Oral metronidazole provides effective treatment against all forms of the disease. It is also used to eradicate the organism from asymptomatic male carriers.

Pneumocystis carinii is an opportunistic pathogen that may colonize the lungs of humans and other animals and, under the right conditions, can cause pneumonia. The organism has long been classified as a protozoan, but recent RNA evidence suggests that it may be more closely related to fungi. At one time, occasional cases of *P. carinii* pneumonia (PCP) were known to occur in premature, undernourished infants and in patients receiving immunosuppressant therapy. The situation changed with the onset of the AIDS epidemic. It is estimated that at least 60% and possibly as high as 85% of patients infected with HIV develop PCP during their lifetimes.

The combination of the antifolate trimethoprim and the sulfonamide sulfamethoxazole constitutes the treatment of choice for PCP. Other effective drugs include pentamidine, atovaquone, and a new antifolate, trimetrexate.

Toxoplasma gondii is an obligate intracellular protozoan that is best known for causing blindness in neonates. Toxoplasmosis, the disseminated form of the disease in which the lymphatic system, skeletal muscles, heart, brain, eye, and placenta may be affected, has become increasingly prevalent in association with HIV infection. A combination of the antifolate pyrimethamine (Chapter 9) and the sulfa drug sulfadiazine constitutes the most effective therapy for toxoplasmosis.

Various forms of trypanosomiasis, chronic tropical diseases caused by pathogenic members of the family Trypanosomidae, occur both in humans and in livestock. The principal disease in humans, sleeping sickness, can be broadly classified into two main geographic and etiological groups: African sleeping sickness caused by *Trypanosoma gam-*

biense (West African), *T. rhodesiense* (East African), or *T. congolense*; and South American sleeping sickness (Chagas' disease) caused by *T. cruzi*. Of the various forms of trypanosomiasis, Chagas' disease is the most serious and generally the most resistant to chemotherapy. Leishmaniasis is a chronic tropical disease caused by various flagellate protozoa of the genus *Leishmania*. The more common visceral form caused by *L. donovani*, called kala-azar, is similar to Chagas' disease. Although these diseases are widespread in tropical areas of Africa and South and Central America, they are of minor importance in the United States, Europe, and Asia.

Chemotherapy of trypanosomiasis and leishmaniasis remains somewhat primitive and is often less than effective. In fact, it is doubtful that these diseases can be controlled by chemotherapeutic measures alone, without successful control of the intermediate hosts and vectors that transmit them. Heavy metal compounds, such as the arsenicals and antimonials, are sometimes effective but frequently toxic. The old standby suramin appears to be of some value in long- and short-term prophylaxis. The nitrofuran derivative nifurtimox may be a major asset in the control of these diseases, but its potential toxicity remains to be fully determined.

Metronidazole, USP. 2-Methyl-5-nitroimidazole-1-ethanol (Flagyl, Protostat, Metro IV) is the most useful of a group of antiprotozoal nitroimidazole derivatives that have been synthesized in various laboratories throughout the world. Metronidazole was first marketed for the topical treatment of *Trichomonas vaginalis* vaginitis. It has since been shown to be effective orally against both the acute and carrier states of the disease. The drug also possesses useful amebicidal activity and is, in fact, effective against both intestinal and hepatic amebiasis. It has also been found of use in the treatment of such other protozoal diseases as giardiasis and balantidiasis.

More recently, metronidazole has been found to possess efficacy against obligate anaerobic bacteria, but it is ineffective against facultative anaerobes or obligate aerobes. It is particularly active against Gram-negative anaerobes, such as *Bacteroides* and *Fusobacterium* spp. It is also effective against Gram-positive anaerobic bacilli (e.g., *Clostridium* spp.) and cocci (e.g., *Peptococcus* and *Peptidostreptococcus* spp.). Because of its bactericidal action, metronidazole has become an important agent for the treatment of serious infections (e.g., septicemia, pneumonia, peritonitis, pelvic infections, abscesses, meningitis) caused by anaerobic bacteria.

The common characteristic of microorganisms (bacteria and protozoa) sensitive to metronidazole is that they are anaerobic. It has been speculated that a reactive intermediate formed in the microbial reduction of the 5-nitro group of metronidazole covalently binds to the DNA of the microorganism, triggering the lethal effect.[89] Potential reactive intermediates include the nitroxide, nitroso, hydroxylamine, and amine. The ability of metronidazole to act as a radiosensitizing agent is also related to its reduction potential.

Metronidazole is a pale yellow crystalline substance that is sparingly soluble in water. It is stable in air but is light sensitive. Despite its low water solubility, metronidazole is well absorbed following oral administration. It has a large apparent volume of distribution and achieves effective concentrations in all body fluids and tissues. Approximately 20% of an oral dose is metabolized to oxidized or conjugated forms. The 2-hydroxy metabolite is active; other metabolites are inactive.

Metronidazole is a weak base that possesses a pK_a of 2.5. Although it is administered parenterally only as the free base by slow intravenous infusion, metronidazole for injection is supplied in two forms: a ready-to-inject 100-mL solution containing 5 mg of base per mL; and a hydrochloride salt as 500 mg of a sterile lyophilized powder. Metronidazole hydrochloride for injection must first be reconstituted with sterile water to yield 5 mL of a solution having a concentration of 100 mg/mL and a pH ranging from 0.5 to 2.0. The resulting solution must then be diluted with either 100 mL of normal saline or 5% dextrose and neutralized with 5 mEq of sodium bicarbonate to provide a final solution of metronidazole base with an approximate concentration of 5 mg/mL and a pH of 6 to 7. Solutions of metronidazole hydrochloride are unsuitable for intravenous administration because of their extreme acidity. Reconstituted metronidazole hydrochloride solutions are stable for 96 hours at 30°C, while ready-to-use solutions of metronidazole base are stable for 24 hours at 30°C. Both solutions should be protected from light.

Diloxanide, USP. Furamide, or eutamide, is the 2-furoate ester of 2,2-dichloro-4′-hydroxy-*N*-methylacetanilide. It was developed as a result of the discovery that various α,α-dichloroacetamides possessed amebicidal activity in vitro. Diloxanide itself and many of its esters are also active, and drug metabolism studies indicate that hydrolysis of the amide is required for the amebicidal effect. Nonpolar esters of diloxanide are more potent than polar ones. Diloxanide furoate has been used in the treatment of asymptomatic carriers of *E. histolytica*. Its effectiveness against acute intestinal amebiasis or hepatic abscesses, however, has not been established. Diloxanide furoate is a white crystalline powder. It is administered orally only as 500-mg tablets and may be obtained in the United States from the CDC in Atlanta, Georgia.

8-Hydroxyquinoline. Oxine, quinophenol, or oxyquinoline is the parent compound from which the antiprotozoal oxyquinolines have been derived. The antibacterial and antifungal properties of oxine and its derivatives, which are believed to result from the ability to chelate metal ions, are well known. Aqueous solutions of acid salts of oxine, particularly the sulfate (Chinosol, Quinosol), in concentrations of 1:3,000 to 1:1,000, have been used as topical antiseptics. The substitution of an iodine atom at the 7 position of 8-hydroxyquinolines yields compounds with broad-spectrum amebicidal properties.

Iodoquinol, USP. 5,7-Diiodo-8-quinolinol, 5,7-diiodo-8-hydroxyquinoline, or diiodohydroxyquin (Yodoxin, Diodoquin, Diquinol) is a yellowish to tan microcrystalline, light-sensitive substance that is insoluble in water. It is recommended for acute and chronic intestinal amebiasis but is not effective in extraintestinal disease. Because a relatively high incidence of topic neuropathy has occurred with its use, iodoquinol should not be used routinely for traveler's diarrhea.

Emetine and Dehydroemetine. The alkaloids emetine and dehydroemetine are obtained by separation from extracts of ipecac. They occur as levorotatory, light-sensitive white powders that are insoluble in water. The alkaloids readily form water-soluble salts. Solutions of the hydrochloride salts intended for intramuscular injection should be adjusted to pH 3.5 and stored in light-resistant containers.

Emetine

Emetine and dehydroemetine exert a direct amebicidal action on various forms of *E. histolytica*. They are protoplasmic poisons that inhibit protein synthesis in protozoal and mammalian cells by preventing protein elongation. Because their effect in intestinal amebiasis is solely symptomatic and the cure rate is only 10 to 15%, they should be used only in combination with other agents. The high concentrations of the alkaloids achieved in the liver and other tissues after intramuscular injection provide the basis for their high effectiveness against hepatic abscesses and other extraintestinal forms of the disease. Toxic effects limit the usefulness of emetine. It causes a high frequency of gastrointestinal distress (especially nausea and diarrhea), cardiovascular effects (hypotension and arrhythmias), and neuromuscular effects (pain and weakness). A lower incidence of cardiotoxicity has been associated with the use of dehydroemetine (Mebadin), which is available from the CDC and is also amebicidal.

Emetine and dehydroemetine have also been used to treat balantidial dysentery and fluke infestations, such as fascioliasis and paragonimiasis.

Pentamidine Isethionate, USP.

4,4'-(Pentamethylenedioxy)dibenzamidine diisethionate (NebuPent, Pentam 300) is a water-soluble crystalline salt that is stable to light and air. The principal use of pentamidine is for the treatment of pneumonia caused by the opportunistic pathogenic protozoan *P. carinii*, a frequent secondary invader associated with AIDS. The drug may be administered by slow intravenous infusion or by deep intramuscular injection for PCP. An aerosol form of pentamidine is used by inhalation for the prevention of PCP in high-risk patients infected with HIV who have a previous history of PCP infection or a low peripheral CD4$^+$ lymphocyte count.

Both the inhalant (aerosol) and parenteral dosage forms of pentamidine isethionate are sterile lyophilized powders that must be made up as sterile aqueous solutions prior to use. Sterile water for injection must be used to reconstitute the aerosol, to avoid precipitation of the pentamidine salt. Adverse reactions to the drug are common. These include cough and bronchospasm (inhalation) and hypertension and hypoglycemia (injection).

Pentamidine has been used for the prophylaxis and treatment of African trypanosomiasis. It also has some value for treating visceral leishmaniasis. Pentamidine rapidly disappears from the plasma after intravenous injection and is distributed to the tissues, where it is stored for a long period. This property probably contributes to the usefulness of the drug as a prophylactic agent.

Atovaquone, USP.

3-[4-(4-Chlorophenyl)-cyclohexyl]-2-hydroxy-1,4-naphthoquinone (Mepron) is a highly lipophilic, water-insoluble analogue of ubiquinone 6, an essential component of the mitochondrial electron transport chain in microorganisms. The structural similarity between atovaquone and ubiquinone suggests that the former may act as an antimetabolite for the latter and thereby interfere with the function of electron transport enzymes.

Atovaquone was originally developed as an antimalarial drug, but *Plasmodium falciparum* was found to develop a rapid tolerance to its action. More recently, the effectiveness of atovaquone against *P. carinii* was discovered. It is a currently recommended alternative to trimethoprim-sulfamethoxazole (TMP-SMX) for the treatment and prophylaxis of PCP in patients intolerant to this combination. Atovaquone was also shown to be effective in eradicating *Toxoplasma gondii* in preclinical animal studies.

The oral absorption of atovaquone is slow and incomplete, in part because of the low water solubility of the drug. Aqueous suspensions provide significantly better absorption than do tablets. Food, especially if it has a high fat content, increases atovaquone absorption. Significant enterohepatic recycling of atovaquone occurs, and most (nearly 95%) of the drug is excreted unchanged in the feces. In vivo, atovaquone is largely confined to the plasma, where it is extensively protein bound (>99.9%). The half-life of the drug ranges from 62 to 80 hours. The primary side effect is gastrointestinal intolerance.

Eflornithine, USP.

DL-2'-Difluoromethylornithine, or DFMO (Ornidyl), an amino acid derivative, is an enzyme-activated inhibitor of ornithine decarboxylase, a pyridoxal phosphate–dependent enzyme responsible for catalyzing the rate-limiting step in the biosynthesis of the diamine putrescine and the polyamines spermine and spermidine. Polyamines are essential for the regulation of DNA synthesis and cell proliferation in animal tissues and microorganisms.

Eflornithine is used for the treatment of West African sleeping sickness, caused by *Trypanosoma brucei gambiense*. It is specifically indicated for the meningoencephalitic stage of the disease. Eflornithine is a myelosuppressive drug that causes high incidences of anemia, leukopenia, and thrombocytopenia. Complete blood cell counts must be monitored during the course of therapy.

The irreversible inactivation of ornithine decarboxylase by eflornithine is accompanied by decarboxylation and release of fluoride ion from the inhibitor,[90] suggesting enzyme-catalyzed activation of the inhibitor. Only the (−) isomer, stereochemically related to L-ornithine, is active.

Eflornithine is supplied as the hydrochloride salt. It may be administered either intravenously or orally. Approximately 80% of the unchanged drug is excreted in the urine. Penetration of eflornithine into the CSF is facilitated by inflammation of the meninges.

Nifurtimox, USP.

Nifurtimox is 4-[(5-nitrofurfurylidene) amino]-3-methylthiomorpholine-1,1-dioxide, or Bayer 2502 (Lampit). The observation that various derivatives of 5-nitrofuraldehyde possessed, in addition to their antibacterial and antifungal properties, significant and potentially useful antiprotozoal activity eventually led to discovery of particular nitrofurans with antitrypanosomal activity.

The most important of such compounds is nifurtimox because of its demonstrated effectiveness against *T. cruzi,* the parasite responsible for South American trypanosomiasis. In fact, use of this drug represents the only clinically proven treatment for both acute and chronic forms of the disease. Nifurtimox is available in the United States from the CDC.

Nifurtimox is administered orally. Oral bioavailability is high, but considerable first-pass metabolism occurs. The half-life of nifurtimox is 2 to 4 hours. The drug is poorly tolerated, with a high incidence of nausea, vomiting, abdominal pain, and anorexia reported. Symptoms of central and peripheral nervous system toxicity also frequently occur with nifurtimox.

Benznidazole, USP.

N-Benzyl-2-nitroimidazole-1-acetamide (Radanil, Rochagan) is a nitroimidazole derivative that is used for the treatment of Chagas' disease. It is not available in the United States but is used extensively in South America. The effectiveness of benznidazole is similar to that of nifurtimox. Therapy for American trypanosomiasis with oral benznidazole requires several weeks and is frequently accompanied by adverse effects such as peripheral neuropathy, bone marrow depression, and allergic-type reactions.

Melarsoprol.

2-*p*-(4,6-Diamino-*s*-triazin-2-yl-amino) phenyl-4-hydroxymethyl-1,3,2-dithiarsoline (Mel B, Arsobal) is prepared by reduction of a corresponding pentavalent arsanilate to the trivalent arsenoxide followed by reaction of the latter with 2,3-dimercapto-1-propanol (British anti-Lewisite, BAL). It has become the drug of choice for the treatment of the later stages of both forms of African trypanosomiasis. Melarsoprol has the advantage of excellent penetration into the CNS and, therefore, is effective against meningoencephalitic forms of *T. gambiense* and *T. rhodesiense*. Trivalent arsenicals tend to be more toxic to the host (as well as the parasites) than the corresponding pentavalent compounds. The bonding of arsenic with sulfur atoms tends to reduce host toxicity, increase chemical stability (to oxidation), and improve distribution of the compound to the arsenoxide. Melarsoprol shares the toxic properties of other arsenicals, however, so its use must be monitored for signs of arsenic toxicity.

Sodium Stibogluconate.

Sodium antimony gluconate (Pentostam) is a pentavalent antimonial compound intended primarily for the treatment of various forms of leishmaniasis. It is available from the CDC as the disodium salt, which is chemically stable and freely soluble in water. The 10% aqueous solution used for either intramuscular or intravenous injection has a pH of ~5.5. Like all antimonial drugs, this drug has a low therapeutic index, and patients undergoing therapy with it should be monitored carefully for signs of heavy metal poisoning. Other organic antimonial compounds are used primarily for the treatment of schistosomiasis and other flukes.

The antileishmanial action of sodium stibogluconate requires its reduction to the trivalent form, which is believed to inhibit phosphofructokinase in the parasite.

Dimercaprol, USP. 2,3-Dimercapto-1-propanol, BAL, or dithioglycerol is a foul-smelling, colorless liquid. It is soluble in water (1:20) and alcohol. It was developed by the British during World War II as an antidote for "Lewisite," hence the name British anti-Lewisite, or BAL. Dimercaprol is effective topically and systematically as an antidote for poisoning caused by arsenic, antimony, mercury, gold, and lead. It can, therefore, also be used to treat arsenic and antimony toxicity associated with overdose or accidental ingestion of organoarsenicals or organoantimonials.

The antidotal properties of BAL are associated with the property of heavy metals to react with sulfhydryl (SH) groups in proteins (e.g., the enzyme pyruvate oxidase) and interfere with their normal function. 1,2-Dithiol compounds such as BAL compete effectively with such proteins for the metal by reversibly forming metal ring compounds of the following type:

These are relatively nontoxic, metabolically conjugated (as glucuronides), and rapidly excreted.

BAL may be applied topically as an ointment or injected intramuscularly as a 5 or 10% solution in peanut oil.

Suramin Sodium. Suramin sodium is a high-molecular-weight bisurea derivative containing six sulfonic acid groups as their sodium salts. It was developed in Germany shortly after World War I as a by-product of research efforts directed toward the development of potential antiparasitic agents from dyestuffs.

The drug has been used for more than half a century for the treatment of early cases of trypanosomiasis. Not until several decades later, however, was suramin discovered to be a long-term prophylactic agent whose effectiveness after a single intravenous injection is maintained for up to 3 months. The drug is tightly bound to plasma proteins, causing its excretion in the urine to be almost negligible.

Tissue penetration of the drug does not occur, apparently because of its high molecular weight and highly ionic character. Thus, an injected dose remains in the plasma for a very long period. Newer, more effective drugs are now available for short-term treatment and prophylaxis of African sleeping sickness. Suramin is also used for prophylaxis of onchocerciasis. It is available from the CDC.

ANTHELMINTICS

Anthelmintics are drugs that have the capability of ridding the body of parasitic worms or helminths. The prevalence of human helminthic infestations is widespread throughout the globe and represents a major world health problem, particularly in Third World countries. Helminths parasitic to humans and other animals are derived from two phyla, Platyhelminthes and Nemathelminthes. Cestodes (tapeworms) and trematodes (flukes) belong to the former, and nematodes or true roundworms belong to the latter. The helminth infestations of major concern on the North American continent are caused by roundworms (i.e., hookworm, pinworm, and *Ascaris* spp.). Human tapeworm and fluke infestations are rarely seen in the United States.

Several classes of chemicals are used as anthelmintics and include phenols and derivatives, piperazine and related compounds, antimalarial compounds (Chapter 9), various heterocyclic compounds, and natural products.

Piperazine, USP. Hexahydropyrazine or diethylenediamine (Arthriticine, Dispermin) occurs as colorless, volatile crystals of the hexahydrate that are freely soluble in water. After the discovery of the anthelmintic properties of a derivative diethylcarbamazine, the activity of piperazine itself was established. Piperazine is still used as an anthelmintic for the treatment of pinworm *(Enterobius [Oxyuris] vermicularis)* and roundworm *(Ascaris lumbricoides)* infestations. It is available in a variety of salt forms, including the citrate (official in the USP) in syrup and tablet forms.

Piperazine blocks the response of the ascaris muscle to acetylcholine, causing flaccid paralysis in the worm, which is dislodged from the intestinal wall and expelled in the feces.

Diethylcarbamazepine Citrate, USP. *N,N*-Diethyl-4-methyl-1-piperazinecarboxamide citrate or 1-diethylcarbamyl-4-methylpiperazine dihydrogen citrate (Hetrazan) is a highly water-soluble crystalline compound that has selective anthelmintic activity. It is effective against various forms of filariasis, including Bancroft's, onchocerciasis, and laviasis. It is also active against ascariasis. Relatively few adverse reactions have been associated with diethylcarbamazine.

Pyrantel Pamoate, USP. *trans*-1,4,5,6,-Tetrahydro-1-methyl-2-[2-(2′-thienyl)ethenyl]pyrimidine pamoate (Antiminth) is a depolarizing neuromuscular blocking agent that causes spastic paralysis in susceptible helminths. It is used in the treatment of infestations caused by pinworms and roundworms (ascariasis). Because its action opposes that of

piperazine, the two anthelmintics should not be used together. Over half of the oral dose is excreted in the feces unchanged. Adverse effects associated with its use are primarily gastrointestinal.

Thiabendazole, USP. 2-(4-Thiazolyl)benzimidazole (Mintezol) occurs as a white crystalline substance that is only slightly soluble in water but is soluble in strong mineral acids. Thiabendazole is a basic compound with a pK_a of 4.7 that forms complexes with metal ions.

Thiabendazole inhibits the helminth-specific enzyme fumarate reductase.[91] It is not known whether metal ions are involved or if the inhibition of the enzyme is related to thiabendazole's anthelmintic effect. Benzimidazole anthelmintic drugs such as thiabendazole and mebendazole also arrest nematode cell division in metaphase by interfering with microtubule assembly.[92] They exhibit a high affinity for tubulin, the precursor protein for microtubule synthesis.

Thiabendazole has broad-spectrum anthelmintic activity. It is used to treat enterobiasis, strongyloidiasis (threadworm infection), ascariasis, uncinariasis (hookworm infection), and trichuriasis (whipworm infection). It has also been used to relieve symptoms associated with cutaneous larva migrans (creeping eruption) and the invasive phase of trichinosis. In addition to its use in human medicine, thiabendazole is widely used in veterinary practice to control intestinal helminths in livestock.

Mebendazole, USP. Methyl 5-benzoyl-2-benzimidazolecarbamate (Vermox) is a broad-spectrum anthelmintic that is effective against a variety of nematode infestations, including whipworm, pinworm, roundworm, and hookworm. Mebendazole irreversibly blocks glucose uptake in susceptible helminths, thereby depleting glycogen stored in the parasite. It apparently does not affect glucose metabolism in the host. It also inhibits cell division in nematodes.[71]

Mebendazole is poorly absorbed by the oral route. Adverse reactions are uncommon and usually consist of abdominal discomfort. It is teratogenic in laboratory animals and, therefore, should not be given during pregnancy.

Albendazole, USP.

Methyl 5-(propylthio)-2-benzimidazolecarbamate (Eskazole, Zentel) is a broad-spectrum anthelmintic that is not currently marketed in North America. It is available from the manufacturer on a compassionate use basis. Albendazole is widely used throughout the world for the treatment of intestinal nematode infection. It is effective as a single-dose treatment for ascariasis, New and Old World hookworm infections, and trichuriasis. Multiple-dose therapy with albendazole can eradicate pinworm, threadworm, capillariasis, clonorchiasis, and hydatid disease. The effectiveness of albendazole against tapeworms (cestodes) is generally more variable and less impressive.

Albendazole occurs as a white crystalline powder that is virtually insoluble in water. The oral absorption of albendazole is enhanced by a fatty meal. The drug undergoes rapid and extensive first-pass metabolism to the sulfoxide, which is the active form in plasma. The elimination half-life of the sulfoxide ranges from 10 to 15 hours. Considerable biliary excretion and enterohepatic recycling of albendazole sulfoxide occurs. Albendazole is generally well tolerated in single-dose therapy for intestinal nematodes. The high-dose, prolonged therapy required for clonorchiasis or echinococcal disease therapy can result in adverse effects such as bone marrow depression, elevation of hepatic enzymes, and alopecia.

Niclosamide, USP.

5-Chloro-N-(2-chloro-4-nitrophenyl)-2-hydroxybenzamide or 2,5′-dichloro-4′-nitrosalicylanilide (Cestocide, Mansonil, Yomesan) occurs as a yellowish white, water-insoluble powder. It is a potent taeniacide that causes rapid disintegration of worm segments and the scolex. Penetration of the drug into various cestodes appears to be facilitated by the digestive juices of the host, in that very little of the drug is absorbed by the worms in vitro. Niclosamide is well tolerated following oral administration, and little or no systemic absorption of it occurs. A saline purge 1 to 2 hours after ingestion of the taeniacide is recommended to remove the damaged scolex and worm segments. This procedure is mandatory in the treatment of pork tapeworm infestation to prevent possible cysticercosis resulting

from release of live ova from worm segments damaged by the drug.

Bithionol.

2,2′-Thiobis(4,6-dichlorophenol), or bis(2-hydroxy-3,5-dichlorophenyl)sulfide (Lorothidol, Bithin), a chlorinated bisphenol, was formerly used in soaps and cosmetics for its antimicrobial properties but was removed from the market for topical use because of reports of contact photodermatitis. Bithionol has useful anthelmintic properties and has been used as a fasciolicide and taeniacide. It is still considered the agent of choice for the treatment of infestations caused by the liver fluke *Fasciola hepatica* and the lung fluke *Paragonimus westermani*. Niclosamide is believed to be superior to it for the treatment of tapeworm infestations.

Oxamniquine, USP.

1,2,3,4-Tetrahydro-2-[(isopropylamino)methyl]-7-nitro-6-quinolinemethanol (Vansil) is an antischistosomal agent that is indicated for the treatment of *S. mansoni* (intestinal schistosomiasis) infection. It has been shown to inhibit DNA, RNA, and protein synthesis in schistosomes.[93] The 6-hydroxymethyl group is critical for activity; metabolic activation of precursor 6-methyl derivatives is critical. The oral bioavailability of oxamniquine is good; effective plasma levels are achieved in 1 to 1.5 hours. The plasma half-life is 1 to 2.5 hours. The drug is extensively metabolized to inactive metabolites, of which the principal one is the 6-carboxy derivative.

The free base occurs as a yellow crystalline solid that is slightly soluble in water but soluble in dilute aqueous mineral acids and soluble in most organic solvents. It is available in capsules containing 250 mg of the drug. Oxamniquine is generally well tolerated. Dizziness and drowsiness are common, but transitory, side effects. Serious reactions, such as epileptiform convulsions, are rare.

Praziquantel, USP. 2-(Cyclohexylcarbonyl)-1,2,3,6,7,11b-hexahydro-4*H*-pyrazino[2,1-*a*]isoquinolin-4-one (Biltricide) is a broad-spectrum agent that is effective against a variety of trematodes (flukes). It has become the agent of choice for the treatment of infections caused by schistosomes (blood flukes). The drug also provides effective treatment for fasciolopsiasis (intestinal fluke), clonorchiasis (Chinese liver fluke), fascioliasis (sheep liver fluke), opisthorchosis (liver fluke), and paragonimiasis (lung fluke). Praziquantel increases cell membrane permeability of susceptible worms, resulting in the loss of extracellular calcium. Massive contractions and ultimate paralysis of the fluke musculature occurs, followed by phagocytosis of the parasite.

Following oral administration, about 80% of the dose is absorbed. Maximal plasma concentrations are achieved in 1 to 3 hours. The drug is rapidly metabolized in the liver in the first pass. It is likely that some of the metabolites are also active. Praziquantel occurs as a white crystalline solid that is insoluble in water. It is available as 600-mg film-coated tablets. The drug is generally well tolerated.

Ivermectin, USP. Ivermectin (Cardomec, Eqvalan, Ivomec) is a mixture of 22,23-dihydro derivatives of avermectins B_{1a} and B_{1b} prepared by catalytic hydrogenation. Avermectins are members of a family of structurally complex antibiotics produced by fermentation with a strain of *Streptomyces avermitilis*. Their discovery resulted from an intensive screening of cultures for anthelmintic agents from natural sources.[94] Ivermectin is active in low dosage against a wide variety of nematodes and arthropods that parasitize animals.[95]

The structures of the avermectins were established by a combination of spectroscopic[96] and x-ray crystallographic[97] techniques to contain pentacyclic 16-membered-ring aglycones glycosidically linked at the 3 position to a disaccharide that comprises two oleandrose sugar residues. The side chain at the 25 position of the aglycone is *sec*-butyl in avermectin B_{1a}, whereas in avermectin B_{1b}, it is isopropyl. Ivermectin contains at least 80% of 22,23-dihydroavermectin B_{1a} and no more than 20% 22,23-dihydroavermectin B_{1b}.

Ivermectin has achieved widespread use in veterinary practice in the United States and many countries throughout the world for the control of endoparasites and ectoparasites in domestic animals.[95] It has been found effective for the treatment of onchocerciasis ("river blindness") in humans,[98] an important disease caused by the roundworm *Oncocerca volvulus*, prevalent in West and Central Africa, the Middle East, and South and Central America. Ivermectin destroys the microfilariae, immature forms of the nematode, which create the skin and tissue nodules that are characteristic of the infestation and can lead to blindness. It also inhibits the release of microfilariae by the adult worms living in the host. Studies on the mechanism of action of ivermectin indicate that it blocks interneuron–motor neuron transmission in nematodes by stimulating the release of the inhibitory neurotransmitter GABA.[95] The drug has been made available by the manufacturer on a humanitarian basis to qualified treatment programs through the World Health Organization.

ANTISCABIOUS AND ANTIPEDICULAR AGENTS

Scabicides (antiscabious agents) are compounds used to control the mite *Sarcoptes scabiei,* an organism that thrives under conditions of poor personal hygiene. The incidence of scabies is believed to be increasing in the United States and worldwide and has, in fact, reached pandemic proportions.[99] Pediculicides (antipedicular agents) are used to eliminate head, body, and crab lice. Ideal scabicides and pediculicides must kill the adult parasites and destroy their eggs.

Benzyl Benzoate, USP. Benzyl benzoate is a naturally occurring ester obtained from Peru balsam and other resins. It is also prepared synthetically from benzyl alcohol and benzoyl chloride. The ester is a clear colorless liquid with a faint aromatic odor. It is insoluble in water but soluble in organic solvents.

Benzyl benzoate is an effective scabicide when applied topically. Immediate relief from itching probably results from a local anesthetic effect; however, a complete cure is frequently achieved with a single application of a 25% emulsion of benzyl benzoate in oleic acid, stabilized with triethanolamine. This preparation has the additional advantage of being essentially odorless, nonstaining, and nonirritating to the skin. It is applied topically as a lotion over the entire dampened body, except the face.

Lindane, USP. Lindane is 1,2,3,4,5,6-hexachlorocyclohexane, γ-benzene hexachloride, or benzene hexachloride (Kwell, Scabene, Kwildane, G-Well). This halogenated hydrocarbon is prepared by the chlorination of benzene. A mixture of isomers is obtained in this process, five of which have been isolated: α, β, γ, δ, and ε. The γ isomer, present to 10 to 13% in the mixture, is responsible for the insecticidal activity. The γ isomer may be separated by a variety of extraction and chromatographic techniques.

Lindane occurs as a light buff to tan powder with a persistent musty odor, and it is bitter. It is insoluble in water but soluble in most organic solvents. It is stable under acidic or neutral conditions but undergoes elimination reactions under alkaline conditions.

The action of lindane against insects is threefold: it is a direct contact poison, it has a fumigant effect, and it acts as a stomach poison. The effect of lindane on insects is similar to that of DDT. Its toxicity in humans is somewhat lower than that of DDT. Because of its lipid solubility properties, however, lindane when ingested tends to accumulate in the body.

Lindane is used locally as a cream, lotion, or shampoo for the treatment of scabies and pediculosis.

Crotamiton, USP. *N*-Ethyl-*N*-(2-methylphenyl)-2-butenamide, or *N*-ethyl-*o*-crotonotoluidide (Eurax), is a colorless, odorless oily liquid. It is virtually insoluble in water but soluble in most organic solvents.

Crotamiton is available in 10% concentration in a lotion and a cream intended for the topical treatment of scabies. Its antipruritic effect is probably due to a local anesthetic action.

Permethrin, USP. Permethrin is 3-(2,2-Dichloroethenyl)-2,2-dimethylcyclopropanecarboxylic acid (3-phenoxyphenyl)methyl ester or 3-(phenoxyphenyl)methyl (±)-*cis, trans*-3-(2,2-dichloroethenyl)-2,2-dimethylcyclopropanecarboxylate (Nix). This synthetic pyrethrinoid compound is more stable chemically than most natural pyrethrins and is at least as active as an insecticide. Of the four isomers present, the *1(R),trans* and *1(R),cis* isomers are primarily responsible for the insecticidal activity. The commercial product is a mixture consisting of 60% *trans* and 40% *cis* racemic isomers. It occurs as colorless to pale yellow lowmelting crystals or as a pale yellow liquid and is insoluble in water but soluble in most organic solvents.

Permethrin exerts a lethal action against lice, ticks, mites, and fleas. It acts on the nerve cell membranes of the parasites to disrupt sodium channel conductance. It is used as a pediculicide for the treatment of head lice. A single application of a 1% solution effects cures in more than 99% of cases. The most frequent side effect is pruritus, which occurred in about 6% of the patients tested.

ANTIBACTERIAL SULFONAMIDES

The sulfonamide antimicrobial drugs were the first effective chemotherapeutic agents that could be used systemically for the cure of bacterial infections in humans. Their introduction led to a sharp decline in the morbidity and mortality of infectious diseases. The rapid development of widespread resistance to the sulfonamides soon after their introduction and the increasing use of the broader-spectrum penicillins in the treatment of infectious disease diminished the usefulness of sulfonamides. Today, they occupy a rather small place in the list of therapeutic agents that can be used for infectious disease. They are not completely outmoded, however. In the mid-1970s, the development of a combination of trimethoprim and sulfamethoxazole and the demonstration of its usefulness in the treatment and prophylaxis of certain opportunistic microbial infections led to resurgence in the use of some sulfonamides.

Fritz Mietzsch and Joseph Klarer of the I. G. Farbenindustrie laboratories systematically synthesized a series of azo dyes, each containing the sulfonamide functional group, as potential antimicrobial agents. Sulfonamide azo dyes were included in the test series because they were readily synthesized and possessed superior staining properties. The Bayer pathologist–bacteriologist who evaluated the new Mietzsch-Klarer dyes was a physician named Gerhard Domagk.[100–102] In 1932, Domagk began to study a brilliant red dye, later named Prontosil. Prontosil was found to protect against, and cure, streptococcal infections in mice.[100] Interestingly, Prontosil was inactive on bacterial cultures. Domagk and others continued to study Prontosil, and in 1933, the first of many cures of severe bacterial infections in humans was reported by Foerster,[103] who treated a 10-month-old infant suffering from staphylococcal septicemia and obtained a dramatic cure. The credit for most of the discoveries relating to Prontosil belongs to Domagk, and for his pioneering work in chemotherapy he was awarded the Nobel Prize in medicine and physiology in 1938. The Gestapo prevented him from actually accepting the award, but after the war, he received it in Stockholm in 1947.

Prontosil is totally inactive in vitro but possesses excellent activity in vivo. This property of the drug attracted much attention and stimulated a large body of research activity into the sulfonamides. In 1935, Trefouel and coinvestigators[104] performed a structure–activity study on the sulfonamide azo dyes and concluded that the azo linkage was reductively cleaved to release the active antibacterial product, sulfanilamide. This finding was confirmed in 1937 when Fuller[105] isolated free sulfanilamide from the blood and urine of patients being treated with Prontosil. Favorable clinical results were reported with Prontosil and the active metabolite itself, sulfanilamide, in puerperal sepsis and meningococcal infections. All of these findings ushered in the modern era of chemotherapy and the concept of the *prodrug*.

Following the dramatic success of Prontosil, a host of sulfanilamide derivatives was synthesized and tested. By 1948, more than 4,500 compounds[106] had been evaluated. Of these, only about two dozen have been used in clinical practice. In the late 1940s, broader experience with sulfonamides had begun to demonstrate toxicity in some patients, and resistance problems brought about by indiscriminate use of sulfonamides limited their use throughout the world. The penicillins were excellent alternatives to the sulfonamides, and they largely replaced the latter in antimicrobial chemotherapy.

Today, there are a few sulfonamides (Table 8-7) and especially sulfonamide-trimethoprim combinations that are used extensively for opportunistic infections in patients with AIDS.[107] A primary infection that is treated with the combination is PCP. The sulfonamide-trimethoprim combination can be used for treatment and prophylaxis. Additionally, cerebral toxoplasmosis can be treated in active infection or prophylactically. Urinary tract infections and burn therapy[107–111] round out the list of therapeutic applications. The sulfonamides are drugs of choice for a few other types of infections, but their use is quite limited in modern antimicrobial chemotherapy.[107–111]

The sulfonamides can be grouped into three classes on the basis of their use: oral absorbable agents, designed to give systemic distribution; *oral nonabsorbable agents* such as sulfasalazine; and topical agents such as sodium sulfacetamide ophthalmic drops.

Nomenclature of Sulfonamides

Sulfonamide is a generic term that denotes three different cases:

1. Antibacterials that are *aniline-substituted sulfonamides* (the "sulfanilamides")

2. *Prodrugs* that react to generate active sulfanilamides (i.e., sulfasalazine)

3. *Nonaniline* sulfonamides (i.e., mafenide acetate)

There are also other commonly used drugs that are sulfonamides or sulfanilamides. Among these are the oral hypoglycemic drug tolbutamide, the diuretic furosemide, and the diuretic chlorthalidone.

In pharmaceutical chemistry, pK_b values are not used to compare compounds that are Lewis bases. Instead, if a pK_a of an amine is given, it refers to its salt acting as the conjugate acid. For example, aniline with a pK_a of 4.6 refers to

TABLE 8–7 Therapy With Sulfonamide Antibacterials

Disease/Infection	Sulfonamides Commonly Used
Relatively Common Use	
Treatment and prophylaxis of *Pneumocystis carinii* pneumonia	Trimethoprim-sulfamethoxazole
Treatment and prophylaxis of cerebral toxoplasmosis	Pyrimethamine-sulfadiazine
First attack of urinary tract infection	Trimethoprim-sulfamethoxazole
Burn therapy: prevention and treatment of bacterial infection	Silver sulfadiazine and mafenide
Conjunctivitis and related superficial ocular infections	Sodium sulfacetamide
Chloroquine-resistant malaria (Chapter 9)	Combinations with quinine, others
	Sulfadoxine
	Sulfalene
Less Common Infections/Diseases	*Drugs of Choice or Alternates*
Nocardiosis	Trimethoprim-sulfamethoxazole
Severe traveler's diarrhea	Trimethoprim-sulfamethoxasole
Meningococcal infections	Sulfonamides, only if proved to be sulfonamide sensitive; otherwise, penicillin G, ampicillin, or (for penicillin-allergic patients) chloramphenicol should be used
Generally Not Useful	
Streptococcal infections	Most are resistant to sulfonamides
Prophylaxis of recurrent rheumatic fever	Most are resistant to sulfonamides
Other bacterial infections	The low cost of penicillin and the widespread resistance to sulfonamides limit their use; sulfonamides are still used in a few countries
Vaginal infections	The FDA and USP-DI find no evidence of efficacy
Reduction of bowel flora	Effectiveness not established
Ulcerative colitis	Corticosteroid therapy often preferred
	Relapses common with sulfonamides
	Salicylazosulfapyridine
	Side effects of the sulfanilamides sometimes mimic ulcerative colitis

It does not refer to

A negative charge on a nitrogen atom is typically not stable unless it can be delocalized by resonance. This is what happens with the sulfanilamides. Therefore, the single pK_a usually given for sulfanilamides refers to the loss of an amide proton (Fig. 8-8).

Mechanism of Action of the Sulfonamides

Folinic acid (N^5-formyltetrahydrofolic acid), N^5,N^{10}-methylenetetrahydrofolic acid, and N^{10}-formyltetrahydrofolic acid are intermediates of several biosynthetic pathways that compose the one-carbon pool in animals, bacteria, and plants. A key reaction involving folate coenzymes is catalyzed by the enzyme thymidylate synthase, which transfers a methyl group from N^5,N^{10}-tetrahydrofolic acid to deoxyuridine monophosphate to form deoxythymidine monophosphate, an important precursor to DNA (Fig. 8-9).

Another key reaction is the generation of formyl groups for the biosynthesis of formylmethionyl tRNA units, the primary building blocks in protein synthesis. The sulfonamides are structural analogues of PABA that competitively inhibit the action of dihydropteroate synthase, preventing the addition of PABA to pteridine diphosphate and blocking the net biosynthesis of folate coenzymes. This action arrests bacterial growth and cell division. The competitive nature of the sulfonamides' action means that the drugs do no permanent damage to a microorganism; hence, they are bacteriostatic. The sulfonamides must be maintained at a minimum effective concentration to arrest the growth of bacteria long enough for the host's immune system to eradicate them.

Folate coenzymes are biosynthesized from dietary folic acid in humans and other animals. Bacteria and protozoa must biosynthesize them from PABA and pteridine diphos-

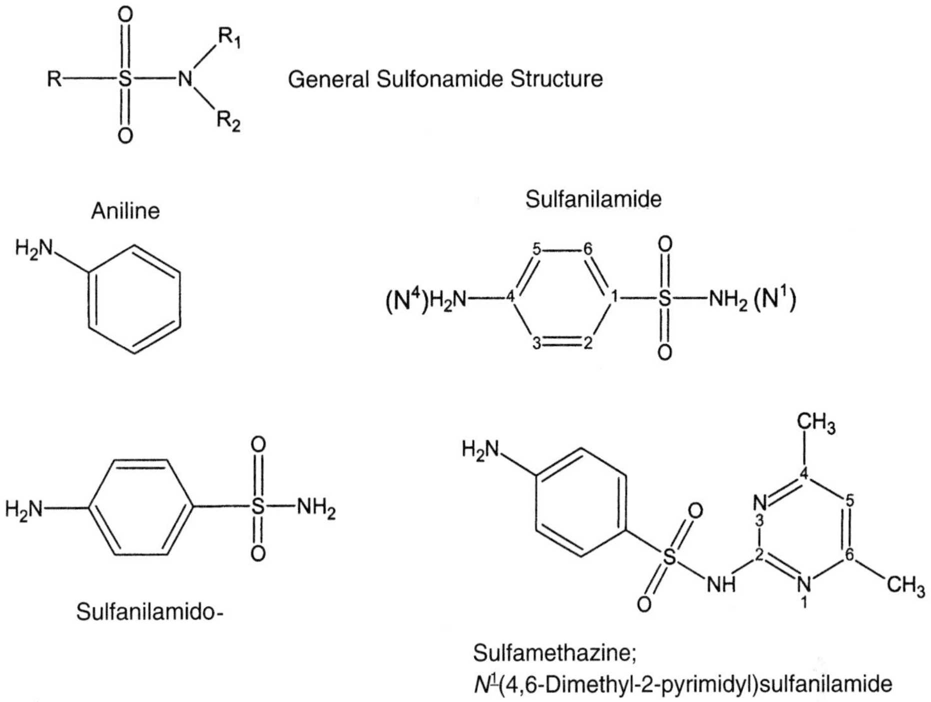

General Sulfonamide Structure

Aniline

Sulfanilamide

Sulfanilamido-

Sulfamethazine;
N^1(4,6-Dimethyl-2-pyrimidyl)sulfanilamide

Figure 8–8 ■ General nomenclature of the sulfonamides.

phate. Microbes cannot assimilate folic acid from the growth medium or from the host. The reasons for this are poorly understood,[102] but one possibility is that bacterial cell walls may be impermeable to folic acid.

Trimethoprim is an inhibitor of dihydrofolate reductase, which is necessary to convert dihydrofolic acid (FAH_2) into tetrahydrofolic acid (FAH_4) in bacteria (Fig. 8-10). Anand has reviewed this biochemistry.[102] Trimethoprim does not have a high affinity for the malaria protozoan's folate reductase, but it does have a high affinity for bacterial folate reductase.

The reverse situation exists for the antimalarial drug pyrimethamine.[112] Trimethoprim does have some affinity for human folate reductase, and this is the cause of some of the toxic effects of the drug.

Spectrum of Action of the Sulfonamides

Sulfonamides inhibit Gram-positive and Gram-negative bacteria, nocardia, *Chlamydia trachomatis*, and some protozoa. Some enteric bacteria, such as *E. coli* and *Klebsiella, Salmonella, Shigella,* and *Enterobacter* spp. are inhibited. Sulfon-

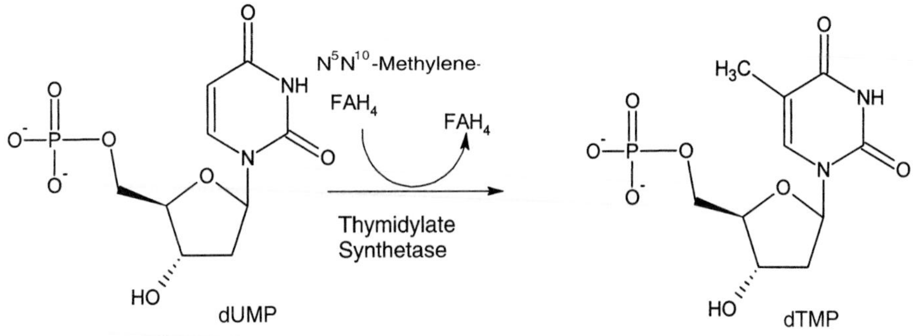

dUMP

N^5N^{10}-Methylene-
FAH_4

FAH_4

Thymidylate
Synthetase

dTMP

Other examples of folate-requiring one-carbon pool reactions:

Coenzyme	Reaction	
N^{10}-Formyl-FAH_4	Met-tRNA	⟶ Formyl-Met-tRNA
N^5N^{10}-Methylene-FAH_4	Glycine	⟶ Serine
N^5-Formyl-FAH_2	Homocysteine	⟶ Methionine

Figure 8–9 ■ The thymidylate synthetase reaction and other reactions representing the one-carbon pool.

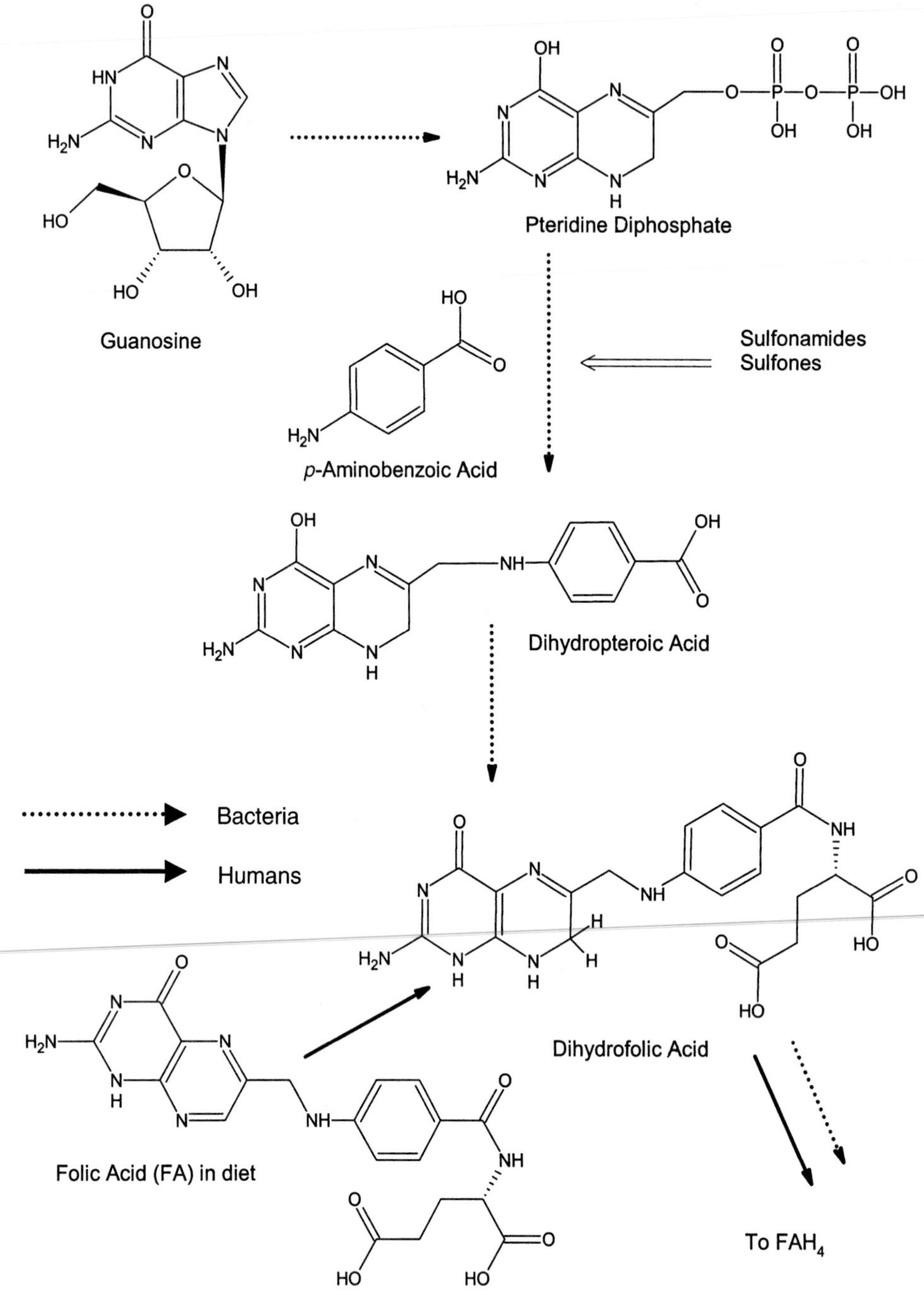

Figure 8–10 ■ Folate pathways in humans and bacteria and the sites of inhibition by sulfonamides and trimethoprim.

amides are infrequently used as single agents. Once drugs of choice for infections such as PCP, toxoplasmosis, nocardiosis, and other bacterial infections, they have been largely replaced by the fixed drug combination TMP-SMX and many other antimicrobials. Many strains of once-susceptible species including meningococci, pneumococci, streptococci, staphylococci, and gonococci are now resistant. Sulfon-

amides are, however, useful in some urinary tract infections because of their high excretion fraction through the kidneys.

Ionization of Sulfonamides

The sulfonamide group, SO_2NH_2, tends to gain stability if it loses a proton, because the resulting negative charge is resonance stabilized.

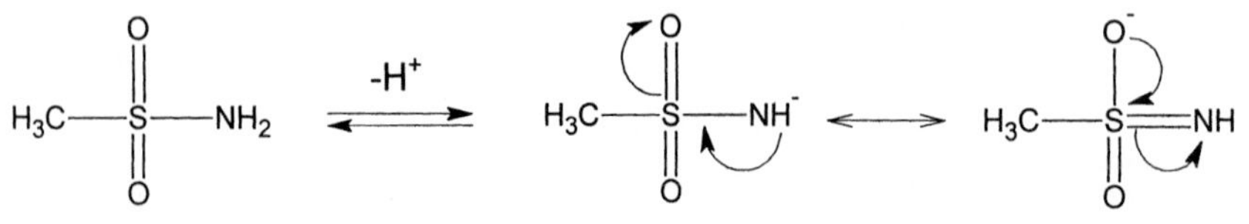

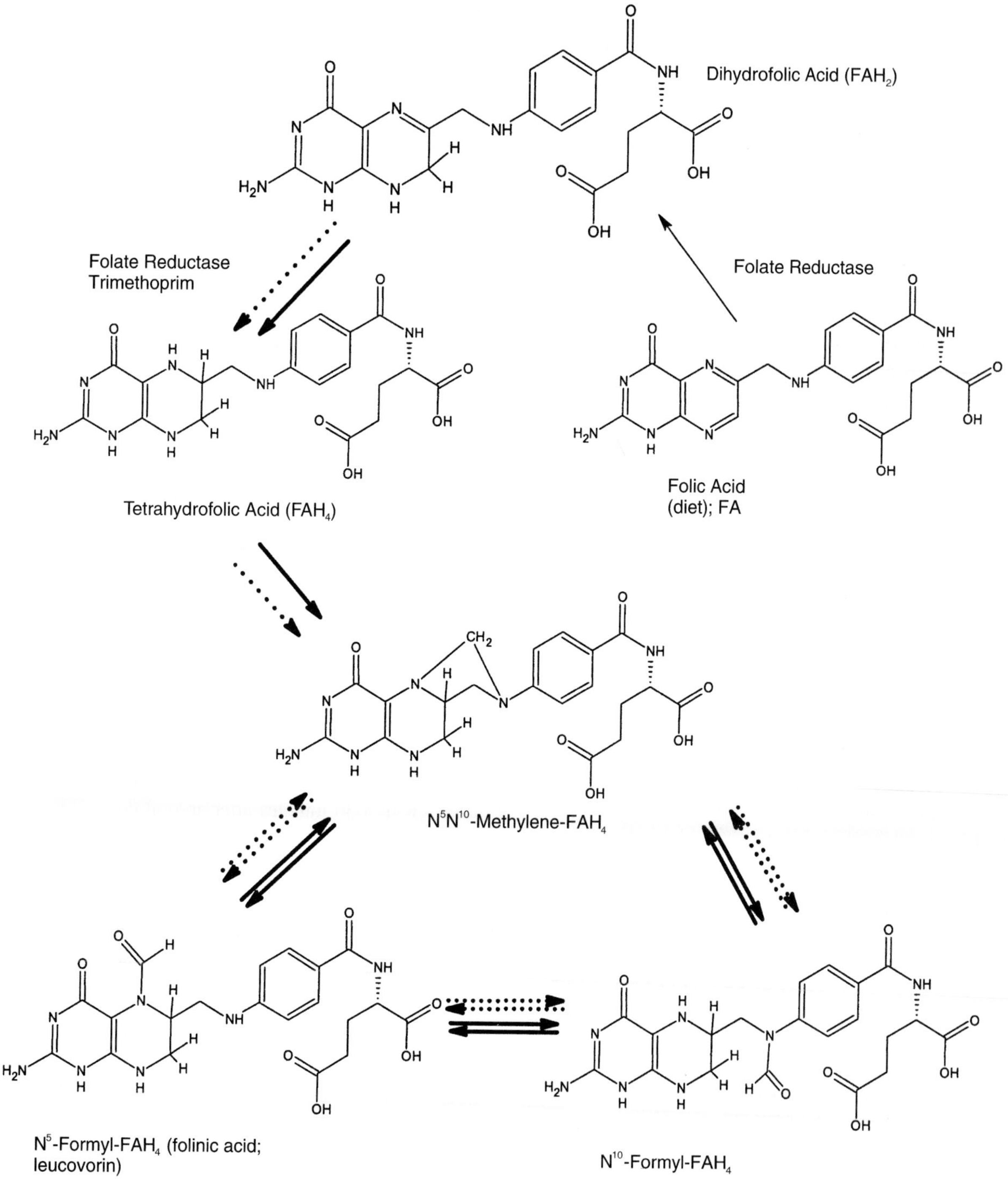

Figure 8–10 ■ *Continued.*

Since the proton-donating form of the functional group is not charged, we can characterize it as an HA acid, along with carboxyl groups, phenols, and thiols. The loss of a proton can be associated with a pK_a for all of the compounds in the series. For example, the pK_a of sulfisoxazole (pK_a 5.0) indicates that the sulfonamide is a slightly weaker acid than acetic acid (pK_a 4.8).

Crystalluria and the pKₐ

Despite the tremendous ability of sulfanilamide to effect cures of pathogenic bacteria, its benefits were often offset by the propensity of the drug to cause severe renal damage by crystallizing in the kidneys. Sulfanilamides and their metabolites (usually acetylated at N^4) are excreted almost entirely in the urine. The pK_a of the sulfonamido group of sulfanilamide is 10.4, so the pH at which the drug is 50% ionized is 10.4. Obviously, unless the pH is above the pK_a, little of the water-soluble salt is present. Because the urine is usually about pH 6 (and potentially lower during bacterial infections), essentially all of the sulfanilamide is in the relatively insoluble, nonionized form in the kidneys. The sulfanilamide coming out of solution in the urine and kidneys causes crystalluria.

Early approaches to adjusting the solubility of sulfanilamide in the urine were

1. Greatly increasing the urine flow. During the early years of sulfonamide use, patients taking the drugs were cautioned to "force fluids." The idea was that if the glomerular filtration rate could be increased, there would be less opportunity for seed crystals to form in the renal tubules.
2. Increasing the pH of the urine. The closer the pH of the urine is to 10.4 (for sulfanilamide itself), the more of the highly water-soluble salt form will be present. Oral sodium bicarbonate sometimes was, and occasionally still is, given to raise urine pH. The bicarbonate was administered before the initial dose of sulfanilamide and then prior to each successive dose.
3. Preparing derivatives of sulfanilamide that have lower pK_a values, closer to the pH of the urine. This approach has been taken with virtually all sulfonamides in clinical use today. Examples of the pK_a values of some ionizable sulfonamides are shown in Table 8-8.
4. Mixing different sulfonamides to achieve an appropriate total dose. The solubilities of the sulfonamides are independent of each other, and more of a mixture of sulfanilamides can stay in water solution at a given pH than can a single sulfonamide. Hence, trisulfapyrimidines, USP (triple sulfa), contain a mixture of sulfadiazine, sulfamerazine, and sulfamethazine. Such mix-

TABLE 8–8 pKₐ Values for Clinically Useful Sulfonamides

Sulfonamide	pKₐ
Sulfadiazine	6.5
Sulfamerazine	7.1
Sulfamethazine	7.4
Sulfisoxazole	5.0
Sulfamethoxazole	6.1

tures are seldom used today, however, because the individual agents have sufficiently low pK_a values to be partially ionized and adequately soluble in the urine, *providing that at least the normal urine flow is maintained*. Patients must be cautioned to maintain a normal fluid intake; forcing fluids, however, is no longer necessary.

The newer, semisynthetic sulfonamides possess lower pK_a values because electron-withdrawing, heterocyclic rings are attached to N^1, providing additional stability for the salt form. Hence, the drugs donate a proton more easily, and the pK_a values are lowered. Simpler electron withdrawing groups were extensively investigated but were found to be too toxic, poorly active, or both.

Metabolism, Protein Binding, and Distribution

Except for the poorly absorbed sulfonamides used for ulcerative colitis and reduction of bowel flora and the topical burn preparations (e.g., mafenide), sulfonamides and trimethoprim tend to be absorbed quickly and distributed well. As Mandell and Petri noted, sulfonamides can be found in the urine "within 30 minutes after an oral dose."[108]

The sulfonamides vary widely in plasma protein binding; for example, sulfisoxazole, 76%; sulfamethoxazole, 60%; sulfamethoxypyridazine, 77%; and sulfadiazine, 38%. (Anand[102] has published an excellent table comparing the percentage of protein binding, lipid solubility, plasma half-life, and N^4 metabolites.) The fraction that is protein bound is not active as an antibacterial, but because the binding is reversible, free, and therefore active, sulfonamide eventually becomes available. Generally, the more lipid soluble a sulfonamide is, at physiological pH, the more of it will be protein bound. Fujita and Hansch[113] have found that among sulfonamides with similar pK_a values, the lipophilicity of the N^1 group has the largest effect on protein binding. N^4-Acetate metabolites of the sulfonamides are more lipid soluble and, therefore, more protein bound than the starting drugs themselves (which have a free 4-amino group that decreases lipid solubility). Surprisingly, the N^4-acetylated metabolites, although more strongly protein bound, are excreted more rapidly than the parent compounds.

Currently, the relationship between plasma protein binding and biological half-life is unclear. Many competing factors are involved, as reflected in sulfadiazine, with a serum half-life of 17 hours, which is much less protein bound than sulfamethoxazole, with a serum half-life of 11 hours.[102]

Sulfonamides are excreted primarily as mixtures of the

parent drug, N^4-acetates, and glucuronides.[114] The N^4-acetates and glucuronides are inactive. For example, sulfisoxazole is excreted about 80% unchanged, and sulfamethoxazole is excreted 20% unchanged. Sulfadimethoxine is about 80% excreted as the glucuronide. The correlation between structure and route of metabolism has not yet been delineated, though progress has been made by Fujita.[113] Vree et al.,[114] however, have described the excretion kinetics and pK_a values of N^1- and N^4-acetylsulfamethoxazole and other sulfonamides.

About 45% of trimethoprim and about 66% of sulfamethoxazole are partially plasma protein bound. Whereas about 80% of excreted trimethoprim and its metabolites are active as antibacterials, only 20% of sulfamethoxazole and its metabolites are active, with most of the activity coming from largely unmetabolized sulfamethoxazole. Six metabolites of trimethoprim are known.[115] It is likely, therefore, that sulfonamide-trimethoprim combinations using a sulfonamide with a higher active urine concentration will be developed in the future for urinary tract infections. Sulfamethoxazole and trimethoprim have similar half-lives, about 10 to 12 hours, but the half-life of the active fraction of sulfamethoxazole is shorter, about 9 hours.[115] (Ranges of half-lives have been summarized by Gleckman et al.,[116] and a detailed summary of pharmacokinetics has been made by Hansen.[115]) In patients with impaired renal function, concentrations of sulfamethoxazole and its metabolites may greatly increase in the plasma. A fixed combination of sulfamethoxazole and trimethoprim should not be used for patients with low creatinine clearances.

Mechanisms of Microbial Resistance to Sulfonamides

As noted above, indiscriminate use of sulfonamides has led to the emergence of many drug-resistant strains of bacteria. Resistance is most likely due to a compensatory increase in the biosynthesis of PABA by resistant bacteria,[117] although other mechanisms such as alterations in the binding strength of sulfonamides to the pathway enzymes, decreased permeability of the cell membrane, and active efflux of the sulfonamide may play a role.[102, 116] As a rule, if a microbe is resistant to one sulfonamide, it is resistant to all. Of note is the finding that sulfonamide resistance can be quickly transferred from a resistant bacterial strain to a previously sensitive one in one or two generations. This resistance propagation is most likely due to R-factor conjugation, as is the case for tetracycline resistance.

Several explanations have been reported to account for bacterial resistance to the dihydrofolate reductase inhibitor trimethoprim, including intrinsic resistance at the enzymatic level, the development of the ability by the bacteria to use the host's 5-deoxythymidine monophosphate (dTMP), and R-factor conjugation.

Synergistic Activities of Sulfonamides and Folate Reductase Inhibitors

If biosynthesis of bacterial (or protozoal) folate coenzymes is blocked at more than one point in the pathway, the result will be a synergistic antimicrobial effect. This is beneficial because the microbe will not develop resistance as readily

as it would with a singly blocked pathway. The synergistic approach is used widely in antibacterial therapy with the combination of sulfamethoxazole and trimethoprim[102, 118–120] (Septra, Bactrim, Co-Trimoxazole) and in antimalarial therapy with pyrimethamine plus a sulfonamide or quinine. Additional combinations with trimethoprim have been investigated (e.g., with rifampin).[121, 122]

Toxicity and Side Effects

A variety of serious toxicity and hypersensitivity problems have been reported with sulfonamide and sulfonamide–trimethoprim combinations. Mandell and Petri[108] note that these problems occur in about 5% of all patients. Hypersensitivity reactions include fever, rash, Stevens-Johnson syndrome, skin eruptions, allergic myocarditis, photosensitization, and related conditions. Hematological side effects also sometimes occur, especially hemolytic anemia in individuals with a deficiency of glucose-6-phosphate dehydrogenase. Other reported hematological side effects include agranulocytosis and aplastic anemia. Crystalluria may occur, even with the modern sulfonamides, when the patient does not maintain normal fluid intake. Nausea and related gastrointestinal side effects are sometimes noted. Detailed summaries of incidences of side effects with trimethoprim-sulfamethoxazole have been published by Wormser and Deutsch[118] and by Gleckman et al.[116]

Structure–Activity Relationships

As noted above in this chapter, several thousand sulfonamides have been investigated as antibacterials (and many as antimalarials). From these efforts, several structure–activity relationships have been proposed, as summarized by Anand.[102] The aniline (N^4) amino group is very important for activity because any modification of it other than to make prodrugs results in a loss of activity. For example, all of the N^4-acetylated metabolites of sulfonamide are inactive.

A variety of studies have shown that the active form of sulfonamide is the N^1-ionized salt. Thus, although many modern sulfonamides are much more active than unsubstituted sulfanilamide, they are only 2 to 6 times more active if equal amounts of N^1-ionized forms are compared.[123] Maximal activity seems to be exhibited by sulfonamides between pK_a 6.6 and 7.4.[123–126] This reflects, in part, the need for enough nonionized (i.e., more lipid soluble) drug to be present at physiological pH to be able to pass through bacterial cell walls.[127] Fujita and Hansch[113] also related pK_a, partition coefficients, and electronic (Hammett) parameters with sulfonamide activity (Table 8-9).

Sulfamethizole, USP. 4-Amino-N-(5-methyl-1,3,4-thiadiazole-2yl)benzenesulfonamide; N^1-(5-methyl-1,3,4-thiadiazol-2-yl)sulfanilamide; 5-methyl-2-sulfanilamido-1,3,4-thiadiazole. Sulfamethizole's plasma half-life is 2.5 hours. This compound is a white crystalline powder soluble 1:2,000 in water.

TABLE 8–9   Characteristics of Absorbable Short- and Intermediate-Acting Sulfonamides

Sulfonamide	Half-Life	Oral Absorption
Sulfisoxazole	Short (6 hours)	Prompt (peak levels in 1–4 hours)
Sulfamethizole	Short (9 hours)	Prompt
Sulfadiazine	Intermediate (10–17 hours)	Slow (peak levels in 4–8 hours)
Sulfamethoxazole	Intermediate (10–12 hours)	Slow
Sulfadoxine	Long (7–9 days)	Intermediate
Pyrimidine		
Trimethoprim	Intermediate (11 hours)	Prompt

Sulfisoxazole, USP.   4-Amino-N-(3,4-dimethyl-5-isoxazolyl)benzenesulfonamide; N^1-(3,4-dimethyl-5-isoxazolyl)sulfanilamide; 5-sulfanilamido-3,4-dimethylisoxazole. Sulfisoxazole's plasma half-life is 6 hours. This compound is a white, odorless, slightly bitter, crystalline powder. Its pK_a is 5.0. At pH 6 this sulfonamide has a water solubility of 350 mg in 100 mL, and its acetyl derivative has a solubility of 110 mg in 100 mL of water.

Sulfisoxazole possesses the action and the uses of other sulfonamides and is used for infections involving sulfonamide-sensitive bacteria. It is claimed to be effective in the treatment of Gram-negative urinary infections.

Sulfisoxazole Acetyl, USP. N-[(4-Aminophenyl)sulfonyl]-N-(3,4-dimethyl-5-isoxazolyl)acetamide; N-(3,4-dimethyl-5-isoxazolyl)-N-sulfanilylacetamide; N^1-acetyl-N^1-(3,4-dimethyl-5-isoxazolyl)sulfanilamide. Sulfisoxazole acetyl shares the actions and uses of the parent compound, sulfisoxazole. The acetyl derivative is tasteless and, therefore, suitable for oral administration, especially in liquid preparations. The acetyl compound is split in the intestinal tract and absorbed as sulfisoxazole; that is, it is a *prodrug* for sulfisoxazole.

Sulfisoxazole Diolamine, USP.   4-Amino-N-(3,5-dimethyl-5-isoxazolyl)benzenesulfonamide compound with 2,2'-iminobis[ethanol](1:1); 2,2'-iminodiethanol salt of N^1-(3,4-dimethyl-5-isoxazolyl)sulfanilamide. This salt is prepared by adding enough diethanolamine to a solution of sulfisoxazole to bring the pH to about 7.5. It is used as a salt to make the drug more soluble in the physiological pH range of 6.0 to 7.5 and is used in solution for systemic administration of the drug by slow intravenous, intramuscular, or subcutaneous injection when high enough blood levels cannot be maintained by oral administration alone. It also is used for instillation of drops or ointment in the eye for the local treatment of susceptible infections.

Sulfamethazine, USP.   4-Amino-N-(4,6-dimethyl-2-pyrimidinyl)benzenesulfonamide; N^1-(4,6-dimethyl-2-pyrimidinyl)sulfanilamide; 2-sulfanilamido-4,6-dimethylpyrimidine. Sulfamethazine's plasma half-life is 7 hours. This compound is similar in chemical properties to sulfamerazine and sulfadiazine but does have greater water solubility than either. Its pK_a is 7.2. Because it is more soluble in acid urine than sulfamerazine is, the possibility of kidney damage from use of the drug is decreased. The human body appears to handle the drug unpredictably; hence, there is some disfavor to its use in this country except in combination sulfa therapy (in trisulfapyrimidines, USP) and in veterinary medicine.

Sulfacetamide. N-[(4-Aminophenyl)sulfonyl]-acetamide; N-sulfanilylacetamide; N^1-acetylsulfanilamide. Sulfacetamide's plasma half-life is 7 hours. This compound is a white crystalline powder, soluble in water (1:62.5 at 37°C) and in alcohol. It is very soluble in hot water, and its water solution is acidic. It has a pK_a of 5.4.

Sulfachloropyridazine. N^1-(6-Chloro-3-pyridazinyl)sulfanilamide. Sulfachloropyridazine's plasma half-life is 8 hours.

Sulfapyridine, USP. 4-Amino-*N*-2-pyridinylbenzene-sulfonamide; *N*[1]-2-pyridylsulfanilamide. Sulfapyridine's plasma half-life is 9 hours. This compound is a white, crystalline, odorless, and tasteless substance. It is stable in air but slowly darkens on exposure to light. It is soluble in water (1:3,500), in alcohol (1:440), and in acetone (1:65) at 25°C. It is freely soluble in dilute mineral acids and aqueous solutions of sodium and potassium hydroxide. The pK$_a$ is 8.4. Its outstanding effect in curing pneumonia was first recognized by Whitby; however, because of its relatively high toxicity, it has been supplanted largely by sulfadiazine and sulfamerazine. Several cases of kidney damage have resulted from acetylsulfapyridine crystals deposited in the kidneys. It also causes severe nausea in most patients. Because of its toxicity, it is used only for dermatitis herpetiformis.

Sulfapyridine was the first drug to have an outstanding curative action on pneumonia. It gave impetus to the study of the whole class of *N*[1] heterocyclically substituted derivatives of sulfanilamide.

Sulfamethoxazole, USP. 4-Amino-*N*-(5-methyl-3-isoxazolyl)benzenesulfonamide; *N*[1]-(5-methyl-3-isoxazolyl) sulfanilamide (Gantanol). Sulfamethoxazole's plasma half-life is 11 hours.

Sulfamethoxazole is a sulfonamide drug closely related to sulfisoxazole in chemical structure and antimicrobial activity. It occurs as a tasteless, odorless, almost white crystalline powder. The solubility of sulfamethoxazole in the pH range of 5.5 to 7.4 is slightly lower than that of sulfisoxazole but higher than that of sulfadiazine, sulfamerazine, or sulfamethazine.

Following oral administration, sulfamethoxazole is not absorbed as completely or as rapidly as sulfisoxazole, and its peak blood level is only about 50% as high.

Sulfadiazine, USP. 4-Amino-*N*-2-pyrimidinyl-benzene-sulfonamide; *N*[1]-2-pyrimidinylsulfanilamide; 2-sulfanilamidopyrimidine. Sulfadiazine's plasma half-life is 17 hours.

It is a white, odorless crystalline powder soluble in water to the extent of 1:8,100 at 37°C and 1:13,000 at 25°C, in human serum to the extent of 1:620 at 37°C, and sparingly soluble in alcohol and acetone. It is readily soluble in dilute mineral acids and bases. Its pK$_a$ is 6.3.

Sulfadiazine Sodium, USP. Soluble sulfadiazine is an anhydrous, white, colorless, crystalline powder soluble in water (1:2) and slightly soluble in alcohol. Its water solutions are alkaline (pH 9 to 10) and absorb carbon dioxide from the air, with precipitation of sulfadiazine. It is administered as a 5% solution in sterile water intravenously for patients requiring an immediately high blood level of the sulfonamide.

Mixed Sulfonamides

The danger of crystal formation in the kidneys from administration of sulfonamides has been greatly reduced through the use of the more soluble sulfonamides, such as sulfisoxazole. This danger may be diminished still further by administering mixtures of sulfonamides. When several sulfonamides are administered together, the antibacterial action of the mixture is the summation of the activity of the total sulfonamide concentration present, but the solubilities are independent of the presence of similar compounds. Thus, by giving a mixture of sulfadiazine, sulfamerazine, and sulfacetamide, the same therapeutic level can be maintained with much less danger of crystalluria, because only one third of the amount of any one compound is present. Descriptions of some of the mixtures used follow.

Trisulfapyrimidines, Oral Suspension. The oral suspension of trisulfapyrimidines contains equal weights of sulfadiazine, USP; sulfamerazine, USP; and sulfamethazine, USP, either with or without an agent to raise the pH of the urine.

Trisulfapyrimidines, Tablets. Trisulfapyrimidine tablets contain essentially equal quantities of sulfadiazine, sulfamerazine, and sulfamethazine.

Sulfadoxine and Pyrimethamine. The mixture of sulfadoxine and pyrimethamine (Fansidar) is used for the treatment of *Plasmodium falciparum* malaria in patients in whom

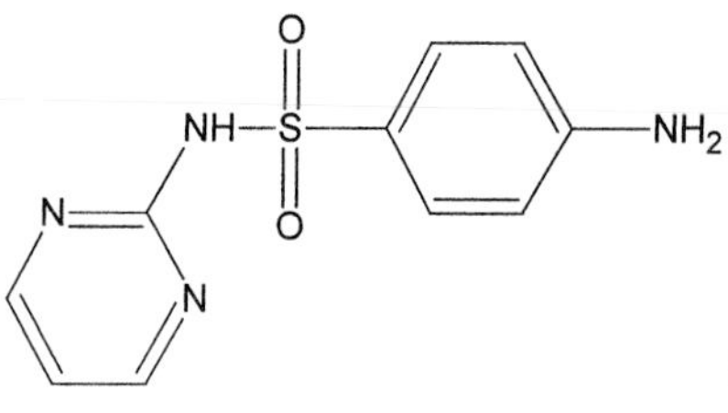

Sulfadiazine

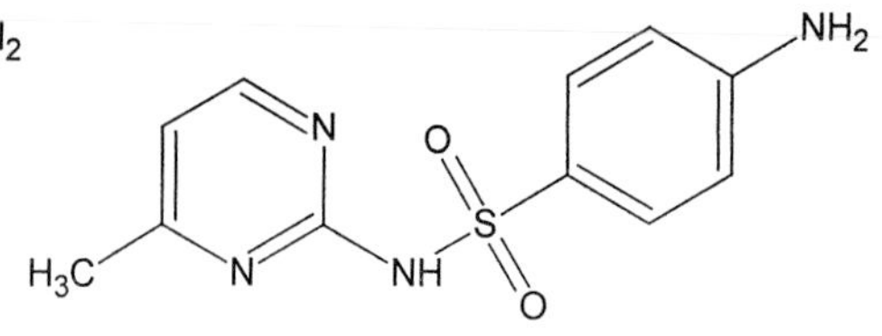

Sulfamerazine

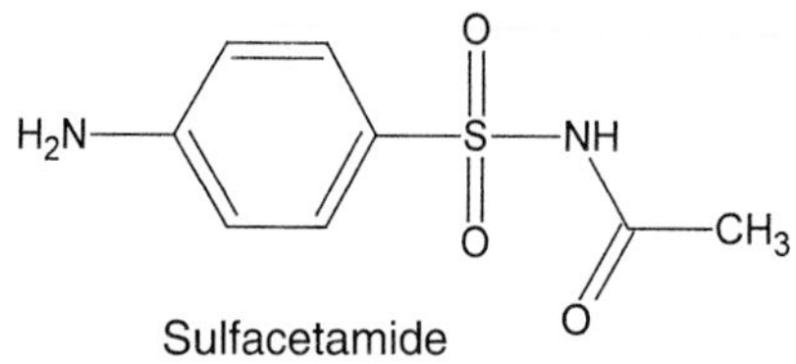

Sulfacetamide

chloroquine resistance is suspected. It is also used for malaria prophylaxis for travelers to areas where chloroquine-resistant malaria is endemic.

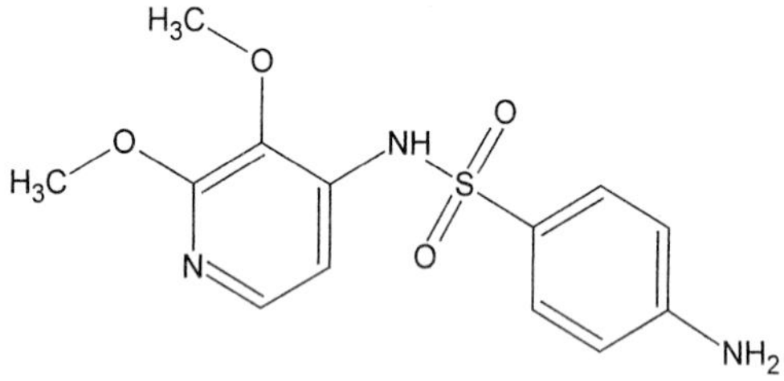

Sulfadoxine

Topical Sulfonamides

Sulfacetamide Sodium, USP. *N*-Sulfanilylacetamide monosodium salt (Sodium Sulamyd) is obtained as the monohydrate and is a white, odorless, bitter, crystalline powder that is very soluble (1:2.5) in water. Because the sodium salt is highly soluble at the physiological pH of 7.4, it is especially suited, as a solution, for repeated topical applications in the local management of ophthalmic infections susceptible to sulfonamide therapy.

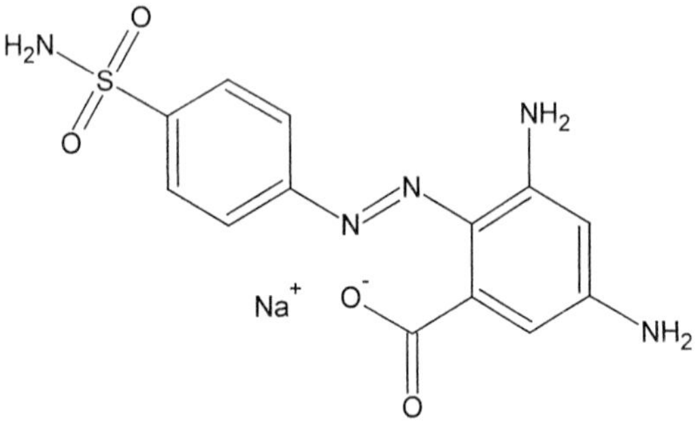

Sulfisoxazole Diolamine, USP. Sulfisoxazole diolamine is described with the short- and intermediate-acting sulfonamides and also used in intravenous and intramuscular preparations.

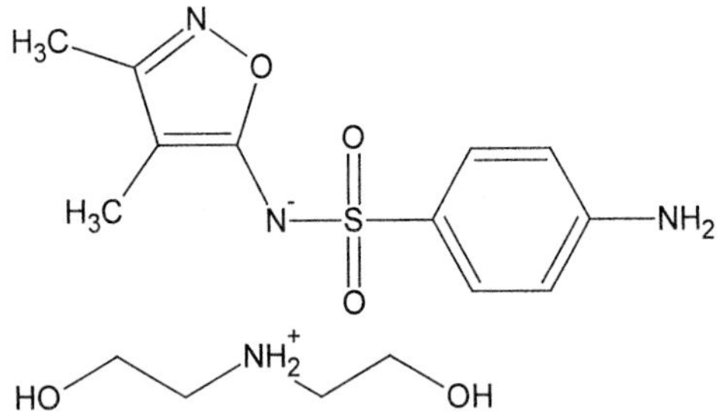

Triple Sulfa. Triple sulfa (sulfabenzamide, sulfacetamide, and sulfathiazole; Femguard) is used as a vaginal cream in the treatment of *Haemophilus vaginalis* vaginitis.

Nonabsorbable Sulfonamides

TOPICAL SULFONAMIDES FOR BURN THERAPY

Mafenide Acetate. 4-(Aminomethyl)benzenesulfonamide acetate (Sulfamylon) is a homologue of the sulfanilamide molecule. It is not a true sulfanilamide-type compound, as it is not inhibited by PABA. Its antibacterial action involves a mechanism that differs from that of true sulfanilamide-type compounds. This compound is particularly effective against *Clostridium welchii* in topical application and was used during World War II by the German army for prophylaxis of wounds. It is not effective orally. It is currently used alone or with antibiotics in the treatment of slow-healing, infected wounds.

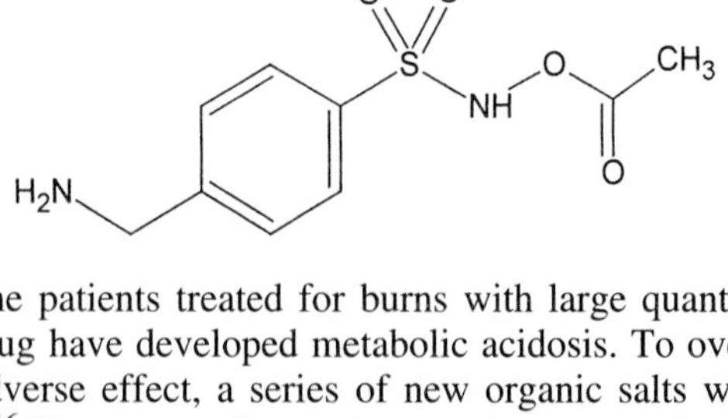

Some patients treated for burns with large quantities of this drug have developed metabolic acidosis. To overcome this adverse effect, a series of new organic salts was prepared.[16] The acetate in an ointment base proved to be the most efficacious.

Silver Sulfadiazine (Silvadene).   The silver salt of sulfadiazine applied in a water-miscible cream base has proved to be an effective topical antimicrobial agent, especially against *Pseudomonas* spp. This is particularly significant in burn therapy because pseudomonads are often responsible for failures in therapy. The salt is only slightly soluble and does not penetrate the cell wall but acts on the external cell structure. Studies using radioactive silver have shown essentially no absorption into body fluids. Sulfadiazine levels in the serum were about 0.5 to 2 mg/100 mL.

This preparation is reported to be easier to use than other standard burn treatments, such as application of freshly prepared dilute silver nitrate solutions or mafenide ointment.

Sulfonamides for Intestinal Infections, Ulcerative Colitis, or Reduction of Bowel Flora

Each of the sulfonamides in this group is a prodrug, which is designed to be poorly absorbable, though usually, in practice, a little is absorbed. Therefore, usual precautions with sulfonamide therapy should be observed. In the large intestine, the N^4-protecting groups are cleaved, releasing the free sulfonamide antibacterial agent. Today, only one example is used clinically, sulfasalazine.

Sulfasalazine, USP.   Sulfasalazine (2-hydroxy-5[[4-[(2-pyridinylamino)sulfonyl]phenyl]azo]benzoic acid or 5-[*p*-(2-pyridylsulfamoyl)phenylazo]salicylic acid) is a brownish yellow, odorless powder, slightly soluble in alcohol but practically insoluble in water, ether, and benzene.

Sulfasalazine is broken down in the body to *m*-aminosalicylic acid and sulfapyridine. The drug is excreted through the kidneys and is detectable colorimetrically in the urine, producing an orange-yellow color when the urine is alkaline and no color when the urine is acid.

DIHYDROFOLATE REDUCTASE INHIBITORS

Trimethoprim, USP.   Trimethoprim (5-[(3,4,5-trimethoxyphenyl)methyl]-2,4-pyrimidinediamine or 2,4-diamino-5-(3,4,5-trimethoxybenzyl)pyrimidine) is closely related to several antimalarials but does not have good antimalarial activity by itself; it is, however, a potent antibacterial. Originally introduced in combination with sulfamethoxazole, it is now available as a single agent.

Approved by the FDA in 1980, trimethoprim as a single agent is used only for the treatment of uncomplicated urinary tract infections. The argument for trimethoprim as a single agent was summarized in 1979 by Wormser and Deutsch.[118] They point out that several studies comparing trimethoprim with TMP-SMX for the treatment of chronic urinary tract infections found no statistically relevant difference between the two courses of therapy. Furthermore, some patients cannot take sulfonamide products for the reasons discussed above in this chapter. The concern is that when used as a single agent, bacteria now susceptible to trimethoprim will rapidly develop resistance. In combination with a sulfonamide, however, the bacteria will be less likely to do so. That is, they will not survive long enough to easily develop resistance to both drugs.

Sulfamethoxazole and Trimethoprim.   The synergistic action of the combination of these two drugs is discussed above in this chapter.

SULFONES

The sulfones are primarily of interest as antibacterial agents, though there are some reports of their use in the treatment of malarial and rickettsial infections. They are less effective than the sulfonamides. PABA partially antagonizes the action of many of the sulfones, suggesting that the mechanism of action is similar to that of the sulfonamides. Further, infections that arise in patients being treated with sulfones are cross-resistant to sulfonamides. Several sulfones have proved useful in the treatment of leprosy, but among them only dapsone is clinically used today.

It has been estimated that there are about 11 million cases of leprosy in the world, of which about 60% are in Asia (with 3.5 million in India alone). The first reports of dapsone resistance prompted the use of multidrug therapy with dapsone, rifampin, and clofazimine combinations in some geographic areas.[128]

The search for antileprotic drugs has been hampered by the inability to cultivate *M. leprae* in artificial media and by the lack of experimental animals susceptible to human leprosy. A method of isolating and growing *M. leprae* in the footpads of mice and in armadillos has been reported and has permitted a much wider range of research. Sulfones were introduced into the treatment of leprosy after it was found that sodium glucosulfone was effective in experimental tuberculosis in guinea pigs.

The parent sulfone, dapsone (4,4'-sulfonyldianiline), is the prototype for a variety of analogues that have been widely studied. Four variations on this structure have given active compounds:

1. Substitution on both the 4- and 4'-amino functions
2. Monosubstitution on only one of the amino functions
3. Nuclear substitution on one of the benzenoid rings
4. Replacement of one of the phenyl rings with a heterocyclic ring

The antibacterial activity and the toxicity of the disubstituted sulfones are thought to be chiefly due to the formation in vivo of dapsone. Hydrolysis of disubstituted derivatives to the parent sulfone apparently occurs readily in the acid medium of the stomach but only to a very limited extent following parenteral administration. Monosubstituted and nuclear-substituted derivatives are believed to act as entire molecules.

Dapsone, USP. Dapsone (4,4'-sulfonylbisbenzeneamine; 4,4'-sulfonyldianiline; *p,p'*-diaminodiphenylsulfone; or DDS [Avlosulfon]) occurs as an odorless, white crystalline powder that is very slightly soluble in water and sparingly soluble in alcohol. The pure compound is light stable, but traces of impurities, including water, make it photosensitive and thus susceptible to discoloration in light. Although no chemical change is detectable following discoloration, the drug should be protected from light.

Dapsone is used in the treatment of both lepromatous and tuberculoid types of leprosy. Dapsone is used widely for all forms of leprosy, often in combination with clofazimine and rifampin. Initial treatment often includes rifampin with dapsone, followed by dapsone alone. It is also used to prevent the occurrence of multibacillary leprosy when given prophylactically.

Dapsone is also the drug of choice for dermatitis herpetiformis and is sometimes used with pyrimethamine for treatment of malaria and with trimethoprim for PCP.

Serious side effects can include hemolytic anemia, methemoglobinemia, and toxic hepatic effects. Hemolytic effects can be pronounced in patients with glucose-6-phosphate dehydrogenase deficiency. During therapy, all patients require frequent blood counts.

REFERENCES

1. Atlas, R. M.: Microbiology, Fundamentals and Applications. New York, Macmillan, 1984, p. 19.
2. Ehrlich, B: United States Patent 986,148.
3. Christiansen, A.: J. Am. Chem. Soc. 42:2402, 1920.
4. Atlas, R.M.: Microbiology, Fundamentals and Applications. New York, Macmillan, 1984, p. 20.
5. Fleming, M., et al.: Ethanol. In Hardman, J. G., Limbird, L. E., and Gilman, A. G. (eds.). Goodman and Gilman's The Pharmacological Basis of Therapeutics. New York, McGraw-Hill, 2001.
6. DuMez, A. G.: J. Am. Pharm. Assoc. 28:416, 1939.
7. Gilbert, G. L.: Appl. Microbiol. 12:496, 1964.
8. Leech, P. N.: J. Am. Med. Assoc. 109:1531, 1937.
9. Miner, N. A., et al.: Am. J. Pharm. 34:376, 1977.
10. United States Food and Drug Administration: Hexachlorophene and Newborns. Bulletin, December 1971.
11. Vasarenesh, A.: Arch. Dermatol. 98:183, 1968
12. Gershenfeld, L.: Milk Food Technol. 18:233, 1955.
13. Domagk, G.: Dtsch. Med. Wochenschr. 61:250, 1935.
14. Rose, F. L., and Swain, G. J.: J. Chem. Soc. 442, 1956.
15. Massey, A. G.: Main Group Elements. Chichester, England, Ellis Horwood Ltd., 1990, p. 160.
16. Garrett, E. R., and Woods, O. R.: J. Am. Pharm. Assoc. (Sci. Ed.) 42:736, 1953.
17. Rippon, J. W. In Burrows, W. (ed.). Textbook of Microbiology. Philadelphia, W. B. Saunders, 1973, p. 683.
18. Friedman, L., et al.: J. Invest. Dermatol. 35:3–5, 1960.
19. Rippon, J. W. In Burrows, W. (ed.). Textbook of Microbiology. Philadelphia, W. B. Saunders, 1973, p. 721.
20. Rippon, J. W. In Burrows, W. (ed.). Textbook of Microbiology. Philadelphia, W. B. Saunders, 1973, p. 734.
21. Goldman, R. C., and Klein, L. L.: Annu. Rep. Med. Chem. 29:155, 1994.
22. Ajello, L.: Science 123:876, 1956.
23. Ajello, L.: Mycopathologia 17:315, 1962.
24. Rebell, G., and Taplin, D.: Dermatophytes. Miami, University of Miami Press, 1970.
25. Rieth, H.: Arzneim. Forsch. 31:1309, 1981.
26. Polak, A., and Scholer, H. J.: Chemotherapy 21:113, 1975.
27. Baginski, M., Resat, H., McCammon, J. A.: Mol. Pharmacol. 52:560, 1997.
28. Baginski, M., Gariboldi, P., Bruni, P., Borowski, E.: Biophys. Chem. 65:91, 1997.
29. Gold, W., et al.: Antibiotics Annual 1955–1956. New York, Medical Encyclopedia, 1956.
30. Mechlinski, W., et al.: Tetrahedron Lett. 3873, 1970.
31. Graybill, J. R.: Ann. Intern. Med. 124:921, 1986.
32. Ianknegkt, R., et al.: Clin. Pharmacokinet. 23:279, 1992.
33. Hazen, E. L., and Brown, R.: Proc. Soc. Exp. Biol. Med. 76:93, 1951.
34. Pandey, R. C., Rinehart, K. L.: J. Antibiot. 29:1035, 1976.
35. Lencelin, J. M., et al.: Tetrahedron Lett. 29:2827, 1988.
36. Struyk, A. P., Hoette, I., Orost, G., et al.: Antibiot. Ann. 878, 1957–1958.
37. Brik, H., et al.: Nystatin. In Florey, K. (ed.). Analytical Profiles of Drug Substances, vol. 10. New York, Academic Press, 1981, p. 513.
38. Oxford, A. E., et al.: Biochem. J. 33:240, 1939.
39. Grove, J. F., et al.: J. Chem. Soc. 3977, 1952.
40. Sloboda, R. D., Van Blaricom, G., Creasey, W. A.: Biochem. Biophys. Res. Commun. 105:882, 1982.
41. Stütz, A., and Petranyi, G.: J. Med. Chem. 27:1539, 1984.
42. Ryder, N. S.: Antimicrob. Agents Chemother. 27:252, 1985.
43. Petranyi, G., et al.: Science 224:1239, 1984.
44. Gupta, M. P., et al.: J. Vet. Med. Mycol. 29:45, 1991.
45. Thomas, A. H.: Antimicrob. Chemother. 17:269, 1986.
46. Hitchcock, C. A.: Biochem. Soc. Trans. 19:782, 1991.
47. Pont, A., et al.: Arch. Intern. Med. 144:2150, 1984.
48. Vanden Bossche, H.: Drug Dev. Res. 8:287, 1986.
49. Rotstein, D. M., Kertesz, D. J., Walker, K. A. M., and Swinney, D. C.: J. Med. Chem. 35:2818, 1992.
50. Dickinson, R. P., et al.: Med. Chem. Lett. 6:2031, 1996.
51. DeBono, M., et al.: J. Med. Chem. 38:3271, 1995.
52. Schwartz, R. E., Masurekar, P. S., and White, R. F.: Clin. Dermatol. 7:375, 1993.
53. Balkovec, J. M.: Annu. Rep. Med. Chem. 33:175, 1998.
54. Jao, E.: Tetrahedron Lett. 37:5661, 1996.
55. Nagiec, M. M., Nagiec, E. E., et al.: J. Biol. Chem. 272:9809, 1997.
56. Shen, L. L., Mitscher, L. A., Sharma, P. N., et al.: Biochemistry 28:3886, 1989.
57. Sreedharan, S., et al.: J. Bacteriol. 172:7260, 1990.
58. Yoshida, H., et al.: Antimicrob. Agents Chemother. 35:1647, 1991.
59. Yoshida, H., et al.: Antimicrob. Agents Chemother. 34:1273, 1990.
60. Bazile, S., et al.: Antimicrob. Agents Chemother. 36:2622, 1992.
61. Domagala, J. M.: J. Antimicrob. Chemother. 33:685, 1994.
62. Ross, D. L., and Riley, C. M.: J. Pharm. Biomed. Anal. 12:1325, 1994.

63. Lee, D.-S., et al.: J. Pharm. Biomed. Anal. 12:157, 1994.
64. Mitscher, L. A., et al.: J. Med. Chem. 30:2283, 1987.
65. Bloom, B. R., and Murray, C. J. L.: Science 257:1055, 1992.
66. Winder, F. G., and Collins, P. B.: J. Gen. Microbiol. 63:41, 1970.
67. Quomard, A., Lacove, C., and LanPelle, G.: Antimicrob. Agents Chemother. 35:1035, 1991.
68. Youatt, J., and Tham, S. H.: Am. Rev. Respir. Dis. 100:25, 1969.
69. Johnsson, K., and Schultz, P. G.: J. Am. Chem. Soc. 116:7425, 1994.
70. Zhang, Y., et al.: Nature 358:591, 1992.
71. Dessen, A., et al.: Science 267:1638, 1995.
72. Banerjee, A., et al.: Science 263:227, 1994.
73. Boxenbaum, H. G., and Riegelman, S.: J. Pharm. Sci. 63:1191, 1974.
74. Heifets, L. B., Flory, M. A., and Lindholm-Levy, P. J.: Antimicrob. Agents Chemother. 33:1252, 1989.
75. Rinehart, K. L.: Acc. Chem. Res. 5:57, 1972.
76. Hartmann, G. R., et al.: Angew. Chem. Int. Ed. Engl. 24:1009, 1985.
77. Katz, E., and Moss, B.: Proc. Natl. Acad. Sci. U. S. A. 66:677, 1970.
78. Werli, W.: Rev. Infect. Dis. 5S:407, 1983.
79. Gallo, G. G., and Radaelli, P.: Rifampin. In Florey, K. (ed.). Analytical Profiles of Drug Substances. New York, Academic Press, 1976.
80. Kuehl, F. A., et al.: J. Am. Chem. Soc. 77:2344, 1955.
81. Hildy, P. H., et al.: J. Am. Chem. Soc. 77:2345, 1955.
82. Stammer, C. H., et al.: J. Am. Chem. Soc. 77:2346, 1955.
83. Smart, J., et al.: Experientia 13:291, 1957.
84. Neuhaus, F. C., and Lynch, J. L.: Biochemistry 3:471, 1964.
85. Rando, R. R.: Biochem. Pharmacol. 24:1153, 1975.
86. Herr, E. B., Pittenger, G. E., and Higgens, C. E.: Indiana Acad. Sci. 69:134, 1960.
87. Bycroft, B. W., et al.: Nature 231:301, 1971.
88. Nomoto, S., et al.: J. Antibiot. 30:955, 1977.
89. Knight, R. C., et al.: Biochem. Pharmacol. 27:2089, 1978.
90. Metcalf, B. W., et al.: J. Am. Chem. Soc. 100:2551, 1978.
91. Prichard, R. K.: Nature 228:684, 1970.
92. Friedman, P. A., and Platzer, E. G.: Biochim. Biophys. Acta 544:605, 1978.
93. Pica-Mattoccia, L., and Cioli, D.: Am. J. Trop. Med Hyg. 34:112, 1985.
94. Burg, R. W., et al.: Antimicrob. Agents Chemother. 15:361, 1979.
95. Campbell, W. C.: Science 221:823, 1983.
96. Albers-Schonberg, G., et al.: J. Am. Chem. Soc. 103:4216, 1981.
97. Springer, J. P., et al.: J. Am. Chem. Soc. 103:4221, 1981.
98. Aziz, M. A., et al.: Lancet 2:171, 1982.
99. Orkin, M., and Maibach, H. I.: N. Engl. J. Med. 298:496, 1978.
100. Domagk, G.: Dtsch. Med. Wochenschr. 61:250, 1935.
101. Baumler, E.: In Search of the Magic Bullet. London, Thames and Hudson, 1965.
102. Anand, N.: Sulfonamides and sulfones. In Wolff, M. E. (ed.). Burger's Medicinal Chemistry, vol. 2, 5th ed. New York, Wiley-Interscience, 1996, Chap. 33.
103. Foerster, J.: Z. Haut. Geschlechtskr. 45:459, 1933.
104. Trefouel, J., et al.: C. R. Seances Soc. Biol. 120:756, 1935.
105. Fuller, A. T.: Lancet 1:194, 1937.
106. Northey, E. H.: The Sulfonamides and Allied Compounds. ACS Monogr. Ser. Washington, DC, American Chemical Society, 1948.
107. MacDonald, L., and Kazanijan, P.: Formulary 31:470, 1996.
108. Petri, W. A.: Antimicrobial agents: Sulfonamides, trimethoprim-sulfamethoxazole, quinolones, and agents for urinary tract infection. In Gilman, A. G., et al. (eds.). The Pharmacological Basis of Therapeutics, 9th ed. New York, Macmillan, 1996.
109. Jawetz, E.: Principles of antimicrobial drug action. In Katzung, B. G. (ed.). Basic and Clinical Pharmacology, 6th ed. Norwalk, CT, Appleton & Lange, 1995.
110. Med. Lett. 30:33, 1988.
111. FDA Drug Bulletin, U.S. Department of Health, Education and Welfare, Food and Drug Administration, Feb., 1980.
112. Med. Lett. 29:53, 1987.
113. Fujita, T., and Hansch, C.: J. Med. Chem. 10:991, 1967.
114. Vree, T. B., et al.: Clin. Pharmacokinet. 4:310, 1979.
115. Hansen, I.: Antibiot. Chemother. 25:217, 1978.
116. Gleckman, R., et al.: Am. J. Hosp. Pharm. 36:893, 1979.
117. Bushby, S. R., and Hitchings, G. H.: Br. J. Pharmacol. Chemother. 33:72, 1968.
118. Wormser, G. P., and Deutsch, G. T.: Ann. Intern. Med. 91:420, 1979.
119. Palminteri, R., and Sassella, D.: Chemotherapy 25:181, 1979.
120. Harvey, R. J.: J. Antimicrob. Chemother. 4:315, 1978.
121. Letters of Burchall, J. J., Then, R., and Poe, M.: Science 197:1300–1301, 1977.
122. Werlin, S. L., and Grand, R. J.: J. Pediatr. 92:450, 1978.
123. Fox, C. L., and Ross, H. M.: Proc. Soc. Exp. Biol. Med. 50:142, 1942.
124. Yamazaki, M., et al.: Chem. Pharm. Bull. (Tokyo) 18:702, 1970.
125. Bell, P. H., and Roblin, R. O.: J. Am. Chem. Soc. 64:2905, 1942.
126. Cowles, P. B.: Yale J. Biol. Med. 14:599, 1942.
127. Brueckner, A. H.: J. Biol. Med. 15:813, 1943.
128. Shepard, C. C.: N. Engl. J. Med. 307:1640, 1982.

SELECTED READING

Bloom, B. R. (ed.): Tuberculosis. Washington, DC, American Society for Microbiology Press, 1994.

Chu, D. T., and Fernandes, P. B.: Recent developments in the field of quinolone antibacterial agents. In Testa, B. (ed.). Advances in Drug Research, vol. 21. New York, Academic Press, 1991.

Como, J. A., and Dismukes, W. E.: Oral azoles as systemic antifungal chemotherapy. N. Engl. J. Med. 330:263, 1994.

Despommier, D. D., and Karapelou, J. W.: Parasitic Life Cycles. New York, Springer-Verlag, 1987.

Goldsmith, R. S., and Heyneman, D. (eds.): Tropical Medicine and Parasitology. New York, Appleton & Lange, 1989.

Hastings, R. C., and Franzblau, S. G.: Chemotherapy of leprosy. Annu. Rev. Pharmacol. Toxicol. 28:231, 1988.

Hooper, D. C., and Wolfson, J. S. (eds.): Quinolone Antimicrobial Agents, 2nd ed. Washington, DC, American Society for Microbiology Press, 1993.

Houston, S., and Fanning, A.: Current and potential treatment of tuberculosis. Drugs 48:689, 1994.

Jernigan, J. A., and Pearson, R. D.: Antiparasitic agents. In Mandell GL, Bennett JE, Dolin R. (eds.). Principles and Practice of Infectious Diseases, vol. 1, 4th ed. New York, Churchill-Livingstone, 1995.

Kreier, J. B., and Baker, J. R. (eds.): Parasitic Protozoa, 2nd ed. San Diego, Academic Press, 1991.

Reed, S.: Amebiasis: an update. Clin. Infect. Dis. 14:385, 1992.

Singh, S. K., and Sherma, S.: Current status of medical research in helminth disease. Med. Res. Rev. 11:581, 1991.

Wang, C. C.: Molecular mechanisms and therapeutic approaches to the treatment of African trypanosomiasis. Annu. Rev. Pharmacol. Toxicol. 35:93, 1995.

Yamaguchi, H., Kobazaski, G. S., and Takahashi, H. (eds.): Recent Advances in Antifungal Chemotherapy. New York, Marcel Dekker, 1992.

Antimalarials

JOHN H. BLOCK

Malaria, one of the most widespread diseases, is caused by a *Plasmodium* parasite. Its name is derived from *mala aria* (bad air), and it has been called ague, intermittent fever, marsh fever, and The Fever.[1, 2] The name is based on the early knowledge that malaria was associated with swamps and badly drained areas. The use of quinine for treating malaria has been known since the 17th century. While malaria is an ancient disease, its upsurge seems to coincide with the advent of farming about 20,000 years ago. The clearing of land provided areas for ponds containing still water. The *Anopheles gambiae* mosquito uses still water that sits in ponds and containers to breed. The gathering of humans in farming communities provided the necessary concentration of people to form a reservoir of hosts for the parasite and "food" for the mosquitos breeding in the ponds.[3-6]

Proof that the *Anopheles* mosquito is the carrier of the causative protozoa was obtained by Dr. Ronald Ross, who was recognized in 1902 with the Nobel Prize in Medicine. In a scenario somewhat similar to that in which definitive proof that yellow fever was transmitted by the *Aedes aegypti* mosquito was required, Dr. Ross strongly argued that malaria was transmitted by an insect vector and finally demonstrated that the parasite was carried in the stomach and salivary glands of the *Anopheles* mosquito. The latter discovery was important because it helped resolve the dispute about whether malaria was spread by the bite of the mosquito or by drinking water containing mosquito eggs and larva.[7]

Because malaria has been eliminated from North America, it only becomes a potential problem when citizens of this continent travel into an area where malaria is endemic. With international travel so common, Americans receive prescriptions to take an antimalarial drug prophylactically when traveling to, and living in, areas where malaria is endemic.[8] Frequently, U. S. citizens returning to the United States from areas where malaria is endemic and citizens of those countries who are coming to the United States have malaria and need antimalaria drugs. In 2002, two cases of malaria were reported in Virginia. Neither patient had any of the risk factors, including international travel, blood transfusion, organ transplantation, or needle sharing. Both lived in the same general geographical area. Examination of ponds in the area found *Anopheles* mosquitoes that initially tested positive for one of the malaria parasites, *Plasmodium vivax* (see below). The hypothesis was that infected mosquitoes had entered the United States through Dulles International Airport or Virginia seaports, possible in cargo. Surveys of surrounding medical facilities showed no recent cases of international travelers who had malaria. Follow-up testing of the mosquitoes, using more precise methods, disputed the initial finding that mosquitoes in the ponds that were tested carried *Plasmodium* spp. This finding is still in dispute.

Malaria, which infects several hundred million people each year, resulting in several million deaths annually, is a complex disease to treat. The causative agent is a group of parasitical protozoa of the *Plasmodium* genus transmitted by the female *Anopheles* mosquito. The impact of malaria on the human species continues to be devastating. The impact of diseases such as smallpox, plague, yellow fever, and polio on human history is fascinating but, fortunately, is mostly historical. The latter three diseases do reappear, but the cases are isolated. Plague is treated effectively with antibiotics, and there are vaccines for yellow fever and polio.

The public is aware of acquired immunodeficiency syndrome (AIDS) because it is a disease that "travels" by human carriers and has infected and killed prominent people who are citizens in economically developed countries. Nevertheless, compare the 2001 figures for AIDS and malaria. After approximately 20 years, 40 million people have been infected with the human immunodeficiency virus (HIV), of whom 5 million were infected and 3 million died in 2001. For North America, 940,000 have become infected in the past 20 years, of whom 45,000 were infected and 20,000 died in 2001. In contrast, approximately 10% of the world's population has malaria (300 to 500 million). Of these, about 1 million will die annually; most are children. In contrast, there are only about 1,500 new cases of malaria annually in the United States, and nearly all of these come from travelers arriving from areas where malaria is endemic. Most prescriptions for antimalarial drugs are for prophylaxis of travelers going to, and coming from, areas of the world where malaria is endemic.

There are three potential ways to control malaria: elimination of the vector, drug therapy, and vaccination. Elimination of the vector currently is the simplest and most cost-effective. Drug therapy has the same challenges as the development of antibiotics (e.g., resistance to the drug). The current antimalarial drugs, while effective against certain species, also have significant adverse reactions, and resistance is increasing. Thus far, no vaccine has been developed that is effective in vivo. The malaria parasite does elicit an immune response, evidenced by the fact that children with an initial exposure are more likely to die than adults who have recurring attacks. A T-cell response that includes both CD4$^+$ and CD8$^+$ T cells, production of interferon gamma, and nitric oxide synthase induction is added evidence that the human immune system does detect the parasite and responds accordingly.[9] An ideal vaccine should, at a minimum, be effective against both *P. falciparum* and *P. vivax,* the two species responsible for 90% of malaria cases.

The *Anopheles* mosquito has adapted very well to human habitats. As pointed out above, it requires still water to lay its eggs, wait for them to hatch, and then let the larvae, which feed on microscopic organisms in still water, mature. Transient still water is ideal because it likely will not contain predators that would feed on the eggs and larvae. In general, mosquitoes need 1 to 2 weeks to develop into mature insects. This usually is enough time before predators begin to populate the still water.

Currently, there are two ways to control the mosquito carrier. One is to prevent contact between humans and the insect. Because the *Anopheles* mosquito is a nocturnal feeder, it is easier to control than the *Aedes aegypti* mosquito, which is a day feeder and carries dengue and yellow fever. Putting screens on windows and using mosquito netting in bedrooms are very effective.

Second, elimination of the *Anopheles* mosquito, usually by application of insecticide and destroying its breeding areas, is the most effective way to eliminate (as opposed to control) malaria. Areas that have been successful at eliminating infected mosquitoes include North America, Europe, and Russia. To do this, the adult female mosquito must be killed, and breeding areas (still water) drained. One of the most effective insecticides has been DDT. Dr. Paul Muller received the 1948 Nobel Prize in Medicine for discovering that DDT kills the malaria-carrying *Anopheles* mosquito. DDT is long lasting and, unfortunately, accumulates in the environment. While being long lasting is beneficial from the standpoint of mosquito control, it also means that these insecticides get into the food chain and can affect both animals and humans. Indeed, use of DDT has been banned in most economically developed countries. Unfortunately, the areas of the world where malaria is endemic are economically poor and cannot *(a)* afford the newer insecticides, which must be reapplied because they degrade; *(b)* fund and maintain the infrastructure to eliminate breeding areas; and *(c)* provide medical facilities, staff, and drugs to treat their citizens.

DDT

New antimalarial drugs must be developed constantly, because the protozoa develop resistance by a variety of mechanisms (see discussions of mechanisms with the different drugs), and there are a wide variety of adverse reactions. The combination of the cost of the drugs and their adverse reactions can make patient compliance difficult. Four different species of protozoa cause malaria, and unfortunately, no one antimalarial drug is effective against all four species. There is a tremendous need for effective antimalarial agents.

STIMULATION OF ANTIMALARIAL RESEARCH BY WAR

From 1941 to 1946 (World War II), more than 15,000 substances were synthesized and screened as possible antimalarial agents by the United States, Australia, and Great Britain. Activity increased again during the Vietnam War, especially because of the increasing problem of resistance to commonly used antimalarials. During the decade 1968 to 1978, more than 250,000 compounds were investigated as part of a U. S. Army research program.[10] Department of Defense funding of this research has continued.

In addition to human intervention, there is evidence for at least five mutations in the human species that provide protection against malaria. These predominate in populations who historically lived and continue to live in areas endemic with malaria. The five mutations are sickling disease (formerly sickle cell anemia), glucose-6-phosphate dehydrogenase deficiency, hemoglobin C, various thalassemias, and increased production of nitric oxide (NO). Sickling disease can be fatal in homozygotes. Heterozygotes usually are asymptomatic and show a 90% decrease in the chance of dying from *P. falciparum*.[11] Homozygotes with hemoglobin C usually are asymptomatic.[12] Erythrocyte glucose-6-phosphate dehydrogenase deficiency (actually, 10 to 15% of normal activity in the erythrocyte) can cause hemolytic anemia and prehepatic jaundice when the patient takes certain drugs or is exposed to some viral infections. Ironically, some of the antimalarial drugs must be used with caution in patients with erythrocytic glucose-6-phosphate dehydrogenase deficiency to minimize the risk of hemolytic anemia. The increased levels of oxidized glutathione in the erythrocytes that are deficient in this enzyme may prevent the parasite from maturing in the erythrocyte. The significance of thalassemia varies with the type of anemia and whether the patient is homozygous or heterozygous.

The most recent of the mutations to be identified is the ability of certain populations to increase their production of NO. The site is in the promoter region of the gene for nitric oxide synthase 2, which generates NO from arginine, and involves a mutation changing a cytosine residue to thymine. The result is higher circulating levels of NO. It is not known how increased NO provides this protection, because there appears to be no significant difference between blood levels of the parasite in individuals with the mutation and those with ''normal'' NO synthase. The protection may be from complications seen with malaria that give the patient's immune system time to respond to the parasite.[13]

Malaria

Malaria is caused by four species of a one-cell protozoan of the *Plasmodium* genus:

P. falciparum: This species is estimated to cause approximately 50% of all malaria. It causes the most severe form and the most debilitating form of the disease, because patients feel ill between acute attacks. One reason why it leaves the patient so weak is that it infects up to 65% of the patient's erythrocytes.

P. vivax: This species is the second most common species, accounting for about 40% of all malaria cases. It can be very chronic, because it can reinfect liver cells.

P. malariae: While causing only 10% of all malarial cases, relapses are very common.

P. ovale: This species is the least common.

Figure 9-1 outlines the stages of the parasite after it is injected into the victim and indicates where drug therapy might be effective. The mosquito stores the sporozoite form of the protozoan in its salivary glands. Upon biting the patient, the sporozoites are injected into the patient's blood.

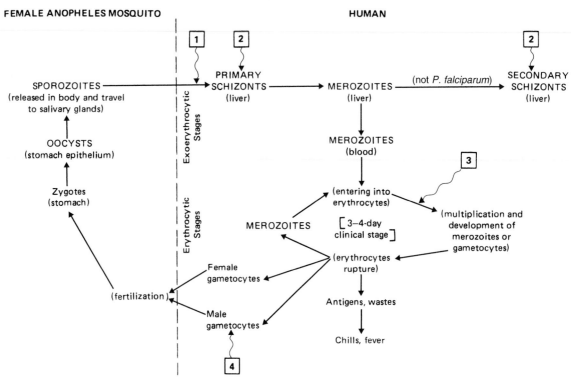

Figure 9–1 ■ Stages of the parasite that causes malaria after injection into its victim. See discussion in the text. □ indicates site of antimalarial drug action in humans.

Ideally, this would be a good site for intervention, before the parasite can infect the liver or erythrocyte. In the case of drug therapy, people living in areas endemic with malaria would need to be taking the drug constantly. Although this would be feasible for people living temporarily in these areas, it is not practical for residents. It is true that antimalarial drugs could be formulated into implanted depot dosage forms, but these are expensive and often require trained medical personnel to implant the drug.

A vaccine would be an excellent way to intercept the newly injected sporozoites. This would be analogous to individuals who have been immunized against mumps having their immune system intercept the virus before it enters target cells. Unfortunately, with all of the effort being expended to develop a vaccine, no vaccine effective in humans has been developed.

Within minutes after being injected into the patient's blood, the sporozoites begin entering hepatocytes, where they become primary schizonts and then merozoites. At this point, there are no symptoms. Depending on the *Plasmodium* species, the merozoites either rupture the infected hepatocytes and enter the systemic circulation or infect other liver cells. The latter process is seen with *P. vivax, P. malariae*, and *P. ovale*, but not *P. falciparum*, and produces secondary schizonts.

This secondary infection of the liver can be very damaging and is one of the sites for possible drug intervention. Killing the secondary schizonts would accomplish two things: protect the liver from further damage and eliminate a reservoir of schizonts that can change to merozoites and enter the systemic circulation. As the protozoan changes from sporozoite to schizont to merozoites, its immunological character

changes. Determination of the *Plasmodium* genome has shown that each form of the parasite produces a different set of proteins. At the same time, once the merozoites have left the hepatocyte and are in the systemic circulation, they are susceptible to attack by the patient's immune system provided it has "learned" to recognize the parasite. Therefore, another site for vaccine development is the merozoite stage. Depending on the *Plasmodium* species, a merozoite vaccine may or may not provide much protection to the liver, but it could reduce subsequent infection of the erythrocytes.

Merozoites in systemic circulation now infect the patient's erythrocytes, where they reside for 3 to 4 days reproducing. The reproduction stage in the erythrocyte can produce either more merozoites or another form, called *gametocytes*. These have different immunological properties from the other forms. Either way, the newly formed merozoites or gametocytes burst out of the infected erythrocytes. The new merozoites infect additional erythrocytes and continue the cycle of reproducing, bursting out of the erythrocytes, and infecting more erythrocytes. The debris from the destroyed erythrocytes is one of the causes of severe fever and chills. Also, the patient's immune system will respond with repeated exposure to the parasite, and this will contribute to the patient's discomfort.

There are four possible sites (Fig. 9-1) for drug therapy at this stage of the disease:

1. Kill the sporozoites injected by the mosquito and/or prevent the sporozoites from entering the liver.
2. Kill the schizonts residing in hepatocytes and/or prevent them from becoming merozoites.
3. Kill the merozoites in the blood and/or prevent them from developing into gametocytes.

4. Kill the gametocytes before they can enter the mosquito and reproduce into zygotes. Some have argued that the focus at this stage should be on the male gametocytes. This would block the female gametocytes from mating.

The conversion of merozoites results in male and female gametocytes. After entering the mosquito, they "mate," producing zygotes in the mosquito stomach. The latter reside in the mosquito's stomach endothelium oocysts. Eventually, they migrate as sporozoites to the mosquito's salivary gland, where the cycle begins again when the mosquito bites a human. So, in effect, there are two reservoirs or vectors for the parasite: the mosquito that infects humans and humans that infect mosquitos. There have been some attempts at developing prophylactic agents that would be in the blood ingested by the mosquito. These drugs would stop further development of the parasite in the mosquito and prevent the insect from being a carrier.

Plasmodium Genome

Just as deciphering the human genome may lead to new therapies, elucidating the genome (genomics) of pathogens and the proteins made by their genes (proteomics) may provide leads for targeting new therapeutic entities. The *P. falciparum* genome consists of 30 million base pairs and 5,000 to 6,000 genes. It is nearly 80% adenine (A)–thymine (T) rich, making it difficult to tally base pairs on the parasite's 14 chromosomes.[14, 15] (In contrast, the human genome is about 59% A–T.) The high A–T content made the *Plasmodium* genome difficult to sequence because *(a)* it was more difficult to slice the chromosomal DNA strands into smaller distinct segments that make it easier to sequence the nucleotides and then reassemble them into chromosome and *(b)* the computer software would fail and had to be modified.[16]

There are at least two goals in decoding the parasite's genome. One is to find a protein that is unique to *Plasmodium* spp. so that a drug is selectively toxic to the protozoan. As seen in the discussion of antimalarial drugs, all have significant adverse reactions. A second goal is to understand the genetic changes that lead to drug resistance. One of the main reasons for the increase in malaria since the late 1990s is the developing resistance to chloroquine, an antimalarial that has been widely used against *P. falciparum*. This resistance is blamed for the increasing mortality rates in Africa and the resurgence of malaria.

Malarial Vaccines

Since the early 1980s, there has been a tremendous effort worldwide to design malaria vaccines, largely based on cell surface proteins of sporozoites, merozoites, or schizonts.[17–31] The use of recombinant DNA techniques to determine the structure of these proteins and to direct their syntheses has been the foundation of most of these studies. Most developmental vaccine work with malaria has centered on *P. falciparum* because it is the primary cause of malaria mortality worldwide.

Three primary lines of research include

- Development of sporozoite–merozoite vaccines to block clinical stages of the disease
- Development of sporozoite vaccines to stop infection and spread of the disease
- Development of vaccines that inactivate or block specific metabolic steps in the parasite after infecting humans

A small field trial of irradiated *P. falciparum* sporozoites produced 90% protection for 10 months. In addition to the fact that plasmodia go through antigenic changes, the parasite is very polymorphic. There is real concern that a vaccine that did not include a spectrum of *Plasmodium* variants could cause development of parasites of even greater virulence.

Polymorphism in the human leukocyte antigen (HLA) system also may be an obstacle to producing an effective vaccine. A potential model for this problem is the observation that T cells, including the cytotoxic T lymphocytes, in patients with HLA-B35 do not respond to certain strains of the parasite. It appears that the combination of certain proteins produced by *Plasmodium* strains with HLA-B35 prevents a normal T-cell response. In other words, the immune system of these patients will respond to some *Plasmodium* strains and not others. The implication is that an effective vaccine will have to be very polyvalent.

That an effective vaccine, even one that only responds to certain *Plasmodium* strains, has not been developed has been puzzling, in that the human immune system does adapt with immunoglobulin-producing B cells and T cells that respond to processed antigen. The innate side of the immune system also responds. In other words, the human immune system responds to the various forms of the *Plasmodium* parasite just as it does to other parasites. It has been suggested that just as the *Plasmodium* genus has adapted to humans, humans have adapted to the parasite. The five human mutations mentioned above are one example. There may be others.

Proper nutrition is important in surviving a malaria attack. The patient must replace the destroyed erythrocytes and, depending on the species of *Plasmodium*, hepatocytes. This requires calories from a high-quality diet that provides essential nutrients including amino acids, lipids, and trace minerals. The severity of malaria is greatest in the areas of the world with malnourishment, poor sanitation, lack of infrastructure to eliminate the mosquito breeding areas, and lack of drugs to treat the sick. The World Health Organization's *2002 World Health Report* scored countries on the basis of their lifestyles and availability of resources. Proper food is one of those resources.[32] In other words, just as the pathology of malaria is complex, so is its control and treatment.

DRUG THERAPY

Antimalarial drugs (see Table 9-1 on pages 296–297) are good examples of anti-infective agents with poor selective toxicity. Contrast them with the antibiotics (Chapter 10). Tetracyclines, chloramphenicol, and aminoglycosides act against bacterial ribosomes, but not mammalian ones. Penicillins and cyclosporines inhibit bacterial cell wall cross-linking, and mammals have cell membranes, not cell walls. The fluoroquinolones inhibit bacterial gyrase, but not mammalian topoisomerases. The biochemistry of *Plasmodium* spp. is similar to that of mammals, making it difficult to design drugs that will not affect the patient adversely. Indeed, some have indications beyond treating and preventing malaria.

CINCHONA ALKALOIDS

The cinchona tree produces four alkaloids that were, until recently, the prototypical molecules on which most antimalarial drugs were based. These alkaloids (Fig. 9-2) are the enantiomeric pair quinine and quinidine and their desmethoxy analogues, cinchonidine (for quinine) and cinchonine (for quinidine). (Unfortunately, the nomenclature for the two series of alkaloids is inconsistent.) Their numbering system is based on rubane. The stereochemistry differs at positions 8 and 9, with quinine and cinchonidine being *S,R* and quinidine (cinchonine) being *R,S*. Historically, quinine was the main treatment for malaria until the advent of World War II, when battle in areas where malaria was endemic led to the search for more effective agents.

Quinine and Quinidine.   Quinine has been used for "fevers" in South America since the 1600s. The pure alkaloids quinine and cinchonine were isolated in 1820. The stereoisomer, quinidine, is a more potent antimalarial, but it also is more toxic (less selectively toxic). Quinine is lethal for all *Plasmodium* schizonts (site 2 in Fig. 9-1) and the gametocytes (site 4) from *P. vivax* and *P. malariae* but not for *P. falciparum*. Today, quinine's spectrum of activity is considered too narrow for prophylactic use, relative to the synthetic agents. The mechanism of action is discussed under "Chloroquine and Chloroquine Phosphate." The mechanism of resistance to quinine is poorly understood and varies with the susceptibility of the parasite to other aminoquinoline antimalarial drugs. Quinine still is indicated for malaria caused by *P. falciparum* resistant to other agents including chloroquine. Many times it is administered in combination with pyrimethamine and sulfadoxine, doxycycline, or mefloquine, depending on the specific form of malaria and geographical location.

Cinchonism is a toxic syndrome. Symptoms start with tinnitus, headache, nausea, and disturbed vision. If administration is not stopped, cinchonism can proceed to involvement of the gastrointestinal tract, nervous and cardiovascular systems, and the skin.

Quinine also is indicated for nocturnal leg cramps, but

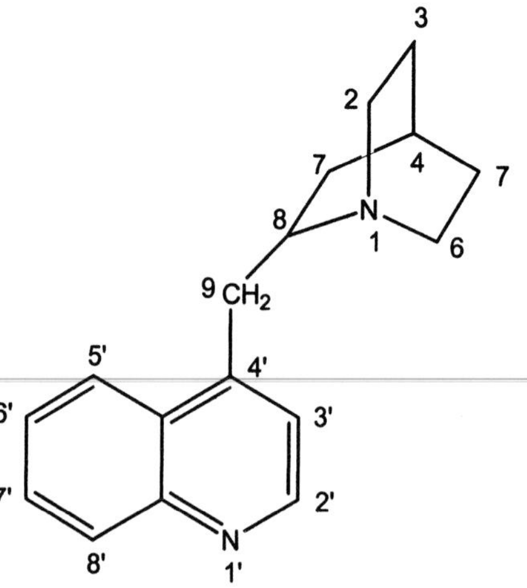

Rubane

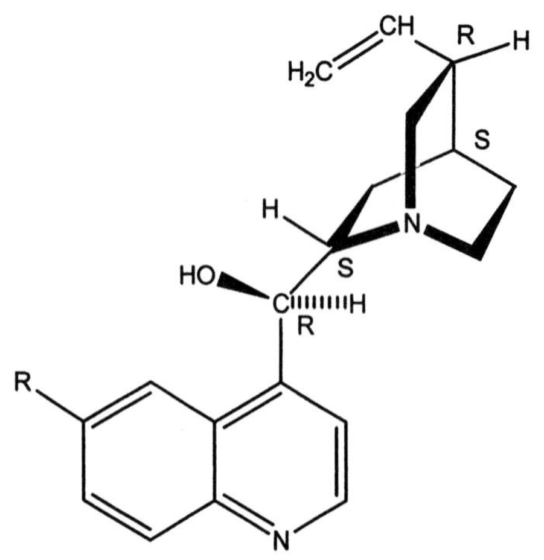

Quinine R = OCH$_3$
Cinchonidine R = H

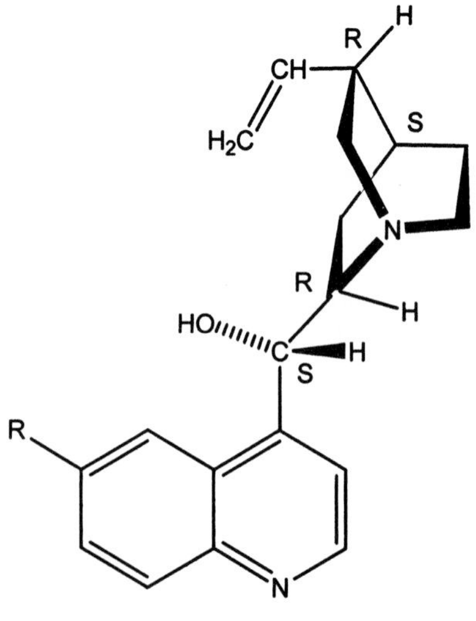

Quinidine R = OCH$_3$
Cinchonine R = H

Figure 9–2 ■ Cinchona alkaloids.

pharmacists must remember that the Food and Drug Administration (FDA) ordered a stop to marketing quinine over the counter for this use because of a lack of proper studies proving its efficacy.

The stereoisomer, quinidine, is schizonticidal, but its primary indication is cardiac arrhythmias. It is a good example of the importance of stereochemistry because it provides a significantly different pharmacological spectrum. Quinidine is discussed further in Chapter 19.

4-Aminoquinolines

The 4-aminoquinolines (Fig. 9-3) are the closest of the antimalarials that are based on the quinine structure. This group is substituted at the same position 4 as quinine and has an asymmetric carbon equivalent to quinine's C-9 position. Just

as with quinine, both isomers are active, and the 4-aminoquinoline racemic mixtures are used. For the newest drug in this series, mefloquine, only the *R,S* isomer is marketed. A significant difference from the commercial cinchona alkaloids is replacing the 6'-methoxy on quinine with a 7-chloro substituent on three of the 4-aminoquinolines. Amodiaquine is no longer used in the United States, and sontoquine has fallen into disuse.

Chloroquine and Chloroquine Phosphate. Chloroquine (Aralen HCl) can be considered the prototypical structure that succeeded quinine and came into use in the mid-1940s. The phosphate salt (Aralen Phosphate) is used in oral dosage forms (tablets), and the hydrochloride salt is administered parenterally. Until recently, chloroquine was

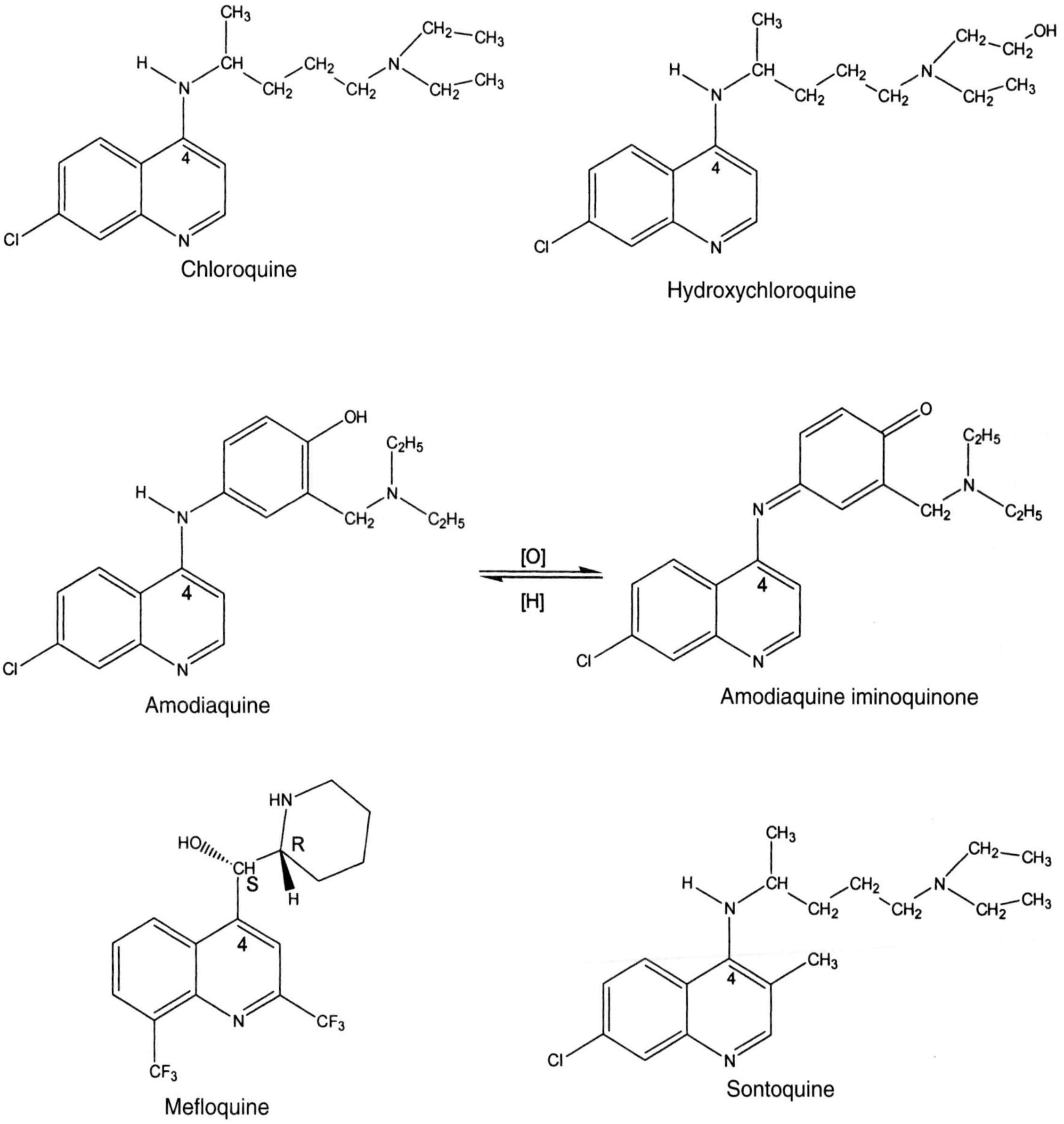

Figure 9–3 ▪ 4-Aminoquinolines.

the main antimalarial drug used both for prophylaxis and treatment. Note that the list of indications for many of the other drugs in this chapter includes *Plasmodium* spp. resistant to chloroquine. It is indicated for *P. vivax, P. malariae, P. ovale,* and susceptible strains of *P. falciparum.* Chloroquine belongs to the 4-aminoquinoline series, of which hundreds have been evaluated, but only about three or four are still in use.

Even though this drug has been used for many years, its mechanism of action is still not known. Its main site of action appears to involve the lysosome of the parasite-infected erythrocyte. The following actions have been suggested on the basis of experimental evidence. A very complex mechanism is based on ferriprotoporphyrin IX, which is released by *Plasmodium*-containing erythrocytes, acting as a chloroquine receptor. The combination of ferriprotoporphyrin IX and chloroquine causes lysis of the parasite's and/or the erythrocyte's membrane. Finally, there is evidence that chloroquine may interfere with *Plasmodium*'s ability to digest the erythrocyte hemoglobin or the parasite's nucleoprotein synthesis. The mechanism is based on the drug entering the erythrocyte's lysosome, which has an acid environment, where it becomes protonated. The protonated (positively charged) chloroquine now is trapped inside the lysosome because the pore that leads out of the lysosome also is positively charged. This leaves chloroquine bound to the patient's hemoglobin, preventing the parasite from processing it properly.[33]

In general, chloroquine and the other 4-aminoquinolines are not effective against exoerythrocytic parasites. Note that each of the mechanisms requires that the parasite be inside the erythrocyte. Therefore, chloroquine does not prevent relapses of *P. vivax* or *P. ovale* malaria. The drug also is indicated for the treatment of extraintestinal amebiasis.

Effective as chloroquine has been, it is a poor example of selective toxicity. Adverse reactions include retinopathy, hemolysis in patients with glucose-6-phosphate dehydrogenase deficiency (same mutation that confers resistance against malaria), muscular weakness, exacerbation of psoriasis and porphyria, and impaired liver function. Further examples of poor selective toxicity include off-label indications such as rheumatoid arthritis, systemic and discoid lupus erythematosus (possibly as an immunosuppressant), and a variety of dermatological conditions.

If the increase in resistance to chloroquine continues, this "reliable" antimalarial drug may no longer be the mainstay of malaria treatment. The increase in *P. falciparum* resistant to chloroquine is considered one of the main reasons for the increases in both incidence and deaths from malaria. Remember that chloroquine resistance is a recent phenomenon that became significant in the mid-1990s. The key *Plasmodium* gene that confers resistance appears to be the *pfcrt* gene, which codes for a transporter protein. The result of the changes in the gene is that the pore through which chloroquine might exit the lysosome no longer is positively charged, allowing protonated chloroquine to exit the lysosome.[33] At least eight mutations have been identified in the *pfcrt* gene, and it is postulated that resistance occurs because of an accumulation of these mutations. Chloroquine remains effective when there are fewer mutations in the *pfcrt* gene. Once the critical number of mutations has occurred, the parasite spreads over a broad geographical area, rendering chloroquine ineffective.[33–35]

Hydroxychloroquine. In most ways, hydroxychloroquine (Plaquenil) parallels chloroquine. Structurally, it differs solely in having a hydroxy moiety on one of the *N*-ethyl groups. Like chloroquine, it remains in the body for over a month, and prophylactic dosing is once weekly. The other indications, both FDA approved and off-label, are very similar.

Amodiaquine. Amodiaquine is listed in USP 25 (2002) but is not covered in the USP-DI for Health Professionals, nor is it on the list of antimalarial drugs recommended by the Centers for Disease Control and Prevention. Mechanistically, it is very similar to chloroquine and does not have any advantages over the other 4-aminoquinoline drugs. When used for prophylaxis of malaria, it was associated with a higher incidence of hepatitis and agranulocytosis than was chloroquine. There is evidence that the hydroquinone (phenol) amine system readily oxidizes to a quinone-imine (Fig. 9-3), antioxidatively and/or metabolically, and this product may contribute to amodiaquine toxicity. The quinone-imine system is similar to the acetaminophen toxic metabolite (Chapters 4 and 22).

Mefloquine HCl. The newest of the 4-aminoquinolines, mefloquine (Lariam), is marketed as the *R,S* isomer. It was developed in the 1960s as part of the U. S. Army's Walter Reed Institute for Medical Research antimalarial research program. It differs significantly from the other agents in this class by having two trifluoromethyl moieties, at positions 2' and 8', and no electronegative substituents at either position 6' (quinine) or 7' (chloroquine). Mefloquine also differs from chloroquine and its analogues by being a schizonticide (site 2 in Fig. 9-1), acting before the parasite can enter the erythrocyte. Some evidence indicates that it acts by raising the pH in the parasite's vesicles, interfering with its ability to process heme. Mefloquine-resistant strains of *P. falciparum* have appeared. Relapse can occur with acute *P. vivax* that has been treated with mefloquine, because the drug does not eliminate the hepatic phase of this species, which can reinfect the liver.

Mefloquine is teratogenic in rats, mice, and rabbits. There is an FDA-required warning that this drug can exacerbate mental disorders, and it is contraindicated in patients with active depression, a recent history of depression, generalized anxiety disorder, psychosis, schizophrenia, and other major psychiatric disorders or a history of convulsions.

8-Aminoquinolines

The other major group of antimalarial drugs based on the cinchona alkaloid quinoline moiety is the substituted 8-aminoquinolines (Fig. 9-4). The first compound introduced in this series was pamaquine. During World War II, pentaquine, isopentaquine, and primaquine became available. Only primaquine, used during the Korean War, is in wide use today. All of the 8-aminoquinolines can cause hemolytic anemia in erythrocytic glucose-6-phosphate dehydrogenase–deficient patients. As pointed out above, this is a common genetic trait found in populations living in areas endemic with malaria, and it provides some resistance to the

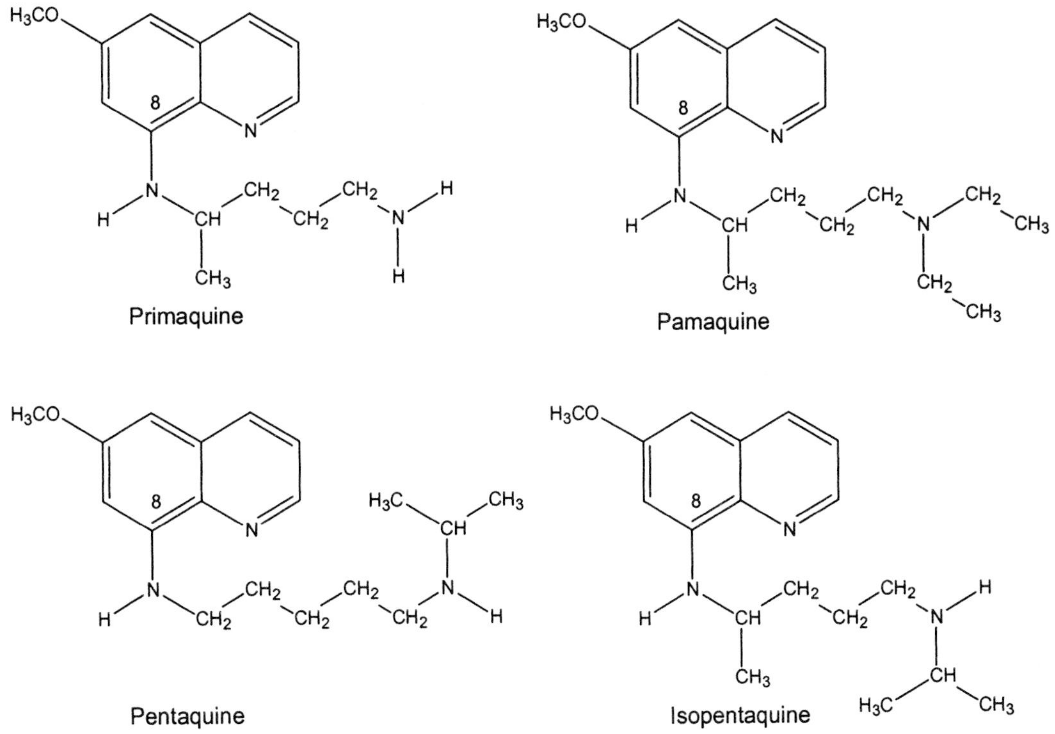

Figure 9–4 ■ 8-Aminoquinolines.

parasite. Its mechanism of action and spectrum of activity are discussed under ''Primaquine.''

Few variations are seen in the structure–activity relationships in this series. All four agents in Figure 9-4 have a 6-methoxy moiety like quinine, but the substituents on quinoline are located at position 8 rather than carbon-4 as found on the cinchona alkaloids. All agents in this series have a four- to five-carbon alkyl linkage or bridge between the two nitrogens. With the exception of pentaquine, the other three 8-aminoquinolines have one asymmetric carbon. While some differences occur in the metabolism of each stereoisomer and type of adverse response, there is little difference in antimalaria activity based on the compounds' stereochemistry.

Primaquine. Primaquine is the only 8-aminoquinoline currently in use for the treatment of malaria. It is not used for prophylaxis. Its spectrum of activity is one of the narrowest of the currently used antimalarial drugs; it is indicated only for exoerythrocytic *P. vivax* malaria (site 2 in Fig. 9-1). To treat endoerythrocytic *P. vivax*, chloroquine or a drug indicated for chloroquine-resistant *P. vivax* is used with primaquine. In addition to its approved indication, it also is active against the exoerythrocytic stages of *P. ovale* and primary exoerythrocytic stages of *P. falciparum*. Primaquine also inhibits the gametocyte stage (site 4 in Fig. 9-1), which eliminates the form required to infect the mosquito carrier. In vitro and in vivo studies indicate that the stereochemistry at the asymmetric carbon is not important for antimalarial activity. There appears to be less toxicity with the levorotatory isomer, but this is dose dependent and may not be that important at the doses used to treat exoerythrocytic *P. vivax* malaria.

Although structurally related to the cinchona alkaloids, the 8-aminoquinolines have a different mechanism of action. Primaquine appears to disrupt the parasite's mitochondria. The result is disruption of several processes, including maturation into the subsequent forms. An advantage is destroying exoerythrocytic forms before the parasite can infect erythrocytes, the step in the infectious process that makes malaria so debilitating.

Fixed Combinations

Because resistance is a frequent problem in the prophylaxis and treatment of malaria, combination therapies that use two

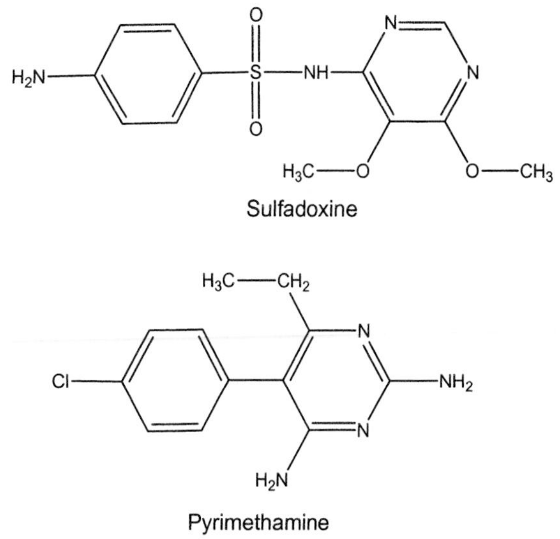

Figure 9–5 ■ Sulfadoxine and pyrimethamine.

distinctly different mechanisms have been developed. One combination inhibits folic acid biosynthesis and dihydrofolate reductase; the other combination acts on the parasite's mitochondria and its dihydrofolate reductase.

Sulfadoxine and Pyrimethamine. The combination of sulfadoxine and pyrimethamine (Fansidar) (Fig. 9-5) uses a drug from the sulfonamide antibacterial group and a pyri-

midinediamine similar to trimethoprim (see Chapter 8). The combination is considered schizonticidal (site 2 in Fig. 9-1). The sulfonamide, sulfadoxine, interferes with the parasite's ability to synthesize folic acid, and the pyrimidinediamine, pyrimethamine, inhibits the reduction of folic acid to its active tetrahydrofolate coenzyme form (Fig. 9-6). Sulfonamides block the incorporation of *p*-aminobenzoic acid (PABA) to form dihydropteroic acid. Note the structures of

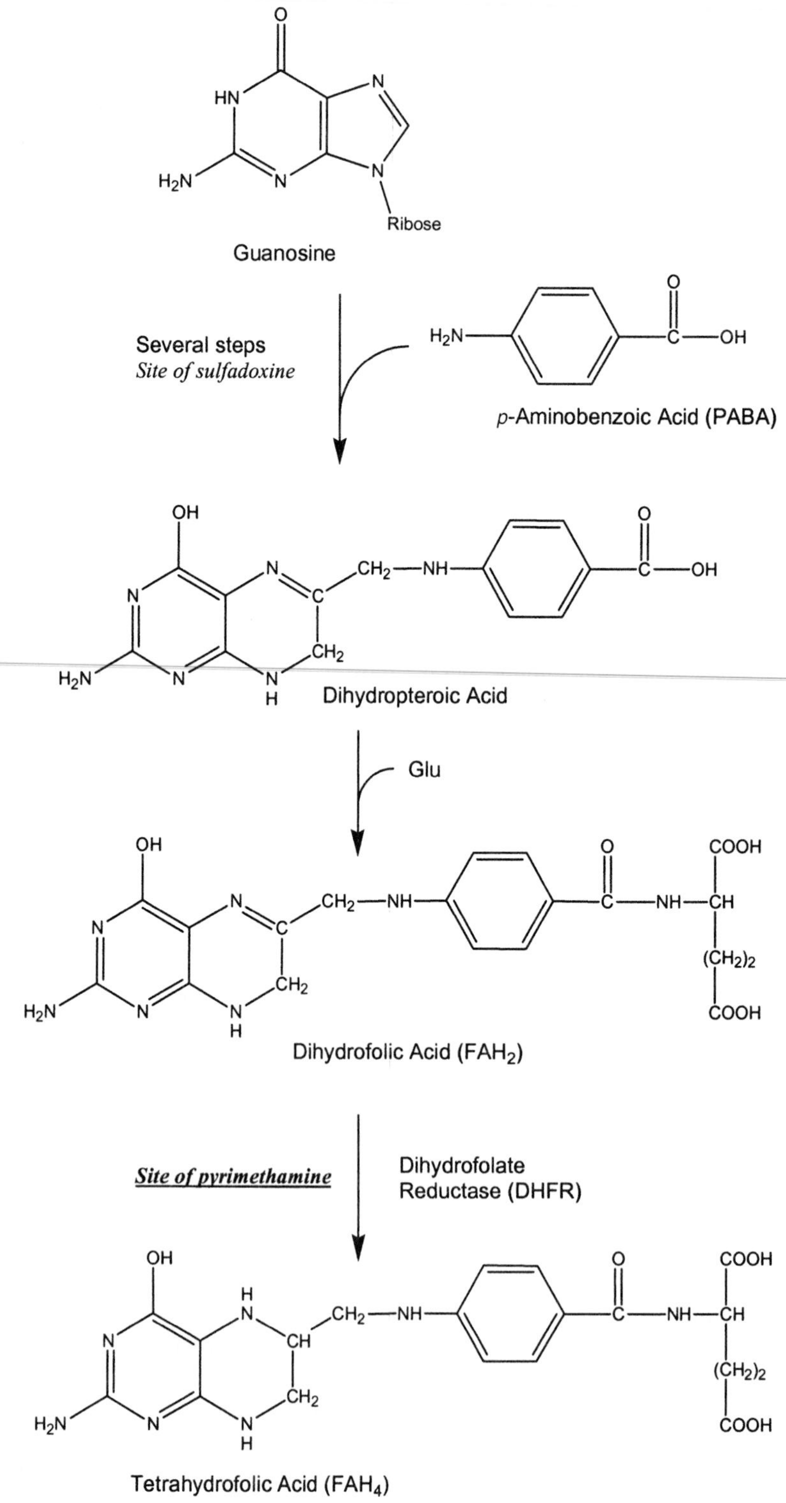

Figure 9–6 ■ Sites where sulfadoxine and pyrimethamine inhibit folate metabolism.

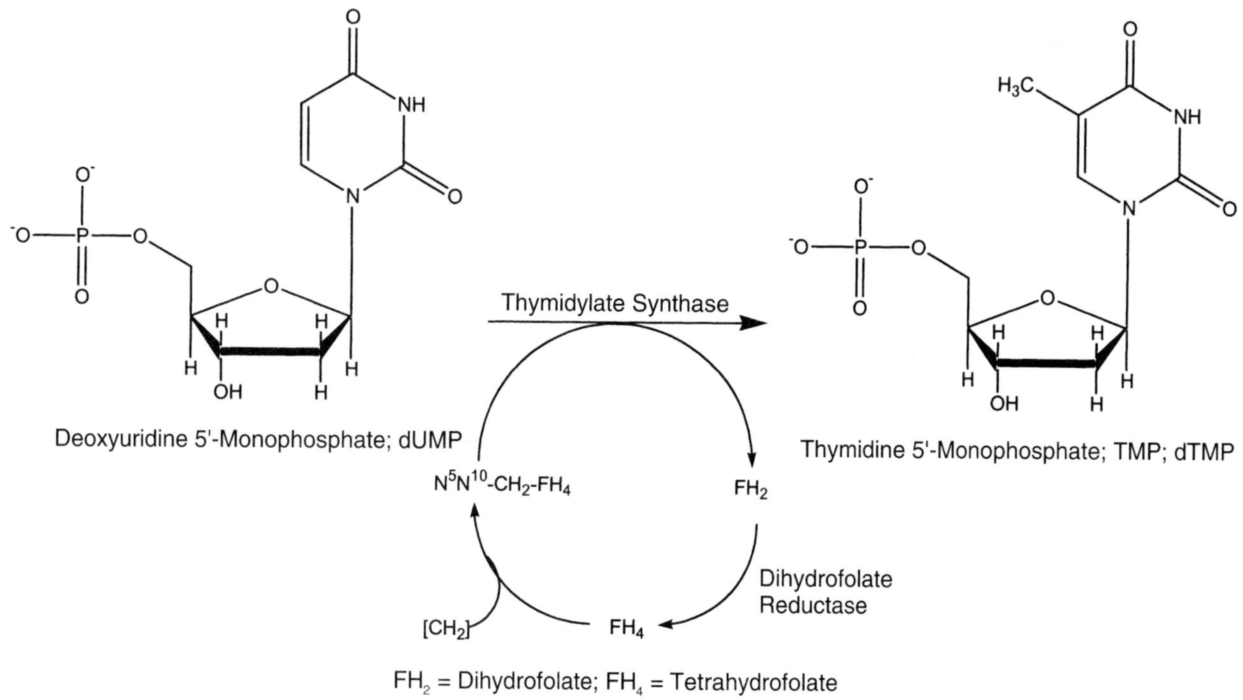

Figure 9–7 ■ Thymidylate synthase.

dihydrofolic acid and tetrahydrofolic acid; PABA is the central part of the folate structure. Normally, sulfonamides exhibit excellent selective toxicity because humans do not synthesize the vitamin folic acid. Nevertheless, there are warnings of severe to fatal occurrences of erythema multiforme, Stevens-Johnson syndrome, toxic epidermal necrolysis, and serum sickness syndromes attributed to the sulfadoxine.

Pyrimethamine, developed in the 1950s, inhibits the reduction of folic acid and dihydrofolic acid to the active tetrahydrofolate coenzyme form. Although the latter is required for many fundamental reactions involving pyrimidine biosynthesis, the focus in the parasite is regeneration of N^5,N^{10}-methylene tetrahydrofolate from dihydrofolate (Fig. 9-7). The synthesis of thymidine 5′-monophosphate from deoxyuridine 5′-monophosphate is a universal reaction in all cells forming DNA. There are enough differences between this enzyme and dihydrofolate reductase found in mammalian, bacterial, and plasmodial cells that folate reductase inhibitors can be developed that show reasonable selective toxicity. In the malaria parasite, the intimate relationship between thymidylate synthase and dihydrofolate reductase means that pyrimethamine can inhibit both enzymes.

This combination is indicated for prophylaxis and treatment of chloroquine-resistant *P. falciparum* and may be used in combination with quinine. Although indicated only for *P. falciparum,* the combination is active against all the asexual erythrocytic forms. It has no activity against the sexual gametocytic form. The fixed combination contains 500 mg of sulfadoxine and 25 mg of pyrimethamine. A wide number of sulfonamides could be used in combination with pyrimethamine. The usual approach is to use a sulfonamide that has pharmacokinetic properties like those of the dihydrofolate reductase inhibitor. For this combination, the peak

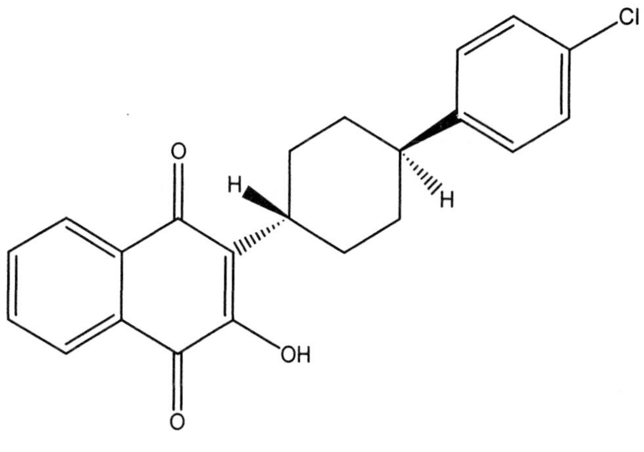

Atovaquone

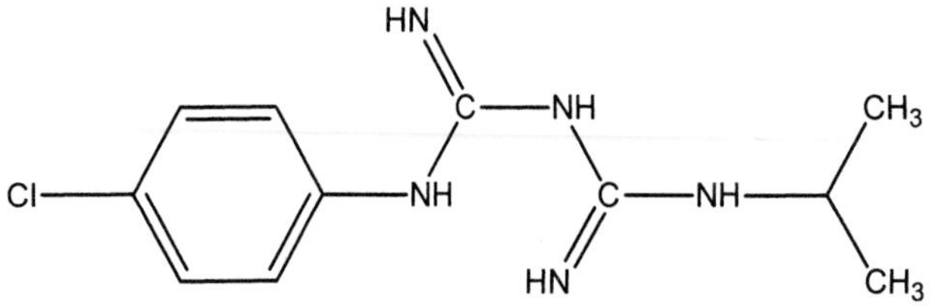

Proguanil

Figure 9–8 ■ Atovaquone and proguanil.

plasma sulfadoxine concentration occurs in 2.5 to 6 hours, and the peak plasma pyrimethamine concentration occurs in 1.5 to 8 hours. Resistance has developed, much of it involving mutations in either or both of the genes coding for dihydrofolate reductase and thymidylate synthase.

Atovaquone and Proguanil HCl. Atovaquone and proguanil HCl (Fig. 9-8) are administered in combination (Malarone) in an atovaquone-to-proguanil HCl ratio of 2.5:1, measured in milligrams (not millimoles). Proguanil, developed in 1945, is an early example of a prodrug. It is metabolized to cycloguanil (Fig. 9-9), primarily by CYP2C19. The polymorphic nature of this hepatic enzyme explains why certain subpopulations do not respond to proguanil; they cannot convert proguanil to the active cycloguanil.

The basis for this combination is two distinct and unrelated mechanisms of action against the parasite. Atovaquone is a selective inhibitor of the *Plasmodium*'s mitochondrial electron transport system, and cycloguanil is a dihydrofolate reductase inhibitor. Atovaquone's chemistry is based on it

being a naphthoquinone that participates in oxidation–reduction reactions as part of its quinone–hydroquinone system. It is patterned after coenzyme Q, found in mitochondrial electron transport chains. The drug selectively interferes with mitochondrial electron transport, particularly at the parasite's cytochrome bc_1 site. This deprives the cell of needed ATP and could cause it to become anaerobic. Resistance to this drug comes from a mutation in the parasite's cytochrome.

Cycloguanil (proguanil) interferes with deoxythymidylate synthesis by inhibiting dihydrofolate reductase (see Fig. 9-6 and the pyrimethamine discussion). Resistance to proguanil/cycloguanil is attributed to amino acid changes near the dihydrofolate reductase binding site. Its elimination half-life (48 to 72 hours) is much shorter than that of the other antimalarial dihydrofolate reductase, pyrimethamine (mean elimination half-life of 111 hours). The combination is effective against both erythrocytic and exoerythrocytic *Plasmodium*. This drug combination is indicated for malaria resistant to chloroquine, halofantrine, mefloquine, and amodiaquine. Its main site is the sporozoite stage (site 1 in Fig. 9-1).

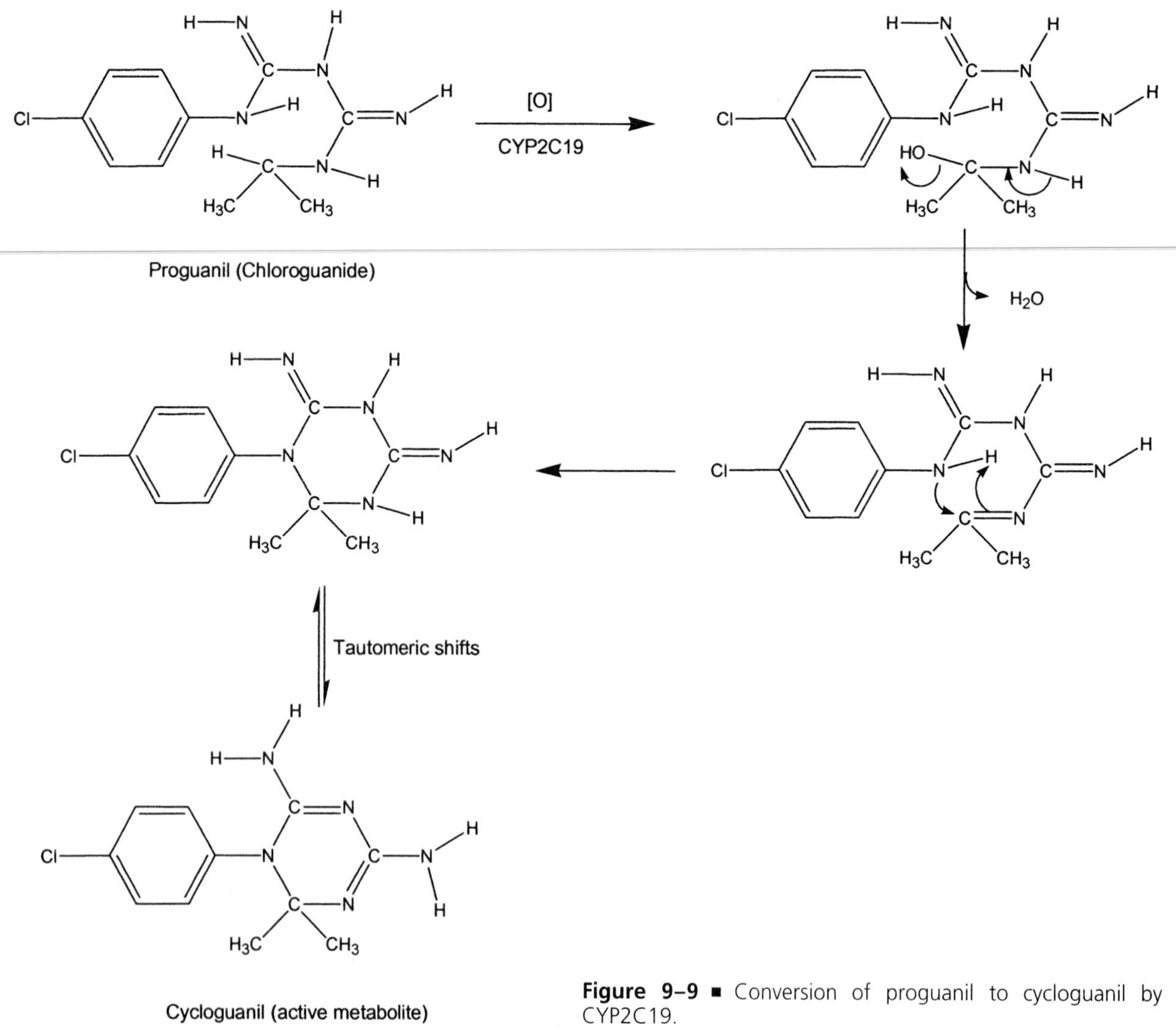

Proguanil (Chloroguanide)

Cycloguanil (active metabolite)

Figure 9–9 ■ Conversion of proguanil to cycloguanil by CYP2C19.

Polycyclic Antimalarial Drugs

Three antimalarial drugs have polycyclic ring systems (Fig. 9-10) in common. The first is the common tetracycline antibiotic, doxycycline. The second is one of the newer drugs indicated for malaria, halofantrine. The third is the discontinued agent used in the South Pacific, aminoacridine.

Doxycycline. Like the other tetracyclines, doxycycline inhibits the pathogen's protein synthesis by reversibly inhibiting the 30S ribosomal subunit. Bacterial and plasmodial ribosomal subunits differ significantly from mammalian ribosomes, and this group of antibiotics does not bind to mammalian ribosomes readily and thus shows good selective toxicity. Although doxycycline is a good antibacterial, its use for malaria is limited to prophylaxis against strains of *P. falciparum* resistant to chloroquine and sulfadoxine–pyrimethamine. This use normally should not exceed 4 months. Because the tetracyclines chelate calcium, they can interfere with development of the permanent teeth in children. Therefore, their use in children definitely should be short term. Also, tetracycline photosensitivity must be kept in mind, particularly since areas where malaria is endemic also are the areas with the greatest sunlight.

Halofantrine. Structurally, halofantrine (Halfan) differs from all other antimalarial drugs. It is a good example of drug design that incorporates bioisosteric principles, as evidenced by the trifluoroethyl moiety. Halofantrine is schiz-

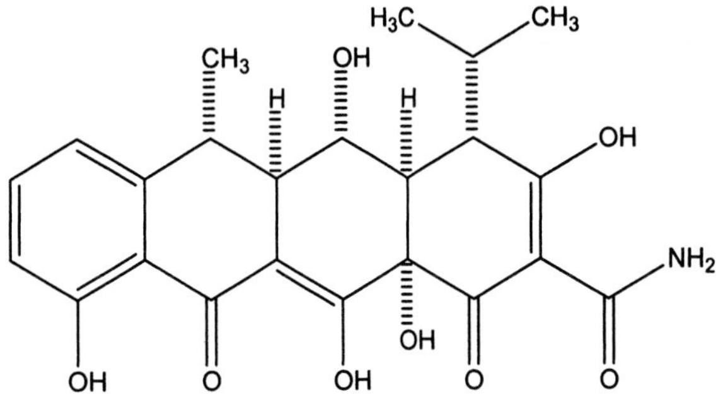

Doxycycline

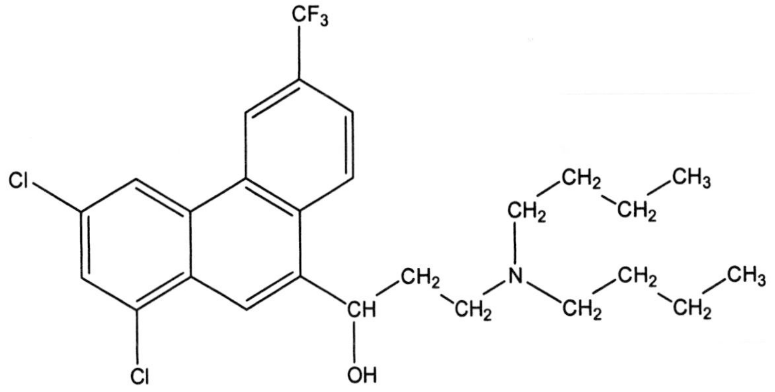

Halofantrine

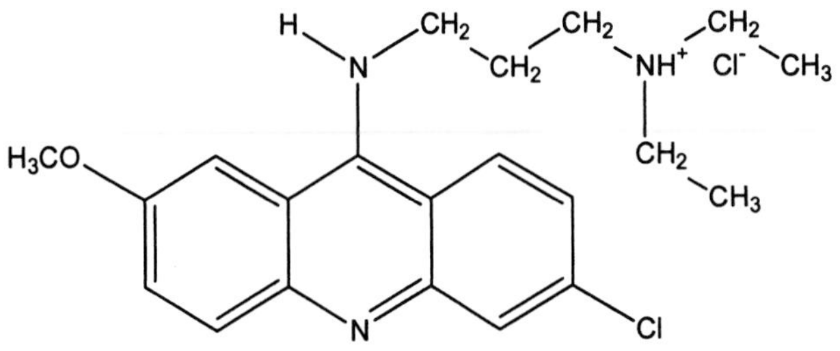

Quinacrine HCl

Figure 9–10 ■ Polycyclic antimalarial drugs.

onticidal (sites 1 and 2 in Fig. 9-1) and has no effect on the sporozoite, gametocyte, or hepatic stages. The parent compound and the *N*-desbutyl metabolite are equally active in vitro. Halofantrine's mechanism of action against the parasite is not known. There is contradictory evidence that its mechanism ranges from requiring heme to disrupting the mitochondria. A prominent warning cautions that halofantrine can affect nerve conduction in cardiac tissue.

Quinacrine HCl.
Quinacrine is no longer available in the United States. It can be considered one of the most toxic of the antimalarial drugs, even though, at one time, it was commonly used. It acts at many sites within the cell, including intercalation of DNA strands, succinic dehydrogenase, mitochondrial electron transport, and cholinesterase. It may be tumorigenic and mutagenic and has been used as a sclerosing agent. Because it is an acridine dye, quinacrine can cause yellow discoloration of the skin and urine.

New Antimalarial Drugs

Artemisinin.
Drugs in the artemisinin series (Fig. 9-11) are the newest of the antimalarial drugs and are structurally unique, compared with the compounds in current use. The parent compound, artemisinin, is a natural product extracted from the dry leaves of *Artemisia annua* (sweet wormwood). The plant must be grown each year from seed because mature plants may lack the active drug. The growing conditions are critical to maximize artemisinin yield. Thus far, the best yields have been obtained from plants grown in North Vietnam, Chongqing region in China, and Tanzania.[36]

All of the structures in Figure 9-11 are active against the *Plasmodium* genera that cause malaria. The key structure characteristic appears to be a "trioxane" consisting of the endoperoxide and doxepin oxygens. This is shown by the somewhat simpler series of 3-aryltrioxanes at the bottom of Figure 9-11, which are active against the parasite. Note that the stereochemistry at position 12 is not critical.[37] While in

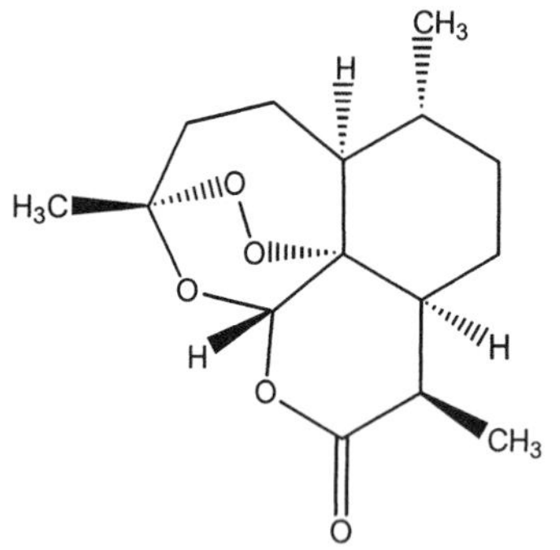

Artemisinin

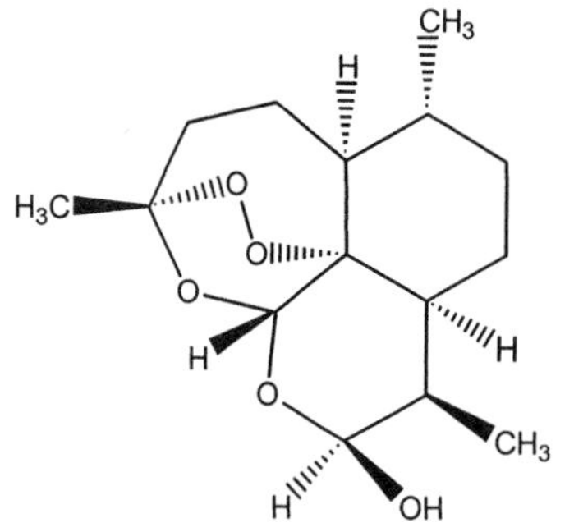

Dihydroartemisinin

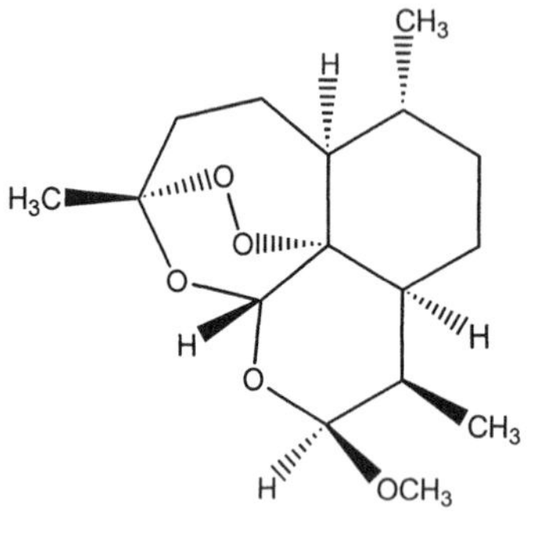

Artemether (oil soluble) R = CH₃
Artemotil (oil soluble) R = CH₂CH₃

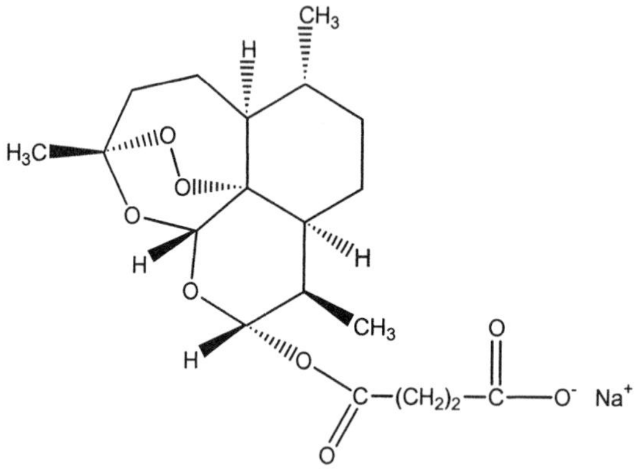

Artesunate (water soluble)

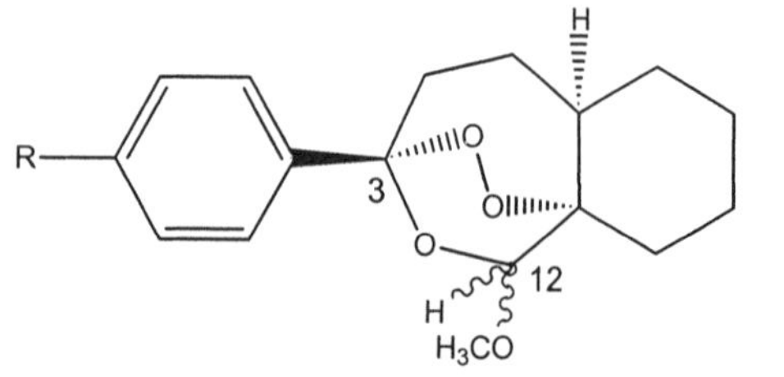

Simplified Aryltrioxanes
R = -F or -COOH

Figure 9–11 ■ Artemisinin and artemisinin-derived compounds.

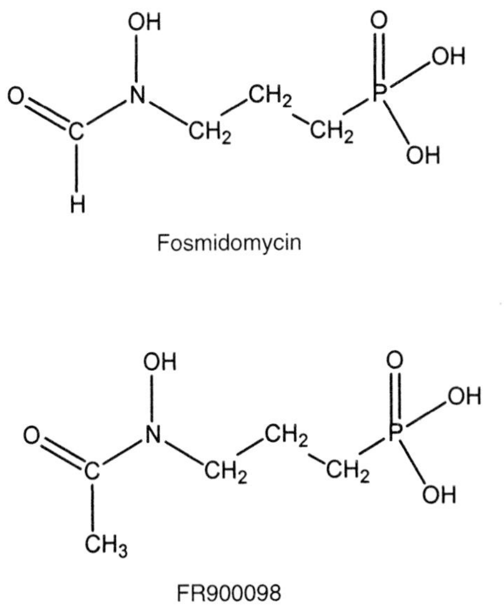

Fosmidomycin

FR900098

Figure 9–12 ▪ Fosmidomycin and a fosmidomycin analogue.

the victim's erythrocyte, the malaria parasite consumes the hemoglobin consisting of ferrous (Fe^{+2}) iron, converting it to toxic hematin containing ferric (Fe^{+3}) iron, then reduced to heme with its ferrous iron. The heme iron reacts with the trioxane moiety, releasing reactive oxygen and carbon radicals and the highly reactive $Fe^{IV}=O$ species. The latter is postulated to be lethal to the parasite.[38, 39]

With the reduction of artemisinin to dihydroartemisinin, an asymmetric carbon forms, and it is possible to form oil-soluble and water-soluble prodrugs. Both stereoisomers are active, just as with the simpler aryltrioxanes. The chemistry forming each of the artemisinin prodrugs results in the predominance of one isomer. The β isomer predominates when producing the nonpolar methyl and ethyl ethers, whereas the α isomer is the predominant product when forming the water-soluble hemisuccinate ester. The latter can be administered as 10-mg rectal capsules for patents who cannot take medication orally and when parenteral treatment is not available.

Fosmidomycin. Fosmidomycin (Fig. 9-12) was isolated from a *Streptomyces* fermentation broth in 1980. Its

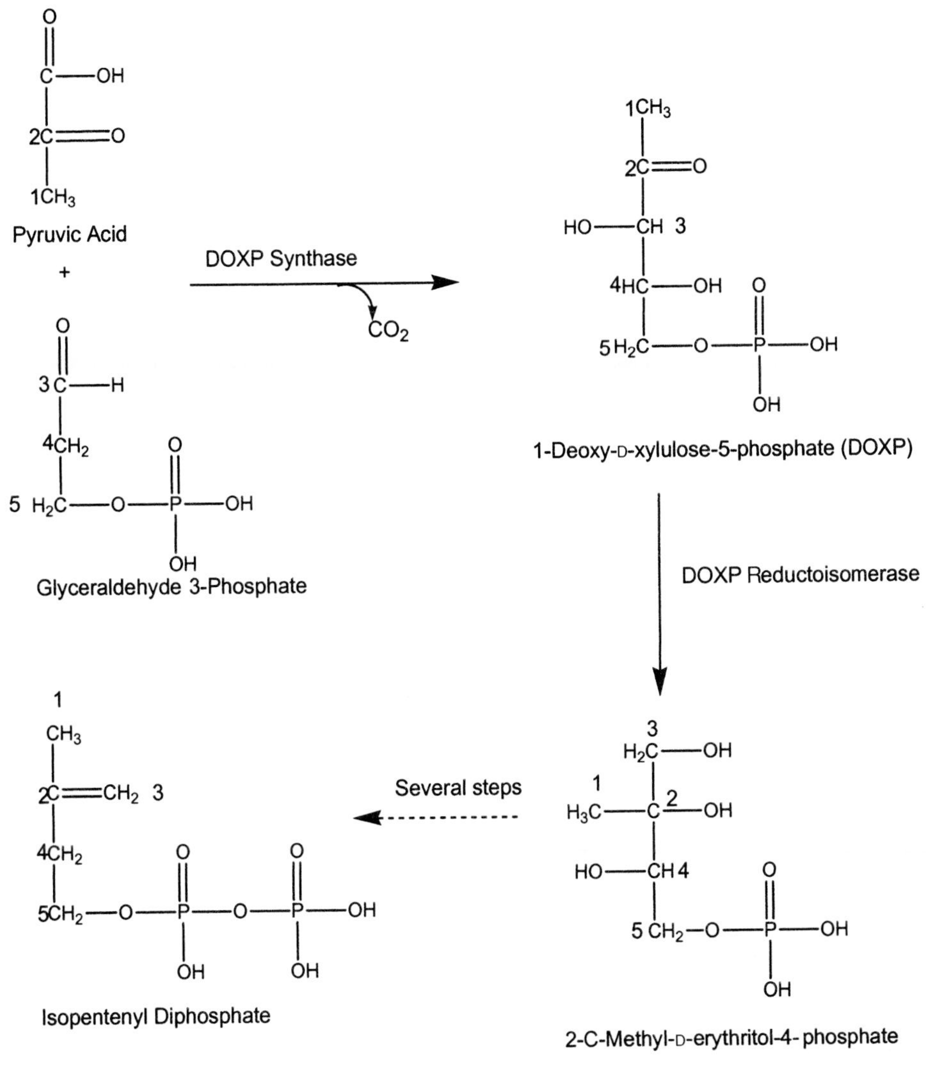

Figure 9–13 ▪ Nonmevalonate pathway.

TABLE 9–1   Summary of Current Drugs Used to Prevent and Treat Malaria

Class	Generic Name	Indications for Malaria	Other Indications	Dosing Ranges for Treatment and Prophylaxis of Malaria
Cinchona alkaloids	Quinine	Chloroquine-resistant *P. falciparum*; combination with other antimalarials; not indicated for prophylaxis	Nocturnal leg cramps (see FDA warnings)	*Adults:* 260–650 mg t.i.d. for 6–12 days *Children:* 10 mg/kg every 8 hours for 5–7 days
	Quinidine	Not indicated for malaria in the United States	Cardiac arrhythmias	
4-Aminoquinolines	Chloroquine	Prophylaxis and treatment of *P. vivax, P. malariae,* and *P. ovale* malaria and susceptible strains of *P. falciparum* malaria	Extraintestinal (liver) amebiasis; the following indications are not approved in the United States: • Forms of hypercalcemia • Rheumatoid arthritis • Discoid and systemic lupus erythematosus • Porphyria cutanea tarda • Solar urticaria	Doses are expressed as chloroquine base equivalent *Prophylaxis for children:* 5 mg/kg weekly up to a maximum of 300 mg *Prophylaxis for adults:* 300 mg weekly See CDC for current recommendations for treatment of acute attacks
	Hydroxychloroquine	Prophylaxis and treatment of *P. vivax, P. malariae,* and *P. ovale* malaria and susceptible strains of *P. falciparum* malaria	Rheumatoid arthritis Discoid and systemic lupus erythematosus The following indications are not approved in the United States: • Forms of hypercalcemia • Porphyria cutanea tarda • Solar urticaria	Doses are expressed as hydroxy chloroquine base equivalent *Prophylaxis for children:* 5 mg/kg weekly up to a maximum adult dose *Prophylaxis for adults:* 310 mg weekly on the same day; begin 1–2 weeks prior to exposure and continue for 4 weeks after leaving the endemic area See CDC for current recommendations for treatment of acute attacks
	Mefloquine	Prophylaxis of *P. falciparum* (including chloroquine-resistant strains) and *P. vivax* malaria; treatment of *P. falciparum* and *P. vivax* malaria	None	*Prophylaxis for children:* 62–250 mg weekly, based on weight starting 1 week before travel and continuing for 4 weeks after leaving the endemic area *Prophylaxis for adults:* 250 mg weekly for 4 weeks, then 250 mg every other week, starting 1 week before travel and continuing for 4 weeks after leaving the endemic area *Treatment for adults:* 1,250 mg as a single dose taken with food and at least 240 mL water
8-Aminoquinolines	Primaquine	Prophylaxis and treatment of *P. vivax*	None	Begin treatment during the past 2 weeks or after stopping therapy with chloroquine or other antimalarial drug *Children:* 0.5 mg/kg per day for 14 days *Adults:* 26.3 mg daily for 14 days

(Continued)

TABLE 9–1—*Continued*

Class	Generic Name	Indications for Malaria	Other Indications	Dosing Ranges for Treatment and Prophylaxis of Malaria
Fixed combinations	Sulfadoxine and pyrimethamine	Prophylaxis and treatment of chloroquine-resistant *P. falciparum*	None	Each tablet contains 500 mg sulfadoxine and 25 mg pyrimethamine
				Prophylaxis: Begin 1–2 days prior to departure and continue for 4–6 weeks after return
				Children: $^1/_4$ to $1^1/_2$ tablets based on age and whether administered once or twice weekly
				Adults: 1–2 tablets once or twice weekly
				Treatment for children: $^1/_2$ to 2 tablets based on age during an attack
				Treatment for adults: 2–3 tablets during an attack
	Atovaquone and proguanil	Prophylaxis and treatment of *P. falciparum* resistant to other antimalarial drugs	None	*Adult tablet:* 250 mg atovaquone and 100 mg proguanil
				Pediatric tablet: 62.5 mg atovaquone and 25 mg proguanil
				Prophylaxis: Begin 1–2 days prior to departure and continue for 7 days after return
				Children: 1–3 pediatric tablets as a single daily dose based on weight
				Adults: 1 adult tablet daily
				Treatment: Take as a single dose for 3 consecutive days
				Children: 1–3 pediatric tablets as a single daily dose based on weight
				Adults: 4 tablets as a single daily dose for 3 consecutive days
Polycyclics	Doxycycline	Prophylaxis against *P. falciparum* strains resistant to chloroquine and sulfadoxine–pyrimethamine	Bacteria infections	Prophylaxis only beginning 1–2 days before travel and for 4 weeks after leaving the area; total use normally does not exceed 4 months
				Children: 2 mg/kg per day up to 100 mg/day
				Adults: 100 mg once daily
	Halofantrine	Treatment of *P. falciparum* and *P. vivax*	None	*Adults:* 500 mg every 6 hours for 3 doses (1,500 mg), repeated 7 days later
				Children: 250–375 mg based on body weight; follow the same schedule as adults
Newest drug	Artemisinin	Appears effective against all *Plasmodium* species including *P. falciparum* and *P. vivax*	None	Not yet specified
Possible new drug	Fosmidomycin and related compounds	Most reports specify *Plasmodium* species that infect rodents	Other microorganisms that have the nonmevalonate pathway	Not yet specified

selective toxicity is based on inhibiting a biochemical pathway not found in humans and mammals in general—the nonmevalonate pathway to form isoprenoids. Mammals, including humans, form their isoprenoids solely by the mevalonic acid pathway. Many microorganisms have both pathways. Whereas the mevalonate pathway starts with three molecules of acetyl-CoA forming 3-hydroxy-3-methylglutaryl coenzyme A (HMG-CoA) followed by reduction to mevalonic acid by HMG-CoA reductase (site of the statin drugs), the nonmevalonate pathway is carbohydrate based (Fig. 9-13). Condensation of pyruvate and glyceraldehyde 3-phosphate by 1-deoxy-D-xylulose-5-phosphate (DOXP) synthase produces the five carbon DOXP, which undergoes a complex reduction and isomerization to form 2-C-methyl-D-erythritol-4-phosphate. The enzyme for this reaction, DOXP reductoisomerase, is inhibited by fosmidomycin. The basic five-carbon isoprene unit, isopentenyl diphosphate, concludes the pathway. The atoms have been numbered to help follow the isomerization of the deoxy-xylulose intermediate to form the erythritol compound. The malarial parasite only has the nonmevalonate pathway, and initial studies show that fosmidomycin is relatively nontoxic in humans.[40] Replacement of fosmidomycin's *N*-aldehyde with an acetate produces a very active antimalarial agent that has been designated FR900098.[41] As this chapter went to press, fosmidomycin and analogues were in phase I and II trials.

REFERENCES

1. Editors: Sci. Am. 286:8, 14, 38–45, 102–103, 2002.
2. Honigsbaum, M.: Men, Money and Malaria. New York, Farrar, Straus & Giroux, 2002.
3. Pennisi, E.: Science 293:416–417, 2001.
4. Tishkoff, S. A., Varkonyi, R., Cahinhinan, N., et al.: Science 293: 455–462, 2001.
5. Luzzatto L., and Notaro R.: Science 293:442–443, 2001.
6. Volkman, S., Barry, A. E., Lyons, E. J, et al.: Science 293:482–484, 2001.
7. Bynum, W. F.: Science 295:47–48, 2002.
8. www.cdc.gov/travel
9. Pombo, D. J., Lawrence, G., Hirunpetcharat, C., et al.: Lancet: 360: 610, 2002.
10. Van den Bossche, H.: Nature 273:626, 1978.
11. Hoffman, S. L.: Science 290:1509, 2000.
12. Pennisi, E.: Science 294:1439, 2001.
13. Hobbs, M. R., Udhayakumar, V., Levesque, M. C., et al.: Lancet 360: 1468, 2002.
14. Enserink, M., and Pennisi, E.: Science 295:207, 2002.
15. Maher, B. A.: Scientist 16:28, 2002.
16. Pennisi, E.: Science 298:33, 2002.
17. Patarroyo, M. E., et al.: Nature 332:58, 1988.
18. Cox, F. E. G.: Nature 333:702, 1988.
19. Certa, U., et al.: Science 240:1036, 1988.
20. Sinigaglia, F., et al.: Nature 336:778, 1988.
21. Cherfas, J.: Science 247:402, 1990.
22. Young, J. F., et al.: Microb. Pathol. 2:237, 1987.
23. Sadoff, J. C., et al.: Science 240:336, 1988.
24. Crisanti, A., et al.: Science 240:1324, 1988.
25. Kaslow, D. C., et al.: Nature 333:74, 1988.
26. Bruce-Chwatt, L. J.: Lancet 1:371, 1987.
27. Hoffman, S. L., et al.: N. Engl. J. Med. 315:601, 1986.
28. Brown, G. V.: Med. J. Aust. 144:703, 1986.
29. McGregor, I.: Parasitol. Today 1:31, 1985.
30. Marx, J. L.: Science 225:607, 1984.
31. Long, C. A., and Hoffman, S. L.: Science 297:345, 2002.
32. World Heath Organization: The World Health Report 2002, available as a PDF file at: http://www.who.int/whr/en/.
33. Warhurst, D. C., Craig, J. C., and Adagu, I. S.: Lancet 360:9345, 2002.
34. Hastings, I. M., Bray, P. G., and Ward, S. A.: Science 298:74, 2002.
35. Sidhu, A. B. S., Verider-Pinard, D., and Fidock, D. A.: Science 298: 210, 2002.
36. http://www.dafra.be/english/artemisinin.html.
37. Posner, G. H., Jeon, H. B., Parker, M. H., et al.: J. Med. Chem. 44: 3054, 2001.
38. Posner, G. H., Cummings, J. N., Ploypradith, P., and Oh, C.: J. Am. Chem. Soc. 117:5885, 1995.
39. Posner, G. H., Park, S. B., González, L., et al.: J. Am. Chem. Soc. 118:3537, 1996.
40. Jomaa, H., Wiesner, J., Sanderbrand, S., et al.: Science 285:1573, 1999.
41. Reichenberg, A., Wiesner, J., Weidemeyer, C., et al.: Bioorg. Med. Chem. Lett. 11:833, 2001.

SELECTED READING

Honigsbaum, M.: The Fever Trail: In Search of the Cure for Malaria. New York, Farrar, Straus & Giroux, 2001.
Science 298(5591), October 4, 2002. (This issue reports the genome of the *Anopheles gambiae* mosquito and includes discussion of how this knowledge might be used to prevent malaria.)
World Heath Organization: The World Health Report 2002, available as a PDF file at: *http://www.who.int/whr/en/*.

C H A P T E R **10**

Antibacterial Antibiotics

JOHN M. BEALE, JR.

HISTORICAL BACKGROUND

Sir Alexander Fleming's accidental discovery of the antibacterial properties of penicillin in 1929[1] is largely credited with initiating the modern antibiotic era. Not until 1938, however, when Florey and Chain introduced penicillin into therapy, did practical medical exploitation of this important discovery begin to be realized. Centuries earlier, humans had learned to use crude preparations empirically for the topical treatment of infections, which we now assume to be effective because of the antibiotic substances present. As early as 500 to 600 BC, molded curd of soybean was used in Chinese folk medicine to treat boils and carbuncles. Moldy cheese had also been used for centuries by Chinese and Ukrainian peasants to treat infected wounds. The discovery by Pasteur and Joubert in 1877 that anthrax bacilli were killed when grown in culture in the presence of certain bacteria, along with similar observations by other microbiologists, led Vuillemin[2] to define *antibiosis* (literally "against life") as the biological concept of survival of the fittest, in which one organism destroys another to preserve itself. The word *antibiotic* was derived from this root. The use of the term by the lay public, as well as the medical and scientific communities, has become so widespread that its original meaning has become obscured.

In 1942, Waksman[3] proposed the widely cited definition that "an antibiotic or antibiotic substance is a substance produced by microorganisms, which has the capacity of inhibiting the growth and even of destroying other microorganisms." Later proposals[4–6] have sought both to expand and to restrict the definition to include any substance produced by a living organism that is capable of inhibiting the growth or survival of one or more species of microorganisms in low concentrations. The advances made by medicinal chemists to modify naturally occurring antibiotics and to prepare synthetic analogues necessitated the inclusion of semisynthetic and synthetic derivatives in the definition. Therefore, a substance is classified as an antibiotic if the following conditions are met:

1. It is a product of metabolism (although it may be duplicated or even have been anticipated by chemical synthesis).
2. It is a synthetic product produced as a structural analogue of a naturally occurring antibiotic.
3. It antagonizes the growth or survival of one or more species of microorganisms.
4. It is effective in low concentrations.

The isolation of the antibacterial antibiotic tyrocidin from the soil bacterium *Bacillus brevis* by Dubois suggested the probable existence of many antibiotic substances in nature and provided the impetus for the search for them. An organized search of the order Actinomycetales led Waksman and associates to isolate streptomycin from *Streptomyces griseus*. The discovery that this antibiotic possessed in vivo activity against *Mycobacterium tuberculosis* in addition to numerous species of Gram-negative bacilli was electrifying. It was now evident that soil microorganisms would provide a rich source of antibiotics. Broad screening programs were instituted to find antibiotics that might be effective in the treatment of infections hitherto resistant to existing chemotherapeutic agents, as well as to provide safer and more effective chemotherapy. The discoveries of broad-spectrum antibacterial antibiotics such as chloramphenicol and the tetracyclines, antifungal antibiotics such as nystatin and griseofulvin (see Chapter 8), and the ever-increasing number of antibiotics that may be used to treat infectious agents that have developed resistance to some of the older antibiotics attest to the spectacular success of this approach as it has been applied in research programs throughout the world.

CURRENT STATUS

Commercial and scientific interest in the antibiotic field has led to the isolation and identification of antibiotic substances that may be numbered in the thousands. Numerous semisynthetic and synthetic derivatives have been added to the total. Very few such compounds have found application in general medical practice, however, because in addition to the ability to combat infections or neoplastic disease, an antibiotic must possess other attributes. First, it must exhibit sufficient selective toxicity to be decisively effective against pathogenic microorganisms or neoplastic tissue, on the one hand, without causing significant toxic effects, on the other. Second, an antibiotic should be chemically stable enough to be isolated, processed, and stored for a reasonable length of time without deterioration of potency. The amenability of an antibiotic for oral or parenteral administration to be converted into suitable dosage forms to provide active drug in vivo is also important. Third, the rates of biotransformation and elimination of the antibiotic should be slow enough to allow a convenient dosing schedule, yet rapid and complete enough to facilitate removal of the drug and its metabolites from the body soon after administration has been discontinued. Some groups of antibiotics, because of certain unique properties, have been designated for specialized uses, such as the treatment of tuberculosis or fungal infections. Others are used for cancer chemotherapy. These antibiotics are described along with other drugs of the same therapeutic class: antifungal and antitubercular antibiotics are discussed in Chapter 8, and antineoplastic antibiotics are discussed in Chapter 12.

The spectacular success of antibiotics in the treatment of

human diseases has prompted the expansion of their use into a number of related fields. Extensive use of their antimicrobial power is made in veterinary medicine. The discovery that low-level administration of antibiotics to meat-producing animals resulted in faster growth, lower mortality, and better quality has led to the use of these products as feed supplements. Several antibiotics are used to control bacterial and fungal diseases of plants. Their use in food preservation is being studied carefully. Indeed, such uses of antibiotics have necessitated careful studies of their long-term effects on humans and their effects on various commercial processes. For example, foods that contain low-level amounts of antibiotics may be able to produce allergic reactions in hypersensitive persons, or the presence of antibiotics in milk may interfere with the manufacture of cheese.

The success of antibiotics in therapy and related fields has made them one of the most important products of the drug industry today. The quantity of antibiotics produced in the United States each year may now be measured in several millions of pounds and valued at billions of dollars. With research activity stimulated to find new substances to treat viral infections that now are combated with only limited success and with the promising discovery that some antibiotics are active against cancers that may be viral in origin, the future development of more antibiotics and the increase in the amounts produced seem to be assured.

COMMERCIAL PRODUCTION

The commercial production of antibiotics for medicinal use follows a general pattern, differing in detail for each antibiotic. The general scheme may be divided into six steps: *(a)* preparation of a pure culture of the desired organism for use in inoculation of the fermentation medium; *(b)* fermentation,

during which the antibiotic is formed; *(c)* isolation of the antibiotic from the culture medium; *(d)* purification; *(e)* assays for potency, sterility, absence of pyrogens, and other necessary data; and *(f)* formulation into acceptable and stable dosage forms.

SPECTRUM OF ACTIVITY

The ability of some antibiotics, such as chloramphenicol and the tetracyclines, to antagonize the growth of numerous pathogens has resulted in their designation as *broad-spectrum* antibiotics. Designations of spectrum of activity are of somewhat limited use to the physician, unless they are based on clinical effectiveness of the antibiotic against specific microorganisms. Many of the broad-spectrum antibiotics are active only in relatively high concentrations against some of the species of microorganisms often included in the "spectrum."

MECHANISMS OF ACTION

The manner in which antibiotics exert their actions against susceptible organisms varies. The mechanisms of action of some of the more common antibiotics are summarized in Table 10-1. In many instances, the mechanism of action is not fully known; for a few (e.g., penicillins), the site of action is known, but precise details of the mechanism are still under investigation. The biochemical processes of microorganisms are a lively subject for research, for an understanding of those mechanisms that are peculiar to the metabolic systems of infectious organisms is the basis for the future development of modern chemotherapeutic agents. Antibiotics that

TABLE 10–1 Mechanisms of Antibiotic Action

Site of Action	Antibiotic	Process Interrupted	Type of Activity
Cell wall	Bacitracin	Mucopeptide synthesis	Bactericidal
	Cephalosporins	Cell wall cross-linking	Bactericidal
	Cycloserine	Synthesis of cell wall peptides	Bactericidal
	Penicillin	Cell wall cross-linking	Bactericidal
	Vancomycin	Mucopeptide synthesis	Bactericidal
Cell membrane	Amphotericin B	Membrane function	Fungicidal
	Nystatin	Membrane function	Fungicidal
	Polymyxins	Membrane integrity	Bactericidal
Ribosomes	Chloramphenicol	Protein synthesis	Bacteriostatic
50S subunit	Erythromycin	Protein synthesis	Bacteriostatic
	Lincomycins	Protein synthesis	Bacteriostatic
30S subunit	Aminoglycosides	Protein synthesis and fidelity	Bactericidal
	Tetracyclines	Protein synthesis	Bacteriostatic
Nucleic acids	Actinomycin	DNA and mRNA synthesis	Pancidal
	Griseofulvin	Cell division, microtubule assembly	Fungistatic
DNA and/or RNA	Mitomycin C	DNA synthesis	Pancidal
	Rifampin	mRNA synthesis	Bactericidal

interfere with the metabolic systems found in microorganisms and not in mammalian cells are the most successful anti-infective agents. For example, antibiotics that interfere with the synthesis of bacterial cell walls have a high potential for selective toxicity. Some antibiotics structurally resemble some essential metabolites of microorganisms, which suggests that competitive antagonism may be the mechanism by which they exert their effects. Thus, cycloserine is believed to be an antimetabolite for D-alanine, a constituent of bacterial cell walls. Many antibiotics selectively interfere with microbial protein synthesis (e.g., the aminoglycosides, tetracyclines, macrolides, chloramphenicol, and lincomycin) or nucleic acid synthesis (e.g., rifampin). Others, such as the polymyxins and the polyenes, are believed to interfere with the integrity and function of microbial cell membranes. The mechanism of action of an antibiotic determines, in general, whether the agent exerts a bactericidal or a bacteriostatic action. The distinction may be important for the treatment of serious, life-threatening infections, particularly if the natural defense mechanisms of the host are either deficient or overwhelmed by the infection. In such situations, a bactericidal agent is obviously indicated. Much work remains to be done in this area, and as mechanisms of action are revealed, the development of improved structural analogues of effective antibiotics probably will continue to increase.

CHEMICAL CLASSIFICATION

The chemistry of antibiotics is so varied that a chemical classification is of limited value. Some similarities can be found, however, indicating that some antibiotics may be the products of similar mechanisms in different organisms and that these structurally similar products may exert their activities in a similar manner. For example, several important antibiotics have in common a macrolide structure, i.e., a large lactone ring. This group includes erythromycin and oleandomycin. The tetracycline family comprises a group of compounds very closely related chemically. Several compounds contain closely related amino sugar moieties, such as those found in streptomycins, kanamycins, neomycins, paromomycins, and gentamicins. The antifungal antibiotics nystatin and the amphotericins (see Chapter 8) are examples of a group of conjugated polyene compounds. The bacitracins, tyrothricin, and polymyxin are among a large group of polypeptides that exhibit antibiotic action. The penicillins and cephalosporins are β-lactam-ring–containing antibiotics derived from amino acids.

MICROBIAL RESISTANCE

The normal biological processes of microbial pathogens are varied and complex. Thus, it seems reasonable to assume that there are many ways in which they may be inhibited and that different microorganisms that elaborate antibiotics antagonistic to a common "foe" produce compounds that are chemically dissimilar and that act on different processes. In fact, nature has produced many chemically different antibiotics that can attack the same microorganism by different pathways. The diversity of antibiotic structure has proved to be of real clinical value. As the pathogenic cell develops drug resistance, another antibiotic, attacking another metabolic process of the resisting cell, remains effective. The development of new and different antibiotics has been very important in providing the means for treating resistant strains of organisms that previously had been susceptible to an older antibiotic. More recently, the elucidation of biochemical mechanisms of microbial resistance to antibiotics, such as the inactivation of penicillins and cephalosporins by β-lactamase-producing bacteria, has stimulated research in the development of semisynthetic analogues that resist microbial biotransformation. The evolution of *nosocomial* (hospital-acquired) strains of staphylococci resistant to penicillin and of Gram-negative bacilli (e.g., *Pseudomonas* and *Klebsiella* spp., *Escherichia coli*, and others) often resistant to several antibiotics has become a serious medical problem. No doubt, the promiscuous and improper use of antibiotics has contributed to the emergence of resistant bacterial strains. The successful control of diseases caused by resistant strains of bacteria will require not only the development of new and improved antibiotics but also the rational use of available agents.

β-LACTAM ANTIBIOTICS

Antibiotics that possess the β-lactam (a four-membered cyclic amide) ring structure are the dominant class of agents currently used for the chemotherapy of bacterial infections. The first antibiotic to be used in therapy, penicillin (penicillin G or benzyl penicillin), and a close biosynthetic relative, phenoxymethyl penicillin (penicillin V), remain the agents of choice for the treatment of infections caused by most species of Gram-positive bacteria. The discovery of a second major group of β-lactam antibiotics, the cephalosporins, and chemical modifications of naturally occurring penicillins and cephalosporins have provided semisynthetic derivatives that are variously effective against bacterial species known to be resistant to penicillin, in particular, penicillinase-producing staphylococci and Gram-negative bacilli. Thus, apart from a few strains that have either inherent or acquired resistance, almost all bacterial species are sensitive to one or more of the available β-lactam antibiotics.

Mechanism of Action

In addition to a broad spectrum of antibacterial action, two properties contribute to the unequaled importance of β-lactam antibiotics in chemotherapy: a potent and rapid bactericidal action against bacteria in the growth phase and a very low frequency of toxic and other adverse reactions in the host. The uniquely lethal antibacterial action of these agents has been attributed to a selective inhibition of bacterial cell wall synthesis.[7] Specifically, the basic mechanism involved is inhibition of the biosynthesis of the dipeptidoglycan that provides strength and rigidity to the cell wall. Penicillins and cephalosporins acylate a specific bacterial D-transpeptidase,[8] thereby rendering it inactive for its role in forming peptide cross-links of two linear peptidoglycan strands by transpeptidation and loss of D-alanine. Bacterial D-alanine carboxypeptidases are also inhibited by β-lactam antibiotics.

Binding studies with tritiated benzyl penicillin have shown that the mechanisms of action of various β-lactam antibiotics are much more complex than previously assumed. Studies in *E. coli* have revealed as many as seven different functional proteins, each with an important role in cell wall biosynthesis.[9] These penicillin-binding proteins (PBPs) have the following functional properties:

- PBPs 1_a and 1_b are transpeptidases involved in peptidoglycan synthesis associated with cell elongation. Inhibition results in spheroplast formation and rapid cell lysis,[9, 10] caused by autolysins (bacterial enzymes that create nicks in the cell wall for attachment of new peptidoglycan units or for separation of daughter cells during cell division[10]).
- PBP 2 is a transpeptidase involved in maintaining the rod shape of bacilli.[11] Inhibition results in ovoid or round forms that undergo delayed lysis.
- PBP 3 is a transpeptidase required for septum formation during cell division.[12] Inhibition results in the formation of filamentous forms containing rod-shaped units that cannot separate. It is not yet clear whether inhibition of PBP 3 is lethal to the bacterium.
- PBPs 4 through 6 are carboxypeptidases responsible for the hydrolysis of D-alanine–D-alanine terminal peptide bonds of the cross-linking peptides. Inhibition of these enzymes is apparently not lethal to the bacterium,[13] even though cleavage of the terminal D-alanine bond is required before peptide cross-linkage.

The various β-lactam antibiotics differ in their affinities for PBPs. Penicillin G binds preferentially to PBP 3, whereas the first-generation cephalosporins bind with higher affinity to PBP 1_a. In contrast to other penicillins and to cephalosporins, which can bind to PBPs 1, 2, and 3, amdinocillin binds only to PBP 2.

THE PENICILLINS

Commercial Production and Unitage

Until 1944, it was assumed that the active principle in penicillin was a single substance and that variation in activity of different products was due to the amount of inert materials in the samples. Now we know that during the biological elaboration of the antibiotic, several closely related compounds may be produced. These compounds differ chemically in the acid moiety of the amide side chain. Variations in this moiety produce differences in antibiotic effect and in physicochemical properties, including stability. Thus, one can speak of penicillins as a group of compounds and identify each penicillin specifically. As each of the different penicillins was first isolated, letter designations were used in the United States; the British used Roman numerals.

Over 30 penicillins have been isolated from fermentation mixtures. Some of these occur naturally; others have been biosynthesized by altering the culture medium to provide certain precursors that may be incorporated as acyl groups. Commercial production of biosynthetic penicillins today depends chiefly on various strains of *Penicillium notatum* and *P. chrysogenum*. In recent years, many more penicillins have been prepared semisynthetically, and undoubtedly, many more will be added to the list in attempts to find superior products.

Because the penicillin first used in chemotherapy was not a pure compound and exhibited varying activity among samples, it was necessary to evaluate it by microbiological assay. The procedure for assay was developed at Oxford, England, and the value became known as the *Oxford unit*: 1 Oxford unit is defined as the smallest amount of penicillin that will

TABLE 10–2 Structure of Penicillins

Generic Name	Chemical Name	R Group
Penicillin G	Benzylpenicillin	
Penicillin V	Phenoxymethylpenicillin	
Methicillin	2,6-Dimethoxyphenyl-penicillin	
Nafcillin	2-Ethoxy-1-naphthyl-penicillin	
Oxacillin	5-Methyl-3-phenyl-4-isoxazolylpenicillin	
Cloxacillin	5-Methyl-3-(2-chlorophenyl)-4-isoxazolylpenicillin	
Dicloxacillin	5-Methyl-3-(2,6-dichlorophenyl)-4-isoxazolylpenicillin	
Ampicillin	D-α-Aminobenzyl-penicillin	
Amoxicillin	D-α-Amino-*p*-hydroxybenzylpenicillin	
Cyclacillin	1-Aminocyclohexyl-penicillin	
Carbenicillin	α-Carboxybenzyl-penicillin	
Ticarcillin	α-Carboxy-3-thienyl-penicillin	

TABLE 10–2—*Continued*

Generic Name	Chemical Name	R Group
Piperacillin	α-(4-Ethyl-2,3-dioxo-1-piperazinylcarbonyl-amino)benzylpenicillin	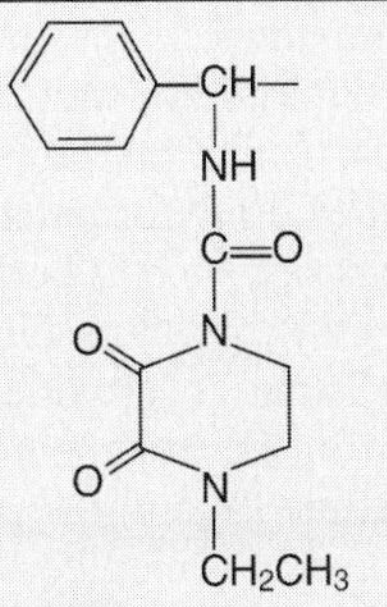
Mezlocillin	α-(1-Methanesulfonyl-2-oxoimidazolidino-carbonylamino)benzyl penicillin	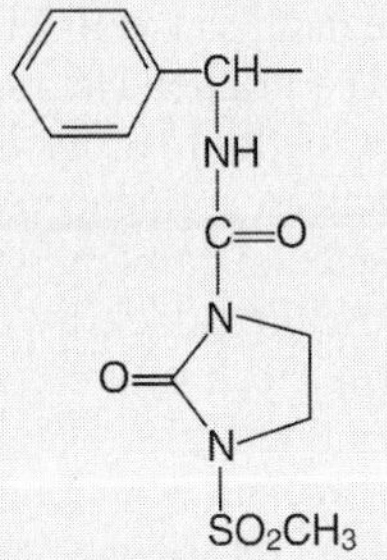

inhibit, in vitro, the growth of a strain of *Staphylococcus* in 50 mL of culture medium under specified conditions. Now that pure crystalline penicillin is available, the *United States Pharmacopoeia* (USP) defines *unit* as the antibiotic activity of 0.6 μg of USP penicillin G sodium reference standard. The weight–unit relationship of the penicillins varies with the acyl substituent and with the salt formed of the free acid: 1 mg of penicillin G sodium is equivalent to 1,667 units, 1 mg of penicillin G procaine is equivalent to 1,009 units, and 1 mg of penicillin G potassium is equivalent to 1,530 units.

The commercial production of penicillin has increased markedly since its introduction. As production increased, the cost dropped correspondingly. When penicillin was first available, 100,000 units sold for $20. Currently, the same quantity costs less than a penny. Fluctuations in the production of penicillins through the years have reflected changes in the relative popularity of broad-spectrum antibiotics and penicillins, the development of penicillin-resistant strains of several pathogens, the more recent introduction of semisynthetic penicillins, the use of penicillins in animal feeds and for veterinary purposes, and the increase in marketing problems in a highly competitive sales area.

Table 10-2 shows the general structure of the penicillins and relates the structure of the more familiar ones to their various designations.

Nomenclature

The nomenclature of penicillins is somewhat complex and very cumbersome. Two numbering systems for the fused bicyclic heterocyclic system exist. The *Chemical Abstracts* system initiates the numbering with the sulfur atom and assigns the ring nitrogen the 4 position. Thus, penicillins are named as 4-thia-l-azabicyclo[3.2.0]heptanes, according to this system. The numbering system adopted by the USP is the reverse of the *Chemical Abstracts* procedure, assigning

number 1 to the nitrogen atom and number 4 to the sulfur atom. Three simplified forms of penicillin nomenclature have been adopted for general use. One uses the name ''penam'' for the unsubstituted bicyclic system, including the amide carbonyl group, with one of the foregoing numbering systems as just described. Thus, penicillins generally are designated according to the *Chemical Abstracts* system as 5-acylamino-2,2-dimethylpenam-3-carboxylic acids. The second, seen more frequently in the medical literature, uses the name ''penicillanic acid'' to describe the ring system with substituents that are generally present (i.e., 2,2-dimethyl and 3-carboxyl). A third form, followed in this chapter, uses trivial nomenclature to name the entire 6-carbonylaminopenicillanic acid portion of the molecule penicillin and then distinguishes compounds on the basis of the R group of the acyl portion of the molecule. Thus, penicillin G is named benzylpenicillin, penicillin V is phenoxymethylpenicillin, methicillin is 2,6-dimethoxyphenylpenicillin, and so on. For the most part, the latter two systems serve well for naming and comparing closely similar penicillin structures, but they are too restrictive to be applied to compounds with unusual substituents or to ring-modified derivatives.

Stereochemistry

The penicillin molecule contains three chiral carbon atoms (C-3, C-5, and C-6). All naturally occurring and microbiologically active synthetic and semisynthetic penicillins have the same absolute configuration about these three centers. The carbon atom bearing the acylamino group (C-6) has the L configuration, whereas the carbon to which the carboxyl group is attached has the D configuration. Thus, the acylamino and carboxyl groups are *trans* to each other, with the former in the α and the latter in the β orientation relative to the penam ring system. The atoms composing the 6-aminopenicillanic acid portion of the structure are derived biosynthetically from two amino acids, L-cysteine (S-1, C-5, C-6, C-7, and 6-amino) and L-valine (2,2-dimethyl, C-2, C-3, N-4, and 3-carboxyl). The absolute stereochemistry of the penicillins is designated 3S:5R:6R, as shown below.

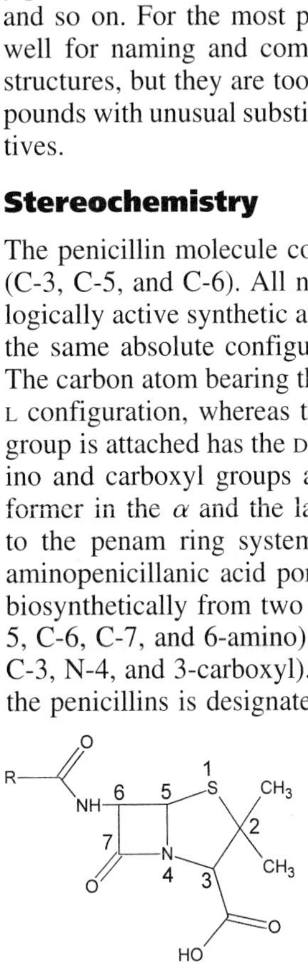

Chemical Abstracts

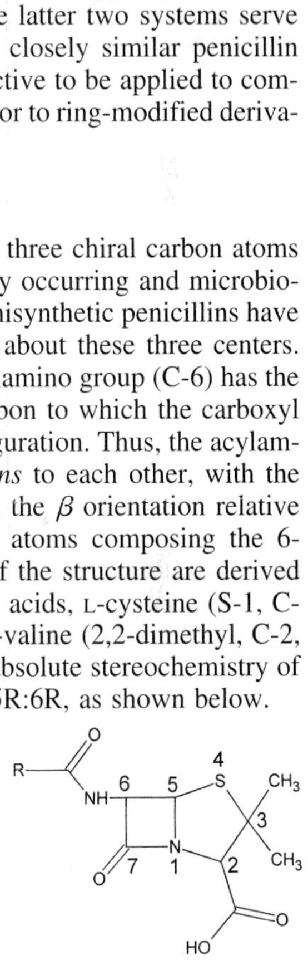

USP

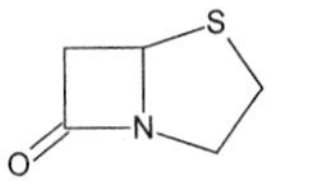

Penam

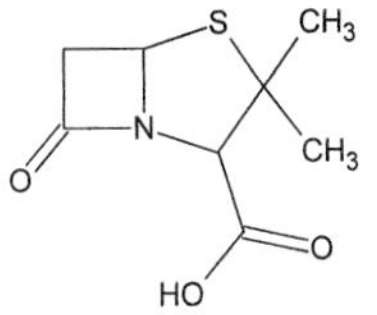

Penicillanic Acid

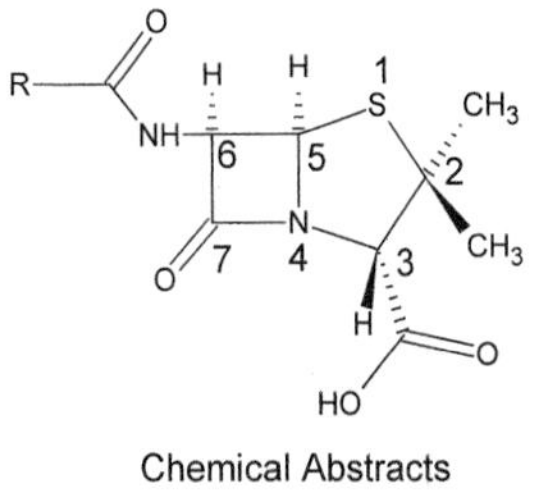

Chemical Abstracts

Synthesis

Examination of the structure of the penicillin molecule shows that it contains a fused ring system of unusual design, the β-lactam thiazolidine structure. The nature of the β-lactam ring delayed elucidation of the structure of penicillin, but its determination resulted from a collaborative research program involving groups in Great Britain and the United States during the years 1943 to 1945.[14] Attempts to synthesize these compounds resulted, at best, in only trace amounts until Sheehan and Henery-Logan[15] adapted techniques developed in peptide synthesis to the synthesis of penicillin V. This procedure is not likely to replace the established fermentation processes because the last step in the reaction series develops only 10 to 12% penicillin. It is of advantage in research because it provides a means of obtaining many new amide chains hitherto not possible to achieve by biosynthetic procedures.

Two other developments have provided additional means for making new penicillins. A group of British scientists, Batchelor et al.,[16] reported the isolation of 6-aminopenicillanic acid from a culture of *P. chrysogenum*. This compound can be converted to penicillins by acylation of the 6-amino group. Sheehan and Ferris[17] provided another route to synthetic penicillins by converting a natural penicillin, such as penicillin G potassium, to an intermediate (Fig. 10-1), from which the acyl side chain has been cleaved and which then can be treated to form biologically active penicillins with a variety of new side chains. By these procedures, new penicillins, superior in activity and stability to those formerly in wide use, were found, and no doubt others will be produced. The first commercial products of these research activities were phenoxyethylpenicillin (phenethicillin) (Fig. 10-2) and dimethoxyphenylpenicillin (methicillin).

Chemical Degradation

The early commercial penicillin was a yellow to brown amorphous powder that was so unstable that refrigeration was required to maintain a reasonable level of activity for a short time. Improved purification procedures provided the white crystalline material in use today. Crystalline penicillin must be protected from moisture, but when kept dry, the salts will remain stable for years without refrigeration. Many penicillins have an unpleasant taste, which must be overcome in the formation of pediatric dosage forms. All of the

natural penicillins are strongly dextrorotatory. The solubility and other physicochemical properties of the penicillins are affected by the nature of the acyl side chain and by the cations used to make salts of the acid. Most penicillins are acids with pK_a values in the range of 2.5 to 3.0, but some are amphoteric. The free acids are not suitable for oral or parenteral administration. The sodium and potassium salts of most penicillins, however, are soluble in water and readily absorbed orally or parenterally. Salts of penicillins with organic bases, such as benzathine, procaine, and hydrabamine, have limited water solubility and are, therefore, useful as depot forms to provide effective blood levels over a long period in the treatment of chronic infections. Some of the crystalline salts of the penicillins are hygroscopic and must be stored in sealed containers.

The main cause of deterioration of penicillin is the reactivity of the strained lactam ring, particularly to hydrolysis. The course of the hydrolysis and the nature of the degradation products are influenced by the pH of the solution.[18, 19] Thus, the β-lactam carbonyl group of penicillin readily undergoes nucleophilic attack by water or (especially) hydroxide ion to form the inactive penicilloic acid, which is reasonably stable in neutral to alkaline solutions but readily undergoes decarboxylation and further hydrolytic reactions in acidic solutions. Other nucleophiles, such as hydroxylamines, alkylamines, and alcohols, open the β-lactam ring to form the corresponding hydroxamic acids, amides, and esters. It has been speculated[20] that one of the causes of penicillin allergy may be the formation of antigenic penicilloyl proteins in vivo by the reaction of nucleophilic groups (e.g., ϵ-amino) on specific body proteins with the β-lactam carbonyl group. In strongly acidic solutions (pH <3), penicillin undergoes a complex series of reactions leading to a variety of inactive degradation products (Fig. 10-3).[19] The first step appears to involve rearrangement to the penicillanic acid. This process is initiated by protonation of the β-lactam nitrogen, followed by nucleophilic attack of the acyl oxygen atom on the β-lactam carbonyl carbon. The subsequent opening of the β-lactam ring destabilizes the thiazoline ring, which then also suffers acid-catalyzed ring opening to form the penicillanic acid. The latter is very unstable and experiences two major degradation pathways. The most easily understood path involves hydrolysis of the oxazolone ring to form the unstable penamaldic acid. Because it is an enamine, penamaldic acid easily hydrolyzes to penicillamine (a major degradation

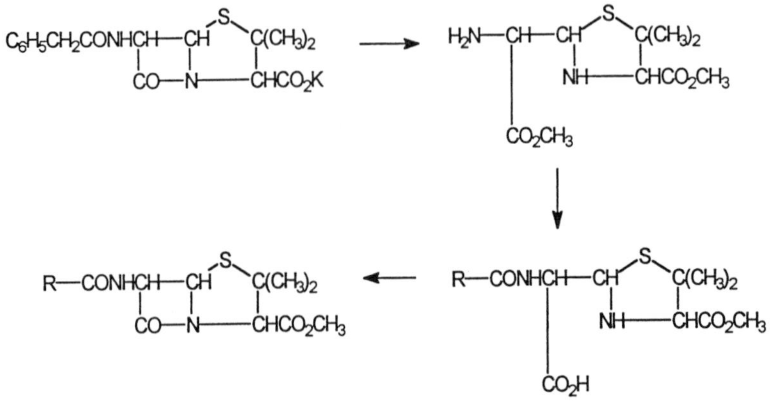

Figure 10-1 ■ Conversion of natural penicillin to synthetic penicillin.

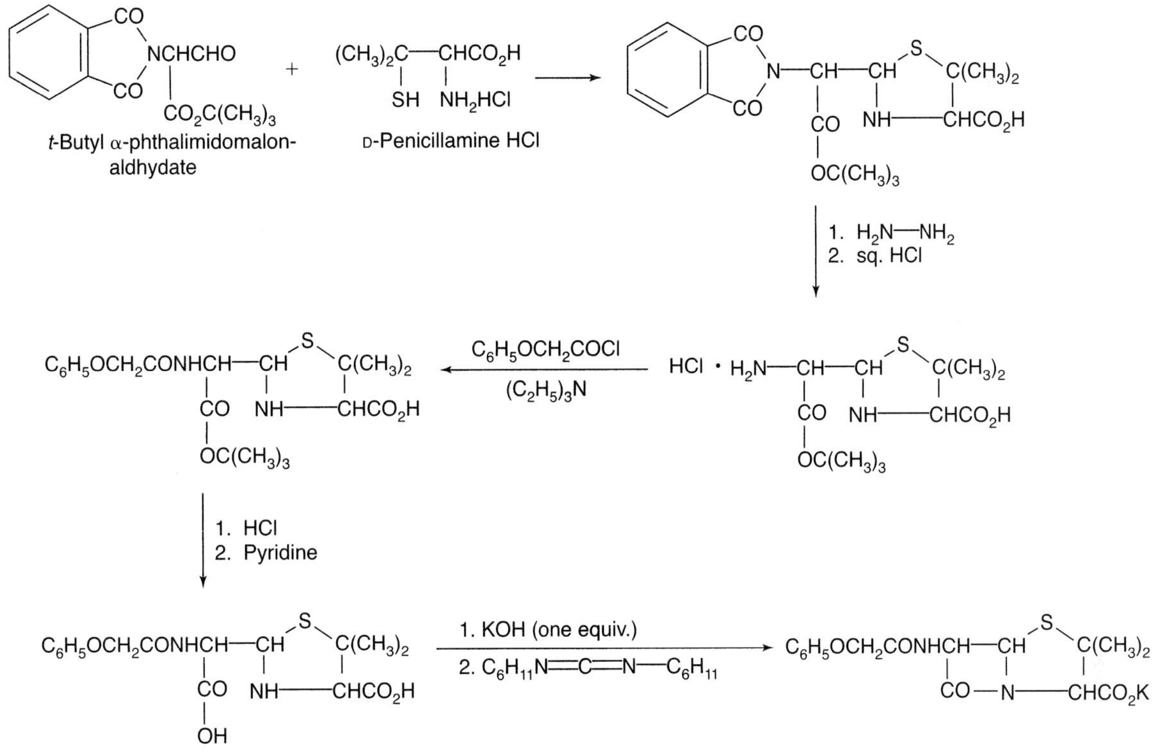

Figure 10–2 ■ Synthesis of phenoxymethylpenicillin.

product) and penaldic acid. The second path involves a complex rearrangement of penicillanic acid to a penillic acid through a series of intramolecular processes that remain to be elucidated completely. Penillic acid (an imidazoline-2-carboxylic acid) readily decarboxylates and suffers hydrolytic ring opening under acidic conditions to form a second major end product of acid-catalyzed penicillin degradation, penilloic acid. Penicilloic acid, the major product formed under weakly acidic to alkaline (as well as enzymatic) hydrolytic conditions, cannot be detected as an intermediate under strongly acidic conditions. It exists in equilibrium with penamaldic acid, however, and undergoes decarboxylation in acid to form penilloic acid. The third major product of the degradation is penicilloaldehyde, formed by decarboxylation of penaldic acid (a derivative of malonaldehyde).

By controlling the pH of aqueous solutions within a range of 6.0 to 6.8 and refrigerating the solutions, aqueous preparations of the soluble penicillins may be stored for up to several weeks. The relationship of these properties to the pharmaceutics of penicillins has been reviewed by Schwartz and Buckwalter.[21] Some buffer systems, particularly phosphates and citrates, exert a favorable effect on penicillin stability, independent of the pH effect. Finholt et al.[22] showed that these buffers may catalyze penicillin degradation, however, if the pH is adjusted to obtain the requisite ions. Hydroalcoholic solutions of penicillin G potassium are about as unstable as aqueous solutions.[23] Because penicillins are inactivated by metal ions such as zinc and copper, it has been suggested that the phosphates and the citrates combine with these metals to prevent their existence as free ions in solution.

Oxidizing agents also inactivate penicillins, but reducing agents have little effect on them. Temperature affects the rate of deterioration; although the dry salts are stable at room temperature and do not require refrigeration, prolonged heating inactivates the penicillins.

Acid-catalyzed degradation in the stomach contributes strongly to the poor oral absorption of penicillin. Thus, efforts to obtain penicillins with improved pharmacokinetic and microbiological properties have focused on acyl functionalities that would minimize sensitivity of the β-lactam ring to acid hydrolysis while maintaining antibacterial activity.

Substitution of an electron-withdrawing group in the α position of benzylpenicillin markedly stabilizes the penicillin to acid-catalyzed hydrolysis. Thus, phenoxymethylpenicillin, α- aminobenzylpenicillin, and α-halobenzylpenicillin are significantly more stable than benzylpenicillin in acid solutions. The increased stability imparted by such electron-withdrawing groups has been attributed to decreased reactivity (nucleophilicity) of the side chain amide carbonyl oxygen atom toward participation in β-lactam ring opening to form penicillenic acid. Obviously, α-aminobenzylpenicillin (ampicillin) exists as the protonated form in acidic (as well as neutral) solutions, and the ammonium group is known to be powerfully electron-withdrawing.

Bacterial Resistance

Some bacteria, in particular most species of Gram-negative bacilli, are naturally resistant to the action of penicillins. Other normally sensitive species can develop penicillin resistance (either through natural selection of resistant individ-

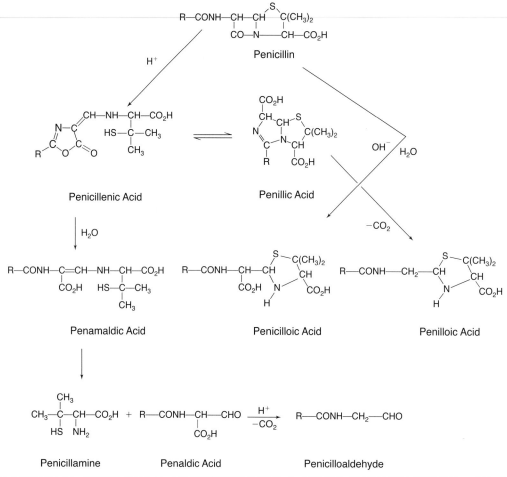

Figure 10–3 ■ Degradation of penicillins.

uals or through mutation). The best understood and, probably, the most important biochemical mechanism of penicillin resistance is the bacterial elaboration of enzymes that inactivate penicillins. Such enzymes, which have been given the nonspecific name *penicillinases,* are of two general types: β-lactamases and acylases. By far the more important of these are the β-lactamases, enzymes that catalyze the hydrolytic opening of the β-lactam ring of penicillins to produce inactive penicilloic acids. Synthesis of bacterial β-lactamases may be under chromosomal or plasmid R factor control and may be either constitutive or inducible (stimulated by the presence of the substrate), depending on the bacterial species. The well-known resistance among strains of *Staphylococcus aureus* is apparently entirely due to the production of an inducible β-lactamase. Resistance among Gram-negative bacilli, however, may result from other, poorly characterized "resistance factors" or constitutive β-lactamase elaboration. β-Lactamases produced by Gram-negative bacilli appear to be cytoplasmic enzymes that remain in the bacterial cell, whereas those elaborated by *S. aureus* are synthesized in the cell wall and released extracellularly. β-Lactamases from different bacterial species may be classified[24–26] by their structure, their substrate and inhib-

itor specificities, their physical properties (pH optimum, isoelectric point, molecular weight, etc.), and their immunological properties.

Specific acylases, enzymes that can hydrolyze the acylamino side chain of penicillins, have been obtained from several species of Gram-negative bacteria, but their possible role in bacterial resistance has not been well defined. These enzymes find some commercial use in the preparation of 6-aminopenicillanic acid (6-APA) for the preparation of semisynthetic penicillins. 6-APA is less active and hydrolyzed more rapidly (enzymatically and nonenzymatically) than penicillin.

Another important resistance mechanism, especially in Gram-negative bacteria, is decreased permeability to penicillins. The cell envelope in most Gram-negative bacteria is more complex than in Gram-positive bacteria. It contains an outer membrane (linked by lipoprotein bridges to the peptidoglycan cell wall) not present in Gram-positive bacteria, which creates a physical barrier to the penetration of antibiotics, especially those that are hydrophobic.[27] Small hydrophilic molecules, however, can traverse the outer membrane through pores formed by proteins called *porins*.[28] Alteration of the number or nature of porins in the cell envelope[28] also could be an important mechanism of antibiotic resistance. Bacterial resistance can result from changes in the affinity of PBPs for penicillins.[29] Altered PBP binding has been demonstrated in non–β-lactamase-producing strains of penicillin-resistant *Neisseria gonorrhoeae*[30] and methicillin-resistant *S. aureus* (MRSA).[31]

Certain strains of bacteria are resistant to the lytic properties of penicillins but remain susceptible to their growth-inhibiting effects. Thus, the action of the antibiotic has been converted from bactericidal to bacteriostatic. This mechanism of resistance is termed *tolerance* and apparently results from impaired autolysin activity in the bacterium.

Penicillinase-Resistant Penicillins

The availability of 6-APA on a commercial scale made possible the synthesis of numerous semisynthetic penicillins modified at the acyl amino side chain. Much of the early work done in the 1960s was directed toward the preparation of derivatives that would resist destruction by β-lactamases, particularly those produced by penicillin-resistant strains of *S. aureus*, which constituted a very serious health problem at that time. In general, increasing the steric hindrance at the α-carbon of the acyl group increased resistance to staphylococcal β-lactamase, with maximal resistance being observed with quaternary substitution.[32] More fruitful from the standpoint of antibacterial potency, however, was the observation that the α-acyl carbon could be part of an aromatic (e.g., phenyl or naphthyl) or heteroaromatic (e.g., 4-isoxazoyl) system.[33] Substitutions at the *ortho* positions of a phenyl ring (e.g., 2,6-dimethoxyl [methicillin]) or the 2 position of a 1-naphthyl system (e.g., 2-ethoxyl [nafcillin]) increase the steric hindrance of the acyl group and confer more β-lactamase resistance than shown by the unsubstituted compounds or those substituted at positions more distant from the α-carbon. Bulkier substituents are required to confer effective β-lactamase resistance among five-membered-ring heterocyclic derivatives.[34] Thus, members of the 4-isoxazoyl penicillin family (e.g., oxacillin, cloxacillin, and dicloxacillin) require both the 3-aryl and 5-methyl (3-methyl and 5-aryl) substituents for effectiveness against β-lactamase-producing *S. aureus*.

Increasing the bulkiness of the acyl group is not without its price, however, because all of the clinically available penicillinase-resistant penicillins are significantly less active than either penicillin G or penicillin V against most non–β-lactamase-producing bacteria normally sensitive to the penicillins. The β-lactamase-resistant penicillins tend to be comparatively lipophilic molecules that do not penetrate well into Gram-negative bacteria. The isoxazoyl penicillins, particularly those with an electronegative substituent in the 3-phenyl group (cloxacillin, dicloxacillin, and floxacillin), are also resistant to acid-catalyzed hydrolysis of the β-lactam, for the reasons described above. Steric factors that confer β-lactamase resistance, however, do not necessarily also confer stability to acid. Accordingly, methicillin, which has electron-donating groups (by resonance) *ortho* to the carbonyl carbon, is even more labile to acid-catalyzed hydrolysis than is penicillin G because of the more rapid formation of the penicillenic acid derivative.

Extended-Spectrum Penicillins

Another highly significant advance arising from the preparation of semisynthetic penicillins was the discovery that the introduction of an ionized or polar group into the α position of the side chain benzyl carbon atom of penicillin G confers activity against Gram-negative bacilli. Hence, derivatives with an ionized α-amino group, such as ampicillin and amoxicillin, are generally effective against such Gram-negative genera as *Escherichia, Klebsiella, Haemophilus, Salmonella, Shigella,* and non–indole-producing *Proteus.* Furthermore, activity against penicillin G–sensitive, Gram-positive species is largely retained. The introduction of an α-amino group in ampicillin (or amoxicillin) creates an additional chiral center. Extension of the antibacterial spectrum brought about by the substituent applies only to the D isomer, which is 2 to 8 times more active than either the L isomer or benzylpenicillin (which are equiactive) against various species of the aforementioned genera of Gram-negative bacilli.

The basis for the expanded spectrum of activity associated with the ampicillin group is not related to β-lactamase inhibition, as ampicillin and amoxicillin are even more labile than penicillin G to the action of β-lactamases elaborated by both *S. aureus* and various species of Gram-negative bacilli, including strains among the ampicillin-sensitive group. Hydrophilic penicillins, such as ampicillin, penetrate Gram-negative bacteria more readily than penicillin G, penicillin V, or methicillin. This selective penetration is believed to take place through the porin channels of the cell membrane.[35]

α-Hydroxy substitution also yields ''expanded-spectrum'' penicillins with activity and stereoselectivity similar to that of the ampicillin group. The α-hydroxybenzylpenicillins are, however, about 2 to 5 times less active than their corresponding α-aminobenzyl counterparts and, unlike the latter, not very stable under acidic conditions.

Incorporation of an acidic substituent at the α-benzyl carbon atom of penicillin G also imparts clinical effectiveness against Gram-negative bacilli and, furthermore, extends the spectrum of activity to include organisms resistant to ampicillin. Thus, α-carboxybenzylpenicillin (carbenicillin) is active against ampicillin-sensitive, Gram-negative species and additional Gram-negative bacilli of the genera *Pseudomonas, Klebsiella, Enterobacter,* indole-producing *Proteus, Serratia,* and *Providencia.* The potency of carbenicillin against most species of penicillin G–sensitive, Gram-positive bacteria is several orders of magnitude lower than that of either penicillin G or ampicillin, presumably because of poorer penetration of a more highly ionized molecule into these bacteria. (Note that α-aminobenzylpenicillins exist as zwitterions over a broad pH range and, as such, are considerably less polar than carbenicillin.) This increased polarity is apparently an advantage for the penetration of carbenicillin through the cell envelope of Gram-negative bacteria via porin channels.[35]

Carbenicillin is active against both β-lactamase-producing and non–β-lactamase-producing strains of Gram-negative bacteria. It is somewhat resistant to a few of the β-lactamases produced by Gram-negative bacteria, especially members of the Enterobacteriaceae family.[36] Resistance to β-lactamases elaborated by Gram-negative bacteria, therefore, may be an important component of carbenicillin's activity against some ampicillin-resistant organisms. β-Lactamases produced by *Pseudomonas* spp., however, readily hydrolyze carbenicillin. Although carbenicillin is also somewhat resistant to staphylococcal β-lactamase, it is considerably less so than methicillin or the isoxazoyl penicillins, and its inherent antistaphylococcal activity is less impressive than that of the penicillinase-resistant penicillins. The penicillinase-resistant penicillins, despite their resistance to most β-lactamases, however, share the lack of activity of penicillin G against Gram-negative bacilli, primarily because of an inability to penetrate the bacterial cell envelope.

Compared with the aminoglycoside antibiotics, the potency of carbenicillin against such Gram-negative bacilli as *Pseudomonas aeruginosa*, *Proteus vulgaris*, and *Klebsiella pneumoniae* is much less impressive. Large parenteral doses are required to achieve bactericidal concentrations in plasma and tissues. The low toxicity of carbenicillin (and the penicillins in general), however, usually permits (in the absence of allergy) the use of such high doses without untoward effects. Furthermore, carbenicillin (and other penicillins), when combined with aminoglycosides, exerts a synergistic bactericidal action against bacterial species sensitive to both agents, frequently allowing the use of a lower dose of the more toxic aminoglycoside than is normally required for treatment of a life-threatening infection. The chemical incompatibility of penicillins and aminoglycosides requires that the two antibiotics be administered separately; otherwise, both are inactivated. Iyengar et al.[37] showed that acylation of amino groups in the aminoglycoside by the β-lactam of the penicillin occurs.

Unlike the situation with ampicillin, the introduction of asymmetry at the α-benzyl carbon in carbenicillin imparts little or no stereoselectivity of antibacterial action; the individual enantiomers are nearly equally active and readily epimerized to the racemate in aqueous solution. Because it is a derivative of phenylmalonic acid, carbenicillin readily decarboxylates to benzylpenicillin in the presence of acid; therefore, it is not active (as carbenicillin) orally and must be administered parenterally. Esterification of the α-carboxyl group (e.g., as the 5-indanyl ester) partially protects the compound from acid-catalyzed destruction and provides an orally active derivative that is hydrolyzed to carbenicillin in the plasma. The plasma levels of free carbenicillin achieved with oral administration of such esters, however, may not suffice for effective treatment of serious infections caused by some species of Gram-negative bacilli, such as *P. aeruginosa*.

A series of α-acylureido-substituted penicillins, exemplified by azlocillin, mezlocillin, and piperacillin, exhibit greater activity against certain Gram-negative bacilli than carbenicillin. Although the acylureidopenicillins are acylated derivatives of ampicillin, the antibacterial spectrum of activity of the group is more like that of carbenicillin. The acylureidopenicillins are, however, superior to carbenicillin against *Klebsiella* spp., *Enterobacter* spp., and *P. aeruginosa*. This enhanced activity is apparently not due to β-lactamase resistance, in that both inducible and plasmid-mediated β-lactamases hydrolyze these penicillins. More facile penetration through the cell envelope of these particular bacterial species is the most likely explanation for the

greater potency. The acylureidopenicillins, unlike ampicillin, are unstable under acidic conditions; therefore, they are not available for oral administration.

Protein Binding

The nature of the acylamino side chain also determines the extent to which penicillins are plasma protein bound. Quantitative structure–activity relationship (QSAR) studies of the binding of penicillins to human serum[38, 39] indicate that hydrophobic groups (positive π dependence) in the side chain appear to be largely responsible for increased binding to serum proteins. Penicillins with polar or ionized substituents in the side chain exhibit low-to-intermediate fractions of protein binding. Accordingly, ampicillin, amoxicillin, and cyclacillin experience 25 to 30% protein binding, and carbenicillin and ticarcillin show 45 to 55% protein binding. Those with nonpolar, lipophilic substituents (nafcillin and isoxazoyl penicillins) are more than 90% protein bound. The penicillins with less complex acyl groups (benzylpenicillin, phenoxymethylpenicillin, and methicillin) fall in the range of 35 to 80%. Protein binding is thought to restrict the tissue availability of drugs if the fraction bound is sufficiently high; thus, the tissue distribution of the penicillins in the highly bound group may be inferior to that of other penicillins. The similarity of biological half-lives for various penicillins, however, indicates that plasma protein binding has little effect on duration of action. All of the commercially available penicillins are secreted actively by the renal active transport system for anions. The reversible nature of protein binding does not compete effectively with the active tubular secretion process.

Allergy to Penicillins

Allergic reactions to various penicillins, ranging in severity from a variety of skin and mucous membrane rashes to drug fever and anaphylaxis, constitute the major problem associated with the use of this class of antibiotics. Estimates place the prevalence of hypersensitivity to penicillin G throughout the world between 1 and 10% of the population. In the United States and other industrialized countries, it is nearer the higher figure, ranking penicillin the most common cause of drug-induced allergy. The penicillins most frequently implicated in allergic reactions are penicillin G and ampicillin. Virtually all commercially available penicillins, however, have been reported to cause such reactions; in fact, cross-sensitivity among most chemical classes of 6-acylaminopenicillanic acid derivatives has been demonstrated.[40]

The chemical mechanisms by which penicillin preparations become antigenic have been studied extensively.[20] Evidence suggests that penicillins or their rearrangement products formed in vivo (e.g., penicillenic acids)[41] react with lysine ϵ-amino groups of proteins to form penicilloyl proteins, which are major antigenic determinants.[42, 43] Early clinical observations with the biosynthetic penicillins G and V indicated a higher incidence of allergic reactions with unpurified, amorphous preparations than with highly purified, crystalline forms, suggesting that small amounts of highly antigenic penicilloyl proteins present in unpurified samples were a cause. Polymeric impurities in ampicillin dosage forms have been implicated as possible antigenic determinants and a possible explanation for the high frequency of allergic reactions with this particular semisynthetic penicillin. Ampicillin is known to undergo pH-dependent polymerization reactions (especially in concentrated solutions) that involve nucleophilic attack of the side chain amino group of one molecule on the β-lactam carbonyl carbon atom of a second molecule, and so on.[44] The high frequency of antigenicity shown by ampicillin polymers together with their isolation and characterization in some ampicillin preparations supports the theory that they can contribute to ampicillin-induced allergy.[45]

Classification

Various designations have been used to classify penicillins, based on their sources, chemistry, pharmacokinetic properties, resistance to enzymatic spectrum of activity, and clinical uses (Table 10-3). Thus, penicillins may be biosynthetic, semisynthetic, or (potentially) synthetic; acid-resistant or not; orally or (only) parenterally active; and resistant to β-lactamases (penicillinases) or not. They may have a narrow, intermediate, broad, or extended spectrum of antibacterial activity and may be intended for multipurpose or limited clinical use. Designations of the activity spectrum as narrow, intermediate, broad, or extended are relative and do not necessarily imply the breadth of therapeutic application. Indeed, the classification of penicillin G as a ''narrow-spectrum'' antibiotic has meaning only relative to other penicillins. Although the β-lactamase-resistant penicillins have a spectrum of activity similar to that of penicillin G, they generally are reserved for the treatment of infections caused by penicillin G–resistant, β-lactamase-producing *S. aureus* because their activity against most penicillin G–sensitive bacteria is significantly inferior. Similarly, carbenicillin and ticarcillin usually are reserved for the treatment of infections caused by ampicillin-resistant, Gram-negative bacilli because they offer no advantage (and have some disadvantages) over ampicillin or penicillin G in infections sensitive to them.

Products

Penicillin G.

For years, the most popular penicillin has been penicillin G, or benzylpenicillin. In fact, with the exception of patients allergic to it, penicillin G remains the agent of choice for the treatment of more different kinds of bacterial infection than any other antibiotic. It was first made available as the water-soluble salts of potassium, sodium, and calcium. These salts of penicillin are inactivated by the gastric juice and are not effective when administered orally unless antacids, such as calcium carbonate, aluminum hydroxide, and magnesium trisilicate, or a strong buffer, such as sodium citrate, is added. Also, because penicillin is absorbed poorly from the intestinal tract, oral doses must be very large, about 5 times the amount necessary with parenteral administration. Only after the production of penicillin had increased enough to make low-priced penicillin available did the oral dosage forms become popular. The water-soluble potassium and sodium salts are used orally and parenterally to achieve high plasma concentrations of penicillin G rapidly. The more water-soluble potassium salt usually is preferred when large doses are required. Situations in which hyperkalemia is a danger, however, as in renal failure, require use of the sodium salt; the potassium salt is preferred for patients on salt-free diets or with congestive heart conditions.

Penicillin G
Benzylpenicillin

The rapid elimination of penicillin from the bloodstream through the kidneys by active tubular secretion and the need to maintain an effective concentration in blood have led to the development of ''repository'' forms of this drug. Suspen-

TABLE 10-3 Classification and Properties of Penicillins

Penicillin	Source	Acid Resistance	Oral Absorption (%)	Plasma Protein Binding (%)	β-Lactamase Resistance (*S. aureus*)	Spectrum of Activity	Clinical Use
Benzylpenicillin	Biosynthetic	Poor	Poor (20)	50–60	No	Intermediate	Multipurpose
Phenoxymethylpenicillin	Biosynthetic	Good	Good (60)	55–80	No	Intermediate	Multipurpose
Methicillin	Semisynthetic	Poor	Nil	30–40	Yes	Narrow	Limited use
Nafcillin	Semisynthetic	Fair	Variable	90	Yes	Narrow	Limited use
Oxacillin	Semisynthetic	Good	Fair (30)	85–94	Yes	Narrow	Limited use
Cloxacillin	Semisynthetic	Good	Good (50)	88–96	Yes	Narrow	Limited use
Dicloxacillin	Semisynthetic	Good	Good (50)	95–98	Yes	Narrow	Limited use
Ampicillin	Semisynthetic	Good	Fair (40)	20–25	No	Broad	Multipurpose
Amoxicillin	Semisynthetic	Good	Good (75)	20–25	No	Broad	Multipurpose
Carbenicillin	Semisynthetic	Poor	Nil	50–60	No	Extended	Limited use
Ticarcillin	Semisynthetic	Poor	Nil	45	No	Extended	Limited use
Mezlocillin	Semisynthetic	Poor	Nil	50	No	Extended	Limited use
Piperacillin	Semisynthetic	Poor	Nil	50	No	Extended	Limited use

sions of penicillin in peanut oil or sesame oil with white beeswax added were first used to prolong the duration of injected forms of penicillin. This dosage form was replaced by a suspension in vegetable oil, to which aluminum monostearate or aluminum distearate was added. Today, most repository forms are suspensions of high-molecular-weight amine salts of penicillin in a similar base.

Penicillin G Procaine, USP. The first widely used amine salt of penicillin G was made with procaine. Penicillin G procaine (Crysticillin, Duracillin, Wycillin) can be made readily from penicillin G sodium by treatment with procaine hydrochloride. This salt is considerably less soluble in water than the alkali metal salts, requiring about 250 mL to dissolve 1 g. Free penicillin is released only as the compound dissolves and dissociates. It has an activity of 1,009 units/mg. A large number of preparations for injection of penicillin G procaine are commercially available. Most of these are either suspensions in water to which a suitable dispersing or suspending agent, a buffer, and a preservative have been added or suspensions in peanut oil or sesame oil that have been gelled by the addition of 2% aluminum monostearate. Some commercial products are mixtures of penicillin G potassium or sodium with penicillin G procaine; the water-soluble salt provides rapid development of a high plasma concentration of penicillin, and the insoluble salt prolongs the duration of effect.

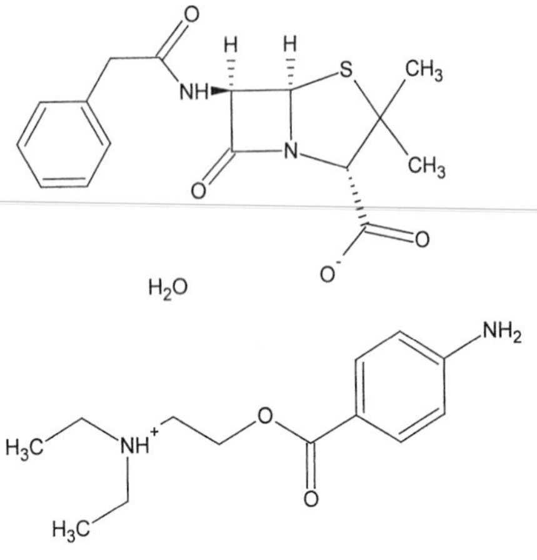

Penicillin G Procaine

Penicillin G Benzathine, USP. Since penicillin G benzathine, *N,N'*-dibenzylethylenediamine dipenicillin G (Bicillin, Permapen), is the salt of a diamine, 2 moles of penicillin are available from each molecule. It is very insoluble in water, requiring about 3,000 mL to dissolve 1 g. This property gives the compound great stability and prolonged duration of effect. At the pH of gastric juice it is quite stable, and food intake does not interfere with its absorption. It is available in tablet form and in a number of parenteral preparations. The activity of penicillin G benzathine is equivalent to 1,211 units/mg.

Several other amines have been used to make penicillin salts, and research is continuing on this subject. Other amines that have been used include 2-chloroprocaine; L-*N*-methyl-1,2-diphenyl-2-hydroxyethylamine (L-ephenamine); dibenzylamine; tripelennamine (Pyribenzamine); and *N,N'*-bis-(dehydroabietyl)ethylenediamine (hydrabamine).

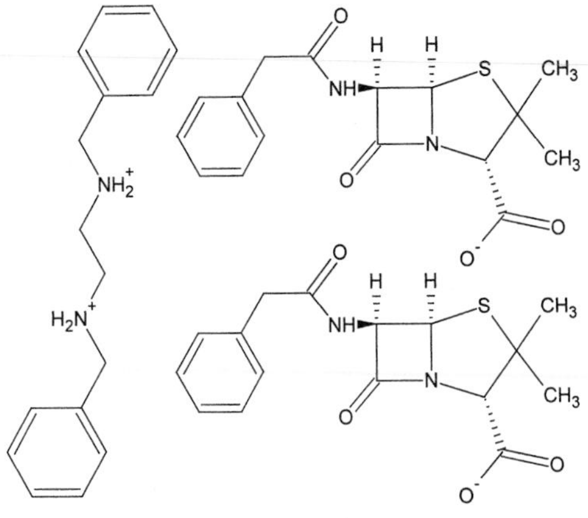

Penicillin G Benzathine

Penicillin V, USP. In 1948, Behrens et al.[46] reported penicillin V, phenoxymethylpenicillin (Pen Vee, V-Cillin) as a biosynthetic product. It was not until 1953, however, that its clinical value was recognized by some European scientists. Since then, it has enjoyed wide use because of its resistance to hydrolysis by gastric juice and its ability to produce uniform concentrations in blood (when administered orally). The free acid requires about 1,200 mL of water to dissolve 1 g, and it has an activity of 1,695 units/mg. For parenteral solutions, the potassium salt is usually used. This salt is very soluble in water. Solutions of it are made from the dry salt at the time of administration. Oral dosage forms of the potassium salt are also available, providing rapid, effective plasma concentrations of this penicillin. The salt of phenoxymethylpenicillin with *N,N'*-bis(dehydroabietyl)ethylenediamine (hydrabamine, Compocillin-V) provides a very long-acting form of this compound. Its high water insolubility makes it a desirable compound for aqueous suspensions used as liquid oral dosage forms.

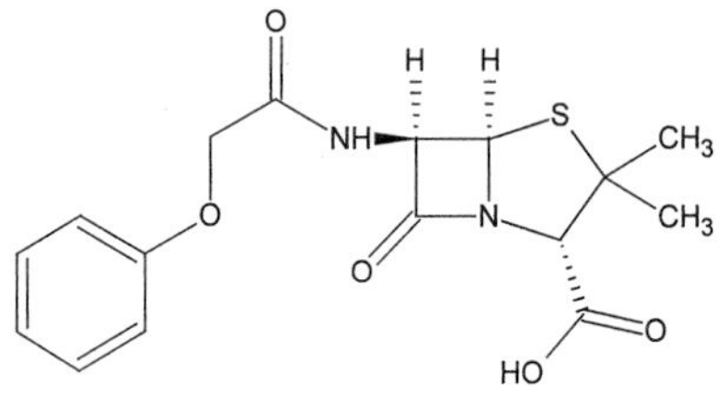

Penicillin V, USP

Methicillin Sodium, USP. During 1960, methicillin sodium, 2,6-dimethoxyphenylpenicillin sodium (Staphcillin), the second penicillin produced as a result of the research that developed synthetic analogues, was introduced for medicinal use.

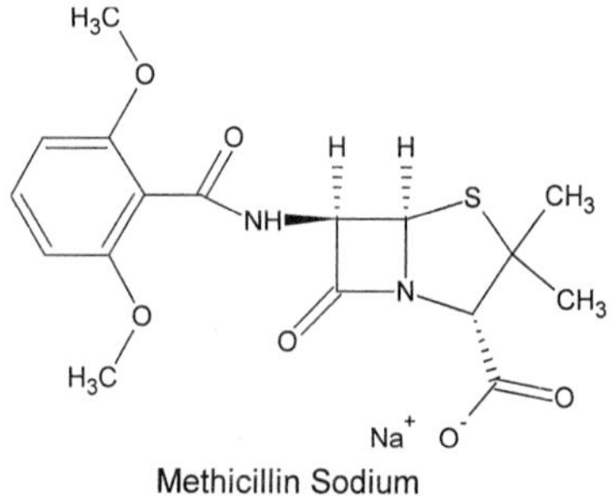

Methicillin Sodium

Reacting 2,6-dimethoxybenzoyl chloride with 6-APA forms 6-(2,6-dimethoxybenzamido)penicillanic acid. The sodium salt is a white, crystalline solid that is extremely soluble in water, forming clear, neutral solutions. As with other penicillins, it is very sensitive to moisture, losing about half of its activity in 5 days at room temperature. Refrigeration at 5°C reduces the loss in activity to about 20% in the same period. Solutions prepared for parenteral use may be kept as long as 24 hours if refrigerated. It is extremely sensitive to acid (a pH of 2 causes 50% loss of activity in 20 minutes); thus, it cannot be used orally.

Methicillin sodium is particularly resistant to inactivation by the penicillinase found in staphylococci and somewhat more resistant than penicillin G to penicillinase from *Bacillus cereus*. Methicillin and many other penicillinase-resistant penicillins induce penicillinase formation, an observation that has implications concerning use of these agents in the treatment of penicillin G–sensitive infections. Clearly, the use of a penicillinase-resistant penicillin should not be followed by penicillin G.

The absence of the benzylmethylene group of penicillin G and the steric protection afforded by the 2- and 6-methoxy groups make this compound particularly resistant to enzymatic hydrolysis.

Methicillin sodium has been introduced for use in the treatment of staphylococcal infections caused by strains resistant to other penicillins. It is recommended that it not be used in general therapy, to avoid the possible widespread development of organisms resistant to it.

The incidence of interstitial nephritis, a probable hypersensitivity reaction, is reportedly higher with methicillin than with other penicillins.

Oxacillin Sodium, USP.   Oxacillin sodium, (5-methyl-3-phenyl-4-isoxazolyl)penicillin sodium monohydrate (Prostaphlin), is the salt of a semisynthetic penicillin that is highly resistant to inactivation by penicillinase. Apparently, the steric effects of the 3-phenyl and 5-methyl groups of the isoxazolyl ring prevent the binding of this penicillin to the β-lactamase active site and, thereby, protect the lactam ring from degradation in much the same way as has been suggested for methicillin. It is also relatively resistant to acid hydrolysis and, therefore, may be administered orally with good effect.

Oxacillin Sodium

Oxacillin sodium, which is available in capsule form, is reasonably well absorbed from the gastrointestinal tract, particularly in fasting patients. Effective plasma levels of oxacillin are obtained in about 1 hour, but despite extensive plasma protein binding, it is excreted rapidly through the kidneys. Oxacillin experiences some first-pass metabolism in the liver to the 5-hydroxymethyl derivative. This metabolite has antibacterial activity comparable to that of oxacillin

but is less avidly protein bound and more rapidly excreted. The halogenated analogues cloxacillin, dicloxacillin, and floxacillin experience less 5-methyl hydroxylation.

The use of oxacillin and other isoxazolylpenicillins should be restricted to the treatment of infections caused by staphylococci resistant to penicillin G. Although their spectrum of activity is similar to that of penicillin G, the isoxazolylpenicillins are, in general, inferior to it and the phenoxymethylpenicillins for the treatment of infections caused by penicillin G–sensitive bacteria. Because they cause allergic reactions similar to those produced by other penicillins, the isoxazolylpenicillins should be used with great caution in patients who are penicillin sensitive.

Cloxacillin Sodium, USP.   The chlorine atom *ortho* to the position of attachment of the phenyl ring to the isoxazole ring enhances the activity of cloxacillin sodium, [3-(o-chlorophenyl)-5-methyl-4-isoxazolyl]penicillin sodium monohydrate (Tegopen), over that of oxacillin, not by increasing its intrinsic antibacterial activity but by enhancing its oral absorption, leading to higher plasma levels. In almost all other respects, it resembles oxacillin.

Cloxacillin Sodium

Dicloxacillin Sodium, USP.   The substitution of chlorine atoms on both carbons *ortho* to the position of attachment of the phenyl ring to the isoxazole ring is presumed to enhance further the stability of the oxacillin congener dicloxacillin sodium, [3-(2,6- dichlorophenyl)-5-methyl-4-isoxazolyl]penicillin sodium monohydrate (Dynapen, Pathocil, Veracillin) and to produce high plasma concentrations of it. Its medicinal properties and use are similar to those of cloxacillin sodium. Progressive halogen substitution, however, also increases the fraction bound to protein in the plasma, potentially reducing the concentration of free antibiotic in plasma and tissues. Its medicinal properties and use are the same as those of cloxacillin sodium.

Dicloxacillin Sodium

Nafcillin Sodium, USP.   Nafcillin sodium, 6-(2-ethoxy-1-naphthyl)penicillin sodium (Unipen), is another semisynthetic penicillin that resulted from the search for penicillinase-resistant compounds. Like methicillin, nafcillin has substituents in positions *ortho* to the point of attachment of the aromatic ring to the carboxamide group of penicillin. No doubt, the ethoxy group and the second ring of the naphthalene group play steric roles in stabilizing nafcillin against penicillinase. Very similar structures have been reported to produce similar results in some substituted 2-biphenylpenicillins.[33]

Nafcillin Sodium

Unlike methicillin, nafcillin is stable enough in acid to permit its use by oral administration. When it is given orally, its absorption is somewhat slow and incomplete, but satisfactory plasma levels may be achieved in about 1 hour. Relatively small amounts are excreted through the kidneys; most is excreted in the bile. Even though some cyclic reabsorption from the gut may occur, nafcillin given orally should be readministered every 4 to 6 hours. This salt is readily soluble in water and may be administered intramuscularly or intravenously to obtain high plasma concentrations quickly for the treatment of serious infections.

Nafcillin sodium may be used in infections caused solely by penicillin G–resistant staphylococci or when streptococci are present also. Although it is recommended that it be used exclusively for such resistant infections, nafcillin is also effective against pneumococci and group A *β*-hemolytic streptococci. Because, like other penicillins, it may cause allergic side effects, it should be administered with care.

Ampicillin, USP. Ampicillin, 6-[D-*α*-aminophenylacetamido]penicillanic acid, D-*α*-aminobenzylpenicillin (Penbriten, Polycillin, Omnipen, Amcill, Principen), meets another goal of the research on semisynthetic penicillins—an antibacterial spectrum broader than that of penicillin G. This product is active against the same Gram-positive organisms that are susceptible to other penicillins, and it is more active against some Gram-negative bacteria and enterococci than are other penicillins. Obviously, the *α*-amino group plays an important role in the broader activity, but the mechanism for its action is unknown. It has been suggested that the amino group confers an ability to cross cell wall barriers that are impenetrable to other penicillins. D-(−)-Ampicillin, prepared from D-(−)-*α*-aminophenylacetic acid, is significantly more active than L-(+)-ampicillin.

Ampicillin, USP

Ampicillin is not resistant to penicillinase, and it produces the allergic reactions and other untoward effects found in penicillin-sensitive patients. Because such reactions are relatively rare, however, it may be used to treat infections caused by Gram-negative bacilli for which a broad-spectrum antibiotic, such as a tetracycline or chloramphenicol, may be indicated but not preferred because of undesirable reactions or lack of bactericidal effect. Ampicillin is not so widely active, however, that it should be used as a broad-spectrum antibiotic in the same manner as the tetracyclines. It is particularly useful for the treatment of acute urinary tract infections caused by *E. coli* or *Proteus mirabilis* and is the agent of choice against *Haemophilus influenzae* infections. Ampicillin together with probenecid, to inhibit its active tubular excretion, has become a treatment of choice for gonorrhea in recent years. *β*-Lactamase-producing strains of Gram-negative bacteria that are highly resistant to ampicillin, however, appear to be increasing in the world population. The threat from such resistant strains is particularly great with *H. influenzae* and *N. gonorrhoeae* because there are few alternative therapies for infections caused by these organisms. Incomplete absorption and excretion of effective concentrations in the bile may contribute to the effectiveness of ampicillin in the treatment of salmonellosis and shigellosis.

Ampicillin is water soluble and stable in acid. The protonated *α*-amino group of ampicillin has a pK_a of 7.3,[46] and thus it is protonated extensively in acidic media, which explains ampicillin's stability to acid hydrolysis and instability to alkaline hydrolysis. It is administered orally and is absorbed from the intestinal tract to produce peak plasma concentrations in about 2 hours. Oral doses must be repeated about every 6 hours because it is excreted rapidly and unchanged through the kidneys. It is available as a white, crystalline, anhydrous powder that is sparingly soluble in water or as the colorless or slightly buff-colored crystalline trihydrate that is soluble in water. Either form may be used for oral administration, in capsules or as a suspension. Earlier claims of higher plasma levels for the anhydrous form than for the trihydrate following oral administration have been disputed.[47, 48] The white, crystalline sodium salt is very soluble in water, and solutions for injections should be administered within 1 hour after being made.

Bacampicillin Hydrochloride, USP. Bacampicillin hydrochloride (Spectrobid) is the hydrochloride salt of the 1-ethoxycarbonyloxyethyl ester of ampicillin. It is a prodrug of ampicillin with no antibacterial activity. After oral absorption, bacampicillin is hydrolyzed rapidly by esterases in the plasma to form ampicillin.

Bacampicillin Hydrochloride

Oral absorption of bacampicillin is more rapid and complete than that of ampicillin and less affected by food. Plasma levels of ampicillin from oral bacampicillin exceed those of oral ampicillin or amoxicillin for the first 2.5 hours but thereafter are the same as for ampicillin and amoxicillin.[49] Effective plasma levels are sustained for 12 hours, allowing twice-a-day dosing.

Amoxicillin, USP. Amoxicillin, 6-[D-(−)-α-amino-*p*-hydroxyphenylacetamido]penicillanic acid (Amoxil, Larotid, Polymox), a semisynthetic penicillin introduced in 1974, is simply the *p*-hydroxy analogue of ampicillin, prepared by acylation of 6-APA with *p*-hydroxyphenylglycine.

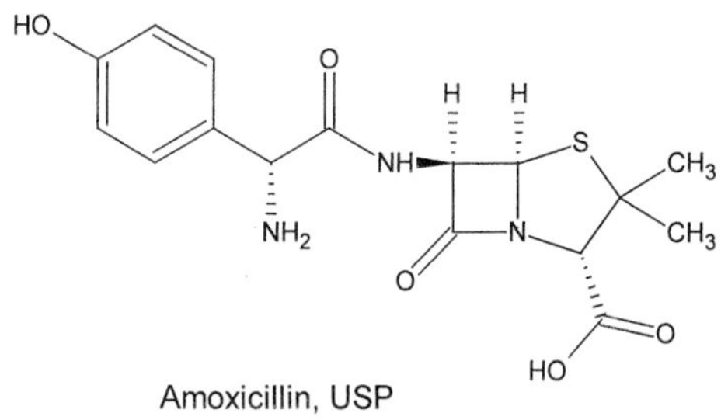

Amoxicillin, USP

Its antibacterial spectrum is nearly identical with that of ampicillin, and like ampicillin, it is resistant to acid, susceptible to alkaline and β-lactamase hydrolysis, and weakly protein bound. Early clinical reports indicated that orally administered amoxicillin possesses significant advantages over ampicillin, including more complete gastrointestinal absorption to give higher plasma and urine levels, less diarrhea, and little or no effect of food on absorption.[50] Thus, amoxicillin has largely replaced ampicillin for the treatment of certain systemic and urinary tract infections for which oral administration is desirable. Amoxicillin is reportedly less effective than ampicillin in the treatment of bacillary dysentery, presumably because of its greater gastrointestinal absorption. Considerable evidence suggests that oral absorption of α-aminobenzyl-substituted penicillins (e.g., ampicillin and amoxicillin) and cephalosporins is, at least in part, carrier mediated,[51] thus explaining their generally superior oral activity.

Amoxicillin is a fine, white to off-white, crystalline powder that is sparingly soluble in water. It is available in a variety of oral dosage forms. Aqueous suspensions are stable for 1 week at room temperature.

Carbenicillin Disodium, Sterile, USP. Carbenicillin disodium, disodium α-carboxybenzylpenicillin (Geopen, Pyopen), is a semisynthetic penicillin released in the United States in 1970, which was introduced in England and first reported by Ancred et al.[52] in 1967. Examination of its structure shows that it differs from ampicillin in having an ionizable carboxyl group rather than an amino group substituted on the α-carbon atom of the benzyl side chain. Carbenicillin has a broad range of antimicrobial activity, broader than any other known penicillin, a property attributed to the unique carboxyl group. It has been proposed that the carboxyl group improves penetration of the molecule through cell wall barriers of Gram-negative bacilli, compared with other penicillins.

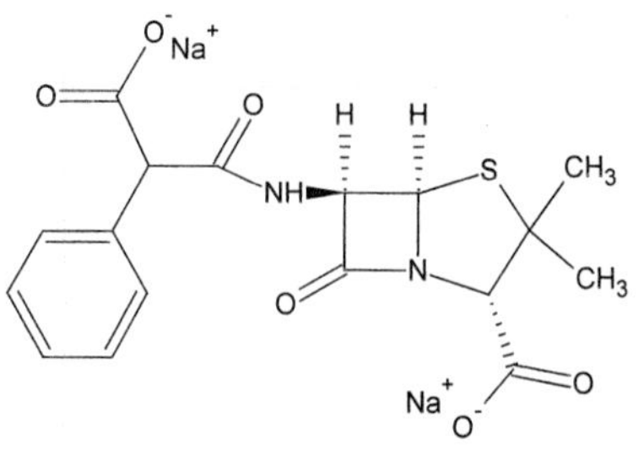

Carbenicillin Disodium, USP

Carbenicillin is not stable in acids and is inactivated by penicillinase. It is a malonic acid derivative and, as such, decarboxylates readily to penicillin G, which is acid labile. Solutions of the disodium salt should be freshly prepared but, when refrigerated, may be kept for 2 weeks. It must be administered by injection and is usually given intravenously.

Carbenicillin has been effective in the treatment of systemic and urinary tract infections caused by *P. aeruginosa*, indole-producing *Proteus* spp., and *Providencia* spp., all of which are resistant to ampicillin. The low toxicity of carbenicillin, with the exception of allergic sensitivity, permits the use of large dosages in serious infections. Most clinicians prefer to use a combination of carbenicillin and gentamicin for serious pseudomonal and mixed coliform infections. The two antibiotics are chemically incompatible, however, and should never be combined in an intravenous solution.

Carbenicillin Indanyl Sodium, USP. Efforts to obtain orally active forms of carbenicillin led to the eventual release of the 5-indanyl ester carbenicillin indanyl, 6-[2-phenyl- 2-(5-indanyloxycarbonyl)acetamido]penicillanic acid (Geocillin), in 1972. Approximately 40% of the usual oral dose of indanyl carbenicillin is absorbed. After absorption, the ester is hydrolyzed rapidly by plasma and tissue esterases to yield carbenicillin. Thus, although the highly lipophilic and highly protein-bound ester has in vitro activity comparable with that of carbenicillin, its activity in vivo is due to carbenicillin. Indanyl carbenicillin thus provides an orally active alternative for the treatment of carbenicillin-sensitive systemic and urinary tract infections caused by *Pseudomonas* spp., indole-positive *Proteus* spp., and selected species of Gram-negative bacilli.

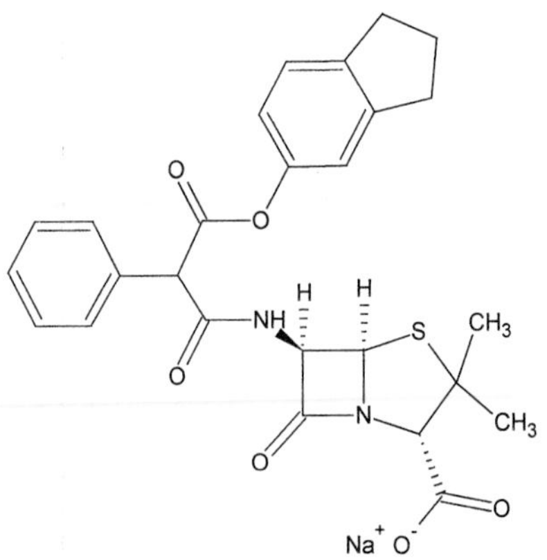

Carbenicillin Indanyl Sodium

Clinical trials with indanyl carbenicillin revealed a relatively high frequency of gastrointestinal symptoms (nausea, occasional vomiting, and diarrhea). It seems doubtful that the high doses required for the treatment of serious systemic infections could be tolerated by most patients. Indanyl carbenicillin occurs as the sodium salt, an off-white, bitter powder that is freely soluble in water. It is stable in acid. It should be protected from moisture to prevent hydrolysis of the ester.

Ticarcillin Disodium, Sterile, USP. Ticarcillin disodium, α-carboxy-3-thienylpenicillin (Ticar), is an isostere of carbenicillin in which the phenyl group is replaced by a thienyl group. This semisynthetic penicillin derivative, like carbenicillin, is unstable in acid and, therefore, must be administered parenterally. It is similar to carbenicillin in antibacterial spectrum and pharmacokinetic properties. Two advantages for ticarcillin are claimed: *(a)* slightly better pharmacokinetic properties, including higher serum levels and a longer duration of action; and *(b)* greater in vitro potency against several species of Gram-negative bacilli, most notably *P. aeruginosa* and *Bacteroides fragilis*. These advantages can be crucial in the treatment of serious infections requiring high-dose therapy.

Ticarcillin Disodium

Mezlocillin Sodium, Sterile, USP. Mezlocillin (Mezlin) is an acylureidopenicillin with an antibacterial spectrum similar to that of carbenicillin and ticarcillin; however, there are some major differences. It is much more active against most *Klebsiella* spp., *P. aeruginosa*, anaerobic bacteria (e.g., *Streptococcus faecalis* and *B. fragilis*), and *H. influenzae*. It is recommended for the treatment of serious infections caused by these organisms.

Mezlocillin Sodium

Mezlocillin is not generally effective against β-lactamase-producing bacteria, nor is it active orally. It is available as a white, crystalline, water-soluble sodium salt for injection. Solutions should be prepared freshly and, if not used within 24 hours, refrigerated. Mezlocillin and other acylureidopenicillins, unlike carbenicillin, exhibit nonlinear pharmacokinetics. Peak plasma levels, half-life, and area under the time curve increase with increased dosage. Mezlocillin has less

effect on bleeding time than carbenicillin, and it is less likely to cause hypokalemia.

Piperacillin Sodium, Sterile, USP. Piperacillin (Pipracil) is the most generally useful of the extended-spectrum acylureidopenicillins. It is more active than mezlocillin against susceptible strains of Gram-negative aerobic bacilli, such as *Serratia marcescens*, *Proteus*, *Enterobacter*, and *Citrobacter* spp., and *P. aeruginosa*. Mezlocillin, however, appears to be more active against *Providencia* spp. and *K. pneumoniae*. Piperacillin is also active against anaerobic bacteria, especially *B. fragilis* and *S. faecalis* (enterococcus). β-lactamase-producing strains of these organisms are, however, resistant to piperacillin, which is hydrolyzed by *S. aureus* β-lactamase. The β-lactamase susceptibility of piperacillin is not absolute because β-lactamase-producing, ampicillin-resistant strains of *N. gonorrhoeae* and *H. influenzae* are susceptible to piperacillin.

Piperacillin Sodium

Piperacillin is destroyed rapidly by stomach acid; therefore, it is active only by intramuscular or intravenous administration. The injectable form is provided as the white, crystalline, water-soluble sodium salt. Its pharmacokinetic properties are very similar to those of the other acylureidopenicillins.

β-LACTAMASE INHIBITORS

The strategy of using a β-lactamase inhibitor in combination with a β-lactamase-sensitive penicillin in the therapy for infections caused by β-lactamase-producing bacterial strains has, until relatively recently, failed to live up to its obvious promise. Early attempts to obtain synergy against such resistant strains, by using combinations consisting of a β-lactamase-resistant penicillin (e.g., methicillin or oxacillin) as a competitive inhibitor and a β-lactamase-sensitive penicillin (e.g., ampicillin or carbenicillin) to kill the organisms, met with limited success. Factors that may contribute to the failure of such combinations to achieve synergy include *(a)* the failure of most lipophilic penicillinase-resistant penicillins to penetrate the cell envelope of Gram-negative bacilli in effective concentrations, *(b)* the reversible binding of penicillinase-resistant penicillins to β-lactamase, requiring high concentrations to prevent substrate binding and hydrolysis, and *(c)* the induction of β-lactamases by some penicillinase-resistant penicillins.

The discovery of the naturally occurring, mechanism-based inhibitor clavulanic acid, which causes potent and progressive inactivation of β-lactamases (Fig. 10-4), has created renewed interest in β-lactam combination therapy. This interest has led to the design and synthesis of additional mechanism-based β-lactamase inhibitors, such as sulbactam and tazobactam, and the isolation of naturally occurring β-lactams, such as the thienamycins, which both inhibit β-lactamases and interact with PBPs.

The chemical events leading to the inactivation of β-lactamases by mechanism-based inhibitors are very complex. In a review of the chemistry of β-lactamase inhibition, Knowles[53] has described two classes of β-lactamase inhibitors: class I inhibitors that have a heteroatom leaving group at position 1 (e.g., clavulanic acid and sulbactam) and class II inhibitors that do not (e.g., the carbapenems). Unlike competitive inhibitors, which bind reversibly to the enzyme they inhibit, mechanism-based inhibitors react with the enzyme in much the same way that the substrate does. With the β-lactamases, an acylenzyme intermediate is formed by reaction of the β-lactam with an active-site serine hydroxyl group of the enzyme. For normal substrates, the acylenzyme intermediate readily undergoes hydrolysis, destroying the substrate and freeing the enzyme to attack more substrate. The acylenzyme intermediate formed when a mechanism-based inhibitor is attacked by the enzyme is diverted by tautomerism to a more stable imine form that hydrolyzes more slowly to eventually free the enzyme (transient inhibition), or for a class I inhibitor, a second group on the enzyme may be attacked to inactivate it. Because these inhibitors are also substrates for the enzymes that they inactivate, they are sometimes referred to as "suicide substrates."

Because they cause prolonged inactivation of certain β-lactamases, class I inhibitors are particularly useful in combination with extended-spectrum, β-lactamase-sensitive penicillins to treat infections caused by β-lactamase-producing bacteria. Three such inhibitors, clavulanic acid, sulbactam, and tazobactam, are currently marketed in the United States for this purpose. A class II inhibitor, the carbapenem derivative imipenem, has potent antibacterial activity in addition to its ability to cause transient inhibition of some β-lactamases. Certain antibacterial cephalosporins with a leaving group at the C-3 position can cause transient inhibition of β-lactamases by forming stabilized acylenzyme intermediates. These are discussed more fully below in this chapter.

The relative susceptibilities of various β-lactamases to inactivation by class I inhibitors appear to be related to the molecular properties of the enzymes.[25, 54, 55] β-Lactamases belonging to group A, a large and somewhat heterogenous group of serine enzymes, some with narrow (e.g., penicillinases or cephalosporinases) and some with broad (i.e., general β-lactamases) specificities, are generally inactivated by class I inhibitors. A large group of chromosomally encoded serine β-lactamases belonging to group C with specificity for cephalosporins are, however, resistant to inactivation by class I inhibitors. A small group of Zn^{2+}-requiring metallo-

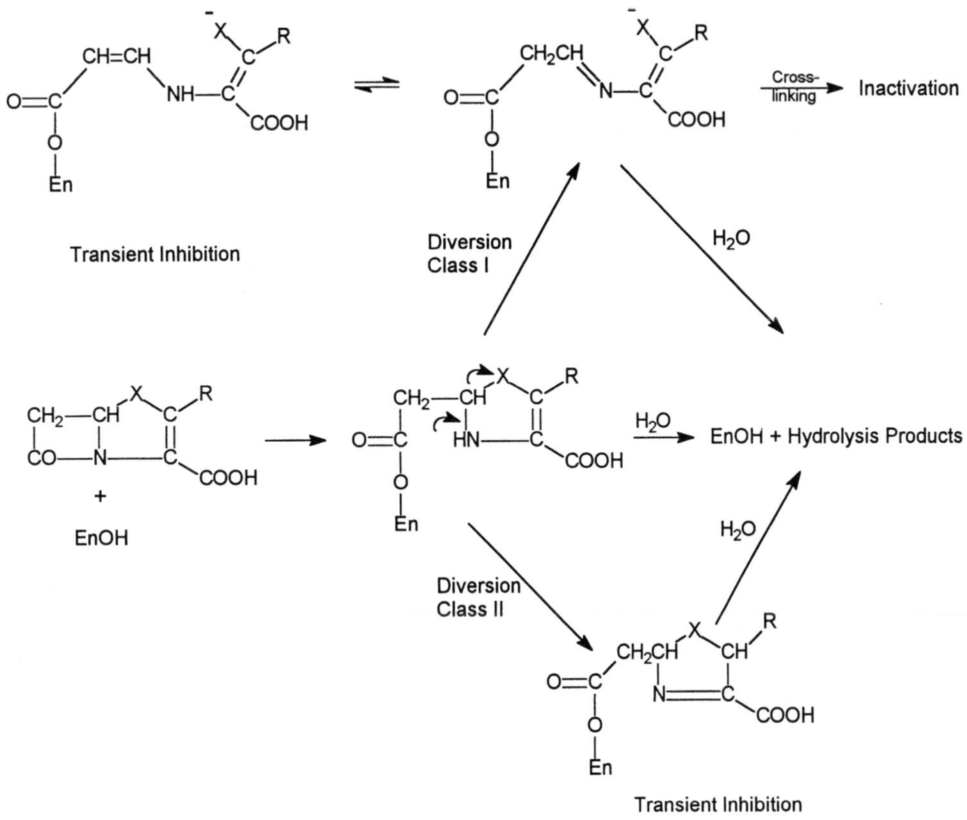

Figure 10–4 ■ Mechanism-based inhibition of β-lactamases.

β-lactamases (group B) with broad substrate specificities[56] are also not inactivated by class I inhibitors.

Products

Clavulanate Potassium, USP. Clavulanic acid is an antibiotic isolated from *Streptomyces clavuligeris*. Structurally, it is a 1-oxopenam lacking the 6-acylamino side chain of penicillins but possessing a 2-hydroxyethylidene moiety at C-2. Clavulanic acid exhibits very weak antibacterial activity, comparable with that of 6-APA and, therefore, is not useful as an antibiotic. It is, however, a potent inhibitor of *S. aureus* β-lactamase and plasmid-mediated β-lactamases elaborated by Gram-negative bacilli.

Clavulanate Potassium

Combinations of amoxicillin and the potassium salt of clavulanic acid are available (Augmentin) in a variety of fixed-dose oral dosage forms intended for the treatment of skin, respiratory, ear, and urinary tract infections caused by β-lactamase-producing bacterial strains. These combinations are effective against β-lactamase-producing strains of *S. aureus, E. coli, K. pneumoniae, Enterobacter, H. influenzae, Moraxella catarrhalis,* and *H. ducreyi,* which are resistant to amoxicillin alone. The oral bioavailability of amoxicillin and potassium clavulanate is similar. Clavulanic acid is acid-stable. It cannot undergo penicillanic acid formation because it lacks an amide side chain.

Potassium clavulanate and the extended-spectrum penicillin ticarcillin have been combined in a fixed-dose, injectable form for the control of serious infections caused by β-lactamase-producing bacterial strains. This combination has been recommended for septicemia, lower respiratory tract infections, and urinary tract infections caused by β-lactamase-producing *Klebsiella* spp., *E. coli, P. aeruginosa* and other *Pseudomonas* spp., *Citrobacter* spp., *Enterobacter* spp., *Serratia marcescens,* and *Staphylococcus aureus.* It also is used in bone and joint infections caused by these organisms. The combination contains 3 g of ticarcillin disodium and 100 mg of potassium clavulanate in a sterile powder for injection (Timentin).

Sulbactam, USP. Sulbactam is penicillanic acid sulfone or 1,1-dioxopenicillanic acid. This synthetic penicillin derivative is a potent inhibitor of *S. aureus* β-lactamase as well as many β-lactamases elaborated by Gram-negative bacilli. Sulbactam has weak intrinsic antibacterial activity but potentiates the activity of ampicillin and carbenicillin against β-lactamase-producing *S. aureus* and members of the Enterobacteriaceae family. It does not, however, synergize with either carbenicillin or ticarcillin against *P. aeruginosa* strains resistant to these agents. Failure of sulbactam to penetrate the cell envelope is a possible explanation for the lack of synergy.

Sulbactam Sodium

Fixed-dose combinations of ampicillin sodium and sulbactam sodium, marketed under the trade name Unasyn as sterile powders for injection, have been approved for use in the United States. These combinations are recommended for the treatment of skin, tissue, intra-abdominal, and gynecological infections caused by β-lactamase-producing strains of *S. aureus, E. coli, Klebsiella* spp., *P. mirabilis, B. fragilis,* and *Enterobacter* and *Acinetobacter* spp.

Tazobactam, USP. Tazobactam is a penicillanic acid sulfone that is similar in structure to sulbactam. It is a more potent β-lactamase inhibitor than sulbactam[57] and has a slightly broader spectrum of activity than clavulanic acid. It has very weak antibacterial activity. Tazobactam is available in fixed-dose, injectable combinations with piperacillin, a broad-spectrum penicillin consisting of an 8:1 ratio of piperacillin sodium to tazobactam sodium by weight and marketed under the trade name Zosyn. The pharmacokinetics of the two drugs are very similar. Both have short half-lives ($t_{1/2} \sim 1$ hour), are minimally protein bound, experience very little metabolism, and are excreted in active forms in the urine in high concentrations.

Tazobactam

Approved indications for the piperacillin–tazobactam combination include the treatment of appendicitis, postpartum endometritis, and pelvic inflammatory disease caused by β-lactamase-producing *E. coli* and *Bacteroides* spp., skin and skin structure infections caused by β-lactamase-producing *S. aureus,* and pneumonia caused by β-lactamase-producing strains of *H. influenzae.*

CARBAPENEMS

Thienamycin. Thienamycin is a novel β-lactam antibiotic first isolated and identified by researchers at Merck[58] from fermentation of cultures of *Streptomyces cattleya*. Its structure and absolute configuration were established both spectroscopically and by total synthesis.[59, 60] Two structural features of thienamycin are shared with the penicillins and cephalosporins: a fused bicyclic ring system containing a β-lactam and an equivalently attached 3-carboxyl group. In other respects, the thienamycins represent a significant departure from the established β-lactam antibiotics. The bicyclic system consists of a carbapenem containing a double bond between C-2 and C-3 (i.e., it is a 2-carbapenem, or Δ^2-carbapenem, system). The double bond in the bicyclic structure creates considerable ring strain and increases the reactivity of the β-lactam to ring-opening reactions. The side chain is unique in two respects: it is a simple 1-hydroxyethyl group instead of the familiar acylamino side chain, and it is oriented to the bicyclic ring system rather than having the usual β orientation of the penicillins and cephalosporins. The remaining feature is a 2-aminoethylthioether function at C-2. The absolute stereochemistry of thienamycin has been determined to be 5*R*:6*S*:8*S*. Several additional structurally related antibiotics have been isolated from various *Streptomyces* spp., including the four epithienamycins, which are isomeric to thienamycin at C-5, C-6, or C-8, and derivatives in which the 2-aminoethylthio side chain is modified.

Thienamycin

Thienamycin displays outstanding broad-spectrum antibacterial properties in vitro.[61] It is highly active against most aerobic and anaerobic Gram-positive and Gram-negative bacteria, including *S. aureus*, *P. aeruginosa*, and *B. fragilis*. Furthermore, it is resistant to inactivation by most β-lactamases elaborated by Gram-negative and Gram-positive bacteria and, therefore, is effective against many strains resistant to penicillins and cephalosporins. Resistance to lactamases appears to be a function of the α-1-hydroxyethyl side chain because this property is lost in the 6-nor derivative and epithienamycins with *S* stereochemistry show variable resistance to the different β-lactamases.

An unfortunate property of thienamycin is its chemical instability in solution. It is more susceptible to hydrolysis in both acidic and alkaline solutions than most β-lactam antibiotics, because of the strained nature of its fused ring system containing an endocyclic double bond. Furthermore, at its optimally stable pH between 6 and 7, thienamycin undergoes concentration-dependent inactivation. This inactivation is believed to result from intermolecular aminolysis of the β-lactam by the cysteamine side chain of a second molecule. Another shortcoming is its susceptibility to hydrolytic inactivation by renal dehydropeptidase-I (DHP-I),[62]

which causes it to have an unacceptably short half-life in vivo.

Imipenem–Cilastatin, USP. Imipenem is *N*-formimidoylthienamycin, the most successful of a series of chemically stable derivatives of thienamycin in which the primary amino group is converted to a nonnucleophilic basic function.[63] Cilastatin is an inhibitor of DHP-I. The combination (Primaxin) provides a chemically and enzymatically stable form of thienamycin that has clinically useful pharmacokinetic properties. The half-life of the drug is nonetheless short ($t_{1/2} \sim 1$ hour) because of renal tubular secretion of imipenem. Imipenem retains the extraordinary broad-spectrum antibacterial properties of thienamycin. Its bactericidal activity results from the inhibition of cell wall synthesis associated with bonding to PBPs 1_b and 2. Imipenem is very stable to most β-lactamases. It is an inhibitor of β-lactamases from certain Gram-negative bacteria resistant to other β-lactam antibiotics, e.g., *P. aeruginosa*, *S. marcescens*, and *Enterobacter* spp.

Imipenem is indicated for the treatment of a wide variety of bacterial infections of the skin and tissues, lower respiratory tract, bones and joints, and genitourinary tract, as well as of septicemia and endocarditis caused by β-lactamase-producing strains of susceptible bacteria. These include aerobic Gram-positive organisms such as *S. aureus*, *S. epidermidis*, enterococci, and viridans streptococci; aerobic Gram-negative bacteria such as *E. coli*, *Klebsiella*, *Serratia*, *Providencia*, *Haemophilus*, *Citrobacter*, and indole-positive *Proteus* spp., *Morganella morganii*, *Acinetobacter* and *Enterobacter* spp., and *P. aeruginosa* and anaerobes such as *B. fragilis* and *Clostridium*, *Peptococcus*, *Peptidostreptococcus*, *Eubacterium*, and *Fusobacterium* spp. Some *Pseudomonas* spp. are resistant, such as *P. maltophilia* and *P. cepacia*, as are some methicillin-resistant staphylococci. Imipenem is effective against non–β-lactamase-producing strains of these and additional bacterial species, but other less expensive and equally effective antibiotics are preferred for the treatment of infections caused by these organisms.

The imipenem–cilastatin combination is marketed as a sterile powder intended for the preparation of solutions for intravenous infusion. Such solutions are stable for 4 hours at 25°C and up to 24 hours when refrigerated. The concomitant

Imipenem-Cilastatin

administration of imipenem and an aminoglycoside antibiotic results in synergistic antibacterial activity in vivo. The two types of antibiotics are, however, chemically incompatible and should never be combined in the same intravenous bottle.

INVESTIGATIONAL CARBAPENEMS

The extended spectrum of antibacterial activity associated with the carbapenems together with their resistance to inactivation by most β-lactamases make this class of β-lactams an attractive target for drug development. In the design of new carbapenems, structural variations are being investigated with the objective of developing analogues with advantages over imipenem. Improvements that are particularly desired include stability to hydrolysis catalyzed by DHP-I,[62] stability to bacterial metallo-β-lactamases ("carbapenemases")[56] that hydrolyze imipenem, activity against MRSA,[31] and increased potency against *P. aeruginosa*, especially imipenem-resistant strains. Enhanced pharmacokinetic properties, such as oral bioavailability and a longer duration of action, have heretofore received little emphasis in carbapenem analogue design.

Early structure–activity studies established the critical importance of the Δ^2 position of the double bond, the 3-carboxyl group, and the 6-α-hydroxyethyl side chain for both broad-spectrum antibacterial activity and β-lactamase stability in carbapenems. Modifications, therefore, have concentrated on variations at positions 1 and 2 of the carbapenem nucleus. The incorporation of a β-methyl group at the 1 position gives the carbapenem stability to hydrolysis by renal DHP-I.[64, 65] Substituents at the 2 position, however, appear to affect primarily the spectrum of antibacterial activity of the carbapenem by influencing penetration into bacteria. The capability of carbapenems to exist as zwitterionic structures (as exemplified by imipenem and biapenem), resulting from the combined features of a basic amine function attached to the 2 position and the 3-carboxyl group, may enable these molecules to enter bacteria via their charged porin channels.

Meropenem. Meropenem is a second-generation carbapenem that, to date, has undergone the most extensive clinical evaluation.[66] It has recently been approved as Merrem for the treatment of infections caused by multiply-resistant bacteria and for empirical therapy for serious infections, such as bacterial meningitis, septicemia, pneumonia, and peritonitis. Meropenem exhibits greater potency against Gram-negative and anaerobic bacteria than does imipenem, but it is slightly less active against most Gram-positive species. It is not effective against MRSA. Meropenem is not hydrolyzed by DHP-I and is resistant to most β-lactamases, including a few carbapenemases that hydrolyze carbapenem.

Like imipenem, meropenem is not active orally. It is provided as a sterile lyophilized powder to be made up in normal saline or 5% dextrose solution for parenteral administration. Approximately 70 to 80% of unchanged meropenem is excreted in the urine following intravenous or intramuscular administration. The remainder is the inactive metabolite formed by hydrolytic cleavage of the β-lactam ring. The lower incidence of nephrotoxicity of meropenem (compared with imipenem) has been correlated with its greater stability to DHP-I and the absence of the DHP-I inhibitor cilastatin in

the preparation. Meropenem appears to be less epileptogenic than imipenem when the two agents are used in the treatment of bacterial meningitis.

Meropenem

Meropenem Metabolite

Biapenem. Biapenem is a newer second-generation carbapenem with chemical and microbiological properties similar to those of meropenem.[67] Thus, it has broad-spectrum antibacterial activity that includes most aerobic Gram-negative and Gram-positive bacteria and anaerobes. Biapenem is stable to DHP-I[67] and resistant to most β-lactamases.[68] It is claimed to be less susceptible to metallo-β-lactamases than either imipenem or meropenem. It is not active orally.

CEPHALOSPORINS

Historical Background

The cephalosporins are β-lactam antibiotics isolated from *Cephalosporium* spp. or prepared semisynthetically. Most of the antibiotics introduced since 1965 have been semisynthetic cephalosporins. Interest in *Cephalosporium* fungi began in 1945 with Giuseppe Brotzu's discovery that cultures of *C. acremonium* inhibited the growth of a wide variety of Gram-positive and Gram-negative bacteria. Abraham and Newton[68a] in Oxford, having been supplied cultures of the fungus in 1948, isolated three principal antibiotic components: cephalosporin Pl, a steroid with minimal antibacterial activity; cephalosporin N, later discovered to be identical with synnematin N (a penicillin derivative now called penicillin N that had earlier been isolated from *C. salmosynnematum*); and cephalosporin C.

Penicillin N

Cephalosporin C

The structure of penicillin N was discovered to be D-(4-amino-4-carboxybutyl)penicillanic acid. The amino acid side chain confers more activity against Gram-negative bacteria, particularly *Salmonella* spp., but less activity against Gram-positive organisms than penicillin G. It has been used successfully in clinical trials for the treatment of typhoid fever but was never released as an approved drug.

Cephalosporin C turned out to be a close congener of penicillin N, containing a dihydrothiazine ring instead of the thiazolidine ring of the penicillins. Despite the observation that cephalosporin C was resistant to *S. aureus* β-lactamase, early interest in it was not great because its antibacterial potency was inferior to that of penicillin N and other penicillins. The discovery that the α-aminoadipoyl side chain could be removed to efficiently produce 7-aminocephalosporanic acid (7-ACA),[69, 70] however, prompted investigations that led to semisynthetic cephalosporins of medicinal value. The relationship of 7-ACA and its acyl derivatives to 6-APA and the semisynthetic penicillins is obvious. Woodward et al.[71] have prepared both cephalosporin C and the clinically useful cephalothin by an elegant synthetic procedure, but the commercially available drugs are obtained from 7-ACA as semisynthetic products.

Nomenclature

The chemical nomenclature of the cephalosporins is slightly more complex than even that of the penicillins because of the presence of a double bond in the dihydrothiazine ring. The fused ring system is designated by *Chemical Abstracts* as 5-thia-1-azabicyclo[4.2.0]oct-2-ene. In this system, cephalothin is 3-(acetoxymethyl)-7-[2-(thienylacetyl)amino]-8-oxo-5-thia-1- azabicyclo[4.2.0]oct-2-ene-2-carboxylic acid. A simplification that retains some of the systematic nature of the *Chemical Abstracts* procedure names the saturated bicyclic ring system with the lactam carbonyl oxygen *cepham* (cf., *penam* for penicillins). According to this system, all commercially available cephalosporins and cephamycins are named *3-cephems* (or *Δ³-cephems*) to designate the position of the double bond. (Interestingly, all known 2-cephems are inactive, presumably because the β-lactam lacks the necessary ring strain to react sufficiently.) The

trivialized forms of nomenclature of the type that have been applied to the penicillins are not consistently applicable to the naming of cephalosporins because of variations in the substituent at the 3 position. Thus, although some cephalosporins are named as derivatives of cephalosporanic acids, this practice applies only to the derivatives that have a 3-acetoxymethyl group.

Cephalosporins

Cepham

Cephalosporanic Acid

Semisynthetic Derivatives

To date, the more useful semisynthetic modifications of the basic 7-ACA nucleus have resulted from acylations of the 7-amino group with different acids or nucleophilic substitution or reduction of the acetoxyl group. Structure–activity relationships (SARs) among the cephalosporins appear to parallel those among the penicillins insofar as the acyl group is concerned. The presence of an allylic acetoxyl function in the 3 position, however, provides a reactive site at which various 7-acylaminocephalosporanic acid structures can easily be varied by nucleophilic displacement reactions. Reduction of the 3-acetoxymethyl to a 3-methyl substituent to prepare 7-aminodesacetylcephalosporanic acid (7-ADCA) derivatives can be accomplished by catalytic hydrogenation, but the process currently used for the commercial synthesis of 7-ADCA derivatives involves the rearrangement of the corresponding penicillin sulfoxide.[72] Perhaps the most noteworthy development thus far is the discovery that 7-phenylglycyl derivatives of 7-ACA and especially 7-ADCA are active orally.

In the preparation of semisynthetic cephalosporins, the following improvements are sought: (*a*) increased acid stability, (*b*) improved pharmacokinetic properties, particularly better oral absorption, (*c*) broadened antimicrobial spectrum, (*d*) increased activity against resistant microorganisms (as a result of resistance to enzymatic destruction, improved penetration, increased receptor affinity, etc.), (*e*) decreased allergenicity, and (*f*) increased tolerance after parenteral administration.

Structures of cephalosporins currently marketed in the United States are shown in Table 10-4.

Chemical Degradation

Cephalosporins experience a variety of hydrolytic degradation reactions whose specific nature depends on the individ-

TABLE 10–4 Structure of Cephalosporins

ORAL CEPHALOSPORINS

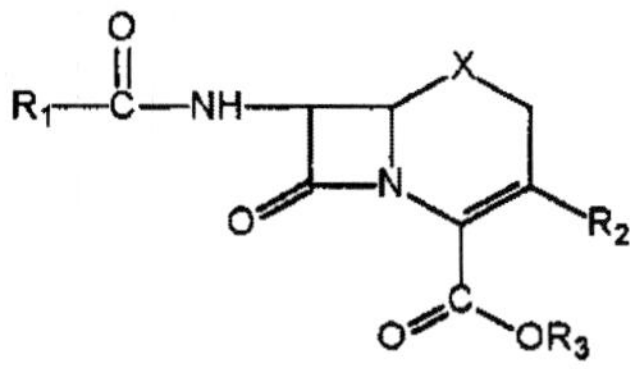

Generic Name	R₁	R₂	R₃	X
Cephalexin		—CH₃	—H	—S—
Cephradine		—CH₃	—H	—S—
Cefadroxil		—CH₃	—H	—S—
Cefachlor	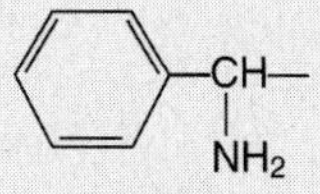	—Cl	—H	—S—
Cefprozil		—CH=CHCH₃	—H	—S—
Loracarbef		—Cl	—H	—CH₂—
Cefuroxime axetil		—CH₂OCNH₂ ($\overset{O}{\|}$)	$-\overset{O}{\overset{\|}{C}}HOCCH_3$ with CH₃	—S—
Cefpodoxime proxetil		—CH₂OCH₃	$-\overset{O}{\overset{\|}{C}}HOCOCH(CH_3)_2$ with CH₃	—S—
Cefixime		—C=CH₂	—H	—S—

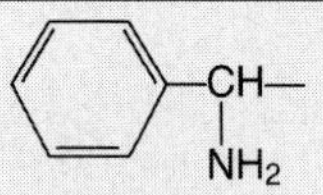

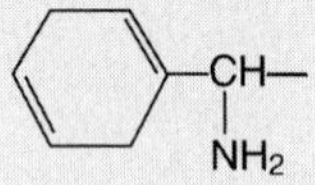

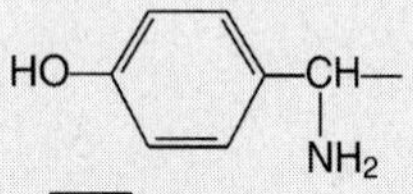

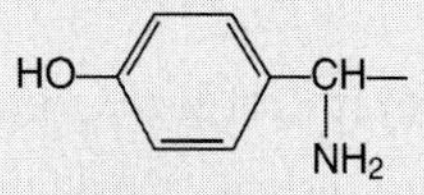

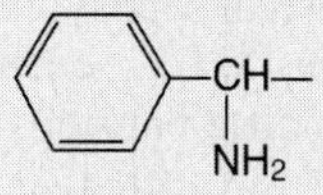

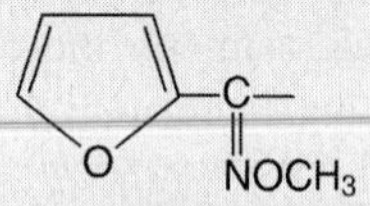

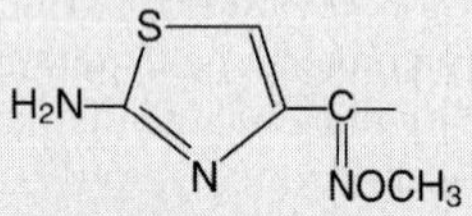

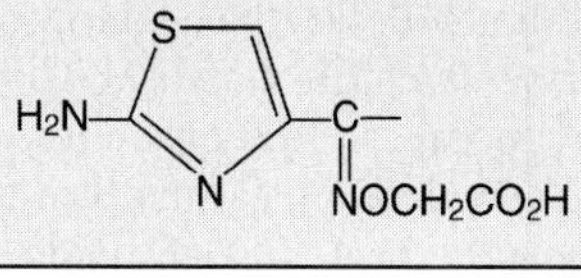

PARENTERAL CEPHALOSPORINS

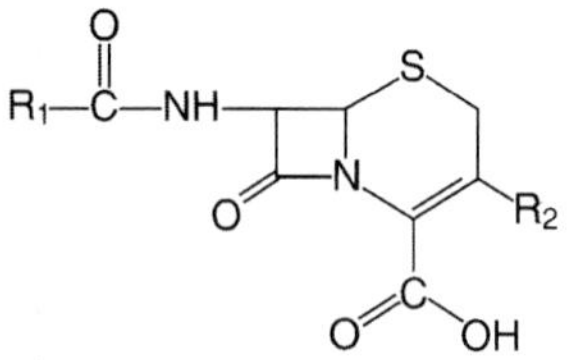

Generic Name	R₁	R₂
Cephalothin		—CH₂OCCH₃ ($\overset{\|}{O}$)
Cephapirin		—CH₂OCCH₃ ($\overset{\|}{O}$)

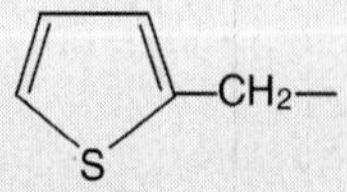

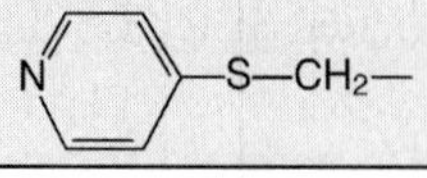

TABLE 10–4—*Continued*

Generic Name	R_1	R_2
Cefazolin	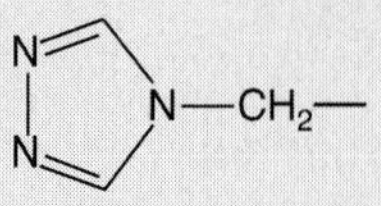	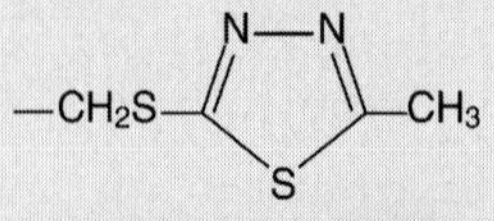
Cefamandole	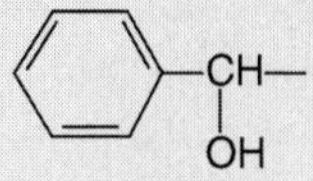	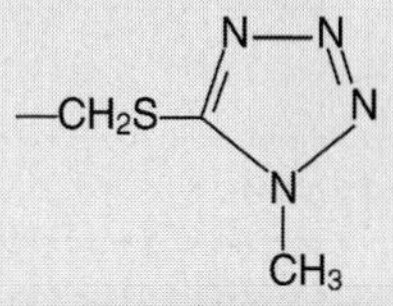
Cefonicid	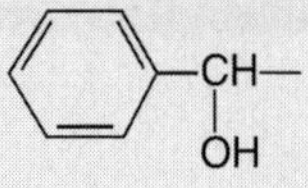	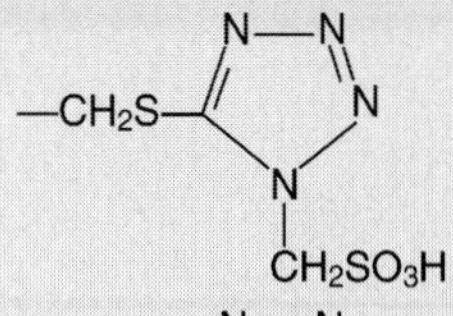
Ceforanide	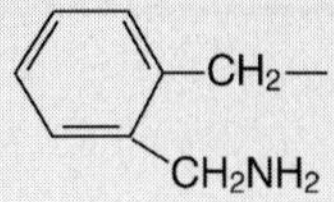	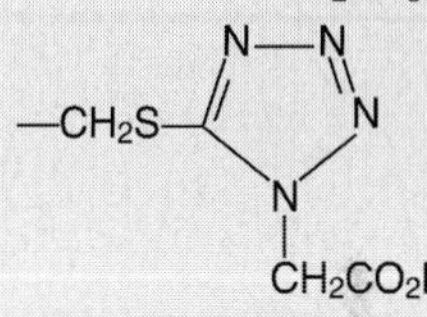
Cefuroxime	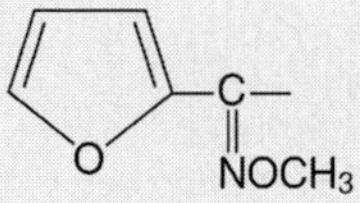	$-CH_2OC(O)NH_2$
Cefotaxime	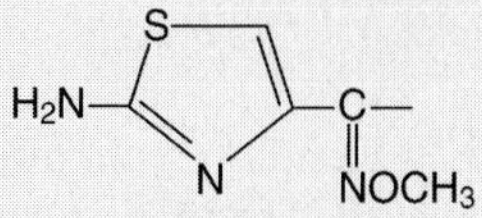	$-CH_2OC(O)CH_3$
Ceftizoxime	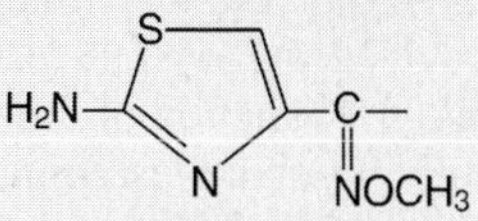	—H
Ceftriaxone	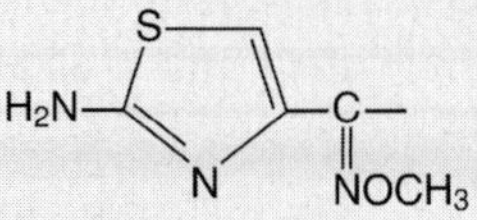	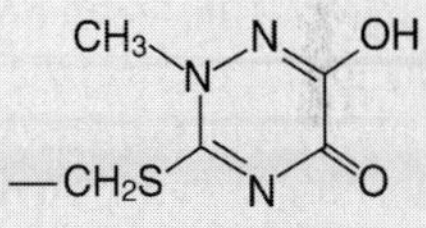
Ceftazidime	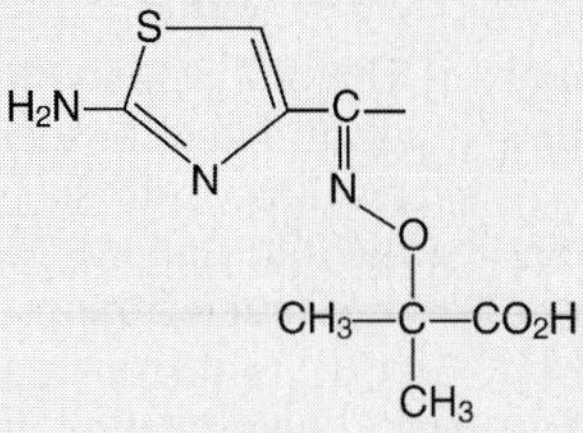	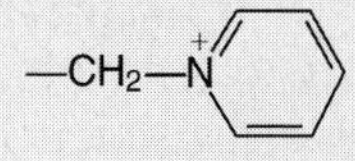
Cefoperazone	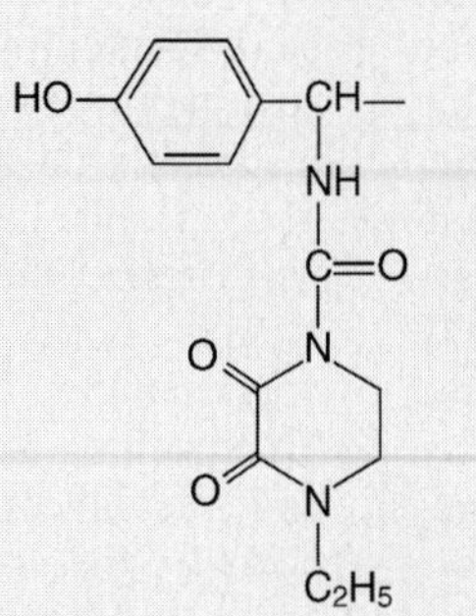	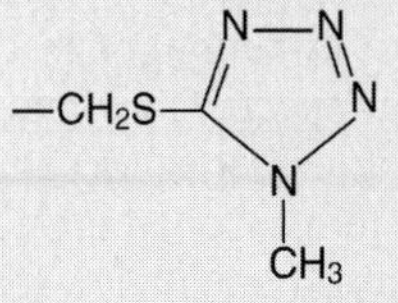

(Continued)

TABLE 10–4 Structure of Cephalosporins—*Continued*

PARENTERAL CEPHAMYCINS

Generic Name	R_1	R_2
Cefoxitin		
Cefotetan		
Cefmetazole		

ual structure (Table 10-4).[73] Among 7-acylaminocephalosporanic acid derivatives, the 3-acetoxylmethyl group is the most reactive site. In addition to its reactivity to nucleophilic displacement reactions, the acetoxyl function of this group readily undergoes solvolysis in strongly acidic solutions to form the desacetylcephalosporin derivatives. The latter lactonize to form the desacetylcephalosporin lactones, which are virtually inactive. The 7-acylamino group of some cephalosporins can also be hydrolyzed under enzymatic (acylases) and, possibly, nonenzymatic conditions to give 7-ACA (or 7-ADCA) derivatives. Following hydrolysis or solvolysis of the 3-acetoxymethyl group, 7-ACA also lactonizes under acidic conditions (Fig. 10-5).

The reactive functionality common to all cephalosporins is the β-lactam. Hydrolysis of the β-lactam of cephalosporins is believed to give initially cephalosporoic acids (in which the R' group is stable, e.g., R' = H or S heterocycle) or possibly anhydrodesacetylcephalosporoic acids (for the 7-acylaminocephalosporanic acids). It has not been possible to isolate either of these initial hydrolysis products in aqueous systems. Apparently, both types of cephalosporanic acid undergo fragmentation reactions that have not been characterized fully. Studies of the in vivo metabolism[74] of orally administered cephalosporins, however, have demonstrated arylacetylglycines and arylacetamidoethanols, which are believed to be formed from the corresponding arylacetylaminoacetaldehydes by metabolic oxidation and reduction, respectively. The aldehydes, no doubt, arise from nonenzymatic hydrolysis of the corresponding cephalosporoic acids. No evidence for the intramolecular opening of the β-lactam ring by the 7-acylamino oxygen to form oxazolones of the penicillanic acid type has been found in the cephalosporins. At neutral to alkaline pH, however, intramolecular

aminolysis of the β-lactam ring by the α-amino group in the 7-ADCA derivatives cephaloglycin, cephradine, and cefadroxil occurs, forming diketopiperazine derivatives.[75, 76] The formation of dimers and, possibly, polymers from 7-ADCA derivatives containing an α-amino group in the acylamino side chain may also occur, especially in concentrated solutions and at alkaline pH values.

Oral Cephalosporins

The oral activity conferred by the phenylglycyl substituent is attributed to increased acid stability of the lactam ring, resulting from the presence of a protonated amino group on the 7-acylamino portion of the molecule. Carrier-mediated transport of these dipeptide-like, zwitterionic cephalosporins[51] is also an important factor in their excellent oral activity. The situation, then, is analogous to that of the α-aminobenzylpenicillins (e.g., ampicillin). Also important for high acid stability (and, therefore, good oral activity) of the cephalosporins is the absence of the leaving group at the 3 position. Thus, despite the presence of the phenylglycyl side chain in its structure, the cephalosporanic acid derivative cephaloglycin is poorly absorbed orally, presumably because of solvolysis of the 3-acetoxyl group in the low pH of the stomach. The resulting 3-hydroxyl derivative undergoes lactonization under acidic conditions. The 3-hydroxyl derivatives and, especially, the corresponding lactones are considerably less active in vitro than the parent cephalosporins. Generally, acyl derivatives of 7-ADCA show lower in vitro antibacterial potencies than the corresponding 7-ACA analogues.

Oral activity can also be conferred in certain cephalosporins by esterification of the 3-carboxylic acid group to form acid-stable, lipophilic esters that undergo hydrolysis in the

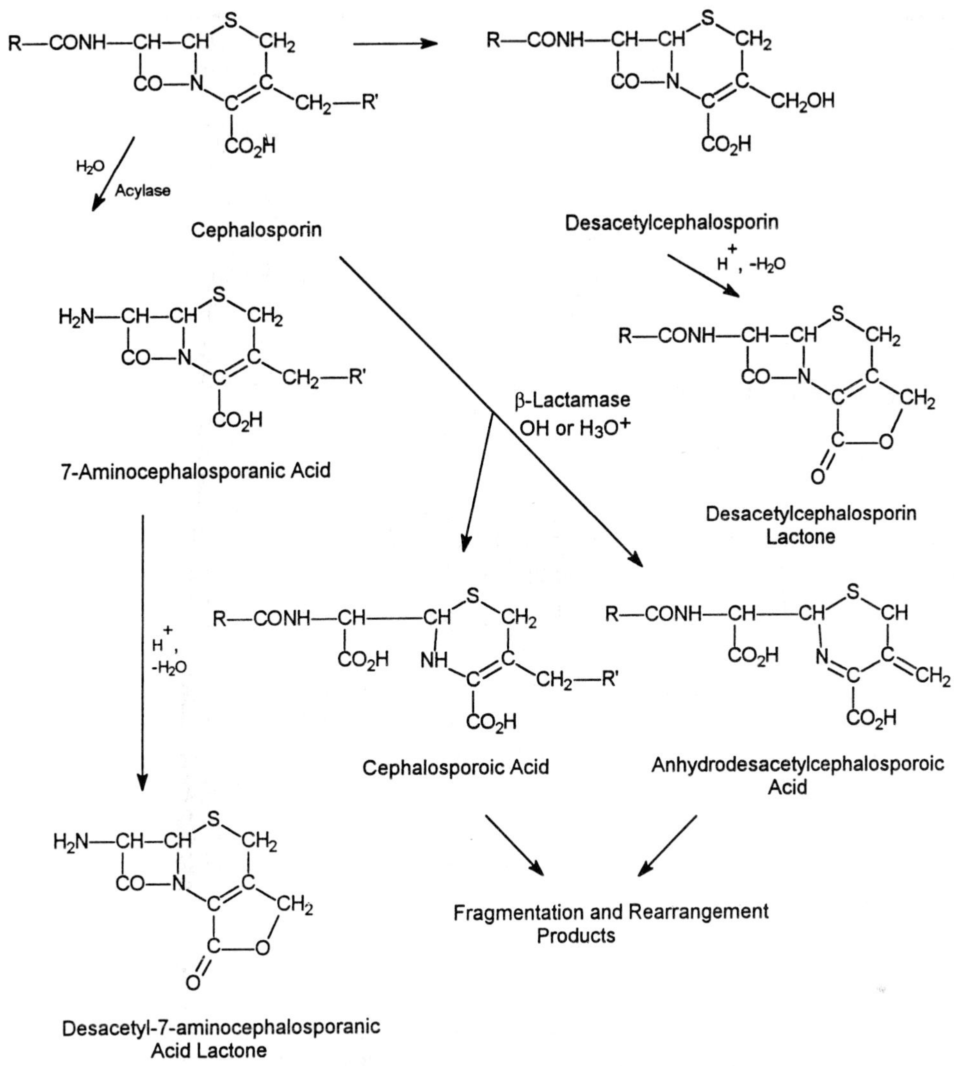

Figure 10–5 ■ Degradation of cephalosporins.

plasma. Cefuroxime axetil and cefpodoxime proxetil are two β-lactamase-resistant alkoximino-cephalosporins that are orally active ester prodrug derivatives of cefuroxime and cefpodoxime, respectively, based on this concept.

Parenteral Cephalosporins

Hydrolysis of the ester function, catalyzed by hepatic and renal esterases, is responsible for some in vivo inactivation of parenteral cephalosporins containing a 3-acetoxymethyl substituent (e.g., cephalothin, cephapirin, and cefotaxime). The extent of such inactivation (20 to 35%) is not large enough to seriously compromise the in vivo effectiveness of acetoxyl cephalosporins. Parenteral cephalosporins lacking a hydrolyzable group at the 3 position are not subject to hydrolysis by esterases. Cephradine is the only cephalosporin that is used both orally and parenterally.

Spectrum of Activity

The cephalosporins are considered broad-spectrum antibiotics with patterns of antibacterial effectiveness comparable to that of ampicillin. Several significant differences exist, however. Cephalosporins are much more resistant to inactivation by β-lactamases, particularly those produced by Gram-positive bacteria, than is ampicillin. Ampicillin, however, is generally more active against non–β-lactamase-producing strains of Gram-positive and Gram-negative bacteria sensitive to both it and the cephalosporins. Cephalosporins, among β-lactam antibiotics, exhibit uniquely potent activity against most species of *Klebsiella*. Differential potencies of cephalosporins, compared with penicillins, against different species of bacteria have been attributed to several variable characteristics of individual bacterial species and strains, the most important of which probably are (*a*) resistance to inactivation by β-lactamases, (*b*) permeability of bacterial cells, and (*c*) intrinsic activity against bacterial enzymes involved in cell wall synthesis and cross-linking.

β-Lactamase Resistance

The susceptibility of cephalosporins to various lactamases varies considerably with the source and properties of these enzymes. Cephalosporins are significantly less sensitive than all but the β-lactamase-resistant penicillins to hydrolysis by the enzymes from *S. aureus* and *Bacillus subtilis*. The "penicillinase" resistance of cephalosporins appears to be a property of the bicyclic cephem ring system rather than of the acyl group. Despite natural resistance to staphylococcal β-lactamase, the different cephalosporins exhibit considerable variation in rates of hydrolysis by the enzyme.[77] Thus, of several cephalosporins tested in vitro, cephalothin and cefoxitin are the most resistant, and cephaloridine and cefazolin are the least resistant. The same acyl functionalities that impart β-lactamase resistance in the penicillins unfortunately render cephalosporins virtually inactive against *S. aureus* and other Gram-positive bacteria.

β-Lactamases elaborated by Gram-negative bacteria present an exceedingly complex picture. Well over 100 different enzymes from various species of Gram-negative bacilli have been identified and characterized,[25] differing widely in specificity for various β-lactam antibiotics. Most of these enzymes hydrolyze penicillin G and ampicillin faster than the cephalosporins. Some inducible β-lactamases belonging to group C, however, are "cephalosporinases," which hydrolyze cephalosporins more rapidly. Inactivation by β-lactamases is an important factor in determining resistance to cephalosporins in many strains of Gram-negative bacilli.

The introduction of polar substituents in the aminoacyl moiety of cephalosporins appears to confer stability to some β-lactamases.[78] Thus, cefamandole and cefonicid, which contain an α-hydroxyphenylacetyl (or mandoyl) group, and ceforanide, which has an o-aminophenyl acetyl group, are resistant to a few β-lactamases. Steric factors also may be important because cefoperazone, an acylureidocepha-

losporin that contains the same 4-ethyl-2,3-dioxo-1-piperazinylcarbonyl group present in piperacillin, is resistant to many β-lactamases. Oddly enough, piperacillin is hydrolyzed by most of these enzymes.

Two structural features confer broadly based resistance to β-lactamases among the cephalosporins: (a) an alkoximino function in the aminoacyl group and (b) a methoxyl substituent at the 7 position of the cephem nucleus having α stereochemistry. The structures of several β-lactamase-resistant cephalosporins, including cefuroxime, cefotaxime, ceftizoxime, and ceftriaxone, feature a methoximino acyl group. β-Lactamase resistance is enhanced modestly if the oximino substituent also features a polar function, as in ceftazidime, which has a 2-methylpropionic acid substituent on the oximino group. Both steric and electronic properties of the alkoximino group may contribute to the β-lactamase resistance conferred by this functionality since *syn* isomers are more potent than *anti* isomers.[78] β-Lactamase-resistant 7α-methoxylcephalosporins, also called cephamycins because they are derived from cephamycin C (an antibiotic isolated from *Streptomyces*), are represented by cefoxitin, cefotetan, cefmetazole, and the 1-oxocephalosporin moxalactam, which is prepared by total synthesis.

Base- or β-lactamase-catalyzed hydrolysis of cephalosporins containing a good leaving group at the 3′ position is accompanied by elimination of the leaving group. The enzymatic process occurs in a stepwise fashion, beginning with the formation of a tetrahedral transition state, which quickly collapses into an acylenzyme intermediate (Fig. 10-6). This intermediate can then either undergo hydrolysis to free the enzyme (path 1) or suffer elimination of the leaving group to form a relatively stable acyl enzyme with a conjugated

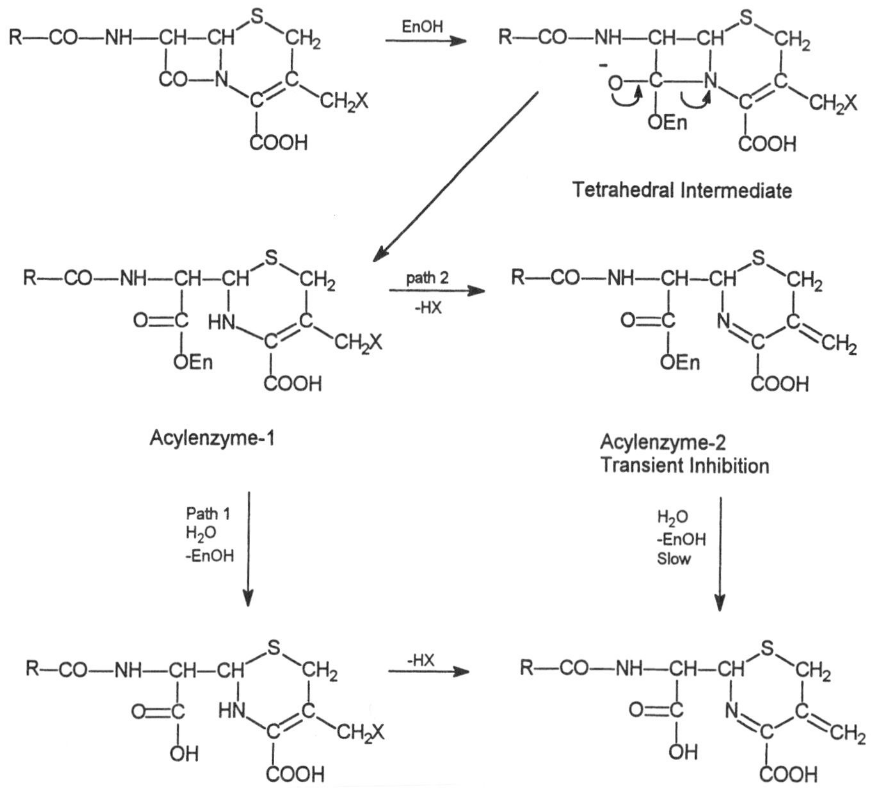

Figure 10–6 ■ Inhibition of β-lactamases by cephalosporins.

imine structure (path 2). Because of the stability of the acyl-enzyme intermediate, path 2 leads to transient inhibition of the enzyme. Faraci and Pratt[79, 79a] have shown that cephalothin and cefoxitin inhibit certain β-lactamases by this mechanism, whereas analogues lacking a 3' leaving group do not.

Antipseudomonal Cephalosporins

Species of *Pseudomonas,* especially *P. aeruginosa,* represent a special public health problem because of their ubiquity in the environment and their propensity to develop resistance to antibiotics, including the β-lactams. The primary mechanisms of β-lactam resistance appear to involve destruction of the antibiotics by β-lactamases and/or interference with their penetration through the cell envelope. Apparently, not all β-lactamase-resistant cephalosporins penetrate the cell envelope of *P. aeruginosa,* as only cefoperazone, moxalactam, cefotaxime, ceftizoxime, ceftriaxone, and ceftazidime have useful antipseudomonal activity. Two cephalosporins, moxalactam and cefoperazone, contain the same polar functionalities (e.g., carboxy and *N*-acylureido) that facilitate penetration into *Pseudomonas* spp. by the penicillins (see carbenicillin, ticarcillin, and piperacillin). Unfortunately, strains of *P. aeruginosa* resistant to cefoperazone and cefotaxime have been found in clinical isolates.

Adverse Reactions and Drug Interactions

Like their close relatives the penicillins, the cephalosporin antibiotics are comparatively nontoxic compounds that, because of their selective actions on cell wall cross-linking enzymes, exhibit highly selective toxicity toward bacteria. The most common adverse reactions to the cephalosporins are allergic and hypersensitivity reactions. These vary from mild rashes to life-threatening anaphylactic reactions. Allergic reactions are believed to occur less frequently with cephalosporins than with penicillins. The issue of cross-sensitivity between the two classes of β-lactams is very complex, but the incidence is considered to be very low (estimated at 3 to 7%). The physician faced with the decision of whether or not to administer a cephalosporin to a patient with a history of penicillin allergy must weigh several factors, including the severity of the illness being treated, the effectiveness and safety of alternative therapies, and the severity of previous allergic responses to penicillins.

Cephalosporins containing an *N*-methyl-5-thiotetrazole (MTT) moiety at the 3 position (e.g., cefamandole, cefotetan, cefmetazole, moxalactam, and cefoperazone) have been implicated in a higher incidence of hypoprothrombinemia than cephalosporins lacking the MTT group. This effect, which is enhanced and can lead to severe bleeding in patients with poor nutritional status, debilitation, recent gastrointestinal surgery, hepatic disease, or renal failure, is apparently due to inhibition of vitamin K–requiring enzymes involved in the carboxylation of glutamic acid residues in clotting factors II, VII, IX, and X to the MTT group.[80] Treatment with vitamin K restores prothrombin time to normal in patients treated with MTT-containing cephalosporins. Weekly vitamin K prophylaxis has been recommended for high-risk patients undergoing therapy with such agents. Cephalosporins containing the MTT group should not be administered to patients receiving oral anticoagulant or heparin therapy because of possible synergism with these drugs.

The MTT group has also been implicated in the intolerance to alcohol associated with certain injectable cephalosporins: cefamandole, cefotetan, cefmetazole, and cefoperazone. Thus, disulfiram-like reactions, attributed to the accumulation of acetaldehyde and resulting from the inhibition of aldehyde dehydrogenase–catalyzed oxidation of ethanol by MTT-containing cephalosporins,[81] may occur in patients who have consumed alcohol before, during, or shortly after the course of therapy.

Classification

Cephalosporins are divided into first-, second-, third-, and fourth-generation agents, based roughly on their time of discovery and their antimicrobial properties (Table 10-5). In general, progression from first to fourth generation is associated with a broadening of the Gram-negative antibacterial spectrum, some reduction in activity against Gram-positive organisms, and enhanced resistance to β-lactamases. Individual cephalosporins differ in their pharmacokinetic properties, especially plasma protein binding and half-life, but the structural bases for these differences are not obvious.

Products

Cephalexin, USP. Cephalexin, 7α-(D-amino-α-phenylacetamido)-3-methylcephemcarboxylic acid (Keflex, Keforal), was designed purposely as an orally active, semisynthetic cephalosporin. The oral inactivation of cephalosporins has been attributed to two causes: instability of the β-lactam ring to acid hydrolysis (cephalothin and cephaloridine) and solvolysis or microbial transformation of the 3-methylacetoxy group (cephalothin, cephaloglycin). The α-amino group of cephalexin renders it acid stable, and reduction of the 3-acetoxymethyl to a methyl group circumvents reaction at that site.

Cephalexin occurs as a white crystalline monohydrate. It is freely soluble in water, resistant to acid, and absorbed well orally. Food does not interfere with its absorption. Because of minimal protein binding and nearly exclusive renal excretion, cephalexin is recommended particularly for the treatment of urinary tract infections. It is also sometimes used for upper respiratory tract infections. Its spectrum of activity is very similar to those of cephalothin and cephaloridine. Cephalexin is somewhat less potent than these two agents after parenteral administration and, therefore, is inferior to them for the treatment of serious systemic infections.

Cephradine, USP. Cephradine (Anspor, Velosef) is the only cephalosporin derivative available in both oral and parenteral dosage forms. It closely resembles cephalexin chemically (it may be regarded as a partially hydrogenated deriva-

TABLE 10–5 Classification and Properties of Cephalosporins

Cephalosporin	Generation	Route of Administration	Acid-Resistant	Plasma Protein Binding (%)	β-Lactamase Resistance	Spectrum of Activity	Antipseudomonal Activity
Cephalexin	First	Oral	Yes	5–15	Poor	Broad	No
Cephradine	First	Oral, parenteral	Yes	8–17	Poor	Broad	No
Cefadroxil	First	Oral	Yes	20	Poor	Broad	No
Cephalothin	First	Parenteral	No	65–80	Poor	Broad	No
Cephapirin	First	Parenteral	No	40–54	Poor	Broad	No
Cefazolin	First	Parenteral	No	70–86	Poor	Broad	No
Cefaclor	Second	Oral	Yes	22–25	Poor	Broad	No
Loracarbef	Second	Oral	Yes	25	Poor	Broad	No
Cefprozil	Second	Oral	Yes	36	Poor	Broad	No
Cefamandole	Second	Parenteral	No	56–78	Poor to average	Extended	No
Cefonicid	Second	Parenteral	No	99	Poor to average	Extended	No
Ceforanide	Second	Parenteral	No	80	Average	Extended	No
Cefoxitin	Second	Parenteral	No	13–22	Good	Extended	No
Cefotetan	Second	Parenteral	No	78–91	Good	Extended	No
Cefmetazole	Second	Parenteral	No	65	Good	Extended	No
Cefuroxime	Second	Oral, parenteral	Yes/no	33–50	Good	Extended	No
Cefpodoxime	Second	Oral	Yes	25	Good	Extended	No
Cefixime	Third	Oral	Yes	65	Good	Extended	No
Cefoperazone	Third	Parenteral	No	82–93	Average to good	Extended	Yes
Cefotaxime	Third	Parenteral	No	30–51	Good	Extended	Yes
Ceftizoxime	Third	Parenteral	No	30	Good	Extended	Yes
Ceftriaxone	Third	Parenteral	No	80–95	Good	Extended	Yes
Ceftazidime	Third	Parenteral	No	80–90	Good	Extended	Yes
Ceftibuten	Third	Oral	Yes	?	Good	Extended	No
Cefepime	Fourth	Parenteral	No	16–19	Good	Extended	Yes
Cefpirome	Fourth	Parenteral	No	—	Good	Extended	Yes

tive of cephalexin) and has very similar antibacterial and pharmacokinetic properties.

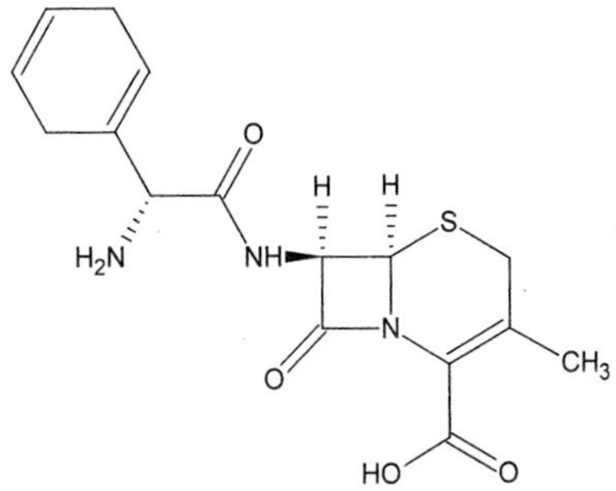

Cephradine

It occurs as a crystalline hydrate that is readily soluble in water. Cephradine is stable to acid and absorbed almost completely after oral administration. It is minimally protein bound and excreted almost exclusively through the kidneys. It is recommended for the treatment of uncomplicated urinary tract and upper respiratory tract infections caused by susceptible organisms. Cephradine is available in both oral and parenteral dosage forms.

Cefadroxil, USP. Cefadroxil (Duricef) is an orally active semisynthetic derivative of 7-ADCA, in which the 7-

acyl group is the D-hydroxylphenylglycyl moiety. This compound is absorbed well after oral administration to give plasma levels that reach 75 to 80% of those of an equal dose of its close structural analogue cephalexin. The main advantage claimed for cefadroxil is its somewhat prolonged duration of action, which permits once-a-day dosing. The prolonged duration of action of this compound is related to relatively slow urinary excretion of the drug compared with other cephalosporins, but the basis for this remains to be explained completely. The antibacterial spectrum of action and therapeutic indications of cefadroxil are very similar to those of cephalexin and cephradine. The D-p-hydroxyphenylglycyl isomer is much more active than the L isomer.

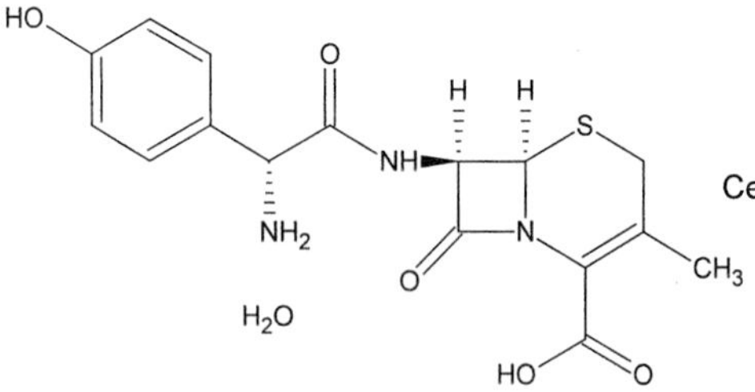

Cefadroxil

Cefaclor, USP. Cefaclor (Ceclor) is an orally active semisynthetic cephalosporin that was introduced in the

American market in 1979. It differs structurally from cephalexin in that the 3-methyl group has been replaced by a chlorine atom. It is synthesized from the corresponding 3-methylenecepham sulfoxide ester by ozonolysis, followed by halogenation of the resulting β-ketoester.[82] The 3-methylenecepham sulfoxide esters are prepared by rearrangement of the corresponding 6-acylaminopenicillanic acid derivative. Cefaclor is moderately stable in acid and achieves enough oral absorption to provide effective plasma levels (equal to about two thirds of those obtained with cephalexin). The compound is apparently unstable in solution, since about 50% of its antimicrobial activity is lost in 2 hours in serum at 37°C.[83] The antibacterial spectrum of activity is similar to that of cephalexin, but it is claimed to be more potent against some species sensitive to both agents. Currently, the drug is recommended for the treatment of non–life-threatening infections caused by *H. influenzae,* particularly strains resistant to ampicillin.

Cefaclor

Cefprozil, USP. Cefprozil (Cefzil) is an orally active second-generation cephalosporin that is similar in structure and antibacterial spectrum to cefadroxil. Oral absorption is excellent (oral bioavailability is about 95%) and is not affected by antacids or histamine-H$_2$ antagonists. Cefprozil exhibits greater in vitro activity against streptococci, *Neisseria* spp., and *S. aureus* than does cefadroxil. It is also more active than the first-generation cephalosporins against members of the Enterobacteriaceae family, such as *E. coli, Klebsiella* spp., *P. mirabilis,* and *Citrobacter* spp. The plasma half-life of 1.2 to 1.4 hours permits twice-a-day dosing for the treatment of most community-acquired respiratory and urinary tract infections caused by susceptible organisms.

Cefprozil

Loracarbef, USP. Loracarbef (Lorabid) is the first of a series of carbacephems prepared by total synthesis to be introduced.[84] Carbacephems are isosteres of the cephalosporin (or Δ³-cephem) antibiotics in which the 1-sulfur atom has been replaced by a methylene (CH$_2$) group. Loracarbef is isosteric with cefaclor and has similar pharmacokinetic and microbiological properties. Thus, the antibacterial spectrum of activity resembles that of cefaclor, but it has some-

what greater potency against *H. influenzae* and *M. catarrhalis,* including β-lactamase-producing strains. Unlike cefaclor, which undergoes degradation in human serum, loracarbef is chemically stable in plasma. It is absorbed well orally. Oral absorption is delayed by food. The half-life in plasma is about 1 hour.

Loracarbef

Cephalothin Sodium, USP. Cephalothin sodium (Keflin) occurs as a white to off-white, crystalline powder that is practically odorless. It is freely soluble in water and insoluble in most organic solvents. Although it has been described as a broad-spectrum antibacterial compound, it is not in the same class as the tetracyclines. Its spectrum of activity is broader than that of penicillin G and more similar to that of ampicillin. Unlike ampicillin, cephalothin is resistant to penicillinase produced by *S. aureus* and provides an alternative to the use of penicillinase-resistant penicillins for the treatment of infections caused by such strains.

Cephalothin Sodium

Cephalothin is absorbed poorly from the gastrointestinal tract and must be administered parenterally for systemic infections. It is relatively nontoxic and acid stable. It is excreted rapidly through the kidneys; about 60% is lost within 6 hours of administration. Pain at the site of intramuscular injection and thrombophlebitis following intravenous injection have been reported. Hypersensitivity reactions have been observed, and there is some evidence of cross-sensitivity in patients noted previously to be penicillin sensitive.

Cefazolin Sodium, Sterile, USP. Cefazolin (Ancef, Kefzol) is one of a series of semisynthetic cephalosporins in which the C-3 acetoxy function has been replaced by a thiol-containing heterocycle—here, 5-methyl-2-thio-1,3,4-thiadiazole. It also contains the somewhat unusual tetrazolylacetyl acylating group. Cefazolin was released in 1973 as a water-soluble sodium salt. It is active only by parenteral administration.

Cefazolin Sodium

Cefazolin provides higher serum levels, slower renal clearance, and a longer half-life than other first-generation cephalosporins. It is approximately 75% protein bound in plasma, a higher value than for most other cephalosporins. Early in vitro and clinical studies suggest that cefazolin is more active against Gram-negative bacilli but less active against Gram-positive cocci than either cephalothin or cephaloridine. Occurrence rates of thrombophlebitis following intravenous injection and pain at the site of intramuscular injection appear to be the lowest of the parenteral cephalosporins.

Cephapirin Sodium, Sterile, USP. Cephapirin (Cefadyl) is a semisynthetic 7-ACA derivative released in the United States in 1974. It closely resembles cephalothin in chemical and pharmacokinetic properties. Like cephalothin, cephapirin is unstable in acid and must be administered parenterally in the form of an aqueous solution of the sodium salt. It is moderately protein bound (45 to 50%) in plasma and cleared rapidly by the kidneys. Cephapirin and cephalothin are very similar in antimicrobial spectrum and potency. Conflicting reports concerning the relative occurrence of pain at the site of injection and thrombophlebitis after intravenous injection of cephapirin and cephalothin are difficult to assess on the basis of available clinical data.

Cephapirin Sodium

Cefamandole Nafate, USP. Cefamandole (Mandol) nafate is the formate ester of cefamandole, a semisynthetic cephalosporin that incorporates D-mandelic acids as the acyl portion and a thiol-containing heterocycle (5-thio-1,2,3,4-tetrazole) in place of the acetoxyl function on the C-3 methylene carbon atom. Esterification of the α-hydroxyl group of the D-mandeloyl function overcomes the instability of cefamandole in solid-state dosage forms[85] and provides satisfactory concentrations of the parent antibiotic in vivo through spontaneous hydrolysis of the ester at neutral to alkaline pH. Cefamandole is the first second-generation cephalosporin to be marketed in the United States.

Cefamandole

The D-mandeloyl moiety of cefamandole appears to confer resistance to a few β-lactamases, since some β-lactamase-producing, Gram-negative bacteria (particularly Enterobacteriaceae) that show resistance to cefazolin and other first-

generation cephalosporins are sensitive to cefamandole. Additionally, it is active against some ampicillin-resistant strains of *Neisseria* and *Haemophilus* spp. Although resistance to β-lactamases may be a factor in determining the sensitivity of individual bacterial strains to cefamandole, an early study[86] indicated that other factors, such as permeability and intrinsic activity, are frequently more important. The L-mandeloyl isomer is significantly less active than the D isomer.

Cefamandole nafate is very unstable in solution and hydrolyzes rapidly to release cefamandole and formate. There is no loss of potency, however, when such solutions are stored for 24 hours at room temperature or up to 96 hours when refrigerated. Air oxidation of the released formate to carbon dioxide can cause pressure to build up in the injection vial.

Cefonicid Sodium, Sterile, USP. Monocid is a second-generation cephalosporin that is structurally similar to cefamandole, except that it contains a methane sulfonic acid group attached to the N-1 position of the tetrazole ring. The antimicrobial spectrum and limited β-lactamase stability of cefonicid are essentially identical with those of cefamandole.

Cefonicid is unique among the second-generation cephalosporins in that it has an unusually long serum half-life of approximately 4.5 hours. High plasma protein binding coupled with slow renal tubular secretion are apparently responsible for the long duration of action. Despite the high fraction of drug bound in plasma, cefonicid is distributed throughout body fluids and tissues, with the exception of the cerebrospinal fluid.

Cefonicid is supplied as a highly water-soluble disodium salt, in the form of a sterile powder to be reconstituted for injection. Solutions are stable for 24 hours at 25°C and for 72 hours when refrigerated.

Cefonicid Sodium

Ceforanide, Sterile, USP. Ceforanide (Precef) was approved for clinical use in the United States in 1984. It is classified as a second-generation cephalosporin because its antimicrobial properties are similar to those of cefamandole. It exhibits excellent potency against most members of the Enterobacteriaceae family, especially *K. pneumoniae*, *E. coli*, *P. mirabilis*, and *Enterobacter cloacae*. It is less active than cefamandole against *H. influenzae*, however.

The duration of action of ceforanide lies between those of cefamandole and cefonicid. It has a serum half-life of

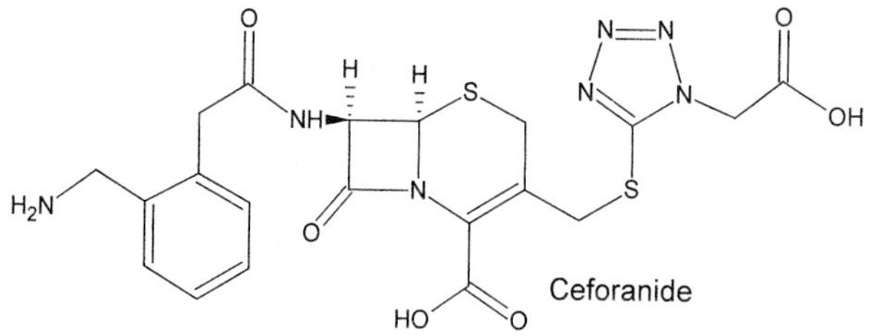

Ceforanide

about 3 hours, permitting twice-a-day dosing for most indications. Ceforanide is supplied as the sterile, crystalline disodium salt. Parenteral solutions are stable for 4 hours at 25°C and for up to 5 days when refrigerated.

Cefoperazone Sodium, Sterile, USP.

Cefoperazone (Cefobid) is a third-generation, antipseudomonal cephalosporin that resembles piperacillin chemically and microbiologically. It is active against many strains of *P. aeruginosa*, indole-positive *Proteus* spp., *Enterobacter* spp., and *S. marcescens* that are resistant to cefamandole. It is less active than cephalothin against Gram-positive bacteria and less active than cefamandole against most of the Enterobacteriaceae. Like piperacillin, cefoperazone is hydrolyzed by many of the β-lactamases that hydrolyze penicillins. Unlike piperacillin, however, it is resistant to some (but not all) of the β-lactamases that hydrolyze cephalosporins.

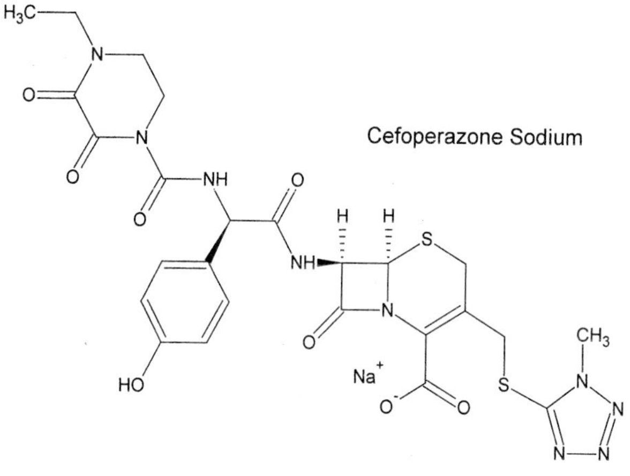

Cefoperazone Sodium

Cefoperazone is excreted primarily in the bile. Hepatic dysfunction can affect its clearance from the body. Although only 25% of the free antibiotic is recovered in the urine, urinary concentrations are high enough to be effective in the management of urinary tract infections caused by susceptible organisms. The relatively long half-life (2 hours) allows dosing twice a day. Solutions prepared from the crystalline sodium salt are stable for up to 4 hours at room temperature. If refrigerated, they will last 5 days without appreciable loss of potency.

Cefoxitin Sodium, Sterile, USP.

Cefoxitin (Mefoxin) is a semisynthetic derivative obtained by modification of cephamycin C, a 7α-methoxy-substituted cephalosporin isolated independently from various *Streptomyces* by research groups in Japan[87] and the United States. Although it is less potent than cephalothin against Gram-positive bacteria and cefamandole against most of the Enterobacteriaceae, cefoxitin is effective against certain strains of Gram-negative ba-

cilli (e.g., *E. coli*, *K. pneumoniae*, *Providencia* spp., *S. marcescens*, indole-positive *Proteus* spp., and *Bacteroides* spp.) that are resistant to these cephalosporins. It is also effective against penicillin-resistant *S. aureus* and *N. gonorrhoeae*.

The activity of cefoxitin and cephamycins, in general, against resistant bacterial strains is due to their resistance to hydrolysis by β-lactamases conferred by the 7α-methoxyl substituent.[88] Cefoxitin is a potent competitive inhibitor of many β-lactamases. It is also a potent inducer of chromosomally mediated β-lactamases. The temptation to exploit the β-lactamase-inhibiting properties of cefoxitin by combining it with β-lactamase-labile β-lactam antibiotics should be tempered by the possibility of antagonism. In fact, cefoxitin antagonizes the action of cefamandole against *E. cloacae* and that of carbenicillin against *P. aeruginosa*.[89] Cefoxitin alone is essentially ineffective against these organisms.

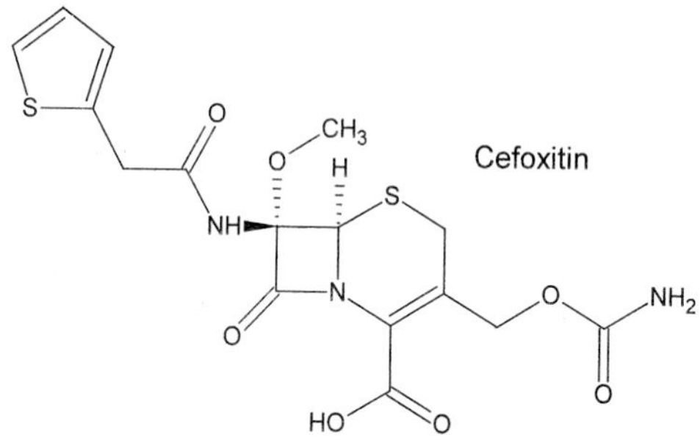

Cefoxitin

The pharmacokinetic properties of cefoxitin resemble those of cefamandole. Because its half-life is relatively short, cefoxitin must be administered 3 or 4 times daily. Solutions of the sodium salt intended for parenteral administration are stable for 24 hours at room temperature and 1 week if refrigerated. 7α-Methoxyl substitution stabilizes, to some extent, the β-lactam to alkaline hydrolysis.

The principal role of cefoxitin in therapy seems to be for the treatment of certain anaerobic and mixed aerobic–anaerobic infections. It is also used to treat gonorrhea caused by β-lactamase-producing strains. It is classified as a second-generation agent because of its spectrum of activity.

Cefotetan Disodium.

Cefotetan (Cefotan) is a third-generation cephalosporin that is structurally similar to cefoxitin. Like cefoxitin, cefotetan is resistant to destruction by β-lactamases. It is also a competitive inhibitor of many β-lactamases and causes transient inactivation of some of these enzymes. Cefotetan is reported to synergize with β-lactamase-sensitive β-lactams but, unlike cefoxitin, does not appear to cause antagonism.[90]

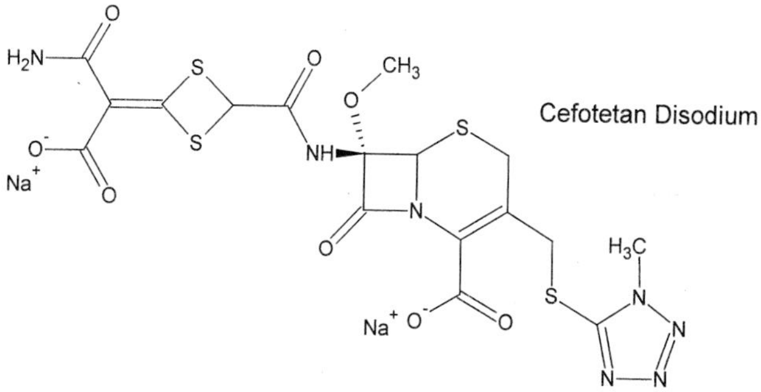

Cefotetan Disodium

The antibacterial spectrum of cefotetan closely resembles that of cefoxitin. It is, however, generally more active against

duration of action of ceftriaxone: high protein binding in the plasma and slow urinary excretion. Ceftriaxone is excreted in both the bile and the urine. Its urinary excretion is not affected by probenecid. Despite its comparatively low volume of distribution, it reaches the cerebrospinal fluid in concentrations that are effective in meningitis. Nonlinear pharmacokinetics are observed.

Ceftriaxone Disodium

Ceftriaxone contains a highly acidic heterocyclic system on the 3-thiomethyl group. This unusual dioxotriazine ring system is believed to confer the unique pharmacokinetic properties of this agent. Ceftriaxone has been associated with sonographically detected "sludge," or pseudolithiasis, in the gallbladder and common bile duct.[93] Symptoms of cholecystitis may occur in susceptible patients, especially those on prolonged or high-dose ceftriaxone therapy. The culprit has been identified as the calcium chelate.

Ceftriaxone exhibits excellent broad-spectrum antibacterial activity against both Gram-positive and Gram-negative organisms. It is highly resistant to most chromosomally and plasmid-mediated β-lactamases. The activity of ceftriaxone against *Enterobacter*, *Citrobacter*, *Serratia*, indole-positive *Proteus*, and *Pseudomonas* spp. is particularly impressive. It is also effective in the treatment of ampicillin-resistant gonorrhea and *H. influenzae* infections but generally less active than cefotaxime against Gram-positive bacteria and *B. fragilis*.

Solutions of ceftriaxone sodium should be used within 24 hours. They may be stored up to 10 days if refrigerated.

Ceftazidime Sodium, Sterile, USP.

Ceftazidime (Fortaz, Tazidime) is a β-lactamase-resistant third-generation cephalosporin that is noted for its antipseudomonal activity. It is active against some strains of *P. aeruginosa* that are resistant to cefoperazone and ceftriaxone. Ceftazidime is also highly effective against β-lactamase-producing strains of the Enterobacteriaceae family. It is generally less active than cefotaxime against Gram-positive bacteria and *B. fragilis*.

Ceftazidime Sodium

The structure of ceftazidime contains two noteworthy fea-

tures: *(a)* a 2-methylpropionicoxaminoacyl group that confers β-lactamase resistance and, possibly, increased permeability through the porin channels of the cell envelope and *(b)* a pyridinium group at the 3' position that confers zwitterionic properties on the molecule.

Ceftazidime is administered parenterally 2 or 3 times daily, depending on the severity of the infection. Its serum half-life is about 1.8 hours. It has been used effectively for the treatment of meningitis caused by *H. influenzae* and *N. meningitidis*.

NEWER CEPHALOSPORINS

Cephalosporins currently undergoing clinical trials or recently being marketed in the United States fall into two categories: *(a)* orally active β-lactamase-resistant cephalosporins and *(b)* parenteral β-lactamase-resistant antipseudomonal cephalosporins. The status of some of these compounds awaits more extensive clinical evaluation. Nonetheless, it appears that any advances they represent will be relatively modest.

Ceftibuten. Ceftibuten (Cedax) is a recently introduced, chemically novel analogue of the oximinocephalosporins in which an olefinic methylene group ($C=CHCH_2-$) with Z stereochemistry has replaced the *syn* oximino ($C=NO-$) group. This isosteric replacement yields a compound that retains resistance to hydrolysis catalyzed by many β-lactamases, has enhanced chemical stability, and is orally active. Oral absorption is rapid and nearly complete. It has the highest oral bioavailability of the third-generation cephalosporins.[94] Ceftibuten is excreted largely unchanged in the urine and has a half-life of about 2.5 hours. Plasma protein binding of this cephalosporin is estimated to be 63%.

Ceftibuten

Ceftibuten possesses excellent potency against most members of the Enterobacteriaceae family, *H. influenzae*, *Neisseria* spp., and *M. catarrhalis*. It is not active against *S. aureus* or *P. aeruginosa* and exhibits modest antistreptococcal activity. Ceftibuten is recommended in the management of community-acquired respiratory tract, urinary tract, and gynecological infections.

Cefpirome. Cefpirome (Cefrom) is a new parenteral, β-lactamase-resistant cephalosporin with a quaternary ammonium group at the 3 position of the cephem nucleus. Because its potency against Gram-positive and Gram-negative bacteria rivals that of the first-generation and third-generation cephalosporins, respectively, cefpirome is being touted as the first fourth-generation cephalosporin.[95] Its broad spectrum includes methicillin-sensitive staphylococci, penicillin-resistant pneumococci, and β-lactamase-producing strains of *E. coli, Enterobacter, Citrobacter,* and *Serratia* spp. Its efficacy against *P. aeruginosa* is comparable with that of ceftazidime. Cefpirome is excreted largely unchanged in the urine with a half-life of 2 hours.

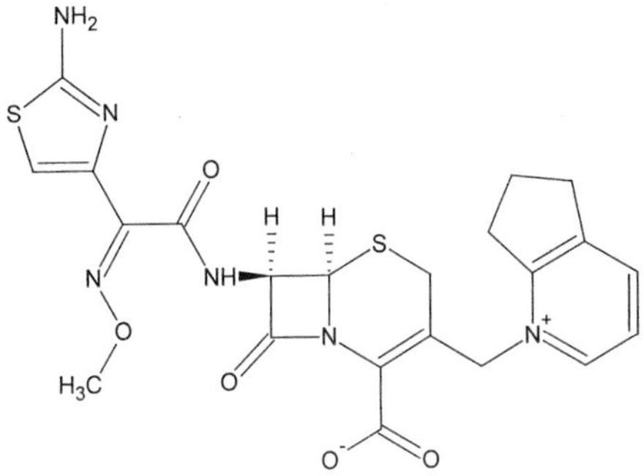

Cefpirome

Cefepime. Cefepime (Maxipime, Axepin) is a parenteral, *β*-lactamase-resistant cephalosporin that is chemically and microbiologically similar to cefpirome. It also has a broad antibacterial spectrum, with significant activity against both Gram-positive and Gram-negative bacteria, including streptococci, staphylococci, *Pseudomonas* spp., and the Enterobacteriaceae. It is active against some bacterial isolates that are resistant to ceftazidime.[96] The efficacy of cefepime has been demonstrated in the treatment of urinary tract infections, lower respiratory tract infections, skin and soft tissue infections, chronic osteomyelitis, and intra-abdominal and biliary infections. It is excreted in the urine with a half-life of 2.1 hours. It is bound minimally to plasma proteins. Cefepime is also a fourth-generation cephalosporin.

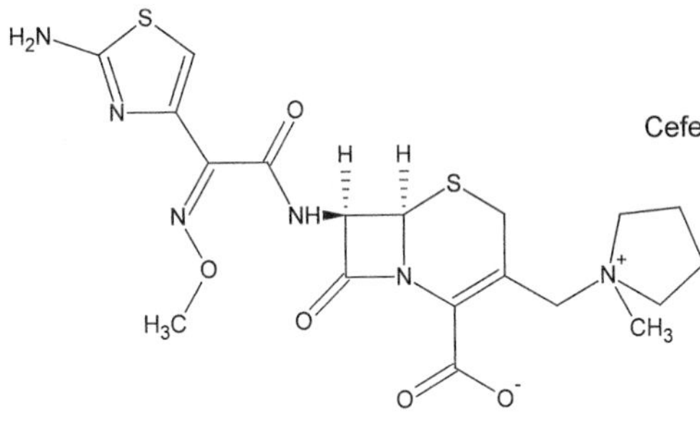

Cefepime

Future Developments in Cephalosporin Design

Recent research efforts in the cephalosporin field have focused primarily on two desired antibiotic properties: *(a)* increased permeability into Gram-negative bacilli, leading to enhanced efficacy against permeability-resistant strains of

Enterobacteriaceae and *P. aeruginosa,* and *(b)* increased affinity for altered PBPs, in particular the PBP 2a (or PBP 2′) of MRSA.[31]

The observation that certain catechol-substituted cephalosporins exhibit marked broad-spectrum antibacterial activity led to the discovery that such compounds and other analogues capable of chelating iron could mimic natural siderophores (iron-chelating peptides) and thus be actively transported into bacterial cells via the *tonB*-dependent iron-transport system.[97, 98] This provides a means of attacking bacterial strains that resist cellular penetration of cephalosporins.

A catechol-containing cephalosporin that exhibits excellent in vitro antibacterial activity against clinical isolates and promising pharmacokinetic properties is GR-69153. GR-69153 is a parenteral *β*-lactamase-resistant cephalosporin with a broad spectrum of activity against Gram-positive and Gram-negative bacteria.

GR-69153

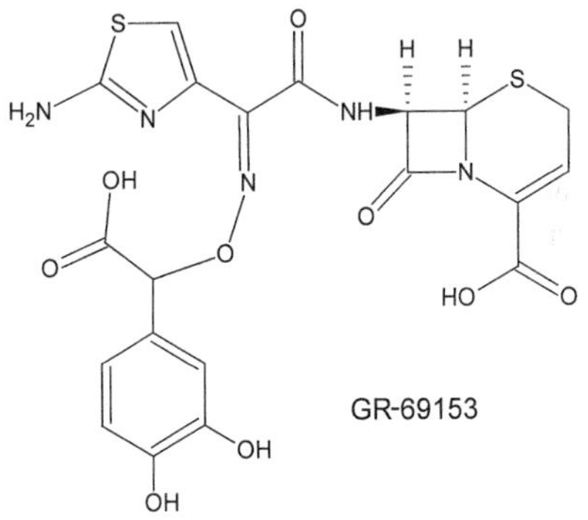

The antibacterial spectrum of GR-69153 includes most members of the Enterobacteriaceae family, *P. aeruginosa, H. influenzae, N. gonorrhoeae, M. catarrhalis,* staphylococci, streptococci, and *Acinetobacter* spp. It was not active against enterococci, *B. fragilis,* or MRSA. The half-life of GR-69153 in human volunteers was determined to be 3.5 hours, suggesting that metabolism by catechol-*O*-methyltransferase may not be an important factor. The relatively long half-life would permit once-a-day parenteral dosing for the treatment of many serious bacterial infections.

An experimental cephalosporin that has exhibited considerable promise against MRSA in preclinical evaluations is TOC-039.

TOC-039 is a parenteral, *β*-lactamase-resistant, hydroxyiminocephalosporin with a vinylthiopyridyl side chain attached to the 3 position of the cephem nucleus. It is a broad-spectrum agent that exhibits good activity against most aerobic Gram-positive and Gram-negative bacteria, including

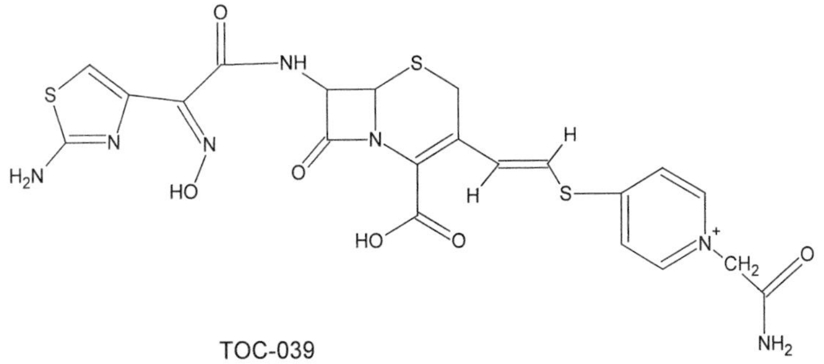

TOC-039

staphylococci, streptococci, enterococci, *H. influenzae, M. catarrhalis,* and most of the Enterobacteriaceae family.[99] A few strains of *P. vulgaris, S. marcescens,* and *Citrobacter freundii* are resistant, and TOC-039 is inactive against *P. aeruginosa.* Although the minimum inhibiting concentration (MIC) of TOC-039 against MRSA is slightly less than that of vancomycin, it is more rapidly bacteriocidal. Future clinical evaluations will determine if TOC-039 has the appropriate pharmacokinetic and antibacterial properties in vivo to be approved for the treatment of bacterial infections in humans.

MONOBACTAMS

The development of useful monobactam antibiotics began with the independent isolation of sulfazecin (SQ 26,445) and other monocyclic β-lactam antibiotics from saprophytic soil bacteria in Japan[100] and the United States.[101] Sulfazecin was found to be weakly active as an antibacterial agent but highly resistant to β-lactamases.

Sulfazecin

Extensive SAR studies[102] eventually led to the development of aztreonam, which has useful properties as an antibacterial agent. Early work established that the 3-methoxy group, which was in part responsible for β-lactamase stability in the series, contributed to the low antibacterial potency and poor chemical stability of these antibiotics. A 4-methyl group, however, increases stability to β-lactamases and activity against Gram-negative bacteria at the same time. Unfortunately, potency against Gram-positive bacteria decreases. 4,4-Gem-dimethyl substitution slightly decreases antibacterial potency after oral administration.

Products

Aztreonam Disodium, USP.   Aztreonam (Azactam) is a monobactam prepared by total synthesis. It binds with high affinity to PBP 3 in Gram-negative bacteria only. It is inactive against Gram-positive bacteria and anaerobes. β-Lactamase resistance is like that of ceftazidime, which has the same isobutyric acid oximinoacyl group. Aztreonam does not induce chromosomally mediated β-lactamases.

Aztreonam Disodium

Aztreonam is particularly active against aerobic Gram-negative bacilli, including *E. coli, K. pneumoniae, K. oxytoca, P. mirabilis, S. marcescens, Citrobacter* spp., and *P. aeruginosa.* It is used to treat urinary and lower respiratory tract infections, intra-abdominal infections, and gynecological infections, as well as septicemias caused by these organisms. Aztreonam is also effective against, but is not currently used to treat, infections caused by *Haemophilus, Neisseria, Salmonella,* indole-positive *Proteus,* and *Yersinia* spp. It is not active against Gram-positive bacteria, anaerobic bacteria, or other species of *Pseudomonas.*

Urinary excretion is about 70% of the administered dose. Some is excreted through the bile. Serum half-life is 1.7 hours, which allows aztreonam to be administered 2 or 3 times daily, depending on the severity of the infection. Less than 1% of an orally administered dose of aztreonam is absorbed, prompting the suggestion that this β-lactam could be used to treat intestinal infections.

The disodium salt of aztreonam is very soluble in water. Solutions for parenteral administration containing 2% or less are stable for 48 hours at room temperature. Refrigerated solutions retain full potency for 1 week.

Tigemonam.   Tigemonam is a newer monobactam that is orally active.[103] It is highly resistant to β-lactamases. The antibacterial spectrum of activity resembles that of aztreonam. It is very active against the Enterobacteriaceae, including *E. coli, Klebsiella, Proteus, Citrobacter, Serratia,* and *Enterobacter* spp. It also exhibits good potency against *H. influenzae* and *N. gonorrhoeae.* Tigemonam is not particularly active against Gram-positive or anaerobic bacteria and is inactive against *P. aeruginosa.*

Tigemonam

In contrast to the poor oral bioavailability of aztreonam, the oral absorption of tigemonam is excellent. It could become a valuable agent for the oral treatment of urinary tract infections and other non–life-threatening infections caused by β-lactamase-producing Gram-negative bacteria.

AMINOGLYCOSIDES

The discovery of streptomycin, the first aminoglycoside antibiotic to be used in chemotherapy, was the result of a planned and deliberate search begun in 1939 and brought to fruition in 1944 by Schatz and associates.[104] This success stimulated worldwide searches for antibiotics from the actinomycetes and, particularly, from the genus *Streptomyces*. Among the many antibiotics isolated from that genus, several are compounds closely related in structure to streptomycin. Six of them—kanamycin, neomycin, paromomycin, gentamicin, tobramycin, and netilmicin—currently are marketed in the United States. Amikacin, a semisynthetic derivative of kanamycin A, has been added, and it is possible that additional aminoglycosides will be introduced in the future.

All aminoglycoside antibiotics are absorbed very poorly (less than 1% under normal circumstances) following oral administration, and some of them (kanamycin, neomycin, and paromomycin) are administered by that route for the treatment of gastrointestinal infections. Because of their potent broad-spectrum antimicrobial activity, they are also used for the treatment of systemic infections. Their undesirable side effects, particularly ototoxicity and nephrotoxicity, have restricted their systemic use to serious infections or infections caused by bacterial strains resistant to other agents. When administered for systemic infections, aminoglycosides must be given parenterally, usually by intramuscular injection. An additional antibiotic obtained from *Streptomyces,* spectinomycin, is also an aminoglycoside but differs chemically and microbiologically from other members of the group. It is used exclusively for the treatment of uncomplicated gonorrhea.

Chemistry

Aminoglycosides are so named because their structures consist of amino sugars linked glycosidically. All have at least one aminohexose, and some have a pentose lacking an amino group (e.g., streptomycin, neomycin, and paromomycin). Additionally, each of the clinically useful aminoglycosides contains a highly substituted 1,3-diaminocyclohexane central ring; in kanamycin, neomycin, gentamicin, and tobramycin, it is deoxystreptamine, and in streptomycin, it is streptadine. The aminoglycosides are thus strongly basic compounds that exist as polycations at physiological pH. Their inorganic acid salts are very soluble in water. All are available as sulfates. Solutions of the aminoglycoside salts are stable to autoclaving. The high water solubility of the aminoglycosides no doubt contributes to their pharmacokinetic properties. They distribute well into most body fluids but not into the central nervous system, bone, or fatty or connective tissues. They tend to concentrate in the kidneys and are excreted by glomerular filtration. Aminoglycosides are apparently not metabolized in vivo.

Spectrum of Activity

Although the aminoglycosides are classified as broad-spectrum antibiotics, their greatest usefulness lies in the treatment of serious systemic infections caused by aerobic Gram-negative bacilli. The choice of agent is generally between kanamycin, gentamicin, tobramycin, netilmicin, and amikacin. Aerobic Gram-negative and Gram-positive cocci (with the exception of staphylococci) tend to be less sensitive; thus, the β-lactams and other antibiotics tend to be preferred for the treatment of infections caused by these organisms. Anaerobic bacteria are invariably resistant to the aminoglycosides. Streptomycin is the most effective of the

group for the chemotherapy of tuberculosis, brucellosis, tularemia, and *Yersinia* infections. Paromomycin is used primarily in the chemotherapy of amebic dysentery. Under certain circumstances, aminoglycoside and β-lactam antibiotics exert a synergistic action in vivo against some bacterial strains when the two are administered jointly. For example, carbenicillin and gentamicin are synergistic against gentamicin-sensitive strains of *P. aeruginosa* and several other species of Gram-negative bacilli, and penicillin G and streptomycin (or gentamicin or kanamycin) tend to be more effective than either agent alone in the treatment of enterococcal endocarditis. The two antibiotic types should not be combined in the same solution because they are chemically incompatible. Damage to the cell wall caused by the β-lactam antibiotic is believed to increase penetration of the aminoglycoside into the bacterial cell.

Mechanism of Action

Most studies concerning the mechanism of antibacterial action of the aminoglycosides were carried out with streptomycin. The specific actions of other aminoglycosides are thought to be qualitatively similar, however. The aminoglycosides act directly on the bacterial ribosome to inhibit the initiation of protein synthesis and to interfere with the fidelity of translation of the genetic message. They bind to the 30S ribosomal subunit to form a complex that cannot initiate proper amino acid polymerization.[105] The binding of streptomycin and other aminoglycosides to ribosomes also causes misreading mutations of the genetic code, apparently resulting from failure of specific aminoacyl RNAs to recognize the proper codons on mRNA and hence incorporation of improper amino acids into the peptide chain.[106] Evidence suggests that the deoxystreptamine-containing aminoglycosides differ quantitatively from streptomycin in causing misreading at lower concentrations than those required to prevent initiation of protein synthesis, whereas streptomycin is equally effective in inhibiting initiation and causing misreading.[107] Spectinomycin prevents the initiation of protein synthesis but apparently does not cause misreading. All of the commercially available aminoglycoside antibiotics are bactericidal, except spectinomycin. The mechanism for the bactericidal action of the aminoglycosides is not known.

Microbial Resistance

The development of strains of Enterobacteriaceae resistant to antibiotics is a well-recognized, serious medical problem. Nosocomial (hospital acquired) infections caused by these organisms are often resistant to antibiotic therapy. Research has established clearly that multidrug resistance among Gram-negative bacilli to a variety of antibiotics occurs and can be transmitted to previously nonresistant strains of the same species and, indeed, to different species of bacteria. Resistance is transferred from one bacterium to another by extrachromosomal R factors (DNA) that self-replicate and are transferred by conjugation (direct contact). The aminoglycoside antibiotics, because of their potent bactericidal action against Gram-negative bacilli, are now preferred for the treatment of many serious infections caused by coliform bacteria. A pattern of bacterial resistance to each of the aminoglycoside antibiotics, however, has developed as their clinical use has become more widespread. Consequently, there are bacterial strains resistant to streptomycin, kanamycin, and gentamicin. Strains carrying R factors for resistance to these antibiotics synthesize enzymes capable of acetylating, phosphorylating, or adenylylating key amino or hydroxyl groups of the aminoglycosides. Much of the recent effort in aminoglycoside research is directed toward identifying new, or modifying existing, antibiotics that are resistant to inactivation by bacterial enzymes.

Resistance of individual aminoglycosides to specific inactivating enzymes can be understood, in large measure, by using chemical principles. First, one can assume that if the target functional group is absent in a position of the structure normally attacked by an inactivating enzyme, then the antibiotic will be resistant to the enzyme. Second, steric factors may confer resistance to attack at functionalities otherwise susceptible to enzymatic attack. For example, conversion of a primary amino group to a secondary amine inhibits N-acetylation by certain aminoglycoside acetyl transferases. At least nine different types of aminoglycoside-inactivating enzymes have been identified and partially characterized.[108] The sites of attack of these enzymes and the biochemistry of the inactivation reactions is described briefly, using the kanamycin B structure (which holds the dubious distinction of being a substrate for all of the enzymes described) for illustrative purposes (Fig. 10-7).

Aminoglycoside-inactivating enzymes include (a) aminoacetyltransferases (designated AAC), which acetylate the 6'-NH_2 of ring I, the 3-NH_2 of ring II, or the 2'-NH_2 of ring I; (b) phosphotransferases (designated APH), which phosphorylate the 3'-OH of ring I or the 2''-OH of ring III; and nucleotidyltransferases (ANT), which adenylate the 2''-OH of ring III, the 4'-OH of ring I, or the 4''-OH of ring III.

The gentamicins and tobramycin lack a 3'-hydroxyl group in ring I (see the section on the individual products for structures) and, consequently, are not inactivated by the phosphotransferase enzymes that phosphorylate that group in the kanamycins. Gentamicin C_1 (but not gentamicins C_{1a} or C_2 or tobramycin) is resistant to the acetyltransferase that acetylates the 6'-amino group in ring I of kanamycin B. All gentamicins are resistant to the nucleotidyltransferase enzyme that adenylylates the secondary equatorial 4''-hydroxyl group of kanamycin B because the 4''-hydroxyl group in the gentamicins is *tertiary* and is oriented axially. Removal of functional groups susceptible to attacking an aminoglycoside occasionally can lead to derivatives that resist enzymatic inactivation and retain activity. For example, the 3'-deoxy-, 4'-deoxy-, and 3',4'-dideoxykanamycins are more similar to the gentamicins and tobramycin in their patterns of activity against clinical isolates that resist one or more of the aminoglycoside-inactivating enzymes.

The most significant breakthrough yet achieved in the search for aminoglycosides resistant to bacterial enzymes has been the development of amikacin, the 1-*N*-L-(-)-amino-α-hydroxybutyric acid (L-AHBA) derivative of kanamycin A. This remarkable compound retains most of the intrinsic potency of kanamycin A and is resistant to virtually all aminoglycoside-inactivating enzymes known, except the aminoacetyltransferase that acetylates the 6'-amino group and the nucleotidyltransferase that adenylylates the 4'-hydroxyl group of ring I.[108, 109] The cause of amikacin's resistance to enzymatic inactivation is not known, but it has been suggested that introduction of the L-AHBA group into kanamycin A markedly decreases its affinity for the inactivating enzymes. The importance of amikacin's resistance to enzymatic inactivation is reflected in the results of an investigation on the comparative effectiveness of amikacin and other aminoglycosides against clinical isolates of bacterial strains known to be resistant to one or more of the aminoglycosides.[110] In this study, amikacin was effective against 91% of the isolates (with a range of 87 to 100%, depending on the species). Of the strains susceptible to other systemically useful aminoglycosides 18% were susceptible to kanamycin, 36% to gentamicin, and 41% to tobramycin.

Low-level resistance associated with diminished aminoglycoside uptake has been observed in certain strains of *P. aeruginosa* isolated from nosocomial infections.[111] Bacterial susceptibility to aminoglycosides requires uptake of the drug by an energy-dependent active process.[112] Uptake is initiated by the binding of the cationic aminoglycoside to anionic phospholipids of the cell membrane. Electron transport-linked transfer of the aminoglycoside through the cell membrane then occurs. Divalent cations such as Ca^{2+} and Mg^{2+} antagonize the transport of aminoglycosides into bacterial cells by interfering with their binding to cell membrane phospholipids. The resistance of anaerobic bacteria to the lethal action of the aminoglycosides is apparently due to the absence of the respiration-driven active-transport process for transporting the antibiotics.

Structure-Activity Relationships

Despite the complexity inherent in various aminoglycoside structures, some conclusions on SARs in this antibiotic class

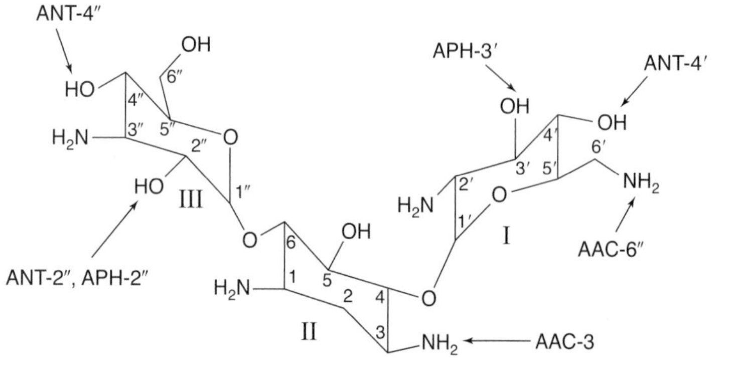

Figure 10-7 ■ Inactivation of kanamycin B by bacterial enzymes.

have been made.[113] Such conclusions have been formulated on the basis of comparisons of naturally occurring aminoglycoside structures, the results of selective semisynthetic modifications, and the elucidation of sites of inactivation by bacterial enzymes. It is convenient to discuss sequentially aminoglycoside SARs in terms of substituents in rings I, II, and III.

Ring I is crucially important for characteristic broad-spectrum antibacterial activity, and it is the primary target for bacterial inactivating enzymes. Amino functions at 6′ and 2′ are particularly important as kanamycin B (6′-amino, 2′-amino) is more active than kanamycin A (6′-amino, 2′-hydroxyl), which in turn is more active than kanamycin C (6′-hydroxyl, 2′-amino). Methylation at either the 6′-carbon or the 6′-amino positions does not lower appreciably antibacterial activity and confers resistance to enzymatic acetylation of the 6′-amino group. Removal of the 3′-hydroxyl or the 4′-hydroxyl group or both in the kanamycins (e.g., 3′,4′-dideoxykanamycin B or dibekacin) does not reduce antibacterial potency. The gentamicins also lack oxygen functions at these positions, as do sisomicin and netilmicin, which also have a 4′,5′-double bond. None of these derivatives is inactivated by phosphotransferase enzymes that phosphorylate the 3′-hydroxyl group. Evidently the 3′-phosphorylated derivatives have very low affinity for aminoglycoside-binding sites in bacterial ribosomes.

Few modifications of ring II (deoxystreptamine) functional groups are possible without appreciable loss of activity in most of the aminoglycosides. The 1-amino group of kanamycin A can be acylated (e.g., amikacin), however, with activity largely retained. Netilmicin (1-*N*-ethylsisomicin) retains the antibacterial potency of sisomicin and is resistant to several additional bacteria-inactivating enzymes. 2″-Hydroxysisomicin is claimed to be resistant to bacterial strains that adenylate the 2″-hydroxyl group of ring III, whereas 3-deaminosisomicin exhibits good activity against bacterial strains that elaborate 3-acetylating enzymes.

Ring III functional groups appear to be somewhat less sensitive to structural changes than those of either ring I or ring II. Although the 2″-deoxygentamicins are significantly less active than their 2″-hydroxyl counterparts, the 2″-amino derivatives (seldomycins) are highly active. The 3″-amino group of gentamicins may be primary or secondary with high antibacterial potency. Furthermore, the 4″-hydroxyl group may be *axial* or *equatorial* with little change in potency.

Despite improvements in antibacterial potency and spectrum among newer naturally occurring and semisynthetic aminoglycoside antibiotics, efforts to find agents with improved margins of safety have been disappointing. The potential for toxicity of these important chemotherapeutic agents continues to restrict their use largely to the hospital environment.

The discovery of agents with higher potency/toxicity ratios remains an important goal of aminoglycoside research. In a now somewhat dated review, however, Price[114] expressed doubt that many significant clinical breakthroughs in aminoglycoside research would occur in the future.

Products

Streptomycin Sulfate, Sterile, USP.
Streptomycin sulfate is a white, odorless powder that is hygroscopic but stable toward light and air. It is freely soluble in water, forming solutions that are slightly acidic or nearly neutral. It is very slightly soluble in alcohol and is insoluble in most other organic solvents. Acid hydrolysis yields streptidine and streptobiosamine, the compound that is a combination of L-streptose and *N*-methyl-L-glucosamine.

Streptomycin

Streptomycin acts as a triacidic base through the effect of its two strongly basic guanidino groups and the more weakly basic methylamino group. Aqueous solutions may be stored at room temperature for 1 week without any loss of potency, but they are most stable if the pH is between 4.5 and 7.0. The solutions decompose if sterilized by heating, so sterile solutions are prepared by adding sterile distilled water to the sterile powder. The early salts of streptomycin contained impurities that were difficult to remove and caused a histamine-like reaction. By forming a complex with calcium chloride, it was possible to free the streptomycin from these impurities and to obtain a product that was generally well tolerated.

The organism that produces streptomycin, *Streptomyces griseus*, also produces several other antibiotic compounds: hydroxystreptomycin, mannisidostreptomycin, and cycloheximide (*q.v.*). Of these, only cycloheximide has achieved importance as a medicinally useful substance. The term *streptomycin A* has been used to refer to what is commonly called streptomycin, and mannisidostreptomycin has been called *streptomycin B*. Hydroxystreptomycin differs from streptomycin in having a hydroxyl group in place of one of the hydrogen atoms of the streptose methyl group. Mannisidostreptomycin has a mannose residue attached in glycosidic linkage through the hydroxyl group at C-4 of the *N*-methyl-L-glucosamine moiety. The work of Dyer and colleagues[115,116] to establish the stereochemical structure of streptomycin has been completed, and confirmed with the total synthesis of streptomycin and dihydrostreptomycin by Japanese scientists.[117]

Clinically, a problem that sometimes occurs with the use of streptomycin is the early development of resistant strains of bacteria, necessitating a change in therapy. Other factors that limit the therapeutic use of streptomycin are chronic toxicities. Neurotoxic reactions have been observed after the use of streptomycin. These are characterized by vertigo, disturbance of equilibrium, and diminished auditory perception. Additionally, nephrotoxicity occurs with some frequency.

Patients undergoing therapy with streptomycin should have frequent checks of renal monitoring parameters. Chronic toxicity reactions may or may not be reversible. Minor toxic effects include rashes, mild malaise, muscular pains, and drug fever.

As a chemotherapeutic agent, streptomycin is active against numerous Gram-negative and Gram-positive bacteria. One of the greatest virtues of streptomycin is its effectiveness against the tubercle bacillus, *Mycobacterium tuberculosis*. By itself, the antibiotic is not a cure, but it is a valuable adjunct to other treatment modalities for tuberculosis. The greatest drawback to the use of streptomycin is the rather rapid development of resistant strains of microorganisms. In infections that may be due to bacteria sensitive to both streptomycin and penicillin, the combined administration of the two antibiotics has been advocated. The possible development of damage to the otic nerve by the continued use of streptomycin-containing preparations has discouraged the use of such products. There has been an increasing tendency to reserve streptomycin products for the treatment of tuberculosis. It remains one of the agents of choice, however, for the treatment of certain "occupational" bacterial infections, such as brucellosis, tularemia, bubonic plague, and glanders. Because streptomycin is not absorbed when given orally or destroyed significantly in the gastrointestinal tract, at one time it was used rather widely in the treatment of infections of the intestinal tract. For systemic action, streptomycin usually is given by intramuscular injection.

Neomycin Sulfate, USP.

In a search for antibiotics less toxic than streptomycin, Waksman and Lechevalier[118] isolated neomycin (Mycifradin, Neobiotic) in 1949 from *Streptomyces fradiae*. Since then, the importance of neomycin has increased steadily, and today, it is considered one of the most useful antibiotics for the treatment of gastrointestinal infections, dermatological infections, and acute bacterial peritonitis. Also, it is used in abdominal surgery to reduce or avoid complications caused by infections from bacterial flora of the bowel. It has broad-spectrum activity against a variety of organisms and shows a low incidence of toxic and hypersensitivity reactions. It is absorbed very slightly from the digestive tract, so its oral use ordinarily does not produce any systemic effect. The development of neomycin-resistant strains of pathogens is rarely reported in those organisms against which neomycin is effective.

Neomycin

Neomycin as the sulfate salt is a white to slightly yellow, crystalline powder that is very soluble in water. It is hygroscopic and photosensitive (but stable over a wide pH range and to autoclaving). Neomycin sulfate contains the equivalent of 60% of the free base.

Neomycin, as produced by *S. fradiae*, is a mixture of closely related substances. Included in the "neomycin complex" is neamine (originally designated *neomycin A*) and neomycins B and C. *S. fradiae* also elaborates another antibiotic, fradicin, which has some antifungal properties but no antibacterial activity. This substance is not present in "pure" neomycin.

The structures of neamine and neomycin B and C are known, and the absolute configurational structures of neamine and neomycin were reported by Hichens and Rinehart.[119] Neamine may be obtained by methanolysis of neomycins B and C, during which the glycosidic link between deoxystreptamine and D-ribose is broken. Therefore, neamine is a combination of deoxystreptamine and neosamine C, linked glycosidically (α) at the 4 position of deoxystreptamine. According to Hichens and Rinehart, neomycin B differs from neomycin C by the nature of the sugar attached terminally to D-ribose. That sugar, called *neosamine B*, differs from neosamine C in its stereochemistry. Rinehart et al.[120] have suggested that in neosamine the configuration is 2,6-diamino-2,6-dideoxy-L-idose, in which the orientation of the 6-aminomethyl group is inverted to the 6-amino-6-deoxy-D-glucosamine in neosamine C. In both instances, the glycosidic links were assumed to be α. Huettenrauch[121] later suggested, however, that both of the diamino sugars in neomycin C have the D-glucose configuration and that the glycosidic link is β in the one attached to D-ribose. The latter stereochemistry has been confirmed by the total synthesis of neomycin C.[122]

Paromomycin Sulfate, USP.

The isolation of paromomycin (Humatin) was reported in 1956 from a fermentation with a *Streptomyces* sp. (PD 04998), a strain said to resemble *S. rimosus* very closely. The parent organism had been obtained from soil samples collected in Colombia. Paromomycin, however, more closely resembles neomycin and streptomycin in antibiotic activity than it does oxytetracycline, the antibiotic obtained from *S. rimosus*.

Neosamine B or C

Paromomycin I: R₁=H; R₂=CH₂NH₂
Paromomycin II: R₁=CH₂NH₂; R₂=H

The general structure of paromomycin was reported by Haskell et al.[123] as one compound. Subsequently, chromatographic determinations have shown paromomycin to consist of two fractions, paromomycin I and paromomycin II. The absolute configurational structures for the paromomycins, as shown in the structural formula, were suggested by Hichens and Rinehart[119] and confirmed by DeJongh et al.[124] by mass spectrometric studies. The structure of paromomycin is the same as that of neomycin B, except that paromomycin contains D-glucosamine instead of the 6-amino-6-deoxy-D-glucosamine found in neomycin B. The same structural relationship is found between paromomycin II and neomycin C. The combination of D-glucosamine and deoxystreptamine is obtained by partial hydrolysis of both paromomycins and is called *paromamine* [4-(2-amino-2-deoxy-α-4-glucosyl)-deoxystreptamine].

Paromomycin has broad-spectrum antibacterial activity and has been used for the treatment of gastrointestinal infections caused by *Salmonella* and *Shigella* spp., and enteropathogenic *E. coli*. Currently, however, its use is restricted largely to the treatment of intestinal amebiasis. Paromomycin is soluble in water and stable to heat over a wide pH range.

Kanamycin Sulfate, USP. Kanamycin (Kantrex) was isolated in 1957 by Umezawa and coworkers[125] from *Streptomyces kanamyceticus*. Its activity against mycobacteria and many intestinal bacteria, as well as a number of pathogens that show resistance to other antibiotics, brought a great deal of attention to this antibiotic. As a result, kanamycin was tested and released for medical use in a very short time.

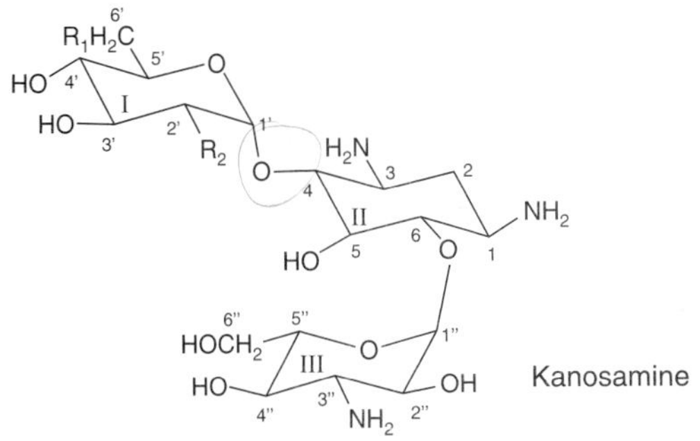

Kanosamine

Kanamycin A: R₁ = NH₂; R₂ = OH
Kanamycin B: R₁ = NH₂; R₂ = NH₂
Kanamycin C: R₁ = OH; R₂ = NH₂

Research activity has been focused intensively on determining the structures of the kanamycins. Chromatography showed that *S. kanamyceticus* elaborates three closely related structures: kanamycins A, B, and C. Commercially available kanamycin is almost pure kanamycin A, the least toxic of the three forms. The kanamycins differ only in the sugar moieties attached to the glycosidic oxygen on the 4 position of the central deoxystreptamine. The absolute configuration of the deoxystreptamine in kanamycins reported by Tatsuoka et al.[126] is shown above. The chemical relationships among the kanamycins, the neomycins, and the paromomycins were reported by Hichens and Rinehart.[119] The kanamycins do not have the D-ribose molecule that is present in neomycins and paromomycins. Perhaps this structural difference is related to the lower toxicity observed with kanamycins. The kanosamine fragment linked glycosidically to the 6 position of deoxystreptamine is 3-amino-3-deoxy-D-glucose (3-D-glucosamine) in all three kanamycins. The structures of the kanamycins have been proved by total synthesis.[127, 128] They differ in the substituted D-glucoses attached glycosidically to the 4 position of the deoxystreptamine ring. Kanamycin A contains 6-amino-6-deoxy-D-glucose; kanamycin B contains 2,6-diamino-2,6-dideoxy-D-

glucose; and kanamycin C contains 2-amino-2-deoxy-D-glucose (see diagram above).

Kanamycin is basic and forms salts of acids through its amino groups. It is water soluble as the free base, but it is used in therapy as the sulfate salt, which is very soluble. It is stable to both heat and chemicals. Solutions resist both acids and alkali within the pH range of 2.0 to 11.0. Because of possible inactivation of either agent, kanamycin and penicillin salts should not be combined in the same solution.

The use of kanamycin in the United States usually is restricted to infections of the intestinal tract (e.g., bacillary dysentery) and to systemic infections arising from Gram-negative bacilli (e.g., *Klebsiella, Proteus, Enterobacter,* and *Serratia* spp.) that have developed resistance to other antibiotics. It has also been recommended for preoperative antisepsis of the bowel. It is absorbed poorly from the intestinal tract; consequently, systemic infections must be treated by intramuscular or (for serious infections) intravenous injections. These injections are rather painful, and the concomitant use of a local anesthetic is indicated. The use of kanamycin in the treatment of tuberculosis has not been widely advocated since the discovery that mycobacteria develop resistance very rapidly. In fact, both clinical experience and experimental work[129] indicate that kanamycin develops cross-resistance in the tubercle bacilli with dihydrostreptomycin, viomycin, and other antitubercular drugs. Like streptomycin, kanamycin may cause decreased or complete loss of hearing. On development of such symptoms, its use should be stopped immediately.

Amikacin, USP. Amikacin, 1-*N*-amino-α-hydroxybutyrylkanamycin A (Amikin), is a semisynthetic aminoglycoside first prepared in Japan. The synthesis formally involves simple acylation of the 1-amino group of the deoxystreptamine ring of kanamycin A with L-AHBA. This particular acyl derivative retains about 50% of the original activity of kanamycin A against sensitive strains of Gram-negative bacilli. The L-AHBA derivative is much more active than the D isomer.[130] The remarkable feature of amikacin is that it resists attack by most bacteria-inactivating enzymes and, therefore, is effective against strains of bacteria that are resistant to other aminoglycosides,[110] including gentamicin and tobramycin. In fact, it is resistant to all known aminoglycoside-inactivating enzymes, except the aminotransferase that acetylates the 6′amino group[109] and the 4′-nucleotidyl transferase that adenylylates the 4′-hydroxyl group of aminoglycosides.[108]

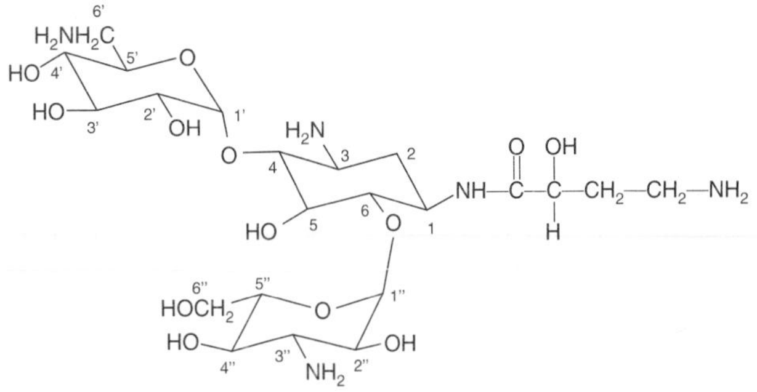

Amikacin

Preliminary studies indicate that amikacin may be less

ototoxic than either kanamycin or gentamicin.[131] Higher dosages of amikacin are generally required, however, for the treatment of most Gram-negative bacillary infections. For this reason, and to discourage the proliferation of bacterial strains resistant to it, amikacin currently is recommended for the treatment of serious infections caused by bacterial strains resistant to other aminoglycosides.

Gentamicin Sulfate, USP. Gentamicin (Garamycin) was isolated in 1958 and reported in 1963 by Weinstein et al.[132] to belong to the streptomycinoid (aminocyclitol) group of antibiotics. It is obtained commercially from *Micromonospora purpurea*. Like the other members of its group, it has a broad spectrum of activity against many common pathogens, both Gram-positive and Gram-negative. Of particular interest is its strong activity against *P. aeruginosa* and other Gram-negative enteric bacilli.

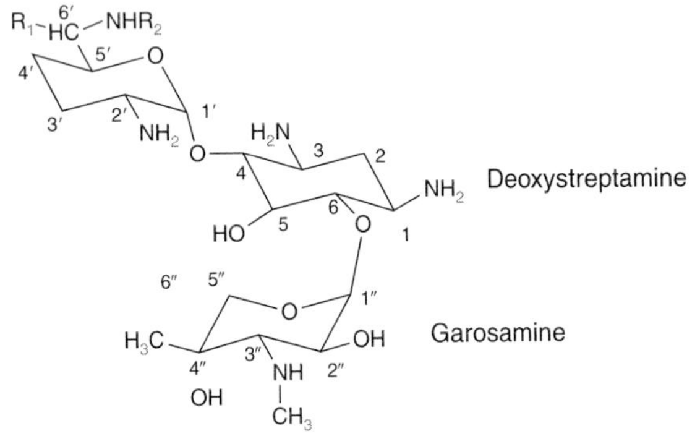

Gentamicin C_1: $R_1 = R_2 = CH_3$
Gentamicin C_2: $R_1 = CH_3$; $R_2 = H$
Gentamicin C_{1a}: $R_1 = R_2 = H$

Gentamicin is effective in the treatment of a variety of skin infections for which a topical cream or ointment may be used. Because it offers no real advantage over topical neomycin in the treatment of all but pseudomonal infections, however, it is recommended that topical gentamicin be reserved for use in such infections and in the treatment of burns complicated by pseudomonemia. An injectable solution containing 40 mg of gentamicin sulfate per milliliter may be used for serious systemic and genitourinary tract infections caused by Gram-negative bacteria, particularly *Pseudomonas, Enterobacter,* and *Serratia* spp. Because of the development of strains of these bacterial species resistant to previously effective broad-spectrum antibiotics, gentamicin has been used for the treatment of hospital-acquired infections caused by such organisms. Resistant bacterial strains that inactivate gentamicin by adenylylation and acetylation, however, appear to be emerging with increasing frequency.

Gentamicin sulfate is a mixture of the salts of compounds identified as gentamicins C_1, C_2, and C_{1a}. These gentamicins were reported by Cooper et al.[133] to have the structures shown in the diagram. The absolute stereochemistries of the sugar components and the geometries of the glycosidic linkages have also been established.[134]

Coproduced, but not a part of the commercial product, are gentamicins A and B. Their structures were reported by Maehr and Schaffner[135] and are closely related to those of the gentamicins C. Although gentamicin molecules are similar in many ways to other aminocyclitols such as streptomycins, they are sufficiently different that their medical effectiveness is significantly greater. Gentamicin sulfate is a white to buff substance that is soluble in water and insoluble in alcohol, acetone, and benzene. Its solutions are stable over a wide pH range and may be autoclaved. It is chemically incompatible with carbenicillin, and the two should not be combined in the same intravenous solution.

Tobramycin Sulfate, USP. Introduced in 1976, tobramycin sulfate (Nebcin) is the most active of the chemically related aminoglycosides called *nebramycins* obtained from a strain of *Streptomyces tenebrarius*. Five members of the nebramycin complex have been identified chemically.[136]

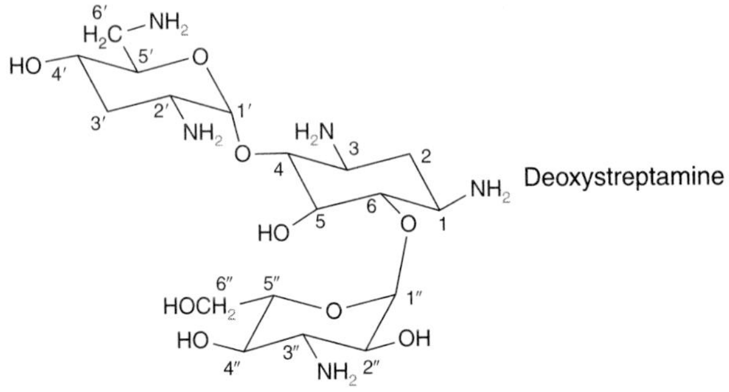

Tobramycin

Factors 4 and 4′ are 6″-*O*-carbamoylkanamycin B and kanamycin B, respectively; factors 5′ and 6 are 6″-*O*-carbamoyltobramycin and tobramycin; and factor 2 is apramycin, a tetracyclic aminoglycoside with an unusual bicyclic central ring structure. Kanamycin B and tobramycin probably do not occur in fermentation broths per se but are formed by hydrolysis of the 6-*O*″-carbamoyl derivatives in the isolation procedure.

The most important property of tobramycin is its activity against most strains of *P. aeruginosa,* exceeding that of gentamicin by two- to fourfold. Some gentamicin-resistant strains of this troublesome organism are sensitive to tobramycin, but others are resistant to both antibiotics.[137] Other Gram-negative bacilli and staphylococci are generally more sensitive to gentamicin. Tobramycin more closely resembles kanamycin B in structure (it is 3′-deoxykanamycin B).

Netilmicin Sulfate, USP. Netilmicin sulfate, 1-*N*-ethyl-sisomicin (Netromycin), is a semisynthetic derivative prepared by reductive ethylation[138] of sisomicin, an aminoglycoside antibiotic obtained from *Micromonospora inyoensis*.[139] Structurally, sisomicin and netilmicin resemble gentamicin C_{1a}, a component of the gentamicin complex.

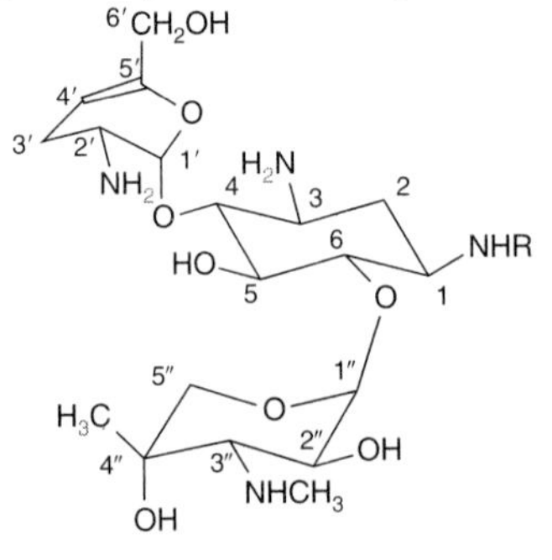

Sisomicin: $R = H$
Netilmicin: $R = C_2H_5$

Against most strains of Enterobacteriaceae, *P. aeruginosa*, and *S. aureus*, sisomicin and netilmicin are comparable to gentamicin in potency.[140] Netilmicin is active, however, against many gentamicin-resistant strains, in particular among *E. coli*, *Enterobacter*, *Klebsiella*, and *Citrobacter* spp. A few strains of gentamicin-resistant *P. aeruginosa*, *S. marcescens*, and indole-positive *Proteus* spp. are also sensitive to netilmicin. Very few gentamicin-resistant bacterial strains are sensitive to sisomicin, however. The potency of netilmicin against certain gentamicin-resistant bacteria is attributed to its resistance to inactivation by bacterial enzymes that adenylylate or phosphorylate gentamicin and sisomicin. Evidently, the introduction of a 1-ethyl group in sisomicin markedly decreases the affinity of these enzymes for the molecule in a manner similar to that observed in the 1-*N*-ε-amino-α-hydroxybutyryl amide of kanamycin A (amikacin). Netilmicin, however, is inactivated by most of the bacterial enzymes that acetylate aminoglycosides, whereas amikacin is resistant to most of these enzymes.

The pharmacokinetic and toxicological properties of netilmicin and gentamicin appear to be similar clinically, though animal studies have indicated greater nephrotoxicity for gentamicin.

Sisomicin Sulfate, USP. Although it has been approved for human use in the United States, sisomicin has not been marketed in this country. Its antibacterial potency and effectiveness against aminoglycoside-inactivating enzymes resemble those of gentamicin. Sisomicin also exhibits pharmacokinetics and pharmacological properties similar to those of gentamicin.

Sisomicin

Spectinomycin Hydrochloride, Sterile, USP. The aminocyclitol antibiotic spectinomycin hydrochloride (Trobicin), isolated from *Streptomyces spectabilis* and once called actinospectocin, was first described by Lewis and Clapp.[141] Its structure and absolute stereochemistry have been confirmed by x-ray crystallography.[142] It occurs as the white, crystalline dihydrochloride pentahydrate, which is stable in the dry form and very soluble in water. Solutions of spectinomycin, a hemiacetal, slowly hydrolyze on standing and should be prepared freshly and used within 24 hours. It is administered by deep intramuscular injection.

Spectinomycin

Spectinomycin is a broad-spectrum antibiotic with moderate activity against many Gram-positive and Gram-negative bacteria. It differs from streptomycin and the streptamine-containing aminoglycosides in chemical and antibacterial properties. Like streptomycin, spectinomycin interferes with the binding of tRNA to the ribosomes and thus with the initiation of protein synthesis. Unlike streptomycin or the streptamine-containing antibiotics, however, it does not cause misreading of the messenger. Spectinomycin exerts a bacteriostatic action and is inferior to other aminoglycosides for most systemic infections. Currently, it is recommended as an alternative to penicillin G salts for the treatment of uncomplicated gonorrhea. A cure rate of more than 90% has been observed in clinical studies for this indication. Many physicians prefer to use a tetracycline or erythromycin for prevention or treatment of suspected gonorrhea in penicillin-sensitive patients because, unlike these agents, spectinomycin is ineffective against syphilis. Furthermore, it is considerably more expensive than erythromycin and most of the tetracyclines.

TETRACYCLINES

Chemistry

Among the most important broad-spectrum antibiotics are members of the tetracycline family. Nine such compounds—tetracycline, rolitetracycline, oxytetracycline, chlortetracycline, demeclocycline, meclocycline, methacycline, doxycycline, and minocycline—have been introduced into medical use. Several others possess antibiotic activity. The tetracyclines are obtained by fermentation procedures from *Streptomyces* spp. or by chemical transformations of the natural products. Their chemical identities have been established by degradation studies and confirmed by the synthesis of three members of the group, oxytetracycline,[143, 144] 6-demethyl-6-deoxytetracycline,[145] and anhydrochlortetracycline,[146] in their (α) forms. The important members of the group are derivatives of an octahydronaphthacene, a hydrocarbon system that comprises four annulated six-membered rings. The group name is derived from this tetracyclic system. The antibiotic spectra and chemical properties of these compounds are very similar but not identical.

The stereochemistry of the tetracyclines is very complex. Carbon atoms 4, 4a, 5, 5a, 6, and 12a are potentially chiral, depending on substitution. Oxytetracycline and doxycycline, each with a 5α-hydroxyl substituent, have six asymmetric centers; the others, lacking chirality at C-5, have only five. Determination of the complete, absolute stereochemistry of the tetracyclines was a difficult problem. Detailed x-ray diffraction analysis[147–149] established the stereochemical formula shown in Table 10-6 as the orientations found in the natural and semisynthetic tetracyclines. These studies also confirmed that conjugated systems exist in the structure from C-10 through C-12 and from C-1 through C-3 and that the formula represents only one of several canonical forms existing in those portions of the molecule.

Structure of Tetracyclines

The tetracyclines are amphoteric compounds, forming salts with either acids or bases. In neutral solutions, these sub-

TABLE 10–6 Structure of Tetracyclines

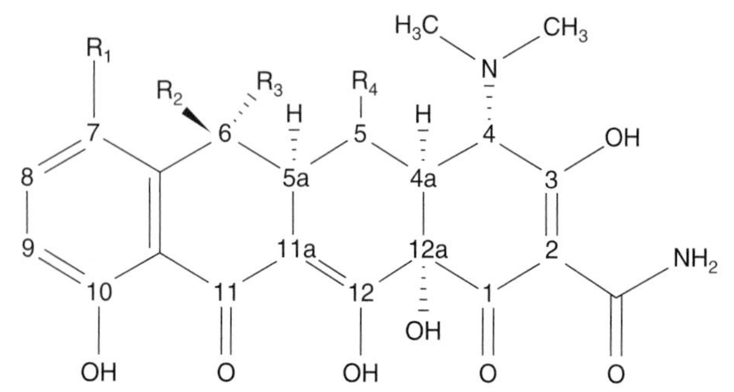

	R_1	R_2	R_3	R_4
Tetracycline	H	CH_3	OH	H
Chlortetracycline	Cl	CH_3	OH	H
Oxytetracycline	H	CH_3	OH	OH
Demeclocycline	Cl	H	OH	H
Methacycline	H	CH_2		OH
Doxycycline	H	H	CH_3	OH
Minocycline	$N(CH_3)_2$	H	H	H

stances exist mainly as zwitterions. The acid salts, which are formed through protonation of the enol group on C-2, exist as crystalline compounds that are very soluble in water. These amphoteric antibiotics will crystallize out of aqueous solutions of their salts, however, unless stabilized by an excess of acid. The hydrochloride salts are used most commonly for oral administration and usually are encapsulated because they are bitter. Water-soluble salts may be obtained also from bases, such as sodium or potassium hydroxides, but they are not stable in aqueous solutions. Water-insoluble salts are formed with divalent and polyvalent metals.

The unusual structural groupings in the tetracyclines produce three acidity constants in aqueous solutions of the acid salts (Table 10-7). The particular functional groups responsible for each of the thermodynamic pK_a values were determined by Leeson et al.[150] as shown in the diagram below. These groupings had been identified previously by Stephens et al.[151] as the sites for protonation, but their earlier assignments, which produced the values responsible for pK_{a2} and

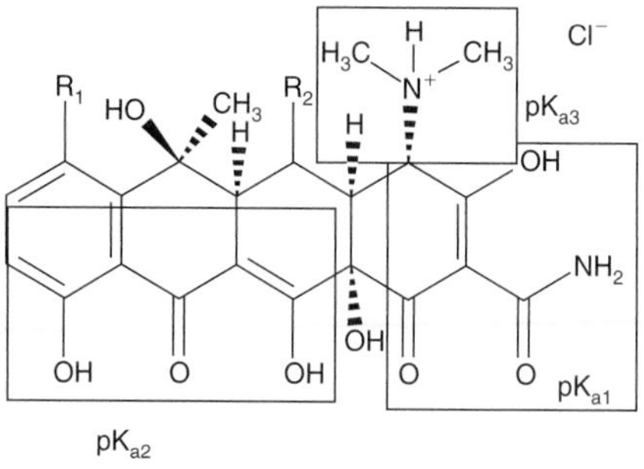

TABLE 10–7 pKa Values (of Hydrochlorides) in Aqueous Solution at 25°C

	pK_{a1}	pK_{a2}	pK_{a3}
Tetracycline	3.3	7.7	9.5
Chlortetracycline	3.3	7.4	9.3
Demeclocycline	3.3	7.2	9.3
Oxytetracycline	3.3	7.3	9.1
Doxycycline	3.4	7.7	9.7
Minocycline	2.8	7.8	9.3

pK_{a3}, were opposite those of Leeson et al.[150] This latter assignment has been substantiated by Rigler et al.[152]

The approximate pK_a values for each of these groups in the six tetracycline salts in common use are shown (Table 10-7). The values are taken from Stephens et al.,[151] Benet and Goyan,[153] and Barringer et al.[154] The pK_a of the 7-dimethylamino group of minocycline (not listed) is 5.0.

An interesting property of the tetracyclines is their ability to undergo epimerization at C-4 in solutions of intermediate pH range. These isomers are called *epitetracyclines*. Under acidic conditions, an equilibrium is established in about 1 day and consists of approximately equal amounts of the isomers. The partial structures below indicate the two forms of the epimeric pair. The 4-epitetracyclines have been isolated and characterized. They exhibit much less activity than the "natural" isomers, thus accounting for the decreased therapeutic value of aged solutions.

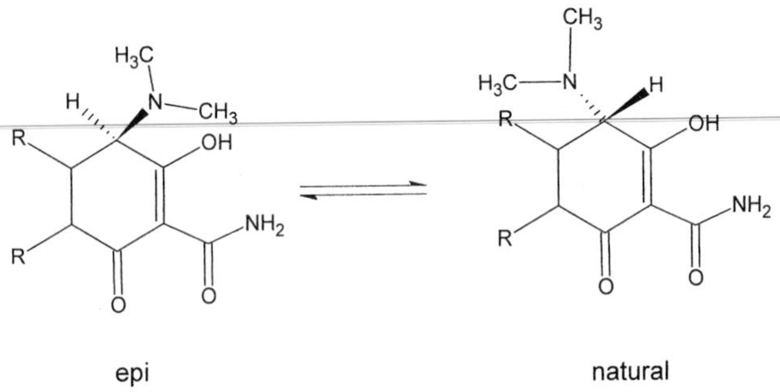

Strong acids and strong bases attack tetracyclines with a hydroxyl group on C-6, causing a loss in activity through modification of the C ring. Strong acids produce dehydration through a reaction involving the 6-hydroxyl group and the 5a-hydrogen. The double bond thus formed between positions 5a and 6 induces a shift in the position of the double bond between C-11a and C-12 to a position between C-11 and C-11a, forming the more energetically favored resonant system of the naphthalene group found in the inactive anhydrotetracyclines. Bases promote a reaction between the 6-hydroxyl group and the ketone group at the 11 position, causing the bond between the 11 and 11a atoms to cleave, forming the lactone ring found in the inactive isotetracycline. These two unfavorable reactions stimulated research that led to the development of the more stable and longer-acting compounds 6-deoxytetracycline, methacycline, doxycycline, and minocycline.

Stable chelate complexes are formed by the tetracyclines with many metals, including calcium, magnesium, and iron. Such chelates are usually very insoluble in water, accounting for the impaired absorption of most (if not all) tetracyclines in the presence of milk; calcium-, magnesium-, and aluminum-containing antacids; and iron salts. Soluble alkalinizers, such as sodium bicarbonate, also decrease the gastrointestinal absorption of the tetracyclines.[155] Deprotonation of tetracyclines to more ionic species and the observed instability of these products in alkaline solutions may account for this observation. The affinity of tetracyclines for calcium causes them to be incorporated into newly forming bones and teeth as tetracycline–calcium orthophosphate complexes. Deposits of these antibiotics in teeth cause a yellow discoloration that darkens (a photochemical reaction) over time. Tetracyclines are distributed into the milk of lactating mothers and will cross the placental barrier into the fetus. The possible effects of these agents on the bones and teeth of the child should be considered before their use during pregnancy or in children under 8 years of age.

Mechanism of Action and Resistance

The strong binding properties of the tetracyclines with metal ions caused Albert[156] to suggest that their antibacterial properties may be due to an ability to remove essential metal ions as chelated compounds. Elucidation of details of the mechanism of action of the tetracyclines,[157] however, has defined more clearly the specific roles of magnesium ions in molecular processes affected by these antibiotics in bacteria. Tetracyclines are specific inhibitors of bacterial protein synthesis. They bind to the 30S ribosomal subunit and, thereby, prevent the binding of aminoacyl tRNA to the mRNA–ribosome complex. Both the binding of aminoacyl tRNA and the binding of tetracyclines at the ribosomal binding site require magnesium ions.[158] Tetracyclines also bind to mammalian ribosomes but with lower affinities, and they apparently do not achieve sufficient intracellular concentrations to interfere with protein synthesis. The selective toxicity of the tetracyclines toward bacteria depends strongly on the self-destructive capacity of bacterial cells to concentrate these agents in the cell. Tetracyclines enter bacterial cells by two processes: passive diffusion and active transport. The active uptake of tetracyclines by bacterial cells is an energy-dependent process that requires adenosine triphosphate (ATP) and magnesium ions.[159]

Three biochemically distinct mechanisms of resistance to tetracyclines have been described in bacteria:[160] (a) efflux mediated by transmembrane-spanning, active-transport proteins that reduces the intracellular tetracycline concentration; (b) ribosomal protection, in which the bacterial protein synthesis apparatus is rendered resistant to the action of tetracyclines by an inducible cytoplasmic protein; and (c) enzymatic oxidation. Efflux mediated by plasmid or chromosomal protein determinants *tet*-A, -E, -G, -H, -K, and -L, and ribosomal protection mediated by the chromosomal protein determinants *tet*-M, -O, and -S are the most frequently encountered and most clinically significant resistance mechanisms for tetracyclines.

Spectrum of Activity

The tetracyclines have the broadest spectrum of activity of any known antibacterial agents. They are active against a wide range of Gram-positive and Gram-negative bacteria, spirochetes, mycoplasma, rickettsiae, and chlamydiae. Their potential indications are, therefore, numerous. Their bacteriostatic action, however, is a disadvantage in the treatment of life-threatening infections such as septicemia, endocarditis, and meningitis; the aminoglycosides and/or cephalosporins usually are preferred for Gram-negative and the penicillins for Gram-positive infections. Because of incomplete absorption and their effectiveness against the natural bacterial flora of the intestine, tetracyclines may induce superin-

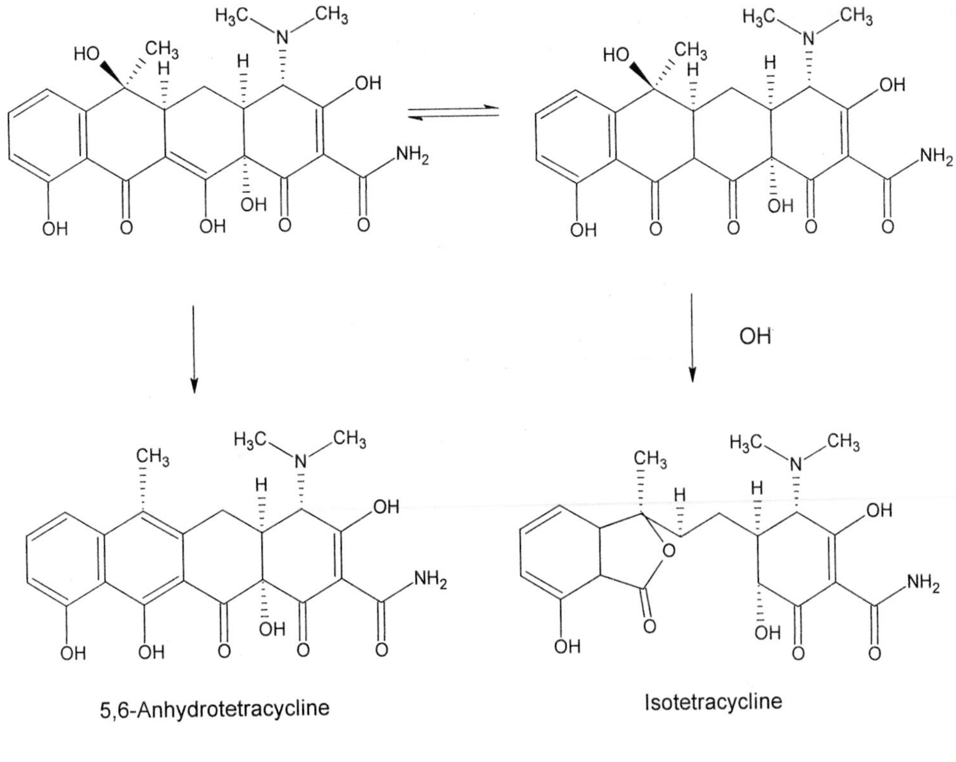

5,6-Anhydrotetracycline

Isotetracycline

fections caused by the pathogenic yeast *Candida albicans*. Resistance to tetracyclines among both Gram-positive and Gram-negative bacteria is relatively common. Superinfections caused by resistant *S. aureus* and *P. aeruginosa* have resulted from the use of these agents over time. Parenteral tetracyclines may cause severe liver damage, especially when given in excessive dosage to pregnant women or to patients with impaired renal function.

Structure–Activity Relationships

The large amount of research carried out to prepare semisynthetic modifications of the tetracyclines and to obtain individual compounds by total synthesis revealed several interesting SARs. Reviews are available that discuss SARs among the tetracyclines in detail,[161–163] their molecular and clinical properties,[164] and their synthesis and chemical properties.[162, 163, 165, 166] Only a brief review of the salient structure–activity features is presented here. All derivatives containing fewer than four rings are inactive or nearly inactive. The simplest tetracycline derivative that retains the characteristic broad-spectrum activity associated with this antibiotic class is 6-demethyl-6-deoxytetracycline. Many of the precise structural features present in this molecule must remain unmodified for derivatives to retain activity. The integrity of substituents at carbon atoms 1, 2, 3, 4, 10, 11, 11a, and 12, representing the hydrophilic "southern and eastern" faces of the molecule, cannot be violated drastically without deleterious effects on the antimicrobial properties of the resulting derivatives.

A-ring substituents can be modified only slightly without dramatic loss of antibacterial potency. The enolized tricarbonylmethane system at C-1 to C-3 must be intact for good activity. Replacement of the amide at C-2 with other functions (e.g., aldehyde or nitrile) reduces or abolishes activity. Monoalkylation of the amide nitrogen reduces activity proportionately to the size of the alkyl group. Aminoalkylation of the amide nitrogen, accomplished by the Mannich reaction, yields derivatives that are substantially more water soluble than the parent tetracycline and are hydrolyzed to it in vivo (e.g., rolitetracycline). The dimethylamino group at the 4 position must have the α orientation: 4-epitetracyclines are very much less active than the natural isomers. Removal of the 4-dimethylamino group reduces activity even further. Activity is largely retained in the primary and *N*-methyl secondary amines but rapidly diminishes in the higher alkylamines. A *cis*-A/B-ring fusion with a β-hydroxyl group at C-12a is apparently also essential. Esters of the C-12a hydroxyl group are inactive, with the exception of the formyl ester, which readily hydrolyzes in aqueous solutions. Alkylation at C-11a also leads to inactive compounds, demonstrating the importance of an enolizable β-diketone functionality at C-11 and C-12. The importance of the shape of the tetracyclic ring system is illustrated further by substantial loss in antibacterial potency resulting from epimerization at C-5a. Dehydrogenation to form a double bond between C-5a and C-11a markedly decreases activity, as does aromatization of ring C to form anhydrotetracyclines.

In contrast, substituents at positions 5, 5a, 6, 7, 8, and 9, representing the largely hydrophobic "northern and western" faces of the molecule, can be modified with varying degrees of success, resulting in retention and, sometimes,

improvement of antibiotic activity. A 5-hydroxyl group, as in oxytetracycline and doxycycline, may influence pharmacokinetic properties but does not change antimicrobial activity. 5a-Epitetracyclines (prepared by total synthesis), although highly active in vitro, are unfortunately much less impressive in vivo. Acid-stable 6-deoxytetracyclines and 6-demethyl-6-deoxytetracyclines have been used to prepare a variety of mono- and disubstituted derivatives by electrophilic substitution reactions at C-7 and C-9 of the D ring. The more useful results have been achieved with the introduction of substituents at C-7. Oddly, strongly electron-withdrawing groups (e.g., chloro lortetracycline] and nitro) and strongly electron-donating groups (e.g., dimethylamino [minocycline]) enhance activity. This unusual circumstance is reflected in QSAR studies of 7- and 9-substituted tetracyclines,[162, 167] which indicated a squared (parabolic) dependence on σ, Hammet's electronic substituent constant, and in vitro inhibition of an *E. coli* strain. The effect of introducing substituents at C-8 has not been studied because this position cannot be substituted directly by classic electrophilic aromatic substitution reactions; thus, 8-substituted derivatives are available only through total synthesis.[168]

The most fruitful site for semisynthetic modification of the tetracyclines has been the 6 position. Neither the 6α-methyl nor the 6β-hydroxyl group is essential for antibacterial activity. In fact, doxycycline and methacycline are more active in vitro than their parent oxytetracycline against most bacterial strains. The conversion of oxytetracycline to doxycycline, which can be accomplished by reduction of methacycline,[169] gives a 1:1 mixture of doxycycline and epidoxycycline (which has a β-oriented methyl group); if the C-11a α-fluoro derivative of methacycline is used, the β-methyl epimer is formed exclusively.[170] 6-Epidoxycycline is much less active than doxycycline. 6-Demethyl-6-deoxytetracycline, synthesized commercially by catalytic hydrogenolysis of the 7-chloro and 6-hydroxyl groups of 7-chloro-6-demethyltetracycline, obtained by fermentation of a mutant strain of *Streptomyces aureofaciens*,[171] is slightly more potent than tetracycline. More successful from a clinical standpoint, however, is 6-demethyl-6-deoxy-7-dimethylaminotetracycline (minocycline)[172] because of its activity against tetracycline-resistant bacterial strains.

6-Deoxytetracyclines also possess important chemical and pharmacokinetic advantages over their 6-oxy counterparts. Unlike the latter, they are incapable of forming anhydrotetracyclines under acidic conditions because they cannot dehydrate at C-5a and C-6. They are also more stable in base because they do not readily undergo β-ketone cleavage, followed by lactonization, to form isotetracyclines. Although it lacks a 6-hydroxyl group, methacycline shares the instability of the 6-oxytetracyclines in strongly acetic conditions. It suffers prototropic rearrangement to the anhydrotetracycline in acid but is stable to β-ketone cleavage followed by lactonization to the isotetracycline in base. Reduction of the 6-hydroxyl group also dramatically changes the solubility properties of tetracyclines. This effect is reflected in significantly higher oil/water partition coefficients of the 6-deoxytetracyclines than of the tetracyclines (Table 10-8).[173, 174] The greater lipid solubility of the 6-deoxy compounds has important pharmacokinetic consequences.[162, 164] Hence, doxycycline and minocycline are absorbed more completely following oral administration, exhibit higher fractions of

TABLE 10–8   Pharmacokinetic Properties[a] of Tetracyclines

| Tetracycline | Substituents | | | | K_{pc} Octanol/ Water pH 5.6[b] | Absorbed Orally (%) | Excreted in Feces (%) | Excreted in Urine (%) | Protein Bound (%) | Volume of Distribution (% body weight) | Renal Clearance (mL/min/ 1.73 m²) | Half-Life (h) |
	C-5α	C-6α	C-6β	C-7								
Tetracycline	H	CH₆	OH	H	0.056	58	20–50	60	24–65	156–306	50–80	10
Oxytetracycline	OH	CH₆	OH	H	0.075	77–80	50	70	20–35	180–305	99–102	9
Chlortetracycline	H	CH₆	OH	Cl	0.41	25–30	>50	18	42–54	149	32	7
Demeclocycline	H	H	OH	Cl	0.25	66	23–72	42	68–77	179	35	15
Doxycycline	OH	CH₆	H	H	0.95	93	20–40	27–39	60–91	63	18–28	15
Minocycline	H	H	H	N(CH₃)₂	1.10	100	40	5–11	55–76	74	5–15	19

[a] Values taken from Brown, J. R., and Ireland, D. S.: Adv. Pharmacol. Chemother. 15:161, 1978.

[b] Values taken from Colazzi, J. L., and Klink, P. R.: J. Pharm. Sci. 58:158, 1969.

plasma protein binding, and have higher volumes of distribution and lower renal clearance rates than the corresponding 6-oxytetracyclines.

Polar substituents (i.e., hydroxyl groups) at C-5 and C-6 decrease lipid versus water solubility of the tetracyclines. The 6 position is, however, considerably more sensitive than the 5 position to this effect. Thus, doxycycline (6-deoxy-5-oxytetracycline) has a much higher partition coefficient than either tetracycline or oxytetracycline. Nonpolar substituents (those with positive σ values; see Chapter 2), for example, 7-dimethylamino, 7-chloro, and 6-methyl, have the opposite effect. Accordingly, the partition coefficient of chlortetracycline is substantially greater than that of tetracycline and slightly greater than that of demeclocycline. Interestingly, minocycline (5-demethyl-6-deoxy-7-dimethylaminotetracycline) has the highest partition coefficient of the commonly used tetracyclines.

The poorer oral absorption of the more water-soluble compounds tetracycline and oxytetracycline can be attributed to several factors. In addition to their comparative difficulty in penetrating lipid membranes, the polar tetracyclines probably experience more complexation with metal ions in the gut and undergo some acid-catalyzed destruction in the stomach. Poorer oral absorption coupled with biliary excretion of some tetracyclines is also thought to cause a higher incidence of superinfections from resistant microbial strains. The more polar tetracyclines, however, are excreted in higher concentrations in the urine (e.g., 60% for tetracycline and 70% for oxytetracycline) than the more lipid-soluble compounds (e.g., 33% for doxycycline and only 11% for minocycline). Significant passive renal tubular reabsorption coupled with higher fractions of protein binding contributes to the lower

renal clearance and longer durations of action of doxycycline and minocycline compared with those of the other tetracyclines, especially tetracycline and oxytetracycline. Minocycline also experiences significant N-dealkylation catalyzed by cytochrome P-450 oxygenases in the liver, which contributes to its comparatively low renal clearance. Although all tetracyclines are distributed widely into tissues, the more polar ones have larger volumes of distribution than the nonpolar compounds. The more lipid-soluble tetracyclines, however, distribute better to poorly vascularized tissue. It is also claimed that the distribution of doxycycline and minocycline into bone is less than that of other tetracyclines.[175]

Products

Tetracycline, USP.   Chemical studies on chlortetracycline revealed that controlled catalytic hydrogenolysis selectively removed the 7-chloro atom and so produced tetracycline (Achromycin, Cyclopar, Panmycin, Tetracyn). This process was patented by Conover[176] in 1955. Later, tetracycline was obtained from fermentations of *Streptomyces* spp., but the commercial supply still chiefly depends on hydrogenolysis of chlortetracycline.

Tetracycline, USP

Tetracycline is 4-dimethylamino-1,4,4a,5,5a,6,11,12a-octahydro-3,6,10,12,12a-pentahydroxy-6-methyl-1,11-dioxo-2-naphthacenecarboxamide. It is a bright yellow, crystalline salt that is stable in air but darkens on exposure to strong sunlight. Tetracycline is stable in acid solutions with a pH above 2. It is somewhat more stable in alkaline solutions than chlortetracycline, but like those of the other tetracyclines, such solutions rapidly lose potency. One gram of the base requires 2,500 mL of water and 50 mL of alcohol to dissolve it. The hydrochloride salt is used most commonly in medicine, though the free base is absorbed from the gastrointestinal tract about equally well. One gram of the hydrochloride salt dissolves in about 10 mL of water and in 100 mL of alcohol. Tetracycline has become the most popular antibiotic of its group, largely because its plasma concentration appears to be higher and more enduring than that of either oxytetracycline or chlortetracycline. Also, it is found in higher concentration in the spinal fluid than the other two compounds.

A number of combinations of tetracycline with agents that increase the rate and the height of plasma concentrations are on the market. One such adjuvant is magnesium chloride hexahydrate (Panmycin). Also, an insoluble tetracycline phosphate complex (Tetrex) is made by mixing a solution of tetracycline, usually as the hydrochloride, with a solution of sodium metaphosphate. There are a variety of claims concerning the efficacy of these adjuvants. The mechanisms of their actions are not clear, but reportedly[177, 178] these agents enhance plasma concentrations over those obtained when tetracycline hydrochloride alone is administered orally. Remmers et al.[179, 180] reported on the effects that selected aluminum–calcium gluconates complexed with some tetracyclines have on plasma concentrations when administered orally, intramuscularly, or intravenously. Such complexes enhanced plasma levels in dogs when injected but not when given orally. They also observed enhanced plasma levels in experimental animals when complexes of tetracyclines with aluminum metaphosphate, aluminum pyrophosphate, or aluminum–calcium phosphinicodilactates were administered orally. As noted above, the tetracyclines can form stable chelate complexes with metal ions such as calcium and magnesium, which retard absorption from the gastrointestinal tract. The complexity of the systems involved has not permitted unequivocal substantiation of the idea that these adjuvants compete with the tetracyclines for substances in the alimentary tract that would otherwise be free to complex with these antibiotics and thereby retard their absorption. Certainly, there is no evidence that the metal ions per se act as buffers, an idea alluded to sometimes in the literature.

Tetracycline hydrochloride is also available in ointments for topical and ophthalmic administration. A topical solution is used for the management of acne vulgaris.

Rolitetracycline, USP.

Rolitetracycline, *N*-(pyrrolidinomethyl)tetracycline (Syntetrin) was introduced for use by intramuscular or intravenous injection. This derivative is made by condensing tetracycline with pyrrolidine and formaldehyde in the presence of *tert*-butyl alcohol. It is very soluble in water (1 g dissolves in about 1 mL) and provides a means of injecting the antibiotic in a small volume of

solution. It has been recommended for cases when the oral dosage forms are not suitable, but it is no longer widely used.

Rolitetracycline, USP

Chlortetracycline Hydrochloride, USP.

Chlortetracycline (Aureomycin hydrochloride) was isolated by Duggar[181] in 1948 from *S. aureofaciens*. This compound, which was produced in an extensive search for new antibiotics, was the first of the group of highly successful tetracyclines. It soon became established as a valuable antibiotic with broad-spectrum activities.

Chlortetracycline Hydrochloride

It is used in medicine chiefly as the acid salt of the compound whose systematic chemical designation is 7-chloro-4-(dimethylamino)-1,4,4a,5,5a,6,11,12a-octahydro-3,6,10,12,12a-pentahydroxy-6-methyl-1,11-dioxo-2-naphthacenecarboxamide. The hydrochloride salt is a crystalline powder with a bright yellow color, which suggested its brand name, Aureomycin. It is stable in air but slightly photosensitive and should be protected from light. It is odorless and bitter. One gram of the hydrochloride salt will dissolve in about 75 mL of water, producing a pH of about 3. It is only slightly soluble in alcohol and practically insoluble in other organic solvents.

Oral and parenteral forms of chlortetracycline are no longer used because of the poor bioavailability and inferior pharmacokinetic properties of the drug. It is still marketed in ointment forms for topical and ophthalmic use.

Oxytetracycline Hydrochloride, USP.

Early in 1950, Finlay et al.[182] reported the isolation of oxytetracycline (Terramycin) from *S. rimosus*. This compound was soon identified as a chemical analogue of chlortetracycline that showed similar antibiotic properties. The structure of oxytetracycline was elucidated by Hochstein et al.,[183] and this work provided the basis for the confirmation of the structure of the other tetracyclines.

Oxytetracycline Hydrochloride

Oxytetracycline hydrochloride is a pale yellow, bitter, crystalline compound. The amphoteric base is only slightly soluble in water and slightly soluble in alcohol. It is odorless and stable in air but darkens on exposure to strong sunlight. The hydrochloride salt is a stable yellow powder that is more bitter than the free base. It is much more soluble in water, 1 g dissolving in 2 mL, and more soluble in alcohol than the free base. Both compounds are inactivated rapidly by alkali hydroxides and by acid solutions below pH 2. Both forms of oxytetracycline are absorbed rapidly and equally well from the digestive tract, so the only real advantage the free base offers over the hydrochloride salt is that it is less bitter. Oxytetracycline hydrochloride is also used for parenteral administration (intravenously and intramuscularly).

Methacycline Hydrochloride, USP. The synthesis of methacycline, 6-deoxy-6-demethyl-6-methylene-5-oxytetracycline hydrochloride (Rondomycin), reported by Blackwood et al.[184] in 1961, was accomplished by chemical modification of oxytetracycline. It has an antibiotic spectrum like that of the other tetracyclines but greater potency; about 600 mg of methacycline is equivalent to 1 g of tetracycline. Its particular value lies in its longer serum half-life; doses of 300 mg produce continuous serum antibacterial activity for 12 hours. Its toxic manifestations and contraindications are similar to those of the other tetracyclines.

The greater stability of methacycline, both in vivo and in vitro, results from modification at C-6. Removal of the 6-hydroxy group markedly increases the stability of ring C to both acids and bases, preventing the formation of isotetracyclines by bases. Anhydrotetracyclines still can form, however, by acid-catalyzed isomerization under strongly acidic conditions. Methacycline hydrochloride is a yellow to dark yellow, crystalline powder that is slightly soluble in water and insoluble in nonpolar solvents. It should be stored in tight, light-resistant containers in a cool place.

Methacycline Hydrochloride

Demeclocycline, USP. Demeclocycline, 7-chloro-6-demethyltetracycline (Declomycin), was isolated in 1957 by McCormick et al.[171] from a mutant strain of *S. aureofaciens*. Chemically, it is 7-chloro-4-(dimethylamino)1,4,4a,5,5a,6,

11,12a-octahydro-3,6,10,12,12a-pentahydroxy1,11-dioxo-2-naphthacenecarboxamide. Thus, it differs from chlortetracycline only in the absence of the methyl group on C-6.

Demeclocycline Hydrochloride

Demeclocycline is a yellow, crystalline powder that is odorless and bitter. It is sparingly soluble in water. A 1% solution has a pH of about 4.8. It has an antibiotic spectrum like that of other tetracyclines, but it is slightly more active than the others against most of the microorganisms for which they are used. This, together with its slower rate of elimination through the kidneys, makes demeclocycline as effective as the other tetracyclines, at about three-fifths of the dose. Like the other tetracyclines, it may cause infrequent photosensitivity reactions that produce erythema after exposure to sunlight. Demeclocycline may produce this reaction somewhat more frequently than the other tetracyclines. The incidence of discoloration and mottling of the teeth in youths from demeclocycline appears to be as low as that from other tetracyclines.

Meclocycline Sulfosalicylate, USP. Meclocycline, 7-chloro-6-deoxy-6-demethyl-6-methylene-5-oxytetracycline sulfosalicylate (Meclan), is a semisynthetic derivative prepared from oxytetracycline.[184] Although meclocycline has been used in Europe for many years, it became available only relatively recently in the United States for a single therapeutic indication, the treatment of acne. It is available as the sulfosalicylate salt in a 1% cream.

Meclocycline Sulfosalicylate

Meclocycline sulfosalicylate is a bright yellow, crystalline powder that is slightly soluble in water and insoluble in organic solvents. It is light sensitive and should be stored in light-resistant containers.

Doxycycline, USP. A more recent addition to the tetracycline group of antibiotics available for antibacterial therapy is doxycycline, α-6-deoxy-5-oxytetracycline (Vibramycin), first reported by Stephens et al.[185] in 1958. It was obtained first in small yields by a chemical transformation of oxytetracycline, but it is now produced by catalytic hydrogenation of methacycline or by reduction of a benzylmercaptan derivative of methacycline with Raney nickel. The latter process produces a nearly pure form of the 6α-methyl epimer. The 6α-methyl epimer is more than 3 times as active as its β-epimer.[169] Apparently, the difference in orientation of the methyl groups, which slightly affects the shapes of the molecules, causes a substantial difference in biological effect. Also, absence of the 6-hydroxyl group produces a compound that is very stable in acids and bases and that has a long biological half-life. In addition, it is absorbed very well from the gastrointestinal tract, thus allowing a smaller dose to be administered. High tissue levels are obtained with it, and unlike other tetracyclines, doxycycline apparently does not accumulate in patients with impaired renal function. Therefore, it is preferred for uremic patients with infections outside the urinary tract. Its low renal clearance may limit its effectiveness, however, in urinary tract infections.

Doxycycline

Doxycycline is available as a hydrate salt, a hydrochloride salt solvated as the hemiethanolate hemihydrate, and a monohydrate. The hydrate form is sparingly soluble in water and is used in a capsule; the monohydrate is water insoluble and is used for aqueous suspensions, which are stable for up to 2 weeks when kept in a cool place.

Minocycline Hydrochloride, USP. Minocycline, 7-dimethylamino-6-demethyl-6-deoxytetracycline (Minocin, Vectrin), the most potent tetracycline currently used in therapy, is obtained by reductive methylation of 7-nitro-6-demethyl-6-deoxytetracycline.[172] It was released for use in the United States in 1971. Because minocycline, like doxycycline, lacks the 6-hydroxyl group, it is stable in acids and does not dehydrate or rearrange to anhydro or lactone forms. Minocycline is well absorbed orally to give high plasma and tissue levels. It has a very long serum half-life, resulting from slow urinary excretion and moderate protein binding. Doxycycline and minocycline, along with oxytetracycline, show the least in vitro calcium binding of the clinically available tetracyclines. The improved distribution properties of the 6-deoxytetracyclines have been attributed to greater lipid solubility.

Minocycline

Perhaps the most outstanding property of minocycline is its activity toward Gram-positive bacteria, especially staphylococci and streptococci. In fact, minocycline has been effective against staphylococcal strains that are resistant to methicillin and all other tetracyclines, including doxycycline.[186] Although it is doubtful that minocycline will replace bactericidal agents for the treatment of life-threatening staphylococcal infections, it may become a useful alternative for the treatment of less serious tissue infections. Minocycline has been recommended for the treatment of chronic bronchitis and other upper respiratory tract infections. Despite its relatively low renal clearance, partially compensated for by high serum and tissue levels, it has been recommended for the treatment of urinary tract infections. It has been effective in the eradication of *N. meningitidis* in asymptomatic carriers.

NEWER TETRACYCLINES

The remarkably broad spectrum of antimicrobial activity of the tetracyclines notwithstanding, the widespread emergence of bacterial genes and plasmids encoding tetracycline resistance has increasingly imposed limitations on the clinical applications of this antibiotic class in recent years.[164] This situation has prompted researchers at Lederle Laboratories to reinvestigate SARs of tetracyclines substituted in the aromatic (D) ring in an effort to discover analogues that might be effective against resistant strains. As a result of these efforts, the glycylcyclines, a class of 9-dimethylglycylamino-(DMG)-substituted tetracyclines exemplified by DMG-minocycline (DMG-MINO) and DMG-6-methyl-6-deoxytetracycline (DMG-DMDOT), were discovered.[187–189]

The glycylcyclines retain the broad spectrum of activity and potency exhibited by the original tetracyclines against tetracycline-sensitive microbial strains and are highly active against bacterial strains that exhibit tetracycline resistance mediated by efflux or ribosomal protection determinants. If ongoing clinical evaluations of the glycylcyclines establish favorable toxicological and pharmacokinetic profiles for these compounds, a new class of "second-generation" tetracyclines could be launched.

X = N(CH₃)₂   9-(Dimethylglycylamino)minocycline (DMG-MINO)
X = H   9-(Dimethylglycylamino)-6-demethyl-6-deoxytetracycline (DMG-DMDOT)

MACROLIDES

Among the many antibiotics isolated from the actinomycetes is the group of chemically related compounds called the *macrolides*. In 1950, picromycin, the first of this group to be identified as a macrolide compound, was first reported. In 1952, erythromycin and carbomycin were reported as new antibiotics, and they were followed in subsequent years by other macrolides. Currently, more than 40 such compounds are known, and new ones are likely to appear in the future. Of all of these, only two, erythromycin and oleandomycin, have been available consistently for medical use in the United States. In recent years, interest has shifted away from novel macrolides isolated from soil samples (e.g., spiramycin, josamycin, and rosamicin), all of which thus far have proved to be clinically inferior to erythromycin and semisynthetic derivatives of erythromycin (e.g., clarithromycin and azithromycin), which have superior pharmacokinetic properties due to their enhanced acid stability and improved distribution properties.

Chemistry

The macrolide antibiotics have three common chemical characteristics: *(a)* a large lactone ring (which prompted the name *macrolide*), *(b)* a ketone group, and *(c)* a glycosidically linked amino sugar. Usually, the lactone ring has 12, 14, or 16 atoms in it, and it is often unsaturated, with an olefinic group conjugated with the ketone function. (The polyene macrocyclic lactones, such as natamycin and amphotericin B; the ansamycins, such as rifampin; and the polypeptide lactones generally are not included among the macrolide antibiotics.) They may have, in addition to the amino sugar, a neutral sugar that is linked glycosidically to the lactone ring (see "Erythromycin," below). Because of the dimethylamino group on the sugar moiety, the macrolides are bases that form salts with pK_a values between 6.0 and 9.0. This feature has been used to make clinically useful salts. The free bases are only slightly soluble in water but dissolve in somewhat polar organic solvents. They are stable in aqueous solutions at or below room temperature but are inactivated by acids, bases, and heat. The chemistry of macrolide antibiotics has been the subject of several reviews.[190, 191]

Mechanisms of Action and Resistance

Some details of the mechanism of antibacterial action of erythromycin are known. It binds selectively to a specific site on the 50S ribosomal subunit to prevent the translocation step of bacterial protein synthesis.[192] It does not bind to mammalian ribosomes. Broadly based, nonspecific resistance to the antibacterial action of erythromycin among many species of Gram-negative bacilli appears to be largely related to the inability of the antibiotic to penetrate the cell walls of these organisms.[193] In fact, the sensitivities of members of the Enterobacteriaceae family are pH dependent, with MICs decreasing as a function of increasing pH. Furthermore, protoplasts from Gram-negative bacilli, which lack cell walls, are sensitive to erythromycin. A highly specific resistance mechanism to the macrolide antibiotics occurs in erythromycin-resistant strains of *S. aureus*.[194, 195] Such strains produce an enzyme that methylates a specific adenine residue at the erythromycin-binding site of the bacterial 50S ribosomal subunit. The methylated ribosomal RNA remains active in protein synthesis but no longer binds erythromycin. Bacterial resistance to the lincomycins apparently also occurs by this mechanism.

Spectrum of Activity

The spectrum of antibacterial activity of the more potent macrolides, such as erythromycin, resembles that of penicillin. They are frequently active against bacterial strains that are resistant to the penicillins. The macrolides are generally effective against most species of Gram-positive bacteria, both cocci and bacilli, and exhibit useful effectiveness against Gram-negative cocci, especially *Neisseria* spp. Many of the macrolides are also effective against *Treponema pallidum*. In contrast to penicillin, macrolides are also effective against *Mycoplasma*, *Chlamydia*, *Campylobacter*, and *Legionella* spp. Their activity against most species of Gram-negative bacilli is generally low and often unpredictable, though some strains of *H. influenzae* and *Brucella* spp. are sensitive.

Products

Erythromycin, USP. Early in 1952, McGuire et al.[196] reported the isolation of erythromycin (E-Mycin, Erythrocin,

Picromycin

Carbomycin A

Ilotycin) from *Streptomyces erythraeus.* It achieved rapid early acceptance as a well-tolerated antibiotic of value for the treatment of a variety of upper respiratory and soft-tissue infections caused by Gram-positive bacteria. It is also effective against many venereal diseases, including gonorrhea and syphilis, and provides a useful alternative for the treatment of many infections in patients allergic to penicillins. More recently, erythromycin was shown to be effective therapy for Eaton agent pneumonia *(Mycoplasma pneumoniae),* venereal diseases caused by chlamydia, bacterial enteritis caused by *Campylobacter jejuni,* and Legionnaires' disease.

Erythromycin

The commercial product is erythromycin A, which differs from its biosynthetic precursor, erythromycin B, in having a hydroxyl group at the 12 position of the aglycone. The chemical structure of erythromycin A was reported by Wiley et al.[197] in 1957 and its stereochemistry by Celmer[198] in 1965. An elegant synthesis of erythronolide A, the aglycone present in erythromycin A, was described by Corey and associates.[199]

The amino sugar attached through a glycosidic link to C-5 is desosamine, a structure found in a number of other macrolide antibiotics. The tertiary amine of desosamine (3,4, 6-trideoxy-3-dimethylamino-D-*xylo*-hexose) confers a basic character to erythromycin and provides the means by which acid salts may be prepared. The other carbohydrate structure linked as a glycoside to C-3 is called *cladinose* (2,3,6-trideoxy-3-methoxy-3-C-methyl-L-*ribo*-hexose) and is unique to the erythromycin molecule.

As is common with other macrolide antibiotics, compounds closely related to erythromycin have been obtained from culture filtrates of *S. erythraeus.* Two such analogues have been found, erythromycins B and C. Erythromycin B differs from erythromycin A only at C-12, at which a hydrogen has replaced the hydroxyl group. The B analogue is more acid stable but has only about 80% of the activity of erythromycin. The C analogue differs from erythromycin by the replacement of the methoxyl group on the cladinose moiety with a hydrogen atom. It appears to be as active as erythromycin but is present in very small amounts in fermentation liquors.

Erythromycin is a very bitter, white or yellow-white, crystalline powder. It is soluble in alcohol and in the other common organic solvents but only slightly soluble in water. The free base has a pK_a of 8.8. Saturated aqueous solutions develop an alkaline pH in the range of 8.0 to 10.5. It is extremely unstable at a pH of 4 or below. The optimum pH for stability of erythromycin is at or near neutrality.

Erythromycin may be used as the free base in oral dosage forms and for topical administration. To overcome its bitterness and irregular oral absorption (resulting from acid destruction and adsorption onto food), various enteric-coated and delayed-release dose forms of erythromycin base have been developed. These forms have been fully successful in overcoming the bitterness but have solved only marginally problems of oral absorption. Erythromycin has been chemically modified with primarily two different goals in mind: *(a)* to increase either its water or lipid solubility for parenteral dosage forms and *(b)* to increase its acid stability (and possibly its lipid solubility) for improved oral absorption. Modified derivatives of the antibiotic are of two types: acid salts of the dimethylamino group of the desosamine moiety (e.g., the glucoheptonate, the lactobionate, and the stearate) and esters of the 2'-hydroxyl group of the desosamine (e.g., the ethylsuccinate and the propionate, available as the lauryl sulfate salt and known as the estolate).

The stearate salt and the ethylsuccinate and propionate esters are used in oral dose forms intended to improve absorption of the antibiotic. The stearate releases erythromycin base in the intestinal tract, which is then absorbed. The ethylsuccinate and the estolate are absorbed largely intact and are hydrolyzed partially by plasma and tissue esterases to give free erythromycin. The question of bioavailability of the antibiotic from its various oral dosage and chemical forms has caused considerable concern and dispute over the past two decades.[200–205] It is generally believed that the 2'-esters per se have little or no intrinsic antibacterial activity[206] and, therefore, must be hydrolyzed to the parent antibiotic in vivo. Although the ethylsuccinate is hydrolyzed more efficiently than the estolate in vivo and, in fact, provides higher levels of erythromycin following intramuscular administration, an equal dose of the estolate gives higher levels of the free antibiotic following oral administration.[201, 205] Superior oral absorption of the estolate is attributed to both its greater acid stability and higher intrinsic absorption than the ethylsuccinate. Also, oral absorption of the estolate, unlike that of both the stearate and the ethylsuccinate, is not affected by food or fluid volume content of the gut. Superior bioavailability of active antibiotic from oral administration of the estolate over the ethylsuccinate, stearate, or erythromycin base cannot necessarily be assumed, however, because the estolate is more extensively protein bound than erythromycin itself.[207] Measured fractions of plasma protein binding for erythromycin-2'-propionate and erythromycin base range from 0.94 to 0.98 for the former and from 0.73 to 0.90 for the latter, indicating a much higher level of free erythromycin in the plasma. Bioavailability studies comparing equivalent doses of the enteric-coated base, the stearate salt, the ethylsuccinate ester, and the estolate ester in human volunteers[203, 204] showed delayed but slightly higher bioavailability for the free base than for the stearate, ethylsuccinate, or estolate.

One study, comparing the clinical effectiveness of recommended doses of the stearate, estolate, ethylsuccinate, and free base in the treatment of respiratory tract infections, failed to demonstrate substantial differences among them.[208] Two other clinical studies, comparing the effectiveness of the ethylsuccinate and the estolate in the treatment of streptococcal pharyngitis, however, found the estolate to be superior.[209, 210]

The water-insoluble ethylsuccinate ester is also available as a suspension for intramuscular injection. The glucoheptonate and lactobionate salts, however, are highly water soluble derivatives that provide high plasma levels of the active antibiotic immediately after intravenous injection. Aqueous solutions of these salts may also be administered by intramuscular injection, but this is not a common practice.

Erythromycin is distributed throughout the body water. It persists in tissues longer than in the blood. The antibiotic is concentrated by the liver and excreted extensively into the bile. Large amounts are excreted in the feces, partly because of poor oral absorption and partly because of biliary excretion. The serum half-life is 1.4 hours. Some cytochrome P-450-catalyzed oxidative demethylation to a less active metabolite may also occur. Erythromycin inhibits cytochrome P-450-requiring oxidases, leading to a variety of potential drug interactions. Thus, toxic effects of theophylline, the hydroxycoumarin anticoagulants, the benzodiazepines alprazolam and midazolam, carbamazepine, cyclosporine, and the antihistaminic drugs terfenadine and astemizole may be potentiated by erythromycin.

The toxicity of erythromycin is comparatively low. Primary adverse reactions to the antibiotic are related to its actions on the gastrointestinal tract and the liver. Erythromycin may stimulate gastrointestinal motility following either oral or parenteral administration.[211] This dose-related, prokinetic effect can cause abdominal cramps, epigastric distress, and diarrhea, especially in children and young adults. Cholestatic hepatitis occurs occasionally with erythromycin, usually in adults and more frequently with the estolate.

Erythromycin Stearate, USP.

Erythromycin stearate (Ethril, Wyamycin S, Erypar) is the stearic acid salt of erythromycin. Like erythromycin base, the stearate is acid labile. It is film coated to protect it from acid degradation in the stomach. In the alkaline pH of the duodenum, the free base is liberated from the stearate and absorbed. Erythromycin stearate is a crystalline powder that is practically insoluble in water but soluble in alcohol and ether.

Erythromycin Ethylsuccinate, USP.

Erythromycin ethylsuccinate (EES, Pediamycin, EryPed) is the ethylsuccinate mixed ester of erythromycin in which the 2′-hydroxyl group of the desosamine is esterified. It is absorbed as the ester and hydrolyzed slowly in the body to form erythromycin. It is somewhat acid labile, and its absorption is enhanced by the presence of food. The ester is insoluble in water but soluble in alcohol and ether.

Erythromycin Estolate, USP.

Erythromycin estolate, erythromycin propionate lauryl sulfate (Ilosone), is the lauryl sulfate salt of the 2′-propionate ester of erythromycin. Erythromycin estolate is acid stable and absorbed as the propionate ester. The ester undergoes slow hydrolysis in vivo. Only the free base binds to bacterial ribosomes. Some evidence, however, suggests that the ester is taken up by bacterial cells more rapidly than the free base and undergoes hydrolysis by bacterial esterases within the cells. The incidence of cholestatic hepatitis is reportedly higher with the estolate than with other erythromycin preparations.

Erythromycin estolate occurs as long needles that are sparingly soluble in water but soluble in organic solvents.

Erythromycin Gluceptate, Sterile, USP.

Erythromycin gluceptate, erythromycin glucoheptonate (Ilotycin Gluceptate), is the glucoheptonic acid salt of erythromycin. It is a crystalline substance that is freely soluble in water and practically insoluble in organic solvents. Erythromycin gluceptate is intended for intravenous administration for the treatment of serious infections, such as Legionnaires' disease, or when oral administration is not possible. Solutions are stable for 1 week when refrigerated.

Erythromycin Lactobionate, USP.

Erythromycin lactobionate is a water-soluble salt prepared by reacting erythromycin base with lactobiono-δ-lactone. It occurs as an amorphous powder that is freely soluble in water and alcohol and slightly soluble in ether. It is intended, after reconstitution in sterile water, for intravenous administration to achieve high plasma levels in the treatment of serious infections.

Clarithromycin USP.

Clarithromycin (Biaxin) is the 6-methyl ether of erythromycin. The simple methylation of the 6-hydroxyl group of erythromycin creates a semisynthetic derivative that fully retains the antibacterial properties of the parent antibiotic, with markedly increased acid stability and oral bioavailability and reduced gastrointestinal side effects associated with erythromycin.[212] Acid-catalyzed dehydration of erythromycin in the stomach initiates as a sequence of reactions, beginning with $\Delta^{6,7}$-bond migration followed by formation of an 8,9-anhydro-6,9-hemiketal and terminating in a 6,9:9,12-spiroketal. Since neither the hemiketal nor the spiroketal exhibits significant antibacterial activity, unprotected erythromycin is inactivated substantially in the stomach. Furthermore, evidence suggests that the hemiketal may be largely responsible for the gastrointestinal (prokinetic) adverse effects associated with oral erythromycin.[211]

Clarithromycin

Clarithromycin is well absorbed following oral administration. Its oral bioavailability is estimated to be 50 to 55%. The presence of food does not significantly affect its absorption. Extensive metabolism of clarithromycin by oxidation and hydrolysis occurs in the liver. The major metabolite is the 14-hydroxyl derivative, which retains antibacterial activity. The amount of clarithromycin excreted in the urine ranges from 20 to 30%, depending on the dose, while 10 to

15% of the 14-hydroxy metabolite is excreted in the urine. Biliary excretion of clarithromycin is much lower than that of erythromycin. Clarithromycin is widely distributed into the tissues, which retain much higher concentrations than the plasma. Protein-binding fractions in the plasma range from 65 to 70%. The plasma half-life of clarithromycin is 4.3 hours.

Some of the microbiological properties of clarithromycin also appear to be superior to those of erythromycin. It exhibits greater potency against *M. pneumoniae, Legionella* spp., *Chlamydia pneumoniae, H. influenzae,* and *M. catarrhalis* than does erythromycin. Clarithromycin also has activity against unusual pathogens such as *Borrelia burgdorferi* (the cause of Lyme disease) and the *Mycobacterium avium* complex (MAC). Clarithromycin is significantly more active than erythromycin against group A streptococci, *S. pneumoniae,* and the viridans group of streptococci in vivo because of its superior oral bioavailability. Clarithromycin is, however, more expensive than erythromycin, which must be weighed against its potentially greater effectiveness.

Adverse reactions to clarithromycin are rare. The most common complaints relate to gastrointestinal symptoms, but these seldom require discontinuance of therapy. Clarithromycin, like erythromycin, inhibits cytochrome P-450 oxidases and, thus, can potentiate the actions of drugs metabolized by these enzymes.

Clarithromycin occurs as a white crystalline solid that is practically insoluble in water, sparingly soluble in alcohol, and freely soluble in acetone. It is provided as 250- and 500-mg oral tablets and as granules for the preparation of aqueous oral suspensions containing 25 or 50 mg/mL.

Azithromycin USP.

Azithromycin (Zithromax) is a semisynthetic derivative of erythromycin, prepared by Beckman rearrangement of the corresponding 6-oxime, followed by N-methylation and reduction of the resulting ring-expanded lactam. It is a prototype of a series of nitrogen-containing, 15-membered ring macrolides known as *azalides*.[213] Removal of the 9-keto group coupled with incorporation of a weakly basic tertiary amine nitrogen function into the macrolide ring increases the stability of azithromycin to acid-catalyzed degradation. These changes also increase the lipid solubility of the molecule, thereby conferring unique pharmacokinetic and microbiological properties.[214]

Azithromycin

The oral bioavailability of azithromycin is good, nearly 40%, provided the antibiotic is administered at least 1 hour before or 2 hours after a meal. Food decreases its absorption by as much as 50%. The pharmacokinetics of azithromycin are characterized by rapid and extensive removal of the drug from the plasma into the tissues followed by a slow release. Tissue levels far exceed plasma concentrations, leading to a highly variable and prolonged elimination half-life of up to 5 days. The fraction of azithromycin bound to plasma proteins is only about 50% and does not exert an important influence on its distribution. Evidence indicates that azithromycin is largely excreted in the feces unchanged, with a small percentage appearing in the urine. Extensive enterohepatic recycling of the drug occurs. Azithromycin apparently is not metabolized to any significant extent. In contrast to the 14-membered ring macrolides, azithromycin does not significantly inhibit cytochrome P-450 enzymes to create potential drug interactions.

The spectrum of antimicrobial activity of azithromycin is similar to that observed for erythromycin and clarithromycin but with some interesting differences. In general, it is more active against Gram-negative bacteria and less active against Gram-positive bacteria than its close relatives. The greater activity of azithromycin against *H. influenzae, M. catarrhalis,* and *M. pneumoniae* coupled with its extended half-life permits a 5-day dosing schedule for the treatment of respiratory tract infections caused by these pathogens. The clinical efficacy of azithromycin in the treatment of urogenital and other sexually transmitted infections caused by *Chlamydia trachomatis, N. gonorrhoeae, Haemophilus ducreyi,* and *Ureaplasma urealyticum* suggests that single-dose therapy with it for uncomplicated urethritis or cervicitis may have advantages over use of other antibiotics.

Dirithromycin.

Dirithromycin (Dynabac) is a more lipid-soluble prodrug derivative of 9S-erythromycyclamine prepared by condensation of the latter with 2-(2-methoxyethoxy)acetaldehyde.[215] The 9N,11O-oxazine ring thus formed is a hemi-aminal that is unstable under both acidic and alkaline aqueous conditions and undergoes spontaneous hydrolysis to form erythromycyclamine. Erythromycyclamine is a semisynthetic derivative of erythromycin in which the 9-keto group of the erythronolide ring has been converted to an amino group. Erythromycyclamine retains the antibacterial properties of erythromycin in vitro but exhibits poor bioavailability following oral administration. The prodrug, dirithromycin, is provided as enteric-coated tablets to protect it from acid-catalyzed hydrolysis in the stomach.

Dirithromycin

Orally administered dirithromycin is absorbed rapidly into the plasma, largely from the small intestine. Spontaneous hydrolysis to erythromycyclamine occurs in the plasma. Oral bioavailability is estimated to be about 10%, but food does not affect absorption of the prodrug.

The low plasma levels and large volume of distribution of erythromycyclamine are believed to result from its rapid distribution into well-perfused tissues, such as lung parenchyma, bronchial mucosa, nasal mucosa, and prostatic tissue. The drug also concentrates in human neutrophils. The elimination half-life is estimated to be 30 to 44 hours. Most of the prodrug and its active metabolite (62 to 81% in normal human subjects) is excreted in the feces, largely via the bile, following either oral or parenteral administration. Urinary excretion accounts for less than 3%.

The incidence and severity of gastrointestinal adverse effects associated with dirithromycin are similar to those seen with oral erythromycin. Preliminary studies indicate that dirithromycin and erythromycyclamine do not interact significantly with cytochrome P-450 oxygenases. Thus, the likelihood of interference in the oxidative metabolism of drugs such as phenytoin, theophylline, and cyclosporine by these enzymes may be less with dirithromycin than with erythromycin.

Dirithromycin is recommended as an alternative to erythromycin for the treatment of bacterial infections of the upper and lower respiratory tracts, such as pharyngitis, tonsillitis, bronchitis, and pneumonia, and for bacterial infections of other soft tissues and the skin. The once-daily dosing schedule for dirithromycin is advantageous in terms of better patient compliance. Its place in therapy remains to be fully assessed.[216]

Troleandomycin. Oleandomycin, as its triacetyl derivative troleandomycin, triacetyloleandomycin (TAO), remains available as an alternative to erythromycin for limited indications permitting use of an oral dosage form. Oleandomycin was isolated by Sobin and associates.[217] The structure of oleandomycin was proposed by Hochstein et al.,[218] and its absolute stereochemistry elucidated by Celmer.[219] The oleandomycin structure consists of two sugars and a 14-member lactone ring designated an *oleandolide*. One of the sugars is desosamine, also present in erythromycin; the other is L-oleandrose. The sugars are linked glycosidically to the 5 and 3 positions, respectively, of oleandolide.

Oleandomycin

Oleandomycin contains three hydroxyl groups that are subject to acylation, one in each of the sugars and one in the oleandolide. The triacetyl derivative retains the in vivo antibacterial activity of the parent antibiotic but possesses superior pharmacokinetic properties. It is hydrolyzed in vivo to oleandomycin. Troleandomycin achieves more rapid and higher plasma concentrations following oral administration than oleandomycin phosphate, and it has the additional advantage of being practically tasteless. Troleandomycin occurs as a white, crystalline solid that is nearly insoluble in water. It is relatively stable in the solid state but undergoes chemical degradation in either aqueous acidic or alkaline conditions.

Because the antibacterial spectrum of activity of oleandomycin is considered inferior to that of erythromycin, the pharmacokinetics of troleandomycin have not been studied extensively. Oral absorption is apparently good, and detectable blood levels of oleandomycin persist up to 12 hours after a 500-mg dose of troleandomycin. Approximately 20% is recovered in the urine, with most excreted in the feces, primarily as a result of biliary excretion. There is some epigastric distress following oral administration, with an incidence similar to that caused by erythromycin. Troleandomycin is the most potent inhibitor of cytochrome P-450 enzymes of the commercially available macrolides. It may potentiate the hepatic toxicity of certain anti-inflammatory steroids and oral contraceptive drugs as well as the toxic effects of theophylline, carbamazepine, and triazolam. Several allergic reactions, including cholestatic hepatitis, have also been reported with the use of troleandomycin.

Approved medical indications for troleandomycin are currently limited to the treatment of upper respiratory infections caused by such organisms as *S. pyogenes* and *S. pneumoniae*. It may be considered an alternative to oral forms of erythromycin. It is available in capsules and as a suspension.

LINCOMYCINS

The lincomycins are sulfur-containing antibiotics isolated from *Streptomyces lincolnensis*. Lincomycin is the most active and medically useful of the compounds obtained from fermentation. Extensive efforts to modify the lincomycin structure to improve its antibacterial and pharmacological properties resulted in the preparation of the 7-chloro-7-deoxy derivative clindamycin. Of the two antibiotics, clindamycin appears to have the greater antibacterial potency and better pharmacokinetic properties. Lincomycins resemble macrolides in antibacterial spectrum and biochemical mechanisms of action. They are primarily active against Gram-positive bacteria, particularly the cocci, but are also effective against non–spore-forming anaerobic bacteria, actinomycetes, mycoplasma, and some species of *Plasmodium*. Lincomycin binds to the 50S ribosomal subunit to inhibit protein synthesis. Its action may be bacteriostatic or bactericidal depending on a variety of factors, including the concentration of the antibiotic. A pattern of bacterial resistance and cross-resistance to lincomycins similar to that observed with the macrolides has been emerging.[195]

Products

Lincomycin Hydrochloride, USP. Lincomycin hydrochloride (Lincocin), which differs chemically from other major antibiotic classes, was isolated by Mason et al.[220] Its chemistry was described by Hoeksema and coworkers,[221] who assigned the structure, later confirmed by Slomp and MacKellar,[222] given in the diagram below. Total syntheses of the antibiotic were accomplished independently in 1970 in England and the United States.[223, 224] The structure contains a basic function, the pyrrolidine nitrogen, by which water-soluble salts with an apparent pK_a of 7.6 may be formed. When subjected to hydrazinolysis, lincomycin is cleaved at its amide bond into *trans*-L-4-*n*-propylhygric acid (the pyrrolidine moiety) and methyl α-thiolincosamide (the sugar moiety). Lincomycin-related antibiotics have been reported by Argoudelis[225] to be produced by *S. lincolnensis*. These antibiotics differ in structure at one or more of three positions of the lincomycin structure: *(a)* the *N*-methyl of the hygric acid moiety is substituted by a hydrogen; *(b)* the *n*-propyl group of the hygric acid moiety is substituted by an ethyl group; and *(c)* the thiomethyl ether of the α-thiolincosamide moiety is substituted by a thioethyl ether.

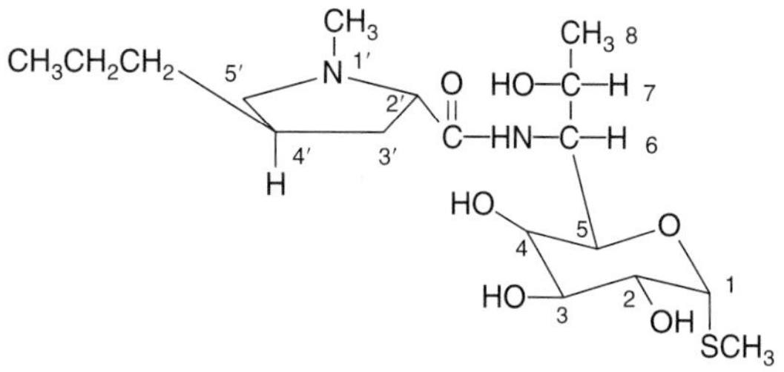

Lincomycin is used for the treatment of infections caused by Gram-positive organisms, notably staphylococci, β-hemolytic streptococci, and pneumococci. It is absorbed moderately well orally and distributed widely in the tissues. Effective concentrations are achieved in bone for the treatment of staphylococcal osteomyelitis but not in the cerebrospinal fluid for the treatment of meningitis. At one time, lincomycin was considered a nontoxic compound, with a low incidence of allergy (rash) and occasional gastrointestinal complaints (nausea, vomiting, and diarrhea) as the only adverse effects. Recent reports of severe diarrhea and the development of pseudomembranous colitis in patients treated with lincomycin (or clindamycin), however, have necessitated reappraisal of the role of these antibiotics in therapy. In any event, clindamycin is superior to lincomycin for the treatment of most infections for which these antibiotics are indicated.

Lincomycin hydrochloride occurs as the monohydrate, a white, crystalline solid that is stable in the dry state. It is readily soluble in water and alcohol, and its aqueous solutions are stable at room temperature. It is degraded slowly in acid solutions but is absorbed well from the gastrointestinal tract. Lincomycin diffuses well into peritoneal and pleural fluids and into bone. It is excreted in the urine and the bile. It is available in capsule form for oral administration and in ampules and vials for parenteral administration.

Clindamycin Hydrochloride, USP.

In 1967, Magerlein et al.[226] reported that replacement of the 7(R)-hydroxy group of lincomycin by chlorine with inversion of configuration resulted in a compound with enhanced antibacterial activity in vitro. Clinical experience with this semisynthetic derivative, clindamycin, 7(S)-chloro-7-deoxylincomycin (Cleocin), released in 1970, has established that its superiority

over lincomycin is even greater in vivo. Improved absorption and higher tissue levels of clindamycin and its greater penetration into bacteria have been attributed to a higher partition coefficient than that of lincomycin. Structural modifications at C-7 (e.g., 7(S)-chloro and 7(R)-OCH$_3$) and of the C-4 alkyl groups of the hygric acid moiety[227] appear to influence activity of congeners more through an effect on the partition coefficient of the molecule than through a stereospecific binding role. Changes in the α-thiolincosamide portion of the molecule seem to decrease activity markedly, however, as evidenced by the marginal activity of 2-deoxylincomycin, its anomer, and 2-O-methyllincomycin.[227, 228] Exceptions to this are fatty acid and phosphate esters of the 2-hydroxyl group of lincomycin and clindamycin, which are hydrolyzed rapidly in vivo to the parent antibiotics.

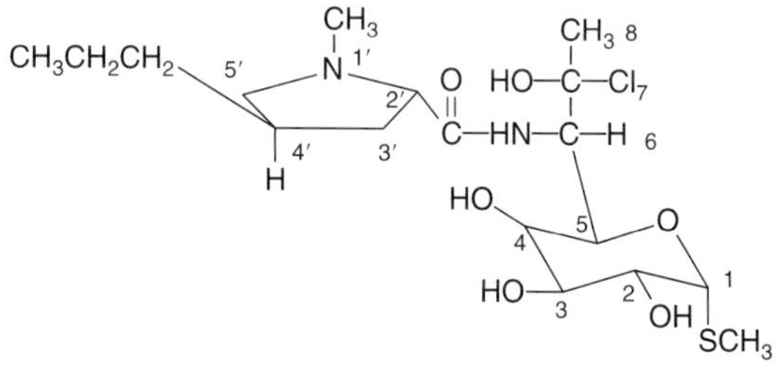

Clindamycin is recommended for the treatment of a wide variety of upper respiratory, skin, and tissue infections caused by susceptible bacteria. Its activity against streptococci, staphylococci, and pneumococci is indisputably high, and it is one of the most potent agents available against some non–spore-forming anaerobic bacteria, the *Bacteroides* spp. in particular. An increasing number of reports of clindamycin-associated gastrointestinal toxicity, which range in severity from diarrhea to an occasionally serious pseudomembranous colitis, have, however, caused some clinical experts to call for a reappraisal of the role of this antibiotic in therapy. Clindamycin- (or lincomycin)-associated colitis may be particularly dangerous in elderly or debilitated patients and has caused deaths in such individuals. The colitis, which is usually reversible when the drug is discontinued, is now believed to result from an overgrowth of a clindamycin-resistant strain of the anaerobic intestinal bacterium *Clostridium difficile*.[229] The intestinal lining is damaged by a glycoprotein endotoxin released by lysis of this organism.

The glycopeptide antibiotic vancomycin has been effective in the treatment of clindamycin-induced pseudomembranous colitis and in the control of the experimentally induced bacterial condition in animals. Clindamycin should be reserved for staphylococcal tissue infections, such as cellulitis and osteomyelitis, in penicillin-allergic patients and for severe anaerobic infections outside the central nervous system. Ordinarily, it should not be used to treat upper respiratory tract infections caused by bacteria sensitive to other, safer antibiotics or in prophylaxis.

Clindamycin is absorbed rapidly from the gastrointestinal tract, even in the presence of food. It is available as the crystalline, water-soluble hydrochloride hydrate (hyclate) and the 2-palmitate ester hydrochloride salts in oral dosage forms and as the 2-phosphate ester in solutions for intramuscular or intravenous injection. All forms are chemically very stable in solution and in the dry state.

Clindamycin Palmitate Hydrochloride, USP. Clindamycin palmitate hydrochloride (Cleocin Pediatric) is the hydrochloride salt of the palmitic acid ester of cleomycin. The ester bond is to the 2-hydroxyl group of the lincosamine sugar. The ester serves as a tasteless prodrug form of the antibiotic, which hydrolyzes to clindamycin in the plasma. The salt form confers water solubility to the ester, which is available as granules for reconstitution into an oral solution for pediatric use. Although absorption of the palmitate is slower than that of the free base, there is little difference in overall bioavailability of the two preparations. Reconstituted solutions of the palmitate hydrochloride are stable for 2 weeks at room temperature. Such solutions should not be refrigerated because thickening occurs that makes the preparation difficult to pour.

Clindamycin Phosphate, USP. Clindamycin phosphate (Cleocin Phosphate) is the 2-phosphate ester of clindamycin. It exists as a zwitterionic structure that is very soluble in water. It is intended for parenteral (intravenous or intramuscular) administration for the treatment of serious infections and instances when oral administration is not feasible. Solutions of clindamycin phosphate are stable at room temperature for 16 days and for up to 32 days when refrigerated.

POLYPEPTIDES

Among the most powerful bactericidal antibiotics are those that possess a polypeptide structure. Many of them have been isolated, but unfortunately, their clinical use has been limited by their undesirable side reactions, particularly renal toxicity. Another limitation is the lack of systemic activity of most peptides following oral administration. A chief source of the medicinally important members of this class has been *Bacillus* spp. The antitubercular antibiotics capreomycin and viomycin (see Chapter 8) and the antitumor antibiotics actinomycin and bleomycin are peptides isolated from *Streptomyces* spp. The glycopeptide antibiotic vancomycin, which has become the most important member of this class, is isolated from a closely related actinomycete, *Amycolatopsis orientalis.*

Polypeptide antibiotics variously possess a number of interesting and often unique characteristics: (a) they frequently consist of several structurally similar but chemically distinct entities isolated from a single source; (b) most of them are cyclic, with a few exceptions (e.g., the gramicidins); (c) they frequently contain D-amino acids and/or "unnatural" amino acids not found in higher plants or animals; and (d) many of them contain non-amino acid moieties, such as heterocycles, fatty acids, sugars, etc. Polypeptide antibiotics may be acidic, basic, zwitterionic, or neutral depending on the number of free carboxyl and amino or guanidino groups in their structures. Initially, it was assumed that neutral compounds, such as the gramicidins, possessed cyclopeptide structures. Later, the gramicidins were determined to be linear, and the neutrality was shown to be due to a combination of the formylation of the terminal amino group and the ethanolamine amidation of the terminal carboxyl group.[230]

Antibiotics of the polypeptide class differ widely in their mechanisms of action and antimicrobial properties. Bacitracin and vancomycin interfere with bacterial cell wall synthesis and are effective only against Gram-positive bacteria. Neither antibiotic apparently can penetrate the outer envelope of Gram-negative bacteria. Both the gramicidins and the polymyxins interfere with cell membrane functions in bacteria. However, the gramicidins are effective primarily against Gram-positive bacteria, while the polymyxins are effective only against Gram-negative species. Gramicidins are neutral compounds that are largely incapable of penetrating the outer envelope of Gram-negative bacteria. Polymyxins are highly basic compounds that penetrate the outer membrane of Gram-negative bacteria through porin channels to act on the inner cell membrane.[231] The much thicker cell wall of Gram-positive bacteria apparently bars penetration by the polymyxins.

Vancomycin Hydrochloride, USP. The isolation of the glycopeptide antibiotic vancomycin (Vancocin, Vancoled) from *Streptomyces orientalis* (renamed *Amycolatopsis orientalis*) was described in 1956 by McCormick et al.[232] The organism originally was obtained from cultures of an Indonesian soil sample and subsequently has been obtained from Indian soil. Vancomycin was introduced in 1958 as an antibiotic active against Gram-positive cocci, particularly streptococci, staphylococci, and pneumococci. It is not active against Gram-negative bacteria, with the exception of *Neisseria* spp. Vancomycin is recommended for use when infections fail to respond to treatment with the more common antibiotics or when the infection is known to be caused by a resistant organism. It is particularly effective for the treatment of endocarditis caused by Gram-positive bacteria.

Vancomycin hydrochloride is a free-flowing, tan to brown powder that is relatively stable in the dry state. It is very soluble in water and insoluble in organic solvents. The salt is quite stable in acidic solutions. The free base is an amphoteric substance, whose structure was determined by a combination of chemical degradation and nuclear magnetic resonance (NMR) studies and x-ray crystallographic analysis of a close analogue.[233] Slight stereochemical and conformational revisions in the originally proposed structure were made later.[234, 235] Vancomycin is a glycopeptide containing two glycosidically linked sugars, glucose and vancosamine, and a complex cyclic peptide aglycon containing aromatic residues linked together in a unique resorcinol ether system.

Vancomycin inhibits cell wall synthesis by preventing the synthesis of cell wall mucopeptide polymer. It does so by binding with the D-alanine-D-alanine terminus of the uridine diphosphate-N-acetylmuramyl peptides required for mucopeptide polymerization.[236] Details of the binding were elucidated by the elegant NMR studies of Williamson et al.[237] The action of vancomycin leads to lysis of the bacterial cell. The antibiotic does not exhibit cross-resistance to β-lactams, bacitracin, or cycloserine, from which it differs in mechanism. Resistance to vancomycin among Gram-positive cocci is rare. High-level resistance in clinical isolates of enterococci has been reported, however. This resistance is in response to the inducible production of a protein, encoded by vancomycin A, that is an altered ligase enzyme that causes the incorporation of a D-alanine-D-lactate depsipeptide instead of the usual D-alanine-D-alanine dipeptide in the peptidoglycan terminus.[238] The resulting peptidoglycan can still undergo cross-linking but no longer binds vancomycin.

Vancomycin hydrochloride is always administered intravenously (never intramuscularly), either by slow injection or by continuous infusion, for the treatment of systemic infections. In short-term therapy, the toxic side reactions are usually slight, but continued use may lead to impaired auditory acuity, renal damage, phlebitis, and rashes. Because it is not absorbed or significantly degraded in the gastrointestinal tract, vancomycin may be administered orally for the treatment of staphylococcal enterocolitis and for pseudomembranous colitis associated with clindamycin therapy. Some conversion to aglucovancomycin likely occurs in the low pH of the stomach. The latter retains about three-fourths of the activity of vancomycin.

Teicoplanin.

Teicoplanin (Teichomycin A$_2$, Targocid) is a mixture of five closely related glycopeptide antibiotics produced by the actinomycete *Actinoplanes teichomyceticus*.[239, 240] The teicoplanin factors differ only in the acyl group in the northernmost of two glucosamines glycosidically linked to the cyclic peptide aglycone. Another sugar, D-mannose is common to all of the teicoplanins. The structures of the teicoplanin factors were determined independently by a combination of chemical degradation[241] and spectroscopic[242, 243] methods in three different groups in 1984.

The teicoplanin complex is similar to vancomycin structurally and microbiologically but has unique physical properties that contribute some potentially useful advantages.[244] While retaining excellent water solubility, teicoplanin has significantly greater lipid solubility than vancomycin. Thus, teicoplanin is distributed rapidly into tissues and penetrates phagocytes well. The complex has a long elimination half-life, ranging from 40 to 70 hours, resulting from a combination of slow tissue release and a high fraction of protein binding in the plasma (approximately 90%). Unlike vancomycin, teicoplanin is not irritating to tissues and may be administered by intramuscular or intravenous injection. Because of its long half-life, teicoplanin may be administered on a once-a-day dosing schedule. Orally administered teicoplanin is not absorbed significantly and is recovered 40% unchanged in the feces.

Teicoplanin exhibits excellent antibacterial activity against Gram-positive organisms, including staphylococci, streptococci, enterococci, *Clostridium* and *Corynebacterium* spp., *Propionibacterium acnes,* and *L. monocytogenes.* It is not active against Gram-negative organisms, including *Neisseria* and *Mycobacterium* spp. Teicoplanin impairs bacterial cell wall synthesis by complexing with the terminal D-alanine-D-alanine dipeptide of the peptidoglycan, thus preventing cross-linking in a manner entirely analogous to the action of vancomycin.

In general, teicoplanin appears to be less toxic than vancomycin. Unlike vancomycin, it does not cause histamine release following intravenous infusion. Teicoplanin apparently also has less potential for causing nephrotoxicity than vancomycin.

Bacitracin, USP.

The organism from which Johnson et al.[245] produced bacitracin in 1945 is a strain of *Bacillus subtilis*. The organism had been isolated from debrided tissue from a compound fracture in 7-year-old Margaret Tracy, hence the name "bacitracin." Bacitracin is now produced from the licheniformis group *(B. subtilis)*. Like tyrothricin, the first useful antibiotic obtained from bacterial cultures, bacitracin is a complex mixture of polypeptides. So far, at least 10 polypeptides have been isolated by countercurrent distribution techniques: A, A^1, B, C, D, E, F$_1$, F$_2$, F$_3$, and G. The commercial product known as bacitracin is a mixture of principally A, with smaller amounts of B, D, E, and F$_{1-3}$.

The official USP product is a white to pale buff powder that is odorless or nearly so. In the dry state, bacitracin is stable, but it rapidly deteriorates in aqueous solutions at room temperature. Because it is hygroscopic, it must be stored in tight containers, preferably under refrigeration. The stability of aqueous solutions of bacitracin is affected by pH and temperature. Slightly acidic or neutral solutions are

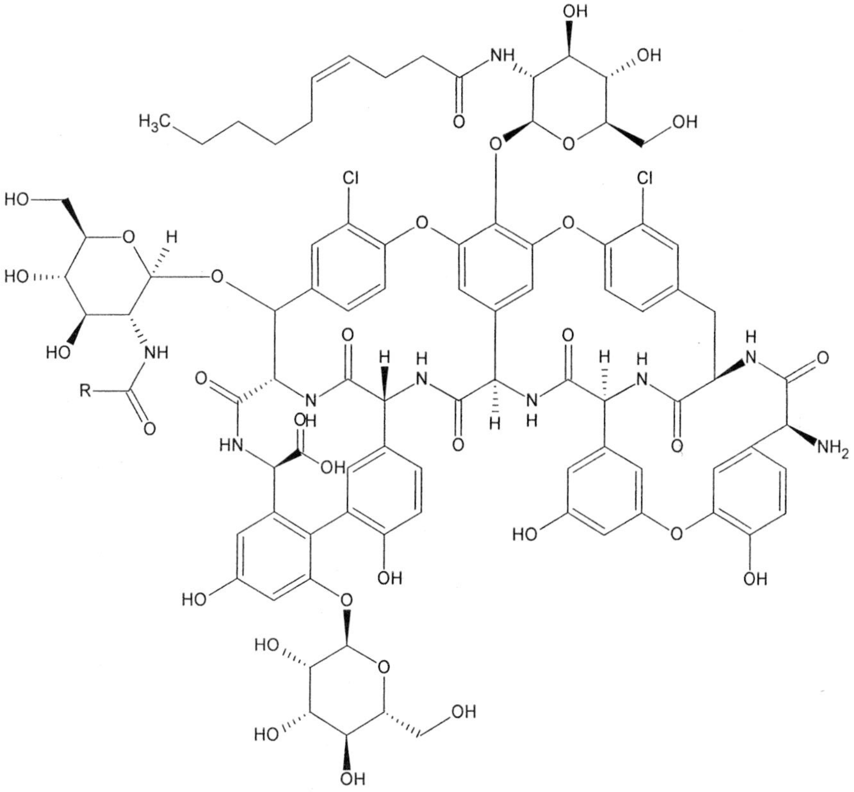

Teicoplanin Factor	R
1	-CH$_2$CH$_2$CH=CH(CH$_2$)$_4$CH$_3$
2	-CH$_2$(CH$_2$)$_5$CH(CH$_3$)$_2$
3	-CH$_2$(CH$_2$)$_7$CH$_3$
4	-CH$_2$(CH$_2$)$_5$CH(CH$_3$)CH$_2$CH$_3$
5	-CH$_2$(CH$_2$)$_6$CH(CH$_3$)$_2$

stable for as long as 1 year if kept at a temperature of 0 to 5°C. If the pH rises above 9, inactivation occurs very rapidly. For greatest stability, the pH of a bacitracin solution is best adjusted to 4 to 5 by the simple addition of acid. The salts of heavy metals precipitate bacitracin from solution, with resulting inactivation. EDTA also inactivates bacitracin, which led to the discovery that a divalent ion (i.e., Zn^{2+}) is required for activity. In addition to being water soluble, bacitracin is soluble in low-molecular-weight alcohols but insoluble in many other organic solvents, including acetone, chloroform, and ether.

The principal work on the chemistry of the bacitracins has been directed toward bacitracin A, the component in which most of the antibacterial activity of crude bacitracin resides. The structure shown in the diagram was proposed by Stoffel and Craig[246] and subsequently confirmed by Ressler and Kashelikar.[247]

The activity of bacitracin is measured in units per milligram. The potency per milligram is not less than 40 USP units/mg except for material prepared for parenteral use, which has a potency of not less than 50 units/mg. It is a bactericidal antibiotic that is active against a wide variety of Gram-positive organisms, very few Gram-negative organisms, and some others. It is believed to exert its bactericidal

effect through inhibition of mucopeptide cell wall synthesis. Its action is enhanced by zinc. Although bacitracin has found its widest use in topical preparations for local infections, it is quite effective in a number of systemic and local infections when administered parenterally. It is not absorbed from the gastrointestinal tract; accordingly, oral administration is without effect, except for the treatment of amebic infections within the alimentary canal.

Polymyxin B Sulfate, USP. Polymyxin (Aerosporin) was discovered in 1947 almost simultaneously in three separate laboratories in the United States and Great Britain.[248–250] As often happens when similar discoveries are made in widely separated laboratories, differences in nomenclature, referring to both the antibiotic-producing organism and the antibiotic itself, appeared in references to the polymyxins. Since the organisms first designated as *Bacillus polymyxa* and *B. aerosporus* Greer were found to be identical species, the name *B. polymyxa* is used to refer to all of the strains that produce the closely related polypeptides called *polymyxins*. Other organisms (e.g., see ''Colistin'' below) also produce polymyxins. Identified so far are polymyxins A, B$_1$, B$_2$, C, D$_1$, D$_2$, M, colistin A (polymyxin E$_1$), colistin B (polymyxin E$_2$), circulins A and B, and polypeptin. The known structures of this group and their properties have been reviewed by Vogler and Studer.[251] Of these, polymyxin B as the sulfate usually is used in medicine because, when used systemically, it causes less kidney damage than the others.

Polymyxin B sulfate is a nearly odorless, white to buff powder. It is freely soluble in water and slightly soluble in alcohol. Its aqueous solutions are slightly acidic or nearly neutral (pH 5 to 7.5) and, when refrigerated, stable for at least 6 months. Alkaline solutions are unstable. Polymyxin B was shown to be a mixture by Hausmann and Craig,[252] who used countercurrent distribution techniques to obtain two fractions that differ in structure only by one fatty acid component. Polymyxin B$_1$ contains (+)-6-methyloctan-1-

oic acid (isopelargonic acid), a fatty acid isolated from all of the other polymyxins. The B$_2$ component contains an isooctanoic acid, C$_8$H$_{16}$O$_2$, of undetermined structure. The structural formula for polymyxin B has been proved by the synthesis by Vogler et al.[253]

Polymyxin B sulfate is useful against many Gram-negative organisms. Its main use in medicine has been in topical applications for local infections in wounds and burns. For such use, it frequently is combined with bacitracin, which is effective against Gram-positive organisms. Polymyxin B sulfate is absorbed poorly from the gastrointestinal tract; therefore, oral administration is of value only in the treatment of intestinal infections such as pseudomonal enteritis

Polymyxin B$_1$

or infections due to *Shigella* spp. It may be given parenterally by intramuscular or intrathecal injection for systemic infections. The dosage of polymyxin is measured in USP units. One milligram contains not less than 6,000 USP units. Some additional confusion on nomenclature for this antibiotic exists because Koyama et al.[254] originally named the product colimycin, and that name is used still. Particularly, it has been the basis for variants used as brand names, such as Coly-Mycin, Colomycin, Colimycine, and Colimicina.

Colistin Sulfate, USP.

In 1950, Koyama and coworkers[254] isolated an antibiotic from *Aerobacillus colistinus* (*B. polymyxa* var. *colistinus*) that was given the name *colistin* (Coly-Mycin S). It was used in Japan and in some European countries for several years before it was made available for medicinal use in the United States. It is recommended especially for the treatment of refractory urinary tract infections caused by Gram-negative organisms such as *Aerobacter, Bordetella, Escherichia, Klebsiella, Pseudomonas, Salmonella,* and *Shigella* spp.

Chemically, colistin is a polypeptide, reported by Suzuki et al.,[255] whose major component is colistin A. They proposed the structure shown below for colistin A, which differs from polymyxin B only by the substitution of D-leucine for D-phenylalanine as one of the amino acid fragments in the cyclic portion of the structure. Wilkinson and Lowe[256] have corroborated the structure and have shown that colistin A is identical with polymyxin E₁.

Two forms of colistin have been made, the sulfate and methanesulfonate, and both forms are available for use in the United States. The sulfate is used to make an oral pediatric suspension; the methanesulfonate is used to make an intramuscular injection. In the dry state, the salts are stable, and their aqueous solutions are relatively stable at acid pH from 2 to 6. Above pH 6, solutions of the salts are much less stable.

Colistimethate Sodium, Sterile, USP.

In colistin, five of the terminal amino groups of the α-aminobutyric acid fragment may be readily alkylated. In colistimethate sodium, pentasodium colistinmethanesulfonate, sodium colistimeth-

anesulfonate (Coly-Mycin M), the methanesulfonate radical is the attached alkyl group, and a sodium salt may be made through each sulfonate. This provides a highly water-soluble compound that is very suitable for injection. In the injectable form, it is given intramuscularly and is surprisingly free from toxic reactions compared with polymyxin B. Colistimethate sodium does not readily induce the development of resistant strains of microorganisms, and there is no evidence of cross-resistance with the common broad-spectrum antibiotics. It is used for the same conditions mentioned for colistin.

Gramicidin, USP.

Gramicidin is obtained from tyrothricin, a mixture of polypeptides usually obtained by extraction of cultures of *Bacillus brevis*. Tyrothricin was isolated in 1939 by Dubos[257] in a planned search to find an organism growing in soil that would have antibiotic activity against human pathogens. With only limited use in therapy now, it is of historical interest as the first in the series of modern antibiotics. Tyrothricin is a white to slightly gray or brown-white powder, with little or no odor or taste. It is practically insoluble in water and is soluble in alcohol and in dilute acids. Suspensions for clinical use can be prepared by adding an alcoholic solution to calculated amounts of distilled water or isotonic saline solutions.

Tyrothricin is a mixture of two groups of antibiotic compounds, the gramicidins and the tyrocidines. Gramicidins are the more active components of tyrothricin, and this fraction, which is 10 to 20% of the mixture, may be separated and used in topical preparations for the antibiotic effect. Five gramicidins, A₂, A₃, B₁, B₂, and C, have been identified. Their structures have been proposed and confirmed through synthesis by Sarges and Witkop.[230] The gramicidins A differ from the gramicidins B by having a tryptophan moiety substituted by an L-phenylalanine moiety. In gramicidin C, a tyrosine moiety substitutes for a tryptophan moiety. In both of the gramicidin A and B pairs, the only difference is the amino acid located at the end of the chain, which has the neutral formyl group on it. If that amino acid is valine, the compound is either valine-gramicidin A or valine-gramicidin B. If that amino acid is isoleucine, the compound is isoleucine-gramicidin, either A or B.

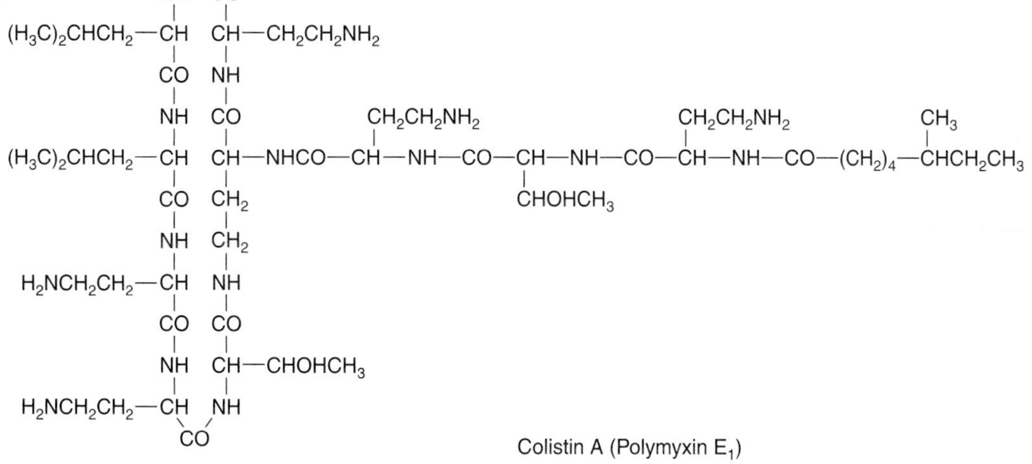

Colistin A (Polymyxin E₁)

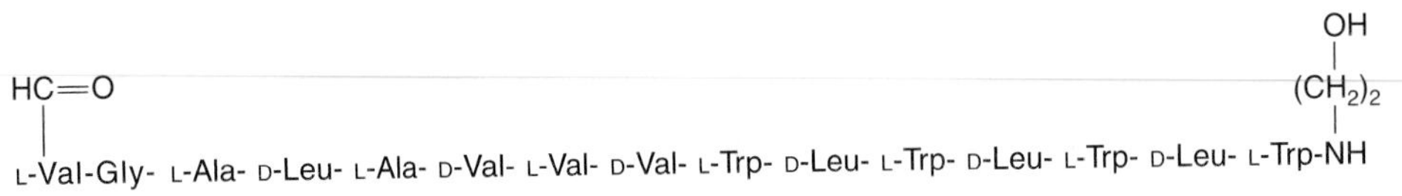

HC=O
     OH
     |
    $(CH_2)_2$

L-Val-Gly- L-Ala- D-Leu- L-Ala- D-Val- L-Val- D-Val- L-Trp- D-Leu- L-Trp- D-Leu- L-Trp- D-Leu- L-Trp-NH

Valine - gramicidin A

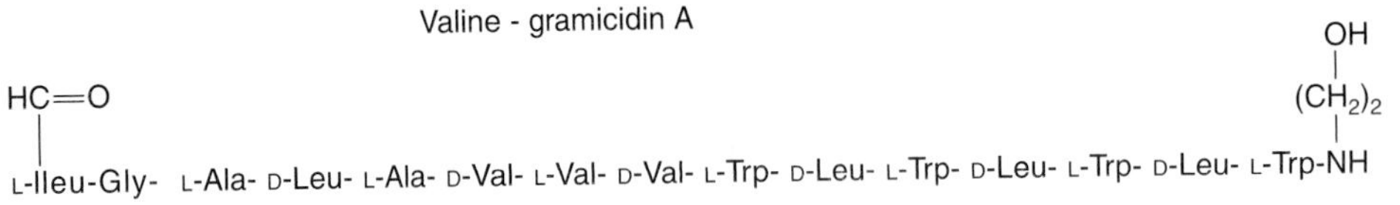

HC=O
     OH
     |
    $(CH_2)_2$

L-Ileu-Gly- L-Ala- D-Leu- L-Ala- D-Val- L-Val- D-Val- L-Trp- D-Leu- L-Trp- D-Leu- L-Trp- D-Leu- L-Trp-NH

Isoleucine - gramicidin A

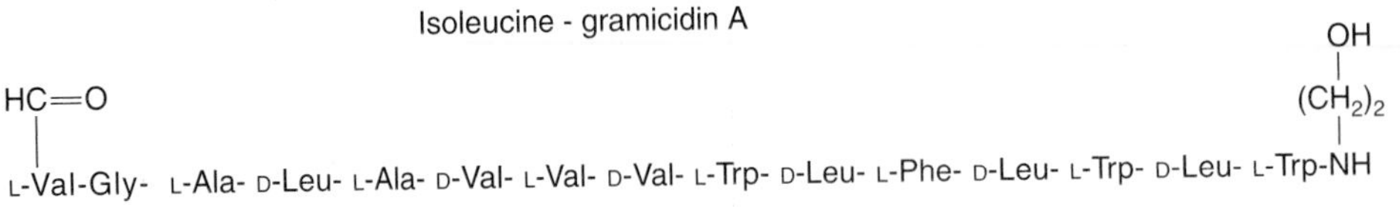

HC=O
     OH
     |
    $(CH_2)_2$

L-Val-Gly- L-Ala- D-Leu- L-Ala- D-Val- L-Val- D-Val- L-Trp- D-Leu- L-Phe- D-Leu- L-Trp- D-Leu- L-Trp-NH

Valine - gramicidin B

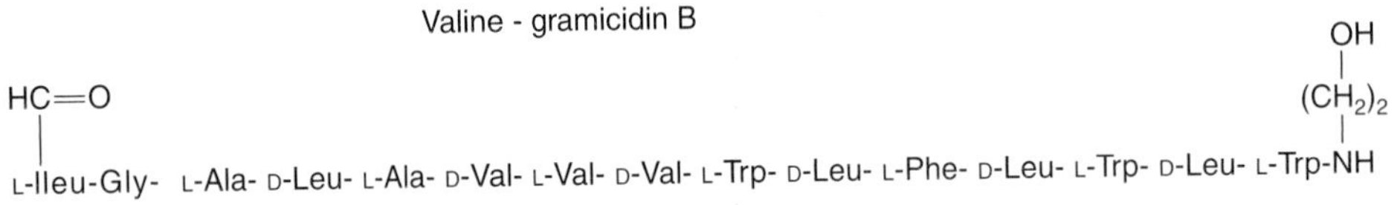

HC=O
     OH
     |
    $(CH_2)_2$

L-Ileu-Gly- L-Ala- D-Leu- L-Ala- D-Val- L-Val- D-Val- L-Trp- D-Leu- L-Phe- D-Leu- L-Trp- D-Leu- L-Trp-NH

Isoleucine - gramicidin B

Tyrocidine is a mixture of tyrocidines A, B, C, and D, whose structures have been determined by Craig and co-workers.[258, 259] The synthesis of tyrocidine A was reported by Ohno et al.[260]

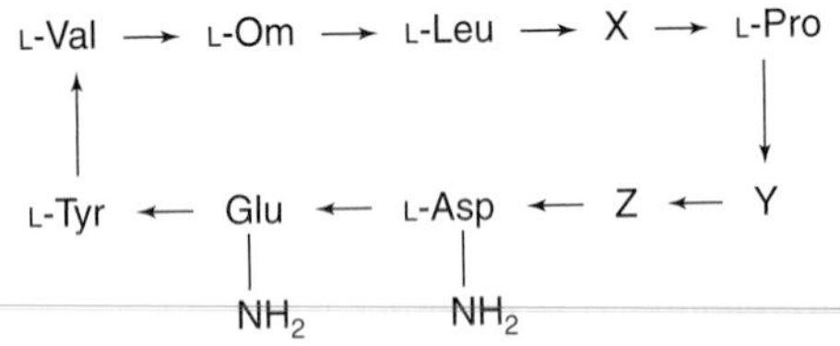

L-Val ⟶ L-Om ⟶ L-Leu ⟶ X ⟶ L-Pro

L-Tyr ⟵ Glu ⟵ L-Asp ⟵ Z ⟵ Y

	X	Y	Z
Tyrocidine A:	D-Phe	D-Phe	D-Phe
Tyrocidine B:	D-Phe	L-Tyr	D-Phe
Tyrocidine C:	D-Tyr	L-Tyr	D-Phe
Tyrocidine D:	D-Tyr	L-Tyr	D-Tyr

Gramicidin acts as an ionophore in bacterial cell membranes to cause the loss of potassium ion from the cell.[261] It is bactericidal.

Tyrothricin and gramicidin are effective primarily against Gram-positive organisms. Their use is restricted to local applications. Tyrothricin can cause lysis of erythrocytes, which makes it unsuitable for the treatment of systemic infections. Its applications should avoid direct contact with the bloodstream through open wounds or abrasions. It is ordinarily safe to use tyrothricin in troches for throat infections, as it is not absorbed from the gastrointestinal tract. Gramicidin is available in a variety of topical preparations containing other antibiotics, such as bacitracin and neomycin.

UNCLASSIFIED ANTIBIOTICS

Among the many hundreds of antibiotics that have been evaluated for activity, several have gained significant clinical attention but do not fall into any of the previously considered groups. Some of these have quite specific activities against a narrow spectrum of microorganisms. Some have found a useful place in therapy as substitutes for other antibiotics to which resistance has developed.

Chloramphenicol, USP. The first of the widely used broad-spectrum antibiotics, chloramphenicol (Chloromycetin, Amphicol) was isolated by Ehrlich et al.[262] in 1947. They obtained it from *Streptomyces venezuelae*, an organism found in a sample of soil collected in Venezuela. Since then, chloramphenicol has been isolated as a product of several organisms found in soil samples from widely separated places. More importantly, its chemical structure was established quickly, and in 1949, Controulis et al.[263] reported its synthesis. This opened the way for the commercial production of chloramphenicol by a totally synthetic route. It was the first and still is the only therapeutically important antibiotic to be so produced in competition with microbiological processes. Diverse synthetic procedures have been developed for chloramphenicol. The commercial process generally used starts with *p*-nitroacetophenone.[264]

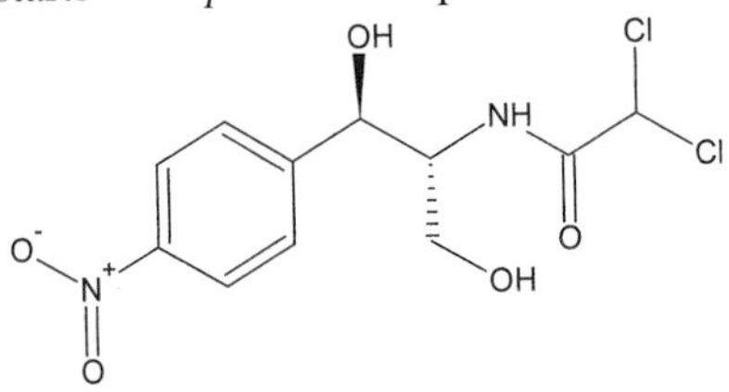

Chloramphenicol

Chloramphenicol is a white, crystalline compound that is very stable. It is very soluble in alcohol and other polar organic solvents but only slightly soluble in water. It has no odor but has a very bitter taste.

Chloramphenicol possesses two chiral carbon atoms in the acylamidopropanediol chain. Biological activity resides almost exclusively in the D-*threo* isomer; the L-*threo* and the D- and L-*erythro* isomers are virtually inactive.

Chloramphenicol is very stable in the bulk state and in solid dosage forms. In solution, however, it slowly undergoes various hydrolytic and light-induced reactions.[265] The rates of these reactions depend on pH, heat, and light. Hydrolytic reactions include general acid–base-catalyzed hydrolysis of the amide to give 1-(p-nitrophenyl)-2-aminopropan-1,3-diol and dichloroacetic acid and alkaline hydrolysis (above pH 7) of the α-chloro groups to form the corresponding α,α-dihydroxy derivative.

The metabolism of chloramphenicol has been investigated thoroughly.[266] The main path involves formation of the 3-O-glucuronide. Minor reactions include reduction of the p-nitro group to the aromatic amine, hydrolysis of the amide, and hydrolysis of the α-chloracetamido group, followed by reduction to give the corresponding α-hydroxyacetyl derivative.

Strains of certain bacterial species are resistant to chloramphenicol by virtue of the ability to produce chloramphenicol acetyltransferase, an enzyme that acetylates the hydroxy groups at the 1 and 3 positions. Both the 3-acetoxy and the 1,3-diacetoxy metabolites lack antibacterial activity.

Numerous structural analogues of chloramphenicol have been synthesized to provide a basis for correlation of structure to antibiotic action. It appears that the p-nitrophenyl group may be replaced by other aryl structures without appreciable loss in activity. Substitution on the phenyl ring with several different types of groups for the nitro group, a very unusual structure in biological products, does not greatly decrease activity. All such compounds yet tested are less active than chloramphenicol. As part of a QSAR study, Hansch et al.[267] reported that the 2-NHCOCF$_3$ derivative is 1.7 times as active as chloramphenicol against *E. coli*. Modification of the side chain shows that it possesses high specificity in structure for antibiotic action. Conversion of the alcohol group on C-1 of the side chain to a keto group causes appreciable loss in activity. The relationship of the structure of chloramphenicol to its antibiotic activity will not be seen clearly until the mode of action of this compound is known. Brock[268] reports on the large amount of research that has been devoted to this problem. Chloramphenicol exerts its bacteriostatic action by a strong inhibition of protein synthesis. The details of such inhibition are as yet undetermined, and the precise point of action is unknown. Some process lying between the attachment of amino acids to sRNA and the final formation of protein appears to be involved.

The broad-spectrum activity of chloramphenicol and its singular effectiveness in the treatment of some infections not amenable to treatment by other drugs made it an extremely popular antibiotic. Unfortunately, instances of serious blood dyscrasias and other toxic reactions have resulted from the promiscuous and widespread use of chloramphenicol in the past. Because of these reactions, it is recommended that it not be used in the treatment of infections for which other antibiotics are as effective and less hazardous. When properly used, with careful observation for untoward reactions, chloramphenicol provides some of the very best therapy for the treatment of serious infections.[269]

Chloramphenicol is recommended specifically for the treatment of serious infections caused by strains of Gram-positive and Gram-negative bacteria that have developed resistance to penicillin G and ampicillin, such as *H. influenzae*,

Salmonella typhi, *S. pneumoniae*, *B. fragilis*, and *N. meningitidis*. Because of its penetration into the central nervous system, chloramphenicol is a particularly important alternative therapy for meningitis. It is not recommended for the treatment of urinary tract infections because 5 to 10% of the unconjugated form is excreted in the urine. Chloramphenicol is also used for the treatment of rickettsial infections, such as Rocky Mountain spotted fever.

Because it is bitter, this antibiotic is administered orally either in capsules or as the palmitate ester. Chloramphenicol palmitate is insoluble in water and may be suspended in aqueous vehicles for liquid dosage forms. The ester forms by reaction with the hydroxyl group on C-3. In the alimentary tract, it is hydrolyzed slowly to the active antibiotic. Chloramphenicol is administered parenterally as an aqueous suspension of very fine crystals or as a solution of the sodium salt of the succinate ester of chloramphenicol. Sterile chloramphenicol sodium succinate has been used to prepare aqueous solutions for intravenous injection.

Chloramphenicol Palmitate, USP. Chloramphenicol palmitate is the palmitic acid ester of chloramphenicol. It is a tasteless prodrug of chloramphenicol intended for pediatric use. The ester must hydrolyze in vivo following oral absorption to provide the active form. Erratic serum levels were associated with early formulations of the palmitate, but the manufacturer claims that the bioavailability of the current preparation is comparable to that of chloramphenicol itself.

Chloramphenicol Sodium Succinate, USP. Chloramphenicol sodium succinate is the water-soluble sodium salt of the hemisuccinate ester of chloramphenicol. Because of the low solubility of chloramphenicol, the sodium succinate is preferred for intravenous administration. The availability of chloramphenicol from the ester following intravenous administration is estimated to be 70 to 75%; the remainder is excreted unchanged.[269, 270] Poor availability of the active form from the ester following intramuscular injection precludes attaining effective plasma levels of the antibiotic by this route. Orally administered chloramphenicol or its palmitate ester actually gives higher plasma levels of the active antibiotic than does intravenously administered chloramphenicol sodium succinate.[270, 271] Nonetheless, effective concentrations are achieved by either route.

Novobiocin Sodium, USP. In the search for new antibiotics, three different research groups independently isolated novobiocin, streptonivicin (Albamycin) from *Streptomyces* spp. It was reported first in 1955 as a product of *S. spheroides* and *S. niveus*. Currently, it is produced from cultures of both species. Until the common identity of the products obtained by the different research groups was ascertained, the naming of this compound was confused. Its chemical identity was established as 7-[4-(carbamoyloxy)tetrahydro-3-hydroxy-5-methoxy-6,6-dimethylpyran-2-yloxyl-4-hydroxy-3-[4-hydroxy-3-(3-methyl-2-butenyl)benzamido]-8-methylcoumarin by Shunk et al.[272] and Hoeksema et al.[273] and confirmed by Spencer et al.[274, 275]

Chemically, novobiocin has a unique structure among antibiotics, though, like several others, it possesses a glycosidic sugar moiety. The sugar in novobiocin, devoid of its carbamate ester, has been named *noviose* and is an aldose with the configuration of L-lyxose. The aglycon moiety has been termed *novobiocic acid*.

Novobiocin is a pale yellow, somewhat photosensitive compound that crystallizes in two chemically identical forms with different melting points (polymorphs). It is soluble in methanol, ethanol, and acetone but is quite insoluble in less polar solvents. Its solubility in water is affected by pH. It is readily soluble in basic solutions, in which it deteriorates, and is precipitated from acidic solutions. It behaves as a diacid, forming two series of salts.

The enolic hydroxyl group on the coumarin moiety behaves as a rather strong acid (pK$_a$ 4.3) and is the group by which the commercially available sodium and calcium salts are formed. The phenolic -OH group on the benzamido moiety also behaves as an acid but is weaker than the former, with a pK$_a$ of 9.1. Disodium salts of novobiocin have been prepared. The sodium salt is stable in dry air but loses activity in the presence of moisture. The calcium salt is quite water insoluble and is used to make aqueous oral suspensions. Because of its acidic characteristics, novobiocin combines to form salt complexes with basic antibiotics. Some of these salts have been investigated for their combined antibiotic effect, but none has been placed on the market, as they offer no advantage.

The action of novobiocin is largely bacteriostatic. Its mode of action is not known with certainty, though it does inhibit bacterial protein and nucleic acid synthesis. Studies indicate that novobiocin and related coumarin-containing antibiotics bind to the subunit of DNA gyrase and possibly interfere with DNA supercoiling[276] and energy transduction in bacteria.[277] The effectiveness of novobiocin is confined largely to Gram-positive bacteria and a few strains of *P. vulgaris*. Its low activity against Gram-negative bacteria is apparently due to poor cellular penetration.

Although cross-resistance to other antibiotics is reported not to develop with novobiocin, resistant *S. aureus* strains are known. Consequently, the medical use of novobiocin is reserved for the treatment of staphylococcal infections resistant to other antibiotics and sulfas and for patients aller-

gic to these drugs. Another shortcoming that limits the usefulness of novobiocin is the relatively high frequency of adverse reactions, such as urticaria, allergic rashes, hepatotoxicity, and blood dyscrasias.

Mupirocin, USP. Mupirocin (pseudomonic acid A, Bactroban) is the major component of a family of structurally related antibiotics, pseudomonic acids A to D, produced by the submerged fermentation of *Pseudomonas fluorescens*. Although the antimicrobial properties of *P. fluorescens* were recorded as early as 1887, it was not until 1971 that Fuller et al.[278] identified the metabolites responsible for this activity. The structure of the major and most potent metabolite, pseudomonic acid A (which represents 90 to 95% of the active fraction from *P. fluorescens*), was later confirmed by chemical synthesis[279] to be the 9-hydroxynonanoic acid ester of monic acid.

The use of mupirocin is confined to external applications.[280] Systemic administration of the antibiotic results in rapid hydrolysis by esterases to monic acid, which is inactive in vivo because of its inability to penetrate bacteria. Mupirocin has been used for the topical treatment of impetigo, eczema, and folliculitis secondarily infected by susceptible bacteria, especially staphylococci and β-hemolytic streptococci. The spectrum of antibacterial activity of mupirocin is confined to Gram-positive and Gram-negative cocci, including staphylococci, streptococci, *Neisseria* spp., and *M. catarrhalis*. The activity of the antibiotic against most Gram-negative and Gram-positive bacilli is generally poor, with the exception of *H. influenzae*. It is not effective against enterococci or anaerobic bacteria.

Mupirocin interferes with RNA synthesis and protein synthesis in susceptible bacteria.[281, 282] It specifically and reversibly binds with bacterial isoleucyl transfer-RNA synthase to prevent the incorporation of isoleucine into bacterial proteins.[282] High-level, plasmid-mediated mupirocin resistance in *S. aureus* has been attributed to the elaboration of a modified isoleucyl tRNA that does not bind mupirocin.[283] Inherent resistance in bacilli is likely due to poor cellular penetration of the antibiotic.[284]

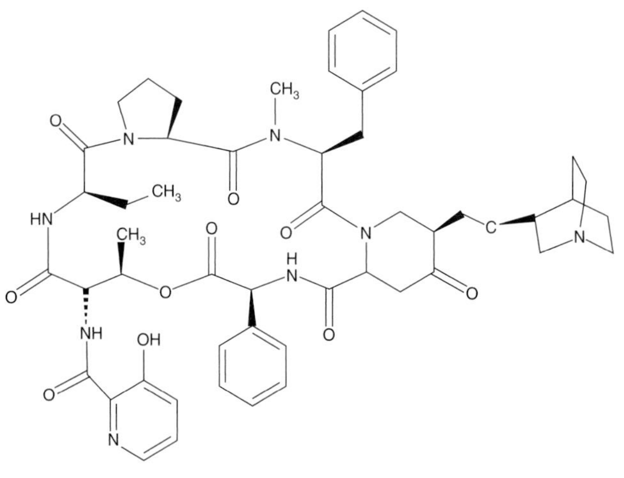

Quinupristin

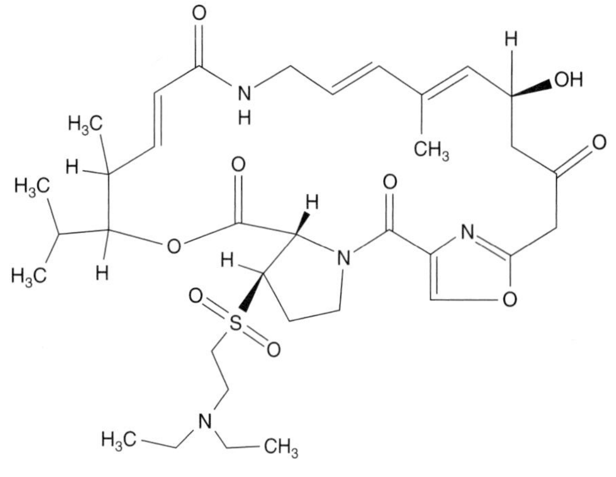

Dalfopristin

Mupirocin is supplied in a water-miscible ointment containing 2% of the antibiotic in polyethylene glycols 400 and 3350.

Quinupristin/Dalfopristin.

Quinupristin/dalfopristin (Synercid) is a combination of the streptogramin B quinupristin with the streptogramin A dalfopristin in a 30:70 ratio.

Both of these compounds are semisynthetic derivatives of two naturally occurring pristinamycins produced in fermentations of *Streptomyces pristinaspiralis*. Quinupristin and dalfopristin are solubilized derivatives of pristinamycin Ia and pristinamycin IIa, respectively, and therefore are suitable for intravenous administration only.

The spectrum of activity of quinupristin/dalfopristin is largely against Gram-positive bacteria. The combination is active against Gram-positive cocci, including *S. pneumoniae*, β-hemolytic and α-hemolytic streptococci, *Enterococcus faecium*, and coagulase-positive and coagulase-negative staphylococci. The combination is mostly inactive against Gram-negative organisms, although *M. catarrhalis* and *Neisseria* spp. are susceptible. The combination is bacteri-

cidal against streptococci and many staphylococci, but bacteriostatic against *E. faecium*.

Quinupristin and dalfopristin are protein synthesis inhibitors that bind to the 50S ribosomal subunit. Quinupristin, a type B streptogramin, binds at the same site as the macrolides and has a similar effect, resulting in inhibition of polypeptide elongation and early termination of protein synthesis. Dalfopristin binds to a site near that of quinupristin. The binding of dalfopristin results in a conformational change in the 50S ribosomal subunit, synergistically enhancing the binding of quinupristin at its target site. In most bacterial species, the cooperative and synergistic binding of these two compounds to the ribosome is bactericidal.

Synercid should be reserved for the treatment of serious infections caused by multidrug-resistant Gram-positive organisms such as vancomycin-resistant *E. faecium*.

Linezolid.

Linezolid (Zyvox) is an oxazolidinedione-type antibacterial agent that inhibits bacterial protein synthesis. It acts in the early translation stage, preventing the formation of a functional initiation complex. Linezolid binds to

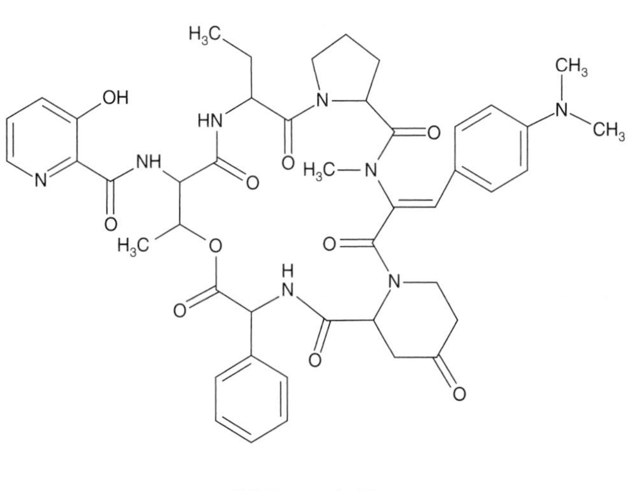

Pristinamycin IA

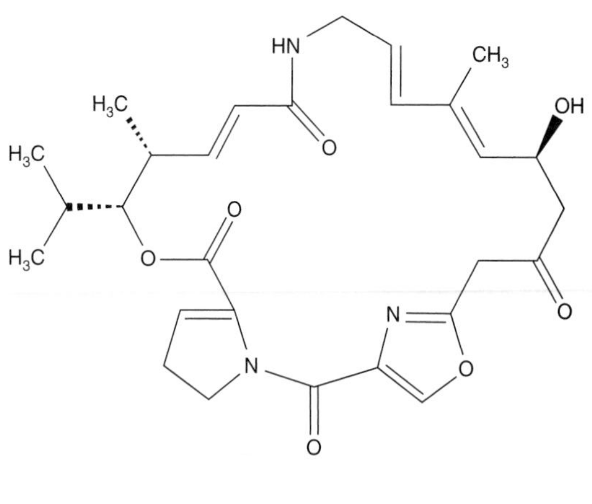

Pristinamycin IIA

the 30S and 70S ribosomal subunits and prevents initiation complexes involving these subunits. Collective data suggest that the oxazolidindiones partition their ribosomal interaction between the two subunits. Formation of the early tRNA^{fMet}-mRNA-70S or 30S is prevented. Linezolid is a newer synthetic agent, and hence, cross-resistance between the antibacterial agent and other inhibitors of bacterial protein synthesis has not been seen.

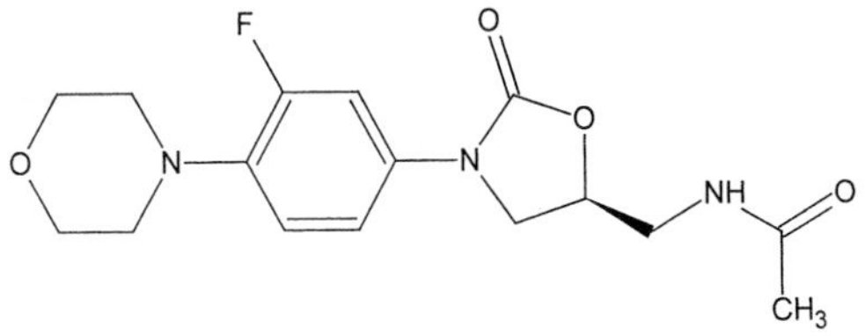

Linezolid

Linezolid possesses a wide spectrum of activity against Gram-positive organisms, including MRSA, penicillin-resistant pneumococci, and vancomycin-resistant *E. faecalis* and *E. faecium*. Anaerobes such as *Clostridium, Peptostreptococcus,* and *Prevotella* spp. are sensitive to linezolid.

Linezolid is a bacteriostatic agent against most susceptible organisms but displays bactericidal activity against some strains of pneumococci, *B. fragilis*, and *Clostridium perfringens*.

The indications for linezolid are for complicated and uncomplicated skin and soft-tissue infections, community- and hospital-acquired pneumonia, and drug-resistant Gram-positive infections.

Fosfomycin Tromethamine. Fosphomycin tromethamine (Monurol) is a phosphonic acid epoxide derivative that was initially isolated from fermentations of *Streptomyces* spp. The structure of the drug is shown below. Making the tromethamine salt greatly expanded the therapeutic utility of this antibacterial because water solubility increased enough to allow oral administration.

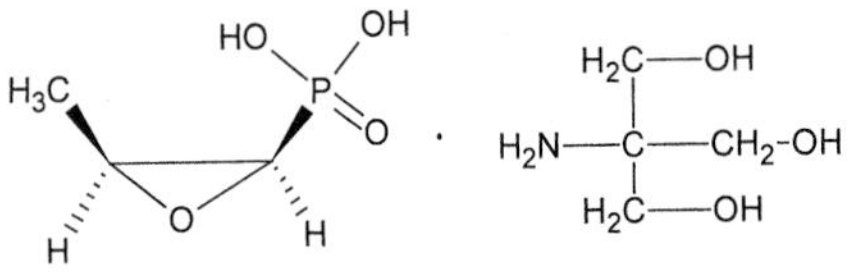

Fosfomycin is a broad-spectrum, bactericidal antibacterial that inhibits the growth of *E. coli, S. aureus,* and *Serratia, Klebsiella, Citrobacter, Enterococcus,* and *Enterobacter* spp. at a concentration less than 64 mg/L. Currently fosfomycin is recommended as single-dose therapy for uncomplicated urinary tract infections. It possesses in vitro efficacy similar to that of norfloxacin and trimethoprim-sulfamethoxazole.

Fosfomycin covalently inactivates the first enzyme in the bacterial cell wall biosynthesis pathway, UDP-*N*-acetylglucosamine enolpyruvyl transferase (MurA) by alkylation of the cysteine-115 residue. The inactivation reaction occurs through nucleophilic opening of the epoxide ring. Resistance to fosfomycin can occur through chromosomal mutations that result in reduced uptake or reduced MurA affinity for the inhibitor. Plasmid-mediated resistance mechanisms involve conjugative bioinactivation of the antibiotic with glutathione. The frequency of resistant mutants in in vitro studies has been low, and there appears to be little cross-resistance between fosfomycin and other antibacterials.

REFERENCES

1. Fleming, A.: Br. J. Exp. Pathol. 10:226, 1929.
2. Vuillemin, P.: Assoc. Fr. Avance Sc.: 2:525, 1889.
3. Waksman, S. A.: Science 110:27, 1949.
4. Benedict, R. G., and Langlykke, A. F.: Annu. Rev. Microbiol. 1:193, 1947.
5. Baron, A. L.: Handbook of Antibiotics. New York, Reinhold, 1950, p. 5.
6. Lancini, G., Parenti, F., and Gallo, G. G.: Antibiotics: An Interdisciplinary Approach, 3rd ed. New York, Plenum Press, 1995, p. 1.
7. Yocum, R. R., et al.: J. Biol. Chem. 255:3977, 1980.
8. Waxman, D. J., and Strominger, J. L.: Annu. Rev. Pharmacol. 52: 825, 1983.
9. Spratt, B. G.: Proc. Natl. Acad. Sci. U. S. A. 72:2999, 1975.
10. Spratt, B. G.: Eur. J. Biochem. 72:341, 1977.
11. Tomasz, A.: Annu. Rev. Microbiol. 33:113, 1979.
12. Spratt, B. G.: Nature 254:516, 1975.
13. Suzuki, H., et al.: Proc. Natl. Acad. Sci. U. S. A. 75:664, 1978.
14. Clarke, H. T., et al.: The Chemistry of Penicillin. Princeton, NJ, Princeton University Press, 1949, p. 454.
15. Sheehan, J. C., and Henery-Logan, K. R.: J. Am. Chem. Soc. 81: 3089, 1959.
16. Batchelor, F. R., et al.: Nature 183:257, 1959.
17. Sheehan, J. C., and Ferris, J. P.: J. Am. Chem. Soc. 81:2912, 1959.
18. Hou, J. P., and Poole, J. W.: J. Pharm. Sci. 60:503, 1971.
19. Blaha, J. M., et al.: J. Pharm. Sci. 65:1165, 1976.
20. Schwartz, M.: J. Pharm. Sci. 58:643, 1969.
21. Schwartz, M. A., and Buckwalter, F. H.: J. Pharm. Sci. 51:1119, 1962.
22. Finholt, P., Jurgensen, G., and Kristiansen, H.: J. Pharm. Sci. 54:387, 1965.
23. Segelman, A. B., and Farnsworth, N. R.: J. Pharm. Sci. 59:725, 1970.
24. Sykes, R. B., and Matthew, M.: J. Antimicrob. Chemother. 2:115, 1976.
25. Bush, K., Jacoby, G. A., and Medeiros, A. A.: Antimicrob. Agents Chemother. 39:1211, 1995.
26. Ambler, R. P.: Phil. Trans. R. Soc. Lond. [B] 289:321, 1980.
27. Zimmerman, W., and Rosselet, A.: Antimicrob. Agents Chemother. 12:368, 1977.
28. Yoshimura, F., and Nikaido, H.: Antimicrob. Agents Chemother. 27: 84, 1985.
29. Malouin, F., and Bryan, L. E.: Antimicrob. Agents Chemother. 30: 1, 1986.
30. Dougherty, et al.: Antimicrob. Agents Chemother. 18:730, 1980.
31. Hartman, B., and Tomasz, A.: Antimicrob. Agents Chemother. 19: 726, 1981.
32. Brain, E. G., et al.: J. Chem. Soc. 1445, 1962.
33. Stedmen, R. J., et al.: J. Med. Chem. 7:251, 1964.
34. Nayler, J. H. C.: Adv. Drug Res. 7:52, 1973.
35. Nikaido, H., Rosenberg, E. Y., and Foulds, J.: J. Bacteriol. 153:232, 1983.
36. Matthew, M.: J. Antimicrob. Chemother. 5:349, 1979.
37. Iyengar, B. S., et al.: J. Med. Chem. 29:611, 1986.
38. Hansch, C., and Deutsch, E. W.: J. Med. Chem. 8:705, 1965.
39. Bird, A. E., and Marshall, A. C.: Biochem. Pharmacol. 16:2275, 1967.
40. Stewart, G. W.: The Penicillin Group of Drugs. Amsterdam, Elsevier, 1965.
41. Corran, P. H., and Waley, S. G.: Biochem. J. 149:357, 1975.
42. Batchelor, F. R., et al.: Nature 206:362, 1965.
43. DeWeck, A. L.: Int. Arch. Allergy 21:20, 1962.
44. Smith, H., and Marshall, A. C.: Nature 232:45, 1974.
45. Monroe, A. C., et al.: Int. Arch. Appl. Immunol. 50:192, 1976.
46. Behrens, O. K., et al.: J. Biol. Chem. 175:793, 1948.
47. Mayersohn, M., and Endrenyi, L.: Can. Med. Assoc. J. 109:989, 1973.
48. Hill, S. A., et al.: J. Pharm. Pharmacol. 27:594, 1975.
49. Neu, H. C.: Rev. Infect. Dis. 3:110, 1981.
50. Neu, H. C.: J. Infect. Dis. 12S:1, 1974.
51. Westphal, J.-F., et al.: Clin. Pharmacol. Ther. 57:257, 1995.
52. Ancred, P., et al.: Nature 215:25, 1967.
53. Knowles, J. R.: Acc. Chem. Res. 18:97, 1985.
54. Bush, K., et al.: Antimicrob. Agents Chemother. 37:429, 1993.
55. Payne, D. J., et al.: Antimicrob. Agents Chemother. 38:767, 1994.
56. Payne, D. J.: J. Med. Microbiol. 39:93, 1993.
57. Micetich, R. G., et al.: J. Med. Chem. 30:1469, 1987.
58. Merck & Co., Inc.: U.S. Patent 3,950,357 (April 12, 1976).

59. Johnston, D. B. R., et al.: J. Am. Chem. Soc. 100:313, 1978.
60. Albers-Schonberg, G., et al.: J. Am. Chem. Soc. 100:6491, 1978.
61. Kahan, J. S., et al.: 16th Conference on Antimicrobial Agents and Chemotherapy, Chicago, 1976, Abstr. 227.
62. Kropp, H., et al.: Antimicrob. Agents Chemother. 22:62, 1982.
63. Leanza, W. J., et al.: J. Med. Chem. 22:1435, 1979.
64. Shih, D. H., et al.: Heterocycles 21:29, 1984.
65. Hikida, M., et al.: J. Antimicrob. Chemother. 30:129, 1992.
66. Wiseman, L. R., et al.: Drugs 50:73, 1995.
67. Petersen, P. J., et al.: Antimicrob. Agents Chemother. 35:203, 1991.
68. Felici, A., et al.: Antimicrob. Agents Chemother. 39:1300, 1995.
68a. Abraham, E. F., and Newton, G. G. F.: Biochem. J. 79:377, 1961.
69. Morin, R. B., et al.: J. Am. Chem. Soc. 84:3400, 1962.
70. Fechtig, B., et al.: Helv. Chim. Acta 51:1108, 1968.
71. Woodward, R. B., et al.: J. Am. Chem. Soc. 88:852, 1966.
72. Morin, R. B., et al.: J. Am. Chem. Soc. 85:1896, 1963.
73. Yamana, T., and Tsuji, A.: J. Pharm. Sci. 65:1563, 1976.
74. Sullivan, H. R., and McMahon, R. E.: Biochem. J. 102:976, 1967.
75. Indelicato, J. M., et al.: J. Med. Chem. 17:523, 1974.
76. Tsuji, A., et al.: J. Pharm. Sci. 70:1120, 1981.
77. Fong, I., et al.: Antimicrob. Agents Chemother. 9:939, 1976.
78. Cimarusti, C. M.: J. Med. Chem. 27:247, 1984.
79. Faraci, W. S., and Pratt, R. F.: Biochemistry 24:903, 1985.
79a. Faraci, W. S., and Pratt, R. F.: Biochemistry 25:2934, 1986.
80. Bechtold, H, et al.: Thromb. Haemost. 51:358, 1984.
81. Buening, M. K., et al.: JAMA 245:2027, 1981.
82. Kukolja, S.: Synthesis of 3-methylenecepham, a key and general intermediate in the preparation of 3-substituted cephalosporins. In Elks, J. (ed.). Recent Advances in the Chemistry of Beta-Lactam Antibiotics. Chichester, Burlington House, 1977, p. 181.
83. Gillett, A. P., et al.: Postgrad. Med. 55(Suppl. 4):9, 1979.
84. Cooper, R. G. D.: Am. J. Med. 92(Suppl. 6A):2S, 1992.
85. Indelicato, J. M., et al.: J. Pharm. Sci. 65:1175, 1976.
86. Ott, J. L., et al.: Antimicrob. Agents Chemother. 15:14, 1979.
87. Nagarajan, R., et al.: J. Am. Chem. Soc. 93:2308, 1971.
88. Stapley, E. O., et al.: Antimicrob. Agents Chemother. 2:122, 1972.
89. Goering, R. V., et al.: Antimicrob. Agents Chemother. 21:963, 1982.
90. Grassi, G. G., et al.: J. Antimicrob. Chemother. 11(Suppl. A):45, 1983.
91. Tsuji, A., et al.: J. Pharm. Pharmacol. 39:272, 1987.
92. Labia, R., et al.: Drugs Exp. Clin. Res. 10:27, 1984.
93. Park, H. Z., Lee, S. P., and Schy, A. L.: Gastroenterology 100:1665, 1991.
94. Fassbender, M., et al.: Clin. Infect. Dis. 16:646, 1993.
95. Schafer, V., et al.: J. Antimicrob. Chemother. 29(Suppl A):7, 1992.
96. Sanders, C. C.: Clin. Infect. Dis. 17:369, 1993.
97. Watanabe, N.-A., et al.: Antimicrob. Agents Chemother. 31:497, 1987.
98. Erwin, M. E., et al.: Antimicrob. Agents Chemother. 35:927, 1991.
99. Hanaki, H., et al.: Antimicrob. Agents Chemother. 39:1120, 1995.
100. Imada, A., et al.: Nature 289:590, 1981.
101. Sykes, R. B., et al.: Nature 291:489, 1981.
102. Bonner, D. B., and Sykes, R. B.: J. Antimicrob. Chemother. 14:313, 1984.
103. Tanaka, S. N., et al.: Antimicrob. Agents Chemother. 31:219, 1987.
104. Schatz, A., et al.: Proc. Soc. Exp. Biol. Med. 55:66, 1944.
105. Weisblum, B., and Davies, J.: Bacteriol. Rev. 32:493, 1968.
106. Davies, J., and Davis, B. D.: J. Biol. Chem. 243:3312, 1968.
107. Lando, D., et al.: Biochemistry 12:4528, 1973.
108. Shah, K. J., et al.: Microbiol. Rev. 57:138, 1993.
109. Chevereau, P. J. L., et al.: Biochemistry 13:598, 1974.
110. Price, K. E., et al.: Antimicrob. Agents Chemother. 5:143, 1974.
111. Bryan, L. E., et al.: J. Antibiot. (Tokyo) 29:743, 1976.
112. Hancock, R. E. W.: J. Antimicrob. Chemother. 8:249, 1981.
113. Cox, D. A., et al.: The aminoglycosides. In Sammes, P. G. (ed.). Topics in Antibiotic Chemistry, vol. 1. Chichester, Ellis Harwood, 1977, p. 44.
114. Price, K. E.: Antimicrob. Agents Chemother. 29:543, 1986.
115. Dyer, J. R., and Todd, A. W.: J. Am. Chem. Soc. 85:3896, 1963.
116. Dyer, J. R., et al.: J. Am. Chem. Soc. 87:654, 1965.
117. Umezawa, S., et al.: J. Antibiot. (Tokyo) 27:997, 1974.
118. Waksman, S. A., and Lechevalier, H. A.: Science 109:305, 1949.
119. Hichens, M., and Rinehart, K. L., Jr.: J. Am. Chem. Soc. 85:1547, 1963.
120. Rinehart, K. L., Jr., et al.: J. Am. Chem. Soc. 84:3218, 1962.
121. Huettenrauch, R.: Pharmazie 19:697, 1964.
122. Umezawa, S., and Nishimura, Y.: J. Antibiot. (Tokyo) 30:189, 1977.
123. Haskell, T. H., et al.: J. Am. Chem. Soc. 81:3482, 1959.
124. DeJongh, D. C., et al.: J. Am. Chem. Soc. 89:3364, 1967.
125. Umezawa, H., et al.: J. Antibiot. [A] 10:181, 1957.
126. Tatsuoka, S., et al.: J. Antibiot. [A] 17:88, 1964.
127. Nakajima, M.: Tetrahedron Lett. 623, 1968.
128. Umezawa, S., et al.: J. Antibiot. (Tokyo) 21:162, 367, 424, 1968.
129. Morikubo, Y.: J. Antibiot. [A] 12:90, 1959.
130. Kawaguchi, H., et al.: J. Antibiot. (Tokyo) 25:695, 1972.
131. Paradelis, A. G., et al.: Antimicrob. Agents Chemother. 14:514, 1978.
132. Weinstein, M. J., et al.: J. Med. Chem. 6:463, 1963.
133. Cooper, D. J., et al.: J. Infect. Dis. 119:342, 1969.
134. Cooper, D. J., et al.: J. Chem. Soc. C 3126, 1971.
135. Maehr, H., and Schaffner, C. P.: J. Am. Chem. Soc. 89:6788, 1968.
136. Koch, K. F., et al.: J. Antibiot. [A] 26:745, 1963.
137. Lockwood, W., et al.: Antimicrob. Agents Chemother. 4:281, 1973.
138. Wright, J. J.: J. Chem. Soc. Chem. Commun. 206, 1976.
139. Wagman, G. M., et al.: J. Antibiot. (Tokyo) 23:555, 1970.
140. Braveny, I., et al.: Arzneimittelforschung 30:491, 1980.
141. Lewis, C., and Clapp, H.: Antibiot. Chemother. 11:127, 1961.
142. Cochran, T. G., and Abraham, D. J.: J. Chem. Soc. Chem. Commun. 494, 1972.
143. Muxfeldt, H., et al.: J. Am. Chem. Soc. 90:6534, 1968.
144. Muxfeldt, H., et al.: J. Am. Chem. Soc. 101:689, 1979.
145. Korst, J. J., et al.: J. Am. Chem. Soc. 90:439, 1968.
146. Muxfeldt, H., et al.: Angew. Chem. Int. Ed. 12:497, 1973.
147. Hirokawa, S., et al.: Z. Krist. 112:439, 1959.
148. Takeuchi, Y., and Buerger, M. J.: Proc. Natl. Acad. Sci. U. S. A. 46: 1366, 1960.
149. Cid-Dresdner, H.: Z. Krist. 121:170, 1965.
150. Leeson, L. J., Krueger, J. E., and Nash, R. A.: Tetrahedron Lett. 1155, 1963.
151. Stephens, C. R., et al.: J. Am. Chem. Soc. 78:4155, 1956.
152. Rigler, N. E., et al.: Anal. Chem. 37:872, 1965.
153. Benet, L. Z., and Goyan, J. E.: J. Pharm. Sci. 55:983, 1965.
154. Barringer, W., et al.: Am. J. Pharm. 146:179, 1974.
155. Barr, W. H., et al.: Clin. Pharmacol. Ther. 12:779, 1971.
156. Albert, A.: Nature 172:201, 1953.
157. Jackson, F. L.: Mode of action of tetracyclines. In Schnitzer, R. J., and Hawking, F. (eds.). Experimental Chemotherapy, vol. 3. New York, Academic Press, 1964, p. 103.
158. Bodley, J. W., and Zieve, P. J.: Biochem. Biophys. Res. Commun. 36:463, 1969.
159. Dockter, M. E., and Magnuson, A.: Biochem. Biophys. Res. Commun. 42:471, 1973.
160. Speer, B. S., Shoemaker, N. B., and Salyers, A. A.: Clin. Microbiol. Rev. 5:387, 1992.
161. Durckheimer, W.: Angew. Chem. Int. Ed. 14:721, 1975.
162. Brown, J. R., and Ireland, D. S.: Adv. Pharmacol. Chemother. 15: 161, 1978.
163. Mitscher, L. A.: The Chemistry of Tetracycline Antibiotics. New York, Marcel Dekker, 1978.
164. Chopra, I., Hawkey, P. M., and Hinton, M.: J. Antimicrob. Chemother. 29:245, 1992.
165. Cline, D. L. J.: Q. Rev. 22:435, 1968.
166. Hlavka, J. J., and Boothe, J. H. (eds.): The Tetracyclines. New York, Springer-Verlag, 1985.
167. Cammarata, A., and Yau, S. J.: J. Med. Chem. 13:93, 1970.
168. Glatz, B., et al.: J. Am. Chem. Soc. 101:2171, 1979.
169. Schach von Wittenau, M., et al.: J. Am. Chem. Soc. 84:2645, 1962.
170. Stephens, C. R., et al.: J. Am. Chem. Soc. 85:2643, 1963.
171. McCormick, J. R. D., et al.: J. Am. Chem. Soc. 79:4561, 1957.
172. Martell, M. J., Jr., and Booth, J. H.: J. Med. Chem. 10:44, 1967.
173. Colazzi, J. L., and Klink, P. R.: J. Pharm. Sci. 58:158, 1969.
174. Schumacher, G. E., and Linn, E. E.: J. Pharm. Sci. 67:1717, 1978.
175. Schach von Wittenau, M.: Chemotherapy 13S:41, 1968.
176. Conover H.: U.S. Patent 2,699,054 (Jan. 11, 1955).
177. Bunn, P. A., and Cronk, G. A.: Antibiot. Med. 5:379, 1958.
178. Gittinger, W. C., and Weinger, H.: Antibiot. Med. 7:22, 1960.
179. Remmers, E. G., et al.: J. Pharm. Sci. 53:1452, 1534, 1964.
180. Remmers, E. G., et al.: J. Pharm. Sci. 54:49, 1965.
181. Duggar, B. B.: Ann. N. Y. Acad. Sci. 51:177, 1948.
182. Finlay, A. C., et al.: Science 111:85, 1950.
183. Hochstein, F. A., et al.: J. Am. Chem. Soc. 75:5455, 1953.
184. Blackwood, R. K., et al.: J. Am. Chem. Soc. 83:2773, 1961.

185. Stephens, C. R., et al.: J. Am. Chem. Soc. 80:5324, 1958.
186. Minuth, J. N.: Antimicrob. Agents Chemother. 6:411, 1964.
187. Goldstein, F. W., Kitzis, M. D., and Acar, J. F.: Antimicrob. Agents Chemother. 38:2218, 1994.
188. Sum, P.-K., et al.: J. Med. Chem. 37:184, 1994.
189. Tally, F. T., Ellestad, G. A., and Testa, R. T.: J. Antimicrob. Chemother. 35:449, 1995.
190. Kirst, H.: Prog. Med. Chem. 31:265, 1994.
191. Lartey, P. A., Nellans, H. N., and Tanaka, S. K.: Adv. Pharmacol. 28:307, 1994.
192. Wilhelm, J. M., et al.: Antimicrob. Agents Chemother. 236, 1967.
193. LeClerq, R., and Courvalin, P.: Antimicrob. Agents Chemother. 35:1273, 1991.
194. Lai, C. J., and Weisblum, B.: Proc. Natl. Acad. Sci. U. S. A. 68:856, 1971.
195. LeClerq, R., and Courvalin, P.: Antimicrob. Agents Chemother. 35:1267, 1991.
196. McGuire, J. M., et al.: Antibiot. Chemother. 2:821, 1952.
197. Wiley, P. F.: J. Am. Chem. Soc. 79:6062, 1957.
198. Celmer, W. D.: J. Am. Chem. Soc. 87:1801, 1965.
199. Corey, E. J., et al.: J. Am. Chem. Soc. 101:7131, 1979.
200. Stephens, C. V., et al.: J. Antibiot. (Tokyo) 22:551, 1969.
201. Bechtol, L. D., et al.: Curr. Ther. Res. 20:610, 1976.
202. Welling, P. G., et al.: J. Pharm. Sci. 68:150, 1979.
203. Yakatan, G. J., et al.: J. Clin. Pharmacol. 20:625, 1980.
204. Tjandramaga, T. B., et al.: Pharmacology 29:305, 1984.
205. Croteau, D., Bergeron, M. G., and Lebel, M.: Antimicrob. Agents Chemother. 32:561, 1989.
206. Tardew, P. L., et al.: Appl. Microbiol. 18:159, 1969.
207. Janicki, R. S., et al.: Clin. Pediatr. (Phila.) 14:1098, 1975.
208. Nicholas, P.: N. Y. State J. Med. 77:2088, 1977.
209. Derrick, W. C., and Dillon, H. C.: Am. J. Dis. Child. 133:1146, 1979.
210. Ginsburg, C. M., et al.: Pediatr. Infect. Dis. 1:384, 1982.
211. Itoh, Z., et al.: Am. J. Physiol. 11:G320, 1985.
212. Sturgill, M. C., and Rapp, R. P.: Ann. Pharmacother. 26:1099, 1992.
213. Bright, G. M., et al.: J. Antibiot. (Tokyo) 41:1029, 1988.
214. Peters, D. H., Friedel, H. A., and McTavish, D.: Drugs 44:750, 1992.
215. Counter, F. T., et al.: Antimicrob. Agents Chemother. 35:1116, 1991.
216. Brogden, R. N., and Peters, D. H.: Drugs 48:599, 1994.
217. Sobin, B. A., et al.: Antibiotics Annual 1954–1955. New York, Medical Encyclopedia, 1955, p. 827.
218. Hochstein, F. A., et al.: J. Am. Chem. Soc. 82:3227, 1960.
219. Celmer, W. D.: J. Am. Chem. Soc. 87:1797, 1965.
220. Mason, D. J., et al.: Antimicrob. Agents Chemother. 544, 1962.
221. Hoeksema, H., et al.: J. Am. Chem. Soc. 86:4223, 1964.
222. Slomp, G., and MacKellar, F. A.: J. Am. Chem. Soc. 89:2454, 1967.
223. Howarth, G. B., et al.: J. Chem. Soc. C 2218, 1970.
224. Magerlein, B. J.: Tetrahedron Lett. 685, 1970.
225. Argoudelis, A. D., et al.: J. Am. Chem. Soc. 86:5044, 1964.
226. Magerlein, B. J., et al.: J. Med. Chem. 10:355, 1967.
227. Bannister, B.: J. Chem. Soc. Perkin Trans. I:1676, 1973.
228. Bannister, B.: J. Chem. Soc. Perkin Trans. I:3025, 1972.
229. Bartlett, J. G.: Rev. Infect. Dis. 1:370, 1979.
230. Sarges, R., and Witkop, B.: J. Am. Chem. Soc. 86:1861, 1964.
231. Storm, D. R., Rosenthal, K. S., and Swanson, P. E.: Annu. Rev. Biochem. 46:723, 1977.
232. McCormick, M. H., et al.: Antibiotics Annual 1955–1956. New York, Medical Encyclopedia, 1956, p. 606.
233. Sheldrick, G. M., et al.: Nature 27:233, 1978.
234. Williamson, M. P., and Williams, D. H.: J. Am. Chem. Soc. 103:6580, 1981.
235. Harris, C. M., et al.: J. Am. Chem. Soc. 105:6915, 1983.
236. Perkins, H. R., Nieto, M.: Ann. N. Y. Acad. Sci. 235:348, 1974.
237. Williamson, M. P., et al.: Tetrahedron Lett. 40:569, 1984.
238. Walsh, C. T.: Science 261:308, 1993.
239. Parenti, F., et al.: J. Antibiot. (Tokyo) 31:276, 1978.
240. Bardone, M. R., Paternoster, M., and Coronelli, C.: J. Antibiot. (Tokyo) 31:170, 1978.
241. Coronelli, C., et al.: J. Antibiot. (Tokyo) 37:621, 1984.
242. Hunt, A. H., et al.: J. Am. Chem. Soc. 106:4891, 1984.
243. Barna, J. C. J., et al.: J. Am. Chem. Soc. 106:4895, 1984.
244. Brogden, R. N., and Peters, D. H.: Drugs 47:823, 1994.
245. Johnson, B. A., et al.: Science 102:376, 1945.
246. Stoffel, W., and Craig, L. C.: J. Am. Chem. Soc. 83:145, 1961.
247. Ressler, C., and Kashelikar, D. V.: J. Am. Chem. Soc. 88:2025, 1966.
248. Benedict, R. G., and Langlykke, A. F.: J. Bacteriol. 54:24, 1947.
249. Stansly, P. J., et al.: Bull. Johns Hopkins Hosp. 81:43, 1947.
250. Ainsworth, G. C., et al.: Nature 160:263, 1947.
251. Vogler, K., and Studer, R. O.: Experientia 22:345, 1966.
252. Hausmann, W., and Craig, L. C.: J. Am. Chem. Soc. 76:4892, 1952.
253. Vogler, K., et al.: Experientia 20:365, 1964.
254. Koyama, Y., et al.: J. Antibiot. [A] 3:457, 1950.
255. Suzuki, T., et al.: J. Biochem. 54:41, 1963.
256. Wilkinson, S., and Lowe, L. A.: J. Chem. Soc. 4107, 1964.
257. Dubos, R. J.: J. Exp. Med. 70:1, 1939.
258. Paladini, A., and Craig, L. C.: J. Am. Chem. Soc. 76:688, 1954.
259. King, T. P., and Craig, L. C.: J. Am. Chem. Soc. 77:627, 1955.
260. Ohno, M., et al.: Bull. Soc. Chem. Jpn. 39:1738, 1966.
261. Finkelstein, A., and Anderson, O. S.: J. Membr. Biol. 59:155, 1981.
262. Ehrlich, J., et al.: Science 106:417, 1947.
263. Controulis, J., et al.: J. Am. Chem. Soc. 71:2463, 1949.
264. Long, L. M., and Troutman, H. D.: J. Am. Chem. Soc. 71:2473, 1949.
265. Szulcewski, D., and Eng, F.: Anal. Profiles Drug Subst. 4:47, 1972.
266. Glazko, A.: Antimicrob. Agents Chemother. 655, 1966.
267. Hansch, C., et al.: J. Med. Chem. 16:917, 1973.
268. Brock, T. D.: Chloramphenicol. In Schnitzer, R. J., and Hawking, F. (eds.). Experimental Chemotherapy, vol. 3. New York, Academic Press, 1964, p. 119.
269. Shalit, I., and Marks, M. I.: Drugs 28:281, 1984.
270. Kauffman, R. E., et al.: J. Pediatr. 99:963, 1981.
271. Kramer, W. G., et al.: J. Clin. Pharmacol. 24:181, 1984.
272. Shunk, C. H., et al.: J. Am. Chem. Soc. 78:1770, 1956.
273. Hoeksema, H., et al.: J. Am. Chem. Soc. 78:2019, 1956.
274. Spencer, C. H., et al.: J. Am. Chem. Soc. 78:2655, 1956.
275. Spencer, C., et al.: J. Am. Chem. Soc. 80:140, 1958.
276. Gellert, M., et al.: Proc. Natl. Acad. Sci. U. S. A. 73:4474, 1976.
277. Sugino, A., et al.: Proc. Natl. Acad. Sci. U. S. A. 75:4842, 1978.
278. Fuller, A. T., et al.: Nature 134:416, 1971.
279. Chain, E. B., and Mellows, G.: J. Chem. Soc. Perkin Trans. I:294, 1977.
280. Pappa, K. A.: J. Am. Acad. Dermatol. 22:873, 1990.
281. Hughes, J., and Mellows, G.: J. Antibiot. (Tokyo) 31:330, 1978.
282. Hughes, J., and Mellows, G.: Biochem. J. 176:305, 1978.
283. Gilbart, J., Perry, C. R., and Slocombe, B.: Antimicrob. Agents Chemother. 37:32, 1993.
284. Capobianco, J. O., Doran, C. C., and Goldman, R. C.: Antimicrob. Agents Chemother. 33:156, 1989.

SELECTED READING

Conte, J. E.: Manual of Antibiotics and Infectious Diseases, 8th ed. Baltimore, Williams & Wilkins, 1995.
Franklin, T. J., and Snow, G. A.: Biochemistry of Antimicrobial Action, 4th ed. London, Chapman & Hall, 1989.
Jawetz, E., et al.: Medical Microbiology, 20th ed. Norwalk, CT, Appleton & Lange, 1995.
Lambert, H. P., and O'Grady, W. D. (eds.): Antibiotic and Chemotherapy, 6th ed. New York, Churchill-Livingstone, 1992.
Lancini, G., Parenti, F., and Gallo, G. G.: Antibiotics, A Multidisciplinary Approach. New York, Plenum Press, 1995.
Mandell, G. L., Bennett, J. E., and Dolin, R. (eds.): Principles and Practice of Infectious Diseases, vol. 1, 4th ed. New York, Churchill-Livingstone, 1995.
Neu, H. C: The crisis of antibiotic resistance. Science 257:1064, 1992.
Page, M. I. (ed.): The Chemistry of Beta Lactams. New York, Chapman & Hall, 1992.
Silver, L. S., and Bostian, K. A: Discovery and development of new antibiotics: The problem of drug resistance. Antimicrob. Agents Chemother. 37:377, 1993.

Antiviral Agents

JOHN M. BEALE, JR.

Viruses are unique organisms. They are the smallest of all self-replicating organisms, able to pass through filters that retain the smallest bacteria.[1] The simplest viruses contain a small amount of DNA or RNA surrounded by an uncomplicated protein coat. Some of the more complex viruses have a lipid bilayer membrane surrounding the nucleic acid.[2] Viruses must replicate in living cells, which has led many to argue that viruses are not even living organisms but that they somehow exist at the interface of the living and the nonliving.[1] The most basic requirement is for the virus to induce either profound or subtle changes in the host cell so that viral genes are replicated and viral proteins are expressed. This will result in the formation of new viruses, usually many more than the number that infected the cell initially. Viruses conduct no metabolic processes on their own; they depend totally on a host cell, which they invade and parasitize to subvert subcellular machinery. They use part of the cell's equipment for replication of viral nucleic acids and expression of viral genes, all of the cell's protein synthesis machinery, and all of the cell's energy stores that are generated by its own metabolic processes. The virus turns the biochemical systems of the host cell to its own purposes, completely subverting the infected cell. An infection that results in the production of more viruses than initiated the infection is called a *productive infection*. The actual number of infectious viruses produced in an infected cell is termed the *burst size*. This number can range from 10 to more than 10,000, depending on the type of cell infected, the nature of the virus, and other factors.[3]

Viruses are known to infect every form of life.[1] A typical DNA virus will enter the nucleus of the host cell, where viral DNA is transcribed into messenger RNA (mRNA) by host cell RNA polymerase. mRNA is then translated into virus-specific proteins that facilitate assembly, maturation, and release of newly formed virus into surrounding tissues. RNA viruses are somewhat different, in that their replication relies on enzymes in the virus itself to synthesize mRNA.

An adult virus possesses only one type of nucleic acid (either a DNA or a RNA genome). This feature differentiates viruses from other intracellular parasites, such as *Chlamydia* (which possesses both DNA and RNA when replicating within a cell) and the *Rickettsiae* (which in addition to DNA and RNA have autonomous energy-generating systems). Viruses are very unlike these other intracellular parasites. Another unique feature of viruses is that their organized structure is completely lost during replication within the host cell; the nucleic acid and proteins exist dispersed in the cytoplasm.

CLASSIFICATION OF VIRUSES

Viruses are classified on the basis of a number of features:

- Nucleic acid content (DNA or RNA)
- Viral morphology (helical, icosahedral)
- Site of replication in cell (cytoplasm or nucleus)
- Coating (enveloped or nonenveloped)
- Serological typing (antigenic signatures)
- Cell types infected (B lymphocytes, T lymphocytes, monocytes)

The Baltimore Classification Scheme[4] (Table 11-1) gives an alternate means of relating the different virus types.

The following lists some virus types together with diseases that they cause:

- RNA viruses: Picornaviruses (polio, hepatitis A, rhinovirus); togavirus (rubella, equine encephalitis); flavivirus (yellow fever, dengue fever, St. Louis encephalitis); bunyaviruses (encephalitis, hemorrhagic fever); rhabdoviruses (vesicular stomatitis); myxoviruses (mumps, measles); reoviruses or rotaviruses (diarrhea); filovirus (Ebola, Marburg); arenaviruses (lymphocytic choriomeningitis); retroviruses (human immunodeficiency syndrome) (HIV)
- DNA viruses: herpesviruses (herpes, cold sores); papovaviruses (polyoma, warts); adenoviruses (respiratory complaints); poxvirus (smallpox); parvovirus (canine distemper)

It has been estimated that viruses cause more than 60% of the infectious diseases that occur in the developing countries. Bacterial infections account for only 15%. Table 11-2 provides a synopsis of virus types with their possible therapeutic modalities.

TARGETS FOR THE PREVENTION OF VIRAL INFECTIONS—CHEMOPROPHYLAXIS

Immunization

Prevention of viral infections by conferring *artificially acquired active immunity* with vaccines is the main approach for preventing most viral diseases. Safe and highly effective vaccines are available for the prevention of polio, rubella, measles, mumps, influenza, yellow fever, encephalitis, rabies, smallpox (now considered to be eradicated worldwide, but still of interest from a biological warfare standpoint), and hepatitis B. Vaccines developed to prevent infection with herpesvirus, Epstein-Barr virus, cytomegalovirus (CMV), respiratory syncytial virus (RSV), and human immunodeficiency virus (HIV) have so far proved ineffective or unreliable. The development of a new vaccine that is effective against a chronic disease-causing virus such as HIV (acquired immunodeficiency syndrome [AIDS]) can be a daunting task. The primary principles of vaccine development apply: The vaccine must be sufficiently antigenic to

TABLE 11–1 Baltimore Classification Scheme for Viruses

I) Single-stranded RNA viruses
- A) Positive sense (virion RNA-like cellular mRNA)
  - 1) Nonenveloped
    - (a) Icosahedral
      - (i) Picornaviruses (polio, hepatitis A, rhinovirus)
      - (ii) Calicivirus
      - (iii) Plant virus relatives of Picornavirus
      - (iv) MS2 bacteriophage
  - 2) Enveloped
    - (a) Icosahedral
      - (i) Togaviruses (rubella, equine encephalitis, Sindbis)
      - (ii) Flaviviruses (yellow fever, dengue fever)
    - (b) Helical
      - (i) Coronavirus
- B) Positive sense but requires RNA to be converted to DNA via a virion-associated enzyme (reverse transcriptase)
  - 1) Enveloped
    - (a) Retroviruses
      - (i) Oncornaviruses
      - (ii) Lentiviruses
- C) Negative-sense RNA (opposite polarity to cellular mRNA, requires a virion-associated enzyme to begin the replication cycle)
  - 1) Enveloped
    - (a) Helical
      - (i) Mononegaviruses (rabies, vesicular stomatitis virus, paramyxovirus, filovirus)
      - (ii) Segmented genome (orthomyxovirus-influenza, bunyavirus, arenavirus)

II) Double-stranded RNA viruses
- A) Nonenveloped
  - 1) Icosahedral
    - (a) Reovirus
    - (b) Rotavirus

III) Single-stranded DNA viruses
- A) Nonenveloped
  - 1) Icosahedral
    - (a) Parvoviruses (canine distemper, adeno-associated virus)
    - (b) Bacteriophage ΦX174

IV) Double-stranded DNA viruses
- A) Nuclear replication
  - 1) Nonenveloped
    - (a) Icosahedral
      - (i) Small circular DNA genome (papoviruses, SV40, polyomaviruses, papillomaviruses)
      - (ii) "Medium" sized, complex morphology, linear DNA (adenovirus)
  - 2) Enveloped-nuclear replicating
    - (a) Icosahedral
      - (i) Herpesviruses (linear DNA)
      - (ii) Hepadnavirus (virion encapsidates RNA that is converted to DNA by reverse transcriptase)
- B) Cytoplasmic replication
  - 1) Icosahedral
    - (a) Iridovirus
  - 2) Complex symmetry
    - (a) Poxvirus
- C) Bacterial viruses
  - 1) Icosahedral with tail
    - (a) T-series bacteriophages
    - (b) Bacteriophage λ

TABLE 11–2   Classification of Viruses Causing Disease in Humans

Family Agent	Disease	Vaccine	Chemotherapy
RNA Viruses			
Picornavirus			
Enterovirus	Polio; three serotypes cause meningitis, paralysis	Live and killed vaccines (very effective)	None
Coxsackie viruses	Variety of symptoms	None	None
Rhinovirus	Common cold, pneumonia (over 100 serotypes)	None	None
Hepatitis A virus	Hepatitis (usually mild and rarely chronic)	Inactivated virus (effective)	None
Calicivirus			
Norwalk virus	Gastroenteritis	None	None
Togavirus			
Alphaviruses (group A arboviruses)	Encephalitis, hemorrhagic fevers	Attenuated virus (generally effective)	None
Rubivirus	Rubella (German measles)	Attenuated virus	None
Flavivirus			
Flaviviruses (group B arboviruses)	Yellow fever, dengue, encephalitis, hemorrhagic fevers	Attenuated virus (generally effective)	None
Hepatitis C virus	Hepatitis	None	None
Coronavirus	Respiratory infection	None	None
Rhabdovirus			
Rabies virus	Rabies	Inactivated virus (effective)	None
Vesicular stomatitis virus		None	None
Filovirus			
Marburg virus	Marburg disease	None	None
Ebola virus	Hemorrhagic fever	None	None
Paramyxovirus			
Parainfluenza virus	Respiratory infection	None	None
Respiratory syncytial virus	Respiratory infection	Attenuated virus (effectiveness uncertain)	Ribavirin
Morbillivirus	Measles (rubeola)	Attenuated virus (90% effective)	None
Mumps virus	Mumps	Attenuated virus	None
Orthomyxovirus			
Influenza virus	Influenza (A, B, C serotypes)	Attenuated virus (70% effective)	Amantadine
Bunyavirus			
Hantavirus	Fever, renal failure	None	None
Arboviruses	Encephalitis, hemorrhagic fever	None	None
Arenavirus			
Lymphocytic choriomeningitis virus	Meningitis	None	None
Junin, Machupo viruses	Hemorrhagic fever	None	None
Lassa virus	Hemorrhagic fever	None	Ribavirin
Reovirus			
Human rotavirus	Gastroenteritis in infants	None	None
Orbivirus	Colorado tick fever	Inactivated virus (effectiveness unknown)	None
Retrovirus			
Human immunodeficiency viruses (HIV-1, HIV-2)	AIDS and AIDS-related complex (ARC)	None	AZT, ddl, ddC, stavudine
Human T-cell lymphotropic viruses (HTLV-1, HTLV-2)	T-cell leukemia, lymphoma	None	None

(Continued)

TABLE 11–2   Classification of Viruses Causing Disease in Humans—Continued

Family Agent	Disease	Vaccine	Chemotherapy
DNA Viruses			
Herpesvirus			
Herpes simplex 1	Stomatitis, eye infections, encephalitis	Inactivated virus (efficacy uncertain)	Iudr, ara-A
Herpes simplex 2	Genital herpes, skin eruptions	None	Acyclovir
Varicella zoster	Chickenpox (children), shingles (adults)	None	Acyclovir
Cytomegalovirus	Infections in the immunocompromised, neonates	None	Ganciclovir, foscarnet
Epstein-Barr virus	Infectious mononucleosis, Burkitt's lymphoma	None	None
Papovavirus			
Papillomavirus	Warts	None	Podophyllin
Polyomavirus (JC virus)	Progressive leukoencephalopathy		None
Adenovirus			
Human adenovirus	Upper respiratory tract and eye infections	None	None
Hepadnavirus			
Hepatitis B virus	Hepatitis (may become chronic)	Inactivated subunit (very effective)	None
Poxvirus			
Variola	Smallpox	Vaccinia (cowpox) (very effective)	Methisazone
Parvovirus			
Human parvovirus B19	Erythema, hemolytic anemia	None	None

induce an effective antibody response, even in very young patients; the vaccine must not cause the disease that it is designed to prevent or cause some other toxic manifestation as the early killed vaccines did; and ideally, the vaccine should produce a lasting form of immunity, with a minimum requirement for booster doses. These requirements are difficult enough to meet for viruses that cause acute infections. The chronic cases are much more complicated. It is difficult to overcome the tendency of some viruses to undergo rapid mutation, leading to multiple antigenic epitopes; this makes development of a broadly effective vaccine much more difficult.

Biochemical Targets for Antiviral Therapy

With the discovery of antibiotics and anti-infective agents, the science of treating bacterial infections moved forward at a rapid rate. The development of useful antiviral agents (antibiotics and antiviral agents), in contrast, has historically lagged behind. There are a number of reasons for this. Unlike bacteria, viruses will not grow in simple synthetic culture media. They must infect human or animal cells to propagate.[5] For example, the most commonly used cell cultures in virology derive from primates (including humans and monkeys), rodents (including hamsters and mice), and birds (especially chickens). These culture methods are very reliable[6] and are in widespread use for the propagation of virus particles, but they are more difficult to perform than their bacterial counterparts. Hence, drug-screening techniques with viruses have taken longer to catch up with those in

bacteria. Another possible reason for the lag in antiviral drug development lies in the comparative biochemical simplicity of viruses vis-à-vis bacteria and their use of the biochemical processes of a host cell. There are fewer specialized targets for potential attack by chemotherapeutic agents. The rapid, spectacular successes of immunization procedures for the prevention of certain viral diseases may have contributed to a relative lack of interest in antiviral chemotherapy. Another feature of mild viral infections, such as the common cold, is that clinical symptoms do not appear until the infection is well established and the immune processes of the host have begun to mount a successful challenge. Thus, for many common viral infections, chemotherapy is simply not an appropriate choice of treatment. Chemotherapeutic agents *are* needed, however, to combat viruses that cause severe or chronic infections, such as encephalitis, AIDS, and herpes, particularly in patients with compromised immune systems.

THE INFECTIOUS PROCESS FOR A VIRUS

Despite their simplicity relative to bacteria, viruses still possess a variety of biochemical targets for potential attack by chemotherapeutic agents. An appropriate chemical compound may interrupt each of these. Hence, a thorough understanding of the specific biochemical events that occur during viral infection of the host cell should guide the discovery of site-specific antiviral agents. The process of viral infection can be sequenced in seven stages:

1. *Adsorption*, attachment[7] of the virus to specific receptors on the surface of the host cells, a specific recognition process.
2. *Entry*, penetration[7] of the virus into the cell.
3. *Uncoating*, release[7] of viral nucleic acid from the protein coat.
4. *Transcription*, production of viral mRNA from the viral genome.[8]
5. *Translation*, synthesis[8] of viral proteins (coat proteins and enzymes for replication) and viral nucleic acid (i.e., the parental genome or complimentary strand). This process uses the host cell processes to express viral genes, resulting in a few or many viral proteins involved in the replication process. The viral proteins modify the host cell and allow the viral genome to replicate by using host and viral enzymes. The mechanisms by which this occurs are complex. This is often the stage at which the cell is irreversibly modified and eventually killed.
6. *Assembly* of the viral particle. New viral coat proteins assemble into capsids (the protein envelope that surrounds nucleic acid and associated molecules in the core) and viral genomes.[8]
7. *Release* of the mature virus from the cell by budding from the cell membrane or rupture of the cell and repeat of the process, from cell to cell or individual to individual.[8] Enveloped viruses typically use budding on the plasma membrane, endoplasmic reticulum, or Golgi membranes. Nonenveloped viruses typically escape by rupture of the host cell.

The initial attachment of viral particles to cells probably involves multiphasic interactions between viral attachment protein(s) and host cell surface receptors. For instance, in the case of the alphaherpesviruses, internalization involves a cascade of events that involve different glycoproteins and different cell surface molecules at different stages. Different cell surface proteins may be used for the initial attachment and entry into target cells and for cell-to-cell spread across closely apposed populations of cells.[9] The pattern of systemic illness produced during an acute viral infection in large part depends on the specific organs infected and in many cases on the capacity of the viruses to infect discrete populations of cells within these organs. This property is called *tissue tropism*.[10, 11] The tissue tropism of a virus is influenced by the interaction between a variety of host and viral factors.

Although the specific viral attachment proteins and specific receptors on target cells are important, a variety of other virus–host interactions can play an important role in determining the tropism of a virus. Increasing attention is being focused on *coreceptors* in mediating viral binding. For instance, entry of HIV-1 into target cells requires the presence of both CD4$^+$ and a second coreceptor protein that belongs to the G-protein–coupled seven-transmembrane receptor family, including the chemokine receptor proteins CCR5 and CXCR4. Cells that express CD4$^+$ but not the coreceptor are resistant to HIV infection. Host cellular receptors can be integrins, heparans, sialic acids, gangliosides, ceramides, phospholipids, and major histocompatibility antigens (to name a few). There is substantial evidence that the cellular receptor for influenza viruses is the peptidoglycan component *N*-acetylmuramic acid, which binds a protein molecule, hemagglutinin, projecting from the viral surface.[12] The binding of *N*-acetylmuramic acid and hemagglutinin sets in motion a sequence of events whereby the viral envelope and the host cell membrane dissolve into each other, and the viral contents enter the cell. Initiation of HIV-1 infection involves the interaction of specific glycoprotein molecules (gp120) that stud the viral cell surface with an antigenic CD4$^+$ receptor molecule on helper T lymphocytes along

with a cytokine coreceptor.[13–16] Substantial evidence indicates that viruses enter cells by *endocytosis,* a process that involves fusion of the viral envelope with the cell membrane, intermixing of components, and dissolution of the membranes of virus and cell. Various receptors and coreceptors facilitate this reaction.[17–19]

Before a virus can begin a replication cycle within a host cell, its outer envelope and capsid must be removed to release its nucleic acid genome. For complex DNA viruses such as vaccinia (its binding receptor is the epidermal growth factor receptor), the uncoating process occurs in two stages[17]:

1. Host cell enzymes partially degrade the envelope and capsid to reveal a portion of the viral DNA, which serves as a template for mRNA synthesis.
2. mRNAs code for the synthesis of viral enzymes, which complete the degradation of the protein coat, allowing the virus to fully enter the host.

The proteins of the viral envelope and capsule are the primary targets for antibodies synthesized in response to immunization techniques. Protein synthesis inhibitors such as cycloheximide and puromycin inhibit the uncoating process, but they are not selective enough to be useful as antiviral agents.

In the critical fourth and fifth stages of infection, the virus usurps the energy-producing and synthetic functions of the host cell to replicate its own genome and to synthesize viral enzymes and structural proteins.[20] Simple RNA viruses conduct both replication and protein synthesis in the cytoplasm of the host cell. These contain specific RNA polymerases (RNA replicases) responsible for replication of the genome. Some single-stranded RNA viruses, such as poliovirus, have a (+)-RNA genome that serves the dual function of messenger for protein synthesis and template for the synthesis of a complementary strand of (–)-RNA, from which the (+)-RNA is replicated. In poliovirus (a picornavirus), the message is translated as a single large open reading frame whose product is cleaved enzymatically into specific viral enzymes and structural proteins.[18, 21] Other RNA viruses, such as influenza viruses, contain (–)-RNA, which serves as the template for the synthesis of a complementary strand of (+)-RNA. The (+)-RNA strand directs viral protein synthesis and provides the template for the replication of the (–)-RNA genome. Certain antibiotics, such as the rifamycins, inhibit viral RNA polymerases in vitro, but none has yet proved clinically useful. Bioactivated forms of the nucleoside analogue ribavirin variously inhibit ribonucleotide synthesis, RNA synthesis, or RNA capping in RNA viruses. Ribavirin has been approved for aerosol treatment of severe lower respiratory infections caused by respiratory syncytial virus (RSV).

Retroviruses constitute a special class of RNA viruses that possess a RNA-dependent DNA polymerase *(reverse transcriptase)* required for viral replication. In these viruses, a single strand of complementary DNA (cDNA) is synthesized on the RNA genome *(reverse transcription),* duplicated, and circularized to a double-stranded proviral DNA. The proviral DNA is then integrated into the host cell chromosomal DNA to form the template *(apovirus* or *virogene)* required for the synthesis of mRNAs and replication of the viral RNA genome. During the process of cDNA biosynthesis, a RNase degrades the RNA strand, leaving only DNA. *Oncogenic* (cancer-causing) viruses, such as the human T-cell leukemia viruses (HTLV) and the related HIV, are retroviruses. Retroviral reverse transcriptase is a good target for chemotherapy, being inhibited by the triphosphates of certain dideoxynucleosides, such as 2',3'-deoxy-3'-azidothymidine (AZT, zidovudine), 2',3'-dideoxycytidine (ddCyd, zalcitabine), and 2',3'-dideoxy-2',3'-didehydro-thymidine (D4T, stavudine), all of which have been approved for the treatment of AIDS. The nomenclature of these agents is straightforward. A 2',3'-dideoxynucleoside is referred to as ddX, while the unsaturated 2',3'-dideoxy-2',3'-didehydronucleosides are named d4X. The dideoxynucleoside triphosphates are incorporated into viral DNA in place of the corresponding 2'-deoxynucleoside (i.e., 2'-deoxy-thymidine, 2'-deoxycytidine, or 2'-deoxyadenosine) triphosphate.[22, 23] This reaction terminates the viral DNA chain, since the incorporated dideoxynucleoside lacks the 3'-hydroxyl group required to form a 3',5'-phosphodiester bond with the next 2'-deoxynucleotide triphosphate to be incorporated.

The DNA viruses constitute a heterogeneous group whose genome is composed of DNA. They replicate in the nucleus of a host cell. Some of the DNA viruses are simple structures, consisting of a single DNA strand and a few enzymes surrounded by a capsule (e.g., parvovirus) or a lipoprotein envelope (e.g., hepatitis B virus). Others, such as the herpesviruses and poxviruses, are large, complex structures with double-stranded DNA genomes and several enzymes encased in a capsule and surrounded by an envelope consisting of several membranes. DNA viruses contain DNA-dependent RNA polymerases *(transcriptases)*, DNA polymerases, and various other enzymes (depending on the complexity of the virus) that may provide targets for antiviral drugs. The most successful chemotherapeutic agents discovered thus far are directed against replication of herpesviruses. The nucleoside analogues idoxuridine, trifluridine, and vidarabine block replication in herpesviruses by three general mechanisms: First, as the monophosphates, they interfere with the biosynthesis of precursor nucleotides required for DNA synthesis; second, as triphosphates, they competitively inhibit DNA polymerase; and third, the triphosphates are incorporated into the growing DNA itself, resulting in DNA that is brittle and does not function normally. Acyclonucleosides (e.g., acycloguanosine) are bioactivated sequentially by viral and host cell kinases to the acyclonucleotide monophosphate and the acyclonucleoside triphosphate, respectively. The latter inhibits viral DNA polymerase and terminates the viral DNA strand, since no 3'-hydroxyl group is available for the subsequent formation of a 3',5'-phosphodiester bond with the next nucleoside triphosphate. The structure of acyclovir with the acyclosugar chain rotated into a pentose configuration (below) shows clearly the absence of the 3'-hydroxyl group.

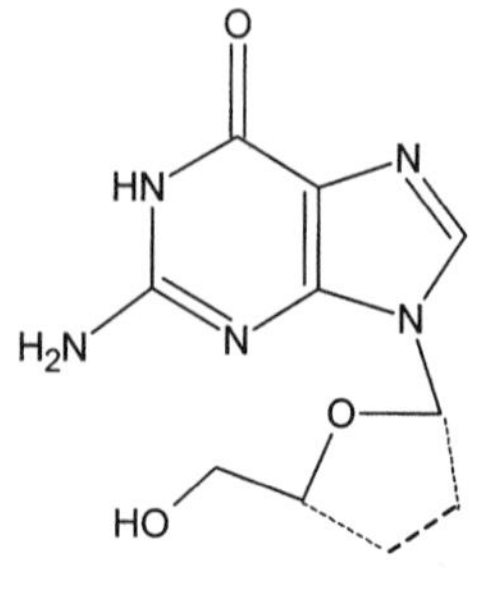

Late stages in viral replication require important virus-specific processing of certain viral proteins by viral or cellular proteases. Retroviruses, such as HIV, express three genes as precursor polyproteins. Two of these gene products, designated the p55gag and p160gag-pol proteins for their location on the genome, undergo cleavage at several sites by a virally encoded protease to form structural (viral coat) proteins (p17, p24, p8, and p7) and enzymes required for replication (reverse transcriptase, integrase, and protease). The demonstration that HIV protease, a member of the aspartyl protease family of enzymes, is essential for the maturation and infectivity of HIV particles[24] has stimulated major research efforts to develop effective inhibitors of this step. These efforts have led to several candidates, some that are on the market and many that are in clinical trials.

To complete the replication cycle, the viral components are assembled into the mature viral particle, or *virion*. For simple, nonenveloped viruses (e.g., the picornavirus poliovirus), the genome and only a few enzymes are encased by capsid proteins to complete the virion. Other, more complex viruses are enveloped by one or more membranes containing carbohydrate and lipoprotein components derived from the host cell membrane.

Once the mature virion has been assembled, it is ready for release from the cell. The release of certain viruses (e.g., poliovirus) is accompanied by lysis of the host cell membrane and cell death. Some of the enveloped viruses, however, are released by *budding* or *exocytosis,* a process involving fusion between the viral envelope and the cell membrane. This process is nearly a reversal of the entry process; the host cell membrane remains intact under these conditions, and the cell may survive.

Chemoprophylaxis is an alternative to active immunization for the prevention of viral infection. With chemoprophylaxis, one uses a chemical agent that interferes with a step in early viral infectivity. The immune system is not directly stimulated by the drug but *is* required to respond to any active infection. It would seem that the most successful chemoprophylactic agents would be those that prevent penetration of the virus into the host cell. In principle, this can be achieved by blocking any of three steps prior to the start of the replication cycle: *(a)* attachment of the virion to the host cell via its receptor complex, *(b)* its entry into the cell via endocytosis, or *(c)* release of the viral nucleic acid from the protein coat. At present, only a single class of agents affects these early stages of replication.[13–16] The adamantanamines (amantadine and rimantadine) have been approved for controlling influenza type A infection. These drugs appear to interfere with two stages of influenza type A viral replication: preventing the early stage of viral uncoating and disturbing the late stage of viral assembly. Clinical studies have shown that amantadine and rimantadine are effective in both prophylaxis and treatment of active influenza type A infection.

Amantadine, USP, and Rimantadine.   Amantadine, 1-adamantanamine hydrochloride (Symmetrel), and its α-methyl derivative rimantadine, α-methyl-1-adamantane methylamine hydrochloride (Flumadine), are unusual caged tricyclic amines with the following structures:

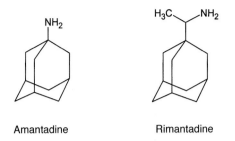

Amantadine   Rimantadine

Amantadine has been used for years as a treatment for Parkinson's disease. Both of these agents will specifically inhibit replication of the influenza type A viruses at low concentrations. Rimantadine is generally 4 to 10 times more active than amantadine. The adamantanamines have two mechanisms in common: *(a)* they inhibit an early step in viral replication, most likely viral uncoating,[25] and *(b)* in some strains they affect a later step that probably involves viral assembly, possibly by interfering with hemagglutinin processing. The main biochemical locus of action is the influenza type A virus M2 protein, which is an integral membrane protein that functions as an ion channel. The M2 channel is a proton transport system. By interfering with the function of the M2 protein, the adamantanamines inhibit acid-mediated dissociation of the ribonucleoprotein complex early in replication. They also interfere with transmembrane proton pumping, maintaining a high intracellular proton concentration relative to the extracellular concentration and enhancing acidic pH-induced conformational changes in the hemagglutinin during its intracellular transport at a later stage. The conformational changes in hemagglutinin prevent transfer of the nascent virus particles to the cell membrane for exocytosis.

Resistant variants of influenza type A have been recovered from amantadine- and rimantadine-treated patients. Resistance with inhibitory concentrations increased more than 100-fold have been associated with single nucleotide changes that lead to amino acid substitutions in the transmembrane domain of M2. Amantadine and rimantadine share cross-susceptibility and resistance.[25, 26]

Amantadine and rimantadine are approved in the United States for prevention and treatment of influenza type A virus infections. Seasonal prophylaxis with either drug is about 70 to 90% protective[27] against influenza type A. The drugs have no effect on influenza type B. The primary side effects are related to the central nervous system and are dopaminergic. This is not surprising, since amantadine is used in the treatment of Parkinson's disease. Rimantadine has significantly fewer side effects, probably because of its extensive biotransformation. Less than 50% of a dose of rimantadine is excreted unchanged, and more than 20% appears in the urine as metabolites.[28] Amantadine is excreted largely unchanged in the urine.

INTERFERONS: INTERFERON ALFA (INTRON A, ROFERON A) AND INTERFERON BETA (BETASERON)

Interferons (IFNs) are extremely potent cytokines that possess antiviral, immunomodulating, and antiproliferative actions.[29] IFNs are synthesized by infected cells in response to various inducers (Fig. 11-1) and, in turn, elicit either an antiviral state in neighboring cells or a natural killer cell response that destroys the initially infected cell (Fig. 11-2). There are three classes of human IFNs that possess significant antiviral activity. These are IFN-α (more than 20 subtypes), IFN-β (2 subtypes), and IFN-γ. IFN-α is used clinically in a recombinant form (called interferon *alfa*). IFN-β (Betaseron) is a recombinant form marketed for the treatment of multiple sclerosis.

IFN-α and IFN-β are produced by almost all cells in response to viral challenge. Interferon production is not limited to viral stimuli, however. A variety of other triggers, including cytokines such as interleukin-1, interleukin-2, and tumor necrosis factor, will elicit the production of IFNs. Both IFN-α and IFN-β are elicited by exposure of a cell to double-stranded viral RNA. IFN-α is produced by lymphocytes and macrophages, while IFN-β is biosynthesized in fibroblasts and epithelial cells. IFN-γ production is restricted to T lymphocytes and natural killer cells responding to antigenic stimuli, mitogens, and specific cytokines. IFN-α and IFN-β bind to the same receptor, and the genes for both are encoded on chromosome 9. The receptor for INF-γ is unique, and only one subtype has been identified. The genes for this molecule are encoded on chromosome 12. INF-γ has less antiviral activity than IFN-α and IFN-β but more potent

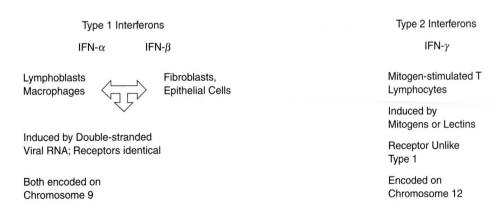

Figure 11-1 ■ Types of interferon.

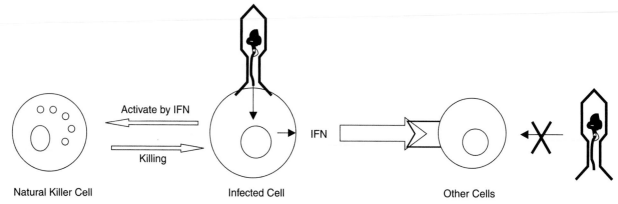

Figure 11–2 ■ Interferon mechanisms.

immunoregulatory effects. INF-γ is especially effective in activating macrophages, stimulating cell membrane expression of class II major histocompatibility complexes (MHCII), and mediating the local inflammatory responses. Most animal viruses are sensitive to the antiviral actions of IFNs. The instances in which a virus is insensitive to IFN typically involve DNA viruses.[13]

On binding to the appropriate cellular receptor, the IFNs induce the synthesis of a cascade of antiviral proteins that contribute to viral resistance. The antiviral effects of the IFNs are mediated through inhibition of [30]

- Viral penetration or uncoating
- Synthesis of mRNA
- The translation of viral proteins
- Viral assembly and release

With most viruses, the IFNs predominantly inhibit protein synthesis. This takes place through the intermediacy of IFN-

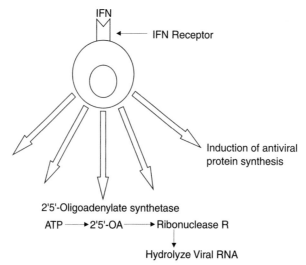

Figure 11–3 ■ IFNs predominantly inhibit protein synthesis.

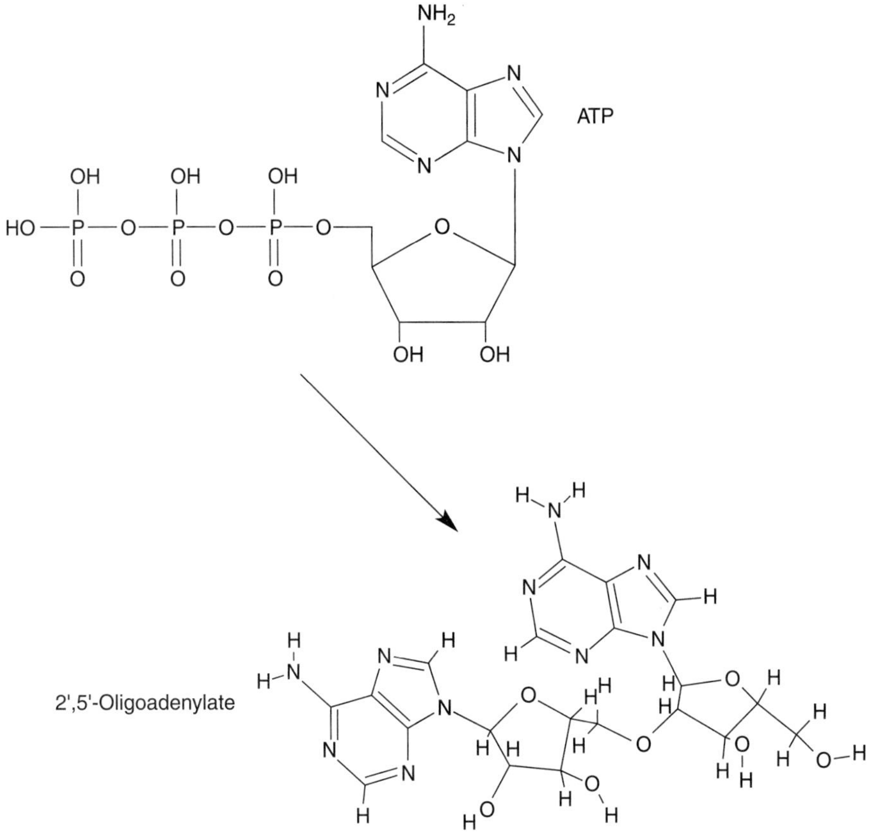

Figure 11–4 ■ Structure of 2′,5′-oligoadenylate.

induced proteins such as 2′,5′-oligoadenylate (2′,5′-OA) synthetases (Fig. 11-3) and a protein kinase, either of which can inhibit viral protein synthesis in the presence of double-stranded RNA. 2′,5′-OA activates a cellular endoribonuclease (RNase) (Fig. 11-4) that cleaves both cellular and viral RNA. The protein kinase selectively phosphorylates and inactivates eukaryotic initiation factor 2 (eIF2), preventing initiation of the mRNA–ribosome complex. IFN also induces a specific phosphodiesterase that cleaves a portion of tRNA molecules and, thereby, interferes with peptide elongation.[30] The infection sequence for a given virus may be inhibited at one or several steps. The *principal* inhibitory effect differs among virus families. Certain viruses can block the production or activity of selected IFN-inducible proteins and thus counter the IFN effect.

IFNs cannot be absorbed orally; to be used therapeutically they must be given intramuscularly or subcutaneously. The biological effects are quite long, so pharmacokinetic parameters are difficult to determine. The antiviral state in peripheral blood mononuclear cells typically peaks 24 hours after a dose of IFN-α and IFN-β, then decreases to baseline in 6 days.[31] Both recombinant and natural INF-α and INF-β are approved for use in the United States for the treatment of condyloma acuminatum (venereal warts), chronic hepatitis C, chronic hepatitis B, Kaposi's sarcoma in HIV-infected patients, other malignancies, and multiple sclerosis.

NUCLEOSIDE ANTIMETABOLITES

Inhibitors of DNA Polymerase

Idoxuridine, USP. Idoxuridine, 5-iodo-2′-deoxyuridine (Stoxil, Herplex), was introduced in 1963 for the treatment of herpes simplex keratitis.[32] The drug is an iodinated analogue of thymidine that inhibits replication of a number of DNA viruses in vitro. The susceptible viruses include the herpesviruses and poxviruses (vaccinia).

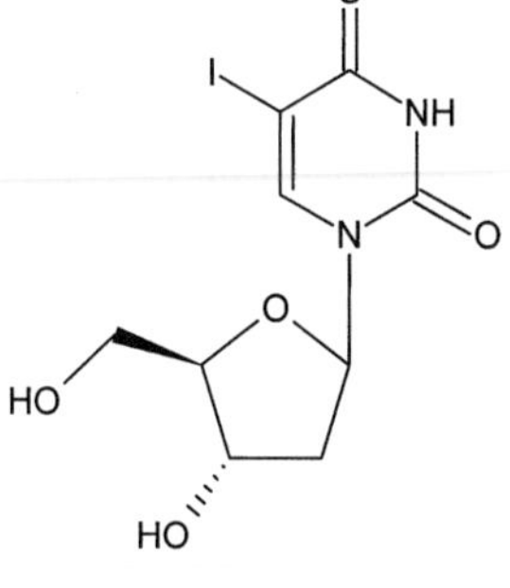

Idoxuridine

The mechanism of action of idoxuridine has not been completely defined, but several steps are involved in the activation of the drug. Idoxuridine enters the cell and is phosphorylated at O-5 by a viral thymidylate kinase to yield a monophosphate, which undergoes further biotransformation to a triphosphate. The triphosphate is believed to be both a substrate and an inhibitor of viral DNA polymerase, causing inhibition of viral DNA synthesis and facilitating the synthesis of DNA that contains the iodinated pyrimidine. The altered DNA is more susceptible to strand breakage and leads to faulty transcription. When the iodinated DNA is transcribed, the results are miscoding errors in RNA and faulty protein synthesis. The ability of idoxuridylic acid to substitute for deoxythymidylic acid in the synthesis of DNA may be due to the similar van der Waals radii of iodine (2.15Å) and the thymidine methyl group (2.00Å).

In the United States, idoxuridine is approved only for the topical treatment of herpes simplex virus (HSV) keratitis, although outside the United States a solution of idoxuridine in dimethyl sulfoxide is available for the treatment of herpes labialis, genitalis, and zoster. The use of idoxuridine is limited because the drug lacks selectivity; low, subtherapeutic concentrations inhibit the growth of uninfected host cells. The effective concentration of idoxuridine is at least 10 times greater than that of acyclovir.

Idoxuridine occurs as a pale yellow, crystalline solid that is soluble in water and alcohol but poorly soluble in most organic solvents. The compound is a weak acid, with a pK_a of 8.25. Aqueous solutions are slightly acidic, yielding a pH of about 6.0. Idoxuridine is light and heat sensitive. It is supplied as a 0.1% ophthalmic solution and a 0.5% ophthalmic ointment.

Trifluridine, USP. Trifluridine, 5-trifluoromethyl-2′-deoxyuridine (Viroptic), is a fluorinated pyrimidine nucleoside that demonstrates in vitro inhibitory activity against HSV 1 and 2, CMV, vaccinia, and some adenoviruses.[33] Trifluridine possesses a trifluoromethyl group instead of an iodine atom at the 5 position of the pyrimidine ring. The van der Waals radius of the trifluoromethyl group is 2.44Å, somewhat larger than that of the iodine atom.

Like idoxuridine, the antiviral mechanism of trifluridine involves inhibition of viral DNA synthesis. Trifluridine monophosphate is an irreversible inhibitor of thymidylate synthetase, and the biologically generated triphosphate competitively inhibits thymidine triphosphate incorporation into DNA by DNA polymerase. In addition, trifluridine in its triphosphate form is incorporated into viral and cellular DNA, creating fragile, poorly functioning DNA.

Trifluridine

Trifluridine is approved in the United States for the treatment of primary keratoconjunctivitis and recurrent epithelial keratitis due to HSV types 1 and 2. Topical trifluridine shows some efficacy in patients with acyclovir-resistant HSV cutaneous infections. Trifluridine solutions are heat sensitive and require refrigeration.

Vidarabine, USP. Chemically, vidarabine (Vira-A), is 9-β-D-arabinofuranosyladenine. The drug is the 2′ epimer of natural adenosine. Introduced in 1960 as a candidate anticancer agent, vidarabine was found to have broad-spectrum activity against DNA viruses.[34] The drug is active against herpesviruses, poxviruses, rhabdoviruses, hepadnavirus, and some RNA tumor viruses. Vidarabine was marketed in the United States in 1977 as an alternative to idoxuridine for the treatment of HSV keratitis and HSV encephalitis. Although the agent was initially prepared chemically, it is now obtained by fermentation with strains of *Streptomyces antibioticus*.

Vidarabine

The antiviral action of vidarabine is completely confined to DNA viruses. Vidarabine inhibits viral DNA synthesis. Enzymes within the cell phosphorylate vidarabine to the triphosphate, which competes with deoxyadenosine triphosphate for viral DNA polymerase. Vidarabine triphosphate is also incorporated into cellular and viral DNA, where it acts as a chain terminator. The triphosphate form of vidarabine also inhibits a set of enzymes that are involved in methylation of uridine to thymidine: ribonucleoside reductase, RNA polyadenylase, and *S*-adenosylhomocysteine hydrolase.

At one time in the United States, intravenous vidarabine was approved for use against HSV encephalitis, neonatal herpes, and herpes or varicella zoster in immunocompromised patients. Acyclovir has supplanted vidarabine as the drug of choice in these cases.

In the treatment of viral encephalitis, vidarabine had to be administered by constant flow intravenous infusion because of its poor water solubility and rapid metabolic conversion to a hypoxanthine derivative in vivo. These problems, coupled with the availability of less toxic and more effective agents, have caused intravenous vidarabine to be withdrawn from the U. S. market.

Vidarabine occurs as a white, crystalline monohydrate that is soluble in water to the extent of 0.45 mg/mL at 25°C. The drug is still available in the United States as a 3% ointment for the treatment of HSV keratitis.

Acyclovir, USP. Acyclovir, 9-[2-(hydroxyethoxy)methyl]-9*H*-guanine (Zovirax), is the most effective of a series of acyclic nucleosides that possess antiviral activity. In contrast with true nucleosides that have a ribose or a deoxyribose sugar attached to a purine or a pyrimidine base, the group attached to the base in acyclovir is similar to an open chain sugar, albeit lacking in hydroxyl groups. The clinically useful antiviral spectrum of acyclovir is limited to herpesviruses. It is most active (in vitro) against HSV type 1, about 2 times less against HSV type 2, and 10 times less potent against varicella-zoster virus. An advantage is that uninfected human cells are unaffected by the drug.

Acyclovir

The ultimate effect of acyclovir is the inhibition of viral DNA synthesis. Transport into the cell and monophosphorylation are accomplished by a thymidine kinase that is encoded by the virus itself.[35] The affinity of acyclovir for the viral thymidine kinase is about 200 times that of the corresponding mammalian enzyme. Hence, some selectivity is attained. Enzymes in the infected cell catalyze the conversion of the monophosphate to acyclovir triphosphate, which is present in 40 to 100 times greater concentrations in HSV-infected than uninfected cells. Acyclovir triphosphate competes for endogenous deoxyguanosine triphosphate (dGTP); hence, acyclovir triphosphate competitively inhibits viral DNA polymerases. The triphosphorylated drug is also incorporated into viral DNA, where it acts as a chain terminator. Because it has no 3′- hydroxyl group, no 3′,5′-phosphodiester bond can form. This mechanism is essentially a suicide inhibition because the terminated DNA template containing acyclovir as a ligand binds to, and irreversibly inactivates, DNA polymerase. Resistance to acyclovir can occur, most often by deficient thymidine kinase activity in HSV isolates. Acyclovir resistance in vesicular stomatitis virus (VSV) isolates is caused by mutations in VSV thymidine kinase or, less often, by mutations in viral DNA polymerase.

Two dosage forms of acyclovir are available for systemic use: oral and parenteral. Oral acyclovir is used in the initial treatment of genital herpes and to control mild recurrent episodes. It has been approved for short-term treatment of shingles and chickenpox caused by varicella-zoster virus (VZV). Intravenous administration is indicated for initial and recurrent infections in immunocompromised patients and for the prevention and treatment of severe episodes. The drug is absorbed slowly and incompletely from the gastrointestinal tract, and its oral bioavailability is only 15 to 30%. Nevertheless, acyclovir is distributed to virtually all body compartments. Less than 30% is bound to protein. Most of the drug is excreted unchanged in the urine, about 10% excreted as the -carboxy metabolite.

Acyclovir occurs as a chemically stable, white, crystalline solid that is slightly soluble in water. Because of its ampho-

teric properties (pK$_a$ values of 2.27 and 9.25), solubility is increased by both strong acids and bases. The injectable form is the sodium salt, which is supplied as a lyophilized powder, equivalent to 50 mg/mL of active acyclovir dissolved in sterile water for injection. Because the solution is strongly alkaline (pH ~ 11), it must be administered by slow, constant intravenous infusion to avoid irritation and thrombophlebitis at the injection site.

Adverse reactions are few. Some patients experience occasional gastrointestinal upset, dizziness, headache, lethargy, and joint pain. An ointment composed of 5% acyclovir in a polyethylene glycol base is available for the treatment of initial, mild episodes of herpes genitalis. The ointment is not an effective preventer of recurrent episodes.

Valacyclovir Hydrochloride. Valacyclovir (Valtrex) is the hydrochloride salt of the L-valyl ester of acyclovir. The compound is a water-soluble crystalline solid, and it is a prodrug intended to increase the bioavailability of acyclovir by increasing lipophilicity. Valacyclovir is hydrolyzed rapidly and almost completely to acyclovir following oral administration. Enzymatic hydrolysis of the prodrug is believed to occur during enterohepatic cycling. The oral bioavailability of valacyclovir is 3 to 5 times that of acyclovir, or about 50%.[36]

Valacyclovir has been approved for the treatment of herpes zoster (shingles) in immunocompromised patients. The side effect profile observed with valacyclovir is comparable in bioequivalent doses of acyclovir. Less than 1% of an administered dose of valacyclovir is recovered in the urine. Most of the dose is eliminated as acyclovir.

Valacyclovir

Ganciclovir. Ganciclovir, 9-[(1,3-dihydroxy-2-propoxy)methyl]guanine) or DHPG (Cytovene), is an analogue of acyclovir, with an additional hydroxymethyl group on the acyclic side chain.

Ganciclovir

This structural modification, while maintaining the activity against HSV and VSV possessed by acyclovir, greatly enhances the activity against CMV infection.

After administration, like acyclovir, ganciclovir is phosphorylated inside the cell by a virally encoded protein kinase to the monophosphate.[37] Host cell enzymes catalyze the formation of the triphosphate, which reaches more than 10-fold higher concentrations in infected cells than in uninfected cells. This selectivity is due to the entry and monophosphorylation step. Further phosphorylation with cellular enzymes occurs, and the triphosphate that is formed selectively inhibits viral DNA polymerase. Ganciclovir triphosphate is also incorporated into viral DNA causing strand breakage and cessation of elongation.[38]

The clinical usefulness of ganciclovir is limited by the toxicity of the drug. Ganciclovir causes myelosuppression, producing neutropenia, thrombocytopenia, and anemia. These effects are probably associated with inhibition of host cell DNA polymerase.[39] Potential central nervous system side effects include headaches, behavioral changes, and convulsions. Ganciclovir is mutagenic, carcinogenic, and teratogenic in animals.

Toxicity limits its therapeutic usefulness to the treatment and suppression of sight-threatening CMV retinitis in immunocompromised patients and to the prevention of life-threatening CMV infections in at-risk transplant patients.[21]

Oral and parenteral dosage forms of ganciclovir are available, but oral bioavailability is poor. Only 5 to 10% of an oral dose is absorbed. Intravenous administration is preferable. More than 90% of the unchanged drug is excreted in the urine. Ganciclovir for injection is available as a lyophilized sodium salt for reconstitution in normal saline, 5% dextrose in water, or lactated Ringer's solution. These solutions are strongly alkaline (pH ~11) and must be administered by slow, constant, intravenous infusion to avoid thrombophlebitis.

Famciclovir and Penciclovir.

Famciclovir is a diacetyl prodrug of penciclovir.[40] As a prodrug, it lacks antiviral activity. Penciclovir, 9-[4-hydroxy-3-hydroxymethylbut-1-yl] guanine, is an acyclic guanine nucleoside analogue. The structure is similar to that of acyclovir, except in penciclovir a side chain oxygen has been replaced by a carbon atom and an extra hydroxymethyl group is present. Inhibitory concentrations for HSV and VSV are typically within twice that of acyclovir. Penciclovir also inhibits the growth of hepatitis B virus.

Penciclovir inhibits viral DNA synthesis. In HSV- or VSV-infected cells, penciclovir is first phosphorylated by viral thymidine kinase[41] and then further elaborated to the triphosphate by host cell kinases. Penciclovir triphosphate is a competitive inhibitor of viral DNA polymerase. The pharmacokinetic parameters of penciclovir are quite different from those of acyclovir. Although penciclovir triphosphate is about 100-fold less potent in inhibiting viral DNA polymerase than acyclovir triphosphate, it is present in the tissues for longer periods and in much higher concentrations than acyclovir. Because it is possible to rotate the side chain of penciclovir into a pseudo-pentose, the triphosphorylated metabolite possesses a 3′-hydroxyl group. This relationship is shown below with guanosine. Penciclovir is not an obligate chain terminator,[41] but it does competitively inhibit DNA elongation. Penciclovir is excreted mostly unchanged in the urine.

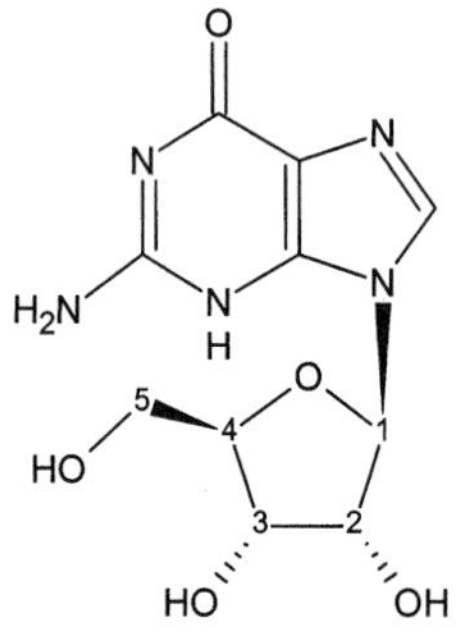

Guanosine 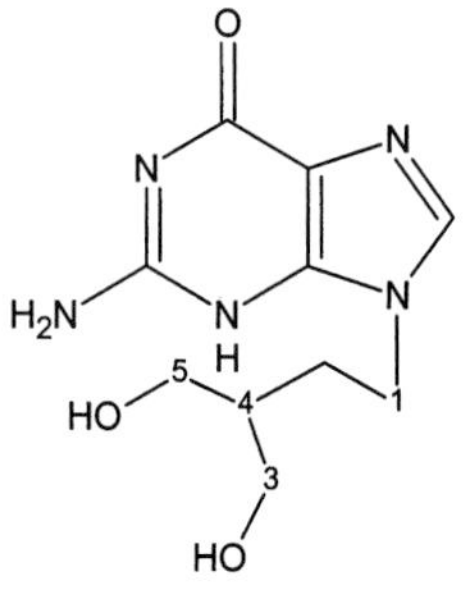   Penciclovir

Penciclovir (Denvir) has been approved for the topical treatment of recurrent herpes labialis (cold sores) in adults. It is effective against HSV-1 and HSV-2.[42] It is available as a cream containing 10% penciclovir.

Cidofovir.

Cidofovir, (S)-3-hydroxy-2-phosphonomethoxypropyl cytosine (HPMPC, Vistide), is an acyclonucleotide analogue that possesses broad-spectrum activity against several DNA viruses. Unlike other nucleotide analogues that are activated to nucleoside phosphates, Cidofovir is a phosphonic acid derivative. The phosphonic acid is not hydrolyzed by phosphatases in vivo but is phosphorylated by cellular kinases to yield a diphosphate. The diphosphate acts as an antimetabolite to deoxycytosine triphosphate (dCTP). Cidofovir diphosphate is a competitive inhibitor of viral DNA[43] polymerase and can be incorporated into the growing viral DNA strand, causing DNA chain termination.

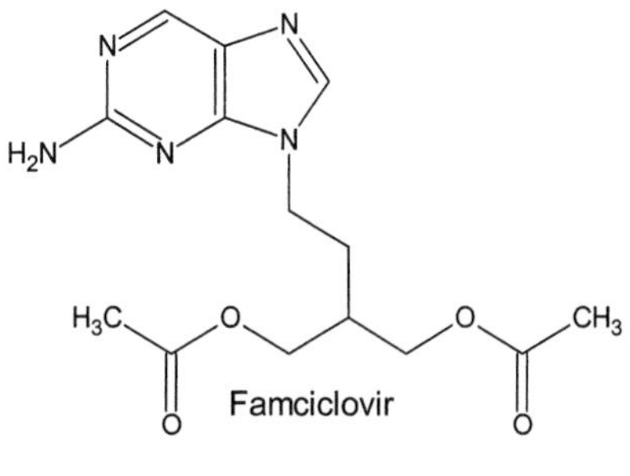

Famciclovir 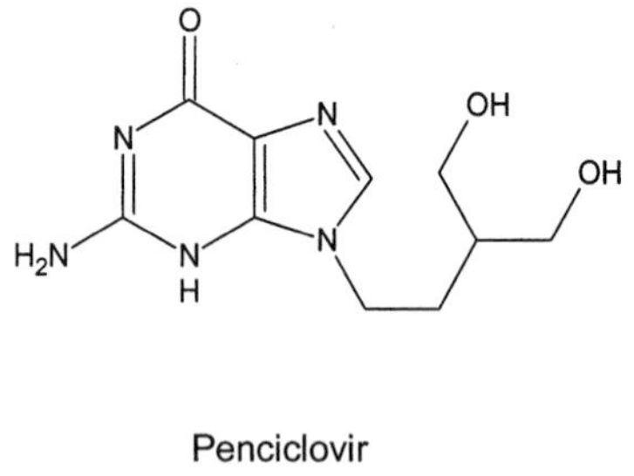   Penciclovir

Cidofovir possesses a high therapeutic index against CMV and has been approved for treating CMV retinitis in AIDS patients. Cidofovir is administered by slow, constant intravenous infusion in a dose of 5 mg/kg over a 1-hour period once a week for 2 weeks. This treatment is followed by a maintenance dose every 2 weeks. About 80% of a dose of Cidofovir is excreted unchanged in the urine, with a $t_{1/2\text{elim}}$ of 2 to 3 hours. The diphosphate antimetabolite, in contrast, has an extremely long half-life (17 to 30 hours).

The main dose-limiting toxicity of cidofovir involves renal impairment. Renal function must be monitored closely. Pretreatment with probenecid and prehydration with intravenous normal saline can be used to reduce the nephrotoxicity of the drug. Patients must be advised that cidofovir is not a cure for CMV retinitis. The disease may progress during or following treatment.

Cidofovir

Foscarnet Sodium. Trisodium phosphonoformate is an inorganic pyrophosphate analogue that inhibits replication in herpesviruses (CMV, HSV, and VSV) and retroviruses (HIV).[44] Foscarnet (Foscavir) is taken up slowly by the cells and does not undergo significant intracellular metabolism. Foscarnet is a reversible, noncompetitive inhibitor at the pyrophosphate-binding site of the viral DNA polymerase and reverse transcriptase. The ultimate effect is inhibition of the cleavage of pyrophosphate from deoxynucleotide triphosphates and a cessation of the incorporation of nucleoside triphosphates into DNA (with the concomitant release of pyrophosphate).[45] Since the inhibition is noncompetitive with respect to nucleoside triphosphate binding, foscarnet can act synergistically with nucleoside triphosphate antimetabolites (e.g., zidovudine and didanosine triphosphates) in the inhibition of viral DNA synthesis. Foscarnet does not require bioactivation by viral or cellular enzymes and, hence, can be effective against resistant viral strains that are deficient in virally encoded nucleoside kinases.[45]

Trisodium Phosphonoformate

Foscarnet is a second-line drug for the treatment of retinitis caused by CMV in AIDS patients. The drug causes metabolic abnormalities including increases or decreases in blood Ca^{2+} levels. Nephrotoxicity is common, and this side effect precludes the use of Foscarnet in other infections caused by herpesvirus or as single-agent therapy for HIV infection. Foscarnet is an excellent ligand for metal ion binding, which undoubtedly contributes to the electrolyte imbalances observed with the use of the drug.[46] Hypocalcemia, hypomagnesemia, hypokalemia, and hypophosphatemia and hyperphosphatemia are observed in patients treated with foscarnet. Side effects such as paresthesias, tetani, seizures, and cardiac arrhythmias may result. Since foscarnet is nephrotoxic, it may augment the toxic effects of other nephrotoxic drugs, such as amphotericin B and pentamidine, which are frequently used to control opportunistic infections in patients with AIDS.

Foscarnet sodium is available as a sterile solution intended for slow intravenous infusion. The solution is compatible with normal saline and 5% dextrose in water but is incompatible with calcium-containing buffers such as lactated Ringer's solution and total parenteral nutrition (TPN) preparations. Foscarnet reacts chemically with acid salts such as midazolam, vancomycin, and pentamidine. Over 80% of an injected dose of foscarnet is excreted unchanged in the urine.[44] The long elimination half-life of foscarnet is thought to result from its reversible sequestration into bone.[46]

Reverse Transcriptase Inhibitors

An early event in the replication of HIV-1 is reverse transcription, whereby genomic RNA from the virus is converted into a cDNA–RNA complex, then into double-stranded DNA ready for integration into the host chromosome. The enzyme that catalyzes this set of reactions is *reverse transcriptase*. Reverse transcriptase actually operates twice prior to the integration step. Its first function is the creation of the cDNA–RNA complex; reverse transcriptase acts alone in this step. In the second step, the RNA chain is digested away by RNase H while reverse transcriptase creates the double-stranded unintegrated DNA.

All of the classical antiretroviral agents are 2′,3′-dideoxynucleoside analogues. These compounds share a common mechanism of action in inhibiting the reverse transcriptase of HIV. Because reverse transcriptase acts early in the viral infection sequence, inhibitors of the enzyme block acute infection of cells but are only weakly active in chronically infected ones. Even though the reverse transcriptase inhibitors share a common mechanism of action, their pharmacological and toxicological profiles differ dramatically.

Zidovudine, USP. Zidovudine, 3′-azido-3′-deoxythymidine or AZT, is an analogue of thymidine that possesses antiviral activity against HIV-1, HIV-2, HTLV-1, and a number of other retroviruses. This nucleoside was synthesized in 1978 by Lin and Prusoff[47] as an intermediate in the preparation of amino acid analogues of thymidine. A screening program directed toward the identification of agents potentially effective for the treatment of AIDS patients led to the discovery of its unique antiviral properties 7 years later.[48] The next year, the clinical effectiveness of AZT in patients with AIDS and AIDS-related complex (ARC) was demonstrated.[49] AZT is active against retroviruses, a group of RNA viruses responsible for AIDS and some kinds of leukemia. Retroviruses possess a reverse transcriptase or a RNA-directed DNA polymerase that directs the synthesis of a DNA copy (proviral DNA) of the viral RNA genome that is duplicated, circularized, and incorporated into the DNA of an infected cell. The drug enters the host cells by diffusion and is phosphorylated by cellular thymidine kinase. Thymidylate kinase then converts the monophosphate into diphosphates and triphosphates. The rate-determining step is conversion to the diphosphate, so high levels of monophosphorylated AZT accumulate in the cell. Low levels of diphosphate and triphosphate are present. Zidovudine triphosphate competitively inhibits reverse transcriptase with respect to thymidine triphosphate. The 3′-azido group prevents formation of a 5′,3′-phosphodiester bond, so AZT causes DNA chain termination, yielding an incomplete proviral DNA.[50] Zidovudine monophosphate also competitively inhibits cellular thymidylate kinase, thus decreasing intracellular levels of thymidine triphosphate. The antiviral selectivity of AZT is due to its greater $(100\times)$[51] affinity for HIV reverse transcriptase than for human DNA polymerases. The human γ-DNA polymerase of mitochondria is more sensitive to zidovudine; this may contribute to the toxicity associated with the drug's use. Resistance is common and is due to point mutations at multiple sites in reverse transcriptase, leading to a lower affinity for the drug.[52]

Zidovudine is recommended for the management of adult patients with symptomatic HIV infection (AIDS or ARC) who have a history of confirmed *Pneumocystis carinii* pneumonia or an absolute CD4$^+$ (T4 or T$_H$ cell) lymphocyte count below 200/mm^3 before therapy. The hematological toxicity of the drug precludes its use in asymptomatic patients. Anemia and granulocytopenia are the most common toxic effects associated with AZT.

For oral administration, AZT is supplied as 100-mg capsules and as a syrup containing 10 mg AZT per mL. The injectable form of AZT contains 10 mg/mL and is injected intravenously. AZT is absorbed rapidly from the gastrointestinal tract and distributes well into body compartments, including the cerebrospinal fluid (CSF). It is metabolized rapidly to an inactive glucuronide in the liver. Only about 15% is excreted unchanged. Because AZT is an aliphatic azide, it is heat and light sensitive. It should be protected from light and stored at 15 to 25°C.

Zidovudine

Didanosine. Didanosine (Videx, ddI) is 2′,3′-dideoxyinosine (ddI), a synthetic purine nucleoside analogue that is bioactivated to 2′,3′-dideoxy-ATP (ddATP) by host cellular enzymes.[53] The metabolite, ddATP, accumulates intracellu-

larly, where it inhibits reverse transcriptase and is incorporated into viral DNA to cause chain termination in HIV-infected cells. The potency of didanosine is 10- to 100-fold less than that of AZT with respect to antiviral activity and cytotoxicity, but the drug causes less myelosuppression than AZT causes.[54]

Didanosine is recommended for the treatment of patients with advanced HIV infection who have received prolonged treatment with AZT but have become intolerant to, or experienced immunosuppression from, the drug. AZT and ddI act synergistically to inhibit HIV replication in vitro, and ddI is effective against some AZT-resistant strains of HIV.[55] Painful peripheral neuropathy (tingling, numbness, and pain in the hands and feet) and pancreatitis (nausea, abdominal pain, elevated amylase) are the major dose-limiting toxicities of didanosine. Didanosine is given orally in the form of buffered chewable tablets or as a solution prepared from the powder. Both oral dosage forms are buffered to prevent acidic decomposition of ddI to hypoxanthine in the stomach. Despite the buffering of the dosage forms, oral bioavailability is quite low and highly variable. Less than 20% of a dose is excreted in the urine, which suggests extensive metabolism.[56] Food interferes with absorption, so the oral drug must be given at least 1 hour before or 2 hours after meals. High-dose therapy can cause hyperuricemia in some patients because of the increased purine load.

Didanosine

Zalcitabine, USP. Zalcitabine, 2′,3′-dideoxycytidine or ddCyd, is an analogue of cytosine that demonstrates activity against HIV-1 and HIV-2, including strains resistant to AZT. The potency (in peripheral blood mononuclear cells) is similar to that of AZT, but the drug is more active in populations of monocytes and macrophages as well as in resting cells.

Zalcitabine enters human cells by carrier-facilitated diffusion and undergoes initial phosphorylation by deoxycytidine kinase. The monophosphorylated compound is further metabolized to the active metabolite, dideoxycytidine-5′-triphosphate (ddCTP), by cellular kinases.[57] ddCTP inhibits reverse transcriptase by competitive inhibition with dCTP. Most likely, ddCTP causes termination of the elongating viral DNA chain.

Zalcitabine inhibits host mitochondrial DNA synthesis at low concentrations. This effect may contribute to its clinical toxicity.[58]

The oral bioavailability of zalcitabine is over 80% in adults and less in children.[59] The major dose-limiting side effect is peripheral neuropathy, characterized by pain, paresthesias, and hypesthesia, beginning in the distal lower extremities. These side effects are typically evident after several months of therapy with zalcitabine. A potentially fatal pancreatitis is another toxic effect of treatment with ddC. The drug has been approved for the treatment of HIV infection in adults with advanced disease who are intolerant to AZT or who have disease progression while receiving AZT. ddC is combined with AZT for the treatment of advanced HIV infection.

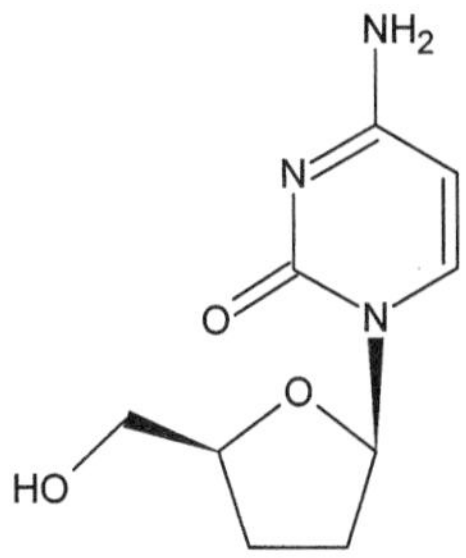

Zalcitabine

Stavudine. Stavudine, 2'3'-didehydro-2'-deoxythymidine (D4T, Zerit), is an unsaturated pyrimidine nucleoside that is related to thymidine. The drug inhibits the replication of HIV by a mechanism similar to that of its close congener, AZT.[60] Stavudine is bioactivated by cellular enzymes to a triphosphate. The triphosphate competitively inhibits the incorporation of thymidine triphosphate (TTP) into retroviral DNA by reverse transcriptase.[61] Stavudine also causes termination of viral DNA elongation through its incorporation into DNA.

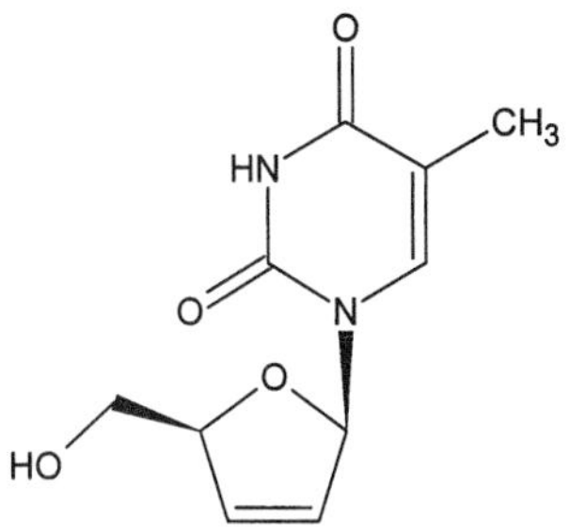

Stavudine

Stavudine is available as capsules for oral administration. The drug is acid stable and well absorbed (about 90%) following oral administration. Stavudine has a short half-life (1 to 2 hours) in plasma and is excreted largely unchanged (85 to 90%) in the urine.[62] As with ddC, the primary dose-limiting effect is peripheral neuropathy. At the recommended dosages, approximately 15 to 20% of patients experience symptoms of peripheral neuropathy. Stavudine is recommended for the treatment of adults with advanced HIV infection who are intolerant of other approved therapies or who have experienced clinical or immunological deterioration while receiving these therapies.

Lamivudine. Lamivudine is (−)-2',3'-dideoxy-3'-thiacytidine, (−)-β-L- (2R,5S)-1,3-oxathiolanylcytosine, 3TC, or (−)-(S)-ddC. Lamivudine is a synthetic nucleoside analogue that differs from 2',3'-dideoxycytidine (ddC) by the substitution of a sulfur atom in place of a methylene group at the 3' position of the ribose ring. In early clinical trials, lamivudine exhibited highly promising antiretroviral activity against HIV and low toxicity in the dosages studied.[63, 64] Preliminary pharmacokinetic studies indicated that it exhibited good oral bioavailability (F = ~80%) and a plasma half-life of 2 to 4 hours.[63]

It is interesting that the unnatural stereoisomer (−)-(S)-ddC exhibits greater antiviral activity against HIV than the natural enantiomer (+)-(S)-ddC.[65] Both enantiomers are bioactivated by cellular kinases to the corresponding triphosphates.[66] Both SddCTP isomers inhibit HIV reverse transcriptase and are incorporated into viral DNA to cause chain termination. (+)-S-ddCTP inhibits cellular DNA polymerases much more strongly than (−)-SddCTP, explaining the greater toxicity associated with (+)-(S)-ddC. Initial metabolic comparison of SddCTP isomers has failed to explain the greater potency of the (−)-isomer against HIV. Therefore, although the intracellular accumulation of (−)-S-ddCTP was twice that of (+)-S-ddCTP, the latter was 1½ times more potent as an inhibitor of HIV reverse transcriptase, and the two isomers were incorporated into viral DNA at comparable rates. The puzzle was solved with the discovery of a cellular 3',5'-exonuclease, which was found to cleave terminal (+)-S-ddCMP incorporated into viral DNA 6 times faster than (−)-S-ddCMP from the viral DNA terminus.

Resistance to lamivudine develops rapidly as a result of a mutation in codon 184 of the gene that encodes HIV-RT when the drug is used as monotherapy for HIV infection.[64] When combined with AZT, however, lamivudine caused substantial increases in CD4$^+$ counts. The elevated counts were sustained over the course of therapy.[67] The codon mutation that causes resistance to lamivudine suppresses AZT resistance,[67] thus increasing the susceptibility of the virus to the drug combination.

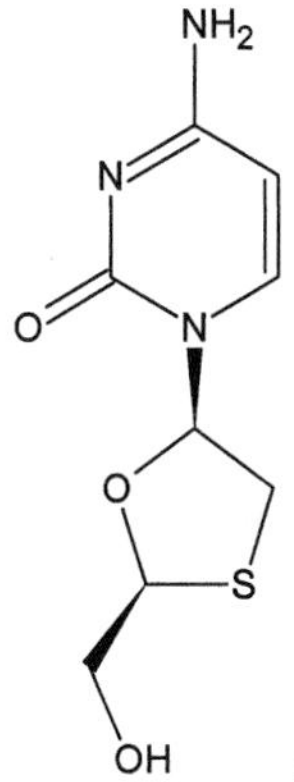

Lamivudine

Miscellaneous Nucleoside Antimetabolites

Ribavirin, USP. Ribavirin is 1-β-D-ribofuranosyl-1,2,4-thiazole-3-carboxamide. The compound is a purine nucleoside analogue with a modified base and a D-ribose sugar moiety. The structure of ribavirin is shown below.

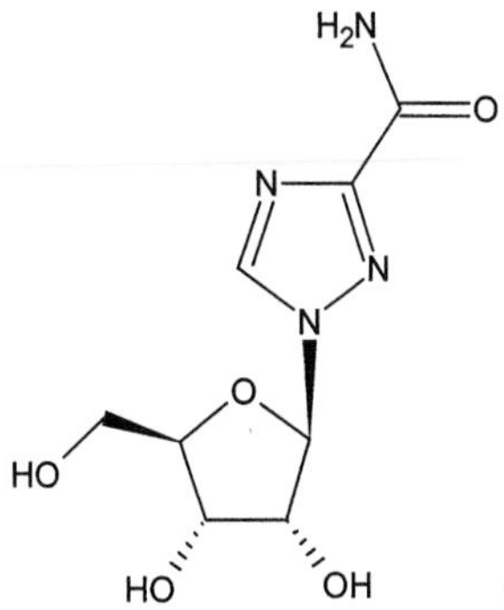

Ribavirin

Ribavirin inhibits the replication of a very wide variety of RNA and DNA viruses,[68] including orthomyxoviruses, paramyxoviruses, arenaviruses, bunyaviruses, herpesviruses, adenoviruses, poxvirus, vaccinia, influenza virus, parainfluenza virus, and rhinovirus. In spite of the broad spectrum of activity of ribavirin, the drug has been approved for only one therapeutic indication—the treatment of severe lower respiratory infections caused by RSV in carefully selected hospitalized infants and young children.

The mechanism of action of ribavirin is not known. The broad antiviral spectrum of ribavirin, however, suggests multiple modes of action.[69] The nucleoside is bioactivated by viral and host cellular kinases to give the monophosphate (RMP) and the triphosphate (RTP). RMP inhibits inosine monophosphate (IMP) dehydrogenase, thereby preventing the conversion of IMP to xanthine monophosphate (XMP). XMP is required for guanosine triphosphate (GTP) synthesis. RTP inhibits viral RNA polymerases. It also prevents the end capping of viral mRNA by inhibiting guanyl-N'-methyltransferase. Emergence of viral resistance to ribavirin has not been documented.

Ribavirin occurs as a white, crystalline, polymorphic solid that is soluble in water and chemically stable. It is supplied as a powder to be reconstituted in an aqueous aerosol containing 20 mg/mL of sterile water. The aerosol is administered with a small-particle aerosol generator (SPAG). Deterioration in respiratory function, bacterial pneumonia, pneumothorax, and apnea have been reported in severely ill infants and children with RSV infection. The role of ribavirin in these events has not been determined. Anemia, headache, abdominal pain, and lethargy have been reported in patients receiving oral ribavirin.

Unlabeled uses of ribavirin include aerosol treatment of influenza types A and B and oral treatment of hepatitis, genital herpes, and Lassa fever. Ribavirin does not protect cells against the cytotoxic effects of the AIDS virus.

NEWER AGENTS FOR THE TREATMENT OF HIV INFECTION

When HIV-1 was characterized and identified as the causative agent of AIDS in 1983,[70, 71] scientists from all over the world joined in the search for a prevention or cure for the disease. Mapping the HIV-1 genome and elucidating the replication cycle of the virus have supplied key information.[72] Biochemical targets, many of which are proteins involved in the replication cycle of the virus, have been cloned and sequenced. These have been used to develop rapid, mechanism-based assays for the virus to complement tissue culture screens for whole virus. Several of the biochemical steps that have been characterized have served as targets for clinical candidates as well as for successfully licensed drugs.[73, 74]

Despite the many advances in the understanding of the HIV virus and its treatment, there is not yet a cure for the infection. Emergent resistance[75] to clinically proven drugs such as the reverse transcriptase inhibitors and the protease inhibitors has complicated the picture of good therapeutic targets. The idea of using a vaccine as a therapeutic tool has

been complicated by the fact that the vaccine apparently can modulate its antigenic structures in its chronic infectious state.[76]

Vaccines. The chronology of vaccine development and use in the 20th century is nothing short of a medical miracle. Diseases such as smallpox and polio, which once ravaged large populations, have become distant memories. The technique of sensitizing a human immune system by exposure to an antigen so that an anamnestic response is generated on subsequent exposure seems quite simple on the surface. Hence, it is natural that a vaccine approach to preventing AIDS be tried. The successes achieved so far have involved live/attenuated or killed whole-cell vaccines and, in more recent times, recombinant coat proteins.

Successes with vaccines of the live/attenuated (low-virulence), killed whole virus or the recombinant coat protein types have primarily involved acute viral diseases in which a natural infection and recovery lead to long-term immunity.

This type of immunity is of the humoral, or antibody-mediated, type, and it is the basis for successes in immunizing the human population. Causative organisms of chronic infections do not respond to vaccines. The AIDS virus causes a chronic disease in which infection persists despite a strong antibody response to the virus (at least initially, HIV can circumvent the humoral response to infection by attacking and killing CD4$^+$ T cells). These T cells, also known as T-helper cells, upregulate the immune response. By eradicating the CD4$^+$ cells, the HIV virus effectively destroys the immune system. Cell-mediated immune responses are critical to the prevention and treatment of HIV infection. To be effective, a vaccine against HIV must elicit an appropriate cellular immune response in addition to a humoral response. In other words, the vaccine must have the potential to act on both branches of the immune system.

The initial work on vaccine development focused on isotypic variants of the HIV envelope glycoprotein gp120 obtained by recombinant DNA techniques. This target was chosen because of concerns about the safety of live/attenuated vaccines. The gp120 glycoprotein is a coat protein, and if great care is taken, a virus-free vaccine is obtainable. Moreover, glycoprotein gp120 is the primary target for neutralizing antibodies associated with the first (attachment) step in HIV infection.[77] Early vaccines were so ineffective that the National Institutes of Health suspended plans for massive clinical trials in high-risk individuals.[78] There are a number of reasons why the vaccine failed.[79] There are multiple subtypes of the virus throughout the world; the virus can infect by means of both cell-free and cell-associated forms; the virus has demonstrated its own immunosuppressive, immunopathological, and infection-enhancing properties of parts of the envelope glycoprotein; and vaccines have not been able to stimulate and maintain high enough levels of immunity to be effective.

The failure of the first generation of AIDS vaccines led to a reexamination of the whole AIDS vaccine effort.[79] As a guide for research efforts, a number of criteria for an "ideal" AIDS vaccine have been developed. The "ideal" AIDS vaccine should (*a*) be safe, (*b*) elicit a protective immune response in a high proportion of vaccinated individuals, (*c*) stimulate both cellular and humoral branches of the immune system, *(d)* protect components against all major HIV subtypes, *(e)* induce long-lasting protection, *(f)* induce local immunity in both genital and rectal mucosa, and *(g)* be practical for worldwide delivery and administration. It is not yet known how well the second-generation AIDS vaccines will satisfy the above criteria or when one might receive approval for widespread use in humans.

A new era in the treatment of AIDS and ARC was ushered in with the advent of some clinically useful, potent inhibitors of HIV. For the first time in the history of AIDS the death rate reversed itself. There are several different classes of drugs that can be used to treat HIV infection. These are the nucleoside reverse transcriptase inhibitors (NRTIs), the nonnucleoside reverse transcriptase inhibitors (NNRTIs), the HIV protease inhibitors (PIs), the HIV entry inhibitors, and the HIV integrase inhibitors (IN). Presently, at least 14 antiretroviral agents belonging to three distinct classes (NRTIs, NNRTIs, PIs) have been licensed for use in patients in the United States. All of these agents are limited by rapid development of resistance and cross-resistance, so commonly three drugs are used at the same time, each acting at a different point in HIV replication. These drugs can effect dramatic reductions in viral load, but eventually, as resistance develops, the virus reasserts itself.

Nonnucleoside Reverse Transcriptase Inhibitors (NNRTIs)

Cloned HIV-1 reverse transcriptase facilitates the study of the effects of a novel compound on the kinetics of the enzyme. Random screening of chemical inventories by the pharmaceutical industry has led to the discovery of several NNRTIs of the enzyme. These inhibitors represent several structurally distinct classes. The NNRTIs share a number of common biochemical and pharmacological properties.[74, 80, 81] Unlike the nucleoside antimetabolites, the NNRTIs do not require bioactivation by kinases to yield phosphate esters. They are not incorporated into the growing DNA chain. Instead, they bind to an allosteric site that is distinct from the substrate (nucleoside triphosphate)-binding site of reverse transcriptase. The inhibitor can combine with either free or substrate-bound enzyme, interfering with the action of both. Such binding distorts the enzyme so that it cannot form the enzyme–substrate complex at its normal rate, and once formed, the complex does not decompose at the normal rate to yield products. Increasing the substrate concentration does not reverse these effects. Hence, NNRTIs exhibit a classical noncompetitive inhibition pattern with the enzyme.

The NNRTIs are extremely potent in in vitro cell culture assays and inhibit HIV-1 at nanomolar concentrations. NNRTIs inhibit reverse transcriptase selectively; they do not inhibit the reverse transcriptases of other retroviruses, including HIV-2 and simian immunodeficiency virus (SIV). The NNRTIs have high therapeutic indices (in contrast to the nucleosides) and do not inhibit mammalian DNA polymerases. The NRTIs and NNRTIs are expected to exhibit a synergistic effect on HIV, since they interact with different mechanisms on the enzyme. The chief problem with the NNRTIs is the rapid emergence of resistance among HIV isolates.[75] Resistance is due to point mutations in the gene coding for the enzyme. Cross-resistance between structurally different NNRTIs is more common than between NNRTIs and NRTIs. In the future, clinical use of the NNRTIs is expected to use combinations with the nucleosides to reduce toxicity to the latter, to take advantage of additive or synergistic effects, and to reduce the emergence of viral resistance.[75, 80] The tricyclic compound nevirapine (Viramune),[82] the bis(heteroacyl)piperazine (BHAP) derivative delavirdine (Rescriptor),[83] and efavirenz[84] have been approved for use in combination with NRTIs such as AZT for the treatment of HIV infection. Numerous others, including the quinoxaline derivative GW-420867X,[84] the tetrahydroimidazobenzodiazpinone (TIBO) analogue R-82913,[85] and calanolide-A[84] are in clinical trials.

Nevirapine. Nevirapine (Viramune)[82] is more than 90% absorbed by the oral route and is widely distributed throughout the body. It distributes well into breast milk and crosses the placenta. Transplacental concentrations are about 50% those of serum. The drug is extensively transformed by cytochrome P-450 to inactive hydroxylated metabolites; it may undergo enterohepatic recycling. The half-life decreases from 45 to 23 hours over a 2- to 4-week period because of autoinduction. Elimination occurs through the kidney, with less than 3% of the parent compound excreted in the urine.[82] Dosage forms are supplied as a 50 mg/5 mL oral suspension and a 200-mg tablet.

Nevirapine

Delavirdine. Delavirdine (Rescriptor)[83] must be used with at least two additional antiretroviral agents to treat HIV-1 infections. The oral absorption of delavirdine is rapid, and peak plasma concentrations develop in 1 hour. Extensive metabolism occurs in the liver by cytochrome P-450 (CYP) isozyme 3A (CYP 3A) or possibly CYP 2D6. Bioavailability is 85%. Unlike nevirapine, which is 48% protein bound, delavirdine is more than 98% protein bound. The half-life is 2 to 11 hours, and elimination is 44% in feces, 51% in urine, and less than 5% unchanged in urine. Delavirdine induces its own metabolism.[83] Oral dosage forms are supplied as a 200-mg capsule and a 100-mg tablet.

Efavirenz. Efavirenz (Sustiva)[84] is also mandated for use with at least two other antiretroviral agents. The compound is more than 99% protein bound, and CSF concentrations exceed the free fraction in the serum. Metabolism occurs in the liver. The half-life of a single dose of efavirenz is 52 to 76 hours, and 40 to 55 after multiple doses (the drug induces its own metabolism). Peak concentration is achieved

Delavirdine

in 3 to 8 hours. Elimination is 14 to 34% in urine (as metabolites) and 16 to 41% in feces (primarily as efavirenz).[84] The oral dosage form is supplied as a capsule.

Efavirenz

HIV Protease Inhibitors

A unique biochemical target in the HIV-1 replication cycle was revealed when HIV protease was cloned and expressed[86, 87] in *Escherichia coli*. HIV protease is an enzyme that cleaves gag-pro propeptides to yield active enzymes that function in the maturation and propagation of new virus. The catalytically active protease is a symmetric dimer of two identical 99 amino acid subunits, each contributing the triad Asp-Thr-Gly to the active site.[86, 87] The homodimer is unlike monomeric aspartyl proteases (renin, pepsin, cathepsin D), which also have different substrate specificities. The designs of some inhibitors[86, 87] for HIV-1 protease exploit the C_2 symmetry of the enzyme. HIV-1 protease has active site specificity for the triad Tyr-Phe-Pro in the unit Ser-(Thr)-Xaa-Xaa-Tyr-Phe-Pro, where Xaa is an arbitrary amino acid.

HIV protease inhibitors are designed to mimic the transition state of hydrolysis at the active site; these compounds are called *analogue inhibitors*. Hydrolysis of a peptide bond proceeds through a transition state that is sp^3 hybridized and, hence, tetrahedral. The analogue inhibitors possess a preexisting sp^3 hybridized center that will be drawn into the active site (one hopes with high affinity) but will not be cleavable by the enzyme. This principle has been used to prepare hundreds of potentially useful transition state inhibitors.[86, 87] Unfortunately, very few of these are likely to be clinically successful candidates for the treatment of HIV infection. Since HIV protease inhibitors are aimed at arresting replication of the virus at the maturation step to prevent the spread of cellular infection, they should possess good oral bioavailability and a relatively long duration of action. A long half-life is also desirable because of the known development of resistance by HIV under selective antiviral pressure.[74, 75] Resistance develops by point mutations.

Most of the early protease inhibitors are high-molecular-weight, dipeptide- or tripeptide-like structures, generally with low water solubility. The bioavailability of these compounds is low, and the half-life of elimination is very short because of hydrolysis or hepatic metabolism.[88] Strategies aimed at increasing water solubility and metabolic stability have led to the development of several highly promising clinical candidates. Saquinavir (Invirase),[81] indinavir (Crixivan),[89] ritonavir (Norvir),[90] nelfinavir (Viracept),[91] and amprenavir (Agenerase)[92] have been approved for the treatment of HIV-infected patients. A number of others are in clinical trials.

There is an important caution for the use of protease inhibitors. As a class, they cause dyslipidemia, which includes elevated cholesterol and triglycerides and a redistribution of body fat centrally to cause the "protease paunch," buffalo hump, facial atrophy, and breast enlargement. These agents also cause hyperglycemia.

Saquinavir. Saquinavir (Invirase)[89] is well tolerated following oral administration. Absorption of saquinavir is poor but is increased with a fatty meal. The drug does not distribute into the CSF, and it is approximately 98% bound to plasma proteins. Saquinavir is extensively metabolized by the first-pass effect. Bioavailability is 4% from a hard capsule and 12 to 15% from a soft capsule. Saquinavir lowers p24 antigen levels in HIV-infected patients, elevates $CD4^+$ counts, and exerts a synergistic antiviral effect when combined with reverse transcriptase inhibitors such as AZT and ddC.[93–95] Although HIV-1 resistance to saquinavir and other HIV protease inhibitors occurs in vivo, it is believed to be less stringent and less frequent than resistance to the reverse transcriptase inhibitors.[96] Nevertheless, cross-resistance between different HIV protease inhibitors appears to be common and additive,[97] suggesting that using combinations of inhibitors from this class would not constitute rational prescribing. The drug should be used in combination with at least two other antiretroviral drugs to minimize resistance. Dosage forms are Invirase (hard capsule) and Fortovase (soft capsule).

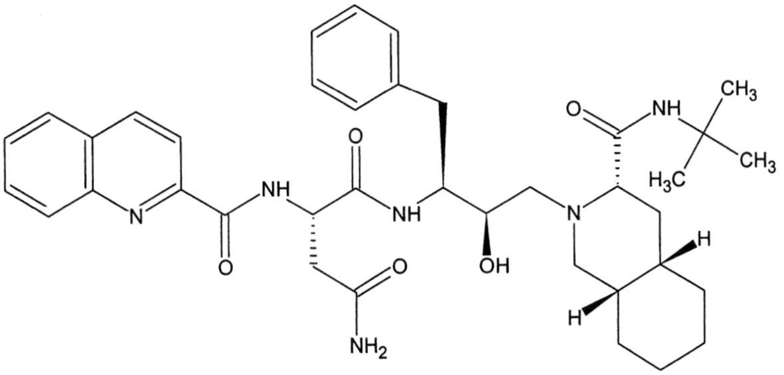

Saquinavir

Indinavir.   When administered with a high fat diet, indinavir (Crixivan)[90] achieves a maximum serum concentration of 77% of the administered dose. The drug is 60% bound in the plasma. It is extensively metabolized by CYP 3A4, and seven metabolites have been identified. Oral bioavailability is good, with a t_{max} of 0.8 ± 0.3 hour. The half-life of elimination is 1.8 hour, and the elimination products are detectable in feces and urine. Indinavir also causes dyslipidemia. The available dosage forms are capsules of 200, 333, and 400 mg.

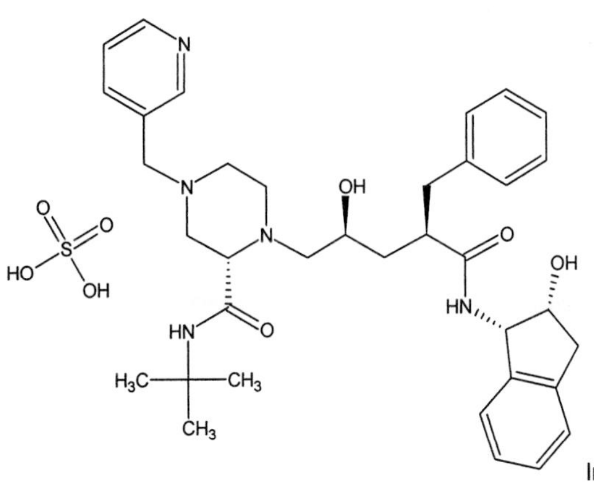

Indinavir

Ritonavir, Amprenavir, and Nelfinavir.   Ritonavir (Norvir),[98] amprenavir (Agenerase),[99] and nelfinavir (Viracept)[100] (see structures on page 386) have similar properties and cautionary statements. All cause dyslipidemia, and they have a host of drug interactions, mainly because they inhibit CYP 3A4. These agents must always be used with at least two other antiretroviral agents. Used properly, the protease inhibitors are an important part of HIV therapy.

A number of nonpeptide inhibitors of HIV protease have been developed as a result of two very different approaches. For example, the C_2 symmetry of the active site of the enzyme was exploited in the structure-based design of the symmetric cyclic urea derivative DMP-323.[101] This inhibitor exhibited potent activity against the protease in vitro, excellent anti-HIV activity in cell culture, and promising bioavailability in experimental animals. In phase I clinical trials, however, the bioavailability of DMP-323 was poor and highly variable, possibly because of its low water solubility and a

high fraction of hepatic metabolism. Subsequent synthesis of nonsymmetric derivatives DMP-850[101] (below) and DMP-851[101] yielded in vitro antiviral potency comparable with that of the already-approved PIs. These were selected as clinical candidates on the basis of their favorable pharmacokinetics in dogs. In a second approach, random screening of chemical inventories yielded the 5,6-dehydropyran-2-one–based inhibitor[102] PD-178390 (below). This compound, in addition to having good potency against HIV protease and good anti-HIV activity in cell culture, exhibits high bioavailability in experimental animals. PD-178390 appears not to share the resistance profile of the other PIs, and no virus resistant to the compound emerged, even during the prolonged in vitro selection.

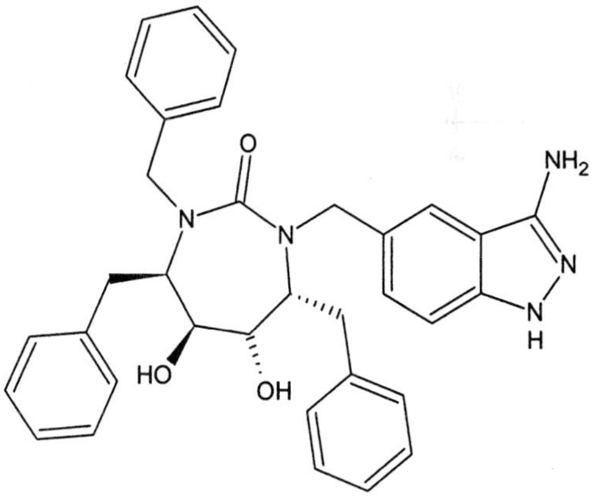

DMP-850

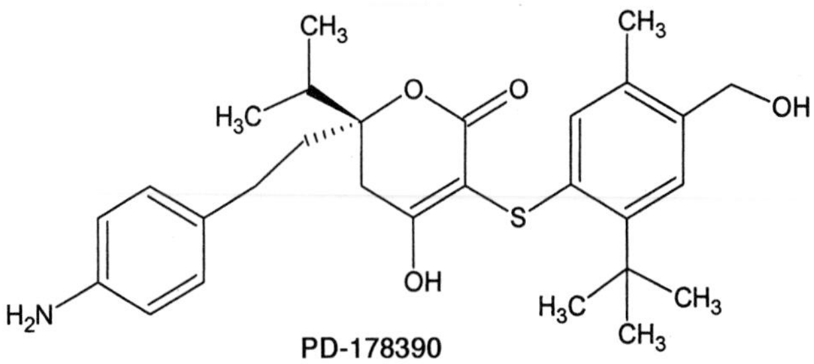

PD-178390

Dipeptide PIs containing 2-hydroxy-3-amino-4-arylbutanoic acid in their scaffold showed promising preclinical results. JE-2147[103] (below), containing the allophenylnorstatin

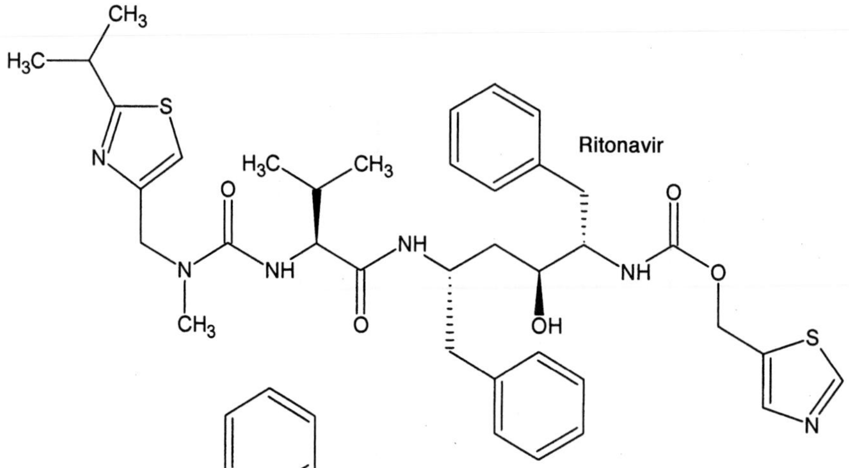

Ritonavir

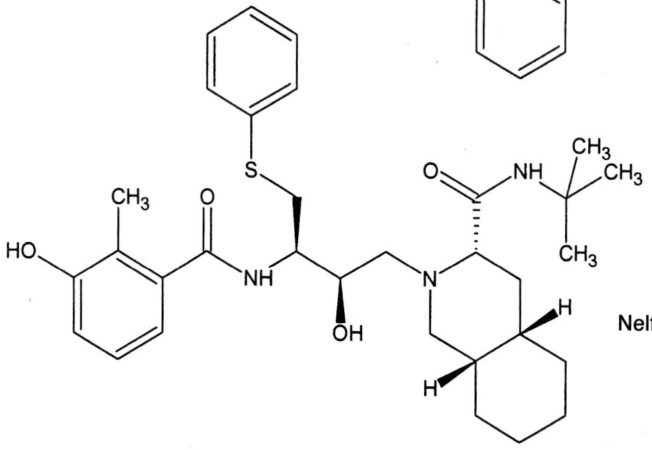

Nelfinavir

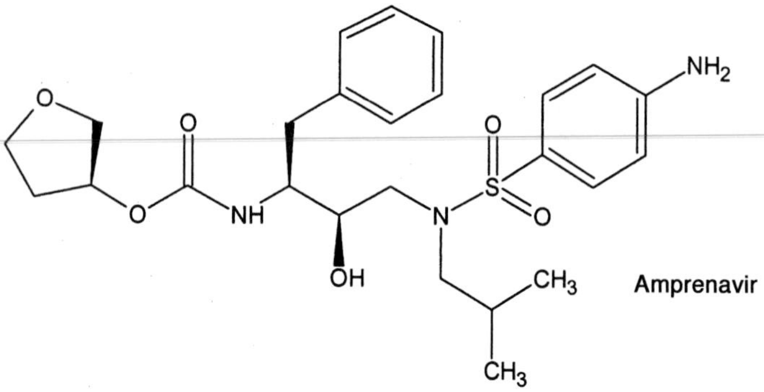

Amprenavir

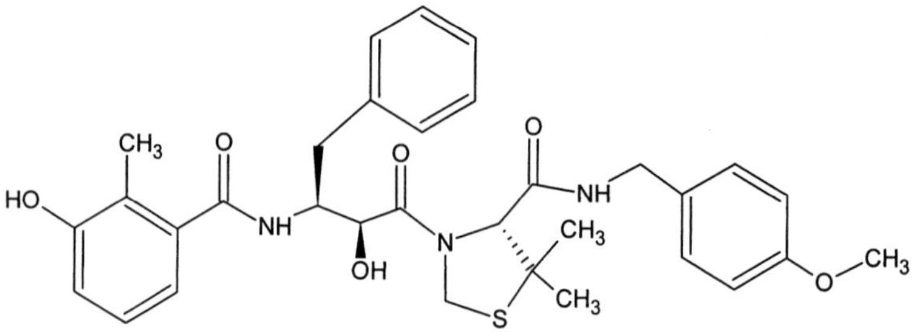

JE-2147

moiety, exhibited potent in vitro anti-HIV activity. JE-2147 appears to fully retain its susceptibility against a variety of HIV strains resistant to multiple approved PIs and exhibits good oral bioavailability and a good pharmacokinetic profile in two animal species. Also, emergence of resistance was considerably delayed with JE-2147.

HIV Entry Inhibitors

Entry of HIV into a cell is a complex process that involves several specific membrane protein interactions. Initially, viral glycoprotein gp120 mediates the virus attachment via its binding to at least two host membrane receptors, CD4$^+$ and the chemokine coreceptor. This bivalent interaction induces a conformational change in the viral fusion protein gp41. Protein gp41 acts as the anchor for gp120 in the virus. With the conformational change, the viral envelope fuses with the host cell membrane. In addition to gp120–chemokine receptor interaction, the fusion activity of gp41 is currently being explored as a novel target for antiretroviral therapy. At least one agent from each class is in clinical testing.

Chemokine Receptor Binders

Most HIV-1 isolates rely on the CCR5 coreceptor for entry (R5 strains). In later stages of the disease, however, more pathogenic selection variants of the virus emerge in about 40% of individuals, which use the CXCR4 coreceptor in addition to CCR5 (R5X4 strains) or the CXCR4 receptor only (X4 strains). Bicyclam compound AMD-3100[104] was the first compound identified as a CXCR4-specific inhibitor that interferes with the replication of X4 but not R5 viruses. The compound is currently in phase II clinical evaluations. It is used as an injectable agent because of its limited bioavailability.

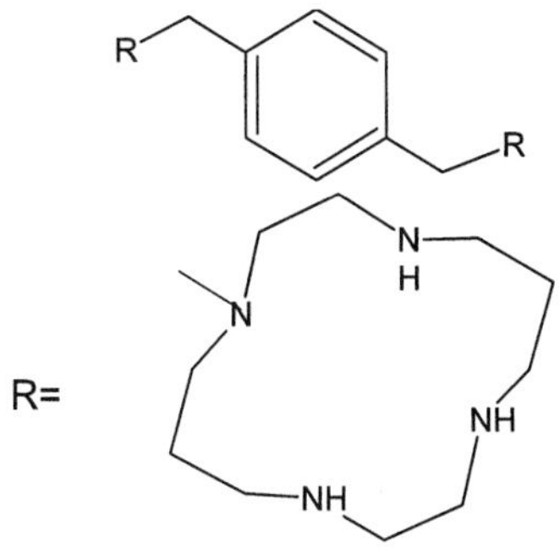

AMD-3100

Several positively charged 9- to14-mer peptides have been described as capable of blocking the CXCR4 coreceptor. A small molecule, TAK-779,[105] exhibits high-affinity binding to the CCR5 coreceptor, specifically blocking R5 isolates.

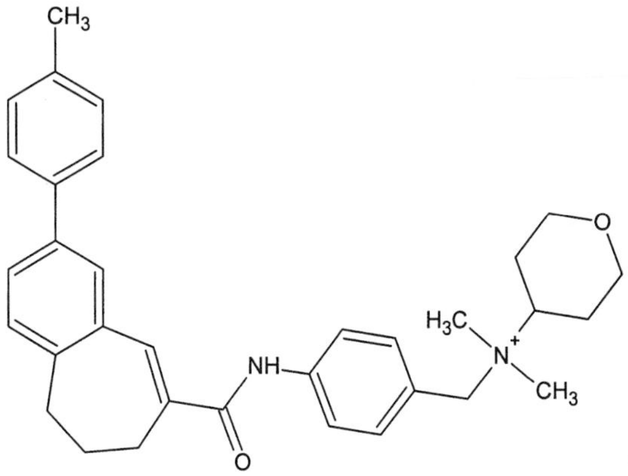

TAK-779

Inhibitors of gp41 Fusion Activity

The fusion of the HIV-1 viral envelope with host plasma membrane is mediated by gp41, a transmembrane subunit of the HIV-1 glycoprotein subunit complex. Pentafuside[106] (T-20) is a 36-mer peptide that is derived from the C-termi-

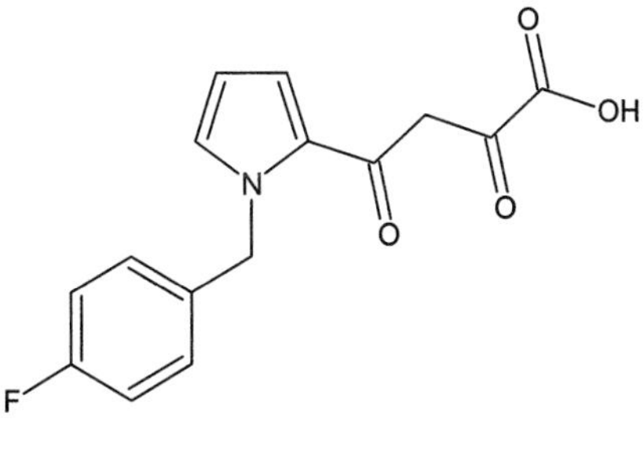

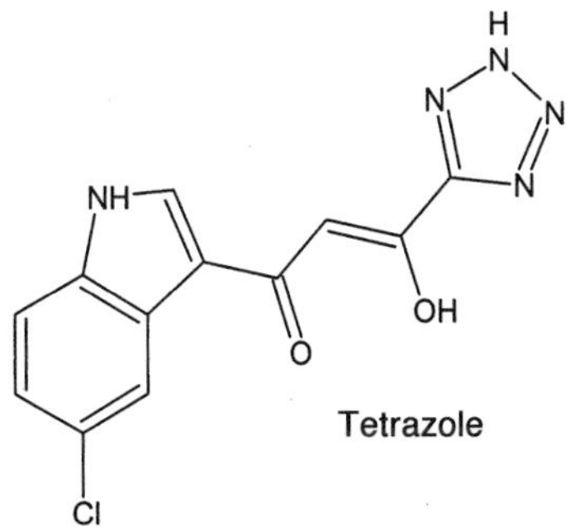

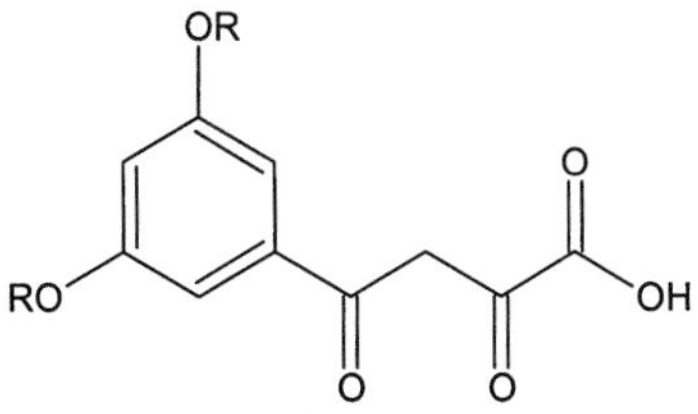

R=benz

Diketo

Tetrazole

nal repeat of gp41. Pentafuside appears to inhibit the formation of the fusion-competent conformation of gp41 by interfering with the interaction between its C- and N-terminal repeat. Pentafuside is a potent inhibitor of HIV-1 clinical isolates, and it is currently in phase II clinical trials.

Integrase (IN) Inhibitors

Two closely related types of small molecules that block strand transfer catalyzed by recombinant integrase have been identified. Both types show in vitro antiviral activity. The diketo acids[107] (above) inhibit strand transfer catalyzed by recombinant integrase with an IC_{50} less than 0.1 μM. Mutations that conferred resistance to the diketo acids mapped near conserved residues in the IN enzyme. This finding demonstrates that the compounds have a highly specific mechanism of action. X-ray crystallography of the bound tetrazole[108] derivative (above) revealed that the inhibitor was centered in the active site of IN near acidic catalytic residues.

Acknowledgment

Portions of this text were taken from Dr. Arnold Martin's chapter in the tenth edition of this book.

REFERENCES

1. Condit, R. C.: Principles of virology. In Knipe, D. M., and Howley, P. M. (eds.). Fundamental Virology, 4th ed. New York, Lippincott Williams & Wilkins, 2001, p. 19.
2. Harrison, S. C.: Principles of viral structure. In Knipe, D. M., and Howley, P. M. (eds.). Fundamental Virology, 4th ed. New York, Lippincott Williams & Wilkins, 2001, p. 53.
3. Wagner, E. K., and Hewlett, M. J. (eds.): Basic Virology. Malden, MA, Blackwell Science, 1999, p. 12.
4. Wagner, E. K., and Hewlett, M. J. (eds.): Basic Virology. Malden, MA, Blackwell Science, 1999, p. 61.
5. Beale, J. M., Jr.: Immunobiologicals. In Block, J. H., and Beale, J. M., Jr. (eds.). Wilson and Gisvold's Textbook of Organic Medicinal and Pharmaceutical Chemistry, 11th ed. Baltimore, Lippincott Williams & Wilkins, 2004, p. 10.
6. Freshney, R. I.: Culture of Animal Cells, 3rd ed. New York, Wiley-Liss, 1994.
7. Young, J. A. T.: Virus entry and uncoating. In Knipe, D. M., and Howley, P. M. (eds.). Fundamental Virology, 4th ed. New York, Lippincott Williams & Wilkins, 2001, p. 87.
8. Hunter, E.: Virus assembly. In Knipe, D. M., and Howley, P. M. (eds.). Fundamental Virology, 4th ed. New York, Lippincott Williams & Wilkins, 2001, p. 171.
9. Lamb, R. A., and Choppin, R. W.: Annu. Rev. Biochem. 52:467, 1983.
10. Cann, A. J.: Principles of Molecular Virology, 3rd ed. New York, Academic Press, 2001, p. 114.
11. Tyler, K. L., and Nathanson, N.: Pathogenesis of viral infections. In Knipe, D. M., and Howley, P. M. (eds.). Fundamental Virology, 4th ed. New York, Lippincott Williams & Wilkins, 2001, pp. 214–220.
12. Dimitrov, R. S.: Cell 91:721, 1997.
13. Dingwell, K. S., Brunetti, C. R., Hendricks, R. L., et al.: J. Virol. 68:834, 1994.
14. Haywood, A. M.: J. Virol. 68:1, 1994.
15. Norkin, L. C.: Clin. Microbiol. Rev. 8:298–315, 1995.
16. Chesebro, B., Buller, R., Portis, J., et al.: J. Virol. 64:215, 1990.
17. Clapham, P. R., Blanc, D., and Weiss, R. A.: Virology 181:703, 1991.
18. Harrington, R. D., and Geballe, A. P.: J. Virol. 67:5939, 1993.
19. Haywood, A. M.: J. Virol. 68:1, 1994.
20. Young, J. A. T.: Virus entry and uncoating. In Knipe, D. M., and Howley, P. M. (eds.). Fundamental Virology, 4th ed. New York, Lippincott Williams & Wilkins, 2001, p. 96

21. Wagner, E. K., and Hewlett, M. J. (eds.): Basic Virology. Malden, MA, Blackwell Science, 1999, p. 257
22. Mitsuya, H., and Broder, S.: Proc. Natl. Acad. Sci. U. S. A. 83:1911, 1986.
23. Johnson, M. A., et al.: J. Biol. Chem. 263:1534, 1988.
24. Kohl, N. E., et al.: Proc. Natl. Acad. Sci. U. S. A. 85:4686, 1988.
25. Hay, A. J.: Semin. Virol. 3:21, 1992.
26. Hayden, F. G., Belsche, R. B., Clover, R. D., et al.: N. Engl. J. Med. 321:1696, 1989.
27. Douglas, R. G.: N. Engl. J. Med. 322:443, 1990.
28. Capparelli, E. V., Stevens, R. C., and Chow, M. S.: Clin. Pharmacol. Ther. 43:536, 1988.
29. Baron, S., et al.: Introduction to the interferon system. In Baron, S., Dianzani, F., Stanton, G. et al. (eds.). Interferon: Principles and Medical Applications. Galveston, University of Texas, Texas Medical Branch, 1992, pp. 1–15.
30. Sen, G. C., and Ransohoff, R. M.: Adv. Virus Res. 42:57, 1993.
31. Bocci, V.: HIV proteases. In Baron, S., Dianzani, F., Stanton, G., et al. (eds.). Interferon: Principles and Medical Applications. Galveston, University of Texas, Texas Medical Branch, 1992, pp. 417–425.
32. Prusoff, W. H.: Idoxuridine or how it all began. In DeClerq, E. (ed.). Clinical Use of Antiviral Drugs. Norwell, MA, Martinus Nijhoff, 1988, pp. 15–24.
33. Birch, et al.: J. Infect. Dis. 166:108, 1992.
34. Pavin-Langston, D., et al.: Adenosine Arabinoside: An Antiviral Agent. New York, Raven Press, 1975.
35. Schaeffer, H. J., et al.: Nature 272:583, 1978.
36. Weller, S., et al.: Clin. Pharmacol. Ther. 54:595, 1993.
37. Sullivan, V., et al.: Nature 358:162, 1992.
38. Clair, M. H., et al.: Antimicrob. Agents Chemother. 25:191, 1984.
39. Faulds, D., and Heel, R. C.: Drugs 39:597, 1990.
40. Vere Hodge, R. A.: Antiviral Chem. Chemother. 4:67, 1993.
41. Earnshaw, D. L., et al.: Antimicrob. Agents Chemother. 36:2747, 1992.
42. Alrabiah, F. A., and Sachs, S. L.: Drugs 52:17, 1996.
43. Xiong, X., et al.: Biochem. Pharmacol. 51:1563, 1996.
44. Chrisp, P., and Chessold, S. P.: Drugs 41:104, 1991.
45. Crumpacker, C. S.: Am. J. Med. 92(Suppl. 2A):25, 1992.
46. Jacobson, M. A., et al.: J. Clin. Endocrinol. Metab. 72:1130, 1991.
47. Lin, T. S., and Prusoff, W. H.: J. Med. Chem. 21:109, 1978.
48. Mitsuya, H., et al.: Proc. Natl. Acad. Sci. U. S. A. 82:7096, 1985.
49. Yarchoan, R., et al.: Lancet 1:575, 1986.
50. Furman, P. A., et al.: Proc. Natl. Acad. Sci. U. S. A. 873:8333, 1986.
51. St. Clair, M. H., et al.: Antimicrob. Agents Chemother. 31:1972, 1987.
52. Richman, D. D., et al.: J. Infect. Dis. 164:1075, 1991.
53. Johnson, M. A., and Fridland, A.: Mol. Pharmacol. 36:291, 1989.
54. McLaren, C., et al.: Antiviral Chem. Chemother. 2:321, 1991.
55. Johnson, V. A., et al.: J. Infect. Dis. 164:646, 1991.
56. Knupp, C. A., et al.: Clin. Pharmacol. Ther. 49:523, 1991.
57. Yarchoan, R., et al.: N. Engl. J. Med. 321:726, 1989.
58. Chen, C., Vazquez-Padua, M., and Cheng, Y.: Mol. Pharmacol. 39:625, 1991.
59. Broder, S.: Am. J. Med. 88(Suppl. 5B):25, 1990.
60. Ho, H. T., and Hitchcock, M. J. M.: Antimicrob. Agents Chemother. 33:844, 1989.
61. Huang, P., Farquhar, D., and Plunkett, W.: J. Biol. Chem. 267:2817, 1992.
62. Browne, M. J., et al.: J. Infect. Dis. 167:21, 1993.
63. Van Leeuwen, R., et al.: J. Infect. Dis. 171:1166, 1995.
64. Pluda, J. M., et al.: J. Infect. Dis. 171:1438, 1995.
65. Coates, J. A. V., et al.: Antimicrob. Agents Chemother. 36:202, 1992.
66. Skalski, V., et al.: J. Biol. Chem. 268:23234, 1993.
67. Larder, B. A., et al.: Science 269:696, 1995.
68. Sidwell, R. W., et al.: Science 177:705, 1972.
69. Robins, R. K.: Chem. Eng. News Jan. 27:28, 1986.
70. Gallo, R. C., et al.: Science 220:865, 1983.
71. Barré-Sinoussi, F., et al.: Science 220:868, 1983.
72. Haseltine, W. A.: FASEB J. 5:2349, 1991.
73. Yarchoan, R., Mitsuya, H., and Broder, S.: Trends Pharmacol. Sci. 14::196, 1993.
74. DeClerq, E.: J. Med. Chem. 38:2491, 1995.
75. Richman, D. D.: Annu. Rev. Pharmacol. Toxicol. 32:149, 1993.
76. Cease, K. B., and Berzofsky, J. A.: Annu. Rev. Immunol. 12:923, 1994.
77. Lasky, L. A., et al.: Science 23:209, 1986.

78. Cohen, J.: Science 264:1839, 1994.
79. Koff, W. C.: Science 266:1335, 1994.
80. Spence, R. A., et al.: Science 267:988, 1995.
81. Vacca, J. P., et al.: Proc. Natl. Acad. Sci. U. S. A. 91:4096, 1994.
82. Merluzzi, U. T., et al.: Science 250:1411, 1990.
83. Romero, D. L.: Drugs Future 19:7, 1994.
84. Pedersen, O., and Pedersen, E.: Antiviral Chem. Chemother. 10:285, 1999.
85. Pialoux, G., et al.: Lancet 338:140, 1991.
86. Wlodawer, R., and Erickson, J. W.: Annu. Rev. Biochem. 62:543, 1993.
87. Chow, Y.-K., et al.: Nature 361:650, 1993.
88. Roberts, N. A., et al.: Science 248:358, 1990.
89. Kun, E. E. et al.: J. Am. Chem. Soc. 117:1181, 1995.
90. Kempf, D. J., et al.: Proc. Natl. Acad. Sci. U. S. A. 92:2484, 1995.
91. Nelfinavir. St. Louis, Facts and Comparisons, 2000, p. 1431.
92. Kageyama, S., et al.: Antimicrob. Agents Chemother. 37:810, 1993.
93. Reich, S. H., et al.: Proc. Natl. Acad. Sci. U. S. A. 92:3298, 1995.
94. Johnson, V. A., Merrill, D. P., Chou, T.-C., and Hirsch, M. S.: J. Infect. Dis. 166:1143, 1992.
95. Craig, J. C., et al.: Antiviral Chem. Chemother. 4:161, 1993.
96. Craig, J. C., et al.: Antiviral Chem. Chemother. 4:335, 1993.
97. Condra, J. H., et al.: Nature 374:569, 1995.
98. Wei, X., et al.: Nature 373:117, 1995.
99. Ho, D. D., et al.: Nature 373:123, 1995.
100. Kageyama, S., et al.: Antimicrob. Agents Chemother. 37:810, 1993.
101. DeLucca, G., et al.: Pharm. Biotechnol. 11:257, 1998.
102. Prasad, J., et al.: Bioorg. Med. Chem. 7:2775, 1999.
103. Yoshimura, K., et al.: Proc. Natl. Acad. Sci. U. S. A. 96:8675, 1999.
104. Hendrix, C., et al.: 6th Conference on Retroviruses and Opportunistic Infections, Abstr. 610, 1999.
105. Baba, M., et al.: Proc. Natl. Acad. Sci. U. S. A. 96:5698, 1999.
106. Wild, C., et al.: Proc. Natl. Acad. Sci. U. S. A. 91:9770, 1994.
107. Hazuda, D., et al.: Science 287:646, 2000.
108. Goldgur, Y. et al.: Proc. Natl. Acad. Sci. U. S. A. 96:13040, 1999.

Antineoplastic Agents

WILLIAM A. REMERS

The chemotherapy of neoplastic disease has become increasingly important in recent years. An indication of this importance is the establishment of a medical specialty in oncology, in which the physician practices various protocols of adjuvant therapy. Most cancer patients now receive some form of chemotherapy, even though it is merely palliative in many cases. The relatively high toxicity of most anticancer drugs has fostered the development of supplementary drugs that may alleviate these toxic effects or stimulate the regrowth of depleted normal cells.

The terms *cancer* and *neoplastic disease* actually encompass more than 100 different tumors, each with its own unique characteristics. Drugs active against a cancer of one tissue often are ineffective against cancers of other tissues. Even cancers of the same apparent type respond widely to a particular therapeutic protocol. Consequently, it has been difficult to make progress on a broad front of neoplastic diseases.

Cancer chemotherapy has received no spectacular breakthrough of the kind that the discovery of penicillin provided for antibacterial chemotherapy. There has been substantial progress in many aspects of cancer research, however. In particular, an increased understanding of tumor biology has led to elucidation of the mechanisms of action for antineoplastic agents. It also has provided a basis for the more rational design of new agents. Recent advances in clinical techniques, including large cooperative studies, are allowing more rapid and reliable evaluation of new drugs. The combination of these advantages with improved preliminary screening systems is enhancing the emergence of newer and more potent compounds.

At present, at least 10 different neoplasms can be ''cured'' by chemotherapy in most patients. *Cure* is defined here as an expectation of normal longevity. These neoplasms are acute leukemia in children, Burkitt's lymphoma, choriocarcinoma in women, Ewing's sarcoma, Hodgkin's disease, lymphosarcoma, mycosis fungoides, rhabdomyosarcoma, retinoblastoma in children, and testicular carcinoma.[1] Unfortunately, only these relatively rare neoplasms are readily curable. Considerable progress is being made in the treatment of breast cancer by combination drug therapy. For carcinoma of the pancreas, colon, liver, or lung (except small cell carcinoma), however, the outlook is bleak. Short-term remissions are the best that can be expected for most patients with these diseases.

There are cogent reasons why cancer is more difficult to cure than bacterial infections. One is that there are qualitative differences between human and bacterial cells. For example, bacterial cells have distinctive cell walls, and their ribosomes differ from those of human cells. In contrast, the differences between normal and neoplastic human cells are mostly quantitative. Another difference is that immune mechanisms and other host defenses are very important in killing bacteria and other foreign cells, whereas they play a lesser role in killing cancer cells. Nevertheless, cancer cells overexpress certain antigens, and antibodies produced by recombinant DNA technology exert a selective cytotoxic effect on them. Quantitative differences in proteins found in signaling pathways that control cell proliferation, differentiation, and the induction of programmed cell death (apoptosis) also provide targets for anticancer drugs.[2] Because cancer cells have overcome the body's surveillance system, chemotherapeutic agents must kill every clonogenic malignant cell, because even one can reestablish the tumor. This kind of kill is extremely difficult to effect because antineoplastic agents kill cells by first-order kinetics. That is, they kill a constant fraction of cells. Suppose that a patient had a trillion leukemia cells. This amount would cause a serious debilitation. A potent anticancer drug might reduce this population 10,000-fold, in which case the symptoms would be alleviated and the patient would be in a state of remission. After cessation of therapy, however, the remaining hundred million leukemia cells could readily increase to the original number. Furthermore, a higher proportion of resistant cells would be present, which would mean that retreatment with the same agent would achieve a lesser response than before. For this reason, multiple drug regimens are used to reduce drastically the number of neoplastic cells. Typical protocols for leukemia contain four different anticancer drugs, usually with different modes of action.

TUMOR CELL PROPERTIES

The basic differences between cancer cells and normal cells are uncontrolled cell proliferation, decreased cellular differentiation, ability to invade surrounding tissue, and ability to establish new growth at ectopic sites (metastasis). Contrary to popular belief, not all tumor cells proliferate rapidly. Proliferation rates vary widely with the cell type. Thus, lymphomas and normal intestinal mucosa both proliferate faster than solid tumors. Acute leukemia cells actually proliferate more slowly than the corresponding precursors in normal bone marrow.

Development and homeostasis in multicellular organisms are controlled by processes of cell division, differentiation, and death. In the adult, the steady-state number of differentiated cells is maintained by a balance between cell proliferation and cell death. Cell death is a complex and actively regulated process known as *apoptosis*. Apoptosis is a defined process of cell shrinkage, membrane blebbing, and nuclear condensation. It differs from necrosis, the cell death induced by severe cellular injury, which is characterized by swelling and lysis.

The process of apoptosis is a complex but carefully orchestrated sequence of events. Scientists disagree on the relative importance of factors such as mitochondrial damage, although many think that when stress factors reach a critical level, the mitochondrial membrane potential changes, and the mitochondria leak or rupture, resulting in their own destruction. This causes the release of factors that trigger proteolytic enzymes called caspases. Other investigators think that the primary apoptotic signals activate caspases directly and then caspases attack mitochondria along with other cellular organelles.

Cancer can be considered a failure of cells to undergo apoptosis. In normal cells, sensors to cell abnormalities lead to withdrawal of survival signals, resulting in cell death. In contrast, cancer cells circumvent the need for survival signals by increasing their abundance of anti-apoptotic proteins. Among these anti-apoptotic proteins, members of the Bcl-2 family, including BAX and BAK, have been identified with the initiation or progression of a variety of tumors. They block the release of cytochrome C and apoptosis-activating factor from mitochondria.

Cells also have a variety of tumor suppressor proteins that respond to DNA damage by shutting down cell division or by inducing apoptosis. One intensively studied protein is p53, which binds to the regulatory sequence of genes and inhibits their transcription. Many mutations produce p53 in a misfolded form, resulting in a conformation unsuitable for binding to regulatory sequences. The development of half of all cancers is thought to result from misfolding of p53. Recent research has produced compounds that restore p53 to its active conformation.

The concept of a cell cycle is based on experiments using [³H]thymidine radiography and flow cytometry. These experiments showed that DNA synthesis, as measured by incorporation of [³H]thymidine, takes place at a specific period, known as the *S phase,* in the life cycle of a dividing cell. Periods between the S phase and cell division (*mitosis* or *M phase*) are termed G_1 and G_2. A circular pictorial model (Fig. 12-1) was derived for the clockwise progression of the cell cycle. The duration of each phase in the cell cycle varies considerably with the cell type and within a single tumor. Typical durations are as follows: S, 10 to 20 hours, G_2, 2 to 10 hours, and M, 0.5 to 1 hour. G_1 is highly variable as the result of another phase, G_0, in which the cell is not active in cell division. Most anticancer drugs block the biosynthesis

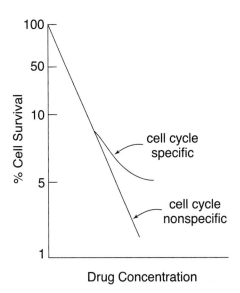

Figure 12–2 ■ Cell cycle specificity.

or transcription of nucleic acids or prevent cell division by interfering with mitotic spindles. Cells in the DNA synthesis or mitosis phases are highly susceptible to these agents. In contrast, cells in the resting state are resistant to many agents. Slow-growing tumors characteristically have many cells in the resting state.[3]

Antitumor agents are classified on the basis of their effects on cell survival as a function of dose. For many drugs, including alkylating agents, cell survival is exponentially related to dose, and a plot of log cell survival against drug concentration (Fig. 12-2) gives a straight line. These drugs exert their cytotoxicity regardless of the cell cycle phase and are termed non–cell cycle phase specific. Other drugs, including antimetabolites and mitotic inhibitors, which act at one phase of the cell cycle (cell cycle phase specific), show a plateau after an initial low-dose exponential region.

The proportion of labeled cells in tissue after a specified interval (usually 1 hour) following injection of [³H]thymidine or 5-bromodeoxyuridine is known as the *labeling index* (LI). Comparison of the LI with the proportion of proliferating cells in DNA synthesis provides the growth fraction. Doubling times for tumor growth are calculated from the growth fraction and cell cycle times. Rarely are they as rapid as predicted because of tumor cell loss through necrosis, metastasis, and differentiation.

The cell-kill hypothesis states that the effects of antitumor drugs on tumor cell populations follow first-order kinetics. This means that the number of cells killed is proportional to the dose. Thus, chemotherapy follows an exponential or log-kill model in which a constant proportion, not a constant number, of cancer cells are killed.[4] Theoretically, the fractional reductions possible with cancer chemotherapy can never reduce tumor populations to zero. Complete eradication requires another effect, such as the immune response. A modified form of the first-order log-kill hypothesis holds that tumor regressions produced by chemotherapy are described by the relative growth fraction present in the tumor at the time of treatment. This idea is consistent with the finding that very small and very large tumors are less responsive than tumors of intermediate size.[5]

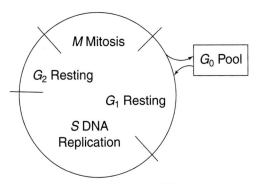

Figure 12–1 ■ The cell life cycle.

Stem cells are the cells of origin of a cell line, which maintain the potential to regenerate the cell population and from which the differentiated cells are derived. They are important in the chemotherapy of human tumors because they must be eradicated completely to effect a cure. Treatments that afford substantial reductions in tumor burdens can produce remissions, but the tumor may recur if some of the stem cells remain. Their eradication is difficult because many are in the G_0 phase of the cell cycle.[6]

Drug resistance to chemotherapy usually involves the selection of certain cell populations. Populations of drug-resistant cells can be produced by clonal evolution or mutation. Drug-resistant cells in tissue culture are generated at a frequency consistent with known rates of genetic mutation. Mutagenic agents increase the frequency of generation of drug-resistant cells. This effect may have clinical importance because many antitumor agents are mutagenic. Intracellular effects that cause drug resistance may be secondary to cellular adaptation or altered enzyme levels or properties. For example, resistance to methotrexate involves increased levels of the target enzyme, dihydrofolate reductase.[7] Other modes of resistance to antimetabolites include reduced drug transport into cells, reduced affinity of the molecular target, stimulation of alternate biosynthetic pathways, and impaired activation or increased metabolism of the drug. A major factor in resistance to alkylating agents is the ability of tumor cells to repair DNA lesions, such as cross-links and breakage of DNA strands caused by alkylation. Cells selected for resistance to one drug may show cross-resistance to other drugs, even if their chemical structures are quite different; most of these drugs are derived from natural products, however. One type of molecular explanation for this form of multiple drug resistance is overexpression of membrane glycoproteins termed *P-glycoproteins,* which function as drug efflux pumps. This overexpression is associated with gene amplification.[2]

Most antineoplastic drugs are highly toxic to the patient and must be administered with extreme caution. Some of them require a clinical setting where supportive care is available. The toxicity usually involves rapidly proliferating tissues, such as bone marrow and the intestinal epithelium. Individual drugs produce distinctive toxic effects on the heart, lungs, kidneys, and other organs, however. Chemotherapy is seldom the initial treatment used against cancer. If the cancer is well defined and accessible, surgery is preferred. Skin cancers and certain localized tumors are treated by radiotherapy. Generally, chemotherapy is important when the tumor is inoperable or has metastasized. Chemotherapy is finding increasing use as an ''adjuvant'' after surgery to ensure that few cells remain to regenerate the parent tumor.

The era of chemotherapy of malignant disease was born in 1941, when Huggins demonstrated that the administration of estrogens produced regressions of metastatic prostate cancer.[8] In the following year, Gilman and others began clinical studies on the nitrogen mustards and discovered that mechlorethamine was effective against Hodgkin's disease and lymphosarcoma.[9] These same two diseases were treated with cortisone acetate in 1949, and dramatic, although temporary, remissions resulted.[10] The next decade was marked by the design and discovery of antimetabolites: methotrexate in

1949, 6-mercaptopurine in 1952, and 5-fluorouracil in 1957. Additional alkylating agents such as melphalan and cyclophosphamide were developed during this period, and the activity of natural products such as actinomycin, mitomycin C, and the vinca alkaloids was discovered. During the 1960s, progress continued in all of these areas with the discovery of cytosine arabinoside, bleomycin, doxorubicin, and carmustine. Novel structures such as procarbazine, dacarbazine, and *cis*-platinum complexes were found to be highly active. In 1965, Kennedy reported that remissions occurred in 30% of postmenopausal women with metastatic breast cancer on treatment with high doses of estrogen.[11]

Much of the leadership and financial support for the development of antineoplastic drugs derives from the National Cancer Institute (NCI). In 1955, this organization established the Cancer Chemotherapy National Service Center (now the Division of Cancer Treatment) to coordinate a national voluntary cooperative cancer chemotherapy development program. By 1958, this effort had evolved into a targeted drug development program. A massive screening system was established to discover new lead compounds, and thousands of samples have been submitted to it. The current highly automated NCI tumor cell culture screening system achieved operational status in 1990. It emphasizes rigorous end points such as net cell killing and tumor regression, rather than earlier growth-inhibitory end points, and it uses a wide variety of specific types of cancer, including many solid tumor models, in the initial stage of screening. New drug candidates are being screened at a rate of about 20,000 per year, with input divided about equally between pure compounds and extracts or fractions from natural products. The present in vitro screening panel contains 60 human tumor cell lines arranged in seven subpanels that represent diverse histologies: leukemia, melanoma, lung, colon, kidney, ovary, and brain. For routine evaluation, each sample is tested in a 2-day continuous drug exposure protocol using five $\log_{10}$-spaced concentrations starting at 10^{-4} M for pure compounds and 100 $\mu g/mL$ for extracts. Antitumor activities are compared at three different levels of response. GI_{50} is the drug concentration that produces 50% inhibition in cell proliferation relative to the control, TGI (tumor growth inhibition) is the drug concentration at which there is no net proliferation, and LC_{50} is the lethal concentration of drug that produces a 50% reduction in the number of tumor cells relative to the control.[12]

The primary NCI screening data are reported in a mean-graph format (Fig. 12-3) in which a vertical reference bar, obtained by averaging the negative $\log_{10} GI_{50}$ values for all of the cell lines tested, is plotted along the drug concentration axis and then horizontal bars are plotted for the individual negative $\log_{10} GI_{50}$s of each line with respect to the vertical reference bar. This graphical representation provides a characteristic fingerprint for a given compound, displaying the individual cell lines that are more sensitive than average (bars to the right of the reference) or less sensitive than average (bars to the left of the reference). Thus, Figure 12-3 shows that colon cancer cell lines are more sensitive than average to 5-fluorouracil (5-FU), whereas central nervous system (CNS) cancer cell lines are more resistant than average to it.[12]

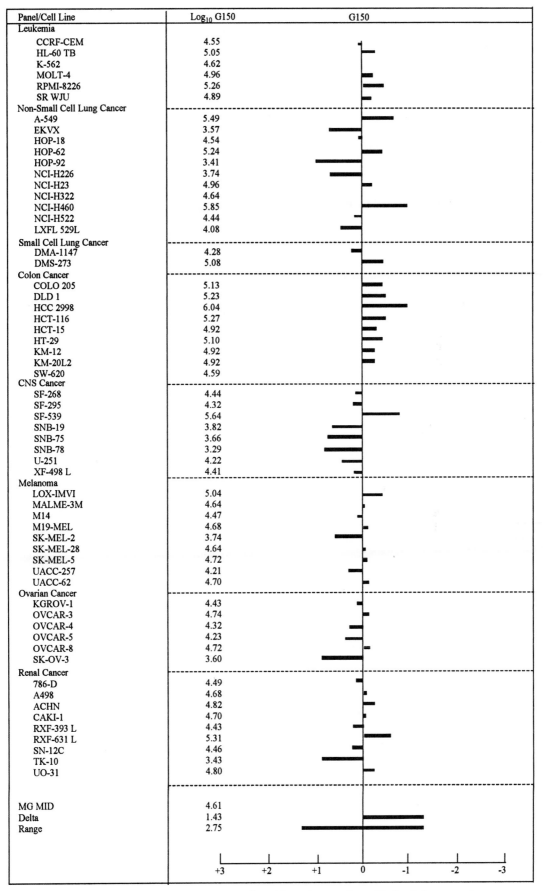

Figure 12–3 ■ National Institutes of Health testing result profile for 5-fluorouracil.

A secondary stage of preliminary screening on selected compounds is performed in vivo in xenograft models by using a subset of cell lines found to be active in the primary in vitro screen. Two xenograft models in current use are the severe combined immunodeficiency (SCID) mouse and the athymic nude mouse. Both of these mouse models have deficient immune responses that permit transplantation of human tumor cells without rejection. Consequently, potential antitumor drugs may be tested against human tumors in an in vivo model. These models predict human clinical tumor responses better than the older allograft models that were based on transplanting mouse tumors such as P388 leukemia into the same strain of mouse (syngeneic tumors). The important antitumor drug paclitaxel was discovered by using a xenograft model.

An in vitro system that is a good predictor of human clinical activity is the human-tumor-colony–forming assay (HTCFA). This system uses fresh human tumor tissue from individual patients.[13] It is valuable in selecting chemotherapeutic agents for individual tumor types and occasionally specific patients, but its use in large-scale primary screening has not been feasible.

Compounds with significant antitumor activity are subjected to preclinical pharmacology and toxicology evaluation in mice and dogs. Clinical trials may be underwritten by the NCI. They involve three discrete phases. Phase I is the clinical pharmacology stage. The dosage schedule is developed, and toxicity parameters are established in it. Phase II involves the determination of activity against a "signal" tumor panel, which includes both solid and hematological types. A broad-based multicenter study is usually undertaken in phase III. It features randomization schemes designed to statistically validate the efficacy of the new drug in comparison to alternative modalities of therapy. As might be anticipated, the design of clinical trials for antineoplastic agents is very complicated, especially in the matter of controls. Ethical considerations do not permit patients to be left untreated if any reasonable therapy is possible.

A number of pharmaceutical industry laboratories and foreign institutions have made significant contributions to the development of anticancer drugs. Organizations such as the United Kingdom's Cancer Research Campaign, the European Organization for Research on the Treatment of Cancer, and the Japanese Foundation for Cancer Research have broadened international cooperation in anticancer drug research.

ALKYLATING AGENTS

Toxic effects of sulfur mustard and ethyleneimine on animals were described in the 19th century.[14] The powerful vesicant action of sulfur mustard led to its use in World War I, and medical examination of the victims revealed that tissues were damaged at sites distant from the area of contact.[15] Such systemic effects included leukopenia, bone marrow aplasia, lymphoid tissue suppression, and ulceration of the gastrointestinal tract. Sulfur mustard was shown to be active against animal tumors, but it was too nonspecific for clinical use. A variety of nitrogen mustards were synthesized between the two world wars. Some of these compounds (e.g.,

mechlorethamine) showed selective toxicity, especially to lymphoid tissue. This observation led to the crucial suggestion that nitrogen mustards be tested against tumors of the lymphoid system in animals. Success in this area was followed by cautious human trials that showed methchlorethamine to be useful against Hodgkin's disease and certain lymphomas. This work was classified during World War II but was finally published in a classical paper by Gilman and Phillips in 1946.[9] This paper described the chemical transformation of nitrogen and sulfur mustards to cyclic "onium" cations and established the nucleus as the locus of their interaction with cancer cells. The now familiar pattern of toxicity to rapidly proliferating cells in bone marrow and the gastrointestinal tract was established.

Alkylation is defined as the replacement of hydrogen on an atom by an alkyl group. The alkylation of nucleic acids or proteins involves a substitution reaction in which a nucleophilic atom (nu) of the biopolymer displaces a leaving group from the alkylating agent.

$$\text{nu-H} + \text{alkyl-Y} \rightarrow \text{alkyl-nu} + \text{H}^+ + \text{Y}^-$$

The reaction rate depends on the nucleophilicity of the atom (S, N, O), which is greatly enhanced if the nucleophile is ionized. Hypothetically, the order of reactivity at physiological pH is ionized thiol, amine, ionized phosphate, and ionized carboxylic acid.[16] Rate differences among various amines would depend on the degree to which they are protonated and their conjugation with other groups. The N-7 position of guanine in DNA (Scheme 12-5, below) is strongly nucleophilic.

Reaction orders depend on the structure of the alkylating agent. Methane sulfonates, epoxides, and aziridines give second-order reactions that depend on concentrations of the alkylating agent and nucleophile. The situation is more complex with β-haloalkylamines (nitrogen mustards) and β-haloalkylsulfides (sulfur mustards), because these molecules undergo neighboring-group reactions in which the nitrogen or sulfur atom displaces the halide to give strained, three-membered "onium" intermediates. These "onium" ions react with nucleophiles in second-order processes. The overall reaction kinetics depend on the relative rates of the two steps, however. In the case of mechlorethamine, the aziridinium ion forms rapidly in water, but reaction with biological nucleophiles is slower. Thus, the kinetics are second order.[17]

In contrast, sulfur mustard forms the less stable episulfonium ion more slowly than this ion reacts with biological nucleophiles. Thus, the neighboring-group reaction is rate limiting, and the kinetics are first order.[18]

Aryl-substituted nitrogen mustards such as chlorambucil are relatively stable to aziridinium ion formation because the aromatic ring decreases the nucleophilicity of the nitrogen atom. These mustards react according to first-order kinetics.[18] The stability of chlorambucil allows it to be taken orally, whereas mechlorethamine is given by intravenous administration of freshly prepared solutions. The requirement for freshly prepared solutions is based on the gradual decomposition of the aziridinium ion by interaction with water.

Ethylene imines and epoxides are strained ring systems, but they do not react as readily as aziridinium or episulfonium ions with nucleophiles. Their reactions are second order and are enhanced by the presence of acid.[16] Examples of antitumor agents containing ethyleneimine groups are triethylenemelamine and thiotepa.

Triethylene Melamine   Thiotepa

Diaziquone is an investigational benzoquinone substituted with ethyleneimine groups and carbamate groups, both of which are cancerostatic.[19] After activation by reduction of the quinone ring to a hydroquinone, the ethyleneimine groups alkylate DNA to produce cross-links. Some DNA–protein cross-links also are formed.

Dlaziquone

The use of epoxides as cross-linking agents in textile chemistry suggested that they be tried in cancer chemotherapy. Simple diepoxides such as 1,2:3,4-diepoxybutane showed clinical activity against Hodgkin's disease,[20] but none of these compounds became an established drug. Dibromomannitol (mitobronitol) gives the corresponding diepoxide on continuous titration at pH 8. This diepoxide (1,2: 5,6-dianhydro-D-mannitol) shows potent alkylating activity against experimental tumors,[21] thus suggesting that dibromomannitol and related compounds such as dibromodulcitol act by way of the diepoxides.

Mitobromitol   Dianhydro-D-mannitol

A somewhat different type of alkylating agent is the *N*-alkyl-*N*-nitrosourea. Compounds of this class are unstable in aqueous solution under physiological conditions. They produce carbonium ions (also called *carbenium ions*) that can alkylate and isocyanates that can carbamoylate. For example, methylnitrosourea decomposes initially to form isocyanic acid and methyldiazohydroxide. The latter species decomposes further to methyldiazonium ion and finally to methyl carbonium ion, the ultimate alkylating species.[22]

Substituents on the nitrogen atoms of the nitrosourea influence the mechanism of decomposition in water, which determines the species generated and controls the biological effects. Carmustine (BCNU) undergoes an abnormal base-catalyzed decomposition in which the urea oxygen displaces chloride to give a cyclic intermediate (Scheme 12-1). This intermediate decomposes to vinyl diazo hydroxide, the precursor to vinyl carbonium ion, and 2-chloroethyl isocyanate. The latter species gives 2-chloroethylamine, an additional alkylating agent.[22]

Some clinically important alkylating agents are not active until they have been transformed by metabolic processes. The leading example of this group is cyclophosphamide,

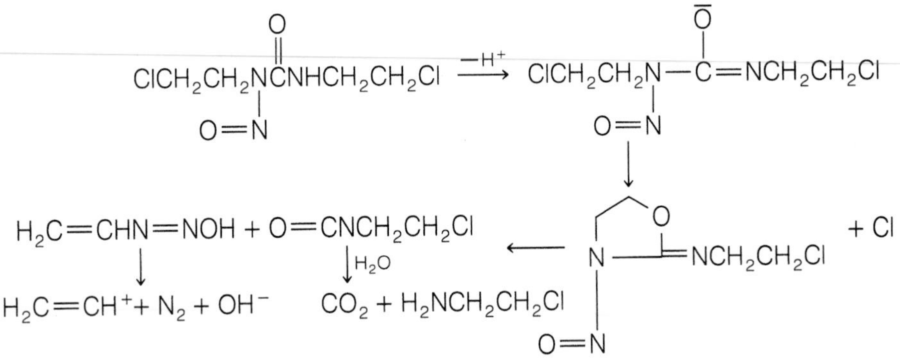

Scheme 12–1 ■ Decomposition of carmustine (BCNU).

which is converted by hepatic cytochrome P-450 into the corresponding 4-hydroxy derivative by way of the 4-hydroperoxy intermediate (Scheme 12-2). The 4-hydroxy derivative is a carbinolamine in equilibrium with the open-chain amino aldehyde form. Nonenzymatic decomposition of the latter form generates phosphoramide mustard and acrolein. Studies based on ^{31}P nuclear magnetic resonance (NMR) have shown that the conjugate base of phosphoramide mustard cyclizes to an aziridinium ion,[23] which is the principal cross-linking alkylator formed from cyclophosphamide. The maximal rate of cyclization occurs at pH 7.4. It was suggested that selective toxicity toward certain neoplastic cells might be based on their abnormally low pH. This would afford slower formation of aziridinium ions, which would persist longer because of decreased inactivation by hydroxide ions.[22]

Cyclophosphamide has been resolved, and the enantiomers have been tested against tumors. The levorotatory form has twice the therapeutic index of the dextrorotatory form.[24]

Ifosfamide, an isomer of cyclophosphamide in which one of the 2-chloroethyl substituents is on the ring nitrogen, also has potent antitumor activity. It requires activation by hepatic enzymes, but its metabolism is slower than that of cyclophosphamide[25] and involves substantially more dechloroethylation, yielding a chloroacetate metabolite.

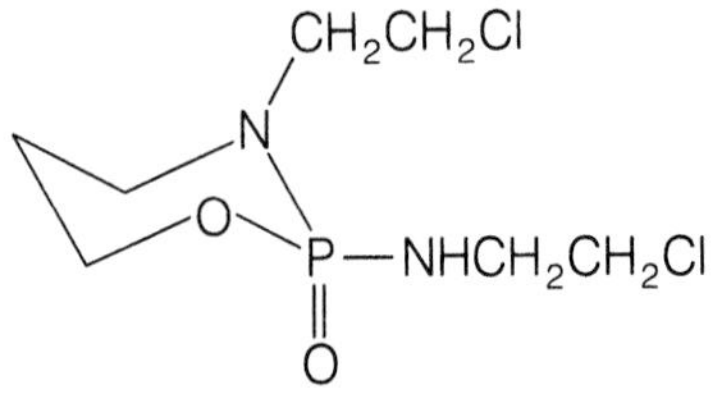

Ifosfamide

Other examples of alkylating species are afforded by carbinolamines as found in maytansine and vinylogous carbinolamines as found in certain pyrrolizine diesters.[26]

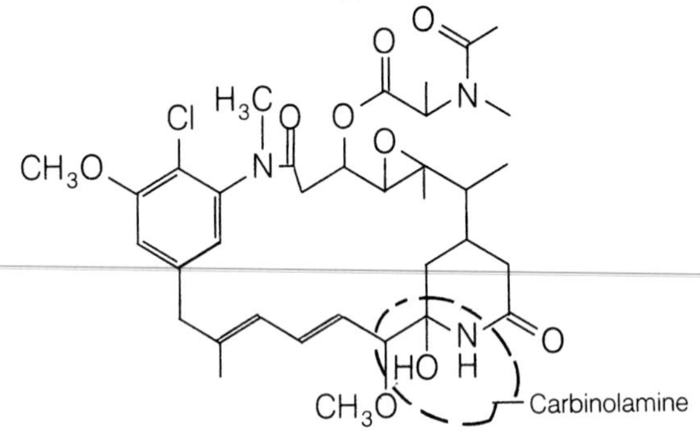

Maytansine

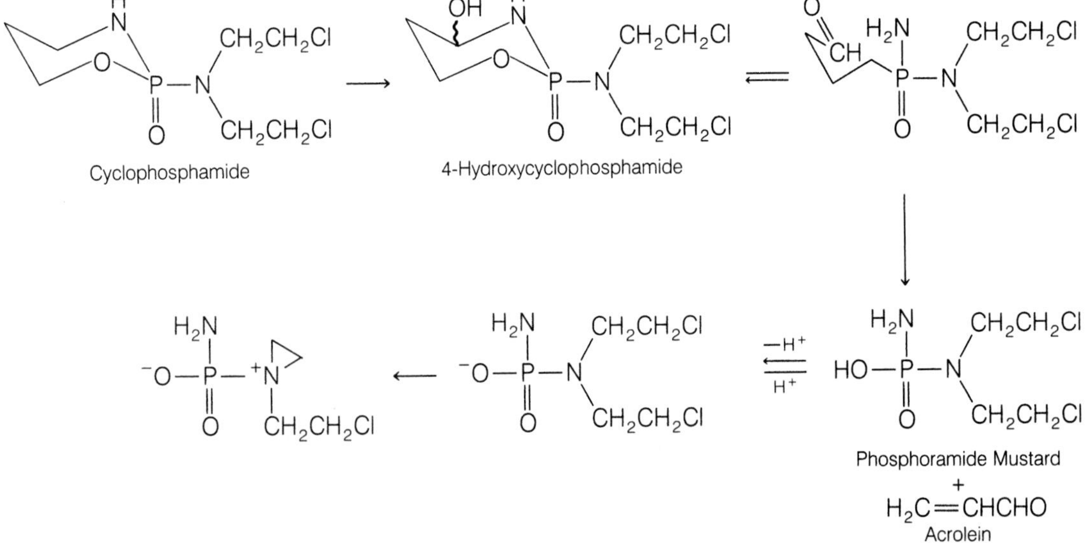

Scheme 12–2 ■ Activation of cyclophosphamide.

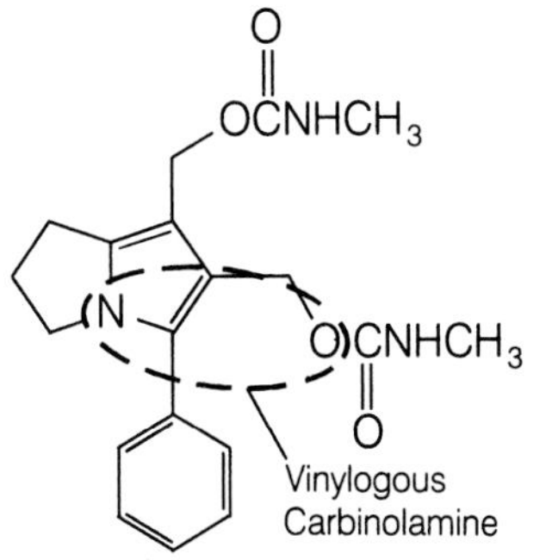

Pyrrolizine Diester

example, the sesquiterpene helenalin has both of these systems.[29]

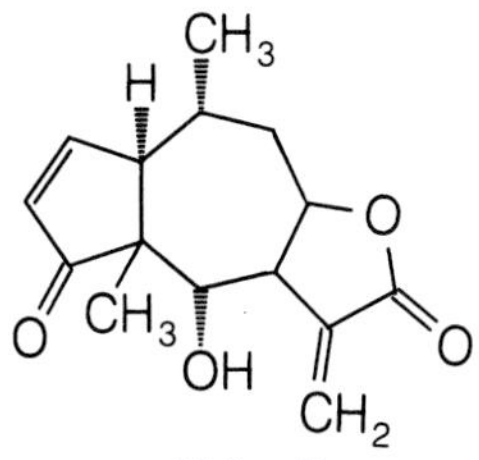

Helenalin

When mitomycin C is reduced enzymatically to its semi-quinone radical, disproportion and spontaneous elimination of methanol afford the vinylogous carbinolamine system. Loss of the carbamoyloxy group from this system gives a stabilized carbonium ion that can alkylate DNA (Scheme 12-3). The first alkylation step results from opening of the aziridine ring, and together with the vinylogous carbinolamine, it allows mitomycin C to cross-link double-helical DNA.[27] Molecules like mitomycin C are said to act by "bioreductive alkylation."[28]

Another type of alkylating species occurs in α,β-unsaturated carbonyl compounds. These compounds can alkylate nucleophiles by conjugate addition. Although there are no established clinical agents of this type, many natural products active against experimental tumors contain α-methylene lactone or α,β-unsaturated ketone functionalities. For

Alkylation can also occur by free radical reactions. The methylhydrazines are a chemical class prone to decomposition in this manner. These compounds were tested as antitumor agents in 1963, and one of them, procarbazine, was found to have a pronounced, but rather specific, effect on Hodgkin's disease.[30] Procarbazine is relatively stable at pH 7, but air oxidation to azoprocarbazine occurs readily in the presence of metalloproteins. Isomerization of this azo compound to the corresponding hydrazone, followed by hydrolysis, gives methylhydrazine and p-formyl-N-isopropyl benzamide. The formation of methylhydrazine from procarbazine has been demonstrated in living organisms.[31] Methylhydrazine is known to be oxidized to methyl diazine, which can decompose to nitrogen, methyl radical, and hydrogen radical.[32] The methyl group of procarbazine is incorporated intact into cytoplasmic RNA.[33] It has not been established conclusively, however, that the methyl radical is the methylating species.

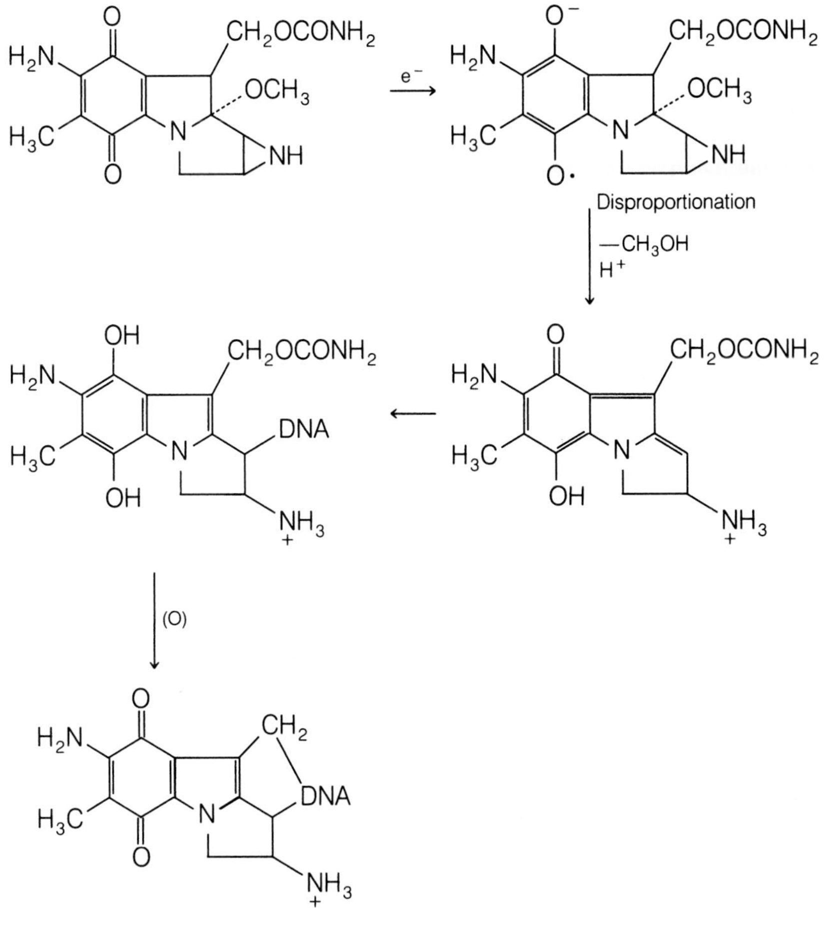

Scheme 12–3 ■ Mitomycin C activation and DNA alkylation.

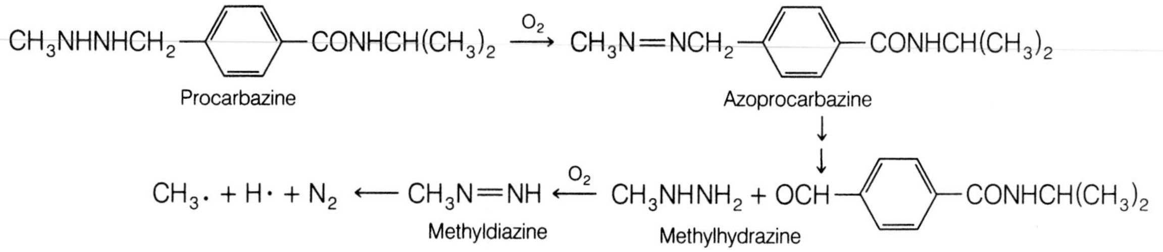

Dacarbazine was originally considered an antimetabolite because of its close resemblance to 5-aminoimidazole-4-carboxamide, an intermediate in purine biosynthesis. It now appears, however, to be an alkylating agent.[34] The isolation of an N-demethyl metabolite suggested that there might be a sequence in which this metabolite was hydrolyzed to methyldiazohydroxide, a precursor to methylcarbonium ion,[35] but it was found that this metabolite was less active than starting material against the Lewis lung tumor. An alternative mode of action was proposed in which dacarbazine undergoes acid-catalyzed hydrolysis to a diazonium ion, which can react in this form or decompose to the corresponding carbonium ion (Scheme 12-4). Support for the latter mechanism was afforded by a correlation between the hydrolysis rates of phenyl-substituted dimethyltriazines and their antitumor activities.[36]

The interaction of alkylating agents with macromolecules such as DNA and RNA has been studied extensively. No mode of action for the lethality to cancer cells has been established conclusively, however. A good working model was developed for the alkylation of bacteria and viruses, but there are uncertainties in extrapolating it to mammalian cells. The present working hypothesis is that most alkylating agents produce cytotoxic, mutagenic, and carcinogenic effects by reacting with cellular DNA. They also react with RNA and proteins, but these effects are thought to be less significant.[37] The most active clinical alkylating agents are bifunctional compounds capable of cross-linking DNA. Agents such as methylnitrosourea that give simple alkylation are highly mutagenic relative to their cytotoxicity. The cross-linking process can be either interstrand or intrastrand. Interstrand links can be verified by a test based on the thermal denaturation and renaturation of DNA. When double-helical DNA is heated in water, it unwinds and the strands separate. Renaturation, in which the strands recombine in the double

helix, is slow and difficult. In contrast, if the two strands are cross-linked, they cannot separate. Hence, they renature rapidly on cooling. Interstrand cross-linking occurs with mechlorethamine and other "two-armed" mustards, but according to this test, busulfan appears to give intrastrand links.[38]

In DNA, the 7 position (nitrogen) of guanine is especially susceptible to alkylation by mechlorethamine and other nitrogen mustards (Scheme 12-5).[39] The alkylated structure has a positive charge in its imidazole ring, which renders the guanine–ribose linkage susceptible to cleavage. This cleavage results in the deletion of guanine, and the resulting "apurinic acid" ribose–phosphate link is readily hydrolyzable. Alkylation of the imidazole ring also activates it to cleavage of the 8,9 bond.[16]

Other consequences of the positively charged purine structure are facile exchange of the 8-hydrogen, which can be used as a probe for 7-alkylation,[40] and a shift to the enolized pyrimidine ring as the preferred tautomer. The latter effect has been cited as a possible basis for abnormal base pairing in DNA replication, but this has not been substantiated. One example in which alkylation of guanine does lead to abnormal base pairing is the 0-6-ethylation produced by ethyl methanesulfonate. This ethyl derivative pairs with thymine, whereas guanine normally pairs with cytosine.[41]

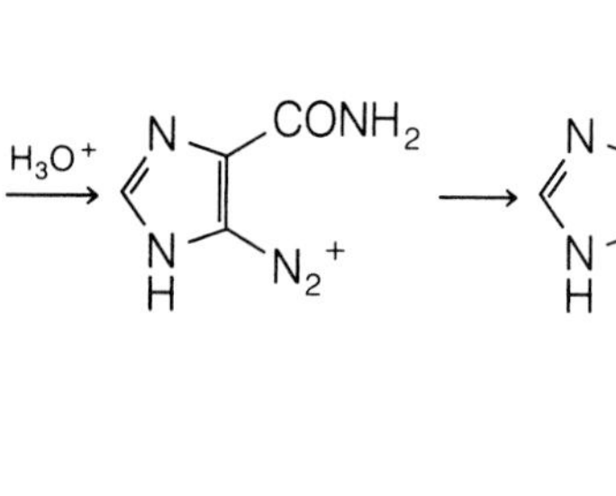

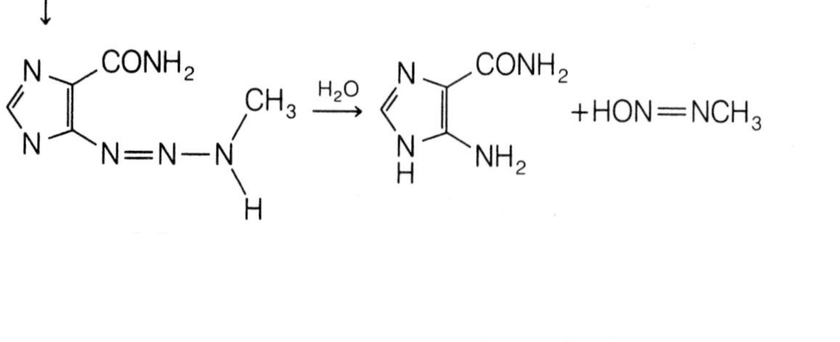

Scheme 12–4 ■ Activation of dacarbazine.

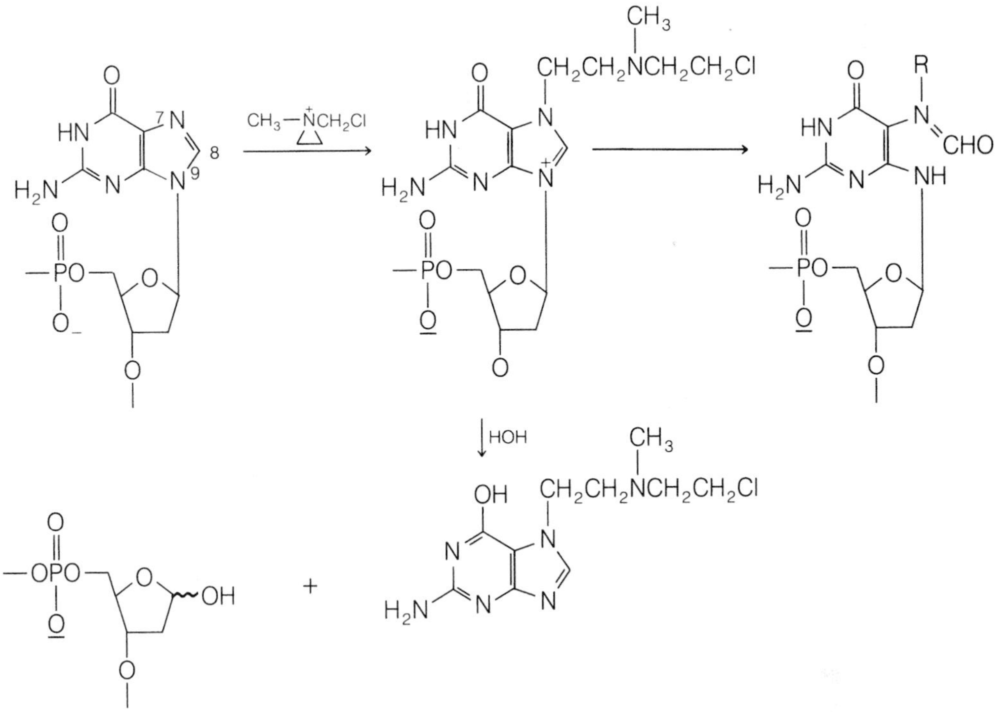

Scheme 12–5 ■ Alkylation of guanine in DNA.

Other base positions of DNA attacked by alkylating agents are N-2 and N-3 of guanine; N-3, N-1, and N-7 of adenine; O-6 of thymine; and N-3 of cytosine. The importance of these minor alkylation reactions is difficult to assess. The phosphate oxygens of DNA are alkylated to an appreciable extent, but the significance of this feature is unknown.[42]

Guanine is also implicated in the cross-linking of double-helical DNA. Di(guanin-7-yl) derivatives have been identified among the products of reaction with mechlorethamine.[43] Busulfan alkylation has given 1′,4′-di(guanin-7-yl)-butane, but this product is considered to have resulted from intrastrand linking.[38] Enzymatic hydrolysis of DNA cross-linked by mitomycin C has given fragments in which the antibiotic is covalently bound to the 2-amino groups of two guanosine residues, presumably from opposite strands of the double helix.[40]

Alkylating agents also interact with enzymes and other proteins. Thus, the repair enzyme DNA nucleotidyltransferase of L1210 leukemia cells is inhibited strongly by BCNU, lomustine (CCNU), and 2-chloroethyl isocyanate. Because 1-(2-chloroethyl)-1-nitrosourea was a poor inhibitor of this enzyme, it was concluded that the main interaction with the enzyme was carbamoylation by the alkyl isocyanates generated in the decomposition of BCNU and CCNU.[44]

Alkylating agents can damage tissues with low mitotic indices, but they are most cytotoxic to rapidly proliferating tissues that have large proportions of cells in cycle. Nucleic acids are especially susceptible to alkylation when their structures are changed or unpaired in the process of replication. Thus, alkylating agents are most effective in the late G_1 or S phases. Some alkylation may occur at any stage in the cell cycle, but the resulting toxicity is usually expressed when cells enter the S phase (Fig. 12-1). Progression through the cycle is blocked at G_2, the premitotic phase, and cell division fails.[45]

If cells can repair damage to their DNA before the next cell division, the effects of alkylation will not be lethal. Cells have developed a complex mechanism to accomplish this repair. Initially, a recognition enzyme discovers an abnormal region in the DNA. This recognition brings about the operation of an endonuclease, which makes a single-strand break in the DNA. An exonuclease then removes a small segment of DNA containing the damaged bases. Finally, the DNA is restored to its original structure by replacing the bases and rejoining the strand.[46] Thus, tumor cells with efficient repair mechanisms will be relatively resistant to alkylating agents. Tumor cells outside the cell cycle, in the resting phase (G_0), will have a rather long time to repair their DNA. Thus, slow-growing tumors should not respond well to alkylating agents, and this is observed clinically.

Products

Mechlorethamine Hydrochloride, USP.

Mechlorethamine hydrochloride, Mustargen, nitrogen mustard, HN$_2$, NSC-762, 2,2-dichloro-N-methyldiethylamine hydrochloride, is prepared by treating 2,2′-(methylimino)diethanol with thionyl chloride.[47] It occurs as hygroscopic leaflets that are very soluble in water. The dry crystals are stable at temperatures up to 40°C. They are very irritating to mucous membranes and harmful to eyes. The compound is supplied in rubber-stoppered vials containing a mixture of 10 mg of mechlorethamine hydrochloride and 90 mg of sodium chloride. It is diluted with 10 mL of sterile water immediately before injection into a rapidly flowing intravenous infusion. Intracavity injections are sometimes given to control malignant effusions.

The aziridinium ion formed from mechlorethamine in body fluids is highly reactive. It acts on various cellular components within minutes of administration. Less than

0.01% is recovered unchanged in the urine, but more than 50% is excreted in urine as inactive metabolites in the first 24 hours.

Mechlorethamine is effective in Hodgkin's disease. Current practice is to give it in combination with other agents. The combination with vincristine (Oncovin), procarbazine, and prednisone, known as the MOPP regimen, was considered the treatment of choice. Other lymphomas and mycosis fungoides can be treated with mechlorethamine. The most serious toxic reaction is bone marrow depression, which results in leukopenia and thrombocytopenia. Emesis is prevalent and lasts about 8 hours. Nausea and anorexia persist longer. These gastrointestinal effects may be prevented by the antiemetic compound ondansetron. Inadvertent extravasation produces intense local reactions at the site of injection. If it occurs, the immediate application of sodium thiosulfate solution can protect the tissues because thiosulfate ion reacts very rapidly with the aziridinium ion formed from mechlorethamine.

Cyclophosphamide, USP.

Cyclophosphamide, Cytoxan, NSC-26271, *N,N*-bis(2-chloroethyl)tetrahydro-2*H*-1,3,2-oxazaphosphorine-2-amine-2-oxide, is prepared by treating bis(2-chloroethyl)-phosphoramide dichloride with propanolamine.[48] The monohydrate is a low-melting solid that is very soluble in water. It is supplied as 25- and 50-mg white tablets, as 50-mg-unit-dose cartons, and as a powder (100, 200, or 500 mg) in sterile vials. For reconstitution, 5 mL/100 mg of Sterile Water for Injection, USP, is added.

The oral dose of cyclophosphamide is 90% bioavailable, with an 8% first-pass loss. It must be metabolized by liver microsomes to become active. Among the metabolites, phosphoramide mustard has antitumor activity, and acrolein is toxic to the urinary bladder. The acrolein toxicity can be decreased by intravenous or oral administration of the sodium salt of 2-mercaptoethane sulfonic acid (mesna), whose sulfhydryl group gives conjugate addition to the double bond of acrolein.[49] In the plasma, mesna forms a disulfide, which is converted selectively to the active sulfhydryl in renal tubules.

Cyclophosphamide has advantages over other alkylating agents in that it is active orally and parenterally and can be given in fractionated doses over prolonged periods. It is active against multiple myeloma, chronic lymphocytic leukemia (CLL), and acute leukemia of children. In combination with other chemotherapeutic agents, it has given complete remissions and even cures in Burkett's lymphoma and acute lymphoblastic leukemia (ALL) in children.[50] The most frequently encountered toxic effects are alopecia, nausea, and vomiting. Leukopenia occurs, but thrombocytopenia is less frequent than with other alkylating agents. Sterile hemorrhagic cystitis may result and even be fatal. Gonadal suppression has been reported in a number of patients.

Ifosfamide.

Ifosfamide, IFEX, Holoxan, NSC-109724, 3-(2-chloroethyl)-2[(2-chloroethyl)amino]-tetrahydro-2*H*-1,3,2-oxazaphosphorine-2-oxide, isophosphamide, is prepared from 3-[(2-chloroethyl)amino]propanol by treatment with phosphorus oxychloride followed by 2-chloroethylamine.[51] It is supplied in 1- and 3-g vials as an off-white lyophilized powder. The intact vials may be stored at room temperature

or under refrigeration for prolonged times. At temperatures above 35°C, it liquifies and decomposition is more rapid.

Ifosfamide usually is administered in a short infusion in 5% dextrose or normal saline. Use within 8 hours of reconstitution is recommended. Pharmacokinetic studies indicate that it is handled in the same way as cyclophosphamide, except that metabolism is less extensive. There is an apparent half-life of 7 hours and a urinary recovery of 73%.[52]

The Food and Drug Administration (FDA)–approved indication for ifosfamide is in combination therapy for germ cell testicular cancer.[53] Combination salvage regimens are effective against soft tissue sarcoma, ovarian and breast carcinomas, and leukemia. Its limiting toxicity is in the urinary tract, especially hemorrhagic cystitis, which results from the excretion of alkylating metabolites in the urinary bladder.[54] Vigorous hydration and/or administration of mesna are needed to prevent bladder damage. Other toxicities include nausea and vomiting, alopecia, and CNS effects.

Melphalan, USP.

Melphalan, Alkeran, L-sarcolysine, L-mustard, NSC-8806, 4-bis(2-chloroethyl)amino-L-phenylalanine, is prepared by treating L-*N*-phthalimido-*p*-aminophenylalanine ethyl ester with ethylene oxide, followed by phosphorus oxychloride, and finally hydrolysis with hydrochloric acid.[55] Scored 2-mg tablets are available for oral administration. Oral absorption is erratic and incomplete, with absolute bioavailability ranging from 25 to 89%. A preparation kit is provided for parenteral formulation. It contains 100 mg of melphalan, which is dissolved in 1 mL of acid-alcohol solution, and then combined with final diluent containing 108 mg of dipotassium phosphate, 5.4 mL of propylene glycol, and Sterile Water for Injection, USP, to give 9 mL of solution. This preparation should be used promptly.

There is no significant first-pass effect with melphalan, but the drug is gradually inactivated by nonenzymatic hydrolysis to monohydroxy and dihydroxy derivatives.[56] Elimination is biphasic, with half-lives of 6 to 8 minutes and 40 to 60 minutes. Most of the drug is cleared by nonrenal mechanisms.

Melphalan is active against multiple myeloma. It also is active against breast, testicular, and ovarian carcinoma.[57] The clinical toxicity is mainly hematological, which means that the blood count must be followed carefully. Nausea and vomiting are infrequent, but alopecia occurs.

Melphalan

Chlorambucil, USP.

Chlorambucil, Leukeran, chloraminophene, NSC-3088, *p*-(di-2-chlorethyl)-aminophenylbutyric acid, is prepared by treating *p*-aminophenylbutyric acid with ethylene oxide, followed by thionyl chloride.[58] Chlorambucil is soluble in ether and aqueous alkali. Its oral absorption is efficient and reliable. Sugar-coated 2-mg tablets are supplied.

Chlorambucil acts most slowly and is the least toxic of any nitrogen mustard derivative in use. It is indicated especially in treatment of CLL and primary macroglobulinemia.

Other indications are lymphosarcoma and Hodgkin's disease.[59] Many patients develop progressive, but reversible, lymphopenia during treatment. Most patients also develop a dose-related and rapidly reversible neutropenia. For these reasons, weekly blood counts are made to determine the total and differential leukocyte levels. The hemoglobin levels are also determined for monitoring both toxicity (low counts) and efficacy in CLL (raised counts).

Busulfan, USP. Busulfan, Myleran, NSC-750, 1,4-di-(methanesulfonyloxy)butane, is synthesized by treating 1,4-butanediol with methanesulfonyl chloride in the presence of pyridine.[60] It is obtained as crystals that are soluble in acetone and alcohol. Although practically insoluble in water, it dissolves slowly on hydrolysis. It is, however, stable in dry form. It is supplied as scored 2-mg tablets.

Busulfan is well absorbed orally and metabolized rapidly. Much of the drug undergoes a process known as "sulfur stripping" in which interaction with thiol compounds such as glutathione or cysteine results in loss of two equivalents of methanesulfonic acid and formation of a cyclic sulfonium intermediate involving the sulfur atom of the thiol.[61] Such sulfonium intermediates are stable in vitro, but in vivo, they are readily converted into the metabolite 3-hydroxythiolane-1,1-dioxide.[62] That the sulfur atom of this thiolane does not come from a methanesulfonyl group was shown by the nearly quantitative isolation of labeled methanesulfonic acid in the urine when busulfan ^{35}S is administered to animals.[63]

Oral doses of busulfan are generally well tolerated. The absorption has zero-order kinetics, with a mean log time of 36 minutes and a 2-hour duration to the end of absorption.[64] Values for mean plasma concentration × time are dose dependent, with peak levels of 24 to 130 ng/mL for 2- to 6-mg doses. The half-life is 2.1 to 2.6 hours.

The main therapeutic use of busulfan is in chronic granulocytic leukemia. Remissions are observed in 85 to 90% of patients after the first course of therapy; it is not curative, however. It is used in preparative regimens (bone marrow ablative) for bone marrow transplantation in patients with various leukemias. Toxic effects are mostly limited to myelosuppression in which the depletion of thrombocytes may lead to hemorrhage. Blood counts should be done at least weekly. The rapid destruction of granulocytes can cause hyperuricemia, which might result in kidney damage. This complication is prevented by using allopurinol, a xanthine oxidase inhibitor.[65]

Carmustine. Carmustine, BiCNU, BCNU, NSC-409962, 1,3-bis(2-chloroethyl)-1-nitrosourea, is synthesized by treating 1,3-bis(2-chloroethyl)urea with sodium nitrite and formic acid.[66] It is a low-melting white powder that changes to an oily liquid at 27°C. This change is considered a sign of decomposition, and such samples should be discarded. Carmustine is most stable in petroleum ether or water at pH 4. It is administered intravenously because metabolism is very rapid. Some of the degradation products, however, have prolonged half-lives in plasma. Carmustine is supplied as 100-mg quantities of lyophilized powder. When it is diluted with 3 mL of the supplied sterile diluent, ethanol, and further diluted with 27 mL of sterile water, a 10% ethanolic solution containing 3.3 mg/mL is obtained.

Biotransformation of carmustine is rapid and extensive, with most of a dose recovered in urine as metabolites. The half-life has an α-phase half-life of 6.1 minutes and a β-phase half-life of 21.5 minutes.[67]

Because of its ability to cross the blood–brain barrier, carmustine is used against brain tumors and other tumors (e.g., leukemias) that have metastasized to the brain.[68] It also is used as secondary therapy in combination with other agents for Hodgkin's disease and other lymphomas. Multiple myeloma responds to a combination of carmustine and prednisone. Delayed myelosuppression is the most frequent and serious toxicity. This condition usually develops 4 to 6 weeks after treatment. Thrombocytopenia is the most pronounced effect, followed by leukopenia. Nausea and vomiting frequently occur about 2 hours after treatment.

Carmustine is given as a single dose by intravenous injection at 100 to 200 mg/m². A repeat course is not given until the blood elements return to normal levels, which requires about 6 weeks.

Lomustine. Lomustine, CeeNU, CCNU, NSC-79037, [1-(2-chlorethyl)]-3-cyclohexyl-l-nitrosourea, is synthesized by treating ethyl 5-(2-chloroethyl)-3-nitrosohydantoate with cyclohexylamine, followed by renitrosation of the resulting intermediate, [1-(2-chloroethyl)]-3-cyclohexyl-urea.[69] It is sufficiently stable to metabolism to be administered orally. The high lipid solubility of lomustine allows it to cross the blood–brain barrier rapidly. Levels in the CSF are 50% higher than those in plasma. Lomustine is supplied in dose packs that contain two each of color-coded 100-, 40-, and 10-mg capsules. The total dose prescribed is obtained by appropriate combination of these capsules.

$$ClCH_2CH_2NCNH \text{—} \bigcirc$$

Lomustine

Oral absorption of lomustine is nearly complete within 30 minutes. It is converted rapidly into *cis*- and *trans*-4-OH metabolites by liver microsomes. The half-life of the parent drug is 1.3 to 2.9 hours, and the peak concentration of metabolites is reached 2 to 4 hours after dosing.

Lomustine is used against both primary and metastatic brain tumors and as secondary therapy in relapsed Hodgkin's disease. The most common adverse reactions are nausea and vomiting, thrombocytopenia, and leukopenia. As in the case of carmustine, the myelosuppression caused by lomustine is delayed.[70]

The recommended dosage of lomustine is 130 mg/m² orally every 6 weeks. A reduced dose is given to patients with compromised bone marrow function.

Thiotepa, USP. Thiotepa, TSPA, NSC-6396, N,N',N''-triethylene-thiophosphoramide, tris(1-aziridinyl)phosphine sulfide, is prepared by treating trichlorophosphine sulfide with aziridine[71] and is obtained as a white powder that is water soluble. It is supplied in vials containing 15 mg of thiotepa, 80 mg of sodium chloride, and 50 mg of sodium bicarbonate. Sterile water is added to make an isotonic solution. Both the vials and solutions must be stored at 2 to 8°C. These solutions may be stored 5 days without loss of potency.

Thiotepa blood levels decline in a rapid biphasic manner. It is converted into TEPA by oxidative desulfurization, and TEPA levels exceed those of thiotepa 2 hours after administration. Aziridine metabolism also occurs, with liberation of ethanolamine.

Thiotepa has been tried against a wide variety of tumors and has given palliation in many types, although with varying frequencies. The most consistent results have been obtained in breast, ovarian, and bronchogenic carcinomas and malignant lymphomas. It is a mainstay of high-dose regimens in treating solid tumors when followed by autologous bone marrow transplantation. It also is used to control intracavity effusions resulting from neoplasms. Thiotepa is highly toxic to bone marrow, and blood counts are necessary during therapy.

Procarbazine Hydrochloride, USP. Procarbazine hydrochloride, Matulane, MIH, NSC-77213, N-isopropyl-α-(2-methylhydrazine)-p-toluamide, is prepared from N-isopropyl-p-toluamide in a process involving condensation with diethyl azodicarboxylate, methylation with methyl iodide and base, and acid hydrolysis.[72] Although soluble in water, it is unstable in solution. Capsules containing the equivalent of 50 mg of procarbazine as its hydrochloride are supplied.

Procarbazine is rapidly and completely absorbed following oral administration. It readily decomposes by chemical and metabolic routes, with a half-life of 7 to 10 minutes, to produce highly reactive species including methyl diazonium ion, methyl radicals, hydrogen peroxide, formaldehyde, and hydroxyl radicals.[73]

Procarbazine has demonstrated activity against Hodgkin's disease. For this condition, it is used in combination with agents such as mechlorethamine, vincristine, and prednisone (MOPP program). Toxic effects, such as leukopenia, thrombocytopenia, nausea, and vomiting, occur in most patients. Neurological and dermatological effects also occur. Concurrent intake of alcohol, certain amine drugs, and foods containing high tyramine levels is contraindicated. The weak monoamine oxidase-inhibiting properties of procarbazine may potentiate catechol amines to produce hypertension.

Dacarbazine. Dacarbazine, DTIC-Dome, DIC, DTIC, NSC-45388, 5-(3,3-dimethyl-1-triazenyl)-1H-imidazole-4-carboxamide, is prepared by treating the diazonium salt, prepared from 5-aminoimidazole-4-carboxamide, with dimethylamine in methanol.[74] It is obtained as a colorless to ivory-colored solid that is very sensitive to light. It does not melt but decomposes explosively when heated above 250°C. Water solubility is good, but solutions must be protected from light. Dacarbazine is supplied in vials containing either 100 or 200 mg. When reconstituted with 9.9 and 19.7 mL, respectively, of sterile water, these samples give solutions containing 10 mg/mL at pH 3.0 to 4.0. Such solutions may be stored at 4°C for 72 hours.

Injected dacarbazine disappears rapidly from plasma because of hepatic metabolism. The half-life is about 40 minutes. Excretion is by the renal tubules, and in the 6-hour excretion fraction, 50% of the drug is intact and 50% is the N-demethylated metabolite.[75]

Dacarbazine is indicated for the treatment of metastatic malignant melanoma.[76, 77] Combination with other antineoplastic drugs is superior to its use as a single agent. Anorexia, nausea, and vomiting are the most frequent toxic reactions. Leukopenia and thrombocytopenia, however, are the most serious effects.[78] Blood counts should be done, and if the counts are too low, therapy should be temporarily suspended. Dacarbazine is also used in combination therapy for Hodgkin's disease.

The recommended daily dosage is 2 to 4.5 mg/kg for 10 days, with repetition at 4-week intervals. Extravasation of the drug during injection may result in severe pain.

ANTIMETABOLITES

Antimetabolites are compounds that prevent the biosynthesis or use of normal cellular metabolites. Nearly all of the clinical agents are related to metabolites and cofactors in the biosynthesis of nucleic acids. They usually are closely related in structure to the metabolite that is antagonized. Many antimetabolites are enzyme inhibitors. They may combine with the active site as if they were the substrate or cofactor.[79] Alternatively, they may bind to an allosteric regulatory site, especially when they resemble the end product of a biosynthetic pathway under feedback control.[16] Sometimes, the antimetabolite must be transformed biosynthetically (anabolized) into the active inhibitor. For example, 6-mercaptopurine is converted into the corresponding ribonucleotide, which is a potent inhibitor of the conversion of 5-phosphoribosylpyrophosphate into 5-phosphoribosylamine, a rate-controlling step in the de novo synthesis of purines[80] (see

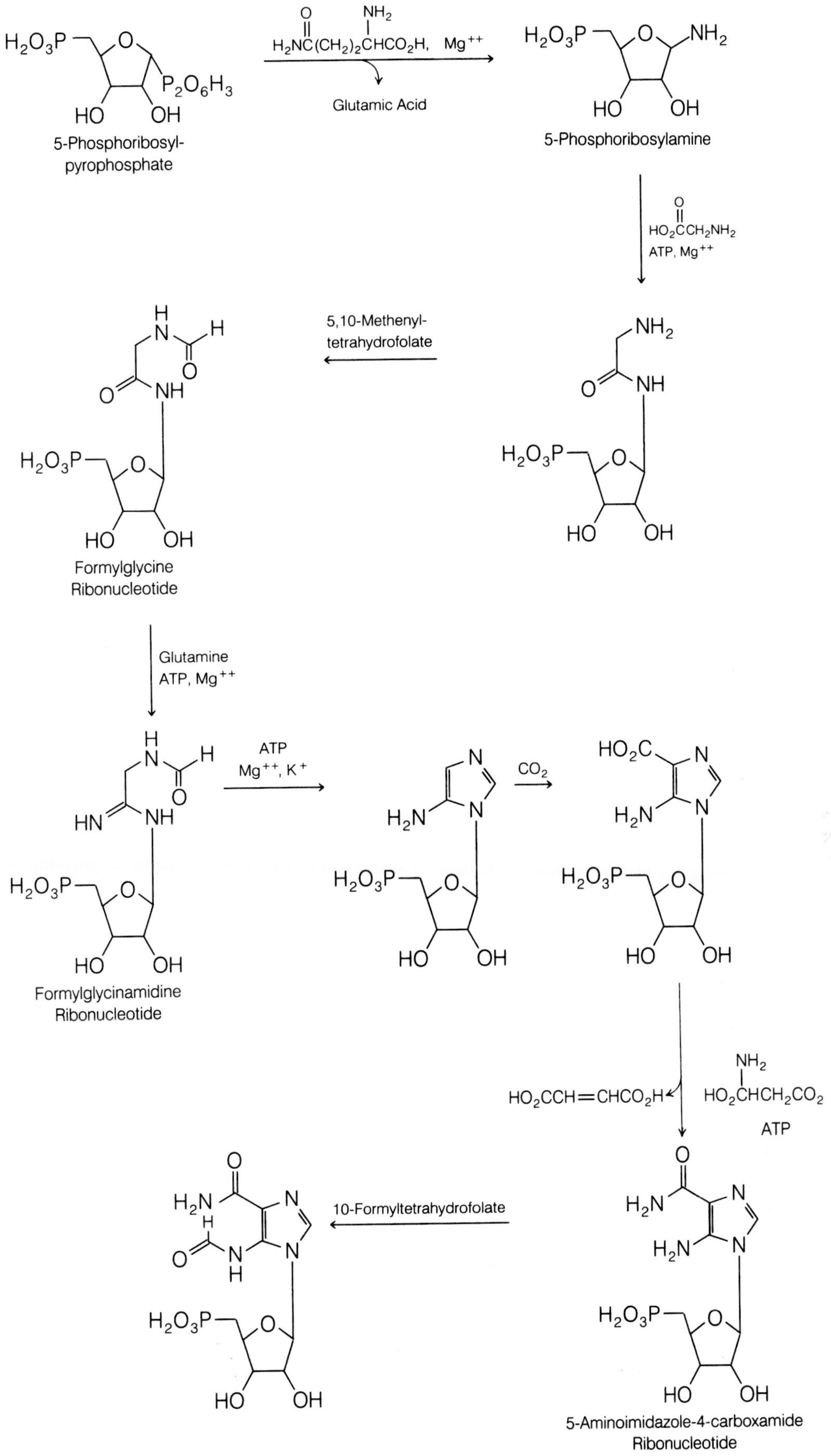

Scheme 12–6 ■ De novo synthesis of purine nucleotides (simplified).

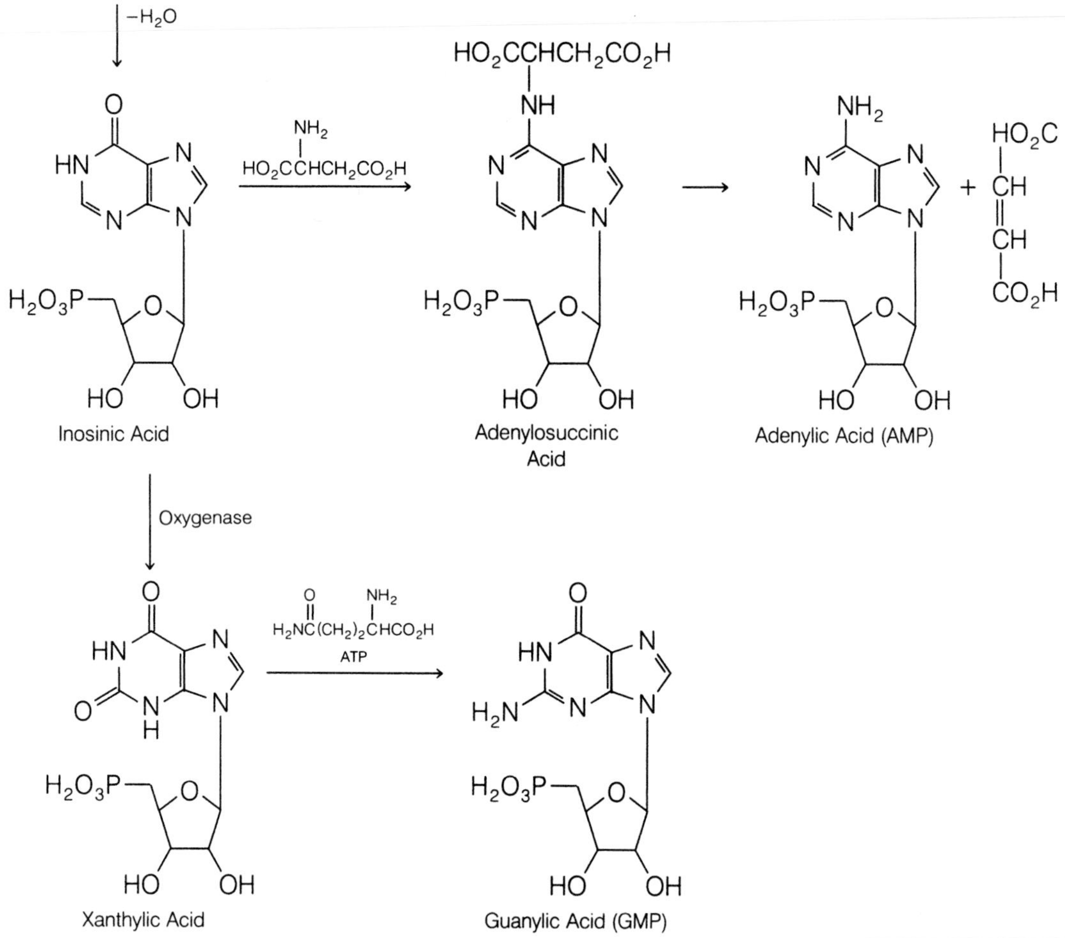

Scheme 12-6 ■ *Continued.*

Scheme 12-6). An antimetabolite and its transformation products may inhibit a number of different enzymes. Thus, 6-mercaptopurine and its anabolites interact with more than 20 enzymes. This multiplicity of effects makes it difficult to decide which ones are crucial to the antitumor activity.

The anabolites of purine and pyrimidine antagonists may be incorporated into nucleic acids. In this event, part of their antitumor effect might result from malfunction of further macromolecular synthesis because of the abnormal nucleic acids.[81]

After the formulation of the antimetabolite theory by Woods and Fildes in 1940,[82, 82a] antimetabolites based on a variety of known nutrients were prepared. The first purine analogue to show antitumor activity in mice, 8-azaguanine, was synthesized by Roblin in 1945.[83] This compound was intro-

duced into clinical trials but was abandoned in favor of newer and more effective agents, such as 6-mercaptopurine and 6-thioguanine, developed by Hitchings and Elion.[84] 6-Mercaptopurine was synthesized in 1952[85] and was shown to be active against human leukemia in the following year.

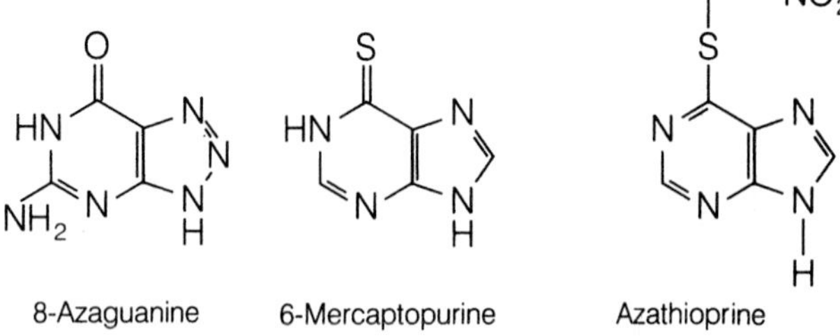

To be active against neoplasms, 6-mercaptopurine must be converted into its ribonucleotide, 6-thioinosinate, by the enzyme hypoxanthine-guanine phosphoribosyltransferase. Neoplasms that lack this enzyme are resistant to the drug.[86] 6-Thioinosinate is a potent inhibitor of the conversion of 5-phosphoribosylpyrophosphate into 5-phosphoribosylamine, as mentioned above. It also inhibits the conversion of inosinic acid to adenylic acid at two stages: (*a*) the reaction of inosinic acid with aspartate to give adenylosuccinic acid and (*b*) the loss of fumaric acid from adenylosuccinic acid to give adenylic acid.[87] Furthermore, it inhibits the oxidation of inosinic acid to xanthylic acid.[88] The mode of action of 6-mercaptopurine is further complicated by the fact that its ribose diphosphate and triphosphate anabolites are also active enzyme inhibitors, and the triphosphate can be incorporated into DNA and RNA to inhibit further chain elongation.[87] Still more complex is the ability of 6-thioinosinate to act as a substrate for a methyl transferase that requires *S*-adenosylmethionine, which converts it into 6-methylthioinosinate. The latter compound is responsible for certain antimetabolite activities of 6-mercaptopurine.[89]

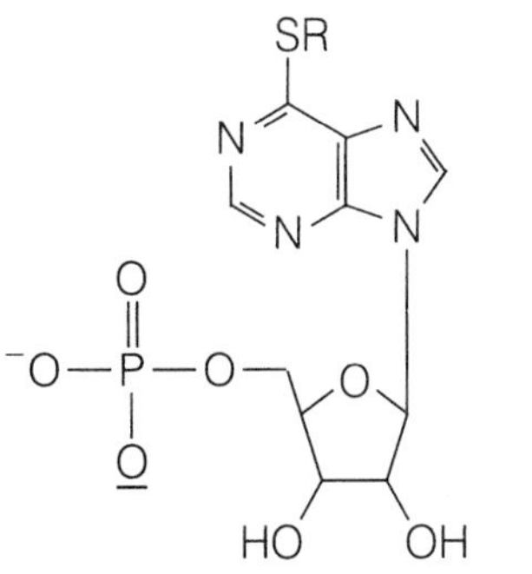

6-Thioinosinate (R = H)
6-Methylthioinosinate (R = CH₃)

Metabolic degradation (catabolism) of 6-mercaptopurine by guanase gives 6-thioxanthine, which is oxidized by xanthine oxidase to yield 6-thiouric acid.[90] Allopurinol, an inhibitor of xanthine oxidase, increases both the potency and the toxicity of 6-mercaptopurine. Its main importance, however, is as an adjuvant to chemotherapy because it prevents the uric acid kidney toxicity caused by the release of purines from destroyed cancer cells. Heterocyclic derivatives of 6-mercaptopurine, such as azathioprine (Imuran), were designed to protect it from catabolic reactions.[91] Although azathioprine has antitumor activity, it is not significantly better than 6-mercaptopurine. It has an important role, however, as an immunosuppressive agent in organ transplants.[84]

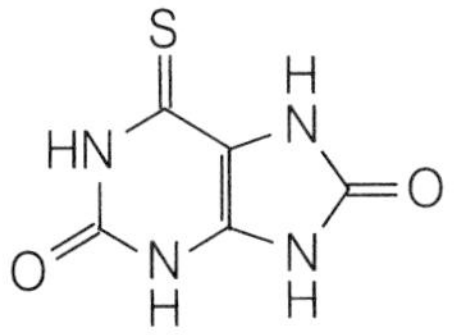

6-Thiouric Acid 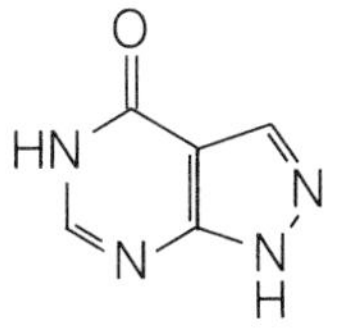   Allopurinol

Thioguanine is converted into its ribonucleotide by the same enzyme that acts on 6-mercaptopurine. It is converted further into the di- and triphosphates.[92] These species inhibit most of the same enzymes that are inhibited by 6-mercaptopurine. Thioguanine is also incorporated into RNA, and its 2′-deoxy metabolite is incorporated into DNA. The significance of these "fraudulent" nucleic acids in lethality to neoplasms is uncertain.[93]

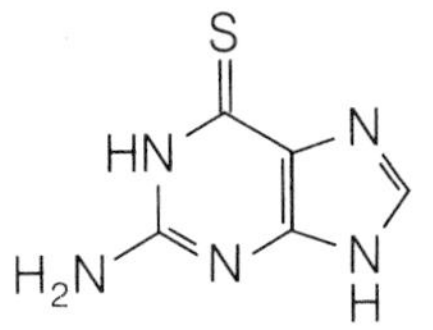

6-Thioguanine

Adenine arabinoside (Vidarabine) was first prepared by chemical synthesis[94] and later isolated from cultures of *Streptomyces antibioticus*.[95] It has a sugar, D-arabinose, which is epimeric with D-ribose at the 2′ position. This structural change makes it a competitive inhibitor of DNA polymerase.[96] In addition to its antineoplastic activity, adenine arabinoside has potent antiviral action. Adenine arabinoside and some of its derivatives are limited in their antitumor effect by susceptibility to adenosine deaminase. This enzyme converts them into hypoxanthine arabinoside derivatives. The resistance of certain tumors correlates with their levels of adenosine deaminase.[97]

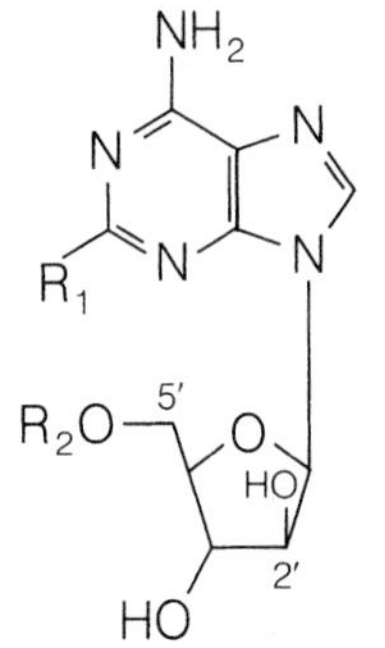

R₁ = R₂ = H; Vidarabine
R₁ = F, R₂ = HOPO₂; Fludarabine

In contrast to the susceptibility of adenosine arabinoside to adenosine deaminase, its 2-fluoro derivative, fludarabine, is stable to this enzyme. Fludarabine is prepared as the 5′-monophosphate. Fludarabine has good activity against CLL. It is converted into the corresponding triphosphate,[98] which inhibits ribonucleotide reductase.[99] 2-Chloro-2′-deoxyadenosine (cladribine) also is resistant to adenosine deaminase. It is phosphorylated in cells to the triphosphate by cytidine kinase, and the triphosphate inhibits enzymes required for DNA repair.[100] Cladribine is highly effective against hairy cell leukemia.

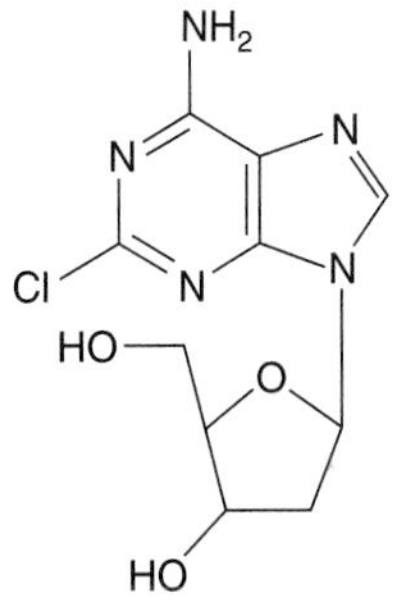

Cladribine

The invention of 5-fluorouracil as an antimetabolite of uracil by Heidelberger in 1957 provided one of our foremost examples of rational drug design.[101] Starting with the observation that in certain tumors uracil was used more than orotic acid, the major precursor for nucleic acid pyrimidine biosynthesis in normal tissue, he decided to synthesize an antimetabolite of uracil with only one modification in the structure. The 5 position was chosen for a substituent to block the conversion of uridylate to thymidylate (Scheme 12-7), thus diminishing DNA biosynthesis. Fluorine was chosen as the substituent because the increased acidity caused by its inductive effect was expected to cause the molecule to bind strongly to enzymes. These choices were well founded, as 5-fluorouracil soon became one of the most widely used antineoplastic agents. It is a mainstay in the therapy of adenocarcinoma of the colon and rectum. Side effects are both dose and schedule dependent. They include myelosuppression on bolus administration and mucositis on prolonged infusions. Otherwise, the drug is well tolerated.

5-Fluorouracil is activated by anabolism to 5-fluoro-2 deoxyuridylic acid. This conversion may proceed by two routes. In one route, 5-fluorouracil reacts with ribose-1 phosphate to give its riboside, which is phosphorylated by uridine kinase.[102] The resulting compound, 5-fluorouridylic acid, is

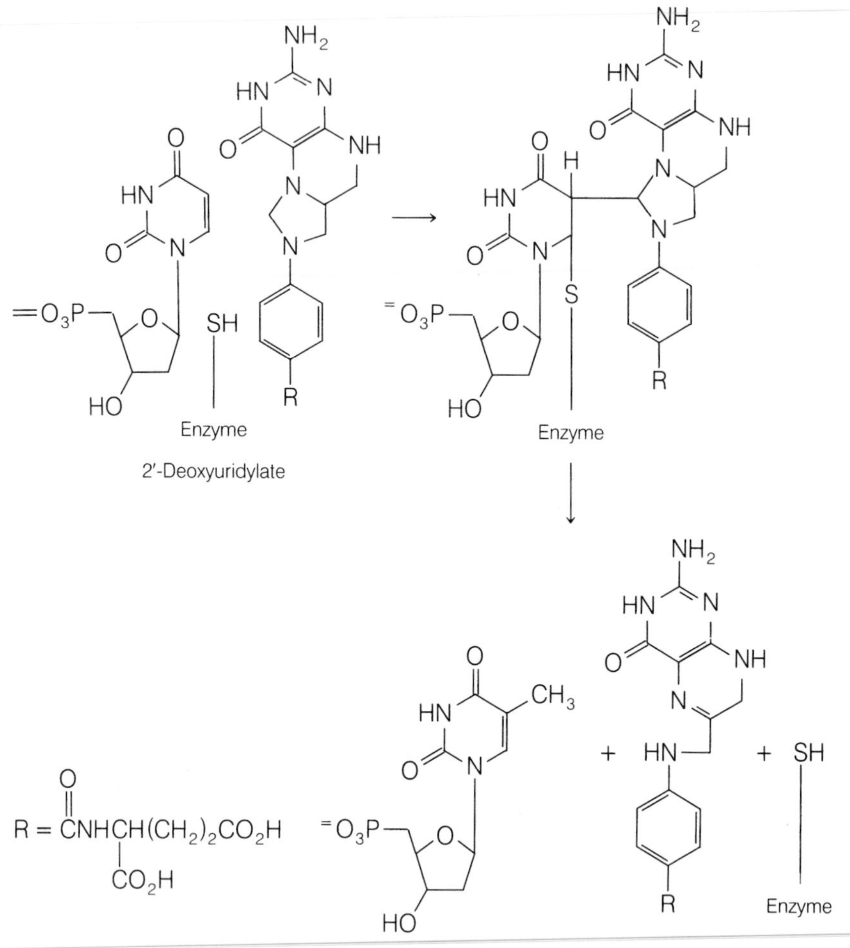

Scheme 12–7 ■ Conversion of uridylate into thymidylate.

converted into its 2′-deoxy derivative by ribonucleotide reductase. 5-Fluorouracil also may be transformed directly into 5-fluorouridylic acid by a phosphoribosyltransferase, which is present in certain tumors.[103] An alternative pharmaceutical based on 5-fluorouracil is its 2-deoxyriboside (floxuridine).[101] This compound is phosphorylated by 2′-deoxyuridine kinase.

5-Fluoro-2′-deoxyuridylic acid is a powerful competitive inhibitor of thymidylate synthetase, the enzyme that converts 2′-deoxyuridylic acid to thymidylic acid. This blockage is probably the main lethal effect of 5-fluorouracil and its metabolites.[104] In the inhibiting reaction, the sulfhydryl group

of a cysteine residue in the enzyme adds to the 6 position of the fluorouracil moiety. The 5 position then binds to the methylene group of 5,10-methylenetetrahydrofolate. Ordinarily, this step would be followed by the transfer of the 5-hydrogen of uracil to the methylene group, resulting in the formation of thymidylate and dihydrofolate; however, the 5-fluorine is stable to transfer, and a terminal product results involving the enzyme, cofactor, and substrate, all covalently bonded. Thus, 5-fluoro-2′-deoxyuridylic acid would be classified as a K_{cat} inhibitor.[105]

The rate-determining enzyme in 5-fluorouracil catabolism is dihydropyrimidine dehydrogenase. Inhibition of this en-

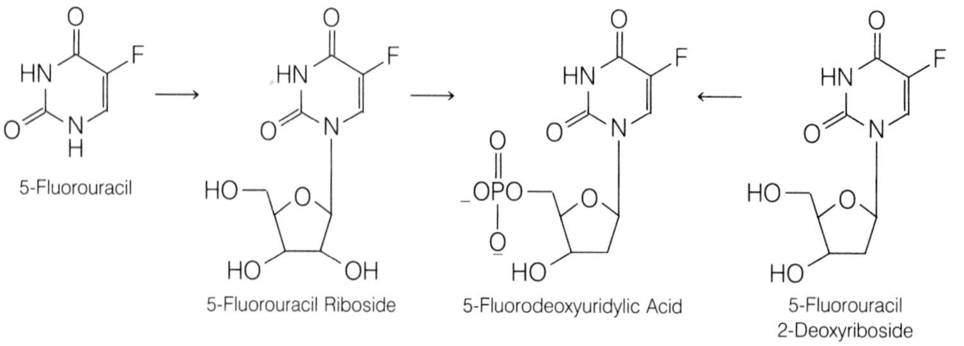

5-Fluorouracil   5-Fluorouracil Riboside   5-Fluorodeoxyuridylic Acid   5-Fluorouracil 2-Deoxyriboside

zyme by 5-ethynyluracil increases the plasma concentration-time curve of 5-fluorouracil enough to raise its therapeutic index two- to fourfold.

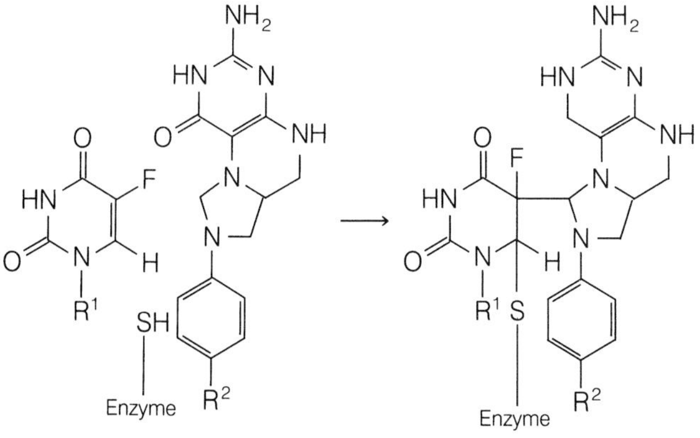

The tetrahydrofuranyl derivative of 5-fluorouracil, tegafur (Ftorafur), was prepared in Russia.[106] It is active in clinical cancer and less myelosuppressive than 5-fluorouracil. It has gastrointestinal and CNS toxicity, however. Tegafur is slowly metabolized to 5-fluorouracil; thus, it may be considered a prodrug.[107]

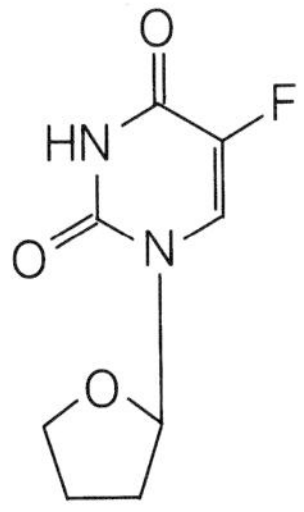

Tegafur
(Ftorafur)

Capecitabine was designed rationally as a tumor-selective and tumor-activated prodrug of 5-fluorouracil, which would be less likely to produce severe diarrhea. It is a carbamate derivative of 5′-deoxy-5-fluorocytidine. On oral administration, it is converted into 5′-deoxy-5-fluorocytidine by cytidine deaminase, which is in higher concentration in many tumors than in most normal tissues, with the notable exception of liver. Activation to cytotoxic species by thymidine phosphorylase occurs preferentially at tumor sites.[108] Despite this complex activation process, capecitabine still exhibits some of the significant toxicities of 5-fluorouracil.

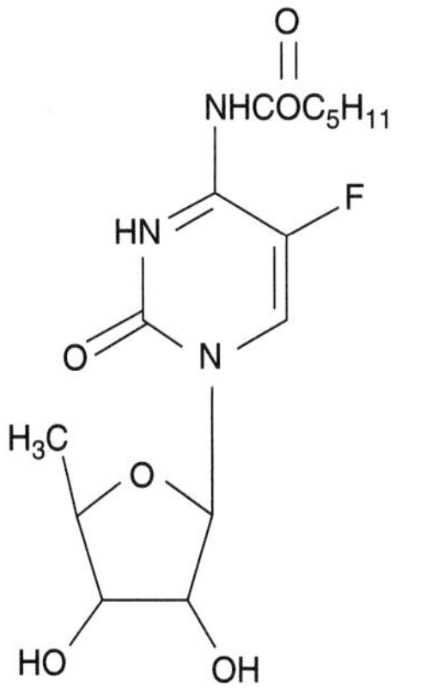

In gemcitabine, fluorine atoms replace the hydroxyl group and the hydrogen atom at the 2′ position of cytidine.[109] After its anabolism to diphosphate and triphosphate metabolites, gemcitabine inhibits ribonucleotide reductase and competes with 2′-deoxycytidine triphosphate for incorporation into DNA. These effects produce cell-cycle-specific cytotoxicity. Gemcitabine has become a first-line treatment for locally advanced and metastatic adenocarcinoma of the pancreas.

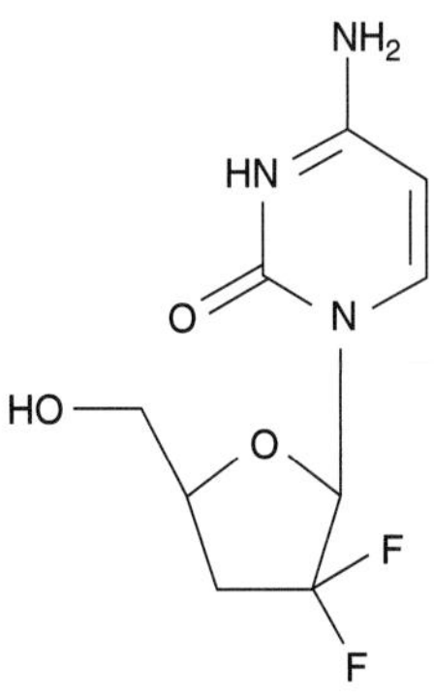

Trifluorothymidine (Trifluridine) was designed by Heidelberger as an antimetabolite of thymine.[101] The riboside is essential because mammalian cells are unable to convert thymine and certain analogues into thymidine and its analogues. Thymidine kinase converts trifluorothymidine into trifluorothymidylic acid, which is a potent inhibitor of thymidylate synthetase.[101] In contrast to the stability of most trifluoromethyl groups, that of trifluorothymidylic acid is extraordinarily labile. It reacts with glycine to give an amide at neutral pH.[110] Kinetic studies have shown that this reaction involves initial nucleophilic attack at position 6, followed by loss of HF to give the highly reactive difluoromethylene group.[111] Glycine then adds to this group and hydrolysis of the remaining two fluorine atoms follows (Scheme 12-8). The interaction of trifluorothymidylic acid with thymidylate synthetase apparently follows a similar course. Thus, after preincubation, it becomes irreversibly bound to the enzyme, and the kinetics are noncompetitive.[101]

Cytosine arabinoside was synthesized in 1959[112] and later found as a fermentation product.[113] Its structure is noteworthy in that the arabinose moiety is epimeric at the 2′ position with ribose. This modification, after anabolism to the triphosphate, causes it to inhibit the conversion of cytidylic acid to 2′-deoxycytidylic acid.[114] For a number of years, this inhibition was believed to be the main mode of action of cytosine arabinoside triphosphate; however, it was shown recently that various deoxyribonucleosides were just as effective as cytosine arabinoside in reducing cellular levels of 2′-deoxycytidylic acid.[115] Other modes of action include the inhibition of DNA-dependent DNA polymerase[116] and miscoding following incorporation into DNA and RNA.[117] Cytosine arabinoside is readily transported into cells and phosphorylated by deoxycytidine kinase. It acts predominantly in the S phase of the cell cycle. Tumor cell resistance is based on low levels of deoxycytidine kinase and the elaboration of deaminases that convert cytosine arabinoside into uridine arabinoside.[118] Partially purified cytidine deaminase is inhibited by tetrahydrouridine.[119]

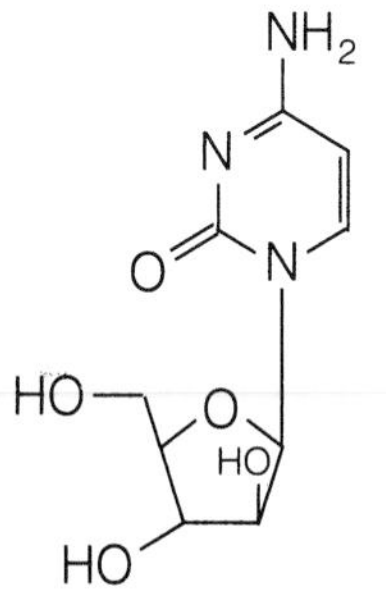

Cytarabine
(Cytosine arabinoside)

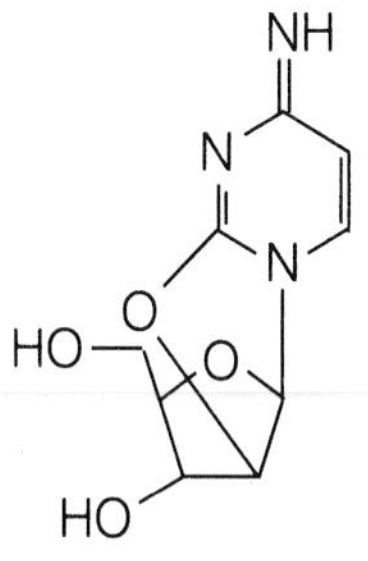

Ancitabine
(Cyclocytidine)

Capecitabine

Gemcitabine

A new analogue of cytosine arabinoside is cyclocytidine (ancitabine). This analogue apparently is a prodrug that is slowly converted into cytosine arabinoside. It is reported to

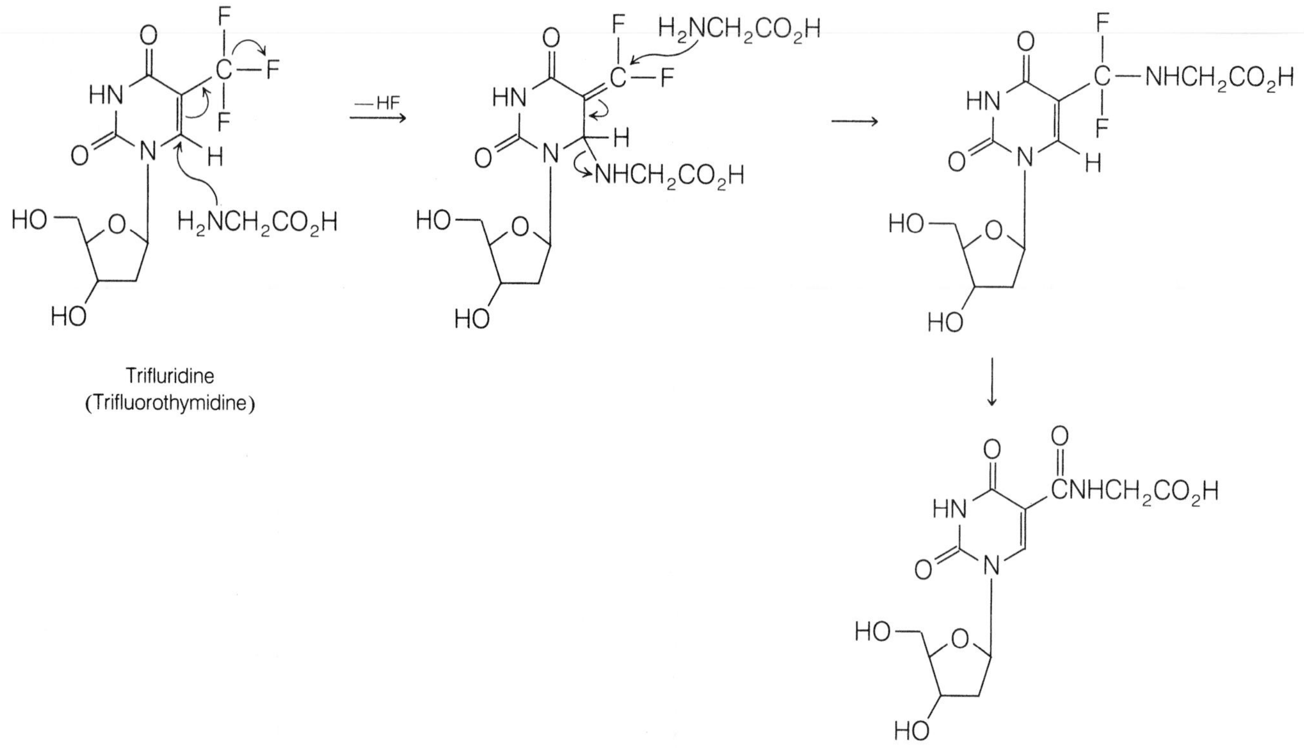

Scheme 12–8 ■ Reaction of trifluorothymidine with glycine.

be resistant to deamination and to have a better therapeutic index than the parent compound.[120]

A number of pyrimidine nucleoside analogues have one more or one less nitrogen in the heterocyclic ring. They are known as azapyrimidine or deazapyrimidine nucleosides. 5-Azacytidine was synthesized in 1964 by Sórm in Czechoslovakia[121] and later was isolated as an antibiotic by Hanka.[122] The mode of action of this compound is complex, involving anabolism to phosphate derivatives and deamination to 5-azauridine. In certain tumor systems, it is incorporated into nucleic acids, which may result in misreading.[123] One of its main effects is the inhibition of orotidylate decarboxylase (Scheme 12-9), which prevents the new synthesis of pyrimidine nucleotides.[124] Tumor resistance is based on decreased phosphorylation of the nucleoside, decreased incorporation into nucleic acids, and increased RNA and DNA polymerase activity.[125] Other pyrimidine nucleoside antagonists that have received clinical study include dihydro-5-azacytidine and 3-deazauridine.[98]

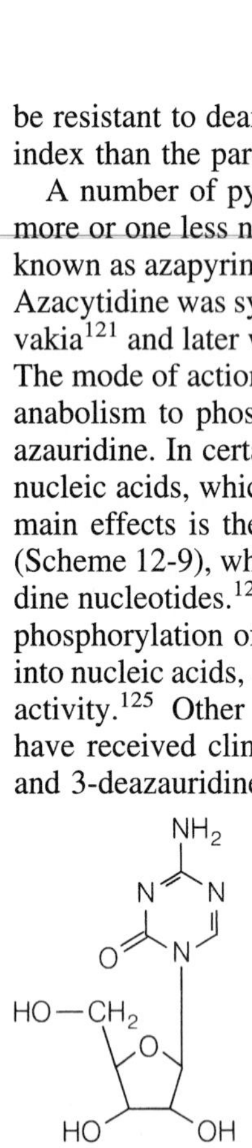

for compounds that might inhibit these deaminases. In theory, a potent deaminase inhibitor would produce a synergistic effect on the antitumor activity of the antimetabolite, even though it might not be active itself. Two types of deaminase inhibitors have emerged recently. One type is the purine analogue in which the pyrimidine ring has been expanded to a seven-membered ring. The first example of this type was 2'-deoxycoformycin (pentostatin), an unusual nucleoside produced in the same cultures as the antibiotic formycin.[126] It strongly synergized the action of formycin against organisms that produce deaminases. In clinical trials it showed a synergistic effect on the activities of adenine arabinoside and cytosine arabinoside. A second type of adenosine deaminase inhibitor has the adenine portion unchanged but is modified in the ribose moiety. Such modifications have been designed to probe the active site of the enzyme and take advantage of strong binding to adjacent lipophilic regions.[127] EHNA is an example of a rationally designed inhibitor.

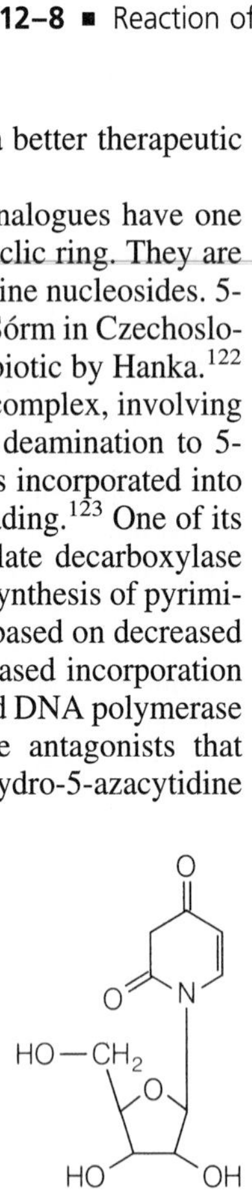

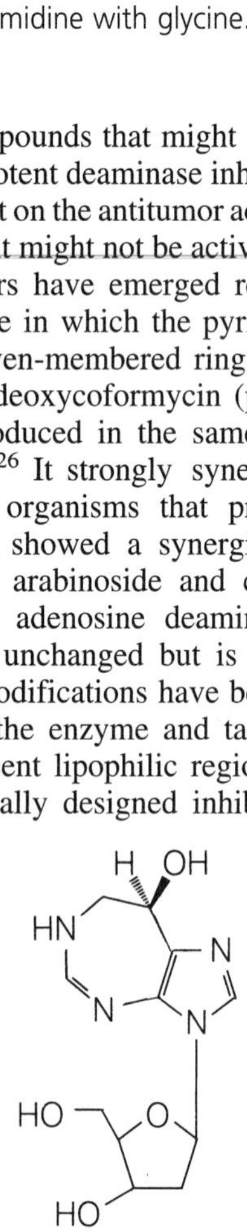

Azacitidine (5-Azacytidine)   Dihydro-5-azacytidine   3-Deazauridine

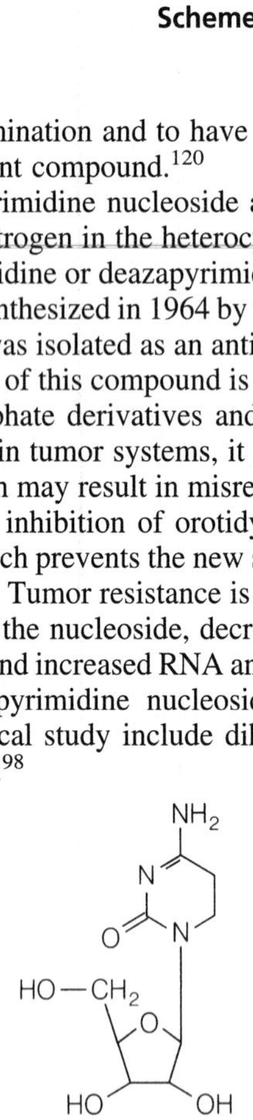

2'-Deoxycoformycin 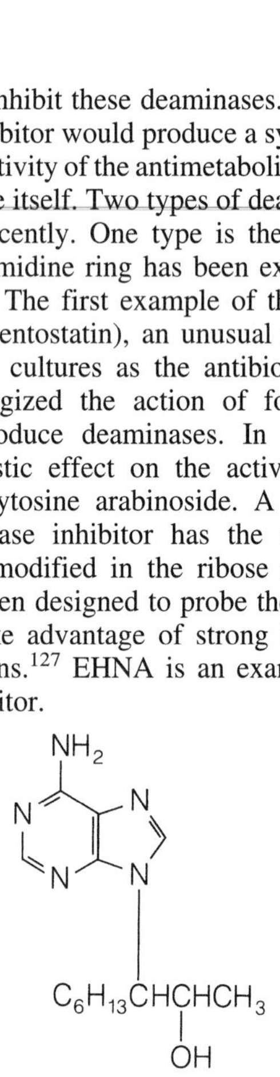   EHNA

Resistance to purine and pyrimidine antimetabolites, such as adenosine arabinoside and cytosine arabinoside, by neoplastic cells that produce deaminases has stimulated a search

After the discovery of folic acid, a number of analogues based on its structure were synthesized and tested as antime-

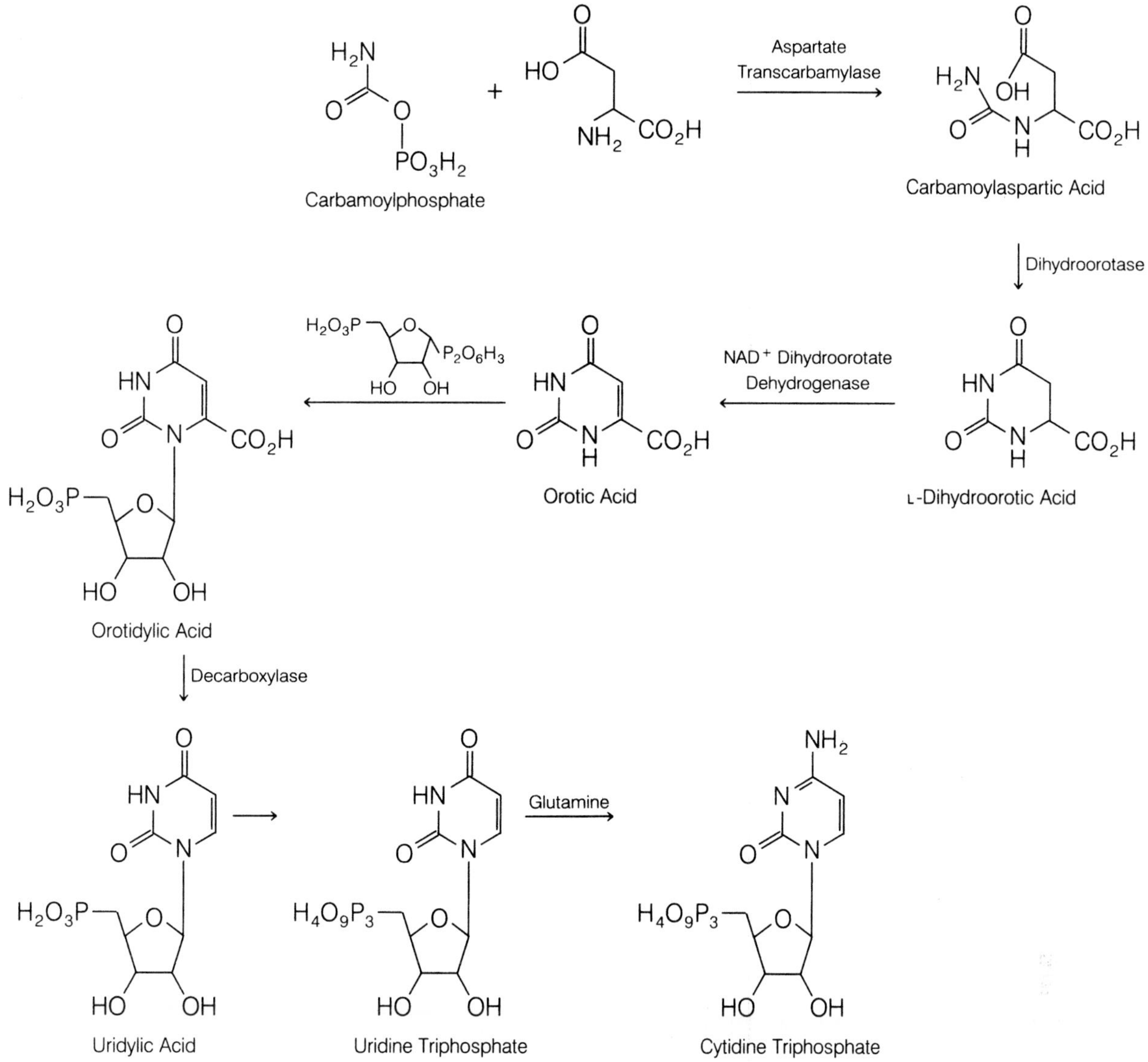

Scheme 12–9 ■ De novo synthesis of pyrimidine nucleotides (simplified).

tabolites. The N^{10}-methyl derivative of folic acid was found to be an antagonist, but it had no antitumor activity. Antitumor activity finally was found for the 4-amino-4-deoxy derivative, aminopterin, and its N^{10}-methyl homologue, methotrexate (amethopterin).[128]

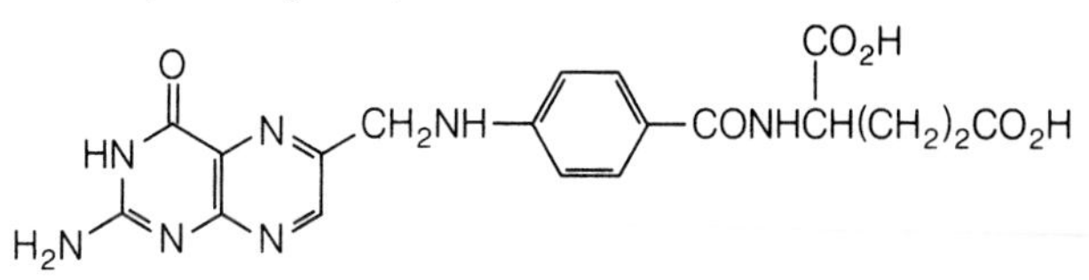

Folic Acid

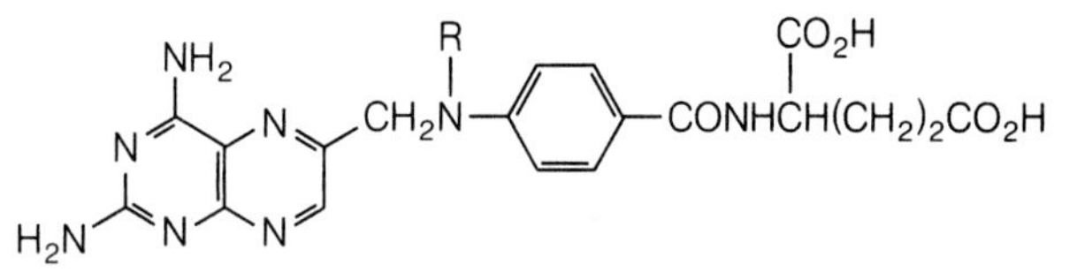

Aminopterin, R = H
Methotrexate, R = CH₃

Methotrexate and related compounds inhibit the enzyme dihydrofolate reductase. They bind so tightly to it that their inhibition has been termed *pseudoirreversible*. The basis of this binding strength is in the diaminopyrimidine ring, which is protonated at physiological pH. At pH 6, methotrexate binds stoichiometrically with dihydrofolate reductase (K_I $10^{-10}M$), but at higher pH the binding is weaker and competitive with the substrate.[129]

Folate acid antagonists kill cells by inhibiting DNA synthesis in the S phase of the cell cycle. Thus, they are most effective in the logarithmic growth phase.[130] Their effect on DNA synthesis results partially from the inhibition of dihydrofolate reductase, which depletes the pool of tetrahydrofolic acid. Folic acid is reduced stepwise to dihydrofolic acid and tetrahydrofolic acid, with dihydrofolic reductase thought to catalyze both steps.[131] As shown in Scheme 12-10, tetrahydrofolic acid accepts the β carbon atom of serine, in a reaction requiring pyridoxal phosphate, to give N^5,N^{10}-methylene tetrahydrofolic acid. The last compound transfers

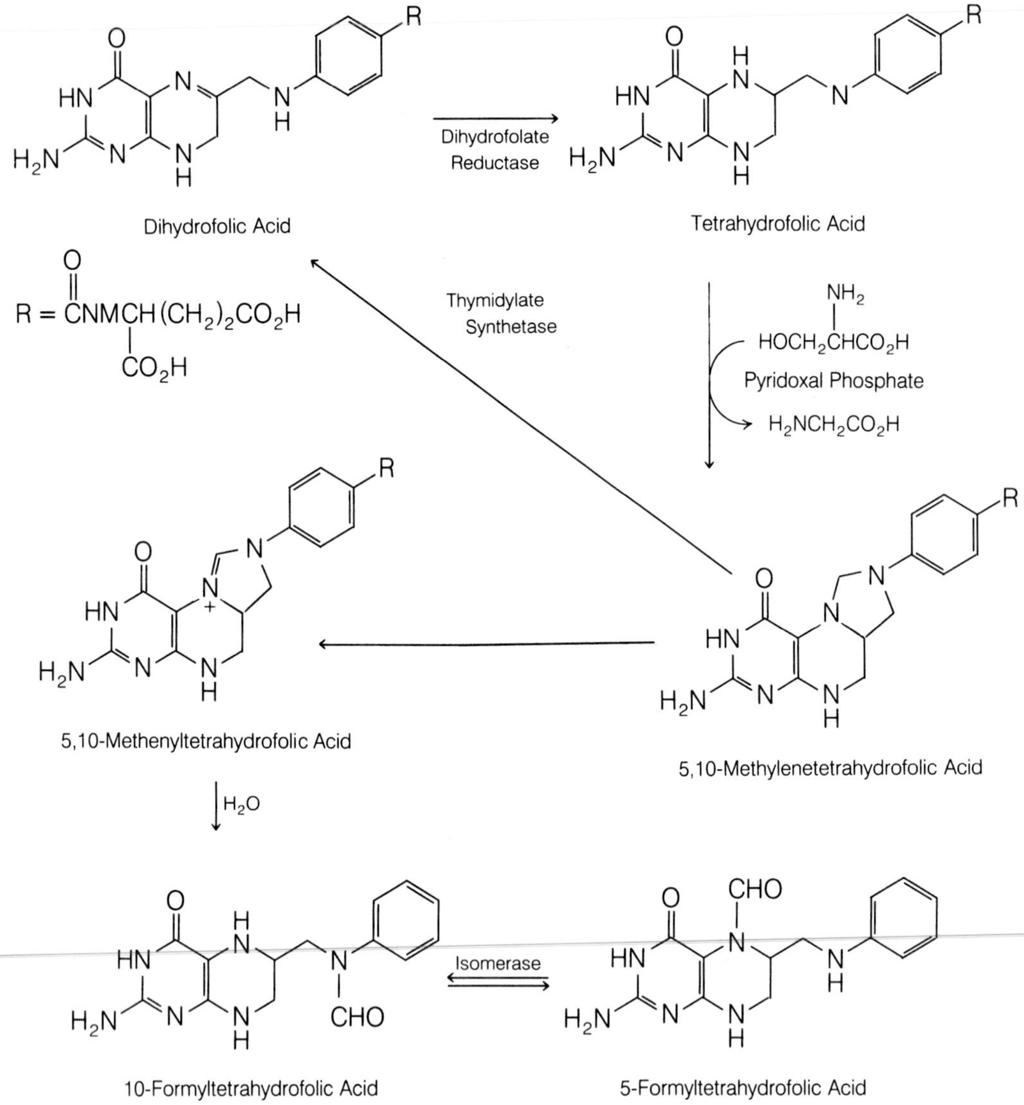

Scheme 12–10 ■ Interconversions of folic acid derivatives.

a methyl group to 2′-deoxyuridylate to give thymidylate in a reaction catalyzed by thymidylate synthetase. Dihydrofolic acid is generated in this reaction, and it must be reduced back to tetrahydrofolic acid before another molecule of thymidylate can be synthesized. It is partly by their effect in limiting thymidylate synthesis that folic acid analogues prevent DNA synthesis and kill cells. This effect has been termed *thymineless death.*[132]

The inhibition of dihydrofolate reductase produces other limitations on nucleic acid biosynthesis. Thus, N^5,N^{10}-methylene tetrahydrofolic acid is oxidized to the corresponding methenyl derivative, which gives N^{10}-formyltetrahydrofolic acid on hydrolysis (Scheme 12-10). The latter compound is a formyl donor to 5-aminoimidazole-4-carboxamide ribonucleotide in the biosynthesis of purines.[133] *N*-Formyltetrahydrofolic acid, also known as leucovorin and citrovorum factor, is interconvertible with the N^{10}-formyl analogue by way of an isomerase-catalyzed reaction. It carries the formimino group for the biosynthesis of formiminoglycine, a precursor of purines (Scheme 12-6). Leucovorin is used in ''rescue

therapy'' with methotrexate. It prevents the lethal effects of methotrexate on normal cells by overcoming the blockade of tetrahydrofolic acid production. In addition, it inhibits the active transport of methotrexate into cells and stimulates its efflux.[134]

Recently, it was shown that giving thymidine with methotrexate to mice bearing L1210 leukemia increased their survival time. This finding contradicts the idea that thymine deficiency is the most lethal effect of methotrexate on tumors. It suggests that the blockade of purine biosynthesis might have greater effects on tumor cells than on normal cells.[135] Consequently, the administration of thymidine might protect the normal cells relative to the tumor cells. Unfortunately, the use of such thymidine rescue in clinical trials was disappointing.[136]

Numerous compounds closely related to methotrexate have been prepared and tested against neoplasms. Most structural variations, such as alkylation of the amino groups, partial reduction, and removal or relocation of heterocyclic nitrogens, lead to decreased activity. Piritrexim and trimetrexate are analogues of methotrexate in which one or two nitrogens in the pyridine ring are replaced by carbons, and the benzoyl glutamic acid chain is replaced by a more lipophilic group. Like methotrexate, both compounds inhibit dihydrofolate reductase; however, they do not interact with the reduced folate transport system used by methotrexate. Consequently, they are active in vitro against some forms of methotrexate resistance. Their increased lipophilicity allows rapid transport by simple diffusion.[137, 138]

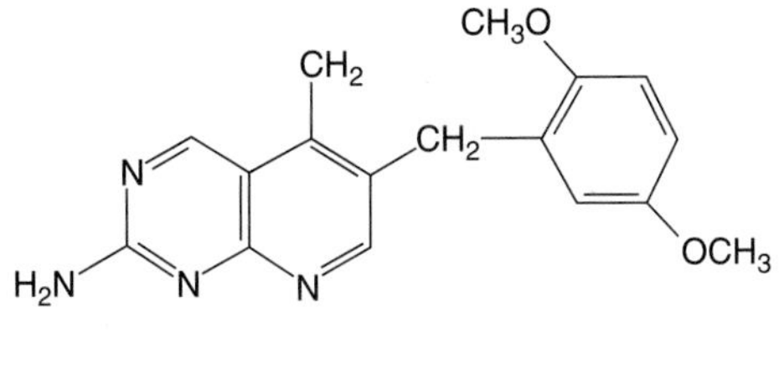

Piritrexim

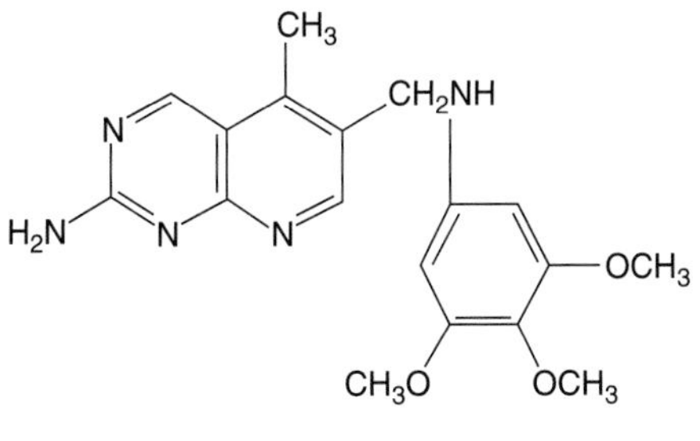

Trimetrexate

Although the active sites of dihydrofolic reductases from normal and neoplastic cells are identical, Baker proposed that regions adjacent to the active sites of these enzymes might differ. He designed inhibitors to take advantage of these differences, thus affording species specificity. One of these inhibitors, known as "Baker's antifol," shows activity against experimental tumors that are resistant to methotrexate.[139]

Glutamine and glutamate are the donors of the three- and nine-nitrogen atoms of purines and the two-amino groups of guanine.[140] They also contribute the three-nitrogen atom and the amino group of cytosine[141] (Schemes 12-6 and 12-9). Thus, they are involved at five different sites of nucleic acid biosynthesis. Although glutamine is not an essential nutrient for normal cells, many tumors depend on exogenous sources of it. This provides a rationale for the selective action of agents that interfere with the uptake, biosynthesis, or functions of glutamine.

In 1954, azaserine was isolated from a *Streptomyces* species.[142] It was found to antagonize many of the metabolic processes involving glutamine, with the most important effect being the conversion of formyl glycine ribonucleotide into formylglycinamidine ribonucleotide (Scheme 12-6).[143] A related compound, 6-diazo-5-oxo-L-norleucine (DON), was isolated in 1956 and found to produce similar antagonism.[144] A study involving incubation with [^{14}C]azaserine followed by digestion with proteolytic enzymes and acid hydrolysis produced S-[^{14}C]carboxymethylcysteine, which showed that azaserine had reacted covalently with a sulfhydryl group of cysteine on the enzyme.[145] DON is a more potent inhibitor than azaserine of this enzyme and of the enzyme that converts uridine nucleosides into cytidine nucleosides.[146] Although both compounds show good antitumor activity in animal models, they have been generally disappointing in clinical trials.

Products

Mercaptopurine, USP. Mercaptopurine, Purinethol, 6-mercaptopurine, 6MP, Leukerin, Mercaleukin, NSC-755, 6-purinethiol, is prepared by treating hypoxanthine with phosphorus pentasulfide[147, 147a] and is obtained as yellow crystals of the monohydrate. Solubility in water is poor. It dissolves in dilute alkali but undergoes slow decomposition. Scored 50-mg tablets are supplied. The injectable formulation is in vials containing 500 mg of the sodium salt of 6-mercaptopurine, which is reconstituted with 49.8 mL of Sterile Water for Injection, USP.

Mercaptopurine is not active until it is anabolized to the phosphorylated nucleotide. In this form, it competes with endogenous ribonucleotides for enzymes that convert inosinic acid into adenine- and xanthine-based ribonucleotides. Furthermore, it is incorporated into RNA, where it inhibits further RNA synthesis. One of its main metabolites is 6-methylmercaptopurine ribonucleotide, which also is a potent inhibitor of the conversion of inosinic acid into purines.[148]

Despite poor absorption, low bioavailability, and first-pass metabolism by the liver, mercaptopurine has oral activity. Peak plasma levels of about 70 ng/mL are reached 1 to

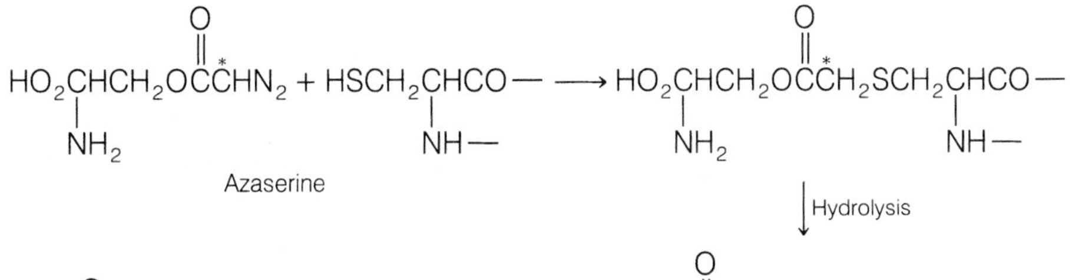

Azaserine

Hydrolysis

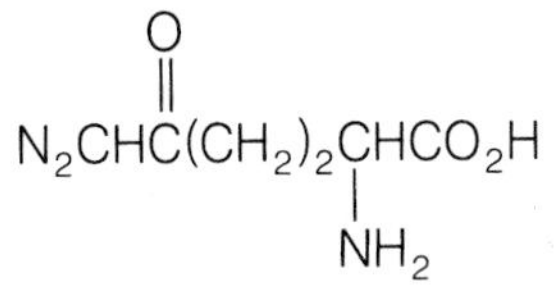

DON

2 hours after ingestion of a 75 mg/m^2 oral dose. After a bolus injection, plasma levels of 5,000 ng/mL are reached within minutes. Renal excretion is rapid. Mercaptopurine is metabolized by S-methylation followed by 8-hydroxylation. It also is oxidized to 6-thiouric acid.

Mercaptopurine is used primarily for treating acute leukemia. Children respond better than adults.[149] The chief toxic effect is leukopenia. Thrombocytopenia and bleeding occur with high doses. Because the leukopenia is delayed, one must discontinue the drug temporarily at the first sign of an abnormally large drop in the white cell count.

The tolerated dose varies with the individual patient. Allopurinol potentiates the effect of mercaptopurine by inhibiting its metabolism. It also increases its toxicity, however. If allopurinol is given for potentiation or reduction of hyperuricemia resulting from the killing of leukemia cells, the doses of mercaptopurine must be decreased.[150]

Thioguanine, USP.   Thioguanine, Thioguanine Tabloic, 6-thioguanine, TG, NSC-752, 2-aminopurine-6-thiol, is prepared by treating guanine with phosphorus pentasulfide in pyridine.[151] Scored 40-mg tablets are supplied. Oral thioguanine is poorly absorbed. An injectable form is supplied in 75-mg vials. It is reconstituted by adding 5 mL of Sodium Chloride for Injection, USP.

Thioguanine is converted by hypoxanthine-guanine phosphoribosyl transferase into a nucleotide form that inhibits a number of reactions in RNA and DNA synthesis, including the activity of phosphoribosyl pyrophosphate amidotransferase, the initial enzyme involved in purine biosynthesis.[152]

The 2′-deoxyribose triphosphate anabolite of thioguanine is extensively incorporated into DNA in place of the natural substrate. Thioguanine is metabolized to methylthioguanine, thiouric acid, methylthioxanthine, and thioxanthine.

Thioguanine is used in treating acute leukemia, especially in combination with cytarabine.[153] Cross-resistance exists between thioguanine and mercaptopurine. The chief toxic effect is delayed bone marrow depression, resulting in leukopenia and eventually thrombocytopenia and bleeding.

The usual initial dose is 2 mg/kg daily by the oral route. If there is no clinical improvement or leukopenia after 4 weeks the dosage is increased to 3 mg/kg daily. In contrast to mercaptopurine, thioguanine may be continued in the usual dose when allopurinol is used to inhibit uric acid formation.

Cladribine.   Cladribine, Leustatin, 2-CdA, NSC-1050 14-F, 2-chlorodeoxyadenosine, 2-chloro-2′-deoxy-β-D-adenosine, is prepared by a multistep procedure from 2,8-dichloroadenine and D-xylose,[154] and is supplied as a 1 mg/mL sterile solution in 0.9% Sodium Chloride for Injection, USP. The desired dose is removed from the vial and diluted with normal saline for infusion over 24 hours. These solutions are stable for 72 hours. Infusion is continued for 5 to 7 days.

Half-lives of 35 minutes (α) and 6.7 hours (β) were found for cladribine.[155] It is completely cleared from plasma in 1 to 3 days after the infusion is stopped. Cladribine is phosphorylated in cells to the active triphosphate by deoxycytidine kinase. It acts by inhibiting several enzymes required for DNA repair, and it is resistant to adenosine deaminase.

The current FDA approval for cladribine is hairy cell leukemia, in which it exhibits a very high percentage of complete responses, even in pretreated patients.[156] It has activity in a variety of other lymphoid malignancies. The limiting toxicity in most patients is a temporary decrease in neutrophils, which commonly leads to infections. There is also a prolonged suppression of helper lymphocytes.

Fludarabine Phosphate.   Fludarabine phosphate, Fludara, 2F-ara-AMP, FLAMP, NSC-312887, 9-β-D-arabinofuranosyl-2-fluoroadenosine 5′-monophosphate. It is prepared by treating fludarabine with triethyl phosphate and phosphorus oxychloride,[157] and it is supplied in 6-mL sterile vials containing 50 mg of fludarabine phosphate, 50 mg of mannitol, and sodium hydroxide to adjust the pH to 7.7. The intact vials should be stored at 2 to 8°C. Each vial is reconstituted with 2 mL of sterile water; this solution is stable for 8 hours at 25°C. It should be discarded after this time because the vial contains no antibacterial agent. Administration is by short intravenous infusion or a rapid loading dose/continuous infusion.

After infusion, fludarabine phosphate is rapidly dephosphorylated by serum phosphatases and converted into 2-fluoroadenosine arabinoside (2-FLAA). The levels of 2-FLAA decline biexponentially, with half-lives of 0.6 and 9.3 hours. 2-FLAA enters cells by a carrier-mediated process and undergoes intracellular phosphorylation by deoxycytidine kinase to the active form, 2-F-ara-ATP.[98]

Fludarabine phosphate has good activity in CLL. In ongoing clinical trials, it also shows activity against low-grade lymphomas and mycosis fungoides. The dose-limiting toxic effect is myelosuppression. Gastrointestinal and CNS toxicity also occur.

Fluorouracil, USP.   Fluorouracil, Fluorouracil Ampuls, Fluoroplex, Efudex, 5-FU, 5-fluoro-2,4(1H,3H)-pyrimidinedione, 2,4-dioxo-5-fluoropyrimidine, is prepared by condensing S-ethylisothiouronium bromide with the potassium salt (enolate) of ethyl 2-fluoro-2-formylacetate.[158] Recently the preparation of fluorouracil by direct fluorination of uracil was demonstrated.[159] Fluorouracil is supplied in 10-mL ampuls containing 500 mg of fluorouracil in a water solution at pH 9. These ampuls should be stored at room temperature and protected from light. Topical formulations of fluorouracil are Efudex Solution, which contains 2 or 5% fluorouracil compounded with propylene glycol, tris(hydroxymethyl)-aminomethane, hydroxypropyl cellulose, methyl and propyl parabens, and disodium edetate and Efudex Cream, which contains 5% fluorouracil in a vanishing cream base consisting of white petrolatum, stearyl alcohol, propylene glycol, polysorbate 60, and methyl and propylparabens.[160]

Fluorouracil is anabolized to its 2′-deoxyribose monophosphate, a potent inhibitor of thymidylate synthetase. It also is converted into fluorouridine triphosphate, which is incorporated into RNA and DNA.[104] There is cell cycle phase-specificity for the S phase.

Plasma levels of fluorouracil are erratic after oral dosing. High plasma levels are obtained after parenteral administration, but the pharmacokinetic characteristics are not linear. Fluorouracil is extensively metabolized in the liver, and the main metabolite is dihydrofluorouracil.[161] Most of an administered dose is excreted in urine as α-fluoro-β-alanine.

Fluorouracil is effective in the palliative management of carcinoma of the breast, colon, pancreas, rectum, and stomach in patients who cannot be cured by surgery or other means.[162] The topical formulations are used with favorable results for the treatment of premalignant keratoses of the skin and superficial basal cell carcinomas.[163] Parenteral administration almost invariably produces toxic effects. Leukopenia usually follows every course of therapy, with the lowest white blood cell counts occurring between days 9 and 14 after the first course. Gastrointestinal hemorrhage may occur and may even be fatal. Stomatitis, esophagopharyngitis, diarrhea, nausea, and vomiting are seen commonly; alopecia and dermatitis also occur. Therapy must be discontinued if leukopenia or gastrointestinal toxicity becomes too severe. Topical administration is contraindicated in patients who develop hypersensitivity. Prolonged exposure to ultraviolet radiation may increase the intensity of topical inflammatory reactions.

Floxuridine, USP. Floxuridine, FUDR, fluorodeoxyuridine, NSC-27640, 2′-deoxy-5-fluorouridine, 1-(2-deoxy-D-ribofuranosyl)-5-fluorouracil. This compound is prepared by condensing monomercuri-5-fluorouracil with 3,5-di-*O-p*-toluyl-2-deoxyribosyl-1-chloride followed by alkaline hydrolysis.[164] It is supplied in 5-mL vials containing 500 mg of floxuridine as sterile powder. Reconstitution is by the addition of 5 mL of sterile water. The resulting solutions should be stored under refrigeration for not more than 2 weeks.

Floxuridine is used for palliation of gastrointestinal adenocarcinoma metastatic to the liver in patients who are considered incurable by surgery or other means.[165] It is administered by continuous regional intra-arterial infusion. When given in this manner, it has significant advantages over fluorouracil. Because floxuridine is catabolized rapidly to fluorouracil, it gives the same toxic reactions as fluorouracil.

Cytarabine, USP. Cytarabine, Cytosar-U, ara-C, cytosine arabinoside, NSC-63878, 1-α-D-arabinofuranosylcytosine. It is synthesized from uracil arabinoside in a route involving acetylation, treatment with phosphorus pentasulfide, and heating with ammonia.[166] It is supplied as the freeze-dried solid in vials containing 100 or 500 mg. The 100-mg sample is reconstituted with 5 mL of sterile water containing 0.9% benzyl alcohol to give 20 mg/mL of cytarabine; the 500-mg sample is reconstituted with 10 mL of sterile water containing 0.9% benzyl alcohol to give 50 mg/mL of cytarabine. These solutions may he stored at room temperature for 48 hours.

Sequential actions of deoxycytidine kinase anabolize cytarabine to the triphosphorylated nucleotide, which acts as a competitive inhibitor of DNA polymerase after incorporation into DNA chains.[167] It is specific for the S phase of the cell cycle. Cytarabine is not orally active because of extensive deamination to inactive uracil arabinoside catalyzed by the enzyme cytidine deaminase.

Plasma levels of 0.01 to 0.15 μg/mL are required for cytotoxic effects of cytarabine, and they are achieved by the use of continuous or sequential bolus doses of 100 to 200 mg/m^2.[168]

Cytarabine is indicated primarily for inducing the remission of acute granulocytic leukemia of adults. It also is used for other acute leukemias of adults and children.[169] Remissions have been brief unless followed by maintenance therapy or given in combination with other antineoplastic agents.[170] Side effects include severe leukopenia, thrombocytopenia, and anemia. Gastrointestinal disturbances also are relatively frequent.

Capecitabine. Capecitabine, Xeloda, N^4-pentyloxycarbonyl-5′-deoxy-5-fluorocytidine, is prepared from 5′-deoxy-5-fluorocytidine and *n*-pentylchloroformate,[171] and supplied as 150- and 500-mg tablets. Absorption in the gastrointestinal tract is rapid, with maximum blood levels obtained in approximately 1.5 hours. This compound is a prodrug of 5′-deoxy-5-fluorouridine, to which it is converted by metabolic oxidation. Further metabolism produces 5-fluoro-2-deoxyuridine monophosphate (F-dUMP) and 5-fluorouracil triphosphate.

The currently approved indication for capecitabine is metastatic breast cancer resistant to paclitaxel and anthracyclines. Significant toxicities include bone marrow depression, diarrhea, mutagenesis in mice, reversible fertility impairment, teratogenicity, hyperbilirubinemia, and hand-mouth syndrome. Drug interactions occur with antacids and leucovorin.[172]

Gemcitabine. Gemcitabine, Gemzar, 2′-deoxy-2,2′-difluorocytidine, is prepared from 2-deoxy-2,2-difluoro-D-ribose and cytosine.[109] It is supplied as a lyophilized powder containing mannitol in 10- and 50-mL vials. Reconstitution provides solutions containing 20 mg/mL of gemcitabine. They are infused intravenously at a dose of 1,000 mg/m^2 over 30 minutes, once weekly, for up to 7 weeks. Clearance half-lives range from 32 to 91 minutes for a 30-minute infusion, or 245 to 638 minutes for longer infusions.

Gemcitabine is a first-line treatment for locally advanced or metastatic adenocarcinoma of the pancreas. It is also used in combination with cisplatin for first-line treatment of inoperable locally advanced or metastatic non–small cell lung cancer. The limiting toxicity is myelosuppression. This toxicity requires a complete blood count before each dose. Other adverse effects include fever, rash, teratogenicity, and mild renal toxicity.[173]

Pentostatin. Pentostatin, 2′-deoxycoformycin. dCF, NSC-218321, (*R*)-3-(2-deoxy-,α-D-erythropentofuranosyl)-3,6,7,8-tetrahydroimidazo[4,5-d][1,3]diazepin-8-ol. This compound is obtained from extracts of *Streptomyces antibioticus*[174] and formulated in 10-mg vials as a lyophilized powder. Mannitol (50 mg) and sodium hydroxide (to adjust pH) are included. It is administered intravenously, usually as short infusions in isotonic solutions. Pentostatin exhibits first-order, two-compartment excretion behavior.[175]

Pentostatin is an irreversible inhibitor of the enzyme adenosine deaminase. The resulting accumulation of deoxyadenosine and its phosphorylated congeners inhibits DNA synthesis. It is most effective against leukemias and lymphomas, especially hairy cell leukemia.[176] The dose-limiting effects include renal dysfunction, neurological toxicity, and reversible granulocytopenia.

Methotrexate, USP. Methotrexate, amethopterin, methyl aminopterin, NSC-740, 4-amino-N^{10}-methyl-pteroylglutamic acid, L-(+)-N-[p-[[(2,4-diamino-6-pteridinyl)-methyl]methylamino]benzoyl]glutamic acid, is prepared by combining 2,4,5,6-tetrahydropyrimidine, 2,3-dibromopropionaldehyde, disodium p-(methylamino)benzoylglutamate, iodine, and potassium iodide, followed by heating with lime water.[128] It is isolated as the monohydrate, a yellow solid. Recent studies indicate that the commercial preparation contains a number of impurities, including 4-amino-N^{10}-methylpteroic acid and N^{10}-methylfolic acid.[177] Methotrexate is soluble in alkaline solutions but decomposes in them. It is supplied as 25-mg tablets and in vials containing either 5 or 50 mg of methotrexate sodium in 2 mL of solution. The 5-mg sample contains 0.90% benzyl alcohol as preservative, 0.63% sodium chloride, and sodium hydroxide to give pH 8.5. The 50-mg sample contains 0.90% benzyl alcohol, 0.26% sodium chloride, and sodium hydroxide to give pH 8.5. A preservative-free lyophilized preparation is recommended for intrathecal administration to prevent or treat tumor cells in the CNS.

After oral administration, methotrexate is rapidly but incompletely absorbed. Approximately 50 to 60% of the absorbed drug is bound to plasma proteins. Cytotoxic levels are found in cerebrospinal fluid when high doses of methotrexate are given. Most of the drug is excreted in the urine unchanged, although some 7-hydroxymethotrexate is found following high-dose therapy. Plasma level decay is biphasic or possibly triphasic.

Methotrexate binds tightly to dihydrofolate reductase, blocking the reduction of dihydrofolate to tetrahydrofolate, the active form of the coenzyme.[178] It is specific for the S phase of the cell cycle. Methotrexate undergoes polyglutamation intracellularly, forming a pool of compounds that is retained for months. Resistance to methotrexate develops by an increase in dihydrofolate reductase, which results from gene amplification, or by defective transport into tumor cells.[179]

Methotrexate was the first drug to produce substantial (although temporary) remissions in leukemia.[180] It is still used for this purpose against acute lymphocytic leukemia and ALL. Because it has some ability to enter the CNS, it is used in the treatment and prophylaxis of meningeal leukemia. The discovery that methotrexate afforded a high percentage of apparently permanent remissions in choriocarcinoma in women justified use of the term *cure* in cancer chemotherapy.[181] Methotrexate is used in combination chemotherapy for palliative management of breast cancer, epidermoid cancers of the head and neck, and lung cancer. It is also used against severe, disabling psoriasis. The most common toxic reactions are ulcerative stomatitis, leukopenia, and abdominal distress. A high dose of methotrexate combined with leucovorin "rescue" produces some responses in osteogenic sarcoma, but it can cause renal failure in some patients. This condition is thought to result from crystallization of the drug or its metabolites in acidic urine, and it is countered by hydration and alkalinization.[182]

Azathioprine, USP. Azathioprine, Imuran, 6-[(1-methyl-4-nitroimidazole-5-yl)thio]purine, is prepared from 6-mercaptopurine and 5-chloro-1-methyl-4-nitroimidazole.[183] It is supplied as 50-mg scored tablets. The injectable

sodium salt is available in 20-mL vials containing 100 mg of azathioprine.

Azathioprine is well absorbed when taken orally. It is converted extensively to 6-mercaptopurine. The main indication for azathioprine is as an adjunct to prevent the rejection of renal heterotransplants. It is contraindicated in patients who show hypersensitivity to it. The chief toxic effects are hematological, expressed as leukopenia, anemia, and thrombocytopenia. Complete blood counts should be performed at least weekly, and the drug should be discontinued if there is a rapid fall or persistent decrease in leukocytes. Patients with impaired renal function might eliminate the drug more slowly, which requires appropriate reduction of the dose. Azathioprine should not be taken with allopurinol, which blocks its metabolism by xanthine oxidase.

ANTIBIOTICS

Nine different antibiotics or their semisynthetic analogues are established clinical anticancer agents, and other antibiotics are undergoing clinical development. Some of these agents have been approved recently; however, others have been known for a long time. For example, dactinomycin (actinomycin D) was first isolated in 1940 by Waksman and Woodruff,[184] although its activity against neoplasms was not described until 1958. Furthermore, plicamycin, originally discovered as aureolic acid in 1953, had to be rediscovered twice before its antitumor activity was established in 1962.[185] These compounds were originally rejected as antibacterial agents because of their cytotoxicity. Only later was it found that this toxicity could be an advantage in the chemotherapy of cancer. The discovery of antitumor activity is much simpler today, and some laboratories routinely screen extracts of microorganism cultures for antitumor activity in cell cultures.

The production of antitumor agents from microbial fermentations has some special advantages and disadvantages over chemical synthesis. Some biosyntheses can be controlled to afford novel analogues. This has been true for actinomycins[186] and bleomycins.[187] Strain selection and fermentation conditions can optimize the formation of a particular component of an antibiotic mixture. Thus, *Streptomyces parvulus* produces dactinomycin almost exclusively, in contrast to other species that form complex mixtures of actinomycins. The fermentation in *Streptomyces caespitosus* has been developed similarly to produce almost all mitomycin C. In some cases, such as with doxorubicin, improving the antibiotic yield has been difficult. This results in an expensive product and intensive research on chemical synthesis.

The actinomycins comprise a large number of closely related structures. All of them contain the same chromophore, a substituted 3-phenoxazone-1,9-dicarboxylic acid known as actinocin. Each of the carboxyl groups is bonded to a pentapeptide lactone by way of the amino group of an L-threonine unit of this pentapeptide. The hydroxyl group of the L-threonine forms part of the lactone along with L-methylvaline, the fifth amino acid from the chromophore. D-Valine or D-alloisoleucine is the second amino acid, and the fourth amino acid usually is sarcosine. The third amino acid is more variable, consisting of L-proline, L-hydroxyproline, L-oxoproline, or others produced by controlled biosynthesis. Actinomycins that have two identical pentapeptide lactones are called *isoactinomycins;* those with different pentapeptide lactones are called *anisoactinomycins.* The individual pentapeptide lactones are designated α and β, depending on their attachment to the 9- or 1-carboxylic acids, respectively. Dactinomycin (actinomycin D, actinomycin C_1) is an isoactinomycin with an amino acid sequence of L-threonine, D-valine, L-proline, sarcosine, and L-*N*-methylvaline. Actinomycin C_3, which is used in Germany, differs from actinomycin D by a D-alloisoleucine unit instead of D-valine in both the α and β chains.[188]

Dactinomycin

The mode of action of actinomycins has been studied extensively, and it now is generally accepted that they intercalate into double-helical DNA. In the intercalation process, the helix unwinds partially to permit the flat phenoxazone chromophore to fit between successive base pairs (Fig. 12-4). Adjacent G-C pairs are especially suitable because the 2-amino groups of the guanines can hydrogen bond with the carbonyl groups of threonines in the actinomycin. This bonding reinforces the π-bonding between the heterocyclic chromophores. Additional stability is conferred by the interaction between the pentapeptide lactone chains and DNA. These chains lie in the minor groove of the double helix, running in opposite directions to each other, and they make numerous van der Waals interactions with the DNA.[189]

Intercalation into DNA changes its physical properties in characteristic ways. The length, viscosity, and melting temperature increase, while the sedimentation coefficient decreases.[190, 191] Changes in substituents on the actinomycins influence their binding to DNA, usually by making it less effective. Opening a lactone ring or changing the stereochemistry of an amino acid abolishes activity, and replacement of the 4- and 6-methyl groups by other substituents reduces it. Replacement of the 2-amino group also reduces activity.[192]

Actinomycins, anthracyclines, and certain other intercalating agents, including mitoxantrone and amsacrine, inhibit the enzyme topoisomerase II. Topoisomerases regulate the topological state of DNA by unwinding and unlinking coiled double-strand DNA molecules. They are thought to be critical for DNA replication and transcription, and they act by cleaving and rejoining one or both strands of the phosphodiester backbone of DNA. Topoisomerase I cuts one of the two DNA strands, allowing the other to act as a swivel

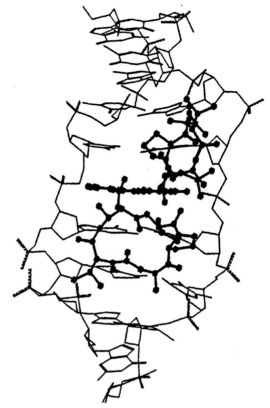

Figure 12–4 ■ Dactinomycin intercalating DNA.

about which the winding or unwinding can take place.[193] In contrast, topoisomerase II cleaves both strands, allowing complete rotation or, as has been suggested, passage of part of the intact double strand through the gap. Drugs that inhibit topoisomerases bind to and trap the covalent complex formed between phosphate groups on the DNA and tyrosine residues on the enzyme, preventing subsequent reclosure of the broken strand or strands. The extent of drug–topoisomerase–DNA complexes formation does not necessarily correlate with cytotoxicity.[193]

Anthracyclines are another large and complex family of antibiotics. Many members of this family were investigated before a useful antitumor agent, daunorubicin, was isolated from *Streptomyces coeruleorubidus* and *S. peucetius.* This significant discovery was made independently in France and Italy in 1963.[194, 195] Daunorubicin proved to be active against acute leukemias, and it became an established clinical agent. It was pushed into the background, however, by the discovery of doxorubicin (Adriamycin) in *S. peucetius* var. *caesius* in 1969.[196] Doxorubicin is active against a broad spectrum of tumors, including both solid and hematological types. It became one of the most widely used antineoplastic agents.[197] A third anthracycline, which was recently approved for clinical use in the United States, is idarubicin. This compound is the 4-demethoxy analogue of daunorubicin. It has enhanced antitumor potency, and it appears to be less cardiotoxic than daunorubicin and doxorubicin. Epirubicin, the 4′-hydroxy epimer of doxorubicin, is available in Europe. It also is considered less toxic than doxorubicin, with equal or greater antitumor activity. The 4-hydroxy analogue of daunorubicin, carminomycin, isolated from *Actinomadura carminata,* has been evaluated in Russia.[198]

Daunorubicin: $R_1 = OCH_3$, $R_2 = H$
Doxorubicin: $R_1 = OCH_3$, $R_2 = OH$
Idarubicin: $R_1 = H$, $R_2 = OH$
Carminomycin: $R_1 = OH$, $R_2 = H$

Many anthracyclines, including all of those with antitumor activity, occur as glycosides of the anthracyclinones. The glycosidic linkage usually involves the 7-hydroxyl group of the anthracyclinone and the β-anomer of a sugar with L configuration. *Anthracyclinone* refers to an aglycone containing the anthraquinone chromophore within a linear hydrocarbon skeleton related to that of the tetracyclines.[199] The anthracyclinones differ from each other in the number and location of phenolic hydroxyl groups, the degree of oxidation of the two-carbon side chain at position 9, and the presence of a carboxylic acid ester at position 10. Thus, daunorubicin is a glycoside formed between daunomycinone and L-daunosamine, and doxorubicin is its 14-hydroxy analogue.[200] In contrast, aclacinomycin A has aklavinone in combination with a trisaccharide chain.[201]

Aclarubicin
(Aclacinomycin A)

Daunorubicin and doxorubicin exhibit biological effects similar to those of actinomycin, and they are thought to intercalate into double-helical DNA and inhibit topoisomerase II.[202] Reduction of doxorubicin followed by intercalation causes DNA strand scission. This scission is thought to result from the attack of hydroxyl radicals generated from redox cycles involving doxorubicin.[203] In contrast to daunorubicin, aclacinomycin and related compounds do not induce lysogenic phage in bacteria. They are believed to interfere more with RNA syntheses than with DNA synthesis. Aclacinomycin lacks the cardiotoxicity shown by daunorubicin and doxorubicin.[201]

In contrast to the actinomycins, anthracyclines are metabolized in the liver. Daunorubicin is readily converted into its 13-hydroxy analogue, daunorubicinol, which is further cleaved to the aglycone.[204] The 14-hydroxyl group of doxorubicin makes it less susceptible to reduction of the 13-carbonyl group. The 13-hydroxy derivative, adriamycinol, however, is found among the metabolites along with the 4-demethyl-4-sulfate. Both daunomycinol and adriamycinol are active against neoplastic cells, but their rates of uptake are low.[205]

Daunomycinol, R = H
Adriamycinol, R = OH

Many analogues of doxorubicin with changes in the sugar moiety have been prepared. They include 4'-deoxydoxorubicin (esorubicin), 4'-epidoxorubicin (epirubicin), and 4'-O-tetrahydropyranyl doxorubicin (pirarubicin). Epirubicin is widely used in Europe, and it is the world's leading anthracycline in sales; however, it is not approved in the United States at this time. Pirarubicin accumulates more rapidly than doxorubicin in tumor cells and shows superior activity in animal models.[206] Valrubicin, a derivative of doxorubicin in which the amino group has a trifluoroacetyl substituent and the 14-hydroxyl group is converted to a valerate ester,[207] has been approved recently for intravesicular therapy of the urinary bladder in patients with carcinoma refractory to BCG.[208] In systemic circulation the valerate ester is hydrolyzed, but the trifluoroacetyl group is stable; however, little metabolism occurs in the 2-hour period valrubicin is in the bladder.

Another anthracycline with significant antitumor activity is nogalamycin, which is obtained from *Streptomyces nogalater*.[209] It differs from other anthracyclines in that the aminosugar is joined to the nucleus by a carbon–carbon bond and a cyclic acetal linkage. There is a nonamino sugar, nogalose, at the usual 7 position, however. Although nogalamycin itself is not an established antineoplastic drug, a semisyn-

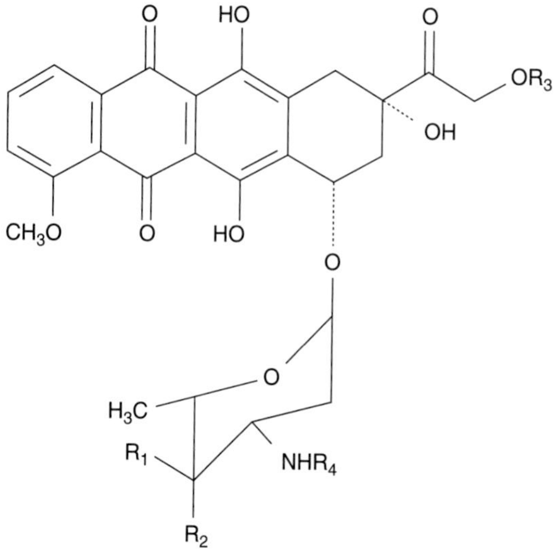

Esorubicin: $R_1 = R_2 = R_3 = R_4 = H$

Epirubicin: $R_1 = OH, = R_2 = R_3 = R_4 = H$

Pirarubicin: $R_1 = H = R_2 = R_4 = H, R_2 = O$

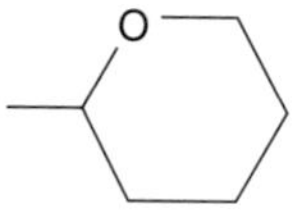

Valrubicin: $_1 = H, R_2 = OH, R_3 = COC_4H_9, R_4 = COCF_3$

Menogaril

Nogalamycin

thetic analogue, menogaril, has received phase II clinical trials and is under consideration for approval. Menogaril has the nogalose moiety replaced by a methoxy group and reversed chirality at the 7 position. It also differs from nogalamycin by the absence of the 10-carbomethoxy group.[210] These structural changes result in a change in the mode of action from intercalation into DNA, as found for nogalamycin, to some other site and type of cytotoxic process. Thus, menogaril localizes in the cytoplasm, rather than the nucleus, and it has very little effect on DNA and RNA synthesis at cytotoxic doses.[211] Menogaril is not more effective than doxorubicin against tumors, but its much lower cardiotoxicity and potential oral activity might offer clinical advantages.

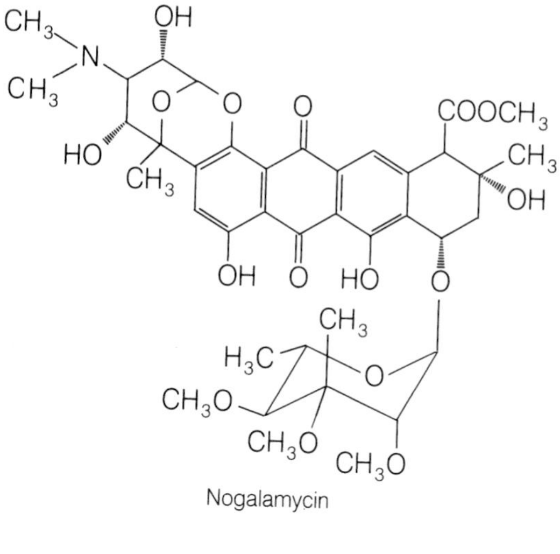

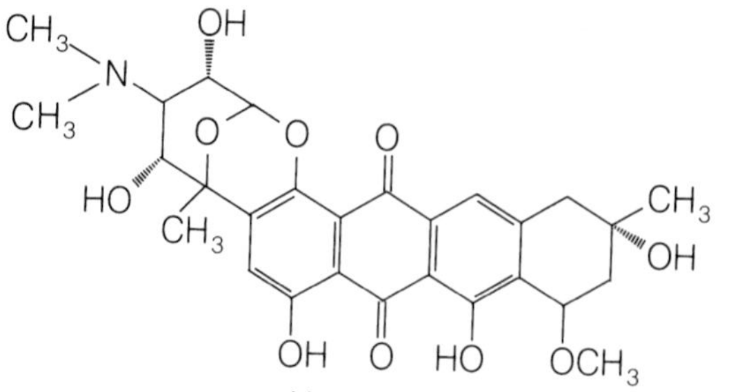

The aureolic acid group of antitumor antibiotics includes aureolic acid (plicamycin, mithramycin), the olivomycins, the chromomycins, variamycin, and related compounds. Plicamycin is the only member approved for clinical use in the United States. It is restricted to testicular carcinoma and hypercalcemia that is resistant to other drugs. Chromomycin A_3 is used in Japan, and olivomycin A is used in Russia.[192] Aureolic acid group compounds have complex structures consisting of an aglycone and two carbohydrate chains. The aglycones are tetrahydroanthracene derivatives with phenolic hydroxyl groups at positions 6, 8, and 9 and a pentanyl side chain that is highly oxygenated. The carbohydrate chains contain either two or three 2,6-dideoxy sugars of novel structures.[212]

Plicamycin and related compounds are weakly acidic owing to the phenolic groups ($pK_a = 5$). They readily form sodium salts that show brilliant yellow fluorescence.[213] The chromophore is responsible for complex formation with divalent metals such as magnesium and calcium. Such complex formation is required before aureolic acids can bind with DNA.[214] The nature of this DNA binding is uncertain at the present time. Intercalation has been suggested, but the evidence for this process is incomplete.[215] Whatever the exact nature of the binding, plicamycin and other aureolic acids inhibit DNA-dependent RNA polymerase, and this effect leads to cell death.[216]

The discovery of bleomycin in 1966 resulted from a program established by H. Umezawa to screen microbial culture filtrates against experimental tumors.[217] Bleomycin is a mixture of closely related compounds that is partly resolved before formulation for clinical use.[218] The presently used commercial product, Blenoxane, contains bleomycins A_2 and B_2. A variety of other antibiotics have structures similar to those of the bleomycins. They include the phleomycins (which differ from bleomycins in having one thiazole ring partly reduced), zorbamycin and the zorbonamycins, antibiotic YA-56, victomycin, the tallysomycins, and the platomycins.[192] New bleomycin analogues also have been prepared from bleomycinic acid by controlled biosynthesis.

Bleomycins and their analogues occur naturally as blue copper chelates. Removal of the copper by chemical reduction or complexing agents affords the antibiotics as white solids.[219, 220] Copper-free bleomycin is the active species for chemotherapy, and it has lower toxicity. Bleomycin complexes readily with metal ions, which is a key factor in its mode of action. Inside the cell, bleomycin forms a chelate with Fe(II) that has square pyramidal geometry.[221] Nitrogen atoms from bleomycin occupy five of the positions in this structure. The sixth position may be occupied by the carboxyl group of the carbamate function, but this group is

Mithramycin

Bleomycinic Acid, R = OH
Bleomycin A$_2$,   R = NH(CH$_2$)$_3$S$^+$(CH$_3$)$_2$
Bleomycin B$_2$,   R = NH(CH$_2$)$_4$NHCNH$_2$
                                          ‖
                                          N—H

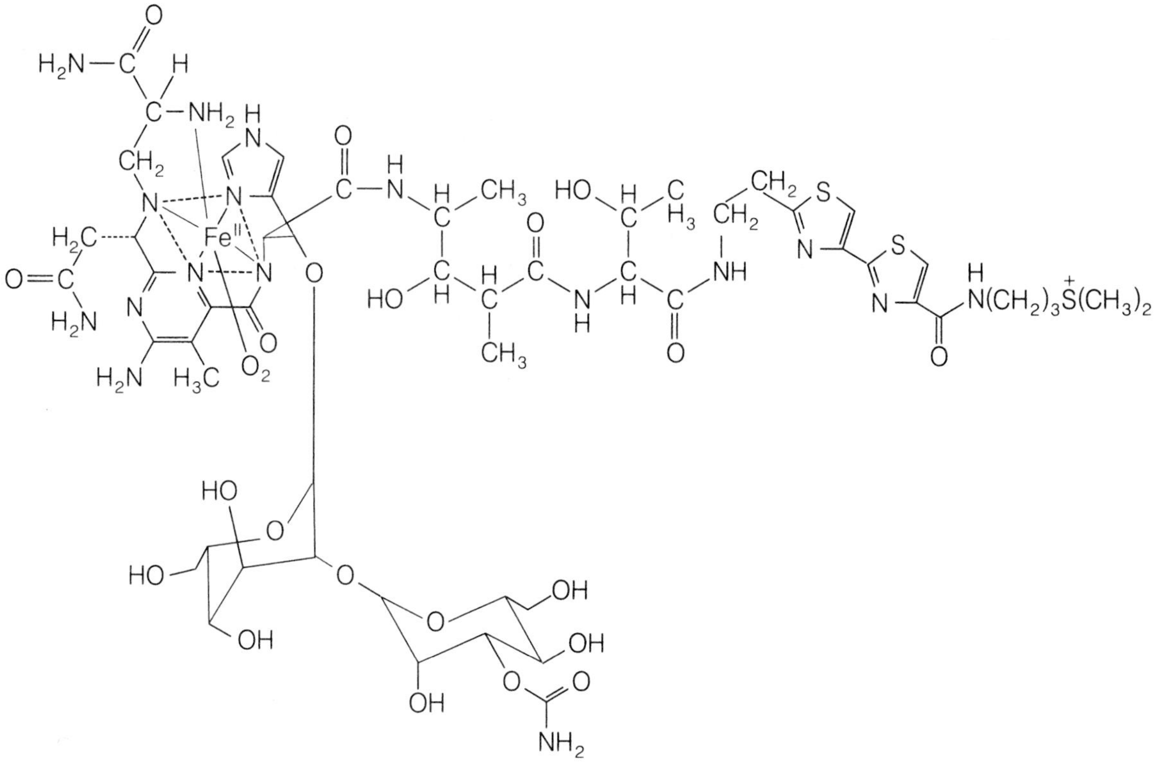

Bleomycin A$_2$ Fe(II) Chelate

readily displaced by molecular oxygen. The resulting complex may give rise to hydroxyl radicals and superoxide radicals. These highly reactive radicals are generated close to the double helix, and they cause cleavage of the phosphodiester bonds. This degradation of DNA strands is thought to be the lethal event in cells.[222]

Bleomycin is inactivated by an intracellular enzyme named *bleomycin hydrolase,* an aminopeptidase that hydrolyzes the carboxamide group of the β-aminoalanine carboxamide residue to the corresponding carboxylate. This structural change increases the pK$_a$ of the α-amino group from 7.3 to 9.4, which results in poorer binding to DNA.[220] Chelation with Fe(II) still occurs, but the production of hydroxyl radicals is drastically reduced.[222] Bleomycin hydrolase levels in tumor cells help to determine their resistance to bleomycin. Thus, squamous cell carcinoma is characterized by ready uptake of bleomycin and low levels of the hydrolase. It is especially sensitive to bleomycin.[223]

Bleomycins undergo two different inactivating reactions under mildly alkaline conditions. One is migration of the carbamoyl group to an adjacent hydroxyl group of the mannose residue. The resulting product is called an *isobleomycin.*[224] Copper-chelated bleomycins do not undergo this reaction. They are, however, slowly transformed into epibleomycins, which are racemized at the carbon atom substituted at the 2 position of the pyrimidine ring.[225] Epibleomycins retain about 25% of the antitumor activity of the parent bleomycins.

Bleomycinic acid is obtained by chemical degradation of bleomycin A or enzymatic degradation of bleomycin B$_2$. It can be transformed readily into semisynthetic bleomycins

such as PEP-bleomycin (peplomycin), which possesses less pulmonary toxicity.[218]

The mitomycins were discovered in Japan in the late 1950s, and one of them, mitomycin C, was rapidly developed as an anticancer drug.[226] Unfortunately, the initial clinical experience with this compound in the United States was disappointing. It was not approved until 1974, following extensive studies and the establishment of satisfactory dosage schedules. Porfiromycin, the N-methyl homologue of mitomycin C, was discovered at the Upjohn Company.[227] It has received clinical study, but it is not yet an approved agent.

Structures of the mitomycins were elucidated at Lederle Laboratories. These compounds have an unusual combination of three different carcinostatic functions: quinone, carbamate, and aziridine.[228] They are arranged in such a way that the molecule is relatively unreactive in its natural state. Chemical or enzymatic reduction to the corresponding hydroquinone is, however, followed by the loss of methanol (water from mitomycin B), and the resulting indolohydroquinone becomes a bifunctional alkylating agent capable of cross-linking double-helical DNA (Scheme 3).[229] Mitomycins bound to DNA may undergo successive redox cycles, each of which results in the generation of hydrogen peroxide. This potent oxidizing agent can cause single-strand cleavage of the DNA.[230]

Mitomycins are unstable in both acids and bases. Mild acid hydrolysis results in opening of the aziridine ring and loss of methanol or water to give mitosenes such as 2,7-diamino-l-hydroxymitosene.[231] Catalytic hydrogenation followed by reoxidation gives aziridinomitosenes, which retain a significant amount of antitumor activity in animals.[232]

Mitomycin A, X = CH$_3$O, Y = H
Mitomycin C, X = H$_2$N, Y = H
Porfiromycin, X = H$_2$N, Y = CH$_3$
BMY-25067, X = O$_2$NC$_6$H$_4$SS(CH$_2$)$_2$NH

Mitomycin B, X = CH$_3$O
Mitomycin D, X = H$_2$N

Many mitomycin analogues have been prepared by partial synthesis, and two of them have received clinical trials.[233–234a] Unexpected toxicity has led to their withdrawal, however. The present clinical candidates, BMY-25067 and KT 6149, contain disulfide substituents on the 7-amino group. Control of the quinone reduction potential is especially stressed in analogue studies, because reduction is the key step in bioactivation of these molecules.[235]

2,7-Diamino-1-hydroxymitosene, R^1 = OH, R^2 = NH$_2$

1,2-Aziridino-7-aminomitosene, R^1, R^2 = >NH

Streptozocin was isolated from *Streptomyces achromogenes* in 1960.[236] It is the nitrosomethylurea derivative of 2-deoxyglucose.[237] The simplicity of its structure and the cost of preparing it by fermentation have led to the development of practical syntheses from 2-amino-2-deoxyglucose.[238] Streptozocin is an alkylating agent similar in reactivity to other nitrosomethylureas, except that its glucose

Streptozocin, R = CH$_3$
Chlorozotocin, R = CH$_2$CH$_2$Cl

moiety causes it to be especially taken up in the pancreas. This effect is detrimental in that it produces diabetes, but it makes the molecule especially effective against malignant insulinomas.[239] It is an approved clinical agent for this specific use. The chloroethyl analogue of streptozotocin, chlorozotocin, shows good antitumor activity in animals and is not diabetogenic.[240]

Acivicin is another antibiotic that has received clinical study. It is obtained from *Streptomyces svicens,* and it functions as an inhibitor of the amidotransferases involved in purine and pyrimidine biosynthesis.[241] The structure of acivicin shows a chlorine atom that can be replaced readily because it is located on an imine group. A cysteine residue at the active site of an amidotransferase replaces this chlorine, affording alkylation and irreversible inhibition of the enzyme. Phase I clinical studies revealed CNS toxicity for acivicin. Conversion of the antibiotic to ibotenic acid, a known CNS toxin found in mushrooms, by exchange of the chlorine for a hydroxyl group, might be responsible for this toxicity.

In 1978, scientists at the Upjohn Company reported the isolation of CC-1065 from *Streptomyces zelensis.*[242] This compound is composed of three pyrrolo[3,2e]indoline units joined by amide bonds. Two of these subunits are virtually identical, but the third has a cyclopropane ring. The structure is curved and twisted in such a manner that it makes a precise fit in the minor groove of double-helical DNA.[243] It prefers DNA sequences rich in adenine and thymine, where the cyclopropane ring can alkylate N(3) of an adenine (Fig. 12-5).[244] CC-1065 has remarkable antitumor potency, but delayed liver toxicity in mice prevented its clinical development. Numerous analogues of CC-1065 were synthesized, and one of them, adozelesin, has been introduced into clinical trials.[245] This analogue retains intact the subunit bearing the cyclopropane ring, but the other two subunits are simplified. It retains significant antitumor activity without the delayed toxicity.

Compounds in the enediyne class of antibiotics show antitumor potencies in the microgram per kilogram range in mice, and they have a remarkable mode of DNA cleavage. Although the gross structures of these compounds differ widely, they have the common feature of a medium-sized ring (9 or 10 carbons) containing one olefinic bond and two acetylenic bonds.[246] On activation, this system is converted

Acivicin

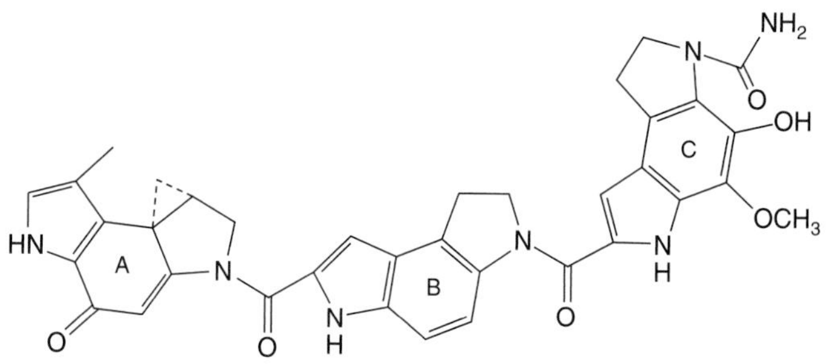

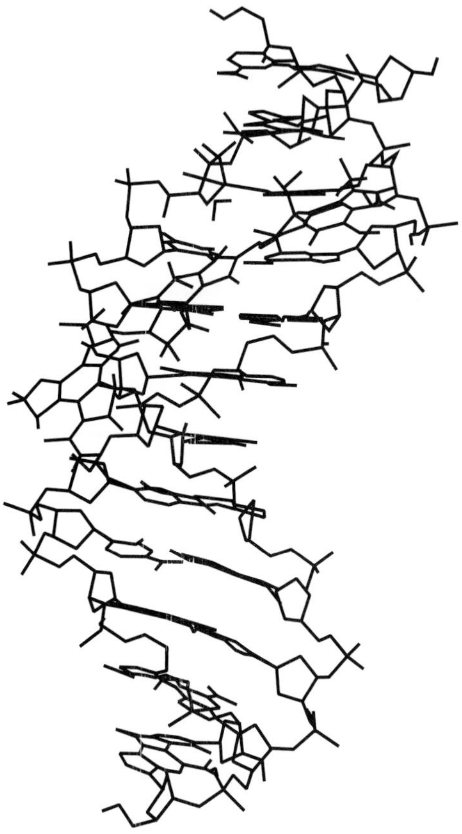

Figure 12–5 ■ CC-1065 binding DNA.

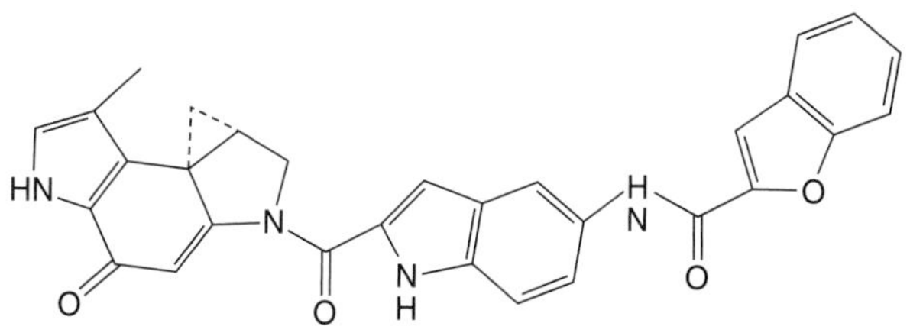

into a benzene diradical, which can simultaneously cleave two strands of double-helical DNA. This process is illustrated for the calicheamicin chromophore in Figure 12-6. Activation begins with the loss of CH₃SS and Michael addition of thiolate to the 1,2-double bond. The resulting loss of strain in the 10-membered ring containing the enediyne system allows Bergman cyclization to a bicyclic system containing a benzene diradical. This diradical can remove hydrogen radicals from the 5′-methylene carbon of 2′-deoxyribose residues in DNA, which leads to cleavage of the strands.[247] Double-strand scission occurs at sites such as TCCT-AGGA, where geometry is favorable; otherwise, only one strand is cleaved.

Calicheamicin is obtained from cultures of *Micromonospora echinospora* ssp. *Calicheansis*.[248] It occurs as a mixture of seven related components, of which calicheamicin γ1ᴵ, the most abundant component, has been investigated extensively. Despite the remarkable potency of calicheamicin, its extreme toxicity has prevented its use. To overcome this limitation, conjugates with monoclonal antibodies have been developed. The conjugate with a humanized monoclonal antibody known as gemtuzumab has been approved for cancer chemotherapy. It is described under monoclonal antibodies. Other enediynes of interest as potential antitumor drugs include dynemycin, esperamicins, and neocarcinostatin.[246]

Products

Dactinomycin, USP. Cosmegen, actinomycin D, actinomycin C₁, actinomycin IV, NSC-3053, is obtained from the fermentation of selected strains of *Streptomyces parvulus*. It is soluble in alcohols and alcohol–water mixtures; however, these solutions are very sensitive to light. Vials containing 0.5 mg of lyophilized powder of the drug and 20 mg of mannitol are supplied. For reconstitution, 1.1 mL of Sterile Water for Injection, USP is added to the vial. The resulting solution is stable for 2 to 5 months at room temperature.

Only minimal metabolism of dactinomycin occurs. Its prolonged half-life may be explained by significant retention in lymphocytes and granulocytes. Dactinomycin intercalates between the base pairs of DNA and inhibits topoisomerase II. It selectively inhibits the synthesis of DNA-dependent ribosomal RNA and messenger RNA.[249]

Dactinomycin is used against rhabdomyosarcoma and Wilms' tumor in children.[250] It can be lifesaving for women with choriocarcinoma resistant to methotrexate. In combination with vincristine and cyclophosphamide, it has received some use in solid tumors in children. Toxic reactions include anorexia, nausea, and vomiting. Bone marrow depression, resulting in pancytopenia, may occur within a week after therapy. Alopecia, erythema, and tissue injury may occur at the injection site.

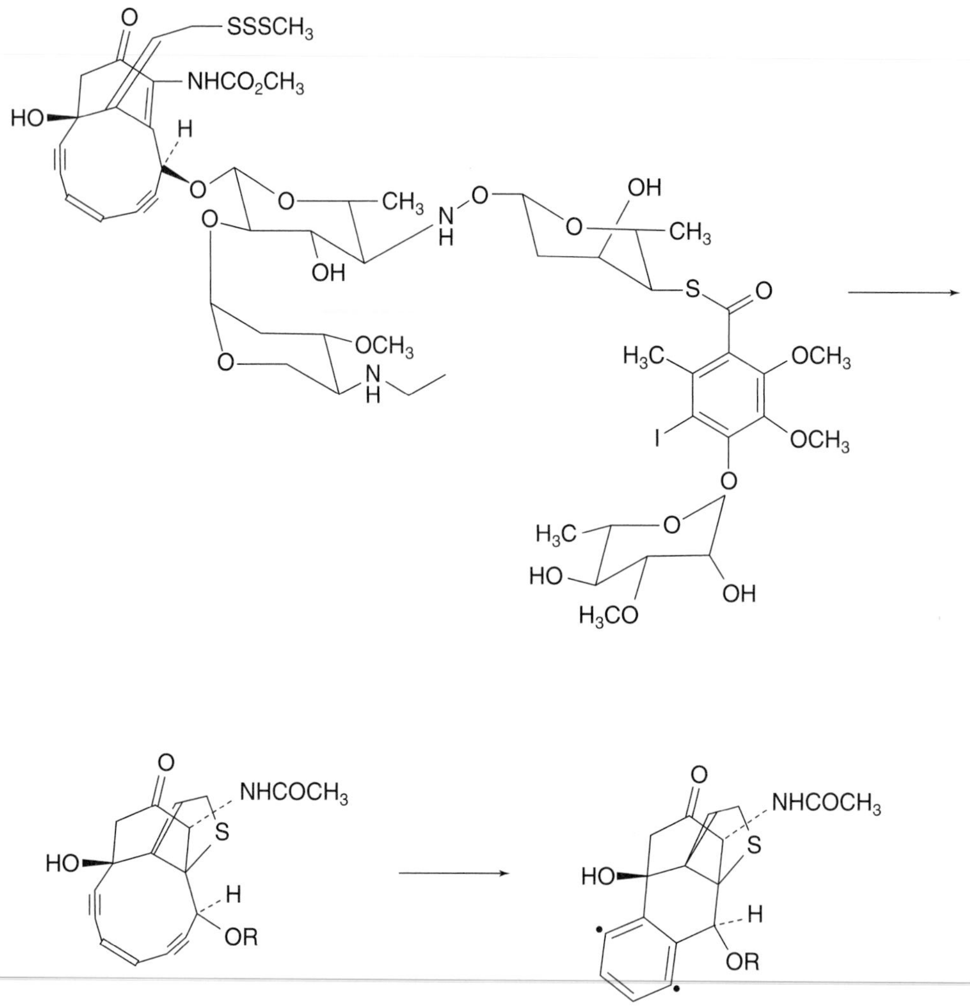

Figure 12–6 ■ Activation of calicheamicin γ^1.

Daunorubicin Hydrochloride. Daunorubicin hydrochloride, Cerubidine, daunomycin, rubidomycin, NSC-82151, is obtained from the fermentation of *Streptomyces peucetius*.[195] The hydrochloride salt is a red crystalline compound that is soluble in water and alcohols. Daunorubicin hydrochloride is available as lyophilized powder in 20-mg vials. In this form, it is stable at room temperature, but after reconstitution with 5 to 10 mL of sterile water it should be used within 6 hours. A new liposomal formulation of daunorubicin known as DaunoXome is in phase II clinical trials. Significantly reduced toxicity, including cardiotoxicity, has been claimed for it.

The long terminal plasma half-life of daunorubicin results from extensive tissue binding. It is readily metabolized to daunorubicinol by reduction of its 13-keto group. This metabolite is one-tenth as active as daunorubicin. The drug and its metabolite are eliminated by hepatobiliary excretion.

A number of cellular lesions may contribute to the antitumor effects of daunorubicin. It intercalates into DNA and inhibits the ligase activity of topoisomerase II, resulting in decreased synthesis of both DNA and RNA. Redox cycling of the quinone functionality generates hydroxyl and superoxide radicals, which peroxidize lipids and damage cellular membranes. This effect may produce cardiotoxicity because heart cells are relatively deficient in antioxidant defenses.[251]

Daunorubicin is used in the treatment of acute lymphocytic and granulocytic leukemias.[252] Toxic effects include bone marrow depression, stomatitis, alopecia, and gastrointestinal disturbances. At higher doses, cardiac toxicity may develop. Severe and progressive congestive heart failure may follow initial tachycardia and arrhythmias.

The usual dose of daunorubicin is 30 to 45 mg/m^2 daily for 3 days. It is administered intravenously, taking care to prevent extravasation.

Doxorubicin Hydrochloride, USP. Doxorubicin hydrochloride, Adriamycin, NSC-123127, 14-hydroxy-daunomycin, is obtained from cultures of *Streptomyces peucetius* var. *caesius*.[253] The orange-red needles are soluble in water and alcohols. Doxorubicin hydrochloride is supplied as a freeze-dried powder in two different sizes: 10 mg plus 50 mg of Lactose, USP, and 50 mg plus 250 mg of Lactose, USP. These amounts are reconstituted with 5 and 25 mL, respectively, of Sodium Chloride Injection, USP.

After administration, doxorubicin is rapidly distributed to body tissues, with about 75% of it binding to plasma proteins. It is extensively metabolized and eliminated primarily as glucuronide conjugates of the parent aglycone or the 13-hydroxyl reduction product, doxorubicinol. A small amount of the 7-deoxyaglycone also is formed. Disposition and elimination can be explained by a two-compartment or a three-compartment model. Liposome-encapsulated doxorubicin (LED) is available in several formulations for clinical trials.

The modes of action of doxorubicin are similar to those described for daunorubicin.

Doxorubicin is one of the most effective antitumor agents. It has been used successfully to produce regressions in acute leukemias, Hodgkin's disease and other lymphomas, Wilms' tumor, neuroblastoma, soft-tissue and bone sarcomas, breast carcinoma, ovarian carcinoma, transitional cell bladder carcinoma, thyroid carcinoma, and small-cell bronchogenic carcinoma.[254] Combination chemotherapy with a variety of other agents is being developed for specific tumors. The dose-limiting toxicities are myelosuppression and cardiotoxicity. There is a high incidence of bone marrow depression, primarily of leukocytes, which usually reaches its nadir at 10 to 14 days. Red blood cells and platelets also may be depressed. Thus, careful blood counts are essential. Acute left ventricular failure has occurred, particularly in patients receiving a total dose exceeding the currently recommended 550 mg/m^2. Cardiomyopathy and congestive heart failure may be encountered several weeks after discontinuing use of Adriamycin. Toxicity is augmented by impaired liver function, because this is the site of metabolism. Thus, evaluation of liver function by conventional laboratory tests is recommended before individual dosing.

The recommended intravenous dosage schedule is 60 to 75 mg/m^2 at 21-day intervals. This dose is decreased if liver function or bone marrow reserves are inadequate. Care must be taken to avoid extravasation.

Idarubicin Hydrochloride.

Idarubicin hydrochloride, Idamycin, IDA, 4-DMR, 4DDM, NSC-256439, 4-demethoxydaunorubicin, has been prepared by a number of synthetic routes.[255] The hydrochloride salt is formulated in single-dose vials containing 5 or 10 mg of orange lyophilized powder and is reconstituted with 5 or 10 mL of Sodium Chloride for Injection. These solutions are stable at least 7 days under refrigeration. Administration is intravenous, with care taken to avoid extravasation because of the potent vesicant action.

Idarubicin differs from daunorubicin by the lack of a methoxy group at the 4 position. Like daunorubicin, it intercalates DNA and inhibits topoisomerase II. Intravenous idarubicin is approved for therapy of acute nonlymphocytic leukemia in combination with cytarabine. It also is active against the blast phase of chronic myelogenous leukemia. The main dose-limiting toxicity is myelosuppression, especially leukopenia. It appears to be less cardiotoxic than doxorubicin and daunorubicin.[256]

Valrubicin.

Valrubicin, Valstar, medeva, *N*-trifluoroacetyldoxorubicin, is prepared by acylation of *N*-trifluoroacetyldoxorubicin.[207] It is supplied as a 40 mg/mL solution in Cremophor EL in 5-mL single-use vials. It should be stored at 2 to 8°C. The usual dose is 800 mg administered intravesically once a week for 6 weeks. Valrubicin is indicated for BCG-refractory carcinoma of the urinary bladder for patients who cannot have cystectomy.

Systemic metabolism gives *N*-trifluoroacetyldoxorubicin; however, the extent of metabolism during the 2-hour retention period in the urinary bladder is negligible. Systemic toxicity is generally low when the drug is instilled into the bladder. Nevertheless, some patients are sensitive to anthracyclines or Cremophor EL. Irritable bladder symptoms are common.[257]

Bleomycin Sulfate, Sterile, USP.

Bleomycin sulfate, Blenoxane, NSC-125066, is a mixture of cytotoxic glycopeptides isolated from a strain of *Streptomyces verticillus*.[258] The main component is bleomycin A$_2$ (~65%), and bleomycin B$_2$ (~20 to 30%) also is present. Bleomycin is a whitish powder that is readily soluble in water. It occurs naturally as a blue copper complex, but the copper is removed from the pharmaceutical form. It is supplied in ampuls containing 15 units of sterile bleomycin sulfate. The bleomycin unit is based on inhibitory activity against *Mycobacterium smegmatis* in culture: 0.1 mg of bleomycin equals 1 unit. Bleomycin sulfate is reconstituted by dissolution in 1 to 5 mL of sterile water, D5W, or Normal Saline for Injection.

Bleomycin undergoes rapid initial distribution with a half-life of 10 to 20 minutes, which is followed by an elimination half-life of 2 to 3 hours. It is inactivated readily in the liver and kidney and excreted in the urine.

The mode of bleomycin action involves binding to DNA followed by single- or double-strand cleavage. Transfer RNA also may be cleaved. This cleavage is caused by active oxygen species that are generated in a stepwise process from bleomycin–iron–oxygen complexes. The process is cell cycle specific, with the main effect in the G$_2$ and M phases.

Resistance to bleomycin is afforded by the cytosolic enzyme bleomycin hydrolase, which removes an amide group from the molecule. This is especially problematic with sarcomas, which have high levels of the hydrolase.

Bleomycin is used for the palliative treatment of squamous cell carcinomas of the head and neck, esophagus, skin, and genitourinary tract, including penis, cervix, and vulva.[259] It also is used against testicular carcinoma, especially in combination with cisplatin and vinblastine.[260] The principal toxicities of bleomycin are in skin and lungs. Other tissues contain an aminopeptidase that rapidly inactivates it. Bleomycin has very little bone marrow toxicity; thus, it may be used in combination with myelosuppressive agents. Pulmonary toxicity is induced in about 10% of treated patients, with pulmonary fibrosis and death occurring in about 1%. Thus, cumulative doses of more than 400 units are not recommended. Skin or mucous membrane toxicity occurs in about half of patients. Anaphylactoid reactions are possible in lymphoma patients.

The recommended dosage is 0.25 to 0.50 units/kg (10 to 20 units/m^2) given intravenously, intramuscularly, or subcutaneously once or twice weekly. For maintenance of Hodgkin's disease patients in remission, a dose of 1 unit daily or 5 units weekly is given. Blenoxane is stable for 24 hours at room temperature in sodium chloride or 5% dextrose solutions for injection.

Mitomycin, USP.

Mitomycin, Mutamycin, mitomycin C, NSC-26980, is obtained from cultures of *Streptomyces caespitosus* as blue-violet crystals.[261] It is soluble in water and polar organic solvents. Vials containing either 5 mg of mitomycin and 10 mg of mannitol or 20 mg of mitomycin and 40 mg of mannitol are supplied. The unreconstituted product is stable at room temperature for at least 2 years. The drug is reconstituted by adding 10 mL of Sterile Water for Injection, USP. Administration is intravenous or intravesical. It is rapidly cleared from the vascular compartment, and liver metabolism is the primary means of elimination.

Although it is a relatively stable compound, mitomycin C is activated by reduction to a bifunctional alkylating agent that cross-links complementary DNA strands, resulting in inhibition of DNA synthesis. The 2-amino groups of guanine residues are alkylated, and the preferred DNA sequence is CpG. There is no cell cycle specificity.[262]

Mitomycin is useful in treating disseminated breast, gastric, pancreatic, or colorectal adenocarcinomas in combination with fluorouracil and Adriamycin (FAM program). It is used in combination with cyclophosphamide and Adriamycin for lung cancer. Complete remissions of superficial transitional cell carcinomas of the bladder have been obtained in 60% of patients given intravesical mitomycin C instillations.[263] The dose-limiting toxicity is myelosuppression, characterized by delayed, cumulative pancytopenia. Fever, anorexia, nausea, and vomiting also occur.

Mitomycin at 10 to 20 mg/m² is given as a single dose by intravenous catheter. No repeat dose should be given until the leukocyte and platelet counts have recovered (~8 weeks).

Plicamycin, USP.   Plicamycin, Mithracin, aureolic acid, mithramycin, NSC-24559, is obtained from *Streptomyces plicatus*[213] or *S. argillaceus* as a yellow solid. It is soluble in polar organic solvents and aqueous alkali; however, it is susceptible to air oxidation in alkali. Mithramycin readily forms complexes with magnesium and other divalent metal ions, and these complexes have drastically altered optical rotations. Vials containing 2.5 mg of mithramycin as a freeze-dried powder, together with 100 mg of mannitol and sufficient disodium phosphate to give pH 7 when diluted with water are supplied. The drug is reconstituted by injecting 4.9 mL of Sterile Water for Injection, USP. Short intravenous infusions are used clinically.

Plicamycin is used in the treatment of advanced embryonal tumors of the testes.[239] It has been largely superseded, however, by newer agents, such as bleomycin and cisplatin. Presently, the main use of mithramycin is in Paget's disease, in which it reduces alkaline phosphatase activity and relieves bone pain.[264] It also is useful in treating patients with severe hypercalcemia or hypercalciuria resulting from advanced metastatic cancer involving bones. Plicamycin may produce severe hemorrhaging. Bone marrow, liver, and kidney toxicity also occur. The lower total dose used for hypercalcemia results in less toxicity.

Streptozocin.   Streptozocin, Zanosar, NSC-85998, 2-(3-methyl-3-nitrosoureido)-2-deoxy-D-glucopyranose, is obtained from cultures of *Streptomyces achromogenes* subsp. *streptozoticus*[265] or synthesized from D-glucosamine.[266] It is readily soluble in water or saline. Vials containing 1.0 g of lyophilized powder are supplied. They should be refrigerated at 35 to 46°F and protected from light. The drug is reconstituted by adding 9.5 mL of either normal saline or Sterile Water for Injection, USP.

Unchanged drug is rapidly cleared from plasma after an intravenous bolus. Metabolites demonstrate triphasic plasma clearance with a short initial phase. Streptozocin undergoes spontaneous decomposition to form methylcarbonium ions, which alkylate DNA and inhibit new DNA synthesis.

Streptozocin is indicated only for metastatic islet cell carcinoma of the pancreas.[267] Therapy is limited to patients with symptomatic or progressive disease, because of inherent renal toxicity of the drug. Up to two-thirds of patients treated with it experience renal toxicity. Adequate hydration is recommended to reduce this toxicity. Nausea and vomiting occur in more than 90% of patients, which occasionally requires discontinuation of drug therapy. Liver dysfunction also occurs. Streptozocin is mutagenic, carcinogenic, and teratogenic in animals. Carcinogenesis following topical exposure is a possible hazard. After rapid injection, unchanged drug is rapidly cleared from the plasma. The half-life is 35 minutes.

PLANT PRODUCTS

The use of higher plants in treating neoplastic disease dates to antiquity. Dioscorides described the use of colchicine for this purpose in the first century. In more recent years, scientists have attempted to select and screen systematically plants reputed to have antitumor activity. If activity is established for one member of a plant family, other members of this family are selected and tested. A major impetus to this research was given by Hartwell at the NCI, who established an extensive system of plant collection, screening, and isolation.[268] More than 100,000 plants have been screened under this program.

Resin of the may apple, *Podophyllum peltatum,* has long been used as a remedy for warts. One of its constituents, podophyllotoxin, has antineoplastic activity, but it is highly toxic.[269] This lignin inhibits mitosis by destroying the structural organization of the mitotic apparatus.[270] Early derivatives of podophyllotoxin showed poor clinical activity, but newer analogues, such as the epipodophyllotoxin derivatives etoposide and teniposide, are much better. Both of these analogues differ from podophyllotoxin in inhibiting topoisomerase II rather than microtubule assembly.[271]

Etoposide,   R = CH₃

Teniposide,   R =

TABLE 12–1 Vinca Alkaloids and Their Analogues

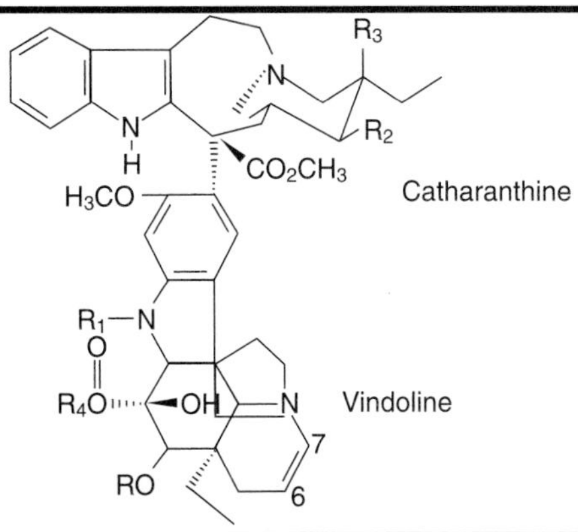

Catharanthine

Vindoline

	R	R₁	R₂	R₃	R₄
Vincristine	CH₃CO	CHO	H	OH	OCH₃
Vinblastine	CH₃CO	CH₃	H	OH	OCH₃
Vinrosidine	CH₃CO	CH₃	OH	H	OCH₃
Vinleurosine	CH₃CO	CH₃	Oxide		OCH₃
Vinglysinate	(CH₃)₂NCH₂CO	CH₃	H	OH	OCH₃
Vindesine	H	CH₃	H	OH	NH₂

The vinca alkaloids are a family of important antitumor agents from plants. These compounds were isolated from the periwinkle *Catharanthus rosea* at the Eli Lilly Company.[272] They have complex structures composed of an indole-containing moiety, catharanthine, and an indoline-containing moiety, vindoline (Table 12-1).[273] Four closely related compounds have antitumor activity: vincristine, vinblastine, vinrosidine, and vinleurosine. Among this group, vincristine and vinblastine are proved clinical agents. These two compounds are used against different types of tumors, despite the similarity of their structures. A number of semisynthetic compounds have been prepared. Among them, vinorelbine is active in advanced lung cancer and was recently approved by the FDA. Vinglycinate and 6,7-dihydrovinblastine show significant antitumor activity.[274] Vindesine is considered to resemble vincristine pharmacologically but to be less neurotoxic.[275]

Vinca alkaloids cause mitotic arrest by promoting the dis-

solution of microtubules in cells. Microtubule crystals containing the alkaloids are formed in the cytoplasm.[276] Vinblastine is the most active compound, whereas vincristine is the only compound to cause irreversible inhibition of mitosis.[277] Cells can resume mitosis following brief exposure to other vinca alkaloids after these compounds are withdrawn.[278]

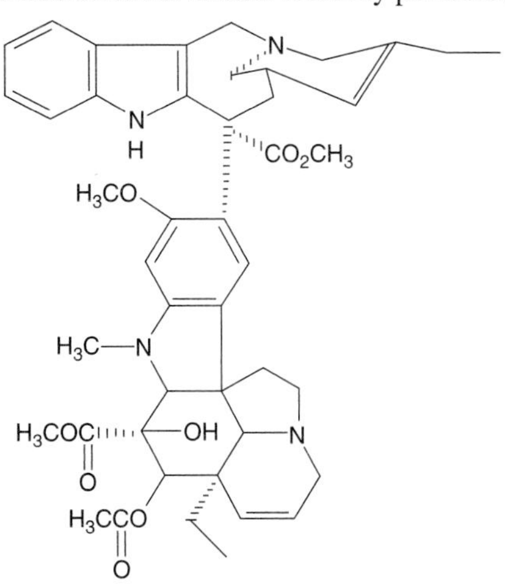

A plant product of high current interest in cancer chemotherapy is paclitaxel (Taxol). This compound was isolated from the bark of the Pacific yew tree *Taxus brevifolia* by Wani et al. in 1971.[279] At that time, it was found to have antitumor activity; however, there was little enthusiasm for its further development until recently, when its potential for human clinical activity was suggested by screening against human tumors in immunodeficient mice. It is now the world's leading antineoplastic agent in terms of sales. Paclitaxel is active against refractory ovarian cancer, metastatic breast cancer, metastatic melanoma, and non–small cell lung cancer.

Paclitaxel inhibits mitosis by acting as a spindle poison; however, it acts by a unique mechanism in promoting the assembly of microtubules and stabilizing them against depolymerization.[280] This mechanism is in contrast to that of compounds like the vinca alkaloids, which prevent the assembly of microtubules.

Initially, paclitaxel was obtained only from the bark of *Taxus brevifolia*, a slow-growing tree containing only a small amount of the drug. This process is expensive and a threat to forest ecology. Consequently, the manufacturer, Bristol-Myers Squibb, developed a route based on partial synthesis from 10-deacetylbaccatin III, which is obtained from the needles of *Taxus baccata*, a European yew tree. Because needles are rapidly regenerated, this is a less destructive method for obtaining paclitaxel. Furthermore, 10-deacetylbaccatin III is an important intermediate for the synthesis of analogues. One such analogue, docetaxel (Taxotere), has been prepared at Rhône-Poulenc Rorer. It is more water soluble than paclitaxel and reported to be more potent against solid tumors, but it is relatively more toxic than paclitaxel.[281] Docetaxel is approved for metastatic breast cancer and for non–small cell lung cancer after patients have failed prior chemotherapy.

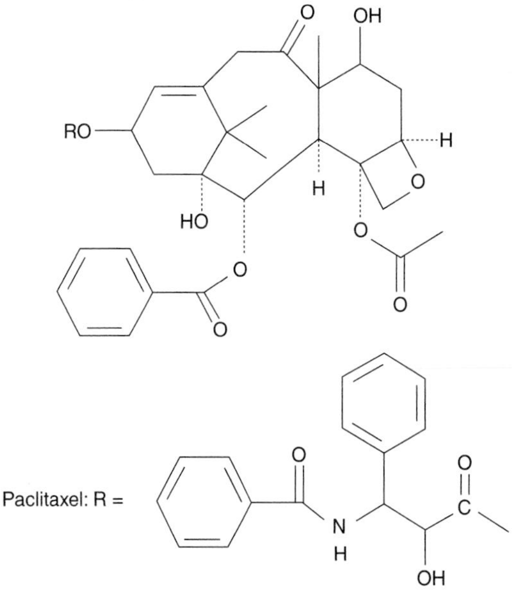

Vinorelbine

Paclitaxel: R =

Docetaxel: R =

As noted above, colchicine, obtained from the crocus *Colchicum autumnale,* has long been known for its antitumor activity. It is currently not used clinically for this purpose, however. Its main use is in terminating acute attacks of gout. Among colchicine derivatives, demecolcine (Colcemid) is active against myelocytic leukemia, but only at near-toxic doses. Colchicines have an unusual tricyclic structure containing a tropolone ring. They inhibit mitosis at metaphase by disorienting the organization of the spindle and asters.[282]

Colchicine, R = COCH$_3$
Colcemid, R = CH$_3$

Irinotecan has been approved recently for first-line therapy, in combination with 5-FU and leucovorin, for patients with metastatic colon or rectal carcinomas. It is a semisynthetic analogue of camptothecan.[283] Camptothecin was isolated from *Camptotheca acuminata,* an ornamental tree found in China.[284] It is very insoluble in water, but its sodium salt, prepared by alkaline hydrolysis of the lactone ring, showed promising antitumor activity. Clinical trials were eventually discontinued because of unpredictable toxic effects. Irinotecan has a basic tertiary amine group, which can be protonated to solubilize the drug. The lactone ring remains intact and increases activity above that of the ring-opened sodium salt. Camptothecin and irinotecan inhibit topoisomerase I. Cytotoxicity is caused by double-strand DNA damage, which occurs during DNA synthesis when replication enzymes interact with the ternary complex formed from DNA, topoisomerase I, and the drug.[285]

Many other plant constituents show significant antitumor activity in animals and have been given clinical evaluation. Some of the more important compounds are homoharringtonine, anguidine, and maytansine.[286]

Products

Etoposide. Etoposide, VePesid, VP-16,213, NSC-141540, is a semisynthetic derivative of podophyllotoxin. It is supplied in 5-mL ampuls containing 20 mg/mL of the drug plus 30 mg of benzyl alcohol, 80 mg of polysorbate 80, 650 mg of polyethylene glycol 300, and absolute alcohol. This mixture is diluted with either 5% dextrose or 0.9% saline to give a final concentration of 0.2 or 0.4 mg/mL. Etoposide also is supplied as 50-mg capsules which also contain sorbitol. They must be stored at 36 to 46°F.

The pharmacokinetics of etoposide fit a two-compartment model. A terminal half-life of 7 hours is independent of the dose and method of administration. About 43% of a dose is recovered in the urine, of which 66% is unchanged drug.[287] The primary metabolites found in plasma are picro hydroxy acids and picro lactone; the major urinary metabolite is 4′-demethylepipodophyllic acid. Oral bioavailability is about 50%.

Etoposide has marked schedule dependence, with cytotoxic effects in the G$_2$ phase. It causes protein-linked DNA strand breaks by inhibiting topoisomerase II. Although etoposide does not bind directly to the DNA, it stabilizes a covalent intermediate form of the DNA–topoisomerase II complex.[288]

Etoposide in combination with other chemotherapeutic agents is the first choice treatment for small cell lung cancer. It also is effective in combination with other agents for refractory testicular tumors, and it has been used alone or in combination against acute nonlymphocytic leukemias, Hodgkin's disease, non-Hodgkin's lymphomas, and Kaposi's sarcoma. It is contraindicated in patients who develop hypersensitivity. Dose-limiting bone marrow suppression is the most significant toxicity, and reversible alopecia occurs frequently. Nausea and vomiting are usually controlled with standard therapy. On intravenous administration, the disposition of etoposide is biphasic, with a distribution half-life of about 1.5 hours and an elimination half-life of 4 to 11 hours.

Teniposide. Teniposide, Vumon, FTP, VM-26, NSC-122819, 4′-de-methylepipodophyllotoxin-β-thenylidine glucoside, is prepared by treating epipodophyllotoxin with thiophene-2-carboxaldehyde.[289] It is supplied in 5-mL ampuls in which each milliliter contains 10 mg of teniposide, 30 mg of benzyl alcohol, 60 mg of *N,N*-dimethylacetamide, 500 mg of Cremophor EL, maleic acid to adjust the pH to 5.1, and absolute alcohol to adjust the total volume to 1 mL. This preparation is stable for 4 years at room temperature. It is diluted with at least five equivalents of sodium chloride solution before intravenous infusion.

Teniposide is highly protein bound to albumin and displays biexponential decay. Most of the urinary excretion is as metabolites.

Camptothecan: R$_1$ = R$_2$ = H

Irinotecan: R$_1$ = C$_2$H$_5$, R$_2$ =

As a single agent, teniposide is active against Kaposi's sarcoma, lymphomas, multiple myeloma, cervical cancer, and small cell lung cancer.[290] It is active in combination with cytarabine against refractory acute lymphocytic leukemia, which is the only indication approved by the FDA. The dose-limiting toxicity is leukopenia. Thrombocytopenia is also observed. Chemical phlebitis at the injection site is common. As with etoposide, prolonged treatment with teniposide may cause secondary acute myelogenous leukemia.[291]

Vinblastine Sulfate, USP.   Vinblastine sulfate, Velban, vincaleucoblastine, VLB, NSC-49842, is an antitumor alkaloid isolated from *Vinca rosea* L., the periwinkle plant.[272] It is soluble in water and alcohol. Vials containing 10 mg of vinblastine sulfate as a lyophilized plug are supplied. It is reconstituted by the addition of sodium chloride solution for injection preserved with phenol or benzyl alcohol.

Intravenous vinblastine is rapidly cleared from plasma and eliminated in a triphasic pattern. The apparent volume of distribution is 3 to 4 times the blood volume. A large portion (73%) is retained in the body, but some is excreted intact in urine and bile.[292] There is some metabolism to deacetyl vinblastine, which is more active than the parent compound.

The mode of action is tubulin binding, which inhibits microtubule assembly and microtubule spindle formation. This binding causes accumulation of cells in metaphase.

Vinblastine has been used for the palliation of a variety of neoplastic diseases. It is one of the most effective single agents against Hodgkin's disease, and it may be used in combination chemotherapy for patients who have relapses after treatment by the MOPP program. Advanced testicular germinal cell tumors respond to vinblastine alone or in combination. Beneficial effects are also obtained against lymphocytic lymphoma, histiocytic lymphoma, mycosis fungoides, Kaposi's sarcoma, Letterer-Siwe disease, resistant choriocarcinoma, and carcinoma of the breast. The limiting toxicity is leukopenia, which reaches its nadir 5 to 10 days after the last dose. Gastrointestinal and neurological symptoms occur and are dose dependent. Extravasation during injection can lead to cellulitis and phlebitis.

Vincristine Sulfate, USP.   Vincristine sulfate, Oncovin, leurocristine VCR, LCR, NSC-67574, is isolated from *Vinca rosea* L.[272] The sulfate is a crystalline solid that is soluble in water. It is supplied in vials containing either 1 mg of vincristine sulfate and 10 mg of lactose, or 5 mg of vincristine and 50 mg of lactose. Each size has an accompanying vial of 10 mL of bacteriostatic sodium chloride solution containing 90 mg of sodium chloride and 0.9% benzyl alcohol. The reconstituted pharmaceutical may be stored 14 days in a refrigerator.

After administration, vincristine is rapidly distributed to tissues and bound to formed blood elements. Elimination is triphasic, with more than half of the drug cleared within 20 minutes. The primary mode of elimination is hepatic extraction with secretion into bile.

Vincristine binds reversibly to tubulin, stopping microtubule assembly, which arrests cell division in metaphase.[293] This temporary arrest causes a cell cycle block called *stathmokinesis*. Resistance to vincristine results from increased cellular levels of P-glycoprotein.

Vincristine is effective against acute leukemia. In combination with prednisone it produces complete remission in 90% of children with ALL.[169] It is used in the MOPP program of combination chemotherapy for Hodgkin's disease.[294] Other tumors that respond to vincristine in combination with other antineoplastic agents include lymphosarcoma, reticulum cell sarcoma, rhabdomyosarcoma, neuroblastoma, and Wilms' tumor. Although the tumor spectra of vinblastine and vincristine are similar, there is a lack of cross-resistance between the two. Because vincristine is less myelosuppressive than vinblastine, it is preferred in combination with myelotoxic agents. The most serious clinical toxicity of vincristine is neurological, with paresthesias, loss of deep tendon reflexes, pain, and muscle weakness. These symptoms can usually be reversed by lowering the dose or suspending therapy. The rapid action of vincristine in destroying cancer cells may result in hyperuricemia. Administration of allopurinol can prevent this complication.

Vinorelbine Tartrate.   Vinorelbine tartrate, Navelbine, is a new semisynthetic vinca alkaloid derived from vinblastine by loss of one carbon from ring C′ and dehydration in ring D′, both in the catharanthine moiety. It is named 3′,4′-didehydro-4′-deoxy-C′-norvincaleukoblastine. Navelbine is supplied in vials containing 10 mg/mL of solution in a volume of 1 mL of Water for Injection or 10 mg/mL of solution in a volume of 5 mL of Water for Injection. Unopened vials are stable at room temperature for up to 72 hours. It is diluted to a concentration of 0.5 to 2 mg/mL with 0.9% Sodium Chloride Injection or 5% Dextrose Injection for intravenous infusion or slow intravenous push administration.

The primary mechanism of action of vinorelbine is binding to tubulin, which inhibits microtubule assembly. It may be more specific than other vinca alkaloids for mitotic microtubules. Vinorelbine has been approved by the FDA for treatment of unresectable advanced non–small cell lung cancer. The most important side effect is granulocytopenia.

Paclitaxel.   Paclitaxel, Taxol, is a diterpene obtained from the needles and bark of the western yew, *Taxus brevifolia*,[279] or by partial synthesis from closely related compounds obtained from similar species. It is formulated as a concentrated sterile solution containing 30 mg of paclitaxel in a 5-mL ampul containing a mixture of 50% polyoxylated castor oil, Cremophor EL, and 50% dehydrated alcohol, USP. It is usually reconstituted in 50 mL of D5W. Solutions should be used within 24 hours of reconstitution. It is administered by intravenous infusion only.

Disposition of paclitaxel from plasma follows a biphasic elimination pattern. Approximately 97.5% of it is bound to plasma proteins. Clearance is triphasic and results mainly from hepatic extraction and biliary excretion. Eleven metabolites have been detected in plasma, but not identified.[295]

Paclitaxel is a mitotic spindle poison that acts by a unique process. It promotes assembly of microtubules and stabilizes them against depolymerization. This process blocks cycle traverse in mitosis.[280] Paclitaxel is highly active against refractory ovarian cancer and effective against metastatic breast cancer, metastatic melanoma, and non–small cell lung cancer. It is used in combinations containing doxorubicin, cisplatin, and filgrastim (a human granulocyte colony-stimulating factor produced by recombinant DNA technology). Hypersensitivity occurs in some patients within 10 minutes of starting an infusion. It has been suggested that the allergen is the Cremophor EL diluent.[296] Reversible peripheral neuropathy is common with prolonged infusions. Bradycardia, gastrointestinal disturbances, flu-like symptoms, and total body alopecia also occur.

Docetaxel.

Docetaxel, Taxotere, RP-56967, NSC-628503, is prepared from a precursor obtained from needles of the yew plant.[297] It is supplied as a 20-mg sample in 0.5 mL of polysorbate 80 or as an 80-mg sample in 2 mL of polysorbate 80, both in single-dose vials with diluent suitable for injection. Samples should be kept at 2 to 8°C and be protected from light. Recommended doses are 60 to 100 mg/m^2 IV over 1 hour every 3 weeks for breast cancer or 75 mg/m^2 for non–small cell lung cancer.

Docetaxel is indicated for breast cancer after failure of prior chemotherapy and for non–small lung carcinoma after failure of platinum-based therapy. Toxic effects include neutropenia, fluid retention, mutagenesis, rash, and neurological symptoms.[298] Peripheral blood counts should be performed because of myelosuppression. Pharmacokinetics indicate a three-compartment model with half-lives of 4 and 36 minutes and 11.1 hours. The drug is 94% protein bound.

MISCELLANEOUS COMPOUNDS

In 1965, Rosenberg investigated the effects of electrical fields on bacteria and found that *Escherichia coli* formed long filaments instead of dividing.[299] He subsequently discovered that this effect was caused not by the electrical current, but by a complex, $[Pt(Cl)_4(NH_3)_2]^0$ formed from the platinum electrode in the presence of ammonium and chloride ions.[300] This discovery was followed by testing a variety of platinum neutral complexes against tumors, with the result that *cis*-dichlorodiammineplatinum II (cisplatin) eventually became established as a clinical agent.[301]

This platinum complex is a potent inhibitor of DNA polymerase. Its activity and toxicity resemble those of the alkylating agents. Considerable evidence has been obtained for DNA binding by the platinum complex, in which the two chlorides are displaced by nitrogen or oxygen atoms of purines. This evidence includes facilitated renaturation, increased sedimentation coefficient, hyperchromicity of the DNA ultraviolet spectrum, and selective reaction of the complex with guanine over other bases.[302]

Many other platinum complexes have been found active against tumors. Generally, they fall into the classification of *cis* isomers in which one pair of ligands are monodentate anions of intermediate leaving ability (e.g., chloride) or bidentate anions (e.g., malonate), and the other pair are mono- or bidentate amines.[303] Among the more significant analogues is carboplatin, the current leader in sales among platinum complexes, which is approved by the FDA for treatment of ovarian cancer and which also is used against lung, genitourinary, and head and neck cancer.[304, 305]

Other platinum complexes of current interest are oxaliplatin, which has oxalate and 1,2-diaminocyclohexane as

ligands,[306] and ormaplatin, a Pt (IV) complex whose six ligands include four chlorides and 1,2-diaminocyclohexane. Ormaplatin must be reduced to dichloro-1,2-diaminocyclohexane Pt (II) for activation.[307]

Cisplatin

Carboplatin

Oxaliplatin

Ormaplatin

Arsenic trioxide has been used in a variety of therapeutic roles including parasitic infections, rheumatism, and asthma. Recently it was found active against promyelocytic leukemia, which is characterized by translocation of *PML/RAR-α* gene expression. The active species is dimethylarsenic acid, which is formed from arsenic trioxide by liver methyltransferase enzymes. This species produces DNA fragmentation characteristic of apoptosis.

Hydroxyurea has been known for more than 100 years, but its antitumor activity was not discovered until 1963. It is active against rapidly proliferating cells in the synthesis phase, during which it prevents the formation of deoxyribonucleotides from ribonucleotides. Its mode of action is inhibition of ribonucleotide diphosphate reductase, an enzyme consisting of two protein subunits.[308] It does this by interfering with the iron-containing portion of one of these subunits.[309]

Hydroxyurea

Guanazole

Another very old compound recently found active against tumors is guanazole.[310] This diaminotriazole resembles hydroxyurea in its ability to limit DNA synthesis by inhibiting the reduction of ribonucleotides. It is clinically active in inducing remissions of acute adult leukemia.[311]

In 1953, Kidd found that injections of guinea pig serum caused regressions of certain transplanted tumors in mice and rats.[312] Subsequent investigation revealed that these tumors required L-asparagine as a nutrient, but the presence of the enzyme L-asparaginase in the guinea pig serum created a deficiency in this amino acid.[313] The practical preparation of L-asparaginase for clinical trials follows the discovery that *E. coli* produces a form of it that has antineoplastic activity.[314] Thus, mass cultures are harvested and treated with ammonium sulfate to rupture the cells, and the liberated enzyme is isolated by solvent extraction and chromatography.

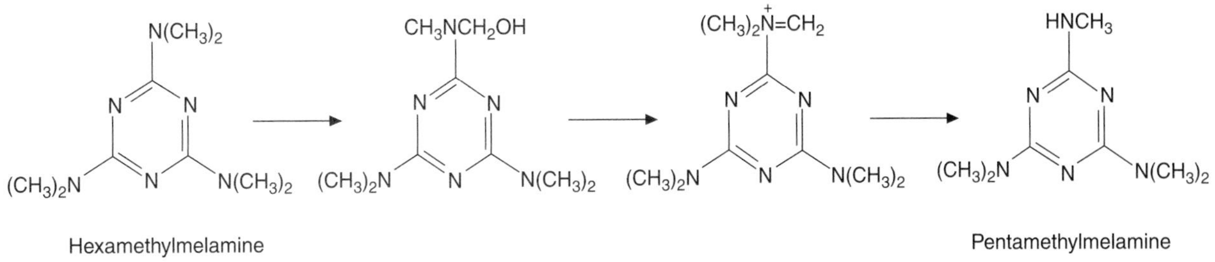

Hexamethylmelamine   Pentamethylmelamine

Very pure material is obtained by gel filtration or affinity chromatography, followed by crystallization. The *E. coli* enzyme has a molecular mass of 120,000 to 141,000 daltons, an isoelectric point of 4.9 to 5.2, and a Km of 1.2×10^{-5}.[315]

Earlier preparations of L-asparaginase contained endotoxins from *E. coli,* but these are absent in the purer new preparations. Clearance of the enzyme from plasma is due to an immunological reaction in which it combines with protein. This reaction may lead to sensitization in some patients. Patients who cannot tolerate L-asparaginase from *E. coli* might be treated by the preparation from *Erwinia caratovora.*[316] Tumor resistance is based on the development of asparagine synthetase by the tumor cells.[317]

Pegaspargase is a modified version of asparaginase in which the enzyme is covalently conjugated with strands of polymeric monomethoxypropylene glycol (PEG), which have molecular weights of about 5,000. It is used in combination chemotherapy of patients with ALL who are sensitive to natural L-asparaginase.

Altretamine (hexamethylmelamine) is approved by the FDA for use as a single agent for resistant ovarian cancer.[318] It is rapidly metabolized to pentamethylmelamine, tetramethylmelamine, and seven other compounds. Pentamethylmelamine also has antitumor activity. A suggested mode of action for altretamine is hydroxylation of one of the methyl groups to give the corresponding hydroxymethyl compound.[319] This compound is a carbinolamine that can lose hydroxide ion to form an immonium ion capable of either alkylation of a macromolecule or hydrolysis to pentamethylmelamine. This process could be repeated in converting pentamethylmelamine to an alkylating agent or to tetramethylmelamine.

Methylglyoxal bis(guanylhydrazone) (mitoguazone) has antitumor activity in humans. It interferes with polyamine synthesis to block nuclear and mitochondrial metabolism.[320] Many of its actions are related to the functions of spermidine, which it resembles in structure. Thus, it competes with spermidine for the transport carrier and intracellular binding site. It also inhibits spermidine biosynthesis. Its antiproliferative effects on cells can be prevented by administering spermidine.[321] Many other bis(guanylhydrazones) have been prepared, but none has proved superior to the methylglyoxal derivative.

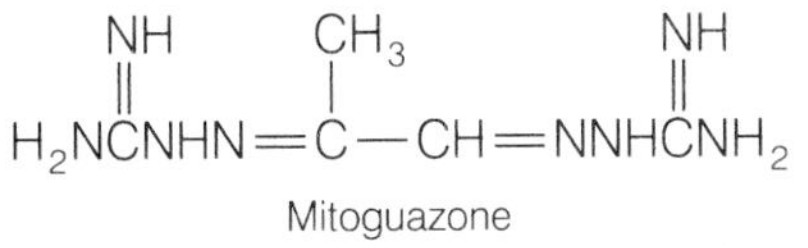

Mitoguazone
[Methylglyoxal Bis(guanylhydrazone)]

$$H_2NCH_2CH_2CH_2NHCH_2CH_2CH_2CH_2NH_2$$
Spermidine

Among the newer antineoplastic drugs, 4-[(9-acridinyl)-amino]methanesulfon-*m*-anisidide (m-AMSA) showed a wide spectrum of activity in early clinical trials. It afforded some remissions in refractory cases of breast cancer, malignant melanoma, and acute myelocytic leukemia. Leukopenia is the limiting toxicity.[322]

m-AMSA (amsacrine) is an acridine derivative that is thought to bind to DNA through intercalation. It does not affect DNA synthesis, however.[323] This compound was rationally designed as one member of a group of acridinylaminomethanesulfonamides.[324] Previously, a number of other acridine derivatives had shown antitumor activity.

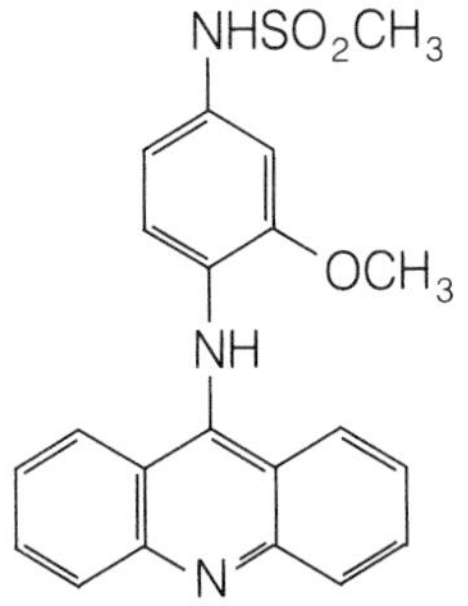

Amsacrine
(m-AMSA)

The clinical importance of anthracyclines stimulated the synthesis and screening of anthraquinones with partial anthracycline structures. One of the best of these analogues is mitoxantrone, which has two hydroxyl and two 2-[(2-hydroxyethylamino)ethyl]amino substituents on the anthraquinone nucleus.[325] Like doxorubicin, mitoxantrone intercalates into DNA and inhibits DNA topoisomerase II[326]; however, it is not a substrate for reductases and does not form oxygen-free radicals in a redox cycling process. Consequently, it is less cardiotoxic than doxorubicin. Mitoxantrone is approved for inducing remissions in acute nonlymphocytic leukemia, usually in combination with cytarabine.

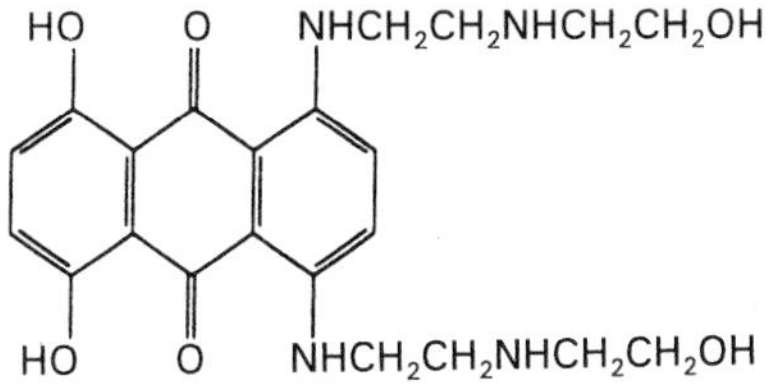

Mitoxantrone

Piroxantrone is an anthrapyrazole structurally related to mitoxantrone in having two phenolic hydroxyls and side chains containing amino groups; however, its quinone ring is modified to form part of a pyrazole ring with a nitrogen atom on the next ring.[327] The mode of action of piroxantrone is intercalation and interference with DNA synthesis by template inhibition. Cardiotoxicity is low because it does not undergo redox cycling.[328] Piroxantrone is presently in clinical trials.

Piroxantrone

The antiparasitic drug suramin sodium (Chapter 8) has long been used to treat trypanosomal and filarial infections. It also inhibits reverse transcriptase in RNA tumor viruses. Antitumor activity was demonstrated in hormonally refractive prostate cancer[329] and advanced ovarian carcinoma. Suramin acts by a variety of biological mechanisms, including inhibition of hyaluronidase, urease, hexokinase, RNA polymerase, DNA topoisomerase II, and lysosomal enzymes.[330] It affects ATP synthesis and degradation and inhibits mitochondrial enzymes. Signal transduction in cells is inhibited by suramin binding to tumor growth factors and protein kinases.[331] Suramin may also inhibit angiogenesis and induce normal cellular differentiation by increasing tissue glycosaminoglycans.[332]

Although antitumor activity was found for gallium nitrate in phase II clinical trials,[333] its approved use is for the treatment of cancer-related hypercalcemia.[334] It has proved superior to calcitonin and etidronate in this use. The clinical material is the nonahydrate of Ga(NO$_3$)$_3$.

Retinoids regulate cellular growth and induce differentiation in a wide variety of preneoplastic and neoplastic cell types, and they induce apoptosis in certain cells. The actions of vitamin A metabolites and of synthetic retinoids on retinoid receptors regulates the expression of specific genes, which control many important cellular proteins that have a pivotal role in cells. Furthermore, retinoids inhibit expression of ornithine decarboxylase and tissue transglutaminase, enzymes highly expressed in certain tumors. Retinoid receptors are classified into two subfamilies: the retinoic acid receptors and the retinoid X receptors, which function as ligand-dependent factors for gene transcription.[335] Each subfamily contains three distinct isoforms.

Tretinoin (*trans*-retinoic acid) is a normal metabolite of retinol (vitamin A). It can induce normal differentiation in a variety of malignant cells, especially acute promyelocytic leukemia cells, and its differentiating effects are augmented by a variety of other agents, including cytotoxic drugs, cytokines, and polar solvents.[336] Topical tretinoin produces regression of basal cell carcinoma in most patients and reduces the size of cutaneous lesions in AIDS-related Kaposi's sarcoma.[337]

Widespread use of tretinoin and related naturally occurring retinoids is limited by undesirable side effects, which probably arise from their activation of multiple receptors. Recently, compounds selective for the retinoid X receptors

have been developed in an effort to limit side effects. One of these selective agents, bexarotene, has been approved for use in patients with cutaneous T-cell lymphoma that is refractory in previous systemic therapy.[338] It is administered orally in gelatin capsules.

Tretinoin

Bexarotene

Sargramostim (GM-CSF, Leukine) is a natural human protein produced by recombinant DNA techniques with yeast or bacteria as the host organism. This partially glycosylated protein contains 120 to 127 amino acids and two internal disulfide bridges. The yeast-derived product is approved by the FDA to promote bone marrow recovery in patients with leukemias or lymphomas who are undergoing autologous bone marrow transplantation.[339]

Filgrastim also promotes the production of neutrophil precursors in the bone marrow. This granulocyte colony-stimulating factor (G-CSF) is a 175-amino acid protein manufactured by recombinant DNA technology. It is identical in sequence with the natural protein except for an N-terminal methionine necessary for expression in *E. coli*. It has no glycosylation because of its production in *E. coli*.

Photodynamic therapy is a two-stage process in which the patient is injected with a photosensitizing agent and then, after this agent has diffused throughout the body, laser light is applied to the tumors. The one antineoplastic photosensitizer approved thus far is porfimer sodium (Photofrin II). It is a polyporphyrin oligomer linked through ether and ester bonds, and it forms aggregates with a combined molecular mass of about 10,000 daltons. When subjected to laser light, it gives an orange-red fluorescence and activates molecular oxygen to form species that attack DNA and produce strand cleavage. This process is used for palliation in patients with completely obstructed esophageal cancer or endobrachial non–small cell lung cancer.[340]

Products

Cisplatin. Cisplatin, Platinol, NSC-119875, CDDP, is prepared by treating potassium chloroplatinite with ammonia.[301] It is a water-soluble white solid supplied in amber vials containing 10 mg of cisplatin as a lyophilized powder. For reconstitution, 10 mL of sterile water is added, and the resulting solution is diluted in 2 L of 5% dextrose in 0.5 or 0.33 N saline containing 37.5 g of mannitol.[341]

Cisplatin has a triphasic disappearance curve with half-lives of 20 minutes, 48 to 70 minutes, and 24 hours. Glomerular filtration and tubular secretion in the kidney removes 90% of the dose.

Interaction with DNA is the primary mode of cisplatin activity. Intrastrand cross-links are produced and cause changes in DNA conformation that affect replication.[342]

Cisplatin is used in combination with bleomycin and vinblastine for metastatic testicular tumors. This combination represents a significant improvement over previous treatments.[343] As a single agent or in combination with doxorubicin, cisplatin is used for the remission of metastatic ovarian tumors. Other tumors that have shown sensitivity to cisplatin include penile cancer, bladder cancer, cervical cancer, head and neck cancer, and small cell cancer of the lung. The major dose-limiting toxicity is cumulative renal insufficiency associated with renal tubular damage. Hydrating patients with intravenous fluids before and during cisplatin treatment reduces the incidence of renal toxicity significantly.[344] Myelosuppression, nausea and vomiting, and ototoxicity also occur frequently.

The usual dosage for metastatic testicular tumors is 20 mg/m^2 intravenously daily for 5 days, once every 3 weeks for three courses. Metastatic ovarian tumors are treated with 50 mg/m^2 intravenously once every 3 weeks. Pretreatment hydration is recommended for both regimens.[341]

Carboplatin.   Carboplatin, Paraplatin, CBDCA, JM8, NSC-241240, *cis*-diammine(1,1-cyclobutanedicarboxalato)platinum (II), is prepared by treatment of *cis*-Pt (NH$_3$)$_2$I$_2$ with silver sulfate followed by the barium salt of 1,1-cyclobutanedicarboxylic acid.[345] It is about 10 times as soluble in water as cisplatin, and its rate of hydrolysis is much slower than that of cisplatin. Hydrolysis of the carboxalato bonds yields transient aquated intermediates that bind to DNA. Carboplatin is supplied in vials containing 50, 150, and 450 mg of sterile lyophilized powder plus an equivalent amount of mannitol. The vials have a shelf life of 3 years. For reconstitution, the drug typically is diluted with 500 mL of Sodium Chloride for Infusion or D5W, and it is administered by infusion.

Plasma clearance of carboplatin is biphasic, with up to 65% excreted in the urine. There is little bound to plasma proteins and no true metabolism.

Carboplatin is approved by the FDA for treatment of advanced ovarian cancer. It is cross resistant with cisplatin in this tumor. Activity also has been reported in non–small cell lung cancer, head and neck cancer, and testicular cancer. The usual dose-limiting toxicity is bone marrow suppression, especially thrombocytopenia. Nephrotoxicity is much less common than with cisplatin.[346]

Hydroxyurea, USP.   Hydroxyurea, Hydrea, hydroxycarbamide, NSC-32065, is prepared from hydroxylamine hydrochloride and potassium cyanide.[347] It is a crystalline solid with good solubility in water. Capsules containing 500 mg of hydroxyurea are supplied.

After passive diffusion into cells, hydroxyurea inhibits ribonucleotide reductase, which results in decreased levels of deoxyribonucleotides.[348] Hydroxyurea may interfere with the function of the enzyme by chelating with its ferrous iron cofactor.

Hydroxyurea is well absorbed after oral administration,

and it produces peak serum levels of 0.3 to 2.0 mM about 1 to 2 hours later. Approximately 50% of a dose is degraded in the liver and excreted as urea and CO$_2$. Acetohydroxamic acid is a major metabolite in humans.

Hydroxyurea is active against melanoma, chronic myelocytic leukemia, and metastatic ovarian carcinoma. It is used in combination with radiotherapy for head and neck cancer. The main toxicity is bone marrow depression expressed as leukopenia, anemia, and, occasionally, thrombocytopenia. Gastrointestinal toxicity and dermatological reactions also occur.

Asparaginase.   L-Asparaginase EC 3.5.1.1, colaspase, L-ASP, L-asnase, L-asparaginase amidohydrolase, NSC-109229 *(E. coli)*, *Erwinia* asparaginase (NSC-106997), is an enzyme isolated commercially from *E. coli* and *E. caratovora*. It has four subunits, each with a molecular weight of 32,000 to 34,000 and one active site per subunit.[349] The isolate is not pure, and the potency varies with the batch. Consequently, batch potencies are rated in terms of the international asparaginase unit (IU), which is the enzyme activity that releases 1 μmol of ammonia from L-asparagine in 1 minute under the test conditions. Lyophilized asparaginase is provided in 10,000-IU vials also containing 80 mg of mannitol *(E. coli)* or 20 mg of dextrose and 0.6 mg of sodium chloride *(E. caratovora)*. It should be stored under refrigeration. Reconstitution is with 2 to 5 mL of normal saline or sterile water.

The reconstituted drug is given by infusion or by intramuscular injection. Allergic reactions can occur in up to 25% of patients. They include life-threatening anaphylactic shock. The manufacturer recommends skin testing before administration. Patients allergic to the *E. coli* preparation may be switched to the *Erwinia* preparation; however, the crossover anaphylactoid rate is about 25% in children. L-Asparaginase conjugated with polyethylene glycol (PEG-Asparaginase) exhibits minimal immunogenicity, although gastrointestinal toxicity may be greater. Asparaginase has very poor extravascular tissue penetration and is slowly and unpredictably cleared from plasma. Elimination is biphasic, with an initial half-life of 4 to 9 hours and a terminal half-life of 1.4 to 1.8 days.[350]

Asparagine is required for the biosynthesis of proteins. Although normal cells can synthesize asparagine, tumors such as ALL lack this ability and depend on exogenous compound. Administration of asparaginase reduces the concentration of asparagine in plasma, making it unavailable to the leukemia cells.[351] Asparaginase is used in combination chemotherapy to induce remissions in ALL, and PEG-asparagine has shown activity in non-Hodgkin's lymphoma. In addition to hypersensitivity, side effects include gastrointestinal damage, hepatic toxicity, and pancreatitis.

Pegaspargase.   Pegaspargase, PEG-L-asparaginase, is a modified version of the enzyme L-asparaginase. It is a covalent conjugate with units of monomethoxypropylene glycol (PEG) with molecular masses of approximately 5,000 daltons. Pegaspargase is supplied as a phosphate-buffered saline solution containing 750 IU/mL. The usual dosage is 2,500 IU/m^2, preferably by IM injection. Generally, it is used in combination with other chemotherapeutic agents in ALL patients who are hypersensitive to L-asparaginase. Toxic effects include allergic reactions such as bronchospasm and anaphylaxis. Depletion of serum proteins and anticoagulants also occurs.

Altretamine. Altretamine, Hexalen, hexamethylmelamine, NSC-13875, N,N,N′,N′,N″,N″-hexamethyl-1,3,5-triazine-2,4,6-triamine, is prepared from dimethylamine and cyanuric chloride[76] and formulated as 50-mg hard gelatin capsules that also contain lactose and calcium stearate. They should be stored at room temperature in a tightly sealed bottle containing a desiccant.

Administration is orally, and there is considerable variation in the bioavailability and pharmacokinetics. It is rapidly metabolized by N-demethylation through hepatic microsomes. The main metabolites include pentamethylmelamine and tetramethylmelamine. A possible mode of action involves hydroxylation of a methyl group to the corresponding hydroxymethyl derivative, a carbinolamine that can lose hydroxide ion to form an immonium ion capable of either alkylation or hydrolysis to the monomethylamine.[77]

The FDA has approved altretamine as a single agent for treatment of resistant ovarian cancer.[78] It also is active in combination regimens against this tumor. Gastrointestinal toxicity, manifested as anorexia, nausea, and vomiting, is dose limiting. Neurotoxicity occurs, but it is usually reversible.

Mitoxantrone Hydrochloride. Mitoxantrone hydrochloride, Novantrone, DHAD, NSC-301739, l-4-dihydroxy-5,8-bis[[2-[(2-hydroxyethyl)amino]ethyl]amino]-9,l0-anthracenedione dihydrochloride, DHAQ (free base), is prepared from 2,3-dihydroxyquinazarine by treatment with 2-(2-amino-ethyl-amino)ethanol followed by chloranil oxidation.[352] It is supplied in vials containing 10, 12.5, or 15 mL of a 2 mg/mL sterile solution that is stable for years at room temperature. Sodium chloride, sodium acetate, and acetic acid are present as inactive ingredients. These preparations are diluted with at least 50 mL of Sodium Chloride for Injection or 5% Dextrose for Injection and administered as an infusion.

Mitoxantrone is bound up to 78% to plasma proteins. The serum concentration-time profile is fit by a three-compartment model that has an α-phase half-life of 2.4 to 15 minutes, corresponding to distribution into formed blood elements; a β-phase half-life of 17 minutes to 3 hours, corresponding to redistribution into blood and various tissues; and a γ-phase half-life of 2.9 to 298 hours.[353] Highest concentrations of the drug are found in the liver, pancreas, thyroid, spleen, heart, and bone marrow. Large amounts of drug may be retained in these organs for prolonged periods.

The mode of action of mitoxantrone involves intercalation and inhibition of topoisomerase II.[354] In contrast to doxorubicin, it does not undergo redox cycling to form oxygen free radicals, because its redox potential is outside the reductive capability of mammalian reductases. Mitoxantrone is approved for remission-induction therapy in acute nonlymphocytic leukemia, where it typically is used with cytarabine.[355] It also is active against other leukemias, breast cancer, and ovarian cancer. The dose-limiting toxic effect is myelosup-pression, which usually involves leukopenia. Other toxic effects include nausea and vomiting. Cardiac toxicity can occur with long-term administration of high doses of mitoxantrone.

Gallium Nitrate. Gallium nitrate, Ganite, NSC-15200, is prepared by the reaction of gallium metal with nitric acid. The clinical material is supplied as 500 mg of the nonahydrate $Ga(NO_3)_3 \cdot 9\ H_2O$ in a 20-mL single-dose flip-top vial. Also present is 28.75 mg of sodium citrate dihydrate and sodium hydroxide for pH adjustment to 6.0 to 7.0. The daily dose is diluted in 1,000 mL of 0.9% Sodium Chloride Injection, USP, or 5% Dextrose Injection, USP, for intravenous infusion.

Gallium nitrate is approved for treating cancer-related hypercalcemia.[334] It showed antitumor activity for patients with lymphoma in phase II trials.[333] Gallium nitrate probably works in hypercalcemia by inhibiting calcium resorption from bone, although the precise mechanism is unknown. Major side effects include hypocalcemia and nephrotoxicity. On continuous infusion, the drug exhibits biphasic elimination with an α half-life of 8.3 to 26 minutes and a β half-life of 6.3 to 96 hours. Between 69 and 91% of the dose was recovered in the urine.[356]

Arsenic Trioxide. Arsenic trioxide, Trisenox, arsenous acid anhydride, As_2O_3 is supplied in solutions containing 1 mg/mL for injection. It is stored at 2.5°C and reconstituted by dilution with 100 to 250 mL of 5% Dextrose for Injection or 0.9% Sodium Chloride for Injection. Administration is by intravenous injection over 2 hours. The usual dose is 0.15 mg/kg per day until bone marrow remission occurs, with the total number of doses limited to 60.

Arsenic trioxide is indicated for patients with acute promyelocytic leukemia characterized by translocation of *PML/RAR-α* gene expression who have relapsed after retinoid and anthracycline therapy. Adverse reactions include leukocytosis, nausea and vomiting, fatigue, edema, hypoglycemia, dyspnea, cough, rashes, headaches, and dizziness. They usually do not prevent continuation of therapy.

Bexarotene. The retinoid class drug bexarotene, Targretin gel, LDG 10069, 4-[1-(5,6,7,8-tetrahydro-3,5,5,8,8,-pentamethyl-2-naphthenyl)propyl]benzoic acid, is supplied in 75-mg soft gelatin capsules. It is stored at 2 to 25°C. The usual dose is 30 mg/m² per day as a single oral dose taken with a meal.

Bexarotine is indicated for cutaneous T-cell lymphoma in patients refractory to prior systemic therapy. After oral administration, it is absorbed with a T_{max} of 2 hours. It is 99% bound to plasma proteins, and the terminal half-life is approximately 7 hours. The metabolites involve oxidation at positions 6 and 7. Adverse reactions include elevated cholesterol and triglycerides, headaches, nausea, rash, and leukopenia.[357]

Sargramostim. Sargramostim, Leukine (yeast-derived, Immunex), Prokine (Hoechst-Roussel), Leucomax (*E. coli*-derived, Schering), granulocyte-macrophage colony-stimulating factor (GM-CSF), is produced by recombinant DNA methods using as host organisms *Saccharomyces cerevisiae* (yeast) or *E. coli.* It contains 120 to 127 amino acids, and the tertiary structure is maintained by two disulfide bridges. Two arginine sites are variably glycosylated in the yeast-derived preparation. Leukine differs from native sargramostim by substitution of leucine at position 23 and by a different carbohydrate makeup. It has a specific activity of about 5 $\times$ 10^7 U/mg of protein. Leukine is available commercially as lyophilized powder in 250- and 500-μg amounts. It is reconstituted with 1.0 mL of Sterile Water for Injection, USP, to yield a clear isotonic solution at pH 7.4. Further dilutions in 0.9% sodium chloride should include 0.1% (v/v) of human serum albumin to reduce adsorption to the glass surface. Vials should be discarded within 6 hours of reconstitution because there is no antibacterial preservative. Prokine also is supplied in 250- and 300-μg vials and is reconstituted like Leukine. Leucomax is available for investigational use from the Schering Corporation. Most doses of sargramostim are administered by infusion, although it is active by the subcutaneous route.

Sargramostim is used to promote bone marrow recovery in patients undergoing autologous bone marrow transplantation.[339] It also reduces the severity and duration of neutropenia following standard chemotherapy with myelosuppressive agents. The mode of action of sargramostim is an interaction with high-affinity cell receptors on neutrophils. Signal transduction may involve coupling to a G protein.[358] After treatment with sargramostim, there is a biphasic increase in circulating leukocytes, including an initial increase that peaks after 4 to 5 days and a second increase over the next 5 days.[359] The dose-limiting toxicities are pericarditis, fluid retention, and venous thromboses. Other side effects include a flu-like syndrome and bone pain. The latter is managed with nonsteroidal anti-inflammatory agents.

Filgrastim. Filgrastim, Neupogen, granulocyte-CSF (G-CSF). This compound is manufactured by recombinant DNA methods using *E. coli* as the host organism. It contains 175 amino acids identical with those in the natural protein except for an N-terminal methionine necessary for expression in *E. coli.* Neupogen is supplied in single-use vials, each containing 300 μg/mL of filgrastim at a specific activity of 1.0 $\pm$ 0.6 $\times$ 10^8 U/mg. It is formulated in 10 mM sodium acetate buffer at pH 4.0 containing 50 mg of mannitol, 0.004% Tween 80, and 1.0 mL of Water for Injection. This formulation is stable for 24 months at 36 to 46°F. The recommended dosage is 5 μg/kg per day, administered subcutaneously or intravenously.

Filgrastim is indicated to decrease the incidence of infection in patients with nonmyeloid malignancies receiving myelosuppressive anticancer drugs associated with a significant incidence of severe neutropenia with fever. A complete blood count and platelet count should be obtained prior to chemotherapy and twice weekly during therapy with filgrastim. The only consistently observed adverse reaction to filgrastim is bone pain.

Absorption and clearance of filgrastim follow first-order kinetics, with a positive linear correlation between the parenteral dose and both the serum concentration and area under the concentration-time curves. The elimination half-life is about 3.5 hours.

Porfimer Sodium. Porfimer sodium, Photofrin II, is a light-sensitive polyporphyrin oligomer linked by ether and ester groups. It is a purified product from hematoporphyrin derivatives, and it exists as aggregates with combined molecular masses of approximately 10,000.[340] The drug is supplied as 75 mg of a freeze-dried cake or powder for injection in vials. Each vial is reconstituted with 31.8 mL of either 5% dextrose or 0.9% Sodium Chloride for Injection. The usual dose is 2 mg/kg by slow injection over 3 to 5 minutes. Illumination by laser light is provided 40 to 50 hours later.

Photodynamic therapy using porfimer sodium is indicated for palliation of symptoms in patients with completely or partially obstructing esophageal cancer or microinvasive small cell lung cancer. Adverse reactions include ocular sensitivity, chest pain, and respiratory distress.

HORMONES

Steroid hormones, including estrogens, androgens, progestins, and glucocorticoids, act on the appropriate target tissues at the level of transcription. Generally, the effect is derepression of genetic template operation, which stimulates the cellular process. Glucocorticoids, however, act in lymphatic tissues to impair glucose uptake and protein synthesis. Target cells contain in their cytoplasm specific protein receptors with very high affinities for the hormones. Binding of the hormone to the receptor transforms the receptor structure, followed by migration of the resulting complex into the nucleus. In the nucleus, the complex interacts with an acceptor site to influence transcription.[360]

Normal and well-differentiated neoplastic target cells have a number of hormone receptors, and they depend on the hormones for stimulation.[361–364] Less differentiated neoplastic cells become independent of hormonal control and lose their specific receptors. Thus, some neoplasms are hormone dependent and responsive to hormone-based therapy, whereas others are independent and unresponsive. Assays of the number of hormone receptors present in the neoplastic cells should be valuable in predicting the probability of a favorable response.

Hormonal effects in breast cancer are complex and not completely understood. The hormone dependency of breast cancer has been known since 1889,[365] and removal of the ovaries of premenopausal women, which decreases estrogen levels, is an established treatment. Some patients who do not respond to this procedure do respond to adrenalectomy, which suggests that the hormone dependence is not simply related to estrogens.[366] Remission after adrenalectomy occurs more often in patients with estrogen receptors than in those lacking receptors. Administration of estrogens to postmenopausal women with metastatic breast cancer resulted in objective remissions in about 30% of cases.[367] This response appears paradoxical, but the estrogen levels resulting from drug treatment are much greater than physiological levels. It has been suggested that high estrogen levels interfere with the peripheral action of prolactin, a pituitary hormone that also stimulates breast tissue.[368] Ethinyl estradiol is given orally in the treatment of breast cancer in postmenopausal women, and estradiol dipropionate or benzoate is used parenterally. Tamoxifen is an antiestrogen that has been used successfully in the treatment of postmenopausal women. It has very low toxicity.[369] Toremifene, an analogue of tamoxifen differing only in the presence of a chlorine substituent on the ethyl group, has been introduced recently. It is similar to tamoxifen in pharmacological properties.

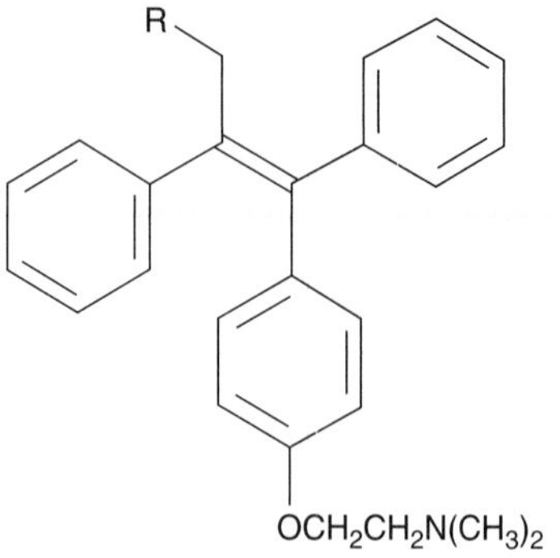

Tamoxifen: R = H

Toremifene: = Cl

Androgens are active against metastatic breast cancer in about 20% of postmenopausal women. Their mode of action is not completely understood. Inhibition of the release of pituitary gonadotrophins has been suggested, but the situation must be more complicated than this because certain androgens are active in hypophysectomized patients.[370] Other useful effects of androgens in advanced breast cancer are stimulation of the hematopoietic system and reversal of bone demineralization. Testosterone propionate is the androgen most frequently used against breast cancer. Other compounds are 2α-methyltestosterone, fluoxymesterone, and 19-nor-17α-methyltestosterone. Testolactone is preferred in some cases because it has no androgenic side effects.

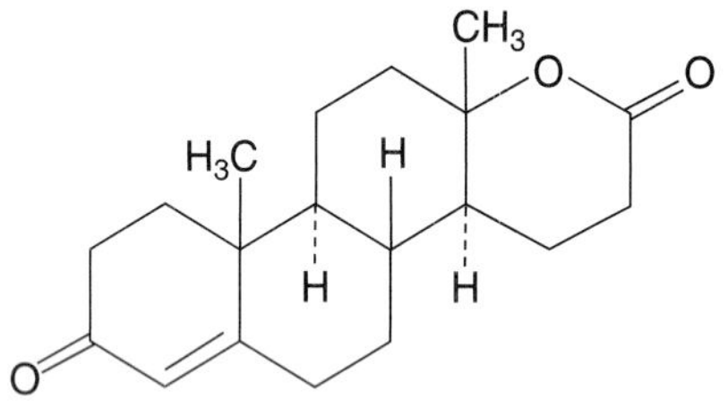

Testolactone

Estrogens can be used to induce remissions of disseminated prostatic cancer. It is not certain whether their effect is due to direct interference with peripheral androgens, inhibition of pituitary gonadotrophin, or both.[371] Diethylstilbestrol is the compound most widely used for advanced prostatic cancer, and it benefits more than 60% of patients. Chlorotrianisene also is used. Estramustine phosphate was designed to carry the nitrogen mustard group selectively into cells with estrogen receptors; however, it does not alkylate them.[372] It appears to act as an antiandrogen, and it promotes microtubule disassembly. The main therapeutic use is in prostate carcinoma.[373]

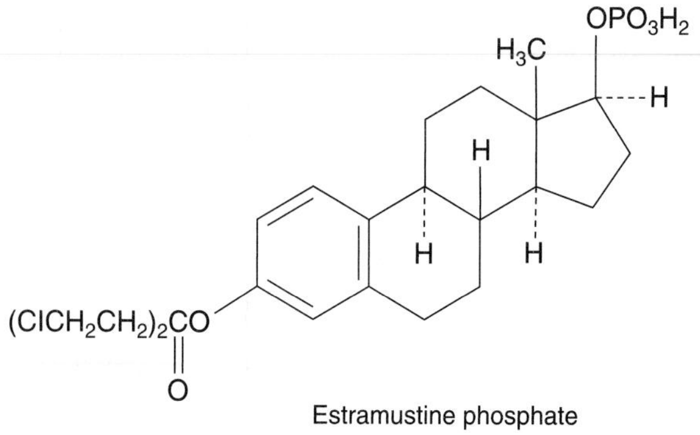

Estramustine phosphate

Three amide derivatives of trifluoromethylaniline have been approved for use in combination therapy of prostate cancer. They are flutamide, nilutamide, and bicalutamide. All of them have an electron-withdrawing group such as nitro or cyano at the 4 position. Substituents on the aniline nitrogen vary from isobutyl in flutamide, to dimethylhydantoin in nilutamide, to a complex functionality containing fluorophenylsulfonyl in bicalutamide. These compounds bind to cytosolic androgen receptors and block the effects of testosterone and other androgens.[374] Their good oral absorption makes them desirable therapeutic agents. Bicalutamide is claimed to be selective for peripheral androgen receptors.[375]

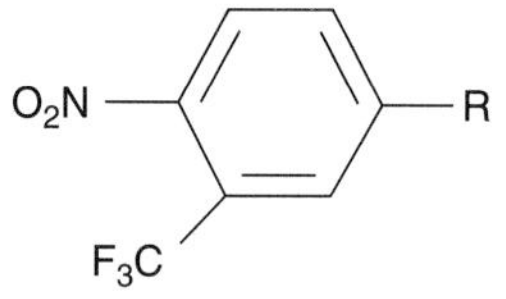

Flutamide: R = NHCOCH(CH₃)₂

Nilutamide: R =

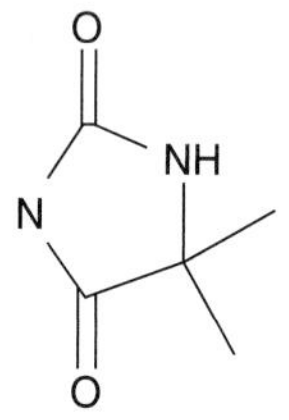

Bicalutamide: R = NHCOCCH₂SO₂—

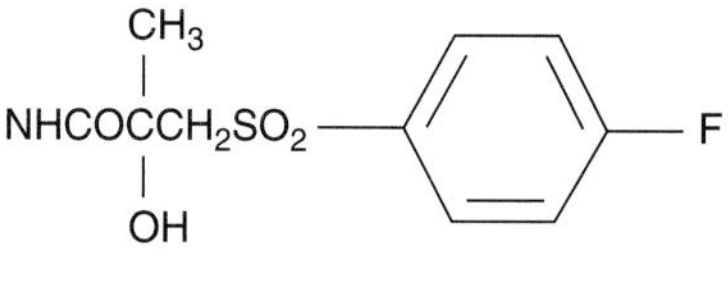

Progesterone and its analogues are active against certain neoplasms that are stimulated by estrogens. They appear to exert antiestrogenic effects of uncertain mechanism. The neoplasms treated by progestins are metastatic endometrial carcinoma and advanced renal cell carcinoma.[376] Progesterone suspensions in oil, megestrol acetate, and medroxyprogesterone acetate are used against endometrial cancer. They provide regressions of several months to 3 years in about 30% of women.[376] Medroxyprogesterone acetate causes regression of renal cell carcinoma in less than 10% of men and women.

Glucocorticoids cause pronounced acute changes in lymphoid tissues. Lymphocytes in the thymus and lymph nodes are dissolved, and lymphopenia occurs in peripheral blood.[377] In lymphocytic tissues, glucocorticoids promote apoptosis by a receptor-mediated active process that induces endonucleolytic cleavage of DNA. This property is used to advantage in the treatment of leukemia and Hodgkin's disease, in which profound temporary regressions are observed following the administration of cortisone derivatives or ACTH.[378] Prednisone is the corticoid usually chosen for this purpose, and it is almost always used in combination with other chemotherapeutic agents, such as mechlorethamine, vincristine, and procarbazine. Such combinations are effective in maintaining the remissions in many cases. Glucocorticoids also are useful in treating metastatic prostate cancer of patients who have relapsed after castration. The rationale for this use is that they inhibit release of ACTH from the pituitary, which leads to adrenal atrophy and decreased adrenal production of androgens.[379] Prednisone and cortisone acetate are used in the treatment of metastatic breast cancer. Their value in this condition derives not from an antineoplastic effect but in alleviating specific complications, such as hypercalcemia and anemia.[380]

Mitotane is unique among antitumor agents in its highly selective effect on one gland, the adrenal cortex. It has a direct cytotoxic action on adrenal cortical cells, in which it damages the mitochondria extensively.[381] This effect leads to cell death and atrophy of the gland. Mitotane is used specifically against adrenocortical carcinoma.[382]

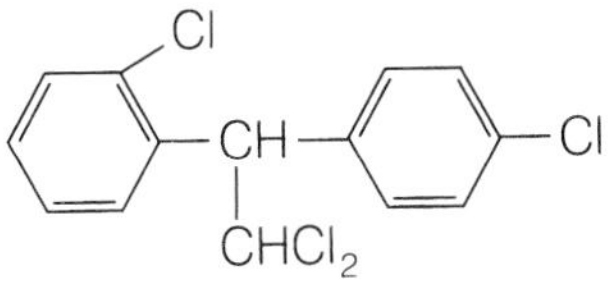

Mitotane

Another way to limit the proliferation of hormone-dependent tumors is to inhibit the release of gonadotropins from the anterior pituitary gland. This release is controlled by gonadotropin-releasing hormone (LH-RH), a nonapeptide, and it can be blocked effectively by continuous administration of certain analogues of this hormone. LH-RH has the amino acid sequence 5-oxoPro-His-Trp-Ser-Tyr-Lys-Leu-Arg-Pro-GluNH$_2$. Synthetic analogues with a D-amino acid at position 6 exhibit reduced degradation and increased duration. They produce a transient surge in LH and follicle-stimulating hormone (FSH), followed by a sustained decrease, which results in markedly reduced testosterone and estrogen secretion.

Leuprolide is a nonapeptide that is identical in structure with LH-RH, except that D-leucine replaces the natural glycine as the sixth amino acid, and the terminal glycine residue is replaced by an ethyl substituent. It is used for palliation of prostatic cancer. Triptoralen differs from LH-RH in that the 6-glycine residue is replaced by D-tryptophan.[383] It is formulated as the pamoate salt, which provides a depot form of 1-month duration when given orally. Goserelin acetate has a D-serine residue substituted with a *t*-butyl group replacing the 6-glycine residue, and a semicarbazide group instead of glycine.[384] It is used for palliation of prostatic carcinoma, and for endometriosis, advanced breast cancer, and endometrial thinning.

An interesting new approach to treating hormone-dependent breast cancer is to selectively decrease the biosynthesis of estrogens. This effect is produced by inhibiting the enzyme aromatase, which controls the conversion of testosterone and androstenedione into estradiol (see Chapter 23). A variety of chemical structures inhibit this enzyme. The triazole derivative anastrozole was the first aromatase inhibitor released in the United States.[385] More recently, the 6-methylene derivative of androstenedione, exemestane, has been approved. Exemestane is an irreversible inhibitor of aromatase. It acts as a false substrate and is processed as an intermediate that binds to the active site of this enzyme.[386] Both anastrazole and exemestane are used in patients in whom tamoxifen is no longer effective. Very recently, the triazole letrozole was claimed to be the first and only aromatase inhibitor to show superiority over tamoxifen in clinical trials.[387]

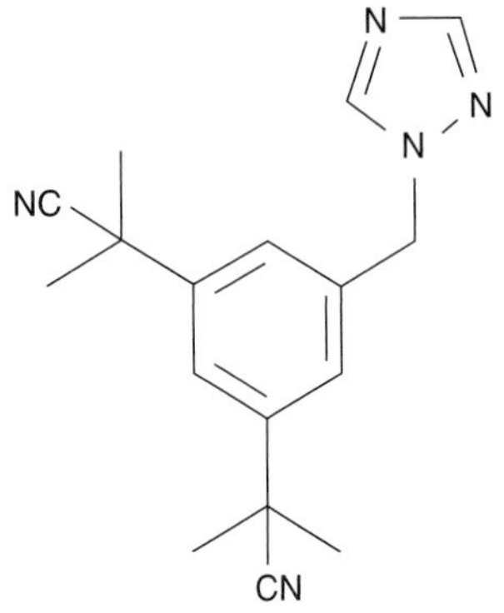

Anastrozole

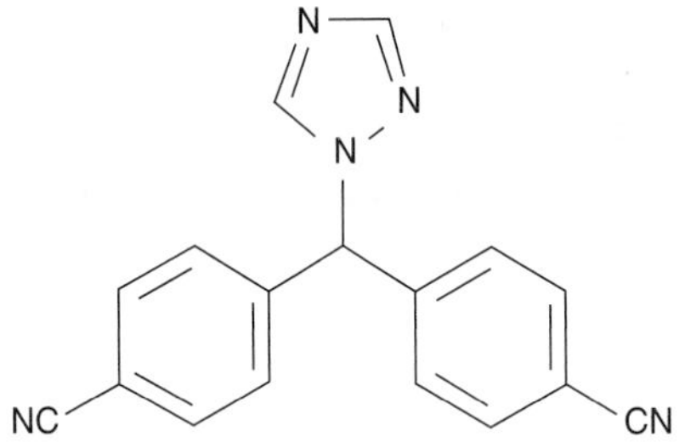

Letrozole

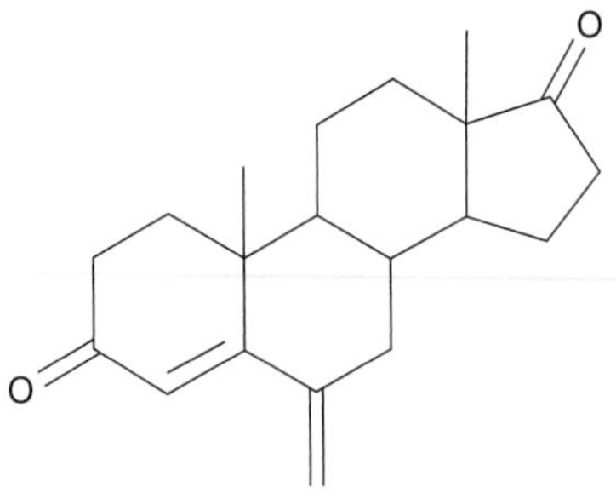

Exemestane

A thorough discussion of the structures, nomenclature, properties, and dose forms of the steroid hormones is presented in Chapter. 23. Only the products not included in detail in that chapter are described below.

Products

Mitotane, USP. Mitotane, Lysodren, *o,p*'-DDD, CB-313, 1,1-dichloro-2-(*o*-chlorophenyl)-2-(*p*-chlorophenyl) ethane, is obtained as a constituent of commercial DDD, which is prepared from 2,2-dichloro-1-(*o*-chlorophenyl) ethanol, chlorobenzene, and sulfuric acid.[388] Isolation from commercial DDD gives mitotane crystals that are soluble in alcohol and other organic solvents.[389] Scored 500-mg tablets are supplied.

About 40% of a single oral dose of mitotane is absorbed. Only 10 to 25% is excreted in urine as an unidentified metabolite, and 60% is excreted unchanged in feces. Most of the remainder is stored in fatty tissues of the body.

Mitotane is indicated only for treating inoperable adrenal cortical carcinoma. Frequently occurring side effects include gastrointestinal disturbances, CNS depression, and skin toxicity.

The usual regimen is 8 to 10 g daily, divided into three or four doses.

Dromostanolone Propionate, USP. The semisynthetic androgen dromostanolone propionate, Drolban, 17*β*-hydroxy-2*α*-methyl-5*α*-androstan-3-one propionate, 2*α*-methyldihydrotestosterone propionate, is prepared from dihydrotestosterone in a route involving condensation with ethyl formate followed by hydrogenation to give the 2*α*-methyl derivative and then reaction with propionic anhydride.[390] The compound is supplied in rubber-stoppered vials containing 500 mg of dromostanolone propionate in 10 mL of sesame oil, with 0.5% phenol as a preservative.

Dromostanolone propionate is used in the palliative treatment of metastatic breast carcinoma in postmenopausal women. It is contraindicated in premenopausal women and in carcinoma of the male breast. The most common side effect is virilism, although this is less intense than that afforded by testosterone propionate. Edema occurs occasionally.

Testolactone, USP. Testolactone, Teslac, D-homo-17*α*-oxa-androsta-1,4-dien-3,17-dione, 1-dehydrotestolactone, is prepared by microbial transformation of progesterone.[391] It is soluble in alcohol and slightly soluble in water. The compound is supplied as a sterile aqueous suspension providing 100 mg/mL of testolactone in multiple-dose vials of 5 mL. Tablets containing 50 mg or 250 mg of testolactone also are supplied.

Testolactone is used in the palliative treatment of advanced or disseminated breast cancer in postmenopausal women. It is contraindicated in breast cancer in men. Testolactone is devoid of androgenic activity in the commonly used doses.

Megestrol Acetate. Megestrol acetate, Megace, 17*α*-acetoxy-6-methyl-pregna-4,6-dien-3,20-dione, is prepared by a multistep synthesis from 17*α*-hydroxy pregnadienolone.[392] It is supplied as light blue scored tablets containing 20 or 40 mg of megestrol acetate.

Megestrol acetate is indicated for the palliative treatment of advanced breast or endometrial carcinoma when other methods of treatment are inappropriate. No serious side effects or adverse reactions have been reported. There is, however, an increased risk of birth defects in children whose mothers take the drug during the first 4 months of pregnancy. In high doses, it can cause weight gain without inducing fluid accumulation. The usual doses are 160 mg/day in four equal doses for breast cancer and 40 to 320 mg/day in divided doses for endometrial cancer.

Tamoxifen Citrate. Tamoxifen Citrate, Nolvadex, (*Z*)-2-[4-(l,2-diphenyl-1-butenyl)phenoxy]-*N,N*-dimethylethanamine citrate, is prepared by treating 2-ethyldeoxybenzoin with 4-[(2-*N,N*-dimethylamino)ethoxy]phenylmagnesium bromide,[393] followed by dehydration and separation of the *E* and *Z* isomers.[394] The citrate salt of the *Z* isomer is soluble in water. Tablets containing 15.2 mg of tamoxifen citrate, which is equivalent to 10 mg of tamoxifen, are supplied. They should be protected from heat and light.

Most of a dose of tamoxifen is excreted in bile as conjugates of metabolites. *N*-Demethyltamoxifen is the primary metabolite, and its long-term levels exceed those of tamoxifen. It is thought to account for a large portion of the antitumor activity.[395]

Tamoxifen is a nonsteroidal agent that has shown potent antiestrogenic properties in animals. In the rat model, it appears to exert its antitumor effects by binding to estrogen receptors.[396] This binding causes a conformational change that decreases DNA transcription. It is cell cycle specific for the mid-G_2 phase. Tamoxifen is useful in the palliative treatment of advanced breast cancer in postmenopausal women. There are no known contraindications. The most frequent side effects are hot flashes, nausea, and vomiting. They are rarely severe enough to require dose reduction. The usual dose is one or two 10-mg tablets twice daily.

Toremifene Citrate. Toremifene citrate, Fareston, (*E*)-1,2-diphenyl-1-[4-(2-dimethylaminoethoxy)phenyl]-4-chlorobutene, is prepared by fractional crystallization of the hydrochloride salts of the mixture of geometrical isomers. It is supplied as 60-mg tablets also containing lactose. The usual dose is 60 mg once daily until disease progression renews. The drug is well absorbed orally and 99.5% bound to serum proteins. Plasma concentrations peak within 3 hours and then follow linear pharmacokinetics, with a clearance rate of 5 L/hour. The volume of distribution is 580 L. The drug is extensively metabolized by N-demethylation.[397]

Toremifene citrate is indicated for metastatic breast cancer in postmenopausal women with estrogen-receptor-positive or estrogen-receptor-unknown tumors. Complete blood counts, calcium levels, and liver function tests should be done before its administration. Side effects include hypercalcemia, hot flashes, sweating, nausea, and vaginal discharge.

Flutamide. Flutamide, Sch-13521, Drogenil, Eulexin, Euflex, Flucinom, Flugerel, Sebatrol, 2-methyl-*N*-[4-nitro-

3-(trifluoro-methyl)phenyl]propanamide, is prepared from 3-trifluoromethyl-4-nitroaniline and isobutyryl chloride.[398] It is supplied as 125-mg capsules that are stable for 5 years when stored at or below 30°C. Administration is oral.

Flutamide is extensively and rapidly metabolized. One hour after dosing, only 2.5% of the drug in plasma is unchanged. The major metabolite in plasma is α-hydroxyflutamide; however, the major metabolite found in urine is 2-amino-5-nitro-4-(trifluoromethyl)phenol, which results from cleavage of the side chain.

Flutamide acts as an androgen receptor antagonist, inhibiting the uptake and binding of testosterone and dihydrotestosterone.[399] It is approved for treatment of advanced prostate cancer when combined with an inhibitor of gonadotropin-releasing hormone, such as leuprolide. The most common side effects are gynecomastia and nipple pain.

Nilutamide.
Nilutamide, Nilandron, 5,5-dimethyl-3-[4-nitro-3-(trifluoromethyl)phenyl]-2,4-imidazolidinedione, is supplied as 50-mg tablets that also contain lactose. The usual daily dose is 300 mg for 30 days, followed by 150 mg daily. Absorption is rapid and complete following oral dosage, and there is moderate binding to plasma proteins. Metabolic oxidation of one of the methyl groups produces D and L isomers, which are equally potent.

Nilutamide is used in combination with surgical castration for metastatic prostate cancer. It blocks testosterone at androgen receptors.[374] Gastrointestinal and endocrine side effects occur, and there are low incidences of interstitial pneumonitis and hepatitis. Chest x-rays should be performed before therapy is initiated. Inhibition of liver cytochrome P-450 isoenzymes may reduce the metabolism of other drugs.

Bicalutamide.
Bicalutamide, Casodex, N-[4-cyano-3-(trifluoromethyl)phenyl]-3-[(4-fluorophenyl)sulfonyl]-2-hydroxy-2-methylpropionamide, is prepared by acylating 3-cyano-4-trifluoromethylaniline with the appropriate acid chloride.[400] It is formulated in 50-mg tablets that also contain lactose. The usual dose is one 50-mg tablet once daily. The drug is well absorbed orally, and the oral clearance is 0.32 L/hour. The peak concentration is 0.77 μg/mL, and the half-life is 5.8 days.

Bicalutamide is formulated as a racemate. The inactive (S) enantiomer is metabolized by glucuronidation; the active (R) enantiomer is oxidized to an inactive metabolite, followed by glucuronidation.

Bicalutamide is approved for combination therapy with an LH-RH analogue for treatment of advanced prostate cancer. Its response is measured by decreased prostate-specific antigen levels. Adverse reactions include gynecomastia, breast pain, and inhibition of spermatogenesis. There is an interaction with coumadin.[401]

Estramustine Phosphate.
Estramustine phosphate, Estrocyte, Emcyt, NSC-89199, estra-1,3,5(10)-triene-3,17 β-diol-3-[bis(2-chloroethyl)carbamate]17-disodium phosphate, is prepared by treating estradiol with sodium hydroxide followed by nitrogen mustard chloroformate.[402] The water-soluble disodium phosphate derivative is made by

using phosphorus oxychloride followed by sodium hydroxide. It is available commercially in 140-mg capsules that are orally active. One to 10 capsules are used daily, and they may be taken with meals to lessen gastrointestinal upset. About 75% of the oral dose is absorbed.[403] The biological half-life is long, and the drug undergoes dephosphorylation to estramustine followed by glucuronide conjugation and elimination in bile and urine. There also is some metabolism of the alkylating functionality.

Estramustine was designed to have an estrogenic molecule carry the alkylating nitrogen mustard functionality selectively into cells with estradiol hormone receptors; however, it may not act as an alkylating agent.[372] It is active in prostate cancer because of its estrogenic (antiandrogenic) effects. Another possible mode of action is binding to microtubule-associated proteins to promote microtubule disassembly.[373] The dose-limiting toxicity is gastrointestinal upset. Gynecomastia also occurs.

Leuprolide Acetate.
Leuprolide acetate, Lupron, is a synthetic nonapeptide analogue of naturally occurring gonadotropin-releasing hormone (LH-RH). It is supplied in 2.8-mL multiple dose vials containing 5 mg/mL of the drug and benzyl alcohol These vials should be refrigerated until dispensed.

Leuprolide is used for palliative treatment of advanced prostatic cancer. There are no known contraindications. Symptoms may worsen during the first few weeks of treatment, with increased bone pain as the usual manifestation. Hot flashes and irritation at the injection site also occur.

Triptoralen Pamoate.
Triptoralen pamoate, Trelstar depot, is a synthetic nonapeptide analogue of LH-RH.[383] It is supplied as microgranules for injection, lyophilized and combined with mannitol in single-dose vials. The amount is equivalent to 3.75 mg of triptoralen free base. Reconstitution is by injection of 2 mL of Sterile Water for Injection into the vial.

Triptoralen pamoate is given by intramuscular injection once monthly. It is indicated for palliation of advanced prostate cancer in patients for whom estrogen and orchiectomy are not indicated.[404] The main adverse effect is hot flashes. Hypersensitivity and anaphylactic reactions have been observed.

Goserelin Acetate.
The synthetic nonapeptide goserelin acetate, Zoladex, is an analogue of LH-RH. It is supplied in preloaded syringes containing 3.6 mg of agent for monthly IM administration or 10.8 mg of agent for 3-monthly administration. The main indication is palliation of advanced prostate carcinoma, and other uses include advanced breast cancer and endometriosis. Adverse reactions include hot flashes and vaginal bleeding, although the drug is generally well tolerated.[405] Pharmacokinetics are determined by release from the depot site. The volume of distribution is 44.1 L in men and 20.3 L in women.

Anastrozole.
The aromatase inhibitor anastrozole, Arimidex, 2,2′-[5-(1H-1,2,4-triazol-1-ylmethyl)-1,3-phenyl-

ene]di(2-methylpropionitrile), is prepared by treating the appropriate 5-bromo compound with sodium triazole.[406] It is supplied as 1-mg tablets that also contain lactose. The usual dose is 1 mg twice daily, continued until tumor progression is apparent. This compound is well absorbed orally and eliminated after hepatic metabolism, which inactivates it. The mean terminal elimination half-life is approximately 50 hours.

Anastrozole is indicated for first-line treatment of locally advanced or metastatic breast carcinoma in postmenopausal women with estrogen-positive or unknown-receptor types.[407] Side effects include vasodilatation, gastrointestinal disturbances, and hot flashes.

Letrozole. The aromatase inhibitor letrozole, Femura, 4-[α-(4-cyanophenyl)-1-(1,2,4-triazolyl)methyl]benzonitrile, is prepared by treating 4-[1-(1,2,4-triazolyl)methyl]-benzonitrile with KOt-Bu and 4-fluorobenzonitrile.[408] It is supplied in 2.5-mg tablets that also contain lactose. The usual dose is 2.5 mg once daily. Oral absorption is rapid and complete, and steady-state plasma concentrations are achieved in 2 to 6 weeks. Pharmacokinetics are nonlinear, and the mean terminal elimination half-life is approximately 2 days. Metabolism produces an inactive compound in which the triazolyl group is replaced by hydroxyl.

Letrozole is indicated for locally advanced or metastatic breast carcinoma in women with positive or unknown estrogen receptors.[387] Adverse reactions include nausea and muscle pain.

Exemestane. Exemestane, Aromasin, is an irreversible aromatase inhibitor related structurally to androstenedione.[409] It is supplied in 25-mg tablets that also contain mannitol, methylparaben, and polyvinyl alcohol. The usual dose is 25 mg once daily after a meal. The drug is rapidly absorbed, bound 90% to plasma proteins, and its blood levels decline exponentially with a mean terminal half-life of about 24 hours. Extensive metabolism includes oxidations of the 6-methylene group and reduction of the 17-keto group.

Exemestane is effective and selective for treating some postmenopausal women with hormone-dependent breast cancer, whose disease has progressed following tamoxifen treatment.[386] Adverse reactions include a low incidence of nausea and fatigue.

SIGNAL TRANSDUCTION INHIBITORS

Cell cycle progression can be viewed as a sequence of events regulated by a cascade of protein kinases. These kinases are controlled by four known mechanisms: protein–protein interactions (cyclin-dependent kinases), phosphorylation, intracellular sequestration, and proteolytic degradation of kinases or their regulatory components. The protein tyrosine kinases phosphorylate specific tyrosine residues of a variety of functional proteins. They provide a common mechanism for transmitting mitogenic signals and regulating numerous cellular processes.

The role of protein tyrosine kinases in tumorigenesis is evident in their ability to transform normal cells into neoplastic phenotypes when expressed in mutated, unregulated forms or when produced in abnormally high levels. Half of the known protooncogenes encode for proteins with protein tyrosine kinase activity.[410] For example, a hybrid gene formed from the *abl* protooncogene from chromosome 9 with the *bcr* gene on chromosome 22 encodes a fusion protein with tyrosine kinase activity. This protein maintains the leukemic phenotype in human chronic myelogenous leukemia.[411] In another example, the *erb*-2 protooncogene encodes a 185-kDa protein that is very similar to the epidermal growth factor receptor (EGFR) and has an extracellular, transmembrane, and cytoplasmic domain. A single point mutation in this gene causes overexpression of the 185-kDa protein, which becomes a factor in a variety of solid tumors.[411]

Development of nontoxic inhibitors of protein tyrosine kinases in tumor cells is a problem because this type of enzyme is present in normal cells. There also are serine protein kinases and other nucleotide-dependent enzymes. Nevertheless, a naturally occurring isoflavone, genestein, inhibits the protein tyrosine kinase of EGFR without significantly affecting serine and threonine kinases. A synthetic compound of the tyrphostin class inhibits the EGFR over insulin receptor tyrosine kinase. Second-generation tyrphostins that lack hydroxyl groups are metabolically stable and active against human tumors in immunodeficient mice.[412]

The microbial product staurosporine is a nonselective protein tyrosine kinase inhibitor of EGFR kinase. A simpler dianilinophthalimide, analogue I, is a potent and selective inhibitor of EGFR kinase.[413]

Genestein

First-generation Tyrphostin

Second-generation Tyrphostin

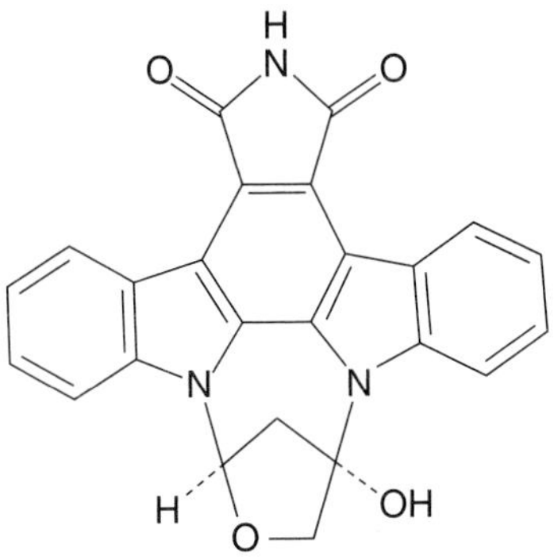

aromatic heterocycle group occupies the adenine pocket of the ATP-binding site.

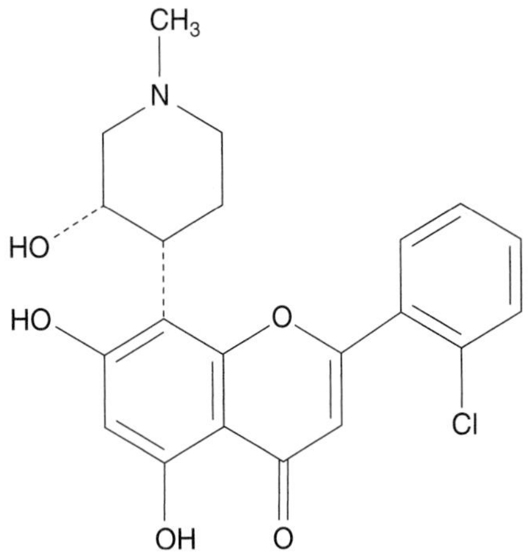

Staurosporine

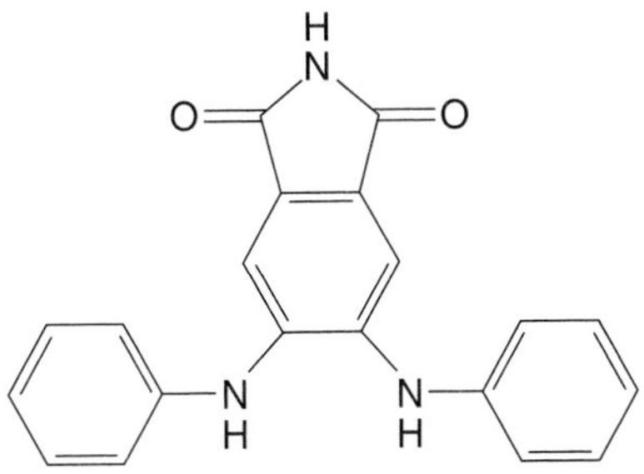

Staurosporine Analogue

Flavopiridol

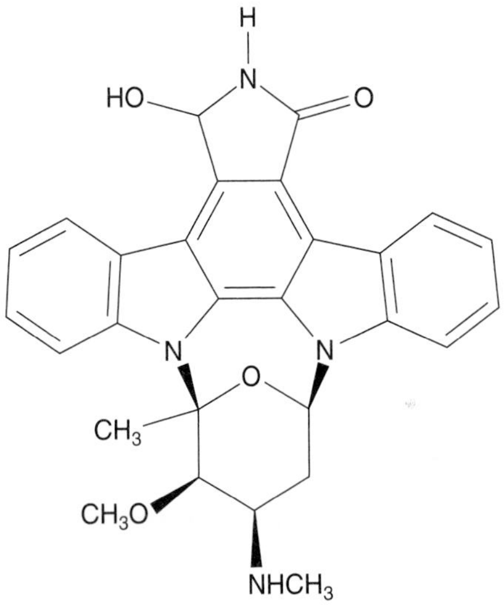

Hydroxystaurospermine (UCN-01)

Considerable progress in obtaining selectivity in receptor tyrosine kinase inhibitors has been made recently at Novartis. Compounds in their series of 2-phenylaminopyrimidines show remarkable selectivity (1,000-fold) against platelet-derived growth factor (PDGF) tyrosine kinase, compared with the EGFRs and other protein kinases.[414] Their newly approved antitumor agent imatinib (Gleevec) inhibits PDGF tyrosine kinase, and it is also highly potent against abl kinase. It produces this effect by binding in the pocket of the enzyme that normally holds the adenosine triphosphate used in phosphorylation. Gleevec also potentiates the activity of retinoic acid. The combined effects make it a useful agent for treatment of chronic myelocytic leukemia.

Two small inhibitors of cyclin-dependent kinases, flavoperidol and UCN-01 (hydroxystaurosporine), are in clinical trials. Flavoperidol is a competitive inhibitor of ATP. Its

Ras protein is central among the many oncogene- or protooncogene-encoded proteins that serve as signal transducers in the pathway from the outer membrane to the nucleus of cells. It acts as a common relay point for signals from various

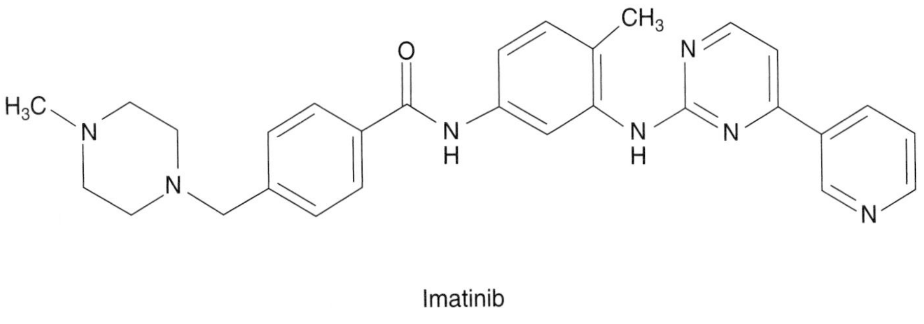

Imatinib

growth factors. Single-base mutations in the gene encoding the 21-kDa ras protein are found in tumors, especially colon and pancreatic carcinomas.[415]

Ras protein is localized at the inner surface of the plasma membrane. It strongly binds guanine nucleotides and hydrolyzes GTP to GDP. The process of cycling between the active GTP-bound form and the inactive GDP-bound form serves as a switch for normal cellular growth and differentiation. Oncogenic ras proteins do not hydrolyze GTP and are, therefore, permanently in the active state.[416] Protein tyrosine kinases at the EGFR initiate a sequence of events that promote GDP release from ras, allowing it to bind ATP and assume an active conformation. Posttranslational modifications of ras, especially the addition of a farnesyl substituent, provide the lipophilicity required for its membrane binding. Farnesylation of ras is a complex process involving initial reaction between farnesyl pyrophosphate and a cysteine residue of ras to form a thioether linkage. The cysteine is located three residues from the end of the COOH terminal residue. These three amino acid residues are cleaved from ras, and the resulting terminal carboxylic acid group on the cysteine is methylated to the corresponding ester.[417]

Current research is focused on inhibiting farnesyl transferase. Certain tetrapeptides, such as CVFM-NH$_2$, show potent inhibition of this enzyme. Further modification of the tetrapeptide structure into a benzodiazepine derivative restored a normal growth pattern in ras-transformed cells.[418] Another research objective is inhibition of methyltransferases that catalyze the esterification of cysteine residues on farnesylated ras. The most potent inhibitor at this time is a farnesylthiosalicyclic acid derivative.[416]

Benzodiazepine Derivative

Farnesylthiosalicyclic Acid

Products

Imatinib. Imatinib, Gleevec, STI571, N-{3-[4-(4-methyl-piperazinomethyl)-benzoylamido]-2-methylphenyl}-4-

(3-pyridyl)-2-pyrimidine-amine, is prepared by a multistep synthesis.[419] It is supplied as the free base in 100-mg capsules. Samples should be stored at 25°C. The usual dosages are 400 mg/day for patients in the chronic phase of the disease and 600 mg/day for patients experiencing a blast crisis. Dosage should be adjusted if severe hepatotoxicity, fluid retention, neutropenia, or thrombocytopenia occur.

Imatinib is indicated for chronic myelocytic leukemia. It acts by inhibiting the tyrosine kinase BRC-ABL, thus preventing it from arresting apoptosis. This agent is well absorbed orally, and the maximum concentration in blood is achieved within 2 to 4 hours. It is 95% bound to serum proteins. The major metabolite results from N-demethylation. Elimination half-times are 18 hours for imatinib and 40 hours for the N-demethyl metabolite. Excretion is mainly in feces.

Adverse reactions include gastrointestinal irritation, fluid retention, neutropenia, thrombocytopenia, musculoskeletal pain, headache, and teratogenicity and fertility impairment in mice.

IMMUNOTHERAPY

Cells of neoplastic potential are continually produced in the human body, and our immune surveillance system destroys them. The development of tumors implies that this system is not functioning properly. Evidence for this factor in carcinogenesis includes *(a)* a high rate of cancer in organ-transplant patients whose immune systems are suppressed by drugs such as azathioprine and *(b)* a high correlation between cancer and immunodeficiency diseases, such as bacterial and viral infections.[420] Stimulation of the body's immune system should provide a valuable method of cancer treatment, because it can eradicate the neoplastic cells completely. Research in this area is expanding rapidly, and some promising leads are emerging.

The first attempt at immunotherapy was made in the 1890s by Coley, who injected bacterial toxins into cancer patients. His results were generally unaccepted because of rather extravagant claims. His techniques have been revived in recent years. Most oncologists now use a live-bacteria tuberculosis vaccine, bacillus Calmette-Guérin (BCG).[421] This vaccine is given to certain patients who show a functioning immune system as determined by sensitivity to dinitrochlorobenzene.[421] Remissions have been obtained in malignant melanoma, breast cancer, and leukemia. Unfortunately, BCG causes a number of undesirable effects, including fever, hypersensitivity, and liver disorders. Other immunostimulants currently under investigation as anticancer agents are the methanol-extracted residue (MER) of BCG, *Corynebacterium parvulum, Bordetella pertussis* vaccine, and synthetic polynucleotides.[422] The activity of these bacterial products is thought to be mediated by a protein known as tumor necrosis factor (TNF). TNF produces hemorrhagic necrosis of sensitive transplanted tumor cells, and it is synergistic with interferons.[423] Unfortunately, TNF does not show activity against primary tumors when used alone. Clinical trials based on expected synergism with interferons are in progress. Potentiation of TNF by agents such as mitomycin C and vinblastine suggest that it might have a role in combination chemotherapy.

One approach to overcoming the difficulties of BCG therapy is to develop simpler chemical structures with immunostimulant properties. One such compound, levamisole, an anthelmintic agent found to be an immunostimulant by Renoux in 1972, is presently under clinical investigation as a potential anticancer drug. It appears to be most effective in patients with small tumor burdens, and it acts by stimulating the responsiveness of lymphocytes to tumor antigens. Advantages of levamisole include oral activity and few adverse reactions. Levamisole may mediate the potentiation of interleukin-2–induced T lymphocyte proliferation.[424] It is used in combination with 5-FU in treating colon cancer.

Levamisole

The induction phase of the immune response of both B and T lymphocytes is regulated by interactions between macrophages and subpopulations of T lymphocytes known as *helper T cells*. This interaction induces the production of soluble glycoproteins, lymphokines, which include interferons, interleukins, and B-cell growth and differentiation factors. Lymphokines in nanomolar to picomolar concentrations cause profound enhancing or suppressing effects on responding precursor cells of the immune system.[425]

Interferons are secreted by cells in response to viral infections or other chemical or biological inducers. Three major classes of interferons—alfa, beta, and gamma—have been identified. They bind to specific high-affinity receptors on cell surfaces, which induces a sequence of intracellular events, including the induction of enzymes. This process produces such effects as release of other cytokines such as interleukin-2 and TNF, enhancement of natural killer cell activity, inhibition of certain oncogenes, and increased specific cytotoxic activity of lymphocytes for target cells.[425] Interferons alfa-2a, alfa-2b, and alfa-n3 promote the immunological response to neoplastic cells, which results in significant cytotoxicity in some instances. They are the drugs of choice for treating hairy cell leukemia.[426] They also are showing responses against renal cell cancer, multiple myeloma, melanoma, and Kaposi's sarcoma in clinical trials.

Another important lymphokine is interleukin-2 (IL-2). This glycoprotein interacts with specific receptors on T-effector cells to activate their cytotoxicity. It also stimulates the activation and proliferation of antigen-nonspecific natural killer cells, which are involved in immune functions associated with tumor surveillance. These effects are thought to be mediated through the induction of interferon gamma. Human IL-2 is now produced by recombinant gene technology, which has permitted extensive clinical trials against a variety of tumors. In some of these trials, IL-2 is given in combination with lymphokine-activated killer cells. Denileuken diftidox is a cytotoxic fusion protein composed of the amino acid sequences for diphtheria toxin fragments A and B followed by the sequences for IL-2. It is produced in an *E. coli* expression system based on recombinant DNA technology. Denileukin is designed to localize the cytotoxic effects of diphtheria toxin to certain leukemias and lymphomas that express the CD25 component of the IL-2 receptor. It is indicated for treating cutaneous T-cell lymphoma in patients whose malignant cells express this receptor.

Products

Interferon Alfa-2a.   Interferon alfa-2a, Roferon-A, rIFN, IFLrA, is a highly purified protein containing 165 amino acids. It is manufactured from a strain of *E. coli* bearing a genetically engineered plasmid containing an interferon alfa-2a gene from human leukocytes.[427] Vials containing 3 million IU with 5 mg of human serum albumin and 3 mg of phenol are supplied. A preparation of 18 million IU also is available. These preparations should be stored at 36 to 48°F.

Interferon alfa-2a is used in patients 18 years old or older for treatment of hairy cell leukemia and chronic myelogenous leukemia. It is contraindicated in persons who develop hypersensitivity. Most patients develop flu-like syndromes consisting of fever, fatigue, myalgias, headache, and chills. Gastrointestinal and CNS symptoms also occur. Caution must be used in administering this drug to patients with renal or hepatic disease, seizure disorders, or cardiac disease. Metabolism occurs by rapid proteolytic degradation during reabsorption in the kidney. The elimination half-life is 3.7 to 8.5 hours.

Interferon Alfa-2b.   Interferon alfa-2b, Interon, IFN-alfa 2, rIFN-α2, α-2-interferon, is a highly purified protein produced by *E. coli* containing a plasmid with an alfa-2b gene. This plasmid is obtained by recombinant DNA technology using human leukocytes.[427] The drug is supplied in vials containing 3, 5, 10, or 25 IU. Sterile water diluent also is supplied. Reconstituted solutions are stable for 1 month at 36 to 48°F.

Hairy cell leukemia is the present indication for interferon alfa-2b. It is also useful in treating malignant melanoma and renal cell carcinoma. Hypersensitivity to this protein has not been observed. Patients develop a flu-like syndrome, CNS effects, and cardiovascular effects, including hypotension, arrhythmia, or tachycardia.

Interferon Alfa-n3.   Interferon alfa-n3 is a glycoprotein produced from cultures of human leucocytes treated with Sendai virus. It is purified initially by chromatography using a mouse monoclonal antibody that binds to multiple species of human interferon. Subsequent purification involves incubation at 4°C and pH 2 to kill viruses and gel filtration chromatography. It then has a specific activity of about 2×108 IU.[427] The drug is supplied in 1-mL vials containing 1 mL of phosphate buffered saline solution, phenol as a preservative, and 1 mg of human serum albumin as a stabilizer. This solution should be kept at 2 to 8°C. Therapeutic indications and side effects of interferon alfa-n3 are similar to those described for interferons alfa-2a and alfa-2b.

Aldesleukin.   IL-2, aldesleukin, Proleukin, Teceleukin, interleukin-2, IL-2, T-cell growth factor, in the human form is produced in mature T lymphocytes. Cleavage of the 20-amino acid signal sequence then results in an active protein containing 133 amino acids. It is glycosylated and has one disulfide bond, which is essential for activity. Recombinant IL-2 is produced by *E. coli* that carries inserted, modified human IL-2 genes. Teceleukin is nonglycosylated but conforms to natural IL-2 in amino acid sequence, except for an additional N-terminal methionine. Proleukin is not glycosylated and differs from the natural protein in lacking the terminal alanine and having serine rather than cysteine for residue 125. IL-2 activity is standardized in IU in an assay based on stimulation of T-cell growth in vitro. Proleukin is available in glass vials containing 1.2 mg of lyophilized powder (22 million IU) plus sodium decyl sulfate. It is reconstituted with 1.2 mL of solution supplied to give 18 million IU/mL. Teceleukin is supplied in vials containing 100 mg of IL-2, 25 mg of human albumin, and 5 mg of mannitol per million IU. It is reconstituted with Sodium Chloride for Injection, USP. All formulations of IL-2 require storage at 4 to 8°C and protection from light.

IL-2 usually is administered intravenously, although the subcutaneous and intramuscular routes are used. The infusion can produce severe hypotension and life-threatening cardiovascular toxicity when given at the maximally tolerated dose. Patients receiving such a dose must be monitored closely, and facilities must be available to treat them for hypotension, tachycardia, pulmonary edema, and (occasionally) delirium. The drug is rapidly cleared from the bloodstream following parenteral administration. The elimination is biphasic for an intravenous bolus injection. The primary route of elimination is renal, with catabolism occurring in the renal tubules.

IL-2 interacts with specific receptors on activated T lymphocytes. The resulting complex is internalized, and signal transduction, possibly involving tyrosine kinase activity, occurs.[428] Effects of IL-2 include stimulation of T cell growth and regulation, proliferation and immunoglobulin production in B lymphocytes, macrophage activity enhancement, and especially generation of lymphokine-activated killer (LAK) cells. The LAK cells generated within tumors, known as *tumor-infiltrating lymphocytes* (TILs), are thought to be the ultimate mediators of IL-2 toxicity. Therapy with IL-2 involves in vitro generation of large quantities of LAK cells, which are then infused with IL-2 to mediate tumor cell lysis.[429] This procedure is known as *adoptive immunotherapy*. Antitumor activity has been observed in metastatic renal cell cancer, chronic 1ymphocytic leukemia, malignant melanoma, malignant lymphoma, and colon cancer. All patients receiving IL-2 experience a flu-like syndrome. The major dose-limiting side effect is pulmonary edema resulting from increased capillary permeability. Other side effects include severe hypotension, which can be fatal, sinus tachycardia, mental state changes, pruritus, nausea and vomiting, and renal toxicity.[430]

Denileukin Diftitox. The cytotoxic protein denileukin diftitox, Ontak, is composed of the amino acid sequences for diphtheria toxin fragments A and B followed by the sequences for IL-2. It is prepared by recombinant DNA technology, and expressed in an *E. coli* system. The dosage form contains 150 μg/mL of drug plus EDTA, supplied as a frozen solution for injection in single-use vials. It is stored frozen. For reconstitution, it is brought to room temperature and diluted to 15 mL with sterile saline in soft plastic IV bags.

The usual dose is 9 or 18 mg/kg per day by IV injection for five consecutive days every 21 days.

Denileukin diftitox is indicated for cutaneous T-cell lymphoma in patients whose malignant cells express IL-2 receptors.[431] After administration, it exhibits two-compartment behavior with a distribution half-life of 2 to 5 minutes and a terminal-phase half-life of 70 to 80 minutes. It is metabolized by proteolytic degradation. Toxic manifestations include hypersensitivity reactions in 69% of patients, which result in hypotension, back pain, dyspnea, rash, chest pain, and tachycardia. Patients also experience vascular leak syndrome, GI toxicity, and infections.

Bacillus Calmette-Guérin (BCG). Two BCG preparations are approved for intravesical treatment of carcinoma in situ of the urinary bladder.[432] Connaught BCG (TheraCys) is a freeze-dried suspension of an attenuated strain of *Mycobacterium bovis* that has been grown on a potato- and glycerin-based medium. It contains 27 mg ($\sim$3.4 $\times$ 10^8 colony-forming units [CFUs]) and 5% monosodium glutamate per vial. The Tice BCG (NSC-116341) is supplied in glass-sealed ampuls that contain 8 $\times$ 10^8 CFU, equivalent to about 50 mg of the drug. The vials should be stored at 2 to 8°C and protected from light. Persons handling BCG preparations should be protected by masks and gloves. After administration, all equipment and material should be considered biohazards.

Intravesical BCG promotes an inflammatory reaction in the urinary bladder that is associated with reduction in carcinoma in situ lesions. The mechanism of action is not known in detail, but a variety of processes that stimulate the immune response have been considered. Toxic effects of BCG include hematuria, dysuria, and bacterial urinary tract infections.

MONOCLONAL ANTIBODIES

The concept of using antibodies for the selective destruction of cancer cells was proposed first by Ehrlich in 1908; however, it could not be realized until Köbler and Milstein demonstrated the practical production of monoclonal antibodies from hybridoma cell lines in 1975.[433] Since then, numerous diagnostic and therapeutic monoclonals have been prepared, although establishing them as clinical agents has been difficult. The first monoclonal antibodies to human cancer cells were developed in mice. They are easy to prepare, but their use in humans results in an immune response leading to human antimouse antibodies (HAMA), which inactivate the monoclonals.[434] Human monoclonals are difficult to prepare and are not internalized into tumor cells. The HAMA problem has been partly solved by the development of chimeric antibodies that contain the variable region of mouse antibodies (which binds with antigens) and the constant region of human antibodies (the effector part of the molecule).[435] A more recent development is the humanized antibody, in which only the complementarity-determining regions of the variable domains are retained from the mouse monoclonals.[436] These antibodies contain only about 5 to 10% of mouse residues and are unlikely to produce the HAMA reaction. The first humanized antibody used in a clinical

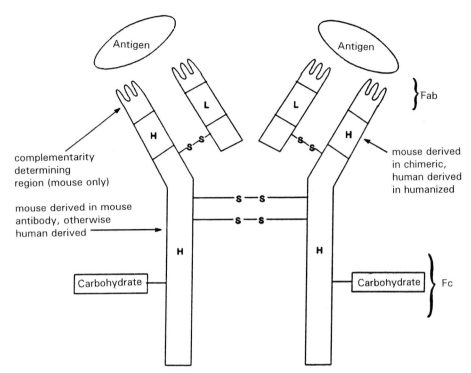

Figure 12–7 ■ Monoclonal antibody.

trial, CAMPATH-IH, induced remission in two non-Hodg-kin's lymphoma patients and showed no detectable HAMA.[437]

As shown in Figure 12-7, antibodies consist of two identical light chains and two identical heavy chains, which form a Y shape. Antigen binding occurs at the ends of the arms of the Y, and each arm is an antigen-binding fragment (Fab). Thus each antibody molecule can bind two antigens. The ends of the arms vary extensively in sequence and provide the binding specificity for the antigen. Each variable domain contains three complementarity-determining regions (CDRs) to give a total of six for binding each antigen molecule (Fig. 12-7).[438]

Two monoclonal antibodies have been approved for cancer chemotherapy. They are humanized monoclonal antibodies in which only the complementarity-determining Fab regions are of mouse origin. Trastuzumab (herceptin) is approved for breast cancer. It selectively binds with high affinity to the extracellular domain of human epidermal growth factor receptor 2 protein (Her 2). This binding inhibits proliferation of cells that overexpress Her and mediates antibody-dependent cytotoxicity.[439]

Rituximab (Rituxan) is directed against the CD20 antigen that is found on the surface of B lymphocytes. This antigen is expressed on more than 90% of B-cell non-Hodgkin's lymphomas but not on normal cells. It regulates early steps in the activation process for cell-cycle initiation and cell differentiation. Administration of rituximab results in rapid depletion of circulating and tissue-bound B cells.

Because monoclonal antibodies by themselves may not be toxic enough to kill cancer cells, extensive efforts have been made to conjugate them with highly toxic substances such as radionuclides, toxins, and anticancer drugs. The radionuclide conjugates also provide diagnostic agents for tu-

mors. Structures of the conjugates typically consist of the monoclonal antibody joined to a linker molecule, which is in turn joined to the cytotoxic agent.[440] Linkers are attached to the ε-amino groups of lysine residues of the monoclonal or to aldehyde groups formed by periodate oxidation of carbohydrate residues on the constant regions of the monoclonal.[441] For radionuclides, the other end of the linker has a chelating group, such as ethylenediaminetetraacetic acid (EDTA), which can bind radioactive metals such as ^{99m}Tc, ^{111}In, and ^{90}Y.[440]

Immunotoxins such as ricin, abrin, and diphtheria toxin are so potent that one molecule can kill a cell. Ricin consists of two subunits, the enzyme-active A chain and the targeting B chain, which are joined by a disulfide bond. Therapeutic agents are designed to have the B chain replaced by a monoclonal antibody targeted to tumor cells, taking advantage of the lability of the disulfide bond.[442] For anticancer drugs, the strategy is to join the drug to the linker molecule through a functional group that can be hydrolyzed. It is expected that the conjugate will be internalized in the cancer cell and then the drug will be released. Gemtuzumab ozogamicin (Mylotarg) is a chemotherapeutic agent composed of a recombinant humanized IgG$_4$ κ antibody conjugated with the antitumor antibiotic calicheamicin (see Fig. 12-6). The antibody portion binds to the CD33 antigen, which is expressed on the surface of leukemic blasts in more than 80% of patients who have acute myelogenous leukemia. The resulting complex is internalized, and the calicheamicin derivative is released inside lysosomes of the leukemia cells where it binds with DNA and produces double-strand breaks.

An alternative strategy for chemotherapy is the use of monoclonal antibodies as carriers for enzymes to tumor cell surfaces. The enzymes convert relatively nontoxic drug precursors (prodrugs) into active anticancer drugs.[443]

Limitations encountered in cancer chemotherapy with monoclonal antibodies and their conjugates include lack of selectivity for tumor cells, heterogeneity of tumor cell antigens, insufficient drug density to kill tumor cells, loss of immunogenicity because drug conjugates block recognition sites, the HAMA effect, and lack of internalization into tumor cells. Internalization is essential with toxins, but less important with radionuclides.[444]

Products

Rituximab.
Rituximab, Rituxan, is a genetically engineered chimeric monoclonal antibody directed to the CD20 antigen on malignant B lymphocytes.[445] It is supplied as solutions containing 10 mg/mL in 10- and 50-mL vials. These solutions should be stored at 2 to 8°C and protected from sunlight. Prior to administration they are diluted to final concentrations of 1 to 4 mg/mL in infusion bags containing 5% dextrose or 0.9% NaCl. The recommended dose is 375 mg/m^2 infused at a rate of 50 mg/hour.

Rituximab is used against malignant B lymphocytes that express the CD20 antigen.[446] The mean serum half-life is 59.8 hours, with variability possibly reflecting the tumor burden. Adverse reactions include hypersensitivity or anaphylactic reactions, cardiac arrhythmias, nausea, fatigue, and urticaria. Fever and chills may occur during infusion.

Gemtuzumab Ozogamicin.
Gemtuzumab ozogamicin, Mylotarg, CMA-676, consists of the antitumor antibiotic calicheamicin conjugated with a recombinant humanized IgG$_4$ κ monoclonal antibody that targets the CD33 receptor in myeloid leukemia cells.[447] It is supplied as 5 mg of a lyophilized powder for injection, which is combined with NaCl and sodium phosphate in 20-mL vials. It is reconstituted with 5 mL of Sterile Water for Injection. Before infusion, the desired volume is injected into 100 mL of 0.9% saline. During these procedures it must be protected from sunlight and direct fluorescent light. The infusion period is 2 hours, and the usual dose is 9 mg/m^2.

Gemtuzumab ozogamicin is indicated in patients who are 60 years of age or older, have CD33-positive acute myeloid leukemia, and are not candidates for other chemotherapy regimens.[448] Binding of the antibody with CD33 antigen forms a complex that is internalized in the tumor cell. The calicheamicin derivative is then released inside the leukemia cell, where it binds to DNA. After infusion of a 9 mg/m^2 dose, the half-lives of total and unconjugated calicheamicin are 45 and 100 hours, respectively. Adverse reactions include severe myelosuppression and mucostatis.

RADIOTHERAPEUTIC AGENTS

The properties of radiation and the use of radionuclides and radiopharmaceuticals for organ imaging are discussed in Chapter 13. Only the radiopharmaceuticals used as antineoplastic agents are described in this chapter. Radiopharmaceuticals used as diagnostic agents are generally chosen for their ability to produce γ-rays, which can penetrate tissues for relatively long distances to reach scintillation cameras. In contrast, radiotherapeutic agents produce β particles (electrons), which travel only short distances (about 3 mm, depending on their energies) to initiate cytotoxicity.

Radiotherapeutic agents are chosen for their ability to concentrate in specific tissues, such as bone and thyroid, as well as their energy and their radiological and biological half-lives. Unfortunately, their cytotoxicity is usually not limited to the targeted tumor, and they generally produce the symptoms of radiation sickness including nausea, vomiting, and diarrhea. Sometimes the toxic effects extend to hair loss and bone marrow damage.

Chromic phosphate P 32 and sodium phosphate P 32 contain the isotope ^{32}P, which decays to ^{32}S by β elimination with mean particle energy of 695 keV. The former is used to reduce peritoneal or plural effusions caused by metastatic disease, whereas the latter is used against hematological cancers such as polycythemia vera, chronic myelocytic leukemia, and CLL. Its selectivity is based on the concentration of phosphorus in rapidly proliferating neoplastic cells.

The ^{131}I in sodium iodide I 131 decays with a half-life of 8 days to emit both β and γ radiation. The β particles account for approximately 90% of local irradiation effects. This radiopharmaceutical is used for both diagnosis and therapy because it concentrates in the thyroid gland and gives the two types of radiation. Its therapeutic use is for palliation in select cases of thyroid carcinoma.

Strontium is a member of the alkaline earth metals and, therefore, similar to calcium in chemical properties including accumulation in bone. The radionuclide ^{89}Sr, supplied as strontium-89 chloride, is a pure β-emitter with a half-life of 50.5 days. It is indicated for relief of bone pain in patients with skeletal metastases.

Samarium belongs to the cerium group of lanthanides. The radionuclide ^{153}Sm is formulated as a chelate with ethylenediamine-tetramethylenephosphonic acid (EDTMP) in the product known as samarium SM 153 lexidronam. This chelate concentrates in areas of bone turnover in association with hydroxyapatite, where it emits β particles of 640, 710, and 810 keV. It is used in patients who have osteoblastic metastatic bone lesions.

Samarium SM 153 Lexidronam

Products

Chromic Phosphate P 32.
Chromic phosphate P 32, Phosphocol P32, Cr^{32}PO$_4$, is supplied as a suspension in 10-mL vials containing NaCl and NaOAc in water with 2% benzyl alcohol. The radioactivity is 15 mCi, with concentration up to 5 mCi/mL. The usual dose is 10 to 20 mCi intraper-

itoneally, 6 to 12 mCi intrapleurally, and 0.1 to 0.5 mCi interstitially.

Chromic phosphate is used for intracavitary instillation to reduce effusions caused by metastatic disease. It decays by β-emission, with a half-life of 14.3 days. Adverse reactions include transitory radiation sickness, bone marrow depression, pleuritis, peritonitis, nausea, and abdominal cramping.

Sodium Phosphate P 32. Sodium phosphate P 32, sodium radiophosphate, is supplied as an aqueous solution of a mixture of $NaH_2{}^{32}PO_4$ and $Na_2H^{32}PO_4$ with a pH range of 5.0 to 6.0. It contains 5 mCi/vial (0.67 mCi/mL) of radioactivity, expressed as a pure β-emitter with a half-life of 14.3 days. Sodium phosphate P 32 is indicated for treatment of polycythemia vera, chronic myelocytic leukemia, and CLL. Depression of leukocytes and platelets requires monitoring of blood and bone marrow at regular intervals.

Sodium iodide I 131. Sodium iodide I 131, sodium radioiodide (^{131}I), Iodotope, Theriodide, is supplied in capsules for oral use, or in aqueous solution for oral or parenteral use. Iodotope capsules contain 1 to 50 mCi, and Iodotope oral solutions contain 7.05 mCi/mL. Sodium iodide I 131 capsules contain 0.7 to 100 mCi, and sodium iodide oral solutions, 3.5 to 150 mCi/vial. Stock solutions are prepared by dilution with Purified Water containing 0.2% sodium thiosulfate as a reducing agent. The dose is individualized for each patient.

Sodium iodide I 131 is used for palliation in selected cases of thyroid carcinoma. The usual toxic effect is radiation sickness.

Strontium 89 Chloride. Strontium 89 chloride, Metastron, $^{89}SrCl_2$, is supplied as a solution in Water for Injection containing 4 mCi of radioactivity (10.9 to 22.6 mg/mL) in 10-mL vials. The usual dose is 4 mCi by slow IV injection. This dose may be repeated after at least 90 days.[449] After injection, the drug is selectively localized in bone mineral. It is a pure β-emitter with a half-life of 50.5 days.

Strontium 89 chloride is used for relief of bone pain for patients with skeletal metastases. Because it is toxic to normal bone, the benefits and risks of its use must be assessed.

Samarium SM 153 Lexidronam. Samarium SM 153 lexidronam, Quadramet, is formed by complexing ^{153}Sm

with EDTMP.[450] This radiopharmaceutical is supplied in 2 or 3 mL of frozen solution contained in 10-mL vials. The radioactivity at calibration is 50 mCi/mL. Prior to administration of the drug, 500 mL of fluid is administered to protect the bladder. Then the drug is administered by IV injection over 1 minute, followed by saline. It is excreted in urine as the intact complex to the extent of 34.5% in the first hour. The total excretion depends on the tumor burden

Samarium SM 153 lexidronam is indicated for relief of pain in patients with osteoblastic metastatic bone lesions.[451] It is also used in ankylosing spondylitis, Paget's disease, and severe rheumatoid arthritis. The main side effect is radiation sickness.

CYTOPROTECTIVE AGENTS

Highly cytotoxic antineoplastic agents produce a variety of serious side effects in patients. This problem has stimulated the search for compounds that protect patients from certain specific toxicities and thus permit the antineoplastic agents to be given in larger doses. The following three widely different cytoprotective agents have been approved for clinical use in the United States.

Mesna is the sodium salt of mercaptoethanesulfonic acid. Although it is oxidized to the corresponding disulfide in blood, it is reduced back to the free thiol in the kidney. There it reacts with urotoxic ifosfamide metabolites including 4-hydroxyifosfamide and acrolein. This property led to its use in preventing hemorrhagic cystitis in patients receiving ifosfamide.

The organic thiophosphate amifostine is used to detoxify the reactive metabolites of cisplatin, especially in the kidney. It is dephosphorylated by alkaline phosphatase to the active free thiol. This transformation occurs selectively in normal tissues because they have higher alkaline phosphatase activity, higher pH, and better vascularity.

Dexrazoxane is the S-($+$)-isomer of razoxane. It is a potent intracellular chelating agent that is used for cardioprotection in patients receiving doxorubicin.[452] Dexrazoxane has two imide groups that open intracellularly to form a compound related to EDTA. This compound complexes with iron and interferes with free radical generation associated with doxorubicin–iron complexes.

$$HSCH_2CH_2SO_3Na$$

Mesna

$$H_2N(CH_2)_3NH(CH_2)_2SPO_3H_2$$

Amiphostine

Dexrazoxane

Products

Mesna. Mesna, Mesnex, sodium mercaptoethanesulfonate, is prepared from sodium bromoethanesulfonate, thiourea, and ammonia.[453] It is supplied in 2-mL ampuls containing 100 mg/mL of the drug plus 0.25 mg/mL of EDTA, and in 10-L multidose vials containing 10.4 mg of benzyl alcohol as preservative. Prior to intravenous administration it is diluted with various mixtures of dextrose and NaCl, or with lactated Ringer's solution to give a final concentration of 20 mg/mL. The diluted solutions are stable for 24 hours at 25°C, but they should be refrigerated and used within 6 hours of reconstitution. Mesna is oxidized to the corresponding disulfide on exposure to oxygen. The usual dosage is 240 mg/m^2, given at the same time as the first ifosfamide injection.

Mesna is indicated for ifosfamide-induced hemorrhagic cystitis. After intravenous administration, it is rapidly oxidized to the disulfide. Once in the kidney, it is reduced to the free thiol, which reacts with urotoxic ifosfamide metabolites including acrolein and 4-hydroxyifosfamide.[454] The half-lives of mesna and its disulfide in blood are 0.36 and 1.17 hours, respectively, and the kinetics are dose dependent. Side effects include diarrhea, limb pain, headache, nausea and fatigue, and bad taste in the mouth. Some patients are hypersensitive.

Amifostine. Amifostine, Ethyol. *S*-[2-(3-aminopropylamino)ethyl] dihydrogen thiophosphate, is prepared by treating 3-(2-bromoethylamino)propylamine with sodium thiophosphate.[455] It is supplied as 500 mg of lyophilized powder in 10-mL single-use vials. Reconstitution is by addition of 9.7 mL of 0.9% NaCl for injection. The usual starting dose is 910 mg/m^2 given once daily as a 15-minute infusion starting 30 minutes before chemotherapy.

Amifostine is indicated for reducing the cumulative toxicity associated with repeated doses of cisplatin. It also reduces the incidence of xerostomia in patients undergoing postoperative radiation treatments in which the parotid glands are exposed. Toxic effects of amifostine include hypotension, severe nausea, and vomiting. Antiemetic medicines including dexamethasone and a serotonin 5-HT$_3$ antagonist are usually administered. Transient hypotension may require interruption of therapy.

Dexrazoxane. Dexrazoxane, (*S*)-1,2-bis(3,5-dioxopiperazinyl)propane or Zinecard, a potent intracellular chelating agent, is prepared by treating (*S*)(+)-propylenediamine tetraacetic tetraamide with sodium dimsylate.[456] It is supplied as 250 mg of lyophilized powder in single-dose vials, together with 25 mL of sodium lactate for injection, or as 500 mg lyophilized powder with 50 mL of M/6 sodium lactate. For reconstitution, it is diluted to 10 mg/mL with 5% dextrose or 0.9% NaCl. Solutions are stored at controlled room temperature. The dose is determined as a 10:1 ratio with doxorubicin. The usual dose is 500 mg/m^2 of dexrazoxane and 50 mg/m^2 of doxorubicin. Administration is by slow IV push or rapid IV drip 30 minutes before doxorubicin is administered. The mean plasma concentration is 31.5 μg/mL after a 15-minute infusion.[452]

Dexrazoxane is indicated for reducing the cumulative cardiotoxicity of doxorubicin. It may add to the myelosuppression caused by this chemotherapeutic agent.

FUTURE ANTINEOPLASTIC AGENTS

Most of the earlier research in antineoplastic drug discovery was related to inhibiting the synthesis and function of DNA. Today, a variety of other targets are under intensive investigation, and they should provide oncologists with significant new approaches to therapy. Although this research has not yet produced an approved agent, many new compounds are in clinical trials. The following new approaches to cancer chemotherapy are of special interest: inhibition of proteases involved in metastasis, angiogenesis inhibitors, antisense technology, and telomerase inhibitors.

Proteases and Metastasis

The ability of cells from primary tumors to colonize secondary sites (metastasis) is the major cause of cancer mortality. Metastasis involves tumor cells entering and leaving the circulation and invading adjacent tissue. It requires degradation of the extracellular matrix by the concerted action of proteases. This process occurs normally, but it is controlled by the elaboration of protease inhibitors. The balance between proteases and inhibitors appears to be regulated abnormally in malignant cells.[457] Matrix protein is degraded by a variety of metalloproteinases, including collagenases, gelatinases, stromelysins, and matrilysins. These metalloproteinases can be activated by a cascade induced by tumor-secreted serine proteases, cysteine proteases, and aspartyl proteinases.[458] Among the synthetic compounds currently under investiga-

E-64

Nafamostat

tion are E-64, an inhibitor of the cysteine proteinase cathepsin B,[459] and nafamostat, a serine protease inhibitor. Suramin blocks melanoma and mammary tumor invasiveness, possibly by inhibiting heparinase, cathepsin D secretion, and urinary plasminogen activator receptor.[458, 460]

Angiogenesis Inhibitors

Angiogenesis is the formation of new blood vessels. It is a necessary but carefully regulated component of normal growth and wound healing. Uncontrolled angiogenesis is a driving factor in solid tumor growth. The process of angiogenesis is complex and requires the coordinated interaction of multiple cell types. Multiple sites for drug intervention are expected.[461] Endogenous angiogenesis inhibitors were sought in tissues such as cartilage, which lack blood vessels. This search afforded a protein named *cartilage-derived inhibitor*.[462] Laminin is a major component of basement membrane. Peptides based on its structure, such as CDPGY-IGSRNH$_2$, inhibit angiogenesis and solid tumor growth.[463] Platelet factor 4, a heparin-binding polypeptide, inhibits human colon cancer cells in mice. Heparin preparations alone promote angiogenesis, but they strongly promote the antiangiogenic activity of small molecules. Synthetic heparin substitutes, including sulfated cyclodextrins[464] and suramin,[465] inhibit angiogenesis, and they are promoted by angiostatic corticosteroids. These corticosteroids are important agents, but their glucocorticoid and mineralocorticoid properties cause serious side effects. Related steroids that lack these side effects include 11α-hydrocortisone, tetrahydrocortisone, and medroxyprogesterone acetate.[466] The antibiotic fumagillin inhibits angiogenesis in tumors, and a more potent analogue, AGM-1470, reduces the growth rate of lung cancer and melanoma in mice.[467]

TNF-α is a powerful stimulant to angiogenesis. The secretion of this factor by macrophages in prostatic cancers is decreased significantly by linomide, a quinoline-3-carboxamide derivative.[468]

Antisense Technology

Single-stranded messenger RNA (mRNA) can undergo sequence-specific, high-affinity binding to a complementary oligonucleotide sequence by Watson-Crick hydrogen bonding. Such a complementary agent is called an *antisense oligomer*. By binding with mRNA, the antisense oligomer can interfere with its translation into protein by ribosomal blockade. Complexes between mRNA and DNA-like antisense oligonucleotides also can activate RNase H, an enzyme that specifically cleaves the RNA strand of a RNA/DNA duplex.[469]

Limitations on the use of antisense oligomers include poor uptake into cells and instability to degradation by nucleases. Cellular uptake has been increased by microinjection and by the addition of lipofectin, a cationic lipid that increases cell permeability.[470] Stability to nucleases is improved by replacement of one phosphate oxygen with sulfur to give phosphorothioate oligonucleotides. The phosphorothioate group is chiral, but racemates are generally used.[471] Other modifications to the oligonucleotide backbone include replacing the phosphate with various amides and acetals, and by using 2'-fluoro-2'-deoxysugars.[472] Peptide nucleic acids in which the sugar-phosphate backbone is replaced by *N*-(2-aminoethyl) glycine units have shown stability in vitro to degradation by nucleases.[467] Novel antisense oligomers have also been prepared with modified pyrimidines, such as 5-(propyn-1-yl)uracil and 6-azathymidine,[473] and modified pu-

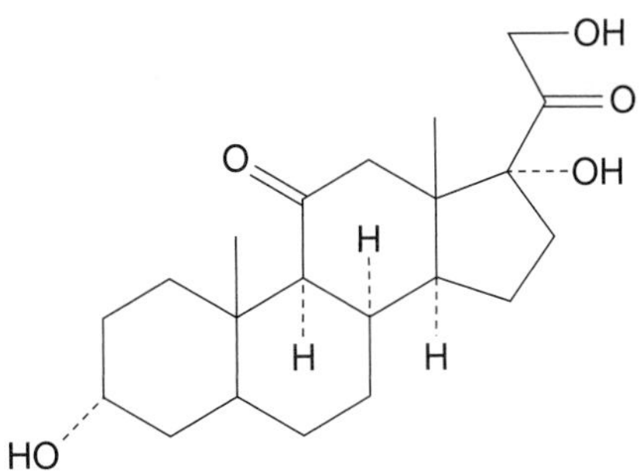

Tetrahydrocortisone

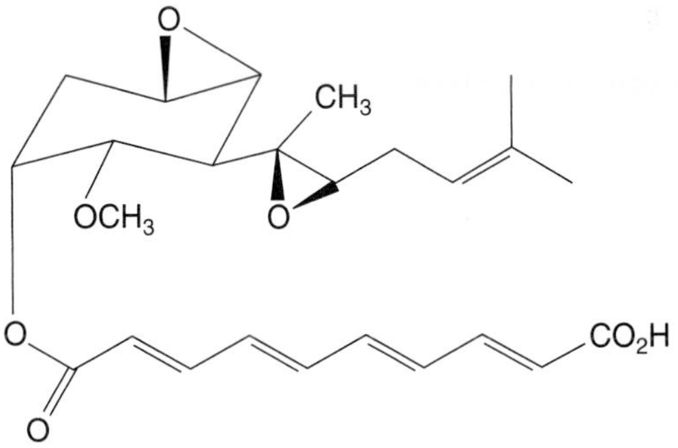

Fumagillin

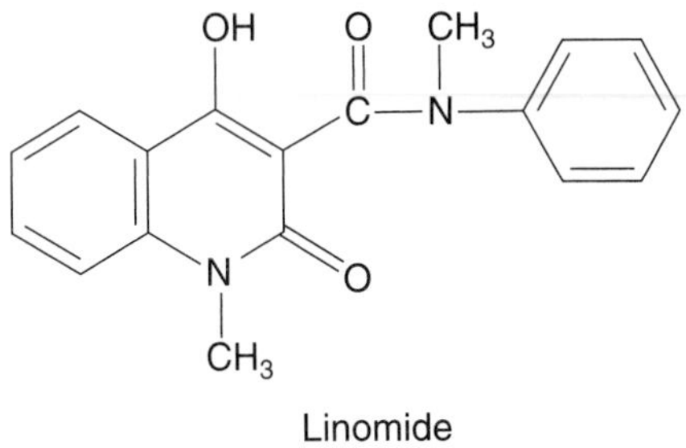

Linomide

rines, such as 3-(1*H*-imidazolyl)propyl guanine.[474] These oligomers also have enhanced stability to nucleases.[475]

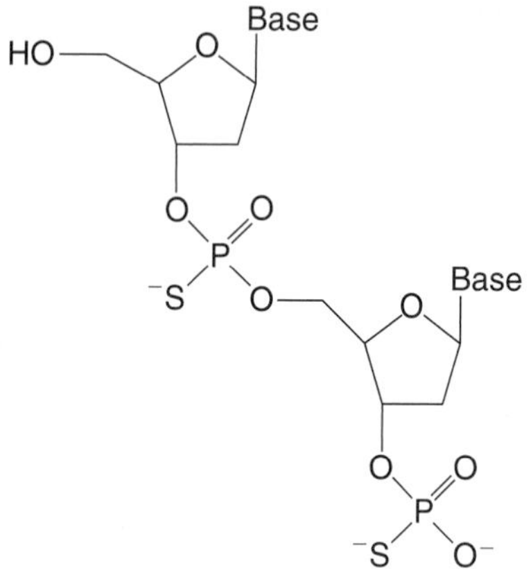

Phosphorothioate

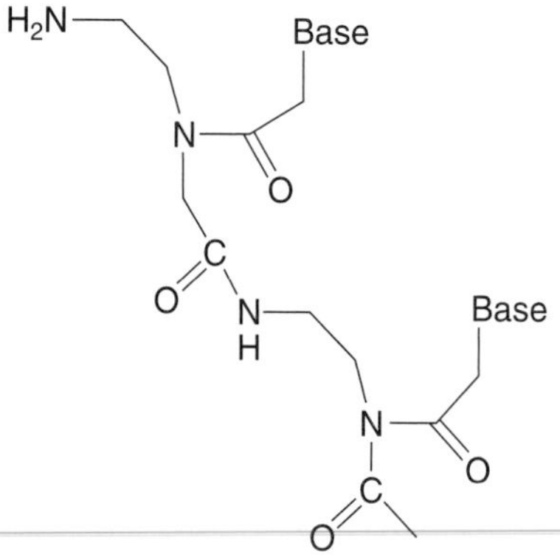

Peptide Nucleic Acid

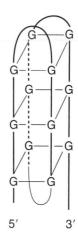

Figure 12–8 ■ Schematic illustration of the G-quadriplex structure formed by four [α TTAGGG]$_4$ oligonucleotides. This repeat sequence occurs in DNA of vertebrates.

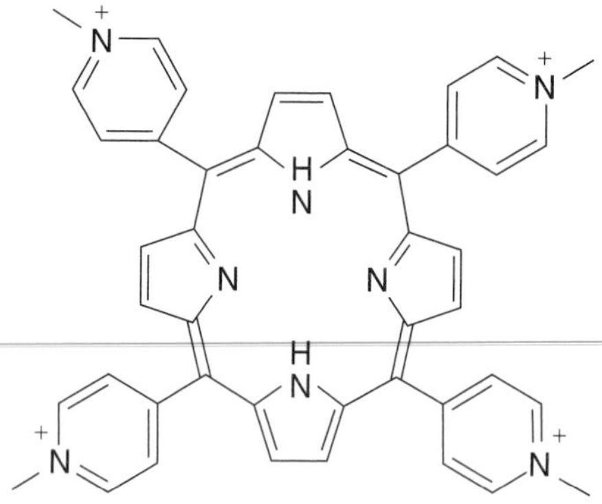

quadriplex of telomeres to stabilize this structure and prevent the action of telomerase.[478] This effectively inhibited human telomerase in HeLa cells. Analogues of 2,6-diaminoanthraquinone also show inhibition of telomerase.[479]

TMPyP4

Telomerase Inhibitors

Telomeres are nucleoprotein structures located at the ends of eucaryotic chromosomes. They protect chromosome ends from fusion and degradation and ensure complete replication of chromosomal DNA. In human somatic cells, telomeres have 1,000 to 3,000 repeats. They gradually shorten with every cell division. This shortening is thought to limit their proliferative capacity. Cancer cells, in contrast, can maintain their telomere length and thus become immortalized. They do this by reactivating telomerase, a specific reverse transcriptase with an endogenous RNA template.[476]

Selective inhibition of telomerase has been recognized as a potentially important new method of cancer chemotherapy because cancer cells have relatively high concentrations of telomerase, and it appears to be essential to their survival, whereas this enzyme is undetectable in normal somatic cells. One approach to telomerase inhibition is to use antisense DNA to target the telomerase RNA component.[477] Another approach takes advantage of the remarkable property of telomeres (and certain other guanine-rich molecules) to form G-quadriplexes (Fig. 12-8). These structures are associated with the telomerase reaction cycle. Hurley's group recently discovered that cationic porphyrins, such as tetramethyl-(*N*-methyl-4-pyridyl)porphine (TMPyP$_4$), can intercalate the G-

POTENTIAL FUTURE DEVELOPMENTS

Recent sequence determinations of the human genome[480, 481] have opened the way to important new advances in the diagnosis and treatment of cancers. They have made it possible to distinguish genetic differences between tumor cells and normal cells and to locate differences within variants of the same tumor type. An important new approach to working with these genomic differences is the technology known as the DNA microarray or ''DNA chip.'' Microarrays consist of slides or chips systematically dotted with thousands of genes that can serve as probes for determining the expression levels of specific genes in different types of cells. This information has been used to specify subtypes of a variety of cancers. In some cases, it has allowed the determination of which cancers are likely to respond to certain current therapies, and which tumors will not respond, thus sparing the patient with a resistant tumor needless exposure to toxic drugs.[482] Changes observed in gene expression on administration of drugs can also be used to predict their toxic effects. Perhaps the most important future use of DNA microarray technology will be to identify new targets for drug therapy. For example, elevated production of a specific protein may be indicated, and antagonists may be developed to inhibit expression of the gene that codes for it. Alternatively, the protein may be directly antagonized. At the present time a number of manufacturers are producing DNA chips for cancer research. Many industrial and academic laboratories are using them in drug discovery research.

Proteomics is a complementary technique to genomics. It is still very new, but laboratories are beginning to determine the entire spectrum of human proteins. This research is important because the number of different mRNAs produced in cells (e.g., as determined by DNA microarray technology) often shows no correlation with the number of different proteins produced in the same cells. Furthermore, after their synthesis, proteins undergo many small chemical changes that can profoundly affect their activity. Techniques for preparing arrays of thousands of proteins on a small glass slide have been devised. These arrays show promise as devices to enable quick screening of potential drugs against protein targets, as well as identifying potentially toxic interactions with proteins not involved in the disease process.[483]

REFERENCES

1. Zubrod, C. G.: Agents of choice in neoplastic disease. In Sartorelli, A. C., and Johns, D. J. (eds.). Handbook of Experimental Pharmacology, vol. 38, part 1. New York, Springer-Verlag, 1974, p. 7.
2. Buick, R. N.: Cellular basis of chemotherapy. In Dorr, R. T., and Von Hoff, D. D. (eds.). Cancer Chemotherapy Handbook. 2nd ed. Norwalk, CT, Appleton & Lange, 1994, pp 3–14.
3. Mackillop, W. J., et al.: J. Natl. Cancer Inst. 70:9, 1983.
4. Schabel, F. M., Jr.: Cancer 35:15, 1975.
5. Norton, L., and Simon, R.: Cancer Treat. Rep. 61:1307, 1977.
6. Schimke, R. T.: Cancer Res. 44:1735, 1984.
7. Bradley, G., et al.: Biochim. Biophys. Acta 948:87, 1988.
8. Huggins, C., and Hodges, C. V.: Cancer Res. 1:293, 1941.
9. Gilman, A., and Phillips, F. S.: Science 103:409, 1946.
10. Pearson, O. H.: Cancer 2:943, 1949.
11. Kennedy, B. J.: Cancer 18:1551, 1965.
12. Boyd, M. R.: The future of new drug development. In Niederhuber, J. E. (ed.). Current Therapy in Oncology. New York, Marcel Dekker, 1993, pp. 11–22.
13. Salmon, S. E., et al.: Cancer Chemother. Pharmacol. 6:103, 1981.
14. Himmelweit, F. (ed.): The collected papers of Paul Ehrlich, vol. 1. London, Pergamon Press, 1956, pp. 596–618.
15. Lynch, V., et al.: J. Pharmacol. Exp. Ther. 12:265, 1918.
16. Montgomery, J. A., et al.: Drugs for neoplastic diseases. In Burger, A. (ed.). Medicinal Chemistry. 3rd ed. New York, Wiley-Interscience, 1970, p. 680.
17. Connors, T. A.: Mechanism of action of 2-chloroethylamine, derivatives, sulfur mustards, epoxides and aziridines. In Sartorelli, A. C., and Johns, D. J. (eds.). Handbook of Experimental Pharmacology, vol. 38, part 2. New York, Springer-Verlag, 1975, p. 19.
18. Price, C. C.: Chemistry of alkylation. In Sartorelli, A. C., and Johns, D. J. (eds.). Handbook of Experimental Pharmacology, vol. 38, part 2. New York, Springer-Verlag, 1975, p. 4.
19. Driscoll, J. S., et al.: J. Pharm. Sci. 68:185, 1979.
20. White, F. R.: Cancer Chemother. Rep. 4:55, 1959.
21. Jarmon, M., and Ross, W. C. J.: Chem. Ind. (Lond.) 1789, 1967.
22. Montgomery, J. A., et al.: J. Med. Chem. 10:668, 1967.
23. Engle, T. W., et al.: J. Med. Chem. 22:897, 1979.
24. Karle, I. L., et al.: J. Am. Chem. Soc. 99:4803, 1977.
25. Ahmann, D. L., et al.: Cancer Chemother. Rep. 58:861, 1974.
26. Anderson, W. K., and Corey, P. F.: J. Med. Chem. 20:812, 1977.
27. Szybalski, W., and Iyer, V. N.: The mitomycins and porfiromysins. In Gottlieb, D., and Shaw, P. D. (eds.). Antibiotics, vol. 1. New York, Springer-Verlag, 1967, p. 221.
28. Lin, A. J., et al.: Cancer Chemother. Rep. 4:23, 1974.
29. Buchi, G., and Rosenthal, D.: J. Am. Chem. Soc. 78:3860, 1956.
30. Bollag, W.: Cancer Chemother. Rep. 33:1, 1963.
31. Chabner, B. A., et al.: Proc. Soc. Exp. Biol. 132:1169, 1969.
32. Tsuji, T., and Kosower, E. M.: J. Am. Chem. Soc. 93:1992, 1971.
33. Kreis, W., and Yen, W.: Experientia 21:284, 1965.
34. Preussmann, R., and Von Hodenberg, A.: Biochem. Pharmacol. 19:1505, 1970.
35. Skibba, J. L., et al.: Cancer Res. 30:147, 1970.
36. Sava, G., et al.: Cancer Treat. Rep. 63:93, 1979.
37. Ludlum, D. B.: Molecular biology of alkylation: An overview. In Sartorelli, A. C., and Johns, D. J. (eds.). Handbook of Experimental Pharmacology, vol. 38, part 2. New York, Springer-Verlag, 1975, p. 7.
38. Kohn, K. W., et al.: J. Mol. Biol. 19:226, 1966.
39. Ross, W. C. J.: Biological Alkylating Agents. London, Butterworths, 1962.
40. Thomasz, M., et al.: Proc. Natl. Acad. Sci. U. S. A. 83:6702, 1986.
41. Lawley, P. D., and Martin, C. M.: Biochem. J. 145:85, 1975.
42. Ludlum, D. B.: Biochim. Biophys. Acta 152:282, 1967.
43. Brooks, P., and Lawley, P. D.: Biochem. J. 80:496, 1961.
44. Wheeler, G. P.: Mechanism of action of nitrosoureas. In Sartorelli, A. C., and Johns, D. J. (eds.). Handbook of Experimental Pharmacology, vol. 38, part 2. New York, Springer-Verlag, 1975, p. 75.
45. Levis, A. G., et al.: Nature 207:608, 1965.
46. Boyce, R. P., and Howard-Flanders, P.: Proc. Natl. Acad. Sci. U. S. A. 51:293, 1964.
47. Prelog, V., and Stepan, V.: Coll. Czech. Chem. Commun. 7:93, 1935.
48. Arnold, H., et al.: Nature 181:931, 1958.
49. Brock, N., et al.: Eur. J. Clin. Oncol. 17:1155, 1981.
50. Zubrod, C. G.: Cancer 21:553, 1968.
51. Arnold, H., et al.: U.S. Patent 3,732,340; Chem. Abstr. 79:18772, 1973.
52. Allen, L. M., et al.: Cancer Treat. Rep. 60:451, 1976.
53. Loehrer, P. J., et al.: J. Clin. Oncol. 4:528, 1986.
54. Creaven, P. J., et al.: Cancer Treat. Rep. 58:455, 1976.
55. Bergel, F., and Stock, J. A.: J. Chem. Soc. 2409, 1954.
56. Evans, T. L., et al.: Cancer Chemother. Pharmacol. 8:175, 1982.
57. Fisher, B., et al.: N. Engl. J. Med. 292:117, 1975.
58. Phillips, A. P., and Mentha, J. W.: U.S. Patent 3,046,301, Oct. 29, 1959.
59. Calabresi, P., and Welch, A. D.: Annu. Rev. Med. 13:147, 1962.
60. Timmis, G. M.: U.S. Patent 2,917,432, Dec. 15, 1959.
61. Parham, W. E., and Wilbur, J. M., Jr.: J. Org. Chem. 26:1569, 1961.
62. Roberts, J. J., and Warwick, G. P.: Biochem. Pharmacol. 6:217, 1961.
63. Warwick, G. P.: Cancer Res. 23:1315, 1963.
64. Ehrsson, H., et al.: Clin. Pharmacol. Ther. 34:86, 1983.
65. Physicians' Desk Reference, 33rd ed. Oradell, NJ, Medical Economics, 1979, p. 746.
66. Johnston, T. P., et al.: J. Med. Chem. 6:669, 1963.
67. DeVita, V. T., et al.: Clin. Pharmacol. Ther. 8:566, 1967.
68. Walker, M. D.: Cancer Chemother. Rep. 4:21, 1973.
69. Johnston, T. P., et al.: J. Med. Chem. 9:892, 1966.
70. Moertel, C. G.: Cancer Chemother. Rep. 4:27, 1973.
71. Kuh, E., and Seeger, D. R.: U.S. Patent 2,670,347, Feb. 23, 1954.
72. Hoffman-LaRoche & Co., A.-G.: Belg. Patent 618,638, Dec. 7, 1962.
73. Weinkam, R. J. and Shiba, D. A.: Life Sci. 22:937, 1978.
74. Shealy, Y. F., et al.: J. Org. Chem. 27:2150, 1962.
75. Leo, T.L., et al.: Cancer Treat. Rep. 60:149, 1976.
76. Bessier-Chretien, Y., and Serne, H.: Bull. Chim. Soc. France 6:2039, 1973.
77. Sanders, M. E., et al.: 184th national meeting of the American Chemical Society, Kansas City, MO, September, 1982. Abstracts MEDI 55.
78. Rosen, G. F., et al.: Gynecol. Oncol. 27:173, 1987.
79. Lyttle, D. A., and Petering, H. F.: J. Am. Chem. Soc. 80:6459, 1958.
80. Lukens, L. N., and Herrington, K. A.: Biochim. Biophys. Acta 24:432, 1957.
81. Patterson, A. R. P., and Tidd, D. M.: 6-Thiopurines. In Sartorelli, A. C., and Johns, D. J. (eds.). Handbook of Experimental Pharmacology, vol. 38, part 2. New York, Springer-Verlag, 1975, p. 384.
82. Woods, D. D.: Br. J. Exp. Pathol. 21:74, 1940.
82a. Fildes, P.: Lancet 1:955, 1940.
83. Roblin, R. O., et al.: J. Am. Chem. Soc. 67:290, 1945.
84. Hitchings, G. H., and Elion, G. B.: Acc. Chem. Res. 2:202, 1969.
85. Elion, G. B., et al.: J. Am. Chem. Soc. 74:411, 1952.
86. Brockman, R. W.: Adv. Cancer Res. 7:129, 1963.

87. Atkison, M. R., et al.: Biochem. J. 92:389, 1964.
88. Salser, J. S., et al.: J. Biol. Chem. 235:429, 1960.
89. Bennett, L. L., Jr., and Allan, P. W.: Cancer Res. 31:152, 1971.
90. Currie, R., et al.: Biochem. J. 104:634, 1967.
91. Elion, G. B.: Fed. Proc. 26:898, 1967.
92. Moor, E. C., and LePage, G. A.: Cancer Res. 18:1075, 1958.
93. LePage, G. A., et al.: Cancer Res. 24:835, 1964.
94. Lee, W. W., et al.: J. Am. Chem. Soc. 82:2648, 1960.
95. Parke-Davis and Co.: Belg. Patent 671,557, 1967.
96. Furth, J. J., and Cohen, S. S.: Cancer Res. 27:1528, 1967.
97. Brink, J. J., and LePage, G. A.: Cancer Res. 24:312, 1964.
98. Brockman, R. W., et al.: Cancer Res. 40:3610, 1980.
99. Tseng, W.-C., et al.: Mol. Pharmacol. 21:474, 1982.
100. Seto, S., et al.: J. Clin. Invest. 75:377, 1985.
101. Heidelberger, C.: Fluorinated pyrimidines and their nucleosides. In Sartorelli, A. C., and Johns, D. J. (eds.). Handbook of Experimental Pharmacology, vol. 38, part 2. New York, Springer-Verlag, 1975, p. 193.
102. Skold, O.: Biochim. Biophys. Acta 29:651, 1958.
103. Reyes, P.: Biochemistry 8:2057, 1969.
104. Cohen, S. S., et al.: Proc. Natl. Acad. Sci. U. S. A. 44:1004, 1958.
105. Santi, D. V., and McHenry, C. S.: Proc. Natl. Acad. Sci. U. S. A. 69:1855, 1972.
106. Hiller, S. A., et al.: Dokl. Akad. Nauk. S. S. S. R. 176:332, 1967.
107. Benvenuto, J., et al.: Cancer Res. 38:3867, 1978.
108. Ishitsuka, H., et al.: Biochem. Pharmacol. 55:1090, 1998.
109. Hertel, L. W., et al.: J. Org. Chem. 53:2406, 1988.
110. Heidelberger, C., et al.: J. Med. Chem. 7:1, 1964.
111. Santi, D. V., and Sakai, T. T.: Biochemistry 10:3598, 1971.
112. Walwick, E. R., et al.: Proc. Chem. Soc. London 84, 1959.
113. Bergmann, W., and Feeney, R. J.: J. Org. Chem. 16:981, 1951.
114. Chu, M. Y., and Fischer, G. G.: Biochem. Pharmacol. 11:423, 1962.
115. Larsson, A., and Reichard, P.: J. Biol. Chem. 241:2540, 1966.
116. Creasey, W. A., et al.: Cancer Res. 28:1074, 1968.
117. Borun, T. W., et al.: Proc. Natl. Acad. Sci. U. S. A. 58:1977, 1967.
118. Creasey, W. A.: Arabinosylcytosine. In Sartorelli, A. C., and Johns, D. J. (eds.). Handbook of Experimental Pharmacology, vol. 38, part 2. New York, Springer-Verlag, 1975, p. 245.
119. Stoller, R. G., et al.: Biochem. Pharmacol. 27:53, 1978.
120. Hoshi, A., et al.: Gann 62:145, 1971.
121. Sórm, F., et al.: Experientia 20:202, 1964.
122. Hanka, L. J., et al.: Antimicrob. Agents Chemother. 6:619, 1966.
123. Paces, V., et al.: Biochim. Biophys. Acta 161:352, 1968.
124. Vesely, J., et al.: Biochem. Pharmacol. 17:519, 1968.
125. Vesely, J., et al.: Cancer Res. 30:2180, 1970.
126. Nakamura, H., et al.: J. Am. Chem. Soc. 96:4327, 1974.
127. Schaeffer, H. J., and Schwender, C. F.: J. Med. Chem. 17:6, 1974.
128. Seeger, D. R., et al.: J. Am. Chem. Soc. 71:1753, 1949.
129. Werkheiser, W.: J. Biol. Chem. 236:888, 1961.
130. Hryniuk, W. M., et al.: Mol. Pharmacol. 5:557, 1969.
131. Zakrzewski, S. F., et al.: Mol. Pharmacol. 2:423, 1969.
132. Cohen, S.: Ann. N. Y. Acad. Sci. 186:292, 1971.
133. Li, M. C., et al.: Proc. Soc. Exp. Biol. 97:29, 1958.
134. Bertino, J. R., et al.: Proc. 5th Int. Congr. Pharmacol. 3:376, 1973.
135. Semon, J. H., and Grindley, G. B.: Cancer Res. 38:2905, 1978.
136. Howell, S. B., et al.: Cancer Res. 38:325, 1978.
137. Grivsky, E. M., et al.: J. Med. Chem. 23:327, 1980.
138. Bertino, J. R., et al.: Biochem. Pharmacol. 28:1983, 1979.
139. Baker, B. R.: Acc. Chem. Res. 2:129, 1969
140. Hartman, S. C.: Purines and pyrimidines. In Greenberg, D. M. (ed.). Metabolic Pathways, vol. 4. New York, Academic Press, 1970, p. 1.
141. Eidinoff, M. L., et al.: Cancer Res. 18:105, 1958.
142. Fusari, S. A., et al.: J. Am. Chem. Soc. 76:2881, 1954.
143. DeWald, H. A., and Moore, A. M.: J. Am. Chem. Soc. 80:3941, 1958.
144. Dion, H. W., et al.: J. Am. Chem. Soc. 78:3075, 1956.
145. French, T. C., et al.: J. Biol. Chem. 238:2186, 1963.
146. Levenberg, B., et al.: J. Biol. Chem. 225:163, 1957.
147. Elion, G. B., et al.: J. Am. Chem. Soc. 74:441, 1952.
147a. Beaman, A. G., and Robbins, R. K.: J. Am. Chem. Soc. 83:4042, 1961.
148. Zimm, S., et al.: Biochem. Pharmacol. 33:4089, 1984.
149. Burchenal, J. H., et al.: Blood 8:965, 1953.
150. Physicians' Desk Reference, 33rd ed. Oradell, NJ, Medical Economics, 1979, p. 749.
151. Elion, G. B., and Hitchings, G. H.: J. Am. Chem. Soc. 77:1676, 1955.
152. Grindley, G. B.: Cancer Treat. Rev. 6:19, 1979.
153. Clarkson, B. D.: Cancer 5:227, 1970.
154. Ikehara, M., and Tada, H.: J. Am. Chem. Soc. 85:2344, 1963.
155. Lilliemark, J., and Juliusson, G.: Cancer Res. 51:5570, 1991.
156. Tallman, M., et al.: Blood 80:2203, 1992.
157. Montgomery, J. A., and Shortnacy, A. T.: U.S. Patent 4,357,324: 1982.
158. Duschinsky, R., et al.: J. Am. Chem. Soc. 79:4559, 1957.
159. Earl, R. A., and Townsend, L. B.: J. Heterocyclic Chem. 9:1141, 1972.
160. Physicians' Desk Reference, 33rd. ed. Oradell, NJ, Medical Economics, 1979, p. 749.
161. Floyd, F. A., et al.: Drug Intell. Clin. Pharm. 16:665, 1982.
162. Moore, G. E., et al.: Cancer Chemother. Rep. 52:641, 1968.
163. Klein, E., et al.: Topical 5-fluorouracil chemotherapy for premalignant and malignant epidermal neoplasms. In Brodsky, I., and Kahn, S. B. (eds.). Cancer Chemotherapy II. New York, Grune & Stratton, 1972, p. 47.
164. Hoffer, M., et al.: J. Am. Chem. Soc. 81:4112, 1959.
165. Sullivan, R. D., and Miller, E.: Cancer Res. 25:1025, 1965.
166. Hunter, J. H.: U.S. Patent 3,116,282, Dec. 31, 1963.
167. Ross, D. D., et al.: Cancer Res. 50:2658, 1974.
168. Wan, S. H., et al.: Cancer Res. 44:5857, 1984.
169. Greenwald, E. S.: Cancer Chemotherapy. Flushing, NY, Medical Examination Publishing, 1973.
170. Clarkson, B. D.: Cancer 30:1572, 1972.
171. Arasaki, M., et al.: European Patent 602454, June 22, 1994.
172. Ishitsuka, H., et al.: Proc. Am. Assoc. Cancer Res. 36:407, 1995.
173. Hertel, R. W., et al.: Cancer Res. 36:407, 1990.
174. Woo, P. W. K., et al.: J. Heterocycl. Chem. 11:641, 1974.
175. Malspies, L., et al.: Cancer Treat. Symp. 2:7, 1984.
176. Johnston, J. B., et al.: Br. J. Hematol. 63:525, 1986.
177. Hignite, C. E., et al.: Cancer Treat. Rep. 62:13, 1978.
178. Goldman, I. D.: Cancer Treat. Rep. 71:549, 1977.
179. Alt, F. W., et al.: J. Biol. Chem. 253:1357, 1978.
180. Farber, S., et al.: N. Engl. J. Med. 238:787, 1948.
181. Hertz, R.: Ann. Intern. Med. 59:931, 1963.
182. Stoller, R. G., et al.: N. Engl. J. Med. 297:630, 1977.
183. Hitchings, G. H., and Elion, G. B.: U.S. Patent 3,056,785, Oct. 2, 1962.
184. Waksman, S. A., and Woodruff, H. B.: Proc. Soc. Exp. Biol. Med. 45:609, 1940.
185. Rao, K. V., et al.: Antibiot. Chemother. 12:182, 1962.
186. Schmidt-Kastner, G.: Naturwissenschaften 43:131, 1956.
187. Umezawa, H.: Bleomycin: discovery, chemistry, and action. In Umezawa, H. (ed.). Bleomycin, Fundamental and Clinical Studies. Tokyo, Gann Monogr. Cancer Res. 1976, p. 3.
188. Brockman, H.: Fortschr. Chem. Org. Naturst. 18:1, 1960.
189. Sobell, H. M., and Jain, S. C.: J. Mol. Biol. 68:21, 1972.
190. Goldberg, I. H., and Friedman, P. A.: Pure Appl. Chem. 28:499, 1971.
191. Wells, R. D., and Larson, J. E.: J. Mol. Biol. 49:319, 1970.
192. Remers, W. A.: The Chemistry of Antitumor Antibiotics, vol. 1. New York, Wiley, 1979.
193. McGovern, J. P.: Pharmacologic principles. In Dorr, R. T., and Von Hoff, D. D. (eds.), Cancer Chemotherapy Handbook. 2nd ed. Norwalk, CT, Appleton & Lange, 1994, pp. 15–34.
194. DuBost, N., et al.: C. R. Acad. Sci. Paris 257:1813, 1963.
195. Grein, A., et al.: Giorn. Microbiol. 11:109, 1963.
196. DiMarco, A., et al.: Cancer Chemother. Rep. 53:33, 1969.
197. Rauscher, F. J., Jr.: Special Communication from the Director, National Cancer Program, June 20, 1975.
198. Gause, G. F., et al.: Antibiotiki 18:675, 1973.
199. Brockman, H.: Fortschr. Chem. Org. Naturst. 21:1, 1963.
200. Arcamone, F., et al.: Tetrahedron Lett. 1968:3349.
201. Oki, T., et al.: J. Antibiot. 28:830, 1975.
202. DiMarco, A.: Daunomycin and related antibiotics. In Gottlieb, D. and Shaw, D. (eds.). Antibiotics, I. New York, Springer-Verlag, 1967, pp. 190–210.
203. Lown, J. W., et al.: Biochem. Biophys. Res. Commun. 76:705, 1979.
204. Bachur, N. R., and Gee, M.: J. Pharmacol. Exp. Ther. 177:567, 1971.
205. Bachur, N. R.: J. Med. Chem. 19:651, 1976.
206. Umezawa, H., et al.: J. Antibiot. 32:1082, 1979.
207. Isreal, M, and Modest, E.: U.S. Patent 4,035,566, July 12, 1977.
208. Steinberg, G., et al.: J. Urol. 163:761, 2000.
209. Bhuyan, B. K., and Dietz, A.: Antimicrob. Agents Chemother. 1965: 836.

210. Eckle, E., et al.: Tetrahedron Lett. 21:507, 1980.
211. McGovren, J. P., et al.: Invest. New Drugs 2:359, 1984.
212. Berlin, Y. A.: Nature 218:193, 1968.
213. Rao, K. V., et al.: Antibiot. Chemother. 12:182, 1962.
214. Nayak, R., et al.: FEBS Lett. 30:157, 1973.
215. Gauze, G. F.: Olivomycin, chromomycin, and mithramycin. In Corcoran, J. W., and Hahn, F. E. (eds.). Antibiotics, III. New York, Springer-Verlag, 1975, pp. 197–202.
216. Kersten, W., and Kersten, H.: Biochem. Z. 341:174, 1965.
217. Umezawa, H., et al.: J. Antibiot. Ser. A. 19:260, 1966.
218. Umezawa, H., et al.: J. Antibiot. Ser. A. 19:210, 1966.
219. Ikekawa, T., et al.: J. Antibiot. Ser. A. 17:194, 1964.
220. Argoudelis, A. A., et al.: J. Antibiot. 24:543, 1971.
221. Takita, T., et al.: J. Antibiot. 31:1073, 1978.
222. Sugiura, Y., and Kikuchi, T.: J. Antibiot. 31:1310, 1978.
223. Umezawa, H., et al.: J. Antibiot. 25:409, 1972.
224. Nakayama, Y., et al.: J. Antibiot. 26:400, 1973.
225. Muraoka, Y., et al.: J. Antibiot. 29:853, 1976.
226. Wakaki, S., et al.: Antibiot. Chemother. 8:288, 1958.
227. DeBoer, C., et al.: Antimicrob. Agents Annu. 1960:17, 1961.
228. Webb, J. S., et al.: J. Am. Chem. Soc. 84:3185, 1962.
229. Iyer, V. N., and Szybalski, W.: Science 145:55, 1964.
230. Tomasz, M.: Chem. Biol. Interactions 13:89, 1976.
231. Taylor, W. G., and Remers, W. A.: J. Med. Chem. 18:307, 1975.
232. Patrick, J. B., et al.: J. Am. Chem. Soc. 86:1889, 1964.
233. Meguro, S., et al.: Invest. New Drugs 2:381, 1984.
234. Bradner, W. T., et al.: Cancer Res. 45:6475, 1985.
234a. Nakatsubo, F., et al.: J. Am. Chem. Soc. 45:8115, 1977.
235. Kinoshita, S., et al.: J. Med. Chem. 14:103, 1971.
236. Vavra, J. J., et al.: Antibiot. Annu. 1960:230, 1960.
237. Herr, R. R., et al.: J. Am. Chem. Soc. 89:4808, 1967.
238. Hessler, E. J., and Jahnke, H. K.: J. Org. Chem. 35:245, 1970.
239. Kennedy, B. J.: Cancer 26:755, 1970.
240. Johnston, T. P., et al.: J. Med. Chem. 18:104, 1975.
241. Jarjaram, H. N., et al.: Cancer Chemother. Rep. Part I 59:481, 1975.
242. Hanka, L. J., et al.: J. Antibiot. 31:1211, 1978.
243. Chidester, G. G., et al.: J. Am. Chem. Soc. 103:7629, 1981.
244. Swensen, D. H., et al.: Proc. Am. Soc. Cancer Res. 24:238, 1983.
245. Li, L. H., et al.: Invest. New Drugs 9:137, 1991.
246. Remers, W. A. and Iyengar, B. S.: Antitumor antibiotics. In Foye, W. W. (ed.). Cancer Chemotherapeutic Agents. Washington, DC, 1995, p. 620.
247. Fujiwara, K., et al.: J. Org. Chem. 56:1688, 1991.
248. Lee, M. M., et al.: J. Antibiot. 42:1070, 1989.
249. Muller, W. and Crothers, D. M.: J. Mol. Biol. 35:251, 1968.
250. Farber, S.: JAMA 198:826, 1966.
251. Doroshow, J. H., et al.: J. Clin. Invest. 65:128, 1980.
252. Livingston, R. B., and Carter, S. K.: Single Agents in Cancer Chemotherapy. New York, Plenum Press, 1970.
253. Arcamone, F., et al.: Tetrahedron Lett. 1969:1007.
254. Chabner, B. A., et al.: N. Engl. J. Med. 292:1107, 1975.
255. Arcamone, F.: Doxorubicin Antibiotics. New York, Academic Press, pp. 259–264.
256. Berman, E., et al.: Blood 77:1666, 1991.
257. Steinberg, G., et al.: J. Urol. 163:761, 2000.
258. Umezawa, H., et al.: J. Antibiot. Ser. A., 19:200, 1966.
259. Blum, R. H., et al.: Cancer 31:903, 1973.
260. Einhorn, L. H., and Donohue, J.: Ann. Intern. Med. 87:293, 1977.
261. Wakaki, S., et al.: Antibiot. Chemother. 8:288, 1958.
262. Tomasz, M., et al.: Proc. Natl. Acad. Sci, U. S. A. 83:6702, 1986.
263. Baker, L. H.: The development of an acute intermittent schedule—mitomycin C. In Carter, S. K., and Crooke, S. T. (eds.). Mitomycin C: Current Status and New Developments. New York, Academic Press, 1969, p. 77.
264. Veldhius, L. D.: Lancet 1:1152, 1978.
265. Vavra, J. J., et al.: Antibiot. Annu. 1959–1960:2330, 1960.
266. Hessler, E. J., and Jahnke, H. K.: J. Am. Chem. Soc. 35:245, 1970.
267. Moertel, C. G., et al.: Cancer Chemother Rep. 55:303, 1971.
268. Hartwell, L. J.: Lloydia 31:71, 1968.
269. Kelley, M. G., and Hartwell, J. L.: J. Natl. Cancer Inst. 14:967, 1953.
270. Sartorelli, A. C., and Creasey, W. A.: Annu. Rev. Pharmacol. 9:51, 1969.
271. Long, B. H., et al.: Cancer Res. 45:3106, 1985.
272. Svoboda, G.: Lloydia 24:173, 1961.
273. Neuss, N., et al.: J. Am. Chem. Soc. 86:1440, 1964.
274. Creasey, W. A.: Vinca alkaloids and colchicine. In Sartorelli, A. C., and Johns, D. J. (eds.). Handbook of Experimental Pharmacology, vol. 38, part 2. New York, Springer-Verlag, 1975, pp. 670–694.
275. Barnett, C. J., et al.: J. Med. Chem. 21:88, 1978.
276. Bensch, K. G., and Malawista, S. E.: J. Cell. Biol. 40:95, 1969.
277. Journey, L. J., et al.: Cancer Chemother. Rep. 52:509, 1968.
278. Krishan, A.: J. Natl. Cancer Inst. 41:581, 1968.
279. Wani, M. C., et al.: J. Am. Chem. Soc. 93:2325, 1971.
280. Schiff, P. B. and Horwitz, S. B.: Proc. Natl. Acad. Sci. U. S. A. 77:1651, 1980.
281. Burris, H., et al.: Proc. Am. Soc. Clin. Oncol. 12:335, 1992.
282. Taylor, E. W.: J. Cell. Biol. 25:145, 1965.
283. Sawada, S., et al.: Chem. Pharm. Bull. 39:1446, 1991.
284. Wall, M., et al.: J. Am. Chem. Soc. 88:3888, 1966.
285. Kingsbury, W. D., et al.: Proc. Am. Soc. Cancer Res. 30:622, 1989.
286. Cassady, J. M. and Duros, J. D.: Anticancer Agents Based on Natural Product Models. New York, Academic Press, 1980.
287. Creaven, P. J. and Allen, L. M.: Clin. Pharmacol. Ther. 18:221, 1975.
288. Ross, W., et al.: Cancer Res. 44:5857, 1984.
289. Keller-Juslen, C., et al.: J. Med. Chem. 14:936, 1971.
290. Dorr, R. T. and Von Hoff, D. D.: Cancer Chemotherapy Handbook. 2nd ed. Norwalk, CT, Appleton & Lange, 1994, p. 883.
291. Pui, C. H., et al.: N. Engl. J. Med. 321:2682, 1991.
292. Owellen, R. J., et al.: Cancer Res. 35:975, 1977.
293. Noble, R. L., and Beir, C. T.: Experimental observations concerning the mode of action of Vinca alkaloids. In Shedden, W. I. H. (ed.). The Vinca Alkaloids in the Chemotherapy of Malignant Disease. Alburcham, England, John Sherrat and Sons, 1986, p. 4.
294. DeVita, V. T., et al.: Cancer 30:1495, 1972.
295. Brown, T., et al.: J. Clin. Oncol. 9:1261, 1991.
296. Weiss, R. B., et al.: J. Clin. Oncol. 8:1263, 1990.
297. Denis, J.: J. Org. Chem. 56:1957, 1990.
298. Piccart, M.: Anti-Cancer Drugs 6:7, 1995.
299. Rosenberg, B., et al.: Nature 205:698, 1965.
300. Rosenberg, B., et al.: J. Bacteriol. 93:716, 1967.
301. Rosenberg, B., et al.: Nature 222:385, 1969.
302. Gale, G. R.: Platinum compounds. In Sartorelli, A. C., and Johns, D. J. (eds.). Handbook of Experimental Pharmacology, vol. 38, part 2. New York, Springer-Verlag, 1975, pp. 829–838.
303. Rozencweig, M., et al.: Cisplatin. In Pinedo, H. M. (ed.). Cancer ChemotherapyAmsterdam, Excerpta Medica, 1979, p. 107.
304. Kennedy, B. J.: Proc. Am. Soc. Clin. Oncol. Annu. Meet., Atlanta, GA, May 17–19, 1986: Abstr. 533.
305. Mathe, G., et al.: Biomed. Pharmacother. 43:237, 1989.
306. Gibbons, G. R., et al.: Cancer Res. 49:1402, 1989.
307. Stearns, B., et al.: J. Med. Chem. 6:201, 1963.
308. Krakoff, I. H., et al.: Cancer Res. 28:1559, 1968.
309. Brown, N. C., et al.: Biochem. Biophys. Res. Commun. 30:522, 1968.
310. Brockman, R. W., et al.: Cancer Res. 30:2358, 1970.
311. Hewlett, J. S.: Proc. Am. Assoc. Cancer Res. 13:119, 1972.
312. Kidd, J. G.: J. Exp. Med. 98:565, 1953.
313. McCoy, T. A., et al.: Cancer Res. 19:591, 1959.
314. Mashburn, L. T., and Wriston, J. C., Jr.: Arch. Biochem. Biophys. 105:450, 1964.
315. Wriston, J. C., Jr.: Enzymes 4:101, 1971.
316. Hrushesky, W. J., et al.: Med. Pediatr. Oncol. 2:441, 1976.
317. Broome, J. D., and Schwartz, J. H.: Biochim. Biophys. Acta 138:637, 1967.
318. Manetta, A., et al.: Gynecol. Oncol. 36:93, 1990.
319. Ames, M. M., et al.: Cancer Res. 43:500, 1983.
320. Pressman, B. C., et al.: J. Biol. Chem. 238:401, 1963.
321. Mihich, E.: Pharmacologist 5:270, 1963.
322. Von Hoff, D. D., et al.: New anticancer drugs. In Pinedo, H. M. (ed.). Cancer Chemotherapy. Amsterdam, Excerpta Medica, 1979, pp. 126–166.
323. Wilson, W. R.: Chem. N. Z. 37:148,1973.
324. Atwell, G. J., et al.: J. Med. Chem. 15:611, 1972.
325. Murdock, K.C., et al.: J. Med. Chem. 22:1024, 1979.
326. Crespi, M. D., et al.: Biochem. Biophys. Res. Commun. 136:521, 1986.
327. Showalter, H. D., et al.: J. Med. Chem. 30:121, 1987.
328. Fry, D. W., et al.: Biochem. Pharmacol. 34:3499, 1985.
329. Myers, C. E., et al.: Proc. Am. Soc. Clin. Oncol. 9:133, 1990.
330. Larsen, A. K., et al.: Proc. Am. Assoc. Cancer Res. 32:338, 1991.
331. McClellan, C. A., et al.: Proc. Am. Assoc. Cancer Res. 33:273, 1992.

332. Folkman, J., and Klagsbrun, M.: Science 235:442, 1987.
333. Keller, J., et al.: Cancer Treat. Rep. 70:1221, 1986.
334. Warrell, R. P, Jr., et al.: Cancer 51:1982, 1983.
335. Boehm, M. F., et al.: J. Med. Chem. 37:2930, 1994.
336. Peck, R., and Bollag, W.: Eur. J. Cancer. 27:53, 1991.
337. Epstein, J.: J. Am. Acad. Dermatol. 15:772, 1986.
338. Agarwalla, V. R., et al.: Cancer Res. 60:6033, 2000.
339. Blazer, B. R., et al.: Blood 73:849, 1989.
340. Dougherty, T. J., et al.: Photoradiation therapy—clinical and drug advances. In Kessel, D., and Daugherty, T. J. (eds.). Photoporphyrin Photosentization, New York, Plenum Press, 1983.
341. Bristol Laboratories: Platinol Product Monograph; Syracuse, NY
342. Reed, F. F., et al.: Proc. Natl. Acad. Sci. U. S. A. 84:5024, 1987.
343. Einhorn, L. H., and Donohue, J.: Ann. Intern. Med. 87:293, 1977.
344. Einhorn, L. H.: Combination chemotherapy with cis-diaminedichloro-platinum, vinblastine, and bleomycin in disseminated testicular cancer. In Carter, S. K, et al. (eds.). Bleomycins: Current Status and New Developments. New York, Academic Press, 1978.
345. Harrison, R. C., et al.: Inorg. Chem. Acta 46:L15, 1980.
346. Dorr, R. T., and Von Hoff, D. D.: Cancer Chemotherapy Handbook. 2nd ed. Norwalk, CT, Appleton & Lange, 1994, p. 260.
347. Hantzsch, A.: Ann. 299:99, 1898.
348. Donehower, R. C.: In Chabner, B. (ed.). Pharmacological Principles of Cancer Treatment. Philadelphia, W.B. Saunders, 1982, pp. 269–275.
349. Jackson, R. C., et al.: Fed. Proc. 28:601, 1969.
350. Haskell, C. M., et al.: N. Engl. Med. 281:1028, 1969.
351. Capizzi, R. L., et al.: Ann. Intern. Med. 24:893, 1971.
352. Murdock, K. C., et al.: J. Med. Chem. 22:1024, 1979.
353. Alberts, D. S., et al.: Cancer Res. 45:1879, 1985.
354. Crespi, M. M., et al.: Biochem. Biophys. Res. Commun. 136:521, 1986.
355. Arlin, Z., et al.: Proc. Am. Soc. Clin. Oncol. 10:223, 1991.
356. Kelsen, D. P., et al.: Cancer 46:2009, 1980.
357. Rizvi, N. A.: Clin. Cancer Res. 5:1658, 1999.
358. McColl, S. R., et al.: Blood 73:588, 1989.
359. Arnaout, M. A., et al.: J. Clin. Invest. 7:597, 1986.
360. Gorski, J., et al.: J. Cell. Comp. Physiol. 66:91, 1965.
361. Jensen, E. V., and Jacobson, H. I.: Recent Prog. Horm. Res. 18: 387,1962.
362. Bruchovsky, N., and Wilson, J. D.: J. Biol. Chem. 243:2012, 1968.
363. Sherman, R. R., et al.: J. Biol. Chem. 245:6085, 1970.
364. Wira, C., and Munck, A.: J. Biol. Chem. 245:3436, 1970.
365. Schinzinger, A.: 18th Kongr. Beilage Centralblatt Chir. 29:5, 1889.
366. Dao, T. L.: Some current thoughts on adrenalectomy. In Segaloff, A., et al. (eds.). Current Concepts of Breast Cancer. Baltimore, Williams & Wilkins, 1967, pp. 189–199.
367. Kennedy, B. J.: Cancer 18:1551, 1965.
368. Pearson, O. H., et al.: Estrogens and prolactin in mammary cancer. In Dao, T. L. (ed.). Estrogen Target Tissues and Neoplasia. Chicago, University of Chicago Press, 1972, pp. 287–305.
369. Heel, R. C., et al.: Drugs 16:1, 1978.
370. Beckett, V. L., and Brennan, M. J.: Surg. Gynecol. Obstet. 109:235, 1959.
371. Dao, T. L.: Pharmacology and clinical utility of hormones in hormone related neoplasms. In Sartorelli, A. C., and Johns, D. J. (eds.). Handbook of Experimental Pharmacology, vol. 38, part 2. New York, Springer-Verlag, 1975, p. 172.
372. Tew, K. D. and Stearns, M. E.: Pharmacol. Ther. 43:299, 1989.
373. Nilsson, T., and Jonnson, G.: Cancer Chemother. Rep. 59:229, 1975.
374. Raynaud, J.-P.: Prostate 5:299, 1984.
375. Fur, B. J. A.: Horm. Res. 32:69, 1989.
376. Bloom, H. J. G.: Br. J. Cancer 25:250, 1971.
377. Kelley, R., and Baker, W.: Clinical observations on the effect of progesterone in the treatment of metastatic endometrial carcinoma. In Pinkus, G., and Vollmer, E. P. (eds.). Biological Activities of Steroids in Relation to Cancer. New York, Academic Press, 1960, pp. 427–443.
378. Dougherty, T. F., and White, A.: Am. J. Anat. 77:81, 1965.
379. Heilmanii, F. R., and Kendall, E. C.: Endocrinology 34:416, 1944.
380. Dao, T. L.: Third National Cancer Conference Proceedings. Philadelphia, J. B. Lippincott, 1957, pp. 292–296.
381. Hart, M. M., and Straw, J. A.: Steroids 17:559, 1971.
382. Bergenstal, D. M., et al.: Ann. Intern. Med. 53:672, 1960.
383. Coy, D. H., et al.: J. Med. Chem. 19:423, 1976.
384. Dutta, A. S., et al.: J. Med. Chem. 21:1018, 1978.
385. Pluorde, P. V., et al.: Breast Cancer Res. Treat. 30:103, 1994.

386. Guidici, D., et al.: J. Steroid Biochem. 30:391, 1998.
387. Bhatreagar, A. S., et al.: J. Steroid Biochem. Mol. Biol. 37:1021, 1990.
388. Haller, H. L., et al.: J. Am. Chem. Soc. 67:1600, 1945.
389. Cueto, C., and Brown, J. H. V.: Endocrinology 62:326, 1958.
390. Ringold, H. E., Batres, E., Halpern, O., and Necoecha, E.: J. Am. Chem. Soc. 81:427, 1959.
391. Fried, J., Thoma, R. W., and Elingsberg, A.: J. Am. Chem. Soc. 75: 5764, 1953.
392. Ringold, H. E., Ruelas, J. P., Batres, E., and Djerassi, C.: J. Am. Chem. Soc. 81:3712, 1959.
393. Imperial Chemical Industries: Belg. Patent 637,389, Mar. 13, 1964.
394. Bedford, G. R., and Richardson, D. N.: Nature 212:733, 1966.
395. Adam, H. K., et al.: Proc. Am. Assoc. Cancer Res. 20:47, 1979.
396. Jordan, V. C., and Jaspan, T.: J. Endocrinol. 68:453, 1976.
397. Kangas, L.: Prog. Cancer Res. Ther. 35:374, 1988.
398. Baker, J. W., et al.: J. Med. Chem. 10:93, 1967.
399. Neri, R., et al.: Endocrinology 91:427, 1972.
400. Tucker, H., et al.: J. Med. Chem. 31:954, 1988.
401. Blackledge, G., et al.: Anti-Cancer Drugs 7:27, 1996.
402. Niculescu-Duvas, I., et al.: J. Med. Chem. 10:172, 1967.
403. Forshell, G. P., et al.: Invest. Urol. 14:128, 1976.
404. Parmer, H., et al.: Lancet 2:1201, 1988.
405. Allen, J. M., et al.: Br. Med. J. 286:1607, 1983.
406. Edwards, P. N., and Lange, M. S.: U.S. Patent 4,935,437, June 19, 1990.
407. Plourde, P. V., et al.: Breast Cancer Res. Treat. 30:103, 1994.
408. Bowman, R. M., et al.: U.S. Patent 4,937, 250, June 26, 1990.
409. Buzder, A.: Anti-Cancer Drugs 11:609, 2000.
410. Yarden, Y. and Ullrich, A.: Annu. Rev. Biochem. 57:443, 1988.
411. Dobrusin, E. M. and Fry, D. W.: Annu. Rep. Med. Chem. 27:169, 1992.
412. Levitzki, A. and Gazit, A.: Science 267:1782, 1995.
413. Buchdinger, E., et al.: Proc. Natl. Acad. Sci. U. S. A. 91:2334, 1994.
414. Buchdinger, E., et al.: Cancer Res. 56:100, 1996.
415. Bolton, G. L., et al.: Annu. Rep. Med. Chem.: 29:165, 1994.
416. Marciano, D., et al.: J. Med. Chem.: 38:1267, 1995.
417. Perez-Sala, D, et al.: Proc. Natl. Acad. Sci. U. S. A. 88:3043, 1991.
418. James, G. L., et al.: Science 260:1937, 1993.
419. Zimmerman, J.: U.S. Patent 5,521,184, May 28, 1996.
420. Morton, D.: Report to the American Association for the Advancement of Science, San Francisco, February, 1974.
421. O'Brien, P. H.: J. S. C. Med. Assoc. 68:466, 1972.
422. Goodnight, J. E., Jr., and Morton, D. L.: Annu. Rev. Med. 29:231, 1978.
423. Sanders, H. J.: Chem. Eng. News. Dec. 23, 1974, p. 74.
424. Hadden, J. W., et al.: Cell. Immunol. 20:98, 1985.
425. Farrar, J. J., et al.: Annu. Rep. Med. Chem. 19:191, 1984.
426. Facts and Comparisons. St. Louis, Facts and Comparisons, 1986, p. 683b.
427. Dorr, R. T. and Von Hoff, D. D.: Cancer Chemotherapy Handbook. 2nd ed. Norwalk, CT., Appleton & Lange, 1994, pp. 564–582,.
428. Bernard, O., et al.: Proc. Natl. Acad. Sci. U. S. A. 84:2125, 1987.
429. Mazumdar, A., and Rosenberg, S. A.: J. Exp. Med. 159:495, 1984.
430. Hanck, J.: Clin. Cancer Res. 5:281, 1999.
431. Potter, M.: Curr. Opin. Oncol. Endocr. Metab. Invest. Drugs 1:291, 1999.
432. Badalament, R. A., et al.: J. Clin. Oncol. 5:441, 1987.
433. Köhler, G., and Milstein, C.: Nature 256:485, 1975.
434. Nisnoff, A.: J. Immunol. 147:2429, 1991.
435. LoBuglio, A. F., et al.: Proc. Natl. Acad. Sci. U. S. A. 86:4220, 1989.
436. Tempest, P. R., et al.: Biotechnology 9:266, 1991.
437. Hale, G., et al.: Lancet 2:1394, 1988.
438. Presta, L.: Annu. Rep. Med. Chem. 29:317, 1994.
439. Carter, P., et al.: Breast Dis. 11:103, 2000.
440. Rodwell, J. D. and McKearn, T. J.: Biotechnology 3:889, 1985.
441. Chua, M. M., et al.: Biochim. Biophys. Acta 800:291, 1984.
442. Pastan, I., and Fiitzgerald, D.: Science 254:1173, 1991.
443. Senter, P. D.: FASEB J. 4:188, 1990.
444. Cattell, L., et al.: Chimicaoggi 1989:51, 1989.
445. Columbat, P., et al.: Blood 97:101, 2001.
446. Foran, J. M., et al.: J. Clin. Oncol. 18:317, 2000.
447. Kunstman, M., et al.: U.S. Patent 5,714,586, Feb. 3, 1998.
448. Radich, J., and Sievers, E.: Oncology 14:125, 2000.
449. Syed, I. B., and Hosain, F.: Toxicol. Appl. Pharmacol. 22:150, 1072.

450. Peck, D. R., and Hudson, D.: Br. Patent. 1.230,121.
451. Goeckler, W. F.: Nucl. Med. Biol. 13:479, 1986.
452. Nolte, D., et al.: Dtsch. Med. Wochenschr. 108:1190, 1978.
453. Schramm, C. H.: J. Am. Chem. Soc. 77:6231, 1955.
454. Brock, N., et al.: Eur. J. Cancer Clin. Oncol. 18:1377, 1982.
455. Piper, J. A., et al.: J. Med. Chem. 12:236, 1969.
456. Miller, W. D.: U.S. Patent 4,764,614, August 16, 1988.
457. Mignatti, P., and Rifkin, D. B.: Physiol. Rev. 73:1. 1993.
458. Henkin, J.: Annu. Rep. Med. Chem. 28:151, 1993.
459. Redwood, S. M., et al.: Cancer 69:1212, 1992.
460. Nakajima, M., et al.: J. Biol. Chem. 266(15):9661, 1991.
461. Eisenstein, R.: Pharmacol. Ther. 49:1, 1991.
462. Moses, M. A., et al.: Science 248:1408, 1990.
463. Sakamoto, N., et al.: Cancer Res. 51:903, 1991.
464. Maione, T. E., et al.: Science 247:77, 1990.
465. Folkman, J., et al.: Science 243:1490, 1989.
466. Wilks, J. W., et al.: Proc. Am. Assoc. Cancer Res. 31:60, 1990.
467. Mitchell, M. A., and Wilks, J. W.: Annu. Rep. Med. Chem. 27:139, 1992.
468. Ingber, D., et al.: Nature 348:555, 1990.
469. Ramanathan, M., et al.: Antisense Res. Dev. 3:3, 1993.
470. Kiely, J. S., Annu. Rep. Med. Chem. 29:297, 1994.
471. Lesnikowski, Z. J.: Biorg. Chem. 21:127, 1993.
472. Varma, R. S.: Syn. Lett. 1993:621, 1993.
473. Froehler, B. C., et al.: Tetrahedron Lett. 34:1003, 1993.
474. Ramasamy, K. S., et al.: Tetrahedron Lett.: 35:215, 1994.
475. Ratajczak, M. Z., et al.: Proc. Natl. Acad. Sci. U. S. A. 89:11823, 1992.
476. Lingner, J., et al.: Science 276:561, 1977.
477. Hamilton, S. E., et al.: Biochemistry 36:11873, 1977.
478. Wheelhouse, R. T., et al.: J. Am. Chem. Soc. 120:3621, 1998.
479. Perry, P. J., et al.: J. Med. Chem. 41:4873, 1998.
480. International Human Genome Sequencing Consortium: Nature 409: 860, 2001.
481. Venter, J. C., et al.: Science 291:1304, 2001.
482. Marx, J.: Science 289:1670, 2000
483. MacBeath, G., and Schreiber, S.: Science 289:1760, 2000.

SELECTED READING

Dorr, R. T., and Von Hoff, D. D.: Cancer Chemotherapy Handbook. Norwalk, CT, Appleton & Lange, 1994.

Foye, W. O. (ed.): Cancer Chemotherapeutic Agents. Washington, DC, American Chemical Society, 1995.

Hall, T. C. (ed.): Prediction of Response to Cancer Chemotherapy. New York, Alan R. Liss, 1988.

Hickman, J. A., and Tritton, T. R.: Cancer Chemotherapy. Oxford, Blackwell Scientific Publications, 1993.

Keppler, B. K. (ed.): Metal Complexes in Cancer Chemotherapy. New York, Weinheim, 1993.

Oldham, R. K. (ed.): Principles of Cancer Biotherapy. New York, Raven Press, 1987.

Pinedo, H. M., and Giaccone, G. (eds.): Drug Resistance in the Treatment of Cancer. Cambridge, United Kingdom, Cambridge University Press, 1998.

Powis, G., and Hacker, M. (eds.): The Toxicity of Anticancer Drugs. New York, Pergamon Press, 1991.

Schilsky, R. L., Milano, G. A., and Ratain, M. J. (eds.): Principles of Antineoplastic Drug Development and Pharmacology. New York, Marcel Dekker, 1996.

Teicher, B. A. (ed.): Cancer Chemotherapeutics. Totowa, N. J., Humana Press, 1997.

Wright, G. L., Jr.: Monoclonal Antibodies and Cancer. New York, Marcel Dekker, 1984.

Agents for Diagnostic Imaging

TIM B. HUNTER, T. KENT WALSH, AND JACK N. HALL

Diagnostic imaging encompasses a group of techniques used in the diagnosis and treatment of disease. These techniques often use chemical agents to improve the information provided in the imaging. This chapter is a discussion of the pharmacology, chemistry, and physics of those agents used in medical imaging.

Medical imaging techniques often present less risk to patients than direct surgical visualization. Also, they often provide information or treatment methods that are simply not available by any other means. What these techniques have in common is that the information is often (but not always) displayed as an image for interpretation by a physician trained to evaluate the meaning of the image in the context of pathophysiology. Also, all of the techniques use physical phenomena (electromagnetic radiation, ultrasonic waves) that can pass through tissue to convey the internal information necessary to create an image. From that point, the techniques of medial imaging diverge in their physical means, methods, and the information that they can provide.

Medical imaging began with Roentgen's discovery of x-rays in 1895, and it has been the domain of diagnostic radiology since then. In its earliest days, the specialty of radiology used x-rays to produce images of the chest and skeleton. At the present time, diagnostic radiology uses ionizing radiation (x-rays), magnetic resonance imaging (MRI) techniques, radionuclides (nuclear medicine), and high-frequency sound waves (ultrasound) to produce diagnostic images of the body. Today, radiologists and other physicians also use diagnostic imaging techniques to guide themselves in interventional procedures, such as organ biopsy or abscess drainage.

INTRODUCTION TO RADIATION

Radiation is the propagation of energy through space or matter. In chemical reactions, only the valence electrons of an atom are affected, and the nucleus remains unchanged. Nuclear reactions may result from bombardment of a stable nucleus with high-energy particles or decomposition of an unstable nucleus. The nuclei of atoms are of two kinds: stable and radioactive. Radioactive nuclei have more internal energy than nuclei with a stable arrangement of protons and neutrons. They obtain stability by emitting energy in the form of particulate and electromagnetic radiation.

Ionizing radiation is radiation that when interacting with matter can cause changes in the atomic or nuclear structure of matter. The first type of ionizing radiation is particulate, which includes alpha (α), beta (β^-), positron (β^+), proton (p), and neutron (n) particles. Radiation is energy in the form of kinetic energy and on the atomic scale is usually measured in electron volts (eV). By definition, an *electron volt* is the

energy needed to accelerate an electron across a potential difference of 1 volt. The second type of ionizing radiation is called *electromagnetic radiation*. Electromagnetic radiation is an electric and magnetic disturbance that is propagated through space at the speed of light. This type of radiation has no mass and is unaffected by either an electrical or magnetic field because it has no charge. These properties are shared by radio waves (10^{10} to 10^{-6} eV), microwaves (10^{-6} to 10^{-2} eV), infrared (10^{-2} to 1 eV), visible light (1 to 2 eV), ultraviolet (2 to 100 eV), or x-rays and gamma (γ) rays (100 to 10^{+7} eV). The various forms of electromagnetic radiation differ in their frequency and, therefore, their energy. The energy of electromagnetic radiation can be calculated in electron volts from the following equation:

$$E = h\nu = \frac{hc}{\lambda}$$

where h is Planck's constant (4.13×10^{-15} eV-sec), ν is the frequency (hertz), c is the speed of light (cm/sec), and λ is the wavelength (cm). The difference between x-rays and γ-rays is based on where they originate; x-rays come from outside the nucleus, while γ-rays originate in the nucleus of an atom. X-rays and γ-rays can exhibit some particulate properties, so they are sometimes called *photons*.

Applying a very high voltage (20,000 to 150,000 volts) to a glass vacuum tube that contains a cathode and a rotating anode produces x-rays used in diagnostic radiology (Fig. 13-1). The cathode is a filament that is heated to a very high temperature, which provides a copious source of electrons. The electrons are accelerated toward the positively charged anode (tungsten). When the accelerated electrons strike the anode (called the *target*), x-rays are produced. The distribution of x-rays is a continuous spectrum, and the low-energy x-rays, which will not travel through the body to the x-ray film, are absorbed by a filter (aluminum). An invaluable modification of the x-ray system is fluoroscopy. This modality allows one to visualize organs in motion, position the patient for spot film exposures, instill contrast media into hollow cavities, and, most importantly, insert catheters into arteries. Figure 13-2 shows a schematic of a fluoroscopic system.

With conventional radiography and with computed tomography (CT) (sometimes called computed axial tomography [CAT]) scanning, organs and tissues are made visible according to how well they attenuate x-rays. The attenuation of x-rays by tissues is a complex process that depends on many factors, including the energy of the x-ray beam and the density of the tissue. Bone has an average density of about 1.16 g/cm^3, which accounts for its ability to absorb most of the radiation it encounters. CT scanning (Fig. 13-3) uses ordinary x-ray energies for imaging but uses complex

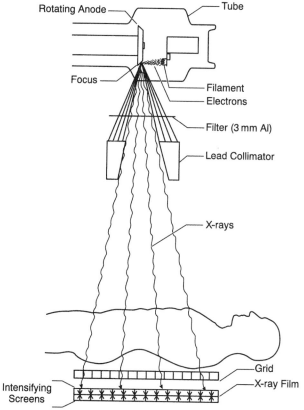

Figure 13–1 ■ Schematic diagram of an x-ray tube producing x-rays that pass through the patient and expose the photographic film. The photographic film will not stop the x-rays, so a plastic screen coated with fluorescent particles that are activated by the x-rays emits light to expose the film within a light-tight film cassette. As x-rays pass through the body, some of them are scattered, so a moving grid device composed of alternating strips of lead and plastic decreases the scattered x-rays that degrade the image.

mathematical reconstructions to produce images of the body in the axial and other planes. In the process, it can increase the visibility of small differences in the radiographic densities between tissues to a far greater extent than ordinary radiographic film can.

Radionuclides undergoing transformation processes, called *radioactive decay,* in most cases involve transmutation of one element into another. A nucleus may undergo several decays before reaching a stable configuration. A nuclear particle, either a proton or a neutron, is called a *nucleon.* A species of atom with a specified number of neutrons and protons in its nucleus is called a *nuclide.* Nuclides with the same number of protons and a different number of neutrons are called *isotopes.* Nuclides with same atomic mass are called *isobars.* Nuclides with the same number of protons and atomic mass but at two energy levels are called *isomers.*

The nucleus has energy levels analogous to the orbital electron shells but at a higher energy. The lower energy level is called the *ground (g) state,* and the highest energy level is called the *metastable (m) state.* Nuclides are all species of elements, of which there are about 265 stable nuclides, 330 naturally occurring radionuclides, and more than 2,500 artificially produced radionuclides. In accordance with a rec-

ommendation of the International Union of Pure and Applied Chemistry, the following notation should be used for the identification of a nuclide:

$$_Z^A X_N^{(valence)} \quad \text{Example: } _{53}^{131}I_{78}^{-1}$$

where X is the symbol of the chemical element to which the nuclide belongs, A represents the atomic mass (number of neutrons plus the number of protons), and Z represents the atomic number (number of protons). The right side of the element is reserved for the oxidation state, and N represents the number of neutrons. For most medical applications, it suffices to indicate the element chemical symbol and the mass number (i.e., ^{131}I, I-131, or iodine-131).

The radionuclide at the beginning of the decay sequence is referred to as the *parent,* and the radionuclide produced by the decay is referred to as the *daughter,* which may be stable or radioactive. There are five types of radioactive decay, distinguished according to the nature of the primary radiation event. A radioactive nucleus may decay by more than one method. The dominant method at any given time depends on such factors as the size of the nucleus and the balance of protons and neutrons. The types of decay described below are in order of how commonly they are used in current diagnostic nuclear medicine practice:

1. **Isomeric transition (IT).** Isomeric transition is a decay process involving neither the emission nor the capture of a particle. The nucleus simply changes from a higher to a lower energy level by emitting γ-rays. Therefore, both mass number and atomic

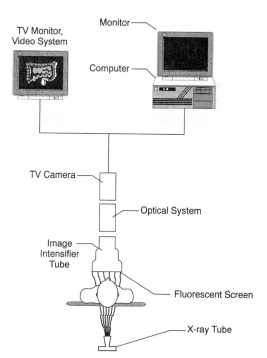

Figure 13–2 ■ Schematic diagram of a fluoroscopic unit with the x-ray tube located behind the patient and a fluorescent screen–image intensifier system positioned on the opposite side. Amplification of the faint fluorescing image by the image intensifier increases brightness level and contrast. The real-time fluoroscopic images can be shown on a television camera for convenient viewing during the examination and stored on videotape, video disk, or computer for later viewing without distortion or destruction of the images.

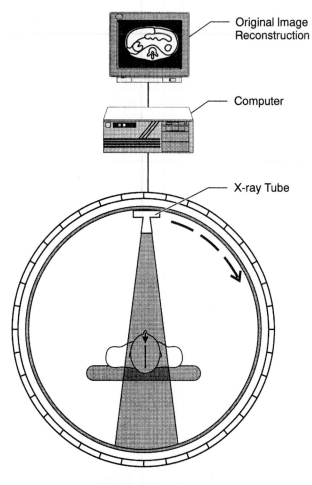

Radiation Detectors

Figure 13–3 ■ Schematic diagram of a computerized axial tomography (CAT) system that produces thin cross-sectional images of the body. An x-ray tube rotates around the patient, and the transmitted x-rays are detected by a circle of moving radiation detectors. The absorptions of x-rays by tissues of different densities are assigned numerical values (CT numbers). The computer uses complex algorithms to reconstruct an anatomical cross-sectional image on a television monitor.

number remain unchanged. The daughter nucleus is the same chemical element as the original nucleus. The original nucleus before the transition is said to be in a metastable (m) state.

$$\text{Example: } ^{99m}_{43}\text{Tc} \rightarrow ^{99}_{43}\text{Tc} + \gamma\text{-ray}$$

2. **Electron capture decay (EC).** The nucleus captures an electron from the electron cloud of the atom (mainly the K shell), and a proton becomes a neutron.

$$\text{Example: } ^{123}_{53}I \xrightarrow{EC} ^{123}_{52}Te + \tilde{a}? \; \rho\alpha\psi \; \gamma\text{-ray}$$

3. **Positron emission (β^+).** The nucleus emits a positive electron when a proton changes to a neutron. A γ-ray may or may not accompany the emission of the positron. A positron (particle of antimatter) emitted from the nucleus loses its kinetic energy, however, by interacting with surrounding atoms. It finally combines with a free electron from one of the surrounding atoms in an interaction in which the rest masses of both particles are given up as 2 γ-rays of 0.511 MeV emitted at 180° to each other. Einstein's theory of relativity states that mass and energy are equivalent and is represented by the following equation:

$$E = mc^2$$

where in the case of an electron, E represents energy equivalent to mass ($m = 9.109 \times 10^{31}$ kg) at rest, and c is the speed of light (3×10^8 m/sec). By using the proper units it can be shown that the mass of an electron is equivalent to 0.511 MeV. This is called *annihilation radiation*. It is used in a specialized imaging technique called *positron emission tomography* (PET).

$$\text{Example: } ^{18}_9F \rightarrow ^{18}_9O + \gamma\text{-ray}$$

$$\beta^+ + e^- \rightarrow 2 \; \gamma\text{-rays (0.511 MeV)}$$

4. **Beta-particle emission (β^-).** The nucleus emits a negative electron when a neutron changes to a proton. A γ-ray may or may not accompany the emission of a β particle.

$$\text{Example: } ^{131}_{53}I \xrightarrow{EC} ^{131}_{54}Xe + \beta^- + \gamma\text{-ray}$$

5. **Alpha-particle emission (α).** The nucleus emits an α particle, which consists of a helium nucleus without the electrons. If the emission of the α particle leaves the nucleus in an excited energy state, the excess energy is liberated in the form of a γ-ray.

$$\text{Example: } ^{226}_{88}Ra \rightarrow ^{222}_{86}Rn + ^4_2He + \gamma\text{-ray}$$

CHARACTERISTICS OF DECAY

It is impossible to predict when an individual atom of a radionuclide will decay. In quantitative terms, however, this transformation occurs at a rate that is characteristic of each specific radionuclide and is expressed as its physical half-life. This is the time in which one-half of the original number of atoms decay. The activity of radionuclides can be expressed in three ways: *(a)* in curies (Ci), millicuries (mCi), or microcuries (μCi); *(b)* in disintegrations per second (dps); and *(c)* in becquerels (Bq; 1 Bq = 1 dps). A curie is the quantity of any radionuclide that decays at a rate of 3.7×10^{10} dps. This number was chosen for a historical reason—this is the number of disintegrations per second in 1 g of radium. The international system of units has adopted the becquerel as the official unit of radioactivity, but the curie is still widely used, and we will use this unit in addition to the official unit. A relevant conversion factor to remember is the following:

$$1 \text{ millicurie (mCi)} = 37 \text{ megabequerels (MBq)}$$

The basic equation for radioactive decay is expressed as follows in terms of atoms:

$$N_t = N_0 \, e^{-\lambda t}$$

N_t (number of atoms at time t) and N_0 (number of atoms at time 0) can be replaced, however, with activities:

$$A_t = A_0 \, e^{-\lambda t}$$

where A_0 is the original activity in Ci, mCi, or μCi, A_t is the activity at time t, λ is the decay constant ($= 0.693/t_{1/2}$, the physical half-life); and $e^{-\lambda t}$ is the decay factor. An example of a radioactive decay calculation follows:

A sample of ^{123}I-sodium iodide had an activity of 200 μCi on May 14 at 12 noon C.S.T. What is the activity on May 15 at 3 PM E.S.T.? (Note: Calculations of elapsed time must also indicate variations in time zones—elapsed time in this case is 26 hours.)

$$(t_{1/2} = 13.2 \text{ hours})$$

$$A = (200 \ \mu\text{Ci}) \ e^{-\left[\dfrac{0.693 \times 26 \text{ hours}}{13.2 \text{ hours}}\right]}$$

$$A = (200 \ \mu\text{Ci}) \ (e^{-1.36})$$

$$A = (200 \ \mu\text{Ci}) \ (0.255)$$

$$A = 51.0 \ \mu\text{Ci}$$

BIOLOGICAL EFFECTS OF RADIATION

The absorption of ionizing radiation by living cells always produces effects potentially harmful to the irradiated organism. An undesirable aspect to the medical use of these types of radiation is that a small number of the atoms in the body tissues will have electrons removed as a result of the energies of these photons. Radiation that does this is often called *ionizing radiation* and is damaging to body tissues. Therefore, in using ionizing radiation, as in using other pharmaceutical agents, the risks must be balanced with the medical benefits provided for the patient.

The amount of radiation energy absorbed by tissue is called *radiation absorbed dose* and is specified in rads or millirads. A dose of 1 rad implies 100 ergs of energy absorbed per gram of any tissue. The unit of exposure for x-rays and γ radiation *in air,* the roentgen, is used to specify radiation levels in the environment. (One roentgen is the amount of radiation that produces 1 electrostatic unit of charge of either sign per 0.001293 g of air at STP.) The international system of units (SI) has adopted the gray (Gy) to replace the rad (1 Gy = 100 rads), but again we will use the more traditional units. In the case of x-rays or γ radiation for medical diagnosis, the roentgen and rad turn out to be numerically equivalent. The major difference between electromagnetic radiation (x-rays or γ-rays) and particulate type radiation (β and α particles) lies in the ability of electromagnetic rays to penetrate matter. Whereas β particles travel only a few millimeters before expending all their energy, x- and γ-rays distribute their energy more diffusely and travel through several centimeters of tissue. Therefore, particles deliver highly localized radiation doses, whereas x- and γ-rays deliver more uniform doses in a less concentrated way throughout the irradiated volume of tissue. The radiation dose of particles is more useful for a therapeutic dose of a radionuclide but not for a diagnostic dose. When cells are irradiated, damage is produced primarily by ionization and free radicals. Particles produce damage by ionization, whereas x-rays and γ-rays produce damage by free radicals. Free radicals are atoms or molecules with an unpaired electron.

The effects of large doses of radiation were derived from epidemiological studies of the atomic bomb survivors at Hiroshima and Nagasaki. Radiobiological damage from large doses of ionizing radiation can be caused by two different mechanisms. One mechanism is the *direct effect* of radiation, in which damage results from absorption of radiation energy directly in a critical biological site or target. The other, called the *indirect effect,* involves aqueous free radicals as intermediaries in the transfer of radiation energy to the biological molecules. All biological systems contain water as the most abundant molecule (70 to 90%), and radiolysis of water is the most likely event in the initiation of biological damage. The absorption of energy by a water molecule results in the ejection of an electron with the formation of a free radical ion ($H_2O^{\cdot+}$). The free radical ion dissociates to yield a hydrogen ion (H^+) and a hydroxyl free radical ($HO\cdot$). The hydroxyl free radicals combine to form hydrogen peroxide (H_2O_2), which is an oxidizing agent. In addition, hydrogen free radicals ($H\cdot$) can form, which can combine with oxygen (O_2) and form a hydroperoxy-free radical ($HO\cdot_2$). These two reaction intermediates are very reactive chemically and can attack and alter chemical bonds. The only significant "target" molecule for biological damage is DNA. Types of DNA damage include single- and double-chain breakage, and intermolecular or intramolecular cross-linking in the double-stranded DNA molecule. With the direct effect of radiation, the damage makes cell replication impossible, and cell death occurs. In the indirect effect of radiation, if the damage is not lethal but changes the genetic sequence or structure, mutations occur that may lead to cancer or birth of genetically damaged offspring. Some effects of radiation may develop within a few hours; others may take years to become apparent. Consequently, the effects of ionizing radiation on human beings may be classified as somatic (affecting the irradiated person) or genetic (affecting progeny).

Radiation dose can only be estimated and its "measurement" is called *radiation dosimetry*. In the case of x-ray exposure, most radiation "doses" in the literature are described as the entrance exposure (in roentgens per minute) to the patient. In diagnostic nuclear medicine procedures, patients are irradiated by radiopharmaceuticals localized in certain organs or distributed throughout their bodies. Since the radionuclides are taken internally, there are many variables, and the radiation absorbed dose (r.a.d. or rad) to individual patients cannot be measured but only estimated by calculation. The methods of calculating the absorbed dose to patients from radiopharmaceuticals were changed in 1964 and then revised by the Medical Internal Radiation Dose (MIRD) Committee under the auspices of the Society of Nuclear Medicine in 1991.

Although the effects of radiation are not totally understood, the benefits associated with low doses of radiation almost always outweigh any potential risks to individual patients. A large number of scientific and advisory groups have published risk estimates for ionizing radiation, but the most widely quoted is report number 5 of the National Academy of Sciences Committee on the Biological Effects of Ionizing Radiation (BEIR-V).[1]

Under normal circumstances, no radiation worker or patient undergoing diagnostic investigation by radiopharmaceutical or radiographic procedures should ever suffer from any acute or long-term injury. Typical radiation doses to patients from radiopharmaceuticals are similar to, or less than, those from radiographic procedures.

The first artificial radionuclide (phosphorus-30) was produced by the French radiochemists Frederic Joliet and Irene Curie. Nuclear medicine became a specialty in 1946 when radionuclides became available from cyclotrons and nuclear reactors. In many medical centers, nuclear medicine is con-

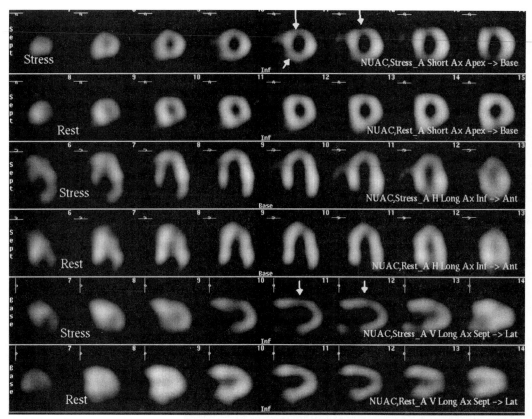

Figure 13–7 ■ SPECT myocardial perfusion study using thallium-201 as the radiotracer. SPECT images are three-dimensional and are often viewed in tomographic slices. The *long arrows* indicate the abnormally diminished myocardial perfusion in the anterior wall of the left ventricle during stress (exercise or pharmacological), compared with that of the same patient during rest. The stress and rest images are matched in spatial location for easier comparison. The *single short arrow* indicates an additional abnormal area in the inferior portion of the left ventricle. The abnormalities indicate that the patient has a high likelihood of significant coronary artery narrowing, which can be confirmed by coronary angiography.

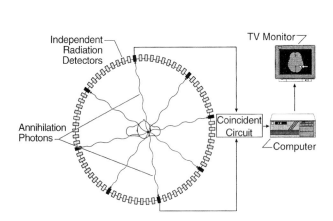

Figure 13–8 ■ Schematic diagram of a PET imaging system with multiple scintillation detectors that localize the positron decay along a line. By using multiple position-sensitive detectors around the patient, the annihilation photons are acquired along many parallel lines and many angles simultaneously with four rings of detectors (only one ring shown). After use of reconstruction algorithms, the internal distribution of the radioactivity can be determined and displayed on a cathode ray tube.

TABLE 13–1   PET Radiotracers

Positron Emitter	Radiotracer
Fluorine-18 (F-18)	F-18-haloperidol
	F-18 fluorodeoxyglucose (FDG)
	F-18 fluorodopa
	F-18 fluroethylspiperone
	F-18 fluorouracil
Nitrogen-13 (N-13)	N-13 ammonia
Carbon-11	C-11 Acetate
	C-11 carfentanil
	C-11 cocaine
	C-11 Depranyl
	C-11 leucine
	C-11 methionine
	C-11 methylspiperone
	C-11 raclopride
Oxygen 15	O-15 water
	O-15 oxygen
	O-15 carbon dioxide
Rubidium-82	Rubidium-82

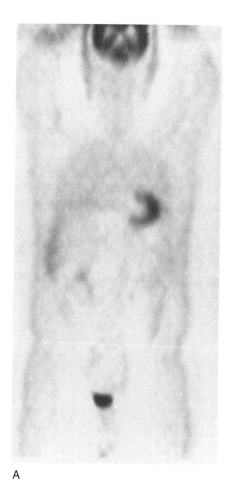

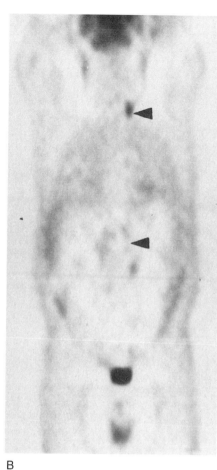

A   B

Figure 13–9 ■ PET whole-body images performed to detect metastases after injection of 4 mCi (148 MBq) of fluorine [¹⁸F]-2-fluoro-2-deoxy-D-glucose (F-18 FDG). **A.** Normal whole-body PET image (coronal view) obtained on a patient with lymphoma after treatment with chemotherapy and radiotherapy. The patient fasted for 12 hours to maintain the blood glucose level between 80 and 140 mg/100 mL. If the blood glucose level is not in that range, F-18 FDG uptake is decreased in the tumors because the mechanism of uptake is an increased rate of glycolysis. (Note increased brain and cardiac uptake because of high glycolytic rates in these organs.) **B.** PET whole-body image obtained with the same technique on a patient with pancreatic carcinoma. Abnormal sites of F-18 FDG uptake are seen in the upper abdomen, posterior mediastinum, and left lower neck *(arrows)* consistent with neoplastic involvement. (Note increased brain, but not cardiac, uptake of F-18 FDG in this patient who had a desirable blood glucose level for tumor imaging.)

clides such as carbon-11 ($t_{1/2}$ = 20 minutes), oxygen-15 ($t_{1/2}$ = 2 minutes), nitrogen-13 ($t_{1/2}$ = 10 minutes), and fluorine-18 ($t_{1/2}$ = 110 minutes). Table 13-1 shows examples of several positron radiotracers that have been investigated in the scientific literature.

Figure 13-9 shows PET whole-body images from patients as a cancer management modality.

RADIONUCLIDE PRODUCTION

The radionuclides used in nuclear medicine are artificially produced. This is accomplished when neutrons, protons, α particles, or other particles impinge on atomic nuclei and initiate a process of nuclear change. The artificial production of a radionuclide requires preparation of a target system, irradiation of the target, and chemical separation of the radionuclide produced from the target material. The radiochemical is converted to the desired radiopharmaceutical and quality assurance of the physical, chemical, and pharmaceutical qualities (i.e., sterility and apyrogenicity) of the final product is obtained. The systems used for practical production of radionuclides are a nuclear reactor, cyclotron, or radioisotope generator.

The shorthand nuclear physics notation of a cyclotron production reaction is as follows:

$$^{112}_{48}\text{Cd (p,2n)}^{111}_{49}\text{In}$$

where Cd-112 is the stable target material, a proton (p) is the bombarding particle, two neutrons (2n) are emitted from the nucleus, and In-111 is the radionuclide produced.

The introduction of radionuclide generators into nuclear medicine arose from the need to administer large doses of a short half-life radionuclide to obtain better statistics in imaging. In consideration of radioactive (parent and daughter) pairs, we can distinguish two general cases, depending on which of two radionuclides has the longer half-life. If the parent has a longer half-life than the daughter, a state of so-called radioactive equilibrium is reached. That is, after a certain time, the ratio of the disintegration rates of parent and daughter become constant. In the second case, if the parent half-life is shorter than that of the daughter, no equilibrium is reached at any time. Therefore, the general principle of the radionuclide generator is that the longer-lived parent is bound to some adsorbent material in a chromatographic ion exchange column and the daughter is eluted from the column with some solvent or gas. There are more than 100 possible generator systems for clinical use, but there is only one in routine use in nuclear medicine (the molybdenum-99/technetium-99m system). All of the molybdenum-99 at the present time is obtained as a fission product of uranium-235 in a nuclear reactor.

$$^{235}_{92}\text{U (n, fission)} \rightarrow ^{99}_{42}\text{Mo} + \text{other radionuclides}$$

By use of elegant inorganic radiochemistry, the molybdenum-99 is separated from the other radionuclides. Molybde-

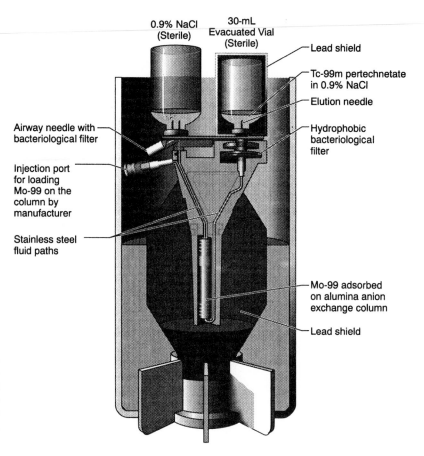

Figure 13–10 ■ Cross section of a radionuclide generator for the production of technetium-99m (Tc-99m) by sterile 0.9% sodium chloride elution of a sterile alumina (Al$_2$O$_3$) column that has molybdenum-99 (Mo-99) adsorbed on it. (Courtesy of Dupont–Pharma, Billerica, MA.)

num-99 ($t_{1/2}$ = 66 hours) decays by β-particle emission to technetium-99m ($t_{1/2}$ = 6 hours), which decays by isomeric transition (IT) to technetium-99 by emission of a γ-ray (140 keV). The anionic molybdate (^{99}MoO$_4^{-2}$) is then loaded on a column of alumina (Fig. 13-10). The molybdate ions adsorb firmly to the alumina, and the generator column is autoclaved to sterilize the system. Then the rest of the generator is assembled under aseptic conditions into its final form in a lead-shielded container. Each generator is eluted with sterile normal saline (0.9% sodium chloride). The column is an inorganic ion exchange column, and the eluate contains sodium pertechnetate, so the chloride ions (Cl$^-$) are exchanging for the pertechnetate ions (^{99m}TcO$_4^-$) but not molybdate ions (MoO$_4^{-2}$). The method for calculating how much daughter is present on the column at any given time is more complex, because it must consider the decay rates of the parent and daughter (Fig. 13-11). The simplified equation for any case in which both the parent and the daughter are radioactive and in equilibrium is as follows:

$$A_d = (A_p)\lambda_d\,[(e^{-\lambda pt} - e^{-\lambda dt})/(\lambda_d - \lambda_p)]$$

where A_p is the activity (mCi) of the parent, A_d is the activity of the daughter, λ_p and λ_d are their respective decay constants, and t is the time since the last elution of the generator. In the case of Mo-99 ($t_{1/2}$ = 66 hours), only 87.2% of the atoms decay to Tc-99m ($t_{1/2}$ = 6 hours), and 12.8% of the atoms decay directly to Tc-99. The generator system can be eluted several times per day to obtain more activity (mCi) per day because the increase in Tc-99m is a logarithmic function.

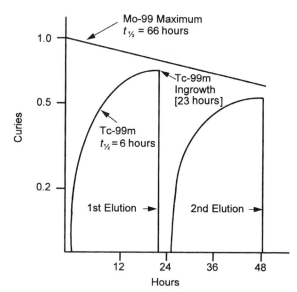

Figure 13–11 ■ Elution graph of radioactivity (exponential) versus time (linear) of the Mo-99m/Tc-99m radionuclide generator with sterile 0.9% sodium chloride for 2 days (actual generator is useful for 12 days postcalibration). The *upper straight line* represents the radioactive decay of the parent (Mo-99) to the daughter (Tc-99m), which reaches equilibrium at four half-lives of the daughter (6 hours × 4 = 24 hours).

TECHNETIUM RADIOCHEMISTRY

Element 43 in the periodic table, technetium, is a transition state metal and is the only "artificial" element with a lower atomic number than uranium. All 22 known isotopes of technetium are radioactive, and there are eight nuclear isomers. Because no stable isotopes of technetium exist, the chemistry has been poorly developed; however, milligram quantities of Tc-99 (a weak β-particle emitter; $t_{1/2} = 2.1 \times 10^5$ years) are now available for determination of the structures of the technetium complexes, and more than 150 structures have been characterized. The chemistry of technetium is similar to that of rhenium and is dominated by forming compounds by bonding between the electron-deficient metal and electronegative groups, which are capable of donating electron pairs. Some examples of these electronegative groups are sulfhydryl, carboxylic acid, amine, phosphate, oxime, hydroxyl, phosphine, and isonitrile.

Basically, all technetium radiopharmaceuticals are metal–electron donor complexes. Compounds that contain two or more electron donor groups and bind to a metal are called *chelating agents*. Technetium as a transition state element can have oxidation states from 1 to $+7$. As a pertechnetate (TcO_4^-) ion, technetium will not form many metal–donor complexes, although it can be reduced to species that will complex with a variety of monodentate, bidentate, or polydentate ligands. The oxidation state of technetium in various complexes and the actual structure are unknown for several of the compounds. Deutsch et al.[2] claim that the oxidation states that are most common in the chemistry of technetium are $+1$, $+3$, and $+5$. Technetium (TcO_4^-) can be reduced by a stannous salt, ascorbic acid, sodium borohydride, and electrolysis. The most common reducing agent is the stannous ion because of water solubility, stability, low toxicity, and effectiveness at room temperature.[3] Reviews of the chemistry of technetium are presented by Hjelstuen[4] and Schwochau,[5] but the stereochemistry of the technetium coordination complexes is not shown. An excellent review by Jurisson et al.[6] covers all coordination compounds used in nuclear medicine, with a special emphasis on Tc-99m complexes.

Tc-99m radiopharmaceuticals are by far the most commonly used radiotracers in day-to-day diagnostic nuclear medicine practice. In fact, most gamma cameras are designed to work most efficiently (crystal thickness and the electronics) with Tc-99m–based radiotracers. Tc-99m radiopharmaceuticals are prepared at the hospital or local nuclear pharmacy by combining $^{99m}TcO_2$ nonradioactive components in a sterile serum reaction vial. The primary chemical substances in the vial are the complexing agent (ligand) and reducing agent, usually some stannous salt (stannous chloride, stannous fluoride, or stannous tartrate). After preparation of the radiopharmaceutical, tests for radiochemical purity should be carried out to ensure that the radiotracer is in the right chemical form. The analytical methods used include paper and thin-layer chromatography, column chromatography, and solvent extraction. Likely radiochemical impurities include sodium pertechnetate ($Na^{99m}TcO_4$), some insoluble compound (i.e., reduced hydrolyzed technetium [TcO_2] or technetium–tin colloid), and a complex different from the one expected (i.e., ^{99m}Tc-monodentate rather than ^{99m}Tc-

bidentate ligand). The sterile serum vials containing the stannous salt and the ligand are lyophilized under a sterile inert gas atmosphere (i.e., nitrogen or argon). The ligand in the reaction vial determines the final chemical structure of the ^{99m}Tc-complex and the biological fate after intravenous injection of the radiopharmaceutical.

Technetium Radiopharmaceuticals

Technetium (^{99m}Tc) Albumin Injection. ^{99m}Tc albumin for injection is a sterile, colorless to pale yellow solution containing human albumin (MW ~60,000) radiolabeled with Tc-99m pertechnetate. The reducing agent is stannous tartrate, which reduces the $^{99m}TcO_4^-$ to an unknown oxidation state and is weakly chelated by the tartrate and possibly forms a complex with sulfhydryl groups on the albumin by ligand exchange. The precise structure of the stannous technetium–albumin complex is currently unknown. The patient receives an intravenous injection of 25 mCi (925 MBq) of Tc-99m albumin.

Multiple images of the blood in the heart are taken by electrocardiogram gating (R-R interval). The rising portion of the R wave coincides with end-diastole. These images are stored in a computer to reconstruct a movie of the beating heart. This procedure is sometimes called a *multigated acquisition* (MUGA) or a *radionuclide ventriculogram*. Information obtained by this technique includes cardiac chamber wall motion and calculation of ejection fraction. Indications for the procedure include evaluation of effects of coronary artery disease, follow-up of coronary artery bypass graft patients, heart failure, heart transplant evaluation (preoperative and postoperative), cardiomyopathies, and effects of cardiotoxic drugs (i.e., doxorubicin).

Technetium (^{99m}Tc) Albumin Aggregated. ^{99m}Tc–albumin aggregated is a sterile white suspension of human albumin aggregates formed by denaturing human albumin by heating at 80°C at pH 4.8 (isoelectric point of albumin). The precise structure of the stannous technetium–albumin aggregated complex is unknown at this time. The particle size and number can be estimated with a hemocytometer grid. The particle size of the suspension should be between 10 and 100 μm, with no particles greater than 150 μm. This agent is used clinically to image the pulmonary microcirculation for pulmonary embolus and to assess regional pulmonary function for surgery (i.e., lung transplants or resection). The patient receives an intravenous injection of 2 to 4 mCi (74 to 148 MBq) of the Tc-99m–albumin aggregates, which lodge in some of the small pulmonary arterioles and capillaries, and the distribution can be imaged. The number of aggregates recommended for good image quality and safety is 100,000 to 500,000 particles; thus, only a small fraction of the 280 billion capillaries are occluded. Multiple images of the lung are obtained to assess lung perfusion. The distribution of the particles in the lung is a function of regional blood flow; consequently, in the normal lung, the particles are distributed uniformly throughout the lung. When blood flow is occluded because of emboli, multiple segmental "cold" (decreased radioactivity) defects are seen. This procedure is almost always combined with a xenon-133 gas lung ventilation scan (should be normal in pulmonary embolism) and same-day chest radiograph x-ray (should be normal).

Technetium (⁹⁹ᵐTc) Albumin Colloid Injection.
⁹⁹ᵐTc–albumin colloid injection is a sterile, opalescent, colorless dispersion of colloidal human albumin labeled with Tc-99m pertechnetate after it is reduced with a stannous salt. The precise structure of the stannous technetium–albumin colloid complex is unknown at this time. The particle size may be examined with a hemocytometer grid. The particle size range of the colloid is 0.1 to 5.0 μm. After the patient receives an intravenous injection of 5 mCi (185 MBq) of Tc-99m–albumin colloid, the agent is cleared from the blood by the reticuloendothelial (RE) cells. These RE cells are located principally in the liver (85%) and spleen (10%), and the remainder are in the bone marrow, kidney, and lung. An initial dynamic flow study may be obtained to determine liver and spleen perfusion in cases of abdominal trauma. Liver and spleen imaging is useful to determine organ size, the presence of hepatic metastases, and the degree of hepatocellular dysfunction in diffuse liver disease (i.e., cirrhosis).

Technetium (⁹⁹ᵐTc) Apcitide. This new radiotracer is a synthetic peptide that binds to the GPIIb/IIIa adhesion-molecule receptors found on activated platelets. This allows the detection of acute venous thrombosis and is Food and Drug Administration (FDA)-approved for detection of acute lower extremity deep venous thrombosis. A lyophilized preparation of 100 μg of bibapcitide in the presence of heat will split and then complex to 20 mCi Tc-99m pertechnetate. Images of area of concern are acquired at 10 and 60 minutes.

Technetium (⁹⁹ᵐTc) Bicisate Injection. A sterile colorless solution of bicisate is complexed with Tc-99m pertechnetate after reduction with a stannous salt. The precise structure of the technetium complex is [N,N'-ethylene-di-L-cysteinato(3-)]oxo [⁹⁹ᵐTc]technetium(V) diethyl ester. This radiopharmaceutical is a neutral and lipophilic complex that crosses the blood–brain barrier and is selectively retained in the brain. Therefore, this radiotracer is used as a brain-perfusion imaging agent. After intravenous injection of 20 mCi (740 MBq) of Tc-99m bicisate, about 5% of the injected dose is localized within the brain cells 5 minutes after injection and demonstrates rapid renal excretion (74% in 24 hours). This radiotracer is used clinically to evaluate dementia, stroke, lack of brain perfusion ("brain death"), cerebral vascular reserve, or risk of stroke (acetazolamide challenge study) and to localize a seizure focus for surgical removal.

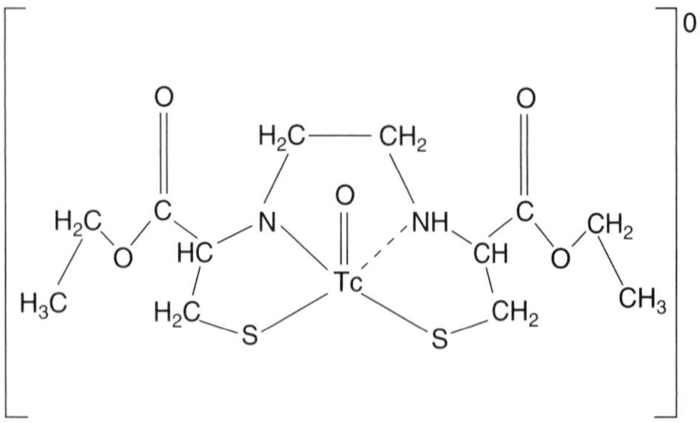

Technetium Bicisate

Technetium (Tc-99m) Depreotide Injection. Technetium depreotide injection is a new radiolabeled synthetic

peptide with high-affinity binding to somatostatin receptors (subtypes 2, 3, and 5) present in many types of cancer, including lung cancer. It is approved for use in patients who are known to have, or are highly suspect for, malignancy and exhibit pulmonary lesions on CT and/or chest x-ray. Over 170,000 new cases of lung cancer are diagnosed each year in the United States alone, and the alternative methods for determining malignancy are needle biopsy, which has an estimated 15% complication rate, and surgery.

The precise structure is cyclo-(L-homocysteinyl-*N*-methyl-L-phenylalanyl-L-tyrosyl-D-tryptophyl-L-lysyl-L-valyl), (1,1')-sulfide with 3-[(mercaptoacetyl)amino]-L-alanyl-L-lysyl-L-cysteinyl-L-lysinamide. A technetium Tc-99m complex of depreotide is formed when sterile, nonpyrogenic sodium pertechnetate Tc-99m (15 to 20 mCi) injection, in 0.9% sodium chloride is added to a nonpyrogenic lyophilized mixture of 50 μg of depreotide, sodium glucoheptonate dihydrate, stannous chloride dihydrate, 100 μg of edetate disodium dihydrate, and enough sodium hydroxide or hydrochloric acid to adjust the pH to 7.4 prior to lyophilization.

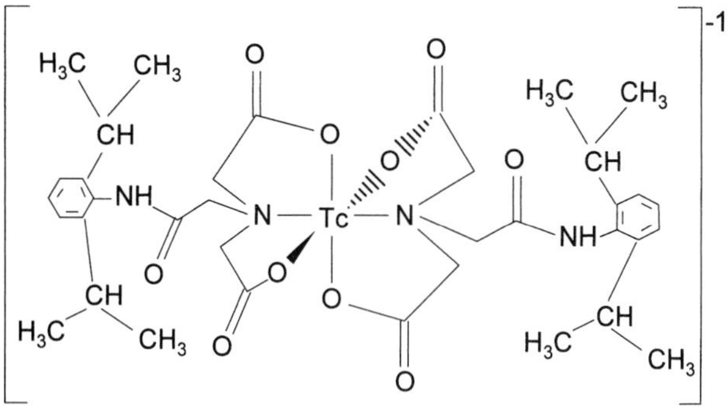

Technetium Disofenin

Technetium (⁹⁹ᵐTc) Disofenin Injection. A sterile colorless solution of disofenin is complexed with Tc-99m pertechnetate after reduction with a stannous salt. The precise structure of the technetium complex is unknown at this time. Costello et al.[7] specify, however, that an analogue of this Tc-99m–lidofenin complex provides a single technetium (III) distorted octahedral (1:2) complex with a coordination number of 6. A newer biliary imaging agent is Tc-99m mebrofenin, which is more lipophilic because it has bromine on the benzene ring. In the presence of high serum bilirubin levels, there is less renal excretion because of its higher lipid solubility. In addition, the product is more stable, which makes it more cost-effective for a centralized nuclear pharmacy.

The patient receives an intravenous injection of 5 mCi (185 MBq) of Tc-99m disofenin, which is taken up by the hepatocytes in the liver by active anionic transport. Then the radiopharmaceutical is excreted in bile, via the biliary canaliculus, into the bile ducts, with accumulation in the gallbladder and finally excretion via the common bile duct into the small bowel. The normal patient exhibits early accumulation of the radiopharmaceutical in the liver and the gallbladder and small bowel can be visualized within 1 to 2 hours after injection. An example is seen in Figure 13-5.

The primary clinical indication for this study is possible acute cholecystitis. In acute cholecystitis, there is obstruction of the cystic duct leading to the gallbladder. The gallbladder is not visualized because the radiotracer cannot enter it. Some other clinical conditions that can be diagnosed by bili-

that disrupt the blood–brain barrier (i.e., tumors, abscesses, strokes). Unlike the iodide ion, the pertechnetate ion is not converted to thyroid hormone but only trapped. Thyroid nodules can appear nonfunctional, with little or no radiotracer present. These nonfunctional nodules have about a 20% probability of being cancerous and generally require biopsy. The patient receives an intravenous injection of 5 to 10 mCi (185 to 370 MBq) of Tc-99m pertechnetate, and images are obtained of the thyroid 0 to 20 minutes after injection. The usual dose for the other imaging procedures is the same for Meckel's diverticulum and salivary glands, and 20 mCi (740 MBq) is used for brain tumor imaging.

Technetium (*99mTc*) Succimer Injection.

A sterile, colorless solution of succimer (2,3-dimercaptosuccinic acid) is complexed with Tc-99m pertechnetate after reduction with a stannous salt at acid pH. The precise structure of Tc-99m (III) succimer is unknown; however, Moretti et al.[11] suggested the possible structure below. Tc-99m succimer is very useful for demonstrating the functioning renal parenchyma, because about 40% of the dose is bound to the renal cortex 1 hour after injection. The patient is injected with 5 mCi (185 MBq) of Tc-99m succimer, and multiple images are taken 2 to 4 hours later. This study can be useful for evaluating renal trauma, renal masses (e.g., tumors, cysts), and renal scarring. Tc-99m succimer is the diagnostic agent of choice in children who have chronic urinary tract infections causing renal scarring. If the pH is adjusted to 8.0 to 8.5, a technetium (V)–succimer complex is formed, which is useful for imaging tumors.[12] Blower et al.[13] have proposed the following structure for Tc-99m (V) succimer.

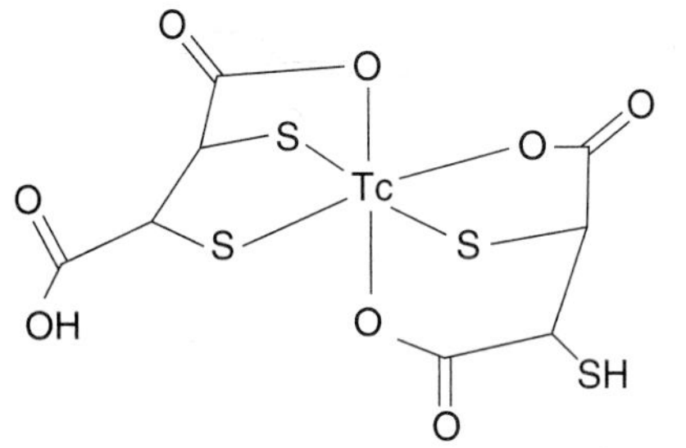

Technetium (III) Succimer

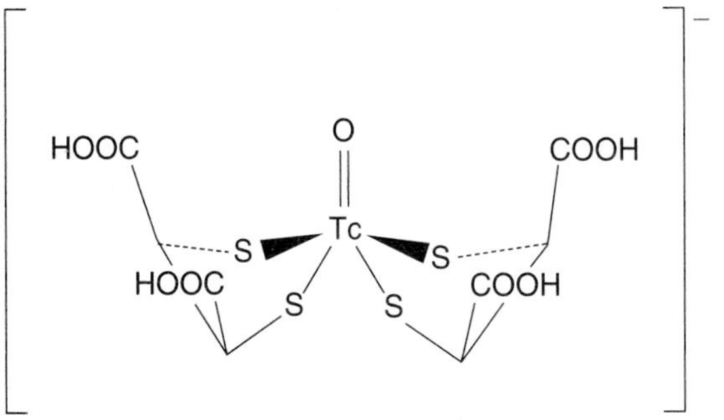

Technetium (V) Succimer

Technetium (*99mTc*) Sulfur Colloid Injection.

Technetium–sulfur colloid injection is a sterile, opalescent colloidal dispersion of sulfur, a unit of structure built up from polymeric molecules and ions (micelles) radiolabeled with Tc-99m pertechnetate formed by heating in dilute hydrochloric acid. The radiocolloid should be stabilized with gelatin A to inhibit clumping of the negatively charged colloidal particles. The particle size of the colloid is 0.1 to 3 μm. After intravenous injection of 5 to 10 mCi (185 to 370 MBq) of Tc-99m sulfur colloid, the radiopharmaceutical is rapidly cleared from the blood by the RE cells of the liver, spleen, and bone marrow. Uptake of the Tc-99m–sulfur colloid depends on the relative blood perfusion rate and the functional capacity of RE cells. In the normal patient, 85% of the radiocolloid is phagocytized by Kupffer cells in the liver, 7.5% by the spleen, and the remainder by the bone marrow, lungs, and kidneys. Bone marrow imaging studies are performed 1 hour after injection of 10 mCi (370 MBq) of Tc-99m–sulfur colloid. Normal bone marrow will take up the radiocolloid, but diseased bone marrow appears as "cold" defects in patients with tumor deposits in the marrow. Tc-99m–sulfur colloid is used as a secondary agent in liver and spleen imaging if Tc-99m–albumin colloid is not available. It is used as the primary agent, however, for GI studies such as gastroesophageal reflux (GER) and gastric emptying of solid food. Gastroesophageal reflux imaging is performed after having the patient swallow acidified orange juice mixed with Tc-99m–sulfur colloid. Normal patients have no GER. This study reportedly has 90% sensitivity in detecting GER. Gastric emptying imaging is performed after the patient swallows solid food (i.e., scrambled eggs or pancakes) radiolabeled with Tc-99m sulfur colloid. In general, the normal gastric emptying half-time is less than 90 minutes for solid food.

Technetium (*99mTc*) Tetrofosmin Injection.

A sterile, colorless solution of tetrofosmin is complexed with Tc-99m pertechnetate after reduction with a stannous salt. The precise structure of the technetium complex is shown below.[14] The formulation contains gluconate to form a weak technetium (V) chelate to keep the technetium in the (V) oxidation state for transchelation to form the technetium (V)–tetrofosmin complex. Technetium (V)–tetrofosmin is another cationic Tc-99m complex that thallous (²⁰¹Tl) chloride accumulates in viable myocardium. Myocardial uptake of this agent in humans is about 1.2% 5 minutes after intravenous injection and decreases to 1.0% at 2 hours. This agent was less specific for detecting ischemia (66%) than Tl-201 chloride (77%) in a small study (252 patients). It appears, however, to have rapid clearance through nontarget organs (liver) and thus fewer high-background imaging problems.

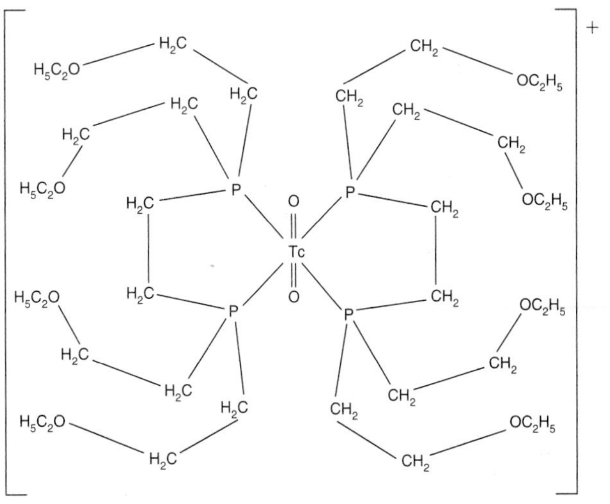

Technetium Tetrofosmin

FLUORINE RADIOCHEMISTRY

The useful radioisotope of fluorine for organ imaging is fluorine-18. Fluorine-18 is produced in a cyclotron by the $^{18}O(p,n)^{18}F$ nuclear reaction. Fluorine-18 ($t_{1/2} = 109$ minutes) decays by electron capture and positron emission to oxygen-18 with γ-ray emissions of 511 keV (194%). Fluorine-18 can be attached to a number of physiologically active molecules and, with the great strength of the C–F bond, appears to be a very useful label for radiopharmaceuticals.[15] Radiotracer production involves relatively complicated synthetic pathways, however, and the preparation of high-specific-activity compounds presents many problems. The short half-life of fluorine-18 makes it necessary to complete the synthetic and purification procedure within 3 hours. Consequently, a separate chemistry system (black box type) is needed for each compound. The chemistry of fluorine is complicated, but some compounds can be fluorinated by $^{18}F^-$ exchange reactions and direct fluorination with elemental fluorine ($^{18}F_2$); also, compounds with an aromatic ring may be fluorinated by several synthetic reactions. For example, partially fluorinated heteroaromatics are readily obtained by the conversion of an amino group on the aromatic ring to fluoride, with use of the Balz-Schiemman and several related reactions.

Fluorine (^{18}F)-2-Fluoro-2-Deoxy-D-Glucose.

The only F-18 radiopharmaceutical presently available is fluorine (^{18}F)-2-fluoro-2-deoxy-D-glucose (F-18 FDG). The precise structure of F-18 FDG is shown below. It is the only PET agent approved by the FDA. Hamacher et al.[16] introduced the current method of synthesis of F-18 FDG by nucleophilic fluorination. Use of this radiotracer for diagnostic imaging in oncology has increased dramatically in the last several years. It is used also as a myocardial viability agent and in evaluation of seizure disorders.[17] The high glycolytic rate of many neoplasms compared with that of the surrounding tissues facilitates tumor imaging with this glucose analogue. Because of the widespread anatomical distribution of metastases, a whole-body imaging technique using a tumor-specific radiopharmaceutical is very useful for tumor detection and mapping to evaluate the extent and relative metabolic activity of the disease.

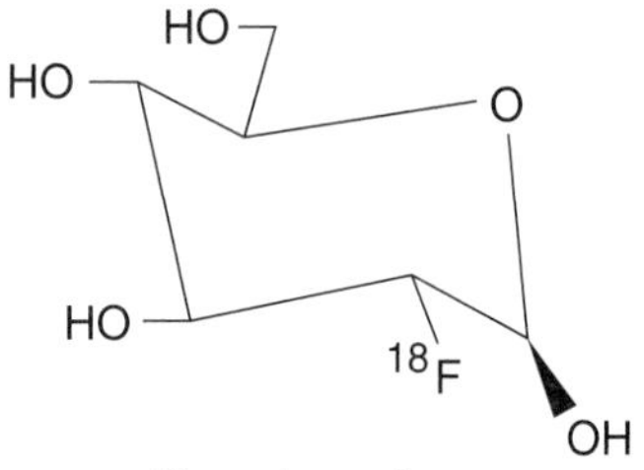

Fluorodeoxyglucose

GALLIUM RADIOCHEMISTRY

The only radioisotope of gallium that is presently used is gallium-67, which is produced in a cyclotron by proton bombardment of a zinc metal target by a $^{68}Zn(p,2n)^{67}Ga$ nuclear reaction. Gallium-67 ($t_{1/2} = 78.2$ hours) decays by electron capture to stable zinc-67 with principal γ-ray emissions of 93 keV (38%), 185 keV (24%), and 300 keV (16%). The radiotracer is isolated by dissolution of the target in hydrochloric acid followed by isopropyl ether extraction of the gallium-67 from the zinc and other impurities. The gallium-67 is back-extracted from the isopropyl ether into 0.2 M hydrochloric acid, evaporated to dryness, and dissolved in sterile, pyrogen-free 0.05 M hydrochloric acid. Gallium is an amphoteric element that acts as a metal at low pH but forms insoluble hydroxides when the pH is raised above 2.0 in the absence of chelating agents. At high pH, gallium hydroxide acts as a nonmetal and dissolves in ammonia to form gallates. Gallium forms compounds of oxidation states $+1$, $+2$, and $+3$; however, only the Ga^{+3} state is stable in aqueous solutions.

Gallium (^{67}Ga) Citrate.

The gallium (III)–citrate complex is formed by adding the required amount of sodium citrate (0.15 M) to gallium (III) chloride and adjusting the pH to 4.5 to 8.0 with sodium hydroxide. The proposed structure of gallium (^{67}Ga) citrate is shown below.[6] The patient receives an intravenous injection of 5 to 10 mCi (185 to 370 MBq) of gallium (^{67}Ga) citrate, and whole-body images are then obtained 24, 48, and 72 hours after injection. Gallium localizes at sites of inflammation or infection as well as a variety of tumors. It is used in clinical practice in the staging and evaluation of recurrence of lymphomas. Gallium localizes normally in the liver and spleen, bone, nasopharynx, lacrimal glands, and breast tissue. There is also some secretion in the bowel; consequently, the patient may require a laxative and/or enemas to evacuate this radioactivity prior to the 48-hour image. As more specific radiotracers have been developed, the nonspecific normal localization of gallium radioactivity has limited its clinical use.

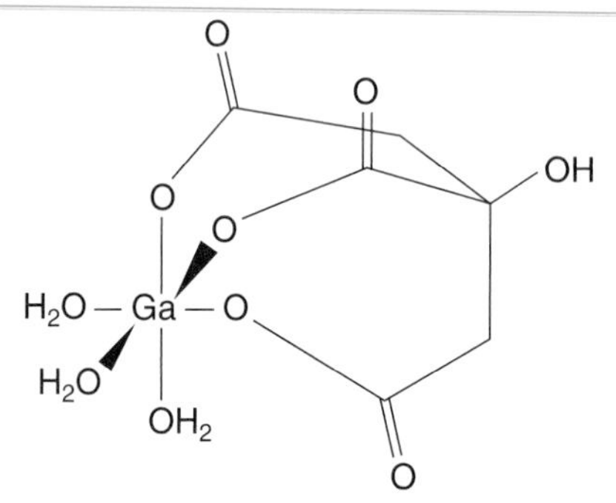

Gallium Citrate

IODINE RADIOCHEMISTRY

The useful radioisotopes of iodine for organ imaging are iodine-131 and iodine-123 because of their desirable physical characteristics. Iodine-131 is obtained from a reactor by production of tellurium-131. It is formed by the nuclear reaction $^{235}U(n,fission)^{131}Te$ or $^{130}Te(n,gamma)^{131}Te$. The tellurium-131 ($t_{1/2} = 25$ minutes) decays by β-particle emission to iodine-131. Iodine-131 ($t_{1/2} = 8.04$ days) transforms by β decay to stable xenon-131, with five significant γ-ray emissions of 80 to 723 keV. The major γ-ray of 364 keV (82%) provides good tissue penetration for organ imaging.

Undesirable properties of iodine-131 are the high radiation dose from the β particles, the long half-life, and the poor image produced by the high-energy γ-rays. Iodine-123 ($t^{1}/_{2}$ = 13.3 hours) decays by electron capture to tellurium-123, with a principal γ-ray emission of 159 keV (83%), which makes it the ideal radioisotope of iodine for organ imaging because of increased detection efficiency and reduced radiation to the patient. Iodine-123 is produced in a cyclotron bombarding an antimony metal target with α particles according to the $^{121}_{51}Sb$ (α,2n)$^{123}_{53}$ reaction or an iodine target with high-energy protons by the $^{127}_{53}I(p,5n)^{123}_{27}$ nuclear reaction. The xenon-123 decays by electron capture to iodine-123. It is, however, relatively expensive to produce and currently has limited availability for radiolabeling compounds. Iodine is in group VIIB with the other halogens (fluorine, chlorine, bromine, and astatine). In aqueous solution, compounds of iodine are known with at least five different oxidation states; however, in nuclear medicine, the −1 and +1 oxidation states are the most significant. The −1 oxidation state represented as sodium iodide (NaI) is important for thyroid studies and, when obtained in a reductant-free solution (no sodium thiosulfate), is the starting compound for the radiolabeling of most iodinated radiopharmaceuticals. The common methods for introducing radioiodine into organic compounds are isotope exchange reactions, electrophilic substitution of hydrogen in activated aromatic systems, nucleophilic substitution, and addition to double bonds.[18] The replacement of aromatic hydrogen in activated aromatic systems is used for protein labeling, and electrophilic iodine (I^+) can be generated by a variety of oxidizing agents, including *(a)* chloramine-T (*N*-chloro-*p*-toluene sulfonamide) sodium, *(b)* enzyme oxidation of I^- (lactoperoxidase), and *(c)* iodogen 1,3,4,6-tetrachlora-3a-6a-diphenylglycoluril). The actual iodinating molecule depends on the oxidizing agent but is probably HOI or H_2OI^+.

Iodine Radiopharmaceuticals

Iobenguane Sulfate (^{131}I) Injection (I-131–Metaiodobenzylguanidine Sulfate).

Iobenguane sulfate is radiolabeled by a Cu^+-catalyzed isotopic nucleophilic exchange reaction. It is a radioiodinated arylalkylguanidine and is similar to the antihypertensive drug guanethidine and to the neurotransmitter norepinephrine. The proposed structure of iobenguane (^{131}I) sulfate is shown below. Iodine-123 is also used to radiolabel this tracer and may have more favorable imaging properties. Functional tumors of the adrenal medulla (pheochromocytomas) and tumors of neuroendocrine origin (neuroblastoma) can be localized on I-131 *meta*-iodobenzylguanidine (^{131}I-MIBG) images, as abnormal tissue that takes up the radiopharmaceutical and exhibits increased activity on the image.[19] Drug intervention studies in animals, using reserpine, have demonstrated that the ^{131}I-MIBG enters adrenergic neurons and chromaffin cells by an active transport mechanism of catecholamine uptake into adrenergic storage granules.

Neuroblastoma is a malignant tumor of the sympathetic nervous system, which occurs most often in children. The tumor is of neural crest origin and consists of cells that form the sympathetic nervous system, called *sympathogonia,* that migrate to the adrenal medulla and many other parts of the body. Metastases may be found in the liver (stage IV) and

in the regional lymph nodes, bone, bone marrow, and soft tissues. After an initial report by Kimmig et al.[20] of ^{131}I-MIBG uptake in neuroblastoma, successful use of this tracer was described by others. The increased uptake of ^{131}I-MIBG is so tissue specific that it can establish the diagnosis of neuroblastoma in a child with a tumor of unknown origin. The patient is treated with Lugol's solution (up to 40 mg/day) 24 hours before and 4 to 7 days after administration of the radiopharmaceutical, to block thyroid uptake of free $^{131}I^-$. The ^{131}I-MIBG is administered by slow intravenous injection 0.3 to 0.5 mCi (11 to 18.5 MBq), and patients are imaged 24, 48, and 72 hours later. Occasionally, the patient receives a renal imaging agent for better localization of the adrenal tumor.

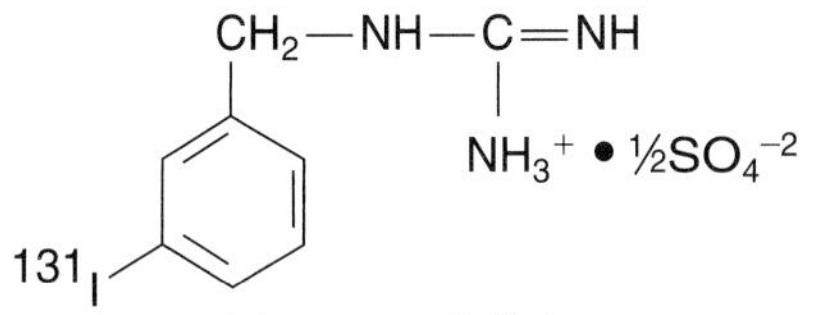

Iobenguane Sulfate

Sodium Iodine (^{123}I) Capsules.

The major indications for thyroid imaging with sodium iodide (^{123}I) are for evaluation of thyroid morphology, for ectopic thyroid tissue (e.g., lingual or mediastinal), and for substernal thyroid tissue. When thyroid nodules are being evaluated for possible thyroid cancer, ^{123}I has an advantage over Tc-99m pertechnetate scans, although I-123 is more expensive. This is because thyroid cancer cells sometimes retain the ability to trap, but not further process, iodine to thyroid hormone. Unlike iodine, Tc-99m pertechnetate is only trapped by the thyroid and in a nodule may give the false impression that a nodule is not cancerous. The patient fasts before receiving the oral dose of 0.4 mCi (15 MBq) of sodium iodine (^{123}I). Images are obtained of the thyroid and surrounding area 4 to 6 hours after ingestion.

Sodium Iodine (^{131}I) Oral (Solution or Capsule).

The thyroid cancer patient receives an oral dose of 5 to 10 mCi (185 to 370 MBq) of sodium iodide (^{131}I), which localizes in residual thyroid tissue after "total" thyroidectomy and functioning thyroid metastasis from thyroid carcinoma. Images of the whole body are obtained 48 to 72 hours later. These metastatic radioiodide surveys are used to detect regional or distant metastases for large-dose 150 mCi (5,550 MBq) inpatient therapy for thyroid carcinoma. Any thyroid hormone medication should be discontinued for 2 weeks (T_3) or 4 weeks (T_4). In addition, the patient should have blood drawn for a thyroid-stimulating hormone (TSH) test to ensure that TSH is elevated before administration of the therapy dose, to permit maximum stimulation of thyroid tissue. The patient should fast before receiving the oral dose of radiotracer.

INDIUM RADIOCHEMISTRY

The most useful radioisotope of indium is indium-111, which is produced in a cyclotron by proton bombardment of a cadmium metal target by a $^{112}Cd(p,2n)^{111}$ nuclear reaction.

Indium-111 ($t_{1/2}$ = 67.4 hours) decays by electron capture to stable cadmium-111 with principal γ-ray emissions of 172 keV (91%) and 247 keV (94%). The radiotracer is isolated by dissolution in hydrochloric acid to form ^{111}In-chloride and separated from cadmium and other impurities by several dissolution and extraction steps. The last extraction is done with isopropyl ether, evaporating to dryness, and dissolving in sterile, pyrogen-free 0.05 M hydrochloric acid. In aqueous solution, lower valence states of indium have been described, but they are unstable and are rapidly oxidized to the trivalent state. In acid solution, indium salts are stable at low pH but are hydrolyzed (above pH 3.5) to form a precipitate of indium hydroxide or trioxide. Indium will remain in solution above pH 3.5, however, if it is complexed with a weak chelating agent such as sodium citrate and stronger chelating agents such as 8-hydroxy quinoline (oxine) or diethylenetriaminepentaacetic acid (DTPA). Monoclonal antibodies or peptides are radiolabeled by indium by using compounds called *bifunctional chelating agents*. Bifunctional chelating agents are molecules that can both bind metal ions and be attached to other molecules; one example is the cyclic anhydride of DTPA.

Indium Radiopharmaceuticals

Indium (^{111}In) Chloride Injection.
Indium (III) chloride is a sterile, colorless solution that is radiolabeled with indium-111 in a hydrochloric acid solution (0.05 M) and has a pH of 1.5. It is primarily used to radiolabel other compounds for use in cisternography and white blood cell labeling studies and is particularly recommended for radiolabeling monoclonal antibodies for metastatic cancer imaging. If this agent is injected intravenously for clinical use, the patient's blood must be drawn into the syringe containing the radiopharmaceutical to buffer the agent to a higher pH to eliminate the burning sensation on injection. When the acidic compound is mixed with blood, the indium-111 chloride binds quickly to transferrin, the iron-binding protein in the plasma. The localization of the indium (III) chloride in bone marrow is probably explained by its ability to behave metabolically like iron and yet not be incorporated into hemoglobin in the RBCs in the bone marrow. The localization of the radiotracer in tumors and abscesses is probably due to increased blood flow and capillary permeability in the area of tissue damage. Transferrin receptors have been suggested as a means of localization but not proved at this time.

Indium (^{111}In) Capromab Pendetide.
Indium capromab pendetide is a new radiotracer for staging patients with newly diagnosed prostate cancer and for those with suspected reoccurrence but a negative localization with a standard evaluation.

Indium (^{111}In) Oncoscint CR/OV (Satumomabpendetide).
The simplified structure of indium (^{111}In) satumomabpendetide is shown below. Antibodies are a heterogeneous group of proteins isolated from human and animal serum and are called *immunoglobulins*. They are divided into classes on the basis of differences in structure and biological properties and are assigned to major classes called IgG (80%), IgM (10%), and IgA, IgD, IgE (<10%). All antibodies have a general structure consisting of two heavy chains (MW ~55,000) and two light chains (MW ~20,000) of glycoproteins, held together by disulfide bonds. Many tumors express antigenic markers on their surfaces that permit detection with radiolabeled antibodies. Antibodies are produced by B lymphocytes and plasma cells sensitized to an antigen. Hybridoma technology permits the manufacture of large quantities of antibody directed against specific antigens. Diagnostic antibodies are of two types: polyclonal and monoclonal. Each chain has a variable region for antigenic binding and a constant region for complement fixation. Polyclonal antibodies include numerous antibody species of varying affinity for the antigen-binding surfaces. Monoclonal antibodies are generated from a clone of a single antibody-producing cell and have uniform affinity for their antigenic determinant.[21] Monoclonal antibodies are produced by immunizing a mouse with purified material from the surface of the human tumor cell. (See Chapter 7 for additional information.) The antigen used in Oncoscint CR/OV is a tumor-associated glycoprotein-72 (TAG-72), a high-molecular-weight glycoprotein expressed by colorectal and ovarian carcinomas.[22] The radiolabeling of Oncoscint CR/OV monoclonal antibody was developed by Rodwell[23] as a site-specific method using a bifunctional chelate. Briefly, carbohydrate moieties on the monoclonal antibody (F-constant region) are oxidized with periodate, and the aldehyde groups on the antibody are reacted with α-amino groups of glycyl-tyrosyl-lysine-*N*-diethylene triaminepentaacetic acid. The Schiff's base form (imine) is stabilized by reduction with sodium cyanoborohydride. In-111 is chelated to a DTPA-carbohydrate molecule attached to the constant region of the monoclonal antibody. The specificity of radiolabeled antibody imaging for tumors exceeds that of gallium (^{67}Ga) citrate studies. Sites of nonspecific uptake have been reported, however, such as recent surgical wounds, an inflamed colon, bone fracture, and normal colostomy stoma. A new method of labeling with Tc-99m has recently been approved by the FDA.

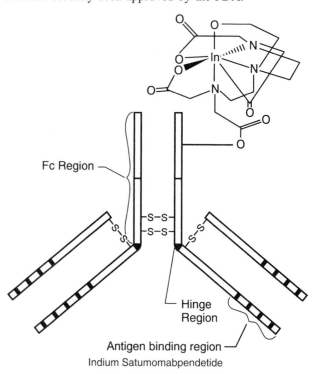

Fc Region

Hinge Region

Antigen binding region

Indium Satumomabpendetide

Indium (¹¹¹In) Oxine (8-Hydroxyquinoline). The indium (III)–oxine complex can be formed by adding the required amount of 8-hydroxyquinoline sulfate to indium (III) chloride and adjusting the pH to 6.5 to 7.5 with HEPES buffer. The precise structure of indium (III) oxine as determined by Green[24] is shown below. The patient has 45 to 90 mL of blood drawn for a 1.5- to 2-hour in vitro process of separating and labeling cellular elements such as leukocytes or platelets. Images are acquired 2 to 48 hours after reinjection of the labeled cells. In the case of indium-111 leukocytes, the procedure is performed to confirm the presence or absence of infection. This technique has replaced gallium (^{67}Ga) citrate imaging for acute infection because of greater specificity and better image quality. Some chronic infections such as osteomyelitis may be imaged better with gallium (^{67}Ga) citrate after a ^{99m}Tc-phosphate bone scan. Another method of radiolabeling leukocytes that has become popular uses Tc-99m-HMPAO (hexamethylpropyleneamine oxime). Finally, indium (^{111}In)-labeled platelets are used to detect thromboses, measure platelet life span, and monitor the success of kidney transplants.

Indium Oxine

Indium (¹¹¹In) Pentetate (¹¹¹In-DTPA). The indium (III)–pentetate complex is formed by adding the required amount of calcium or sodium pentetate (DTPA) to the indium (III) chloride and adjusting the pH to 7.0 to 8.0 with sodium hydroxide and/or hydrochloric acid. A proposed structure of indium (III) pentetate is shown below.[6] The patient undergoes a lumbar puncture under sterile conditions and receives an intrathecal injection of 0.5 to 1.0 mCi (18.5 to 37.0 MBq) of indium (^{111}In) pentetate, which distributes into the cerebrospinal fluid (CSF). Initial images are obtained to ensure a good intrathecal injection. Images of the spinal canal and CSF spaces of the brain are acquired at 0 to 72 hours to assess CSF flow or leakage from the normal CSF space. The normal CSF flow pattern shows that the radiopharmaceutical ascends to the basilar cisterns in 2 to 4 hours and flows over the cerebral convexities in 24 hours. From 24 to 72 hours, there should be a gradual clearance from the CSF via the choroid plexus. Cisternography is helpful in evaluating for communicating hydrocephalus because there is abnormal CSF flow into the lateral ventricles of the brain in this disease. There is also an MRI method for evaluating this type of hydrocephalus. This disease may be treated surgically by shunting CSF to other areas of the body, such as the peritoneal space, and this radiotracer can be used to assess the possibility of a blockage of such a shunt.

Another indication for this technique is evaluation for a CSF leak after surgery or trauma. One variation of evaluating for a leak is to put cotton pledgets in the nostrils for 24 hours and check for abnormal radioactivity on the pledgets.

Indium Pentetate

Indium (¹¹¹In) Pentreotide Injection. A proposed structure of indium (^{111}In) pentreotide is shown below.[25] Pentreotide has a bifunctional chelating agent, DTPA, linked to octreotide, which is a long-acting analogue of the human hormone somatostatin. Somatostatin is a peptide hormone consisting of 14 amino acids. It is present in the GI tract, pancreas, cerebral cortex, brainstem, and hypothalamus. Somatostatin receptors have been found on many cells of neuroendocrine origin. Neuroendocrine tumors are small and slow growing, which makes them hard to detect by CT or MRI. Somatostatin receptors are expressed in nearly all tumors of neuroendocrine origin and can be imaged with the DTPA-octreotide analogue, which chelates indium (III) chloride.

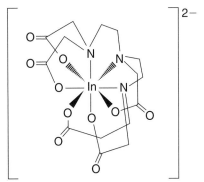

Indium Pentreotide

Indium (^{111}In) pentreotide binds to somatostatin receptors on many cell surfaces throughout the body. The patient receives an intravenous injection of 5 mCi (185 MBq) of ^{111}In-pentreotide, and within an hour, the radiopharmaceutical diffuses into the extracellular fluid space and concentrates in tumors containing a large number of somatostatin receptors. Whole-body images are obtained 4 to 48 hours after injection to localize the primary tumor and sites of metastases. Normally, the pituitary gland, thyroid gland, liver, spleen, kidneys, urinary bladder, and, in most patients, the bowel are visualized on the image.

THALLIUM RADIOCHEMISTRY

The only useful radioisotope of thallium is thallium-201, which is produced in a cyclotron by proton bombardment of a thallium metal target by a $^{203}Tl(p,3n)^{201}Pb$ nuclear reaction. The lead-201 ($t_{1/2} = 9.4$ hours) is allowed to decay by electron capture to Tl-201. Thallium-201 ($t_{1/2} = 73.0$ hours) decays by electron capture to stable mercury-201, with principal γ-ray emissions of 135 keV (2%) and 167 keV (8%), and mercury-201 daughter x-rays of 68 to 80 keV (94.5%), all of which can be used for organ imaging. The thallium target is dissolved in hydrochloric acid, and the Pb-201 is isolated from the thallium-203 by ion exchange column chromatography. The lead-201 (^{201}Pb) is allowed to decay on the column to thallium-201. The thallium-201 (^{201}Tl) is removed from the column by ion exchange, and the chloride salt is formed by adding hydrochloric acid and evaporating to dryness. Then the pH is adjusted to 4.5 to 7.0 with sodium hydroxide and the salt is sterilized. The solution is made isotonic with sodium chloride containing benzyl alcohol as a preservative.

Thallium Radiopharmaceuticals

Thallium (²⁰¹Tl) Chloride. Thallium chloride is the only radiopharmaceutical of thallium-201 currently in use. The most common clinical uses of this radiotracer are for the evaluation of myocardial perfusion and myocardial viability. In recent years, thallium-201 has also been used to evaluate a variety of types of cancer as well as hyperparathyroidism.

Research using radiolabeled microspheres with human volunteers demonstrated that the myocardial distribution of thallous (I) chloride correlates with regional blood perfusion. Thallium (^{201}Tl) chloride accumulation in myocytes requires an intact sodium–potassium pump mechanism within the cell membrane. Accumulation in the myocardial tissue therefore reflects viable tissue as well as blood flow to the myocardial tissue. Conversely, in clinical imaging studies, the areas of myocardial infarction (not viable scar) are visualized as nonperfused ("cold") areas. Although the Tc-99m–based myocardial perfusion radiotracers (sestamibi and tetrofosmin) are mostly bound in the heart cell, Tl-201 is continually, passively moving back out of the cells. This phenomenon is called *thallium redistribution*.

Currently, the most commonly performed test in all of nuclear medicine is the evaluation for significant narrowing of the coronary arteries. To do this, the patient submits to either physiological "stress" (treadmill exercise) or pharmacological "stress" with an intravenous infusion of a vasodilator (dipyridamole or adenosine), depending on physical condition. At maximum stress, the patient is injected with 2.0 to 4.0 mCi (74 to 148 MBq) of thallous (I) chloride, which localizes in the heart muscle (myocardium) in proportion to regional blood flow and cell viability. The "stress test" accentuates the myocardial perfusion abnormality because areas of significant arterial narrowing cannot respond to the increased blood flow demands of the stress as well as the normal arteries can. Images of the heart are obtained immediately after stress, and the damaged myocardium shows less Tl-201 chloride uptake than surrounding normal heart muscle. Four hours after stress, the resting patient is injected with 1.0 mCi (37 MBq) of Tl-201 chloride to provide information under normal conditions. An example is shown in Figure 13-7.

XENON RADIOCHEMISTRY

The useful radioisotope of xenon for organ imaging is xenon-133. Xenon-133 is produced in a nuclear reactor as a byproduct of uranium fission by the nuclear reaction $^{235}U(n, fission)^{133}Xe$. Xenon-133 ($t_{1/2} = 5.3$ days) decays by β-particle emission to cesium-133, with γ-ray emissions of 81 keV (36%). Gases used in lung ventilation studies must be chemically inert and, at the concentrations used, be physiologically inert. Xenon-133 is chemically inert and insoluble in water, which makes it insoluble in body fluids. Unfavorable physical characteristics of xenon-133 include poor image quality because of the low tissue penetration of the low-energy γ-ray, increased patient dose due to β-particle emission, and the low γ-ray emission (36 γ-rays/100 disintegrations). An alternative would be xenon-127, which is unavailable and not cost-effective.

Xenon Radiopharmaceuticals

Xenon (¹³³Xe) Gas. Radioactive xenon gas is supplied at standard pressure and room temperature in a septum-sealed glass vial (2 mL) in doses of 10 to 20 mCi (370 to 740 MBq). The glass vial can contain atmospheric air or a mixture of 5% xenon and 95% carbon dioxide and is suitable for inhalation by the patient for diagnostic evaluation of pulmonary function and imaging. The general procedure involves mixing the xenon-133 gas in air or oxygen in a closed-circuit spirometer system that delivers the radioactive gas and rebreathing the gas mixture. The inhalation study consists of equilibrium and washout phases, with the patient sitting or supine. In the washout study, the patient exhales the xenon-133 gas into an activated charcoal trap to prevent exposure of the technologist. Images are obtained continuously for approximately 10 minutes with the gamma (γ-ray) camera. In the normal equilibrium study, there is an initial homogeneous distribution of the radioactive gas throughout the lungs. In the washout phase, the xenon-133 gas clears readily from the lungs. In the abnormal study, the initial flow into the lungs of xenon-133 gas is delayed, and the outflow is also delayed. These abnormal lung ventilation findings add significant information in the evaluation of pulmonary embolism (blood clots in the lungs) when combined with the results of a lung blood perfusion study with Tc-99m aggregated albumin.

RADIOLOGICAL CONTRAST AGENTS

A photographic film containing a radiographic image is properly called a *radiograph,* although it is commonly referred to as an *x-ray* or a *film.* The relative difference between the light and dark areas on a radiographic image reflects what is called *radiographic contrast.* Traditional radiographic images of the body, such as skeletal, abdominal, and chest x-rays, have five radiographic densities: air (gas) density, fat density, fluid (soft tissue) density, bone (calcium) density, and metallic density.

Whereas traditional radiological "film" studies have been used since 1895 and continue to be a mainstay of diagnostic medical imaging, they have their limitations. Many organs and tissues of the body do not show up well on traditional radiographic images. For example, the liver, spleen, kidneys, intestines, bladder, and abdominal musculature all have very similar radiographic densities and are difficult, if not impossible, to distinguish from each other.

From the earliest days of radiology, much effort has been devoted to developing compounds that if swallowed or injected would increase the radiographic contrast between various tissues and organs. Injection of air or other gases into a GI tube in the esophagus, stomach, or duodenum or into a rectal tube in the colon provides increased radiographic contrast for evaluating the gut; however, the information obtained by this technique is limited, and more opaque substances have been developed.

Any agent or compound administered to a patient to improve the visualization of an organ or tissue is called a *contrast agent*. Contrast agents can be classified as negative or positive. Air and other gases are negative contrast agents because they render a structure, such as the gut, more translucent. An agent that increases the radiographic opacity of an organ or tissue is a positive contrast agent. The majority of contrast agents used in diagnostic radiology are positive contrast agents.

An ideal contrast agent should have the following properties: *(a)* ready availability and low cost; *(b)* excellent x-ray absorption characteristics at the x-ray energies used in diagnostic radiology; *(c)* minimal toxicity and ready patient acceptance; *(d)* chemical stability; *(e)* high water solubility with low viscosity and no significant osmotic effects; and *(f)* the ability to be administered for selective tissue uptake and excretion.

No compound has all of these characteristics. Barium sulfate and a variety of iodine compounds, however, produce excellent radiological contrast with low patient toxicity and relatively low cost. The use of barium and iodine compounds as radiological contrast agents is based on their radiographic appearance and their distribution and elimination from the body. Contrast media are used in very large quantities and are usually administered over a short time.

Barium sulfate is a nearly ideal contrast agent for oral and rectal studies of the GI tract. It produces a metal-like density on radiological studies, is readily available at low cost, and, when used properly, has minimal patient morbidity and mortality. Many water-soluble barium compounds are quite toxic, but barium sulfate is an insoluble white power that is formulated in water as a colloidal suspension.

The majority of contrast agents used to opacify blood vessels and increase contrast in solid organs such as the liver are water-soluble organic iodides. Iodine absorbs x-rays effectively at many energy levels and produces a type of "calcific" or "bone" density on radiographic studies. Its density, somewhat less than that of barium sulfate, is quite acceptable.

Until the 1980s, most water-soluble contrast agents consisted of triiodinated benzoic acid salts. In solution, they dissociate into two particles, a triiodinated anion and a cation, which consists of either a sodium or methylglucamine

(meglumine) ion. These compounds (Table 13-2), known as *high-osmolar contrast media* (HOCM), have in effect three iodine atoms for every two ions in solution, a 3:2 ratio. They are often called *ionic ratio 1.5 contrast agents* or *triiodinated monomers*.[26] They are mainly represented by diatrizoate and iothalamate compounds and find frequent use in urography and contrast-enhanced CT studies.

One must administer the water-soluble iodinated organic compounds in fairly high concentrations to achieve satisfactory radiological contrast. It is not unusual to administer 100 mL or more of a 60% solution of one of these compounds intravenously for urography. A typical concentration used for intravascular studies has an osmolality 5 to 7 times greater than that of normal plasma. Therefore, administration of these agents can be associated with osmotoxic effects, such as local pain, flushing, nausea, and vomiting. The common triiodinated contrast agents listed in Table 13-2 represent what are commonly called *ionic* or *high-osmolar* agents. They are relatively inexpensive and have been in use since the 1960s.

Much research has gone into developing water-soluble compounds with a higher ratio of iodine to osmotic particles. The first commercially available nonionic contrast agent was metrizamide, which dissolves in water in a nondissociated form, giving three iodine atoms for every molecule in solution and is referred to as a *ratio-3 contrast agent*. Metrizamide was mainly used for myelographic studies of the spinal canal and has been largely replaced by newer agents. This has led to the development of ionic hexaiodinated dimers, such as ioxaglate (Hexabrix), and nonionic water-soluble contrast agents (Table 13-2).

Metrizamide

Ioxaglate

Iopamidol, iohexol, and ioversol are newer "low-osmolar, nonionic" contrast agents (Table 13-2) and are heavily used around the world for many types of radiological studies. These types of agents, known as *low osmolar contrast media* (LOCM), produce far fewer osmotoxic effects, such as local arm pain, flushing, and nausea and vomiting. They are generally considered safer than the common ionic triiodinated contrast agents and, in many locales, have replaced them in daily practice. They are very expensive, however, compared with the ionic agents. In the United States, they may cost up to 10 to 20 times as much as the ionic agents.[27, 28]

TABLE 13–2   Diagnostic Imaging Agents and Procedures

Common Contrast Agents

High-osmolality (1,400 to 2,938 mOsm/kg) ("ionic") agents,

  Conray 60 (60% meglumine iothalamate)

  Conray 400 (66.8% sodium iothalamate)

  Hypaque 50 (50% sodium diatrizoate)

  Hypaque 60 (60% sodium diatrizoate)

  Hypaque 76 (76% sodium diatrizoate)

  Hypaque M 90 (60% meglumine diatrizoate, 30% sodium diatrizoate)

  Renografin 60 (52% meglumine diatrizoate, 8% sodium diatrizoate)

  Renografin 76 (66% meglumine diatrizoate, 10% sodium diatrizoate)

  Reno-M-60 (60% meglumine diatrizoate)

Low-osmolality ("nonionic") agents (290 to 862 mOsm/kg)

  Amipaque (metrizamide)

  Hexabrix (ioxaglate; this is an ionic hexaiodinated dimer)-Guerbet, S.A.

  Isovue (iopamidol)—Bracco Diagnostics

  Omnipaque (iohexol)—Nycomed

  Optiray (ioversol)—Mallinckrodt

  Oxilan (ioxilan)—Cook Imaging

  Ultravist (iopromide)—Berlex Laboratories

  Visipaque (Iodixanol)—Nycomed

  Xenetrix (iobitridol)

Miscellaneous infrequently used biliary contrast agents

  Cistobil, Colepax, Telepaque, Teletrast (iopanoic acid)

  Cholebrine, Cholimil (iocetamic acid)

  Bilopac, Bilopaque, Lumopaque, Tyropaque (tyropanoate sodium)

  Bilimiro, Bilimiron, Oravue, Videobil (iopronic acid)

Oily and fat-soluble contrast agents (water-insoluble agents)

  Ethiodol (ethyl diiodostearate/ethyl monoiodostearate)

  Dionosil (propyliodone)

  Lipiodol (iodinated poppy-seed oil)

Gadolinium-based magnetic resonance imaging (MRI) agents

  Dotarem (gadoterate meglumine)

  Eovist (gadoxetic acid)

  Gadovist (gadobutrol)

  Magnevist (gadopentetate dimeglumine)

  MultiHance (gadobenate dimeglumine)

  Omniscan (gadodiamide)

  ProHance (gadoteridol)

  OptiMark (gadoversetamide)

Radiological Procedures

Plain film radiography—Routine chest, abdomen, and skeletal studies

Contrast studies

  Barium studies—Esophagram, UGI examination, SBFT, BE, and other specialized GI tract examinations

  Water-insoluble contrast studies—Lymphangiography, and formerly, bronchography and myelography

  Gallbladder studies—Abdominal ultrasound, oral cholecystography, intravenous cholangiography

  Studies using water-soluble contrast agents—Excretory urography (IVP), venography, arteriography, contrast-enhanced CT and MRI, arthrography, hysterosalpingography, and myelography

Cross-sectional imaging studies

  Ultrasound examinations

  CT studies

  MRI studies

Data are from Mitchell, D. G.: MRI Principles. Philadelphia, W. B. Saunders, 1999; Franken, E. A., Jr.: Proceedings of the Contrast Media Research Symposium, Kyoto, Japan, May 18–22, 1997. Acad. Radiol. 5:S1, 1998; Katzberg, R. W.: Urography into the 21st century: New contrast media, renal handling, imaging.

Iopamidol

Iohexol

Ioversol

In general, high or moderate osmolality and high viscosity are the hallmarks of all iodinated contrast media. Because of this, considerable hemodynamic and subjective effects are caused by administration of these agents. Initially, water shifts rapidly from the interstitial and cellular spaces into the plasma after injection of an iodinated contrast agent. This is typically accompanied by vasodilatation, local pain and warmth, a metallic taste in the mouth, and flushing. Later, there is an osmotic diuresis as these agents are excreted by the kidneys.

All of the water-soluble iodinated contrast media are clear, colorless liquids with no visible precipitates. They are viscous and, when spilled, produce a somewhat sticky mess. Even though they are clear liquids, they are often called "dyes" when their administration is being explained to patients. The sodium salts are slightly less viscous than the meglumine salts. Contrast media viscosity can also be reduced by heating them to body temperature prior to administration.

The water-soluble iodinated contrast media have relatively small molecular sizes and low chemical reactivity with body fluids and tissues. Agents of this class include diatrizoate meglumine, diatrizoate sodium, iocetamic acid, iodipamide meglumine, iopanoic acid, iopronic acid, iothalamate sodium, ipodate sodium, and tyropanoate sodium. Their pharmaceutical characteristics are similar to those of extracellular tracers. They have low lipid solubility and distribute throughout the extracellular space. They do not penetrate significantly into the intracellular space. The water-soluble iodinated contrast agents are cleared from the body by glomerular filtration. They are neither reabsorbed nor secreted by the renal tubules. When renal function is compromised, these contrast agents are eliminated in part or totally through the liver and gut. This vicarious excretion occurs at a much slower rate than elimination by normal glomerular filtration in a healthy person. The half-time for the renal clearance portion of a water-soluble contrast agent is 1 to 2 hours in a patient with normal renal function. The water-soluble organic iodides are the largest group of radiological contrast agents, and the importance of their clinical use is only approached by barium sulfate.

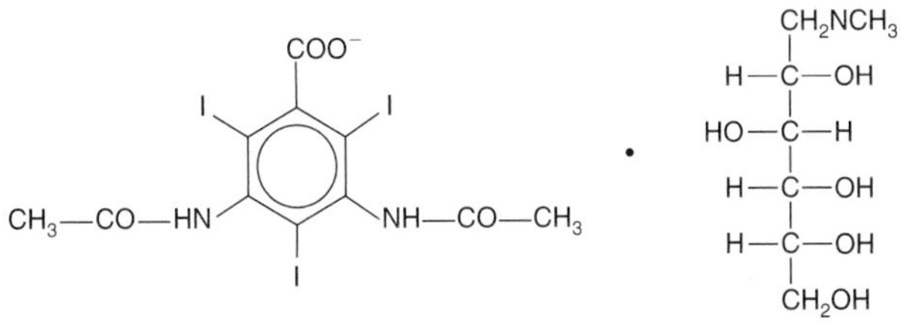

Diatrizoate Meglumine

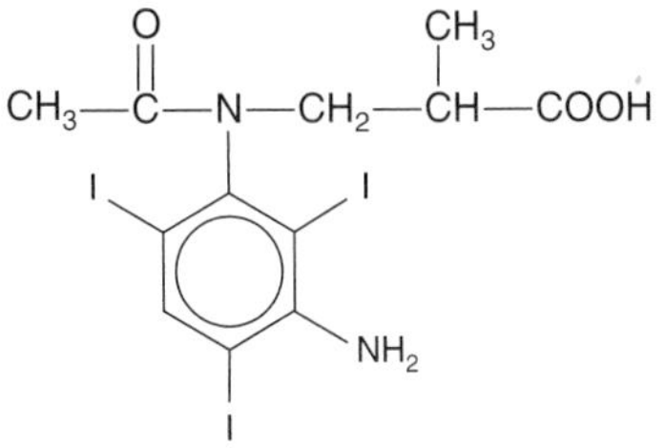

Iocetamic Acid

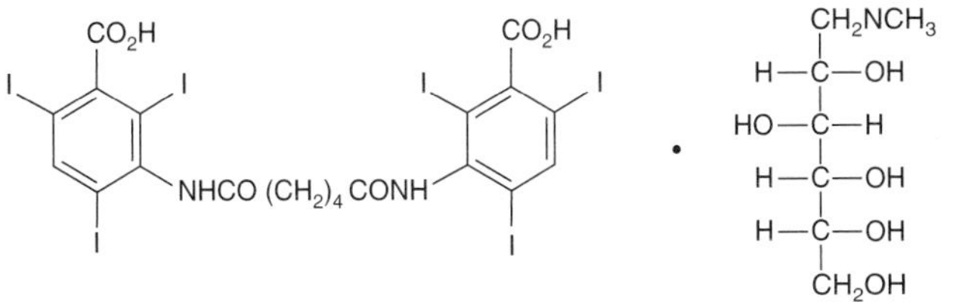

Iodipamide Meglumine

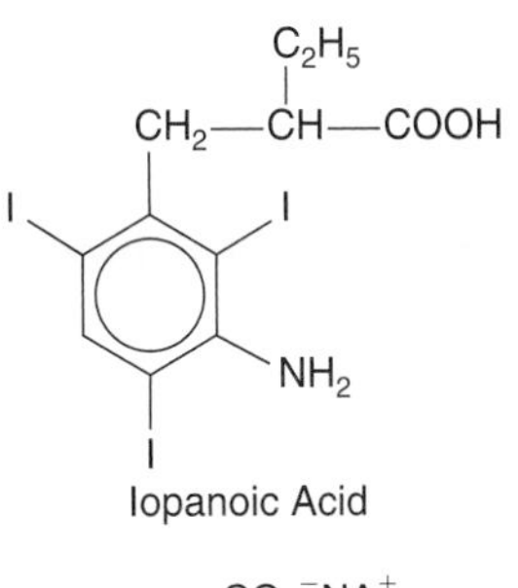

Iopanoic Acid

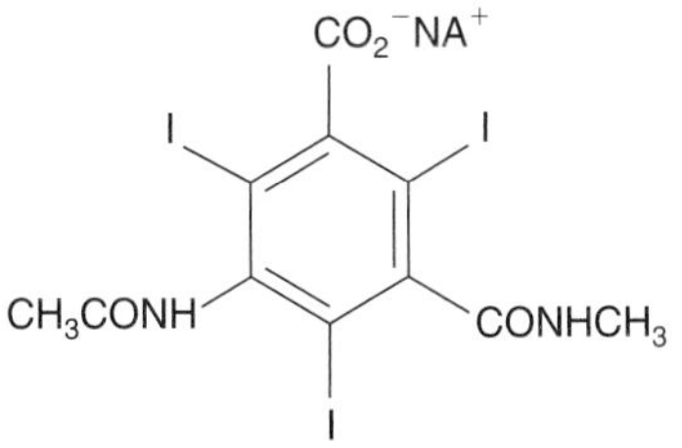

Iothalamate Sodium

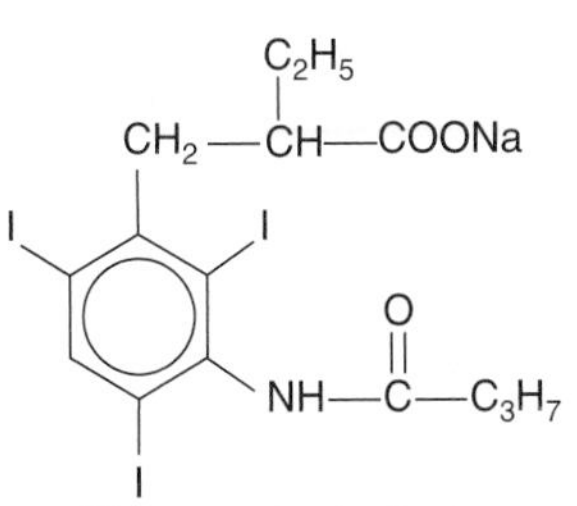

Tyropanoate Sodium

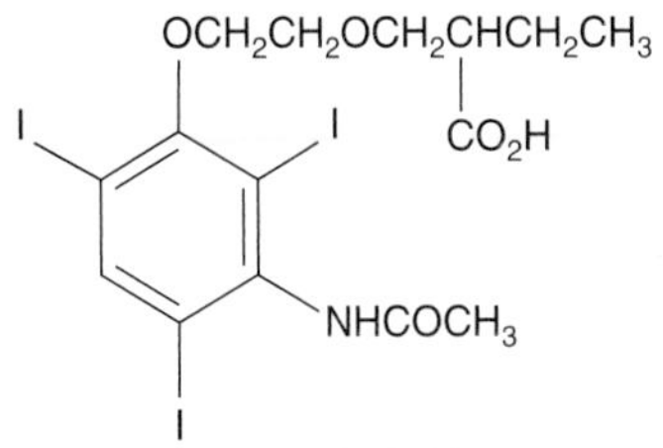

Iopronic Acid

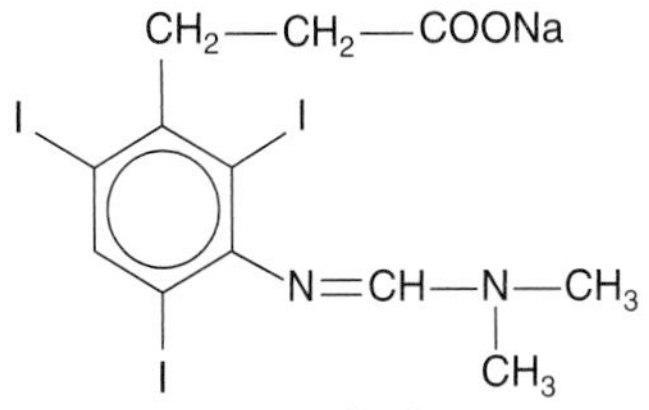

Ipodate Sodium

On the other hand, there is a heterogenous group of water-insoluble compounds of iodine that only rarely find use as radiological contrast agents. These compounds consist of ester derivatives of iodinated vegetable (poppy-seed) oils and iodinated pyridones such as propyliodone (Table 13-2). In the case of iodized oils, unsaturated vegetable fatty acid moieties are iodinated by addition across double bonds and are then converted into various esters. Some water-insoluble aromatic iodides have also been used occasionally as radiological contrast agents. These substances are more resistant to breakdown from exposure to light and air, but like the iodized oils, they cannot be used intravascularly.

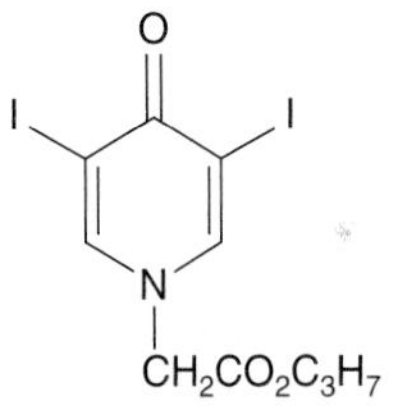

Propyliodone

PARAMAGNETIC COMPOUNDS

MRI is a unique method of medical imaging (Fig. 13-12). When a patient is placed in a large, strong, uniform magnetic field, one can use smaller, well-directed gradient fields to selectively excite hydrogen nuclei (protons) in a selected small volume of the patient's body. The excitation is done by use of radiofrequency fields, and once the excitation fields are removed, the excited protons lose the energy they gained. They emit a weak, but detectable, radio wave, whose strength and manner of decay can be used to generate diagnostic medical images. The tesla (T) has been adopted as the official unit of magnetic field strength for the international system of units. The conventional unit, the gauss (G), is 10,000 times smaller. MRI is normally performed at 0.5 to 1.5 T.

The images produced by MRI are superficially similar to the cross-sectional images of the body produced by CT. MRI, however, has the added advantage of not using ionizing radiation, such as x-rays or γ-rays, and easily produces exquisite soft tissue images of the body in any desired plane (coronal, axial, sagittal, oblique, etc.). With MRI, image con-

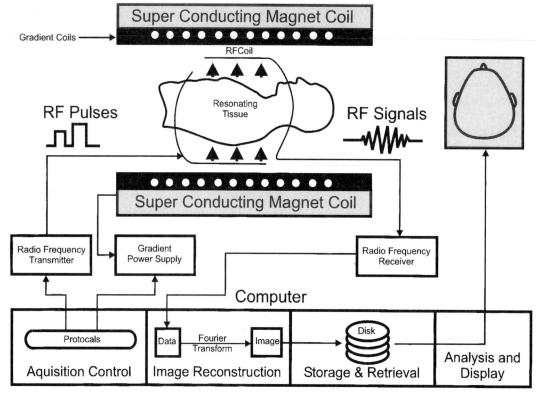

Figure 13–12 ■ Schematic diagram of an MRI system. MRI uses radiofrequency waves to image a patient in a strong magnetic field. Subsequent image information is reconstructed with computer techniques similar to those for CT. MRI can produce images in any desired plane (axial, coronal, sagittal, or oblique).

trast is determined by many physical parameters, whereas with conventional radiography and CT scanning, only a single tissue parameter, x-ray beam attenuation, is important. The three most important parameters in MRI are water content (proton density), blood flow, and relaxation times (T_1 and T_2). T_1 is a measure of the proton's ability to exchange energy with its environment, and T_2 portrays how quickly a tissue loses its magnetism.

When a compound is placed in a magnetic field, it displays a certain susceptibility to becoming magnetized and an ability to alter the magnetic field into which it has been placed. The ability of a substance to produce additional magnetism within a magnetic field is known as its *susceptibility*. A vacuum has a susceptibility defined as zero in comparison with water. Air and many nonmetallic solid materials are said to be *diamagnetic,* because they have negative susceptibility and induce weaker magnetic fields than water. Such substances have fully paired electrons. Materials with unpaired electrons are said to be *paramagnetic,* because they strengthen magnetic fields in their vicinity. A substance with many unpaired electrons will be *superparamagnetic,* because it produces a strong supplementary magnetic field. A *ferromagnetic* material has a very large number of unpaired electrons and produces a large supplementary magnetization that remains when the magnetic field has been removed.

Contrast agents developed for MRI thus far have relied on the use of paramagnetic ions. There are two ways to categorize MR contrast agents. *One classification system groups them into paramagnetic agents and iron oxides.* The paramagnetic agents predominantly decrease tissue T_1 relax-

ation time, which increases (brightens) tissue intensity on T_1-weighted images. Iron oxides in various formulations, on the other hand, are used primarily to decrease (darken) tissue signal intensity on T_2 images, because they primarily decrease T_2 relaxation times, which decreases signal intensity. *Another way to classify MRI agents is to categorize them as either extracellular or intracellular agents.*

The MR contrast agents most commonly used for clinical imaging are the extracellular paramagnetic agents. The primary paramagnetic metal ion used for MRI is gadolinium, which is a rare earth element. Gadolinium (Gd) forms the Gd(III) ion when prepared in 0.05 M hydrochloric acid, and it is extremely effective for enhancing water proton relaxation rates. It is, however, toxic for human use because of its biological half-life of several weeks. When the acidic Gd(III) ion is used intravenously, it quickly binds to Fe(III) protein-binding sites, most notably plasma transferrin. In addition, Gd(III) ions form insoluble compounds readily by interacting with endogenous ions, including phosphate, carbonate, and hydroxide.[29] Consequently, the development of Gd(III) contrast agents has mainly focused on chelated compounds that clear rapidly from the body through the kidneys and exhibit minimal toxicity. Many extracellular gadolinium chelates are being used or explored as potential MRI contrast agents. These include: gadoteridol (ProHance), gadopentetate dimeglumine (Magnevist), gadodiamide (Omniscan), gadoterate meglumine (Dotarem), gadobutrol (Gadovist), and gadoversetamide (Optimark).

Much research is taking place in all phases of MRI, including development of new contrast agents. Several MR contrast agents have been introduced or proposed to provide selective imaging of various organs and tissues, such as the liver, the RE system, the lymphatic system, and the blood pool. For example, gadobenate dimeglumine (MultiHance) and gadoxetic acid (Eovist) accumulate in the interstitial space and the urine. They are eliminated by both the renal and hepatobiliary routes, and therefore, they can be used as selective hepatocyte and biliary excretion contrast agents.

Manganese (Mn^{2+}) is strongly paramagnetic, but it is toxic if used as a free ion. To make it safe for use in humans, various manganese complexes have been developed as MRI contrast agents. At this time, the only parenteral manganese compound used in humans is mangafodipir trisodium. This compound is delivered to tissues with active metabolism, such as the pancreas, renal cortex, GI tract, heart, and adrenal glands.

Specially designed parenteral particulate agents can be used to examine the RE system. One way to do this is to incorporate a paramagnetic material into a hollow structure composed of surrounding lipid layers. The size of these lipid complexes (liposomes) is then manipulated so that they will be selectively filtered by the RE system, producing MRI contrast enhancement of the liver, spleen, and lymph nodes, depending on the liposome size and other characteristics. Polysaccharide-coated superparamagnetic iron oxide particles (SPIO) can be specifically designed with useful properties. These contain a crystalline core composed of iron oxide complexes with ferrous (Fe^{2+}) and ferric (F^{3+}) ions. The core is coated with dextran or another large polysaccharide. Their size is between 1 and 10 μm, and their biological characteristics can be manipulated by changing their polysaccharide coating. Large particles accumulate in the liver and spleen, while smaller particles remain in the circulation longer and tend to aggregate in lymph nodes. Ferumoxides (Feridex or AMI-25), ferrixan (Resovist), and ferumoxtran (Combidex or AMI 227) are three examples of such agents. Because main MRI effect of the iron oxide particles is on T2 images, they darken the tissue in which they accumulate.

Oral MRI contrast agents are being developed for improved visualization of the GI tract. One method of improving bowel visibility is to displace the bowel contents with air or liquids. Air is not widely used, because it requires intubation of the stomach or the rectum, and it has unpleasant aftereffects. Perfluorocarbon compounds have the same magnetic susceptibility as water and will displace bowel contents for improved imaging. They are, however, expensive and not widely used.

Clays, such as the formulation used in Kaopectate, superparamagnetic iron oxide particles (SPIOs), some natural foods or nutritional supplements, also may be used as gastrointestinal MRI contrast agents because of their distinct effects on the T_1 or T_2 relaxation times of bowel contents. Bananas and blueberries, for example, contain high amounts of manganese. Although all of these agents are potentially useful, they are generally reserved for special imaging situations. There are no generally accepted MRI contrast agents used for imaging the bowel contents. All of them have some type of disadvantage that limits their use, such as terrible taste, excessive cost, unpleasant aftereffects, or the production of excessive imaging artifacts on some imaging sequences. The most universally accepted bowel contrast agent is tap water. It gives the bowel a low signal intensity on T1 images and a high signal intensity on T2 images. Tap water is inexpensive, readily available, and readily accepted by patients. Unfortunately, its ability to image bowel contents and to contrast the bowel with surrounding organs and with pathological processes is not always good.

ULTRASOUND CONTRAST AGENTS

Diagnostic ultrasound imaging uses high-frequency sound waves from 1 to 12 MHz to produce cross-sectional images of the body. A small handheld transducer connected to a larger electronic box is used to scan the body part of interest (e.g., the abdomen), and the resultant images are displayed on a computer screen. They may be later printed on film or stored digitally. Various body tissues reflect the sound waves in characteristic fashion, and diagnostic ultrasound is similar to the sonar imaging used by aquatic mammals and submarines. Differing tissues (e.g., the liver and the right kidney) have different acoustic properties. At the interface between tissues with different acoustic properties, the sound waves are reflected back to the transducer and are displayed on the screen, showing the interface and the tissues at the interface. Unfortunately, gas-containing structures (lungs, bowel) and bones either absorb or scatter most of the sound waves and are not usually imaged satisfactorily by ultrasound. Solid organs (liver, spleen, kidneys), organs containing fluid (heart, gallbladder, urinary bladder), blood vessels, fatty tissue, and muscles, however, are usually amenable to diagnostic sonographic imaging.

Ultrasound finds widespread application in diagnostic radiology, obstetrics, gynecology, and cardiology because it produces diagnostic results comparable or even superior in some cases to other imaging techniques that require the use of ionizing radiation. Ultrasound machines are often portable and may be taken to the patient's bedside. Moreover, diagnostic ultrasound has no known harmful effects.

Contrast agents are not used for most diagnostic ultrasound examinations. Much research is being conducted, however, to develop safe, inexpensive ultrasound contrast agents that may be ingested orally or injected intravenously. Ultrasound relies on the detection of acoustic energy (sound waves) reflected at tissue interfaces within the body. Gases create prominent acoustic interfaces with body tissues and can be adapted as contrast agents. Microbubbles containing air or other gases introduced into the bloodstream may act as a contrast agent by increasing the ultrasound signal reflected from the vessel contents or from the structures fed by the vessels. Agents relying on microbubbles may be classified as *(a)* stabilized or encapsulated microbubbles, *(b)* polymer microballoons and gaseous liposomes, or *(c)* colloidal suspensions and emulsions. These agents allow visualization of small vessels, identification of tumor vascularity, improved contrast visualization of solid organs, and improved visualization of the heart chambers and vascular grafts and conduits and are generally very safe. They are designed so no large bubbles form in the body, and they have relatively short life spans and then break down and dissipate. The problems generally encountered with them are their instability during passage through the heart and lungs and their limited time of action. Research into ultrasound contrast agents is in its infancy and will no doubt produce useful products in the near future.

Gadoteridol

Gadopentetate Dimeglumine

Gadodiamide

RADIOLOGICAL PROCEDURES

Modern radiology has many imaging procedures that use contrast agents (Table 13-2). Some of the more common procedures are discussed below and illustrated with examples to show the usefulness of contrast agents. Although it is traditional to think of radiological studies as using film, except in the case of CT or MRI, one should realize that the digital revolution has come to diagnostic imaging. Many traditional radiographic studies, such as chest radiology, no longer use traditional radiographic film. Instead, x-rays are used to "expose" an imaging plate instead of a piece of film. This imaging plate can create a digital signal if properly processed. The electronic signals from digital imaging plates are then used to create radiological images that are read from computer monitors instead of film view boxes. Thus, imaging studies can be stored, manipulated, and transported worldwide digitally over local area networks or over wide area networks. Diagnostic radiologists, however, perform the same type of studies and use the same contrast agents whether the studies are film based or computer based.

Intravenous Pyelography, Intravenous Urography, Excretory Urography, and Computed Tomography

The intravenous pyelogram (IVP) is one of the oldest and most fundamental diagnostic radiological studies using contrast material. It is a mainstay of genitourinary (GU) radiology and delineates the kidneys and the urinary tract (renal calices, pelvis, and ureters) as well as the bladder (Fig. 13-13). A more modern name and one that better describes the relevant physiology involved in the study is *excretory urography*. Nevertheless, the term *IVP* has been in common use for so long that it still is the name used most frequently. Excretory urography is based on the rapid renal clearance of water-soluble iodinated benzoic acid compounds (whether they are low-osmolar or high-osmolar agents) after they are injected intravenously. In normal individuals, the ionic and nonionic water-soluble iodinated contrast agents are all excreted by glomerular filtration.

Many body and head CT studies (Figs. 13-14 and 13-15) use intravenous contrast material to improve the quality of the study. The type of contrast material and their doses are similar to those in excretory urography except that higher volumes of contrast and a more rapid injection system are often used. The contrast material increases the relative contrast between space-occupying lesions (tumors, cysts, and abscesses) and normal body tissues. It also frequently shows blood vessels to better advantage.

Arteriography and Venography

Angiography refers to the radiographic visualization of blood vessels by contrast injection directly into an artery (arteriography) (Fig. 13-16) or a vein (venography). There are many types of arteriograms, including those from cerebral angiography (visualization of head and neck vessels),

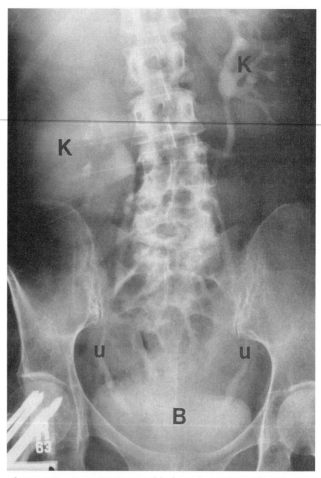

Figure 13-13 ■ IVP in an elderly patient. Note the contrast visualization of the kidneys (*K*), ureters (*U*), and bladder (*B*). The patient also has fixation screws in her right hip from past surgery to stabilize a hip fracture.

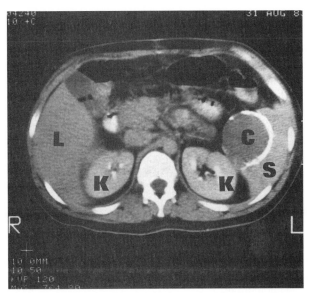

Figure 13–14 ■ CT scan of the upper abdomen in a middle-aged adult. The image is an axial view of the patient's upper abdomen viewed as if looking up from the patient's feet. The patient's right side is on the left side of the image. The liver *(L)*, kidneys *(K)*, and spleen *(S)* are partially visualized. There is a large cyst *(C)* in the spleen, with a calcified rim.

coronary angiography (visualization of the coronary arteries), aortography (visualization of the abdominal or thoracic aorta), and peripheral arteriography (visualization of the major arteries of the upper and lower extremities).

Arteriography is widely practiced for diagnosing vessel

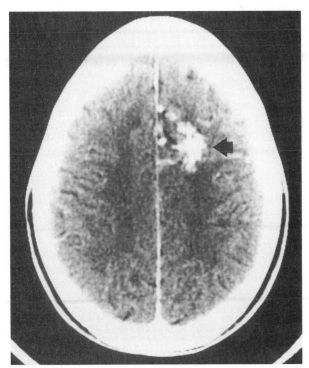

Figure 13–15 ■ Axial CT scan of the brain of a patient with an arteriovenous malformation (AVM), after injection of an intravenous iodinated contrast agent *(arrow)*.

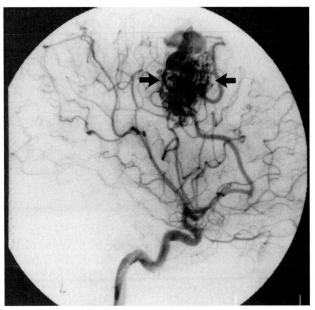

Figure 13–16 ■ Same patient as shown in Figure 13-15. A cerebral arteriogram was performed to delineate the vascular anatomy of the patient's AVM. In this case, a digital subtraction technique was used in which digital images obtained prior to injection of the contrast agent were subtracted from the contrast agent images by computer.

narrowing or blockage, aneurysm formation, and sites of bleeding. The type of contrast used depends on the vessel being injected and the preferences of the physician performing the study. Venography, the contrast opacification of venous structures, is performed less commonly than arteriography. The main indication for venography is to diagnose deep venous thrombosis in the lower extremities, based on changes in ultrasound by a moving reflector (blood).

High-quality modern diagnostic ultrasonography coupled with Doppler imaging techniques has largely replaced venography in the workup of suspected deep venous thromboses. Sonography is easy to perform, is much safer than venography, and causes much less patient discomfort. Venography is still used in selected cases, particularly when sonography is equivocal or there is a past history of documented venous thrombosis that requires detailed evaluation of the venous anatomy.

Cholecystography and Cholangiography

Cholecystography refers to contrast visualization of the gallbladder. Modern gallbladder visualization and diagnosis rely mainly on abdominal ultrasonography or nuclear medicine and rarely use traditional radiological techniques.

Oral cholecystographic agents consist of analogues of 2,4,6-triiodinated alkylbenzoic acids. They have various substituents in the 1 and 3 positions and are absorbed orally, followed by hepatic excretion. Oral cholecystographic agents include iopanoic acid, iocetamic acid, sodium tyropanoate, and sodium ipodate. In general, these agents are bound to serum albumin and converted by the liver into water-soluble glucuronide conjugates. These conjugates are excreted in the bile and stored in the gallbladder, thus facilitating gallbladder visualization.

Iodipamide meglumine (Cholografin) is the main agent used for intravenous cholangiography. Under ideal circumstances, iodipamide meglumine produces excellent visualization of the intrahepatic and extrahepatic bile ducts as well as the gallbladder. Oral cholecystography generally produces better visualization of the gallbladder itself but poorer visualization of the bile ducts than intravenous cholangiography.

Myelography

Myelography involves injection of contrast material into the subarachnoid space, usually in the lower lumbar region, for visualization of the spinal cord, nerve roots, and subarachnoid space. It has been somewhat superseded by modern MRI and CT imaging of the spinal canal, and it can be performed by itself or in conjunction with a subsequent CT study of the spinal canal. Until the advent of the low-osmolar contrast agents, iophendylate (Pantopaque) was the standard agent used for myelography. It was first replaced by metrizamide, which has now been largely supplanted by iohexol and similar agents, which give improved image detail and have lower toxicity.

Great care must be taken when performing contrast injection into the subarachnoid space. Improper technique could lead to a devastating infection or spinal injury, and the use of the wrong contrast agent can also have devastating results such as convulsions and subsequent, severe arachnoid inflammation.

Hysterosalpingography

Hysterosalpingography refers to visualization of the uterine cavity and fallopian tubes (Fig. 13-17). Contrast material is injected into the uterus through the cervical canal to assess uterine anatomy and the patency of the fallopian tubes. Most practitioners use some type of water-soluble contrast material for hysterosalpingography, though in the past the use of oily agents such as Ethiodol was popular. One popular agent

(Salpix) consists of a water-soluble gel that is a 2:1 mixture of diatrizoate meglumine and iodipamide meglumine. Iohexol and other low-osmolar agents are also used for hysterosalpingography, and they may produce slightly lower incidence of abdominal pain and discomfort after the procedure.

Gastrointestinal Studies

Traditional GI tract studies have used various preparations of barium sulfate to opacify the hypopharynx and esophagus (barium swallow); the lower esophagus, stomach, and duodenum (upper gastrointestinal tract; UGI); the small bowel (small bowel follow-through; SBFT); and the colon (barium enema; BE) (Fig. 13-18). In the BE, the barium is administered per rectum as an enema, usually with the intention of visualizing the entirety of the colon and the terminal-most portion of the ileum. Gastrointestinal tract studies are used to diagnose peptic acid disease (ulcers), benign and malignant tumors, and such conditions as GER and inflammatory bowel conditions.

If there is a possibility of a GI tract perforation, a water-soluble agent is used in place of a barium sulfate preparation. If there is leakage of contrast from the GI tract into the peritoneum, retroperitoneum, or mediastinum, water-soluble agents are generally rapidly absorbed by these tissues with no untoward patient effects. Barium preparations are particulate and will not be easily cleared from these spaces. Barium mixed with feces may produce severe peritonitis and be life-threatening.

Oral contrast material is often used as part of an abdominal

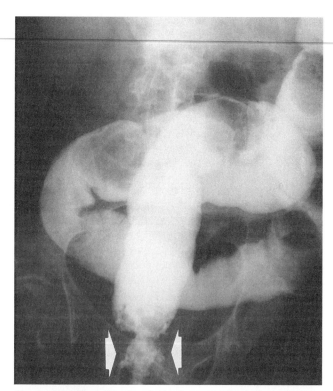

Figure 13–18 ■ Results of a barium enema performed on an elderly man. Barium absorbs x-rays very well and has a white appearance that shows the rectum and sigmoid portions of the colon. In the rectum, a large tumor *(arrows)* encircles the rectum and narrows the barium column.

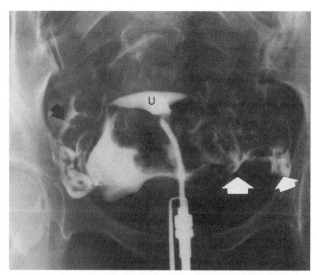

Figure 13–17 ■ Normal hysterosalpingogram performed in a young woman as part of an infertility workup. The contrast material outlines the uterus *(U)* and has traveled through patent fallopian tubes to spill into her peritoneum *(arrows)*.

CT study to opacify the bowel. A relatively dilute barium sulfate mixture or a dilute solution of ionic contrast material mixed with a flavoring agent are commonly used.

Arthrography

Arthrography is radiographic visualization of the internal structure of a joint. The shoulder, hip, knee, and wrist are joints commonly visualized by arthrography, although the procedure may be applied to other joints, such as the elbow or ankle. Some forms of arthrography, especially knee arthrography, have been completely replaced by MRI studies. An arthrogram is obtained by injecting a small amount (1 to 10 mL) of water-soluble, usually low-osmolar, contrast material into the joint space. The contrast agent may be mixed with a local anesthetic to reduce patient discomfort, and air or carbon dioxide may also be injected to produce a double-contrast effect. In the latter case, the water-soluble contrast material outlines the surface of the joint, including the joint capsule and cartilage surfaces, whereas the gas produces a negative-contrast effect as it distends the joint space.

Adverse Reactions

Radiological contrast agents can be taken orally in large amounts, and some of them are injected intravascularly in gram amounts with no ill effects. Nevertheless, any radiological contrast material may produce an untoward patient reaction, even sudden death.[30–33] Untoward patient events occur when contrast material is aspirated or when it leaks from the GI tract. Hypertonic ionic water-soluble contrast agents are potentially dangerous if aspirated into the tracheobronchial tree. They are very irritating and reportedly have caused pulmonary edema. Any contrast material that leaks out of the bowel into the abdomen, pelvis, or chest is potentially quite dangerous, especially barium sulfate. Barium sulfate is insoluble, and its particulate nature means it is poorly cleared from the mediastinum, peritoneum, and retroperitoneum. Water-soluble agents, on the other hand, are rapidly absorbed from the mediastinum, peritoneum, and retroperitoneum, almost as quickly as if they had been injected intravenously. In general, water-soluble agents that leak from the GI tract cause no significant problems beyond a transient inflammation.

The intravenous or intra-arterial injection of iodinated contrast material for pyelography, contrast-enhanced CT studies, and angiographic studies opens the door to a diverse assortment of contrast reactions, most of which are minor and easily treated. Minor reactions include arm pain, a feeling of general body warmth and discomfort, mild nausea and vomiting, a strong metallic taste in the mouth, and mild urticaria (hives). Minor reactions dissipate in a few minutes with patient reassurance and observation.

Intermediate or moderate reactions are those that require some form of therapy but are not life threatening. Depending on the contrast agent used and on how contrast reactions are defined in a given institution, moderate reactions occur in approximately 1% of contrast injections. They include difficulty breathing, severe hives, severe nausea and vomiting, mild hypotension, wheezing, and other similar reactions. Treatment ranges from administration of intravenous fluids to the use of intravenous diphenhydramine for hives. Epi-

nephrine may be administered, and atropine is used if there is a vasovagal reaction with hypotension and bradycardia.

Severe reactions are those that are life threatening. They include sudden cardiovascular collapse and death, as well as severe hypotension; severe shortness of breath, wheezing, or laryngoedema; loss of consciousness; massive hives and angioneurotic edema; ventricular cardiac arrhythmias; angina; and myocardial infarction. Their treatment depends on the patient's signs and symptoms and includes intravenous fluids, oxygen, various drugs (including epinephrine, diphenhydramine, and atropine), and possible cardiopulmonary resuscitation (CPR).

The incidence of adverse reactions to radiopharmaceuticals is estimated to be less than 0.006%. Most reactions are allergic and occur within minutes after intravenous injection. In the case of radiolabeled murine antibodies, an anaphylactic reaction may occur, although serious reactions of this type have not been reported.

Selected Products

Barium Sulfate. The many commercial preparations of barium sulfate differ in their density and their ability to coat the bowel wall. These characteristics are determined by the particle size of the barium suspension, its viscosity, and its pH, which in turn are determined by the addition of small amounts of flavoring agents, suspending agents, and so forth. These additives are the proprietary secret of the manufacturer and do improve the diagnostic properties of the barium colloidal suspension for GI radiological studies.

Barium sulfate preparations are used to study the esophagus, stomach, and duodenum as part of an esophagram or UGI series and are given orally. Most patients find the taste of these dense mixtures acceptable (they are usually given a strawberry or lemon flavor), but they dislike the heavy texture of the barium. Barium sulfate suspensions are also given orally to study the entire small bowel (SBFT) or rectally to examine the colon (BE) (Fig. 13-18).

Typical barium suspensions range from 30 to more than 120% weight/volume (w/v), and because they are colloidal suspensions, they cannot be given intravascularly; the colloidal particles would produce fatal pulmonary embolism. The barium suspensions used for UGI or BE studies are too dense to be used for gut opacification during CT studies of the abdomen, because they produce unacceptable radiographic artifacts. Instead, commercial barium preparations are diluted to 1 to 4% w/v.

Diatrizoate. Diatrizoate is classified as an ionic monomeric contrast agent and is available in the meglumine, sodium, or combination of meglumine and sodium salts of the fully substituted triiodobenzoic acid. It has a molecular weight of 614, and the organically bound iodine content is 62%. Its salts are used mainly for angiography and excretory urography. The diatrizoate meglumine (66%) and diatrizoate sodium (10%) combination may be used orally or rectally to delineate the GI tract. This preparation is indicated when the use of barium sulfate is potentially dangerous (i.e., whenever a suspected perforation of the GI tract exists), because water-soluble contrast agents are quickly absorbed through the peritoneal surface. The high osmolality prevents water absorption and leads to rapid transit through the GI tract.

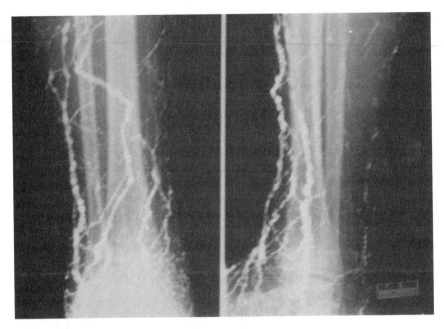

Figure 13–19 ■ Lymphangiogram of a normal leg after Ethiodol administration.

The meglumine salt dilute solution (18% w/v) is used for cystography after sterile catheterization of the bladder.

Ethiodol. Ethiodol is a sterile preparation containing ethyl esters of the iodinated fatty acids of poppy-seed oil and it is used for lymphangiography. It contains 35 to 39% of organically bound iodine that has been added to the double bonds of the fatty acids. Because Ethiodol is an oily substance and not miscible with plasma, it cannot be administered intravascularly. For lymphangiography, it is injected into tiny lymphatics of the web space of the hand or foot. The lymphatics carry tiny globules of Ethiodol to regional lymph nodes, where they are partially filtered by the nodes and localized in them. The iodine in the Ethiodol makes the nodes sufficiently radiopaque to be visualized on plain film radiographs. A lymphangiogram typically is used to evaluate lymph nodes in the groin, pelvis, and abdomen in patients with Hodgkin's disease and sometimes other malignancies. A typical normal lymphangiogram of the lower leg is illustrated in Figure 13-19.

Iobitridol. Iobitridol is a low-osmolar nonionic monomeric contrast agent. It is similar to the other agents in its class and finds use in excretory urography, angiography, and CT.

Iocetamic Acid. Iocetamic acid is a high-osmolar ionic monomeric contrast agent and is used as an oral cholecystographic agent for the radiographic visualization of the biliary tract and gallbladder. It has a molecular weight of 614 and an organically bound iodine content of about 62%. A dose of 3.0 to 4.5 g is given orally 10 to 15 hours before radiographic examination, and about 60% of this dose is excreted in the urine within 48 hours. A typical radiograph of a gallbladder is illustrated in Figure 13-20.

Iohexol. Iohexol is a low-osmolar nonionic monomeric contrast agent. It finds widespread use in excretory urography, CT, myelography, and angiographic procedures.

Iodipamide Meglumine. Iodipamide meglumine is an ionic dimeric contrast agent and is given as the meglumine salt, which is highly water soluble. It has a molecular weight of 1,530 and an organically bound iodine content of 49.9%. Iodipamide meglumine is very strongly bound to serum albu-

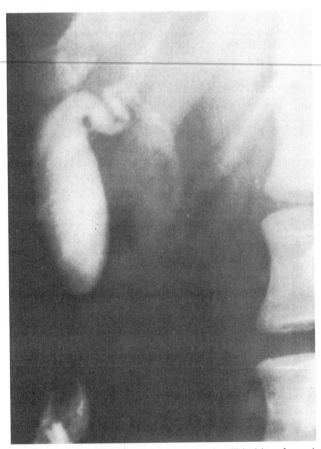

Figure 13–20 ■ Radiograph of a normal gallbladder after administration of iopanoic acid.

min and is excreted by the liver into the biliary system unmodified. Unfortunately, iodipamide meglumine produces a high incidence of adverse patient reactions, such as urticaria and hypotension, and intravenous cholangiography has generally been discontinued. Modern ultrafast helical (spiral) CT scanners, however, can produce exquisite high-contrast studies of the liver and biliary system, and these sophisticated CT scanning techniques have renewed interest in the use of intravenous cholangiography.

Iodixanol. Iodixanol is a low-osmolar nonionic *dimeric* contrast agent. It is designed for intravascular injection and is used for excretory urography, angiography, and CT.

Iopamidol. Iopamidol is a low-osmolar nonionic monomeric contrast agent. It has a molecular weight of 777 and an organically bound iodine content of 49%. Although the osmolality is much lower than that of the ionic contrast agents, the viscosity is very similar. It is used for a variety of angiographic procedures, excretory urography, arthrography, and oral and rectal visualization of the GI tract. It is available in solutions containing 30.6 to 75.5% iopamidol.

Iopanoic Acid. Iopanoic acid is an ionic monomeric contrast agent. It has a molecular weight of 571 and an organically bound iodine content of 66.7%. It is used as an oral cholecystographic agent for the radiographic visualization of the biliary tract and gallbladder. A dose of 3 g is given by mouth with ample water about 10 to 14 hours before radiographic examination. It frequently produces mild GI discomfort.

Iopromide. Iopromide is a low-osmolar nonionic monomeric contrast agent. It has a molecular weight of 791 and an organically bound iodine content of 48.12%. It is designed for intravascular injection.

Iotrol. Iotrol is a low-osmolar nonionic *dimeric* contrast agent. It has a molecular weight of 1,626 and contains six iodine atoms per particle in solution. It is designed for intravascular injection.

Ioversol. Ioversol is a low-osmolar nonionic monomeric contrast agent. It has a molecular weight of 807 and an iodine content of 47.2%. Its main uses are in angiography and excretory urography.

Ioxaglate. Ioxaglate is a *low-osmolal ionic dimeric* contrast agent that is formulated as a combined solution of its meglumine and sodium salts. It has a molecular weight of 1,269 and an organically bound iodine content of 60%. Ioxaglate is used in angiography, arthrography, urography, venography, and hysterosalpingography. This agent is not suitable for myelography.

Ioxilan. Ioxilan is a low-osmolar nonionic monomeric contrast agent. Like other agents in its class, it is mainly used by intravascular injection in excretory urography, angiography, and CT.

Metrizamide. Metrizamide is a low-osmolar nonionic monomeric contrast agent. It has a molecular weight of 789

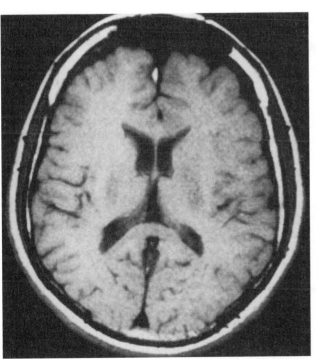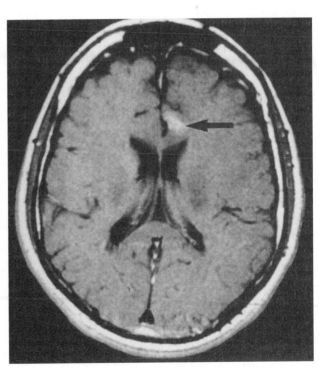

A   B

Figure 13–21 ■ MRI of the brain of a 36-year-old patient with a single episode of acute weakness. **A.** T₁-weighted axial image without contrast agent taken 3 days later. **B.** T₁-weighted image after intravenous injection of gadopentetate dimeglumine, which has concentrated in the left frontal lobe *(arrow)*. The patient was diagnosed as having a cerebrovascular accident. (Courtesy of Berlex Laboratories, Inc.)

and an organically bound iodine content of 48.2%. It is used mainly in the radiographic examination of the spinal cord and central nervous system (i.e., myelography, cisternography, and ventriculography). The most frequent adverse effects are headache, nausea, and vomiting. Metrizamide was the first commercially available nonionic contrast agent. On-site reconstitution of the lyophilized powder is necessary because of the instability of metrizamide in solution. It has largely been replaced in daily practice by the newer low-osmolar contrast agents.

MRI Agents.

There are many types of MRI contrast agents. At the present time, only the extracellular gadolinium chelates have found widespread use. These agents, in general, are highly soluble in water and can be administered by intravenous injection. They are classified as ionic or nonionic, and they are either linear or macrocyclic chelates. Gadolinium-based contrast agents are administered in a typical dose of 0.1 mmol/kg, which can be increased to a total dose of 0.3 mmol/kg for the nonionic agent gadoteridol in patients who have poorly enhancing tumors or equivocal scans. Figure 13-21 illustrates an MRI study of a brain before and after injection of gadopentetate dimeglumine.

Propyliodone.

Dionosil, a commercial preparation of propyliodone, a pyridone ester, was once popular for use in bronchography. It consists of a white powder suspended in an oily medium and was used for bronchography and laryngography (examination of the larynx). Other methods of imaging, such as CT, ultrasonography, and MRI, as well as modern fiber optic bronchoscopy have largely replaced bronchography.

Tyropanoate Sodium.

Tyropanoate sodium is a high-osmolar ionic monomeric contrast agent that is given by mouth for the radiographic visualization of the biliary tract and gallbladder. It has a molecular weight of 633 and an organically bound iodine content of 57.4%. A dose of 3.0 g is given with water 10 to 12 hours before radiographic examination. This agent is not recommended for children under 12 years of age.

REFERENCES

1. National Research Council (U.S.) Committee on the Biological Effects of Ionizing Radiation. Health Effects of Exposure to Low Levels of Ionizing Radiation: BEIRV. Washington, D.C., National Academy Press, 1990.
2. Deutsch, E., et al.: Technetium chemistry and technetium radiopharmaceuticals. In Lippard S. J. (ed.). Progress in Inorganic Chemistry. New York, John Wiley & Sons, 1983.
3. Nowotnik, D. P.: Physico-chemical concepts in the preparation of technetium radiopharmaceuticals. In Sampson C. B. (ed.). Textbook of Radiopharmacy: Theory and Practice, 2nd ed. New York, Gordon & Breach, 1994.
4. Hjelstuen, O. K.: Analyst 120:863, 1995.
5. Schwochau, K.: Angew. Chem. Int. Ed. Engl. 33:2258, 1994.
6. Jurisson, S., et al.: Chem. Rev. 93:1137, 1993.
7. Costello, C. E., et al.: J. Nucl. Med. 24:353, 1983.
8. Jurisson, S., et al.: Inorg. Chem. 25:543, 1986.
9. Libson, K., et al.: J. Am. Chem. Soc. 102:2476, 1980.
10. de Ligny, C. L., et al.: Nucl. Med. Biol. 17:161, 1990.
11. Moretti, J. L., et al.: Int. J. Nucl. Med. Biol. 11:270, 1984.
12. Ohta, H., et al.: Clin. Nucl. Med. 10:508, 1984.
13. Blower, P. J., Singh, J., and Clarke, S.: J. Nucl. Med. 32:845, 1991.
14. Forster, A. M., et al.: J. Nucl. Med. 33:850, 1992.
15. Palmer, A. J., Clark, J. C., and Goulding, R. W.: Int. J. Appl. Radiat. Isotopes 28:53, 1977.
16. Hamacher, K., Coenen, H. H., and Stocklin, G.: J. Nucl. Med. 27:235, 1986.
17. Hawkins, R. A., and Hoh, C. K.: Nucl. Med. Biol. 21:739, 1994.
18. Baldwin, R. N.: Int. J. Appl. Radiat. Isotopes 37:817, 1986.
19. Sisson, J. C., et al.: N. Engl. J. Med. 305:12, 1981.
20. Kimmig, B., et al.: J. Nucl. Med. 25:773, 1984.
21. Kohler, G. P., and Milstein, C.: Nature 256:495, 1975.
22. Colcher, D., et al.: Proc. Natl. Acad. Sci. U. S. A. 78:3199, 1981.
23. Rodwell, J. D., et al.: Proc. Natl. Acad. Sci. U. S. A. 83:2632, 1986.
24. Green, M. A., and Huffman, J. C.: J. Nucl. Med. 29:417, 1988.
25. Bakker, W. H., et al.: Life Sci. 49:1583, 1991.
26. Fisher, H. W.: Radiology 159:561, 1986.
27. Wolf, G. L.: Radiology 159:557, 1986.
28. White, R. I., and Holden, W. J.: Radiology 159:559, 1986.
29. Tweedle, M. F., et al.: Invest. Radiol. 30:372, 1995.
30. Katayama, H., et al.: Radiology 175:621, 1990.
31. Wold, G. L., et al.: Invest. Radiol. 26:404, 1991.
32. Bush, W. H., McClennan, B. L., and Swanson, D. P.: Postgrad. Radiol. 13:137, 1993.
33. Lasser, E. C., and Berry, C.: Invest. Radiol. 26:402, 1991.

SELECTED READING

Bushberg, J. T., Seibert, J. A., Leidholdt, E. M., and Boone, J. M.: The Essential Physics of Medical Imaging. Baltimore, Williams & Wilkins, 1995.
Committee on Drugs and Contrast Media, Commission on Education, American College of Radiology: Manual on Iodinated Contrast Media. Reston, VA, American College of Radiology, 1991.
Committee on the Biological Effects of Ionizing Radiations (BEIR V): Health Effects of Exposure to Low Levels of Ionizing Radiation, National Research Council. Washington, DC, National Academy Press, 1990.
Eisenberg, R. L.: Radiology. An Illustrated History. St. Louis, Mosby–Year Book, 1992.
Elgazzar A. The Pathophysiologic Basis of Nuclear Medicine. New York, Springer-Verlag, 2001.
Katzberg, R. W. (ed.): The Contrast Media Manual. Baltimore, Williams & Wilkins, 1992.
Kowalsky, R. J., and Perry, J. R.: Radiopharmaceuticals in Nuclear Medicine Practice. Norwalk, CT, Appleton & Lange, 1987.
Kuroda, S., Kamiyama, H., Abe, H., et al.: Acetazolamide test in detecting reduced cerebral perfusion reserve and predicting long-term prognosis in patients with internal carotid artery occlusion. Neurosurgery 32: 912–918, 1993.
Lister-James, J., and Dean, R. T.: Tc-99m P829: Characterization of a Technetium-99-labeled somatostatin receptor-binding peptide.
Loevinger, R., Budinger, T., and Watson E.: MIRD Primer for Absorbed Dose Calculations. Rev. ed. New York, Society of Nuclear Medicine, 1991, *www.snm.org*.
Loevinger, R., Budinger, T. F., and Watson, E. E.: MIRD Primer for Absorbed Dose Calculation. Reston, VA, Society of Nuclear Medicine, 1988.
Nicolini, M, and Mazzi, U. (eds.): Technetium, Rhenium and Other Metals in Chemistry and Nuclear Medicine. Padua, SGEditoriali, 1999:473-478, 769–774.
Palmer, E., Scott, J., and Strauss, H. W.: Practical Nuclear Medicine. Philadelphia, W. B. Saunders, 1992.
Putman, C. E., and Ravin, C. E.: Textbook of Diagnostic Imaging, 2nd ed. Philadelphia, W. B. Saunders, 1994.
Runge, V. M. (ed.): Contrast Media in Magnetic Resonance Imaging: A Clinical Approach. Philadelphia, J. B. Lippincott, 1992.
Sprawls, P., Jr.: Physical Principles of Medical Imaging, 2nd ed. Gaithersburg, MD, Aspen Publishers, 1993.
Steigman, J., and Eckelman, W. C.: The Chemistry of Technetium in Medicine. Washington, DC, National Academy Press, 1992.
Swanson, D. P., Chilton, H. M., and Thrall, J.: Pharmaceuticals in Medical Imaging. New York, Macmillan, 1990.
University Hospital Consortium: Technology Assessment: Low-Osmolality Contrast Media. Oakbrook, IL, 1993.

Central Nervous System Depressants

EUGENE I. ISAACSON

The common denominator of the drug classes considered in this chapter is depression of neuronal activity in the central nervous system (CNS), that is, the brain and spinal cord. In most cases the brain is the intended target. In a few cases, as in skeletal muscle relaxants, the cord is also targeted.

The drug classes are the anxiolytics, sedative–hypnotics, general anesthetics, anticonvulsants, and antipsychotics. The primary clinical indication for anxiolytic drugs is in the treatment of the anxiety disorders, which are conditions characterized by excessive or inappropriate anxiety. Examples of these disorders are posttraumatic stress disorder, generalized anxiety disorder, panic attacks, social phobia, and obsessive-compulsive disorder. The major clinical indication for the sedative–hypnotic drugs is in the treatment of some of the insomnias, which are failures to get adequate sleep.

General anesthetic agents are used to produce unconsciousness and loss of perception to painful surgical procedures. Anticonvulsant drugs are used to prevent or lessen the sudden excessive electrical activity in brain neurons that is a characteristic of the epilepsies. Antipsychotics are used in the thought disorders (psychoses), most notably the schizophrenias.

The first four classes of drugs often have a number of structural features in common and likewise often share at least one mode of action, positive modulation of the action of γ-aminobutyric acid (GABA) at $GABA_A$ receptors. Additionally, many anticonvulsants also have an overall bottle-stopper shape that has been associated with neuronal voltage-gated sodium channel block, leading to decreased neuronal excitation. Channel block of other inorganic cations, most notably Ca^{2+}, may contribute significantly to overall action in some instances. Antipsychotics are grouped into typical and atypical categories. Both categories share a common feature, a dopamine-like structure, often hydrophobically substituted. This feature can be related to the most commonly cited action of these agents, competitive antagonism of dopamine (DA) at D_2 and D_3 receptors in the limbic system. In recombinant D_2 receptor cultures, antipsychotic drugs have been observed to act as inverse agonists. For inverse agonism to be a significant mode of action, there must be proof that there is a baseline level of dopaminergic activation in the limbic system. Preliminary indicators suggest that baseline activation will be found; so, inverse agonism is a clinical possibility.[1] The structures of present-day antipsychotics are not inconsistent with inverse antagonism of DA as a mode of antipsychotic action. A defective gating mechanism in the processing of incoming environmental stimuli by the limbic system appears to characterize schizophrenia. The resulting inability to distinguish relevant from irrelevant stimuli evokes the positive symptoms (e.g., illogical and disordered thought, delusions, and hallucinations).

The defective mechanism appears to result from excessive limbic D_2 and D_3 activation.

The fundamental differences between typical and atypical antipsychotics reportedly are that the atypical agents are *(a)* less prone to produce extrapyramidal symptoms (EPS), because they are less able to block striata D_2 receptors vis-a-vis limbic D_2 and D_3 receptors, and *(b)* more active against negative symptoms (social withdrawal, apathy, anhedonia). These differences are examined in a greater detail under the heading, Antipsychotics.

The foregoing introductory condensation may be useful in organizing and clarifying major structural and biological activity relationships throughout this chapter. More details about, and some exceptions to, these generalizations are presented under the discussion headings that follow.

GENERAL ANESTHETICS

The classical inhalation anesthetics, the general anesthetic alcohols, the anesthetic phenol Diprivan, the barbiturates, the neurosteroids, and the benzodiazepines are positive modulators of the action of GABA on $GABA_A$ receptors by binding to allosteric binding sites (different sites exist for each drug group listed).[2, 3] A unifying theory of anesthesia proposes that general anesthetics act by facilitation of $GABA_A$ receptors to promote chloride ion conductance,[2] and at anesthetic concentrations, at least some of the agents (ethanol, phenobarbital) depress the function of ionotropic glutamate receptors (excitatory), which may contribute to the overall anesthetic effect in those cases.[4]

Lipid and protein components of neuronal cell membranes have long been implicated as the site(s) of action in the various theories of how the structurally diverse chemical agents produce general anesthesia. Implicating allosteric binding sites on $GABA_A$ receptors as important in anesthesia does not mean that other proposed sites of action should be ignored. By their nature, many of the simple anesthetic agents could affect a broad range of neuronal components. Also, none of the existing theories of anesthesia is refuted. Inhibition of sodium ion channels by structurally disruptive hydrophobic binding to channel protein is considered likely by many investigators. Still, it is intriguing that the apolar sites of action implied by the Meyer-Overton relationship,[5] theorized as long ago as Johnson and Eyring[6] to be sites of a bioactive protein, might significantly be allosteric modulatory sites of the protein of $GABA_A$ receptors.

Clinically, general anesthesia for surgery uses multiple drug regimens. Some drugs may be used to augment the general anesthetic agent (e.g., neuroleptics and opioid analgesics). Other drugs may add an action (e.g., the skeletal muscle relaxants). Also, drugs such as anticholinergics may be used to decrease adverse effects. Consult a current medical textbook for the ways in which these agents are used together. Our purpose is to consider only the general anesthetic agent.

General anesthetic agents can be broadly categorized as those useful by the inhalation route and those useful by the intravenous (IV) route. These are dictated by the physical state of the agents.

Inhalation Anesthetics

The inhalation anesthetics in use are halothane, enflurane, isoflurane, methoxyflurane, sevoflurane, desflurane, and nitrous oxide. Older agents such as ethylene and cyclopropane are obsolete because of a fundamental chemical property—they are explosive and flammable when mixed with oxygen. This adds an unacceptable level of danger to the production of anesthesia.

Halothane, USP. Halothane, 2-bromo-2-chloro-1,1,1-trifluoroethane (Fluothane), $CH(Cl)CF_3$, a volatile liquid-halogenated hydrocarbon (bp, 50°C), was introduced in 1956 and gained rapid acceptance, largely because of its nonflammability. Additionally, the drug has high potency and a relatively low blood/gas partition coefficient. Accordingly, induction of and recovery from anesthesia are relatively rapid. In actual practice, intravenous sodium thiopental is usually used to induce anesthesia.

Most of halothane is eliminated intact in the expired air. There is sufficient reactivity to oxidative processes, however, to allow up to 20% of the administered compound to undergo metabolism. The trifluoromethyl group is quite stable; the C–H bond, however, is destabilized and is the probable site of metabolic entry. Metabolites are chloride and bromide ions and trifluoroacetate. Additionally, loss of HF yields the olefin 1,1-difluoro-2-chloro-2-bromoethylene, which reacts with the SH group of glutathione.

A low incidence of hepatic necrosis is associated with halothane. This has greatly reduced its use. It is suggested that the olefin might lead to metabolites that produce an immunoreactive response.[7, 8] Halothane has a narrow margin of safety. Respiratory depression is notable, and mechanical ventilation and increased oxygen concentrations are often required. Opioids or nitrous oxide are often needed to obtain adequate surgical analgesia. Overall, halothane is not much used today.

Methoxyflurane, USP. Methoxyflurane, 2,2-dichloro-1,1-difluoroethyl methyl ether, $CHCl_2CF_2$-O-CH_3 (Penthrane), is a volatile liquid (bp, 105°C). The agent does not have a high vapor pressure at room temperature, so concentrations in the inspired air are low. This, together with a large blood/gas partition coefficient, produces a slow induction of anesthesia, featuring an excitatory phase. Accordingly, induction may be made with intravenous sodium thiopental. The compound is very soluble in lipids; consequently, recovery is slow. The agent produces excellent analgesia and good muscle relaxation.

Methoxyflurane is as much as 70% metabolized. Apparently, all labile sites are attacked. Metabolites include dichloroacetate, difluoromethoxyacetate, oxalate, and fluoride

ions. The fluoride ion especially and oxalate are responsible for the renal damage the agent produces when used to produce deep anesthesia over prolonged periods. Because of the potential for renal damage, it has restricted application as an anesthetic.[9] It is said to be safe when used by intermittent inhalation as an analgesic during labor.

Enflurane, USP. Enflurane, 2-chloro-1,1,2-trifluoroethyl difluoromethyl ether, HF_2COCF_2CHFCl (Ethrane), is a volatile liquid with a vapor pressure at room temperature about three-fourths that of halothane and a blood/gas partition coefficient also about three-fourths that of halothane. Consequently, induction is relatively easy, although an ultrashort-acting barbiturate is generally used for this purpose. Enflurane is said to be relatively easy to work with and to have a relatively low frequency of adverse cardiovascular effects. Respiration is depressed, so mechanical ventilation and oxygen supplementation are used. At high doses in a small percentage of patients, tonic–clonic convulsive activity is seen. Accordingly, enflurane should not be used in patients with epileptic foci.

As much as 5% of administered drug is metabolized. Difluoromethoxydifluoroacetate and fluoride ion have been reported as metabolites. The fluoride concentration, however, is generally thought to lie within safe limits.[10]

Isoflurane, USP. Isoflurane, 1-chloro-,2,2,2-trifluoroethyl difluoromethyl ether, $F_3CC(H)ClOCF_3$ (Forane), is a close structural relative of enflurane and shares many properties with it, although changes in the electroencephalogram (EEG) and tonic–clonic activity are not reported. It does differ considerably in extent of metabolism; only about 0.2% is metabolized.[11] Metabolites are fluoride ion and trifluoroacetate. Neither kidney nor liver damage has been reported for the drug.

Desflurane. Desflurane (Suprane), $FC(H_2)$-O-$C(H)F$-$C(H)F_2$, has an oil/gas partition coefficient about one-fifth and a blood/gas partition coefficient one-third that of isoflurane. Its physical properties confer pharmacokinetic properties claimed to be superior to those of isoflurane. Desflurane and isoflurane are metabolized to about the same extent.

Sevoflurane. Sevoflurane, $FC(H)_2$-O-$CH(CF_3)_2$, has an oil/gas partition coefficient about one-half that of isoflurane, and the blood/gas partition coefficient is about one-third that of isoflurane. Pharmacokinetically, it reportedly has the advantages of rapid uptake and rapid elimination. It is metabolized to about the same extent as enflurane.

Nitrous Oxide, USP. Nitrous oxide, nitrogen monoxide, N_2O, is a gas at room temperature and is supplied as a liquid under pressure in metal cylinders. It is a good analgesic, but such high concentrations are required in the inspired mixture (up to 80%) to achieve anesthesia that attendant dangers of hypoxia exist. Accordingly, it is rarely used as the sole anesthetic agent. It is often used in combination with other agents, permitting their use at lower concentrations. It has analgesic effects that have been reported to result from a general depressant effect on synaptic transmission of pain messages.[12] It is a positive modulator of GABA on $GABA_A$

receptors, which would constitute a basis for its general anesthetic action.[3]

Intravenous Anesthetics

The sodium salts of the ultra-short-acting barbiturates may be administered intravenously in aqueous solutions to induce anesthesia. Thereafter, the maintaining volatile anesthetic with or without nitrous oxide is used. Respiratory depression is marked with the barbiturates at anesthetic doses; consequently, these agents are not used to maintain surgical anesthesia. Unconsciousness is produced within seconds of intravenous injection, and the duration of action is about 30 minutes. The rapid onset of action is attributed to rapid partitioning from the blood, across the blood–brain barrier, into the sites of action in the brain. Thiobarbiturates (thiamylal, thiopental) have an exceptionally high lipid/water partition coefficient, which is considered to be the basis of this rapid partitioning. The very short duration of action is attributed to repartitioning from the brain into peripheral tissues—initially to well-perfused tissues and subsequently to body fat. Methohexital is not a thiobarbiturate, but its structure confers properties that produce an ultra-short action (see the discussion under the heading, Methohexital Sodium). The structures of the compounds are given in Table 14-1.

Methohexital Sodium. Methohexital, sodium-($\pm$)-1-methyl-5-allyl-5-(1-methyl-2-pentynyl) barbiturate (Brevital Sodium), is an *N*-methyl barbiturate with a pK_a of 8.4, versus about 7.6 for the non–*N*-methylated compounds. This pK_a change increases the concentration of the lipid-soluble free acid form at physiological hydrogen ion concentrations. The compound also has extensive hydrophobic character (total of nine hydrocarbon carbons); consequently, the lipid/water partition coefficient of the free acid form is high. Finally, it has an accessible site of metabolic inactivation, the CH_2 α to the triple bond. Overall, the compound has the properties to rapidly penetrate the CNS after intravenous injection and then redistribute rapidly to other body sites and also undergo rapid metabolic inactivation.

Thiamylal Sodium. Thiamylal, sodium 5-allyl-5-(1-methylbutyl)-2-thiobarbiturate (Surital Sodium), is a highly hydrophobic thiobarbiturate that has structural features closely related to those of thiopental. It has biological properties similar to those of thiopental. Intravenous administration induces unconsciousness within seconds, and consciousness is regained within 30 minutes.

Thiopental Sodium, USP. Thiopental sodium, sodium 5-ethyl-5-(1-methylbutyl)-2-thiobarbiturate (Pentothal Sodium), is the most widely used ultra-short-acting anesthetic barbiturate. Additionally, the compound is the prototype for the ultra-short-acting barbiturates. Most discussions of how structure influences duration of action in this group of agents relate specifically to it. The compound's onset of action is about equal to the time required for it to travel to the brain from the site of administration. Consciousness is regained within 30 minutes.

Benzodiazepines. Benzodiazepines alone cannot produce surgical anesthesia. Some of the more CNS-depressant benzodiazepines (e.g., diazepam and midazolam), however, are used intravenously to induce anesthesia. Diazepam has a very high lipid/water partition coefficient and, consequently, is highly depotized and very long acting. So, it is usually not chosen for induction for short-term anesthetic procedures. Midazolam has a lower lipid/water partition coefficient, which improves pharmacokinetic properties. It has a marked amnesiac effect that is valued in this use. Its physical and biological properties make it a frequent choice for induction anesthesia. The sedative effect of these compounds can be reversed by flumazenil.

Etomidate. Etomidate (Amidate) contains a 4-carboxylic acid ester–substituted imidazole moiety, which is also present in a number of compounds that are structural variations of the triazolo and imidazolo benzodiazepines. It is a positive allosteric modulator of GABA$_A$ receptors. Since it is a hydrophobically substituted imidazole, a side effect of

TABLE 14–1 Ultra-Short-Acting Barbiturates Used to Produce General Anasthesia

General Structure

Generic Name Proprietary Name	R$_5$	R'$_5$	R$_1$	R$_2$
				Substituents
Methohexital sodium *Brevital Sodium*	$CH_2{=}CH{-}CH_2{-}$	$CH_3CH_2C{\equiv}C{-}\overset{\underset{\mid}{CH_3}}{CH}{-}$	CH_3	O
Thiamylal sodium *Surital Sodium*	$CH_2{=}CH{-}CH_2{-}$	$CH_3CH_2CH_2\overset{\underset{\mid}{CH_3}}{CH}{-}$	H	S
Thiopental sodium *Pentothal Sodium*	$CH_3CH_2{-}$	$CH_3CH_2CH_2\overset{\underset{\mid}{CH_3}}{CH}{-}$	H	S

the drug that can have serious clinical consequences is depression of steroidogenesis. The compound is a base, and water-soluble salts can be made for intravenous administration.

Etomidate

Propofol. Simple phenols are rarely seen among useful CNS depressants, possibly because of tissue destruction and general toxicity largely due to the phenolic hydroxy group. It is likely that the 2,6-isopropyl groups of propofol (Diprivan) favorably influence the biological properties of the hydroxyl group. Propofol is useful for induction and maintenance of anesthesia. It is not water soluble, so an emulsion is given intravenously. Penetration into the brain is rapid, as is redistribution to other tissues, characteristics of compounds with a high lipid/water partition coefficient. The drug binds allosterically to $GABA_A$ receptors at a site different from the benzodiazepine site.[2]

Propofol

Alphaxalone. Alphaxalone, 5α-pregnane-3α-ol,11,20-dione, is a long- discontinued anesthetic, but it may be instructive. It was introduced into the clinic as a consequence of research begun after recognition of the anesthetic properties of cholesterol and then a number of 3-hydroxy steroidal metabolites. After the discontinuation of alphaxalone use, it was found that a number of such compounds, some endogenously produced, are positive allosteric modulators at $GABA_A$ receptors. Negative allosteric modulating steroids are also known, and some steroids are positive or negative modulators, depending on their concentration. It is believed that modulation of $GABA_A$ function may be a normal physiological role of such steroids. Collectively, they are called neurosteroids. Research in the area continues.

Ketamine Hydrochloride, USP. Ketamine, ($\pm$)-2-(*o*-chlorophenyl)-2-methylaminocyclohexanone hydrochloride (Ketalar), has a different mode of action from the other anesthetic agents in this review. Ketamine was designed as a structural relative of the medically discontinued agent phencyclidine (PCP) (see Chapter 15), with which it shares a number of biological properties. Blockage of glutamic acid *N*-methyl-D-aspartate (NMDA) receptors explains many of the actions of the two compounds. The incidence of hallucinations is much lower with ketamine than with phencyclidine. Ketamine produces a sense of dissociation from events being experienced, followed by anesthesia, analgesia, and sometimes amnesia. The anesthetic state produced by ketamine has also been described as cataleptic anesthesia. It is

also called *dissociative anesthesia*.[2] The prevalence of hallucinations and excitement is higher in adults than in children. The drug may be used as the sole agent (mainly for minor surgical procedures in children), or it can be used to induce anesthesia that is then maintained by one of the potent inhalation agents, or it and nitrous oxide may be used together for general anesthesia.

Ketamine Hydrochloride

ANXIOLYTIC, SEDATIVE, AND HYPNOTIC AGENTS

The list of anxiolytic, sedative, and hypnotic drugs is a short one—benzodiazepines, barbiturates, and a miscellaneous group. In addition to the short list of agents reviewed, a number of drugs belonging to other pharmacological classes may possess one or more of the anxiolytic, sedative, and hypnotic properties. These classes include H_1-antihistamines, antiadrenergics, antipsychotics, and anticonvulsants as prominent examples. Additionally, other areas are being explored for sleep-promoting agents. Adenosine-2A receptor (A_{2A}) agonists and melatonin-2 receptor (MT_2) agonists are under study.[13] Both adenosine and melatonin are thought to be involved in natural mediation of sleep. Adenosine is considered a possible endogenous sleep-producing agent. Melatonin affects circadian rhythms and may be a weak sedative–hypnotic.

Linoleamide and 9,10-octadecenoamide have also been implicated recently as possible endogenous sleep-producing agents. They are positive modulators of $GABA_A$ receptors.[14] Anandamide (and other endogenous cannabinoids) presumably do not bind to $GABA_A$ receptors. Some of their roles in the CNS function are discussed in Chapter 15. Further work should clarify the exact role and importance in sleep of linoleamide and 9,10-octadecenoamide. As we review the agents classed as anxiolytics, sedatives, and hypnotics, note that these groups of CNS depressants have an especially close relationship with anticonvulsants. Strong evidence indicates that in many cases the neuronal effects associated with anxiolytic, sedative, and hypnotic effects, especially positive modulation of $GABA_A$ receptors, also relate to anticonvulsant effects. In addition, other mechanisms of action, such as sodium channel blockade and calcium T channel blockade, may predominate among anticonvulsants; so, it is appropriate to discuss them separately.

Benzodiazepines and Related Compounds

Benzodiazepines and benzodiazepine-like drugs bind to a benzodiazepine recognition site, one of several allosteric sites that modulate the effect of GABA binding to $GABA_A$ receptors.[2, 3, 15] The $GABA_A$ receptor is a ligand-gated chloride ion channel. It is a protein anchored in the cell membrane and is pentomeric, as are other ligand-gated ion channels. The five polypeptide subunits that together make up its structure come from the subunit families α, β, δ, ϵ, π, ρ, and θ. There are six iso forms of the α polypeptide (α_1 to α_6), four of the β with two splice variants, and three of the γ with two variants. Presently, one form of each of the others is known. Each subunit has an extracellular N-terminal domain, then three membrane-spanning domains, an intracellular loop, a fourth membrane-spanning domain, and an extracellular C terminus.

At least 16 different $GABA_A$ receptors have so far been identified in rodent brain. The subunit composition of the receptors has great bearing on the response to benzodiazepines and other ligands. Most receptors consist of α, β, and γ combinations. Of these, α_1, β_2, and γ_2 are most common. Other highly expressed combinations are α_2, β_2, γ_2 and α_2, β_3, γ_2.

The benzodiazepine recognition site is in the extracellular N terminus of the α_1, α_2, α_3, and α_5 subunits. $GABA_A$ receptors with α_4 or α_6 subunits do not respond to benzodiazepines. α_4 and α_6 subunits have an arginine residue replacing histidine at position 101 of the extracellular N-terminal domain; α_1 subunits are required for sedative and hypnotic effects, and to a lesser extent, anticonvulsant effects of benzodiazepines; α_2 subunits are required for the anxiolytic effects of benzodiazepines; and α_3 and α_5 subunits may be involved in other actions of benzodiazepines. If an arginine replaces histidine in an α_2 subunit of the GABA receptor, the receptor is resistant to the sedative effects of benzodiazepines and zolpidem. If arginine replaces histidine in an α_2 subunit, the anxiolytic effect of benzodiazepines is lost.[15]

Although the binding domain of the benzodiazepines is considered to be in the N-terminal domain of the α unit, the benzodiazepines also require a γ_2 subunit for most positive allosteric effects. Amino acid residues in the α_1 subunit that have been identified as key binding sites within the benzodiazepine binding site are Tyr 161, Thr 162, Gly 200, Ser 204, Thr 206, and Val 211. In the γ subunit, Phe 77 has been identified.[14–21]

A number of compounds that have structural characteristics broadly related to the benzodiazepines, including neuroactive flavanoids, imidazopyridines, and pyrazolopyrimidines, can act as positive modulators at the benzodiazepine recognition site on one or more of the $GABA_A$ receptor subtypes. Compounds may produce all the characteristic actions of benzodiazepines or be selective, as are, for example, anxiolytic flavanoids or the sedative–hypnotics zolpidem and zalephon.

Most classical benzodiazepines are positive modulators, many probably nonselectively for all the receptor subtypes that respond to benzodiazepines. Some have been claimed to be relatively selective as anticonvulsants. Such drugs, with only part of the spectrum of all possible benzodiazepine actions have been called *partial agonists*. This term can mislead, since in this use, it applies to drugs that do not have all the possible qualitative actions, rather than being at a point on a single activity scale between an agonist and an antagonist.

Some β-carbolines are negative modulators at benzodiazepine modulatory sites. Additionally, there are $GABA_A$ receptor subtypes that recognize benzodiazepines but not β-carbolines and subtypes that recognize β-carbolines but not

benzodiazepines. Negative modulators diminish the positive effect of GABA on chloride flux. In whole animals, they appear to increase anxiety, produce panic attacks, and improve memory. β-Carbolines were once suspected of being the endogenous modulators of benzodiazepine binding sites. Now, this is not considered likely. Many experts in the field now think that there is no endogenous ligand for the benzodiazepine recognition site (allosteric modulatory site).

There are also compounds that can occupy benzodiazepine modulatory sites, have no effect on chloride flux themselves, and block positive and negative modulators. They have been called variously *antagonists, zero modulators,* and *neutralizing allosteric modulators.* One such compound, flumazenil, is used clinically to counteract the sedative effect of benzodiazepines.

Flumazenil

As noted under the heading of general anesthetics, there are other allosteric sites that recognize respectively, neurosteroids, barbiturates, inhalation anesthetics, alcohols and the phenol Diprivan (separate sites). The convulsants picrotoxin and pentylenetetrazole have definite binding sites on GABA receptors.

The field of benzodiazepines was opened with the synthesis of chlordiazepoxide by Sternbach and the discovery of its unique pharmacological properties by Randall.[22] Chlordiazepoxide (see the discussion of individual compounds) is a 2-amino benzodiazepine, and other amino compounds have been synthesized. When it was discovered that chlordiazepoxide is rapidly metabolized to a series of active benzodiazpin-2-ones (see the general scheme of metabolic relationships), however, emphasis shifted to the synthesis and testing of the latter group. Empirical structure–activity relationships (SARs) for antianxiety activity have been tabulated for this group (analogous statements apply for the older 2-amino group).[22, 23] The following general structure helps to visualize them.

An electronegative substituent at position 7 is required for activity, and the more electronegative it is, the higher the activity. Positions 6, 8, and 9 should not be substituted. A phenyl at position 5 promotes activity. If this phenyl group is *ortho* (2′) or di*ortho* (2′,6′) substituted with electron-attracting substituents, activity is increased. On the other hand, *para* substitution decreases activity greatly. Saturation of the 4,5 double bond or a shift of it to the 3,4 position decreases activity. Alkyl substitution at the 3 position decreases activity; substitution with a hydroxy does not. The presence or absence of the 3-hydroxyl is important pharmacokinetically. Compounds without the hydroxyl are nonpolar, have long half-lives, and undergo hepatic oxidation. Compounds with the hydroxyl are much more polar and are readily converted to the excreted glucuronide (see the overall metabolic relationship scheme). The 2-carbonyl function is optimal for activity, as is the nitrogen atom at position 1. The N-substituent should be small.

Additional research yielded compounds with a fused triazolo ring, represented by triazolam and alprazolam. Midazolam, with a fused imidazolo ring, also followed. These compounds are metabolized mainly by hydroxylation of the methyl substituent on the triazolo or imidazolo ring. The resulting hydroxy compound is active but is quickly conjugated. The compounds are also metabolized by 3-hydroxylation of the benzodiazepine ring. Interestingly, an electron-attracting group at position 7 is not required for activity in these compounds.

The metabolism of benzodiazepines has received much study.[24, 25] Some of the major metabolic relationships are shown in the scheme below.

The benzodiazepines generally are well absorbed from the gastrointestinal (GI) tract, although the more polar compounds (e.g., those with a hydroxyl at the 3-position) tend to be absorbed more slowly than the more nonpolar compounds.

The drugs tend to be highly bound to plasma proteins; in general, the more nonpolar the drug, the greater the binding. They are also very effectively distributed to the brain. Generally, the more nonpolar the compound, the greater the distribution to the brain, at least initially. When diazepam is used as an anesthetic, it initially distributes to the brain and then redistributes to sites outside the brain.

Compounds without the 3-hydroxyl group usually have long half-lives and undergo conversion to the 3-hydroxy compounds by hepatic oxidation. Compounds with the 3-hydroxyl group have short half-lives because of rapid conjugation to the 3-glucuronide, which undergoes urinary excretion.

In addition to lower abuse potential, and a much greater margin of safety than the barbiturates, the drugs have fewer drug interactions. Especially noteworthy is that they do not promote the metabolism of other drugs.

Chlordiazepoxide Hydrochloride, USP. Chlordiazepoxide hydrochloride, 7-chloro-2-(methylamino)-5-phenyl-3*H*-1,4-benzodiazepine 4-oxide monohydrochloride (Librium), is absorbed well from the GI tract. Peak plasma levels are reached in 2 to 4 hours. N-demethylation and hydrolysis of the condensed amidino group are rapid and extensive, producing demoxepam as a major metabolite. Demoxepam, in turn, is converted principally to nordazepam. Nordazepam, in turn, is converted principally to oxepam, which undergoes conjugation to the excreted glucuronide. Other routes of metabolism can occur, for example, opening of the seven-membered ring by hydrolysis of the lactam group.

Chlordiazepoxide Hydrochloride

Diazepam, USP. Diazepam, 7-chloro-1,3-dihydro-1-methyl-5-phenyl-2*H*-1,4-benzodiazpin-2-one (Valium), was

Oxazepam Glucuronide

the first member of the benzodiazpin-2-one group to be introduced. It is very nonpolar and is rapidly absorbed. Diazepam is metabolized by N-demethylation to nordazepam, which is then metabolized according to the general scheme. It is widely used for several anxiety states and has an additional wide range of uses (e.g., as an anticonvulsant, a premedication in anesthesiology, and in various spastic disorders).

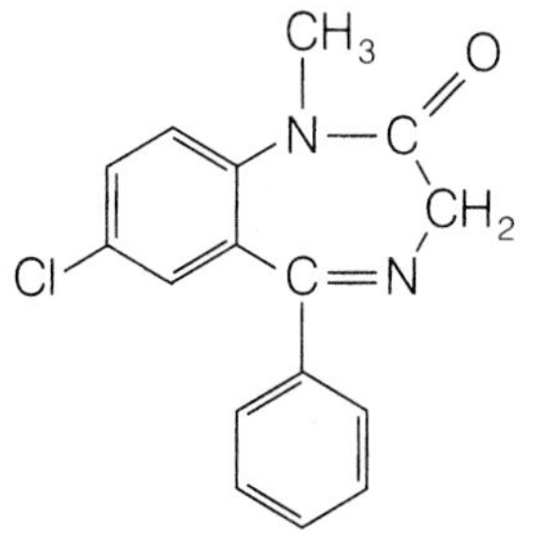

Diazepam

Oxazepam, USP. Oxazepam, 7-chloro-1,3-dihydro-3-hydroxy-5-phenyl-2*H*-1,4-benzodiazpin-2-one (Serax), can be considered a prototype for the 3-hydroxy compounds. For the stereochemistry of this and other 3-hydroxy compounds, see the chapter dealing with metabolism. It is much more polar than diazepam, for example. Metabolism is relatively uncomplicated, and the duration of action is short.

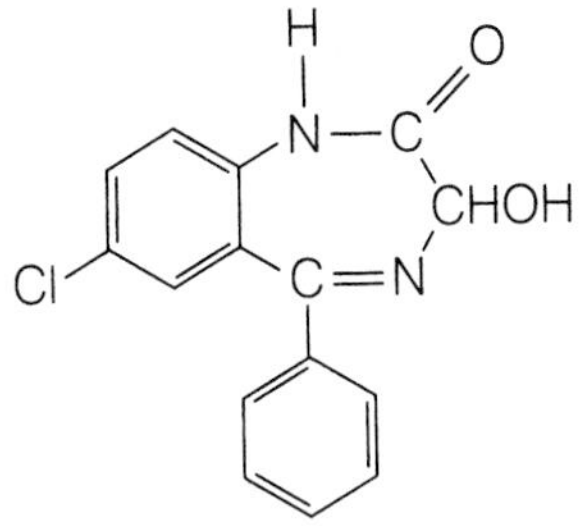

Oxazepam

Clorazepate Dipotassium. Clorazepate dipotassium, 7-chloro-2,3-dihydro-2-oxo-5-phenyl-1*H*-1,4-benzodiazepine-3-carboxylic acid dipotassium salt monohydrate (Tranxene), can be considered a prodrug. Inactive itself, it undergoes rapid loss of water and then decarboxylation to nordazepam, which has a long half-life and undergoes hepatic conversion to oxazepam. Despite the polar character of the drug as administered, because it is quickly converted in the GI tract to a nonpolar compound, it has an overall long half-life.

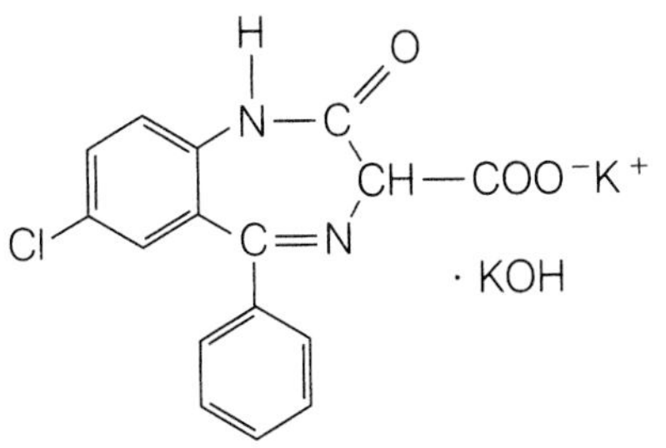

Clorazepate Dipotassium

Prazepam, USP. Prazepam, 7-chloro-1-(cyclopropylmethyl)-1,3-dihydro-5-phenyl-2*H*-1,4-benzodiazpin-2-one (Verstran), has a long overall half-life. Extensive N-dealkyl-

ation occurs to yield nordazepam. 3-Hydroxylation of both prazepam and nordazepam occurs.

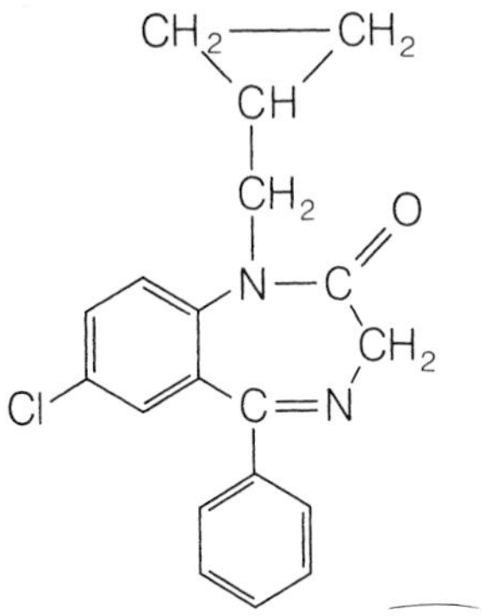

Prazepam

Lorazepam, USP. Lorazepam, 7-chloro-5-(2-chlorophenyl)-3-dihydro-3-hydroxy-2*H*-1,4-benzodiazpin-2-one (Ativan), can be recognized as the 2'-chloro substituted analogue of oxazepam. In keeping with overall SARs, the 2'-chloro substituent increases activity. Metabolism is relatively rapid and uncomplicated because of the 3-hydroxyl group in the compound.

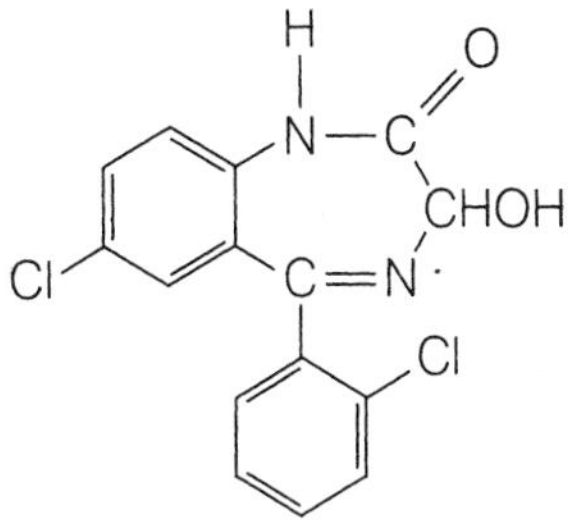

Lorazepam

Halazepam, USP. Halazepam, 7-chloro-1,3-dihydro-5-phenyl-1(2,2,2-trifluoroethyl)-2*H*-1,4-benzodiazpin-2-one (Paxipam), is well absorbed. It is active and present in plasma, but much of its activity is due to the major metabolites nordazepam and oxazepam. The drug is marketed as an anxiolytic.

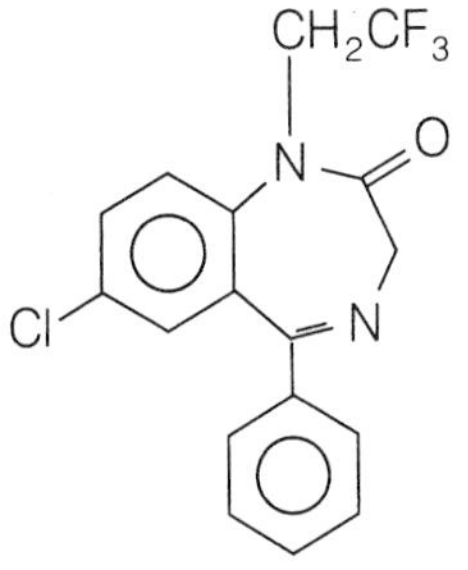

Halazepam

Temazepam. Temazepam, 7-chloro-1,3-dihydro-3-hydroxy-1-methyl-5-phenyl -2*H*-1,4-benzodiazpin-2-one (Restoril), also occurs as a minor metabolite of diazepam. It can be visualized as *N*-methyl oxazepam. A small amount of N-demethylation occurs. Metabolism proceeds mainly through conjugation of the 3-hydroxyl group, however. The duration of action is short. It is marketed as a hypnotic said to have little or no residual effect.

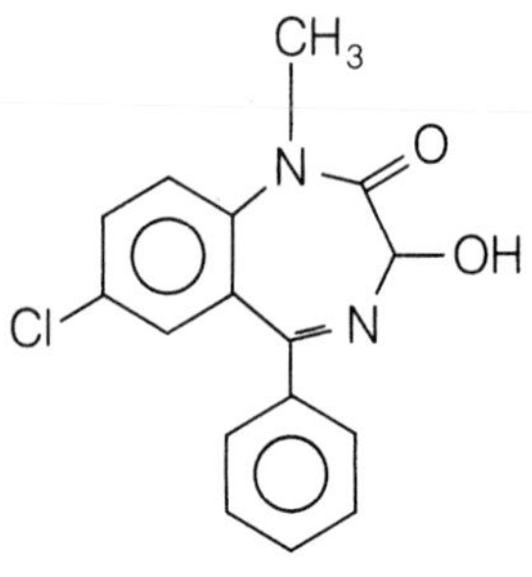

Temazepam

Triazolam

Flurazepam Hydrochloride, USP. Flurazepam hydrochloride, 7-chloro-1-[2-(diethylamino)ethyl]-5-(2-fluorophenyl)-1, 3-dihydro-2*H*-1, 4-benzodiazpin-2-one dihydrochloride (Dalmane), is notable as a benzodiazepine marketed almost exclusively for use in insomnia. Metabolism of the dialkyl aminoalkyl side chain is extensive. A major metabolite is N^1-dealkyl flurazepam, which has a very long half-life and persists for several days after administration.

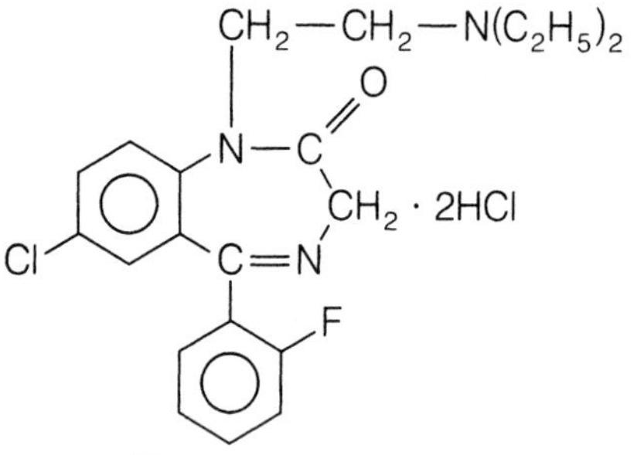

Flurazepam Hydrochloride

Alprazolam, USP. Alprazolam, 8-chloro-1-methyl-6-phenyl-4*H*-*s*-triazolo[4,3-a][1,4]benzodiazepine (Xanax), is rapidly absorbed from the GI tract. Protein binding is lower (~70%) than with most benzodiazepines. Oxidative metabolism of the methyl group to the methyl alcohol followed by conjugation is rapid; consequently, the duration of action is short. The drug is a highly potent anxiolytic on a milligram basis.

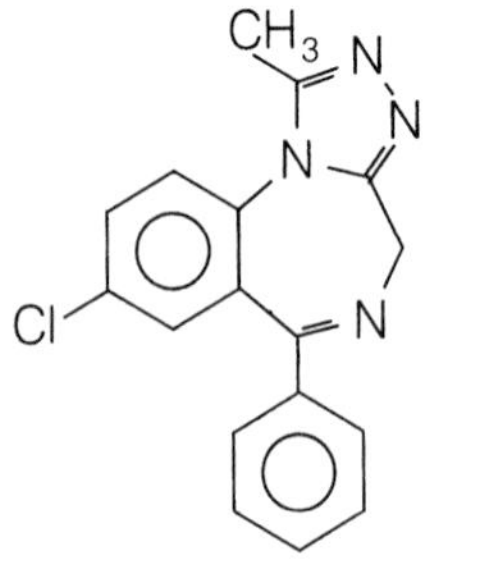

Alprazolam

Triazolam, USP. Triazolam, 8-chloro-6-(*o*-chlorophenyl)-1-methyl-4*H*-*s*-triazolo[4,3-a][1,4] benzodiazepine (Halcion), has all of the characteristic benzodiazepine pharmacological actions. It is marketed as a sedative–hypnotic drug said to impair little, if any, daytime function. It is rapidly metabolized to the 1-methyl alcohol, which is then conjugated and excreted.

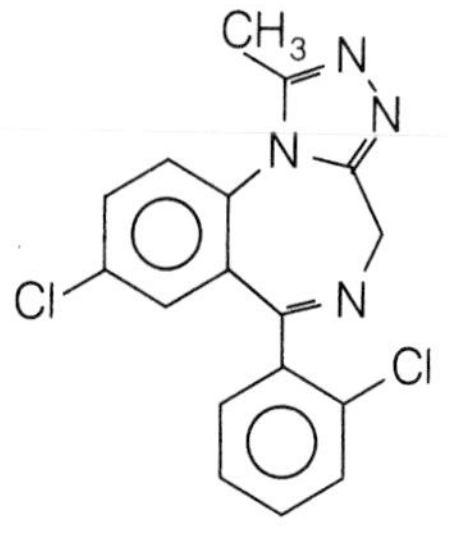

Midazolam. This drug is used intravenously as a sedative–hypnotic and as an induction anesthetic. Further information can be found in the section on anesthetics.

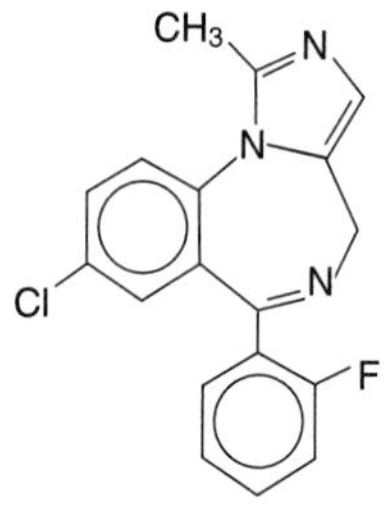

Midazolam

Quazepam. Quazepam (Doral) and its active metabolites reportedly are relatively selective for the benzodiazepine modulatory site on (ω-1) type 1 GABA$_A$ receptors (i.e., receptors with an α_1 subunit) and are hypnotic agents. Quazepam is metabolized by oxidation to the 2-oxo compound and then N-dealkylation. Both metabolites are active, the first reportedly is the more potent and selective. Thereafter, 3-hydroxylation and glucuronidation occur.

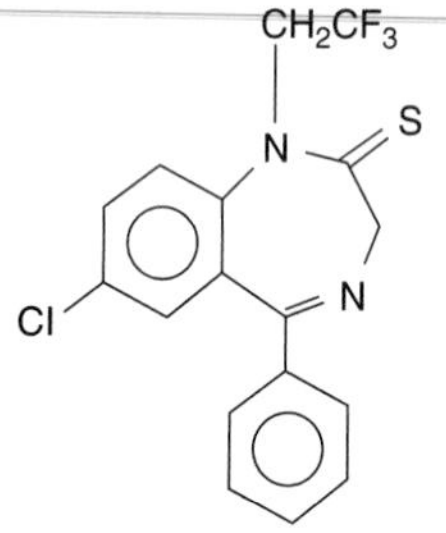

Zolpidem. Zolpidem (Ambien) has attracted attention as a relatively selective positive modulator at the ω-1 benzodiazepine binding site. As such, it is a hypnotic. It is said to be relatively fast in action and to produce no active metabolites. Metabolism of the aryl methyl groups would be expected; however, the resulting compounds would not be long-lived.

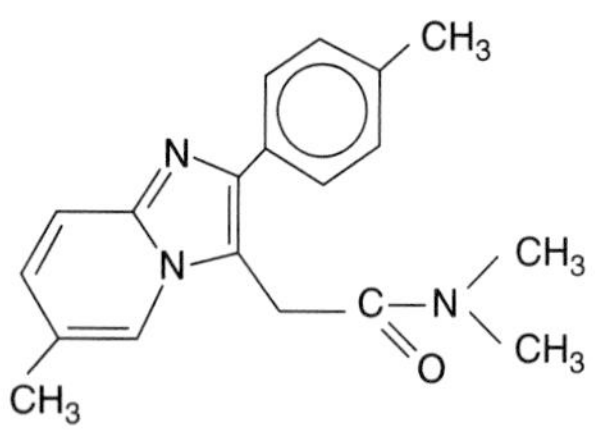

Zaleplon. Zaleplon (Sonata) is another ω-1 sedative hypnotic with overall biological properties resembling those of zolpidem. It may have a more rapid onset and termination of action than zolpidem.

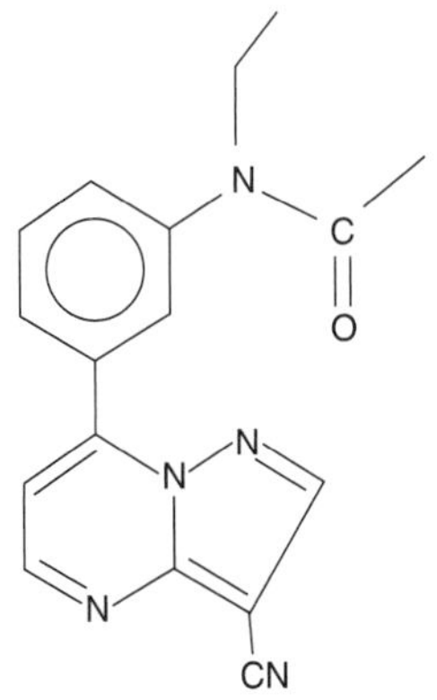

Zaleplon

Metabolism involves the aldehyde dehydrogenase and the cytochrome system.

Barbiturates

The barbiturates appear to exert most of their characteristic CNS effects by binding to an allosteric recognition site on GABA$_A$ receptors that positively modulates the effect of the GABA$_A$–GABA combination. In addition, by attaching to the barbiturate modulatory site, barbiturates can increase chloride ion flux without GABA attaching to its receptor site on GABA$_A$. This has been termed a *GABA mimetic effect*. It is thought to be related to the profound CNS depression that barbiturates can produce.

The first historical sedative–hypnotic barbiturate, 5,5-diethylbarbituric acid, was introduced in 1903. With time, many members were added, and the barbiturates dominated the sedative–hypnotic field until the advent of the benzodiazepines. The benzodiazepines are much safer to use and have replaced the barbiturates as the most broadly useful agents in sedative–hypnotic applications.

The barbiturates are 5,5-disubstituted barbituric acids. The following scheme shows how the 5,5-dialkyl compounds are synthesized. Substitution of thiourea for urea in the reaction produces the 2-thiobarbiturates, useful as induction anesthetics.

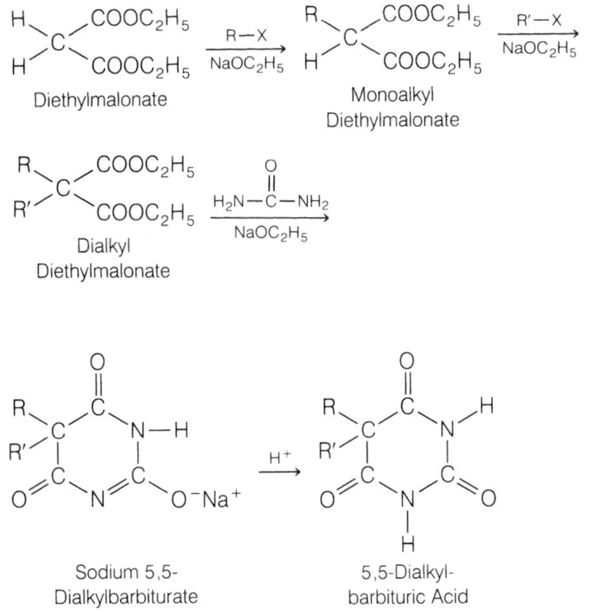

Diethylmalonate

Monoalkyl Diethylmalonate

Dialkyl Diethylmalonate

Sodium 5,5-Dialkylbarbiturate

5,5-Dialkyl-barbituric Acid

Consideration of the structure of 5,5-disubstituted barbituric acids reveals their acidic character. Those without methyl substituents on the nitrogen have pK$_a$s of about 7.6; those with a methyl substituent have pK$_a$s of about 8.4. The free acids have poor water solubility and good lipid solubility (the latter largely a function of the two hydrocarbon substituents on the 5 position, although in the 2-thiobarbiturates the sulfur atom increases lipid solubility).

Sodium salts of the barbiturates are readily prepared and are water soluble. Their aqueous solutions generate an alkaline pH. A classic incompatibility is the addition of an agent with an acidic pH in solution, which results in formation and precipitation of the free water-insoluble disubstituted barbituric acid. Sodium salts of barbiturates in aqueous solution decompose at varying rates by base-catalyzed hydrolysis, generating ring-opened salts of carboxylic acids.

The names of many barbiturates end in *al* (e.g., phenobarbital), appearing to denote an aldehydic compound, because chloral hydrate was widely recognized as a sedative–hypnotic agent when the first barbiturates were introduced. Hence, the suffix was an effort to indicate a therapeutic, not a chemical, class.

Structure–Activity Relationships

Extensive synthesis and testing of the barbiturates over a long time span have produced well-defined SARs, which have been summarized.[26]

Both hydrogen atoms at the 5 position of barbituric acid must be replaced. This may be because if one hydrogen is available at position 5, tautomerization to a highly acidic trihydroxypyrimidine (pK$_a$ ~ 4) can occur. Consequently, the compound is largely in the anionic form at physiological pHs, with little nonionic lipid-soluble compound available to cross the blood–brain barrier.

Beginning with lower alkyls, there is an increase in onset and a decrease in duration of action with increasing hydrocarbon content up to about seven to nine total carbon atoms substituted on the 5 position. Lipophilicity and an ability to penetrate the brain in the first case and an ability to penetrate liver microsomes in the second may be involved. Also, for more hydrophobic compounds, partitioning out of the brain to other sites can be involved in the second instance. There is an inverse correlation between the total number of carbon atoms substituted on the 5 position and the duration of action, which is even better when the character of these substituents is taken into account, for example, the relatively polar character of a phenyl substituent (approximates a three- to four-carbon aliphatic chain), branching of alkyls, presence of an isolated double or triple bond, and so on. Additionally, these groups can influence the ease of oxidative metabolism by effects on bond strengths as well as by influencing partitioning.

Metabolism of the barbiturates is discussed in Chapter 4. Suffice it to say that increasing the lipid/water partition coefficient generally increases the rate of metabolism, except for compounds with an extremely high lipid/water partition coefficient (e.g., thiopental), which tend to depotize and are thus relatively unavailable for metabolism. Metabolism generally follows an ultimate (ω) or penultimate (ω-1) oxidation pattern. Ring-opening reactions are usually minor. N-methylation decreases duration of action, in large part, probably, by increasing the concentration of the lipid-soluble free barbituric acid. 2-Thiobarbiturates have a very short duration of action because the lipid/water partition coefficient is extremely high, promoting depotization. Barbiturates find use as sedatives, as hypnotics, for induction of anesthesia, and as anticonvulsants. Absorption from the GI tract is good. Binding to blood proteins is substantial. Compounds with low lipid/water partition coefficients may be excreted intact in the urine. Those with higher lipid/water partition coefficients are excreted after metabolism to polar metabolites.

Some of the more frequently used barbiturates are described briefly in the following sections. For the structures, the usual dosages required to produce sedation and hypnosis, the times of onset, and the duration of action, see Table 14-2.

BARBITURATES WITH A LONG DURATION OF ACTION (OVER 6 HOURS)

Barbital. Barbital, 5,5-diethylbarbituric acid, although discontinued as a sedative–hypnotic, is interesting because of the biological consequence of its low lipid/water partition coefficient. It is slowly eliminated, mostly intact, by the kidney.

Phenobarbital, USP. Phenobarbital, 5-ethyl-5-phenyl-barbituric acid (Luminal), is a long-acting sedative and hypnotic. It is also a valuable anticonvulsant, especially in generalized tonic–clonic and partial seizures (see the discussion on anticonvulsants). Metabolism to the *p*-hydroxy compound followed by glucuronidation accounts for about 90% of a dose.

Mephobarbital, USP. Mephobarbital, 3-methyl-5-ethyl-5-phenylbarbituric acid (Metharbital), is metabolically N-dealkylated to phenobarbital, which many consider to account for almost all of the activity. Its principal use is as an anticonvulsant.

BARBITURATES WITH AN INTERMEDIATE DURATION OF ACTION (3 TO 6 HOURS)

Barbiturates with an intermediate duration of action are used principally as sedative–hypnotics. They include **Amobarbital, USP,** 5-ethyl-5-isopentylbarbituric acid (Amytal), and its water-soluble sodium salt, **Amobarbital Sodium, USP,** 5-allyl-5-isopropylbarbituric acid (aprobarbital, Alurate); **Butabarbital Sodium, USP,** the water-soluble sodium salt of 5-*sec*-butyl-5-ethylbarbituric acid (Butisol Sodium).

TABLE 14–2 Barbiturates Used as Sedatives and Hypnotics

General Structure

Generic Name Proprietary Name	Substituents			Sedative Dose (mg)	Hypnotic Dose (mg)	Usual Onset of Action (min)
	R$_5$	R'$_5$	R$_1$			
A. Long Duration of Action (more than 6 hours)						
Mephobarbital, USP *Mebaral*	C$_2$H$_5$	(phenyl)	CH$_3$	30–100[a]	100	30–60
Phenobarbital, USP *Luminal*	C$_2$H$_5$	(phenyl)	H	15–30[a]	100	20–40
B. Intermediate Duration of Action (3 to 6 hours)						
Amobarbital, USP *Amytal*	CH$_3$CH$_2$—	(CH$_3$)$_2$CHCH$_2$CH$_2$—	H	20–40	100	20–30
Butabarbital Sodium, USP *Butisol Sodium*	CH$_3$CH$_2$—	CH$_3$CH$_2$CH— with CH$_3$	H	15–30	100	20–30
C. Short Duration of Action (less than 3 hours)						
Pentobarbital Sodium, USP *Nembutal Sodium*	CH$_3$CH$_2$—	CH$_3$CH$_2$CH$_2$CH— with CH$_3$	H	30	100	20–30
Secobarbital, USP *Seconal*	CH$_2$=CHCH$_2$—	CH$_3$CH$_2$CH$_2$CH— with CH$_3$	H	15–30	100	20–30

[a]Daytime sedative and anticonvulsant.

BARBITURATES WITH A SHORT DURATION OF ACTION (UNDER 3 HOURS)

Barbiturates that have substituents in the 5 position promoting more rapid metabolism (e.g., by increasing the lipid/water partition coefficient) than the intermediate group include **Pentobarbital-Sodium, USP,** sodium 5-ethyl-5-(1-methylbutyl)barbiturate (Nembutal); **Secobarbital, USP,** 5-allyl-5-(1-methylbutyl)barbituric acid (Seconal); and the sodium salt sodium secobarbital.

Barbiturates with an ultra-short duration of action are discussed under anesthetic agents.

Miscellaneous Sedative–Hypnotics

A wide range of chemical structures (e.g., imides, amides, alcohols) can produce sedation and hypnosis resembling those produced by the barbiturates. Despite this apparent structural diversity, the compounds have generally similar structural characteristics and chemical properties: a hydrophobic portion and a semipolar portion that can participate in H bonding. In some cases, modes of action are undetermined. As a working hypothesis, most of the agents can be envisioned to act by mechanisms similar to those proposed for barbiturates and alcohols.

AMIDES AND IMIDES

Glutethimide, USP. Glutethimide, 2-ethyl-2-phenylglutarimide (Doriden), has many structural relationships with the barbiturates and resembles them in many respects biologically. It is an effective sedative–hypnotic. It is very hydrophobic, and absorption from the GI tract is somewhat erratic. Metabolism is extensive, and the drug is an enzyme inducer. In the therapeutic dosage range, adverse effects tend to be infrequent. Toxic effects in overdose are as severe as, and possibly more troublesome than, those of the barbiturates.

Glutethimide

Alcohols and Their Carbamate Derivatives

The very simple alcohol ethanol has a long history of use as a sedative and hypnotic. Its modes of action were described under the anesthetic heading and are said to apply to other alcohols. It is widely used in self-medication as a sedative–hypnotic. Because this use has so many hazards, it is seldom a preferred agent medically.

As the homologous series of normal alcohols is ascended from ethanol, CNS depressant potency increases up to eight carbon atoms, with activity decreasing thereafter (the Meyer-Overton parabola, Chapter 2). Branching of the alkyl chain increases depressant activity and, in an isometric series, the order of potency is tertiary > secondary > primary. In part,

this may be because tertiary and secondary alcohols are not metabolized by oxidation to the corresponding carboxylic acids. Replacement of a hydrogen atom in the alkyl group by a halogen increases the alkyl portion and, accordingly, for the lower-molecular-weight compounds, increases potency. Carbamylation of alcohols generally increases depressant potency. Carbamate groups are generally much more resistant to metabolic inactivation than hydroxyl functions. Most of the alcohols and carbamates have been superseded as sedative–hypnotics. A number of difunctional compounds (e.g. diol carbamates) have depressant action on the cord in addition to the brain and are retained principally for their skeletal muscle relaxant properties.

Ethchlorvynol, USP. Ethchlorvynol, 1-chloro-3-ethyl-1-penten-4-yn-3-ol (Placidyl), is a sedative–hypnotic with a rapid onset and short duration of action. Metabolism, probably involving the hydroxyl group, accounts for about 90% of a dose. Acute overdose shares several features with barbiturate overdose.

Ethchlorvynol

Meprobamate, USP. Meprobamate, 2-methyl-2-propyltrimethylene dicarbamate, 2-methyl-2-propyl-1,3-propanediol dicarbamate (Equanil, Miltown), is officially indicated as an antianxiety agent. It is also a sedative–hypnotic agent. It has a number of overall pharmacological properties resembling those of benzodiazepines and barbiturates. The mechanism of action underlying anxiolytic effects is unknown but may involve effects on conductivity in specific brain areas.[27] It does not appear to act through effects on GABAergic systems. The drug is effective against absence seizures and may worsen generalized tonic–clonic seizures.

Meprobamate is also a centrally acting skeletal muscle relaxant. The agents in this group find use in a number of conditions, such as strains and sprains that may produce acute muscle spasm. They have interneuronal blocking properties at the level of the spinal cord, which are said to be partly responsible for skeletal muscle relaxation.[27] Also, the general CNS depressant properties they possess may contribute to, or be mainly responsible for, the skeletal muscle relaxant activity. Dihydric compounds and their carbamate (urethane) derivatives, as described above in the discussion of meprobamate, are prominent members of the group.

Meprobamate: R = H
Carisoprodol: R = —CH(CH$_3$)$_2$

Chlorphenesin Carbamate. Chlorphenesin carbamate, 3-(*p*-chlorophenoxy)-1,2-propanediol 1-carbamate (Maolate), is the *p*-chloro substituted and 1-carbamate derivative of the lead compound in the development of this group of agents, mephenesin.

Mephenesin is weakly active and short-lived because of facile metabolism of the primary hydroxyl group. Carbamylation of this group increases activity. p-Chlorination increases the lipid/water partition coefficient and seals off the *para* position from hydroxylation.

Metabolism, still fairly rapid, involves glucuronidation of the secondary hydroxyl group. The biological half-life in humans is 3.5 hours.

Chlorphenesin Carbamate

Methocarbamol, USP. Methocarbamol, 3-(*o*-methoxyphenoxy)-1,2-propanediol 1-carbamate (Robaxin), is said to be more sustained in effect than mephenesin. Likely sites for metabolic attack include the secondary hydroxyl group and the two ring positions opposite the ether functions. The dihydric parent compound, guaifenesin, is used as an expectorant.

Guaifenesin: R = H

Methocarbamol: R = —$\overset{\text{O}}{\overset{\|}{\text{C}}}$—NH$_2$

Carisoprodol, USP. Carisoprodol, *N*-isopropyl-2-methyl-2-propyl-1,3-propanediol dicarbamate, 2-methyl-2-propyl-1,3-propanediol carbamate isopropylcarbamate (Soma), is the mono-*N*-isopropyl–substituted relative of meprobamate. The structure is given in the discussion of meprobamate. It is indicated in acute skeletomuscular conditions characterized by pain, stiffness, and spasm. As can be expected, a major side effect of the drug is drowsiness.

ALDEHYDES AND THEIR DERIVATIVES

For chemical reasons that are easily rationalized, few aldehydes are valuable hypnotic drugs. The aldehyde in use, chloral (as the hydrate), is thought to act principally through a metabolite, trichloroethanol. Acetaldehyde is used as the cyclic trimer derivative, paraldehyde, which could also be grouped as an ether.

Chloral Hydrate, USP. Chloral hydrate, trichloroacetaldehyde monohydrate, CCl$_3$CH(OH)$_2$ (Noctec), is an aldehyde hydrate stable enough to be isolated. The relative stability of this *gem*-diol is largely due to an unfavorable dipole–dipole repulsion between the trichloromethyl carbon and the carbonyl carbon present in the parent carbonyl compound.[28]

Chloral hydrate is unstable in alkaline solutions, undergoing the last step of the haloform reaction to yield chloroform

and formate ion. In hydroalcoholic solutions, it forms the hemiacetal with ethanol. Whether or not this compound is the basis for the notorious and potentially lethal effect of the combination of ethanol and chloral hydrate (the "Mickey Finn") is controversial. Synergism between two different CNS depressants also could be involved. Additionally, ethanol, by increasing the concentration of NADH, enhances the reduction of chloral to the more active metabolite trichloroethanol, and chloral can inhibit the metabolism of alcohol because it inhibits alcohol dehydrogenase. Although it is suggested that chloral hydrate per se may act as a hypnotic,[29] chloral hydrate is very quickly converted to trichloroethanol, which is generally assumed to account for almost all of the hypnotic effect. It appears to have potent barbiturate-like binding to GABA$_A$ receptors.

Triclofos Sodium. Triclofos sodium, 2,2,2,-trichloroethanol dihydrogen phosphate monosodium salt (Triclos), is irritating to the GI mucosa. Its active metabolite, trichloroethanol, also has unpleasant GI effects when given orally. Triclofos is the nonirritating sodium salt of the phosphate ester of trichloroethanol and is readily converted to trichloroethanol. Accordingly, triclofos sodium produces CNS effects similar to those of oral chloral hydrate.

Triclofos Sodium

Paraldehyde, USP. Paraldehyde, 2,4,6-trimethyl-*s*-trioxane; paracetaldehyde, is recognizable as the cyclic trimer of acetaldehyde. It is a liquid with a strong characteristic odor detectable in the expired air and an unpleasant taste. These properties limit its use almost exclusively to an institutional setting (e.g., in the treatment of delirium tremens). In the past, when containers were opened and air admitted and then reclosed and allowed to stand, fatalities occurred because of oxidation of paraldehyde to glacial acetic acid.

Paraldehyde

ANTIPSYCHOTICS

Antipsychotics are drugs that ameliorate mental aberrations that are characteristic of the psychoses. The psychoses differ from the milder behavioral disorders, such as the anxiety disorders, in that thinking tends to be illogical, bizarre, and loosely organized. Importantly, patients have difficulty understanding reality and their own conditions. There are often hallucinations (usually auditory) and delusions.

In the schizophrenias, in addition to these symptoms,

called *positive symptoms,* there are negative symptoms represented by apathy, social withdrawal, and anhedonia. Cognitive deficits may also be observed.

Psychoses can be organic and related to a specific toxic chemical (e.g., delirium produced by central anticholinergic agents), an NMDA antagonist (e.g., phencyclidine), a definite disease process (e.g., dementia) or they can be idiopathic. Idiopathic psychoses may be acute or chronic. Idiopathic acute psychotic reactions have been reported to follow extremely severe short-term stress. Schizophrenia is a group of chronic idiopathic psychotic disorders with the overall symptomology described above.

The term *antipsychotic* was slow in gaining acceptance. Now it is widely acknowledged that antipsychotics actually diminish the underlying thought disorder that is the chief characteristic of the schizophrenias. The agents often have a calming effect in agitated psychotic patients; hence, they also have been referred to as *major tranquilizers.* Finally, because they lessen reactivity to emotional stimuli, with little effect on consciousness, they are referred to as *neuroleptics.*

The most frequent uses of these agents are in manic disorders and the schizophrenias. In the manic disorders, the agents may block DA at limbic D_2 and D_3 receptors, reducing euphoria, delusional thinking, and hyperactivity. In the chronic idiopathic psychoses (schizophrenias), both conventional (typical) and newer (most are atypical) antipsychotics appear to act to benefit positive symptoms by blocking DA at D_2 and D_3 limbic receptors.[1] The bases of the atypical group's activity against negative symptoms may be serotonin-2_A receptor (5-HT$_{2A}$) block, block at receptors yet to be determined, and possibly decreased striatal D_2 block.[1, 30] A classic competitive antagonism has been demonstrated at D_2 and D_3 receptors. Also, in recombinantly expressed receptors, inverse agonism has been demonstrated. For this to apply in vivo, a ground state of dopaminergic activity must be shown. Some preliminary signs indicate this is likely.[1]

In the schizophrenias, which have an extremely complex and multifactored etiology,[31, 32] the fundamental lesion appears to be a defect in the brain's informational gating mechanism. A slight abnormality in the startle response may be observed in infancy, but the disease does not emerge until late in the second decade or in the third decade of life. Basically the gating system has difficulty discriminating between relevant and irrelevant stimuli. Perception is illogical. Proceeding from this, thought and actions become illogical. Although the actual structural or anatomical lesions are not known, the basic defect appears to involve overactivity of dopaminergic neurons in the mesolimbic system. Some investigators suggest that this is the cause of most, if not all, of the common symptoms of the disease. Negative symptoms (e.g., social withdrawal) may be considered secondary symptoms. Others argue that all or part of the foregoing is excessively reductionist, and that other lesions cause some or all of the symptoms.

A major reason for the recent interest in the negative symptoms of schizophrenia has been the introduction of atypical, as opposed to typical, antipsychotics. Typical antipsychotics began with the serendipitous discovery of the antipsychotic activity of chlorpromazine. Many compounds were synthesized, usually with chlorpromazine as the model, and the antipsychotic potential assessed. A clear association between the ability to block DA at mesolimbic D_2 receptors

was established. During the same time, amphetamine-induced psychosis was determined to be caused by overactivation of mesolimbic D_2 receptors and judged to be the closest of the various chemically induced model psychoses to the schizophrenias.

The conventional typical antipsychotics are characterized by the production of EPS, roughly approximating the symptoms of Parkinson's disease. These are reversible on discontinuing or decreasing the dose of the drug and are associated with blockade of DA at D_2 striatal receptors. After sustained high-dose therapy with antipsychotics, a late-appearing EPS, tardive dyskinesia, may occur. The overall symptomatology resembles the symptoms of Huntington's chorea. The condition is thought to arise from biological compensation (increased D_2 activity) for the striatal D_2 block of antipsychotic drugs.

Atypical antipsychotics date from the discovery of clozapine, its antipsychotic properties and its much lower production of EPS. Some investigators express concern that typical antipsychotics, especially by producing EPS, introduce drug-induced effects that are hard to distinguish from negative symptoms. This leads to the view that diminishing EPS can account for perceived decreased negative symptoms. It is, however, reportedly also more active against negative symptoms of schizophrenia, independent of reduced EPS, and has a unique, notably expanded, receptor-blocking profile. Compounds are now under synthesis and being tested at the various CNS receptors at which clozapine acts to determine the role of these receptors in schizophrenia.

Also contributing to the development of typical antipsychotics was the introduction of risperidone. It has reduced EPS, has increased activity against negative symptoms, and, in addition to its DA blocking ability, is a 5-HT$_{2A}$ antagonist. One view of the drug is that it combines structurally the features of an antidepressant and an antipsychotic, and so the two drug effects are attained. Related to this is the view that at least some negative symptoms (e.g., depression, withdrawal) are secondary to the positive symptoms. The view has also been advanced, however, that 5-HT$_{2A}$ receptors are involved in part (the negative symptoms) or wholly in schizophrenia. So far, the evidence appears to be that 5-HT$_{2A}$ blocking agents do not relieve positive effects of schizophrenia.[30] The view that 5-HT$_{2A}$ overactivity is the source of negative symptoms (part of the basis psychosis) is not disproved at present, though some say it has been weakened.[30]

One result of the development of atypical antipsychotics has been a renewed interest in models of psychosis other than the amphetamine model. In line with possible dual involvement of 5-HT and DA, the lysergic acid diethylamide model has been cited as better fitting schizophrenias than the amphetamine model. But, this has been disputed. Interest in serotoninergic involvement is still high and involves elucidating the roles of 5-HT$_6$ and 5-HT$_7$ receptors.

Interest remains in understanding the psychosis produced by several central anticholinergics. Muscarinic (M_1 and M_4) agonists appear to offer the best approach at this time.[33] The role of the M_5 receptor awaits synthesis of M_5-specific drugs.[34]

Phencyclidine-induced psychosis has been proposed as a superior model for schizophrenia because it presents both positive and negative symptoms.[30] It suggests that deficits in glutaminergic function occur in schizophrenia. Results of agonists of NMDA receptors overall have not been productive because of the excitatory and neurotoxic effects of the agents tested. Identification of susceptible receptor subtypes as targets, using glycine modulation or group II metabotropic receptor agonists to modulate NMDA receptors, has been proposed to circumvent the problems associated with the NMDA agonists.

The ionotropic glutamic acid α-amino-3-hydroxy-5-methyl-4-isoxazole propionic acid (AMPA) receptors are activated by brain-penetrating ampakines. There are suggestions that these agents exert some antipsychotic actions by increasing glutaminergic activity.

The individual antipsychotic compounds are now considered. The substituted dopamine motif is useful as an organizational device. Atypical antipsychotics are indicated when they occur. Future growth in this area should be interesting.

Phenothiazines

Many potentially useful phenothiazine derivatives have been synthesized and evaluated pharmacologically. Consequently, the large body of information permits accurate statements about the structural features associated with activity. Many of the features were summarized and interpreted by Gordon et al.[35] The best position for substitution is the 2 position. Activity increases (with some exceptions) as electron-withdrawing ability of the substituent increases. Another possibly important structural feature in the more potent compounds is the presence of an unshared electron pair on an atom or atoms of the 2 substituent. Substitution at the 3 position can improve activity over nonsubstituted compounds but not as significantly as substitution at the 2 position. Substitution at position 1 has a deleterious effect on antipsychotic activity, as does (to a lesser extent) substitution at the 4 position.

Phenothiazine Antipsychotic
Agents–General Structure

The significance of these substituent effects could be that the hydrogen atom of the protonated amino group of the side chain H bonds with an electron pair of an atom of the 2 substituent to develop a DA-like arrangement. Horn and Snyder, from x-ray crystallography, proposed that the chlorine-substituted ring of chlorpromazine base could be superimposed on the aromatic ring of dopamine base with the sulfur atom aligned with the *p*-hydroxyl of dopamine and the aliphatic amino groups of the two compounds also aligned.[36] The model used here is based on the interpretation of the SARs by Gordon et al.[35] and on the Horn and Snyder proposal[36] but involves the protonated species rather than the free base. The effect of the substituent at the 1 position might be to interfere with the side chain's ability to bring the protonated amino group into proximity with the 2 substituent. In the Horn and Snyder scheme,[36] the sulfur atom at

position 5 is in a position analogous to the *p*-hydroxyl of dopamine, and it was also assigned a receptor-binding function by Gordon et al.[35] A substituent at position 4 might interfere with receptor binding by the sulfur atom.

The three-atom chain between position 10 and the amino nitrogen is required. Shortening or lengthening the chain at this position drastically decreases activity. The three-atom chain length may be necessary to bring the protonated amino nitrogen into proximity with the 2-substituent.

As expected, branching with large groups (e.g., phenyl) decreases activity, as does branching with polar groups. Methyl branching on the β position has a variable effect on activity. More importantly, the antipsychotic potency of *levo* (the more active) and *dextro* isomers differs greatly. This has long been taken to suggest that a precise fit (i.e., receptor site occupancy) is involved in the action of these compounds.

Decreases in size from a dimethylamino group (e.g., going to a monomethylamino) greatly decrease activity, as do effective size increases, such as the one that occurs with *N,N*-diethylamino. Once the fundamental requirement of an *effective* size of about that equivalent to a dimethylamino is maintained, as in fusing *N,N*-diethyl substituents to generate a pyrrolidino group, activity can be enhanced with increasing chain length, as in N₂-substituted piperizino compounds.

The critical size of groups on the amino atom suggests the importance of the amino group (here protonated) for receptor attachment. The effect of the added chain length, once the critical size requirement is met, could be increased affinity. It appears to have been reasonably proved that the protonated species of the phenothiazines can bind to DA receptors.[37]

Metabolism of the phenothiazines is complex in detail, but simple overall. A major route is hydroxylation of the tricyclic system. The usual pattern, for which there are good chemical reasons, is hydroxylation *para* to the 10-nitrogen atom of the ring other than the ring bearing the electron-attracting substituent at the 2 position. Thus, the major initial metabolite is frequently the 7-hydroxy compound. This compound is further metabolized by conjugation with glucuronic acid, and the conjugate is excreted. Detailed reviews of the metabolites of phenothiazines (as well as SARs and pharmacokinetic factors) are available.[38]

PRODUCTS

The structures of the phenothiazine derivatives described below are given in Table 14-3.

Promazine. Promazine, 10-[3-(dimethylamino) propyl-(phenothiazine monohydrochloride (Sparine), was introduced into antipsychotic therapy after its 2-chloro-substituted relative. The 2H substituent *vis-a-vis* the 2Cl substituent gives a milligram potency decrease as an antipsychotic, as encompassed in Gordon's rule. Tendency to EPS is also lessened, which may be significant, especially if it is decreased less than antipsychotic potency.

Chlorpromazine Hydrochloride, USP. Chlorpromazine hydrochloride, 2-chloro-10-[3-(dimethylamino)propyl]phenothiazine monohydrochloride (Thorazine), was the first phenothiazine compound introduced into therapy. It is

TABLE 14–3 Phenothiazine Derivatives

Generic Name *Proprietary Name*	R10	R2
Propyl Dialkylamino Side Chain		
Promazine hydrochloride, USP *Sparine*	—(CH2)3N(CH3)2 · HCl	H
Chlorpromazine hydrochloride, USP *Thorazine*	—(CH2)3N(CH3)2 · HCl	Cl
Triflupromazine hydrochloride, USP *Vesprin*	—(CH2)3N(CH3)2 · HCl	CF3
Akyl Piperidyl Side Chain		
Thioridazine hydrochloride, USP *Mellaril*	—(CH2)2— [piperidine N-CH3] · HCl	SCH3
Mesoridazine besylate, USP *Serentil*	—(CH2)2— [piperidine N-CH3] · C6H5SO3H	O↑SCH3
Propyl Piperazine Side Chain		
Prochlorperazine maleate, USP *Compazine*	—(CH2)3—N[piperazine]N—CH3 · 2C4H4O4	Cl
Trifluoperazine hydrochloride, USP *Stelazine*	—(CH2)3—N[piperazine]N—CH3 · 2HCl	CF3
Perphenazine, USP *Trilafon*	—(CH2)3—N[piperazine]N—CH2—CH2—OH	Cl
Fluphenazine hydrochloride, USP *Permitil, Prolixin*	—(CH2)3—N[piperazine]N—CH2—CH2—OH · 2HCl	CF3

still useful as an antipsychotic. Other uses are in nausea and vomiting and hiccough. It is the reference compound in activity comparisons, that is, the compound to which others are compared. The drug has significant sedative and hypotensive properties, possibly reflecting central and peripheral α_1-noradrenergic blocking activity, respectively. Effects of peripheral anticholinergic activity are common. As with the other phenothiazines, the effects of other CNS-depressant drugs, such as sedatives and anesthetics, can be potentiated.

Triflupromazine Hydrochloride, USP. Triflupromazine hydrochloride, 10-[3-(dimethylamino)propyl]-2-(trifluoromethyl)phenothiazine monohydrochloride (Vesprin), has lower sedative and hypotensive effects than chlorpromazine

and a greater milligram potency as an antipsychotic. EPS are higher. The 2-CF3 versus the 2-Cl is associated with these changes. Overall, the drug has uses analogous to those of chlorpromazine.

Thioridazine Hydrochloride, USP. Thioridazine hydrochloride, 10-[2-(1-methyl-2-piperidyl)ethyl]-2-(methylthio)phenothiazine monohydrochloride (Mellaril), is a member of the piperidine subgroup of the phenothiazines. The drug has a relatively low tendency to produce EPS. The drug has high anticholinergic activity, and this activity in the striatum, counterbalancing a striatal DA block, may be responsible for the low EPS. It also has been suggested that there may be increased DA receptor selectivity, which may be responsible. The drug has sedative and hypotensive activity in common with chlorpromazine and less antiemetic activity. At high doses, pigmentary retinopathy has been observed. A metabolite of the drug is mesoridazine (discussed next).

Mesoridazine Besylate, USP. Mesoridazine besylate, 10-[2-(methyl-2-piperidyl)ethyl]-2-(methylsulfinyl)phenothiazine monobenzenesulfonate (Serentil), shares many properties with thioridazine. No pigmentary retinopathy has been reported, however.

Prochlorperazine Maleate, USP. Prochlorperazine maleate, 2-chloro-10-[3-(4-methyl-1-piperazinyl)propyl]-phenothiazine maleate (Compazine), is in the piperazine subgroup of the phenothiazines, characterized by high milligram antipsychotic potency, a high prevalence of EPS, and low sedative and autonomic effects. Prochlorperazine is more potent on a milligram basis than its alkylamino counterpart, chlorpromazine. Because of the high prevalence of EPS, however, it is used mainly for its antiemetic effect, not for its antipsychotic effect.

Perphenazine, USP. Perphenazine, 4-[3-(2-chlorophenothiazine-10-yl)propyl]piperazineethanol; 2-chloro-10-[3-[4-(2-hydroxyethyl)piperazinyl]propyl]phenothiazine (Trilafon), is an effective antipsychotic and antiemetic.

Fluphenazine Hydrochloride, USP. The member of the piperazine subgroup with a trifluoromethyl group at the 2-position of the phenothiazine system and the most potent antipsychotic phenothiazine on a milligram basis is fluphenazine hydrochloride, 4-[3-[2-(trifluoromethyl)phenazin-10-yl]propyl]-1-piperazineethanol dihydrochloride, 10[3-[4-(2-hydroxyethyl)piperazinyl]propyl]-2-trifluoromethylphenothiazine dihydrochloride (Permitil, Prolixin). It is also available as two lipid-soluble esters for depot intramuscular injection, the enanthate (heptanoic acid ester) and the decanoate ester. These long-acting preparations have use in treating psychotic patients who do not take their medication or are subject to frequent relapse.

Ring Analogues of Phenothiazines: Thioxanthenes, Dibenzoxazepines, and Dibenzodiazepines

The ring analogues of phenothiazines are structural relatives of the phenothiazine antipsychotics. Most share many clinical properties with the phenothiazines. The dibenzodiazepine clozapine has some important differences, however, notably low production of EPS and reduction of negative symptoms. It is an important atypical antipsychotic.

Thioxanthene, USP. The thioxanthene system differs from the phenothiazine system by replacement of the N-H moiety with a carbon atom doubly bonded to the propylidene side chain. With the substituent in the 2 position, Z and E isomers are produced. In accordance with the concept that the presently useful antipsychotics can be superimposed on DA, the Z isomers are the more active antipsychotic isomers. The compounds of the group are very similar in pharmaco-

logical properties to the corresponding phenothiazines. Thus, thiothixene (Z-N-dimethyl-9-[3-(4-methyl-1-piperazinyl)propylidene]thioxanthene-2-sulfonamide (Navane), displays properties similar to those of the piperazine subgroup of the phenothiazines.

Thiothixene

A dibenzoxazepine derivative in use is **loxapine succinate**, 2-chloro-11-(4-methyl-1-piperazinyl)dibenz[b, f][1, 4]oxazepine succinate (Daxolin). The structural relationship to the phenothiazine antipsychotics is apparent. It is an effective antipsychotic and has side effects similar to those reported for the phenothiazines.

Loxapine Succinate

The dibenzodiazepine derivative is **clozapine** (Clozaril). It is not a potent antipsychotic on a milligram basis (note the orientation of the N-methyl piperazino group relative to the chlorine atom). It is effective against both positive and negative symptoms of schizophrenia and has a low tendency to produce EPS. There are legal restrictions on its use because of a relatively high frequency of agranulocytosis. As a rule, two other antipsychotics are tried before recourse to therapy with clozapine.

Clozapine

Fluorobutyrophenones

The fluorobutyrophenones belong to a much-studied group of compounds, many of which possess high antipsychotic activity. Only a few of these are used in the United States, which can be misleading about the importance of the group and its evolved relatives. The structural requirements for antipsychotic activity in the group are well worked out.[39] General features are expressed in the following structure.

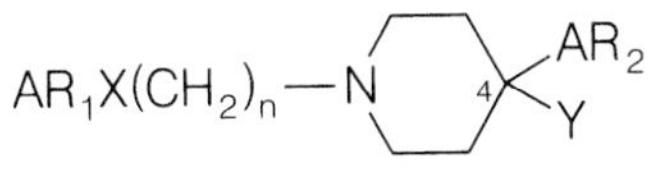

$$AR_1X(CH_2)_n - N \underset{4}{\diagup} \overset{AR_2}{\underset{Y}{\diagdown}}$$

Optimal activity is seen when AR_1 is an aromatic system. A *p*-fluoro substituent aids activity. When X = C = O, optimal activity is seen, although other groups, C(H)OH and C(H)aryl, also give good activity. When n = 3, activity is optimal; longer or shorter chains decrease activity. The aliphatic amino nitrogen is required, and highest activity is seen when it is incorporated into a cyclic form. AR_2 is an aromatic ring and is needed. It should be attached directly to the 4 position or (occasionally) separated from it by one intervening atom. The Y group can vary and assist activity. An example is the hydroxyl group of haloperidol.

The empirical SARs could be construed to suggest that the 4-aryl piperidino moiety is superimposable on the 2-phenylethylamino moiety of dopamine and, accordingly, could promote affinity for D_2 and D_3 receptors. The long *N*-alkyl substituent could help promote receptor affinity and produce receptor antagonism activity and/or inverse agonism..

Some members of the class are extremely potent antipsychotic agents and D_2 and D_3 receptor antagonists. EPS are extremely marked in some members of this class, which may, in part, be due to a potent DA block in the striatum and almost no compensatory striatal anticholinergic block. Most of the compounds do not have the structural features associated with effective anticholinergic activity.

Haloperidol, USP. Haloperidol, 4[4-(*p*-chlorophenyl)-4-hydroxypiperidone]-4′-*n*-fluorobutyrophenone (Haldol), is a potent antipsychotic useful in schizophrenia and in psychoses associated with brain damage. It is frequently chosen as the agent to terminate mania and often used in therapy for Gilles de la Tourette's syndrome.

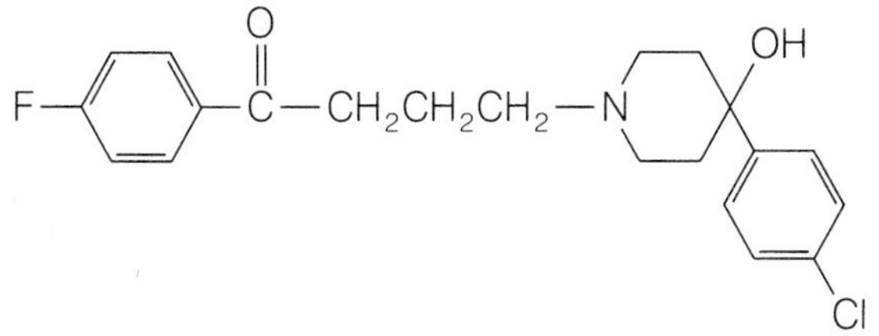

Haloperidol

Droperidol, USP. Droperidol, 1-{1-[3-(*p*-fluorobenzoyl)propyl]-1,2, 3,6-tetrahydro-4-pyridyl-2-benzimidazolinone (Inapsine), may be used alone as a preanesthetic neuroleptic or as an antiemetic. Its most frequent use is in combination (Innovar) with the narcotic agent fentanyl (Sublimaze) preanesthetically.

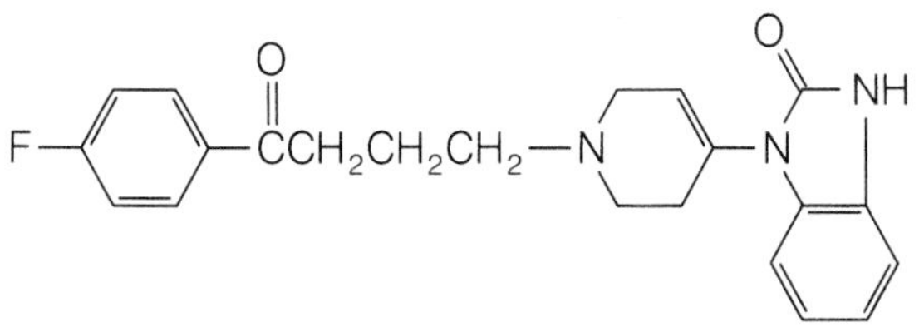

Droperidol

Risperidone. Risperidone (Risperdal) has the structural features of a hybrid molecule between a butyrophenone antipsychotic and a trazodone-like antidepressant. It benefited refractory psychotic patients, with parkinsonism controlled at one-tenth the dose of antiparkinsonian drugs used with haloperidol.[40] Coexisting anxiety and depressive syndromes were also lessened. It is reported to decrease the negative (e.g., withdrawal, apathy) as well as the positive (e.g., delusions, hallucinations) symptoms of schizophrenia. This is reportedly a consequence of the compound's combination $5\text{-HT}_2\text{-D}_2$ receptor antagonistic properties.[41] Overall the reasons for the decreased EPS and effectiveness against negative symptom are still under investigation. It is an important atypical antipsychotic.

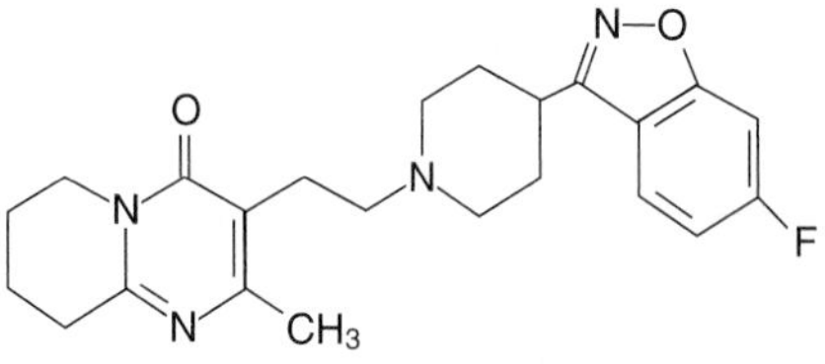

Risperidone

The diphenylbutylpiperidine class can be considered a modification of the fluorobutyrophenone class. Because of their high hydrophobic character, the compounds are inherently long acting. Penfluridol has undergone clinical trials in the United States, and pimozide has been approved for antipsychotic use. Overall, side effects for the two compounds resemble those produced by the fluorobutyrophenones.

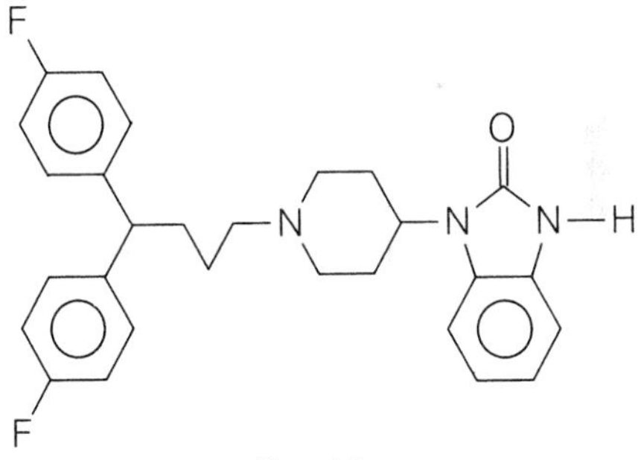

Pimozide

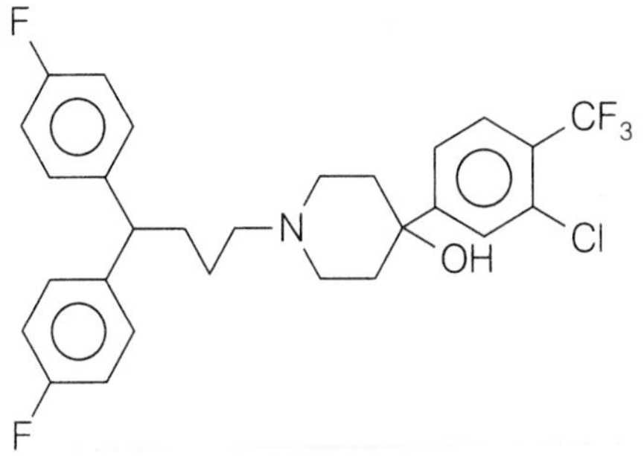

Penfluridol

β-Aminoketones

Several β-aminoketones have been examined as antipsychotics.[38] They evolved out of research on the alkaloid lobeline. The overall structural features associated with activity can be seen in the structure of molindone. In addition to the β-aminoketone group, there must be an aryl group positioned as in molindone. It might be conjectured that the proton on the protonated amino group in these compounds H-bonds with the electrons of the carbonyl oxygen atom. This would produce a cationic center, two-atom distance, and an aryl group that could be superimposed on the analogous features of protonated dopamine.

Molindone Hydrochloride.

Molindone hydrochloride, 3-ethyl-6,7-dihydro-2-methyl-5-morpholinomethyl)indole-4(5H)-one monohydrochloride (Moban), is about as potent an antipsychotic as trifluoperazine. Overall, side effects resemble those of the phenothiazines.

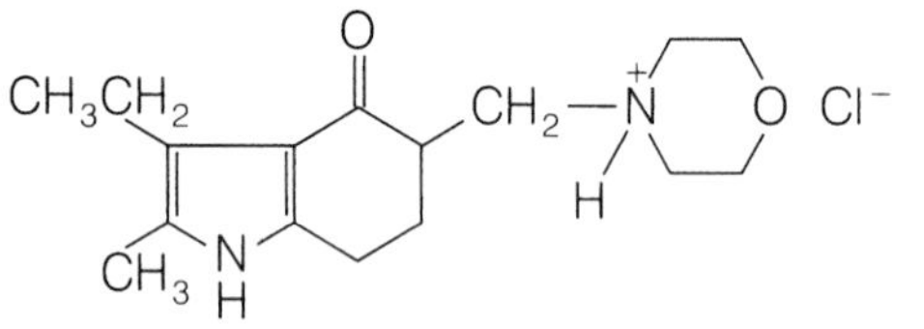

Molindone Hydrochloride

Benzamides

The benzamides evolved from observations that the gastroprokinetic and antiemetic agent metoclopramide has antipsychotic activity related to D_2 receptor block. It was hoped that the group might yield compounds with diminished EPS liability. This expectation appears to have been met. A H bond between the amido H and the unshared electrons of the methoxy group to generate a pseudo ring is considered important for antipsychotic activity in these compounds. Presumably, when the protonated amine is superimposed on that of protonated dopamine, this pseudo ring would superimpose on dopamine's aromatic ring.[42] These features can be seen in sulpiride and remoxipride.

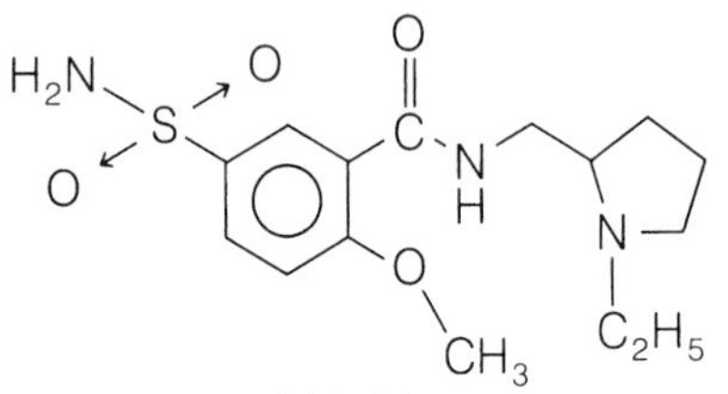

Sulpieride

Remoxipride (Roxiam).

Remoxipride is a D_2 receptor blocker.[40] It is said to be as effective as haloperidol with fewer EPS. Negative symptoms of schizophrenia are diminished. The drug is classed as an atypical antipsychotic. The substituents on the aliphatic amino nitrogen and the substituents on the aromatic ring are interesting.

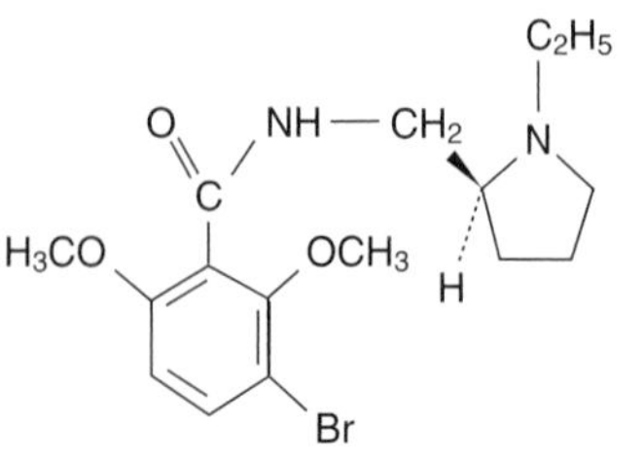

Remoxipride

Olanzapine and Quetiapine.

Olanzapine (Zyprexa) and quetiapine (Seroquel) possess tricyclic systems with greater electron density than chlorpromazine. They thus resemble clozapine. The drugs are atypical antipsychotics.

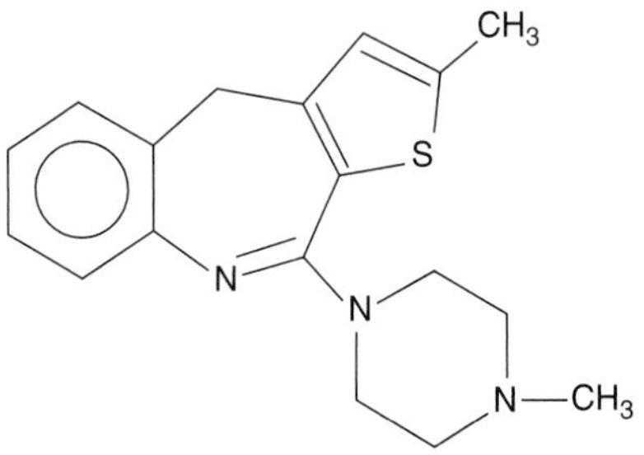

Olanzapine

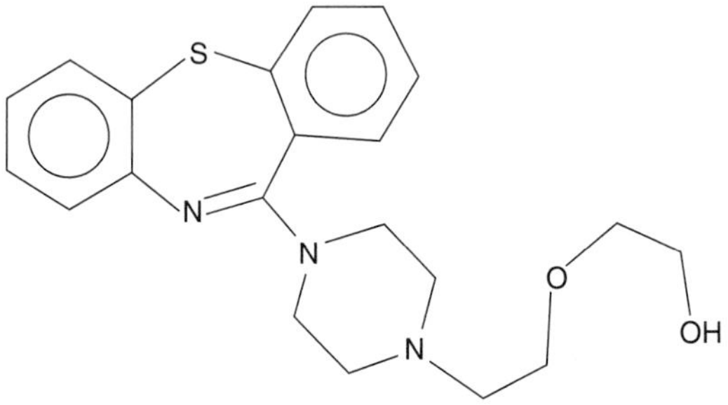

Quetiapine

Overall, these two compounds should bind less strongly to D_2 receptors and permit more receptor selectivity among receptor subtypes than typical antipsychotics. This could account for decreased striatal D_2-blocking activity, which would produce less discomfort in patients. It would be interesting to see testing results of these drugs' activities over a broad range of receptors, as are presently being accumulated for clozapine.

With respect to the atypical antipsychotics, two events long in the past may shed some light on the events of today. The field of reuptake-inhibiting antidepressants arose when only a very small structural change was made in an antipsychotic drug, and the new activity noted. (The antipsychotic activity remained.) So, small changes in structure can produce antipsychotics that are active against depressive symptoms. Likewise, small changes in structure could provide selectivity among D_2 receptors.

Almost 40 years ago, it was noted that thioridazine was far less unpleasant for patients than its relatives.[43] Its tricyclic system is far more nucleophilic than that of most other drugs. The emphasis at the time, however, was to increase milligram potency by increasing D_2 receptor affinity by lowering tricyclic electron density. The experience of clozapine, with increased electron density of the receptor-binding rings and thus lower affinity, appears to validate the observation about thioridazine and appears to allow more selectivity among D_2 receptors. Lessening blocks on, for example, striatal D_2 receptors, and possibly mesocortical D_2 receptors as well could produce drugs that are much less unpleasant for the patient. Additionally, a less intense D_2 block could allow the effects of other blocks to make up more of the drug's total action (e.g., 5-HT transporter block). Several atypical antipsychotics have rings with enhanced nucleophility. Of course, other structural features could be influencing receptor selectivity, for example, increasing steric hindrance to receptor binding by the protonated amino group or to the ring binding.

Antimanic Agents

LITHIUM SALTS

The lithium salts used in the United States are the carbonate (tetrahydrate) and the citrate. Lithium chloride is not used because of its hygroscopic nature and because it is more irritating than the carbonate or citrate to the GI tract.

The active species in these salts is the lithium ion. The classic explanation for its antimanic activity is that it resembles the sodium ion (as well as potassium, magnesium, and calcium ions) and can occupy the sodium pump. Unlike the sodium ion, it cannot maintain membrane potentials. Accordingly, it might prevent excessive release of neurotransmitters (e.g., dopamine) that characterize the manic state. Many of the actions of lithium ion have been reviewed.[44] The indications for lithium salts are acute mania (often with a potent neuroleptic agent for immediate control, since lithium is slow to take effect) and as a prophylactic to prevent occurrence of the mania of bipolar manic–depressive illness. Lithium salts are also used in severe recurrent unipolar depression. One effect of the drug that might be pertinent is an increase in the synthesis of presynaptic serotonin. Some have speculated that simply evening out transmission, preventing downward mood swing, for example, could be a basis for antidepressant action.

Because of its water solubility, the lithium ion is extensively distributed in body water. It tends to become involved in the many physiological processes involving sodium, potassium, calcium, and magnesium ions, hence, many side effects and potential drug interactions exist. The margin of safety is low; therefore lithium should be used only when plasma levels can be monitored routinely. In the desired dose range, side effects can be adequately controlled.

Because of the toxicity of lithium, there is substantial interest in design of safer compounds. As more is learned about lithium's specific actions, the likelihood of successful design of compounds designed to act on specific targets is increased. Actually, carbamazepine and valproic acid, which target sodium channels, are proving to be effective.[45] These two drugs are discussed in the anticonvulsant section.

Lithium Carbonate, USP, and Lithium Citrate. Lithium carbonate (Eskalith, Lithane) and lithium citrate (Cibalith-S) are the salts commercially available in the United States.

ANTICONVULSANT OR ANTIEPILEPTIC DRUGS

As is customary, the terms *anticonvulsant* and *antiepileptic* are used interchangeably in this discussion. Strictly speaking, however, an anticonvulsant is an agent that blocks experimentally produced seizures in laboratory animals, and

an antiepileptic drug is a drug used medically to control the epilepsies, not all of which are convulsive, in humans.

A classification of the types of epilepsy has been widely accepted because its accuracy facilitates diagnosis, drug selection, and precise discussion of seizure disorders.[46, 47] The major classification types are *(a)* generalized seizures, which essentially involve the entire brain and do not have an apparent local onset; *(b)* unilateral seizures, which involve one entire side of the body; *(c)* partial (or focal) seizures that have a focus (i.e., begin locally); *(d)* erratic seizures of the newborn; and *(e)* unclassified seizures (severe seizures associated with high mortality such that time does not permit a precise categorization).

Two major types of generalized seizures are the generalized tonic–clonic seizure (grand mal) and the nonconvulsive seizures or absence (petit mal) seizures. The typical generalized tonic–clonic seizure is often preceded by a series of bilateral muscular jerks; followed by loss of consciousness, which in turn is followed by a series of tonic and then clonic spasms. The typical absence seizure (classic petit mal) consists of a sudden brief loss of consciousness, sometimes with no motor activity, although often some minor clonic motor activity exists.

Major types of focal (partial) epilepsy are simple focal and complex focal seizures. A prototypic simple partial seizure is jacksonian motor epilepsy in which the jacksonian march may be seen. As the abnormal discharge proceeds over the cortical site involved, the visible seizure progresses over the area of the body controlled by the cortical site. The complex partial seizure is represented by the psychomotor or temporal lobe seizure. There is an aura, then a confused or bizarre but seemingly purposeful behavior lasting 2 to 3 minutes, often with no memory of the event. The seizure may be misdiagnosed as a psychotic episode. This is an extremely difficult epilepsy to treat. Much effort has been made in recent years to develop drugs to control it.

For broad consideration of how structure relates to antiepileptic activity, the classification of the epilepsies is traditionally further condensed (generalized tonic–clonic seizures, simple partial seizures, complex partial seizures, and absence seizures). The broad general pattern of structural features associated with antigeneralized tonic–clonic seizure activity is discernible for barbiturates, hydantoins, oxazolidinediones, and succinimides. This SAR also applies to simple partial seizures. It applies with less certainty to complex partial seizures, which are relatively resistant to treatment. With fewer effective drug entities, overall structural conclusions are more tenuous. The other general seizure type for which a broad SAR pattern among the cited compounds can be seen is the absence seizure. These features are cited under the heading, SARs Among Anticonvulsants.

Likewise, animal models characteristically discern three types of activity: activity against electrically induced convulsions correlates with activity against generalized tonic–clonic and partial seizures, and activity against pentylenetetrazole (PTZ)-induced seizures correlates with antiabsence activity. Of late, a fourth model, activity against pilocarpine and kainic acid seizures, is said to predict protection against temporal lobe epilepsy (a complex partial seizure).

Each of the epilepsy types is characterized by a typical abnormal pattern in the EEG. The EEG indicates sudden, excessive electrical activity in the brain. Antiepileptic drugs act to prevent, stop, or lessen this activity. The precise causes of the sudden, excessive electrical discharges may be many, and not all are understood. A working hypothesis is that there is a site or focus of damaged or abnormal and, consequently, hyperexcitable neurons in the brain. These can fire excessively and sometimes recruit adjacent neurons that in turn induce other neurons to fire. The location and the extent of the abnormal firing determine the epilepsy. An addition to this theory is based on the kindling model.[48] Experimentally, a brief and very localized electrical stimulus is applied to a site in the brain, with long intervals between applications. As the process is repeated, neuronal afterdischarges grow both longer and more intense at the original site and at new sites far from the original site. It is thought that changes occur in neurons at the discharge site, and these neurons in turn induce changes in neurons far from the site. Progressively more severe seizures can be induced, and these can arise from secondary foci that have been kindled far from the site of stimulation.

A major mode of action of anticonvulsants can be positive allosteric modulation of $GABA_A$ receptors. This is probably the mode of action of benzodiazepines and a major mode of action of barbiturates. On the basis of the structure of barbiturates, some inorganic cation blocking action would be expected as well—voltage-gated sodium channel for phenobarbital and calcium T channel block for 5,5-dialkyl members. Oxazolidine-2,4-diones (only trimethadione remains) and succinimides appear to act via calcium T-type channel block. Some sodium channel block could be expected among phenyl-substituted succinimides. The major mode of action for phenytoin (and probably monophenyl substituted hydantoins), carbamazepine, oxcarbazepine, valproic acid, felbamate, topiramate, lamotrigine and zonisamide is reported to be voltage-gated sodium channel block and is in accord with their structures. This does not exclude other expected actions in some of the examples.

Direct block of ionotropic glutamate receptors has so far not yielded clinically useful drugs. Some voltage-gated sodium channel drugs are reported to be antiglutamate as well by blocking glutamate release. Side effects of direct ionotropic glutamic acid receptor blocking has been a serious problem. Because of this, present approaches are to use the modulatory route. That is, lessen ionotropic glutamate activity by *(a)* using drugs that act at the glycine modulatory site on NMDA and *(b)* developing antagonists of members group II and group III metabotropic receptors and agonists of metabotropic group I glutamic acid receptors. These drugs would lower ionotropic glutaminergic activity.

Adenosine, which may be an endogenous anticonvulsant, continues to serve as a model but, for reasons such as poor brain distribution and an array of cardiovascular effects of agonists, has not yet yielded useful drugs. Elaboration of roles of receptor subtypes may give leads for drug design.

SARs Among Anticonvulsants

Several major groups of drugs have the common structure shown below.

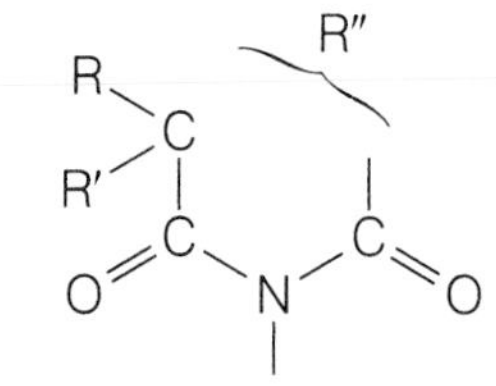

Structure common to anticonvulsant drugs.

R''	
$\overset{O}{\underset{}{\overset{\|}{C}}}$—NH	Barbiturates
—NH	Hydantoins
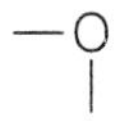 —O	Oxazolidinediones
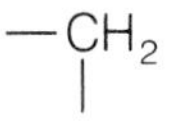 —CH$_2$	Succinimides

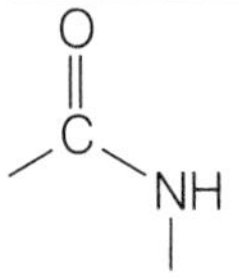

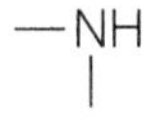

An overall pattern in the foregoing is that R and R' should both be hydrocarbon radicals. If both R and R' are lower alkyls, the tendency is to be active against absence seizures (petit mal) and not active against generalized tonic–clonic (grand mal) or partial seizures. If one of the hydrocarbon substituents is an aryl group, activity tends to be directed toward generalized tonic–clonic and partial seizures and not antiabsence activity.[49]

A conformational analysis of the aryl-containing antigeneralized tonic–clonic agents indicates that the conformational arrangement of the hydrophobic groups is important.[50]

Barbiturates

Although sedative–hypnotic barbiturates commonly display anticonvulsant properties, only phenobarbital and mephobarbital display enough anticonvulsant selectivity for use as antiepileptics. For the structures of these agents, consult Table 14-2, and for discussion of chemical properties see the section on barbiturates under sedative–hypnotic–anxiolytic agents. The metabolism of phenobarbital involves p-hydroxylation, followed by conjugation.

Mephobarbital is extensively N-demethylated in vivo and is thought to owe most of its activity to the metabolite phenobarbital. In keeping with their structures, both agents are effective against generalized tonic–clonic and partial seizures.

Hydantoins

The hydantoins are close structural relatives of the barbiturates, differing in lacking the 6-oxo group. They are cyclic monoacylureas rather than cyclic diacylureas. As a consequence of losing a carbonyl group, they are weaker organic acids than the barbiturates (e.g., phenytoin $pK_a = 8.3$). Thus, aqueous solutions of sodium salts, such as of phenytoin sodium, generate strongly alkaline solutions.

TABLE 14–4 Anticonvulsant Hydantoin Derivatives

Generic Name	Substituents		
Proprietary Name	R_5	R'_5	R_3
Phenytoin, USP *Dilantin, Diphentoin*	phenyl	phenyl	H
Mephenytoin, USP *Mesantoin*	phenyl	$CH_3{-}CH_2{-}$	$CH_3{-}$
Ethotoin *Peganone*	phenyl	H	$CH_3{-}CH_2{-}$

The compounds have a trophism toward antigeneralized tonic–clonic rather than antiabsence activity. This is not an intrinsic activity of the hydantoin ring system. All of the clinically useful antigeneralized tonic–clonic compounds (Table 14-4) possess an aryl substituent on the 5 position, corresponding to the branched atom of the general pharmacophore. Hydantoins with lower alkyl substituents reportedly have antiabsence activity.

Phenytoin and Phenytoin Sodium, USP. Phenytoin, 5,5-diphenylhydantoin (Dilantin), is the first anticonvulsant in which it was clearly demonstrated that anticonvulsant activity could definitely be separated from sedative–hypnotic activity. It is often cited as the prime example of an anticonvulsant acting as a sodium channel blocker.[13, 51] One effect of neuronal sodium channel block is to decrease presynaptic glutamic acid release, giving anticonvulsant activity.[50, 51] Another consequence is to reduce glutamate-induced ischemic damage to neurons.[51, 52] The drug is useful against all seizure types except absence. It is sometimes noted that the drug is incompletely or erratically absorbed from sites of administration. This is due to its very low water solubility. Metabolism proceeds by stereospecific p-hydroxylation of an aromatic ring, followed by conjugation.

Mephenytoin, USP. Mephenytoin, 5-ethyl-3-methyl-5-phenyl-hydantoin (Mesantoin), is metabolically N-dealkylated to 5-ethyl-5-phenylhydantoin, believed to be the active agent. Interestingly, 5-ethyl-5-phenylhydantoin, the hydantoin counterpart of phenobarbital, was one of the first hydantoins introduced into therapy. It was introduced as a sedative–hypnotic and anticonvulsant under the name Nirvanol, but it was withdrawn because of toxicity. Presumably, mephenytoin may be considered a prodrug that ameliorates some of the toxicity—serious skin and blood disorders—of the delivered active drug.

Metabolic inactivation of mephenytoin and its demethyl metabolite is by p-hydroxylation and then conjugation of the hydroxyl group. The drug has a spectrum of activity similar to that of phenytoin. It may worsen absence seizures.

Ethotoin. Ethotoin, 3-ethyl-5-phenylhydantoin (Peganone), is N-dealkylated and p-hydroxylated; the *N*-dealkyl metabolite, presumably the active compound, is likewise metabolized by p-hydroxylation. The hydroxyl group is then conjugated.

The compound is used against generalized seizures, but usually on an adjunctive basis, owing to its low potency. In general, agents that are not completely branched on the appropriate carbon have lower potency than their more completely branched counterparts.

Oxazolidinediones

Replacement of the N-H group at position 1 of the hydantoin system with an oxygen atom yields the oxazolidine-2,4-dione system. The oxazolidinedione system is sometimes equated with antiabsence activity, but this trophism probably is more dictated by the fact that the requisite branched atom of these compounds is substituted with lower alkyls. Aryl-substituted oxazolidine-2,4-diones have shown activity against generalized tonic–clonic seizures. The oxazolidinedione group of anticonvulsants used clinically has shrunk to one clinically useful member. Toxicities associated with the group may be the problem.

Trimethadione, USP. Trimethadione, 3,5,5-trimethyl-2,4-oxazolidinedione, 3,5,5-trimethadione (Tridione), was the first drug introduced specifically for treating absence seizures. It is important as a prototype structure for antiabsence compounds. Dermatological and hematological toxicities limit its clinical use.

The drug is metabolized by N-demethylation to the putative active metabolite dimethadione.[53] Dimethadione is a calcium T channel blocker. Dimethadione is a water-soluble and lowly lipophilic compound and thus is excreted as such without further metabolism.

Trimethadione $R_5 = R'_5 = CH_3$

Succinimides

In view of the activity of antiepileptic agents such as the oxazolidine-2,4-diones, substituted succinimides (CH_2 replaces O) were a logical choice for synthesis and evaluation. Three are now in clinical use.

Phensuximide, USP. Some trophism toward antiabsence activity is attributed to the succinimide system. The $-CH_2-$ could be viewed as an α-alkyl branch condensed into the ring. Phensuximide, N-methyl-2-phenylsuccinimide (Milontin), is used primarily against absence seizures, but it has low potency and is relegated to secondary status. The phenyl substituent confers some activity against generalized tonic–clonic and partial seizures. N-demethylation occurs to yield the putative active metabolite. Both phensuximide and the N-demethyl metabolite are inactivated by p-hydroxylation and conjugation.

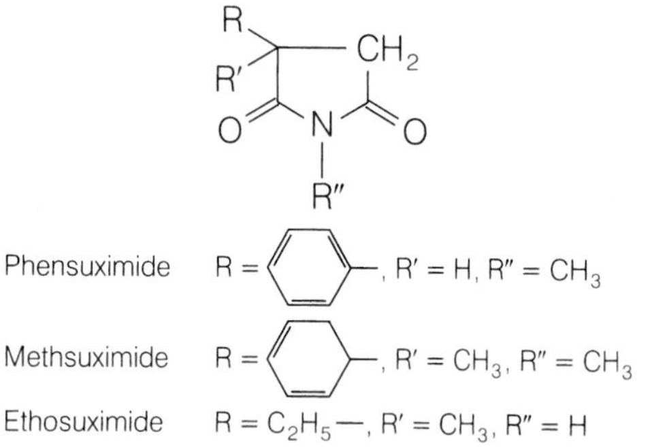

Phensuximide   R = (phenyl), R' = H, R'' = CH₃

Methsuximide   R = (phenyl), R' = CH₃, R'' = CH₃

Ethosuximide   R = C₂H₅—, R' = CH₃, R'' = H

Methsuximide.   N-demethylation and p-hydroxylation of parent and metabolite occur. Methsuximide, *N*,2-dimethyl-2-phenylsuccinimide (Celontin), has some use against absence and complex partial seizures.

Ethosuximide, USP.   Ethosuximide, 2-ethyl-2-methylsuccinimide (Zarontin), conforms very well to the general structural pattern for antiabsence activity. The drug is more active and less toxic than trimethadione. It is a calcium T channel–blocking drug. Toxicity primarily involves the skin and blood.

Some of the drug is excreted intact. The major metabolite is produced by oxidation of the ethyl group.

Ureas and Monoacylureas

The two chemical classes, ureas and monoacylureas, have a long history of producing compounds with anticonvulsant activity. The numerical yield of clinically useful compounds has not been great, however. Most of the simpler compounds have gone by the way. For convenience of grouping, carbamazepine and oxcarbazepine can be considered N,N-diacylureas.

Carbamazepine, USP.   Carbamazepine, 5*H*-dibenz[b,-f]lazepine-5-carboxamide (Tegretol), for SAR discussion purposes, can be viewed either as an ethylene-bridged 1,1-diphenylurea or an amido-substituted tricyclic system. The two phenyls substituted on the urea nitrogen fit the pattern of antigeneralized tonic activity. The overall shape of the molecule suggests the mode of action, sodium channel block. Carbamazepine is useful in generalized tonic–clonic and partial seizures.

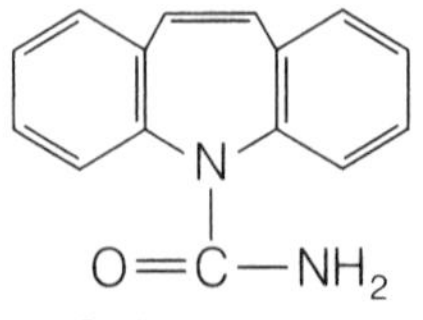

Carbamazepine

The drug has the potential for serious hematological toxicity, and it is used with caution.

Metabolism proceeds largely through the epoxide formed at the *(Z)cis*-stilbene double bond. In humans, the epoxide reportedly is converted largely to the 10*S*,11*S*-*trans*-diol.[54] The epoxide is a suspect in the idiosyncratic reactions carbamazepine may produce (e.g., aplastic anemia). With this in mind, compounds designed to avoid the epoxide such as oxcarbazepine (Trileptal) were developed.

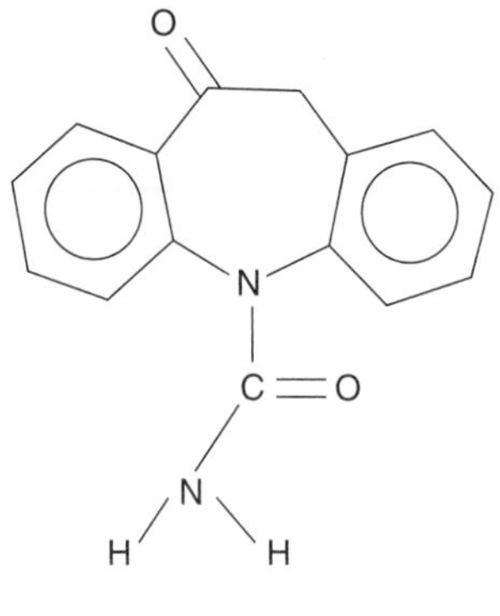

Oxcarbazepine

Oxcarbazepine is reduced to the monohydroxy compound, undoubtedly stereospecifically. The monohydroxy compound is considered the major active metabolite. The drug is used against partial seizures. The major mechanism of action is sodium channel block.

Miscellaneous Agents

Primidone.   Primidone, 5-ethyldihydro-5-phenyl-4,6-(1*H*,5*H*)-pyrimidinedione (Mysoline), is sometimes described as a 2-deoxybarbiturate. It appears to act as such and through conversion to phenobarbital and to phenylethylmalonyldiamide (PEMA).[55] The efficacy is against all types of seizures except absence. The agent has good overall safety, but rare serious toxic effects do occur.

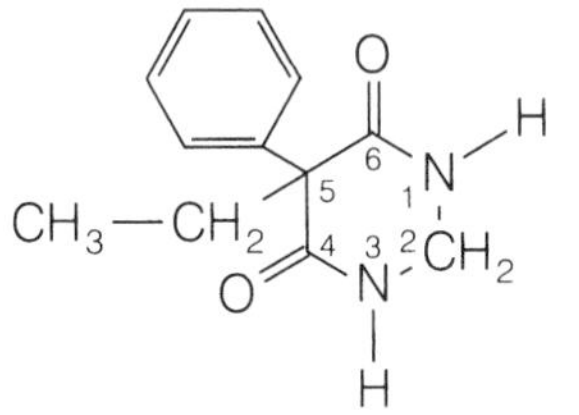

Primidone

Valproic Acid.   Many carboxylic acids have anticonvulsant activity, although often of low potency, possibly in part because extensive dissociation at physiological pH produces poor partitioning across the blood–brain barrier. Valproic acid, 2-propylpentanoic acid (Depakene), has good potency and is used against several seizure types. They include typical and atypical absence seizures and absence seizure with generalized tonic–clonic seizure. Mechanistically, the drug is a sodium channel blocker. This is in accordance with its structural features. It is also reported to increase GABA levels, again in conformity with its structure. Metabolism is by conjugation of the carboxylic acid group and oxidation of one of the hydrocarbon chains. Many of the side effects are mild. A rare, but potentially fatal, fulminate hepatitis has caused concern, however. One tends to look to the hydrogen atom α to the carboxyl acid as being labile and generating a toxiphore.

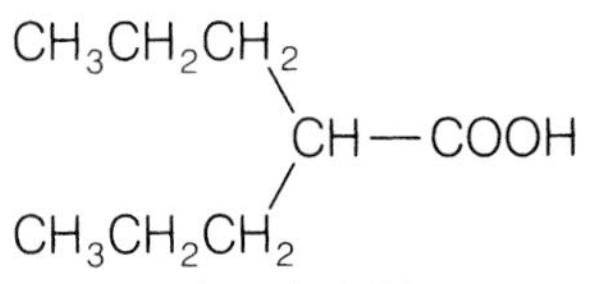

Valproic Acid

Gabapentin. Despite the fact that gabapentin (Neurontin) is a relative of GABA with increased hydrophobic character, its mechanism of action does not appear to involve an interaction with GABA$_A$ receptors. A binding site on calcium channels has been identified, but the mode of action of the drug is considered unclear. The drug is said to have a good pharmacokinetic profile and to cross the blood–brain barrier well. It was introduced for adjunctive therapy of refractory partial seizures and, secondarily, generalized tonic–clonic seizures. It was studied as a single drug therapy for various seizures.[56]

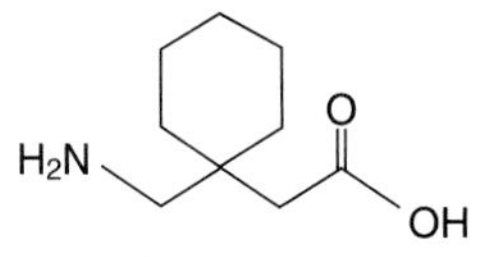

Gabapentin

Tiagabine (Gabitril). A glance at tiagabine's structure suggests an uptake inhibitor. Reportedly, it blocks GABA reuptake as a major mode of its anticonvulsant activity. Its use is against partial seizures.

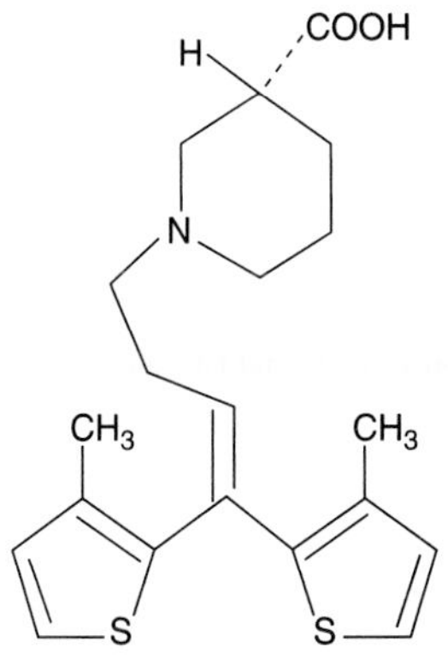

Tiagabine

Felbamate. Felbamate (Felbatol) has been used successfully in refractory patients with generalized tonic–clonic seizures and complex partial seizures. The mechanism of action may involve an interaction with the strychnine-insensitive receptor on the NMDA receptor.[56] It is also a sodium channel blocker. The drug is associated with a serious risk of aplastic anemia. It is used with extreme caution after other anticonvulsants have been tried and a careful risk-to-benefit assessment has been made.

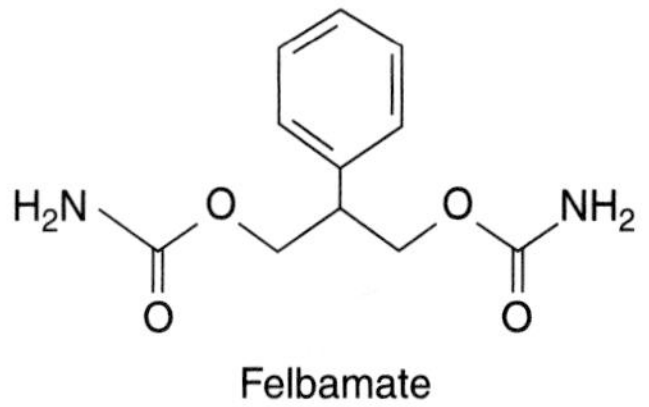

Felbamate

Lamotrigine. Lamotrigine (Lamictal) has been found effective against refractory partial seizures. It is said to act by blocking sodium channels and preventing glutamate release.[52] It is a member of a group of drugs that reduce glutamate release and thus reduce neuronal cell death in ischemia. One trial with lamotrigine did not detect slowing of the progression of amyotrophic lateral sclerosis (ALS). Another member of the group (sodium channel blockers with antiglutamate effect), riluzole (Rilutek) (2-amino-6-(trifuroethoxy)-benzothiazole) is used to slow progression. The bottle-stopper shape of both drugs is readily apparent.

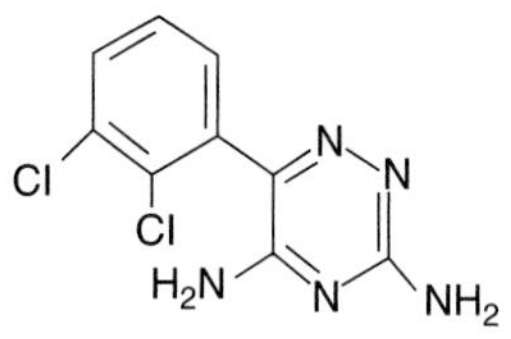

Lamotrigine

Zonisamide (Zonegran) and Topiramate (Topamax). Zonisamide and Topiramate have, respectively, the sulfonamide and sulfate amido as the small diameter end polar group and an extensive hydrophobic group as the large diameter end of the bottle stopper. Both are sodium channel blockers. Zonisamide also blocks calcium-T channels and Topamax increases the effect of GABA and antagonizes glutamate kainic acid/AMPA receptors. Each of the drugs is employed adjunctively against partial seizures.

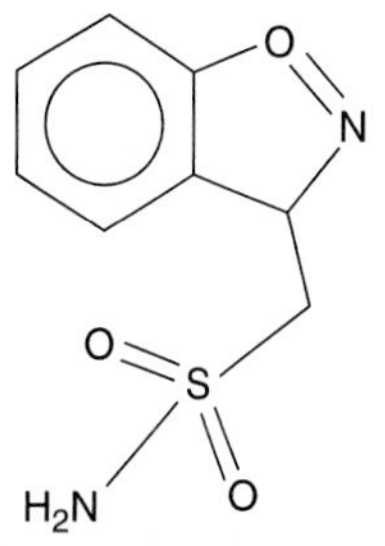

Zonisamide

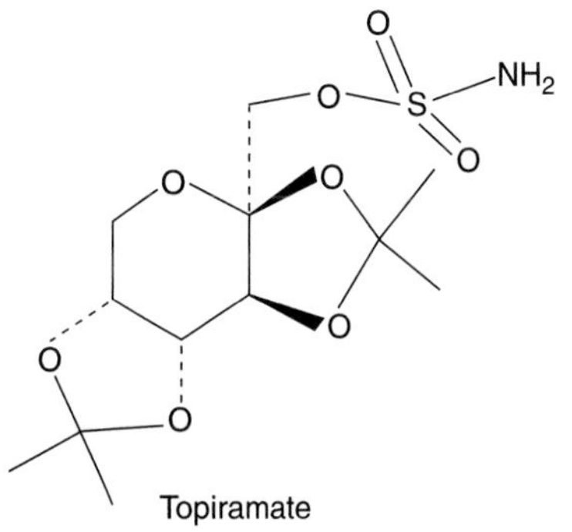

Topiramate

Benzodiazepines

For details of the chemistry and SARs of the benzodiazepines, see the discussion of anxiolytic–sedative–hypnotic drugs. Among the present clinically useful drugs, the structural features associated with anticonvulsant activity are identical with those associated with anxiolytic–sedative–hypnotic activity.[22] Animal models predict that benzodiazepines are modestly effective against generalized tonic–clonic and partial seizures and very highly active against absence seizures. This difference in seizure control tropism differs markedly from that of the barbiturates, hydantoins, and most other chemical compounds when they are aryl- or diaryl-substituted. Despite the high effectiveness of benzodiazepines as a group in animal models, only a few benzodiazepines have achieved established positions in anticonvulsant therapy. Because selective anticonvulsants should be attainable among agents acting at GABA$_A$ benzodiazepine allosteric modulatory sites, the number may increase in the future. A problem with the benzodiazepines has been decreased effectiveness over time. When physiological adaptation of this type occurs, it usually happens with sedative agents. If sedation were divorced from anticonvulsant action, possibly the latter might be sustained.

Clonazepam, USP. Clonazepam 5-(2-chlorophenyl)-3-dihydro-7-nitro-2*H*-1,4-benzodiazpin-2-one (Klonopin), partially selective at benzodiazepine allosteric binding sites on GABA$_A$ receptors, is useful in absence seizures and in myoclonic seizures. Tolerance to the anticonvulsant effect often develops, a common problem with the benzodiazepines. Metabolism involves hydroxylation of the 3 position, followed by glucuronidation and nitro group reduction, followed by acetylation.

Clonazepam

Diazepam. For details on diazepam (Valium) see its discussion under anxiolytics and sedative–hypnotic agents. The drug is mainly useful in treating generalized tonic–clonic status epilepticus, which is an ongoing and potentially fatal generalized tonic–clonic seizure.

Chlorazepate. See the detailed discussion of chlorazepate (Tranxene) in the sedative–hypnotic–anxiolytic section. Its principal anticonvulsant use is adjunctively in complex partial seizures.

Conclusion

Overall, there has been progress in recent years in the introduction of antiseizure drugs. Most of the progress has involved voltage-gated sodium channel blocking drugs.[56] Good reviews are available.[57, 58]

REFERENCES

1. Strange, P. G.: Pharmacol. Rev. 53:119, 2001.
2. Longoni, B., and Olsen, R. W.: Studies on the mechanism of interaction of anesthetics with GABA$_A$ receptors. Adv. Biochem. Psychopharmacol. 47:365, 1992.
3. Chebib, M., and Johnston, G. A. R.: J. Med. Chem. 43:1427, 2000.
4. Weight, F. F., Aguayo, L. G., White, G., et al.: GABA- and glutamate-gated ion channels as molecular sites of alcohol and anesthetic action. Adv. Biochem. Psychopharmacol. 47:335, 1992.
5. Miller, K. W.: General anesthetics. In Wolff, M. D. (ed.). Burger's Medicinal Chemistry, part III, 4th ed. New York, John Wiley & Sons, 1981, p. 623 (and references therein).
6. Johnson, F. H., Eyring, H., and Polissar, M. J.: The Kinetic Basis of Molecular Biology. New York, John Wiley & Sons, 1954.
7. Cohen, E. N.: Br. J. Anaesth. 50:665, 1978.
8. Stock, J. G. L., and Strunin, L.: Anesthesiology 63:424, 1985.
9. Cousins, M. J., and Mazze, R. L.: JAMA 225:1611, 1973.
10. Hitt, B. A., et al.: J. Pharmacol. Exp. Ther. 203:193, 1977.
11. Holliday, J. C., et al.: Anesthesiology 43:325, 1975.
12. Willer, J. C., Bergeret, S., Gaudy, J. H., and Dauthier, C.: Anesthesiology 63:467, 1985.
13. Takaki, K. S., and Epperson, J. R.: Annu. Rep. Med. Chem. 34:41, 1999.
14. Huang, J.-K., and Jan, C.-R.: Life Sci. 68:611, 2000.
15. Weinberger, D. R.: N. Engl. J. Med. 344:1247, 2001.
16. Xue, H., et al.: J. Med. Chem. 44:1883, 2001.
17. Xue, H., et al.: J. Mol. Biol. 296:739, 2000.
18. Renard, S., et al.: J. Biol. Chem. 274:13370, 1999.
19. Buhr, A., et al.: Mol. Pharmacol. 49:1080, 1996.
20. Buhr, A., et al.: Mol. Pharmacol. 52:672, 1997.
21. Buhr, A., et al.: J. Neurochem. 74:1310, 2000.
22. Sternbach, L. H.: In Garattini, S., Mussini, E., and Randall, L. O. (eds.). The Benzodiazepines. New York, Raven Press, 1972, p. 1.
23. Childress, S. J.: Antianxiety agents. In Wolff, M. E. (ed.). Burger's Medicinal Chemistry, part III, 4th ed. New York, John Wiley and Sons, 1981, p. 981.
24. Greenblatt, D. J., and Shader, R. I.: Benzodiazepines in Clinical Practice. New York, Raven Press, 1974, p. 17 (and references therein).
25. Greenblatt, D. J., Shader, R. I., and Abernethy, D. R.: N. Engl. J. Med. 309:345, 410, 1983.
26. Daniels, T. C., and Jorgensen, E. C.: Central nervous system depressants. In Doerge, R. F. (ed.). Wilson and Gisvold's Textbook of Organic Medicinal and Pharmaceutical Chemistry, 8th ed. Philadelphia, J. B. Lippincott, 1982, p. 335.
27. Berger, F. M.: Meprobamate and other glycol derivatives. In Usdin, E., and Forrest, I. S. (eds.). Psychotherapeutic Drugs, part II. New York, Marcel Dekker, 1977, p. 1089.
28. Cram, D. J., and Hammond, G. S.: Organic Chemistry, 2nd ed. New York, McGraw-Hill, 1964, p. 295.
29. Mackay, F. J., and Cooper, J. R.: J. Pharmacol. Exp. Ther. 135:271, 1962.
30. Rowley, M., Bristow, L. J., and Hutson, P. H.: J. Med. Chem. 44:477, 2001.
31. Karlsson, H., et al.: Proc. Natl. Acad. Sci. U. S. A. 98:4634, 2001.
32. Lewis, D. A.: Proc. Natl. Acad. Sci. U. S. A. 98:4293, 2000.
33. Felder, C. C.: Life Sci. 68:2605, 2001.
34. Yeomans, J., et al.: Life Sci. 68:2449, 2001.
35. Gordon, M., Cook, L., Tedeschi, D. H., and Tedeshi, R. E.: Arzneim. Forsch. 13:318, 1963.
36. Horn, A. S., and Snyder, S. H.: Proc. Natl. Acad. Sci. U. S. A. 68:2325, 1971.
37. Miller, D. D., et al.: J. Med. Chem. 30:163, 1987.
38. Kaiser, C., and Setler, P.: Antipsychotic agents. In Wolff, M. E. (ed.). Burger's Medicinal Chemistry, part III, 4th ed. New York, John Wiley and Sons, 1981, p. 859.
39. Janssen, P. A. J., and Van Bever, W. F. M.: Butyrophenones and diphenylbutylamines. In Usdin, E., and Forrest, I. S. (eds.). Psychotherapeutic Drugs, part II. New York, Marcel Dekker, 1977, p. 869.
40. Howard, H. R., and Seeger, T. F.: Annu. Rep. Med. Chem. 28:39, 1993 (and references therein).
41. Chen, X.-M.: Annu. Rep. Med. Chem. 29:331, 1994.
42. van de Waterbeemd, H., and Testa, B.: J. Med. Chem. 26:203, 1983.
43. Potter, W. Z., and Hollister, L. E.: Antipsychotic agents and lithium. In Katzung, B. G. (ed.). Basic and Clinical Pharmacology, 8th ed. New York, Lange Medical Books/McGraw-Hill, Medical Publishing Division, 2001, p. 478.
44. Emrich, H. M., Aldenhoff, J. B., and Lux, H. D. (eds.): Basic Mechanisms in the Action of Lithium. Symposium Proceedings. Amsterdam, Excerpta Medica, 1981.
45. Leysen, D., and Pinder, R. M.: Annu. Rep. Med. Chem. 29:1, 1994.
46. Gastaut, H., and Broughton, R.: In Radouco-Thomas, C. (ed.): Anticon-

vulsant Drugs, vol. 1. International Encyclopedia of Pharmacology and Therapeutics. New York, Pergamon, 1973, p. 3.

47. Commission on Classification and Terminology of the International League Against Epilepsy: Epilepsia 22:489, 1981.
48. Wada, J. A. (ed.): Symposium: Kindling 2. New York, Raven Press, 1981.
49. Close, W. J., and Spielman, M. A.: In Hartung, W. H. (ed.). Medicinal Chemistry, vol. 5. New York, John Wiley & Sons, 1961, p. 1.
50. Wong, M. G., Defina, J. A., and Andrews, P. R.: J. Med. Chem. 29: 562, 1986.
51. Bigge, C. F., and Boxer, P. A.: Annu. Rep. Med. Chem. 29:13, 1994.
52. Knöpfel, T., Kuhn, R., and Allgeier, H.: J. Med. Chem. 38:1417, 1995.
53. Frey, H. H., and Dretschmer, B. H.: Arch. Int. Pharmacodyn. Ther. 193:181, 1971.
54. Bellucci, G., Berti, G., Chiappe, C., et al.: J. Med. Chem. 30:768, 1987.
55. Spinks, A., and Waring, W. S.: In Ellis, G. P., and West, G. B. (eds.). Progress in Medicinal Chemistry, vol. 3. Washington, DC, Butterworth, 1963, p. 261.
56. Cosford, N. D. P., et al.: Annu. Rep. Med. Chem. 33:61, 1998.
57. Madge, D. J.: Annu. Rep. Med. Chem 33:51, 1998.
58. Anger, T., Madge, D. J., Mulla, M., and Riddall, D.: J. Med. Chem. 44:115, 2001.

SELECTED READING

Chebib, M., and Johnston, G. A. R.: GABA-activated ligand gated ion channels, medicinal chemistry and molecular biology. J. Med. Chem. 43:1427, 2000.

Cosford, N. D. P., McDonald, I. A., and Schweiger, E. J.: Recent progress in antiepileptic drug research. Annu. Rep. Med. Chem. 33:61, 1998.

Roweley, M., Bristow, L. J., and Hutson, P. H.: Current and novel approaches to the drug treatment of schizophrenia. J. Med. Chem. 44: 477, 2001.

Strange, P. G.: Antipsychotic drugs: importance of dopamine receptors for mechanisms of therapeutic actions and side effects. Pharmacol. Rev. 53:119, 2001.

Weinberger, D. R.: Anxiety at the frontier of molecular medicine. N. Engl. J. Med. 344:1247, 2001.

CHAPTER 15

Central Nervous System Stimulants

EUGENE I. ISAACSON

This chapter discusses a broad range of agents that stimulate the central nervous system (CNS). The *analeptics* classically are a group of agents with a limited range of use because of the general nature of their effects. The *methylxanthines* have potent stimulatory properties, mainly cortical at low doses but with more general effects as the dose is increased. The *central sympathomimetic agents* amphetamine and close relatives have alerting and antidepressant properties but medically are used more often as anorexiants. The *antidepressant drugs* are used most frequently in depressive disorders and can be broadly grouped into the monoamine oxidase inhibitors (MAOIs), the monoamine reuptake inhibitors, and agents acting on autoreceptors. A small group of miscellaneously acting drugs, which includes a number of hallucinogens, cocaine, and cannabinoids, concludes the chapter.

ANALEPTICS

The traditional analeptics are a group of potent and relatively nonselective CNS stimulants. The convulsive dose lies near their analeptic dose. They can be illustrated by picrotoxinin and pentylenetetrazole. Both are obsolete as drugs but remain valuable research tools in determining how drugs act. Newer agents, modafinil and doxapram, are more selective and have use in narcolepsy and as respiratory stimulants.

Picrotoxin. Picrotoxinin, the active ingredient of picrotoxin, has the following structure:

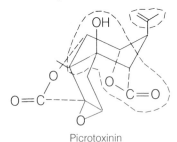

Picrotoxinin

According to Jarboe et al.,[1] the encircled hydroxylactonyl moiety is mandatory for activity, with the encircled 2-propenyl group assisting. Picrotoxinin exerts its effects by interfering with the inhibitory effects of γ-aminobutyric acid (GABA) at the level of the GABA$_A$ receptor's chloride channel. The drug is obsolete medically. Pharmacologically, it has been useful in determining mechanisms of action of sedative–hypnotics and anticonvulsants. Butyrolactones bind to the picrotoxinin site.

Pentylenetetrazole. Pentylenetetrazole, 6,7,8,9-tetrahydro-5*H*-tetrazolo*[1,5-a]*azepine, 1,5-pentamethylenetetrazole (Metrazol), has been used in conjunction with the electroencephalograph to help locate epileptic foci. It is used as a laboratory tool in determining potencies of potential anticonvulsant drugs in experimental animals. The drug acts as a convulsant by interfering with chloride conductance.[2] It binds to an allosteric site on the GABA$_A$ receptor and acts as a negative modulator. Overall, it appears to share similar effects on chloride conductance with several other convulsive drugs, including picrotoxinin.

Pentylenetetrazole

Modafinil. Modafinil (Provigil) has overall wakefulness-promoting properties similar to those of central sympathomimetics. It is considered an atypical α_1-norepinephrine (NE) receptor stimulant and is used to treat daytime sleepiness in narcolepsy patients. Adverse reactions at therapeutic doses are reportedly not severe and may include nervousness, anxiety, and insomnia.

Modafinil

Doxapram Hydrochloride, USP. Doxapram, 1-ethyl-4-(2-morpholinoethyl)-3,3-diphenyl-2-pyrolidinone hydrochloride hydrate (Dopram), has an obscure molecular mechanism of action. Overall, it stimulates respiration by action on peripheral carotid chemoreceptors. It has use as a respiratory stimulant postanesthetically, after CNS depressant drug overdose, in chronic obstructive pulmonary diseases, and in the apneas.

Doxapram Hydrochloride

METHYLXANTHINES

The naturally occurring methylxanthines are caffeine, theophylline, and theobromine. See Table 15-1 for their structures and occurrence and Table 15-2 for their relative potencies.

Caffeine is a widely used CNS stimulant. Theophylline has some medical use as a CNS stimulant, but its CNS-stimulant properties are encountered more often as sometimes severe, and potentially life-threatening, side effects of its use in bronchial asthma therapy. Theobromine has very little CNS activity (probably because of poor physicochemical properties for distribution to the CNS).

Caffeine is often used as it occurs in brewed coffee, brewed tea, and cola beverages. In most subjects, a dosage of 85 to 250 mg of caffeine acts as a cortical stimulant and facilitates clear thinking and wakefulness, promotes an ability to concentrate on the task at hand, and lessens fatigue. As the dose is increased, side effects indicating excessive stimulation (e.g., restlessness, anxiety, nervousness, and tremulousness) become more marked. (They may be present in varying degrees at lower dose levels.) With further increases in dosage, convulsions can occur. A review of the actions of caffeine in the brain with special reference to factors that contribute to its widespread use appears to be definitive.[3]

The CNS effects of theophylline at low dose levels have been little studied. At high doses, the tendency to produce convulsions is greater for theophylline than for caffeine. In addition to being cortical stimulants, theophylline and caffeine are medullary stimulants, and both are used as such. Caffeine may be used in treating poisoning from CNS-depressant drugs, though it is not a preferred drug.

The important use of theophylline and its preparations in bronchial asthma is discussed elsewhere. Caffeine also is reported to have valuable bronchodilating properties in asthma. Finally, because of central vasoconstrictive effects, caffeine has value in treating migraine and tension headaches and may have actual analgesic properties in the latter use.

The CNS-stimulating effects of the methylxanthines were once attributed to their phosphodiesterase-inhibiting ability. This action is probably irrelevant at therapeutic doses. Evidence indicates that the overall CNS-stimulant action is related more to the ability of these compounds to antagonize adenosine at A_1 and A_{2A} receptors.[3–6] All of the roles of these receptors are still under study. The adenosine receptor subtypes and their pharmacology have been reviewed.[3, 7–9] Problems with the present compounds, such as caffeine and theophylline, are lack of receptor selectivity and the ubiquitous nature of the various receptor subtypes.

Caffeine and theophylline have pharmaceutically important chemical properties. Both are weak Brønsted bases. The reported pK_a values are 0.8 and 0.6 for caffeine and 0.7 for theophylline. These values represent the basicity of the imino nitrogen at position 9. As acids, caffeine has a pK_a above 14, and theophylline, a pK_a of 8.8. In theophylline, a proton can be donated from position 7 (i.e., it can act as a Brønsted acid). Caffeine cannot donate a proton from position 7 and does not act as a Brønsted acid at pH values under 14. Caffeine does have electrophilic sites at positions 1, 3, and 7. In addition to its Brønsted acid site at 7, theophylline has electrophilic sites at 1 and 3. In condensed terms, both compounds are electron-pair donors, but only theophylline is a proton donor in most pharmaceutical systems.

Although both compounds are quite soluble in hot water (e.g., caffeine 1:6 at 80°C), neither is very soluble in water at room temperature (caffeine about 1:40, theophylline about 1:120). Consequently, a variety of mixtures or complexes designed to increase solubility are available (e.g., citrated caffeine, caffeine and sodium benzoate, and theophylline ethylenediamine compound [aminophylline]).

Caffeine in blood is not highly protein bound; theophylline is about 50% bound. Differences in the substituent at the 7 position may be involved. Additionally, caffeine is

TABLE 15–1 Xanthine Alkaloids

Xanthine
(R, R′ & R″ = H)

Compound	R	R′	R″	Common Source
Caffeine	CH_3	CH_3	CH_3	Coffee, tea
Theophylline	CH_3	CH_3	H	Tea
Theobromine	H	CH_3	CH_3	Cocoa

TABLE 15–2 Relative Pharmacological Potencies of the Xanthines

Xanthine	CNS Stimulation	Respiratory Stimulation	Diuresis	Coronary Dilatation	Cardiac Stimulation	Skeletal Muscle Stimulation
Caffeine	1[a]	1	3	3	3	1
Theophylline	2	2	1	1	1	2
Theobromine	3	3	2	2	2	3

[a]1, most potent.

more lipophilic than theophylline and reputedly achieves higher brain concentrations. The half-life of caffeine is 5 to 8 hours, and that of theophylline, about 3.5 hours. About 1% of each compound is excreted unchanged. The compounds are metabolized in the liver. The major metabolite of caffeine is 1-methyluric acid, and that of theophylline, 1,3-dimethyluric acid.[10] Neither compound is metabolized to uric acid, and they are not contraindicated in gout.

CENTRAL SYMPATHOMIMETIC AGENTS (PSYCHOMOTOR STIMULANTS)

Sympathomimetic agents, whose effects are manifested mainly in the periphery, are discussed in Chapter 16. A few simple structural changes in these peripheral agents produce compounds that are more resistant to metabolism, more non-polar, and better able to cross the blood–brain barrier. These effects increase the ratio of central to peripheral activity, and the agents are designated, somewhat arbitrarily, as *central sympathomimetic agents*.

In addition to CNS-stimulating effects, manifested as excitation and increased wakefulness, many central sympathomimetics exert an anorexiant effect. Central sympathomimetic (noradrenergic) action is often the basis for these effects. Other central effects, notably dopaminergic and serotoninergic effects, can be operative, however.[11] In some agents, the ratio of excitation and increased wakefulness to anorexiant effects is decreased, and the agents are marketed as anorexiants. Representative structures of this group of compounds are given in Table 15-3. The structures of the anorexiants phendimetrazine and sibutramine and the alerting agents methylphenidate and pemoline, useful in attention-deficient disorders, are given in the text.

Structural features for many of the agents can be visualized easily by considering that within their structure they

TABLE 15–3 Sympathomimetics With Significant Central Stimilant Activity

Generic Name	Base Structure		
Amphetamine	H	CH₃	NH / H / H
Methamphetamine	H	H	CH₃
Phentermine	H	CH₃	H
Benzphetamine	H	H	CH₃ / CH₂C₆H₅
Diethylpropion	Oᵃ	H	C₂H₅ / C₂H₅
Fenfluramine			

ᵃCarbonyl.

contain a β-phenethylamine moiety, and this grouping can give some selectivity for presynaptic or postsynaptic nora-drenergic systems. β-Phenethylamine, given peripherally, lacks central activity. Facile metabolic inactivation by mono-amine oxidases (MAOs) is held responsible. Branching with lower alkyl groups on the carbon atom adjacent (α) to the amino nitrogen increases CNS rather than peripheral activity (e.g., amphetamine, presumably by retarding metabolism). The α branching generates a chiral center. The *dextro(S)* isomer of amphetamine is up to 10 times as potent as the *levo(R)* isomer for alerting activity and about twice as active as a psychotomimetic agent. Hydroxylation of the ring or hydroxylation on the β carbon (to the nitrogen) decreases activity, largely by decreasing the ability to cross the blood–brain barrier. For example, phenylpropanolamine, with a β-OH, has about 1/100th the ability to cross the blood–brain barrier of its deoxy congener, amphetamine.

Halogenation (F, Cl, Br) of the aromatic ring decreases sympathomimetic activity. Other activities may increase. *p*-Chloroamphetamine has strong central serotoninergic activity (and is a neurotoxin, destroying serotoninergic neurons in experimental animals).[12, 13]

Methoxyl or methylenedioxy substitution on the ring tends to produce psychotomimetic agents, suggesting tropism for dopaminergic (D₂) receptors.

N-methylation increases activity (e.g., compare metham-phetamine with dextroamphetamine). Di-N-methylation decreases activity. Mono-N substituents larger than methyl decrease excitatory properties, but many compounds retain anorexiant properties. Consequently, some of these agents are used as anorexiants, reportedly with less abuse potential than amphetamine.

There can be some departure from the basic β-phenethyl-amine structure when compounds act by indirect noradrener-gic mechanisms. A β-phenethylamine-like structure, how-ever, can be visualized in such compounds.

The abuse potential of the more euphoriant and stimulatory of the amphetamines and amphetamine-like drugs is well documented. They produce an exceedingly destructive addiction. Apparently, both a euphoric "high" (possibly related to effects on hedonistic D₂ receptors) and a posteuphoric depression (especially among amine-depleting drugs) contribute to compulsive use of these agents. Abuse of these drugs (especially methamphetamine) in recent years has reached disastrous proportions.

Recognized medical indications for dextroamphetamine and some very close congeners include narcolepsy, Parkinson's disease, attention-deficient disorders, and, although not the preferred agents for obesity, appetite suppression. In some conditions, such as Parkinson's disease, for which its main use is to decrease rigidity, the antidepressant effects of dextroamphetamine can be beneficial. It is also reportedly an effective antidepressant in terminal malignancies. In almost all cases of depression, and especially in major depressive disorders of the unipolar type, however, dextroamphetamine has long been superseded by other agents, notably the MAOIs and the monoamine reuptake inhibiting antidepressants.

The compounds and their metabolites can have complex, multiple actions. In a fundamental sense, the structural basis for action is quite simple. The compounds and their metabolites resemble NE and can participate in the various neuronal and postsynaptic processes involving NE, such as synthesis, release, reuptake, and presynaptic and postsynaptic receptor activation. Also, because dopamine (DA) and, to a lesser extent, serotonin (5-hydroxytryptamine [5-HT]) bear a structural resemblance to NE, processes in DA- and 5-HT-activated systems can be affected. To illustrate the potential complexity, the receptor activations that can be associated with just one parameter, reduction in food intake, reportedly are α_1, β_1, β_2, $5HT_{1B}$, $5HT_{2A}$, $5HT_{2C}$, D_1, and D_2.

PRODUCTS

Amphetamine Sulfate, USP. Amphetamine, ($\pm$)-1-phenyl-2-aminopropane (Benzedrine), as the racemic mixture has a higher proportion of cardiovascular effects than the *dextro* isomer. For most medical uses, the dextrorotatory isomer is preferred.

Dextroamphetamine Sulfate, USP, and Dextroamphetamine Phosphate. Dextroamphetamine, ($+$)-(S)-methylphenethylamine, forms salts with sulfuric acid (Dexedrine) and with phosphoric acids. The phosphate is the more water-soluble salt and is preferred if parenteral administration is required. The dextrorotatory isomer has the *(S)* configuration and fewer cardiovascular effects than the levorotatory *(R)* isomer. Additionally, it may be up to 10 times as potent as the *(R)* isomer as an alerting agent and about twice as potent a psychotomimetic agent. Although it is a more potent psychotomimetic agent than the *(R)* isomer, it has a better ratio of alerting to psychotomimetic effects.

The major mode of action of dextroamphetamine is release of NE from the mobile pool of the nerve terminal. Other mechanisms, such as inhibition of uptake, may make a small contribution to the overall effects. The alerting actions relate to increased NE available to interact with postsynaptic receptors (α_1). Central β-receptor activation has classically been considered the basis for most of the anorexiant effect.

The psychotomimetic effects are linked to release of DA and activation of postsynaptic receptors. D_2 and mesolimbic D_3 receptors would be involved. Effects on 5-HT systems also have been linked to some behavioral effects of dextroamphetamine. Effects via 5-HT receptors would include $5HT_{1A}$ receptors and, theoretically, all additional receptors through $5HT_7$.

Dextroamphetamine is a strongly basic amine, with values from 9.77 to 9.94 reported. Absorption from the gastrointestinal tract occurs as the lipid-soluble amine. The drug is not extensively protein bound. Varying amounts of the drug are excreted intact under ordinary conditions. The amount is insignificant under conditions of alkaline urine. Under conditions producing systemic acidosis, 60 to 70% of the drug can be excreted unchanged. This fact can be used to advantage in treating drug overdose.

The α-methyl group retards, but does not terminate, metabolism by MAO. Under most conditions, the bulk of a dose of dextroamphetamine is metabolized by N-dealkylation to phenylacetone and ammonia. Phenylacetone is degraded further to benzoic acid.

In experimental animals, about 5% of a dose accumulates in the brain, especially the cerebral cortex, the thalamus, and the corpus callosum. It is first p-hydroxylated and then β-hydroxylated to produce p-hydroxynorephedrine, which has

been reported to be the major active metabolite involved in NE and DA release.[14]

Methamphetamine Hydrochloride. Methamphetamine, ($+$)-1-phenyl-2-methylaminopropane hydrochloride desoxyephedrine hydrochloride (Desoxyn), is the *N*-methyl analogue of dextroamphetamine. It has more marked central and less peripheral action than dextroamphetamine. It has a very high abuse potential, and by the intravenous route, its salts are known as "speed." The overall abuse problem presented by the drug is a national disaster. Medicinally acceptable uses of methamphetamine are analogous to those of dextroamphetamine.

Phentermine Ion-Exchange Resin and Phentermine Hydrochloride, USP. The free base is α,α-dimethylphenethylamine, 1-phenyl-2-methylaminopropane. In the resin preparation (Ionamin), the base is bound with an ion-exchange resin to yield a slow-release product; the hydrochloride (Wilpowr) is a water-soluble salt.

Phentermine has a quaternary carbon atom with one methyl oriented like the methyl of *(S)*-amphetamine and one methyl oriented like the methyl of *(R)*-amphetamine, and it reportedly has pharmacological properties of both the *(R)* and *(S)* isomers of amphetamine. The compound is used as an appetite suppressant and is a Schedule IV agent, indicating less abuse potential than dextroamphetamine.

Benzphetamine Hydrochloride. Benzphetamine hydrochloride, ($+$)-*N*-benzyl-*N*,α-dimethylphenethylamine hydrochloride, ($+$)-1-phenyl-2-(*N*-methyl-*N*-benzylamine)-propane hydrochloride (Didrex), is *N*-benzyl-substituted methamphetamine. The large (benzyl) N-substituent decreases excitatory properties, in keeping with the general structure–activity relationship (SAR) for the group. Anorexiant properties are retained. Classically, amphetamine-like drugs with larger than *N*-methyl substituents are cited as anorexiant through central β agonism. No claims for selectivity among β-receptor subtypes have been made in such citations. The compound shares mechanism-of-action characteristics with methylphenidate. Overall, it is said to reduce appetite with fewer CNS excitatory effects than dextroamphetamine.

Diethylpropion Hydrochloride, USP. Because it has two large (relative to H or methyl) *N*-alkyl substituents, diethylpropion hydrochloride, 1-phenyl-2-diethylaminopropan-1-one hydrochloride (Tenuate, Tepanil), has fewer sympathomimetic, cardiovascular, and CNS-stimulatory effects than amphetamine. It is reportedly an anorexiant agent that can be used for the treatment of obesity in patients with hypertension and cardiovascular disease. According to the generalization long used for this group of drugs, increasing *N*-alkyl size reduces central α_1 effects and increases β effects, even though the effects are likely mediated principally by indirect NE release.

Fenfluramine Hydrochloride. Fenfluramine hydrochloride, ($\pm$)*N*-ethyl-α-methyl-*m*-(trifluoromethyl)phenethylamine hydrochloride (Pondimin), is unique in this group of drugs, in that it tends to produce sedation rather than excitation. Effects are said to be mediated principally by central serotoninergic, rather than central noradrenergic, mechanisms. In large doses in experimental animals, the drug is a serotonin neurotoxin.[15] It was withdrawn from human use after reports of heart valve damage and pulmonary hypertension. From its structure, more apolar or hydrophobic character than amphetamine, tropism for serotoninergic neurons would be expected. Likewise, the structure suggests an indirect mechanism. If an indirect mechanism were operative, then all postsynaptic 5-HT receptors could be activated. Evidence from several studies indicates that the $5HT_{1B}$ and the $5HT_{2C}$ receptors are most responsible for the satiety effects of 5-HT. 5-HT may also influence the type of food selected (e.g., lower fatter food intake).[11] The (+) isomer, dexfenfluramine (Redux), has a greater tropism for 5-HT systems than the racemic mixture. It, too, was withdrawn because of toxicity.

Phendimetrazine Tartrate, USP. The optically pure compound phendimetrazine tartrate, (2S,3S)-3,4-dimethyl-2-phenylmorpholine-L-(+)-tartrate (Plegine), is considered an effective anorexiant that is less abuse prone than amphetamine. The stereochemistry of (+)phendimetrazine is as shown.[16]

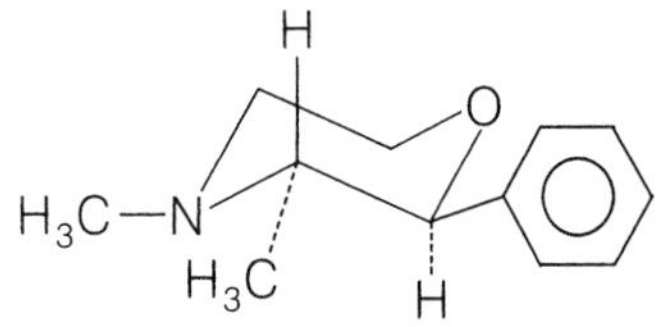

Phendimetrazine Tartrate

Sibutramine. Sibutramine (Meridia) is said to be an uptake inhibitor of NE and 5-HT. These mechanisms fit its structure. It is reportedly an antidepressant and an anorexiant drug. This mechanism implies that activation of all presynaptic and postsynaptic receptors in NE and 5-HT systems is possible. The data are not completely clear, but studies to date indicate that the receptors principally involved are α_1, β_1, and $5HT_{2C}$.[11]

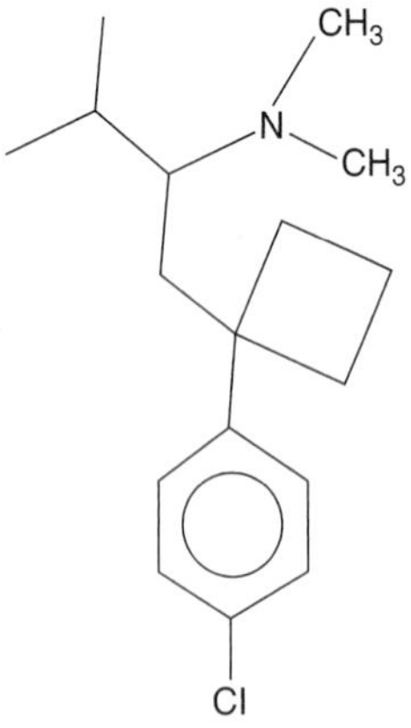

Sibutramine

Methylphenidate Hydrochloride, USP. Because methylphenidate (Ritalin) has two asymmetric centers, there are four possible isomers. The *threo* racemate is the mar-

keted compound and is about 400 times as potent as the *erythro* racemate.[17] The absolute configuration of each of the *threo*-methylphenidate isomers has been determined.[18] Considering that the structure is fairly complex (relative to amphetamine), it is likely that one of the two components of the *threo* racemate contains most of the activity. Evidence indicates that the (+)-(2R,2′R)*threo* isomer is involved principally in the behavioral and pressor effects of the racemate.[19] As is likely with many central psychomotor stimulants, there are multiple modes of action.

Methylphenidate, probably largely via its *p*-hydroxy metabolite, blocks NE reuptake, acts as a postsynaptic agonist, depletes the same NE pools as reserpine, and has effects on dopaminergic systems, such as blocking DA reuptake.

Methylphenidate is an ester drug with interesting pharmacokinetic properties arising from its structure. The pK_a values are 8.5 and 8.8. The protonated form in the stomach reportedly resists ester hydrolysis. Absorption of the intact drug is very good. After absorption from the gastrointestinal tract, however, 80 to 90% of the drug is hydrolyzed rapidly to inactive ritalinic acid.[20] (The extent of hydrolysis may be about 5 times that for (+) versus (−).[21]) Another 2 to 5% of the racemate is oxidized by liver microsomes to the inactive cyclic amide. About 4% of a dose of the racemate reportedly reaches the brain in experimental animals and there is p-hydroxylated to yield the putative active metabolite.

Methylphenidate is a potent CNS stimulant. Indications include narcolepsy and attention-deficit disorder. The structure of the (2R,2′R) isomer of the *threo* racemic mixture is shown.

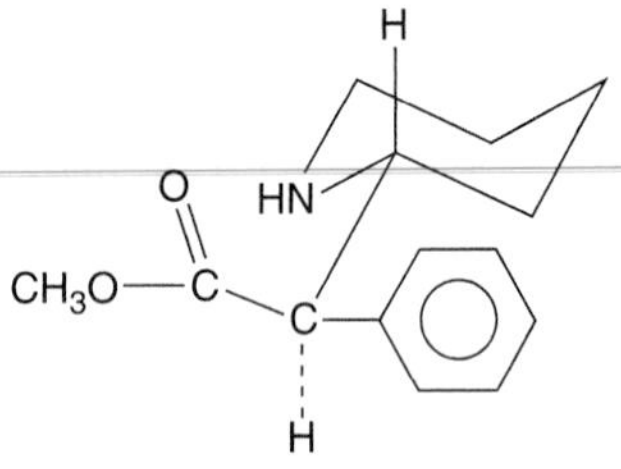

Methylphenidate Hydrochloride

Pemoline. The unique structure of pemoline, 2-amino-5-phenyl-4(5H)-oxazolone (Cylert), is shown below.

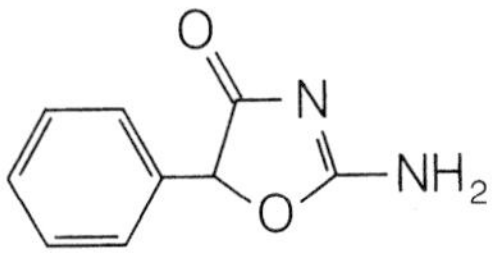

Pemoline

The compound is described as having an overall effect on the CNS like that of methylphenidate. Pemoline requires 3 to 4 weeks of administration, however, to take effect. A partial explanation for the delayed effect may be that one of the actions of the agent, as observed in rats, is to increase the rate of synthesis of DA.

ANTIDEPRESSANTS

Monoamine Oxidase Inhibitors (MAOIs)

Antidepressant therapy usually implies therapy directed against major depressive disorders of the unipolar type and is centered around three groups of chemical agents: the MAOIs, the monoamine reuptake inhibitors, and autoreceptor desensitizers and antagonists. Electroshock therapy is another option. The highest cure or remission rate is achieved with electroshock therapy. In some patients, especially those who are suicidal, this may be the preferred therapy. MAOIs and monoamine reuptake inhibitors have about the same response rate (~60 to 70%). In the United States, the latter group is usually chosen over MAOIs for antidepressant therapy.

A severe problem associated with the MAOIs that has been a major factor in relegating them to second-line drug status is that the original compounds inhibit liver MAOs irreversibly in addition to brain MAOs, thereby allowing dietary pressor amines that normally would be inactivated to exert their effects systemically. A number of severe hypertensive responses, some fatal, have followed ingestion of foods high in pressor amines. It was hoped that the development of agents such as selegiline that presumably spare liver MAO might solve this problem. The approach of using MAO selectivity did solve the hypertensive problem, but the compound was not an antidepressant (it is useful in Parkinson's disease). Another approach using a reversible MAOI has yielded antidepressants that lacked the hypertensive "cheese" effect. Another prominent side effect of MAOIs is orthostatic hypotension, said to arise from a block of NE released in the periphery. Actually, one MAOI, pargyline, was used clinically for its hypotensive action. Finally, some of the first compounds produced serious hepatotoxicity. Compounds available today reportedly are safer in this regard but suffer the stigma of association with the older compounds.

The history of MAOI development illustrates the role of serendipity. Isoniazid is an effective antitubercular agent but is a very polar compound. To gain better penetration into the *Mycobacterium tuberculosis* organism, a more hydrophobic compound, isoniazid substituted with an isopropyl group on the basic nitrogen (iproniazid), was designed and synthesized. It was introduced into clinical practice as an effective antitubercular agent. CNS stimulation was noted, however, and the drug was withdrawn. Later, it was determined in experimental animals and in vitro experiments with a purified MAO that MAO inhibition, resulting in higher synaptic levels of NE and 5-HT, could account for the CNS effects. The compound was then reintroduced into therapy as an antidepressant agent. It stimulated an intense interest in hydrazines and hydrazides as antidepressants and inaugurated effective drug treatment of depression.[22] It continued to be used in therapy for several years but eventually was withdrawn because of hepatotoxicity.

The present clinically useful irreversible inactivators can be considered mechanism-based inhibitors of MAO.[23] They are converted by MAO to agents that inhibit the enzyme. They can form reactants that bond covalently with the enzyme or its cofactor. A consequence of irreversible inactivation is that the action of the agents may continue for up to 2 weeks after administration is discontinued. Consequently, many drugs degraded by MAO or drugs that elevate levels of MAO substrates cannot be administered during that time.

For a long time, because the agents that opened the field and then dominated it were irreversible inactivator, MAO

inhibition was almost always regarded as irreversible. From the beginning, however, it was known that it was possible to have agents that act exclusively by competitive enzyme inhibition. For example, it has long been known that the harmala alkaloids harmine and harmaline act as CNS stimulants by competitive inhibition of MAO. Reversible (competitive) inhibitors selective for each of the two major MAO subtypes (A and B) are reportedly forthcoming.

Moclobemide

Moclobemide has received considerable attention abroad. A reversible inhibitor of MAO-A, it is considered an effective antidepressant and permits metabolism of dietary tyramine.[24] Metabolites of the drug are implicated in the activity. Reversible inhibitors of MAO-A (RIMAs) reportedly are antidepressant without producing hypertensive crises. Reversible inhibitors of MAO-B have also been studied. Presently, selective MAO-B inhibition has failed to correlate positively with antidepressant activity; selegiline, however, has value in treating Parkinson's disease.

The clinically useful MAOI antidepressants are nonselective between inhibiting metabolism of NE and 5-HT. Agents selective for a MAO that degrades 5-HT have been under study for some time. The structures of phenelzine and tranylcypromine are given in Table 15-4

Phenelzine Sulfate, USP. Phenelzine sulfate, 2-(phenylethyl)hydrazine sulfate (Nardil), is an effective antidepressant agent. A mechanism-based inactivator, it irreversibly inactivates the enzyme or its cofactor, presumably after oxidation to the diazine, which can then break up into molecular nitrogen, a hydrogen atom, and a phenethyl free radical. The latter would be the active species in irreversible inhibition.[25]

Tranylcypromine Sulfate, USP. Tranylcypromine sulfate, (±)-*trans*-2-phenylcyclopropylamine sulfate (Parnate), was synthesized to be an amphetamine analogue (visualize the α-methyl of amphetamine condensed onto the β-carbon atom).[26] It does have some amphetamine-like properties, which may be why it has more immediate CNS stimulant effects than agents that act by MAO inhibition alone. For MAO inhibition, there may be two components to the

TABLE 15–4   Monoamine Oxidase Inhibitors

Generic Name / Proprietary Name	Structure
Phenelzine sulfate, USP / Nardil	
Tranylcypromine sulfate, USP / Parnate	

action of this agent. One is thought to arise because tranylcypromine has structural features (the basic nitrogen and the quasi-π character of the α- and β-cyclopropane carbon atoms) that approximate the transition state in a route of metabolism of β-arylamines.[27, 28] As α- and β-hydrogen atoms are removed from the normal substrate of the enzyme, the quasi-π character develops over the α,β-carbon system. Duplication of the transition state permits extremely strong, but reversible, attachment to the enzyme. Additionally, tranylcypromine is a mechanism-based inactivator. It is metabolized by MAO, with one electron of the nitrogen pair lost to flavin. This, in turn, produces homolytic fission of a carbon–carbon bond of cyclopropane, with one electron from the fission pairing with the remaining lone nitrogen electron to generate an imine (protonated) and with the other residing on a methylene carbon. Thus, a free radical is formed that reacts to form a covalent bond with the enzyme or with reduced flavin to inactivate the enzyme.[29]

Monoamine Reuptake Inhibitors

Originally, the monoamine reuptake inhibitors were a group of closely related agents, the tricyclic antidepressants, but now they are quite diverse chemically. Almost all of the agents block neuronal reuptake of NE or 5-HT or both (i.e., are selective).

Reuptake inhibition by these agents is at the level of the respective monoamine transporter via competitive inhibition of binding of the monoamine to the substrate-binding compartment. Probably the same site on the protein is involved for inhibitor and monoamine, but this has not yet been proved. The mechanism of reuptake by monoamine transporters has been reviewed.[30]

The net effect of the drug is to increase the level of the monoamine in the synapse. Sustained high synaptic levels of 5-HT, NE, or both appear to be the basis for the antidepressant effect of these agents. There is a time lag of 2 or more weeks before antidepressant action develops. It is considered that (in the case of 5-HT) $5HT_{1A}$ receptors and (in the case of NE) α_2 receptors undergo desensitization and transmitter release is maintained. Of course activation of postsynaptic receptors and sustained transmission is the ultimate result of sustained synaptic levels of neurotransmitter.[31]

Tricyclic Antidepressants

The SARs for the TCAs are compiled in detail in the eighth edition of this text.[32] The interested reader is referred to this compilation. In summary, there is a large, bulky group encompassing two aromatic rings, preferably held in a skewed arrangement by a third central ring, and a three- or, sometimes, two-atom chain to an aliphatic amino group that is monomethyl- or dimethyl-substituted. The features can be visualized by consulting the structures of imipramine and desipramine as examples. The overall arrangement has features that approximate a fully extended *trans* conformation of the β-arylamines. To relate these features to the mechanism of action, reuptake block, visualize that the basic arrangement is the same as that found in the β-arylamines, plus an extra aryl bulky group that enhances affinity for

the substrate-binding compartment of the transporter. The overall concept of a β-arylamine-like system with added structural bulk, usually an aryl group, appears to be applicable to many newer compounds—selective serotonin reuptake inhibitors (SSRIs), selective norepinephrine reuptake inhibitors (SNERIs)—that do not have a tricyclic grouping.

The TCAs are structurally related to each other and, consequently, possess related biological properties that can be summarized as characteristic of the group. The dimethylamino compounds tend to be sedative, whereas the monomethyl relatives tend to be stimulatory. The dimethyl compounds tend toward higher 5-HT to NE reuptake block ratios: in the monomethyl compounds, the proportion of NE uptake block tends to be higher and in some cases is considered selective NE reuptake. The compounds have anticholinergic properties, usually higher in the dimethylamino compounds. When treatment is begun with a dimethyl compound, a significant accumulation of the monomethyl compound develops as N-demethylation proceeds.

The TCAs are extremely lipophilic and, accordingly, very highly tissue bound outside the CNS. Since they have anticholinergic and noradrenergic effects, both central and peripheral side effects are often unpleasant and sometimes dangerous. In overdose, the combination of effects, as well as a quinidine-like cardiac depressant effect, can be lethal. Overdose is complicated because the agents are so highly protein bound that dialysis is ineffective.

PRODUCTS

Imipramine Hydrochloride, USP. Imipramine hydrochloride, 5-[3-(dimethylamino)propyl]-10,11-dihydro-5*H*-dibenz[*b,f*]azepine monohydrochloride (Tofranil), is the lead compound of the TCAs. It is also a close relative of the antipsychotic phenothiazines (replace the 10–11 bridge with sulfur, and the compound is the antipsychotic agent promazine). It has weaker D_2 postsynaptic blocking activity than promazine and mainly affects amines (5-HT, NE, and DA) via the transporters. As is typical of dimethylamino compounds, anticholinergic and sedative (central H_1 block) effects tend to be marked. The compound per se has a tendency toward a high 5-HT-to-NE uptake block ratio and probably can be called a serotonin transport inhibitor (SERTI). Metabolic inactivation proceeds mainly by oxidative hydroxylation in the 2 position, followed by conjugation with glucuronic acid of the conjugate. Urinary excretion predominates (about 75%), but some biliary excretion (up to 25%) can occur, probably because of the large nonpolar grouping. Oxidative hydroxylation is not as rapid or complete as that of the more nucleophilic ring phenothiazine antipsychotics; consequently, appreciable N-demethylation occurs, with a buildup of norimipramine (or desimipramine).

The demethylated metabolite is less anticholinergic, less sedative, and more stimulatory and is a SNERI.[31] Consequently, a patient treated with imipramine has two compounds that contribute to activity. Overall, the effect is nonselective 5-HT versus NE reuptake. The activity of des- or norimipramine is terminated by 2-hydroxylation, followed by conjugation and excretion. A second N-demethylation can occur, which in turn is followed by 2-hydroxylation, conjugation, and excretion.

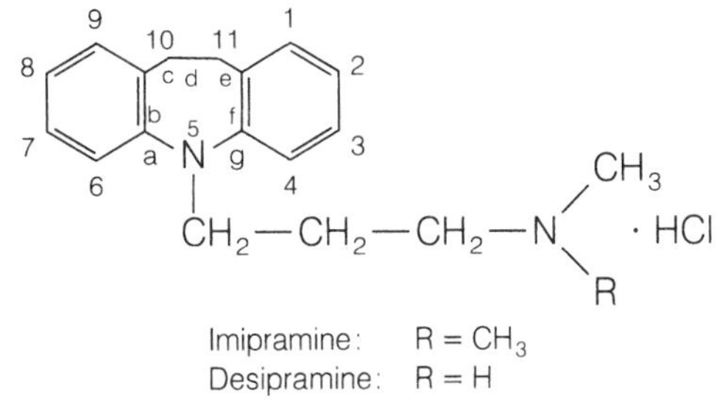

Imipramine: R = CH₃
Desipramine: R = H

Desipramine Hydrochloride, USP.

The structure and salient properties of desipramine hydrochloride, 10,11-dihydro-*N*-methyl-5*H*-dibenz[*b,f*]azepine-5-propanamine monohydrochloride, 5-(3-methylaminopropyl)-10,11-dihydro-5*H*-dibenz[*b,f*]azepine hydrochloride (Norpramin, Pertofrane), are discussed under the heading, Imipramine, above. Among tricyclics, desipramine would be considered when few anticholinergic effects or a low level of sedation are important. It is a SNERI.[31]

Clomipramine Hydrochloride.

Clomipramine (Anafranil) is up to 50 times as potent as imipramine in some bioassays. This does not imply clinical superiority, but it might be informative about tricyclic and, possibly, other reuptake inhibitors. The chloro replacing the H substituent could increase potency by increasing distribution to the CNS, but it is unlikely that this would give the potency magnitude seen. It might be conjectured that a H bond between the protonated amino group (as in vivo) and the unshared electrons of the chloro substituent might stabilize a β-arylamine-like shape and give more efficient competition for the transporter. The drug is an antidepressant. It is used in obsessive-compulsive disorder, an anxiety disorder that may have an element of depression.

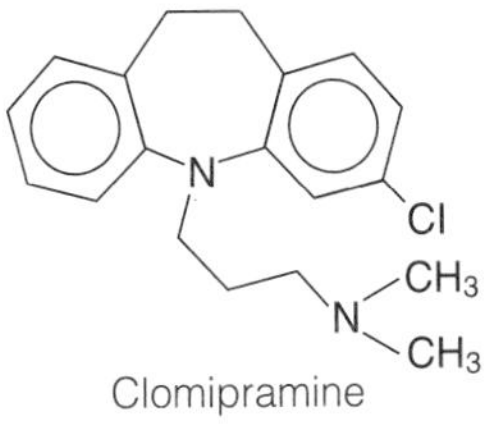

Clomipramine

Amitriptyline Hydrochloride, USP.

Amitriptyline, 3-(10,11-dihydro-5*H*-dibenzo[*a,d*]cyclohepten-5-ylidene)-*N*,*N*-dimethyl-1-propanamine hydrochloride, 5-(3-dimethylaminopropylidene)-10,11-dihydro-5*H*-dibenzo[*a,d*]cycloheptene hydrochloride (Elavil), is one of the most anticholinergic and sedative of the TCAs. Because it lacks the ring electron–enriching nitrogen atom of imipramine, metabolic inactivation mainly proceeds not at the analogous 2 position but at the benzylic 10 position (i.e., toluene-like metabolism predominates). Because of the 5-exocyclic double bond, *E*- and *Z*-hydroxy isomers are produced by oxidation metabolism. Conjugation produces excretable metabolites. As is typical of the dimethyl compounds, N-demethylation occurs, and nortriptyline is produced, which has a less anticholinergic, less sedative, and more stimulant action than amitripty-

line. Nortriptyline is a SNERI[31]; the composite action of drug and metabolite is nonselective.

Nortriptyline Hydrochloride, USP.

Pertinent biological and chemical properties for nortriptyline, 3-(10,11-dihydro-5*H*-dibenzo[*a,d*]cyclohepten-5-ylidene)*N*-methyl-1-propanamine hydrochloride, 5-(3-methyl-aminopropylidene)-10,11-hydro-5*H*-dibenzo[*a,d*]cycloheptene hydrochloride (Aventyl, Pamelor), are given above in the discussion of amitriptyline. Metabolic inactivation and elimination are like those of amitriptyline. Nortriptyline is a selective NE transporter (NET) inhibitor.[31]

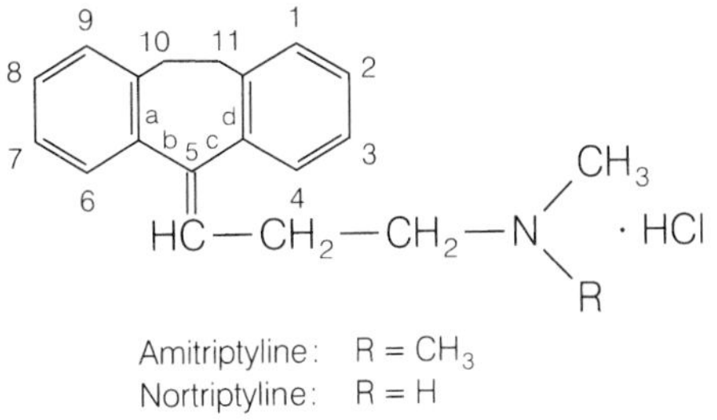

Amitriptyline: R = CH₃
Nortriptyline: R = H

Protriptyline Hydrochloride, USP.

Protriptyline hydrochloride, *N*-methyl-5*H*-dibenzo[*a,d*]cycloheptene-5-propylamine hydrochloride, 5-(3-methylaminopropyl)-5*H*-dibenzo[*a,d*]cycloheptene hydrochloride (Vivactil), like the other compounds under consideration, is an effective antidepressant. The basis for its chemical naming can be seen by consulting the naming and the structure of imipramine. Protriptyline is a structural isomer of nortriptyline. Inactivation can be expected to involve the relatively localized double bond. Because it is a monomethyl compound, its sedative potential is low.

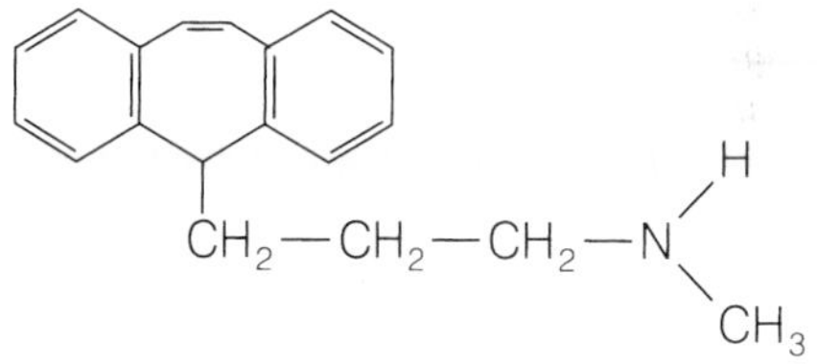

Protriptyline

Trimipramine Maleate.

For details of chemical nomenclature, consult the description of imipramine. Replacement of hydrogen with an α-methyl substituent produces a chiral carbon, and trimipramine (Surmontil) is used as the racemic mixture. Biological properties reportedly resemble those of imipramine.

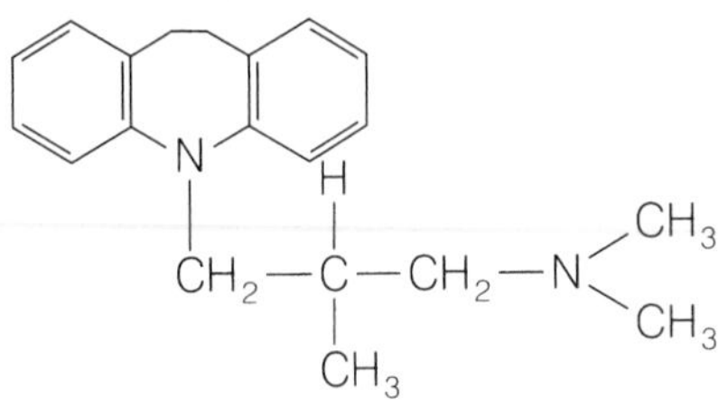

Trimipramine

Doxepin Hydrochloride, USP.

Doxepin, 3-dibenz-[*b,e*]-oxepin-11(6*H*)ylidine-*N*,*N*-dimethyl-1-propanamine hydrochloride, *N,N*-dimethyl-3-(dibenz[*b,e*]oxepin-11(6*H*)-ylidene)propylamine (Sinequan, Adapin), is an oxa congener of amitriptyline, as can be seen from its structure.

The oxygen is interestingly placed and should influence oxidative metabolism as well as postsynaptic and presynaptic binding affinities. The (*Z*) isomer is the more active, although the drug is marketed as the mixture of isomers. The drug overall is a NE and 5-HT reuptake blocker with significant anticholinergic and sedative properties. It can be anticipated that the nor- or des- metabolite will contribute to the overall activity pattern.

Doxepin Hydrochloride

Maprotiline Hydrochloride, USP.

Maprotiline hydrochloride, *N*-methyl-9,10-ethanoanthracene-9(10*H*)-propanamine hydrochloride (Ludiomil), is sometimes described as a tetracyclic rather than a tricyclic antidepressant. The description is chemically accurate, but the compound, nonetheless, conforms to the overall TCA pharmacophore. It is a dibenzobicyclooctadiene and can be viewed as a TCA with an ethylene-bridged central ring. The compound is not strongly anticholinergic and has stimulant properties. It can have effects on the cardiovascular system. It is a SNERI.[31]

Maprotiline Hydrochloride

Amoxapine.

Consideration of the structure of amoxapine, 2-chloro-11-(1-piperazinyl)dibenz-[*b,f*] [1,4]oxazepine (Asendin), reinforces the fact that many antidepressants are very closely related to antipsychotics. Indeed, some, including amoxapine, have significant effects at D₂ receptors. The *N*-methyl-substituted relative of amoxapine is the antipsychotic loxapine (Loxitane). The 8-hydroxy metabolite of amoxapine is reportedly active as an antidepressant and as a D₂ receptor blocker.

Amoxapine

Selective Serotonin Reuptake Inhibitors

Structurally, the SSRIs differ from the tricyclics, in that the tricyclic system has been taken apart in the center. (This abolishes the center ring, and one ring is moved slightly forward from the tricyclic "all-in-a-row" arrangement.) The net effect is that the *β*-arylamine-like grouping is present, as in the tricyclics, and the compounds can compete for the substrate-binding site of the serotonin transporter protein (SERT). As in the tricyclics, the extra aryl group can add extra affinity and give favorable competition with the substrate, serotonin.

Many of the dimethylamino tricyclics are, in fact, SSRIs. Since they are extensively N-demethylated in vivo to nor-compounds, which are usually SNERIs, however, the overall effect is not selective. Breaking up the tricyclic system breaks up an anticholinergic pharmacophoric group and gives compounds with diminished anticholinergic effects. Overall, this diminishes unpleasant CNS effects and increases cardiovascular safety. Instead, side effects related to serotonin predominate.

Fluoxetine.

In fluoxetine (Prozac), protonated in vivo, the protonated amino group can H-bond to the ether oxygen electrons, which can generate the *β*-arylamino-like group, with the other aryl serving as the characteristic "extra" aryl. The *S* isomer is much more selective for SERT than for NET. The major metabolite is the *N*-demethyl compound, which is as potent as the parent and more selective (SERT versus NET).

Therapy for 2 or more weeks is required for the antidepressant effect. Somatodendritic 5HT₁ₐ autoreceptor desensitization with chronic exposure to high levels of 5-HT is the accepted explanation for the delayed effect for this and other serotonin reuptake inhibitors.

To illustrate a difference between selectivity for a SERT and a NET, if the *para* substituent is moved to the *ortho* position (and is less hydrophobic, typically), a NET is obtained. This and other SERTs have anxiolytic activity. One of several possible mechanisms would be agonism of 5HT₁ₐ receptors, diminishing synaptic 5-HT. Presumably, synaptic levels of 5-HT might be high in an anxious state.

Fluoxetine

Paroxetine.

In the structure of paroxetine (Paxil), an amino group, protonated in vivo could H-bond with the —CH₂—O— unshared electrons. A *β*-arylamine-like structure with an extra aryl group results. The compound is a very highly selective SERT. As expected, it is an effective antidepressant and anxiolytic.

Paroxetine

Sertraline. Inspection of sertraline (Zoloft) (1*S*,4*S*) reveals the pharmacophore for SERT inhibition. The Cl substituents also predict tropism for a 5-HT system. The depicted stereochemistry is important for activity.

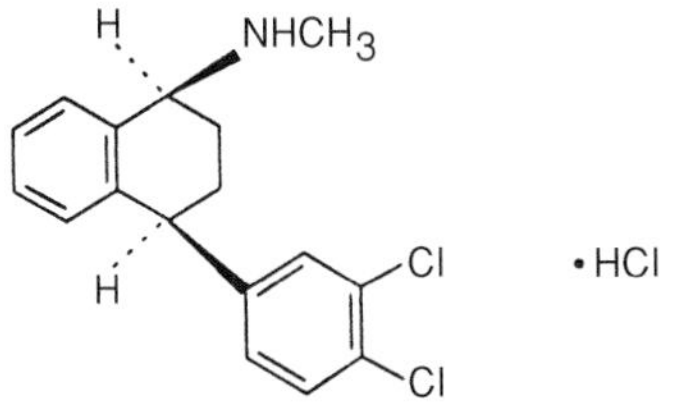

Sertraline

Fluvoxamine. The *E* isomer of fluvoxamine (Luvox) (shown) can fold after protonation to the *β*-arylamine-like grouping. Here the "extra" hydrophobic group is aliphatic.

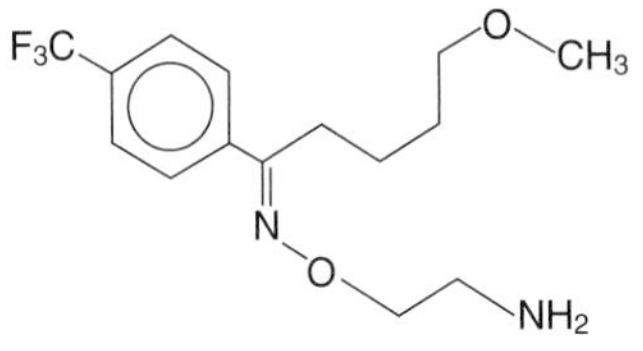

Fluvoxamine

Citalopram. Citalopram (Celexa) is a racemic mixture and is very SERT selective. The N-monodemethylated compound is slightly less potent but is as selective. The aryl substituents are important for activity. The ether function is important and probably interacts with the protonated amino group to give a suitable shape for SERT binding.

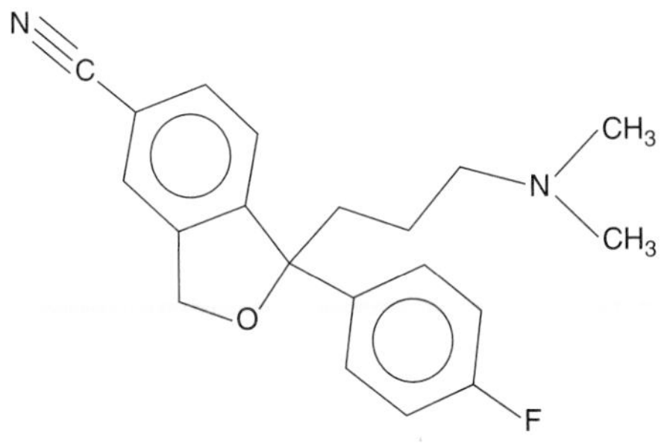

Citalopram

Selective Norepinephrine Reuptake Inhibitors

The discussion of fluoxetine opened the subject of SNERIs. That is, movement of a *para* substituent of fluoxetine (and relatives) to an *ortho* position produces a SNERI.

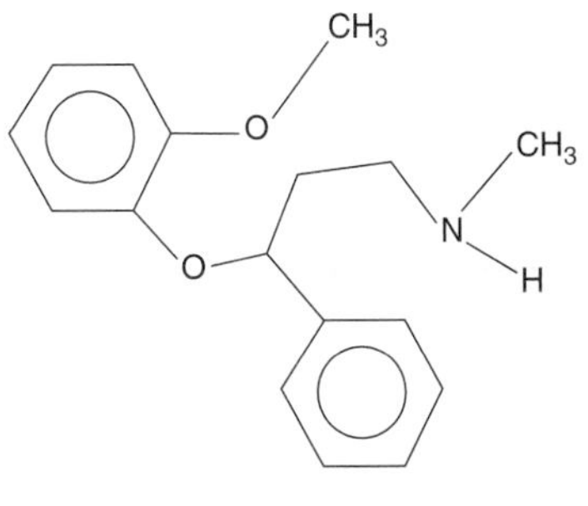

Nisoxetine

Nisoxetine is a SNERI and is an antidepressant. Most activity resides in the *β* isomer.

Reboxetine. Most of the activity of reboxetine resides in the *S,S* isomer (The marketed compound is *RR* and *SS*.) It is claimed to be superior to fluoxetine in severe depression. It is marketed in Europe. At least three tricyclic compounds, desipramine, nortriptyline, and the technically tetracyclic maprotiline are SNERIs. They, of course, have typical characteristic TCA side effects but lower anticholinergic and H$_1$-antihistaminic (sedative) effects than dimethyl compounds. SNERIs are clinically effective antidepressants.

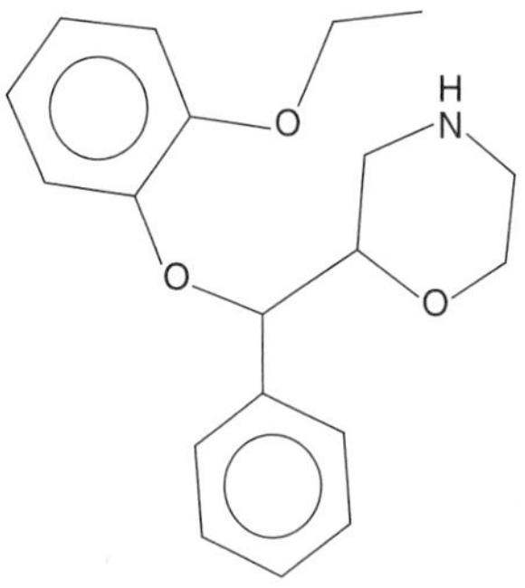

Reboxetine

It would be expected that in the case of SNERIs, α_2 presynaptic receptors would be desensitized, after which sustained NE transmission would be via one or more postsynaptic receptors; α_1, β_1, and β_2 receptors are possibilities.

Newer (Nontricyclic) Nonselective 5-HT and NE Reuptake Inhibitors

Presently, one such compound is clinically used in the United States.

Venlafaxine. The structure and activity of venlafaxine (Effexor) are in accord with the general SARs for the group. As expected, it is an effective antidepressant.

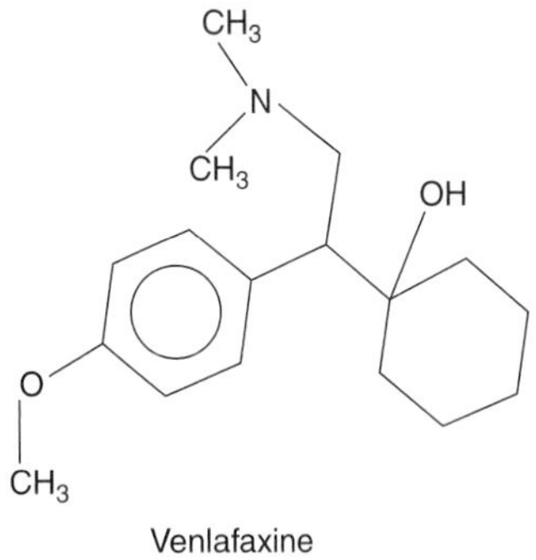

Venlafaxine

Selective Serotoninergic Reuptake Inhibitors and 5HT$_{2A}$ Antagonists

The SSRIs and 5HT$_{2A}$ antagonists are represented by trazodone (Desyrel) and nefazodone (Serzone).

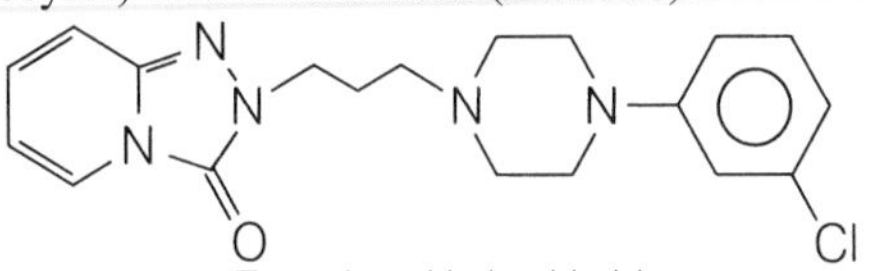

Trazodone Hydrochloride

The structures of these two compounds derive from those of the fluorobutyrophenone antipsychotics. They have *β*-arylamine-like structures that permit binding to the SERT

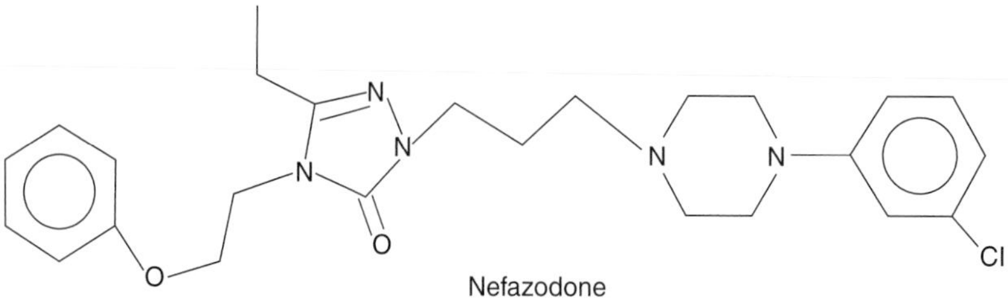

Nefazodone

and inhibit 5-HT reuptake. In these compounds, the additional hydrophobic substituent can be viewed as being attached to the nitrogen of the β-arylamine-like group. Additionally, they are 5HT$_{2A}$ antagonists. That antagonism may or may not afford antipsychotic effectiveness is discussed under antipsychotics. 5HT$_{2A}$ antagonists appear to have antidepressant and anxiolytic activities. They may act, at least in part, by enhancing 5HT$_{1A}$ activities.[33] Also, some of the effects may be mediated through 5HT$_{2C}$ agonism (perhaps generally so for 5-HT-acting antidepressants.) Some of the side effects of SSRIs are considered to be mediated through 5HT$_{2A}$ receptors, so a 5HT$_{2A}$ blocker would reduce them.[33] The two compounds yield the same compound on N-dealkylation. It is a serotonin reuptake inhibitor.

5HT$_{1A}$ Agonists and Partial Agonists

Buspirone. The initial compound in this series, buspirone (BuSpar), has anxiolytic and antidepressant activities and is a partial 5HT$_{1A}$ agonist. Its anxiolytic activity is reportedly due to its ability to diminish 5-HT release (via 5HT$_{1A}$ agonism). High short-term synaptic levels of 5-HT are characteristic of anxiety. Also, since it is a partial agonist, it can stimulate postsynaptic receptors when 5-HT levels are low in the synapse, as is the case in depression. A number of other spirones are in development as anxiolytics and antidepressants.[34]

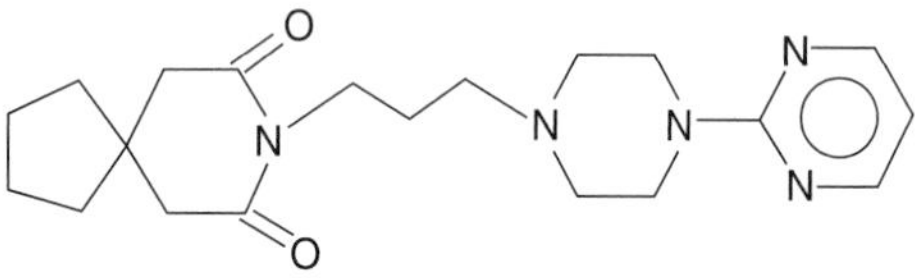

Buspirone

α_2 Antagonists

Mirtazapine. Mirtazapine (Remeron) was recently introduced for clinical use in the United States; its parent mianserin (pyridyl N replaced with C-H) was long known to be an antidepressant. It is reported to be faster acting and more potent than certain SSRIs. The mode of action gives increased NE release via α_2-NE receptor antagonism and increased 5-HT release via antagonism of NE α_2 heteroreceptors located on serotoninergic neurons.[33, 34]

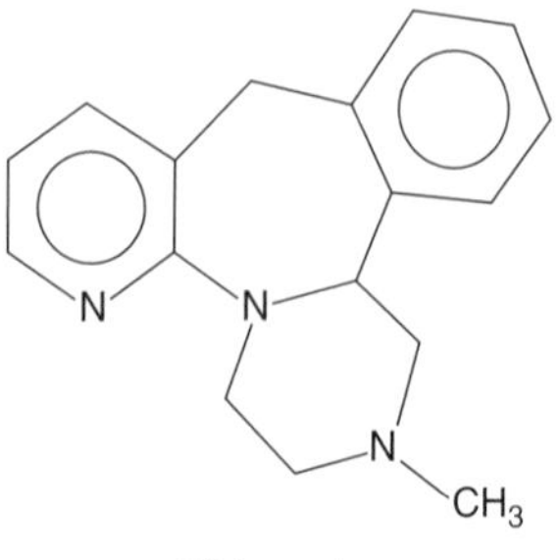

Mirtazapine

Miscellaneous Antidepressants

Bupropion. The mechanism of action of bupropion (Wellbutrin) is considered complex and reportedly involves a block of DA reuptake via the dopamine transporter (DAT), but the overall antidepressant action is noradrenergic. A metabolite that contributes to the overall action and its formation can be easily rationalized.

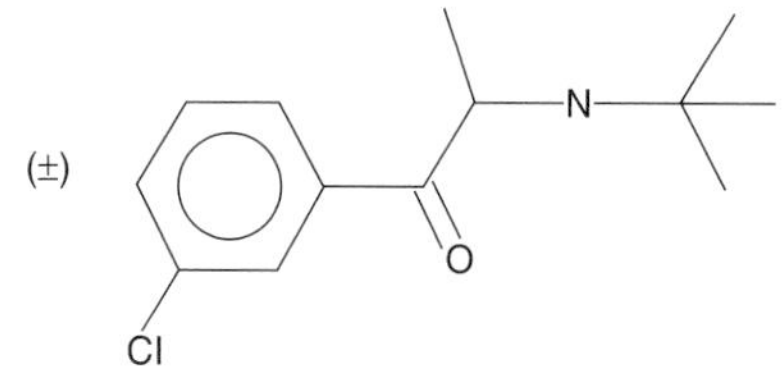

(±)

Bupropion

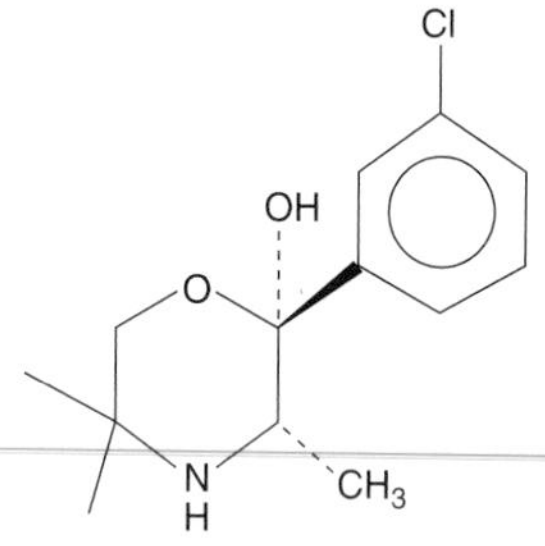

Metabolite

MISCELLANEOUS CNS-ACTING DRUGS

This section deals with a collection of drugs that do not fit easily under other topic headings in this chapter or the chapter on CNS depressants. All of the drugs are drugs of abuse and could be organized under that heading.

The β-arylamino hallucinogens arose because of interest in the naturally occurring hallucinogens psilocin and mescaline and in modifying the amphetamines, which were popular drugs at the time. Lysergic acid diethylamide was accidentally discovered during research on ergot alkaloids. It is of scientific interest because it serves as one model for clinical psychosis. Phencyclidine is scientifically interesting because it gives information about the ionotropic *N*-methyl-D-aspartate glutamic acid receptor, and its CNS effects serve as a model for schizophrenia.

Cocaine as a CNS stimulant is a pernicious drug of abuse. Research on why it is so strongly addictive and on drug measures that might mitigate its effects has been intense in the past two decades.

Δ^1-Tetrahydrocannabinol and its relatives were studied for many years to determine the SARs. The field was given stimulus with the discovery of the endogenous cannabinoid receptors. Presently, the endogenous cannabinoid system is under investigation.

1β-Arylamino Hallucinogens

A property of the 1β-arylamino hallucinogens is alteration of the perception of stimuli. Reality is distorted, and the user may undergo depersonalization. Literally, the effects are those of a psychosis. Additionally, the drugs can produce anxiety, fear, panic, frank hallucinations, and additional symptoms that may be found in a psychosis. Accordingly, they are classed as hallucinogens and psychotomimetics.

This group can be subgrouped into those that possess an indolethylamine moiety, those that possess a phenylethylamine moiety, and those with both. In the first group, there is a structural resemblance to the central neurotransmitter 5-HT, and in the second, there is a structural resemblance to NE and DA. This resemblance is suggestive, and there may be some selectivity of effects on the respective transmitter systems. With structures of the complexity found in many of these agents, however, a given structure may possibly affect not just the closest structurally related neurotransmitter systems but other systems as well. Thus, a phenethylamine system could affect not only NE and DA systems but also 5-HT systems, and an indolethylamine system could affect not only 5-HT but also NE and DA systems.

INDOLETHYLAMINES

Dimethyltryptamine.   Dimethyltryptamine is a very weak hallucinogen, active only by inhalation or injection, with a short duration of action. It possesses pronounced sympathomimetic (NE) side effects.

Psilocybin and Psilocin.   Psilocybin is the phosphoric acid ester of psilocin and appears to be converted to psilocin as the active species in vivo. It occurs in a mushroom, *Psilocybe mexicana*. Both drugs are active orally, with a short duration of action.

Synthetic α-methyl-substituted relatives have a much longer duration of action and enhanced oral potency.[35] This suggests that psilocin is metabolized by MAOs.

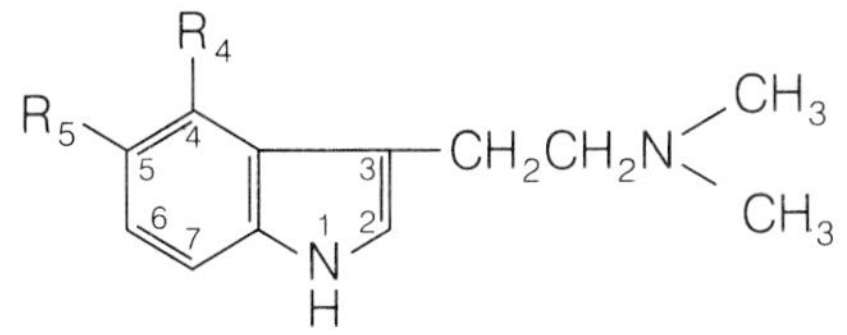

Dimethyltryptamine:	$R_4 = R_5 = H$
Psilocybin:	$R_4 = OPO(OH)_2$; $R_5 = H$
Psilocin:	$R_4 = OH$; $R_5 = H$

2-PHENYLETHYLAMINES

Mescaline.   Mescaline, 3,4,5-trimethoxyphenethylamine, is a much-studied hallucinogen with many complex effects on the CNS. It occurs in the peyote cactus. The oral dose required for its hallucinogenic effects is very high, as much as 500 mg of the sulfate salt. The low oral potency probably results from facile metabolism by MAO. α-Methylation increases CNS activity. Synthetic α-methyl-substituted relatives are more potent.[35, 36] The drugs DOM, MDA, and DMDA (ecstasy) are extremely potent, dangerous drugs of abuse.

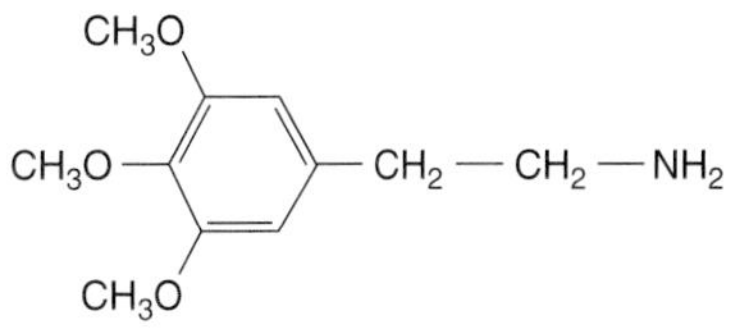

Mescaline

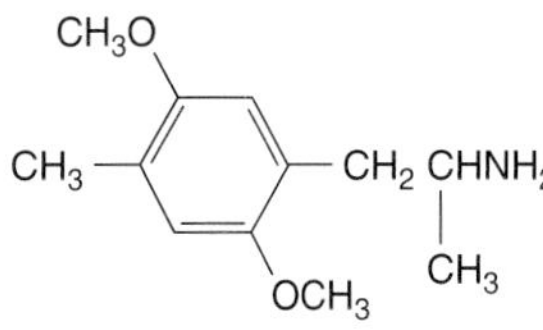

1-(2,5-Dimethoxy-4-methyphenyl)-2-aminopropane
(DOM, STP)

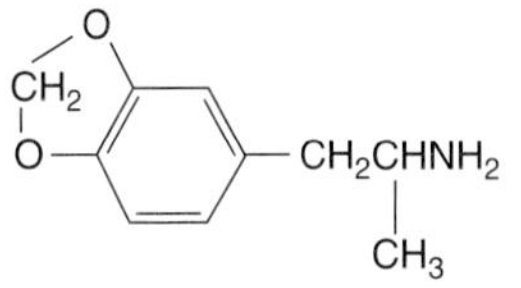

3,4-Methylenedioxyamphetamine
(MDA)

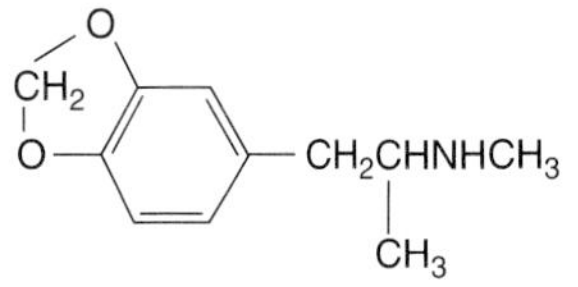

DMDA (ecstasy)

The presence of methoxyl or dioxymethylene (methylenedioxy) substituents on a 2-phenethylamine system is a characteristic of many psychotomimetic compounds and strongly suggests DA involvement.

AGENT POSSESSING BOTH AN INDOLETHYLAMINE AND A PHENYLETHYLAMINE MOIETY

(+)-Lysergic Acid Diethylamide.   Both an indolethylamine group and a phenylethylamine group can be seen in the structure of the extraordinarily potent hallucinogen lysergic acid diethylamide (LSD). The stereochemistry is exceedingly important. Chirality, as shown, must be maintained or activity is lost; likewise, the location of the double bond, as shown, is required.[37] Experimentally, LSD has marked effects on serotoninergic and dopaminergic neurons. The bases for all of its complex CNS actions are not completely understood, however. Recently, its actions have been suggested as being more typical of schizophrenic psychotic reactions than the model based on amphetamine. For more on this, see the discussion of atypical antipsychotics (Chapter 14).

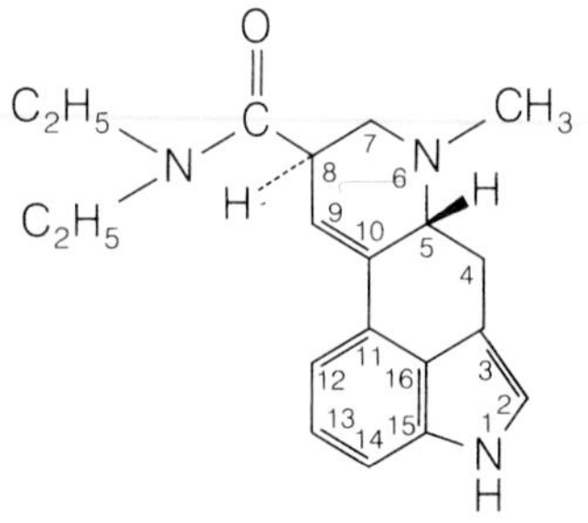

Lysergic Acid Diethylamide

Dissociative Agents

Phencyclidine.   Phencyclidine (PCP) was introduced as a dissociative anesthetic for animals. Its close structural relative ketamine is still so used and may be used in humans (Chapter 14). In humans, PCP produces a sense of intoxication, hallucinogenic experiences not unlike those produced by the anticholinergic hallucinogens, and often amnesia.

The drug affects many systems, including those of NE, DA, and 5-HT. It has been proposed that PCP (and certain other psychotomimetics) produces a unique pattern of activation of ventral tegumental area dopaminergic neurons.[38] It blocks glutaminergic *N*-methyl-D-aspartate receptors.[39] This action is the basis for many of its CNS effects. PCP itself appears to be the active agent. The psychotic state produced by this drug is also cited as a better model than amphetamine psychosis for the psychotic state of schizophrenia.[40]

Phencyclidine Hydrochloride

Euphoriant–Stimulant

Cocaine.   Cocaine as a euphoriant–stimulant, psychotomimetic, and drug of abuse could as well be discussed with amphetamine and methamphetamine, with which it shares many biological properties. At low doses, it produces feelings of well-being, decreased fatigue, and increased alertness. Cocaine tends to produce compulsive drug-seeking behavior, and a full-blown toxic psychosis may emerge. Many of these effects appear to be related to the effects of increased availability of DA for interaction with postsynaptic receptors (D_2 and D_3 receptors are pertinent). Cocaine is a potent DA reuptake blocker, acting by competitive inhibition of the DAT. A phenethylamine moiety with added steric bulk may suffice for this action. An interaction between a hydrogen atom on the nitrogen of the protonated form of cocaine and an oxygen of the benzoyl ester group, or alternatively, an interaction between the unshared electron pair of the free-base nitrogen and the carbonyl of the benzoyl ester group, could approximate this moiety.

Cocaine

Considerable research on drugs affecting the DAT has been published in recent years. A review of pharmacotherapeutic agents for cocaine abuse is available.[41]

Depressant–Intoxicant

Δ^1-Tetrahydrocannabinol or Δ^9-THC.   There are two conventions for numbering THC: that arising from terpenoid chemistry produces Δ^1-THC, and that based on the dibenzopyran system results in a Δ^9-THC designation. The terpenoid convention is used here.

$(-)$-Δ^1-*trans*-Tetrahydrocannabinol

THC is a depressant with apparent stimulant sensations arising from depression of higher centers. Many effects, reputedly subjectively construed as pleasant, are evident at low doses. The interested reader may consult a pharmacology text for a detailed account. At higher doses, psychotomimetic actions, including dysphoria, hallucinations, and paranoia, can be marked. Structural features associated with activity among cannabis-derived compounds have been reviewed.[42] Notably, the phenolic OH is required for activity. Certain SARs (especially separation of potency between enantiomers) for cannabinoids suggested action at receptors.[43] Two receptors for THC have been discovered. The relevant receptor for CNS actions is CB_1.[44] CB_2 occurs in immune tissues. The first natural ligand found for the receptor is the amide derivative of arachidonic acid, anandamide.[45] Other natural cannabinoids are arachidonic acid 2-glycerol ester and 2-arachidonyl glycerol ether.[46] The endogenous cannabinoid system appears to function as a retrograde messenger system at both stimulatory synapses and depressant synapses. The synaptic transmitter causes postsynaptic syntheses of endocannabinoids that are then transported to CB_1 receptors located presynaptically where they fine-tune both excitatory and inhibitory neurons.[47–51] Because CB_1 receptors appear to be present in all brain areas and affect both excitatory and inhibitory systems, the prospect of developing selective cannabinoid drugs acting at receptors is considered not good. Designing drugs to affect the transporter is considered the most promising research route.

Endocannabinoids, as regulated by leptin, are also involved in maintaining food intake and in other behaviors.[52, 53]

REFERENCES

1. Jarboe, C. H., Porter, L. A., and Buckler, R. T.: J. Med. Chem. 11: 729, 1968.
2. Pellmar, T. C., and Wilson, W. A.: Science 197:912, 1977.
3. Fredholm, B. B., et al.: Pharmacol. Rev. 51:83, 1999.
4. Daly, J. W.: J. Med. Chem. 25:197, 1982.
5. Williams, M., and Huff, J. R.: Annu. Rep. Med. Chem. 18:1, 1983.
6. Snyder, S. H., et al.: Proc. Natl. Acad. Sci. U. S. A. 78:3260, 1981.
7. Tucker, A. L., and Linden, J.: Cardiovasc. Res. 27:62, 1993.
8. Erion, M. D.: Annu. Rep. Med. Chem. 28:295, 1993.
9. DeNinno, M. P.: Annu. Rep. Med. Chem. 33:111, 1998.
10. Arnaud, M. J.: Products of metabolism of caffeine. In Dews, P. B. (ed.). Caffeine, Perspectives From Recent Research. New York, Springer-Verlag, 1984, p. 3.

11. Halford, J. C. G., and Blundell, J. E.: Prog. Drug Res. 54:25, 2000.
12. Fuller, R. W.: Ann. N. Y. Acad. Sci. 305:147, 1978.
13. Harvey, J. A.: Ann. N. Y. Acad. Sci. 305:289, 1978.
14. Groppetti, A., and Costa, E.: Life Sci. 8:635, 1969.
15. Clineschmidt, B. V., et al.: Ann. N. Y. Acad. Sci. 305:222, 1987.
16. Dvornik, D., and Schilling, G.: J. Med. Chem. 8:466, 1965.
17. Weisz, I., and Dudas, A.: Monatsh. Chem. 91:840, 1960.
18. Shaffi'ee, A., and Hite, G.: J. Med. Chem. 12:266, 1969.
19. Patrick, K. S., et al.: J. Pharmacol. Exp. Ther. 241:152, 1987.
20. Perel, J. M., and Dayton, P. G.: Methylphenidate. In Usdin, E., and Forrest, I. S. (eds.). Psychotherapeutic Drugs, part II. New York, Marcel Dekker, 1977, p. 1287.
21. Srinvas, N. R., et al.: J. Pharmacol. Exp. Ther. 241:300, 1987.
22. Whitelock, O. V. (ed.): Ann. N. Y. Acad. Sci., 80:000–000, 1959.
23. Richards, L. E., and Burger, A.: Prog. Drug Res. 30:205, 1986.
24. Strupczewski, J. D., Ellis, D. B., and Allen, R. C.: Annu. Rep. Med. Chem. 26:297, 1991.
25. Green, A. L.: Biochem. Pharmacol. 13:249, 1964.
26. Burger, A.: J. Med. Pharm. Chem. 4:571, 1961.
27. Belleau, B., and Moran, J. F.: J. Am. Chem. Soc. 82:5752, 1960.
28. Belleau, B., and Moran, J. F.: J. Med. Pharm. Chem. 5:215, 1962.
29. Silverman, R. B.: J. Biol. Chem. 258:14766, 1983.
30. Rudnick, G., and Clark, J.: Biochim. Biophys. Acta 1144:249, 1993.
31. Olivier, B.: Prog. Drug Res. 54:59, 2000.
32. Daniels, T. C., and Jorgensen, E. C.: Central nervous system stimulants. In Doerge, R. F. (ed.). Wilson and Gisvold's Textbook of Organic Medicinal and Pharmaceutical Chemistry, 8th ed. Philadelphia, J. B. Lippincott, 1982, p. 383.
33. Evrad, D. A., and Harrison, B. L.: Annu. Rep. Med. Chem. 34:1, 1999.
34. Olivier, B., et al.: Prog. Drug Res. 52:103, 1999.
35. Murphree, H. B., et al.: Clin. Pharmacol. Ther. 2:722, 1961.
36. Shulgin, A. T.: Nature 201:120, 1964.
37. Stoll, A., and Hofmann, A.: Helv. Chim. Acta 38:421, 1955.
38. Bowers, M. B., Bannon, M. J., and Hoffman, F. J., Jr.: Psychopharmacology 93:133, 1987.
39. Foster, A. C., and Fogg, G. E.: Nature 329:395, 1987.
40. Rowley, M., Bristow, L. J., and Hutson, P. H.: J. Med. Chem 44:477, 2001.
41. Carroll, F. I., Howell, L. L., and Kuhov, M. J.: J. Med. Chem. 42:2721, 2000.
42. Edery, H., et al.: Ann. N. Y. Acad. Sci. 191:40, 1971.
43. Hollister, L. E., Gillespie, H. K., and Srebnik, M.: Psychopharmacology 92:505, 1987.
44. Matsuda, L. A., et al.: Nature 346:561, 1990.
45. Davanne, W. A., et al.: Science 258:1946, 1992.
46. Mechoulam, R., et al.: Proc. Natl. Acad. Sci. U. S. A. 98:3602, 2001.
47. Egertova, M., et al.: Proc. R. Soc. London B 265:208, 1998.
48. Wilson, R. I. and Nicoll, R. A.: Nature 410:588, 2001.
49. Ohn-Shosaku, T., Maejqma, T., and Kano, N.: Neuron 29:729, 2001.
50. Kreitzer, A. C., and Regehr, W. G.: Neuron 29:717, 2001.
51. Christie, M. J., and Vaughn, C. W.: Nature 410:527, 2001.
52. DiMarzo, V., et al.: Nature 410:822, 2001.
53. Mechoulam, R., and Fride, E.: Nature 410:763, 2001.

SELECTED READING

Carrol, F. I., Howell, F. I., and Kuhar, M. J.: Pharmacotherapies for treatment of cocaine abuse: Preclinical aspects. J. Med. Chem. 42:2721, 2000.

Fredholm, B. B., Battig K., Holmen, J., et al.: Actions of caffeine in the brain with special reference to factors that contribute to its widespread use. Pharmacol. Rev. 51:83, 1999.

Halford, J. C. G., and Blundell, J. E.: Pharmacology of appetite suppression. Prog. Drug. Res. 54:25, 2000.

Olivier, B., Soudijn, W., and van Wijngaarden, I.: Serotonin, dopamine and norepinephrine transporters in the central nervous system and their inhibitors. Prog. Drug. Res. 54:59, 2000.

Xiang, J.-N., and Lee, J. C.: Pharmacology of cannabinoid receptor agonists and antagonists. Annu. Rep. Med. Chem. 54:199, 2000.

CHAPTER 16

Adrenergic Agents

RODNEY L. JOHNSON

Adrenergic drugs are chemical agents that exert their principal pharmacological and therapeutic effects by either enhancing or reducing the activity of the various components of the sympathetic division of the autonomic nervous system. In general, substances that produce effects similar to stimulation of sympathetic nervous activity are known as *sympathomimetics* or *adrenergic stimulants*. Those that decrease sympathetic activity are referred to as *sympatholytics, antiadrenergics,* or *adrenergic-blocking agents*. Because of the important role that the sympathetic nervous system plays in the normal functioning of the body, adrenergic drugs find wide use in the treatment of a number of diseases. In addition to their effects on sympathetic nerve activity, a number of adrenergic agents produce important effects on the central nervous system (CNS). In this chapter, those agents that affect adrenergic neurotransmission and those that act directly on the various types of adrenergic receptors are discussed.

ADRENERGIC NEUROTRANSMITTERS

Structure and Physicochemical Properties

Norepinephrine (NE) is the neurotransmitter of the postganglionic sympathetic neurons. As a result of sympathetic nerve stimulation, it is released from sympathetic nerve endings into the synaptic cleft, where it interacts with specific presynaptic and postsynaptic adrenergic receptors. Another endogenous adrenergic receptor agonist is epinephrine. This compound is not released from peripheral sympathetic nerve endings, as is NE. Rather, it is synthesized and stored in the adrenal medulla, from which it is released into the circulation. Thus, epinephrine is often referred to as a neurohormone. Epinephrine is also biosynthesized in certain neurons of the CNS, where both it and NE serve as neurotransmitters.

Norepinephrine: R = H

Epinephrine: R = CH$_3$

Epinephrine and NE belong to the chemical class of substances known as the *catecholamines*. This name was given to these compounds because they contain an amino group attached to an aromatic ring that contains two hydroxyl groups situated *ortho* to each other, the same arrangement of hydroxyl groups as found in catechol. Aromatic compounds that contain such an arrangement of hydroxyl substituents are highly susceptible to oxidation. Catecholamines, such as epinephrine and NE, undergo oxidation in the presence of oxygen (air) or other oxidizing agents to produce *ortho*-quinone-like compounds, which undergo further reactions to give mixtures of colored products. Hence, solutions of catecholamine drugs often are stabilized by the addition of an antioxidant (reducing agent) such as ascorbic acid or sodium bisulfite.

Catechol   *ortho*-Quinone

Epinephrine and NE each possess a chiral carbon atom; thus, each can exist as an enantiomeric pair of isomers. The enantiomer with the *(R)* configuration is biosynthesized by the body and possesses the biological activity.

Catecholamines are polar substances that contain both acidic (the aromatic hydroxyls) and basic (the aliphatic amine) functional groups. For example, the pK$_a$ values for the epinephrine cation are 8.7 and 9.9 and are attributed to the phenolic hydroxyl group and the protonated amino group, respectively. Ganellin[1] calculated the relative populations of the various ionized and nonionized species of NE and epinephrine at pH 7.4 and found that the cation form (Fig. 16-1A) is present to an extent slightly greater than 95% for both catecholamines. The zwitterionic form (Fig. 16-1B), in which the aliphatic amine is protonated and one of the phenolic hydroxyl groups is ionized, is present to about 3%. Thus, at physiological pH, less than 2% of either epinephrine or NE exists in the nonionized form. This largely accounts for the high water solubility of these compounds as well as other catecholamines, such as isoproterenol and dopamine.

Biosynthesis

The biosynthesis of the catecholamines dopamine, NE, and epinephrine involves a sequence of enzymatic reactions,[2] as illustrated in Figure 16-2. Catecholamine biosynthesis takes place in adrenergic and dopaminergic neurons in the CNS, in sympathetic neurons of the autonomic nervous system, and in the adrenal medulla. The amino acid L-tyrosine serves as the precursor for the catecholamines. It is transported actively into the axoplasm, where it is acted on by tyrosine-3-monooxygenase (tyrosine hydroxylase) to form L-dihydroxyphenylalanine (L-dopa). Tyrosine hydroxylase is an Fe^{2+}-containing enzyme that requires molecular oxygen and

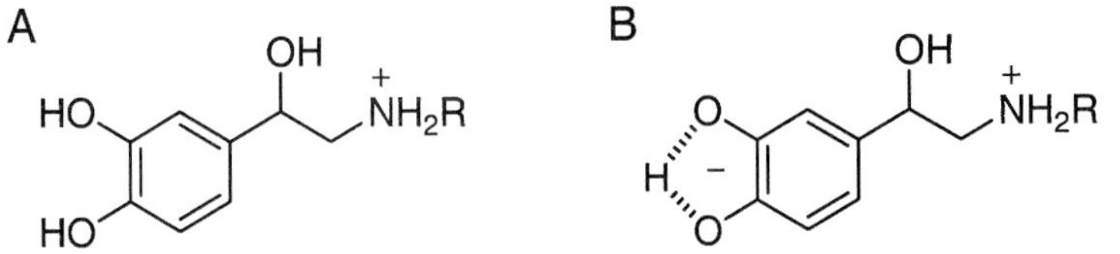

Figure 16–1 ■ Cationic **(A)** and zwitterionic **(B)** forms of norepinephrine (R = H) and epinephrine (R = CH$_3$).

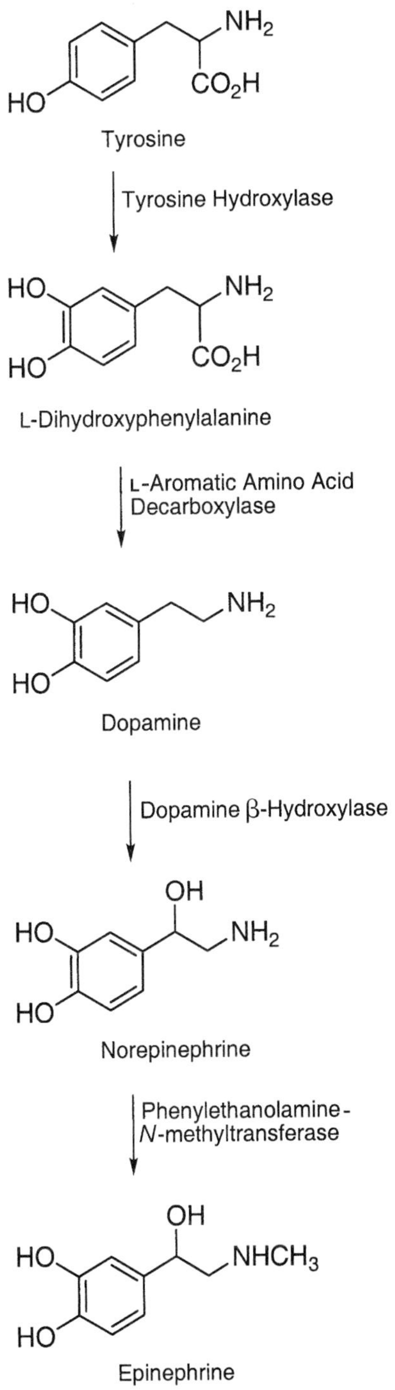

uses tetrahydrobiopterin as a cofactor. The enzyme plays a key role in the regulation of catecholamine biosynthesis, as it is the rate-limiting step. For example, adrenergic nerve stimulation leads to activation of a protein kinase that phosphorylates tyrosine hydroxylase, thereby increasing its activity.[3] In addition, through end-product inhibition, NE markedly reduces tyrosine hydroxylase activity. The basis of this feedback inhibition is believed to be a competition between the catecholamine product and the pterin cofactor.

The second enzymatic step in catecholamine biosynthesis is the decarboxylation of L-dopa to give dopamine. The enzyme that carries out this transformation is L-aromatic amino acid decarboxylase (dopa decarboxylase). It is a cytoplasmic enzyme that uses pyridoxal phosphate as a cofactor. In addition to being found in catecholaminergic neurons, L-aromatic amino acid decarboxylase is found in high concentrations in many other tissues, including the liver and kidneys. It exhibits broad substrate specificity, in that aromatic amino acids, such as L-tyrosine, L-phenylalanine, L-histidine, and L-tryptophan, in addition to L-dopa and L-5-hydroxytryptophan, serve as substrates.

The dopamine formed in the cytoplasm of the neuron is actively transported into storage vesicles, where it is hydroxylated stereospecifically by the Cu^{2+}-containing enzyme dopamine β-monooxygenase (dopamine β-hydroxylase) to give NE. Dopamine β-hydroxylase requires molecular oxygen and uses ascorbic acid as a cofactor. It exhibits rather wide substrate specificity. The NE formed is stored in the vesicles until depolarization of the neuron initiates the process of vesicle fusion with the plasma membrane and extrusion of NE into the synaptic cleft. Adenosine triphosphate (ATP) and the protein chromogranin A are released along with NE.

In the adrenal medulla, NE is converted to epinephrine. This reaction, which involves the transfer of a methyl group from *S*-adenosyl methionine to NE, is catalyzed by phenylethanolamine-*N*-methyltransferase (PNMT). It occurs in the cytoplasm, and the epinephrine formed is transported into the storage granules of the chromaffin cells. Although PNMT is highly localized in the adrenal medulla, it is also present in small amounts in heart and brain tissues.

Uptake and Metabolism

The action of NE at adrenergic receptors is terminated by a combination of processes, including uptake into the neuron and into extraneuronal tissues, diffusion away from the synapse, and metabolism. Usually, the primary mechanism for termination of the action of NE is reuptake of the catecholamine into the nerve terminal. This process is termed *uptake-1* and involves a Na$^+$/Cl$^-$-dependent transmembrane transporter that has a high affinity for NE.[4] This uptake system also transports certain amines other than NE into the

Figure 16–2 ■ Biosynthesis of the catecholamines dopamine, norepinephrine, and epinephrine.

nerve terminal, and it can be blocked by such drugs as cocaine and some of the tricyclic antidepressants. Some of the NE that reenters the sympathetic neuron is transported into storage granules, where it is held in a stable complex with ATP and protein until sympathetic nerve activity or some other stimulus causes it to be released into the synaptic cleft. The transport of NE from the cytoplasm into the storage granules is carried out by an H^+-dependent transmembrane vesicular transporter.[5]

In addition to the neuronal uptake of NE discussed above, there exists an extraneuronal uptake process, uptake-2. This uptake process is present in a wide variety of cells, including glial, hepatic, and myocardial cells. It has relatively low affinity for NE. Although its physiological significance is unknown, it may play a role in the disposition of circulating catecholamines, since catecholamines that are taken up into extraneuronal tissues are metabolized rapidly.

The two principal enzymes involved in catecholamine metabolism are monoamine oxidase (MAO) and catechol-*O*-methyltransferase (COMT).[6, 7] Both of these enzymes are distributed throughout the body, with high concentrations found in the liver and kidneys. MAO is associated primarily with the outer membrane of the mitochondria, while COMT is found primarily in the cytoplasm. The wide tissue distribution of MAO and COMT indicates that both act on catecholamines that enter the circulation and the extraneuronal tissues after being released from nerves or the adrenal gland or after being administered exogenously. In addition, the fact that COMT is not present in sympathetic neurons whereas the neuronal mitochondria do contain MAO indicates that MAO also has a role in the metabolism of intraneuronal catecholamines.

Neither COMT nor MAO exhibits high substrate specificity. MAO oxidatively deaminates a variety of compounds that contain an amino group attached to a terminal carbon. There are two types of MAOs, and these exhibit different substrate selectivity.[8] For example, MAO-A shows substrate preference for NE and serotonin, while MAO-B shows substrate selectivity for β-phenylethylamine and benzylamine. Similarly, COMT catalyzes the methylation of a variety of catechol-containing molecules. The lack of substrate specificity of COMT and MAO is manifested in the metabolic disposition of NE and epinephrine, shown in Figure 16-3. Not only do both MAO and COMT use NE and epinephrine

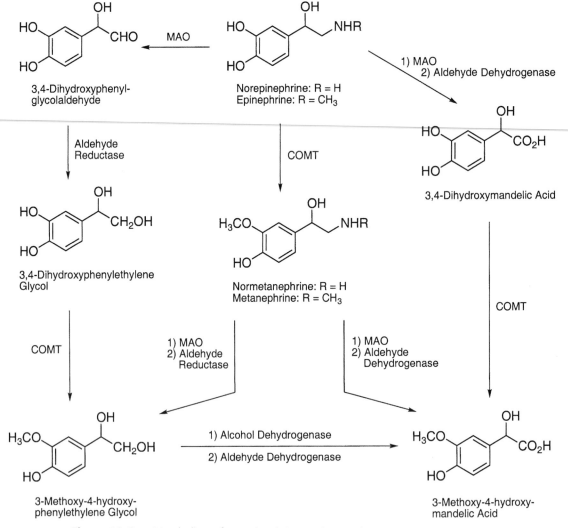

Figure 16–3 ■ Metabolism of norepinephrine and epinephrine by MAO and COMT.

as substrates, but each also acts on the metabolites produced by the other.

The results of extensive research on catecholamine metabolism indicate that in the adrenergic neurons of human brain and peripheral tissues, NE is deaminated oxidatively by MAO to give 3,4-dihydroxyphenylglycolaldehyde, which then is reduced by aldehyde reductase to 3,4-dihydroxyphenylethylene glycol. It is primarily this glycol metabolite that is released into the circulation, where it undergoes methylation by the COMT that it encounters in nonneuronal tissues. The product of methylation, 3-methoxy-4-hydroxyphenylethylene glycol, is oxidized by alcohol dehydrogenase and aldehyde dehydrogenase to give 3-methoxy-4-hydroxymandelic acid. This metabolite commonly is referred to as vanillylmandelic acid (VMA), and although it can be the end product of several pathways of NE metabolism, 3-methoxy-4-hydroxyphenylethylene glycol is its principal precursor. In the oxidative deamination of NE and epinephrine at extraneuronal sites such as the liver, the aldehyde that is formed is oxidized usually by aldehyde dehydrogenase to give 3,4-dihydroxymandelic acid.

Methylation by COMT occurs almost exclusively on the *meta*-hydroxyl group of the catechol, regardless of whether the catechol is NE, epinephrine, or one of the metabolic products. For example, the action of COMT on NE and epinephrine gives normetanephrine and metanephrine, respectively. A converging pattern of NE metabolism of NE and epinephrine in which 3-methoxy-4-hydroxymandelic acid and 3-methoxy-4-hydroxyphenylethylene glycol are common end products thus occurs, regardless of whether the first metabolic step is oxidation by MAO or methylation by COMT.

Under normal circumstances, 3-methoxy-4-hydroxymandelic acid is the principal urinary metabolite of NE, though substantial amounts of 3-methoxy-4-hydroxyphenylethylene glycol are excreted along with varying quantities of other metabolites, both in the free form and as sulfate or glucuronide conjugates. Endogenous epinephrine is excreted primarily as metanephrine and 3-methoxy-4-hydroxymandelic acid.

ADRENERGIC RECEPTORS

α-Adrenergic Receptors

Ahlquist[9] was the first to propose the existence of two general types of adrenergic receptors (adrenoceptors) in mammalian tissues. He designated these adrenergic receptors α and β. His hypothesis was based on the differing relative potencies of a series of adrenergic receptor agonists on various smooth muscle preparations. In the early 1970s, the discovery that certain adrenergic agonists and antagonists exhibited various degrees of selectivity for presynaptic and postsynaptic α-adrenergic receptors led to the proposal that postsynaptic α receptors be designated α_1 and that presynaptic α receptors be referred to as α_2.[10] Later, a functional classification of the α receptors was proposed wherein α_1 receptors were designated as those that were excitatory, while α_2 receptors purportedly mediated inhibitory responses.[11] Further developments revealed, however, that both α_1 and α_2 receptors could be either presynaptic or post-

synaptic and either excitatory or inhibitory in their responses. Thus, it became clear that neither an anatomical nor a functional classification system was as generally useful in classifying adrenergic receptors as a pharmacological classification based on the relative potency of a series of receptor agonists and antagonists.[12] Pharmacological and molecular biological methods have shown that it is possible to subdivide the α_1 and α_2 receptors into additional subtypes. Although the subtyping of adrenergic receptors continues to evolve, at present, the α_1 and α_2 receptors each have been divided into at least three subtypes, which have been designated α_{1A}, α_{1B}, α_{1D} and α_{2A}, α_{2B}, α_{2C}, respectively.[13-15]

The molecular basis by which activation of α-adrenergic receptors produces the appropriate tissue responses has been studied extensively. Both receptor subtypes belong to a superfamily of membrane receptors whose general structure consists of seven transmembrane α-helical segments and whose signal-transduction mechanisms involve coupling to guanine nucleotide-regulatory proteins (G proteins). They differ from each other, however, in the second-messenger system that is affected.[16, 17] The α_1-adrenergic receptor is coupled to the enzyme phospholipase C via a G protein, G_q. When stimulated by activation of the α_1-adrenergic receptor, phospholipase C hydrolyzes phosphatidylinositol-4,5-bisphosphate to give the second messengers inositol-1,4,5-triphosphate $[Ins(1,4,5)P_3]$ and 1,2-diacylglycerol (DAG). $Ins(1,4,5)P_3$ stimulates the release of Ca^{2+} from the sarcoplasmic reticulum, while DAG activates protein kinase C, an enzyme that phosphorylates proteins. α_1-Receptor activation also can increase the influx of extracellular Ca^{2+} via voltage-dependent as well as non–voltage-dependent Ca^{2+} channels. Activation of α_2-adrenergic receptors leads to a reduction in the catalytic activity of adenylyl cyclase, which in turn results in a lowering of intracellular levels of cyclic-3,5-adenosine monophosphate (cAMP). The α_2-adrenergic receptor–mediated inhibition of adenylyl cyclase is regulated by the G protein G_i.

α-Adrenergic receptors of the CNS and in peripheral tissues affect a number of important physiological functions.[16] In particular, α receptors are involved in control of the cardiovascular system. For example, constriction of vascular smooth muscle is mediated by both postjunctional α_1- and α_2-adrenergic receptors, though the predominant receptor mediating this effect is α_1.[18] In the heart, activation of α_1 receptors results in a selective inotropic response with little or no change in heart rate.[19] This is in contrast to the β_1 receptor, which is the predominant postjunctional receptor in the heart, mediating both inotropic and chronotropic effects. In the brain, activation of postjunctional α_2 receptors reduces sympathetic outflow from the CNS, which in turn causes a lowering of blood pressure.[20] The prototypical α_2 receptor is the presynaptic α receptor found on the terminus of the sympathetic neuron.[10, 11, 21] Interaction of this receptor with agonists such as NE and epinephrine results in inhibition of NE release from the neuron. The α_2 receptors not only play a role in the regulation of NE release but also regulate the release of other neurotransmitters, such as acetylcholine and serotonin. Both α_1- and α_2-adrenergic receptors also play an important role in the regulation of a number of metabolic processes, such as insulin secretion and glycogenolysis.[22]

β-Adrenergic Receptors

In 1967, almost 20 years after Ahlquist's landmark paper proposing the existence of α- and β-adrenergic receptors, Lands et al.[23] suggested that β receptors also could be subdivided into β_1 and β_2 types. Seventeen years later, Arch et al.[24] identified a third subtype of β receptor in brown adipose tissue. They initially referred to this as an atypical β receptor, but it later became designated the β_3 subtype.[13] These β-adrenergic receptor subtypes differ in terms of the rank order of potency of the adrenergic receptor agonists NE, epinephrine, and isoproterenol. The β_1 receptors exhibit the agonist potency order isoproterenol > epinephrine = NE, while β_2 receptors exhibit the agonist potency order isoproterenol > epinephrine >> NE. For the β_3 receptor, the agonist potency order is isoproterenol = NE > epinephrine.

The β receptors are located mainly in the heart, where they mediate the positive inotropic and chronotropic effects of the catecholamines. They are also found on the juxtaglomerular cells of the kidney, where they are involved in increasing renin secretion. The β_2 receptors are located on smooth muscle throughout the body, where they are involved in relaxation of the smooth muscle, producing such effects as bronchodilation and vasodilation. They are also found in the liver, where they promote glycogenolysis. The β_3 receptor is located on brown adipose tissue and is involved in the stimulation of lipolysis.

Like the α_1-adrenergic receptors, the β-adrenergic receptors belong to the superfamily of membrane receptors whose general structure consists of seven transmembrane α-helical segments and whose signal-transduction mechanisms involve coupling to G proteins. All three β-receptors are coupled to adenylyl cyclase, which catalyzes the conversion of ATP to cAMP. This coupling is via the guanine nucleotide protein G_s.[25, 26] In the absence of agonist, guanosine diphosphate (GDP) is bound reversibly to the G_s protein. Interaction of the agonist with the receptor is believed to bring about a conformational change in the protein receptor, which causes a reduction in the affinity of the G_s protein for GDP and a concomitant increase in affinity for guanosine triphosphate (GTP). The α_s subunit of the G_s protein, with GTP bound to it, dissociates from the receptor–G protein ternary complex, binds to adenylyl cyclase, and activates the enzyme. The bound GTP then undergoes hydrolysis to GDP, and the receptor–G_s protein complex returns to the basal state.

The intracellular function of the second-messenger cAMP appears to be activation of protein kinases, which phosphorylate specific proteins, thereby altering their function. Thus, the phosphorylated proteins mediate the actions of cAMP, which functions as the mediator of the action of the drug or neurotransmitter that originally interacted with the β-receptor.[27] The action of cAMP is terminated by a class of enzymes known as phosphodiesterases, which catalyze the hydrolysis of cAMP to AMP.

Cloning of the gene and complementary DNA (cDNA) for the mammalian β-adrenergic receptor has made it possible to explore through single point mutations and the construction of chimeric receptors the structure–function relationships of the receptor.[28] Through such studies, it has been proposed that the adrenergic agonist-binding site is within the transmembrane-spanning regions, while the cytoplasmic regions of the receptor interact with the G_s protein. Specifically, aspartic acid residue 113 in transmembrane region III acts as the counterion to the cationic amino group of the adrenergic agonist, while two serine residues, at positions 204 and 207 in transmembrane region V, form hydrogen bonds with the catechol hydroxyls of the adrenergic agonists. The β-hydroxyl group of adrenergic agonists is thought to form a hydrogen bond with the side chain of asparagine 293 in transmembrane region VI, while the phenylalanine residue at position 290 in the same transmembrane region is believed to interact with the catechol ring. Information such as this will no doubt aid in the future design and synthesis of new and improved adrenergic receptor agonists and antagonists.

Molecular biological techniques have shown the existence of adrenergic receptor polymorphism for both the α- and β-adrenergic receptors. It is postulated that such polymorphisms may be an important factor behind individual differences in responses to drugs acting at these receptors. Also, there may be an association between the polymorphisms of adrenergic receptor genes and disease states.[29] This will certainly be an active area of research in the future, and the results could have a great impact on the development and therapeutic use of not only the current adrenergic agents but also those that are yet to be developed.

DRUGS AFFECTING ADRENERGIC NEUROTRANSMISSION

Drugs Affecting Catecholamine Biosynthesis

Metyrosine. Many agents that affect catecholamine biosynthesis are known, but only a few are used as therapeutic agents. Metyrosine (α-methyl-*p*-tyrosine, Demser) is one example of a catecholamine-biosynthesis inhibitor in clinical use.[30] Metyrosine differs structurally from tyrosine only in the presence of an α-methyl group. It is a competitive inhibitor of tyrosine hydroxylase, the first and rate-limiting step in catecholamine biosynthesis. As such, metyrosine is a much more effective inhibitor of epinephrine and NE production than agents that inhibit any of the other enzymes involved in catecholamine biosynthesis. Although metyrosine is used as a racemic mixture, it is the (−) isomer that possesses the inhibitory activity. Metyrosine, which is given orally in dosages ranging from 1 to 4 g/day, is used principally for the preoperative management of pheochromocytoma. This condition involves chromaffin cell tumors that produce large amounts of NE and epinephrine. Although these tumors, which occur in the adrenal medulla, are often benign, patients frequently suffer hypertensive episodes. Metyrosine reduces the frequency and severity of these episodes by significantly lowering catecholamine production (35 to 80%). The drug is excreted mainly unchanged in the urine. Because of its limited solubility in water, crystalluria is a potential serious side effect. Sedation is the most common side effect of metyrosine.

Metyrosine

Drugs Affecting Catecholamine Storage and Release

Reserpine. Reserpine is the prototypical drug affecting the vesicle storage of NE in sympathetic neurons and neurons of the CNS and of epinephrine in the adrenal medulla. Its actions are not limited to NE and epinephrine, however, as it also affects the storage of serotonin and dopamine in their respective neurons in the brain. Reserpine is an indole alkaloid obtained from the root of *Rauwolfia serpentina,* a climbing shrub found in India. Other alkaloid constituents of this plant that possess pharmacological activity similar to that of reserpine are **deserpidine** and **rescinnamine**. Reserpine binds extremely tightly with the ATP-driven monoamine transporter that transports NE and other biogenic amines from the cytoplasm into the storage vesicles.[31] This binding leads to a blockade of the transporter. Thus in sympathetic neurons, NE, which normally is transported into the storage vesicles, is instead metabolized by mitochondrial MAO in the cytoplasm. In addition, there is a gradual loss of vesicle-stored NE as it is used up by release resulting from sympathetic nerve activity. It is thought that the storage vesicles eventually become dysfunctional. The end result is a depletion of NE in the sympathetic neuron. Analogous effects are seen in the adrenal medulla with epinephrine and in serotonergic neurons.

Reserpine: R^1 = OCH$_3$, R^2 =

Deserpidine: R^1 = H, R^2 =

Rescinnamine: R^1 = OCH$_3$, R^2 = —CH=CH—

When reserpine is given orally, it maximum effect is seen after a couple of weeks. A sustained effect up to several weeks is seen after the last dose has been given. Reserpine is extensively metabolized through hydrolysis of the ester function at position 18. This yields methyl reserpate and 3,4,5-trimethoxybenzoic acid. As is typical of many indole alkaloids, reserpine is susceptible to decomposition by light and oxidation. Both the pure alkaloid and the powdered whole root of *R. serpentina* are used in the treatment of hypertension. Preparations in which reserpine is combined with a diuretic also are available, as diuretics increase the efficacy of reserpine.

Guanethidine and Guanadrel. Neuronal blocking agents are drugs that produce their pharmacological effects primarily by preventing the release of NE from sympathetic nerve terminals. Drugs of this type enter the adrenergic neuron by way of the uptake-1 process and accumulate within the neuronal storage vesicles. There, they stabilize the neuronal storage vesicle membranes, making them less responsive to nerve impulses. The ability of the vesicles to fuse with the neuronal membrane is diminished, resulting in inhibition of NE release into the synaptic cleft. Some of these agents on long-term administration also can produce a depletion of NE stores in sympathetic neurons.

Structurally, the neuronal blocking drugs typically possess a guanidino moiety [CNHC(=NH)NH$_2$], which is attached to either an alicyclic or an aromatic lipophilic group. These structural features are seen in guanethidine (Ismelin) and guanadrel (Hylorel), which are used clinically in the treatment of hypertension. The presence of the very basic guanidino group (pK$_a$ > 12) in these drugs means that at physiological pH they are essentially completely protonated. Thus, these agents do not get into the CNS.

Guanethidine

Guanadrel

Although guanethidine and guanadrel have virtually the same mechanism of action on sympathetic neurons, they differ in their pharmacokinetic properties. For example, while guanethidine is absorbed incompletely after oral administration (3 to 50%), guanadrel is well absorbed, with a bioavailability of 85%.[32] These two agents also differ in terms of half-life: Guanethidine has a half-life of about 5 days, whereas guanadrel has a half-life of 12 hours. Both agents are partially metabolized (~50%) by the liver, and both are used to treat moderate-to-severe hypertension, either alone or in combination with another antihypertensive agent.

Bretylium Tosylate. Another neuronal blocking agent is the aromatic quaternary ammonium compound bretylium tosylate (Bretylol). This agent is used as an antiarrhythmic drug. Its antiarrhythmic actions are not believed to be due to its neuronal blocking effects, however. This agent is discussed in more detail in Chapter 19.

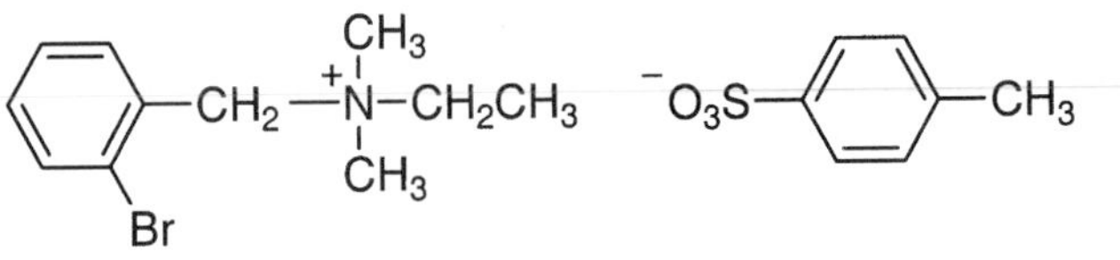

Bretylium Tosylate

SYMPATHOMIMETIC AGENTS

Sympathomimetic agents produce effects resembling those produced by stimulation of the sympathetic nervous system. They may be classified as agents that produce effects by a direct, indirect, or mixed mechanism of action. Direct-acting agents elicit a sympathomimetic response by interacting directly with adrenergic receptors. Indirect-acting agents produce effects primarily by causing the release of NE from adrenergic nerve terminals; the NE that is released by the indirect-acting agent activates the receptors to produce the response. Compounds with a mixed mechanism of action interact directly with adrenergic receptors and cause the release of NE. As described below, the mechanism by which an agent produces its sympathomimetic effect is related intimately to its chemical structure.

Direct-Acting Sympathomimetics

STRUCTURE–ACTIVITY RELATIONSHIPS

Structure–activity relationships for α- and β-adrenergic receptor agonists have been reviewed.[33–35] The parent structure for many of the sympathomimetic drugs is β-phenylethylamine. The manner in which β-phenylethylamine is substituted on the *meta* and *para* positions of the aromatic ring and on the amino, α, and β positions of the ethylamine side chain influences not only the mechanism of sympathomimetic action but also the receptor selectivity of the drug. For the direct-acting sympathomimetic amines, maximal activity is seen in β-phenylethylamine derivatives containing hydroxyl groups in the *meta* and *para* positions of the aromatic ring (a catechol) and a β-hydroxyl group of the correct stereochemical configuration on the ethylamine portion of the molecule. Such structural features are seen in the prototypical direct-acting compounds NE, epinephrine, and isoproterenol.

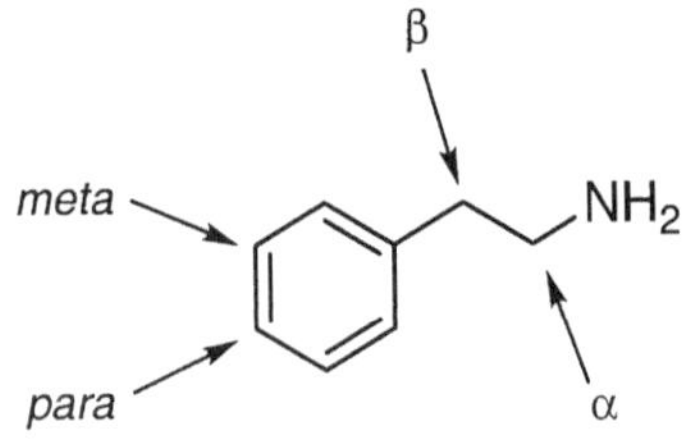

β-Phenylethylamine

A critical factor in the interaction of adrenergic agonists with their receptors is stereoselectivity. Direct-acting sympathomimetics that exhibit chirality by virtue of the presence of a β-hydroxyl group (phenylethanolamines) invariably exhibit high stereoselectivity in producing their agonistic effects; that is, one enantiomeric form of the drug has greater

affinity for the receptor than the other form has. This is true for both α- and β-receptor agonists. For epinephrine, NE, and related compounds, the more potent enantiomer has the *(R)* configuration. This enantiomer is typically several 100-fold more potent than the enantiomer with the *(S)* configuration. It appears that for all direct-acting, β-phenylethylamine-derived agonists that are structurally similar to NE, the more potent enantiomer is capable of assuming a conformation that results in the arrangement in space of the catechol group, the amino group, and the β-hydroxyl group in a fashion resembling that of $(-)$-(R)-NE. This explanation of stereoselectivity is based on the presumed interaction of these three critical pharmacophoric groups with three complementary binding areas on the receptor and is known as the Easson-Stedman hypothesis.[17, 36] This three-point interaction is supported by recent site-directed mutagenesis studies[28] on the adrenergic receptor and is illustrated in Figure 16-4.

The presence of the amino group in phenylethylamines is important for direct agonist activity. The amino group should be separated from the aromatic ring by two carbon atoms for optimal activity. Both primary and secondary amines are found among the potent direct-acting agonists, but tertiary or quaternary amines tend to be poor direct agonists. The nature of the amino substituent dramatically affects the receptor selectivity of the compound. In general, as the bulk of the nitrogen substituent increases, α-receptor agonist activity decreases and β-receptor activity increases. Thus NE, which is an effective β_1-receptor agonist, is also a potent α agonist, while epinephrine is a potent agonist at α, β_1, and β_2 receptors. Isoproterenol, however, is a potent β_1- and β_2-receptor agonist but has little affinity for α receptors. The nature of the substituent can also affect β_1- and β_2-receptor selectivity. In several instances, it has been shown that an *N-tert*-butyl

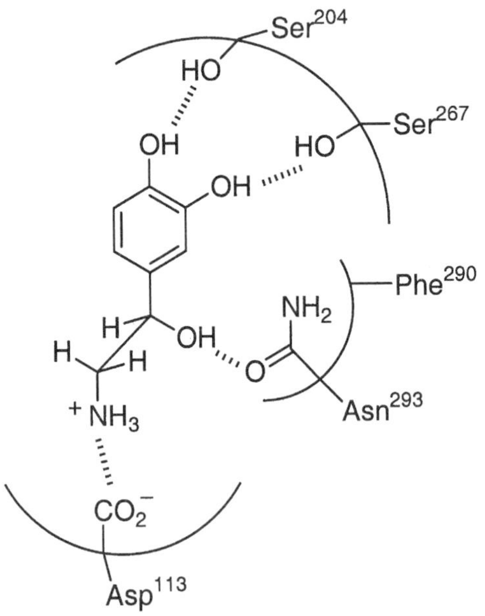

Figure 16–4 ■ Illustration of the Easson-Stedman hypothesis representing the interaction of three critical pharmacophoric groups of norepinephrine with the complementary binding areas on the adrenergic receptor as suggested by site-directed mutagenesis studies.

group enhances β_2 selectivity. For example, *N-tert*-butylnor-epinephrine (Colterol) is 9 to 10 times as potent an agonist at tracheal β_2 receptors than at cardiac β_1 receptors. Large substituents on the amino group also protect the amino group from undergoing oxidative deamination by MAO.

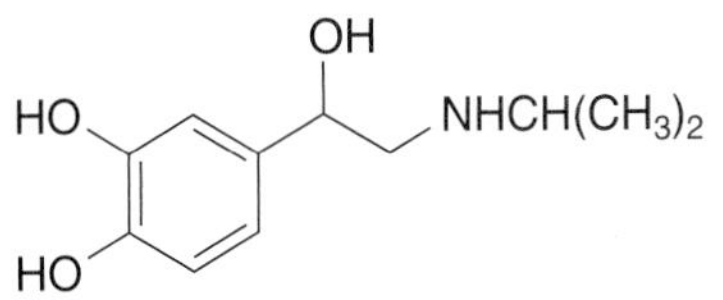

Isoproterenol

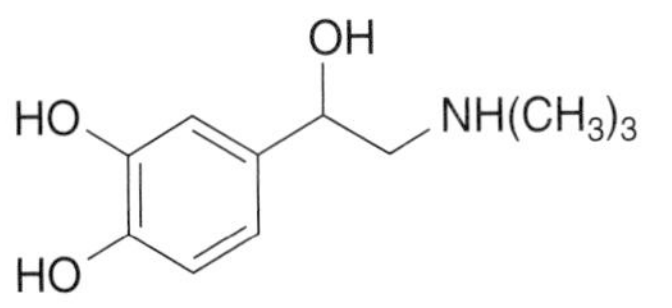

N-tert-Butylnorepinephrine (Colterol)

Methyl or ethyl substitution on the α-carbon of the eth-ylamine side chain reduces direct receptor agonist activity at both α and β receptors. Importantly, however, an α-alkyl group increases the duration of action of the phenylethylam-ine agonist by making the compound resistant to metabolic deamination by MAO. Such compounds often exhibit en-hanced oral effectiveness and greater CNS activity than their counterparts that do not contain an α-alkyl group. α-Substi-tution also significantly affects receptor selectivity. In the case of β receptors, for example, α-methyl or ethyl substitu-tion results in compounds with selectivity toward the β_2 receptor, while in the case of α receptors, α-methyl substitu-tion gives compounds with selectivity toward the α_2 recep-tor. Another effect of α-substitution is the introduction of a chiral center, which has pronounced effects on the stereo-chemical requirements for activity. For example, with α-methylnorepinephrine, it is the *erythro* (1*R*,2*S*) isomer that possesses significant activity at α receptors.

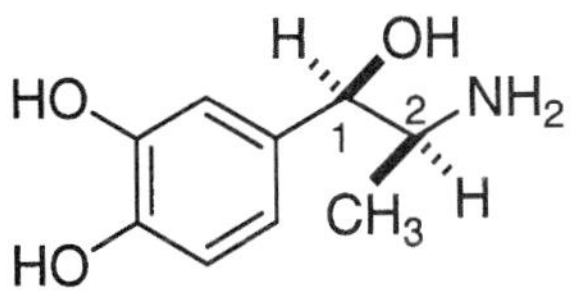

(1*R*,2*S*)-α-Methylnorepinephrine

Although the catechol moiety is an important structural feature in terms of yielding compounds with maximal ago-nist activity at adrenergic receptors, it can be replaced with other substituted phenyl moieties to provide selective adren-ergic agonists. In particular, this approach has been used in the design of selective β_2-receptor agonists. For example, replacement of the catechol function of isoproterenol with the resorcinol structure gives the drug metaproterenol, which is a selective β_2-receptor agonist. Furthermore, since the resorcinol ring is not a substrate for COMT, β agonists that contain this ring structure tend to have better absorption characteristics and a longer duration of action than their cate-chol-containing counterparts. In another approach, replace-ment of the *meta*-hydroxyl of the catechol structure with a hydroxymethyl group gives agents, such as albuterol, which

show selectivity to the β_2 receptor. As in the case of the resorcinol modification, this type of substitution gives agents that are not metabolized by COMT and thus show improved oral bioavailability.

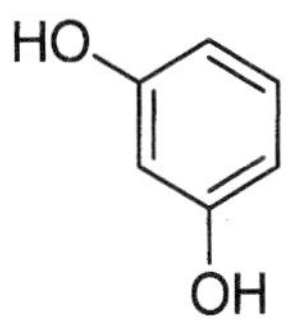

Resorcinal

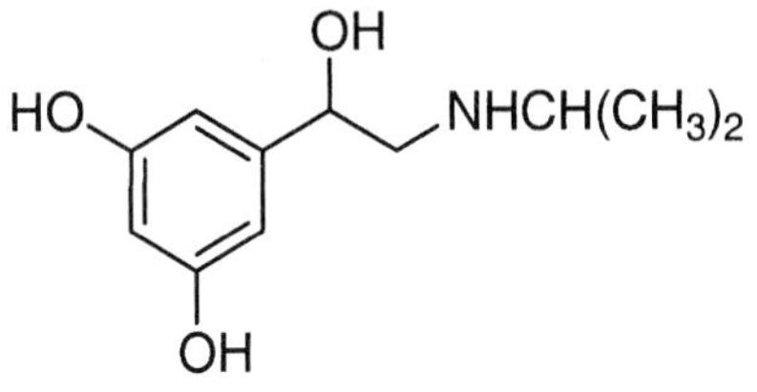

Metaproterenol

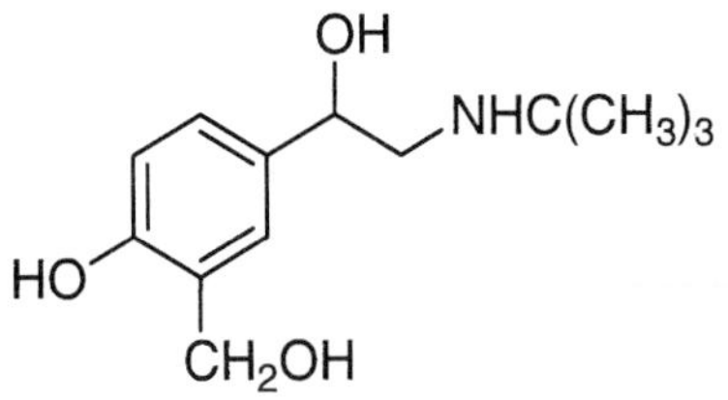

Albuterol

Modification of the catechol ring can also bring about selectivity at α receptors as it appears that the catechol moiety is more important for agonist activity at α_2 receptors than at α_1 receptors. For example, removal of the *p*-hydroxyl group from epinephrine gives phenylephrine, which, in con-trast to epinephrine, is selective for the α_1-adrenergic re-ceptor.

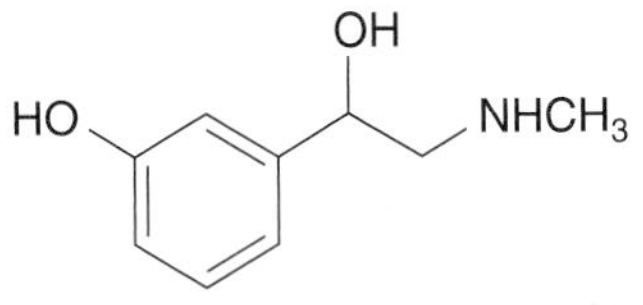

Phenylephrine

In addition to the β-phenylethylamine class of adrenergic receptor agonists, there is a second chemical class of com-pounds, the imidazolines, that give rise to α-adrenergic re-ceptor agonists. These imidazolines can be nonselective, or they can be selective for either the α_1- or α_2-adrenergic re-ceptors. Structurally, imidazolines for the most part have the heterocyclic imidazoline nucleus linked to a substituted aromatic moiety via some type of bridging unit (Fig. 16-5).[34] Although modification of the imidazoline ring gener-ally results in compounds with significantly reduced agonist activity, there are examples of so-called open-ring imidazo-lines that are highly active. The optimum bridging unit (X) is usually a single amino or methylene group. The nature of the aromatic moiety, as well as how it is substituted, is quite

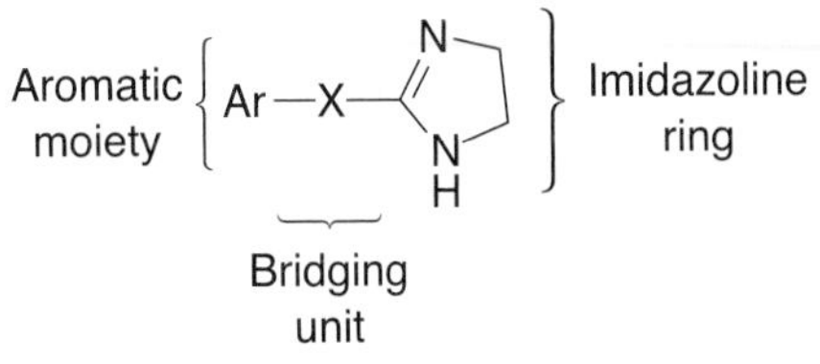

Figure 16-5 ■ General structural features of the imidazoline α-adrenergic receptor agonists.

flexible. However, agonist activity is enhanced when the aromatic ring is substituted with halogen substituents like Cl or small alkyl groups like methyl, particularly when they are placed in the two *ortho* positions. Since the structure–activity relationships of the imidazolines are quite different from those of the β-phenylethylamines, it has been postulated that the imidazolines interact with α-adrenergic receptors differently from the way the β-phenylethylamines do, particularly with regard to the aromatic moiety.[37]

ENDOGENOUS CATECHOLAMINES

The three naturally occurring catecholamines dopamine, NE, and epinephrine are used as therapeutic agents.

Dopamine. Dopamine is used in the treatment of shock. It is ineffective orally, in large part because it is a substrate for both MAO and COMT. Thus, it is used intravenously. In contrast with the catecholamines NE and epinephrine, dopamine increases blood flow to the kidney in doses that have no chronotropic effect on the heart or that cause no increase in blood pressure. The increased blood flow to the kidneys enhances glomerular filtration rate, Na^+ excretion, and, in turn, urinary output. The dilation of renal blood vessels produced by dopamine is the result of its agonist action on the D_1-dopamine receptor.

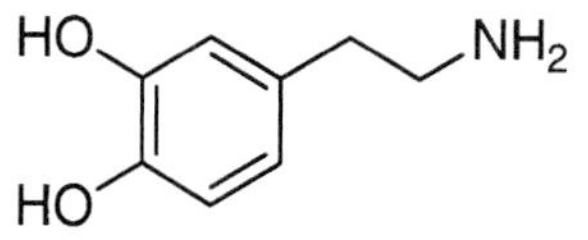

Dopamine

In doses slightly higher than those required to increase renal blood flow, dopamine stimulates the β_1 receptors of the heart to increase cardiac output. Some of the effects of dopamine on the heart are also due to NE release. Infusion at a rate greater than 10 μg/kg per minute results in stimulation of α_1 receptors, leading to vasoconstriction and an increase in arterial blood pressure.

Norepinephrine (NE). NE (Levophed) is used to maintain blood pressure in acute hypotensive states resulting from surgical or nonsurgical trauma, central vasomotor depression, and hemorrhage. Like the other endogenous catecholamines, it is a substrate for both MAO and COMT and thus is not effective by the oral route of administration. It is given by intravenous injection.

Epinephrine. Epinephrine (Adrenalin) finds use in a number of situations because of its potent stimulatory effects on both α- and β-adrenergic receptors. Like the other catecholamines, epinephrine is light sensitive and easily oxidized on exposure to air because of the catechol ring system. The development of a pink to brown color indicates oxidative breakdown. To minimize oxidation, solutions of the drug are stabilized by the addition of reducing agents such as sodium bisulfite. As the free amine, it is used in aqueous solution for inhalation. Like other amines, it forms salts with acids; for example, those now used include the hydrochloride and the bitartrate. Epinephrine is destroyed readily in alkaline solutions and by metals (e.g., Cu, Fe, Zn), weak oxidizing agents, and oxygen of the air. It is not effective by the oral route because of poor absorption and rapid metabolism by MAO and COMT.

Although intravenous infusion of epinephrine has pronounced effects on the cardiovascular system, its use in the treatment of heart block or circulatory collapse is limited because of its tendency to induce cardiac arrhythmias. It increases systolic pressure by increasing cardiac output, and it lowers diastolic pressure by causing an overall decrease in peripheral resistance; the net result is little change in mean blood pressure.

Epinephrine is of value as a constrictor in hemorrhage or nasal congestion. Also, it is used to enhance the activity of local anesthetics. Its use in these two situations takes advantage of the drug's potent stimulatory effects on α receptors. The ability of epinephrine to stimulate β_2 receptors has led to its use by injection and by inhalation to relax bronchial smooth muscle in asthma and in anaphylactic reactions. Several over-the-counter preparations (e.g., Primatene, Bronkaid) used for treating bronchial asthma use epinephrine.

Epinephrine is used in the treatment of open-angle glaucoma, where it apparently reduces intraocular pressure by increasing the rate of outflow of aqueous humor from the anterior chamber of the eye. The irritation often experienced on instillation of epinephrine into the eye has led to the development of other preparations of the drug that potentially are not as irritating. One such example is dipivefrin.

Dipivefrin. Dipivefrin (dipivalyl epinephrine, Propine) is a prodrug of epinephrine that is formed by the esterification of the catechol hydroxyl groups of epinephrine with pivalic acid. Dipivefrin is much more lipophilic than epinephrine, and it achieves much better penetration of the eye when administered topically as an aqueous solution for the treatment of primary open-angle glaucoma. It is converted to epinephrine by esterases in the cornea and anterior chamber. Dipivefrin offers the advantage of being less irritating to the eye than epinephrine, and because of its more efficient transport into the eye, it can be used in lower concentrations than epinephrine.

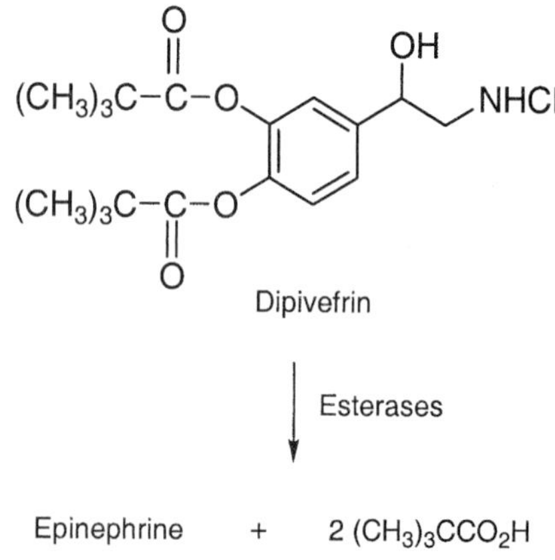

Dipivefrin

Esterases

Epinephrine + 2 $(CH_3)_3CCO_2H$

α-ADRENERGIC RECEPTOR AGONISTS

Phenylephrine. Phenylephrine (Neo-Synephrine, structure shown above under "Structure–Activity Relationships") is the prototypical selective direct-acting α_1-receptor agonist. It is a potent vasoconstrictor but is less potent than epinephrine and norepinephrine (NE). It is active when given orally, and its duration of action is about twice that of epinephrine. It is metabolized by MAO, but since it lacks the catechol moiety, it is not metabolized by COMT. It is relatively nontoxic and produces little CNS stimulation. When applied to mucous membranes, it reduces congestion and swelling by constricting the blood vessels of the membranes. Thus, one of its main uses is in the relief of nasal congestion. In the eye, it is used to dilate the pupil and to treat open-angle glaucoma. It also is used in spinal anesthesia, to prolong the anesthesia and to prevent a drop in blood pressure during the procedure. Another use is in the treatment of severe hypotension resulting from either shock or drug administration.

Methoxamine. Another selective direct-acting α_1-receptor agonist used therapeutically is methoxamine (Vasoxyl). This drug is a vasoconstrictor that has no stimulant action on the heart. In fact, it tends to slow the ventricular rate because of activation of the carotid sinus reflex. It is less potent than phenylephrine as a vasoconstrictor. Methoxamine is used primarily during surgery to maintain adequate arterial blood pressure, especially in conjunction with spinal anesthesia. It does not stimulate the CNS.

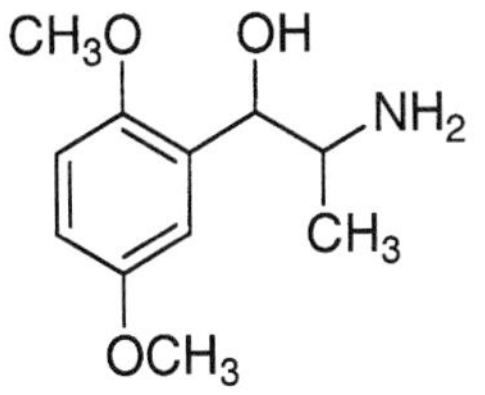

Methoxamine

Midodrine. Midodrine (ProAmatine) represents another example of a dimethoxy-β-phenylethylamine derivative that is used therapeutically for its vasoconstrictor properties. Specifically, it is used in the treatment of symptomatic orthostatic hypotension. Midodrine is the *N*-glycyl prodrug of the selective α_1-receptor agonist desglymidodrine. Removal of the *N*-glycyl moiety from midodrine occurs readily in the liver as well as throughout the body, presumably by amidases.

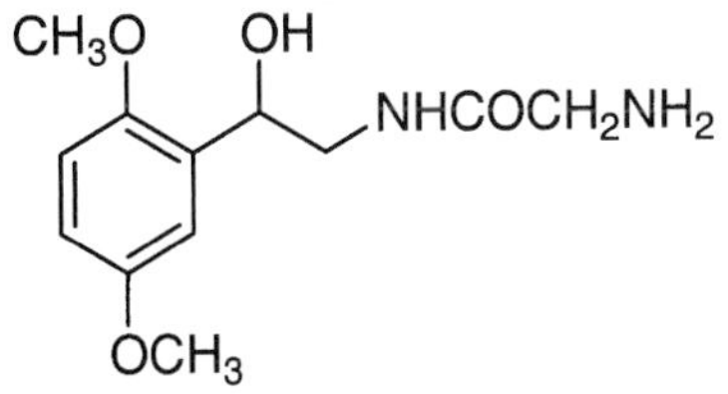

Midodrine

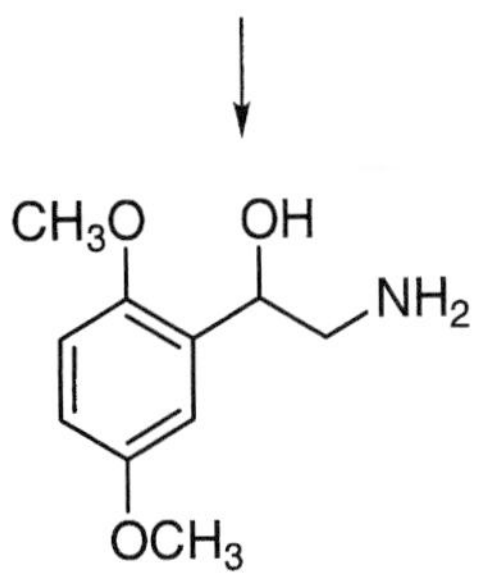

Desglymidodrine

Naphazoline, Tetrahydrozoline, Xylometazoline, and Oxymetazoline. The 2-aralkylimidazolines naphazoline (Privine), tetrahydrozoline (Tyzine, Visine), xylometazoline (Otrivin), and oxymetazoline (Afrin) are agonists at both α_1- and α_2-adrenergic receptors. These agents are used for their vasoconstrictive effects as nasal and ophthalmic decongestants. They have limited access to the CNS, since they essentially exist in an ionized form at physiological pH because of the very basic nature of the imidazoline ring (pK_a 9 to 10).

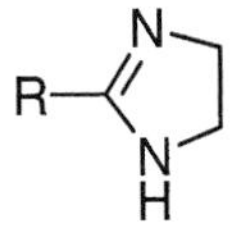

Naphazoline: R = —CH_2—

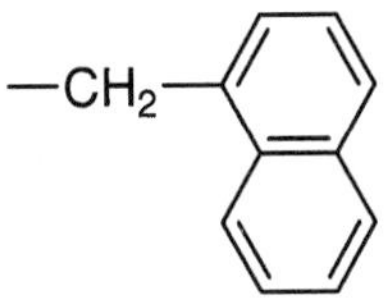

Tetrahydrozoline: R =

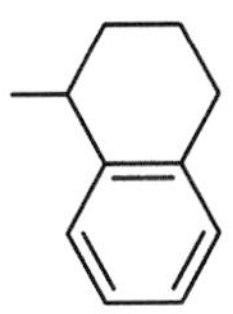

Oxymetazoline: R = —CH_2—

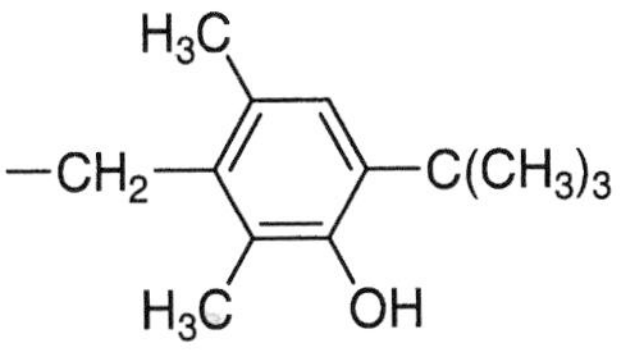

Xylometazoline: R = —CH_2—

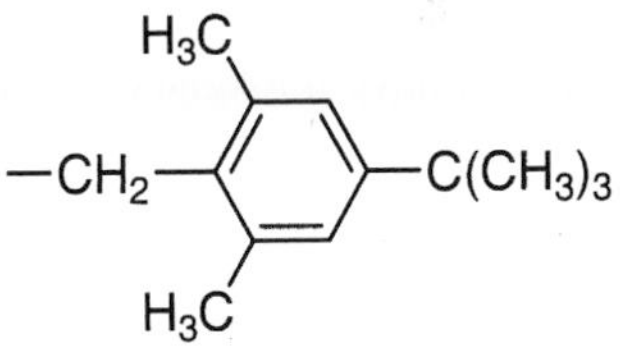

Clonidine. Clonidine (Catapres) is an example of a (phenylimino)imidazolidine derivative that possesses selectivity for the α_2-adrenergic receptor. The $\alpha1:\alpha2$ ratio is 300:1. Under certain conditions, such as intravenous infusion, clonidine can briefly exhibit vasoconstrictive activity as a result of stimulation of peripheral α-adrenergic receptors. However, this hypertensive effect, if it occurs, is followed by a much longer lasting hypotensive effect as a result of the ability of clonidine to enter into the CNS and stimulate α_2 receptors located in regions of the brain, such as the nucleus tractus solitarius. Stimulation of these α_2 receptors brings about a decrease in sympathetic outflow from the CNS, which in turn leads to decreases in peripheral vascular resistance and blood pressure.[20, 38] Bradycardia is also produced by clonidine as a result of a centrally induced facilitation of the vagus nerve and stimulation of cardiac prejunctional α_2-adrenergic receptors.[39] These pharmacological actions have made clonidine quite useful in the treatment of hypertension.

Clonidine: R = H

4-Hydroxyclonidine: R = OH

Apraclonidine: R = NH$_2$

The ability of clonidine and its analogues to exert an antihypertensive effect depends on the ability of these compounds not only to interact with the α_2 receptor but also to gain entry into the CNS. For example, in the case of clonidine, the basicity of the guanidine group (typically pK$_a$ 13.6) is decreased to 8.0 (the pK$_a$ of clonidine) because of its direct attachment to the dichlorophenyl ring. Thus, at physiological pH, clonidine will exist to a significant extent in the nonionized form required for passage into the CNS.

Substitutions on the aromatic ring also affect the ability of clonidine and its analogues to gain entry into the CNS to produce an antihypertensive effect. Although various halogen and alkyl substitutions can be placed at the two *ortho* positions of the (phenylimino)imidazolidine nucleus without affecting the affinity of the derivatives toward α_2 receptors, such substitutions have a marked effect on the lipophilicity of the compound. Halogen substituents such as chlorine seem to provide the optimal characteristics in this regard.[40] This distributive phenomenon is seen with one of the metabolites of clonidine, 4-hydroxyclonidine. This compound has good affinity for α_2 receptors, but since it is too polar to get into the CNS, it is not an effective antihypertensive agent.

In addition to binding to the α_2 adrenergic receptor, clonidine, as well as some other imidazolines, shows high affinity for what has been termed the ''imidazoline'' receptor.[41, 42] Some studies have implicated a role for the imidazoline receptors in the antihypertensive effects of clonidine.[43, 44] However, other studies involving both site-directed mutagenesis of the α_{2A}-adrenergic receptor subtype and genetically engineered knockout mice deficient in either the α_{2B}- or α_{2A}-adrenergic receptor subtypes provide evidence that the hypotensive response of the α_2-receptor agonists like clonidine primarily involves the α_{2A}-adrenergic receptor subtype.[45, 46]

Guanabenz and Guanfacine.

Two analogues of clonidine, guanabenz (Wytensin) and guanfacine (Tenex), are also used as antihypertensive drugs. Their mechanism of action is the same as that of clonidine. Structurally, these two compounds can be considered ''open-ring imidazolidines.'' In these compounds, the 2,6-dichlorophenyl moiety found in clonidine is connected to a guanidino group by a two-atom bridge. In the case of guanabenz, this bridge is a –CH=N– group, while for guanfacine it is a –CH$_2$CO– moiety. For both compounds, conjugation of the guanidino moiety with the bridging moiety helps to decrease the pK$_a$ of this normally very basic group so that at physiological pH a significant portion of each drug exists in its nonionized form. Differences between clonidine and its two analogues are seen in their elimination half-life values and in their metabolism and urinary excretion patterns. The elimination

half-life of clonidine ranges from 20 to 25 hours, while that for guanfacine is about 17 hours. Guanabenz has the shortest duration of action of these three agents, with a half-life of about 6 hours. Clonidine and guanfacine are excreted unchanged in the urine to the extent of 60 and 50%, respectively. Very little of guanabenz is excreted unchanged in the urine.

Guanabenz

Guanfacine

Apraclonidine and Brimonidine.

In addition to its therapeutic use as an antihypertensive agent, clonidine has been found to provide beneficial effects in a number of other situations.[47] These include migraine prophylaxis, glaucoma, opiate withdrawal syndrome, and anesthesia. This has prompted the development of analogues of clonidine for specific use in some of the above areas. Two such examples are apraclonidine (Iopidine) and brimonidine (Alphagan). Both are selective α_2-receptor agonists with $\alpha1$:$\alpha2$ ratios of 30:1 and 1,000:1, respectively. They both lower intraocular pressure by decreasing aqueous humor production and increasing aqueous humor outflow. Apraclonidine is used specifically to control elevations in intraocular pressure that can occur during laser surgery on the eye. Brimonidine also is used in such a manner; in addition, it is approved for use in treating glaucoma. Another example is **tizanidine** (Zanaflex), which finds use in treating spasticity associated with multiple sclerosis or spinal cord injury. By stimulating α_2-adrenergic receptors, it is believed to decrease the release of excitatory amino acid neurotransmitters from spinal cord interneurons.[48]

Brimonidine

Tizanidine

Methyldopa. A phenylethylamine derivative that shows selectivity toward the α_2 receptor is α-methylnorepinephrine (Fig. 16-6). As discussed above under ''Structure–Activity Relationships,'' the presence of an α-methyl group in the correct configuration on the phenylethylamine nucleus yields compounds with increased potency at α_2 receptors and decreased potency at α_1 receptors. Although α-methylnorepinephrine is not given as a drug, it is the metabolic product of the drug methyldopa (L-α-methyl-3,4-dihydroxyphenylalanine, Aldomet). Since methyldopa is a close structural analogue of L-dopa, it is treated as an alternate substrate by the enzyme L-aromatic amino acid decarboxylase. The product of this initial enzymatic reaction is α-methyldopamine. This intermediate, in turn, is acted on by dopamine β-hydroxylase to give the diastereoisomer of α-methylnorepinephrine, which possesses the *(R)* configuration at the carbon with the β-hydroxyl group and the *(S)* configuration at the carbon with the α-methyl substituent (Fig. 16-6). It is postulated that α-methylnorepinephrine acts on α_2 receptors in the CNS in the same manner as clonidine, to decrease sympathetic outflow and lower blood pressure.[38] Since methyldopa serves as an alternate substrate to L-aromatic amino acid decarboxylase, it ultimately decreases the concentration of dopamine, NE, epinephrine, and serotonin in the CNS and periphery.

Methyldopa is used only by oral administration since its zwitterionic character limits its solubility. Absorption can range from 8 to 62% and appears to involve an amino acid transporter. Absorption is affected by food, and about 40% of that absorbed is converted to methyldopa-*O*-sulfate by the mucosal intestinal cells. Entry into the CNS also appears to involve an active transport process. The ester hydrochloride salt of methyldopa, **methyldopate** (Aldomet ester), was developed as a highly water-soluble derivative that could be used to make parenteral preparations. Methyldopate is converted to methyldopa in the body through the action of esterases (Fig. 16-6).

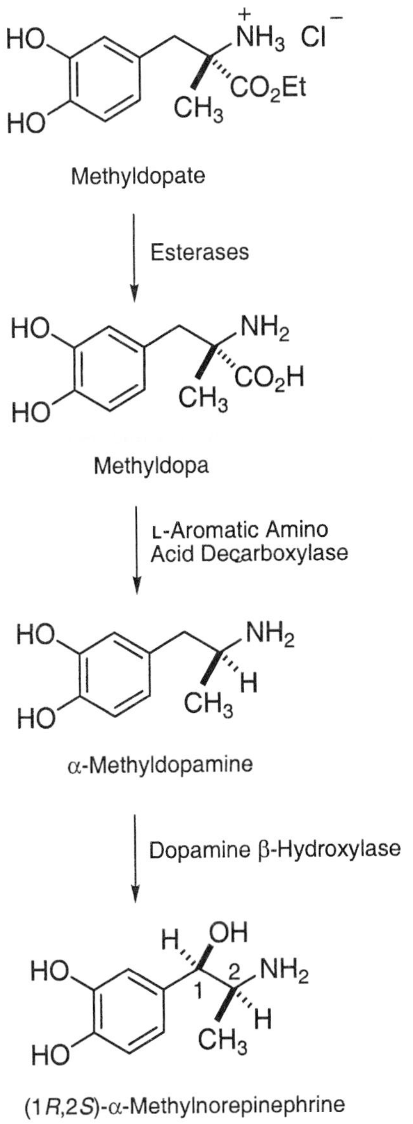

DUAL α- AND β-ADRENERGIC RECEPTOR AGONISTS

Dobutamine. There are synthetic direct-acting sympathomimetics whose therapeutic use relies on their ability to act at both α- and β-adrenergic receptors. One example is dobutamine (Dobutrex). Structurally, dobutamine can be viewed as an analogue of dopamine in which a 1-(methyl)-3-(4-hydroxyphenyl)propyl substituent has been placed on the amino group. This substitution gives a compound that possesses an asymmetric carbon atom. Thus, dobutamine exists as a pair of enantiomers, with each enantiomer possessing a distinct pharmacology.[49] The (+) enantiomer is a potent full agonist at both β_1 and β_2 receptors. In contrast, the (–) enantiomer is some 10 times less potent at β_1 and β_2 receptors. The (–) enantiomer is, however, a potent agonist at α_1 receptors. Dobutamine does not act as an agonist at the dopaminergic receptors that mediate renal vasodilation.

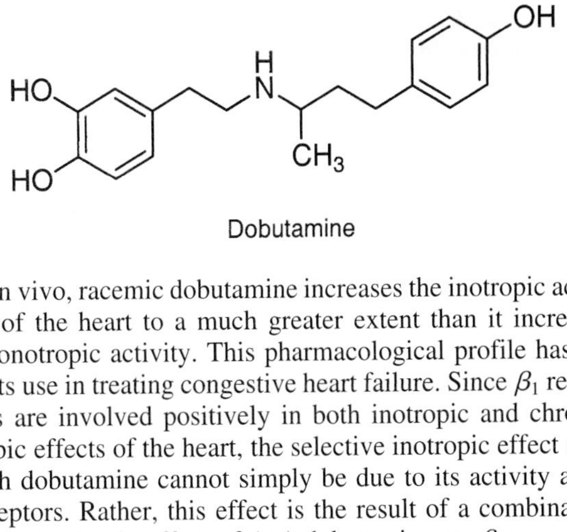

Dobutamine

Figure 16–6 ■ Metabolic conversion of methyldopate and methyldopa to α-methylnorepinephrine.

In vivo, racemic dobutamine increases the inotropic activity of the heart to a much greater extent than it increases chronotropic activity. This pharmacological profile has led to its use in treating congestive heart failure. Since β_1 receptors are involved positively in both inotropic and chronotropic effects of the heart, the selective inotropic effect seen with dobutamine cannot simply be due to its activity at β_1 receptors. Rather, this effect is the result of a combination of the inotropic effect of (+)-dobutamine on β_1 receptors and that of (–)-dobutamine mediated through α_1 receptors.[50] Thus, this is a case where a racemic mixture provides a more desirable pharmacological and therapeutic effect than would either enantiomer alone.

Dobutamine is given by intravenous infusion, since it is not effective orally. Solutions of the drug can exhibit a slight pink color as a result of oxidation of the catechol function. It has a plasma half-life of about 2 minutes. It is metabolized by COMT and conjugation but not by MAO.

β-ADRENERGIC RECEPTOR AGONISTS

Isoproterenol.

Isoproterenol (Isuprel, structure shown above under "Structure–Activity Relationships") is the prototypical β-adrenergic receptor agonist. Because of an isopropyl substitution on the nitrogen atom, it has virtually no effect on α receptors. However, it does act on both $β_1$ and $β_2$ receptors. It thus can produce an increase in cardiac output by stimulating cardiac $β_1$ receptors and can bring about bronchodilation through stimulation of $β_2$ receptors in the respiratory tract. It also produces the metabolic effects expected of a potent β agonist. Isoproterenol is available for use by inhalation and injection. Its principal clinical use is for the relief of bronchospasms associated with bronchial asthma. In fact, it is one of the most potent bronchodilators available. Cardiac stimulation is an occasionally dangerous adverse effect in its use. This effect of isoproterenol on the heart is sometimes made use of in the treatment of heart block.

After oral administration, the absorption of isoproterenol is rather erratic and undependable. The drug has a duration of action of 1 to 3 hours after inhalation. The principal reason for its poor absorption characteristics and relatively short duration of action is its facile metabolic transformation by sulfate and glucuronide conjugation of the ring hydroxyls and methylation by COMT. Unlike epinephrine and NE, isoproterenol does not appear to undergo oxidative deamination by MAO. Since it is a catechol, it is sensitive to light and air. Aqueous solutions become pink on standing.

The problems of lack of β-receptor selectivity and rapid metabolic inactivation associated with isoproterenol have been overcome at least partially by the design and development of a number of selective $β_2$-adrenergic receptor agonists. These agents relax smooth muscle of the bronchi, uterus, and skeletal muscle vascular supply. They find their primary use as bronchodilators in the treatment of acute and chronic bronchial asthma and other obstructive pulmonary diseases.

Metaproterenol and Terbutaline.

As pointed out in the discussion of structure–activity relationships, modification of the catechol portion of a β agonist has resulted in the development of selective $β_2$-receptor agonists. For example, metaproterenol (Alupent, structure shown above under "Structure–Activity Relationships") and terbutaline (Bricanyl, Brethine) are resorcinol derivatives that are $β_2$ selective. Metaproterenol is less $β_2$ selective than either terbutaline or albuterol. Although these agents have a lower affinity for $β_2$ receptors than isoproterenol, they are much more effective when given orally, and they have a longer duration of action. This is because they are not metabolized by either COMT or MAO. Instead, their metabolism primarily involves glucuronide conjugation. Although both metaproterenol and terbutaline exhibit significant $β_2$-receptor selectivity, the common cardiovascular effects associated with other adrenergic agents can also be seen with these drugs when high doses are used.

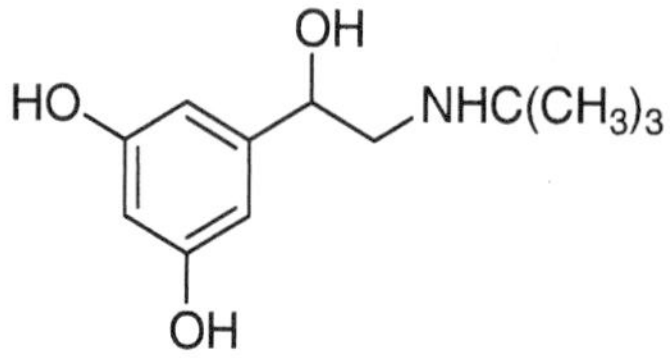

Terbutaline

Albuterol, Pirbuterol, and Salmeterol.

Albuterol (Proventil, Ventolin, structure shown above under "Structure–Activity Relationships"), pirbuterol (Maxair), and salmeterol (Serevent) are examples of selective $β_2$-receptor agonists whose selectivity results from replacement of the *meta*-hydroxyl group of the catechol ring with a hydroxymethyl moiety. Pirbuterol is closely related structurally to albuterol; the only difference between the two is that pirbuterol contains a pyridine ring instead of a benzene ring. As in the case of metaproterenol and terbutaline, these drugs are not metabolized by either COMT or MAO. Instead, they are conjugated with sulfate. They thus are active orally, and they exhibit a longer duration of action than isoproterenol. The duration of action of terbutaline, albuterol, and pirbuterol is in the range of 3 to 6 hours.

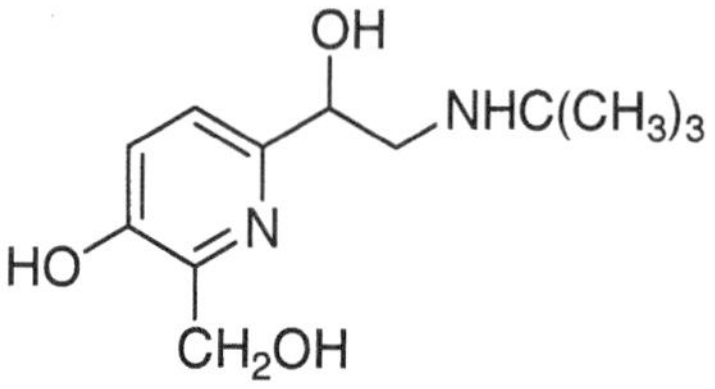

Pirbuterol

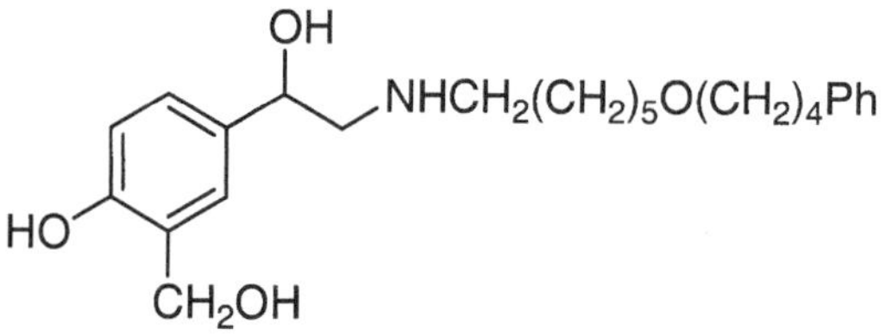

Salmeterol

Salmeterol is a partial agonist at $β_2$ receptors and has a potency similar to that of isoproterenol. It is very long acting (12 hours), an effect attributed to the lipophilic phenylalkyl substituent on the nitrogen atom, which is believed to interact with a site outside but adjacent to the active site. This agent associates with the $β_2$ receptor slowly and dissociates from the receptor at an even slower rate.[51]

Formoterol and Levalbuterol.

Another long-acting $β_2$-receptor agonist is Formoterol (Foradil). Its long duration of action, which is comparable to that of salmeterol, has been suggested to result from its association with the membrane lipid bilayer.[52] Formoterol has a much faster onset of action than does salmeterol. Both of these long-acting drugs are used by inhalation and are recommended for maintenance treatment of asthma, usually in conjunction with an inhaled corticosteroid.

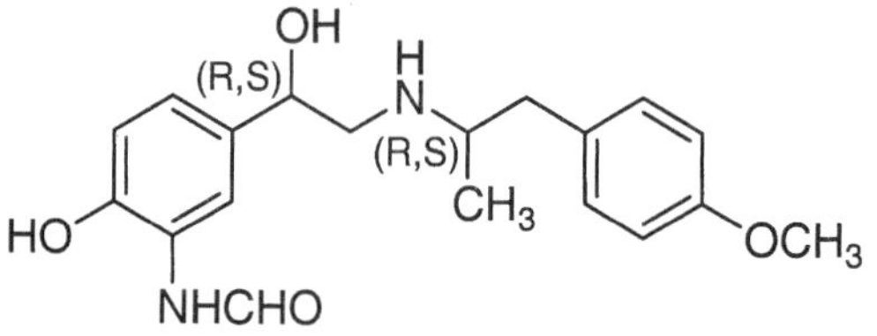

Formoterol

All of the above $β_2$-receptor agonists possess at least one chiral center and are used as racemic mixtures. Formoterol possesses two chiral centers and is used as the racemic mixture of the *(R,R)* and *(S,S)* enantiomers. As mentioned above, it is the *(R)* isomer of the phenylethanolamines that possesses the pharmacological activity. Concerns have been raised about the use of such racemic mixtures under the belief that the inactive *(S)* isomer may be responsible for some of the adverse effects seen with these agents. Levalbuterol (Xopenex), the *(R)* isomer of racemic albuterol, represents the first attempt to address this issue.

Isoetharine. Another sympathomimetic drug that finds use as a bronchodilator is the *α*-ethyl catecholamine, isoetharine. This agent is weaker than isoproterenol at stimulating *β₂* receptors. In addition, its *β₂* selectivity is not as great as that seen with drugs such as terbutaline or albuterol. Because of the presence of the *α*-ethyl group, isoetharine is not metabolized by MAO. Because it contains the catechol ring system, however, it is metabolized quite effectively by COMT. It also is *O*-sulfated quite effectively. Isoetharine has a duration of action similar to that of isoproterenol.

Isoetharine

Bitolterol. Bitolterol (Tornalate) is a prodrug of the *β₂*-selective adrenergic agonist colterol, the *N-tert*-butyl analogue of NE. The presence of the two *p*-toluic acid esters in bitolterol makes it considerably more lipophilic than colterol. Bitolterol is administered by inhalation for bronchial asthma and reversible bronchospasm. It is hydrolyzed by esterases in the lung and other tissues to produce the active agent, colterol. Bitolterol has a longer duration of action than isoproterenol (5 to 8 hours) and is metabolized, after hydrolysis of the esters, by COMT and conjugation.

Bitolterol

Colterol   *p*-Toluic Acid

Ritodrine. Ritodrine (Yutopar) is a selective *β₂*-receptor agonist used to control premature labor and to reverse

fetal distress caused by excessive uterine activity. Its uterine inhibitory effects are more sustained than its effects on the cardiovascular system, which are minimal compared with those caused by nonselective *β* agonists. The cardiovascular effects usually associated with its administration are mild tachycardia and slight diastolic pressure decrease. Usually, it is administered initially by intravenous infusion to stop premature labor. Subsequently, it may be given orally.

Ritodrine

β₃-Adrenergic Receptor Agonists. Selective direct-acting agonists for the *β₃*-adrenergic receptor have been developed, but they have not been approved for therapeutic use.[53] Because stimulation of the *β₃* receptor promotes lipolysis, these agents may have potential as antiobesity drugs and as drugs for the treatment of non–insulin-dependent diabetes.

Indirect-Acting Sympathomimetics

Indirect-acting sympathomimetics act by releasing endogenous NE. They enter the nerve ending by way of the active-uptake process and displace NE from its storage granules. Certain structural characteristics tend to impart indirect sympathomimetic activity to phenylethylamines. As with the direct-acting agents, the presence of the catechol hydroxyls enhances the potency of indirect-acting phenylethylamines. However, the indirect-acting drugs that are used therapeutically are not catechol derivatives and, in most cases, do not even contain a hydroxyl moiety. In contrast with the direct-acting agents, the presence of a *β*-hydroxyl group decreases, and an *α*-methyl group increases, the effectiveness of indirect-acting agents. The presence of nitrogen substituents decreases indirect activity, with substituents larger than methyl rendering the compound virtually inactive. Phenylethylamines that contain a tertiary amino group are also ineffective as NE-releasing agents. Given the foregoing structure–activity considerations, it is easy to understand why amphetamine and *p*-tyramine are often cited as prototypical indirect-acting sympathomimetics. Since amphetamine-type drugs exert their primary effects on the CNS, they are discussed in more detail in Chapter 15. This chapter discusses those agents that exert their effects primarily on the periphery.

Amphetamine   *p*-Tyramine

Hydroxyamphetamine. Although *p*-tyramine is not a clinically useful agent, its *α*-methylated derivative, hydroxyamphetamine (Paredrine), is an effective, indirect-acting sympathomimetic drug. Hydroxyamphetamine has little or no ephedrine-like, CNS-stimulating action. It is used to dilate the pupil for diagnostic eye examinations and for surgical procedures on the eye. It is used sometimes with cholinergic blocking drugs like atropine to produce a mydriatic effect, which is more pronounced than that produced by either drug alone.

Hydroxyamphetamine

L-(+)-Pseudoephedrine.   L-(+)-Pseudoephedrine (Sudafed, Afrinol, Drixoral) is the *(S,S)* diastereoisomer of ephedrine. It is a naturally occurring alkaloid from the *Ephedra* species. Whereas ephedrine has a mixed mechanism of action, pseudoephedrine acts principally by an indirect mechanism. The structural basis for this difference in mechanism is the stereochemistry of the carbon atom possessing the β-hydroxyl group. In pseudoephedrine, this carbon atom possesses the *(S)* configuration, which is the wrong stereochemistry at this center for a direct-acting effect at adrenergic receptors. This agent is found in many over-the-counter nasal decongestant and cold medications. Although it is less prone to increase blood pressure than ephedrine, it should be used with caution in hypertensive individuals, and it should not be used in combination with MAO inhibitors.

L-(+)-Pseudoephedrine

Propylhexedrine.   Propylhexedrine (Benzedrex) is an analogue of amphetamine in which the aromatic ring has been replaced with a cyclohexane ring. This drug produces vasoconstriction and a decongestant effect on the nasal membranes, but it has only about one-half the pressor effect of amphetamine and produces decidedly fewer effects on the CNS. Its major use is for a local vasoconstrictive effect on nasal mucosa in the symptomatic relief of nasal congestion caused by the common cold, allergic rhinitis, or sinusitis.

Propylhexedrine

Sympathomimetics With a Mixed Mechanism of Action

Those phenylethylamines considered to have a mixed mechanism of action usually have no hydroxyls on the aromatic ring but do have a β-hydroxyl group.

D-(-)-Ephedrine.   D-(-)-Ephedrine is the classic example of a sympathomimetic with a mixed mechanism of action. This drug is an alkaloid that can be obtained from the

TABLE 16–1   Relative Pressor Activity of the Isomers of Ephedrine

Isomer	Relative Activity
D-(−)-Ephedrine	36
DL-(±)-Ephedrine	26
L-(+)-Ephedrine	11
L-(+)-Pseudoephedrine	7
DL-(±)-Pseudoephedrine	4
D-(−)-Pseudoephedrine	1

stems of various species of *Ephedra*. Mahuang, the plant containing ephedrine, was known to the Chinese in 2,000 BC, but the active principle, ephedrine, was not isolated until 1885.

Ephedrine has two asymmetric carbon atoms; thus, there are four optically active forms. The *erythro* racemate is called "ephedrine," and the *threo* racemate is known as "pseudoephedrine" (ψ-ephedrine). Natural ephedrine is the D(−) isomer, and it is the most active of the four isomers as a pressor amine (Table 16-1). This is largely due to the fact that this isomer has the correct *(R)* configuration at the carbon atom bearing the hydroxyl group and the desired *(S)* configuration at the carbon bearing the methyl group for optimal direct action at adrenergic receptors.

D-(-)-Ephedrine

Ephedrine decomposes gradually and darkens when exposed to light. The free alkaloid is a strong base, and an aqueous solution of the free alkaloid has a pH above 10. The salt form has a pK_a of 9.6.

The pharmacological activity of ephedrine resembles that of epinephrine. The drug acts on both α- and β-adrenergic receptors. Although it is less potent than epinephrine, its pressor and local vasoconstrictive actions are of greater duration. It also causes more pronounced stimulation of the CNS than epinephrine, and it is effective when given orally. The drug is not metabolized by either MAO or COMT. Rather, it is p-hydroxylated and N-demethylated by cytochrome P-450 mixed-function oxidases.

Ephedrine and its salts are used orally, intravenously, intramuscularly, and topically for a variety of conditions, such as allergic disorders, colds, hypotensive conditions, and narcolepsy. It is used locally to constrict the nasal mucosa and cause decongestion and to dilate the pupil or the bronchi. Systemically, it is effective for asthma, hay fever, and urticaria.

Phenylpropanolamine.   Phenylpropanolamine (Propadrine) is similar in structure to ephedrine except that it is a primary instead of a secondary amine. This modification gives an agent that has slightly higher vasopressive action and lower central stimulatory action than ephedrine. Its action as a nasal decongestant is more prolonged than that of ephedrine. It is effective when given orally. Phenylpropanolamine was a common active component in over-the-counter appetite suppressants and cough and cold medications until 2001, when the Food and Drug Administration (FDA) recommended its removal from such medications because studies showed an increased risk of hemorrhagic stroke in young women who took the drug.

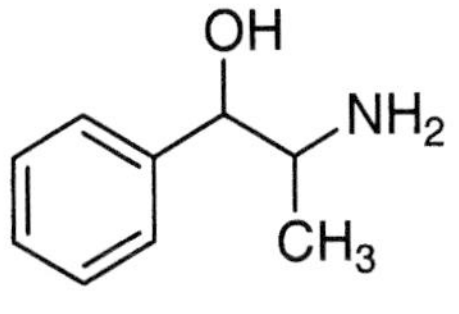

Phenylpropanolamine

Metaraminol.   Metaraminol (Aramine) is structurally similar to phenylephrine except that it is a primary instead of a secondary amine. It possesses a mixed mechanism of action, with its direct-acting effects mainly on α-adrenergic receptors. It is used parenterally as a vasopressor in the treatment and prevention of the acute hypotensive state occurring with spinal anesthesia. It also has been used to treat severe hypotension brought on by other traumas that induce shock.

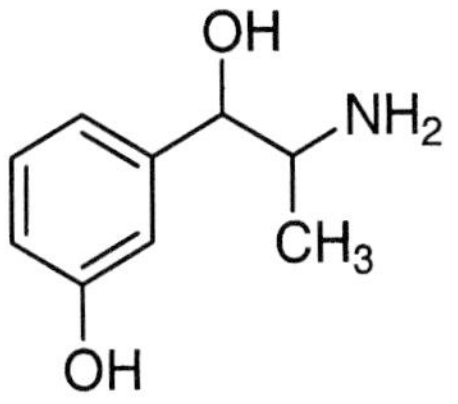

Metaraminol

ADRENERGIC RECEPTOR ANTAGONISTS

α-Adrenergic Receptor Antagonists

Unlike the β-adrenergic receptor antagonists, which bear clear structural similarities to the adrenergic agonists NE, epinephrine, and isoproterenol, the α-adrenergic receptor antagonists consist of a number of compounds of diverse chemical structure that bear little obvious resemblance to the α-adrenergic receptor agonists.[34]

NONSELECTIVE α-RECEPTOR ANTAGONISTS

Tolazoline and Phentolamine.   The agents in this class are structurally similar to the imidazoline α-agonists, such as naphazoline, tetrahydrozoline, and xylometazoline. The type of group attached to the imidazoline ring dictates whether an imidazoline is an agonist or an antagonist. The two representatives of the imidazoline α antagonists that are used therapeutically are tolazoline (Priscoline) and phentolamine (Regitine). Both are competitive (reversible) blocking agents. Phentolamine is the more effective α antagonist, but neither drug is useful in treating essential hypertension. Theoretically, the vasodilatory effects of an α-antagonist should be beneficial in the management of hypertension. Tolazoline and phentolamine, however, have both α_1- and α_2-antagonistic activity and produce tachycardia. Presum-

ably, the antagonistic actions of these agents at presynaptic α_2 receptors contribute to their cardiac stimulant effects by enhancing the release of NE. Both agents have a direct vasodilatory action on vascular smooth muscle that may be more prominent than their α-receptor antagonistic effects.

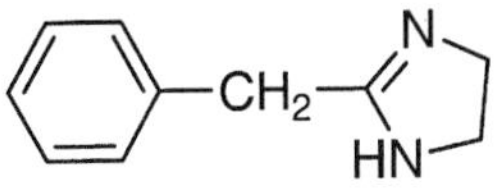

Tolazoline

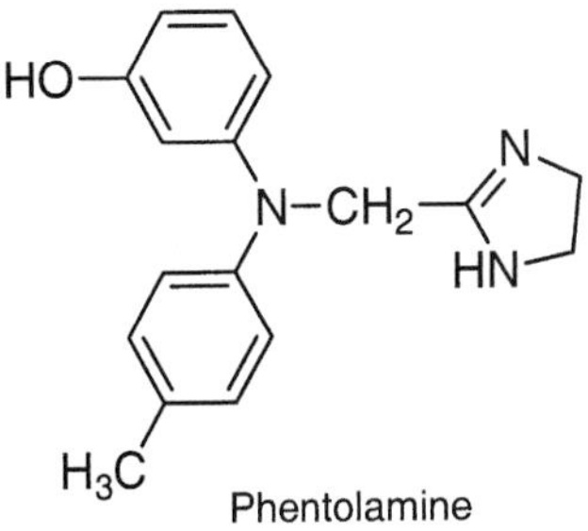

Phentolamine

The antagonistic action of tolazoline is relatively weak, but its histamine-like and acetylcholine-like agonistic actions probably contribute to its vasodilatory activity. Its histamine-like effects include stimulation of gastric acid secretion, rendering it inappropriate for administration to patients who have gastric or peptic ulcers. It has been used to treat Raynaud's syndrome and other conditions involving peripheral vasospasm. Tolazoline is available in an injectable form and is indicated for use in persistent pulmonary hypertension of the newborn when supportive measures are not successful.

Phentolamine is used to prevent or control hypertensive episodes that occur in patients with pheochromocytoma. It can be used as an aid in the diagnosis of pheochromocytoma, but measurement of catecholamine levels is a safer and more reliable method of diagnosis. It also has been used in combination with papaverine to treat impotence.

IRREVERSIBLE α-RECEPTOR BLOCKERS

Agents in this class, when given in adequate doses, produce a slowly developing, prolonged adrenergic blockade that is not overcome by epinephrine. In essence, they are irreversible blockers of the α-adrenergic receptor. Chemically, they are β-haloalkylamines. Although dibenamine is the prototypical agent in this class, it is phenoxybenzamine that is used therapeutically today.

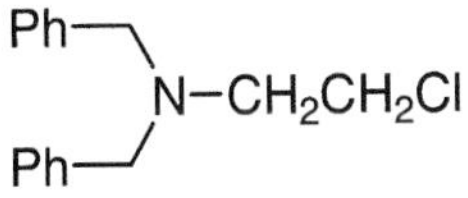

Dibenamine

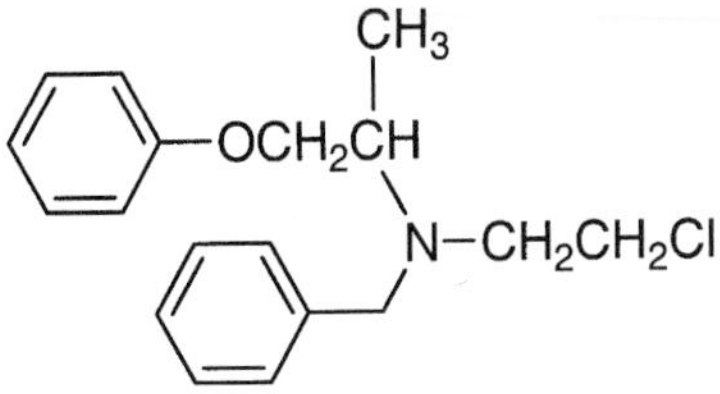

Phenoxybenzamine

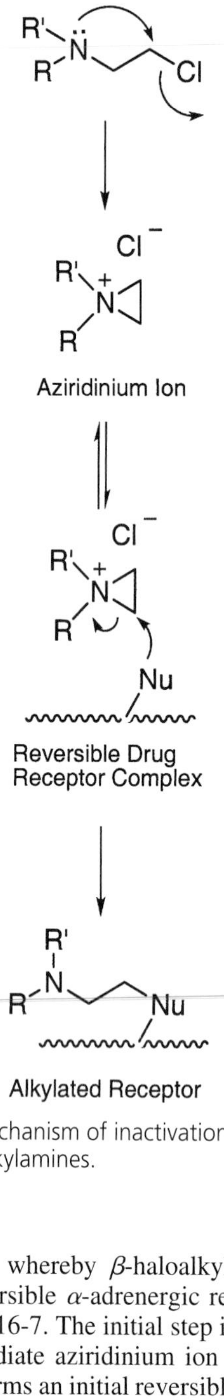

Figure 16–7 ■ Mechanism of inactivation of α-adrenergic receptors by β-haloalkylamines.

The mechanism whereby β-haloalkylamines produce a long-lasting, irreversible α-adrenergic receptor blockade is depicted in Figure 16-7. The initial step involves the formation of an intermediate aziridinium ion (ethylene iminium ion), which then forms an initial reversible complex with the receptor. The positively charged aziridinium ion electrophile then reacts with a nucleophilic group on the receptor, resulting in the formation of a covalent bond between the drug and the receptor. Although the aziridinium ion intermediate has long been believed to be the active receptor-alkylating species, it was not until 1976 that it was demonstrated unequivocally that the aziridinium ions derived from dibenamine and phenoxybenamine are capable of α-receptor alkylation.[54]

Phenoxybenzamine. The action of phenoxybenzamine (Dibenzyline) has been described as representing a ''chemical sympathectomy'' because of its selective blockade of the excitatory responses of smooth muscle and of the heart muscle. Although phenoxybenzamine is capable of blocking acetylcholine, histamine, and serotonin receptors, its primary pharmacological effects, especially vasodilation, may be attributed to its α-adrenergic blocking capability. As would be expected of a drug that produces such a profound α blockade, administration is frequently associated with reflex tachycardia, increased cardiac output, and postural hypotension. There is also evidence indicating that blockade of presynaptic α_2 receptors contributes to the increased heart rate produced by phenoxybenzamine.

The onset of action of phenoxybenzamine is slow, but the effects of a single dose of drug may last 3 to 4 days, since essentially new receptors need to be made to replace those that have been inhibited irreversibly. The principal effects following its administration are an increase in peripheral blood flow, an increase in skin temperature, and a lowering of blood pressure. It has no effect on the parasympathetic system and little effect on the gastrointestinal tract. The most common side effects are miosis, tachycardia, nasal stuffiness, and postural hypotension, all of which are related to the production of adrenergic blockade.

Oral phenoxybenzamine is used for the preoperative management of patients with pheochromocytoma and in the chronic management of patients whose tumors are not amenable to surgery. Only about 20 to 30% of an oral dose is absorbed.

SELECTIVE α_1-RECEPTOR ANTAGONISTS

Prazosin, Terazosin, Doxazosin. One group of highly selective α_1-receptor antagonists are the quinazolines. Examples include prazosin (Minipress), terazosin (Hytrin), and doxazosin (Cardura). Structurally, these three agents consist of three components: the quinazoline ring, the piperazine ring, and the acyl moiety. The 4-amino group on the quinazoline ring is very important for α_1-receptor affinity. Although prazosin, terazosin, and doxazosin possess a piperazine moiety attached to the quinazoline ring, this group can be replaced with other heterocyclic moieties (e.g., piperidine moiety) without loss of affinity. The nature of the acyl group has a significant effect on the pharmacokinetic properties.[55]

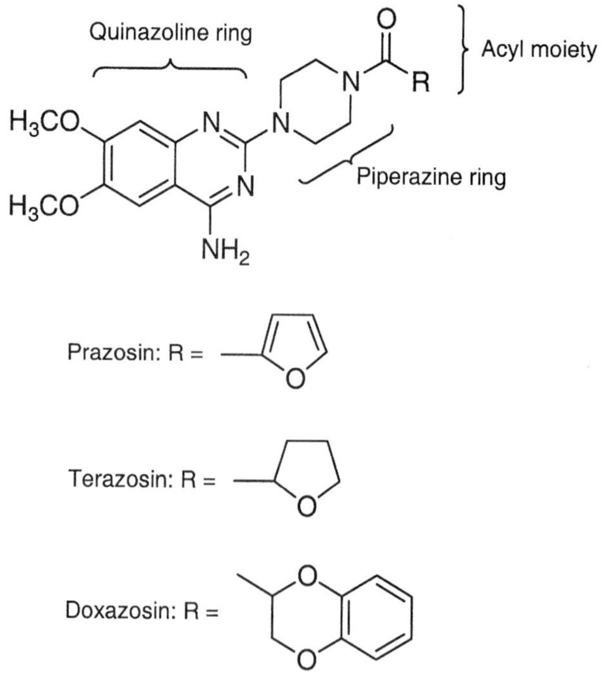

These drugs are used in the treatment of hypertension. They dilate both arterioles and veins. Agents in this class offer distinct advantages over the other α-blockers because they produce peripheral vasodilation without an increase in heart rate or cardiac output. This advantage, at least in part, is attributed to the fact that prazosin blocks postjunctional α_1 receptors selectively without blocking presynaptic α_2 receptors. These agents also find use in the treatment of benign prostatic hyperplasia, where they help improve urine flow rates.

Although the adverse effects of these drugs are usually minimal, the most frequent one, known as the *first-dose phenomenon,* is sometimes severe. This is a dose-dependent effect characterized by marked excessive postural hypotension and syncope. This phenomenon can be minimized by giving an initial low dose at bedtime.

The main difference between prazosin, terazosin, and doxazosin lies in their pharmacokinetic properties. As mentioned above, these differences are dictated by the nature of the acyl moiety attached to the piperazine ring. A comparison of these three agents with respect to their oral bioavailability, half-life, and duration of action is shown in Table 16-2. These drugs are metabolized extensively, with the metabolites excreted in the bile.

Tamsulosin.   The aryl sulfonamide tamsulosin (Flomax) represents the first in the class of subtype selective α_1-receptor antagonists. It is selective for the α_{1A}-adrenergic receptor, which seems to predominate in the prostate. It is approved for treating benign prostatic hyperplasia, for which it is administered once daily. Orthostatic hypotension may not be as great with this agent as with the nonselective quinazolines.

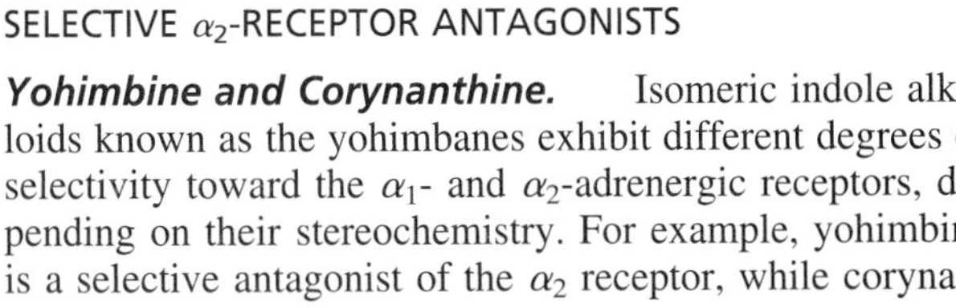

Tamsulosin

SELECTIVE α_2-RECEPTOR ANTAGONISTS

Yohimbine and Corynanthine.   Isomeric indole alkaloids known as the yohimbanes exhibit different degrees of selectivity toward the α_1- and α_2-adrenergic receptors, depending on their stereochemistry. For example, yohimbine is a selective antagonist of the α_2 receptor, while corynan-

thine is a selective antagonist of the α_1 receptor. The only difference between these two compounds is the relative stereochemistry of the carbon containing the carbomethoxy substituent. In yohimbine, this group lies in the plane of the alkaloid ring system, while in corynanthine, it lies in an axial position and thus is out of the plane of the rings.[56]

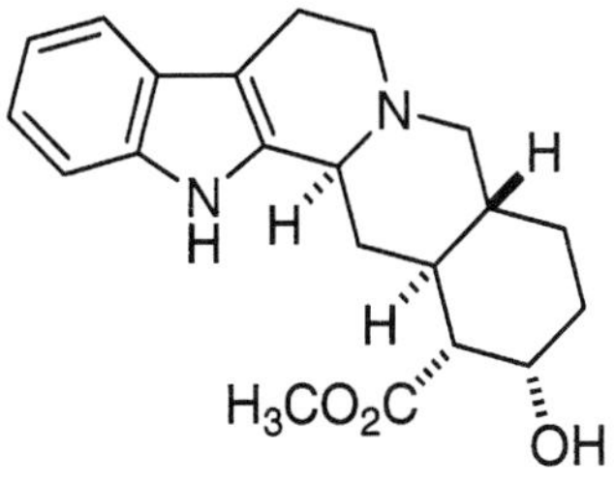

Yohimbine

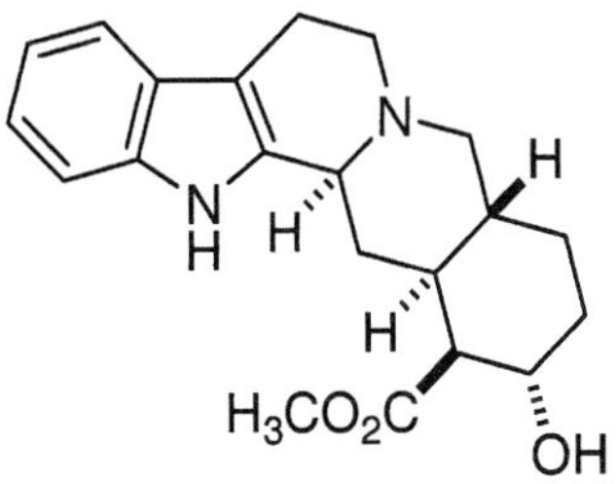

Corynanthine

Yohimbine increases heart rate and blood pressure as a result of its blockade of α_2 receptors in the CNS. It has been used experimentally to treat male erectile impotence.

Mirtazapine.   The tetracyclic mirtazapine (Remeron) is another example of an α-antagonist that shows selectivity for α_2 receptors versus α_1 receptors.[57] Blockade of central α_2 receptors results in an increased release of norepinephrine and serotonin. This has prompted its use as an antidepressant. This agent also has activity at nonadrenergic receptors. It is a potent blocker of 5-HT$_2$ and 5-HT$_3$ serotonin receptors and at histamine H$_1$ receptors.

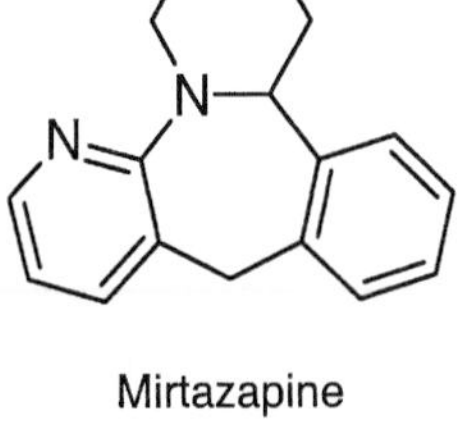

Mirtazapine

β-Adrenergic Receptor Antagonists

STRUCTURE–ACTIVITY RELATIONSHIPS

The first β blocker was not reported until 1958, when Powell and Slater[58] described the activity of dichloroisoproterenol (DCI). The structure of DCI is like that of isoproterenol, except that the catechol hydroxyl groups have been replaced by two chloro groups. This simple structural modification, involving the replacement of the aromatic hydroxyl groups,

TABLE 16–2   Pharmacokinetic Properties of Prazosin, Terazosin, and Doxazosin

Agent	Bioavailability (%)	Half-life (hours)	Duration of Action (hours)
Prazosin	50–70	2–3	4–6
Terazosin	90	9–12	18
Doxazosin	65	22	36

has provided the basis for nearly all of the approaches used in subsequent efforts to design and synthesize therapeutically useful β-receptor antagonists.[35] Unfortunately, DCI is not a pure antagonist but a partial agonist. The substantial direct sympathomimetic action of DCI precluded its development as a clinically useful drug.

Dichloroisoproterenol

Pronethalol was the next important β antagonist to be described. Although it had much less intrinsic sympathomimetic activity than DCI, it was withdrawn from clinical testing because of reports that it caused thymic tumors in mice. Within 2 years of this report, however, Black and Stephenson[59] described the β-blocking actions of propranolol, a close structural relative of pronethalol. Propranolol has become one of the most thoroughly studied and widely used drugs in the therapeutic armamentarium. It is the standard against which all other β antagonists are compared.

Pronethalol

Propranolol

Propranolol belongs to the group of β-blocking agents known as *aryloxypropanolamines*. This term reflects the fact that an –OCH₂– group has been incorporated into the molecule between the aromatic ring and the ethylamino side chain. Because this structural feature is frequently found in β antagonists, the assumption is made that the –OCH₂– group is responsible for the antagonistic properties of the molecules. However, this is not true; in fact, the –OCH₂– group is present in several compounds that are potent β agonists.[60] This latter fact again leads to the conclusion that it is the nature of the aromatic ring and its substituents that is the primary determinant of β-antagonistic activity. The aryl group also affects the absorption, excretion, and metabolism of the β blockers.[61]

The nature of the aromatic ring is also a determinant in the β₁ selectivity of the antagonists. One common structural feature of many cardioselective antagonists is the presence of a *para* substituent of sufficient size on the aromatic ring along with the absence of *meta* substituents. Practolol is the prototypical example of a β₁ antagonist of this structural

type. Although it was not released for use in the United States, it was the first cardioselective β₁ antagonist to be used extensively in humans. Because it produced several toxic effects, however, it is no longer in general use in most countries.

Practolol

As in the sympathomimetics, bulky aliphatic groups, such as the *tert*-butyl and isopropyl groups, are normally found on the amino function of the aryloxypropanolamine β-receptor antagonists. It must be a secondary amine for optimal activity.

The β-blocking agents exhibit high stereoselectivity in the production of their β-blocking effects. As with the sympathomimetic agents, the configuration of the hydroxyl-bearing carbon of the aryloxypropanolamine side chain plays a critical role in the interaction of β-antagonist drugs with β receptors. This carbon must possess the (S) configuration for optimal affinity to the β receptor. The enantiomer with the (R) configuration is typically 100 times less potent. The available data indicate that the pharmacologically more active enantiomer interacts with the receptor recognition site in a manner analogous to that of the agonists. The structural features of the aromatic portion of the antagonist, however, appear to perturb the receptor or to interact with it in a manner that inhibits activation. In spite of the fact that nearly all of the β-antagonistic activity resides in one enantiomer, propranolol and most other β blockers are used clinically as racemic mixtures. The only exceptions are levobunolol, timolol, and penbutolol, with which the (S) enantiomer is used.

NONSELECTIVE β BLOCKERS

Propranolol. Propranolol (Inderal) is the prototypical β-adrenergic receptor antagonist. It is nonselective in that it blocks the β₁ and β₂ receptors equally well. Propranolol, like the other β-receptor antagonists that are discussed, is a competitive antagonist whose receptor-blocking actions can be reversed with sufficient concentrations of β agonists. Currently, propranolol is approved for use in the United States for hypertension, cardiac arrhythmias, angina pectoris, postmyocardial infarction, hypertrophic cardiomyopathy, pheochromocytoma, migraine prophylaxis, and essential tremor. In addition, propranolol is under investigation for the treatment of a variety of other conditions, including anxiety, schizophrenia, alcohol withdrawal syndrome, and aggressive behavior.

Some of the most prominent effects of propranolol are on the cardiovascular system. By blocking the β receptors of the heart, propranolol slows the heart, reduces the force of contraction, and reduces cardiac output. Because of reflex sympathetic activity and blockade of vascular β₂ receptors, administration may result in increased peripheral resistance. The antihypertensive action, at least in part, may be attributed to its ability to reduce cardiac output, as well as to its suppression of renin release from the kidney. Because it exhibits no selectivity for β_1 receptors, it is contraindicated in the presence of conditions such as asthma and bronchitis.

A facet of the pharmacological action of propranolol that has received a good deal of attention is its so-called membrane-stabilizing activity. This is a nonspecific effect (i.e., not mediated by a specific receptor), which is also referred to as a *local anesthetic effect* or a *quinidine-like effect*. Both enantiomers possess membrane-stabilizing activity. Since the concentrations required to produce this effect far exceed those obtained with normal therapeutic doses of propranolol and related β-blocking drugs, it is most unlikely that the nonspecific membrane-stabilizing activity plays any role in the clinical efficacy of β-blocking agents.

The metabolism of propranolol has received intense study. Propranolol is well absorbed after oral administration, but it undergoes extensive first-pass metabolism before it reaches the systemic circulation. Lower doses are extracted more efficiently than higher doses, indicating that the extraction process may become saturated at higher doses. In addition, the active enantiomer is cleared more slowly than the inactive enantiomer.[62]

Numerous metabolites of propranolol have been identified, but the major metabolite in people, after a single oral dose, is naphthoxylactic acid, which is formed by a series of metabolic reactions involving N-dealkylation, deamination, and oxidation of the resultant aldehyde. One metabolite of particular interest is 4-hydroxypropranolol. This compound is a potent β antagonist that has some intrinsic sympathomimetic activity. It is not known what contribution, if any, 4-hydroxypropranolol makes to the pharmacological effects seen after administration of propranolol. The half-life of propranolol after a single oral dose is 3 to 4 hours, which increases to 4 to 6 hours after long-term therapy.

Naphthoxylactic Acid

4-Hydroxypropranolol

Other Nonselective β Blockers. Several other nonselective β blockers are used clinically. These include **nadolol** (Corgard), **pindolol** (Visken), **penbutolol** (Levatol), **carteo-**

lol (Cartrol, Ocupress), **timolol** (Blocadren, Timoptic), **levobunolol** (Betagan), **sotalol** (Betapace) and **metipranolol** (OptiPranolol). Structures of these compounds are shown in Figure 16-8. The first five of these agents are used to treat hypertension. Nadolol is also used in the long-term management of angina pectoris, while timolol finds use in the prophylaxis of migraine headaches and in the therapy following myocardial infarction. Sotalol is used as an antiarrhythmic in treating ventricular arrhythmias and atrial fibrillation because in addition to its β-adrenergic blocking activity, this agent blocks the inward K^+ current that delays cardiac repolarization.

Carteolol, timolol, levobunolol, and metipranolol are used topically to treat open-angle glaucoma. These agents lower intraocular pressure with virtually no effect on pupil size or accommodation. They thus offer an advantage over many of the other drugs used in the treatment of glaucoma. Although the precise mechanism whereby β blockers lower intraocular pressure is not known with certainty, it is believed that they may reduce the production of aqueous humor. Even though these agents are administered into the eye, systemic absorption can occur, producing such adverse effects as bradycardia and acute bronchospasm in patients with bronchospastic disease.

Pindolol possesses modest membrane-stabilizing activity and significant intrinsic β-agonistic activity. Penbutolol and carteolol also have partial agonistic activity but not to the degree that pindolol does. The β antagonists with partial agonistic activity cause less slowing of the resting heart rate than do agents without this capability. The partial agonistic activity may be beneficial in patients who are likely to exhibit severe bradycardia or who have little cardiac reserve.

Timolol, pindolol, penbutolol, and carteolol have half-life values in the same range as propranolol. The half-life of nadolol, however, is about 20 hours, making it one of the longest-acting β blockers. Timolol undergoes first-pass metabolism but not to the same extent that propranolol does. Timolol and penbutolol are metabolized extensively, with little or no unchanged drug excreted in the urine. Pindolol is metabolized by the liver to the extent of 60%, with the remaining 40% being excreted in the urine unchanged. In contrast, nadolol undergoes very little hepatic metabolism. Most of this drug is excreted unchanged in the urine.

β_1-SELECTIVE BLOCKERS

The discovery that β-blocking agents are useful in the treatment of cardiovascular disease, such as hypertension, stimulated a search for cardioselective β blockers. Cardioselective β antagonists are drugs that have a greater affinity for the β_1 receptors of the heart than for β_2 receptors in other tissues. Such cardioselective agents should provide two important therapeutic advantages. The first advantage should be the lack of an antagonistic effect on the β_2 receptors in the bronchi. Theoretically, this would make β_1 blockers safe for use in patients who have bronchitis or bronchial asthma. The second advantage should be the absence of blockade of the vascular β_2 receptors, which mediate vasodilation. This would be expected to reduce or eliminate the increase in peripheral resistance that sometimes occurs after the administration of nonselective β antagonists. Unfortunately, cardi-

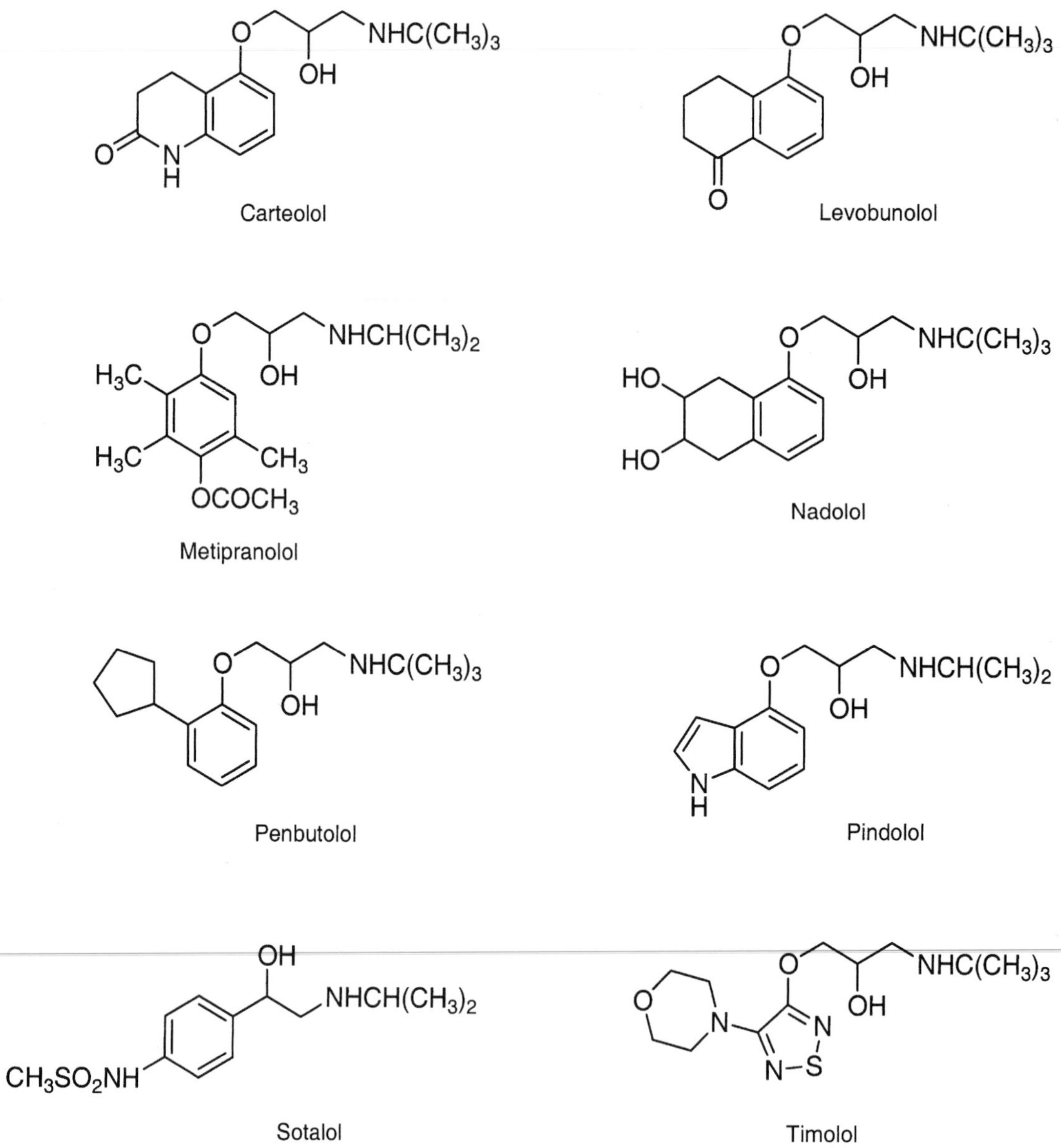

Figure 16–8 ■ Nonselective β blockers.

oselectivity is usually observed with β_1 antagonists at only relatively low doses. At normal therapeutic doses, much of the selectivity is lost.

At present, the following β_1-selective agents are used therapeutically: **acebutolol** (Sectral), **atenolol** (Tenormin), **betaxolol** (Kerlone, Betoptic), **bisoprolol** (Zebeta), **esmolol** (Brevibloc), and **metoprolol** (Lopressor). Structures of these agents are depicted in Figure 16-9. All of these agents except esmolol are indicated for the treatment of hypertension. Atenolol and metoprolol are also approved for use in treating angina pectoris and in therapy following myocardial infarction. Betaxolol is the only β_1-selective blocker indicated for the treatment of glaucoma.

Acebutolol and esmolol are indicated for treating certain cardiac arrhythmias. Esmolol was designed specifically to possess a very short duration of action; it has an elimination half-life of 9 minutes. This agent is administered by continuous intravenous infusion for control of ventricular rate in

patients with atrial flutter, atrial fibrillation, or sinus tachycardia. Its rapid onset and short duration of action render it useful during surgery, after an operation, or during emergency situations for short-term control of heart rates. Its effects disappear within 20 to 30 minutes after the infusion is discontinued. Esmolol must be diluted with an injection solution before administration; it is incompatible with sodium bicarbonate.

The short duration of action of esmolol is the result of rapid hydrolysis of its ester functionality by esterases present in erythrocytes (Fig. 16-10). The resultant carboxylic acid is an extremely weak β antagonist that does not appear to exhibit clinically significant effects. The acid metabolite has an elimination half-life of 3 to 4 hours and is excreted primarily by the kidneys.

In the class of β_1-selective blockers, only acebutolol possesses intrinsic sympathomimetic activity. This activity is very weak, however. Acebutolol and betaxolol possess

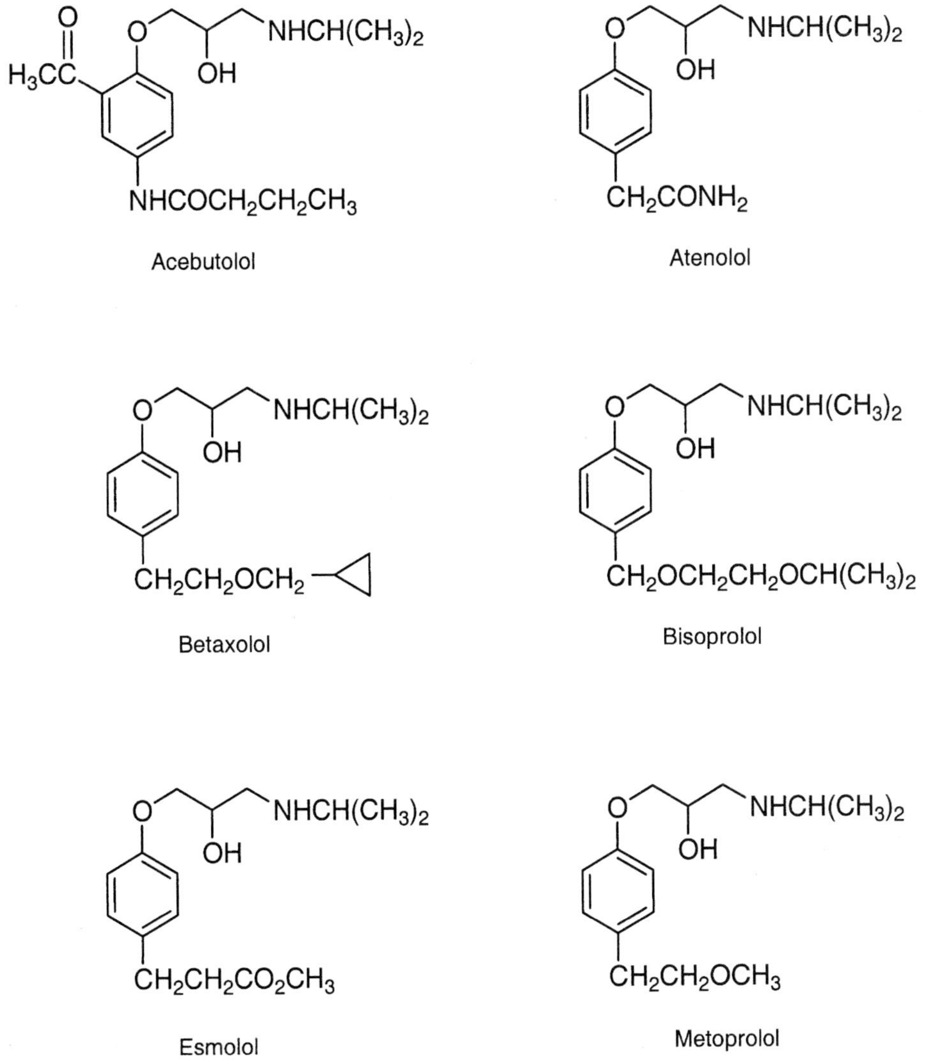

Acebutolol

Atenolol

Betaxolol

Bisoprolol

Esmolol

Metoprolol

Figure 16–9 ■ β_1-Selective blockers.

membrane-stabilizing activity, but the activity is much weaker than that seen with propranolol.

The half-life values of acebutolol and metoprolol are comparable to that seen with propranolol, and those of atenolol and bisoprolol are about twice that of propranolol. Betaxolol,

Esmolol

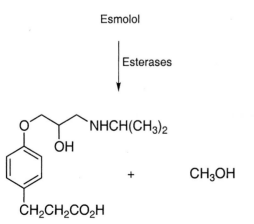

Esterases

+ CH$_3$OH

Figure 16–10 ■ Metabolism of esmolol.

with a half-life ranging between 14 and 22 hours, has the longest duration of action of the β_1-selective blockers. Like propranolol, metoprolol has low bioavailability because of significant first-pass metabolism. Although the bioavailability of betaxolol is very high, it is metabolized extensively by the liver, with very little unchanged drug excreted in the urine. Atenolol, like nadolol, has low lipid solubility and does not readily cross the blood–brain barrier. It is absorbed incompletely from the gastrointestinal tract, the oral bioavailability being approximately 50%. Little of the absorbed portion of the dose is metabolized; most of it is excreted unchanged in the urine. In the case of bisoprolol, about 50% of a dose undergoes hepatic metabolism, while the remaining 50% is excreted in the urine unchanged.

Acebutolol is one of the very few β blockers whose metabolite plays a significant role in its pharmacological actions. This drug is absorbed well from the gastrointestinal tract, but it undergoes extensive first-pass metabolic conversion to diacetolol. Diacetolol is formed by hydrolytic conversion of the amide group to the amine, followed by acetylation of the amine (Fig. 16-11). After oral administration, plasma levels of diacetolol are higher than those of acebutolol. Diacetolol is also a selective β_1-receptor antagonist with partial

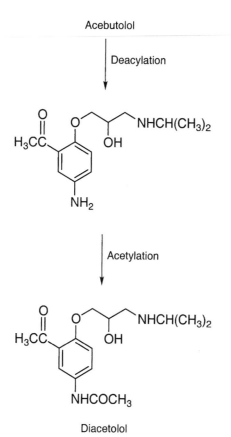

Figure 16–11 ■ Metabolism of acebutolol.

agonistic activity; it has little membrane-stabilizing activity. It has a longer half-life (8 to 12 hours) than the parent drug and is excreted by the kidneys.

β BLOCKERS WITH α_1-RECEPTOR ANTAGONIST ACTIVITY

Several drugs have been developed that possess both β- and α-receptor–blocking activities within the same molecule. Two examples of such molecules are labetalol (Normodyne) and carvedilol (Coreg).

Labetalol.

Labetalol (Normodyne) is a phenylethanol-amine derivative that is a competitive inhibitor at both β_1- and β_2-adrenergic receptors and at the α_1-adrenergic receptor. It is a more potent β antagonist than α antagonist. Since it has two asymmetric carbon atoms (1 and 1′), it exists as a mixture of four isomers. It is this mixture that is used clinically in treating hypertension. The different isomers, however, possess different α- and β-antagonistic activities. The β-blocking activity resides solely in the (1R,1′R) isomer, while the α_1-antagonistic activity is seen in the (1S,1′R) and (1S,1′S) isomers, with the (1S,1′R) isomer possessing the greater activity.[63] Labetalol is a clinically useful antihypertensive agent. The rationale for its use in the management of hypertension is that its α-receptor–blocking effects produce vasodilation and its β-receptor–blocking effects prevent the reflex tachycardia usually associated with vasodilation. Although labetalol is very well absorbed, it undergoes extensive first-pass metabolism.

Carvedilol.

Carvedilol (Coreg), like labetalol, is a β blocker that possesses α_1-adrenergic receptor-blocking activity. Only the (S) enantiomer possesses the β-blocking activity, while both enantiomers are antagonists of the α_1-adrenergic receptor.[64] This drug is also unique in that it possesses antioxidant activity and an antiproliferative effect on vascular smooth muscle cells. It thus has a neuroprotective effect and the ability to provide major cardiovascular organ protection.[65] It is used in treating hypertension and congestive heart failure.

REFERENCES

1. Ganellin, C. R.: J. Med. Chem. 20:579, 1977.
2. Musacchio, J. M.: Enzymes involved in the biosynthesis and degradation of catecholamines. In Iversen, L. L., Iversen, S. D., and Snyder, S. H. (eds.). Handbook of Psychopharmacology, vol. 3, Biochemistry of Biogenic Amines. New York, Plenum Press, 1975.
3. Masserano, J. M., et al.: The role of tyrosine hydroxylase in the regulation of catecholamine synthesis. In Trendelenburg, U., and Weiner, N. (eds.). Handbook of Experimental Pharmacology, vol. 90/II, Catecholamines II. Berlin, Springer-Verlag, 1989.
4. Borowsky, B., and Hoffman, B. J.: Int. Rev. Neurobiol. 38:139, 1995.
5. Schuldiner, S.: J. Neurochem. 62:2067, 1994.
6. Kopin, I. J.: Pharmacol. Rev. 37:333, 1985.
7. Dostert, P. L., Benedetti, M. S., and Tipton, K. F.: Med. Res. Rev. 9: 45, 1989.
8. Boulton, A. A., and Eisenhofer, G.: Adv. Pharmacol. 42:273, 1998.
9. Ahlquist, R. P.: Am. J. Physiol. 153:586, 1948.
10. Langer, S. Z.: Biochem. Pharmacol. 23:1793, 1974.
11. Berthelsen, S., and Pettinger, W. A.: Life Sci. 21:595, 1977.
12. McGrath, J. C.: Biochem. Pharmacol. 31:467, 1982.
13. Bylund, D. B., et al.: Pharmacol. Rev. 46:121, 1994.
14. Hieble, J. P., et al.: Pharmacol. Rev. 47:267, 1995.
15. Hieble, J. P., and Ruffolo, R. R., Jr.: Prog. Drug Res. 47:81, 1996.
16. Ruffolo, R. R., Jr., and Hieble, J. P.: Pharmacol. Ther. 61:1, 1994.
17. Ruffolo, R. R., Jr., Stadel, J. M., and Hieble, J. P.: Med. Res. Rev. 14: 229, 1994.
18. Ruffolo, R. R., Jr., Nichols, A. J., and Hieble, J. P.: Functions mediated by alpha-2 adrenergic receptors. In Limbird, L. E. (ed.). The Alpha-2 Adrenergic Receptor. Clifton, NJ, Humana Press, 1988, p. 187.
19. Broadley, K. J.: J. Auton. Pharmacol. 2:119, 1982.
20. Timmermans, P. B. M. W. M.: Centrally acting hypotensive drugs. In van Zwieten, P. A. (ed.). Handbook of Hypertension, vol 3. Pharmacology of Antihypertensive Drugs. Amsterdam, Elsevier, 1984, p. 102.
21. Langer, S. Z., and Hicks, P. E.: J. Cardiovasc. Pharmacol. 6(Suppl. 4): S547, 1984.
22. Ruffolo, R. R., Jr., Nichols, A. J., and Hieble, J. P.: Life Sci. 49:171, 1991.

23. Lands, A. M., et al.: Nature 214:597, 1967.
24. Arch, J. R., et al.: Nature 309:163, 1984.
25. Gilman, A. G.: Annu. Rev. Biochem. 56:615, 1987.
26. Lefkowitz, R. J., et al.: Trends Pharmacol. Sci. 7:444, 1986.
27. Nestor, E. J., Walaas, S. I., and Greengard, P.: Science 225:1357, 1984.
28. Ostrowski, J., et al.: Annu. Rev. Pharmacol. Toxicol. 32:167, 1992.
29. Buscher, R., Herrmann, V., and Insel, P. A.: Trends Pharmacol. Sci. 20:94, 1999.
30. Brogden, R. N., et al.: Drugs 21:81, 1981.
31. Rudnick, G., et al.: Biochemistry 29:603, 1990.
32. Palmer, J. D., and Nugent, C. A.: Pharmacotherapy 3:220, 1983.
33. Triggle, D. J.: Adrenergics: catecholamines and related agents. In Wolff, M. E. (ed.). Burger's Medicinal Chemistry, 4th ed., part III. New York, John Wiley & Sons, 1981.
34. Nichols, A. J., and Ruffolo, R. R., Jr.: Structure–activity relationships for α-adrenoreceptor agonists and antagonists. In Ruffolo, R. R., Jr. (ed.). α-Adrenoceptors: Molecular Biology, Biochemistry, and Pharmacology. Progress in Basic Clinical Pharmacology, vol. 8. Basel, Karger, 1991, p. 75.
35. Hieble, J. P.: Structure–activity relationships for activation and blockade of β-adrenoceptors. In Ruffolo, R. R., Jr. (ed.). β-Adrenoceptors: Molecular Biology, Biochemistry, and Pharmacology. Progress in Basic Clinical Pharmacology, vol. 7. Basel, Karger, 1991, p. 105.
36. Easson, L. H., and Stedman, E.: Biochem. J. 27:1257, 1933.
37. Ruffolo, R. R., Jr., and Waddel, J. E.: J. Pharmacol. Exp. Ther. 224: 559, 1983.
38. Langer, S. Z., Cavero, I., and Massingham, R.: Hypertension 2:372, 1980.
39. de Jonge, A., Timmermans, P. B. M. W. M., and van Zwieten, P. A.: Naunyn-Schmiedebergs Arch. Pharmacol. 317:8, 1981.
40. Comer, W. T., and Matier, W. L.: Antihypertensive agents. In Wolff, M. E. (ed.). Burger's Medicinal Chemistry, 4th ed., part III. New York, John Wiley & Sons, 1981, p. 285.
41. Bricca, G., et al.: Eur. J. Pharmacol. 266:25, 1994.
42. French, N.: Pharmacol. Ther. 68:175, 1995.
43. Bousquet, P., et al.: Ann. N. Y. Acad. Sci. 881:272, 1999.
44. Head, G. A.: Ann. N. Y. Acad. Sci. 881:279, 1999.
45. MacMillan, L. B., et al.: Science 273:801, 1996.
46. Link, R. E., et al.: Science 273:803, 1996.
47. Ruffolo, R. R., Jr., et al.: Annu. Rev. Pharmacol. Toxicol. 33:243, 1993.
48. Davies, J., and Quinlan, J. E.: Neuroscience 16:673, 1985.
49. Ruffolo, R. R., Jr., et al.: J. Pharmacol. Exp. Ther. 219:447, 1981.
50. Majerus, T. C., et al.: Pharmacotherapy 9:245, 1989.
51. Clark, R. B., et al.: Mol. Pharmacol. 49:182, 1996.
52. Anderson, G. P., Linden, A., and Rabe, K. F.: Eur. Respir. J. 7:569, 1994.
53. Weber, A. E.: Annu. Rep. Med. Chem. 33:193, 1998.
54. Henkel, J. G., and Portoghese, P. S.: J. Med. Chem. 19:6, 1976.
55. Honkanen, E., et al.: J. Med. Chem. 26:1433, 1983.
56. Ferry, N., et al.: Br. J. Pharmacol. 78:359, 1983.
57. Holm, K. J. and Markham, A.: Drugs 57:607, 1999.
58. Powell, C. E., and Slater, I. H.: J. Pharmacol. Exp. Ther. 122:480, 1958.
59. Black, J. W. and Stephenson, J. S.: Lancet 2:311, 1962.
60. Kaiser, C., et al.: J. Med. Chem. 20:687, 1977.
61. Riddell, J. G., Harron, D. W. G., and Shank, R. G.: Clin. Pharmacokinet. 12:305, 1987.
62. Walle, T., et al.: Biochem. Pharmacol. 37:115, 1988.
63. Gold, E. H., et al.: J. Med. Chem. 25:1363, 1982.
64. Nichols, A. J., et al.: Chirality 1:265, 1989.
65. Lysko, P. G., Feuerstein, G. Z., and Ruffolo, R. R., Jr.: Pharm. News 2:12, 1995.

SELECTED READING

Cooper, J. R., Bloom, F. E., and Roth, R. H.: The Biochemical Basis of Neuropharmacology, 7th ed. New York, Oxford University Press, 1996.

Goldstein, D. S., Eosenhofer, G., and McCarthy, R (eds.): Catecholamines: Bridging Basic Science with Clinical Medicine, vol. 42. In Advances in Pharmacology. San Diego, Academic Press, 1998.

Hieble, J. P., Bondinell, W. E., and Ruffolo, R. R., Jr.: α- and β-Adrenoceptors: From the Gene to the Clinic. 1. Molecular Biology and Adrenoceptor Subclassification. J. Med. Chem. 38:3415, 1995.

Hoffman, B. B.: Catecholamines, sympathetic drugs, and adrenergic receptors antagonists. In Hardman, J. G., and Limbird, L. E. (eds.). The Pharmacological Basis of Therapeutics, 10th ed. New York, McGraw-Hill, 2001, p. 215.

Lefkowitz, R. J., Hoffman, B. B., and Taylor, P.: Neurotransmission: The autonomic and somatic motor nervous systems. In Hardman, J. G., and Limbird, L. E. (eds.). The Pharmacological Basis of Therapeutics, 10th ed. New York, McGraw-Hill, 2001, p. 115.

Main, B. G.: β-Adrenergic receptors. In Hansch, C., Sammes, P. G., and Taylor, J. B. (eds.). Comprehensive Medicinal Chemistry, vol. 3, Membranes and Receptors. Oxford, Pergamon Press, 1990, p. 187.

Ruffolo, R. R., Jr., Bondinell, W., and Hieble, J. P.: α- and β-Adrenoceptors: From the Gene to the Clinic. 2. Structure-Activity Relationships and Therapeutic Applications. J. Med. Chem. 38:3681, 1995.

Timmermans, P. B. M. W. M., Chiu, A. T., and Thoolen, M. J. M. C.: α-Adrenergic receptors. In Hansch, C., Sammes, P. G., and Taylor, J. B. (eds.). Comprehensive Medicinal Chemistry, vol. 3, Membranes and Receptors. Oxford, Pergamon Press, 1990, p. 133.

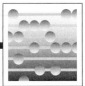

Cholinergic Drugs and Related Agents

GEORGE H. COCOLAS AND STEPHEN J. CUTLER

Few systems, if any, have been studied as extensively as those innervated by neurons that release acetylcholine (ACh) at their endings. Since the classic studies of Dale,[1] who described the actions of the esters and ethers of choline on isolated organs and their relationship to muscarine, pharmacologists, physiologists, chemists, and biochemists have applied their knowledge to understand the actions of the cholinergic nerve and its neurotransmitter. Advances in the applications of biotechnology and chemistry have developed probes that have uncovered the complexity of the action of ACh on cholinergic neurons and receptors, unknown when ACh was first demonstrated in the frog heart in 1921 by Loewi as the substance released by vagus nerve stimulation.[2]

This chapter includes the drugs and chemicals that act on cholinergic nerves or the tissues they innervate to either mimic or block the action of ACh. Drugs that mimic the action of ACh do so either by acting directly on the cholinergic receptors in the tissue or by inhibiting acetylcholinesterase (AChE), the enzyme that inactivates ACh at the nerve terminal. Chemicals that bind or compete with ACh for binding to the receptor may block cholinergic neurotransmission.

$$H_3C-\underset{\underset{CH_3}{|}}{\overset{\overset{CH_3}{|}}{N^+}}-\underset{\alpha}{CH_2}-\underset{\beta}{CH_2}-O-\overset{\overset{O}{||}}{C}-CH_3$$

Acetylcholine

Cholinergic nerves are found in the peripheral nervous system and central nervous system (CNS) of humans. Its presence in the CNS is currently receiving the most attention, as researchers are beginning to unlock the mysteries surrounding cognitive impairment and, most particularly, Alzheimer's disease. Synaptic terminals in the cerebral cortex, corpus striatum, hippocampus, and several other regions in the CNS are rich in ACh and in the enzymes that synthesize and hydrolyze this neurotransmitter. Many experiments show that agonists and antagonists of cholinergic receptors can modify the output of neurotransmitters, including ACh, from brain preparations. Although the function of ACh in the brain and brainstem is not clear, it has been implicated in memory and behavioral activity in humans.[3] The *peripheral nervous system* consists of those nerves outside the cerebrospinal axis and includes the somatic nerves and the autonomic nervous system. The *somatic nerves* are made up of a sensory (afferent) nerve and a motor (efferent) nerve. The *motor nerves* arise from the spinal cord and project uninterrupted throughout the body to all skeletal muscle. ACh mediates transmission of impulses from the motor nerve to skeletal muscle (i.e., neuromuscular junction).

The *autonomic nervous system* is composed of two divisions: *sympathetic* and *parasympathetic*. ACh serves as a neurotransmitter at both sympathetic and parasympathetic preganglionic nerve endings, postganglionic nerve fibers in the parasympathetic division, and some postganglionic fibers (e.g., salivary and sweat glands) in the sympathetic division of the autonomic nervous system. The autonomic nervous system regulates the activities of smooth muscle and glandular secretions. These, as a rule, function below the level of consciousness (e.g., respiration, circulation, digestion, body temperature, metabolism). The two divisions have contrasting effects on the internal environment of the body. The sympathetic division frequently discharges as a unit, especially during conditions of rage or fright, and expends energy. The parasympathetic division is organized for discrete and localized discharge and stores and conserves energy.

Drugs and chemicals that cause the parasympathetic division to react are termed *parasympathomimetic,* whereas those blocking the actions are called *parasympatholytic.* Agents that mimic the sympathetic division are *sympathomimetic,* and those that block the actions are *sympatholytic.* Another classification used to describe drugs and chemicals acting on the nervous system or the structures that the fibers innervate is based on the neurotransmitter released at the nerve ending. Drugs acting on the autonomic nervous system are divided into *adrenergic,* for those postganglionic sympathetic fibers that release norepinephrine and epinephrine, and *cholinergic,* for the remaining fibers in the autonomic nervous system and the motor fibers of the somatic nerves that release ACh.

CHOLINERGIC RECEPTORS

There are two distinct receptor types for ACh that differ in composition, location, and pharmacological function and have specific agonists and antagonists. Cholinergic receptors have been characterized as *nicotinic* and *muscarinic* on the basis of their ability to be bound by the naturally occurring alkaloids nicotine and muscarine, respectively. Receptor subtypes that differ in location and specificity to agonists and antagonists have been identified for both the nicotinic and muscarinic receptors.

Nicotinic Receptors

Nicotinic receptors are coupled directly to ion channels and, when activated by Ach, mediate very rapid responses. Ion

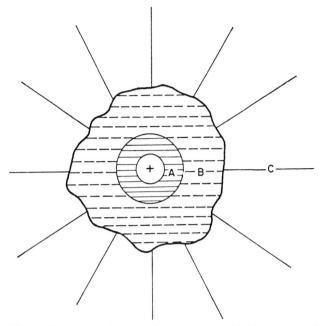

Figure 17–1 ■ Hydrated cation showing a highly structured shell of water around the cation *(A)*, a less structured layer surrounding the inner water shell *(B)*, and water in a "normal" state *(C)*. (With permission from the author and the Royal Society of Chemistry.)

TABLE 17–1   Radii of Alkali and Alkali Earth Cations

Ion	Ionic Radius (Å)	Effective Hydrated Radius (Å)
Li^+	0.60	4.5
Na^+	0.95	3.4
K^+	1.33	2.2
Rb^+	1.48	1.9
Cs^+	1.69	1.9
Mg^{2+}	0.65	5.9
Ca^{2+}	0.99	4.5
Sr^{2+}	1.13	3.7
Ba^{2+}	1.35	3.7

From Triggle, D. J.: Neurotransmitter-Receptor Interactions. San Diego, Academic Press, 1971.

channels are responsible for the electrical excitability of nerve and muscle cells and for the sensitivity of sensory cells. The channels are pores that open or close in an all-or-nothing fashion on time scales ranging from 0.1 to 10 milliseconds to provide aqueous pathways through the plasma membrane that ions can transverse. Factors affecting selectivity of ion pores include both the charge and size of the ion. Ions in aqueous solution are hydrated. The water around the ion is characterized by the presence of two distinct water structures: a tightly bound, highly ordered layer immediately surrounding the ion and a second, less structured layer[4] (Fig. 17-1). Ion transport through a channel requires some denuding of the surrounding water shell. The degree of organization of the water structure determines the energy required to remove the hydration shell and is a factor

in the selectivity of that ion channel.[5] Table 17-1 lists the effective radii of alkali and alkaline earth cations.

The nicotinic ACh receptor was the first neurotransmitter isolated and purified in an active form.[6] It is a glycoprotein embedded into the polysynaptic membrane that can be obtained from the electric organs of the marine ray *Torpedo california* and the electric eel *Electrophorus electricus*. The receptor is pictured as a cylindrical protein of about 250,000 Da and consists of five-subunit polypeptide chains, of which two appear to be identical.[7, 8] The subunit stoichiometry of the polypeptide units from the *Torpedo* receptor is $\alpha_2, \beta, \gamma, \delta$.[9] The peptide chains of the receptor are arranged to form an opening in the center, which is the ion channel. Each α chain contains a negatively charged binding site for the quaternary ammonium group of ACh. The receptor appears to exist as a dimer of the two five-subunit polypeptide chain monomers linked through a disulfide bond between δ chains. A structural protein of molecular weight 43,000 binds the nicotinic receptor to the membrane (Fig. 17-2). With so many variables in the subunits, many combinations of nicotinic subtype receptors are available.

When the neurotransmitter ACh binds to the nicotinic receptor, it causes a change in the permeability of the membrane to allow passage of small cations Ca^{2+}, Na^+, and

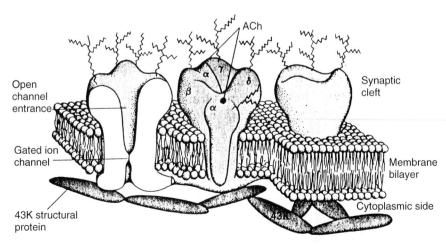

Figure 17–2 ■ Model of the nicotinic receptor consisting of five protein subunits embedded in a cell membrane, based on electron microscopy and neutron scattering data. *Jagged lines* represent oligosaccharide chains on the upper part of the receptor. A 43K protein is bound to the receptor on the cytosolic side of the cell membrane. The ACh-binding sites are shown on the two-subunit proteins. (Reprinted with permission from Lindstrom, J. M., et al.: Cold Spring Harbor Symp. Quant. Biol. 48:93, 1983.)

K^+. The physiological effect is to temporarily depolarize the end plate. This depolarization results in muscular contraction at a neuromuscular junction or, as occurs in autonomic ganglia, continuation of the nerve impulse. Neuromuscular nicotinic ACh receptors are of interest as targets for autoimmune antibodies in myasthenia gravis and for muscle relaxants used during the course of surgical procedures. Nicotinic receptors in autonomic ganglia, when blocked by drugs, can play a role in the control of hypertension.

NICOTINIC RECEPTOR SUBTYPES

Nicotinic receptors located in the neuromuscular junction differ from those on neurons, such as those in the CNS and autonomic ganglia, in that they have different ligand specificities. Nicotinic receptors at the neuromuscular junction (N_1) are blocked by succinylcholine, *d*-tubocurarine, and decamethonium and stimulated by phenyltrimethylammonium. N_2 nicotinic receptors are found in autonomic ganglia. They are blocked by hexamethonium and trimethaphan but stimulated by tetramethylammonium and dimethyl-4-phenylpiperazinium (DMPP). Nicotinic receptor subtypes have also been identified in many regions of the CNS; however, their pharmacological function is not yet fully understood.[10] Even so, great attempts are being made to understand the role of so many receptor subtypes, particularly those found in the CNS.[11, 12]

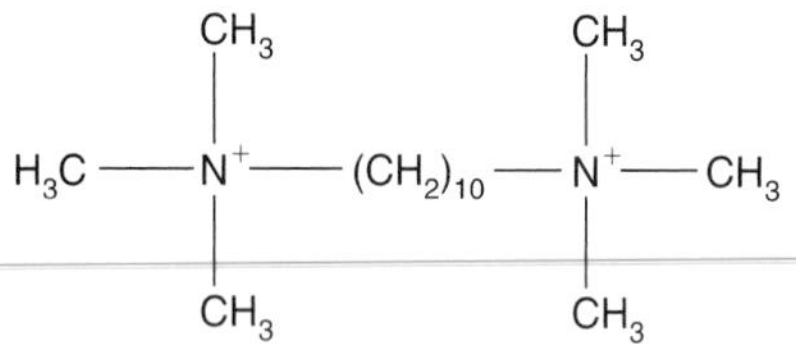

Decamethonium

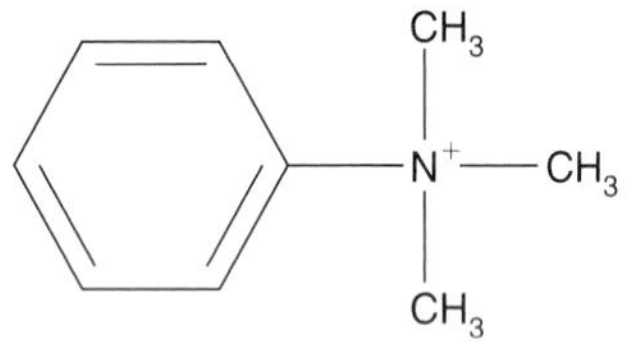

Phenyltrimethylammonium

Muscarinic Receptors

Muscarinic receptors play an essential role in regulating the functions of organs innervated by the autonomic nervous system to maintain homeostasis of the organism. The action of ACh on muscarinic receptors can result in stimulation or inhibition of the organ system affected. ACh stimulates secretions from salivary and sweat glands, secretions and contraction of the gut, and constriction of the airways of the respiratory tract. It inhibits contraction of the heart and relaxes smooth muscle of blood vessels.

As early as 1980, it became apparent that a single muscar-

inic receptor type could not mediate the actions of ACh. Research on cholinergic receptors has increased since the 1980s, as these receptors represent potential targets for useful drugs for disease states that are becoming more prevalent because of our increasing population of aged persons. The outcome of these studies has been the discovery of several muscarinic receptor subtypes.

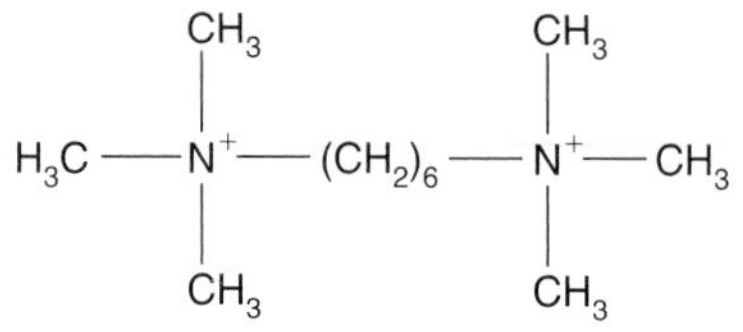

Hexamethonium

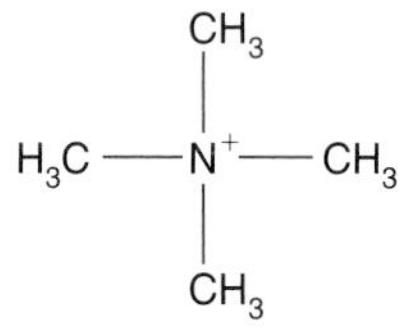

Tetramethylammonium

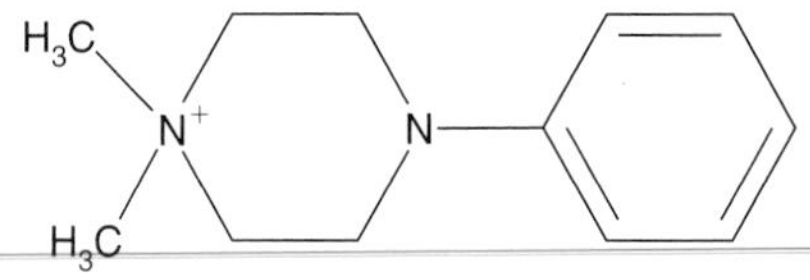

DMPP

Muscarinic receptors mediate their effects by activating guanosine triphosphate (GTP)-binding proteins (G proteins). These receptors have seven protein helixes that transcend the plasma membrane, creating four extracellular domains and four intracellular domains (Fig. 17-3). The extracellular domain of the receptor contains the binding site for ACh. The intracellular domain couples with G proteins to initiate biochemical changes that result in pharmacological action from receptor activation.

MUSCARINIC RECEPTOR SUBTYPES

Evidence from both pharmacological and biochemical studies shows that subtypes of muscarinic receptors are located in the CNS and peripheral nervous system.[13, 14] Molecular cloning studies have revealed the existence of five different molecular mammalian muscarinic receptor proteins. The cloned receptors have been identified as m_1 to m_5. In another method of identification, muscarinic receptor subtypes have been defined on the basis of their affinity for selective agonists and antagonists and the pharmacological effects they cause. These receptors are designated with capital letters and subscript numbers as M_1 to M_5. The nomenclature convention adopted for these receptors is that the pharmacologically defined subtypes M_1, M_2, and M_3 correspond to the geneti-

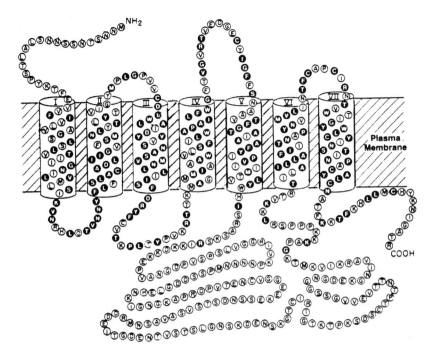

Figure 17–3 ■ Hypothetical model of a muscarinic receptor showing the location of the transmembrane helical protein domains and the extracellular and intracellular domains connecting the seven α-helical proteins in the membrane. (Reprinted from Goyal, R. K.: N. Engl. J. Med. 321:1024, 1989, with permission from the author and the Massachusetts Medical Society.)

cally defined subtypes m_1, m_2, and m_3. The m_4 gene-derived protein is referred to as the M_4 subtype and has many pharmacological properties similar to those of the M_2 subtype. The m_5 receptor gene product does not have an equivalent pharmacological profile.

M₁ Receptors. Even though molecules do not have exclusive selectivity on muscarinic receptor subtypes, M_1 receptors have been defined as those with high affinity for pirenzepine and low affinity for compounds such as AF-DX 116. They have been termed *neural* because of their distribution within particular brain structures. In addition to the CNS, M_1 receptors are located in exocrine glands and autonomic ganglia. In humans, these receptors seem to affect arousal attention, rapid eye movement (REM) sleep, emotional responses, affective disorders including depression, and modulation of stress. They are believed to participate in higher brain functions, such as memory and learning. Alzheimer's disease research has implicated cholinergic neurons and receptors, but evidence does not show conclusively that these are the primary causes of the disease. M_1 receptors have been identified in submucosal glands and some smooth muscle. They are located in parietal cells in the gastrointestinal (GI) tract and in peripheral autonomic ganglia, such as the intramural ganglia of the stomach wall. When stimulated, M_1 receptors cause gastric secretion.[15] Although McN-A-343 is a selective agonist, pirenzepine HCl acts as an antago-

nist and has been used outside the United States for the treatment of peptic ulcer disease.

M₂ Receptors. M_2 receptors are identified by their high affinity for methoctramine, a polyamine, and by their low affinity for pirenzepine. M_2 receptors are also called *cardiac* muscarinic receptors because they are located in the atria and conducting tissue of the heart. Their stimulation causes a decrease in the strength and rate of cardiac muscle contraction. These effects may be produced by affecting intracellular K^+ and Ca^{2+} levels in heart tissue. M_2 receptors activate K^+ channels to cause hyperpolarization of cardiac cells, resulting in bradycardia. These receptors may also act through an inhibitory G protein (G_i) to reduce adenylate cyclase activity and lower cyclic 3′,5′-adenosine monophosphate (cAMP) levels in cardiac cells. Lower cAMP levels decrease the amount of free Ca^{2+} in cardiac cells and slow down the heart rate.[16] M_2 receptors can also serve as autoreceptors on presynaptic terminals of postganglionic cholinergic nerves to inhibit ACh release. The balance of the effects of multiple muscarinic receptor subtypes determines the size of the airway of the smooth muscle in the bronchioles. Contraction is primarily the result of the action of ACh on M_3 receptors (see below) following stimulation of the vagus. At the same time, ACh stimulates inhibitor M_2 autoreceptors located on nerve endings to limit release of ACh. In asthmatics, neuronal M_2 receptors in the lungs do not function normally.[17]

McN-A-343

M₃ Receptors.   M₃ receptors, referred to as *glandular* muscarinic receptors, are located in exocrine glands and smooth muscle. Their effect on these organ systems is mostly stimulatory. Glandular secretions from lacrimal, salivary, bronchial, pancreatic, and mucosal cells in the GI tract are characteristic of M₃ receptor activation. Contraction of visceral smooth muscle is also a result of M₃ receptor stimulation. These stimulant effects are mediated through G protein activation of phospholipase C (PLC) to form the second messengers inositol triphosphate (IP₃) and diacylglycerol (DAG). Discoveries in the past decade have revealed that the endothelium can control the tone of vascular smooth muscle by the synthesis of a potent relaxant, endothelium-derived relaxing factor (EDRF), now identified as nitric oxide (NO), and a vasoconstrictor substance, endothelium-derived contracting factor (EDCF). The synthesis and release of these substances contribute to the tone of the vascular epithelium. M₃ receptors, when activated in endothelial cells, cause the release of EDRF and contribute to vasodilation.[18]

M₄ Receptors.   M₄ receptors, like M₂ receptors, act through G_i protein to inhibit adenylate cyclase. They also function by a direct regulatory action on K^+ and Ca^{2+} ion channels. M₄ receptors in tracheal smooth muscle, when stimulated, inhibit the release of ACh[19] in the same manner that M₂ receptors do.

M₅ Receptors.   A great deal of research remains to be performed on the M₅ subclass of receptors. Since the M₅ receptor messenger RNA (mRNA) is found in the substantia nigra, it has been suggested that M₅ receptors may regulate dopamine release at terminals within the striatum.

BIOCHEMICAL EFFECTS OF MUSCARINIC RECEPTOR STIMULATION

Transmission at the synapse involving second messengers is much slower, about 100 milliseconds, compared with the few milliseconds at synapses where ion channels are activated directly. The delayed reaction to receptor stimulation is due to a cascade of biochemical events that must occur to cause the pharmacological response (Fig. 17-4). The sequence of events in these second-messenger systems begins with activation of the receptors by an agonist and involves the activation of G proteins that are bound to a portion of the intracellular domain of the muscarinic receptor.[20] G proteins are so called because of their interaction with the guanine nucleotides GTP and guanosine diphosphate (GDP). They translate drug–receptor interactions at the surface of the cell to components inside the cell to create the biological response. G proteins consist of three subunits, α, β, and γ. When the receptor is occupied, the α subunit, which has enzymatic activity, catalyzes the conversion of GTP to GDP. The α subunit bound with GTP is the active form of the G protein that can associate with various enzymes (i.e., PLC and adenylate cyclase) and ion channels (K^+ and Ca^{2+}). G proteins are varied, and the α subunit may cause activation (G_s) or inactivation (G_i) of the enzymes or channels. Recent studies suggest that β and γ subunits also contribute to pharmacological effects.[21]

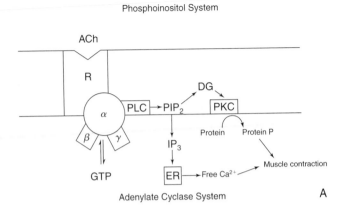

Phosphoinositol System

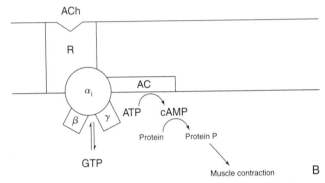

Adenylate Cyclase System

Figure 17–4 ■ Proposed biochemical mechanisms of cholinergic receptor action. **A.** ACh activates a G protein (α, β, γ) in the phospholipase system to activate the membrane enzyme phospholipase C (PLC), enhancing muscle contraction. **B.** Inhibition of adenylate cyclase system through an inhibitory G protein (α₁) to cause muscle relaxation.

A single drug–receptor complex can activate several G protein molecules, and each in turn can remain associated with a target molecule, e.g., an enzyme, and cause the production of many molecules, amplifying the result of the initial drug–receptor combination. M₁, M₃, and M₅ receptors activate PLC, causing the release of IP₃ and DAG, which in turn release intracellular Ca^{2+} and activate protein kinases, respectively. M₂ and M₄ receptors produce inhibition of adenylate cyclase.

Phosphoinositol System.   The phosphoinositol system requires the breakdown of membrane-bound phosphatidylinositol 4,5-diphosphate (PIP₂) by PLC to IP₃ and DAG, which serve as second messengers in the cell. IP₃ mobilizes Ca^{2+} from intracellular stores in the endoplasmic reticulum to elevate cytosolic free Ca^{2+}. The Ca^{2+} activates Ca^{2+}-dependent kinases (e.g., troponin C in muscle) directly or binds to the Ca^{2+}-binding protein calmodulin, which activates calmodulin-dependent kinases. These kinases phosphorylate cell-specific enzymes to cause muscle contraction. DAG is lipid-like and acts in the plane of the membrane through activation of protein kinase C to cause the phosphorylation of cellular proteins, also leading to muscle contraction (Fig. 17-4).[22, 23]

Adenylate Cyclase. Adenylate cyclase, a membrane enzyme, is another target of muscarinic receptor activation. The second messenger cAMP is synthesized within the cell from adenosine triphosphate (ATP) by the action of adenylate cyclase. The regulatory effects of cAMP are many, as it can activate a variety of protein kinases. Protein kinases catalyze the phosphorylation of enzymes and ion channels, altering the amount of calcium entering the cell and thus affecting muscle contraction. Muscarinic receptor activation causes lower levels of cAMP, reducing cAMP protein-dependent kinase activity, and a relaxation of muscle contraction. Some have suggested that a GTP-inhibitory protein (G_i) reduces the activity of adenylate cyclase, causing smooth muscle relaxation (Fig. 17-4).[20, 24]

Ion Channels. In addition to the action of protein kinases that phosphorylate ion channels and modify ion conductance, G proteins are coupled directly to ion channels to regulate their action.[24] The Ca^{2+} channel on the cell membrane is activated by G proteins without the need of a second messenger to allow Ca^{2+} to enter the cell. The α subunit of the G protein in heart tissue acts directly to open the K^+ channel, producing hyperpolarization of the membrane and slowing the heart rate.

CHOLINERGIC NEUROCHEMISTRY

Cholinergic neurons synthesize, store, and release ACh (Fig. 17-5). The neurons also form choline acetyltransferase (ChAT) and AChE. These enzymes are synthesized in the soma of the neuron and distributed throughout the neuron by axoplasmic flow. AChE is also located outside the neuron and is associated with the neuroglial cells in the synaptic cleft. ACh is prepared in the nerve ending by the transfer of an acetyl group from acetyl-coenzyme A (CoA) to choline. The reaction is catalyzed by ChAT. Cell fractionation studies show that much of the ACh is contained in synaptic vesicles in the nerve ending but that some is also free in the cytosol. Choline is the limiting substrate for the synthesis

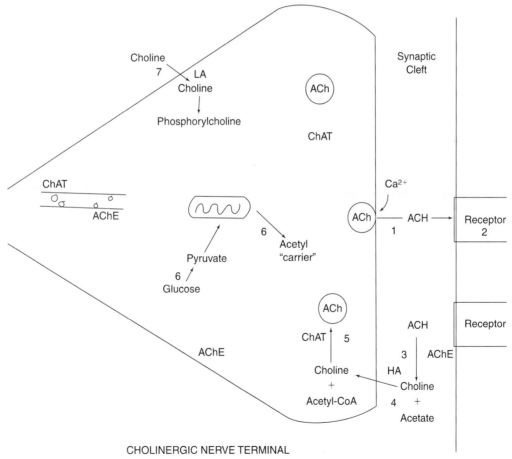

CHOLINERGIC NERVE TERMINAL

Figure 17–5 ■ Hypothetical model of synthesis, storage, and release of ACh. *(1)* ACh is released from storage granules under the influence of the nerve action potential and Ca^{2+}. *(2)* ACh acts on postsynaptic cholinergic receptors. *(3)* Hydrolysis of ACh by AChE occurs in the synaptic cleft. *(4)* A high-affinity uptake system returns choline to the cytosol. *(5)* ChAT synthesizes ACh in the cytosol, and the ACh is stored in granules. *(6)* Glucose is converted to pyruvate, which is converted to acetyl-CoA in the mitochondria. Acetyl-CoA is released from the mitochondria by an acetyl carrier. *(7)* Choline is also taken up into the neuron by a low-affinity uptake system and converted partly to phosphorylcholine.

Hemicholinium (HC-3)

2-Hydroxethyltriethylammonium

of ACh. Most choline for ACh synthesis comes from the hydrolysis of ACh in the synapse. Choline is recaptured by the presynaptic terminal as part of a high-affinity uptake system under the influence of sodium ions[25] to synthesize ACh.

Several quaternary ammonium bases act as competitive inhibitors of choline uptake. Hemicholinium (HC-3), a bisquaternary cyclic hemiacetal, and the triethyl analogue of choline, 2-hydroxyethyltriethylammonium, act at the presynaptic membrane to inhibit the high-affinity uptake of choline into the neuron. These compounds cause a delayed paralysis at repetitively activated cholinergic synapses and can produce respiratory paralysis in test animals. The delayed block is due to the depletion of stored ACh, which may be reversed by choline. The acetyl group used for the synthesis of ACh is obtained by conversion of glucose to pyruvate in the cytosol of the neuron and eventual formation of acetyl-CoA. Because of the impermeability of the mitochondrial membrane to acetyl-CoA, this substrate is brought into the cytosol by the aid of an acetyl ''carrier.''

The synthesis of ACh from choline and acetyl-CoA is catalyzed by ChAT. Transfer of the acetyl group from acetyl-CoA to choline may be by a random or an ordered reaction of the Theorell-Chance type. In the ordered sequence, acetyl-CoA first binds to the enzyme, forming a complex (EA) that then binds to choline. The acetyl group is transferred, and the ACh formed dissociates from the enzyme active site. The CoA is then released from the enzyme complex, EQ,

to regenerate the free enzyme. The scheme is diagrammed in Figure 17-6. ChAT is inhibited in vitro by *trans-N*-methyl-4-(1-naphthylvinyl)pyridinium iodide[26]; however, its inhibitory activity in whole animals is unreliable.[27]

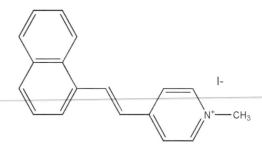

trans-N-Methyl-4-(1-napthylvinyl)pyridinium iodide

Newly formed ACh is released from the presynaptic membrane when a nerve action potential invades a presynaptic nerve terminal.[28] The release of ACh results from depolarization of the nerve terminal by the action potential, which alters membrane permeability to Ca^{2+}. Calcium enters the nerve terminal and causes release of the contents of several synaptic vesicles containing ACh into the synaptic cleft. This burst, or quantal release, of ACh causes depolarization of the postsynaptic membrane. The number of quanta of ACh released may be as high as several hundred at a neuromuscular junction, with each quantum containing between 12,000 and 60,000 molecules. ACh is also released spontaneously in small amounts from presynaptic membranes. This small amount of neurotransmitter maintains muscle tone by acting on the cholinergic receptors on the postsynaptic membrane.

After ACh has been released into the synaptic cleft, its concentration decreases rapidly. It is generally accepted that there is enough AChE at nerve endings to hydrolyze into choline and acetate any ACh that has been liberated. For example, there is sufficient AChE in the nerve junction of rat intercostal muscle to hydrolyze about 2.7×10^8 ACh molecules in 1 millisecond; this far exceeds the 3×10^6 molecules released by one nerve impulse.[29]

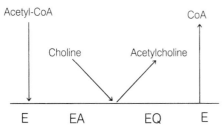

Figure 17–6 ■ Ordered synthesis of acetylcholine (ACh) by choline acetyltransferase (ChAT).

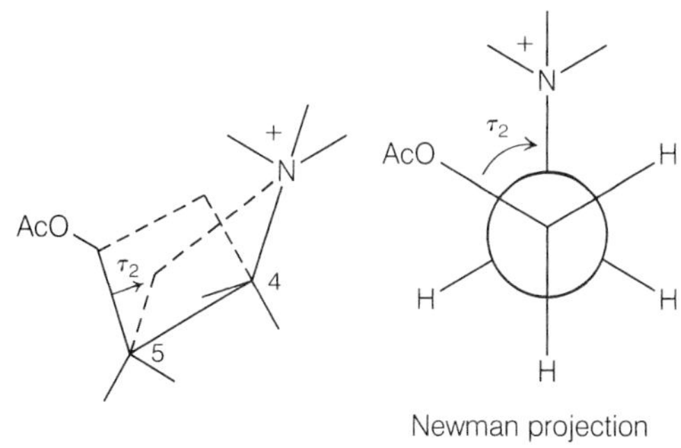

Figure 17–7 ■ Spatial orientation of O1–C5–C4–N atoms in ACh.

CHOLINERGIC AGONISTS

Cholinergic Stereochemistry

Three techniques have been used to study the conformational properties of ACh and other cholinergic chemicals: x-ray crystallography, nuclear magnetic resonance (NMR), and molecular modeling by computation. Each of these methods may report the spatial distribution of atoms in a molecule in terms of torsion angles. A *torsion angle* is defined as the angle formed between two planes, for example, by the O1–C5–C4–N atoms in ACh. The angle between the oxygen and nitrogen atoms is best depicted by means of Newman projections (Fig. 17-7). A torsion angle has a positive sign when the bond of the front atom is rotated to the right to eclipse the bond of the rear atom. The spatial orientation of ACh is described by four torsion angles (Fig. 17-8).

The conformation of the choline moiety of ACh has drawn the most attention in studies relating structure and pharmacological activity. The torsion angle (τ_2) determines the spatial orientation of the cationic head of ACh to the ester group. X-ray diffraction studies have shown that the torsion angle (τ_2) on ACh has a value of $+77°$. Many compounds that are muscarinic receptor agonists containing a choline component—e.g., O-C-C-N$^+$(CH$_3$)$_3$—have a preferred synclinal (gauche) conformation, with τ_2 values ranging from 68 to 89° (Table 17-2). Intermolecular packing forces in the crystal as well as electrostatic interactions between the charged nitrogen group and the ether oxygen of the ester group are probably the two dominant factors that lead to a preference for the synclinal conformation in the crystal state. Some choline esters display an antiperiplanar *(trans)* conformation between the onium and ester groups. For example, carbamoyl choline chloride (τ_2, $+178°$) is stabilized in this *trans* conformation by several hydrogen bonds. Acetylthiocholine iodide (τ_2, $+171°$) is in this conformation because of the presence of the bulkier and less electronegative sulfur

TABLE 17–2   Conformational Properties of Some Cholinergic Agents

Compound	O1-C5-C4-N Torsion Angle
Acetylcholine bromide	+77
Acetylcholine chloride	+85
(+)-2S,3R,5S-Muscarine iodide	+73
Methylfurmethide iodide	+83
(+)-Acetyl-(S)-β-methylcholine iodide	+85
(−)-Acetyl-(R)-α-methylcholine iodide	
Crystal form A	+89
Crystal form B	−150
(+)-cis(2S)-Methyl-(4R)-trimethylammonium-1,3-dioxolane iodide	+68
(+)-trans(1S, 2S)-Acetoxycyclopropyltrimethyl ammonium iodide	+137
Carbamoylcholine bromide	+178
Acetylthiocholine bromide	+171
Acetyl-(Rα, Sβ)-dimethylcholine iodide (*erythro*)	+76

From Shefter, E.: Structural variations in cholinergic legends. In Triggle, D. J., Moran, J. F., and Barnard, E. A. (eds.). Cholinergic Ligand Interactions. New York, Academic Press, 1971, pp. 87–89.

atom, and (+) *trans*-(1S,2S)-acetoxycyclopropyltrimethylammonium iodide (τ_2, $+137°$) is fixed in this conformation by the rigidity of the cyclopropyl ring.

NMR spectroscopy of cholinergic molecules in solution is more limited than crystallography in delineating the conformation of compounds and is restricted to determining the torsion angle O1–C5–C4–N. Most NMR data are in agreement with the results of x-ray diffraction studies. NMR studies indicate that ACh and methacholine apparently are not in their most stable *trans* conformation but exist in one of two gauche conformers[30] (Fig. 17-9). This may result from strong intramolecular interactions that stabilize the conformation of these molecules in solution.[31]

Molecular orbital calculations based on the principles of quantum mechanics may be used to determine energy minima of rotating bonds and to predict preferred conformations for the molecule. By means of molecular mechanics, theoretical conformational analysis has found that ACh has an energy minimum for the τ_2 torsion angle at about 84° and that the preferred conformation of ACh corresponds closely in aqueous solution to that found in the crystal state.

The study of interactions between bimolecules and small

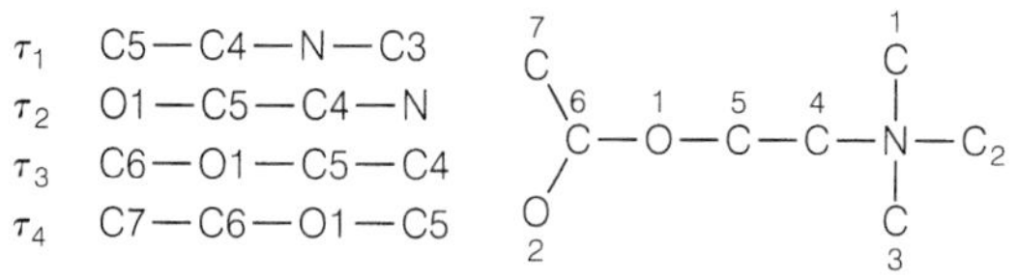

τ_1 C5—C4—N—C3
τ_2 O1—C5—C4—N
τ_3 C6—O1—C5—C4
τ_4 C7—C6—O1—C5

Figure 17–8 ■ ACh torsion angles.

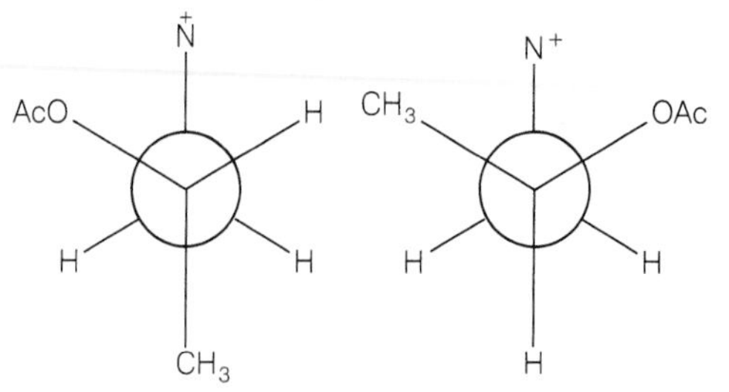

Figure 17–9 ■ Gauche conformers of methacholine.

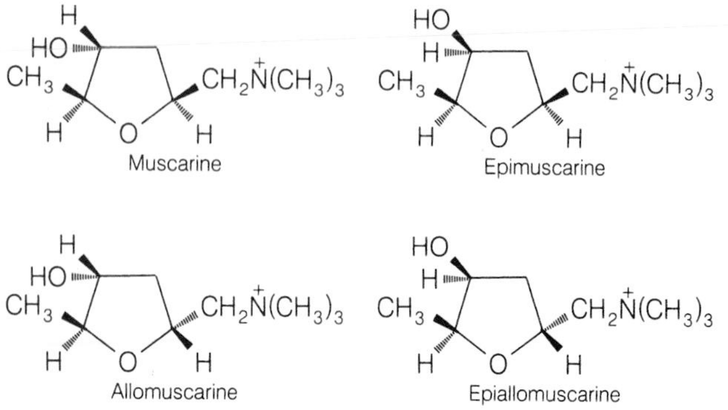

Figure 17–10 ■ Geometric isomers of muscarine.

molecules is of great interest and importance toward the understanding of drug action. These studies are challenging because of the large size of at least one molecule. For the first time, the conformation of a neurotransmitter has been determined for a molecule in the bound state. ACh is transformed from the gauche conformation in the free state to a nearly *trans* conformation when bound to the nicotinic receptor.[32] The active conformation of muscarinic agonists on their receptor has a dihedral angle of τ_2 between 110 and 117°.[33]

The parasympathomimetic effects of muscarine were first reported in 1869,[34] but its structure was not elucidated until 1957.[35] Muscarine has four geometric isomers: muscarine, epimuscarine, allomuscarine, and epiallomuscarine (Fig. 17-10). None has a center or plane of symmetry. Each geometric isomer can exist as an enantiomeric pair. The activity of muscarine, a nonselective muscarinic receptor agonist, resides primarily in the naturally occurring (+)-muscarine enantiomer. It is essentially free of nicotinic activity and apparently has the optimal stereochemistry to act on the muscarinic receptor subtypes. Synthetic molecules with a substituent on the carbon atom that corresponds to the β carbon of ACh also show great differences in muscarinic activity between their isomers. Acetyl-(+)-(*S*)-β-methylcholine, (+)-*cis*-(2*S*)-methyl-(4*R*)-trimethylammonium-

1,3-dioxolane, (+)-*trans*-(1*S*,2*S*)-acetoxycyclopropyltrimethylammonium, and naturally occurring (+)-(2*S*,3*R*,5*S*)-muscarine are more potent than their enantiomers and have very high ratios of activity between the (*S*) and (*R*) isomers (Table 17-3). A similar observation may be made of (+)-acetyl-(*S*)-β-methylcholine, (+)-*cis*-(2*S*)-methyl-(4*R*)-trimethylammonium-1,3-dioxolane, and (+)-*trans*-(1*S*,2*S*)-acetoxycyclopropyltrimethylammonium, all of which have an (*S*) configuration at the carbon atom that corresponds to the β carbon of ACh. Each of these active muscarinic molecules may be deployed on the receptor in the same manner as ACh and (+)-muscarine. Their (*S*)/(*R*) ratios (Table 17-3) show the greatest stereoselectivity of the muscarinic receptor in guinea pig ileum for the configuration at the carbon adjacent to the ester group. In contrast, the nicotinic receptors are not considered as highly stereoselective as their muscarinic counterparts.

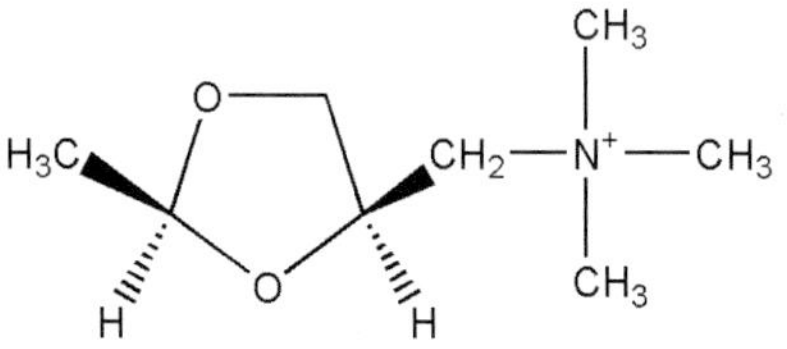

cis-2-Methyl-4-trimethylammonium-1,3-dioxolane

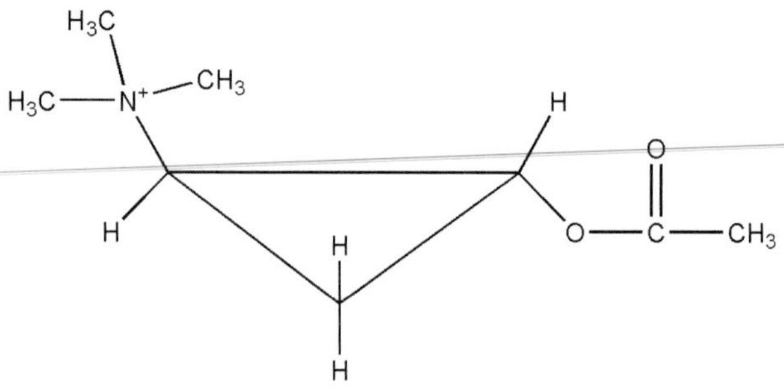

trans-2-Acetoxycyclopropyltrimethylammonium

TABLE 17–3   Equipotent Molar Ratios of Isomers on Guinea Pig Ileum: Ratios Relative to Acetylcholine

Compound	Guinea Pig Ileum	(*S*)/(*R*) Ratio
(+)-Acetyl-(*S*)-β-methylcholine chloride	1.0[a]	24
(−)-Acetyl-(*R*)-β-methylcholine chloride	24.0[a]	
(+)-(2*S*,3*R*,5*S*)-Muscarine iodide	0.33[b]	394
(−)-(2*R*,3*S*,5*R*)-Muscarine iodide	130[b]	
(+)-*cis*(2*S*)-Methyl-(4*R*)-trimethylammonium-1,3-dioxolane iodide	6.00[c]	100
(−)-*cis*(2*R*)-Methyl-(4*S*)-trimethylammonium-1,3-dioxolane iodide	0.06[c]	
(+)-*trans*(1*S*,2*S*)-Acetoxycyclopropyltrimethylammonium iodide	00.88[d]	517
(−)-*trans*(1*R*,2*R*)-Acetoxycyclopropyltrimethylammonium iodide	455[d]	

[a] Beckett, A. H., et al. Nature 189:671, 1961.
[b] Waser, P. I.: Pharmacol. Rev. 13:465, 1961.
[c] Belleau, B., and Puranen, J.: J. Med. Chem. 6:235–328, 1963.
[d] Armstrong, P. D., Cannon, J. G., and Long, J. P.: Nature 220:65–66, 1968.

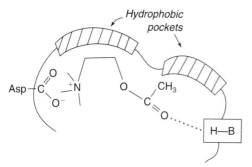

Figure 17–11 ■ Hypothetical structure of the muscarinic receptor.

Structure–Activity Relationships

Although muscarinic receptors have been cloned and the amino acid sequences are known, their three-dimensional structures remain unresolved. Thus, it is not possible to use this information alone to design specific drug molecules. Scientists still use pharmacological and biochemical tests to determine optimal structural requirements for activity. ACh is a relatively simple molecule. The chemistry and ease of testing for ACh biological activity have allowed numerous chemical derivatives to be made and studied. Alterations on the molecule may be divided into three categories: the onium group, the ester function, and the choline moiety.

The onium group is essential for intrinsic activity and contributes to the affinity of the molecule for the receptors, partially through the binding energy and partially because of its action as a detecting and directing group. Molecular modeling data show the binding site to be a negatively charged aspartic acid residue in the third of the seven trans-

membrane helixes of the muscarinic receptor.[36] Hydrophobic pockets are located in helices 4, 5, 6, and 7 of the muscarinic receptor (Fig. 17-11).[37] The trimethylammonium group is the optimal functional moiety for activity, though some significant exceptions are known (e.g., pilocarpine, arecoline, nicotine, and oxotremorine). Phosphonium, sulfonium, arsenonium isosteres, or substituents larger than methyl on the nitrogen increase the size of the onium moiety, produce diffusion of the positive charge, and interfere sterically with proper drug–receptor interaction, resulting in decreased activity (Table 17-4).

The ester group in ACh contributes to the binding of the compound to the muscarinic receptor because of hydrogen bond formation with threonine and asparagine residues at the receptor site. A comparison of the cholinergic activity of a series of alkyltrimethylammonium compounds [R-N$^+$(CH$_3$), R = C$_1$–C$_9$] shows *n*-amyltrimethylammonium,[38] which may be considered to have a size and mass similar to those of ACh and to be one magnitude weaker as a muscarinic agonist. The presence of the acetyl group in ACh is not as critical as the size of the molecule. Studying a series of *n*-alkyltrimethylammonium salts revealed[39] that for maximal muscarinic activity, the quaternary ammonium group should be followed by a chain of five atoms; this has been referred to as the *five-atom rule*.

Shortening or lengthening the chain of atoms that separates the ester group from the onium moiety reduces muscarinic activity. An α substitution on the choline moiety decreases both nicotinic and muscarinic activity, but muscarinic activity is decreased to a greater extent. Nicotinic activity is decreased to a greater degree by substitution on the β carbon. Therefore, acetyl α-methylcholine, although less potent than ACh, has more nicotinic than muscarinic activity, while acetyl-β-methylcholine (methacholine) exhibits

---

TABLE 17–4   Activity of Acetoxyethyl Onium Salts: Equipotent Molar Ratios Relative to Acetylcholine

CH$_3$COOCH$_2$CH$_2$	Cat Blood Pressure	Intestine	Frog Heart
N$_+$Me$_3$	1	1 (Rabbit)	1
N$^+$Me$_2$H	50	40	50
N$^+$MeH$_2$	500	1000	500
N$^+$H$_3$	2000	20,000	40,000
N$^+$Me$_2$Et	3	2.5 (Guinea pig)	2
N$^+$MeEt$_2$	400	700	1500
N$^+$Et$_3$	2000	1700	10,000[a]
N$^+$PMe$_3$	13	12 (Rabbit)	12
As$^+$Me$_3$	66	90	83
S$^+$Me$_2$	50	30 (Guinea pig)	96
N	d = 1.47 Å	d' = 2.4 Å	
P	1.87	3.05	
S	1.82	—	
As	1.98	3.23	

Data are from Barlow, R. B.: Introduction to Chemical Pharmacology, London, Methuen and Co., 1964. Welsh, A. D., and Roepke, M. H.: J. Pharmacol. Exp. Ther. 55:118, 1935; Stehle, K. L., Melville, K. J., and Oldham, F. K.: J. Pharmacol. Exp. Ther. 56:473, 1936; Holton, P., and Ing, H. R.: Br. J. Pharmacol. 4:190, 1949; Ing, H. R., Kordik, P., and Tudor Williams, D. P. H.: Br. J. Pharmacol. 7:103, 1952.
[a] Reduces effect of acetylcholine.

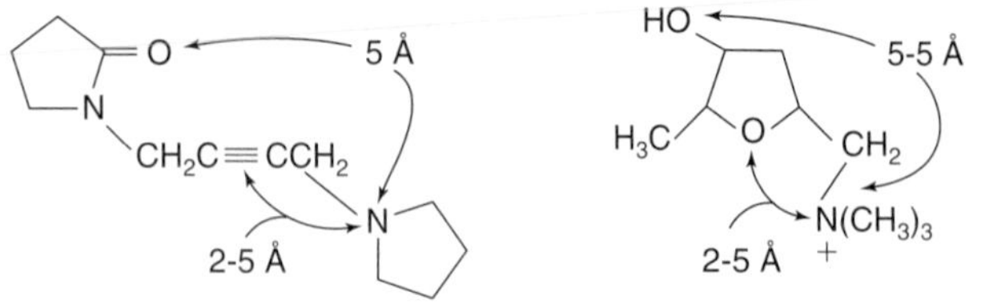

Figure 17–12 ■ Comparison of the geometries of oxotremorine and muscarine.

more muscarinic than nicotinic activity. Hydrolysis by AChE is more affected by substitutions on the β than the α carbon. The hydrolysis rate of racemic acetyl β-methylacetylcholine is about 50% of that of ACh; racemic acetyl α-ACh is hydrolyzed about 90% as fast.

Oxotremorine. Oxotremorine [1-(-pyrrolidono)-4-pyrrolidino-2-butyne] has been regarded as a CNS muscarinic stimulant. Its action on the brain produces tremors in experimental animals. It increases ACh brain levels in rats up to 40% and has been studied as a drug in the treatment of Alzheimer's disease. Although earlier studies suggested that this approach of elevating levels of ACh to treat Alzheimer's disease is useful, this belief was highly disputed by many researchers. Nevertheless, oxotremorine, as a cholinergic agonist, facilitates memory storage.[40] These findings have served as important leads in the development of agents useful in treating Alzheimer's disease. Although it possesses groups that do not occur in other highly active muscarinic agents, oxotremorine's *trans* conformation shows that distances between possible active centers correspond with (+)-muscarine (Fig. 17-12).[41]

Arecoline. Arecoline is an alkaloid obtained from the seeds of the betel nut *(Areca catechu)*. For many years, natives of the East Indies have consumed the betel nut as a source of a euphoria-creating substance.

CHOLINERGIC RECEPTOR ANTAGONISTS

Characterization of muscarinic receptors can now be extended beyond the pharmacological observations on organ systems (e.g., smooth muscle, heart) to determine structure–activity relationships. Dissociation constants of antagonists from radioligand-binding experiments on the various muscarinic receptors have played a major role in identifying these receptors and the selectivity of antagonists to the five muscarinic receptor subtypes. Antagonists with high affinity for one receptor and a low affinity for the other four receptor types are very few, however, and many antagonists bind to several subtypes with equal affinity. M_1 receptors have been identified as those with high affinity for pirenzepine and low affinity for a compound such as AF-DX 116. Pirenzepine can distinguish between M_1 and M_2, M_3, or M_5 but has significant affinity for M_4 receptors. Himbacine can distinguish between M_1 and M_4 receptors. Methoctramine, a polymethylenetetramine, not only discriminates between

M_1 and M_2 receptors but also has good selectivity for M_2 muscarinic receptors. M_2 receptors bind to AF-DX 116 and gallamine, a neuromuscular blocking agent. M_3 receptors have a high affinity for 4-diphenylacetoxy-N-methylpiperidine (4-DAMP) and hexahydrosiladifenidol (HHSiD) but also exhibit affinity for M_1 and M_2 receptors.[21] Tropicamide has been reported to be a putative M_4 receptor antagonist. Figure 17-13 includes structures of some receptor subtype antagonists.

Products

Acetylcholine Chloride. ACh chloride exerts a powerful stimulant effect on the parasympathetic nervous system. Attempts have been made to use it as a cholinergic agent, but its duration of action is too short for sustained effects, because of rapid hydrolysis by esterases and lack of specificity when administered for systemic effects. It is a cardiac depressant and an effective vasodilator. Stimulation of the vagus and the parasympathetic nervous system produces a tonic action on smooth muscle and induces a flow from the salivary and lacrimal glands. Its cardiac-depressant effect results from *(a)* a negative chronotropic effect that causes a decrease in heart rate and *(b)* a negative inotropic action on heart muscle that produces a decrease in the force of myocardial contractions. The vasodilatory action of ACh is primarily on the arteries and the arterioles, with distinct effect on the peripheral vascular system. Bronchial constriction is a characteristic side effect when the drug is given systemically.

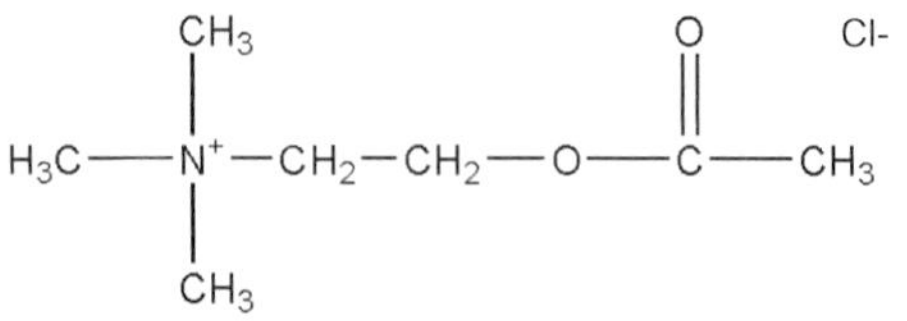

Acetylcholine Chloride

One of the most effective antagonists to the action of ACh is atropine, a nonselective muscarinic antagonist. Atropine blocks the depressant effect of ACh on cardiac muscle and its production of peripheral vasodilation (i.e., muscarinic effects) but does not affect the skeletal muscle contraction (i.e., nicotinic effect) produced.

ACh chloride is a hygroscopic powder that is available in an admixture with mannitol to be dissolved in sterile water for injection shortly before use. It is a short-acting miotic when introduced into the anterior chamber of the eye and is especially useful after cataract surgery during the placement of sutures. When applied topically to the eye, it has little therapeutic value because of poor corneal penetration and rapid hydrolysis by AChE.

Methacholine Chloride, USP. Methacholine chloride, acetyl-β-methylcholine chloride or (2-hydroxypropyl)trimethylammonium chloride acetate, is the acetyl ester of β-methylcholine. Unlike ACh, methacholine has sufficient stability in the body to give sustained parasympathetic stimula-

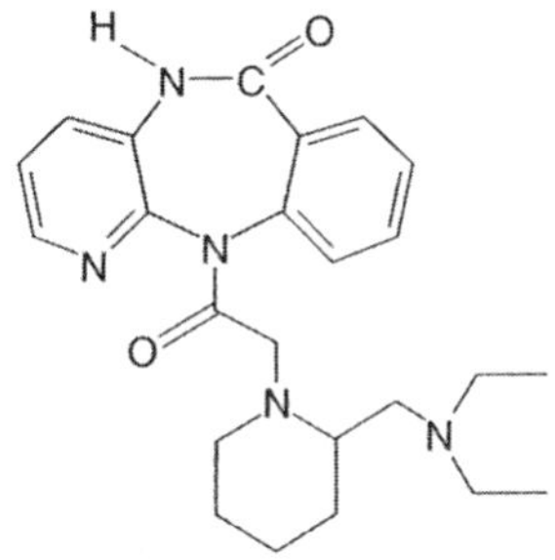

AF—DX 116

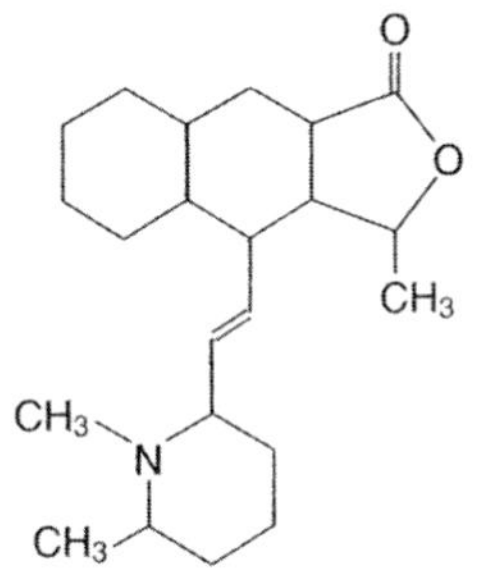

Himbacine

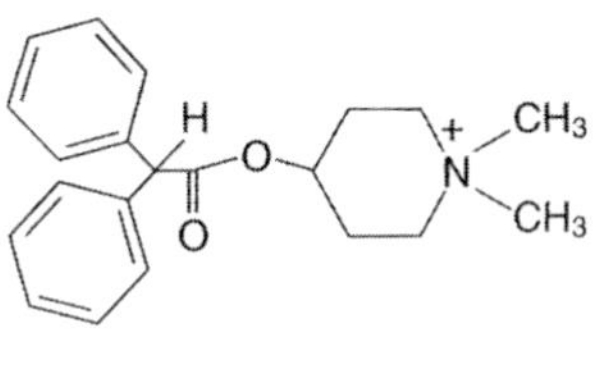

4-DAMP

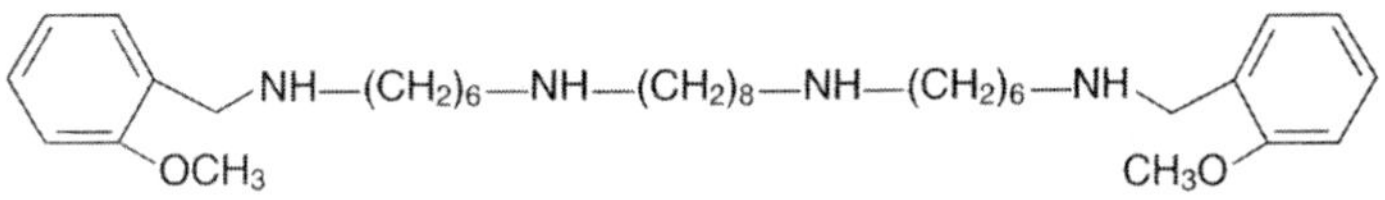

Methoctramine

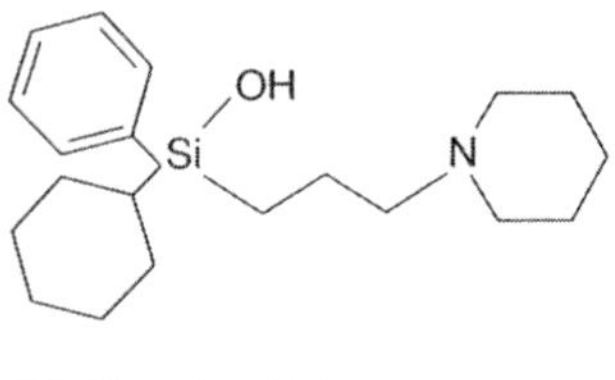

Hexahydrosiladiphenidol

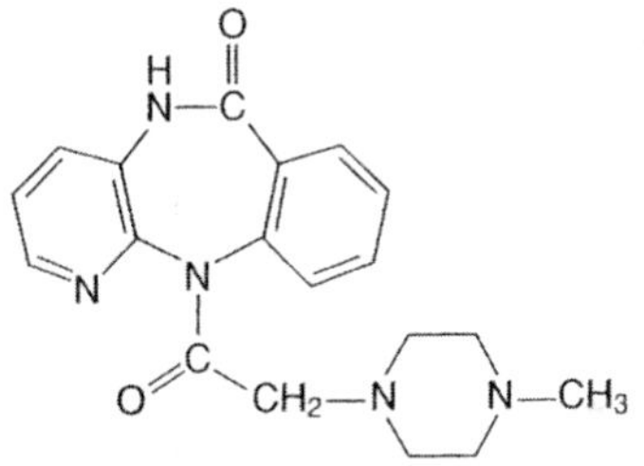

Pirenzepine

Figure 17–13 ■ Chemical structures of partially selective muscarinic antagonists.

tion. This action is accompanied by little (1/1000 that of ACh) or no nicotinic effect.

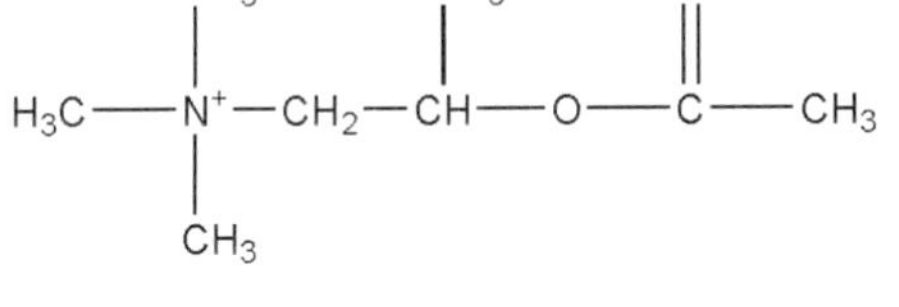

Methacholine Chloride

Methacholine can exist as (*S*) and (*R*) enantiomers. Although the chemical is used as the racemic mixture, its muscarinic activity resides principally in the (*S*) isomer. The (*S*)/(*R*) ratio of muscarinic potency for these enantiomers is 240:1.

(+)-Acetyl-(*S*)-β-methylcholine is hydrolyzed by AChE, whereas the (*R*)(–) isomer is not. (–)-Acetyl-(*R*)-β-methylcholine is a weak competitive inhibitor (K_i, 4×10^{-4} M) of AChE obtained from the electric organ of the eel (*Electrophorus electricus*). The hydrolysis rate of the (*S*)(+) isomer is about 54% that of ACh. This rate probably compensates for any decreased association (affinity) owing to the β-methyl group with the muscarinic receptor site and may account for the fact that ACh and (+)-acetyl-β-methylcholine have equimolar muscarinic potencies in vivo. (–)-Acetyl-(*R*)-β-methylcholine weakly inhibits AChE and slightly reinforces the muscarinic activity of the (*S*)(+) isomer in the racemic mixture of acetyl-β-methylcholine.

In the hydrolysis of the acetyl α- and β-methylcholines, the greatest stereochemical inhibitory effects occur when the choline is substituted in the β position. This also appears to be true of organophosphorous inhibitors. The (*R*)(–) and (*S*)(+) isomers of acetyl-α-methylcholine are hydrolyzed at 78 and 97% of the rate of ACh, respectively.

Methacholine chloride occurs as colorless or white crystals or as a white crystalline powder. It is odorless or has a slight odor and is very deliquescent. It is freely soluble in water, alcohol, or chloroform, and its aqueous solution is neutral to litmus and bitter. It is hydrolyzed rapidly in alkaline solutions. Solutions are relatively stable to heat and will keep for at least 2 or 3 weeks when refrigerated to delay growth of molds.

Carbachol. Choline chloride carbamate is nonspecific in its action on muscarinic receptor subtypes. The pharmacological activity of carbachol is similar to that of ACh. It is an ester of choline and thus possesses both muscarinic and nicotinic properties by cholinergic receptor stimulation. It can also act indirectly by promoting release of ACh and by its weak anticholinesterase activity. Carbachol forms a carbamyl ester in the active site of AChE, which is hydrolyzed more slowly than an acetyl ester. This slower hydrolysis rate reduces the amount of free enzyme and prolongs the duration of ACh in the synapse. Carbachol also stimulates the autonomic ganglia and causes contraction of skeletal muscle but differs from a true muscarinic agent in that it does not have cardiovascular activity despite the fact that it seems to affect M_2 receptors.[42]

Carbachol is a miotic and has been used to reduce the intraocular tension of glaucoma when a response cannot be obtained with pilocarpine or neostigmine. Penetration of the cornea is poor but can be enhanced by the use of a wetting agent in the ophthalmic solution. In addition to its topical use for glaucoma, carbachol is used during ocular surgery, when a more prolonged miosis is required than can be obtained with ACh chloride.

Carbachol Chloride

Carbachol differs chemically from ACh in its stability to hydrolysis. The carbamyl group of carbachol decreases the electrophilicity of the carbonyl and, thus, can form resonance structures more easily than ACh can. The result is that carbachol is less susceptible to hydrolysis and, therefore, more stable in aqueous solutions.

Bethanechol Chloride, USP.   Bethanechol, β-methylcholine chloride carbamate, (2-hydroxypropyl)trimethylammonium chloride carbamate, carbamylmethylcholine chloride (Urecholine), is nonspecific in its action on muscarinic receptor subtypes but appears to be more effective at eliciting pharmacological action of M_3 receptors.[43] It has pharmacological properties similar to those of methacholine. Both are esters of β-methylcholine and have feeble nicotinic activity. Bethanechol is inactivated more slowly by AChE in vivo than is methacholine. It is a carbamyl ester and is expected to have stability in aqueous solutions similar to that of carbachol.

The main use of bethanechol chloride is in the relief of urinary retention and abdominal distention after surgery. The drug is used orally and by subcutaneous injection. It must never be administered by intramuscular or intravenous injection because of the danger from cholinergic overstimulation and loss of selective action. Proper administration of the drug is associated with low toxicity and no serious side effects. Bethanechol chloride should be used with caution in asthmatic patients; when used for glaucoma, it produces frontal headaches from the constriction of the sphincter muscle in the eye and from ciliary muscle spasms. Its duration of action is 1 hour.

Bethanechol Chloride

Pilocarpine Hydrochloride, USP.   Pilocarpine monohydrochloride is the hydrochloride of an alkaloid obtained from the dried leaflets of *Pilocarpus jaborandi* or *P. microphyllus*, in which it occurs to the extent of about 0.5% together with other alkaloids.

Pilocarpine Hydrochloride

It occurs as colorless, translucent, odorless, faintly bitter crystals that are soluble in water (1:0.3), alcohol (1:3), and chloroform (1:360). (In this chapter, a solubility expressed as 1:360 indicates that 1 g is soluble in 360 mL of the solvent at 25°C. Solubilities at other temperatures are so indicated.) It is hygroscopic and affected by light; its solutions are acid to litmus and may be sterilized by autoclaving. Alkalies saponify the lactone group to give the pharmacologically inactive hydroxy acid (pilocarpic acid). Base-catalyzed epimerization at the ethyl group position occurs to an appreciable extent and is another major pathway of degradation.[44] Both routes result in loss of pharmacological activity.

Pilocarpine is a nonselective agonist on the muscarinic receptors. Despite this, it reportedly acts on M_3 receptors in smooth muscle to cause contractions in the gut, trachea, and eye.[45, 46] In the eye, it produces pupillary constriction (miosis) and a spasm of accommodation. These effects are valuable in the treatment of glaucoma. The pupil constriction and spasm of the ciliary muscle reduce intraocular tension by establishing better drainage of ocular fluid through the canal of Schlemm, located near the corner of the iris and cornea. Pilocarpine is used as a 0.5 to 0.6% solution (i.e., of the salts) in treating glaucoma. Systemic effects include copious sweating, salivation, and gastric secretion.

Pilocarpine Nitrate, USP.   Pilocarpine mononitrate occurs as shining white crystals that are not hygroscopic but are light sensitive. It is soluble in water (1:4) and alcohol (1:75) but insoluble in chloroform and ether. Aqueous solutions are slightly acid to litmus and may be sterilized in the autoclave. The alkaloid is incompatible with alkalies, iodides, silver nitrate, and reagents that precipitate alkaloids.

Cholinesterase Inhibitors

There are two types of cholinesterases in humans, AChE and butyrylcholinesterase (BuChE). The cholinesterases differ in their location in the body and their substrate specificity.

TABLE 17–5 Hydrolysis of Various Substrates by AChE and BuChE

	AChE		BuChE	
Enzyme Substrate	Source	Relative Rate[a]	Source	Relative Rate[a]
Acetylcholine	Human or bovine RBC	100	Human or horse plasma	100
Acetylthiocholine	Bovine RBC	149	Horse plasma	407
Acetyl-β-methylcholine	Bovine RBC	18	Horse plasma	0
Propionylcholine	Human RBC	80	Horse plasma	170
Butyrylcholine	Human RBC	2.5	Horse plasma	250
Butyrylthiocholine	Bovine RBC	0	Horse plasma	590
Benzoylcholine	Bovine RBC	0	Horse plasma	67
Ethyl acetate	Human RBC	2	Human plasma	1
3,3-Dimethylbutyl acetate	Human RBC	60	Human plasma	35
2-Chloroethyl acetate	Human RBC	37	Human plasma	10
Isoamyl acetate	Human RBC	24	Horse plasma	7
Isoamyl propionate	Human RBC	10	Horse plasma	13
Isoamyl butyrate	Human RBC	1	Horse plasma	14

Adapted from Heath, D. F.: Organophosphorus Poisons—Anticholinesterases and Related Compounds. New York, Pergamon Press, 1961.
[a] Relative rates at approximately optimal substrate concentration; rate with acetylcholine = 100.

AChE is associated with the outside surface of glial cells in the synapse and catalyzes the hydrolysis of ACh to choline and acetic acid. Inhibition of AChE prolongs the duration of the neurotransmitter in the junction and produces pharmacological effects similar to those observed when ACh is administered. These inhibitors are indirect-acting cholinergic agonists. AChE inhibitors have been used in the treatment of myasthenia gravis, atony in the GI tract, and glaucoma. They have also been used as agricultural insecticides and nerve gases. More recently, they have received attention as symptomatic drug treatments in patients suffering from Alzheimer's disease.[47]

BuChE (pseudocholinesterase) is located in human plasma. Although its biological function is not clear, it has catalytic properties similar to those of AChE. The substrate specificity is broader (Table 17-5), and it may hydrolyze dietary esters and drug molecules in the blood.

Three different chemical groupings, acetyl, carbamyl, and phosphoryl, may react with the esteratic site of AChE. Although the chemical reactions are similar, the kinetic parameters for each type of substrate differ and result in differences between toxicity and usefulness.

The initial step in the hydrolysis of ACh by AChE is a reversible enzyme–substrate complex formation. The association rate (k_{+1}) and dissociation rate (k_{-1}) are relatively large. The enzyme–substrate complex, E_A–ACh, may also form an acetyl-enzyme intermediate at a rate (k_2) that is slower than either the association or dissociation rates. Choline is released from this complex with the formation of the acetyl-enzyme intermediate, EA. This intermediate is then hydrolyzed to regenerate the free enzyme and acetic acid. The acetylation rate, k_2, is the slowest step in this sequence and is rate-limiting (see discussion below).

Kinetic studies with different substrates and inhibitors suggest that the active center of AChE consists of several major domains: an anionic site, to which the trimethylammonium group binds; an esteratic site, which causes hydrolysis of the ester portion of ACh; and hydrophobic sites, which bind aryl substrates, other uncharged ligands, and the alkyl portion of the acyl moiety of ACh. There is also a peripheral anionic site, removed by at least 20 Å from this active center, which allosterically regulates activity at the esteratic site.[48] The anionic site was believed to have been formed by the γ-carboxylate group of a glutamic acid residue,[49] but more

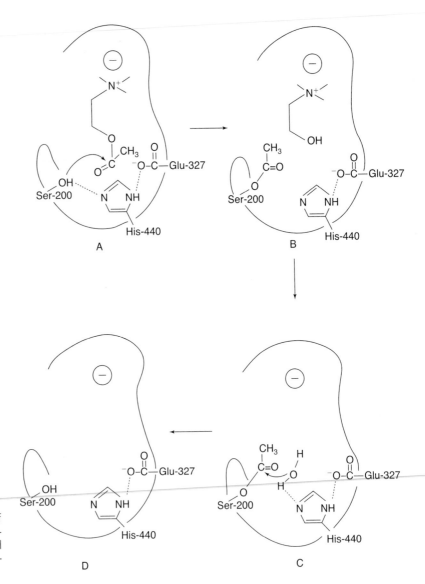

Figure 17–14 ■ Mechanism of hydrolysis of ACh by AChE. **A.** ACh–AChE reversible complex. **B.** Acetylation of esteratic site. **C.** General base-catalyzed hydrolysis of acetylated enzyme. **D.** Free enzyme.

recent studies suggest that the aromatic moieties of tryptophan and phenylalanine residues bind the quaternary ammonium group of ACh in the anionic site through cation–π interactions.[50] The location and spatial organization in the esteratic site by serine, histidine, and glutamic acid residues constitute the esteratic site. The triad of these amino acid residues contributes to the high catalytic efficiency of AChE (Fig. 17-14).[51]

AChE attacks the ester substrate through a serine hydroxyl, forming a covalent acyl–enzyme complex. The serine is activated as a nucleophile by the glutamic acid and histidine residues that serve as the proton sink to attack the carbonyl carbon of ACh. Choline is released, leaving the acetylated serine residue on the enzyme. The acetyl-enzyme intermedi-

ate is cleaved by a general base catalysis mechanism to regenerate the free enzyme. The rate of the deacetylation step is indicated by k_3.

Carbamates such as carbachol are also able to serve as substrates for AChE, forming a carbamylated enzyme intermediate (E–C). The rate of carbamylation (k_2) is slower than the rate of acetylation. Hydrolysis (k_3, decarbamylation) of the carbamyl-enzyme intermediate is 10^7 times slower than that of its acetyl counterpart. The slower hydrolysis rate limits the optimal functional capacity of AChE, allowing carbamate substrates to be semireversible inhibitors of AChE.

In the mechanism above, k_3 is rate-limiting. The rate k_2 depends not only on the nature of the alcohol moiety of the

$$E + ACh \underset{k_{-1}}{\overset{k_{+1}}{\rightleftharpoons}} E\text{-}ACh \xrightarrow[-\text{ choline}]{k_2} E\text{—}A \xrightarrow[H_2O]{k_3} E + H\text{—}O\text{—}\overset{\overset{\displaystyle O}{\|}}{C}\text{—}CH_3$$

$$E + CX \underset{k_{-1}}{\overset{k_{+1}}{\rightleftharpoons}} E\text{-}CX \overset{k_2}{\underset{X}{\searrow}} E\text{---}C \overset{k_3}{\longrightarrow} E + C$$

where CX = carbamylating substrate

ester but also on the type of carbamyl ester. Esters of carbamic acid

$$R\text{---}O\text{---}\overset{\overset{\displaystyle O}{\|}}{C}\text{---}NH_2$$

are better carbamylating agents of AChE than the methylcarbamyl

$$R\text{---}O\text{---}\overset{\overset{\displaystyle O}{\|}}{C}\text{---}NHCH_3$$

and dimethylcarbamyl analogues.[52]

$$R\text{---}O\text{---}\overset{\overset{\displaystyle O}{\|}}{C}\text{---}N(CH_3)_3$$

Organophosphate esters of selected compounds can also esterify the serine residue in the active site of AChE. The hydrolysis rate (k_3) of the phosphorylated serine is extremely slow, and hydrolysis to the free enzyme and phosphoric acid derivative is so limited that the inhibition is considered irreversible. These organophosphorous compounds are used in the treatment of glaucoma, as agricultural insecticides, and, at times, as nerve gases in warfare and bioterrorism. Finally, some have either been or are currently being evaluated for use against Alzheimer's disease. Table 17-6 shows the relative potencies of several AChE inhibitors.

Reversible Inhibitors

Physostigmine, USP. Physostigmine is an alkaloid obtained from the dried ripe seed of *Physostigma venenosum*. It occurs as a white, odorless, microcrystalline powder that is slightly soluble in water and freely soluble in alcohol, chloroform, and the fixed oils. The alkaloid, as the free base, is quite sensitive to heat, light, moisture, and bases, undergoing rapid decomposition. In solution it is hydrolyzed to methyl carbamic acid and eseroline, neither of which inhibits AChE. Eseroline is oxidized to a red compound, rubreserine,[53] and then further decomposed to eserine blue and eserine brown. Addition of sulfite or ascorbic acid prevents oxidation of the phenol, eseroline, to rubreserine. Hydrolysis does take place, however, and the physostigmine is inactivated. Solutions are most stable at pH 6 and should never be sterilized by heat.

TABLE 17–6 Inhibition Constants for Anticholinesterase Potency of Acetylcholinesterase Inhibitors

Reversible and Semireversible Inhibitors	K_1 (M)
Ambenonium	4.0×10^{-8}
Carbachol	1.0×10^{-4}
Demecarium	1.0×10^{-10}
Edrophonium	3.0×10^{-7}
Neostigmine	1.0×10^{-7}
Physostigmine	1.0×10^{-8}
Pyridostigmine	4.0×10^{-7}

Irreversible Inhibitors	K_2 **(mol/min)**
Isoflurophate	1.9×10^4
Echothiophate	1.2×10^5
Paraoxon	1.1×10^6
Sarin	6.3×10^7
Tetraethylpyrophosphate	2.1×10^8

Physostigmine is a relatively poor carbamylating agent of AChE and is often considered a reversible inhibitor of the enzyme. Its cholinesterase-inhibiting properties vary with the pH of the medium (Fig. 17-15). The conjugate acid of physostigmine has a pK_a of about 8, and as the pH of the solution is lowered, more is present in the protonated form. Inhibition of cholinesterase is greater in acid media, suggesting that the protonated form makes a contribution to the inhibitory activity well as its carbamylation of the enzyme.

Physostigmine was used first as a topical application in the treatment of glaucoma. Its lipid solubility properties permit adequate absorption from ointment bases. It is used systemically as an antidote for atropine poisoning and other anticholinergic drugs by increasing the duration of action of ACh at cholinergic sites through inhibition of AChE. Physostigmine, along with other cholinomimetic drugs acting in the CNS, has been studied for use in the treatment of Alzheimer's disease.[54] Cholinomimetics that are currently used or which have been recently evaluated in the treatment of Alzheimer's disease include donepezil, galantamine, metrifo-

$$E + PX \underset{k_{-1}}{\overset{k_{+1}}{\rightleftharpoons}} E\text{-}PX \overset{k_2}{\underset{X}{\searrow}} E\text{---}P \overset{k_3}{\longrightarrow} E + P$$

where PX = phosphorylating substrate

Physostigmine

Eseroline

Rubreserine

nate, rivastigmine, and tacrine.[47] It is anticipated that this list will continue to grow as the etiology of this disease becomes better understood.

Physostigmine Salicylate, USP. The salicylate of physostigmine (eserine salicylate) may be prepared by neutralizing an ethereal solution of the alkaloid with an ethereal solution of salicylic acid. Excess salicylic acid is removed from the precipitated product by washing it with ether. The salicylate is less deliquescent than the sulfate.

Physostigmine salicylate occurs as a white, shining, odorless crystal or white powder that is soluble in water (1:75), alcohol (1:16), or chloroform (1:6) but much less soluble in ether (1:250). On prolonged exposure to air and light, the

crystals turn red. The red may be removed by washing the crystals with alcohol, although this causes loss of the compound as well. Aqueous solutions are neutral or slightly acidic and take on a red coloration after a period. The coloration may be taken as an index of the loss of activity of physostigmine solutions.

Physostigmine Salicylate

Solutions of physostigmine salicylate are incompatible with the usual reagents that precipitate alkaloids (alkalies) and with iron salts. Incompatibility also occurs with benzalkonium chloride and related wetting agents because of the salicylate ion.

Physostigmine Sulfate, USP. Physostigmine sulfate occurs as a white, odorless, microcrystalline powder that is deliquescent in moist air. It is soluble in water (1:4), alcohol (1:0.4), and ether (1:1200). It has the advantage over the salicylate salt of being compatible in solution with benzalkonium chloride and related compounds.

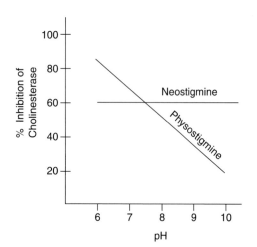

Figure 17–15 ■ Effect of pH on inhibition of cholinesterase by physostigmine and neostigmine.

Neostigmine Bromide. Neostigmine bromide, (*m*-hydroxyphenyl)trimethylammonium bromide dimethylcarbamate or the dimethylcarbamic ester of 3-hydroxyphenyltrimethylammonium bromide (Prostigmin bromide), is used as an antidote to nondepolarizing neuromuscular blocking drugs and in the treatment of myasthenia gravis. It occurs as a bitter, odorless, white, crystalline powder. It is soluble in water and alcohol. The crystals are much less hygroscopic than those of neostigmine methylsulfate and thus may be used in tablets. Solutions are stable and may be sterilized by boiling. Aqueous solutions are neutral to litmus.

Neostigmine Bromide

Use of physostigmine, as a prototype of an indirect-acting parasympathomimetic drug, facilitated the development of stigmine, in which a trimethylamine group was placed *para* to a dimethylcarbamate group in benzene. Better inhibition of cholinesterase was observed when these groups were placed *meta* to each other as in neostigmine, a more active and useful agent. Although physostigmine contains a methylcarbamate functional group, greater chemical stability toward hydrolysis was obtained with the dimethylcarbamyl group in neostigmine.[55]

Neostigmine has a half-life of about 50 minutes after oral or intravenous administration. About 80% of a single intramuscular dose is excreted in the urine within 24 hours; approximately 40% is excreted unchanged, and the remainder is excreted as metabolites. Of the neostigmine that reaches the liver, 98% is metabolized in 10 minutes to 3-hydroxyphenyltrimethyl ammonium, which has activity similar to, but weaker than, neostigmine. Its transfer from plasma to liver cells and then to bile is probably passive. Because cellular membranes permit the passage of plasma proteins synthesized in the liver into the bloodstream through capillary walls or lymphatic vessels, they may not present a barrier to the diffusion of quaternary amines such as neostigmine. The rapid hepatic metabolism of neostigmine may provide a downhill gradient for the continual diffusion of this compound.[56] A certain amount is hydrolyzed slowly by plasma cholinesterase.

Neostigmine has a mechanism of action quite similar to that of physostigmine. It effectively inhibits cholinesterase at about 10^{-6} M concentration. Its activity does not vary with pH, and at all ranges it exhibits similar cationic properties (Fig. 17-15). Skeletal muscle is also stimulated by neostigmine, a property that physostigmine does not have.

The uses of neostigmine are similar to those of physostigmine but differ in exhibiting greater miotic activity, fewer and less unpleasant local and systemic manifestations, and greater chemical stability. The most frequent application of neostigmine is to prevent atony of the intestinal, skeletal, and bladder musculature. An important use is in the treatment of myasthenia gravis, a condition caused by an autoimmune mechanism that requires an increase in ACh concentration in the neuromuscular junction to sustain normal muscular activity.

Neostigmine Methylsulfate.

Neostigmine methylsulfate, (*m*-hydroxyphenyl)trimethylammonium methylsulfate dimethylcarbamate or the dimethylcarbamic ester of 3-hydroxyphenyltrimethylammonium methylsulfate (Prostigmin methylsulfate), is a bitter, odorless, white, crystalline powder. It is very soluble in water and soluble in alcohol. Solutions are stable and can be sterilized by boiling. The compound is too hygroscopic for use in a solid form and thus is always used as an injection. Aqueous solutions are neutral to litmus.

Neostigmine Methylsulfate

The methylsulfate salt is used postoperatively as a urinary stimulant and in the diagnosis and treatment of myasthenia gravis.

Pyridostigmine Bromide, USP.

Pyridostigmine bromide, 3-hydroxy-1-methylpyridinium bromide dimethylcarbamate or pyridostigmine bromide (Mestinon), occurs as a white, hygroscopic, crystalline powder with an agreeable, characteristic odor. It is freely soluble in water, alcohol, and chloroform.

Pyridostigmine Bromide

Pyridostigmine bromide is about one-fifth as toxic as neostigmine. It appears to function in a manner similar to that of neostigmine and is the most widely used anticholinesterase agent for treating myasthenia gravis. The liver enzymes and plasma cholinesterase metabolize the drug. The principal metabolite is 3-hydroxy-*N*-methylpyridinium. Orally administered pyridostigmine has a half-life of 90 minutes and a duration of action of between 3 and 6 hours.

Ambenonium Chloride.

Ambenonium chloride, [oxalylbis(iminoethylene)]bis[(*o*-chlorobenzyl)diethylammon-

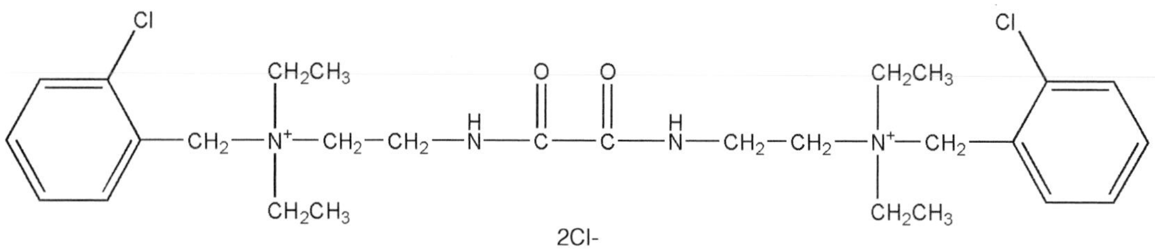

Ambenonium Chloride

ium] dichloride (Mytelase chloride), is a white, odorless powder, soluble in water and alcohol, slightly soluble in chloroform, and practically insoluble in ether and acetone. Ambenonium chloride is used for the treatment of myasthenia gravis in patients who do not respond satisfactorily to neostigmine or pyridostigmine.

This drug acts by suppressing the activity of AChE. It possesses a relatively prolonged duration of action and causes fewer side effects in the GI tract than the other anticholinesterase agents. The dosage requirements vary considerably, and the dosage must be individualized according to the response and tolerance of the patient. Because of its quaternary ammonium structure, ambenonium chloride is absorbed poorly from the GI tract. In moderate doses, the drug does not cross the blood–brain barrier. Ambenonium chloride is not hydrolyzed by cholinesterases.

Demecarium Bromide, USP. Demecarium bromide, (*m*-hydroxyphenyl)trimethylammonium bromide, decamethylenebis[methylcarbamate] (Humorsol), is the diester of (*m*-hydroxyphenyl)trimethylammonium bromide with de-

camethylene bis(methylcarbamic acid) and thus is comparable to a bis-prostigmine molecule.

It occurs as a slightly hygroscopic powder that is freely soluble in water or alcohol. Ophthalmic solutions of the drug have a pH of 5 to 7.5. Aqueous solutions are stable and may be sterilized by heat. Its efficacy and toxicity are comparable to those of other potent anticholinesterase inhibitor drugs. It is a long-acting miotic used to treat wide-angle glaucoma and accommodative esotropia. Maximal effect occurs hours after administration, and the effect may persist for days.

Donepezil. Donepezil, (±)-2,3-dihydro-5,6-dimethoxy-2-[[1-(phenylmethyl)-4-piperidinyl]methyl]-1*H*-inden-1-one (Aricept), commonly referred to in the literature as E2020, is a reversible inhibitor of AChE. It is indicated for the treatment of symptoms of mild-to-moderate Alzheimer's disease. Donepezil is approximately 96% bound to plasma proteins, with an elimination half-life of 70 hours. It is metabolized principally by the 2D6 and 3A4 isozymes of the P-450 system.

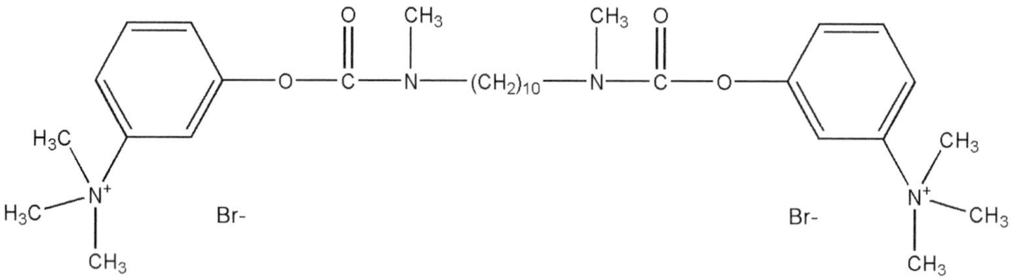

Demecarium Bromide

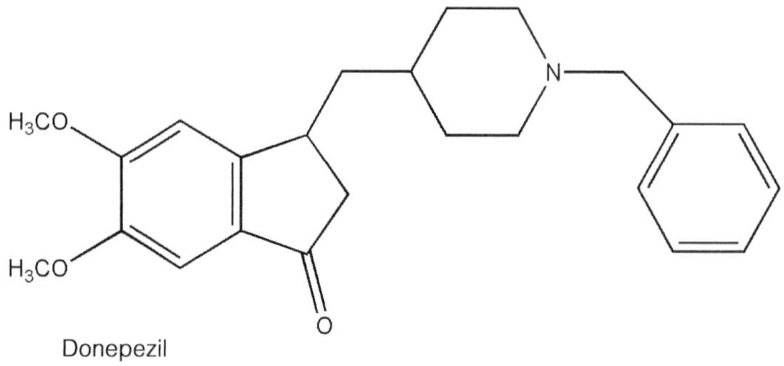

Donepezil

Edrophonium Chloride, USP. Edrophonium chloride, ethyl(*m*-hydroxyphenyl)dimethylammonium chloride (Tensilon), is a reversible anticholinesterase agent. It is bitter and very soluble in water and alcohol. Edrophonium chloride injection has a pH of 5.2 to 5.5. On parenteral administration, edrophonium has a more rapid onset and shorter duration of action than neostigmine, pyridostigmine, or ambenonium. It is a specific anticurare agent and acts within 1 minute to alleviate overdose of *d*-tubocurarine, dimethyl *d*-tubocurarine, or gallamine triethiodide. The drug is also used to terminate the action of any one of these drugs when the physician so desires. It is of no value, however, in terminating the action of the depolarizing (i.e., noncompetitive) blocking agents, such as decamethonium and succinylcholine. In addition to inhibiting AChE, edrophonium chloride has a direct cholinomimetic effect on skeletal muscle, which is greater than that of most other anticholinesterase drugs.

Edrophonium Chloride

Edrophonium chloride is structurally related to neostigmine methylsulfate and has been used as a potential diagnostic agent for myasthenia gravis. This is the only degenerative neuromuscular disease that can be temporarily improved by administration of an anticholinesterase agent. Edrophonium chloride brings about a rapid increase in muscle strength without significant side effects.

Galantamine. Galantamine, 4a,5,9,10,11,12-hexahydro-3-methoxy-11-methyl-6*H*-benzofuro-[3a,3,2,ef][2]-benzazepin-6-ol (Nivalin, Reminyl), is an alkaloid extracted from the tuberous plant *Leucojum aestivum* (L.) belonging to the Amaryllidaceae family and from the bulbs of the daffodil, *Narcissus pseudonarcissus*. It is a reversible cholinesterase inhibitor that appears to have no effect on butyrylcholinesterase. In addition, it acts at allosteric nicotinic sites, further enhancing its cholinergic activity. Galantamine undergoes slow and minor biotransformation with approximately 5 to 6% undergoing demethylation. It is primarily excreted in the urine.

Galantamine

Metrifonate. Metrifonate is an organophosphate that was originally developed to treat schistosomiasis under the trade name Bilarcil. It is an irreversible cholinesterase inhibitor with some selectivity for BuChE over AChE. It achieves sustained cholinesterase inhibition by its nonenzymatic metabolite dichlorvos (DDVP), a long-acting organophosphate. Its use in mild- to-moderate Alzheimer's disease was suspended recently because of adverse effects experienced by several patients during the clinical evaluation of this product. Toxicity at the neuromuscular junction is probably attributable to the inhibition by the drug of neurotoxic esterase, a common feature of organophosphates.

Rivastigmine. Rivastigmine (Exelon, EA 713) is a pseudoirreversible noncompetitive carbamate inhibitor of AChE. Although the half-life is approximately 2 hours, the inhibitory properties of this agent last for 10 hours because of the slow dissociation of the drug from the enzyme. The FDA approved its use in mild-to-moderate Alzheimer's disease in April 2000.

Rivastigmine

Tacrine Hydrochloride. Tacrine hydrochloride, 1,2,3,4-tetrahydro-9-aminoacridine hydrochloride (THA, Cognex), is a reversible cholinesterase inhibitor that has been used in the treatment of Alzheimer's disease for several years. The drug has been used to increase the levels of ACh in these patients on the basis of observations from autopsies that concentrations of ChAT and AChE are markedly reduced in the brain, while the number of muscarinic receptors is almost normal. The use of the drug is not without controversy, as conflicting results on efficacy have been reported.[57, 58] The drug has been used in mild-to-moderate Alzheimer's dementia.

Tacrine Hydrochloride

Irreversible Inhibitors

Both AChE and BuChE are inhibited irreversibly by a group of phosphate esters that are highly toxic (LD_{50} for humans is 0.1 to 0.001 mg/kg). These chemicals are nerve poisons and have been used in warfare, in bioterrorism, and as agricultural insecticides. They permit ACh to accumulate at nerve endings and exacerbate ACh-like actions. The compounds belong to a class of organophosphorous esters. A general formula for such compounds follows:

where R_1 = alkoxy
R_2 = alkoxyl, alkyl, or tertiary amine
X = a good leaving group
(e.g., F, CN, thiomalate, p-nitrophenyl)

A is usually oxygen or sulfur but may also be selenium. When *A* is other than oxygen, biological activation is required before the compound becomes effective as an inhibitor of cholinesterases. Phosphorothionates $[R_1R_2P(S)X]$ have much poorer electrophilic character than their oxygen analogues and are much weaker hydrogen bond–forming molecules because of the sulfur atom.[59] Their anticholinesterase activity is 10^5-fold weaker than their oxygen analogues. *X* is the leaving group when the molecule reacts with the enzyme. Typical leaving groups include fluoride, nitrile, and *p*-nitrophenoxy. The *R* groups may be alkyl, alkoxy, aryl, aryloxy, or amino. The *R* moiety imparts lipophilicity to the molecule and contributes to its absorption through the skin.

Inhibition of AChE by organophosphorous compounds takes place in two steps, association of enzyme and inhibitor and the phosphorylation step, completely analogous to acylation by the substrate (Fig. 17-16). Stereospecificity is mainly due to interactions of enzyme and inhibitor at the esteratic site.

The serine residue at the esteratic site forms a stable phosphoryl ester with the organophosphorous inhibitors. This stability permits labeling studies[60] to be carried out on this and other enzymes (e.g., trypsin, chymotrypsin) that have the serine hydroxyl as part of their active site.

Although insecticides and nerve gases are irreversible inhibitors of cholinesterases by forming a phosphorylated ser-

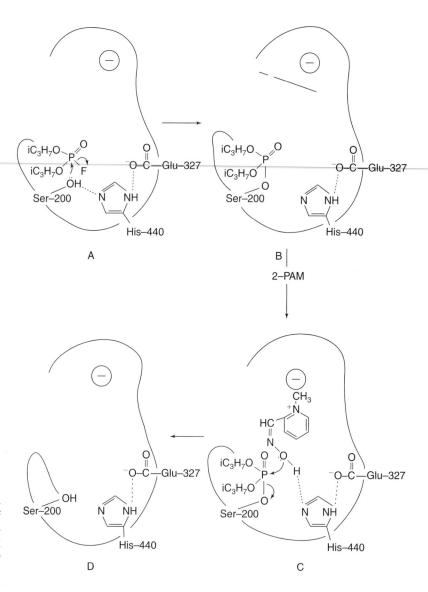

Figure 17–16 ■ Phosphorylation and reactivation of cholinesterase. **A.** Phosphorylation of serine by isofluorphate. **B.** Phosphorylated serine at the esteratic site. **C.** Nucleophilic attack on phosphorylated residue by 2-PAM. **D.** Free enzyme.

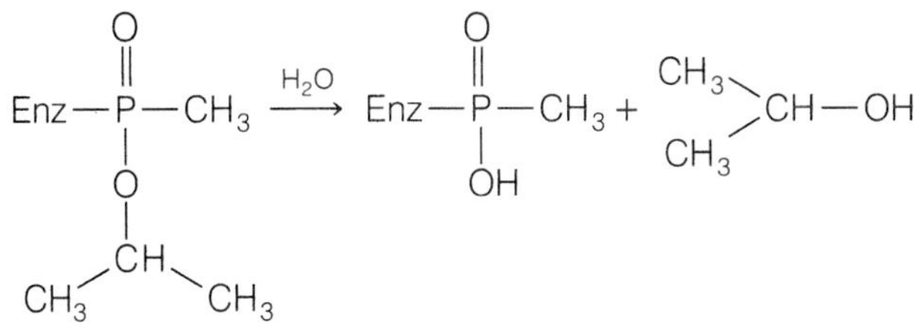

Figure 17–17 ■ Aging of phosphorylated enzyme.

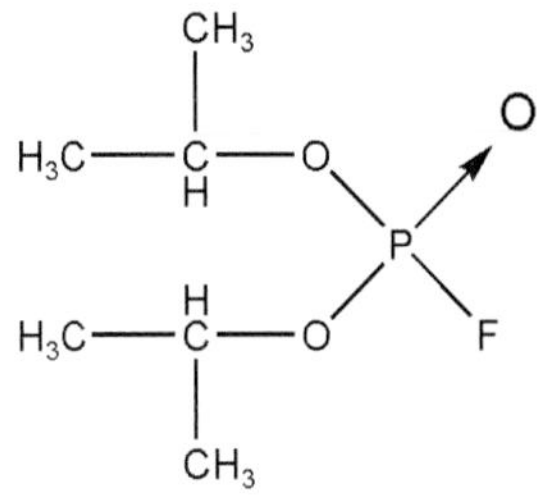

Isofluorphate

ine at the esteratic site of the enzyme, it is possible to reactivate the enzyme if action is taken soon after exposure to these poisons. Several compounds can provide a nucleophilic attack on the phosphorylated enzyme and cause regeneration of the free enzyme. Substances such as choline, hydroxylamine, and hydroxamic acid have led to the development of more effective cholinesterase reactivators, such as nicotinic hydroxamic acid and pyridine-2-aldoxime methiodide (2-PAM). A proposed mode of action for the reactivation of cholinesterase that has been inactivated by isoflurophate by 2-PAM is shown in Figure 17-16.

Cholinesterases that have been exposed to phosphorylating agents (e.g., sarin) become refractory to reactivation by cholinesterase reactivators. The process is called *aging* and occurs both in vivo and in vitro with AChE and BuChE. Aging occurs by partial hydrolysis of the phosphorylated moiety that is attached to the serine residue at the esteratic site of the enzyme (Fig. 17-17).

Phosphate esters used as insecticidal agents are toxic and must be handled with extreme caution. Symptoms of toxicity are nausea, vomiting, excessive sweating, salivation, miosis, bradycardia, low blood pressure, and respiratory difficulty, which is the usual cause of death.

The organophosphate insecticides of low toxicity, such as malathion, generally cause poisoning only by ingestion of relatively large doses. Parathion or methylparathion, however, cause poisoning by inhalation or dermal absorption. Because these compounds are so long acting, cumulative and serious toxic manifestations may result after several small exposures.

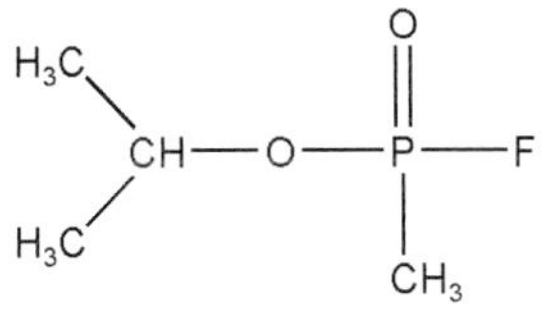

Sarin

Products

Isofluorphate, USP. Isofluorphate, diisopropylphosphorofluoridate (Floropryl), is a colorless liquid soluble in water to the extent of 1.54% at 25°C, which decomposes to give a pH of 2.5. It is soluble in alcohol and to some extent in peanut oil. It is stable in peanut oil for a period of 1 year but decomposes in water in a few days. Solutions in peanut oil can be sterilized by autoclaving. The compound should be stored in hard glass containers. Continued contact with soft glass is said to hasten decomposition, as evidenced by discoloration.

Isofluorphate must be handled with extreme caution. Contact with eyes, nose, mouth, and even skin should be avoided because it can be absorbed readily through intact epidermis and more so through mucous tissues.

Since isofluorphate irreversibly[61] inhibits cholinesterase, its activity lasts for days or even weeks. During this period, new cholinesterase may be synthesized in plasma, erythrocytes, and other cells.

A combination of atropine sulfate and magnesium sulfate protects rabbits against the toxic effects of isofluorphate. Atropine sulfate counteracts the muscarinic effect, and magnesium sulfate counteracts the nicotinic effect of the drug.[62] Isofluorphate has been used in the treatment of glaucoma.

Echothiophate Iodide, USP. Echothiophate iodide, (2-mercaptoethyl)trimethylammonium iodide, *S*-ester with *O,O*-diethylphosphorothioate (Phospholine Iodide), occurs as a white, crystalline, hygroscopic solid that has a slight mercaptan-like odor. It is soluble in water (1:1) and dehydrated alcohol (1:25); aqueous solutions have a pH of about 4 and are stable at room temperature for about 1 month.

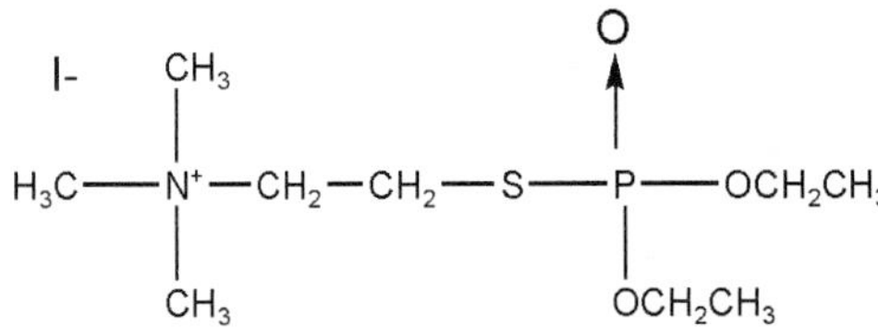

Echothiophate Iodide

Echothiophate iodide is a long-lasting cholinesterase inhibitor of the irreversible type, as is isofluorphate. Unlike the latter, however, it is a quaternary salt, and when applied locally, its distribution in tissues is limited, which can be very desirable. It is used as a long-acting anticholinesterase agent in the treatment of glaucoma.

Hexaethyltetraphosphate (HETP) and Tetraethylpyrophosphate (TEPP). HETP and TEPP are compounds that also show anticholinesterase activity. HETP was developed by the Germans during World War II and is used as an insecticide against aphids. When used as insecticides, these compounds have the advantage of being hydrolyzed rapidly to the relatively nontoxic, water-soluble compounds phosphoric acid and ethyl alcohol. Fruit trees or vegetables sprayed with this type of compound retain no harmful residue after a period of a few days or weeks, depending on the weather conditions. Workers spraying with these agents should use extreme caution so that the vapors are not breathed and none of the vapor or liquid comes in contact with the eyes or skin.

Tetraethylpyrophosphate

Malathion. Malathion, 2-[(dimethoxyphosphinothioyl)-thio]butanedioic acid diethyl ester, is a water-insoluble phosphodithioate ester that has been used as an agricultural insecticide. Malathion is a poor inhibitor of cholinesterases. Its effectiveness as a safe insecticide is due to the different rates at which humans and insects metabolize the chemical. Microsomal oxidation, which causes desulfuration, occurs slowly to form the phosphothioate (malaoxon), which is 10,000 times more active than the phosphodithioate (malathion) as a cholinesterase inhibitor. Insects detoxify the phosphothioate by a phosphatase, forming dimethyl phosphorothioate, which is inactive as an inhibitor. Humans, however, can rapidly hydrolyze malathion by a carboxyesterase en-

zyme, yielding malathion acid, a still poorer inhibitor of AChE. Phosphatases and carboxyesterases further metabolize malathion acid to dimethylphosphothioate. The metabolic reactions are shown in Figure 17-18.

Parathion. Parathion, *O,O*-diethyl *O-p*-nitrophenyl phosphorothioate (Thiophos), is a yellow liquid that is freely soluble in aromatic hydrocarbons, ethers, ketones, esters, and alcohols but practically insoluble in water, petroleum ether, kerosene, and the usual spray oils. It is decomposed at a pH above 7.5. Parathion is used as an agricultural insecticide. It is a relatively weak inhibitor of cholinesterase; however, enzymes present in liver microsomes and insect tissues convert parathion ($pI_{50} <4$) to paraoxon, a more potent inhibitor of cholinesterase ($pI_{50} >8$).[63] Parathion is also metabolized by liver microsomes to yield *p*-nitrophenol and diethylphosphate; the latter is inactive as an irreversible cholinesterase inhibitor.[64]

Schradan. Schradan, octamethyl pyrophosphoramide, OMPA, *bis*[bisdimethylaminophosphonous] anhydride (Pestox III), is a viscous liquid that is miscible with water and soluble in most organic solvents. It is not hydrolyzed by alkalies or water but is hydrolyzed by acids. Schradan is used as a systemic insecticide for plants, being absorbed by

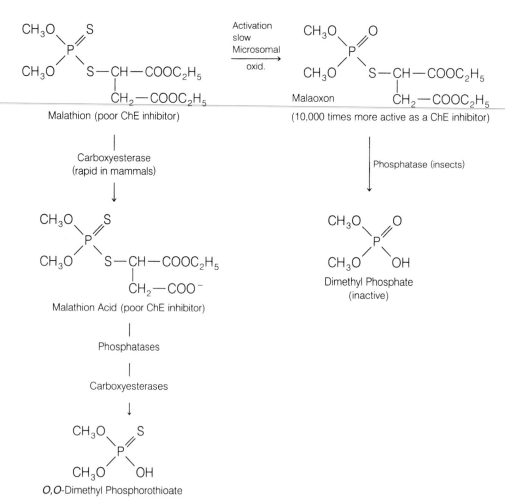

Figure 17-18 ■ Comparison of metabolism of malathion by mammals and insects.

Parathion
(low anti-AChE activity)

Paraoxon
(high anti-AChE activity)

the plants without appreciable injury. Insects feeding on the plant are incapacitated.

Schradan is a weak inhibitor of cholinesterases in vitro. In vivo, it is metabolized to the very strong inhibitor hydroxymethyl OMPA. Hydroxymethyl OMPA is not stable and is metabolized further to the *N*-methoxide, which is a weak inhibitor of cholinesterase.[65]

Pralidoxime Chloride, USP. Pralidoxime chloride, 2-formyl-1-methylpyridinium chloride oxime, 2-PAM chlo-

ride, or 2-pyridine aldoxime methyl chloride (Protopam chloride), is a white, nonhygroscopic, crystalline powder that is soluble in water, 1 g in less than 1 mL.

Pralidoxime chloride is used as an antidote for poisoning by parathion and related pesticides. It may be effective against some phosphates that have a quaternary nitrogen. It is also an effective antagonist for some carbamates, such as neostigmine methylsulfate and pyridostigmine bromide. The mode of action of pralidoxime chloride is described in Figure 17-16.

OMPA
(weak cholinesterase inhibitor)

Hydroxymethyl OMPA
(strong cholinesterase inhibitor)

OMPA-*N*-methoxide
(strong cholinesterase inhibitor)

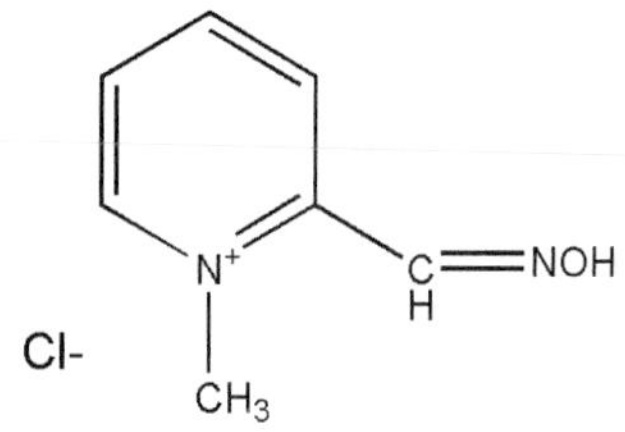

Pralidoxime Chloride

The biological half-life of pralidoxime chloride in humans is about 2 hours, and its effectiveness is a function of its concentration in plasma, which reaches a maximum 2 to 3 hours after oral administration.

Pralidoxime chloride, a quaternary ammonium compound, is most effective by intramuscular, subcutaneous, or intravenous administration. Treatment of poisoning by an anticholinesterase will be most effective if given within a few hours. Little will be accomplished if the drug is used more than 36 hours after parathion poisoning has occurred.

CHOLINERGIC BLOCKING AGENTS

A wide variety of tissues respond to ACh released by the neuron or exogenously administered chemicals to mimic this neurotransmitter's action. Peripheral cholinergic receptors are located at parasympathetic postganglionic nerve endings in smooth muscle, sympathetic and parasympathetic ganglia, and neuromuscular junctions in skeletal muscle. Although ACh activates these receptors, there are antagonists that are selective for each. Atropine is an effective blocking agent at parasympathetic postganglionic terminals. Like most classic blocking agents, it acts on all muscarinic receptor subtypes. *d*-Tubocurarine blocks the effect of ACh on skeletal muscle, which is activated by N_1 nicotinic receptors. Hexamethonium blocks transition at N_2 nicotinic receptors located in autonomic ganglia.

Anticholinergic action by drugs and chemicals apparently depends on their ability to reduce the number of free receptors that can interact with ACh. The theories of Stephenson[66] and Ariens[67] have explained the relationship between drug–receptor interactions and the observed biological response (see Chapter 2). These theories indicate that the amount of drug–receptor complex formed at a given time depends on the affinity of the drug for the receptor and that a drug that acts as an agonist must also possess another property, called *efficacy* or *intrinsic activity*. Another explanation of drug–receptor interactions, the Paton rate theory,[68] defines a biological stimulus as proportional to the rate of drug–receptor interactions (see Chapter 2). Both of these theories are compatible with the concept that a blocking agent that has high affinity for the receptor may decrease the number of available free receptors and the efficiency of the endogenous neurotransmitter.

Structure–Activity Relationships

A wide variety of compounds possess anticholinergic activity. The development of such compounds has been largely empiric and based principally on atropine as the prototype.

Nevertheless, structural permutations have resulted in compounds that do not have obvious relationships to the parent molecule. The following classification delineates the major chemical types encountered:

- Solanaceous alkaloids and synthetic analogues
- Synthetic aminoalcohol esters
- Aminoalcohol ethers
- Aminoalcohols
- Aminoamides
- Miscellaneous
- Papaveraceous

The chemical classification of anticholinergics acting on parasympathetic postganglionic nerve endings is complicated somewhat because some agents, especially the quaternary ammonium derivatives, act on the ganglia that have a muscarinic component to their stimulation pattern and, at high doses, at the neuromuscular junction in skeletal muscle.

There are several ways in which the structure–activity relationship could be considered, but in this discussion we follow, in general, the considerations of Long et al.,[69] who based their postulations on the 1-hyoscyamine molecule being one of the most active anticholinergics and, therefore, having an optimal arrangement of groups.

Anticholinergic compounds may be considered chemicals that have some similarity to ACh but contain additional substituents that enhance their binding to the cholinergic receptor.

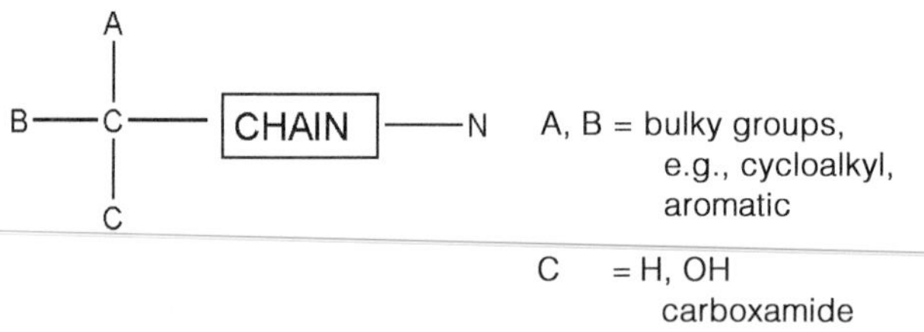

A, B = bulky groups, e.g., cycloalkyl, aromatic

C = H, OH carboxamide

As depicted above, an anticholinergic agent may contain a quaternary ammonium function or a tertiary amine that is protonated in the biophase to form a cationic species. The nitrogen is separated from a pivotal carbon atom by a chain that may include an ester, ether, or hydrocarbon moiety. The substituent groups *A* and *B* contain at least one aromatic moiety capable of van der Waals' interactions to the receptor surface and one cycloaliphatic or other hydrocarbon moiety for hydrophobic bonding interactions. *C* may be hydroxyl or carboxamide to undergo hydrogen bonding with the receptor.

THE CATIONIC HEAD

It is generally considered that the anticholinergic molecules have a primary point of attachment to cholinergic sites through the *cationic head* (i.e., the positively charged nitrogen). For quaternary ammonium compounds, there is no question of what is implied, but for tertiary amines, one assumes, with good reason, that the cationic head is achieved by protonation of the amine at physiological pH. The nature of the substituents on this cationic head is critical insofar as a parasympathomimetic response is concerned. Steric factors that cause diffusion of the onium charge or produce a less-than-optimal drug–receptor interaction result in a decrease of parasympathomimetic properties and allow the drug to act as an antagonist because of other bonding interactions. Ariens[67] has shown that carbocholines (e.g., benzilylcarbocholine) engage in a typical competitive action with ACh, though they are less effective than the corresponding compounds possessing a cationic head, suggesting that hydrophobic bonding may play an important role in these drug–receptor interactions.

Benzilylcarbocholine

THE HYDROXYL GROUP

Although not requisite for activity, a suitably placed alcoholic hydroxyl group enhances antimuscarinic activity over that of a similar compound without the hydroxyl group. The position of the hydroxyl group relative to the nitrogen appears to be fairly critical, with the diameter of the receptive area estimated to be about 2 to 3 Å. It is assumed that the hydroxyl group contributes to the strength of binding, probably by hydrogen bonding to an electron-rich portion of the receptor surface.

THE ESTERATIC GROUP

Many of the highly potent antimuscarinic compounds possess an ester grouping, and this may be a contributing feature for effective binding. This is reasonable because the agonist (i.e., ACh) possesses a similar function for binding to the same site. An esteratic function is not necessary for activity, since several types of compounds do not possess such a group (e.g., ethers, aminoalcohols).

CYCLIC SUBSTITUTION

Examination of the active compounds discussed in the following sections reveals that at least one cyclic substituent (phenyl, thienyl, or other) is a common feature in almost all anticholinergic molecules. Aromatic substitution is often used in connection with the acidic moiety of the ester function. Virtually all acids used, however, are of the aryl-substituted acetic acid variety. Use of aromatic acids leads to low activity of these compounds as anticholinergics but potential activity as local anesthetics.

In connection with the apparent need for a cyclic group, Ariens[67] points out that the "mimetic" molecules, richly endowed with polar groups, undoubtedly require a complementary polar receptor area for effective binding. As a consequence, it is implied that a relatively nonpolar area surrounds such sites. Thus, increasing the binding of the molecule in this peripheral area by introducing flat, nonpolar groups (e.g., aromatic rings) should achieve compounds with

excellent affinity but without intrinsic activity. This postulate is consistent with most antimuscarinic drugs, whether they possess an ester group or not.

PARASYMPATHETIC POSTGANGLIONIC BLOCKING AGENTS

Parasympathetic postganglionic blocking agents are also known as antimuscarinic, anticholinergic, parasympatholytic, or cholinolytic drugs. Antimuscarinic drugs act by competitive antagonism of ACh binding to muscarinic receptors. Endogenous neurotransmitters, including ACh, are relatively small molecules. Ariens[67] noted that competitive reversible antagonists generally are larger molecules capable of additional binding to the receptor surface. The most potent anticholinergic drugs are derived from muscarinic agonists that contain one or sometimes two large or bulky groups. Ariens[67] suggested that molecules that act as competitive reversible antagonists generally are capable of binding to the active site of the receptor but have an additional binding interaction that increases receptor affinity but does not contribute to the intrinsic activity (efficacy) of the drug. Several three-dimensional models of G-protein–coupled receptors, including the muscarinic receptor, have been reported. Despite knowledge of their amino acid sequences, it is not yet possible to provide an unambiguous description of the docking of molecules to these receptors. The concepts of Ariens[67] and others, however, appear consistent with the binding site models proposed. Bebbington and Brimblecombe[41] proposed in 1965 that there is a relatively large area lying outside the agonist–receptor binding site, where van der Waals' interactions can take place between the agonist and the receptor area. This, too, is not inconsistent with contemporary theories on cholinergic receptor interaction with small molecules.

Therapeutic Actions

Organs controlled by the autonomic nervous system usually are innervated by both the sympathetic and the parasympathetic systems. There is a continual state of dynamic balance between the two systems. Theoretically, one should achieve the same end result by either stimulation of one of the systems or blockade of the other. Unfortunately, there is usually a limitation to this type of generalization. There are, however, three predictable and clinically useful results from blocking the muscarinic effects of ACh.

1. *Mydriatic effect:* dilation of the pupil of the eye; and *cycloplegia,* a paralysis of the ciliary structure of the eye, resulting in a paralysis of accommodation for near vision
2. *Antispasmodic effect:* lowered tone and motility of the GI tract and the genitourinary tract
3. *Antisecretory effect:* reduced salivation *(antisialagogue),* reduced perspiration *(anhidrotic),* and reduced acid and gastric secretion

These three general effects of parasympatholytics can be expected in some degree from any of the known drugs, though occasionally one must administer rather heroic doses to demonstrate the effect. The mydriatic and cycloplegic effects, when produced by topical application, are not subject to any greatly undesirable side effects because of limited systemic absorption. This is not true for the systemic antispasmodic effects obtained by oral or parenteral administration. Drugs with effective blocking action on the GI tract are seldom free of adverse effects on the other organs. The same is probably true of drugs used for their antisecretory effects. Perhaps the most common side effects experienced from the oral use of these drugs, under ordinary conditions, are dryness of the mouth, mydriasis, and urinary retention.

Mydriatic and cycloplegic drugs are generally prescribed or used in the office by ophthalmologists. Their principal use is for refraction studies in the process of fitting lenses. This permits the physician to examine the eye retina for possible abnormalities and diseases and provides controlled conditions for the proper fitting of glasses. Because of the inability of the iris to contract under the influence of these drugs, there is a definite danger to the patient's eyes during the period of drug activity unless they are protected from strong light by the use of dark glasses. These drugs also are used to treat inflammation of the cornea (keratitis), inflammation of the iris and the ciliary organs (iritis and iridocyclitis), and inflammation of the choroid (choroiditis). A dark-colored iris appears to be more difficult to dilate than a light-colored one and may require more concentrated solutions. Caution in the use of mydriatics is advisable because of their demonstrated effect in raising the intraocular pressure. Pupil dilation tends to cause the iris to restrict drainage of fluid through the canal of Schlemm by crowding the angular space, thereby leading to increased intraocular pressure. This is particularly true for patients with glaucomatous conditions.

Atropine is used widely as an antispasmodic because of its marked depressant effect on parasympathetically innervated smooth muscle. It appears to block all muscarinic receptor subtypes. Atropine is, however, the standard by which other similar drugs are measured. Also, atropine has a blocking action on the transmission of the nerve impulse, rather than a depressant effect directly on the musculature. This action is termed *neurotropic,* in contrast with the action of an antispasmodic such as papaverine, which appears to act by depression of the muscle cells and is termed *musculotropic.*

Papaverine is the standard for comparison of musculotropic antispasmodics and, although not strictly a parasympatholytic, is treated together with its synthetic analogues below in this chapter. The synthetic antispasmodics appear to combine neurotropic and musculotropic effects in greater or lesser measure, together with a certain amount of ganglion-blocking activity for the quaternary derivatives.

Anticholinergic drugs have a minor role in the management of peptic ulcer disease.[70] For the present, the most rational therapy involving anticholinergic drugs seems to be a combination of a nonirritating diet to reduce acid secretion, antacid therapy, and reduction of emotional stress. Most of the anticholinergic drugs are offered either as the chemical alone, or in combination with a CNS depressant such as phenobarbital, or with a neuroleptic drug to reduce the CNS contribution to parasympathetic hyperactivity. In addition to the antisecretory effects of anticholinergics on hydrochloric acid and gastric acid secretion, there have been some efforts to use them as antisialagogues and anhidrotics.

Paralysis agitans or parkinsonism (Parkinson's disease), first described by the English physician James Parkinson in 1817, is another condition that is often treated with anticholinergic drugs. It is characterized by tremor, "pill rolling," cogwheel rigidity, festinating gait, sialorrhea, and mask-like facies. Fundamentally, it represents a malfunction of the extrapyramidal system. Parkinsonism is characterized by progressive and selective degeneration of dopaminergic neurons, which originate in the substantia nigra of the midbrain and terminate in the basal ganglia (i.e., caudate nucleus, putamen, and pallidum). Skeletal muscle movement is controlled to a great degree by patterns of excitation and inhibition resulting from the feedback of information to the cortex and mediated through the pyramidal and extrapyramidal pathways. The basal ganglia structures, such as the pallidum, corpus striatum, and substantia nigra, serve as data processors for the pyramidal pathways and the structures through which the extrapyramidal pathways pass on their way from the spinal cord to the cortex. Lesions of the pyramidal pathways lead to a persistent increase in muscle tone, resulting in an excess of spontaneous involuntary movements, along with changes in the reflexes. Thus the basal ganglia are functional in maintaining normal motor control. In parkinsonism, there is degeneration of the substantia nigra and corpus striatum, which are involved with controlled integration of muscle movement. The neurons in the substantia nigra and basal ganglia use the neurotransmitter dopamine and interact with short cholinergic interneurons. When dopamine neurons degenerate, the balance between them is altered. The inhibitory influence of dopamine is reduced, and the activity of cholinergic neurons is increased. The principal goal of anticholinergic drugs in the treatment of parkinsonism is to decrease the activity of cholinergic neurons in the basal ganglia.

The usefulness of the belladonna group of alkaloids for the treatment of parkinsonism was an empiric discovery. Since then, chemists have prepared many synthetic analogues of atropine in an effort to retain the useful antitremor and antirigidity effects of the belladonna alkaloid while reducing the adverse effects. In this process, it was discovered that antihistamine drugs (e.g., diphenhydramine) reduced tremor and rigidity. The antiparkinsonian-like activity of antihistamines has been attributed to their anticholinergic properties. The activity of these drugs is confined to those that can pass through the blood–brain barrier.

SOLANACEOUS ALKALOIDS AND ANALOGUES

The solanaceous alkaloids, represented by (−)-hyoscyamine, atropine [(−)-hyoscyamine], and scopolamine (hyoscine), are the forerunners of the class of antimuscarinic drugs. These alkaloids are found principally in henbane *(Hyoscyamus niger)*, deadly nightshade *(Atropa belladonna)*, and jimson weed *(Datura stramonium)*. There are other alkaloids that are members of the solanaceous group (e.g., apoatropine, noratropine, belladonnine, tigloidine, meteloidine) but lack sufficient therapeutic value to be considered in this text.

Crude drugs containing these alkaloids have been used since early times for their marked medicinal properties, which depend largely on inhibition of the parasympathetic nervous system and stimulation of the higher nervous centers. Belladonna, probably as a consequence of the weak local anesthetic activity of atropine, has been used topically for its analgesic effect on hemorrhoids, certain skin infections, and various itching dermatoses. Application of sufficient amounts of belladonna or its alkaloids results in mydriasis. Internally, the drug causes diminution of secretions, increases the heart rate (by depression of the vagus nerve), depresses the motility of the GI tract, and acts as an antispasmodic on various smooth muscles (ureter, bladder, and biliary tract). In addition, it directly stimulates the respiratory center. The multiplicity of actions exerted by the drug is looked on with some disfavor, because the physician seeking one type of response unavoidably also obtains the others. The action of scopolamine-containing drugs differs from those containing hyoscyamine and atropine in having no CNS stimulation; rather, a narcotic or sedative effect predominates. The use of this group of drugs is accompanied by a fairly high incidence of reactions because of individual idiosyncrasies; death from overdosage usually results from respiratory failure. A complete treatment of the pharmacology and uses of these drugs is not within the scope of this text. The introductory pages of this chapter briefly review some of the more pertinent points in connection with the major activities of these drug types.

Structural Considerations

All of the solanaceous alkaloids are esters of the bicyclic aminoalcohol 3-hydroxytropane or of related aminoalcohols. The structural formulas that follow show the piperidine ring system in the commonly accepted chair conformation because this form has the lowest energy requirement. The alternate boat form can exist under certain conditions, however, because the energy barrier is not great. Inspection of the 3-hydroxytropane formula also indicates that even though there is no optical activity because of the plane of symmetry, two stereoisomeric forms (tropine and pseudotropine) can exist because of the rigidity imparted to the molecule through the ethylene chain across the 1,5 positions.

In tropine, the axially oriented hydroxyl group, *trans* to the nitrogen bridge, is designated α, and the alternate *cis* equatorially oriented hydroxyl group is designated β. The aminoalcohol derived from scopolamine, namely scopine, has the axial orientation of the 3-hydroxyl group but, in addition, a β-oriented epoxy group bridged across the 6,7 positions, as shown. Of the several different solanaceous alkaloids known, it has been indicated that (−)-hyoscyamine, atropine, and scopolamine are the most important. Their structures are shown, but antimuscarinic activity is associated with all of the solanaceous alkaloids that possess the tropine-like axial orientation of the esterified hydroxyl group. Studying the formulas reveals that in each case tropic acid is the esterifying acid. Tropic acid contains an easily racemized asymmetric carbon atom, the moiety accounting for optical activity in these compounds in the absence of racemization. The proper enantiomorph is necessary for high antimuscarinic activity, as illustrated by the potent (−)-hyoscyamine in comparison with the weakly active (+)-hyoscyamine. The racemate, atropine, has intermediate activity. The marked difference in antimuscarinic potency of the optical enantiomorphs apparently does not extend to the action

on the CNS, inasmuch as both seem to have the same degree of activity.[71]

The solanaceous alkaloids have been modified by preparing other esters of 3-α-tropanol or making a quaternary of the nitrogen in tropanol or scopine with a methyl halide. These compounds represent some of the initial attempts to separate the varied actions of atropine and scopolamine. Few aminoalcohols have been found that impart the same degree of neurotropic activity as that exhibited by the ester formed by combination of tropine with tropic acid. Similarly, the tropic acid portion is highly specific for the anticholinergic action, and substitution by other acids decreases neurotropic potency, though the musculotropic action may increase. The earliest attempts to modify the atropine molecule retained the tropine portion and substituted various acids for tropic acid.

Besides changing the acid residue, other changes have been directed toward the quaternization of the nitrogen. Examples of this type of compound are methscopolamine bromide, homatropine methylbromide, and anisotropine methylbromide. Quaternization of the tertiary amine produces variable effects in terms of increasing potency. Decreases in activity are apparent in comparing atropine with methylatropine (no longer used) and scopolamine with methscopolamine. Ariens et al.[72] ascribed decreased activity, especially when the groups attached to nitrogen are larger than methyl, to a possible decrease in affinity for the anionic site on the cholinergic receptor. They attributed this decreased affinity to a combination of greater electron repulsion by such groups and greater steric interference to the approach of the cationic head to the anionic site. In general, quaternization reduces parasympathomimetic action much more than parasympatholytic action. This may be partially due to the additional blocking at the parasympathetic ganglion induced by quaternization, which could offset the decreased affinity at the postganglionic site. However, quaternization increases the curariform activity of these alkaloids and aminoesters, a usual consequence of quaternizing alkaloids. Another disadvantage in converting an alkaloidal base to the quaternary form is that the quaternized base is absorbed more poorly through the intestinal wall, so that the activity becomes erratic and, in some instances, unpredictable. Bases (such as alkaloids) are absorbed through the lipoidal gut wall only in the dissociated form, which can be expected to exist for a tertiary base, in the small intestine. Quaternary nitrogen bases cannot revert to an undissociated form, even in basic media and, presumably, may have difficulty passing through the gut wall. Since quaternary compounds can be absorbed, other less efficient mechanisms for absorption probably prevail. Quaternary ammonium compounds combine reversibly with endogenous substances in the gut, such as mucin, to form neutral ion-pair complexes. These complexes penetrate the lipid membrane by passive diffusion.

Products

Atropine, USP. Atropine is the tropine ester of racemic tropic acid and is optically inactive. It possibly occurs naturally in various Solanaceae, though some claim, with justification, that whatever atropine is isolated from natural sources results from racemization of (−)-hyoscyamine during the isolation process. Conventional methods of alkaloid

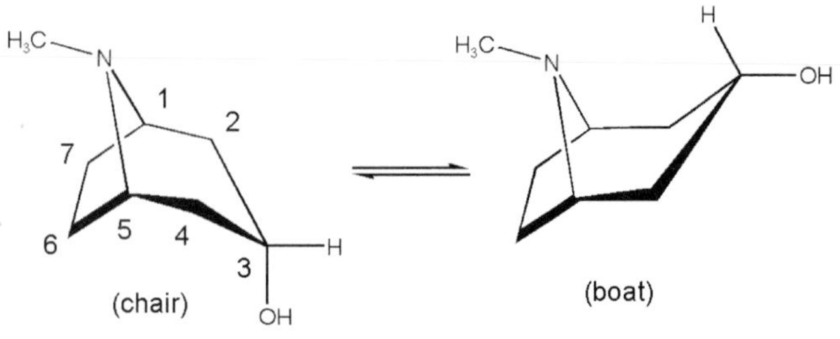

TROPINE
(3α-Hydroxytropane or
3α-Tropanol)

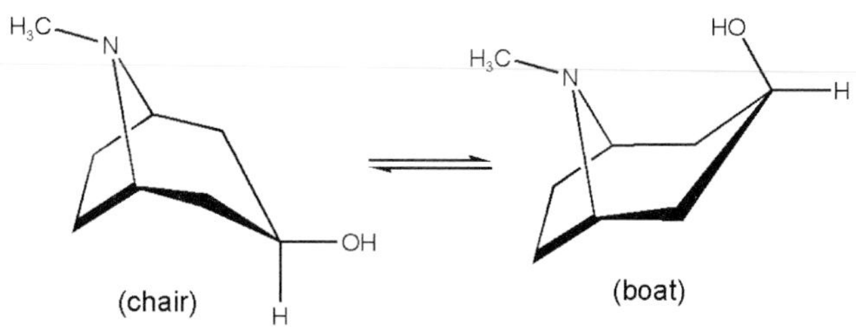

PSEUDOTROPINE
(3β-Hydroxytropane or
3β-Tropanol)

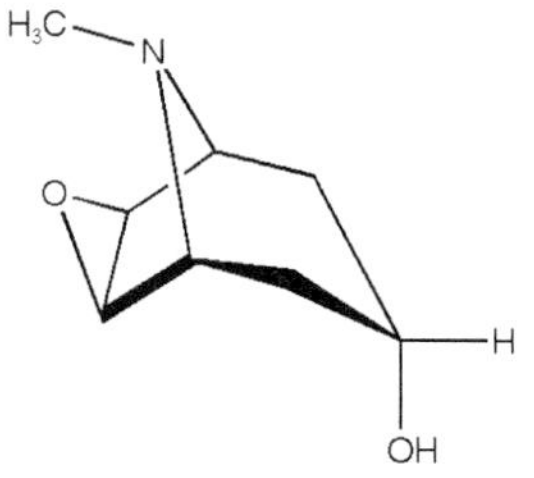

SCOPINE
(6:7 β-Epoxy-3-α-hydroxytropane
or 6:7 β-Epoxy-3-α-tropanol

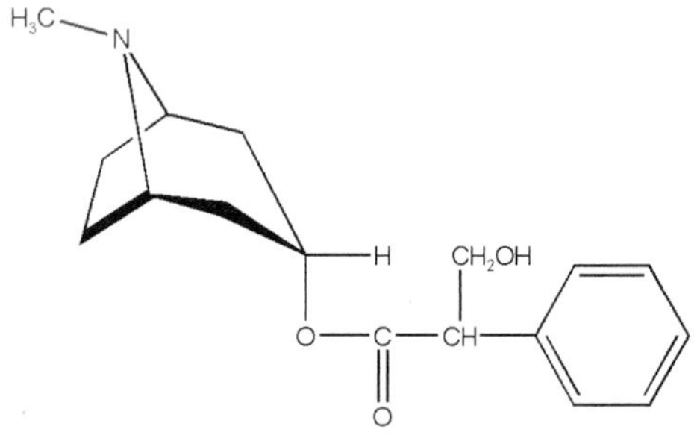

ATROPINE
(or hyoscyamine)

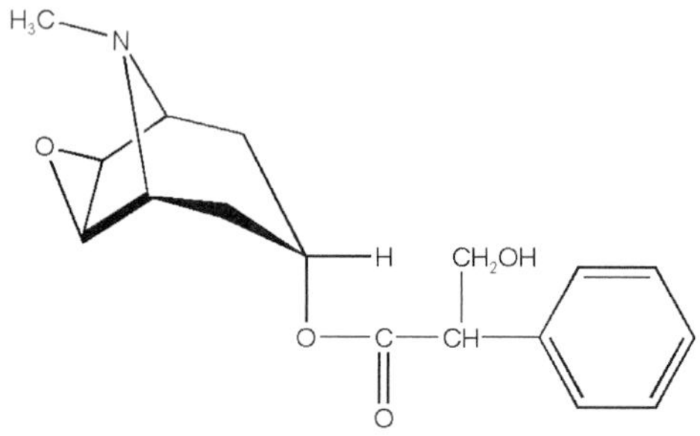

SCOPOLAMINE
(or hyoscine)

isolation are used to obtain a crude mixture of atropine and hyoscyamine from the plant material. This crude mixture is racemized to atropine by refluxing in chloroform or by treatment with cold dilute alkali. Because the racemization process makes atropine, an official limit is set on the hyoscyamine content by restricting atropine to a maximum levorotation under specified conditions.

Atropine occurs in the form of optically inactive, white, odorless crystals possessing a bitter taste. It is not very soluble in water (1:460, 1:90 at 80°C) but is more soluble in alcohol (1:2, 1:1.2 at 60°C). It is soluble in glycerin (1:27),

in chloroform (1:1), and in ether (1:25). Saturated aqueous solutions are alkaline in reaction (pH ~9.5). The free base is useful when nonaqueous solutions are to be made, such as in oily vehicles and ointment bases. Atropine has a plasma half-life of about 2 to 3 hours. It is metabolized in the liver to several products, including tropic acid and tropine.

Atropine Sulfate, USP. Atropine sulfate (Atropisol) is prepared by neutralizing atropine in acetone or ether solution with an alcoholic solution of sulfuric acid, with care used to prevent hydrolysis. The salt occurs as colorless crystals or as a white, crystalline powder. It is efflorescent in dry air and should be protected from light to prevent decomposition.

Atropine sulfate is freely soluble in water (1:0.5), in alcohol (1:5, 1:2.5 at boiling point), and in glycerin (1:2.5). Aqueous solutions are not very stable, though solutions may be sterilized at 120°C (15 lb pressure) in an autoclave if the pH is kept below 6. Sterilization probably is best effected by the use of aseptic techniques and a bacteriological filter. It has been suggested that no more than a 30-day supply of an aqueous solution should be made and that for small quantities the best procedure is to use hypodermic tablets and sterile distilled water.[72] Kondritzer and Zvirblis[73] have studied the kinetics of alkaline and proton-catalyzed hydrolyses of atropine in aqueous solution. The region of maximal stability lies between pH 3 and approximately 5. They have also proposed an equation to predict the half-life of atropine undergoing hydrolysis at constant pH and temperature.

The action of atropine or its salts is the same. It produces a mydriatic effect by paralyzing the iris and the ciliary muscles and, for this reason, is used by the oculist in iritis and corneal inflammations and lesions. Its use is rational in these conditions because one of the first rules in the treatment of inflammation is rest, which, of course, is accomplished by the paralysis of muscular motion. Its use in the eye (0.5 to 1% solutions or gelatin disks) for fitting glasses is widespread. Atropine is administered in small doses before general anesthesia to lessen oral and air passage secretions and, when administered with morphine, to lessen the respiratory depression induced by morphine.

Atropine causes restlessness, prolonged pupillary dilation, and loss of visual accommodation and, furthermore, gives rise to arrhythmias such as atrioventricular dissociation, ventricular extrasystoles, and even ventricular fibrillation. Even though ether has been gradually replaced by other anesthetics, thereby eliminating problems with respiratory secretions caused by ether and thus requiring atropine, surgeons and anesthesiologists today continue to use it as an anesthetic premedicant to reduce excessive salivary and airway secretions and to prevent vagal reflexes.

Its ability to dry secretions has also been used in the so-called rhinitis tablets for symptomatic relief in colds. In cathartic preparations, atropine or belladonna has been used as an antispasmodic to lessen the smooth muscle spasm (griping) often associated with catharsis.

Atropine may be used to treat some types of arrhythmias. It increases the heart rate by blocking the effects of ACh on the vagus. In this context, it is used to treat certain reversible bradyarrhythmias that may accompany acute myocardial infarction. It is also used as an adjunct to anesthesia to protect against bradycardia, hypotension, and even cardiac arrest induced by the skeletal muscle relaxant succinylcholine chloride.

Another use for atropine sulfate emerged following the development of the organophosphates, which are potent inhibitors of AChE. Atropine is a specific antidote to prevent the muscarinic effects of ACh accumulation, such as vomiting, abdominal cramps, diarrhea, salivation, sweating, bronchoconstriction, and excessive bronchial secretions. It is used intravenously but does not protect against respiratory failure caused by depression of the respiratory center and the muscles of respiration.

Hyoscyamine, USP. Hyoscyamine is a levorotatory alkaloid obtained from various solanaceous species. One of the commercial sources is Egyptian henbane (*Hyoscyamus muticus*), in which it occurs to the extent of about 0.5%. Usually, it is prepared from the crude drug in a manner similar to that used for atropine and is purified as the oxalate. The free base is obtained easily from this salt.

It occurs as white needles that are sparingly soluble in water (1:281), more soluble in ether (1:69) or benzene (1:150), very soluble in chloroform (1:1), and freely soluble in alcohol. It is used as the sulfate and hydrobromide. The principal reason for the popularity of the hydrobromide has been its nondeliquescent nature. The salts have the advantage over the free base in being quite water soluble.

Hyoscyamine is the *levo* form of the racemic mixture known as atropine. The *dextro* form does not exist naturally but has been synthesized. Cushny[74] compared the activities of (−)-hyoscyamine, (+)-hyoscyamine, and the racemate (atropine) in 1904 and found greater peripheral potency for the (−) isomer and twice the potency of the racemate. All later studies have essentially confirmed that the (+) isomer is only weakly active and that the (−) isomer is, in effect, the active portion of atropine. Inspection of the relative doses of atropine sulfate and hyoscyamine sulfate illustrates the differences very nicely. The principal criticism offered against the use of hyoscyamine sulfate exclusively is that it tends to racemize to atropine sulfate rather easily in solution, so that atropine sulfate then becomes the more stable of the two. All of the isomers behave very much the same in the CNS.

Hyoscyamine is used to treat disorders of the urinary tract more so than any other antispasmodic, though there is no evidence that it has any advantages over the other belladonna preparations and the synthetic anticholinergics. It is used to treat spasms of the bladder and, in this manner, serves as a urinary stimulant. It is used together with a narcotic to counteract the spasm produced by the narcotic when the latter is used to relieve the pain of urethral colic. Hyoscyamine preparations are also used as antispasmodics in the therapy of peptic ulcers.

Hyoscyamine Sulfate, USP. Hyoscyamine sulfate (Levsin sulfate) is a white, odorless, crystalline compound of a deliquescent nature that also is affected by light. It is soluble in water (1:0.5) and alcohol (1:5) but almost insoluble in ether. Solutions of hyoscyamine sulfate are acidic to litmus.

This drug is used as an anticholinergic in the same manner and for the same indications as atropine and hyoscyamine, but it possesses the disadvantage of being deliquescent.

Scopolamine. Scopolamine (hyoscine) is found in various members of the Solanaceae (e.g., *H. niger, Duboisia myoporoides, Scopolia* spp., and *Datura metel*). Scopolamine usually is isolated from the mother liquor remaining from the isolation of hyoscyamine.

Hyoscine is the older name for this alkaloid, though *scopolamine* is the accepted name in the United States. Scopolamine is the *levo* component of the racemic mixture that is known as *atroscine*. The alkaloid is racemized readily in the presence of dilute alkali.

The alkaloid occurs in the form of a levorotatory, viscous liquid that is only slightly soluble in water but very soluble in alcohol, chloroform, or ether. It forms crystalline salts with most acids, with the hydrobromide being the most stable and the most popularly accepted. An aqueous solution of the hydrobromide containing 10% mannitol is said to be less prone to decomposition than unprotected solutions. The commercially available transdermal system of scopolamine comprises an outer layer of polymer film and a drug reservoir containing scopolamine, polyisobutylene, and mineral oil, which is interfaced with a microporous membrane to control diffusion of the drug. In this dosage form, scopolamine is effective in preventing motion sickness. The action is believed to be on the cortex or the vestibular apparatus. Whereas atropine stimulates the CNS, causing restlessness and talkativeness, scopolamine usually acts as a CNS depressant.

Scopolamine Hydrobromide, USP.

Scopolamine hydrobromide (hyoscine hydrobromide) occurs as white or colorless crystals or as a white, granular powder. It is odorless and tends to effloresce in dry air. It is freely soluble in water (1:1.5), soluble in alcohol (1:20), only slightly soluble in chloroform, and insoluble in ether.

Scopolamine is a competitive blocking agent of the parasympathetic nervous system as is atropine, but it differs markedly from atropine in its action on the higher nerve centers. Both drugs readily cross the blood–brain barrier and, even in therapeutic doses, cause confusion, particularly in the elderly.

A sufficiently large dose of scopolamine will cause an individual to sink into a restful, dreamless sleep for about 8 hours, followed by a period of approximately the same length in which the patient is in a semiconscious state. During this time, the patient does not remember events that take place. When scopolamine is administered with morphine, this temporary amnesia is termed *twilight sleep*.

Homatropine Hydrobromide, USP.

Homatropine hydrobromide, 1αH,5αH-tropan-3α-ol mandelate (ester) hydrobromide (Homatrocel), occurs as white crystals or as a white, crystalline powder that is affected by light. It is soluble in water (1:6) and alcohol (1:40), less soluble in chloroform (1:420), and insoluble in ether.

Solutions are incompatible with alkaline substances, which precipitate the free base, and with the common reagents that precipitate alkaloids. As with atropine, solutions are sterilized best by filtration through a bacteriological filter.

Homatropine hydrobromide is used topically to paralyze the ciliary structure of the eye (cycloplegia) and to effect mydriasis. It behaves very much like atropine but is weaker and less toxic. In the eye, it acts more rapidly but less persistently than atropine. Dilation of the pupil takes place in about 15 to 20 minutes, and the action subsides in about 24 hours. By using a miotic, such as physostigmine, it is possible to restore the pupil to normality in a few hours.

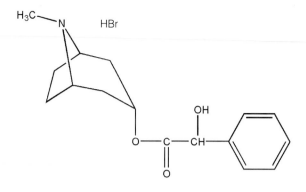

Homatropine Hydrobromide

Homatropine Methylbromide, USP.

Homatropine methylbromide, 3α-hydroxy-8-methyl-1αH,5αH-tropanium bromide mandelate (Novatropine, Mesopin), occurs as a bitter, white, odorless powder and is affected by light. The compound is readily soluble in water and alcohol but insoluble in ether. The pH of a 1% solution is 5.9 and that of a 10% solution is 4.5. Although a solution of the compound yields a precipitate with alkaloidal reagents, such as mercuric potassium iodide test solution, addition of alkali hydroxides or carbonates does not cause the precipitate that occurs with nonquaternary nitrogen salts (e.g., atropine, homatropine).

Homatropine Methylbromide

Homatropine methylbromide is transported poorly across the blood–brain barrier because of its quaternary ammonium group and, therefore, has far fewer stimulant properties than atropine. It does have all the characteristic peripheral parasympathetic depressant properties of atropine and is used to reduce oversecretion and to relieve GI spasms.

Ipratropium Bromide.

Ipratropium bromide, 3-(3-hydroxy-1-oxo-2-phenylpropoxy)-8-methyl-8-(1-methylethyl)-8-azoniabicyclo[3.2.1]octane bromide (Atrovent), is a quaternary ammonium derivative of atropine. It is freely soluble in water and ethanol but insoluble in chloroform and ether. The salt is stable in neutral and acidic solutions but rapidly hydrolyzed in alkaline solutions.

Ipratropium Bromide

Ipratropium bromide is used in inhalation therapy to produce dilation of bronchial smooth muscle for acute asthmatic attacks. The drug produces bronchodilation by competitive inhibition of cholinergic receptors bound to smooth muscle of the bronchioles. Ipratropium may also act on the surface of mast cells to inhibit ACh-enhanced release of chemical mediators. The drug has a slow onset of action, within 5 to 15 minutes after being administered by inhalation, and should not be used alone for acute asthmatic attacks. The peak therapeutic effect from one dose is observed between 1 and 2 hours. The effects of the drug last for about 6 hours. It has a half-life of 3.5 hours.

SYNTHETIC CHOLINERGIC BLOCKING AGENTS

Aminoalcohol Esters

The solanaceous alkaloids are generally agreed to be potent parasympatholytics, but they have the undesirable property of producing a wide range of effects through their nonspecific blockade of autonomic functions. Efforts to use the antispasmodic effect of the alkaloids most often result in side effects such as dryness of the mouth and fluctuations in pulse rate. Therefore, synthesis of compounds possessing specific cholinolytic actions has been a very desirable field of study. Few prototypical drugs were as avidly dissected in the minds of researchers as atropine in attempts to modify its structure to separate the numerous useful activities (i.e., antispasmodic, antisecretory, mydriatic, and cycloplegic). Most early research was carried out in the pre– and post–World War II era before muscarinic receptor subtypes were known.

Efforts at synthesis started with rather minor deviations from the atropine molecule, but a review of the commonly used drugs today indicates a marked departure from the rigid tropane aminoalcohols and tropic acid residues. Examination of the structures of antispasmodics shows that the acid portion has been designed to provide a large hydrophobic moiety rather than the stereospecific requirement of (*S*)-tropic acid in (−)-hyoscyamine that was once considered important. One of the major developments in the field of aminoalcohol esters was the successful introduction of the quaternary ammonium derivatives as contrasted with the tertiary amine–type esters synthesized originally. Although some effective tertiary amine esters are in use today, the quaternaries, as a group, represent the more popular type and appear to be slightly more potent than their tertiary amine counterparts.

The accompanying formula shows the portion of the atropine molecule (enclosed in the curved dotted line) believed to be responsible for its major activity. This is sometimes called the *spasmophoric* group and compares with the *anesthesiophoric* group obtained by similar dissection of the cocaine molecule. The validity of this conclusion has been amply borne out by the many active compounds having only a simple diethylaminoethyl residue replacing the tropine portion.

Tropic Acid   Tropine

The aminoalcohol portion of eucatropine may be considered a simplification of the atropine molecule. In eucatropine, the bicyclic tropine has been replaced by a monocyclic aminoalcohol and mandelic acid replaces tropic acid (see under ''Products'').

Although simplification of the aminoalcohol portion of the atropine prototype has been a guiding principle in most research, many of the anticholinergics now used still include a cyclic aminoalcohol moiety. The aminoalcohol ester anticholinergics are used primarily as antispasmodics or mydriatics, and cholinolytic compounds classed as aminoalcohol or aminoalcohol ether analogues of atropine are, with few exceptions, used as antiparkinsonian drugs.

Another important feature in many of the synthetic anticholinergics used as antispasmodics is that they contain a quaternary nitrogen, presumably to enhance activity. The initial synthetic quaternary compound methantheline bromide has served as a forerunner for many others. These compounds combine anticholinergic activity of the antimuscarinic type with some ganglionic blockade to reinforce the parasympathetic blockade. Formation of a quaternary ammonium moiety, however, introduces the possibility of blockade of voluntary synapses (curariform activity); this can become evident with sufficiently high doses.

Products

The antimuscarinic compounds now in use are described in the following monographs.

Clidinium Bromide, USP. Clidinium bromide, 3-hydroxy-1-methylquinuclidinium bromide benzilate (Quarzan), is a white or nearly white, almost odorless, crystalline powder that is optically inactive. It is soluble in water and alcohol but only very slightly soluble in ether and benzene.

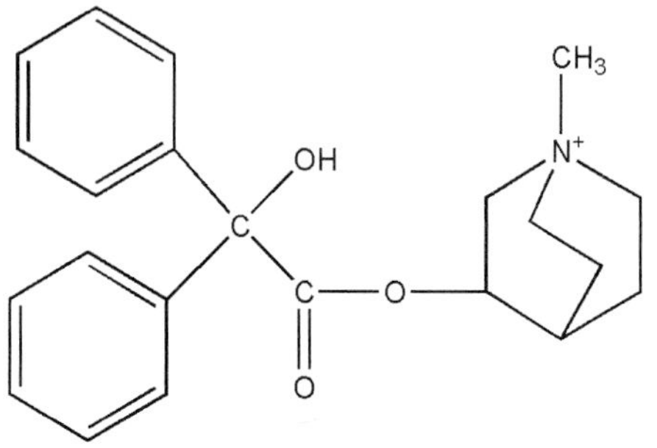

Clidinium Bromide

This anticholinergic agent is marketed alone and in combination with the minor tranquilizer chlordiazepoxide (Librium) in a product known as Librax. The rationale of the combination for the treatment of GI complaints is the use of an anxiety-reducing agent together with an anticholinergic agent, based on the recognized contribution of anxiety to the development of the diseased condition. It is suggested for peptic ulcer, hyperchlorhydria, ulcerative or spastic colon, anxiety states with GI manifestations, nervous stomach, irritable or spastic colon, and others. Clidinium bromide is contraindicated in glaucoma and other conditions that may be aggravated by the parasympatholytic action, such as prostatic hypertrophy in elderly men, which could lead to urinary retention.

Cyclopentolate Hydrochloride, USP. Cyclopentolate hydrochloride, 2-dimethylaminoethyl 1-hydroxy-α-phenyl-cyclopentaneacetate hydrochloride (Cyclogyl), is a crystalline, white, odorless solid that is very soluble in water, easily soluble in alcohol, and only slightly soluble in ether. A 1% solution has a pH of 5.0 to 5.4.

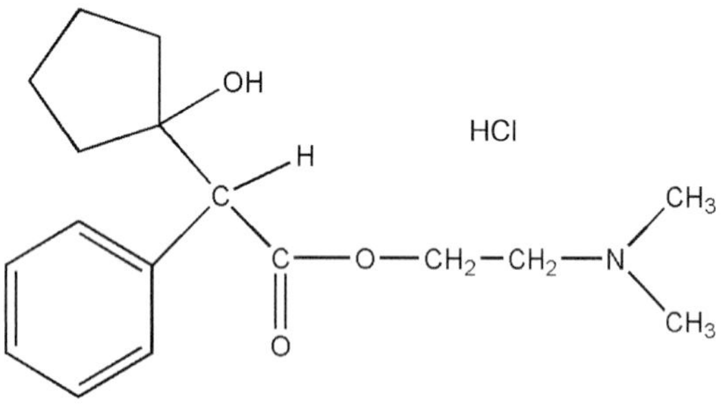

Cyclopentolate Hydrochloride

It is used only for its effects on the eye, where it acts as a parasympatholytic. When placed in the eye, it quickly produces cycloplegia and mydriasis. Its primary field of usefulness is in refraction studies. Cyclopentolate hydrochloride can be used, however, as a mydriatic in the management of iritis, iridocyclitis, keratitis, and choroiditis. Although it does not seem to affect intraocular tension significantly, it is best to be very cautious with patients with high intraocular pressure and with elderly patients with possible unrecognized glaucomatous changes.

Cyclopentolate hydrochloride has one half of the antispas-modic activity of atropine and is nonirritating when instilled repeatedly into the eye. If not neutralized after the refraction studies, its effect dissipates within 24 hours. Neutralization with a few drops of pilocarpine nitrate solution, 1 to 2%, often results in complete recovery in 6 hours. It is supplied as a ready-made ophthalmic solution in concentrations of either 0.5 or 2%.

Dicyclomine Hydrochloride, USP. Dicyclomine hydrochloride, 2-(diethylamino)ethyl bicyclohexyl-1-carboxylate hydrochloride (Bentyl), has some muscarinic receptor subtype selectivity. It binds more firmly to M_1 and M_3 than to M_2 and M_4 receptors.[75]

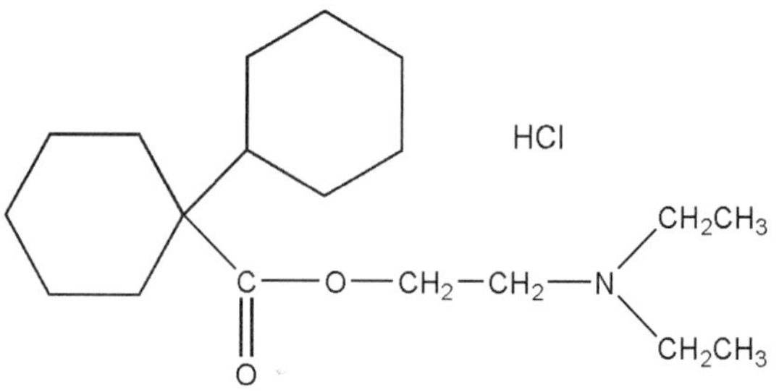

Dicyclomine Hydrochloride

Dicyclomine hydrochloride has one eighth of the neurotropic activity of atropine and approximately twice the musculotropic activity of papaverine. This preparation, first introduced in 1950, has minimized the adverse effects associated with the atropine-type compounds. It is used for its spasmolytic effect on various smooth muscle spasms, particularly those associated with the GI tract. It is also useful in dysmenorrhea, pylorospasm, and biliary dysfunction.

Eucatropine Hydrochloride, USP. Eucatropine hydrochloride, euphthalmine hydrochloride or 1,2,2,6-tetramethyl-4-piperidyl mandelate hydrochloride, possesses the aminoalcohol moiety characteristic of one of the early local anesthetics (e.g., β-eucaine) but differs in the acidic portion of the ester by being a mandelate instead of a benzoate. The salt is an odorless, white, granular powder, providing solutions that are neutral to litmus. It is very soluble in water, freely soluble in alcohol and chloroform, but almost insoluble in ether.

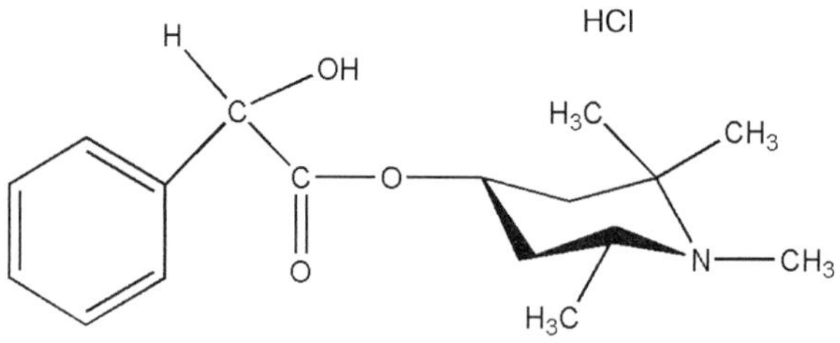

Eucatropine Hydrochloride

The action of eucatropine hydrochloride closely parallels that of atropine, though it is much less potent than the latter. It is used topically in a 0.1 mL dose as a mydriatic in 2% solution or in the form of small tablets. Use of concentrations from 5 to 10% is, however, not uncommon. Dilation, with little impairment of accommodation, takes place in about 30 minutes, and the eye returns to normal in 2 to 3 hours.

Glycopyrrolate, USP.

Glycopyrrolate, 3-hydroxy-1,1-dimethylpyrrolidinium bromide α-cyclopentylmandelate (Robinul), occurs as a white, crystalline powder that is soluble in water or alcohol but practically insoluble in chloroform or ether.

Glycopyrrolate

Glycopyrrolate is a typical anticholinergic and possesses, at adequate dosage levels, the atropine-like effects characteristic of this class of drugs. It has a spasmolytic effect on the musculature of the GI tract as well as the genitourinary tract. It diminishes gastric and pancreatic secretions and the quantity of perspiration and saliva. Its side effects are typically atropine-like also (i.e., dryness of the mouth, urinary retention, blurred vision, constipation). Glycopyrrolate is a more potent antagonist on M_1 than on M_2 and M_3 receptors. The low affinity of M_2 receptors may, in part, explain the low incidence of tachycardia during use of this drug as an antispasmodic.[76] Because of its quaternary ammonium character, glycopyrrolate rarely causes CNS disturbances, though in sufficiently high dosage it can bring about ganglionic and myoneural junction block.

The drug is used as an adjunct in the management of peptic ulcer and other GI ailments associated with hyperacidity, hypermotility, and spasm. In common with other anticholinergics, its use does not preclude dietary restrictions or use of antacids and sedatives if these are indicated.

Mepenzolate Bromide.

Mepenzolate bromide, 3-hydroxy-1,1-dimethylpiperidinium bromide benzilate (Cantil), has an activity about one-half that of atropine in reducing ACh-induced spasms of the guinea pig ileum. The selective action on colonic hypermotility is said to relieve pain, cramps, and bloating and to help curb diarrhea.

Mepenzolate Bromide

Methantheline Bromide, USP.

Methantheline bromide, diethyl(2-hydroxyethyl)methylammonium bromide xanthene-9-carboxylate (Banthine Bromide), is a white, slightly hygroscopic, crystalline salt that is soluble in water to produce solutions with a pH of about 5. Aqueous solutions are not stable and hydrolyze in a few days. The bromide form is preferable to the very hygroscopic chloride.

Methantheline Bromide

This drug, introduced in 1950, is a potent anticholinergic agent and acts at the nicotinic cholinergic receptors of the sympathetic and parasympathetic systems, as well as at the myoneural junction of the postganglionic cholinergic fibers. Like other quaternary ammonium drugs, methantheline bromide is absorbed incompletely from the GI tract.

Among the conditions for which methantheline bromide is indicated are gastritis, intestinal hypermotility, bladder irritability, cholinergic spasm, pancreatitis, hyperhidrosis, and peptic ulcer, all of which are manifestations of parasympathotonia.

Side reactions are atropine-like (mydriasis, cycloplegia, dryness of mouth). The drug is contraindicated in glaucoma. Toxic doses may bring about a curare-like action, a not too surprising fact when it is considered that ACh is the mediating factor for neural transmission at the somatic myoneural junction. This side effect can be counteracted with neostigmine methylsulfate.

Oxyphencyclimine Hydrochloride.

Oxyphencyclimine hydrochloride, 1,4,5,6-tetrahydro-1-methyl-2-pyrimidinyl)methyl α-phenylcyclohexaneglycolate monohydrochloride (Daricon, Vistrax), was introduced in 1958 and promoted as a peripheral anticholinergic–antisecretory agent, with little or no curare-like activity and little or no ganglionic blocking activity. These activities are probably absent because of the tertiary character of the molecule. This activity is in contrast with that of compounds that couple antimuscarinic action with ganglionic blocking action. The tertiary character of the nitrogen promotes intestinal absorption of the molecule. Perhaps the most significant activity of this compound is its marked ability to reduce both the volume and the acid content of the gastric juices, a desirable action in view of the more recent hypotheses pertaining to peptic ulcer therapy. Another important feature of this compound is its low toxicity in comparison with many of the other available anticholinergics. Oxyphencyclimine hydrochloride is hydrolyzed in the presence of excessive moisture and heat. It is absorbed from the GI tract and has a duration of action of up to 12 hours.

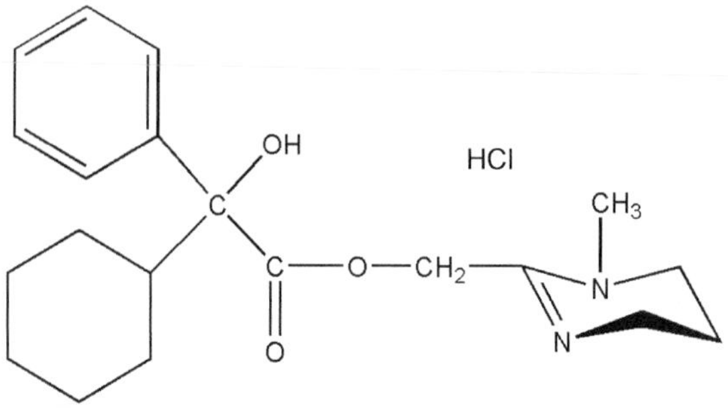

Oxyphencyclimine Hydrochloride

Oxyphencyclimine hydrochloride is suggested for use in peptic ulcer, pylorospasm, and functional bowel syndrome. It is contraindicated, as are other anticholinergics, in patients with prostatic hypertrophy and glaucoma.

Propantheline Bromide, USP. Propantheline bromide, 2-hydroxy-ethyl)diisopropylmethylammonium bromide xanthene-9-carboxylate (Pro-Banthine), is prepared in a manner exactly analogous to that used for methantheline bromide. It is a white, water-soluble, crystalline substance, with properties quite similar to those of methantheline bromide. Its chief difference from methantheline bromide is in its potency, which has been estimated variously to be 2 to 5 times as great.

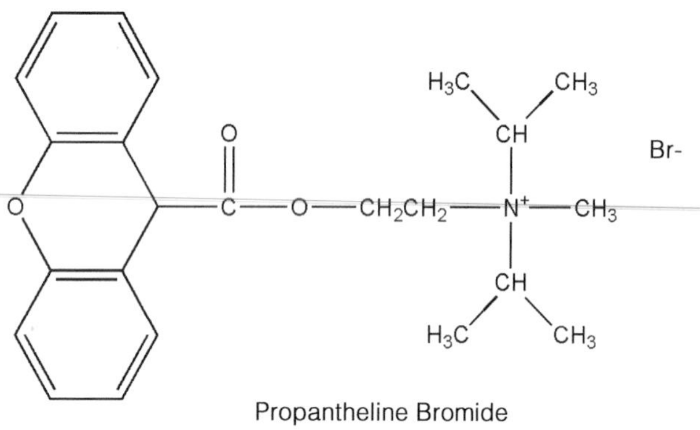

Propantheline Bromide

Aminoalcohol Ethers

The aminoalcohol ethers thus far introduced have been used as antiparkinsonian drugs rather than as conventional anticholinergics (i.e., as spasmolytics or mydriatics). In general, they may be considered closely related to the antihistaminics and, indeed, do possess substantial antihistaminic properties. In turn, the antihistamines possess anticholinergic activity and have been used as antiparkinsonian agents. Comparison of chlorphenoxamine and orphenadrine with the antihistaminic diphenhydramine illustrates the close similarity of structure. The use of diphenhydramine in parkinsonism has been cited above. Benztropine may also be considered a structural relative of diphenhydramine, though the aminoalcohol portion is tropine and, therefore, more distantly related than chlorphenoxamine and orphenadrine. In the structure of benztropine, a three-carbon chain intervenes between the nitrogen and oxygen functions, whereas the others evince a two-carbon chain. However, the rigid ring structure possibly orients the nitrogen and oxygen functions into more nearly

the two-carbon chain interprosthetic distance than is apparent at first glance. This, combined with the flexibility of the alicyclic chain, would help to minimize the distance discrepancy.

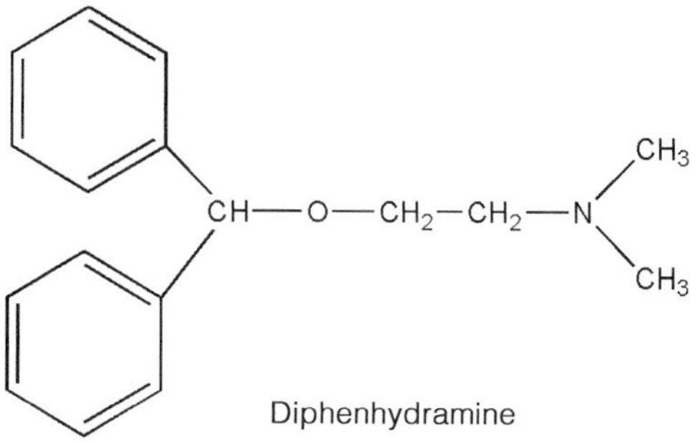

Diphenhydramine

Benztropine Mesylate, USP. Benztropine mesylate, 3α-(diphenylmethoxy)-1αH,5αH-tropane methanesulfonate (Cogentin), has anticholinergic, antihistaminic, and local anesthetic properties. Its anticholinergic effect makes it applicable as an antiparkinsonian agent. It is about as potent an anticholinergic as atropine and shares some of the side effects of this drug, such as mydriasis and dryness of mouth. Importantly, however, it does not produce central stimulation but instead exerts the characteristic sedative effect of the antihistamines.

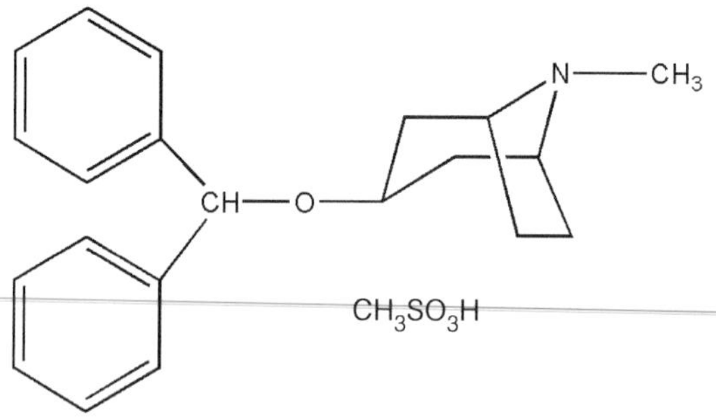

Benztropine Mesylate

The tremor and rigidity characteristic of parkinsonism are relieved by benztropine mesylate, and it is particularly valuable for those patients who cannot tolerate central excitation (e.g., aged patients). It may also have a useful effect in minimizing drooling, sialorrhea, mask-like facies, oculogyric crises, and muscular cramps.

The usual caution exercised with any anticholinergic in glaucoma and prostatic hypertrophy is observed with this drug.

Orphenadrine Citrate. Orphenadrine citrate, *N,N*-dimethyl-2-(*o*-methyl-α-phenylbenzyloxy)ethylamine citrate (1:1) (Norflex), introduced in 1957, is closely related to diphenhydramine structurally but has much lower antihistaminic activity and much higher anticholinergic action. Likewise, it lacks the sedative effects characteristic of diphenhydramine. Pharmacological testing indicates that it is not primarily a peripherally acting anticholinergic because it has only weak effects on smooth muscle, on the eye, and on secretory glands. It does reduce voluntary muscle spasm, however, by a central inhibitory action on cerebral motor areas, a central effect similar to that of atropine.

Orphenadrine Citrate

This drug is used for the symptomatic treatment of Parkinson's disease. It relieves rigidity better than it does tremor, and in certain cases, it may accentuate the latter. The drug combats mental sluggishness, akinesia, adynamia, and lack of mobility, but this effect seems to diminish rather rapidly with prolonged use. It is best used as an adjunct to the other agents, such as benztropine, procyclidine, cycrimine, and trihexyphenidyl, in the treatment of paralysis agitans. Orphenadrine citrate is also used as an adjunct to rest, physiotherapy, and other measures to relieve pain of local muscle spasm (e.g., nocturnal leg cramps).

The drug has a low incidence of the usual side effects for this group, namely, dryness of mouth, nausea, and mild excitation.

Aminoalcohols

The development of aminoalcohols as parasympatholytics took place in the 1940s. It was soon established, however, that these antispasmodics were equally efficacious in parkinsonism.

Several of the drugs in this class of antimuscarinic agents possess bulky groups in the vicinity of hydroxyl and cyclic amino functional groups. These compounds are similar to the classic aminoester anticholinergic compounds derived from atropine. The presence of the alcohol group seems to substitute adequately as a prosthetic group for the carboxyl function in creating an effective parasympathetic blocking agent. The aminoester group, per se, is not a necessary adjunct to cholinolytic activity, provided that other polar groupings, such as the hydroxyl, can substitute as a prosthetic group for the carboxyl function. Another structural feature common to all aminoalcohol anticholinergics is the γ-aminopropanol arrangement, with three carbons intervening between the hydroxyl and amino functions. All of the aminoalcohols used for paralysis agitans are tertiary amines. Because the desired locus of action is central, formation of a quaternary ammonium moiety destroys the antiparkinsonian properties. These aminoalcohols have been quaternized, however, to enhance the anticholinergic activity to produce an antispasmodic and antisecretory compound, such as tridihexethyl chloride.

Biperiden, USP. Biperiden, α-5-norbornen-2-yl-α-phenyl-1-piperidinepropanol (Akineton), introduced in

1959, has a relatively weak visceral anticholinergic, but a strong nicotinolytic, action in terms of its ability to block nicotine-induced convulsions. Therefore, its neurotropic action is rather low on intestinal musculature and blood vessels. It has a relatively strong musculotropic action, which is about equal to that of papaverine, in comparison with most synthetic anticholinergic drugs. Its action on the eye, although mydriatic, is much lower than that of atropine. These weak anticholinergic effects add to its usefulness in Parkinson's syndrome by minimizing side effects.

Biperiden

The drug is used in all types of Parkinson's disease (postencephalitic, idiopathic, arteriosclerotic) and helps to eliminate akinesia, rigidity, and tremor. It is also used in drug-induced extrapyramidal disorders to eliminate symptoms and permit continued use of tranquilizers. Biperiden is also of value in spastic disorders not related to parkinsonism, such as multiple sclerosis, spinal cord injury, and cerebral palsy. It is contraindicated in all forms of epilepsy.

Biperiden Hydrochloride, USP. Biperiden hydrochloride, α-5-norbornen-2-yl-α-phenyl-1-piperidinepropanol hydrochloride (Akineton hydrochloride), is a white, optically inactive, crystalline, odorless powder that is slightly soluble in water, ether, alcohol, and chloroform and sparingly soluble in methanol.

Biperiden hydrochloride has all of the actions described for biperiden. The hydrochloride is used for tablets because it is better suited to this dosage form than is the lactate salt. As with the free base and the lactate salt, xerostomia (dryness of the mouth) and blurred vision may occur.

Procyclidine Hydrochloride, USP. Procyclidine hydrochloride, α-cyclohexyl-α-phenyl-1-pyrrolidinepropanol hydrochloride (Kemadrin), was introduced in 1956. Although it is an effective peripheral anticholinergic and, indeed, has been used for peripheral effects similar to its methochloride (i.e., tricyclamol chloride), its clinical usefulness lies in its ability to relieve voluntary muscle spasticity by its central action. Therefore, it has been used with success in the treatment of Parkinson's syndrome. It is said to be as effective as trihexyphenidyl and is used to reduce muscle rigidity in postencephalitic, arteriosclerotic, and idiopathic types of the disease. Its effect on tremor is not predictable and probably should be supplemented by combination with other similar drugs.

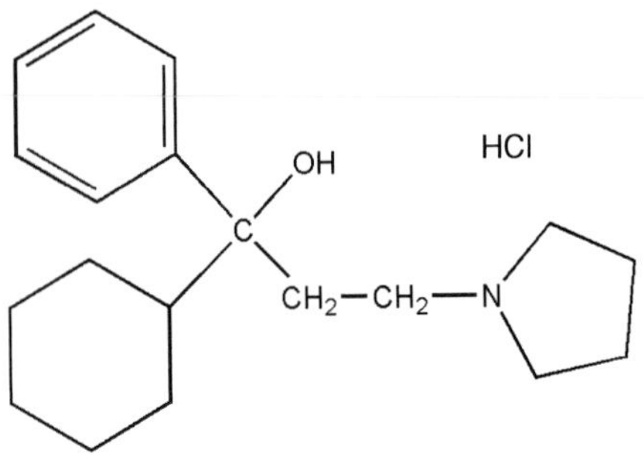

Procyclidine Hydrochloride

The toxicity of the drug is low, but when the dosage of the drug is high, side effects are noticeable. At therapeutic dosage levels, dry mouth is the most common side effect. The same care should be exercised with this drug as with all other anticholinergics when it is administered to patients with glaucoma, tachycardia, or prostatic hypertrophy.

Tridihexethyl Chloride, USP.   Tridihexethyl chloride, 3-cyclohexyl-3-hydroxy-3-phenylpropyl)triethylammonium chloride (Pathilon), is a white, bitter, crystalline powder with a characteristic odor. The compound is freely soluble in water and alcohol, with aqueous solutions being nearly neutral in reaction.

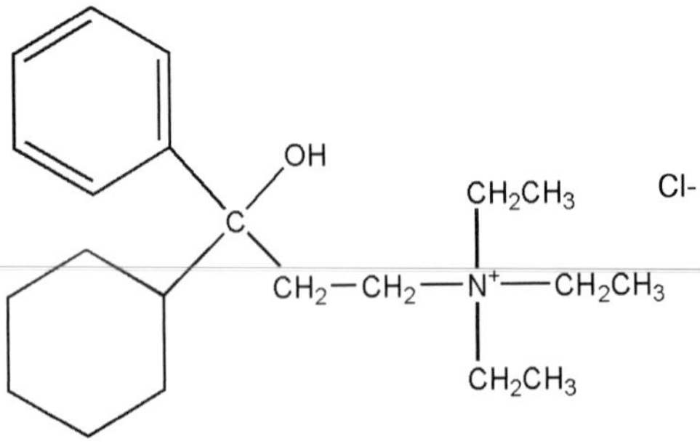

Tridihexethyl Chloride

Although this drug, introduced in 1958, has ganglion-blocking activity, its peripheral atropine-like activity predominates; therefore, its therapeutic application has been based on the latter activity. It possesses the antispasmodic and the antisecretory activities characteristic of this group, but because of its quaternary character, it is valueless in relieving Parkinson's syndrome.

The drug is useful for adjunctive therapy in a wide variety of GI diseases, such as peptic ulcer, gastric hyperacidity, and hypermotility and spastic conditions, such as spastic colon, functional diarrhea, pylorospasm, and other related conditions. Because its action is predominantly antisecretory, it is more effective in gastric hypersecretion than in hypermotility and spasm. It is best administered intravenously for the latter conditions.

The side effects usually found with effective anticholinergic therapy occur with the use of this drug. These are dryness of mouth, mydriasis, and such. As with other anticholinergics, care should be exercised when administering the drug to patients with glaucomatous conditions, cardiac decompensation, and coronary insufficiency. It is contraindicated

in patients with obstruction at the bladder neck, prostatic hypertrophy, stenosing gastric and duodenal ulcers, or pyloric or duodenal obstruction.

Trihexyphenidyl Hydrochloride, USP.   Trihexyphenidyl hydrochloride, α-cyclohexyl-α-phenyl-1-piperidinepropanol hydrochloride (Artane, Tremin, Pipanol), introduced in 1949, is approximately half as active as atropine as an antispasmodic but is claimed to have milder side effects, such as mydriasis, drying of secretions, and cardioacceleration. It has a good margin of safety, though it is about as toxic as atropine. It has found a place in the treatment of parkinsonism and is claimed to provide some measure of relief from the mental depression often associated with this condition. It does, however, exhibit some of the side effects typical of the parasympatholytic-type preparation, though adjusting the dose carefully may often eliminate these.

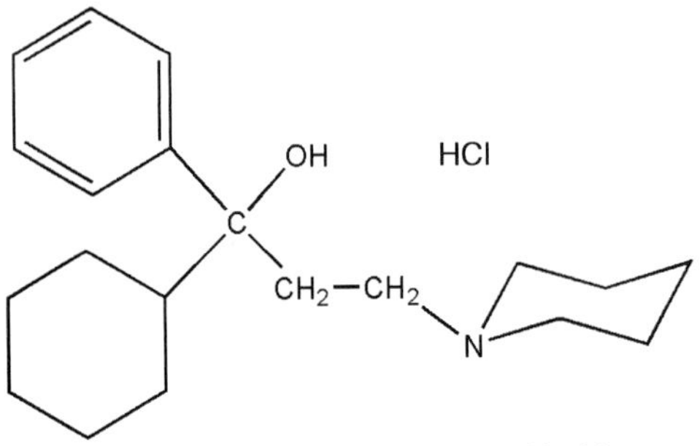

Trihexyphenidyl Hydrochloride

Aminoamides

From a structural standpoint, the aminoamide type of anticholinergic represents the same type of molecule as the aminoalcohol group, with the important exception that the polar amide group replaces the corresponding polar hydroxyl group. Aminoamides retain the same bulky structural features found at one end of the molecule or the other in all of the active anticholinergics. Isopropamide iodide is the only drug of this class currently in use.

Another amide-type structure is that of tropicamide, formerly known as bis-tropamide, a compound with some of the atropine features.

Isopropamide Iodide, USP.   Isopropamide iodide, 3-carbamoyl-3,3-diphenylpropyl)diisopropylmethylammonium iodide (Darbid), occurs as a bitter, white to pale yellow, crystalline powder that is only sparingly soluble in water but freely soluble in chloroform and alcohol.

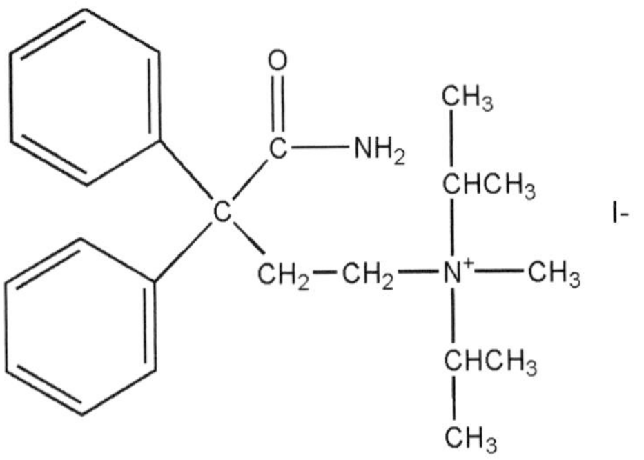

Isopropamide Iodide

This drug, introduced in 1957, is a potent anticholinergic, producing atropine-like effects peripherally. Even with its quaternary nature, it does not cause sympathetic blockade at the ganglionic level except at high dosages. Its principal distinguishing feature is its long duration of action. A single dose can provide antispasmodic and antisecretory effects for as long as 12 hours.

It is used as adjunctive therapy in the treatment of peptic ulcer and other conditions of the GI tract associated with hypermotility and hyperacidity. It has the usual side effects of anticholinergics (dryness of mouth, mydriasis, difficult urination) and is contraindicated in glaucoma, prostatic hypertrophy, etc.

Tropicamide, USP. Tropicamide, *N*-ethyl-2-phenyl-*N*-(4-pyridylmethyl)hydracrylamide (Mydriacyl), is an effective anticholinergic for ophthalmic use when mydriasis is produced by relaxation of the sphincter muscle of the iris, allowing adrenergic innervation of the radial muscle to dilate the pupil. Its maximum effect is achieved in about 20 to 25 minutes and lasts for about 20 minutes, with complete recovery in about 6 hours. Its action is more rapid in onset and wears off more rapidly than that of most other mydriatics. To achieve mydriasis, either 0.5 or 1.0% concentration may be used, though cycloplegia is achieved only with the stronger solution. Its uses are much the same as those described above for mydriatics in general, but opinions differ on whether the drug is as effective as homatropine, for example, in achieving cycloplegia. For mydriatic use, however, in examination of the fundus and treatment of acute iritis, iridocyclitis, and keratitis, it is quite adequate; and because of its shorter duration of action, it is less prone to initiate a rise in intraocular pressure than the more potent, longer-lasting drugs. As with other mydriatics, however, pupil dilation can lead to increased intraocular pressure. In common with other mydriatics, it is contraindicated in patients with glaucoma, either known or suspected, and should not be used in the presence of a shallow anterior chamber. Thus far, no allergic reactions or ocular damage has been observed with this drug. The ability to clone the various muscarinic receptor subtypes has allowed the observation that tropicamide has modest selectivity for the M_4 receptor.[77]

Tropicamide

Miscellaneous

Further structural modification of classic antimuscarinic agents can be found in the drugs described below. Each of them has the typical bulky group characteristic of the usual anticholinergic molecule. One modification is represented by the diphenylmethylene moiety (e.g., diphemanil); a sec-ond, by a phenothiazine (e.g., ethopropazine); and a third, by a thioxanthene structure (e.g., methixene).

Diphemanil Methylsulfate, USP. Diphemanil methyl-sulfate, 4-(diphenylmethylene)-1,1-dimethylpiperidinium methylsulfate (Prantal), or diphemanil methylsulfate is a potent cholinergic blocking agent. In the usual dosage range, it acts as an effective parasympatholytic by blocking nerve impulses at the parasympathetic ganglia, but it does not invoke a sympathetic ganglionic blockade. It is claimed to be highly specific in its action on those innervations that activate gastric secretion and GI motility. Although this drug can produce atropine-like side effects, they rarely occur at recommended doses. The highly specific nature of its action on gastric functions makes the drug useful in the treatment of peptic ulcer, and its lack of atropine-like effects makes its use much less distressing than other antispasmodic drugs. In addition to its action in decreasing gastric hypermotility, diphemanil methylsulfate is valuable in hyperhidrosis in low doses (50 mg twice daily) or topically. The drug is not well absorbed from the GI tract, particularly in the presence of food, and should be administered between meals. The methylsulfate salt was chosen as the best because the chloride is hygroscopic and the bromide and iodide ions have exhibited toxic manifestations in clinical use.

Diphemanil Methylsulfate

Ethopropazine Hydrochloride, USP. Ethopropazine hydrochloride, 10-[2-(diethylamino)propyl]phenothiazine monohydrochloride (Parsidol), introduced to therapy in 1954, has antimuscarinic activity and is especially useful in the symptomatic treatment of parkinsonism. In this capacity, it has value in controlling rigidity, and it also has a favorable effect on tremor, sialorrhea, and oculogyric crises. It is used often in conjunction with other antiparkinsonian drugs for complementary activity.

Ethopropazine Hydrochloride

Side effects are common with this drug but are usually not severe. Drowsiness and dizziness are the most common side effects at ordinary dosage levels, and as the dose increases, xerostomia, mydriasis, and others become evident. It is contraindicated in conditions such as glaucoma because of its mydriatic effect.

Papaverine Hydrochloride, USP. Papaverine hydrochloride, 6,7-dimethoxy-1-veratrylisoquinoline hydrochloride, was isolated by Merck in 1848 from opium, in which it occurs to the extent of about 1%. Although its natural origin is closely related to morphine, the pharmacological actions of papaverine hydrochloride are unlike those of morphine. Its main effect is as a spasmolytic on smooth muscle, acting as a direct, nonspecific relaxant on vascular, cardiac, and other smooth muscle. Because of its broad antispasmodic action on ACh muscarinic receptors, it is often called a nonspecific antagonist. Papaverine hydrochloride has been used in the treatment of peripheral vascular disorders, but its use is limited by lack of potency.

Papaverine hydrochloride interferes with the mechanism of muscle contraction by inhibiting the cyclic nucleotide phosphodiesterases in smooth muscle cells responsible for converting cAMP and cyclic guanosine monophosphate (cGMP) to $5'$-AMP and $5'$-GMP, respectively. The increased levels of cAMP and cGMP are associated with muscle relaxation through their phosphorylation of myosin light-chain kinase.

Papaverine Hydrochloride

GANGLIONIC BLOCKING AGENTS

Autonomic ganglia have been the subject of interest for many years in the study of interactions between drugs and nervous tissues. The first important account[78] was given by Langley and described the stimulating and blocking actions of nicotine on sympathetic ganglia. It was found that small amounts of nicotine stimulated ganglia and then produced a blockade of ganglionic transmission because of persistent depolarization. From these experiments, Langley was able to outline the general pattern of innervation of organs by the autonomic nervous system. *Parasympathetic* ganglia usually

are located near the organ they innervate and have preganglionic fibers that stem from the cervical and thoracic regions of the spinal cord. *Sympathetic* ganglia consist of 22 pairs that lie on either side of the vertebral column to form lateral chains. These ganglia are connected both to each other by nerve trunks and to the lumbar or sacral regions of the spinal cord.

Nicotine

Using the sympathetic cervical ganglion as a model revealed that transmission in the autonomic ganglion is more complex than formerly believed. Traditionally, stimulation of autonomic ganglia by ACh was considered to be the nicotinic action of the neurotransmitter. It is now understood that stimulation by ACh produces a triphasic response in sympathetic ganglia. Impulse transmission through the ganglion occurs when ACh is released from preganglionic fibers and activates the N_2 nicotinic receptors of the neuronal membrane. This triggers an increase in sodium and potassium conductances of a subsynaptic membrane, resulting in an initial excitatory postsynaptic potential (EPSP) with a latency of 1 millisecond, followed by an inhibitory postsynaptic potential (IPSP) with a latency of 35 milliseconds, and, finally, a slowly generating EPSP with a latency of several hundred milliseconds. The ACh released by preganglionic fibers also activates M_1 muscarinic receptors of the ganglion and probably of the small-intensity fluorescent (SIF) cell. This results in the appearance of a slow IPSP and a slow EPSP in the neurons of the ganglion.[79] The initial EPSP is blocked by conventional competitive nondepolarizing ganglionic blocking agents, such as hexamethonium, and is considered the primary pathway for ganglionic transmission.[80] The slowly generating or late EPSP is blocked by atropine but not by the traditional ganglionic blocking agents. This receptor has muscarinic properties because methacholine causes generation of the late EPSP without causing the initial spike characteristic of ACh. Atropine also blocks the late EPSP produced by methacholine. There may be more than one type of muscarinic receptor in sympathetic ganglia. Atropine blocks both high-affinity (M_1) and low-affinity (M_2) muscarinic receptors in the ganglion.[81] In addition to the cholinergic pathways, the cervical sympathetic ganglion has a neuron that contains a catecholamine.[82] These neuronal cells, identified initially by fluorescence histochemical studies and shown to be smaller than the postganglionic neurons, are now referred to as SIF cells. Dopamine has been identified as the fluorescent catecholamine in the SIF cells that are common to many other sympathetic ganglia. Dopamine apparently mediates an increase in cAMP, which causes hyperpolarization of postganglionic neurons (Fig. 17-19). The IPSP phase of the transmission of sympathetic ganglia following ACh administration can be blocked by both atropine and α-adrenergic blocking agents.[79]

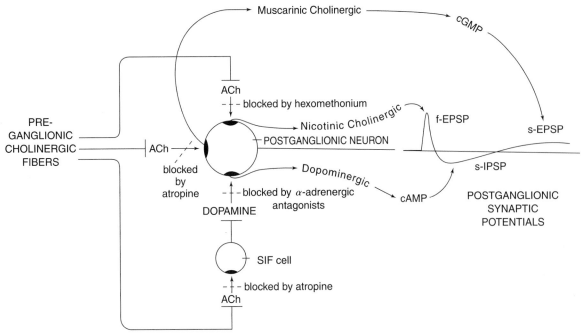

Figure 17–19 ■ Neurotransmission at the sympathetic cervical ganglion.

If a similar nontraditional type of ganglionic transmission occurs in the parasympathetic ganglia, it has not yet become evident. With the anatomical and physiological differences between sympathetic and parasympathetic ganglia, it should be no surprise that ganglionic agents may show some selectivity between the two types of ganglia. Although we do not have drug classifications such as ''parasympathetic ganglionic blockers'' and ''sympathetic ganglionic blockers,'' we do find that certain ganglia have a predominant effect over certain organs and tissues and that a nondiscriminant blockade of autonomic ganglia results in a change in the effect of the autonomic nervous system on that organ (Table 17-7). None of the commonly known ganglionic blockers has yet

been identified as a selective blocker of parasympathetic ganglia.

Van Rossum[83, 84] has reviewed the mechanisms of ganglionic synaptic transmission, the mode of action of ganglionic stimulants, and the mode of action of ganglionic blocking agents. They have been classified as blocking agents in the following manner.

Depolarizing Ganglionic Blocking Agents

Depolarizing blocking agents are actually ganglionic stimulants. Thus, for nicotine, small doses give an action similar to that of the natural neuroeffector ACh, an action known as

TABLE 17–7   Results of Ganglionic Blockers on Organs

Organ	Predominant System	Results of Ganglionic Blockade
Cardiovascular system		
Heart	Parasympathetic	Tachycardia
Arterioles	Sympathetic	Vasodilation
Veins	Sympathetic	Dilation
Eye		
Iris	Parasympathetic	Mydriasis
Ciliary muscle	Parasympathetic	Cycloplegia
GI tract	Parasympathetic	Relaxation
Urinary bladder	Parasympathetic	Urinary retention
Salivary glands	Parasympathetic	Dry mouth
Sweat glands	Sympathetic[a]	Anhidrosis

Adapted from Goth, A.: Medical Pharmacology, 9th ed. St. Louis, C. V. Mosby, 1978.
[a] Neurotransmitter is ACh.

the "nicotinic effect of ACh." Larger amounts of nicotine, however, bring about a ganglionic block characterized initially by depolarization, followed by a typical competitive antagonism. To conduct nerve impulses, the cell must be able to carry out a polarization and depolarization process, and if the depolarized condition is maintained without repolarization, obviously no conduction occurs. ACh itself, in high concentration, will bring about an autoinhibition. Chemicals that cause this type of ganglionic block are not of therapeutic significance. The classes of ganglionic blocking agents that are described are therapeutically useful.

Nondepolarizing Competitive Ganglionic Blocking Agents

Compounds in the class of nondepolarizing competitive ganglionic blocking agents possess the necessary affinity to attach to the nicotinic receptor sites that are specific for ACh, but they lack the intrinsic activity necessary for impulse transmission (i.e., they cannot effect depolarization of the cell). Under experimental conditions, in the presence of a fixed concentration of blocking agent of this type, a large enough concentration of ACh can offset the blocking action by competing successfully for the specific receptors. When such a concentration of ACh is administered to a ganglion preparation, it appears that the intrinsic activity of the ACh is as great as it was when no antagonist was present, the only difference being in the larger concentration of ACh required. It is evident, then, that such blocking agents are "competitive" with ACh for the specific receptors involved and that either the agonist or the antagonist, if present in sufficient concentration, can displace the other. Drugs falling into this class are tetraethylammonium salts, hexamethonium, and trimethaphan. Mecamylamine possesses a competitive component in its action but is also noncompetitive, a so-called dual antagonist.

Nondepolarizing Noncompetitive Ganglionic Blocking Agents

Nondepolarizing noncompetitive ganglionic blocking agents produce their effect not at the specific ACh receptor site but at some point farther along the chain of events that is necessary for transmission of the nerve impulse. When the block has been imposed, increasing the concentration of ACh has no effect; thus, apparently, ACh does not act competitively with the blocking agent at the same receptors. Theoretically, a pure noncompetitive blocker should have a high specific affinity for the noncompetitive receptors in the ganglia and a very low affinity for other cholinergic synapses, together with no intrinsic activity. Mecamylamine, as mentioned above, has a noncompetitive component but is also a competitive blocking agent.

The first ganglionic blocking agents used in therapy were tetraethylammonium chloride and bromide. Although one might assume that curariform activity would be a deterrent to their use, the curariform activity of the tetraethyl compound is less than 1% of that of the corresponding tetramethylammonium compound. A few years after the introduction of the tetraethylammonium compounds, Paton and Zaimis[85] investigated the usefulness of the bis-trimethylammonium polymethylene salts:

n = 5 or 6, active as ganglionic blockers (feeble curariform activity)

n = 9 to 12, weak ganglionic blockers (strong curariform activity)

As shown, their findings indicate that there is a critical distance of about five to six carbon atoms between the onium centers for good ganglionic blocking action. Interestingly, the pentamethylene and hexamethylene compounds are effective antidotes against the curare effect of the decamethylene compound. Hexamethonium bromide and hexamethonium chloride emerged from this research as clinically useful products.

Trimethaphan camphorsulfonate, a monosulfonium compound, bears some similarity to the quaternary ammonium types because it, too, is a completely ionic compound. Although it produces a prompt ganglion-blocking action on parenteral injection, its action is short, and it is used only for controlled hypotension during surgery. Almost simultaneously with the introduction of chlorisondamine (now long removed from the market), announcement was made of the powerful ganglionic blocking action of mecamylamine, a secondary amine *without* quaternary ammonium character. As expected, the latter compound showed uniform and predictable absorption from the GI tract as well as a longer duration of action. Its action was similar to that of hexamethonium.

Drugs of this class have limited usefulness as diagnostic and therapeutic agents in the management of peripheral vascular diseases (e.g., thromboangiitis obliterans, Raynaud's disease, diabetic gangrene). The principal therapeutic application has been in the treatment of hypertension through blockade of the sympathetic pathways. Unfortunately, the action is nonspecific, and the parasympathetic ganglia, unavoidably, are blocked simultaneously to a greater or lesser extent, causing visual disturbances, dryness of the mouth, impotence, urinary retention, and constipation. Constipation, in particular, probably caused by unabsorbed drug in the intestine (poor absorption), has been a drawback because the condition can proceed to a paralytic ileus if extreme care is not exercised. For this reason, cathartics or a parasympathomimetic (e.g., pilocarpine nitrate) is frequently administered simultaneously. Another adverse effect is the production of orthostatic (postural) hypotension (i.e., dizziness when the patient stands up in an erect position). Prolonged administration of the ganglionic blocking agents results in diminished effectiveness because of a buildup of tolerance, though some are more prone to this than others. Because of the many serious side effects, more effective hypotensive agents have replaced this group of drugs.

In addition to these adverse effects, there are several limitations to the use of these drugs. For instance, they are contraindicated in disorders characterized by severe reduction of blood flow to a vital organ (e.g., severe coronary insufficiency, recent myocardial infarction, retinal and cerebral thrombosis) as well as situations in which there have been large reductions in blood volume. In the latter, the contraindication exists because the drugs block the normal vasoconstrictor compensatory mechanisms necessary for homeostasis. A potentially serious complication, especially in older male patients with prostatic hypertrophy, is urinary retention. These drugs should be used with care or not at all in the presence of renal insufficiency, glaucoma, uremia, and organic pyloric stenosis.

Trimethaphan Camsylate, USP. Trimethaphan camsylate, (+)-1,3-dibenzyldecahydro2-oxoimidazo[4,5-*c*]thieno[1,2- *α*]-thiolium 2-oxo-10-bornanesulfonate (1:1) (Arfonad), consists of white crystals or a crystalline powder with a bitter taste and a slight odor. It is soluble in water and alcohol but only slightly soluble in acetone and ether. The pH of a 1% aqueous solution is 5.0 to 6.0.

This ganglionic blocking agent is short acting and is used for certain neurosurgical procedures in which excessive bleeding obscures the operative field. Certain craniotomies are included among these operations. The action of the drug is direct vasodilation, and because of its transient action, it is subject to minute-by-minute control. This fleeting action, however, makes it useless for hypertensive control. The drug is ineffective when given orally. The usual route of administration is intravenous. Trimethaphan camsylate is indicated in the treatment of hypertensive emergencies to reduce blood pressure rapidly. These emergencies may include pulmonary hypertension associated with systemic hypertension and acute dissecting aneurysm.

Trimethaphan Camsylate

Mecamylamine Hydrochloride. The secondary amine mecamylamine hydrochloride, *N*,2,3,3-tetramethyl-2-norbornanamine hydrochloride (Inversine), has a powerful ganglionic blocking effect that is almost identical to that of hexamethonium. It has an advantage over most of the ganglionic blocking agents in being absorbed readily and smoothly from the GI tract. It is rarely used, however, for the treatment of moderate-to-severe hypertension because severe orthostatic hypotension occurs when the drug blocks sympathetic ganglia.

Mecamylamine Hydrochloride

NEUROMUSCULAR BLOCKING AGENTS

Agents that block the transmission of ACh at the motor end plate are called *neuromuscular blocking agents*. The therapeutic use of these compounds is primarily as adjuvants in surgical anesthesia to obtain relaxation of skeletal muscle. They also are used in various orthopedic procedures, such as alignment of fractures and correction of dislocations.

The therapeutically useful compounds in this group sometimes are referred to as possessing *curariform* or *curarimimetic* activity in reference to the original representatives of the class, which were obtained from curare. Since then, synthetic compounds have been prepared with similar activity. Although all of the compounds falling into this category, natural and synthetic alike, bring about substantially the same end result (i.e., voluntary-muscle relaxation), there are some significant differences in mechanisms.

The possible existence of a junction between muscle and nerve was suggested as early as 1856, when Claude Bernard observed that the site of action of curare was neither the nerve nor the muscle. Since that time, it has been agreed that ACh mediates transmission at the neuromuscular junction by a sequence of events described above in this chapter. The neuromuscular junction consists of the axon impinging onto a specialized area of the muscle known as the muscle end plate. The axon is covered with a myelin sheath, containing the nodes of Ranvier, but is bare at the ending. The nerve terminal is separated from the end plate by a gap of 200 Å. The subsynaptic membrane of the end plate contains the cholinergic receptor, the ion-conducting channels (which are opened under the influence of ACh), and AChE.

One of the anatomical differences between the neuromuscular junction and other ACh-responsive sites is the absence in the former of a membrane barrier or sheath that envelopes the ganglia or constitutes the blood–brain barrier. This is important in the accessibility of the site of action to drugs, particularly quaternary ammonium compounds, because they pass through living membranes with considerably greater difficulty and selectivity than do compounds that can exist in a nonionized species. The essentially bare nature (i.e., lack of lipophilic barriers) of the myoneural junction permits ready access by quaternary ammonium compounds. In addition, compounds with considerable molecular dimensions are accessible to the receptors in the myoneural junction. As a result of this property, variations in the chemical structure of quaternaries have little influence on the potential ability of the molecule to reach the cholinergic receptor in the neuromuscular junction. Thus, the following types of neuromuscular junction blockers have been noted.

Nondepolarizing Blocking Agents

Traditionally, *nondepolarizing blocking agents* is a term applied to categorize drugs that compete with ACh for the recognition site on the nicotinic receptor by preventing depolarization of the end plate by the neurotransmitter. Thus, by decreasing the effective ACh–receptor combinations, the end plate potential becomes too small to initiate the propagated action potential. This results in paralysis of neuromuscular transmission. The action of these drugs is quite analogous to that of atropine at the muscarinic receptor sites of ACh. Many experiments suggest that the agonist (ACh) and the antagonist compete on a one-to-one basis for the end plate receptors. Drugs in this class are tubocurarine, dimethyltubocurarine, pancuronium, and gallamine.

Depolarizing Blocking Agents

Drugs in the category of depolarizing blocking agents depolarize the membrane of the muscle end plate. This depolarization is quite similar to that produced by ACh itself at ganglia and neuromuscular junctions (i.e., its so-called nicotinic effect), with the result that the drug, if in sufficient concentration, eventually will produce a block. Either smooth or voluntary muscle, when challenged repeatedly with a depolarizing agent, eventually becomes insensitive. This phenomenon is known as *tachyphylaxis,* or *desensitization,* and is demonstrated convincingly under suitable experimental conditions with repeated applications of ACh itself, the results indicating that within a few minutes the end plate becomes insensitive to ACh. The statements above may imply that a blocking action of this type is clear-cut, but under experimental conditions, it is not quite so unambiguous, because a block that begins with depolarization may regain the polarized state even before the block. Furthermore, depolarization induced by increasing the potassium ion concentration does not prevent impulse transmission. For these and other reasons, it is probably best to consider the blocking action a desensitization until a clearer picture emerges. Drugs falling in this class are decamethonium and succinylcholine.

Curare and Curare Alkaloids

Originally *curare* was a term used to describe collectively the very potent arrow poisons used since early times by the South American Indians. The arrow poisons were prepared from numerous botanic sources and often were mixtures of several different plant extracts. Some were poisonous by virtue of a convulsant action and others by a paralyzant action. Only the latter type is of value in therapeutics and is spoken of ordinarily as curare.

Chemical investigations of the curares were not especially successful because of difficulties in obtaining authentic samples with definite botanic origin. Not until 1935 was a pure crystalline alkaloid, *d*-tubocurarine chloride, possessing in great measure the paralyzing action of the original curare, isolated from a plant. Wintersteiner and Dutcher,[86] in 1943, isolated the same alkaloid. They showed, however, that the botanic source was *Chondodendron tomentosum* (Menispermaceae) and, thus, provided a known source of the drug.

Following the development of quantitative bioassay methods for determining the potency of curare extracts, a purified and standardized curare was developed and marketed under the trade name Intocostrin (purified *C. tomentosum* extract), the solid content of which consisted of almost one-half (+)-tubocurarine solids. Following these essentially pioneering developments, (+)-tubocurarine chloride and dimethyltubocurarine iodide appeared on the market as pure entities.

Tubocurarine Chloride, USP. Tubocurarine chloride, (+)-tubocurarine chloride hydrochloride pentahydrate, is prepared from crude curare by a process of purification and crystallization. Tubocurarine chloride occurs as a white or yellowish white to grayish white, odorless, crystalline powder that is soluble in water. Aqueous solutions of it are stable to heat sterilization.

The structural formula for (+)-tubocurarine was long thought to be that of Ia (see structure diagram). Through the work of Everett et al.,[87] the structure is now known to be that of Ib. The monoquaternary nature of Ib thus revealed has caused some reassessment of thinking concerning the theoretical basis for the blocking action, because all had previously assumed a diquaternary structure (i.e., Ia). Nevertheless, this does not negate the earlier conclusions that a diquaternary nature of the molecule provides better blocking action than does a monoquaternary nature (e.g., Ib is approximately fourfold less potent than dimethyl tubocurarine iodide). Further, (+)-isotubocurarine chloride (Ic) has twice the activity of Ib in the particular test used.

(Ia) $R_1 = R_2 = CH_3$
(Ib) $R_1 = H$; $R_2 = CH_3$
(Ic) $R_1 = CH_3$; $R_2 = H$

Tubocurarine is a nondepolarizing blocking agent used for its paralyzing action on voluntary muscles, the site of action being the neuromuscular junction. Its action is inhibited or reversed by the administration of AChE inhibitors, such as neostigmine, or by edrophonium chloride (Tensilon). Such inhibition of its action is necessitated in respiratory embarrassment caused by overdosage. Additionally, in somewhat higher concentrations, *d*-tubocurarine may enter the open ion channel and add a noncompetitive blockade. Cholinesterase inhibitors do not restore this latter action easily or fully. Often, adjunctive artificial respiration is needed until the maximal curare action has passed. The drug is inactive orally because of inadequate absorption through lipoidal membranes in the GI tract, and when used therapeutically, it usually is injected intravenously.

d-Tubocurarine binds for only 1 millisecond to the receptor, yet its pharmacological effect of muscle paralysis, produced by administration of the drug intravenously during surgery, lasts for up to 2 hours. The basis of this action is the pharmacokinetics of the drug. *d*-Tubocurarine is given intravenously, and although 30 to 77% is bound to plasma proteins, the drug is distributed rapidly to central body compartments, including neuromuscular junctions. About 45%

of *d*-tubocurarine is eliminated unchanged by the kidneys. Its half-life is 89 minutes.

Tubocurarine, in the form of a purified extract, was used first in 1943 as a muscle relaxant in shock therapy for mental disorders. Its use markedly reduced the incidence of bone and spine fractures and dislocations from convulsions due to shock. Following this, it was used as an adjunct in general anesthesia to obtain complete muscle relaxation, a use that persists to this day. Before its use began, satisfactory muscle relaxation in various surgical procedures (e.g., abdominal operations) was obtainable only with "deep" anesthesia with the ordinary general anesthetics. Tubocurarine permits a lighter plane of anesthesia, with no sacrifice in the muscle relaxation so important to the surgeon. A reduced dose of tubocurarine is administered with ether because ether itself has curare-like action.

Metocurine Iodide, USP. Metocurine iodide, (+)-*O,O'*-dimethylchondrocurarine diiodide (Metubine iodide), is prepared from natural crude curare by extracting the curare with methanolic potassium hydroxide. When the extract is treated with an excess of methyl iodide, the (+)-tubocurarine is converted to the diquaternary dimethyl ether and crystallizes out as the iodide (see "Tubocurarine Chloride," above). Other ethers besides the dimethyl ether have been made and tested. For example, the dibenzyl ether was one-third as active as tubocurarine chloride, and the diisopropyl compound had only one-half the activity. For comparison, the dimethyl ether has approximately 4 times the activity of tubocurarine chloride.

The pharmacological action of this compound is the same as that of tubocurarine chloride, namely, a nondepolarizing competitive blocking effect on the motor end plate of skeletal muscles. It is considerably more potent than *d*-tubocurarine, however, and has the added advantage of exerting much less effect on respiration. The effect on respiration is not a significant factor in therapeutic doses. Accidental overdosage is counteracted best by forced respiration.

Synthetic Compounds With Curariform Activity

Curare, until relatively recent times, remained the only useful curarizing agent; and it, too, suffered from a lack of standardization. The original pronouncement in 1935 of the structure of (+)-tubocurarine chloride, unchallenged for 35 years, led other workers to hope for activity in synthetic substances of less complexity. The quaternary ammonium character of the curare alkaloids coupled with the known activity of the various simple onium compounds hardly seemed to be coincidental, and it was natural for research to follow along these lines. One of the synthetic compounds discovered was marketed in 1951 as Flaxedil (gallamine triethiodide). A variety of other neuromuscular blocking agents have followed.

Atracurium Besylate. Atracurium besylate, 2-(2-carboxyethyl)-1,2,3,4-tetrahydro-6,7-dimethoxy-2-methyl-1-veratrylisoquinolinium benzenesulfonate pentamethylene ester (Tracrium), is a nondepolarizing neuromuscular blocking agent that is approximately 2.5 times more potent than *d*-tubocurarine. Its duration of action (half-life, 0.33 hours) is much shorter than that of *d*-tubocurarine. The drug is metabolized rapidly and nonenzymatically to yield laudanosine and a smaller quaternary compound (Fig. 17-20), which do not have neuromuscular blocking activity. In vitro experiments show that atracurium besylate breaks down at pH 7.4 and 37°C by a Hoffman elimination reaction.[88] Atracurium besylate undergoes enzymatic decomposition of its ester function to yield an inactive quaternary alcohol and quaternary acid. AChE inhibitors such as neostigmine, edrophonium, and pyridostigmine antagonize paralysis by atracurium besylate.

Doxacurium Chloride. The molecular structure of doxacurium chloride, 1,2,3,4-tetrahydro-2-(3-hydroxypropyl)-6,7,8-trimethoxy2-methyl-1-(3,4,5-trimethoxybenzyl) isoquinolinium chloride succinate (Nuromax), provides the

Atracurium Besylate

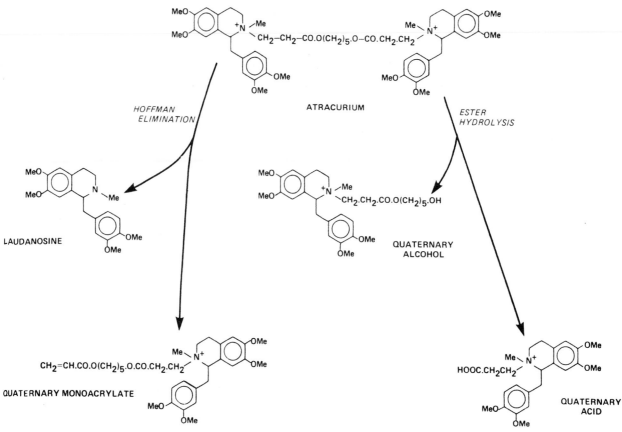

Figure 17–20 ■ Hoffman elimination and hydrolysis reactions of atracurium.

possibility for 10 stereoisomers: 4 *d,l* pairs and two *meso* forms. Of the 10 stereoisomers, 3 are all-*trans* configuration, and these are the only active ones.[89] Doxacurium chloride is a long-acting nondepolarizing blocking agent. The drug differs from drugs such as gallium and pancuronium in that it has no vagolytic activity. It is used as a skeletal muscle relaxant in surgical procedures expected to last longer than 90 minutes.

Gallamine Triethiodide, USP. Gallamine triethiodide, [*v*-phenenyl-tris(oxyethylene)]tris[triethylammonium] triio-

dide (Flaxedil), is a skeletal muscle relaxant that works by blocking neuromuscular transmission in a manner similar to that of *d*-tubocurarine (i.e., a nondepolarizing blocking agent). It does have some differences, however. It has a strong vagolytic effect and a persistent decrease in neuromuscular function after successive doses that cannot be overcome by cholinesterase inhibitors. Gallamine triethiodide also has muscarinic antagonistic properties and binds with greater affinity to the M_2 receptors than to the M_1 receptor. This latter characteristic may cause its strong vagolytic action.[89, 90]

Doxacurium Chloride

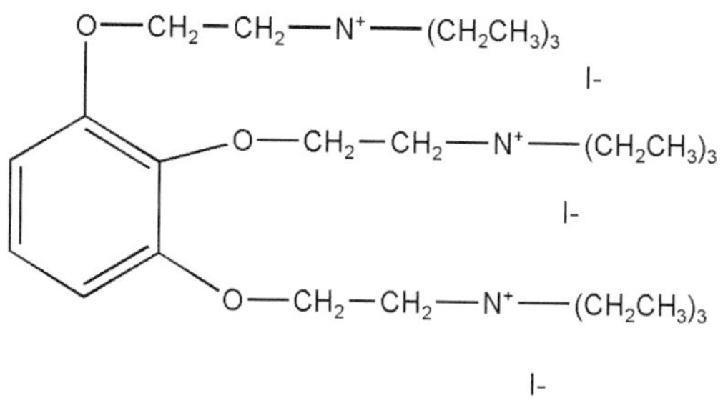

Gallamine Triethiodide

The drug is contraindicated in patients with myasthenia gravis, and one should remember that its action is cumulative, as with curare. The antidote for gallamine triethiodide is neostigmine.

Mivacurium Chloride.   Mivacurium chloride, 1,2,3,4-tetrahydro-2-(3-hydroxypropyl)-6,7-dimethoxy-2-methyl-1-(3,4,5-trimethoxybenzyl)isoquinolinium chloride, (E)-4-octandioate (Mivacron), is a mixture of three stereoisomers, the *trans-trans, cis-trans,* and *cis-cis* diesters, each of which has neuromuscular blocking properties. The *cis-cis* isomer is about one-tenth as potent as the other isomers. Mivacurium chloride is a short-acting nondepolarizing drug used as an adjunct to anesthesia to relax skeletal muscle. The drug is hydrolyzed by plasma esterases, and it is likely that anticholinesterase agents used as antidotes could prolong rather than reverse the effects of the drug.

Pancuronium Bromide.   Although pancuronium bromide, 2β,16β-dipiperidino-5α-androstane-3α,17β-diol diacetate dimethobromide (Pavulon), is a synthetic product, it is based on the naturally occurring alkaloid malouetine, found in arrow poisons used by primitive Africans. Pancuronium bromide acts on the nicotinic receptor and in the ion channel, inhibiting normal ion fluxes.

This blocking agent is soluble in water and is marketed in concentrations of 1 or 2 mg/mL for intravenous administration. It is a typical nondepolarizing blocker, with a potency approximately 5 times that of (+)-tubocurarine chloride and a duration of action approximately equal to the latter. Studies indicate that it has little or no histamine-releasing potential or ganglion-blocking activity and that it has little effect on the circulatory system, except for causing a slight rise in the pulse rate. As one might expect, ACh, anticholinesterases, and potassium ion competitively antagonize it, whereas its action is increased by inhalation anesthetics such as ether, halothane, enflurane, and methoxyflurane. The latter enhancement in activity is especially important to the anesthetist because the drug is frequently administered as an adjunct to the anesthetic procedure to relax the skeletal muscle. Perhaps the most frequent adverse reaction to this agent is occasional prolongation of the neuromuscular block beyond the usual time course, a situation that can usually be controlled with neostigmine or by manual or mechanical ventilation, since respiratory difficulty is a prominent manifestation of the prolonged blocking action.

As indicated, the principal use of pancuronium bromide is as an adjunct to anesthesia, to induce relaxation of skeletal muscle, but it is also used to facilitate the management of patients undergoing mechanical ventilation. Only experienced clinicians equipped with facilities for applying artificial respiration should administer it, and the dosage should be adjusted and controlled carefully.

Pipecurium Bromide.   Pipecurium bromide, 4,4'-(3α, 17β-dihydroxy-5α-androstan-2β,16β-ylene)bis(1,1-dimethylpiperazinium)dibromide diacetate (Arduan), is a nondepolarizing muscle relaxant similar, both chemically and clinically, to pancuronium bromide. It is a long-acting drug indicated as an adjunct to anesthesia and in patients undergoing mechanical ventilation.

Vecuronium Bromide.   Vecuronium bromide, 1-(3α, 17β-dihydroxy-2β-piperidino-5α-androstan-16β-yl)-1-methylpiperidinium bromide diacetate (Norcuron), is the monoquaternary analogue of pancuronium bromide. It belongs to the class of nondepolarizing neuromuscular blocking agents and produces effects similar to those of drugs in this class. It is unstable in the presence of acids and undergoes gradual hydrolysis of its ester functions in aqueous solution. Aqueous solutions have a pH of about 4.0. This drug is used mainly to produce skeletal muscle relaxation during surgery and to assist in controlled respiration after general anesthesia has been induced.

Succinylcholine Chloride, USP.   Succinylcholine chloride, choline chloride succinate (2:1) (Anectine, Sucostrin), is a white odorless crystalline substance that is freely soluble in water to give solutions with a pH of about 4. It is stable

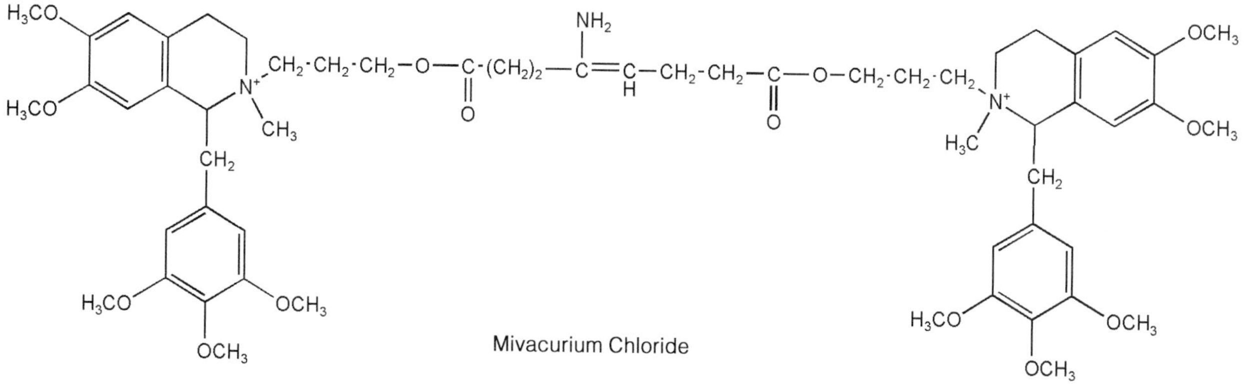

Mivacurium Chloride

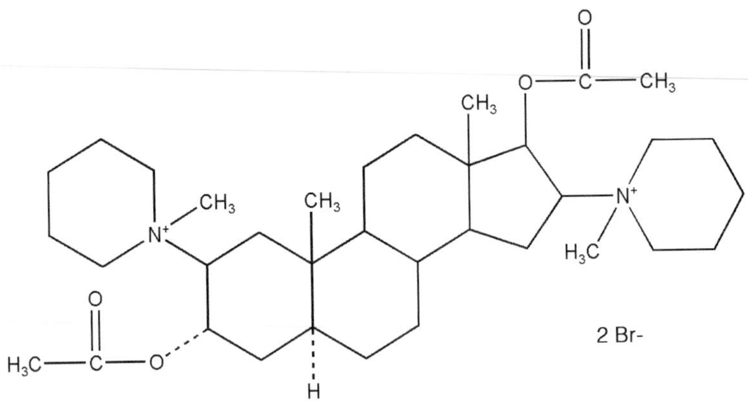

Pancuronium Bromide

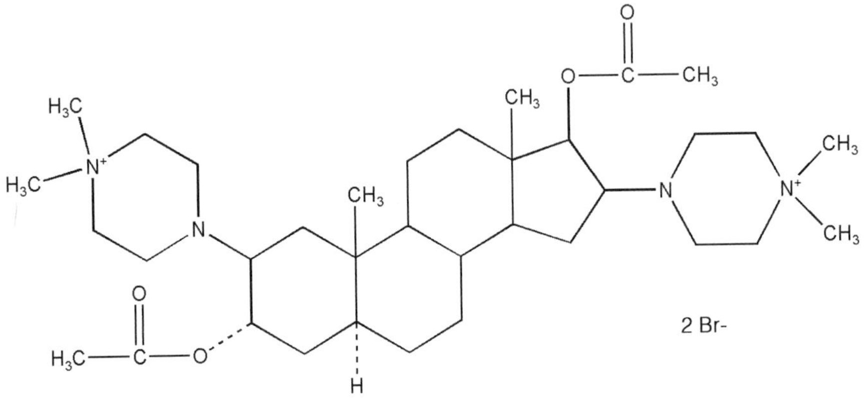

Pipecurium Bromide

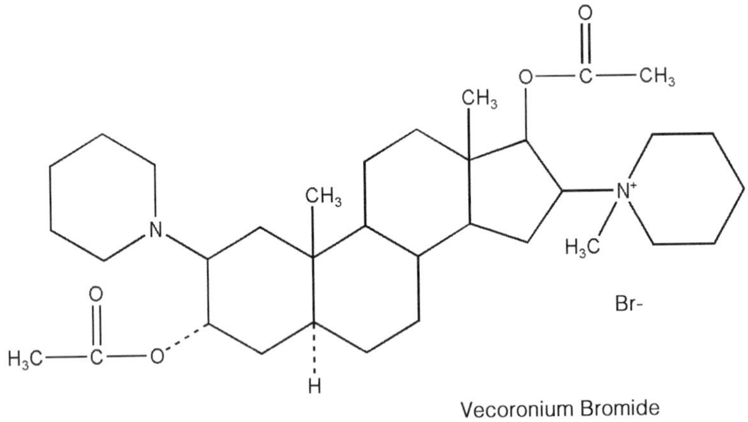

Vecoronium Bromide

in acidic solutions but unstable in alkali. Aqueous solutions should be refrigerated to ensure stability.

Succinylcholine chloride is characterized by a very short duration of action and a quick recovery because of its rapid hydrolysis after injection. It brings about the typical muscular paralysis caused by blocking nervous transmission at the myoneural junction. Large doses may cause temporary respiratory depression, as with similar agents. Its action, in contrast with that of (+)-tubocurarine, is not antagonized by neostigmine, physostigmine, or edrophonium chloride.

These anticholinesterase drugs actually prolong the action of succinylcholine chloride, which suggests that the drug is probably hydrolyzed by cholinesterases. The brief duration of action of this curare-like agent is said to render an antidote unnecessary if the proper supportive measures are available. Succinylcholine chloride has a disadvantage, however, in that the usual antidotes cannot terminate its action promptly.

It is used as a muscle relaxant for the same indications as other curare agents. It may be used for either short or long periods of relaxation, depending on whether one or several injections are given. In addition, it is suitable for continuous intravenous drip administration.

Succinylcholine chloride should not be used with thiopental sodium because of the high alkalinity of the latter. If used together, they should be administered immediately after mixing; however, separate injection is preferable.

REFERENCES

1. Dale, H. H.: J. Pharmacol. Exp. Ther. 6:147, 1914.
2. Loewi, O.: Arch. Gesamte. Physiol. (Pfluegers) 189:239, 1921.
3. Zola-Morgan, S., and Squire, L. R.: Annu. Rev. Neurosci. 16:547, 1994.
4. Frank, H. S., and Wen, W-Y.: Discuss. Faraday Soc. 24:133, 1957.
5. Hille, B.: Annu. Rev. Physiol. 38:139, 1976.
6. Karlin, A.: In Cotman, C. U., Poste, G., and Nicolson, G. L. (eds.). Cell Surface and Neuronal Function. Amsterdam, Elsevier Biomedical, 1980, p. 191.
7. Changeaux, J. P., Devillers-Thiery, A., and Chermoulli, P.: Science 225:1335, 1984.
8. Anholt, R., et al.: In Martonosi, A. N. (ed.). The Enzymes of Biological Membranes, vol. 3. New York, Plenum Press, 1985.
9. Raftery, M. A., et al.: Science 208:1445, 1980.
10. Sargent, P. B.: Neuroscience 16:403, 1994.
11. Dani, J. A.: Biol. Psychiatry 49:166, 2001.
12. Rattray, M. Biol. Psychiatry 49:185, 2001.
13. Goyal, R. K.: N. Engl. J. Med. 321:1022, 1989.
14. Birdsall, N. J. M., et al.: Pharmacology 37(Suppl.):22, 1988.
15. Mutschlur, E., et al.: Prog. Pharmacol. Clin. Pharmacol. 7:13, 1989.
16. Doods, H. N., et al.: Prog. Pharmacol. Clin. Pharmacol. 7:47, 1989.
17. Barnes, P. J.: Life Sci. 52:521, 1993.
18. Rubanyi, G. M.: J. Cell Biol. 46:27, 1991.
19. Kilbinger, H., Dietricht, C., and von Bardeleben, R. S.: J. Physiol. Paris 87:77, 1993.
20. Linder, M. E., and Gilman, A. E.: Sci. Am. 27:56, 1992.
21. Caufield, M. P.: Pharmacol. Ther. 58:319, 1993.
22. Berridge, M. J., and Irvine, R. F.: Nature 312:315, 1984.
23. Berridge, M. J.: Annu. Rev. Biochem. 56:159, 1987.
24. Clapham, D. E.: Annu. Rev. Neurosci. 17:441, 1994.
25. Haga, T., and Nada, H.: Biochim. Biophys. Acta 291:564, 1973.
26. Cavallito, C. J., et al.: J. Med. Chem. 12:134, 1969.
27. Aquilonius, S. M., et al.: Acta Pharmacol. Toxicol. 30:129, 1979.
28. Whittaker, V. P.: Trends Pharmacol. Sci. 7:312, 1986.
29. Namba, T., and Grob, D.: J. Neurochem. 15:1445, 1968.
30. Partington, P., Feeney, J., and Burgen, A. S. V.: Mol. Pharmacol. 8:269, 1972.
31. Casey, A. F.: Prog. Med. Chem. 11:1, 1975.
32. Behling, R. W., et al.: Proc. Natl. Acad. Sci. U. S. A. 85:6721, 1988.
33. Nordvall, G., and Hacksell, U.: J. Med. Chem. 36:967, 1993.
34. Schmeideberg, O., and Koppe, R.: Das Muscarine, das Giftege Alka id des Fiielgenpiltzes. Leipzig, Vogel, 1869.
35. Hardegger, E., and Lohse, F.: Helv. Chim. Acta 40:2383, 1957.
36. Trumpp-Kallmeyer, S., et al.: J. Med. Chem. 35:3448, 1992.
37. Triggle, D. J., et al.: J. Med. Chem. 34:3164, 1991.
38. Ariens, E. J., and Simonis, A. M.: In deJong, H. (ed.). Quantitative Methods in Pharmacology. Amsterdam, Elsevier, 1969.
39. Ing, H. R.: Science 109:264, 1949.
40. Hernandez, M., et al.: Br. J. Pharmacol. 110:1413, 1993.
41. Bebbington, A., and Brimblecombe, R. W.: Adv. Drug Res. 2:143, 1965.
42. Ren, L. N., Nakane, T., and Chiba, S.: J. Cardiovasc. Pharmacol. 22:841, 1993.
43. Morrison, K. J., and Vanhoutte, P. M.: Br. J. Pharmacol. 106:672, 1992.
44. Nunes, M. A., and Brochmann-Hanssen, E. J.: J. Pharm. Sci. 63:716, 1974.
45. Williams, P. D., et al.: Pharmacology 23:177, 1992.
46. Gabelt, B. T., and Kaufman, P. L.: J. Pharmacol. Exp. Ther. 263:1133, 1992.
47. Mallarkey, G.: Cholinesterase Inhibitors in Alzheimer's Disease. Auckland, Adis International, 1999.
48. Berman, A. H., Yguerabide, J., and Taylor, P.: Biochemistry 19:2226, 1980.
49. Englehard, N., Prchal, K., and Nenner, M.: Angew. Chem. Int. Ed. 6:615, 1967.
50. Ordentlich, A., et al.: J. Biol. Chem. 268:17083, 1993.
51. Shafferman, A., et al.: J. Biol. Chem. 267:17640, 1992.
52. Wilson, I. B., Harrison, M. A., and Ginsberg, S.: J. Biol. Chem. 236:1498, 1961.
53. Ellis, S., Krayer, O., and Plachte, F. L.: J. Pharmacol. Exp. Ther. 79:309, 1943.
54. Enz, A., et al.: Prog. Brain Res. 98:431, 1993.
55. O'Brien, R. D.: Mol. Pharmacol. 4:121, 1968.
56. Calvey, H. T.: Biochem. Pharmacol. 16:1989, 1967.
57. Summers, W. K., et al.: N. Engl. J. Med. 315:1241, 1986.
58. Molloy, D. W., et al.: Can. Med. Assoc. J. 144:29, 1991.
59. Heath, D. F.: Organophosphorus Poisons. Oxford, Pergamon Press, 1961.
60. Oosterban, R. A., and Cohen, J. A. The active site of esterases. In Goodwin, T. W., Harris, I. J., and Hartley, B. S. (eds.). Structure and Activity of Enzymes. New York, Academic Press, 1964.
61. Linn, J. G., and Tomarelli, R. C.: Am. J. Ophthalmol. 35:46, 1952.
62. Comroe, J. H., et al.: J. Pharmacol. Exp. Ther. 87:281, 1946.
63. Gage, J. C.: Biochem. J. 54:426, 1953.
64. Nakatsugawa, T., Tolman, N. M., and Dahm, P. A.: Biochem. Pharmacol. 17:1517, 1968.
65. Mountner, L. A., and Cheatam, R. M.: Enzymologia 25:215, 1963.
66. Stephenson, R. P.: Br. J. Pharmacol. Chemother. 11:379, 1956.
67. Ariens, E. J.: Adv. Drug Res. 3:235, 1966.
68. Paton, W. D. M.: Proc. R. Soc. Lond. B 154:21, 1961.
69. Long, J. P., et al.: J. Pharmacol. Exp. Ther. 117:29, 1956.
70. AMA Drug Evaluations Annual 1994. Chicago, American Medical Association, 1994, p. 894.
71. Gyermek, L., and Nador, K.: J. Pharm. Pharmacol. 9:209, 1957.
72. Ariens, E. J., Simonis, A. M., and Van Rossum, J. M.: In Ariens, E. J. (ed.). Molecular Pharmacology. New York, Academic Press, 1964, p. 205.
73. Kondritzer, A. A., and Zvirblis, P.: J. Am. Pharm. Assoc. Sci. Ed. 46:531, 1957.
74. Cushny, A. R.: J. Physiol. 30:176, 1904.
75. Doods, H. N., et al.: Eur. J. Pharmacol. 250:223, 1993.
76. Fuder, M., and Meincke, M.: Naunyn-Schmiedebergs Arch. Pharmakol. 347:591, 1993.
77. Lazareno, S., and Birdsall, N. J.: Br. J. Pharmacol. 109:1120, 1993.
78. Karczmar, A. G. (ed.): International Encyclopedia of Pharmacology and Therapeutics, Sect. 12, Ganglionic Blocking and Stimulating Agents, vol. 1. Berlin, Springer-Verlag, 1980.
79. Skok, V. I.: In Karkevich, D. A. (ed.). Pharmacology of Ganglionic Transmission. Berlin, Springer-Verlag, 1980, p. 7.
80. Greengard, P., and Kebabian, J. W.: Fed. Proc. 33:1059, 1974.
81. Hammer, R., and Giachetti, A.: Life Sci. 31:2291, 1982.
82. Volle, R. L., and Hancock, J. C.: Fed. Proc. 29:1913, 1970.
83. Van Rossum, J. M.: Int. J. Neuropharmacol. 1:97, 1962.
84. Van Rossum, J. M.: Int. J. Neuropharmacol. 1:403, 1962.
85. Paton, W. D. M., and Zaimis, E. J.: Br. J. Pharmacol. 4:381, 1949.
86. Wintersteiner, O., and Dutcher, J. D.: Science 97:467, 1943.
87. Everett, A. J., Lowe, L. A., and Wilkinson, S.: Chem. Commun. 1020, 1970.
88. Stenlake, J. B., et al.: Br. J. Anaesth. 55:3S, 1983.
89. USAN and the USP Dictionary of Drug Names. Rockville, MD, United States Pharmacopeial Convention, 1994, p. 231.
90. Burke, R. E.: Mol. Pharmacol. 30:58, 1986.

CHAPTER 18

Diuretics

DANIEL A. KOECHEL

A *diuretic* is defined as a chemical that increases the rate of urine formation. The *primary action* of most diuretics is the direct inhibition of Na^+ transport at one or more of the four major anatomical sites along the nephron where Na^+ reabsorption takes place. Because the Na^+ transport systems at each of these locations are unique, there is a different set of relatively rigid structural features that a diuretic must possess to inhibit Na^+ reabsorption at each site. Of additional importance are the *secondary (or indirect) events* that are triggered as a result of the diuretic's primary action. The nature and magnitude of many of the observed secondary effects depend on the locus of action of the diuretic and the response of nephron sites "downstream" to an enhanced delivery of fluid, Na^+, or other solutes. The secondary events are quite characteristic for each class of diuretics and are often highly predictable if the reader has an understanding of normal renal physiological processes. Collectively, the primary and secondary effects induced by a diuretic determine its electrolyte excretion pattern. A diuretic usually possesses some combination of *natriuretic, chloruretic, saluretic, kaliuretic, bicarbonaturetic, or calciuretic properties,* depending on whether it enhances the renal excretion of Na^+, Cl^-, Na^+/Cl^-, K^+, HCO_3^-, or Ca^{2+}, respectively.

In this chapter, the normal function of the nephron is presented, including the four major reabsorptive sites for Na^+ and other important solutes and the renal physiological events that occur when Na^+ and water reabsorption are altered by the patient's state of hydration, disease, or intake of diuretics. This is followed by a discussion of each class of diuretics in current use. A knowledge of the important structural features and the site(s) of action of each class of diuretics should give the reader a better understanding of the factors that dictate the nature and magnitude of the anticipated diuresis and the associated secondary effects.

ANATOMY AND PHYSIOLOGY OF THE NEPHRON

The functional unit of the kidney is the nephron with its accompanying glomerulus (Fig. 18-1). There are approximately a million nephrons in each kidney. The blood (or, more appropriately, the plasma), from which all urine is formed, is brought to each nephron within the glomerular capillary network (Fig. 18-2). Many plasma components are filtered into Bowman's space. During the process of urine formation, the resulting glomerular filtrate flows through the convoluted and straight portions of the proximal tubule, descending limb of Henle's loop, thin and thick portions of the ascending limb of Henle's loop, area of the macula densa

cells, distal convoluted tubule (also referred to as the *early distal tubule*), connecting tubule (also referred to as the *late distal tubule*), and the cortical and medullary collecting tubules. Each of these nephron segments consists of ultrastructurally and functionally unique cell types. The physiological role of the glomerulus and each nephron segment is discussed below as it relates to the handling of important solutes and water in normally hydrated (normovolemic) and dehydrated (hypovolemic) persons and in patients afflicted with various edematous disorders (e.g., congestive heart failure, cirrhosis of the liver with ascites, and the nephrotic syndrome).

FUNCTION

Function of the Nephron When the Plasma Volume Is Normal (Normovolemia or Euvolemia)

As blood is delivered to each glomerulus, many (but not all) of its components are filtered into Bowman's space through the "pores" in the glomerular capillary loops. Several physicochemical properties of each blood component dictate the extent to which it is removed from the blood by glomerular filtration. These include the component's relative molecular mass (M_r), overall charge (applies primarily to large molecules), and degree and nature of binding to plasma proteins. For example, plasma proteins with an M_r in excess of 50,000 Da and red blood cells are not readily filtered, whereas low-M_r, non–protein-bound components (e.g., Na^+, K^+, Cl^-, HCO_3^-, glucose, and amino acids) are readily filtered.[1]

The *rate* of filtration of plasma components that possess an M_r of less than 50,000 Da and are not bound to plasma proteins

- Depends directly on the hydraulic (hydrostatic) pressure in the renal vasculature (created by the pumping heart), which tends to drive water and solutes out of the glomerular capillaries into Bowman's space
- Relates inversely to the plasma oncotic pressure (the osmotic pressure created by the plasma proteins within the vasculature), which tends to hold or prevent the filtration of water and solutes across the glomerular capillaries into Bowman's space[1]
- Follows the intrarenal signals that allow each nephron to adjust the filtration rate through its own glomerular capillary network (i.e., tubuloglomerular feedback)[2]

Clearly, the cardiovascular and renal functional status of an individual will also affect the rate of filtration of plasma components through the glomeruli. In addition, neonates and the elderly usually have a reduced glomerular filtration rate (GFR), though for different reasons.[3, 4]

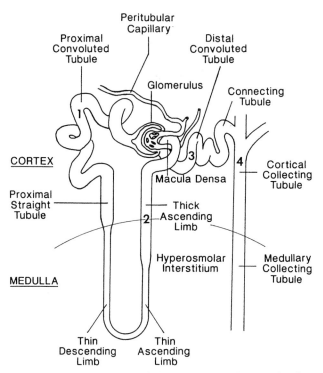

Figure 18–1 ■ Anatomy of the nephron, indicating the four major sites of sodium reabsorption (*1–4*).

The *fraction* of the total renal plasma flow that is filtered collectively by the glomeruli per unit time (i.e., the filtration fraction) is about one fifth.[2] This means that only one fifth (or 20%) of the plasma presented to the kidneys in a given period undergoes filtration at the glomeruli (i.e., about 650 mL of plasma flow through the kidneys each minute, approximately 125 mL/minute of which is filtered through the glomerular capillaries). The remaining four fifths (or 80%) of

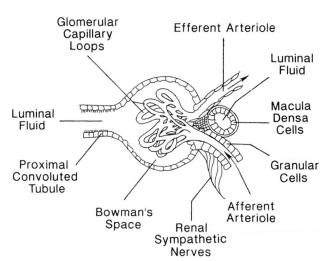

Figure 18–2 ■ Juxtaglomerular apparatus (JGA). Urine is formed from the filtration of plasma through the glomerular capillary loops into Bowman's space. The JGA is of paramount importance for the operation of the tubuloglomerular feedback mechanism, which allows a nephron to regulate the glomerular filtration rate of its own glomerulus.

the renal plasma flow is directed into the peritubular capillaries (Fig. 18-1). Each minute only 1 mL of urine is formed from the 125 mL of glomerular filtrate.[5] Thus, approximately 99% of the glomerular filtrate is normally reabsorbed.

The *absolute quantity* of each filtrable plasma component that reaches Bowman's space—the *filtered load* of a substance—depends directly on the GFR and the concentration in plasma of the portion of the filtrable substance that is not bound to plasma proteins. That is, the filtered load of a substance equals the GFR (in milliliters per minute) times the concentration of unbound, filtrable substance in plasma (in amount per milliliter).[5] The glomerular filtrate that houses the filtered load of a given solute is referred to below as the *luminal fluid,* since it enters the lumen of each nephron immediately upon leaving Bowman's space. In the following discussion, attention focuses on the percentage of the filtered load of Na^+ and other key solutes that is reabsorbed (i.e., transported from the luminal fluid into renal tubule cells, with subsequent passage into the interstitium and ultimately into the renal vasculature) at various nephron sites.

There are four major anatomical sites along the nephron that are responsible for the bulk of Na^+ reabsorption[6] (Fig. 18-1): *site 1,* the convoluted and straight portions of the proximal tubule; *site 2,* the thick ascending limb of Henle's loop; *site 3,* the distal convoluted tubule; and *site 4,* the connecting tubule and the cortical collecting tubule. The actual transport processes involved in Na^+ reabsorption at each of these sites are highlighted in Figures 18-3 through 18-6 and are discussed in order.

SITE 1

The convoluted and straight portions of the proximal tubule are responsible for the reabsorption of

- About 65% of the filtered loads of Na^+, Cl^-, Ca^{2+}, and water[6, 7]
- 80 to 90% of the filtered loads of HCO_3^-,[6, 8] phosphate,[7] and urate[9]
- Essentially 100% of the filtered loads of glucose, amino acids, and low-M_r proteins[10]

Thus, under normal circumstances, the proximal tubule has a tremendous reabsorptive capacity. There are primarily two driving forces for this high reabsorptive activity. First, because the plasma in the peritubular capillaries (Fig. 18-1) has a lower hydraulic pressure and a higher oncotic pressure than the luminal fluid or the plasma delivered to the glomerulus (because of the removal of water but not protein from plasma during glomerular filtration), there is a net movement of the luminal fluid contents in a reabsorptive direction.[1] Second, the Na^+/K^+-ATPase, strategically located on the antiluminal membrane (sometimes referred to as the *basolateral, peritubular,* or *contraluminal membrane*) of the proximal tubule cells, catalyzes the countertransport of intracellular Na^+ into the interstitium and extracellular K^+ into the proximal tubule cells[10] (Fig. 18-3). The stoichiometry for this countertransport is 3 Na^+:2 K^+. This activity creates a deficit of intracellular Na^+, a surfeit of intracellular K^+, and a voltage oriented negatively inside proximal tubule cells.[10]

In response to the action of the Na^+/K^+-ATPase, Na^+

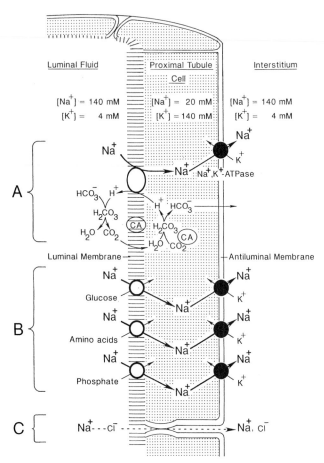

Figure 18–3 ■ Site 1: The Na^+ transport systems responsible for the reabsorption of Na^+ and associated solutes in the proximal tubule. **A.** Transcellular reabsorption of Na^+/HCO_3^-, which is controlled by carbonic anhydrase *(CA)*. Acetazolamide and other CA inhibitors block Na^+ reabsorption by this route. **B.** Transcellular reabsorption of Na^+ coupled to glucose, amino acids, and phosphate. **C.** Paracellular transport of Na^+/Cl^-. No commercially available agents inhibit Na^+ reabsorption by routes B or C. Na^+/K^+-ATPase is indicated by *filled circles* on the antiluminal membrane.

in the luminal fluid moves down the concentration gradient into proximal tubule cells by a combination of at least three distinct processes (labeled *A, B,* and *C* in Fig. 18-3). The first mechanism of Na^+ reabsorption at site 1 involves carbonic anhydrase (CA), which is located in the cytoplasm and on the brush border of proximal tubule cells (Fig. 18-3A). H^+, generated as the result of the action of intracellular CA, is exchanged (i.e., countertransported) for the filtered Na^+ in the luminal fluid. The Na^+ that enters proximal tubule cells during the exchange for H^+ is then pumped into the interstitium by the Na^+/K^+-ATPase in the antiluminal membrane. The H^+ secreted (i.e., transported uphill or against its gradient) into the luminal fluid reacts there with the filtered HCO_3^- to generate carbonic acid. The carbonic acid decomposes, both spontaneously and with the aid of the brush border–bound CA, to carbon dioxide and water. The carbon dioxide diffuses into the proximal tubule cells and is converted back into HCO_3^-, which subsequently passes from the proximal tubule cells, across the antiluminal membrane,

and into the interstitium by way of an Na^+/HCO_3^- symporter in the antiluminal membrane. CA is very plentiful in the convoluted portion of the human proximal tubule but is nonexistent in the straight portion.[8] Thus, the processes just described occur primarily in the convoluted portion of the proximal tubule and account for the reabsorption of about 20 to 25% of the filtered load of Na^+ (or about one third of the filtered load of Na^+ that is reabsorbed at site 1) and about 80 to 90% of the filtered load of HCO_3^-.[8, 11]

The second mechanism by which Na^+ moves out of the luminal fluid at site 1 involves its cotransport into proximal tubule cells along with glucose, amino acids, or phosphate[10] (Fig. 18-3B). The latter three solutes enter proximal tubule cells against their concentration gradients. The reabsorption of the Na^+ that enters proximal tubular cells by these processes is completed when it is subsequently pumped into the interstitium by the antiluminal membrane–bound Na^+/K^+-ATPase and then passes into the adjacent peritubular capillaries. The amount of Na^+ reabsorbed by this type of cotransport varies and depends on the filtered loads of the three solutes. Such cotransport, however, is the mechanism by which 100% of the filtered loads of glucose and amino acids and 80 to 90% of the filtered load of phosphate are normally removed from the luminal fluid and subsequently reabsorbed.

Third, Na^+ is reabsorbed at site 1 along with Cl^- (Fig. 18-3C).[10] As the reabsorption of Na^+ occurs in the early proximal convoluted tubule accompanied by bicarbonate, glucose, amino acids, and phosphate, the concentration of Cl^- within the luminal fluid tends to rise. As a result, the concentration of Cl^- in the mid to late proximal tubule luminal fluid exceeds that in the interstitium, and Cl^- moves *paracellularly* (i.e., between the proximal tubular cells) into the interstitium; Na^+ follows. Additional Na^+/Cl^- is reabsorbed *transcellularly* (i.e., through cells) in the proximal tubule by the combination of a Na^+/H^+ antiporter and one or more Cl^-/anion antiporters (not shown).[10]

Collectively, these site 1 Na^+-transporting processes remove 65% of the filtered load of Na^+ from the luminal fluid, and they do so *isosmotically* (i.e., the osmolality of the luminal fluid entering the descending limb of Henle's loop is similar to that of the initial glomerular filtrate).

As the luminal fluid moves through the descending limb of Henle's loop, the high *osmolality* (i.e., concentration of solutes) in the surrounding medullary interstitium draws approximately 15% of the filtered load of water out of the luminal fluid by osmosis and allows a small amount of Na^+ from the interstitium to be added to the luminal fluid. In other words, the luminal fluid is concentrated as it flows through the descending limb of Henle's loop.[12]

SITE 2

When the luminal fluid enters the thick ascending limb of Henle's loop, it comes into contact with tubule cells that are impermeable to water and possess a capacious luminal membrane–bound transport system for Na^+ (Fig. 18-4). Here, as at site 1, the major driving force for the reabsorption of Na^+ is the creation of an intracellular deficit of Na^+ by the antiluminal membrane–bound Na^+/K^+-ATPase. The electroneutral sodium/potassium/chloride cotransport system located on the luminal membrane of thick ascending

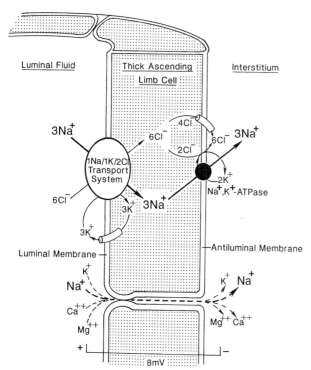

Figure 18–4 ■ Site 2: The Na$^+$ transport systems responsible for the reabsorption of Na$^+$ and associated solutes in the water-impermeable cortical and medullary portions of the thick ascending limb of Henle's loop. The collective actions of the antiluminal membrane–bound Na$^+$/K$^+$-ATPase and the luminal membrane–bound 1Na$^+$/1K$^+$/2Cl$^-$ cotransport system account for *transcellular* reabsorption of Na$^+$/Cl$^-$, in a Na$^+$/Cl$^-$ ratio of 3:6, and the generation of a lumen-positive potential that drives the reabsorption of Na$^+$ and other cations via the *paracellular* pathway *(dashed line)*. Diuretic agents that block Na$^+$ reabsorption in the thick ascending limb by inhibition of the luminal membrane–bound 1Na$^+$/1K$^+$/2Cl$^-$ cotransport system include furosemide, bumetanide, torsemide, ethacrynic acid, and a number of miscellaneous agents cited in Figure 18-13.

limb cells then transports Na$^+$, along with K$^+$ and Cl$^-$, from the luminal fluid into the cells of the thick ascending limb in a ratio of 1 Na$^+$:1 K$^+$:2 Cl$^-$.[10] Reabsorption of the Na$^+$ that enters thick ascending limb cells by this mechanism is completed when it is pumped actively into the interstitium by the antiluminal membrane–bound Na$^+$/K$^+$-ATPase and then passes into the surrounding vasculature. Cl$^-$ enters the interstitium through Cl$^-$ channels in the antiluminal membrane and by cotransport with K$^+$. The luminal K$^+$ that accompanies Na$^+$ and Cl$^-$ into the thick ascending limb cells recycles passively downhill back into the luminal fluid. The K$^+$ that enters the thick ascending limb cells by way of the antiluminal membrane–bound Na$^+$/K$^+$-ATPase recycles back into the interstitium via cotransport with Cl$^-$. Hence, the net result is the transport of 3 Na$^+$ and 6 Cl$^-$ from the luminal fluid into the interstitium. This results in the generation of a lumen-positive transepithelial voltage. This positive luminal environment drives more cations (Na$^+$, K$^+$, Ca^{2+}, Mg^{2+}) from the lumen into the interstitium paracellularly (i.e., between the thick ascending limb cells).[10, 13] The combined activities of the Na$^+$/K$^+$-ATPase

countertransport system on the antiluminal membrane and the 1Na$^+$/1K$^+$/2Cl$^-$ cotransport system on the luminal membrane of the thick ascending limb cells normally account for the reabsorption of up to 30% of the filtered load of Na$^+$,[6, 10] the reabsorption of up to 20 to 30% of the filtered load of Ca^{2+},[10] the maintenance of the high osmolality of the medullary interstitium (which is absolutely critical for the normal functioning of the human nephron),[12] and the ability of this nephron segment to reabsorb more Na$^+$ and other solutes than usual when proximal tubule Na$^+$ transport has been inhibited.[6, 14] This latter compensatory phenomenon explains why diuretics that act primarily at site 1 are not particularly efficacious.

The descending limb of Henle's loop is responsible for the concentration of luminal fluid (i.e., removal of water and addition of Na$^+$), while the thick ascending limb is responsible for the dilution of luminal fluid (i.e., removal of solute from the luminal fluid without concomitant removal of water). Hence, collectively, these two nephron segments produce a massive overall reduction of luminal fluid volume and solute content. Interestingly, the osmolality of the luminal fluid in the terminal portion of the thick ascending limb of Henle's loop is not much different from that of the fluid that enters the descending portion of the loop (though drastic changes take place in between).

As the luminal fluid leaves the thick ascending limb of Henle's loop, it comes into contact with the *macula densa cells*, a specialized group of tubule cells that communicate with the granular cells of the afferent arteriole belonging to the same nephron[15] (Fig. 18-2). The macula densa cells are like the thick ascending limb cells, in that they house both the antiluminal membrane–bound Na$^+$/K$^+$-ATPase and the luminal membrane–bound 1Na$^+$/1K$^+$/2Cl$^-$ cotransport system. Their uniqueness lies in their ability to detect changes in either the rate of luminal fluid flow or the solute composition of the luminal fluid, which in part dictates how much solute they remove from the luminal fluid. Signals are then transmitted by way of the granular cells to the afferent arteriole associated with that nephron.[2] When fluid/solute delivery past the macula densa cells increases, a macula densa–derived substance mediates constriction of the afferent arteriole supplying that particular nephron and a reduction in GFR ensues. This is commonly referred to as *tubuloglomerular feedback*. On the other hand, when fluid/solute delivery past the macula densa cells decreases, a signal is transmitted from these cells to the granular cells surrounding the afferent arteriole, which results in the release of renin.[2]

SITE 3

Following its sojourn past the macula densa cells, the luminal fluid comes into contact with the third major site for the reabsorption of Na$^+$, the relatively short, water-impermeable, distal convoluted tubule (Fig. 18-5). Again, the major driving force for Na$^+$ reabsorption from the luminal fluid at site 3 involves the deficit of intracellular Na$^+$ produced by the action of the antiluminal membrane–bound Na$^+$/K$^+$-ATPase. In this instance, the luminal membrane–bound Na$^+$/Cl$^-$ cotransport system moves luminal fluid Na$^+$ downhill and luminal fluid Cl$^-$ uphill into distal convoluted tubule cells. The reabsorption of Na$^+$ is completed when the antiluminal membrane–bound Na$^+$/K$^+$-ATPase ac-

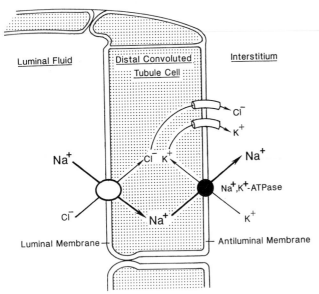

Figure 18–5 ■ Site 3: The Na^+ transport systems responsible for the reabsorption of Na^+ and Cl^- in the water-impermeable distal convoluted tubule. Inhibitors of the luminal membrane–bound Na^+/Cl^- cotransport system include the thiazide and thiazide-like diuretics.

tively pumps it into the interstitium with subsequent passage into the surrounding vasculature; intracellular Cl^- enters the interstitium through channels in the antiluminal membrane. Approximately 5 to 8% of the filtered load of Na^+ is reabsorbed at site 3.[6, 11]

SITE 4

The connecting tubule (i.e., late distal tubule) and the cortical collecting tubule house the fourth and final major site for the reabsorption of Na^+ from the luminal fluid[6] (Fig. 18-6). This portion of the nephron is composed of two distinct cell types, the *principal cells* and the *intercalated cells*. The principal cells are important for Na^+ reabsorption and K^+ secretion, whereas the intercalated cells (subtype A) are important for the generation and secretion of H^+. The intercalated cells possess only small quantities of the Na^+/K^+-ATPase on their antiluminal membranes, but they contain abundant quantities of intracellular CA, which catalyzes the formation of carbonic acid from CO_2 and water. The carbonic acid ionizes, yielding H^+ and HCO_3^-. The H^+ is then pumped actively into the luminal fluid by the luminal membrane–bound H^+-ATPase. The driving force for the reabsorption of Na^+ in the principal cells is once again the deficit of intracellular Na^+ created by the Na^+/K^+-ATPase on the antiluminal membrane, which countertransports 3 Na^+ uphill from the principal cells into the interstitium and 2 K^+ uphill from the interstitium into the principal cells. In response to the deficit of Na^+ in the principal cells, the Na^+ in the luminal fluid moves downhill into the principal cells through Na^+ channels in the luminal membrane and is subsequently pumped actively into the interstitium by the antiluminal membrane–bound Na^+/K^+-ATPase. These events create a lumen-negative transepithelial voltage. In response to this voltage difference, some combination of the following three processes occurs:

- Cl^- moves paracellularly from the lumen into the interstitium (not shown)
- K^+ in the principal cells moves downhill into the luminal fluid through K^+ channels in the luminal membrane
- H^+ generated in the intercalated cells moves into the luminal fluid by way of the H^+-ATPase[10]

Because the latter two processes predominate, one may view the activities at site 4 as an exchange of luminal fluid Na^+ for principal cell K^+ and intercalated cell H^+. The exchange of luminal fluid Na^+ for intracellular H^+ or K^+ normally is associated with the reabsorption of only 2 to 3% of the filtered load of Na^+,[6] and the distal location of this exchange system dictates the final acidity and K^+ content of the urine.

The amount of Na^+ reabsorbed at site 4 and, therefore, the amount of H^+ and K^+ present in the final urine are modulated by

- Plasma and renal levels of mineralocorticoids like aldosterone—the higher the levels of circulating aldosterone, the greater the Na^+ reabsorption and K^+ and H^+ excretion
- Luminal fluid flow rate and the percentage of the filtered load of Na^+ presented to the exchange sites—the greater the flow rate and the load of Na^+, the greater the amount of exchange
- Acid–base status of the individual—acidosis favors exchange of Na^+ and H^+, whereas alkalosis favors exchange of Na^+ and K^+ [6, 16]

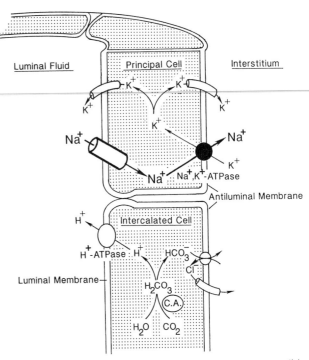

Figure 18–6 ■ Site 4: The Na^+ transport systems responsible for the reabsorption of Na^+ in the connecting and cortical collecting tubules. Na^+ reabsorption and K^+ secretion take place in the principal cells; H^+ formation and secretion occur in the intercalated cells. Spironolactone inhibits Na^+ reabsorption by competitively antagonizing the effects of aldosterone on the principal cells. Triamterene and amiloride "plug" the Na^+ channels in the luminal membrane of the principal cells, thereby preventing Na^+ reabsorption and K^+ and H^+ secretion. Thus, while producing a modest natriuresis, these drugs prevent K^+ loss and are commonly referred to as K^+-sparing diuretics.

The classes of diuretics that inhibit the reabsorption of Na^+ at sites 1, 2, or 3 (i.e., sites proximal to site 4) ultimately increase, to varying degrees, the luminal fluid flow rate and the percentage of the filtered load of Na^+ delivered to site 4. Thus, many diuretics acutely enhance the urinary loss of K^+ and may be associated with the induction of hypokalemia (i.e., abnormally low levels of K^+ in the circulating blood).

Function of the Nephron During Reduced Plasma Volume (Hypovolemia)

When a patient's plasma volume decreases below normal (hypovolemia) because of such events as hemorrhage, diarrhea, vomiting, excessive sweating, or overzealous use of diuretics, a cascade of intrarenal and extrarenal signals that decreases urine and electrolyte output occurs in an attempt to restore the plasma volume and mean arterial pressure.[2, 17] The many signals result in

- Decreased renal blood flow and GFR
- Increased proximal tubule reabsorption of solutes and water[14, 17]
- Increased renin secretion from the renal granular cells, which leads to increased circulating levels of angiotensin II (a potent vasoconstrictor) and aldosterone
- Increased secretion of antidiuretic hormone (ADH), which acts on the collecting tubules to increase water reabsorption

When hypovolemia is the result of overzealous use of diuretics, the compensatory reductions in urinary water and electrolyte output that occur are commonly referred to as the ''*diuretic braking phenomenon.*'' The compensatory cascade of events mentioned above has basically put on the brakes to continued diuretic-induced increases in water and electrolyte excretion. Thus, the efficacy of the diuretic is blunted significantly. No diuretic induces the loss of urine that has the same composition as extracellular fluid; therefore, overzealous use of these agents results in hypovolemic patients who are frequently left with electrolyte and/or acid–base derangements.

Function of the Nephron During Disease States Associated With Retention of Body Fluids (Edematous States)

Frequently, the kidneys of individuals with congestive heart failure, cirrhosis of the liver with ascites, or the nephrotic syndrome receive signals that are interpreted to mean that they are being hypoperfused. This may occur whether or not there is an actual plasma volume reduction. The kidneys attempt to retain body fluids and solutes by a combination of the processes discussed in the previous paragraph. Ultimately, edema ensues.[18]

INTRODUCTION TO THE DIURETICS

Before embarking on a discussion of the various classes of diuretics, one must understand the difference between the terms *potency* and *efficacy* as they relate to diuretics, the major determinants of diuretic efficacy, and the shortcomings of many of the previous structure–activity relationship (SAR) studies that have involved diuretics.

A clear distinction must be made between the use of the terms *potency* and *efficacy*.[19] The *potency* of a diuretic is related to the absolute amount of drug (e.g., milligrams or milligrams per kilogram) required to produce an effect. The *relative potency* is a convenient means of comparing two diuretics and is expressed as a ratio of equieffective doses. The potency of a diuretic is influenced by its absorption, distribution, biotransformation, excretion, and inherent ability to combine with its receptor (i.e., its intrinsic activity). The potency of a diuretic is important for establishing its dosage but is otherwise a relatively unimportant characteristic. *Efficacy* relates to the maximal diuretic effect attainable (usually measured in terms of urine volume per unit of time or urinary loss of Na^+ or NaCl per unit of time).

Numerous factors contribute to the efficacy of a diuretic. First, the anatomical site of action and the capacity of the Na^+-reabsorbing sites downstream play major roles in determining the overall efficacy. That is, a diuretic's efficacy is determined in part by whether it acts at site 1, 2, 3, or 4. Diuretics that inhibit the reabsorption of Na^+ at the same anatomical site are usually equiefficacious (i.e., evoke similar maximal responses) but may vary in potency (i.e., the amount of diuretic necessary to produce similar effects). Diuretics that act at site 1 by inhibiting CA may inhibit the reabsorption of 20 to 25% of the filtered load of Na^+ but are not as efficacious as one might think, because the three major sites of Na^+ reabsorption downstream (sites 2, 3, and 4) compensate by reabsorbing most of the extra Na^+ presented to them. Diuretics that inhibit the reabsorption of Na^+ at site 2 are the most efficacious because site 2 is normally responsible for the reabsorption of up to 30% of the filtered load of Na^+, and the two Na^+ reabsorptive sites downstream (sites 3 and 4) are relatively low capacity sites. Diuretics that act at site 2 frequently are referred to as *high-ceiling* or *loop* diuretics. Diuretics that act at sites 3 or 4 are less efficacious because these two sites are responsible for the reabsorption of only 5 to 8% and 2 to 3% of the filtered load of Na^+, respectively.

Second, the efficacy of a diuretic depends on its concentration at the site where it inhibits Na^+ transport. In all but a few cases, diuretics interfere with the processes responsible for the reabsorption of Na^+ that are located on the luminal membrane, and hence, their intraluminal concentration is of critical importance. The concentration of a diuretic agent that ultimately is presented to a luminal site is determined by how well it is filtered at the glomerulus, whether it undergoes active tubular secretion in proximal tubules, and whether it undergoes nonionic back diffusion in the distal nephron segments. All diuretics enter luminal fluid by the process of glomerular filtration but to varying degrees. The amount that enters the luminal fluid by the filtration process depends on the GFR, the plasma concentration of the diuretic agent, and the extent to which the diuretic is bound to the predominant unfiltrable plasma protein, albumin. In addition, all but a few of the diuretics attain relatively high concentrations in the luminal fluid of the proximal tubule by a two-step process commonly referred to as *active tubular secretion*[20] (Fig. 18-7). The antiluminal membrane of the proximal tubule houses a set of bidirectional active transport systems that participate in the first step of active tubular secretion of a

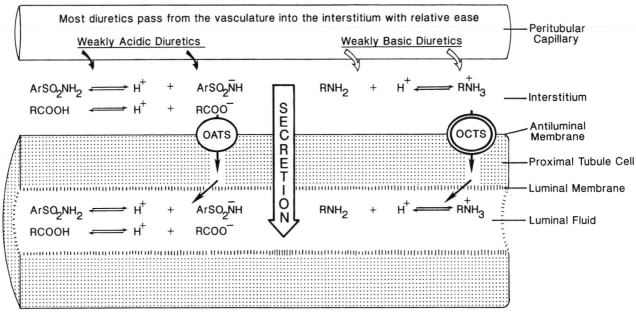

Figure 18–7 ■ Active tubular secretion of a drug is a two-step process that is localized only in the proximal tubule area of the nephron. The first step involves the active transport of a drug that can exist as an organic anion or an organic cation from the interstitium into proximal tubule cells by way of the organic anion transport system (OATS) or the organic cation transport system (OCTS), respectively. These systems are located on the antiluminal membrane of proximal tubule cells. The second step involves some combination of passive diffusion of the uncharged drug species or active transport of the charged drug species from the proximal tubule cells into the luminal fluid. Active tubular secretion contributes in a major way to the high luminal fluid levels of most diuretics.

diuretic. The organic anion transport system (OATS) transports endogenous and exogenous organic anions; the organic cation transport system (OCTS) handles endogenous and exogenous organic cations. Because most diuretics are weak organic acids (e.g., carboxylic acids or sulfonamides) or weak organic bases (e.g., amines), they exist as organic anions and cations, respectively, and are likely to be handled by the OATS or the OCTS. Although the OATS and OCTS are bidirectional, they transport diuretics primarily in a secretory direction (i.e., from the interstitium into proximal tubule cells). Even diuretics that are extensively bound to plasma proteins may be secreted avidly. Importantly, neither the OATS nor the OCTS possesses rigid structural requirements for the respective organic anion or cation being transported. The second step of active tubular secretion of a diuretic involves its passage from proximal tubule cells into the luminal fluid, probably by a combination of passive diffusion and active transport.

In addition to the filtration and secretion processes, the concentration of a diuretic in the luminal fluid of the more distal segments of the tubule is determined by the agent's lipid/water partition coefficient and pK_a, as well as the pH of the distal luminal fluid. These factors modulate the concentration of diuretic at sites 3 and 4. Weakly acidic diuretics, whose undissociated forms possess a favorable balance of lipid and water solubility, may undergo pH-dependent diffusion (referred to as *nonionic back diffusion*) from the distal tubular luminal fluid back into the bloodstream. This frequently decreases the luminal fluid concentration and the renal excretion rate of the diuretic but prolongs its plasma half-life. Diuretics that are weak bases

follow a similar course if the urinary pH is on the alkaline side, which favors the presence of the uncharged drug species. Weak organic acids or bases, whose uncharged forms possess an unfavorable lipid/water partition coefficient, will not undergo nonionic back diffusion. These diuretics will be retained within the luminal fluid and, ultimately, will be excreted. Thus, diuretic agents may reach high concentrations in luminal fluid following glomerular filtration, active tubular secretion, and little or no subsequent nonionic back diffusion. Diuretics that act at sites 2 and 3 as well as some that act at site 4 inhibit Na^+ transport processes on the luminal membrane and must attain relatively high luminal fluid concentrations. In contrast, the CA-inhibiting diuretics that act at site 1 must attain adequate concentrations within luminal fluid as well as intracellularly, and the aldosterone antagonist spironolactone must attain adequate intracellular concentrations at site 4.

Finally, the efficacy of a diuretic is also determined by the patient's plasma volume and renal function status, concurrently administered drugs that reduce the GFR, and concurrently administered drugs that bind competitively to the OATS or OCTS and reduce the active tubular secretion and luminal fluid concentration of the diuretic.

Many of the past SAR studies involving diuretics were conducted in whole animals, and the results may be misinterpreted unless caution is exercised. Generally, compounds of varied chemical structure are administered to animals and ranked according to their ability to produce changes in urine volume or Na^+ output over a prescribed period. Conclusions are then drawn about which functional groups are the most important for optimal diuretic activity. The novice must remember that the results from such studies cannot necessarily be interpreted as a ranking of the intrinsic activity of the agents under study. Diuretic SAR studies conducted in whole animals yield results that are a composite of differences in the absorption, plasma protein binding, distribution, biotransformation, excretion, active tubular secretion, intrinsic activity, and secondary effects (e.g., changes in the GFR) of the various agents. Unfortunately, most, if not all, of these variables are neglected during initial diuretic screening procedures; therefore, it may be assumed erroneously that differences in diuretic activity are due to differences in intrinsic activity. If one is interested in the intrinsic activity of the members of a group of diuretics, a closer approximation can be achieved by examining the agents on isolated nephron segments on which related or prototypic diuretics are known to act. Several such studies have been conducted.[21, 22] It should not be a surprise when results from in vivo and in vitro SAR studies differ. This occurs because of the interplay between numerous parameters in the in vivo studies (i.e., absorption, distribution, and such) that can be eliminated in a properly designed in vitro study. Almost all structure–activity data cited in the upcoming portion of this chapter came from whole animal and human investigations.

SITE 1 DIURETICS: CARBONIC ANHYDRASE INHIBITORS

Although the available CA inhibitors are used infrequently as diuretics, they not only played an important role in the development of other major classes of diuretics that are currently in widespread use but also aided in our understanding of basic renal physiology. Shortly after its introduction for the treatment of bacterial infections, sulfanilamide (Fig. 18-8) was observed to produce a mild diuresis characterized by the presence of urinary Na^+ and a substantial amount of HCO_3^-.[23] It was subsequently shown that it induced this effect through inhibition of renal CA.[24, 25] However, it was a relatively weak inhibitor of renal CA, and the dose needed to exert adequate diuresis was associated with severe adverse effects. To improve on the CA-inhibitory property of sulfanilamide, many sulfamoyl-containing compounds ($-SO_2NH_2$) were synthesized and screened for their diuretic activity in vivo and their ability to inhibit CA in vitro. Two groups of CA inhibitors emerged: simple heterocyclic sulfonamides and *meta*-disulfamoylbenzene derivatives (Fig. 18-8).

STRUCTURE–ACTIVITY RELATIONSHIPS

SAR studies involving the *simple heterocyclic sulfonamides* yielded the prototypic CA inhibitor, acetazolamide[26–30] (Fig. 18-8). The sulfamoyl group is essential for in vitro CA-inhibitory activity and for diuresis production in vivo. The sulfamoyl nitrogen atom must remain unsubstituted to retain both in vivo and in vitro activities. This feature explains why all antibacterial sulfonamides except sulfanilamide are incapable of inhibiting CA or exerting diuresis. In contrast, substitution of a methyl group on one of acetazolamide's ring nitrogens yields methazolamide (Fig. 18-8), a product

that retains CA-inhibitory activity. The moiety to which the sulfamoyl group is attached must possess aromatic character. In addition, within a given series of heterocyclic sulfonamides, the derivatives with the highest lipid/water partition coefficients and the lowest pK_a values have the greatest CA-inhibitory and diuretic activities.

The SAR studies involving the *meta-disulfamoylbenzenes* revealed that the parent 1,3-disulfamoylbenzene lacked diuretic activity, but key substitutions (summarized in Fig. 18-8) led to compounds with diuretic activity.[31] The first commercially available analogue, dichlorphenamide (Fig. 18-8), is similar to acetazolamide in its CA-inhibitory activity, but it is also a chloruretic agent. Subsequently, chloraminophenamide (Fig. 18-8) when given by the intravenous route was shown to possess less CA-inhibitory activity but more chloruretic activity. Poor diuretic activity following the oral administration of chloraminophenamide precluded its marketing.

PHARMACOKINETICS

The clinically available CA inhibitors are absorbed well from the gastrointestinal tract, are distributed to the sites of major importance for CA inhibition, undergo little, if any, biotransformation, and are excreted primarily by the kidneys. All CA inhibitors attain relatively high concentrations in renal luminal fluid (by a combination of glomerular filtration and active tubular secretion) and in proximal tubule cells.

SITE AND MECHANISM OF ACTION

CA is located both intracellularly (type II CA) and in the luminal brush border membrane (type IV CA) of proximal convoluted tubule cells (Fig. 18-3A). Both of these site 1 locations are major targets of the CA inhibitors.[8] This group of diuretics also inhibits intracellular CA in the intercalated cells of the connecting and cortical collecting tubules (i.e., site 4; Fig. 18-6).

During the first 4 to 7 days of continuous therapy with a CA inhibitor, several noteworthy events occur that lead to an increase in Na^+ and HCO_3^- excretion: *(a)* inhibition of the intracellular CA in proximal tubule cells decreases the available H^+ normally exchanged for luminal fluid Na^+, thus decreasing proximal tubule reabsorption of Na^+ (Fig. 18-3); and *(b)* inhibition of CA on the luminal brush border membrane of proximal tubule cells causes a decrease in the production of carbon dioxide within the luminal fluid and a decrease in the proximal tubule uptake of carbon dioxide. The net result is a decrease in the reabsorption of HCO_3^-. One might assume that a massive diuresis would follow inhibition of the portion of proximal tubule Na^+ reabsorption under the control of CA (i.e., one third of the 65% of the filtered load of Na^+ normally reabsorbed from the proximal luminal fluid, or about 22% of the filtered load of Na^+). However, Na^+ reabsorption sites downstream (especially site 2) compensate for such an action by reabsorbing much of the additional Na^+ presented to them.[6, 11, 13] Some of the luminal fluid HCO_3^- is reabsorbed downstream by a non–CA-mediated system.[32] Thus, the actions of the CA inhibitors ultimately result in the urinary loss of only 2 to

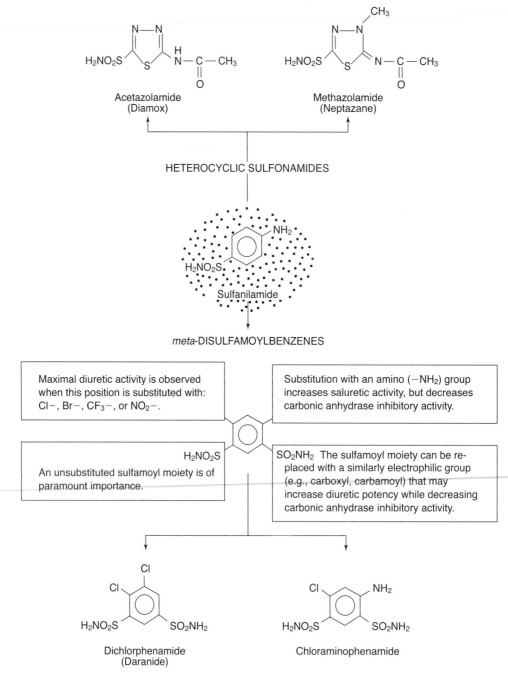

Figure 18–8 ■ Development of two classes of carbonic anhydrase inhibitors based on the actions of sulfanilamide.

5% of the filtered load of Na⁺ and up to 30% of the filtered load of HCO_3^-.

Secondarily, the CA inhibitors enhance the urinary excretion of a substantial amount of K⁺.[11, 33] The urinary loss of K⁺ increases because the proximal tubule actions of CA inhibitors present a greater percentage of the filtered load of Na⁺ to site 4, increase the flow rate of luminal fluid through the distal convoluted tubule and collecting tubule, and decrease the availability of intracellular H⁺ at site 4. All three changes favor enhanced exchange of luminal fluid Na⁺ for intracellular K⁺ at site 4. The urinary concentration of Cl⁻ actually decreases after the administration of CA in-

hibitors.[32] Hence, CA inhibitors are primarily natriuretic, bicarbonaturetic, and kaliuretic agents.

Toward the end of the first week of continuous therapy with a CA inhibitor, resistance develops to its diuretic effect.[34] This is primarily due to two factors. First, there is a marked reduction in the filtered load of HCO_3^- because the CA inhibitors produce both a 20% reduction in the GFR, via the tubuloglomerular feedback mechanism, and a reduction in the plasma concentration of HCO_3^-. When there is less HCO_3^- present in the luminal fluid, there is less HCO_3^- reabsorption to inhibit. Second, the metabolic acidosis created by these diuretics provides a sufficient amount of non–CA-generated intracellular H^+ to exchange for the luminal fluid Na^+. The Na^+ reabsorption at site 1 progressively returns to a near-normal rate, and diuresis wanes.

ADVERSE EFFECTS

Four highly predictable adverse effects are associated with the CA inhibitors:

1. Development of metabolic acidosis due to the renal loss of HCO_3^-
2. Hypokalemia due to the renal loss of K^+
3. Up to a 20% reduction in the GFR, which appears to be mediated via the juxtaglomerular apparatus because of either the increased flow rate of luminal fluid past the macula densa cells or the increased reabsorption of the additional solute presented to the macula cells (i.e., tubuloglomerular feedback)[33, 35]
4. Typical sulfonamide-associated hypersensitivity reactions, such as urticaria, drug fever, blood dyscrasias, and interstitial nephritis

CA inhibitors may also be associated with the production of paresthesias (tingling in the extremities), drowsiness, fatigue, anorexia, gastrointestinal disturbances, and urinary calculi. The latter occur because of a reduction in the urinary excretion rate of citrate, a normal urinary component that assists in maintaining urinary Ca^{2+} salts in a solubilized form.[32, 33]

CA inhibitors can exacerbate the symptoms associated with cirrhosis of the liver.[32, 36] Consequently, their use should be avoided in patients with this disorder. CA inhibitor–induced alkalinization of the urine decreases the normal luminal fluid trapping of ammonia (NH_3) in the form of ammonium ions (NH_4^+). This leads to a subsequent reduction in the urinary excretion of ammonium ions. Under these circumstances the highly diffusible ammonia is diverted from the luminal fluid into the systemic circulation, where it may contribute to the development of hepatic encephalopathy.

USES

The major use of the CA inhibitors is in the treatment of glaucoma.[36] CA is a functionally important enzyme in the eye, where it plays a key role in the formation of aqueous humor. Inhibition of this ocular enzyme reduces the rate of formation of the aqueous humor, thereby reducing the intraocular pressure associated with glaucoma. Interestingly, a reduction in the intraocular pressure usually persists at a time when resistance has developed to the renal effects of the CA inhibitors.[33] CA inhibitors have been used prophylactically to counteract acute mountain sickness,[36] to act as adjuvants for the treatment of epilepsy, and to create an alkaline urine in an attempt to hasten the renal excretion of certain noxious weak acids or to maintain the urinary solubility of certain poorly water soluble, endogenous weak acids (e.g., uric acid).[36]

PRODUCTS

Acetazolamide, USP.   Acetazolamide, *N*-[5-(aminosulfonyl)-1,3,4-thiadiazol-2-yl]acetamide (Diamox) (Fig. 18-8), was introduced in 1953 as the first orally effective, nonmercurial diuretic available to the physician. It has a rela-

tively restricted use today because of its limited efficacy and the refractoriness that develops to its diuretic action within the first week of continuous therapy. However, it remains the most important CA inhibitor available and serves as the prototypic agent in its class. Acetazolamide is absorbed extremely well from the gastrointestinal tract, is bound extensively to plasma proteins, and is not biotransformed. Peak plasma levels are attained within 2 to 4 hours. Its onset of action is about 1 hour, and its duration of action ranges from 6 to 12 hours. Acetazolamide is removed totally from the plasma by the kidneys within 24 hours. The renal handling of acetazolamide involves its filtration at the glomeruli, active tubular secretion exclusively in the proximal tubules, and a varying degree of pH-dependent nonionic back diffusion in the distal segments of the nephron.

Methazolamide, USP.   Although in vitro studies have shown methazolamide, *N*-[5-(aminosulfonyl)-3-methyl-1,3,4-thiadiazol-2(3H)-ylidene]acetamide (Neptazane) (Fig. 18-8), to be a more potent CA inhibitor than the prototypic acetazolamide, it is seldom used as a diuretic (for the same reasons stated for acetazolamide). Methazolamide displays improved penetration into the eye,[28] a property that contributes to its usefulness in the treatment of glaucoma.

Dichlorphenamide, USP.   Like the other CA inhibitors, dichlorphenamide, 4,5-dichloro-1,3-benzenedisulfonamide (Daranide) (Fig. 18-8), is seldom used as a diuretic. Little is known about its pharmacokinetics. Like other CA inhibitors, it reduces intraocular pressure and may be useful in the treatment of glaucoma. The importance of dichlorphenamide and chloraminophenamide is that they ultimately served as stepping stones away from the "pure" CA-inhibiting diuretics and toward the development of the thiazide and thiazide-like diuretics, which are effective natriuretic and chloruretic agents with minimal CA-inhibitory activity.[28, 30]

SITE 3 DIURETICS: THIAZIDE AND THIAZIDE-LIKE DIURETICS

Chloraminophenamide became a logical key intermediate in the development of diuretics that lacked the undesirable properties of the CA inhibitors. When chloraminophenamide was treated with acylating reagents, cyclization resulted in the formation of 1,2,4-benzothiadiazine-1,1-dioxides[28] (Fig. 18-9). The use of aldehydes or ketones in place of the acylating reagents yielded the corresponding dihydro derivatives. The products of these reactions became known as thiazides and hydrothiazides, respectively. Hereafter, they are referred to collectively as the *thiazide diuretics*. The thiazides were the first orally effective saluretic agents whose diuretic activity was not influenced by the patient's acid–base status.

STRUCTURE–ACTIVITY RELATIONSHIPS

Exhaustive SAR studies have been conducted with the thiazide diuretics[28, 30] (see Fig. 18-9 for the numbering of the thiazide ring positions). Briefly, the 2 position can tolerate the presence of relatively small alkyl groups, such as CH_3^-. The 3 position is an extremely important site of molecular

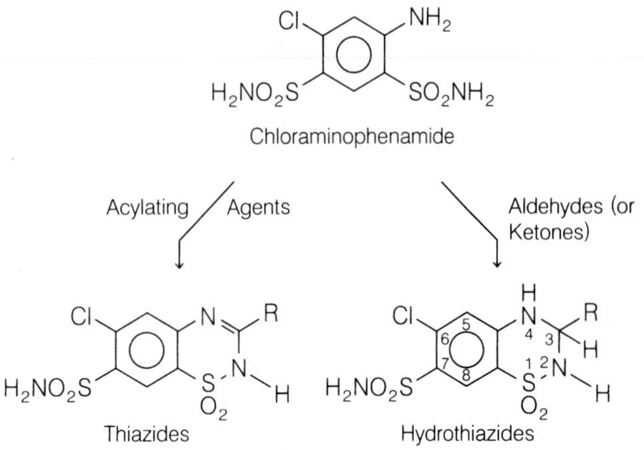

Figure 18–9 ■ Development of thiazide and hydrothiazide diuretics from chloraminophenamide.

modification. Substituents in the 3 position play a dominant role in determining the potency and duration of action of the thiazide diuretics. In addition, certain substituents in the 3 position have yielded compounds that are relatively specific inhibitors of the diuretic action of the thiazides.[37–40] Loss of the carbon–carbon double bond between the 3 and 4 positions of the benzothiadiazine-1,1-dioxide nucleus increases the potency of this class of diuretics approximately 3- to 10-fold. Direct substitution of the 4, 5, or 8 position with an alkyl group usually diminishes diuretic activity. Substitution at the 6 position with an "activating" group is essential for diuretic activity. The best substituents include Cl-, Br-, CF_3-, and NO_2-groups. The sulfamoyl group in the 7 position is a prerequisite for diuretic activity. Table 18-1 depicts the commercially available diuretics derived from the many alterations performed on the benzothiadiazine-1,1-dioxide nucleus.

When it was discovered that the sulfamoyl group *para* to the activating group in the *meta*-disulfamoylbenzenes could be replaced by several other electronegative groups with re-

TABLE 18–1 Thiazide and Hydrothiazide Diuretics

Thiazide Diuretics

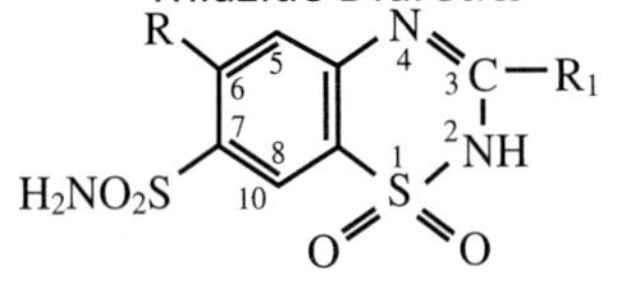

Generic Name	Proprietary Name	R	R₁
Chlorothiazide, USP	Diuril	—Cl	—H
Benzthiazide, USP	Exna, Hydrex	—Cl	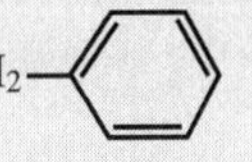 —CH₂—S—CH₂—⟨phenyl⟩

Hydrothiazide Diuretics

Generic Name	Proprietary Name	R	R₁	R₂
Hydrochlorothiazide, USP	HydroDIURIL, Esidrix, Oretic	—Cl	—H	—H
Hydroflumethiazide, USP	Saluron, Diucardin	—CF₃	—H	—H
Bendroflumethiazide, USP	Naturetin	—CF₃	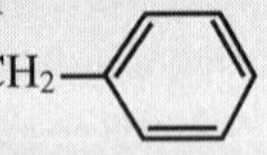 —CH₂—⟨phenyl⟩	—H
Trichlormethiazide, USP	Naqua, Metahydrin	—Cl	—CHCl₂	—H
Methyclothiazide, USP	Enduron, Aquatensen	—Cl	—CH₂Cl	—CH₃
Polythiazide, USP	Renese	—Cl	—CH₂—S—CH₂—CF₃	—CH₃
Cyclothiazide, USP	Anhydron	—Cl	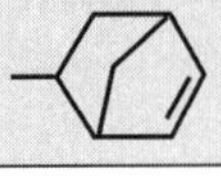 ⟨bicyclic alkenyl⟩	—H

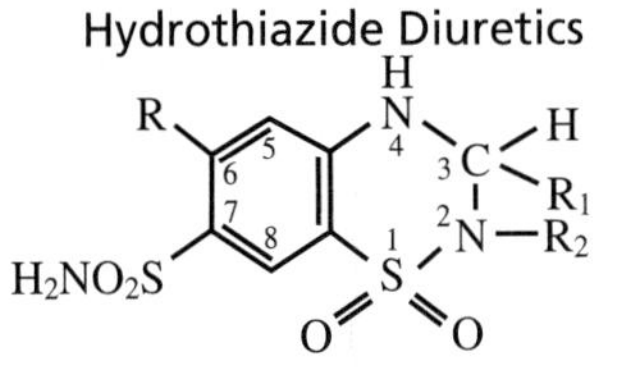

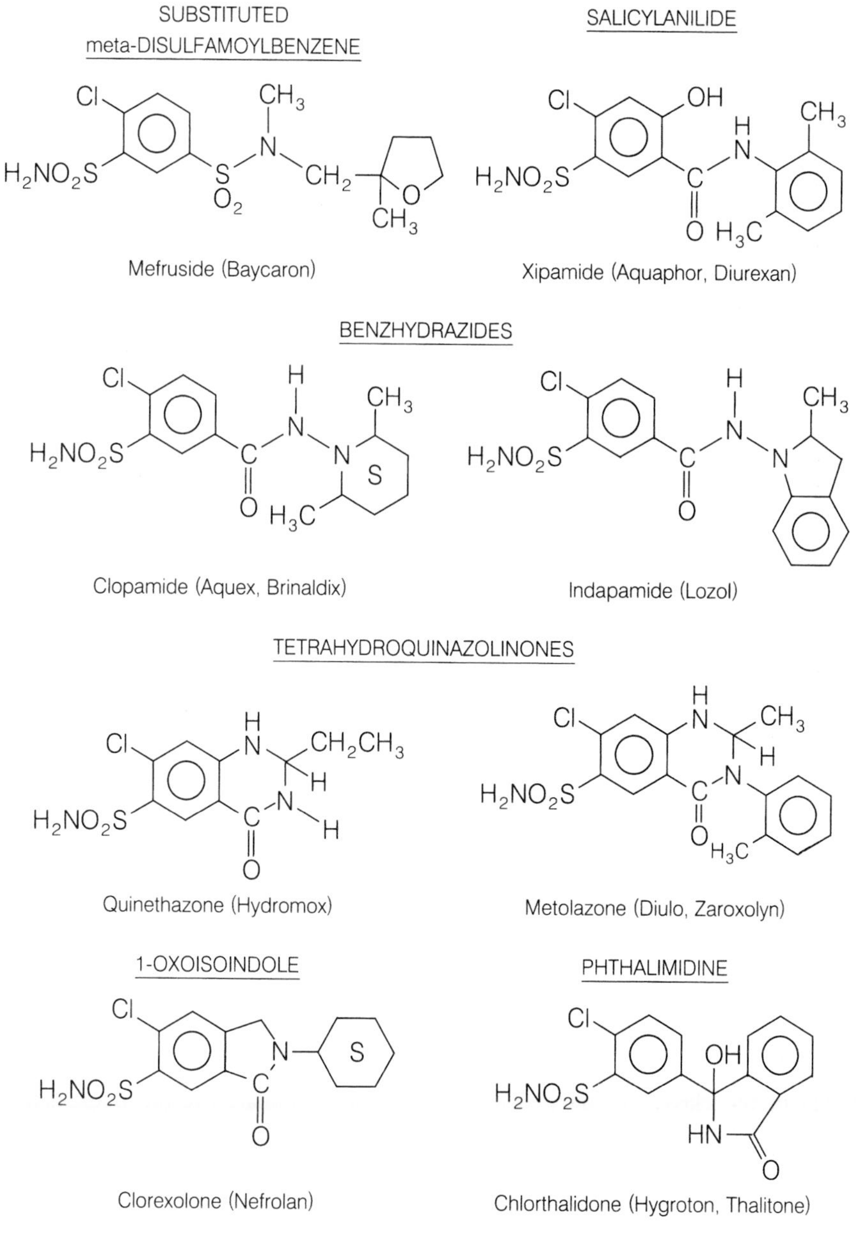

SUBSTITUTED
meta-DISULFAMOYLBENZENE

Mefruside (Baycaron)

SALICYLANILIDE

Xipamide (Aquaphor, Diurexan)

BENZHYDRAZIDES

Clopamide (Aquex, Brinaldix)

Indapamide (Lozol)

TETRAHYDROQUINAZOLINONES

Quinethazone (Hydromox)

Metolazone (Diulo, Zaroxolyn)

1-OXOISOINDOLE

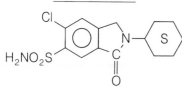

Clorexolone (Nefrolan)

PHTHALIMIDINE

Chlorthalidone (Hygroton, Thalitone)

Figure 18–10 ■ Representatives from six classes of thiazide-like diuretics. These diuretics were developed as an outgrowth of the thiazide research that involved molecular modification of aromatic sulfamoyl-containing compounds.

tention of diuretic activity (Fig. 18-8), a host of diuretics emerged that have become known as *thiazide-like diuretics*. The diuretics shown in Figure 18-10 represent the most active member(s) of each series. Clearly, these diuretics are not benzothiadiazines, but their sites of action, efficacies, electrolyte excretion patterns, and adverse effects resemble those of the thiazides. For these reasons, the thiazide and thiazide-like diuretics are discussed as a group.

PHARMACOKINETICS

Most of the thiazide and thiazide-like diuretics are absorbed well after oral administration, except chlorothiazide (only about 10% of which is absorbed).[32] Their onset of action usually occurs within 1 to 2 hours, and their peak diuretic effect is expressed within 3 to 6 hours.[41] Most diuretics in this class are bound extensively to plasma proteins (or to red blood cell CA for chlorthalidone and metolazone[32, 42]),

undergo little, if any, biotransformation (except mefruside and metolazone[42]), and are excreted primarily by the kidneys.[32, 42, 43] Relatively high luminal fluid concentrations of these diuretics are attained, usually by a combination of glomerular filtration and active tubular secretion by the OATS in the proximal tubule (Fig. 18-7). The luminal fluid concentration of these diuretics is critical for elicitation of diuresis.[44]

The diuretics in this class differ primarily in potency and duration of action.[32, 41, 43, 45, 46] The differences in potency (which are reflected in their dosages) are determined mainly by the chemical nature of the moiety attached to the 3 position of the benzothiadiazine nucleus, which modulates the overall lipophilicity of the diuretic.[28, 30] The differences in duration of action are dictated primarily by the degree of plasma protein binding (or red blood cell binding) and their lipid/water partition coefficients.[45, 47] The latter values along with the pK_a of the drug and the pH of the luminal fluid

TABLE 18–2 Important Pharmacological Parameters of the Thiazide Diuretics

Thiazide or Hydrothiazide (Trade Name)	Partition Coefficient (Ether/H$_2$O)[47]	Plasma Protein Binding (%)[32,42]	Usual Daily Adult Oral Dosage Range (mg)		Diuretic Effect			% Parent Drug Excreted in Urine[32,42]
			Optimal Diuresis[32]	Hypertension[46]	Onset (hours)[41]	Peak (hours)[41]	Duration (hours)[41,43,45]	
Chlorothiazide, USP (Diuril)	0.08	88–96	500–2000	125–500	2	4	6–12	92
Benzthiazide, USP (Exna, Hydrex)			50–200	12.5–50	2	4–6	12–18	
Hydrochlorothiazide, USP (HydroDIURIL, Esidrix, Oretic)	0.37	64	25–100	12.5–25^a	2	4	6–12	95 (IV)
Hydroflumethiazide, USP (Diucardin, Saluron)		95	25–200	12.5–50	1–2	3–4	18–24	65 (oral) 85 (IV)
Trichlormethiazide, USP (Metahydrin, Naqua)	1.53		1–4	1–4	2	6	up to 24	62–70
Bendroflumethiazide, USP (Naturetin)		93	2.5–15	2.5–5	1–2	4	6–12	
Methyclothiazide, USP (Aquatensen, Enduron)			2.5–10	2.5–5	2	6	>24	
Polythiazide, USP (Renese)		83.5	1–4	1–4	2	6	24–48	25 (oral) 83 (IV)
Cyclothiazide, USP (Anhydron)			1–2	1–2	2–4	7–12	18–24	

^{a} Data are from Oates, J. A., and Brown, N. J.: Antihypertensive agents and the drug therapy of hypertension. In Hardman, J. G., and Limbird, L. E. (eds.). Goodman & Gilman's The Pharmacological Basis of Therapeutics, 10th ed. New York, McGraw-Hill, 2001, p. 873.

determine the extent to which each member of the class undergoes reabsorption in the distal convoluted tubule by nonionic back diffusion. Many of the diuretics in this class have long half-lives, in part because they undergo significant nonionic back diffusion. Pertinent pharmacological data on the thiazide and thiazide-like diuretics are presented in Tables 18-2 and 18-3, respectively.

SITE AND MECHANISM OF ACTION

The site of action of the thiazide and thiazide-like diuretics differs slightly from one species to another. In humans, however, it appears safe to conclude that all of these diuretics block the reabsorption of Na$^+$ (and, thereby, the reabsorption of Cl$^-$) in the distal convoluted tubules by inhibiting the luminal membrane–bound Na$^+$/Cl$^-$ cotransport system[6, 44, 48, 49] (Fig. 18-5). Thus, all diuretics in this class are responsible for the urinary loss of about 5 to 8% of the filtered load of Na$^+$. Although they differ in their potencies (i.e., the amount of drug needed to produce a given diuretic response), they are equally efficacious (i.e., they can all exert a similar maximal diuretic response).[28, 30, 50]

As a result of their action at site 3, the thiazide and thiazide-like diuretics secondarily alter the renal excretion rate of important ions other than Na$^+$ and Cl$^-$. Inhibition of Na$^+$

and Cl$^-$ reabsorption at site 3 ultimately results in the delivery of more of the filtered load of Na$^+$ to site 4. As a result, there is enhanced exchange of luminal fluid Na$^+$ for principal cell K$^+$, which results in an increase in the urinary excretion of K$^+$. Most of the thiazide and thiazide-like diuretics possess residual CA-inhibitory activity that can be associated with a slight increase in the renal excretion rate of HCO$_3^-$. Unlike the "pure" CA inhibitors, the thiazide and thiazide-like diuretics usually do not evoke development of resistance due to drug-induced derangements in acid–base balance. Hence, diuretics in this class may be referred to as *natriuretic, chloruretic, saluretic, kaliuretic,* and extremely weak *bicarbonaturetic agents*. Importantly, short-term therapy with a thiazide or thiazide-like diuretic results in little or no change in Ca^{2+} excretion; however, long-term therapy with these agents may lead to reduced Ca^{2+} excretion.[36]

ADVERSE EFFECTS

Four of the adverse effects associated with the thiazide and thiazide-like diuretics are highly predictable because of their chemical makeup or their site of action along the nephron.

1. All of these diuretics possess a sulfamoyl moiety, which has been associated with hypersensitivity reactions such as urticaria,

TABLE 18–3   Important Pharmacological Parameters of the Thiazide-Like Diuretics

Thiazide-Like Diuretic (Trade Name)	Partition Coefficient (Octanol/ H₂O PO₄ Buffer)[30]	Plasma Protein Binding (%)[42]	Usual Daily Adult Oral Dosage Range (mg)		Diuretic Effect			% Parent Drug Excreted in Urine[42]
			Optimal Diuresis[32]	Hypertension[46]	Onset (hours)[41]	Peak (hours)[41]	Duration (hours)[32,41,43,45]	
Mefruside (Baycaron)								0.3–1.1
Xipamide (Aquaphor, Diurexan)		99						
Clopamide (Aquex, Brinaldix)	6.8	46						27
Indapamide (Lozol)	31.7	71–79	2.5–5	1.25–5			24–36	5–7
Quinethazone, USP (Hydromox)			50–200	25–100	2	6	18–24	
Metolazone (Diulo, Zaroxolyn, Mykrox)		50–70 (RBC)	2.5–20	1.25–5^a	1–2	2	12–24	80–95
Clorexolone (Nefrolan)								
Chlorthalidone, USP (Hygroton, Thalitone)	5.0	94–99 (RBC)	25–200	12.5–50	2	2	48–72	44 (oral) 65 (IV)

^{a}Mykrox dose is 0.5–1 mg.

drug fever, blood dyscrasias, and interstitial nephritis. Persons who are hypersensitive to one of the agents in this class will probably be hypersensitive to all of them. Cross-hypersensitivity also may occur between the thiazide and thiazide-like diuretics, CA inhibitors, and the sulfamoyl-containing loop diuretics such as furosemide and bumetanide.

2. Hypokalemia is a product of the diuretic-induced increase in the renal excretion of K^+.

3. Initially, these diuretics produce a slight reduction in the cardiac output. Slight reductions in plasma volume and blood pressure occur with continued use. These latter changes are frequently associated with increases in the proximal tubule reabsorption of water and solutes, renin release, angiotensin II formation, and aldosterone secretion. The combination of the events is frequently referred to as the *diuretic braking phenomenon*. These changes usually help mitigate the diuretic effect, but the blood pressure reduction persists.[51]

4. Occasionally, a patient may experience hypercalcemia or hyperuricemia after long-term use of a thiazide or thiazide-like diuretic. This results from diuretic-induced reduction of the patient's plasma volume and a concomitant compensatory increase in the proximal tubule reabsorption of luminal fluid and solutes. In such a situation, more Ca^{2+} and uric acid than usual will be reabsorbed proximally.[36] The seriousness of these two adverse effects depends in part on the duration and extent of the plasma volume reduction.

The precise mechanisms behind some of the adverse effects of the thiazide and thiazide-like diuretics are not well understood. These include an acute reduction in the GFR (especially after intravenous administration[32]) and hyperglycemia. It is unlikely that the reduced GFR is related to the tubuloglomerular feedback mechanism, because the major site of action of these diuretics is distal to the macula densa cells. Some investigators have suggested that the thiazide and thiazide-like diuretics act directly on the renal vascula-

ture to depress the GFR.[32, 43] Nonetheless, the acute reduction in the GFR involves all diuretics in this class, with the possible exceptions of metolazone and indapamide.[52] This is particularly important to individuals with preexisting impaired renal function who require diuretic therapy. Thiazide and thiazide-like drugs are frequently ineffective in individuals who have a GFR below 15 to 25 mL/minute. Metolazone[43, 45, 46, 53, 54] and indapamide[52] may be useful in such circumstances.

Thiazide and thiazide-like diuretics can be involved in several potentially serious drug interactions. The first of these may occur if unadjusted doses of Li^+ are administered to individuals on long-term thiazide or thiazide-like diuretic therapy. The proximal tubule handles Li^+ and Na^+ similarly. During long-term thiazide treatment, the resulting reduction in plasma volume triggers a compensatory increase in the proximal tubule reabsorption of fluid and solutes. Thus, more Li^+ is reabsorbed than would be in normovolemic individuals. The resulting elevated plasma levels of Li^+ may provoke serious Li^+ toxicity.[45] Second, concurrent administration of a thiazide or thiazide-like diuretic with large doses of Ca^{2+}-containing substances may result in hypercalcemia because of the Ca^{2+}-retaining property of these diuretics. Third, concurrent use of thiazides and thiazide-like diuretics and nonsteroidal anti-inflammatory drugs (NSAIDs), which inhibit prostaglandin synthesis, can result in the NSAIDs antagonizing the induced diuresis. In addition, NSAIDs can increase the risk of renal failure in patients whose marginal renal function is being maintained by the intrarenal release of prostaglandins. Fourth, when thiazide and thiazide-like diuretics are used along with cardiac glycosides (e.g., digoxin or digitoxin) in the treatment of congestive heart failure, serious toxicity can result if hypokalemia occurs (see discussion below).

USES

Thiazide and thiazide-like diuretics are extremely useful in the treatment of edema associated with mild-to-moderate congestive heart failure, cirrhosis of the liver, or the nephrotic syndrome. Because edema is a symptom of an underlying disease and not a disease itself, the underlying disease should be treated first if possible. If treatment of the underlying disease does not remove the edema fluid, then diuretic therapy may be indicated. Caution is always necessary when thiazide or thiazide-like diuretics are coadministered with cardiac glycosides for the treatment of edema associated with congestive heart failure. These diuretics tend to promote hypokalemia, a condition that enhances the general toxicity of the cardiac glycosides.[36, 45] Combination diuretic therapy (i.e., a thiazide or thiazide-like diuretic plus a K^+-sparing diuretic) may prevent K^+ loss under these circumstances. If combination diuretic therapy is instituted, the recipient should be advised not to take K^+ supplements, to avoid serious hyperkalemia.[32]

Thiazide and thiazide-like diuretics are also useful in the treatment of certain nonedematous disorders. These include hypertension, diabetes insipidus (either the nephrogenic or the neurohypophyseal form), type II renal tubular acidosis, and hypercalciuria. These diuretics are primary agents in the treatment of hypertension—either alone or in combination with other drugs, depending on the severity of the condition. Thiazides generally lower blood pressure 10 to 15 mm Hg within the first 3 to 4 days of continuous treatment.[55] After approximately a week of continuous treatment (about when there is a concomitant reduction in plasma volume), the kidneys readjust to the initial effects of the diuretic, and the diuretic effect wanes while the blood pressure reduction is maintained.[51] This readjustment occurs provided Na^+ intake is not increased.

Some individuals with hypercalciuria (an elevated urinary concentration of calcium) are prone to the formation of Ca^{2+}-containing stones within the urinary tract. Because long-term use of thiazide and thiazide-like diuretics decreases the urinary excretion rate of Ca^{2+}, they may help prevent Ca^{2+}-containing stone formation.[36, 56]

SITE 2 DIURETICS: HIGH-CEILING OR LOOP DIURETICS

The diuretics in this class have extremely diverse chemical structures.[57] Although brief mention is made of the organomercurial diuretics, primary attention is focused on the agents with clinical utility: for example, furosemide (a 5-sulfamoyl-2-aminobenzoic acid or anthranilic acid derivative), bumetanide (a 5-sulfamoyl-3-aminobenzoic acid or metanilic acid derivative), torsemide (a 4-amino-3-pyridinesulfonylurea), and ethacrynic acid (a phenoxyacetic acid derivative).

Organomercurials

The organomercurials were the mainstay of diuretic therapy from 1920 to the early 1950s.[28] They elicit diuresis by inhibiting Na^+ reabsorption at site 2,[58] and they blunt the subsequent exchange of Na^+ for K^+ at site 4.[59] Thus, they are natriuretic and chloruretic and minimally kaliuretic. Although these properties are true attributes for any class of diuretics, the organomercurials have a number of serious limitations. First, when given orally they cannot be relied on to elicit diuresis because of poor and erratic absorption. Second, after parenteral administration there is a 1- to 2-hour lag in the onset of diuresis.[60] Third, their ability to trigger a diuretic response depends on the acid–base status of the individual (i.e., they are ineffective when the urine is alkaline).[61, 62] Fourth, they are cardiotoxic and nephrotoxic. The organomercurials became obsolete with the introduction of the thiazides and thiazide-like diuretics, furosemide, bumetanide, and ethacrynic acid. All of the latter agents are orally effective, equally effective in both acidotic and alkalotic conditions, capable of inducing relatively rapid diuresis when given parenterally, and relatively nontoxic.

5-Sulfamoyl-2-aminobenzoic Acid and 5-Sulfamoyl-3-aminobenzoic Acid Derivatives

Bumetanide, USP. The structure of bumetanide, 3-(butylamino)-4-phenoxy-5-sulfamoylbenzoic acid (Bumex), is shown in Figure 18-11.

Furosemide, USP. The structure of furosemide, 4-chloro-*N*-furfuryl-5-sulfamoylanthranilic acid (Lasix), is shown in Figure 18-11.

STRUCTURE–ACTIVITY RELATIONSHIPS

The development of the loop diuretics is an outgrowth of the research involving the thiazide and thiazide-like diuretics.[30] There are important structural requirements that are common to the 5-sulfamoyl-2-aminobenzoic acid derivatives and the 5-sulfamoyl-3-aminobenzoic acid derivatives (Fig. 18-11). First, the substituent at the 1 position must be acidic. The carboxyl group provides optimal diuretic activity, but other groups, such as a tetrazole, may impart respectable diuretic activity. Second, a sulfamoyl group in the 5 position is a prerequisite for optimal high-ceiling diuretic activity. Third, the "activating" group (-X) in the 4 position can be Cl^- or CF_3^-, as was the case with the thiazides and thiazide-like diuretics, or better yet, a phenoxy, alkoxy, anilino, benzyl, or benzoyl group. Interestingly, substitution of one of the latter five functional groups for the Cl^- or CF_3^- group in the thiazides or thiazide-like diuretics decreases their diuretic activity.

These two series of 5-sulfamoylbenzoic acids differ greatly in the nature of the functional groups that can be substituted into the 2 and 3 positions with retention of maximal diuretic activity (Fig. 18-11). The substituents that can be tolerated on the 2-amino group of the 5-sulfamoyl-2-aminobenzoic acids are extremely limited, and no acceptable deviations are allowed on the few moieties. For example, only the furfuryl, benzyl, and thienylmethyl (in decreasing order) moieties yield derivatives with maximal diuretic activity. The substituents allowable on the 3-amino group of the 5-sulfamoyl-3-aminobenzoic acids can vary widely, however, without jeopardizing optimal diuretic activity. High-ceiling diuretics that have emerged from the 5-sulfamoyl-2-aminobenzoic acid series include furosemide and azosemide, those from the 5-sulfamoyl-3-aminobenzoic acid series include bumetanide and piretanide. Only furosemide

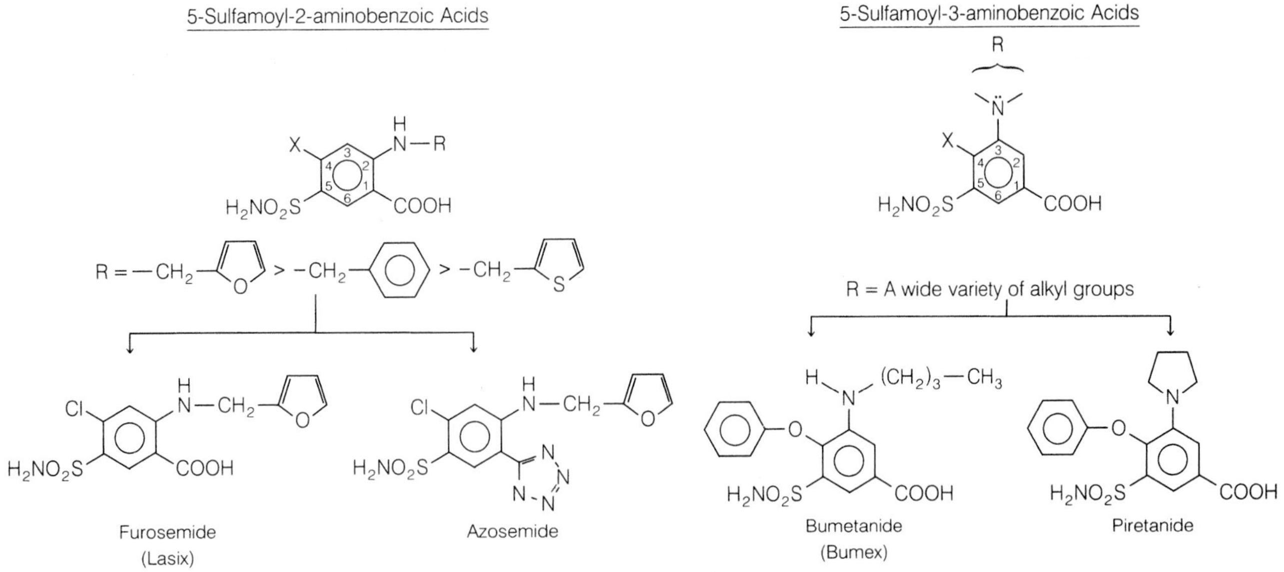

Figure 18–11 ■ Results from structure–activity relationship studies that led to the development of furosemide and bumetanide.

and bumetanide are commercially available in the United States.

PHARMACOKINETICS

Furosemide and bumetanide differ pharmacologically primarily in their potencies and bioavailabilities. Bumetanide is more potent than furosemide; it produces an equieffective diuresis in about 1/40th the dose.[63, 64] The bioavailability of furosemide when administered orally is about 60 to 69% in normal subjects but only 43 to 46% in individuals with end-stage renal disease.[45] The bioavailability of bumetanide in normal individuals is 80 to 90%.[63]

After parenteral administration, both furosemide and bumetanide have an extremely rapid onset of action (3 to 5 minutes). Duration of action following parenteral therapy is 2 hours for furosemide and 3.5 to 4 hours for bumetanide. Both diuretics have an onset of action of approximately 30 to 60 minutes after oral therapy, but furosemide has a slightly longer duration of action than bumetanide (6 to 8 hours versus 4 to 6 hours).[41] Once these agents reach the bloodstream, they are extensively bound to plasma proteins (93 to 95%).[63] This degree of plasma protein binding severely limits the amount of each drug that can be removed from the plasma by glomerular filtration, but it does not prevent either drug from attaining high renal luminal fluid concentrations by active tubular secretion. Both diuretics are weak organic acids and are secreted avidly into the luminal fluid of the proximal tubule (Fig. 18-7).[20, 65] This is important for two reasons. First, it is responsible for the relatively rapid renal excretion (hence, the short duration of action) of both diuretics; and second, it provides for the delivery of substantial amounts of each diuretic to their luminal site of action.

The factors discussed above that determine the luminal concentration of diuretics are critical when these agents are used in individuals with uremia. Uremic individuals frequently have a low GFR and high circulating levels of endogenous weak organic acids, both of which lower the luminal fluid concentrations of the loop diuretics. The endogenous weak organic acids compete with the weakly acidic diuretics for active tubular secretion into proximal tubule luminal fluid. Often, the effects of the endogenous weak acids can be overridden by increasing the dose of these diuretics. Caution must be exercised, however, because an increased incidence of adverse effects is likely to accompany higher doses.

A small percentage of furosemide is converted to the corresponding glucuronide, and 88% of the administered drug is excreted by the kidneys. Bumetanide undergoes more extensive biotransformation in the human, and 81% of it is excreted in the urine (45% as unchanged drug).[41]

SITE AND MECHANISM OF ACTION

The events that contribute to the tremendous efficacy of furosemide and bumetanide are multifaceted. *First,* these diuretics inhibit the $1Na^+/1K^+/2Cl^-$ cotransport system located on the luminal membrane of cells of the thick ascending limb of Henle's loop[21, 57] (Fig. 18-4). Importantly, the carboxylate moieties of furosemide and bumetanide are thought to compete with Cl^- for the Cl^--binding site on the $1Na^+/1K^+/2Cl^-$ cotransport system. Because site 2 is such a high-capacity site for Na^+ reabsorption, up to 30% of the filtered load of Na^+ that is normally reabsorbed in this nephron segment may be excreted in the urine. In addition, reabsorption of this 30% of the filtered load of Na^+ (and Cl^-) is required to maintain the hypertonicity of the medullary interstitium.[12] The hypertonic medullary interstitium allows us to produce concentrated urine by drawing water out of the descending limb of Henle's loop by osmosis and out of the collecting duct by osmosis when ADH is present. Thus, when these diuretics inhibit the reabsorption of up to 30% of the filtered load of Na^+ at site 2, within minutes they also destroy the hypertonicity of the medullary interstitium.[6] The net result is that when Na^+ and Cl^- are not reabsorbed at site 2, water is no longer removed by osmosis from the luminal fluid in the descending limb of Henle's loop or from the collecting tubule. Large amounts of water, Na^+, and Cl^- are excreted. *Second,* high concentrations of furosemide and bumetanide are attained in proximal luminal fluid by way of the OATS and delivered to the $1Na^+/1K^+/2Cl^-$ cotransport system at site 2. *Third,* although these diuretics increase the flow rate of luminal fluid past the macula densa cells, the expected reduction in GFR (which normally would mitigate the diuresis) does not occur. This is because these efficacious diuretics inhibit the $1Na^+/1K^+/2Cl^-$ cotransport system in the luminal membrane of the macula densa cells and so decrease the uptake of these solutes, which in turn inhibits the tubuloglomerular feedback mechanism from decreasing the GFR.[66] *Fourth,* these diuretics also transiently increase total renal blood flow by enhancing the intrarenal release of vasodilatory prostaglandins. *Fifth,* they induce a redistribution of intrarenal blood flow that is thought to participate in a positive way toward the magnitude of the diuresis.[57]

All diuretics that act at site 2 are equally efficacious and far more efficacious than diuretics that act at sites 1, 3, or 4. As mentioned above, because of their site of action and efficacy, these agents are commonly referred to as *loop* and *high-ceiling diuretics.*[57]

High-ceiling diuretics secondarily enhance the urinary loss of K^+ and H^+. First, by inhibiting the $1Na^+/1K^+/2Cl^-$ cotransport complex at site 2, they prevent the generation of a lumen-positive transepithelial voltage and, therefore, the paracellular reabsorption of K^+ and other cations. Second, inhibition of Na^+ reabsorption at site 2 ultimately delivers more of the filtered load of Na^+, at a faster rate, to site 4. This leads to an enhanced exchange of the Na^+ in the luminal fluid for the K^+ in the principal cells and the H^+ in the intercalated cells (Fig. 18-6).

When the loop diuretics are used in "submaximal" doses for the treatment of hypertension, they are intended to create a diuresis similar in magnitude to that produced by the thiazide and thiazide-like diuretics. Under these circumstances, loop diuretics usually are associated with a lower frequency of hypokalemia than the thiazide and thiazide-like diuretics because their duration of action is shorter, and the kidneys have more time to readjust.[30, 67] When the loop diuretics are used to treat acute edema, however, higher dosages are frequently used, and the Na^+ and K^+ losses exceed those accompanying thiazide therapy.[30]

When the loop diuretics inhibit the $1Na^+/1K^+/2Cl^-$ cotransport system in the luminal membrane of thick ascending limb cells, they in turn decrease the lumen-positive transepithelial voltage that promotes the paracellular movement of luminal fluid cations such as Ca^{2+} into the interstitium (Fig. 18-4). Hence, loop diuretics may induce the renal excretion of up to 20 to 30% of the filtered load of Ca^{2+}, provided the plasma volume is not allowed to decrease.[10] If plasma volume decreases as a result of the diuresis, there is an accompanying compensatory increase in the proximal tubule reabsorption of fluid and solutes. About 60% of the filtered load of Ca^{2+} is reabsorbed in the proximal tubule during normovolemia, and the percentage of proximally reabsorbed Ca^{2+} will increase in a state of plasma volume reduction. Therefore, during diuretic-induced hypovolemia, less Ca^{2+} is delivered to the thick ascending limb for the loop diuretics to inhibit, which will blunt the loop diuretic's calciuretic effect.

ADVERSE EFFECTS

Four highly predictable adverse effects are associated with furosemide and bumetanide:

1. Hypokalemic alkalosis results from the enhanced exchange of luminal fluid Na^+ for intracellular K^+ or H^+ ions at site 4. Caution should be exercised when concurrent therapy with loop diuretics and cardiac glycosides is instituted because hypokalemia intensifies the toxicity of the cardiac glycosides.[41]
2. In the short term, fluid and electrolyte losses may not be accompanied by changes in the GFR because of the effect of these agents on the tubuloglomerular feedback mechanism. The long-term use of these diuretics, however, may reduce plasma volume. If this condition is allowed to persist, the above-mentioned compensatory changes take place, one of which is a reduction in GFR.
3. Because diuretic-induced plasma volume reduction leads to increased reabsorption of solutes normally handled by the proximal tubule (e.g., uric acid), some borderline hyperuricemic individuals may develop symptoms of gout on long-term loop diuretic therapy. For similar reasons, concurrent administration of loop diuretics and unadjusted doses of Li^+ may lead to severe Li^+ toxicity.[41]
4. Furosemide and bumetanide are similar to the CA inhibitors, thiazides, and thiazide-like diuretics in possessing a sulfamoyl moiety. This functional group has been associated with hypersensitivity reactions such as urticaria, drug fever, blood dyscrasias, and interstitial nephritis.

Several unforeseen adverse effects are associated with the loop diuretics. For example, they are unique among diuretics in producing ototoxicity. Usually, hearing loss is temporary, but it may be permanent. Ototoxicity may be associated directly with rising plasma concentrations of the loop diuretics. Accordingly, individuals with impaired renal function appear to be at increased risk because they have a reduced ability to excrete these efficacious diuretics.[45] Although the milligram dose of bumetanide is 1/40th that of furosemide, these agents appear to be quite similar in their ototoxic potential. Caution is needed if loop diuretics are administered to patients who are receiving any of the available aminoglycoside antibiotics. The ototoxicity of these two classes of drugs may be additive.[41] Other adverse effects of furosemide and bumetanide include hyperglycemia, nausea, vomiting, and myalgia.

NSAIDs, which inhibit prostaglandin synthesis, may blunt the natriuresis produced by loop diuretics. In patients with preexisting impaired renal function who are on diuretic therapy, NSAIDs may increase the risk of renal failure by blocking the intrarenal synthesis of vasodilatory prostaglandins, the one thing that may be sustaining renal blood flow in these patients.[41]

USES

High-ceiling diuretics are effective for the treatment of edema that may accompany congestive heart failure, cirrhosis of the liver, and the nephrotic syndrome. A most important use of furosemide or bumetanide is in the treatment of pulmonary edema associated with congestive heart failure. No group of diuretics is more effective than the loop diuretics in this situation, but they must be used with extreme caution. Overzealous use may reduce plasma volume so severely that the resulting decreased venous return and cardiac output exacerbate the heart failure.[68]

Loop diuretics may be used for the treatment of certain nonedematous disorders. Symptomatic hypercalcemia may be treated with a loop diuretic, provided no reduction in plasma volume occurs and the fluid used for replacement of the urinary losses is calcium free.[69] In addition, furosemide has been used for the treatment of hypertension. Some investigators believe, however, that because of its relatively short duration of action, it may be less effective than the thiazide or thiazide-like diuretics. It has been suggested that furosemide be reserved for hypertensive patients with fluid retention refractory to thiazides or patients with impaired renal function.[46]

In general, furosemide or bumetanide is preferred over ethacrynic acid (another site 2 diuretic) because they have a broader dose–response curve, less ototoxicity, and less gastrointestinal toxicity.[45]

4-Amino-3-Pyridinesulfonylureas

Torsemide. The structure of torsemide, 1-isopropyl-3-{[4-(3-methylphenylamino)pyridine]-3-sulfonyl}urea (Demadex), is shown below.

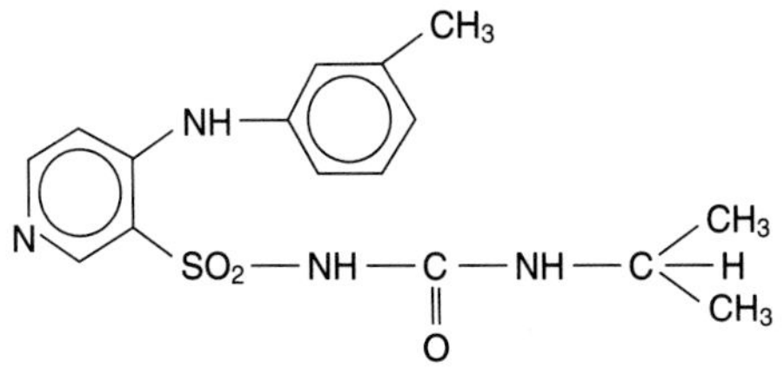

Torsemide

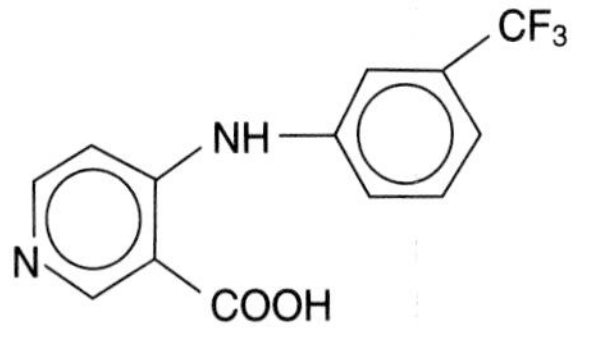

Triflocin

STRUCTURE–ACTIVITY RELATIONSHIPS

Initial screening of many 4-amino-3-pyridinesulfonylureas revealed that maximum diuretic activity was attained with torsemide.[70] Torsemide is closely related structurally to triflocin, a loop diuretic that was studied extensively in the late 1960s and early 1970s but abandoned because it produced transitional cell carcinoma in the urinary bladders of over 50% of the rats that had received high doses over an 18- to 22-month period.

PHARMACOKINETICS

Torsemide is approximately 80% bioavailable after oral administration. Its extensive plasma protein binding (98 to 99%) is similar to that of other loop diuretics. Peak serum concentrations are generally attained within 1 hour, and the half-life is 3 to 4 hours, somewhat longer than that of furosemide (2 hours) and bumetanide (1 to 1.5 hours). Torsemide is metabolized by the hepatic cytochrome P-450 system. The primary products result from the oxidation of the aromatic methyl group to hydroxy and carboxyl derivatives and *para* hydroxylation of the methylphenylamino moiety.

Approximately 20% of the dose is excreted unchanged in the urine.[71, 72]

SITE AND MECHANISM OF ACTION

Like furosemide and bumetanide, torsemide induces diuresis by inhibition of the $1Na^+/1K^+/2Cl^-$ cotransport system on the luminal membrane of thick ascending limb cells (Fig. 18-4). Thus, torsemide must reach adequate levels in the luminal fluid. Higher doses, which have been studied in isolated nephron segments, also inhibit the efflux of Cl^- from the thick ascending limb cells by the Cl^- channels on the basolateral membrane.[73] Whether this second site of action is clinically relevant remains to be determined.

ADVERSE EFFECTS

Torsemide may produce fatigue, dizziness, muscle cramps, nausea, and orthostatic hypotension. At this early date, no evidence of ototoxicity has appeared in humans, but studies in cats have shown torsemide to be similar to furosemide in ototoxic potential.[74]

USES

Torsemide is useful in the treatment of mild-to-moderate hypertension in doses of 2.5 to 5 mg given once daily. These doses lower blood pressure as effectively as 25 mg of hydrochlorothiazide but without producing diuresis. Higher doses of torsemide (10 to 20 mg) are associated with significant diuresis and are effective in treating edema associated with congestive heart failure and cirrhosis of the liver.[71, 75]

Phenoxyacetic Acids

The phenoxyacetic acid group of high-ceiling diuretics was developed and introduced into clinical use about the same time as furosemide.

Ethacrynic Acid, USP. The structure of ethacrynic acid, [2,3-dichloro-4-(2-methylene-1-oxobutyl)phenoxy]acetic acid (Edecrin), is shown in Figure 18-12.

STRUCTURE–ACTIVITY RELATIONSHIPS

As mentioned above, certain organomercurials can elicit a diuretic response, but because of their heavy metal content, they are too toxic for widespread use. Consequently, a search was undertaken for a non–mercury-containing compound that like the organomercurials would react with sulfhydryl-containing receptors in renal tissue but be devoid of heavy metal-type toxicity. Because one of the commercially available organomercurials (mersalyl, Salyrgan) possessed a phenoxyacetic acid moiety, the phenoxyacetic acids served as the chemical root for development of new non–mercury-containing diuretics. Hundreds of phenoxyacetic acids were examined.[76, 77]

Within the phenoxyacetic acid series (Fig. 18-12), optimal diuretic activity is achieved when *(a)* an oxyacetic acid moiety is placed in the 1 position on the benzene ring, *(b)* a sulfhydryl-reactive acryloyl moiety is located *para* to the oxyacetic acid group, *(c)* activating groups (i.e., Cl- or CH_3-) occupy either the 3 position or the 2 and 3 positions,

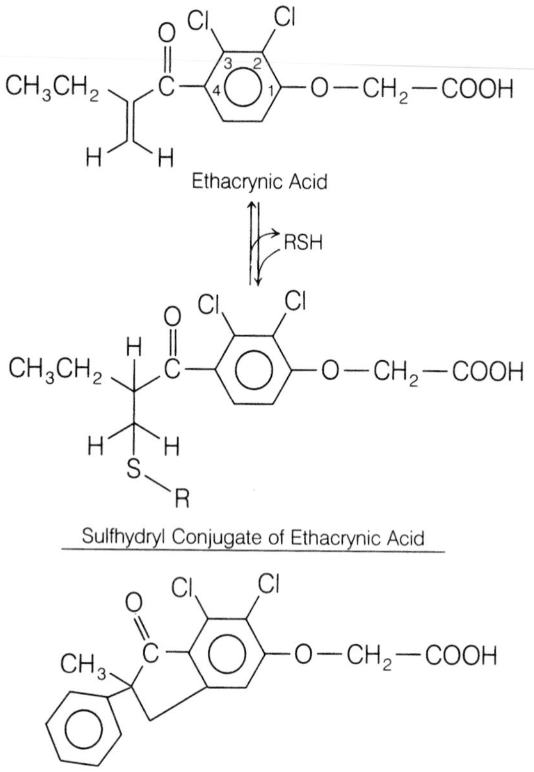

Ethacrynic Acid

RSH

Sulfhydryl Conjugate of Ethacrynic Acid

Indacrinone

Figure 18–12 ■ Ethacrynic acid is a high-ceiling diuretic that readily reacts with many sulfhydryl-containing nucleophiles *(top)*. Indacrinone, a structurally related high-ceiling diuretic, lacks sulfhydryl reactivity *(bottom)*.

(d) alkyl substituents of two to four carbon atoms in length occupy the position α to the carbonyl on the acryloyl moiety, and *(e)* hydrogen atoms occupy the terminal position of the carbon–carbon double bond of the acryloyl moiety. These structural features seemed to maximize both the diuretic activity and the in vitro rate of reaction with various sulfhydryl-containing nucleophiles. The correlation between diuretic activity and chemical reactivity within this series of diuretics was strengthened by the finding that reduction or epoxidation of the carbon–carbon double bond in the acryloyl moiety yielded compounds with little or no diuretic activity or chemical reactivity.[78, 79] The design and synthesis of ethacrynic acid appeared to be the ultimate in terms of "the rational approach to drug design." The need for designing a diuretic with high sulfhydryl reactivity was foiled, however, when indacrinone was found to be a highly efficacious diuretic, incapable of reacting with sulfhydryl-containing nucleophiles (Fig. 18-12).[80] Indacrinone was withdrawn from clinical trials because some individuals developed abnormal liver function test results.

PHARMACOKINETICS

In spite of ethacrynic acid's unique chemical structure and avid reactivity toward various nucleophiles, it has many pharmacological features in common with the sulfamoyl-containing loop diuretics. After oral administration, onset of action is about 30 minutes, and duration of action is 6 to 8 hours. After parenteral administration, onset of action and

duration of action are 3 to 5 minutes and 2 to 3 hours, respectively. Ethacrynic acid is highly bound to plasma proteins (>95%). Ethacrynic acid is handled and excreted predominately by the kidneys. Very little of the drug is removed from the plasma by glomerular filtration because of its extensive binding to unfiltrable plasma proteins such as albumin. However, the drug is secreted avidly into the luminal fluid of the proximal tubule with the assistance of the OATS (Fig. 18-7).[65, 81, 82] High luminal fluid concentrations of ethacrynic acid are essential for its diuretic action and ultimate excretion.

Ethacrynic acid is biotransformed by a pathway completely different from that of furosemide or bumetanide. Ethacrynic acid alkylates the thiol group of glutathione in vivo (Fig. 18-12; RSH = glutathione), and the resulting conjugate subsequently is converted to the ethacrynic acid–cysteine and ethacrynic acid–N-acetylcysteine (the mercapturic acid) conjugates. Ethacrynic acid–cysteine is quite unstable in vivo and in vitro; it readily releases cysteine and ethacrynic acid. Ethacrynic acid, ethacrynic acid–glutathione, and ethacrynic acid–cysteine are equiefficacious diuretics because of the aforementioned interconversions.[76] Approximately two thirds of the ethacrynic acid appears in the urine in the various forms cited; the remaining one third is found in the bile.

SITE AND MECHANISM OF ACTION

Like furosemide and bumetanide, ethacrynic acid

- Blocks reabsorption of up to 30% of the filtered load of Na^+ at site 2 by inhibiting the $1Na^+/1K^+/2Cl^-$ cotransport system located on the luminal membrane of cells in the thick ascending limb of Henle's loop and in the macula densa cells[21] (Fig. 18-4)
- Reaches high levels in luminal fluid because of its active tubular secretion by the OATS in proximal tubular cells
- Blocks the tubuloglomerular feedback mechanism that normally would result in an acute reduction of the GFR when the flow of luminal fluid is increased through the nephron segment possessing the macula densa cells[83]
- Increases total renal blood flow transiently by enhancing the intrarenal release of vasodilatory prostaglandins[84]
- Induces a transient redistribution of intrarenal blood flow, which contributes in a positive way toward the magnitude of the diuresis[85]

Because ethacrynic acid induces a short-term increase in the renal excretion rate of Na^+, Cl^-, K^+, and Ca^{2+}, it is a natriuretic, chloruretic, saluretic, kaliuretic, and calciuretic agent.

ADVERSE EFFECTS

Ethacrynic acid may produce all of the adverse effects noted with furosemide and bumetanide except those related to the presence of a sulfamoyl group. Use of ethacrynic acid has waned because it is more ototoxic than furosemide and bumetanide and it produces more serious gastrointestinal effects (i.e., gastrointestinal hemorrhage) than the sulfamoyl-containing loop diuretics. In addition, as with furosemide and bumetanide, serious drug interactions may occur when ethacrynic acid is used concurrently with Li^+, cardiac glycosides, aminoglycoside antibiotics, or NSAIDs (see discussion above of adverse effects of furosemide and bumetanide).

USES

Ethacrynic acid has the indications cited for furosemide and bumetanide. However, when a high-ceiling diuretic is indicated in the treatment of an individual who has a known hypersensitivity to sulfamoyl-containing drugs, ethacrynic acid may be an appropriate substitute.

Miscellaneous Site 2 Diuretics

Three nondiuretic agents are biotransformed to high-ceiling diuretics in vivo by sulfation of their –OH moieties (Fig. 18-13). The sulfated metabolites exert a diuresis by inhibition of the $1Na^+/1K^+/2Cl^-$ cotransport system on the luminal membrane of thick ascending limb cells (Fig. 18-4). These agents include 2-(p-fluorophenoxy), 1-(o-hydroxy-

phenyl)ethane (CRE 10904) [86]; 2-(aminomethyl)-4-(1,1-dimethylethyl)-4-iodophenol (MK-447) [87]; and 6-chloro-2,3-dihydro-1-(1-oxopropyl)-4(H)-quinolinone 4-oxime (M12285).[88]

In each case the sulfated metabolite undergoes active tubular secretion by the OATS in proximal tubular cells and, hence, attains high levels in luminal fluid. The negatively charged sulfate moiety probably binds to the Cl⁻-binding site on the luminal membrane–bound $1Na^+/1K^+/2Cl^-$ cotransport system of thick ascending limb and macula densa cells.

In addition, etozoline (only after being hydrolyzed in vivo to ozolinone, a carboxylic acid) and muzolimine possess diuretic activity by virtue of their actions on the transport processes in the cells of the thick ascending limb of Henle's loop. Ozolinone is secreted actively into proximal tubule luminal fluid by the OATS. The high concentrations of ozolinone delivered to the thick ascending limb cells of Henle's

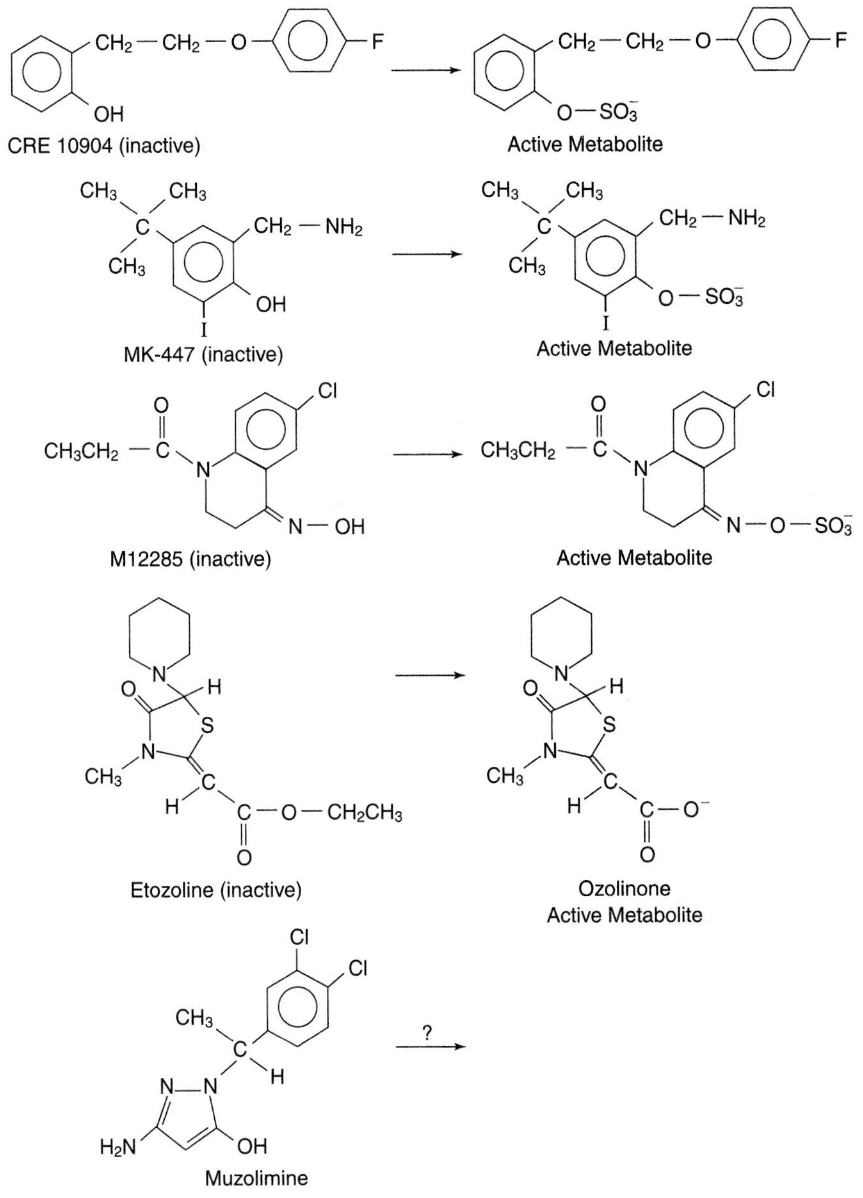

Figure 18–13 ■ Various seemingly unrelated agents that block Na⁺ reabsorption in the thick ascending limb of Henle's loop. The precise mechanism of action of muzolimine is unknown. All of the other agents are inactive as such and must be biotransformed to active metabolites before their diuretic activity can be expressed. In each case, like furosemide, bumetanide, torsemide, and ethacrynic acid, the active metabolites have an anionic moiety that may permit binding to the Cl⁻-binding site on the $1Na^+/1K^+/2Cl^-$ cotransport system in thick ascending limb cells.

loop inhibit the luminal membrane–bound $1Na^+/1K^+/2Cl^-$ cotransport system[89, 90] (Fig. 18-4). The precise mechanism(s) by which muzolimine exerts a diuresis remains to be determined.[91] It has been suggested, however, that muzolimine inhibits the K^+/Cl^- cotransport system on the basolateral membrane of the thick ascending limb cells, which in turn inhibits the $1Na^+/1K^+/2Cl^-$ cotransport system.[92] None of these miscellaneous site 2 agents has been marketed in the United States.

SITE 4 DIURETICS: POTASSIUM-SPARING DIURETICS

A negative feature of all of the above-discussed classes of diuretics in current use is that they increase the renal excretion rate of K^+ and thus can induce hypokalemia. Over the years, three chemically distinct diuretics have emerged that increase Na^+ and Cl^- excretion without a concomitant increase in the urinary excretion rate of K^+. These agents are known as *potassium-sparing diuretics* or *antikaliuretic agents*. Although the K^+-sparing diuretics are derived from completely different chemical roots, they act at site 4 (though not all by the same mechanism), have similar efficacies and electrolyte excretion patterns, and share certain adverse effects. The K^+-sparing diuretics include spironolactone (a spirolactone), triamterene (a 2,4,7-triamino-6-arylpteridine), and amiloride (a pyrazinoylguanidine). A recently approved spirolactone, eplerenone, is discussed later in this chapter.

Spirolactones, Aldosterone Antagonists

Spironolactone, USP. The structure of spironolactone, 7α-(acetylthio)-17β-hydroxy-3-oxopregn-4-ene-21-carboxylic acid γ-lactone (Aldactone), is shown in Figure 18-14.

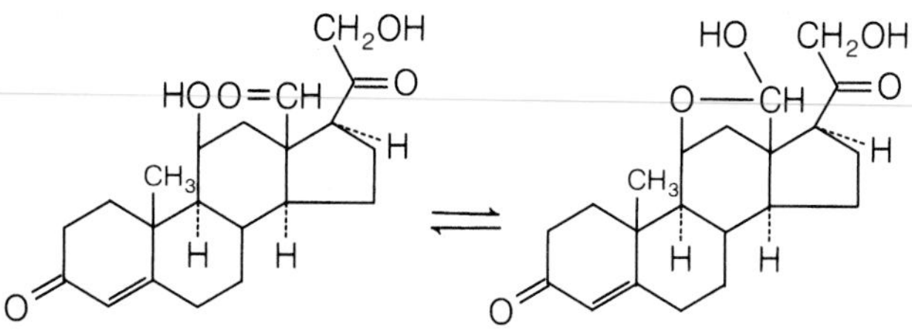

(Aldehyde Form) Aldosterone (Hemiacetal Form)

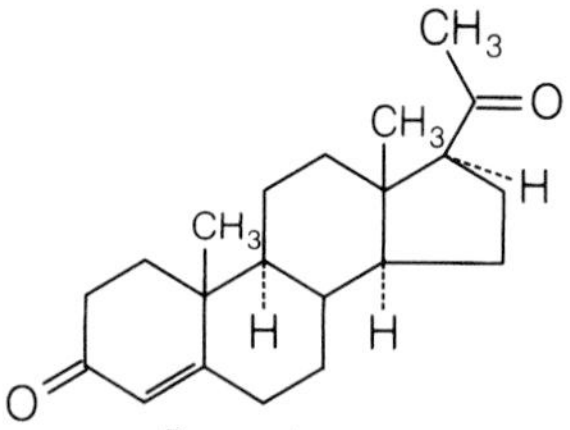

Progesterone

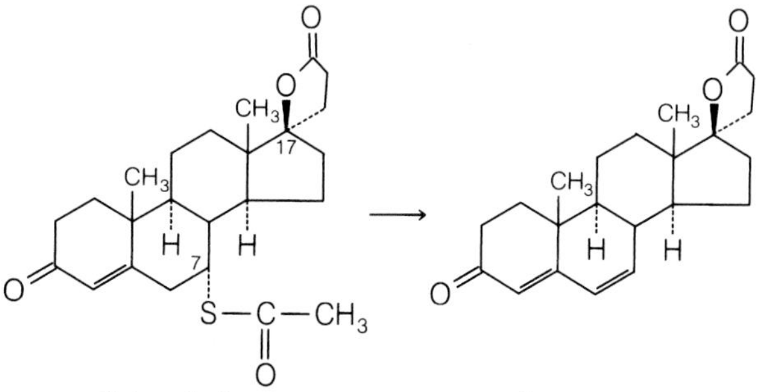

Spironolactone (Aldactone)

Canrenone (a major metabolite) (an active aldosterone antagonist)

Figure 18–14 ■ Aldosterone enhances the passage of Na^+ from the luminal fluid into tubular cells and the passage of intracellular K^+ into the luminal fluid at site 4. Progesterone inhibits these actions of aldosterone but has undesirable hormonal side effects. Spironolactone and canrenone also competitively inhibit the actions of aldosterone at site 4 and are associated with a lower frequency of hormonal side effects.

STRUCTURE–ACTIVITY RELATIONSHIPS

In the mid-1950s, it was observed that progesterone inhibited the antinatriuretic and kaliuretic effects of aldosterone, the primary mineralocorticoid in humans.[93, 94] An intensive effort was launched to develop steroidal derivatives that possessed only the antimineralocorticoid activity of progesterone.[95–98] Spironolactone was selected from a host of derivatives for further examination.[97]

PHARMACOKINETICS

Spironolactone is absorbed well after oral administration (bioavailability, >90%), biotransformed rapidly and extensively by the liver (~80%) to canrenone, an active metabolite (Fig. 18-14), bound extensively to plasma proteins (most likely as canrenone), and excreted primarily as metabolites in the urine. Some biliary excretion of metabolites also occurs. Its onset of action is slow (12 to 72 hours),[99] and its duration of action is quite long (2 to 3 days).[41]

SITE AND MECHANISM OF ACTION

Spironolactone inhibits the reabsorption of 2 to 3% of the filtered load of Na^+ at site 4 by competitively inhibiting the actions of aldosterone[6, 36] (Fig. 18-6). Under normal circumstances, aldosterone enters the principal cells of the connecting tubule (i.e., the late distal tubule) and the cortical collecting tubule, where it combines with a cytosolic receptor. The complex moves into the nucleus, where it turns on the synthesis of additional quantities of the Na^+/K^+-ATPase,[100–101] and luminal membrane channels that are involved in the exchange of Na^+ for K^+. Intercalated cell H^+-ATPase that actively pumps H^+ into the luminal fluid at site 4 is also affected. Thus, passage of luminal fluid Na^+ into, and K^+ and H^+ out of, the connecting tubule cells and the cortical collecting tubule cells is enhanced. Increased intracellular levels of Na^+ elicited by the actions of aldosterone stimulate the basolateral membrane–bound Na^+/K^+-ATPase.[11] Because spironolactone competitively inhibits these actions of aldosterone,[101] it enhances water, Na^+, and Cl^- excretion. Therefore, spironolactone is a natriuretic, chloruretic, saluretic, and antikaliuretic agent. *Unlike the other K^+-sparing diuretics, spironolactone requires the presence of endogenous aldosterone to exert its diuretic action.* Because it inhibits the reabsorption of only 2 to 3% of the filtered load of Na^+, it (and the site 4 K^+-sparing diuretics) has relatively low efficacy.

ADVERSE EFFECTS

One might anticipate that inhibition of the exchange of luminal fluid Na^+ for intracellular K^+ and H^+ would lead to retention of the latter two ions in certain individuals. Important adverse effects of spironolactone include hyperkalemia and mild metabolic acidosis, especially in individuals with poor renal function.[6, 36] Therefore, patients taking spironolactone should be warned not to take K^+ supplements. Caution must also be exercised when administering spironolactone with other drugs, such as angiotensin-converting enzyme (ACE) inhibitors, angiotensin II receptor antagonists, and β-adrenergic blockers, that may also evoke increases in $[K^+]_{plasma}$. In addition, spironolactone may produce gynecomastia in men and breast tenderness and menstrual disturbances in women because of its residual hormonal activity.[102] Gynecomastia occurs in approximately 6 to 10% of males given 50 mg/day or less and in up to 52% in doses above 150 mg/day. Other adverse effects include minor gastrointestinal symptoms and rashes.[32, 45]

USES

Spironolactone may be used alone as an extremely mild diuretic to remove edema fluid in individuals with congestive heart failure, cirrhosis of the liver with ascites, or the nephrotic syndrome or as an antihypertensive agent. Its primary use, however, has been in combination with diuretics that act at site 2 or 3 in an attempt to reduce the urinary K^+ loss associated with these latter groups of diuretics.

2,4,7-Triamino-6-arylpteridines

Triamterene, USP. The structure of triamterene, 2,4,7-triamino-6-phenylpteridine (Dyrenium), is shown below.

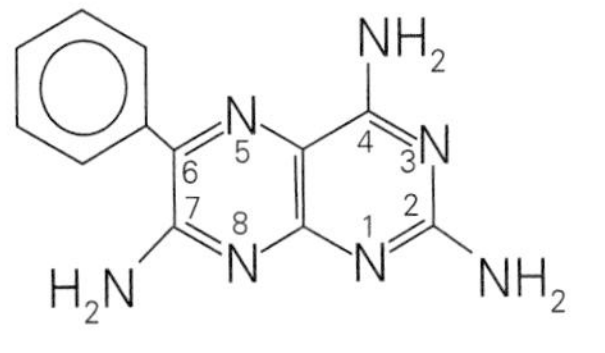

Triamterene

STRUCTURE–ACTIVITY RELATIONSHIPS

Triamterene is the primary compound selected from a host of synthetic pteridine analogues.[103] Although it bears a structural resemblance to folic acid and certain dihydrofolate reductase inhibitors, it has little, if any, of their activities.[32]

PHARMACOKINETICS

Triamterene is absorbed rapidly but incompletely (30 to 70%) from the gastrointestinal tract,[41] bound to plasma proteins to the extent of about 60%, biotransformed extensively in the liver, and excreted primarily by the biliary route and secondarily via the renal route as unchanged drug (20%) and metabolites (80%). It enters the luminal fluid of the nephrons by glomerular filtration and active tubular secretion in the proximal tubule. Because it is a weak organic base, it is assumed to be handled by the proximal tubule OCTS[32] (Fig. 18-7). Its onset of action following a single oral dose is 2 to 4 hours, and its duration of action is 7 to 9 hours.[41]

SITE AND MECHANISM OF ACTION

Triamterene "plugs" the Na^+ channels in the luminal membrane of the principal cells at site 4 and thereby inhibits the electrogenic entry of 2 to 3% of the filtered load of Na^+ into these cells[6, 11] (Fig. 18-6). As triamterene's action decreases the principal cell concentration of Na^+, the antiluminal membrane–bound Na^+/K^+-ATPase activity also decreases. This leads to decreases in the cellular extrusion of Na^+ and the cellular uptake of K^+. Because the secretion of K^+ and H^+ at site 4 is linked to Na^+ reabsorption, a concomitant reduction in the excretion rate of K^+ and H^+ occurs. *Unlike spironolactone, triamterene's diuretic action does not depend on the presence of aldosterone.* Triamterene, like the other K^+-sparing diuretics, has a low efficacy and is a mild natriuretic, chloruretic, saluretic, and antikaliuretic agent.

ADVERSE EFFECTS

Like the other K^+-sparing diuretics whose primary actions are elicited at site 4, triamterene's major adverse effect is hyperkalemia.[36] Therefore, patients taking triamterene should be warned not to take K^+ supplements. Caution is also needed when administering triamterene along with other drugs, such as ACE inhibitors, angiotensin II receptor antagonists, and β-adrenergic blockers, that may also give rise to increases in $[K^+]_{plasma}$. In addition, it appears to be unique among the K^+-sparing diuretics in being associated with the formation of renal stones. Approximately 1 of 1,500 individuals taking a triamterene-containing diuretic experiences nephrolithiasis.[104, 105] The stones consist of triamterene (with or without its metabolite) or triamterene along with calcium oxalate or uric acid. It also may produce nausea, vomiting, leg cramps, and dizziness.[32]

USES

Triamterene may be used alone in the treatment of mild edema associated with congestive heart failure or cirrhosis of the liver with ascites, but it should not be given to patients with impaired renal function.[106] It is not to be used alone in the treatment of hypertension.[46, 106] Its primary use is in combination with hydrochlorothiazide (or other diuretics that act at site 2 or 3) to prevent the hypokalemia associated with the latter diuretics.

Pyrazinoylguanidines

Amiloride Hydrochloride, USP. The structure of amiloride hydrochloride, 3,5-diamino-N-(aminoiminomethyl)-6-chloropyrazinecarboxamide monohydrochloride dihydrate (Midamor), is shown below.

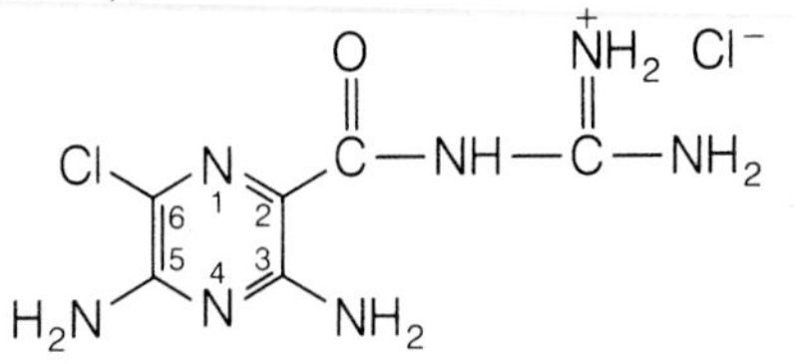

Amiloride Hydrochloride

STRUCTURE–ACTIVITY RELATIONSHIPS

An extensive screening procedure that examined over 25,000 agents was undertaken in an attempt to discover an antikaliuretic agent that did not have overlapping hormonal activity like that of spironolactone.[107] Promising activity was noted with appropriately substituted pyrazinoylguanidines. Optimal diuretic activity in this series is observed when the 6 position is substituted with chlorine, the amino groups in the 3 and 5 positions are unsubstituted, and the guanidino nitrogens are not multiply substituted with alkyl groups. Amiloride emerged as the most active compound in the series.

PHARMACOKINETICS

Amiloride contains the strongly basic guanidine moiety and possesses a pK_a of 8.7. Thus, it exists predominantly as the charged guanidinium ion in the pH range of most body tissues and fluids. It is not surprising that amiloride is absorbed incompletely and erratically (15 to 20%) from the gastrointestinal tract, an event that occurs by passive diffusion of the uncharged form of most drugs. Amiloride is bound to plasma proteins to a moderate degree, is not biotransformed, and is excreted in the urine (20 to 50%) and in the feces (40%). The fecal content may represent unabsorbed drug. Amiloride reaches the luminal fluid by glomerular filtration and active tubular secretion. The proximal tubule OCTS (Fig. 18-7) is involved in the latter process.[32] Onset of action occurs within 2 hours after oral administration, and duration of action may extend to 24 hours.[41]

SITE AND MECHANISM OF ACTION

Like triamterene, amiloride inhibits the electrogenic entry of 2 to 3% of the filtered load of Na^+ into the principal cells of the connecting tubule and cortical collecting tubule (i.e., site 4) by "plugging" the sodium channels in the luminal membrane (Fig. 18-6). In turn, the driving force for K^+ secretion is reduced or eliminated.[6, 11, 36] *Like triamterene, amiloride does not require the presence of aldosterone to produce diuresis.* It induces the urinary loss of Na^+, Cl^-, and water and, therefore, is a natriuretic, chloruretic, saluretic, and antikaliuretic agent, though with low efficacy.

ADVERSE EFFECTS

The major adverse effect of amiloride is hyperkalemia, which also may be observed with the other K^+-sparing diuretics that act at site 4. Therefore, patients taking amiloride should be warned not to take K^+ supplements. Caution is also needed when administering amiloride along with other drugs, such as ACE inhibitors, angiotensin II receptor antagonists, and β-adrenergic blockers, that may also give rise to increases in $[K^+]_{plasma}$. Nausea, vomiting, diarrhea, and headache may also accompany the use of amiloride.[32]

USES

Amiloride may be used alone in the treatment of mild edema associated with congestive heart failure, cirrhosis of the liver with ascites, or the nephrotic syndrome or in the treatment of hypertension. Its most common use is in combination with diuretics that act at sites 2 or 3, to circumvent the renal loss of K^+ commonly associated with the latter agents.

MISCELLANEOUS DIURETICS

Mannitol, USP. The prototypic osmotic diuretic D-mannitol is a water-soluble, lipid-insoluble, hexahydroxy alcohol. Because of its lack of lipid solubility, mannitol does not diffuse across the gastrointestinal epithelium and must be given by the intravenous route to obtain systemic effects. Once it enters the bloodstream, little, if any, is bound to plasma albumin; its distribution is confined to extracellular fluids, and it is not biotransformed. It enters renal luminal fluid only by glomerular filtration; it is neither secreted nor reabsorbed. The net result of its renal handling is twofold. First, it is excreted primarily by the kidneys; up to 80% of a 100-g intravenous dose appears in the urine within a 3-hour period.[41] Second, high luminal fluid concentrations of mannitol create an osmotic effect, and a great deal of the water in the luminal fluid is retained within the lumens of the nephrons. This osmotic effect prevents the reabsorption of up to 28% of the filtered load of water.[99] Mannitol, therefore, may be used prophylactically in a hospital setting to keep the nephrons open (i.e., prevent them from collapsing) in an attempt to avoid acute renal failure in certain circumstances. It has also been useful for the reduction of cerebrospinal fluid volume and pressure. Because intravenous solutions of mannitol may expand the extracellular fluid volume, they should not be used in patients with severe renal disease or cardiac decompensation who may not be able to excrete the additional fluid load and may subsequently develop pulmonary edema. Aqueous solutions are available in a range of concentrations for intravenous use. The adult dosage range for the induction of diuresis is from 50 to 200 g/24 hours.

Theophylline. The prototypic xanthine, theophylline, is known to promote a weak diuresis by stimulation of cardiac function and by a direct action on the nephron. Although it is infrequently used as a diuretic, diuresis may be an observed side effect when it is used as a bronchodilator.

EMERGING DEVELOPMENTS IN THE USE OF DIURETICS TO TREAT HYPERTENSION AND CONGESTIVE HEART FAILURE

Although the precise mechanism(s) by which the thiazide, thiazide-like, and loop diuretics lower blood pressure in hypertensive patients is not known, it is thought to involve slight reductions in plasma volume and cardiac output as well as direct relaxation of the vasculature. Over the years, the adverse effects associated with these drugs were considered relatively mild. Recently, however, several of the well-known adverse effects of these drugs have attracted attention because they appear to be more troubling than previously thought. First, diuretic-induced increased K^+ excretion leads not only to varying degrees of hypokalemia, but also to decreased cardiac and skeletal muscle $[K^+]$. Such changes in [K^+] impair cardiac performance and damage heart, brain, and kidney vessels.[108] Second, diuretic-induced reductions in plasma volume trigger increased sympathetic tone and increased renal secretion of renin and, ultimately, increased plasma levels of angiotensin II. In addition to being a potent vasoconstrictor, angiotensin II stimulates aldosterone secretion. Although the mechanism of aldosterone's actions at site 4 in the nephron have been known for a long time, its extrarenal actions have largely been ignored. Recently, it has been observed that diuretic-induced increased aldosterone levels not only cause changes in electrolyte transport at site 4 with ultimate damaging hypokalemia but also produce effects at extrarenal aldosterone receptors in the vasculature, which lead to vascular damage, and in the heart, which lead to cardiac fibrosis.[109] These observations help to explain why diuretic-induced reductions in blood pressure do not necessarily protect some hypertensive individuals from other cardiovascular problems.

Laragh and Sealey[108, 110] have amassed clinical evidence that spironolactone, a *nonselective aldosterone antagonist*, when used alone is as effective as the thiazides in treating mild hypertension without inducing hypokalemia or increased secretion of aldosterone. Furthermore, when spironolactone is used in combination with a thiazide, thiazide-like, or loop diuretic, it markedly blunts the renal and extrarenal actions of the elevated levels of aldosterone brought about by these latter diuretics.

In the past, spironolactone has not enjoyed widespread use for several well-documented reasons.[108, 110] First, its maximal effectiveness is usually not observed for 3 to 5 weeks. Second, its residual hormonal side effects have produced unacceptable rates of gynecomastia in males and menstrual irregularities in females, especially when doses exceeded 50 to 100 mg/day. These hormonal side effects can be largely avoided by giving spironolactone in doses of 12.5 to 25 mg/day.

Eplerenone, a *specific aldosterone antagonist* recently approved by the Food and Drug Administration, appears to have a much lower affinity for androgen and progesterone receptors than spironolactone and a reduced incidence of sexual disturbances.[109] If this finding is confirmed in additional clinical studies, eplerenone or another drug with the specificity of eplerenone may emerge as a very useful agent and improve the treatment of hypertension (and congestive heart failure) when used alone or in combination with other diuretics or ACE inhibitors.

Eplerenone

SUMMARY

The major driving force for the reabsorption of Na^+ at all four Na^+ reabsorption sites is the deficit of intracellular Na^+ created by the activity of the basolateral membrane–bound Na^+/K^+-ATPase. In response, the luminal fluid Na^+ moves into the Na^+-deficient cells by a luminal membrane–bound Na^+ transport system that is unique to each of the four sites. Most diuretics must attain sufficient concentration in luminal fluid to inhibit a luminal membrane–bound Na^+ transport system; this is usually accomplished by a combination of glomerular filtration and active tubular secretion. The chemical structure of a diuretic dictates which of the four Na^+-transporting sites will be inhibited. The site that is inhibited is one of the major determinants of the efficacy of the diuretic. The historical development of many diuretics has involved molecular modification of the chemical structure of sulfamoyl-containing compounds. This has yielded CA inhibitors, which inhibit the reabsorption of Na^+/HCO_3^- at site 1; the thiazide and thiazide-like diuretics, which inhibit the reabsorption of Na^+/Cl^- at site 3; and the high-ceiling diuretics, which block $Na^+/Cl^-/K^+/Ca^{2+}/Mg^{2+}$ reabsorption at site 2. Diuretic efficacy has increased with the corresponding changes in the site of action of each of the three classes of diuretics. Predictable secondary effects that depend on a diuretic's site of action have also surfaced.

DIURETIC PREPARATIONS[41]

Carbonic Anhydrase Inhibitors
Acetazolamide, USP (Diamox, Generic)
   Oral: 125-, 250-mg tablets; 500-mg extended-release capsules
   Parenteral: 500-mg powder (as the sodium salt)
Dichlorphenamide, USP (Daranide)
   Oral: 50-mg tablets
Methazolamide, USP (Neptazane, Generic)
   Oral: 25-, 50-mg tablets

Thiazide and Thiazide-Like Diuretics
Bendroflumethiazide, USP (Naturetin)
   Oral: 5-, 10-mg tablets

Benzthiazide (Exna, Hydrex)
   Oral: 50-mg tablets
Chlorothiazide, USP (Diuril, Generic)
   Oral: 250-, 500-mg tablets; 50-mg/mL oral suspension
   Parenteral: 500-mg base for injection
Chlorthalidone, USP (Hygroton, Thalitone, Generic)
   Oral: 25-, 50-, 100-mg tablets
Clopamide (Aquex, Brinaldix)
   Not available in the United States
Clorexolone (Nefrolan)
   Not available in the United States

Cyclothiazide (Anhydron)
Oral: 2-mg tablets
Hydrochlorothiazide, USP (Esidrix, HydroDIURIL, Oretic, Generic)
Oral: 25-, 50-, 100-mg tablets; 12.5-mg capsules (Microzide); 10-, 100-mg/mL oral solutions
Hydroflumethiazide, USP (Diucardin, Saluron, Generic)
Oral: 50-mg tablets
Indapamide (Lozol, Generic)
Oral: 1.25-, 2.5-mg tablets
Mefruside (Baycaron)
Not available in the United States
Methyclothiazide, USP (Aquatensen, Enduron, Generic)
Oral: 2.5-, 5-mg tablets
Metolazone
Oral: 2.5-, 5-, 10-mg extended tablets (Diulo, Zaroxolyn); 0.5-mg prompt tablets (Mykrox)
Polythiazide, USP (Renese)
Oral: 1-, 2-, 4-mg tablets
Quinethazone, USP (Hydromox)
Oral: 50-mg tablets
Trichlormethiazide, USP (Metahydrin, Naqua, Generic)
Oral: 2-, 4-mg tablets
Xipamide (Aquaphor, Diurexan)
Not available in the United States

Loop or High-Ceiling Diuretics
Bumetanide, USP (Bumex, Generic)
Oral: 0.5-, 1-, 2-mg tablets
Parenteral: 0.25 mg/mL for IV or IM use
Ethacrynic Acid, USP (Edecrin)
Oral: 25-, 50-mg tablets
Parenteral: 50-mg (base) for IV use
Furosemide, USP (Lasix, Generic)

Oral: 20-, 40-, 80-mg tablets; 8-, 10-mg/mL oral solution
Parenteral: 10 mg/mL for IV or IM use
Torsemide (Demadex)
Oral: 5-, 10-, 20-, 100-mg tablets
Parenteral: 10 mg/mL for IV use

K⁺-Sparing Diuretics
Amiloride Hydrochloride, USP (Midamor, Generic)
Oral: 5-mg tablets
Eplerenone (Inspra)
Oral: 25-, 50-, 100-mg tablets
Spironolactone, USP (Aldactone, Generic)
Oral: 25-, 50-, 100-mg tablets
Triamterene (Dyrenium)
Oral: 50-, 100-mg tablets; 50-, 100-mg capsules

Diuretic Combinations
Amiloride/Hydrochlorothiazide, USP (Moduretic, Generic)
Oral: 5 mg amiloride hydrochloride/50 mg hydrochlorothiazide
Spironolactone/Hydrochlorothiazide, USP (Aldactazide)
Oral:
25 mg spironolactone/25 mg hydrochlorothiazide
50 mg spironolactone/50 mg hydrochlorothiazide
Triamterene/Hydrochlorothiazide, USP (Dyazide, Maxzide)
Oral—capsules:
37.5 mg triamterene/25 mg hydrochlorothiazide (Dyazide)
50 mg triamterene/25 mg hydrochlorothiazide (Generic)
75 mg triamterene/50 mg hydrochlorothiazide (Generic)
Oral—tablets:
37.5 mg triamterene/25 mg hydrochlorothiazide (Maxzide)
75 mg triamterene/50 mg hydrochlorothiazide (Maxzide)

Osmotic Diuretics
Mannitol (Osmitrol, Generic)
Parenteral: 5, 10, 15, 20, 25% for IV use

REFERENCES

1. Brenner, B. M., and Beeuwkes, R. III: Hosp. Pract. 13:35, 1978.
2. Vander, A. J.: Renal blood flow and glomerular filtration. In Vander, A. J. (ed.). Renal Physiology, 5th ed. New York, McGraw-Hill, 1995, pp. 24–50.
3. Cafruny, E. J.: Am. J. Med. 62:490, 1977.
4. Holliday, M. A.: Hosp. Pract. 13:101, 1978.
5. Valtin, H.: Sodium and water transport. Sodium balance. In Valtin, H. (ed.). Renal Function, Mechanisms Preserving Fluid and Solute Balance in Health. Boston, Little, Brown & Co., 1983, pp. 119–159.
6. Puschett, J. B.: Am. J. Cardiol. 57:6A, 1986.
7. Sullivan, L. P., and Grantham, J. J. (eds.): Physiology of the Kidney, 2nd ed. Philadelphia, Lea & Febiger, 1982, pp. 213–215.
8. DuBose, T. D., Jr.: Ann. N. Y. Acad. Sci. 429:528, 1984.
9. Sullivan, L. P., and Grantham, J. J. (eds.): Physiology of the Kidney, 2nd ed. Philadelphia, Lea & Febiger, 1982, pp. 114–115.
10. Moe, O. W., Berry, C. A., and Rector, F. C., Jr.: Renal transport of glucose, amino acids, sodium, chloride, and water. In Brenner, B. M. (ed.). Brenner & Rector's The Kidney, vol. 1, 6th ed. Philadelphia, W. B. Saunders, 2000, pp. 375–415.
11. Steinmetz, P. R., and Koeppen, B. M.: Hosp. Pract. 19:125, 1984.
12. Sullivan, L. P., and Grantham, J. J. (eds.): Physiology of the Kidney, 2nd ed. Philadelphia, Lea & Febiger, 1982, pp. 135–137.
13. Koeppen, B. M., and Stanton, B. A.: Renal transport mechanisms: NaCl and water reabsorption along the nephron. In Koeppen, B. M., and Stanton, B. A. (eds.). Renal Physiology, 2nd ed. St. Louis, Mosby 1997, pp. 53–76.
14. Buckalew, V. M., Jr., et al.: J. Clin. Invest. 49:2336, 1970.
15. Vander, A. J.: Renal functions, anatomy, and basic processes. In Vander, A. J. (ed.). Renal Physiology, 5th ed. New York, McGraw-Hill, 1995, p. 14.
16. Eknoyan, G.: Drug Ther. (Hosp.) 6:87, 1981.
17. Vander, A. J.: Control of sodium and water excretion: Regulation of plasma volume and osmolarity. In Vander, A. J. (ed.). Renal Physiology, 5th ed. New York, McGraw-Hill, 1995, pp. 116–144.
18. Levy, M.: Hosp. Pract. 13:95, 1978.
19. Ross, E. M., and Gilman, A. G.: Pharmacodynamics: Mechanisms of drug action and the relationship between drug concentration and effect. In Gilman, A. G., et al. (eds.). The Pharmacological Basis of Therapeutics, 7th ed. New York, Macmillan, 1985, pp. 35–48.
20. Møller, J. V., and Sheikh, M. I.: Pharmacol. Rev. 34:315, 1983.
21. Schlatter, E., Greger, R., and Weidtke, C.: Pflugers Arch. 396:210, 1983.
22. Wittner, M., et al.: Pflugers Arch. 408:54, 1987.
23. Strauss, M. B., and Southworth, H.: Bull. Johns Hopkins Hosp. 63: 41, 1938.
24. Mann, T., and Keilin, K.: Nature 146:164, 1940.
25. Beckman, W. W., et al.: J. Clin. Invest. 19:635, 1940.
26. Miller, W. H., Dessert, A. M., and Roblin, R. O.: J. Am. Chem. Soc. 72:4893, 1950.
27. Roblin, R. O., and Clapp, J. W.: J. Am. Chem. Soc. 72:4890, 1950.
28. Sprague, J. M.: In Gould, R. F. (ed.). Molecular Modification in Drug Design, Advances in Chemistry Series 45. Washington, DC, American Chemical Society, 1964, pp. 87–101.
29. Maren, T. H.: Physiol. Rev. 47:595, 1967.
30. Allen, R. C.: In Cragoe, E. J. (ed.). Diuretics—Chemistry, Pharmacology and Medicine. New York, John Wiley & Sons, 1983, pp. 49–200.
31. Beyer, K. H., and Baer, J. E.: Pharmacol. Rev. 13:517, 1961.
32. Weiner, I. M., and Mudge, G. H.: Diuretics and other agents employed in the mobilization of edema fluid. In Gilman, A. G., et al. (eds.). The Pharmacological Basis of Therapeutics, 7th ed. New York, Macmillan, 1985, pp. 887–907.
33. Leaf, A., and Cotran, R. S.: Diuretics. In Leaf, A., and Cotran, R. S. (eds.). Renal Pathophysiology, 2nd ed. New York, Oxford University Press, 1980, pp. 145–161.
34. Whelton, A.: Am. J. Cardiol. 57:2A, 1986.
35. Erik, A. Persson, G., and Wright, F. S.: Acta Physiol. Scand. 114:1, 1982.
36. Wilcox, C. S.: Diuretics. In Brenner, B. M. (ed.). Brenner & Rector's The Kidney, vol. 2, 6th ed. Philadelphia, W. B. Saunders, 2000, pp. 2219–2252.
37. Ross, C. R., and Cafruny, E. J.: J. Pharmacol. Exp. Ther. 140:125, 1963.
38. Yeary, R. A., Brahm, C. A., and Miller, D. L.: Toxicol. Appl. Pharmacol. 7:598, 1965.

39. Terry, B., Hirsch, G., and Hook, J. B.: Eur. J. Pharmacol. 4:289, 1968.
40. Belair, E. J., Borrelli, A. R., and Yelnosky, J.: Proc. Soc. Exp. Biol. Med. 131:327, 1969.
41. Diuretics. In United States Pharmacopeia Dispensing Information (USP DI), vol. 1. 21st ed. Englewood, CO, Micromedex, 2001, pp. 791–796, 1266–1290, 1708–1710.
42. Ings, R. M. J., and Stevens, L. A.: Prog. Drug Metab. 7:57, 1983.
43. Am. J. Hosp. Pharm. 32:473, 1975.
44. Shimizu, T., et al.: J. Clin. Invest. 82:721, 1988.
45. AMA Drug Evaluations Annual 1995. Chicago, American Medical Association, 1995, pp. 837–856.
46. Med. Lett. 37:45, 1995 and 41:23, 1999.
47. Beyer, K. H., Jr., and Baer, J. E.: Med. Clin. North Am. 59:735, 1975.
48. Kunau, R. T., Weller, D. R., Jr., and Webb, H. L.: J. Clin. Invest. 56:401, 1975.
49. Hropot, M., et al.: Kidney Int. 28:477, 1985.
50. Fuchs, M., Moyer, J. H., and Newman, B. E.: Ann. N. Y. Acad. Sci. 88:795, 1960.
51. Tobian, L.: Annu. Rev. Pharmacol. 7:399, 1967.
52. Greenberg, A.: Am. Fam. Physician 33:200, 1986.
53. Bennett, W. M., and Porter, G. A.: J. Clin. Pharmacol. 13:357, 1973.
54. Craswell, P. W., et al.: Nephron 12:63, 1973.
55. Med. Lett. 16:65, 1974.
56. Preminger, G. M.: Urol. Clin. North Am. 14:325, 1987.
57. Imbs, J. L., Schmidt, M., and Giessen-Crouse, E.: Pharmacology of loop diuretics: State of the art. In Grunfeld, J.-P., et al. (eds.). Advances in Nephrology, vol. 16. Chicago, Year Book Medical, 1987, pp. 137–158.
58. Burg, M., and Green, N.: Kidney Int. 4:245, 1973.
59. Cafruny, E. J.: Geriatrics, 22:107, 1967.
60. Cafruny, E. J., Cho, K. C., and Gussin, R. Z.: Ann. N. Y. Acad. Sci. 139:362, 1966.
61. Ethridge, C. B., Myers, D. W., and Fulton, M. N.: Arch. Intern. Med. 57:714, 1936.
62. Weiner, I. M., Levy, R. I., and Mudge, G. H.: J. Pharmacol. Exp. Ther. 138:96, 1962.
63. Ward, A., and Heel, R. C.: Drugs 28:426, 1984.
64. Feig, P. U.: Am. J. Cardiol. 57:14A, 1986.
65. Odlind, B.: J. Pharmacol. Exp. Ther. 211:238, 1979.
66. Gutsche, H.-U., et al.: Can. J. Physiol. Pharmacol. 62:412, 1984.
67. Finnerty, F. A., Jr., et al.: Angiology 28:125, 1977.
68. Reineck, H. J., and Stein, J. H.: Mechanisms of action and clinical uses of diuretics. In Brenner, B. M., and Rector, F. C., Jr. (eds.). The Kidney, vol. 1, 2nd ed. Philadelphia, W. B. Saunders, 1981, pp. 1097–1131.
69. Suki, W. N., et al.: N. Engl. J. Med. 283:836, 1970.
70. Delarge, J.: Arzneimittelforschung 38:144, 1988.
71. Med. Lett. 36:73, 1994.
72. Schwartz, S., et al.: Clin. Pharmacol. Ther. 54:90, 1993.
73. Greger, R.: Arzneimittelforschung 38:151, 1988.
74. Klinke, R., and Mertens, M.: Arzneimittelforschung 38:153, 1988.
75. Dunn, C. J., Fitton, A., and Brogden, R. N.: Drugs 49:121, 1995.
76. Koechel, D. A.: Annu. Rev. Pharmacol. Toxicol. 21:265, 1981.
77. Cragoe, E. J., Jr.: The (aryloxy)acetic acid family of diuretics. In Cragoe, E. J., Jr. (ed.). Diuretics—Chemistry, Pharmacology and Medicine. New York, John Wiley & Sons, 1983, pp. 201–266.
78. Koechel, D. A., Gisvold, O., and Cafruny, E. J.: J. Med. Chem. 14:628, 1971.
79. Koechel, D. A., Smith, S. A., and Cafruny, E. J.: J. Pharmacol. Exp. Ther. 203:272, 1977.
80. deSolm, S. J., et al.: J. Med. Chem. 21:437, 1978.
81. Beyer, K. H., et al.: J. Pharmacol. Exp. Ther, 147:1, 1964.
82. Gussin, R. Z., and Cafruny, E. J.: J. Pharmacol. Exp. Ther. 153:148, 1966.
83. Schnermann, J.: Influence of diuretics on the tubuloglomerular feedback mechanism, XII Symposium of the Nephrology Society, Sept. 28–Oct. 1, 1977, Bonn, West Germany.
84. Williamson, H., Bourland, W., and Marchand, G.: Prostaglandins 8:297, 1974.
85. Birtch, A. G., et al.: Circ. Res. 24:869, 1967.
86. Garay, R. P., et al.: J. Pharmacol. Exp. Ther. 255:415, 1990.
87. Garay, R. P., Nazaret, C., and Cragoe, E. J., Jr.: Eur. J. Pharmacol. 200:141, 1991.
88. Shinkawa, T., et al.: Eur. J. Pharmacol. 238:317, 1993.
89. Greven, J., Klein, H., and Heidenreich, O.: Naunyn Schmiedebergs Arch. Pharmacol. 304:289, 1978.
90. Benabe, J. E., Pedraza-Chaverri, J., and Martinez-Maldonado, M.: Am. J. Hypertens. 6:701, 1993.
91. Wangemann, P. H., Braitsch, R., and Greger, R.: Pflugers Arch. 410:674, 1987.
92. Breyer, J., and Jacobson, H. R.: Annu. Rev. Med. 41:265, 1990.
93. Landau, R. L., et al.: J. Clin. Endocrinol. 15:1194, 1955.
94. Rosemberg, E., and Engel, I.: Endocrinology 69:496, 1961.
95. Cella, J. A., and Kagawa, C. M.: J. Org. Chem. 79:4808, 1957.
96. Cella, J. A., Brown, E. A., and Burtner, R. R.: J. Org. Chem. 24:743, 1959.
97. Cella, J. A., and Tweit, R. C.: J. Org. Chem. 24:1109, 1959.
98. Brown, E. A., Muir, R. D., and Cella, J. A.: J. Org. Chem. 25:96, 1960.
99. Henry, D. A., and Coburn, J. W.: Diuretics. In Bevan, J. A., and Thompson, J. H. (eds.). Essentials of Pharmacology, 3rd ed. Philadelphia, Harper & Row, 1983, pp. 410–422.
100. Geering, K., et al.: J. Biol. Chem. 257:10338, 1982.
101. Verrey, F., et al.: J. Cell. Biol. 104:1231, 1987.
102. Smith, R. L.: Endogenous agents affecting kidney function: Their interrelationships, modulation, and control. In Cragoe, E. J., Jr. (ed.). Diuretics—Chemistry, Pharmacology and Medicine. New York, John Wiley & Sons, 1983, pp. 571–651.
103. Wiebelhaus, V. D., et al.: J. Pharmacol. Exp. Ther. 149:397, 1965.
104. Carey, R. A., et al.: Clin. Ther. 6:302, 1984.
105. Sorgel, F., Ettinger, B., and Benet, L. Z.: J. Pharm. Sci. 75:129, 1986.
106. Berndt, W. O., and Friedman, P. A.: Diuretic Drugs. In Craig, C. R., and Stitzel, R. E. (eds). Modern Pharmacology with Clinical Applications, 5th ed. Boston, Little, Brown and Co., 1997, pp. 253–268.
107. Cragoe, E. J., Jr.: Pyrazine Diuretics. In Cragoe, E. J., Jr. (ed.). Diuretics—Chemistry, Pharmacology and Medicine. New York, John Wiley & Sons, 1983, pp. 303–341.
108. Laragh, J. H., and Sealey, J. E.: Hypertension 37(part 2):806, 2001.
109. Epstein, M.: Am. J. Kidney Dis. 37:677, 2001.
110. Laragh, J. H.: Am. J. Hypertens. 14:84, 2001.

SELECTED READING

Brenner, B. M., and Beeuwkes, R. III: Hosp. Pract. 13:35–46, 1978.
Breyer, J., and Jacobson, H. R.: Annu. Rev. Med. 41:265, 1990.
Greenberg, A.: Am. Fam. Physician 33:200–212, 1986.
Imbs, J.-L., Schmidt, M., and Giessen-Crouse, E.: Pharmacology of loop diuretics: State of the art. Adv. Nephrol. 16:137–158, 1987.
Koeppen, B. M., and Stanton, B. A.: Renal transport mechanisms: NaCl and water reabsorption along the nephron. In Koeppen, B. M., and Stanton, B. A. (eds.). Renal Physiology, 2nd ed. St. Louis, Mosby 1997, pp. 53–76.
Puschett, J. B.: Am. J. Cardiol. 57:6A–13A, 1986.
Steinmetz, P. R., and Koeppen, B. M.: Hosp. Pract. 19:125–134, 1984.
Weiner, I. M., and Mudge, G. H.: Diuretics and other agents employed in the mobilization of edema fluid. In Gilman, A. G., et al. (eds.). The Pharmacological Basis of Therapeutics, 7th ed. New York, Macmillan, 1985, pp. 887–907.
Wilcox, C. S.: Diuretics. In Brenner, B. M. (ed.). Brenner & Rector's The Kidney, vol. 2, 6th ed. Philadelphia, W. B. Saunders, 2000, pp. 2219–2252.

Cardiovascular Agents

STEPHEN J. CUTLER AND GEORGE H. COCOLAS

The treatment and therapy of cardiovascular disease have undergone dramatic changes since the 1950s. Data show that since 1968 and continuing through the 1990s, there has been a noticeable decline in mortality from cardiovascular disease. The bases for advances in the control of heart disease have been *(a)* a better understanding of the disease state, *(b)* the development of effective therapeutic agents, and *(c)* innovative medical intervention techniques to treat problems of the cardiovascular system.

The drugs discussed in this chapter are used for their action on the heart or other parts of the vascular system, to modify the total output of the heart or the distribution of blood to the circulatory system. These drugs are used in the treatment of angina, cardiac arrhythmias, hypertension, hyperlipidemias, and disorders of blood coagulation. This chapter also includes a discussion of hypoglycemic agents, thyroid hormones, and antithyroid drugs.

ANTIANGINAL AGENTS AND VASODILATORS

Most coronary artery disease conditions are due to deposits of atheromas in the intima of large and medium-sized arteries serving the heart. The process is characterized by an insidious onset of episodes of cardiac discomfort caused by ischemia from inadequate blood supply to the tissues. Angina pectoris (angina), the principal symptom of ischemic heart disease, is characterized by a severe constricting pain in the chest, often radiating from the precordium to the left shoulder and down the arm. The syndrome has been described since 1772 but not until 1867 was amyl nitrite introduced for the symptomatic relief of angina pectoris.[1] It was believed at that time that anginal pain was precipitated by an increase in blood pressure and that the use of amyl nitrite reduced both blood pressure and, concomitantly, the work required of the heart. Later, it was generally accepted that nitrites relieved angina pectoris by dilating the coronary arteries and that changes in the work of the heart were of only secondary importance. We now know that the coronary blood vessels in the atherosclerotic heart already are dilated and that ordinary doses of dilator drugs do not significantly increase blood supply to the heart; instead, anginal pain is relieved by a reduction of cardiac consumption of oxygen.[2]

Although vasodilators are used in the treatment of angina, a more sophisticated understanding of the hemodynamic response to these agents has broadened their clinical usefulness to other cardiovascular conditions. Because of their ability to reduce peripheral vascular resistance, vasodilators, including organonitrates, angiotensin-converting enzyme (ACE) inhibitors, and angiotensin receptor–blocking agents, are used to improve cardiac output in some patients with congestive heart failure (CHF).

The coronary circulation supplies blood to the myocardial tissues to maintain cardiac function. It can react to the changing demands of the heart by dilating its blood vessels to provide sufficient oxygen and other nutrients and to remove metabolites. Myocardial metabolism is almost exclusively aerobic, which makes blood flow critical to the support of metabolic processes of the heart. This demand is met effectively by the normal heart because it extracts a relatively large proportion of the oxygen delivered to it by the coronary circulation. The coronary blood flow depends strongly on myocardial metabolism, which in turn is affected by work done by the heart and the efficiency of the heart. The coronary system normally has a reserve capacity that allows it to respond by vasodilation to satisfy the needs of the heart during strenuous activity by the body.

Coronary atherosclerosis, one of the more prevalent cardiovascular diseases, develops with increasing age and may lead to a reduction of the reserve capacity of the coronary system. It most often results in multiple stenosis and makes it difficult for the coronary system to meet adequately the oxygen needs of the heart that occur during physical exercise or emotional duress. Insufficient coronary blood flow *(myocardial ischemia)* in the face of increased oxygen demand produces angina pectoris.

The principal goal in the prevention and relief of angina is to limit the oxygen requirement of the heart so that the amount of blood supplied by the stenosed arteries is adequate. Nitrate esters, such as nitroglycerin, lower arterial blood pressure and, in turn, reduce the work of the left ventricle. This action is produced by the powerful vasodilating effect of the nitrates on the arterial system and, to an even greater extent, on the venous system. The result is reduced cardiac filling pressure and ventricular size. This reduces the work required of the ventricle and decreases the oxygen requirements, allowing the coronary system to satisfy the oxygen demands of myocardial tissue and relieve anginal pain.

Intermediary Myocardial Metabolism

Energy metabolism by heart tissue provides an adequate supply of high-energy phosphate compounds to replace the adenosine triphosphate (ATP) that is continually being consumed in contraction, ion exchange across membranes, and other energy-demanding processes. Because of the high

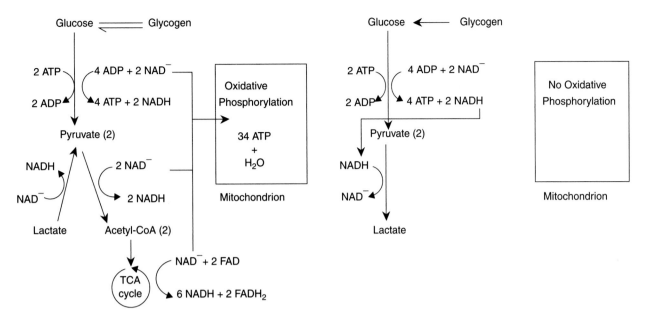

Figure 19–1 ■ Normal and ischemic myocardial metabolism of glucose. A total production of 36 moles of ATP results from the aerobic catabolism of 1 mole of glucose and use of NADH and $FADH_2$ in the oxidative phosphorylation process in mitochondria. When oxygen is not available, NADH and $FADH_2$ levels rise and shut off the tricarboxylic acid (TCA) cycle. Pyruvate is converted to lactate. Only 2 moles of ATP are formed from anaerobic catabolism of 1 mole of glucose. (Adapted from Giuliani, E. R., et al.: Cardiology: Fundamentals and Practice, 2nd ed. By permission of the Mayo Foundation, Rochester, MN.)

turnover rate of ATP in heart muscle, a correspondingly high rate of ATP production in the mitochondria is required.

Normal myocardial metabolism is aerobic, and the rate of oxygen use parallels the amount of ATP synthesized by the cells.[3] Free fatty acids (FFAs) are the principal fuel for myocardial tissue, but lactate, acetate, acetoacetate, and glucose are also oxidized to CO_2 and water. A large volume of the myocardial cell consists of mitochondria in which two-carbon fragments from FFA breakdown are metabolized through the Krebs cycle. The reduced flavin and nicotinamide dinucleotides formed by this metabolism are reoxidized by the electron-transport chain because of the presence of oxygen (Fig. 19-1). In the hypoxic or ischemic heart, the lack of oxygen inhibits the electron-transport chain function and causes an accumulation of reduced flavin and nicotinamide coenzymes. As a result, fatty acids are converted to lipids rather than being oxidized. To compensate for this, glucose use and glycogenolysis increase, but the resulting pyruvate cannot be oxidized; instead, it is converted to lactate. A great loss of efficiency occurs as a result of the change of myocardial metabolism from aerobic to anaerobic pathways. Normally, 36 moles of ATP are formed from the oxidation of 1 mole of glucose, but only 2 moles are formed from its glycolysis. This great loss of high-energy stores during hypoxia thus limits the functional capacity of the heart during stressful conditions and is reflected by the production of anginal pain.

Nitrovasodilators

SMOOTH MUSCLE RELAXATION

The contractile activity of all types of muscle (smooth, skeletal) is regulated primarily by the reversible phosphorylation of myosin. Myosin of smooth muscle consists of two heavy chains (MW 200,000 each) that are coiled to produce a filamentous tail. Each heavy chain is associated with two pairs of light chains (MW 20,000 and 16,000) that serve as substrates for calcium- and calmodulin-dependent protein kinases in the contraction process. Together with actin (MW 43,000) they participate in a cascade of biochemical events that are part of the processes of muscle contraction and relaxation (Fig. 19-2).

Cyclic nucleotides, cyclic adenosine monophosphate (cAMP), and, especially, cyclic guanosine monophosphate (cGMP) play important roles in the regulation of smooth muscle tension. cAMP is the mediator associated with the smooth muscle relaxant properties of drugs such as β-adrenergic agonists. It activates the protein kinases that phosphorylate myosin light-chain kinase (MLCK). Phosphorylation of MLCK inactivates this kinase and prevents its action with Ca^{2+} and calmodulin to phosphorylate myosin, which interacts with actin to cause contraction of smooth muscle (Fig. 19-2).

The activity of cGMP in smooth muscle relaxation is affected by exogenous and endogenous agents. It is suggested[4] that nitrovasodilators undergo metabolic transformation in

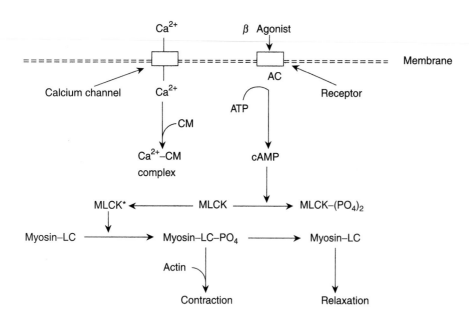

Figure 19-2 ■ Regulation of smooth muscle contraction. Contraction is triggered by an influx of Ca^{2+}. The increase of free Ca^{2+} causes binding to calmodulin (CM). The Ca^{2+}–CM complex binds to myosin light-chain kinase (MLCK) and causes its activation (MLCK*). MLCK* phosphorylates myosin, which combines with actin to produce contraction of smooth muscle. Myosin is dephosphorylated in the presence of myosin phosphatase to cause muscle relaxation. The β agonists activate adenylate cyclase (AC) to raise levels of cAMP, which in turn activates kinases that phosphorylate MLCK, inactivating it to prevent muscle contraction.

vascular smooth muscle cells to form nitric oxide (NO). NO mediates smooth muscle relaxation by activating guanylate cyclase to increase intracellular concentrations of cGMP. cGMP activates protein kinases that can regulate free Ca^{2+} levels in the muscle cell and cause relaxation of smooth muscle by phosphorylating MLCK.

A short-lived free radical gas, NO is widely distributed in the body and plays an important role by its effect through cGMP on the smooth muscle vasculature. It is synthesized in the vascular endothelial cell from the semiessential amino acid L-arginine by NO synthase. After production in the cell, it diffuses to the smooth muscle cell, where it activates the enzyme guanylate cyclase, which leads to an increase in cGMP and then muscle relaxation (Fig. 19-3). Endothelium-derived relaxing factor (EDRF), released from the endothelial cell to mediate its smooth muscle–relaxing properties through cGMP, is identical with NO.

Inhibitors of phosphodiesterases of cAMP and cGMP also cause smooth muscle relaxation. These inhibitors increase cellular levels of cAMP and cGMP by preventing their hy-drolysis to AMP and GMP, respectively. Drugs such as papaverine (see Chapter 17) and theophylline (see Chapter 18), which relax smooth muscle, do so in part by inhibiting phosphodiesterases.

METABOLISM OF NITROVASODILATORS

After oral administration, organic nitrates are metabolized rapidly by the liver, kidney, lungs, intestinal mucosa, and vascular tissue. Buccal absorption reduces the immediate hepatic destruction of the organic nitrates because only 15% of the cardiac output is delivered to the liver; this allows a transient but effective circulating level of the intact organic nitrate before it is inactivated.[5]

Organic nitrates, nitrites, nitroso compounds, and a variety of other nitrogen-containing substances, such as sodium nitroprusside, for the most part cause their pharmacological effects by generating or releasing NO in situ. In some ways, these drugs are viewed as "replacement agents" for the endogenous NO generated by the NO synthase pathway from arginine. The mechanisms by which vasodilatory drugs release NO have become better understood recently. Table 19-1 shows the oxidation state of various nitrosyl compounds that are common in nitrovasodilatory drugs. A common feature of these drugs is that they release nitrogen in the form of NO and contain nitrogen in an oxidation state higher than +3 (as would occur in ammonia, amines, amides, and most biological nitrogen compounds). The nitrogen in NO has an oxidation state of +2. Compounds such as nitroprusside, nitrosoamines, and nitrothiols with oxidation states of +3 release NO nonenzymatically. Although their spontaneous liberation of NO is by an unknown mechanism, it involves only a one-electron reduction, which may occur on exposure of these chemicals to the variety of reducing agents in the tissue of vascular smooth muscle membranes. Organic nitrites such as amyl nitrite react with available thiol groups to form unstable S-nitrosothiols, which rapidly decompose to NO by homolytic cleavage of their S–N bond. In mammalian smooth muscle, this will occur almost exclusively with glutathione as the most abundant thiol compound.[6]

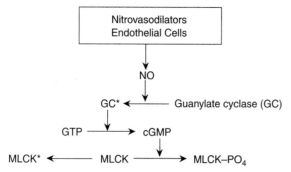

Figure 19-3 ■ Mechanism of nitrovasodilators. Nitric oxide (NO) formed in smooth muscle from nitrovasodilators or from endothelial cells (EDRF) activates guanylate cyclase (GC*). GC* activates cGMP-dependent protein kinases that phosphorylate myosin light-chain kinase (MLCK), causing its inactivation and subsequent muscle relaxation (see also Fig. 19-2).

TABLE 19–1 Nitrosyl Vasodilatory Substances and Their Oxidation State

Nitrosyl Compound	Structure	Nitrogen Oxidation State
Nitric oxide	N=O	+2
Nitrite	–ONO	+3
Nitrate	–ONO$_2$	+5
Organic nitrite	R–O–N=O	+3
Nitrosothiol	R–S–N=O	+3
Organic nitrate	R–O–NO$_2$	+5
Thionitrate	R–S–NO$_2$	+5
Nitroprusside	[(CN)$_5$Fe–N=O]^2	+3

The pharmacodynamic action of nitroglycerin is preceded by metabolic changes that follow a variety of paths. Biotransformation of nitroglycerin to the dinitrates and the increase of intracellular cGMP precede vascular relaxation. Sulfhydryl-containing compounds, such as cysteine, react chemically with organic nitrates to form inorganic nitrite ions. The release of NO from an organic nitrate, such as nitroglycerin, appears to occur in a stepwise fashion involving nonenzymatic and enzymatic steps. Because nitroglycerin requires a three-electron reduction to release NO, thiols may be involved in the process. Nitroglycerin may decompose nonenzymatically by interaction with a variety of thiols, such as cysteine or *N*-acetylcysteine, which may be present in tissue, to form a nitrosothiol intermediate before undergoing enzymatic transformation to release NO. Nitroglycerin also readily releases NO by acting on an enzyme system attached to the cellular surface membrane of smooth muscle. The process may include glutathione-*S*-transferases, which convert nitroglycerin to a vasoinactive nitrite, which then may release NO nonenzymatically.[7]

ESTERS OF NITROUS AND NITRIC ACIDS

Inorganic acids, like organic acids, will form esters with an alcohol. Pharmaceutically, the important ones are sulfate, nitrite, and nitrate. Sulfuric acid forms organic sulfates, of which methyl sulfate and ethyl sulfate are examples.

Nitrous acid (HNO$_2$) esters may be formed readily from an alcohol and nitrous acid. The usual procedure is to mix sodium nitrite, sulfuric acid, and the alcohol. Organic nitrites are generally very volatile liquids that are only slightly soluble in water but soluble in alcohol. Preparations containing water are very unstable because of hydrolysis.

The organic nitrates and nitrites and the inorganic nitrites have their primary utility in the prophylaxis and treatment of angina pectoris. They have a more limited application in treating asthma, gastrointestinal spasm, and certain cases of migraine headache. Their application may be regarded as causal therapy, since they act by substituting an endogenous factor, the production or release of NO, which may be impaired under pathophysiological circumstances associated with dysfunction of the endothelial tissue. Nitroglycerin (glyceryl trinitrate) was one of the first members of this group to be introduced into medicine and remains an important member of the group. Varying the chemical structure of the organic nitrates yields differences in speed of onset, duration of action, and potency (Table 19-2). Although the number of nitrate ester groups may vary from two to six or more, depending on the compound, there is no direct relationship between the number of nitrate groups and the level of activity.

It appears that the higher the oil/water partition coefficient of the drug, the greater the potency. The orientation of the groups within the molecule also may affect potency. Lipophilicity of the nitrogen oxide–containing compound produces a much longer response of vasodilatory action. The highly lipophilic ester nitroglycerin permeates the cell membrane, allowing continual formation of NO within the cell. The same effect appears to occur for sodium nitroprusside, nitroso compounds, and other organic nitrate and nitrite esters.[4]

ANTIANGINAL ACTION OF NITROVASODILATORS

The action of short-acting sublingual nitrates in the relief of angina pectoris is complex. Although the sublingual nitrates relax vascular smooth muscle and dilate the coronary arteries of normal humans, there is little improvement of coronary blood flow when these chemicals are administered to individuals with coronary artery disease. Nitroglycerin is an effective antianginal agent because it causes redistribution of coronary blood flow to the ischemic regions of the heart and reduces myocardial oxygen demand. This latter effect

TABLE 19–2 Relationship Between Speed and Duration of Action of Sodium Nitrite and Certain Inorganic Esters

Compound	Action Begins (minutes)	Maximum Effect (minutes)	Duration of Action (minutes)
Amyl nitrite	0.25	0.5	1
Nitroglycerin	2	8	30
Isosorbide dinitrate	3	15	60
Sodium nitrite	10	25	60
Erythrityl tetranitrate	15	32	180
Pentaerythritol tetranitrate	20	70	330

is produced by a reduction of venous tone resulting from the nitrate vasodilating effect and a pooling of blood in the peripheral veins, which results in a reduction in ventricular volume, stroke volume, and cardiac output. It also causes reduction of peripheral resistance during myocardial contractions. The combined vasodilatory effects cause a decrease in cardiac work and reduce oxygen demand.

PRODUCTS

Amyl Nitrite, USP. Amyl nitrite, isopentyl nitrite [$(CH_3)_2CHCH_2CH_2ONO$], is a mixture of isomeric amyl nitrites but is principally isoamyl nitrite. It may be prepared from amyl alcohol and nitrous acid by several procedures. Usually, amyl nitrite is dispensed in ampul form and used by inhalation or orally in alcohol solution. Currently, it is recommended for treating cyanide poisoning; although not the best antidote, it does not require intravenous injections.

Amyl nitrite is a yellowish liquid with an ethereal odor and a pungent taste. It is volatile and inflammable at room temperature. Amyl nitrite vapor forms an explosive mixture in air or oxygen. Inhalation of the vapor may involve definite explosion hazards if a source of ignition is present, as both room and body temperatures are within the flammability range of amyl nitrite mixtures with either air or oxygen. It is nearly insoluble in water but is miscible with organic solvents. The nitrite also will decompose into valeric acid and nitric acid.

Nitroglycerin. Glyceryl trinitrate is the trinitrate ester of glycerol and is listed as available in tablet form in the *United States Pharmacopoeia*. It is prepared by carefully adding glycerin to a mixture of nitric and fuming sulfuric acids. This reaction is exothermic, and the reaction mixture must be cooled to between 10 and 20°C.

The ester is a colorless oil, with a sweet, burning taste. It is only slightly soluble in water, but it is soluble in organic solvents.

$$H_2C-ONO_2$$
$$|$$
$$HC-ONO_2$$
$$|$$
$$H_2C-ONO_2$$

Nitroglycerin

Transmucosal	Nitrogard
Translingual	Nitrolingual
Oral	Nitrobid
	Nitroglyn
Ointment	Nitroglyn
Injection	Nitrobid IV
	Tridil
Transdermal	Nitrodur
	Nitrodisc
	Minitran
	Deponit
	Transderm-Nitro

Nitroglycerin is used extensively as an explosive in dynamite. A solution of the ester, if spilled or allowed to evaporate, will leave a residue of nitroglycerin. To prevent an explosion of the residue, the ester must be decomposed by the addition of alkali. Even so, the material dispensed is so dilute that the risk of explosions does not exist. It has a strong

vasodilating action and, because it is absorbed through the skin, is prone to cause headaches among workers associated with its manufacture. This transdermal penetration is why nitroglycerin is useful in a patch formulation. In medicine, it has the action typical of nitrites, but its action develops more slowly and is of longer duration. Of all the known coronary vasodilatory drugs, nitroglycerin is the only one capable of stimulating the production of coronary collateral circulation and the only one able to prevent experimental myocardial infarction by coronary occlusion.

Previously, the nitrates were thought to be hydrolyzed and reduced in the body to nitrites, which then lowered the blood pressure. This is not true, however. The mechanism of vasodilation of nitroglycerin through its formation of NO is described above.

Nitroglycerin tablet instability was reported in molded sublingual tablets.[8] The tablets, although uniform when manufactured, lost potency both because of volatilization of nitroglycerin into the surrounding materials in the container and intertablet migration of the active ingredient. Nitroglycerin may be stabilized in molded tablets by incorporating a "fixing" agent such as polyethylene glycol 400 or polyethylene glycol 4000.[9] In addition to sublingual tablets, the drug has been formulated into an equally effective lingual aerosol for patients who have problems with dissolution of sublingual preparations because of dry mucous membranes. Transdermal nitroglycerin preparations appear to be less effective than other long-acting nitrates, as absorption from the skin is variable.

Diluted Erythrityl Tetranitrate, USP. Erythritol tetranitrate, 1,2,3,4-butanetetrol, tetranitrate (*R**, *S**)-(Cardilate), is the tetranitrate ester of erythritol and nitric acid. It is prepared in a manner analogous to that used for nitroglycerin. The result is a solid, crystalline material. This ester is also very explosive and is diluted with lactose or other suitable inert diluents to permit safe handling; it is slightly soluble in water and soluble in organic solvents.

$$H_2C-ONO_2$$
$$|$$
$$HC-ONO_2$$
$$|$$
$$HC-ONO_2$$
$$|$$
$$H_2C-ONO_2$$

Erythrityl Tetranitrate
(Cardilate)

Erythrityl tetranitrate requires slightly more time than nitroglycerin to produce its effect, which is of longer duration. It is useful when mild, gradual, and prolonged vascular dilation is warranted. The drug is used in the treatment of, and as prophylaxis against, attacks of angina pectoris and to reduce blood pressure in arterial hypertonia.

Erythrityl tetranitrate produces a reduction of cardiac preload as a result of pooling blood on the venous side of the circulatory system by its vasodilating action. This action results in a reduction of blood pressure on the arterial side during stressful situations and is an important factor in preventing the precipitation of anginal attacks.

Diluted Pentaerythritol Tetranitrate, USP. Pentaerythritol tetranitrate, 2,2-bis (hydroxymethyl)-1,3-propanediol tetranitrate (Peritrate, Pentritol), is a white, crystalline material with a melting point of 140°C. It is insoluble in water, slightly soluble in alcohol, and readily soluble in acetone. The drug is a nitric acid ester of the tetrahydric alcohol pentaerythritol and is a powerful explosive. Accordingly, it is diluted with lactose, mannitol, or other suitable inert diluents to permit safe handling.

Pentaerythritol Tetranitrate
(Peritrate)
(Pentritol)

It relaxes smooth muscle of smaller vessels in the coronary vascular tree. Pentaerythritol tetranitrate is used prophylactically to reduce the severity and frequency of anginal attacks and is usually administered in sustained-release preparations to increase its duration of action.

Diluted Isosorbide Dinitrate, USP. Isosorbide dinitrate, 1,4:3,6-dianhydro-D-glucitol dinitrate (Isordil, Sorbitrate), occurs as a white, crystalline powder. Its water solubility is about 1 mg/mL.

Isosorbide Dinitrate
(Isordil)

Isosorbide Mononitrate
(ISMO Imdur)
This molecule is lacking one of the nitro substitutions

Isosorbide dinitrate, as a sublingual or chewable tablet, is effective in the treatment or prophylaxis of acute anginal attacks. When it is given sublingually, the effect begins in about 2 minutes, with a shorter duration of action than when it is given orally. Oral tablets are not effective in acute anginal episodes; the onset of action ranges from 15 to 30 minutes. The major route of metabolism involves denitration to isosorbide 5-mononitrate. This metabolite has a much longer half-life than the parent isosorbide dinitrate. As such, this particular metabolite is marketed in a tablet form that has excellent bioavailability with much less first-pass metabolism than isosorbide dinitrate.

Calcium Antagonists

EXCITATION–CONTRACTION COUPLING MUSCLE

Stimulation of the cardiac cell initiates the process of excitation, which has been related to ion fluxes through the cell membrane. Depolarization of the tissue in the atria of the

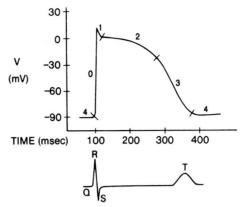

Figure 19–4 ■ Diagrammatic representation of the membrane action potential, as recorded from a Purkinje fiber, and an electrogram recorded from an isolated ventricular fiber. The membrane resting potential is 90 mV relative to the exterior of the fiber. At the point of depolarization, there is a rapid change (phase 0) to a more positive value. *0–4* indicate the phases of depolarization and repolarization. Note that phases 0 and 3 of the membrane action potential correspond in time to the inscription of the QRS and T waves, respectively, of the local electrogram.

heart is mediated by two inwardly directed ionic currents. When the cardiac cell potential reaches its threshold, ion channels in the membrane are opened, and Na^+ enters the cell through ion channels. These channels give rise to the fast sodium current that is responsible for the rapidly rising phase, phase 0, of the ventricular action potential (Fig. 19-4). The second current is caused by the slow activation of an L-type Ca^{2+} ion channel that allows the movement of Ca^{2+} into the cell. This "slow channel" contributes to the maintenance of the plateau phase (phase 2) of the cardiac action potential. We now understand that the Ca^{2+} that enters with the action potential initiates a second and larger release of Ca^{2+} from the sarcoplasmic reticulum in the cell. This secondary release of Ca^{2+} is sufficient to initiate the contractile process of cardiac muscle.

Contraction of cardiac and other muscle occurs from a reaction between actin and myosin. In contrast to smooth vascular muscle, the contractile process in cardiac muscle involves a complex of proteins (troponins I, C, and T and tropomyosin) attached to myosin, which modulates the interaction between actin and myosin. Free Ca^{2+} ions bind to troponin C, uncovering binding sites on the actin molecule and allowing interaction with myosin, causing contraction of the muscle. The schematic diagram in Figure 19-5 shows the sequence of events.[10] Contraction of vascular smooth muscle, like that of cardiac muscle, is regulated by the concentration of cytoplasmic Ca^{2+} ions. The mechanism by which the contraction is effected, however, includes a calcium- and calmodulin-dependent kinase as opposed to a Ca^{2+}-sensitive troponin–tropomyosin complex (Fig. 19-2). The activating effect depends on a different type of reaction. The elevated free cytosolic Ca^{2+} in vascular smooth muscle cells binds to a high-affinity binding protein, calmodulin.

ION CHANNELS AND CALCIUM

Calcium ions play an important role in the regulation of many cellular processes, such as synaptic transmission and

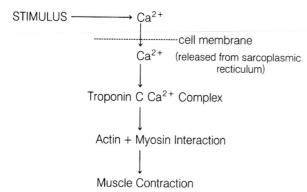

STIMULUS ⟶ Ca^{2+}

--------------cell membrane

Ca^{2+} (released from sarcoplasmic recticulum)

Troponin C Ca^{2+} Complex

Actin + Myosin Interaction

Muscle Contraction

Figure 19–5 ■ Sequence of events showing excitation–contraction coupling in cardiac muscle.

muscle contraction. The role of calcium in these cellular functions is as a second messenger, for example, regulating enzymes and ion channels. The entry of extracellular Ca^{2+} into the cytosol of myocardial cells and the release of Ca^{2+} from intracellular storage sites is important for initiating contractions of the myocardium. Normally, the concentration of Ca^{2+} in the extracellular fluid is in the millimolar range, whereas the intracellular concentration of free Ca^{2+} is less than 10^{-7} M, even though the total cellular concentration may be 10^{-3} M or higher. Most of the Ca^{2+} is stored within intracellular organelles or tightly bound to intracellular proteins. The free Ca^{2+} needed to satisfy the requirements of a contraction resulting from a stimulus may result from activation of calcium channels on the cell membrane and/or the release of calcium from bound internal stores. Each of these methods of increasing free cytosolic Ca^{2+} involves channels that are selective for the calcium ion. Calcium channel blockers reduce or prevent the increase of free cytosolic calcium ions by interfering with the transport of calcium ions through these pores.

Calcium is one of the most common elements on earth. Most calcium involved in biological systems occurs as hydroxyapatite, a static, stabilizing structure like that found in bone. The remaining calcium is ionic (Ca^{2+}). Ionic calcium functions as a biochemical regulator, more often within the cell. The importance of calcium ions to physiological functions was realized first by Ringer, who observed in 1883 the role of Ca^{2+} in cardiac contractility.

The ionic composition of the cytosol in excitable cells, including cardiac and smooth muscle cells, is controlled to a large extent by the plasma membrane, which prevents the free movement of ions across this barrier. Present in the membranes are ion-carrying channels that open in response to either a change in membrane potential or binding of a ligand. Calcium-sensitive channels include *(a)* Na^+ to Ca^{2+} exchanger, which transports three Na^+ ions in return for one Ca^{2+}; *(b)* a voltage-dependent Ca^{2+} channel, which provides the route for entry of Ca^{2+} for excitation and contraction in cardiac and smooth muscle cells and is the focus of the channel-blocking agents used in medicine; and *(c)* receptor-operated Ca^{2+} channels mediated by ligand binding to membrane receptors as in the action of epinephrine on the α-adrenergic receptor. The membrane of the sarcolemma within the cell also has ion-conducting channels that facili-

tate movement of Ca^{2+} ions from storage loci in the sarcoplasmic reticulum.

Four types of calcium channels, differing in location and function, have been identified: *(a)* L type, located in skeletal, cardiac, and smooth muscles, causing contraction of muscle cells; *(b)* T type, found in pacemaker cells, causing Ca^{2+} entry, inactivated at more negative potentials and more rapidly than the L type; *(c)* N type, found in neurons and acting in transmitter release; and *(d)* P type, located in Purkinje cells but whose function is unknown at this time.

Calcium antagonists act only on the L-type channel to produce their pharmacological effects. The L channels are so called because once the membrane has been depolarized, their action is long lasting. Once the membrane has been depolarized, L channels must be phosphorylated to open. Although there are similarities between L-type calcium channels that exist in cardiac and smooth muscle, there are distinct differences between the two. Cardiac L channels are activated through β-adrenergic stimulation via a cAMP-dependent phosphorylation process,[11] while L channels in smooth muscle may be regulated by the inositol phosphate system linked to G-protein–coupled, receptor-linked phospholipase C activation.[12]

CALCIUM CHANNEL BLOCKERS

The L-type calcium channel, acted on by calcium channel blockers, consists of five different subunits, designated α_1, α_2, β, γ, and δ. The α_1 subunit provides the central pore of the channel (Fig. 19-6). Calcium channel blockers can be divided conveniently into the three different chemical classes of the prototype drugs that have been used: phenylalkylamines (verapamil), 1,4-dihydropyridines (nifedipine), and benzothiazepines (diltiazem). These prototype compounds sometimes are termed the "first generation" of calcium channel blockers because two of the groups of drug classes have been expanded by the introduction of a "second" generation of more potent analogues (Table 19-3).

The specific Ca^{2+} channel antagonists verapamil, nifedipine, and diltiazem interact at specific sites on the calcium channel protein. These blockers do not occlude the channel physically but bind to sites in the channel, as they can promote both channel activation and antagonism. Affinity for binding sites on the channel varies, depending on the status of the channel. The channel can exist in either an open (O), resting (R), or inactivated (I) state, and the equilibrium between them is determined by stimulus frequency and mem-

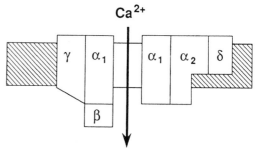

Ca^{2+}

Figure 19–6 ■ Schematic representation of an L-type Ca^{2+} channel.

TABLE 19-3 First- and Second-Generation Calcium Channel Blockers

Chemical Classification	First Generation	Second Generation
Phenylalkylamines	Verapamil	Anipamil
		Bepridil
1,4-Dihydropyridine	Nifedipine	Amlodipine
		Felodipine
		Isradipine
		Nicardipine
		Nimodipine
Benzothiazepine	Diltiazem	—

brane potential (Fig. 19-7). Verapamil and diltiazem do not bind to a channel in the resting state, only after the channel has been opened. They are ionized, water-soluble Ca^{2+}-entry blockers that reach their binding sites by the hydrophilic pathway when the channel is open. Verapamil and diltiazem are use dependent (i.e., their Ca^{2+}-blocking activity is a function of the frequency of contractions). An increase in contraction frequency causes a reduction, rather than an augmentation, of contractions. Nifedipine is a neutral molecule at physiological pH and can cause interference with the Ca^{2+} in the open or closed state. In the closed state, nifedipine can traverse the phospholipid bilayer to reach its binding site because of its lipid solubility.

CARDIOVASCULAR EFFECTS OF CALCIUM ION CHANNEL BLOCKERS

All Ca^{2+} antagonists yet developed are vasodilators. Vasodilation is due to the uncoupling of the contractile mechanism of vascular smooth muscle, which requires Ca^{2+}. Coronary artery muscle tone is reduced in healthy humans but is particularly pronounced in a condition of coronary spasm. Peripheral arteriole resistance is reduced more than venous beds. The vasodilatory effect of these drugs is the basis for their use in the control of angina and hypertension.[13]

Although verapamil, nifedipine, and diltiazem can cause vasodilation, they are not equally effective at blocking the Ca^{2+} channels found in various tissues. The phenylalkylamine verapamil and the benzothiazepine diltiazem have both cardiac and vascular actions. These drugs have antiar-

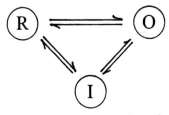

Figure 19-7 ■ Schematic representation of an ion channel existing in an equilibrium of resting (*R*), open (*O*), and inactivated (*I*) states.

rhythmic, antianginal, and antihypertensive activity. They depress the cardiac neural network, and so slow sinus node automaticity, prolong atrioventricular (AV) nodal conductance, and depress myocardial contractility, as well as reduce peripheral vascular resistance to prevent a coronary vascular spasm. Nifedipine and other 1,4-dihydropyridines are more effective at causing vasodilation than affecting pacemaker and tension responses in the heart. This is especially important because selectivity occurs as a consequence of disease states. Hypertensive smooth muscle is more sensitive to Ca^{2+} channel blockers than is normotensive tissue.[14] This makes verapamil and diltiazem more useful in ischemic conditions, as they have a more profound effect on cardiac muscle calcium channels.[15]

The inhibition of Ca^{2+} influx into cardiac tissue by Ca^{2+} antagonists is also the basis for the use of these drugs as antiarrhythmic agents. The Ca^{2+} channel blockers dampen Ca^{2+}-dependent automaticity in the regular pacemaker cells in the sinoatrial (SA) node and depress the origination of ectopic foci. Calcium antagonists can block reentry pathways in myocardial tissue, an integral component of arrhythmias. Numerous side effects in the heart, such as bradycardia, decreased cardiac contractility, and reduced AV conductance, are traced to Ca^{2+} channel–blocking activity.

PRODUCTS

Verapamil. Verapamil, 5-[3,4-dimethoxyphenethyl)-methylamino]-2-(3,4-dimethoxyphenyl)-2-isopropylvaleronitrile (Calan, Isoptin), was introduced in 1962 as a coronary vasodilator and is the prototype of the Ca^{2+} antagonists used in cardiovascular diseases. It is used in the treatment of angina pectoris, arrhythmias from ischemic myocardial syndromes, and supraventricular arrhythmias.

Verapamil's major effect is on the slow Ca^{2+} channel. The result is a slowing of AV conduction and the sinus rate. This inhibition of the action potential inhibits one limb of the reentry circuit believed to underlie most paroxysmal supraventricular tachycardias that use the AV node as a reentry point. It is categorized as a class IV antiarrhythmic drug (see "Classes of Antiarrhythmic Drugs" below). Hemodynamically, verapamil causes a change in the preload, afterload, contractility, heart rate, and coronary blood flow. The drug reduces systemic vascular resistance and mean blood pressure, with minor effects on cardiac output.

Verapamil is a synthetic compound possessing slight structural similarity to papaverine. It can be separated into its optically active isomers, of which the levorotatory enantiomer is the most potent. It is absorbed rapidly after oral administration. The drug is metabolized quickly and, as a result, has low bioavailability. The liver is the main site of first-pass metabolism, forming several products. The preferential metabolic step involves N-dealkylation, followed by O-demethylation, and subsequent conjugation of the product before elimination. The metabolites have no significant biological activity. Verapamil has an elimination half-life of approximately 5 hours.

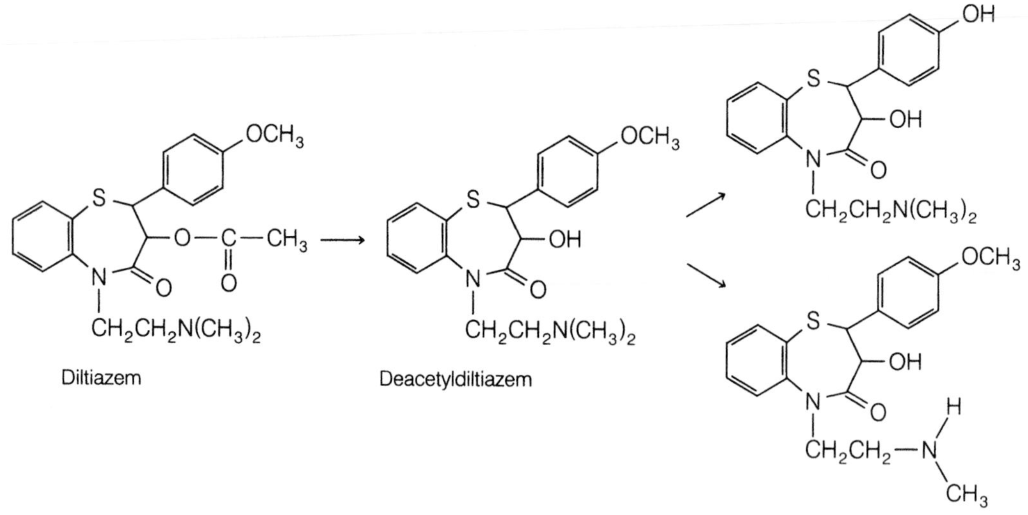

Figure 19–8 ■ Biotransformations of diltiazem.

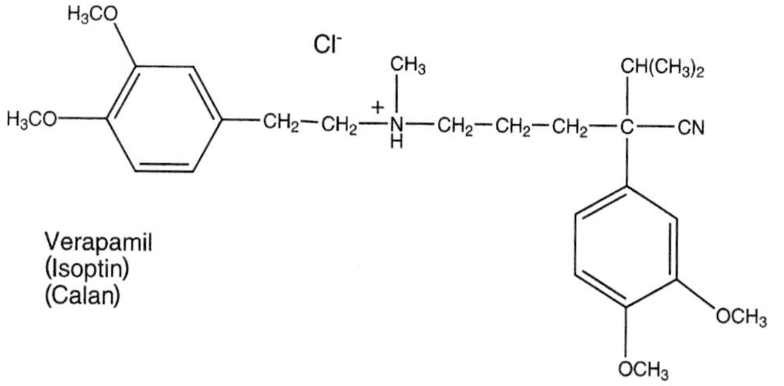

The route traveled by a Ca^{2+} channel blocker, such as verapamil, to its receptor site parallels that observed with many local anesthetic-like antiarrhythmic agents. It is believed that verapamil, like most of the Ca^{2+} channel blockers, crosses the cell membrane in an uncharged form to gain access to its site of action on the intracellular side of the membrane. Data show a greater affinity of verapamil and other Ca^{2+} channel blockers to the inactivated state of the channel.[16]

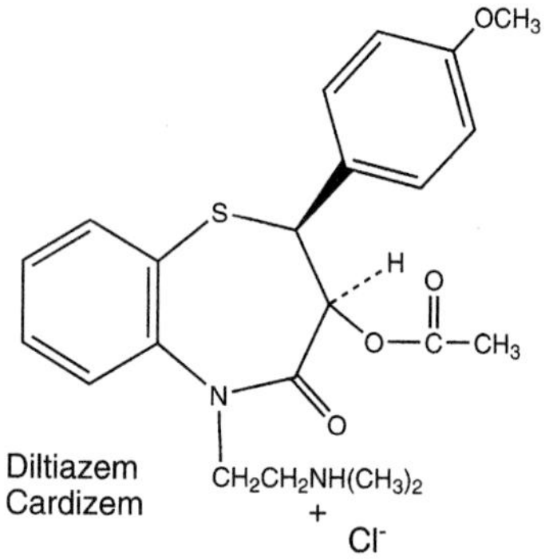

Diltiazem Hydrochloride. Diltiazem hydrochloride, (+)-*cis*-3-(acetoxy)-5-[2(dimethylamino)ethyl]-2,3-dihydro-2-(4-methoxyphenyl)1,5-benzothiazepin-4(5*H*)one hydrochloride (Cardizem), was developed and introduced in Japan as a cardiovascular agent to treat angina pectoris. It was observed to dilate peripheral arteries and arterioles. The drug increases myocardial oxygen supply by relieving coronary artery spasm and reduces myocardial oxygen demand by decreasing heart rate and reducing overload. Diltiazem hydrochloride is used in patients with variant angina. The drug has electrophysiological properties similar to those of verapamil and is used in clinically similar treatment conditions as an antiarrhythmic agent, but it is less potent.

The drug is absorbed rapidly and almost completely from the digestive tract. It reaches peak plasma levels within 1 hour after administration in gelatin capsules. Oral formulations on the market are sustained-release preparations providing peak plasma levels 3 to 4 hours after administration.

Diltiazem hydrochloride is metabolized extensively after oral dosing, by first-pass metabolism. As a result, the bioavailability is about 40% of the administered dose. The drug undergoes several biotransformations, including deacetylation, oxidative O- and N-demethylations, and conjugation of the phenolic metabolites. Of the various metabolites (Fig. 19-8), only the primary metabolite, deacetyldiltiazem, is pharmacologically active. Deacetyldiltiazem has about 40 to 50% of the potency of the parent compound.

Nifedipine. Nifedipine, 1,4-dihydro-2, 6-dimethyl-4-(2-nitrophenyl)-3,5-pyridinedicarboxylate dimethyl ester (Adalat, Procardia), is a dihydropyridine derivative that bears no structural resemblance to the other calcium antagonists. It is not a nitrate, but its nitro group is essential for its antianginal effect.[17] As a class, the dihydropyridines possess a central pyridine ring that is partially saturated. To this, positions 2 and 6 are substituted with an alkyl group that may play a role in the agent's duration of action. Also, position 3 and 4 are carboxylic groups that must be protected with an ester functional group. Depending on the type of ester used at these sites, the agent can be distributed to various parts of the body. Finally, position 4 requires an aromatic substitution possessing an electron-withdrawing group (i.e., Cl or NO_2) in the *ortho* and/or *meta* position.

The prototype of this class, nifedipine, has potent peripheral vasodilatory properties. It inhibits the voltage-dependent calcium channel in the vascular smooth muscle but has little or no direct depressant effect on the SA or AV nodes, even though it inhibits calcium current in normal and isolated

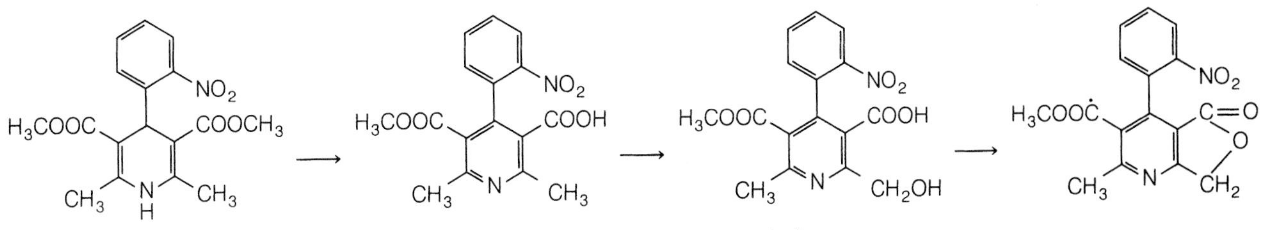

Figure 19-9 ■ Nifedipine metabolism.

cardiac tissues. Nifedipine is more effective in patients whose anginal episodes are due to coronary vasospasm and is used in the treatment of vasospastic angina as well as classic angina pectoris. Because of its strong vasodilatory properties, it is used in selected patients to treat hypertension.

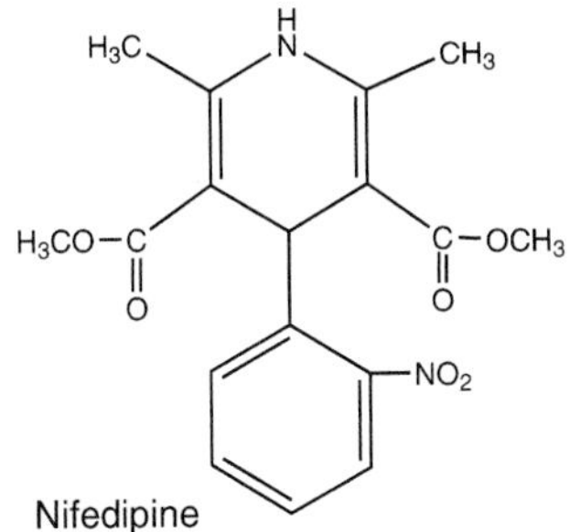

Nifedipine
(Procardia)
(Adalat)

Nifedipine is absorbed efficiently on oral or buccal administration. A substantial amount (90%) is protein bound. Systemic availability of an oral dose of the drug may be approximately 65%. Two inactive metabolites are the major products of nifedipine metabolism and are found in equilibrium with each other (Fig. 19-9). Only a trace of unchanged nifedipine is found in the urine.[18]

Amlodipine. Amlodipine, 2-[(2-aminoethoxy)methyl]-4-(2-chlorophenyl)-1,4-dihydro-6-methyl-3,5-pyridinedicarboxylic acid 3-ethyl 5-methyl ester (Norvasc), is a second-generation 1,4-dihyropyridine derivative of the prototypical molecule nifedipine. Like most of the second-generation dihydropyridine derivatives, it has greater selectivity for the vascular smooth muscle than myocardial tissue, a longer half-life (34 hours), and less negative inotropy than the prototypical nifedipine. Amlodipine is used in the treatment of chronic stable angina and in the management of mild-to-moderate essential hypertension. It is marketed as the benzene sulfonic acid salt (besylate).

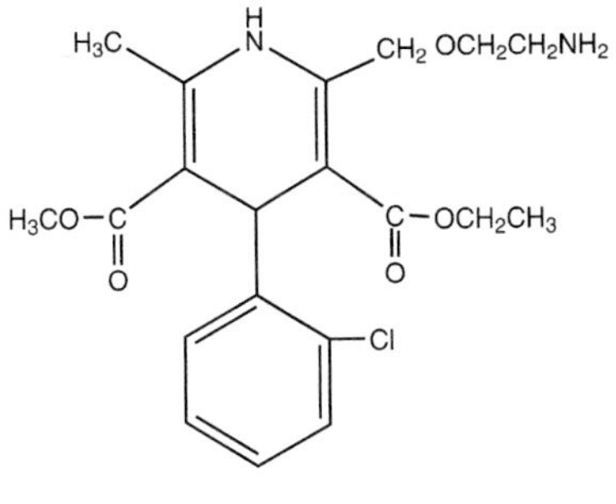

Amlodipine
(Norvasc)

Felodipine. Felodipine, 3,5-pyridinedicarboxylic acid, 4-(2,3-dichlorophenyl)1,4-dihydro-2,6-dimethyl-, ethyl methyl ester (Plendil), is a second-generation dihydropyridine channel blocker of the nifedipine type. It is more selective for vascular smooth muscle than for myocardial tissue and serves as an effective vasodilator. The drug is used in the treatment of angina and mild-to-moderate essential hypertension. Felodipine, like most of the dihydropyridines, exhibits a high degree of protein binding and has a half-life ranging from 10 to 18 hours.

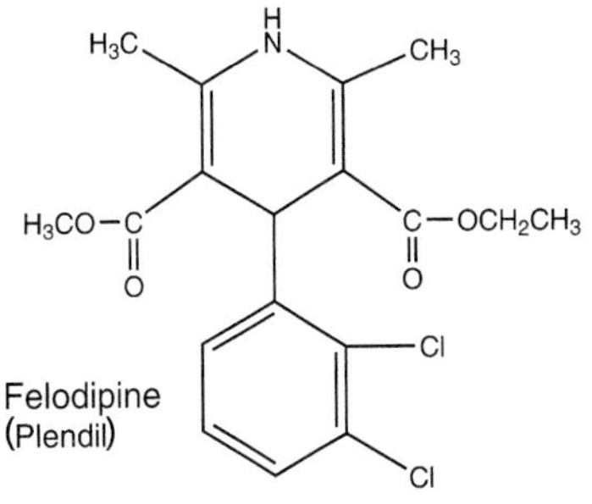

Felodipine
(Plendil)

Isradipine. Isradipine, 4-(4-benzofuranazyl)-1,4-dihydro-2,6-dimethyl-3,5-pyridinecarboxylic acid methyl 1-methylethyl ester (DynaCirc), is another second-generation dihydropyridine-type channel blocker. This drug, like the other second-generation analogues, is more selective for vascular smooth muscle than for myocardial tissue. It is effective in the treatment of stable angina, reducing the frequency of anginal attacks and the need to use nitroglycerin.

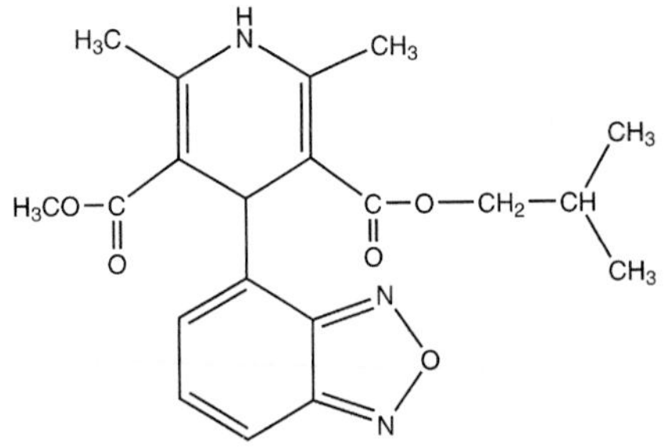

Isradipine
(DynaCirc)

Nicardipine Hydrochloride. Nicardipine hydrochloride, 1,4-dihydro-2,6-dimethyl-4-(3-nitrophenyl)-3,5-pyridinedicarboxylic acid methyl 2-[methyl(phenylmethyl)amino]ethyl ester hydrochloride (Cardene), is a more potent vasodilator of the systemic, coronary, cerebral, and renal vasculature and has been used in the treatment of mild, moderate, and severe hypertension. The drug is also used in the management of stable angina.

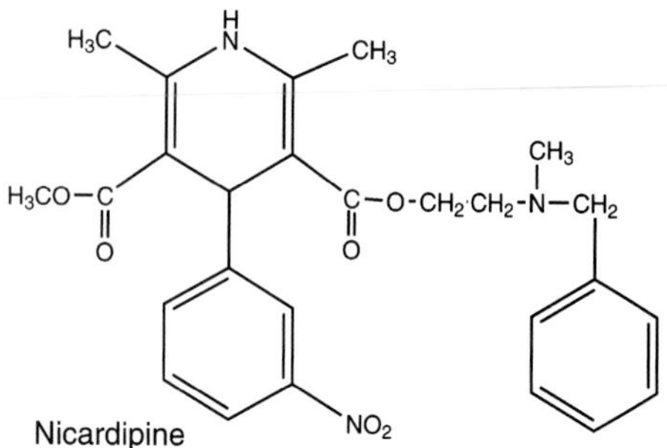

Nicardipine
(Cardene)

Nimodipine. Nimodipine, 1,4-dihydro-2,6-dimethyl-4-(3-nitrophenyl)- 3,5-pyridinedicarboxylic acid 2-methoxyethyl 1-methylethyl ester (Nimotop), is another dihydropyridine calcium channel blocker but differs in that it dilates the cerebral blood vessels more effectively than do the other dihydropyridine derivatives. This drug is indicated for treatment of subarachnoid hemorrhage-associated neurological deficits.

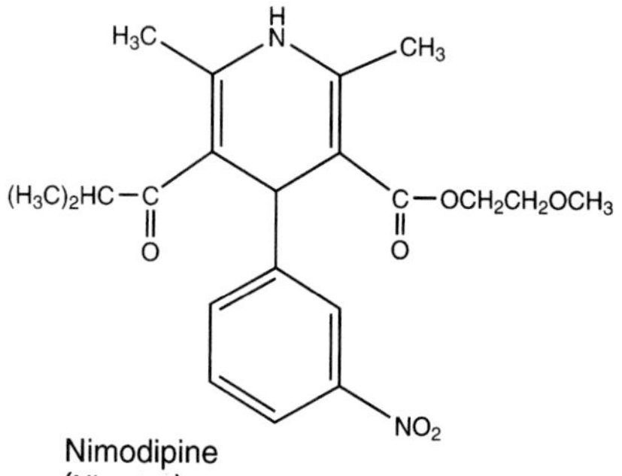

Nimodipine
(Nimotop)

Nisoldipine. In vitro studies show that the effects of nisoldipine, 1,4-dihydro-2, 6-dimethyl-4-(3-nitrophenyl)-3,5-pyridinecarboxylic acid methyl 2-methylpropyl ester (Sular), on contractile processes are selective, with greater potency on vascular smooth muscle than on cardiac muscle.

Nisoldipine is highly metabolized, with five major metabolites identified. As with most of the dihydropyridines, the cytochrome P-450 (CYP) 3A4 isozyme is mainly responsible for the metabolism of nisoldipine. The major biotransformation pathway appears to involve the hydroxylation of the isobutyl ester side chain. This particular metabolite has approximately 10% of the activity of the parent compound.

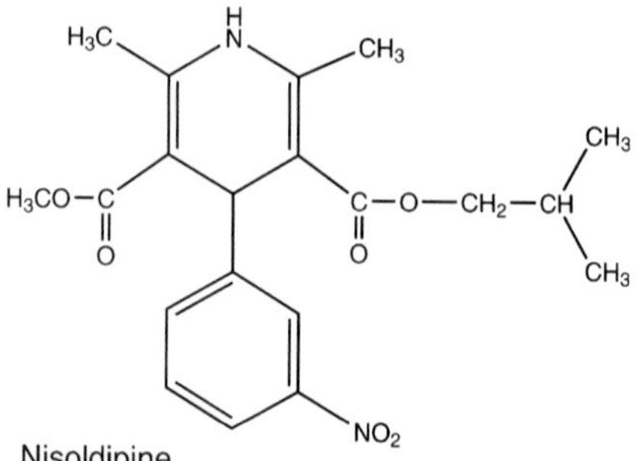

Nisoldipine
(Sular)

Nitrendipine. Nitrendipine, 1,4-dihydro-2,6-dimethyl-4-(3-nitrophenyl)-3,5-pyridinecarboxylic acid methyl ethyl

ester (Baypress), is a second-generation dihydropyridine channel blocker of the nifedipine type. It is more selective for vascular smooth muscle than for myocardial tissue and serves as an effective vasodilator. The drug is used in the treatment of mild-to-moderate essential hypertension.

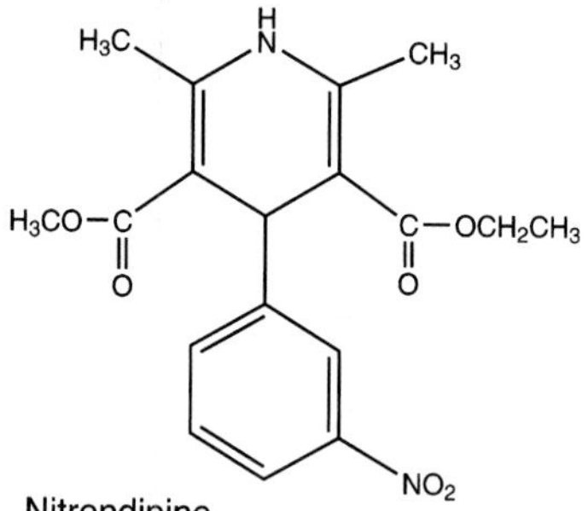

Nitrendipine
(Baypress)

Bepridil Hydrochloride. Bepridil hydrochloride, β-[(2-methylpropoxy)methyl]-*N*-phenyl-*N*-(phenylmethyl)-1-pyrrolidineethylamine hydrochloride (Vascor), is a second-generation alkylamine-type channel blocker, structurally unrelated to the dihydropyridines. Its actions are less specific than those of the three prototypical channel blockers, verapamil, diltiazem, and nifedipine. In addition to being a Ca^{2+} channel blocker, it inhibits sodium flow into the heart tissue and lengthens cardiac repolarization, causing bradycardia. Caution should be used if it is given to a patient with hypokalemia. Bepridil hydrochloride is used for stable angina. The drug has a half-life of 33 hours and is highly bound to protein (99%).

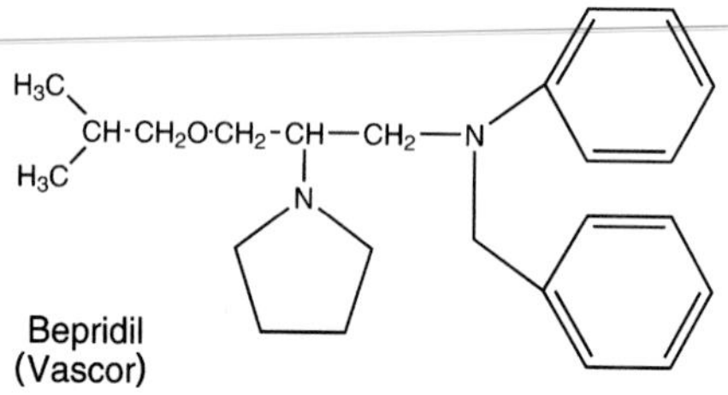

Bepridil
(Vascor)

Antithrombotic Agents

Platelet activation and platelet aggregation play an important role in the pathogenesis of thromboses. These, in turn, play an important role in unstable angina, myocardial infarction, stroke, and peripheral vascular thromboses. Since many cardiovascular diseases are associated with platelet activation, many agents possessing antiplatelet or antithrombotic effects have been investigated. This has revolutionized cardiovascular medicine, in which vascular stenting or angioplasty can be used without compromising normal hemostasis or wound healing. Although most of these agents act by different mechanisms, many of the newer agents are being developed to antagonize the GPIIb/IIIa receptors of platelets.

Aspirin. Aspirin, acetylsalicylic acid, has an inhibitory effect on platelet aggregation not only because of its ability to inhibit cyclooxygenase but also because of its ability to acetylate the enzyme. Aspirin irreversibly inhibits cyclooxygenase (COX) (prostaglandin H synthase), which is the enzyme involved in converting arachidonate to prostaglandin

G_2 and ultimately thromboxane 2, an inducer of platelet aggregation. Aspirin's mechanism of action includes not only the inhibition in the biosynthesis of thromboxane 2, but also its ability to acetylate the serine residue (529) in the polypeptide chain of platelet prostaglandin H synthetase-1. This explains why other nonsteroidal anti-inflammatory agents that are capable of inhibiting the COX enzyme do not act as antithrombotics—they aren't capable of acetylating this enzyme. Since platelets cannot synthesize new enzymes, aspirin's ability to acetylate COX lasts for the life of the platelet (7 to 10 days) and is, thus, irreversible.

Aspirin

Dipyridamole. Dipyridamole, 2,2′,2″,2‴-[(4,8-di-1-piperidinylpyrimido[5,4-*d*]pyrimidine-2,6-diyl)dinitrilo]-tetrakisethanol (Persantine), may be used for coronary and myocardial insufficiency. Its biggest use today, however, is as an antithrombotic in patients with prosthetic heart valves. It is a bitter, yellow, crystalline powder, soluble in dilute acids, methanol, or chloroform. A formulation containing dipyridamole and aspirin (Aggrenox) is currently being marketed as an antithromobotic.

Dipyridamole is a long-acting vasodilator. Its vasodilating action is selective for the coronary system; it is indicated for long-term therapy of chronic angina pectoris. The drug also inhibits adenosine deaminase in erythrocytes and interferes with the uptake of the vasodilator adenosine by erythrocytes. These actions potentiate the effect of prostacyclin (PGI_2), which acts as an inhibitor to platelet aggregation.

Dipyridamole
(Persantine
with ASA Aggrenox)

Clopidrogel. Clopidrogel, methyl (+)-(*S*)-α-(2-chlorophenyl)-6,7-dihydrothieno[3,2-c] pyridine-5(4H)-acetate . sulfate (Plavix), is useful for the preventative management of secondary ischemic events, including myocardial infarction, stroke, and vascular deaths. It may be classified as a thienopyridine because of its heterocyclic system. Several agents

possessing this system have been evaluated as potential antithrombotic agents. These agents have a unique mechanism, in that they inhibit the purinergic receptor located on platelets. Normally, nucleotides act as agonists on these receptors, which include the P2Y type. Two P2Y receptor subtypes (P2Y1 and P2Y2) found on platelets, when stimulated by ADP, cause platelet aggregation. Clopidrogel acts as an antagonist to the P2Y2 receptor. It is probably a prodrug that requires metabolic activation, since in vitro studies do not interfere with platelet aggregation. Although platelet aggregation is not normally seen in the first 8 to 11 days after administration to a patient, the effect lasts for several days after the drug therapy is discontinued. Unlike other thienopyridines currently used, clopidrogel does not seriously reduce the number of white cells in the blood, and therefore, routine monitoring of the white blood cell count is not necessary during treatment.

Clopidrogel
(Plavix)

Ticlopidine. Ticlopidine, 5-[(2-chlorophenyl)methyl]-4,5,6,7-tetrahydrothieno [3,2-c]pyridine hydrochloride (Ticlid), is useful in reducing cardiac events in patients with unstable angina and cerebrovascular events in secondary prevention of stroke. It belongs to the thienopyridine class and facilitated the development of clopidrogel. One of the drawbacks to this agent is its side effect profile, which includes neutropenia, and patients receiving this antithrombotic should have their blood levels monitored. Its mechanism of action is similar to that of clopidrogel, in that it inhibits the purinergic receptors on platelets.

Ticlopidine
(Ticlid)

GPIIB/IIIA RECEPTORS

Located on platelets is a site that serves to recognize and bind fibrinogen. This site is a dimeric glycoprotein that allows fibrinogen to bind, leading to the final step of platelet aggregation. The receptor must be activated before it will associate with fibrinogen, and this may be accomplished by thrombin, collagen, or thromboxane A_2. Once the receptor is activated, fibrinogen most likely binds to the platelet through the arginine-glycine-aspartic acid (RGD) sequences at residues 95-96-97 and 572-573-574 of the α chain of fibrinogen. This particular feature has been used in the design of nonpeptide

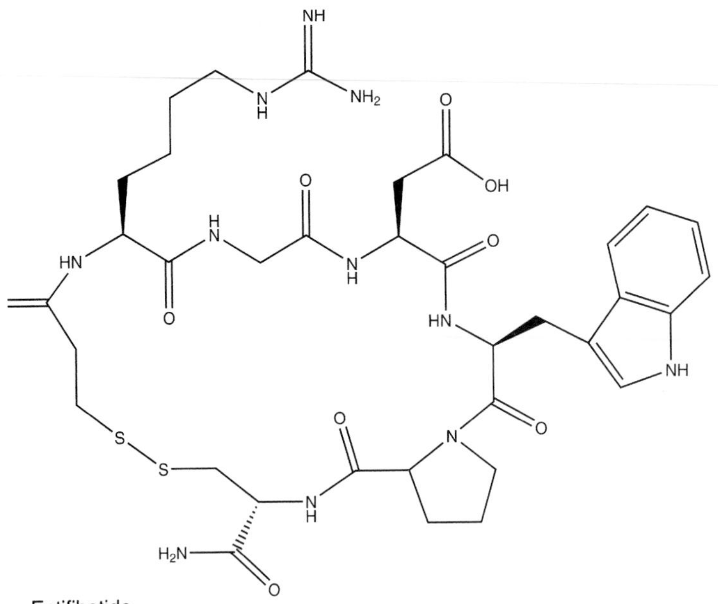

Eptifibatide
(Integrilin)

antagonists that mimic the RGD system in which a distance of 15 to 17Å (16 to 18 atoms) separates the amine group of arginine and the carbonyl oxygen of aspartic acid.

Eptifibatide.   Eptifibatide (Integrilin) is a synthetic cyclic heptapeptide that acts as a GPIIb/IIIa receptor antagonist, thus causing inhibition of platelet aggregation. Its structure is based on the natural product barbourin, a peptide isolated from the venom of a pygmy rattlesnake *(Sistrurus milarud barbouri)*. As part of the structure, there is a sequence arginine-glycine-aspartic acid (RGD) that can bind to the RGD receptor found on platelets and block its ability to bind with fibrinogen. This agent is used in the treatment of unstable angina and for angioplastic coronary interventions.

Tirofiban.   Tirofiban is a nonpeptide that appears unrelated chemically to eptifibatide, but actually has many similarities. The chemical architecture incorporates a system that is mimicking the arginine-glycine-aspartic acid (RGD) moiety that is present in eptifibatide. This can be seen in the distance between the nitrogen of the piperidine ring, which mimics the basic nitrogen of arginine in the RGD sequence, and the carboxylic acid, which mimics the acid of aspartate in the RGD sequence. The basic nitrogen and the carboxylic acid of tirofiban are separated by approximately 15 to 17Å (16 to 18 atoms). This is the optimum distance seen in the RGD sequence of the platelet receptor. Tirofiban is useful in treating non–Q wave myocardial infarction and unstable angina.

Abciximab.   Abciximab (ReoPro) is a chimeric Fab fragment monoclonal antibody that can bind to the GPIIa/IIIb receptor of platelets and block the ability of fibrinogen to associate with the platelet. This results in less platelet aggregation. Abciximab is useful in treating unstable angina and as an adjunct to percutaneous coronary intervention (PCI). The half-life of abciximab is about 30 minutes, while its effects when bound to the GPIIa/IIIb may last up to 24 hours. A significant drawback to using abciximab lies in its cost, which is approximately $1,500 for a single dose.

ANTIARRHYTHMIC DRUGS

Cardiac arrhythmias are caused by a disturbance in the conduction of the impulse through the myocardial tissue, by disorders of impulse formation, or by a combination of these factors. The antiarrhythmic agents used most commonly affect impulse conduction by altering conduction velocity and the duration of the refractory period of heart muscle tissue. They also depress spontaneous diastolic depolarization, causing a reduction of automaticity by ectopic foci.

Many pharmacological agents are available for the treatment of cardiac arrhythmias. Agents such as oxygen, potassium, and sodium bicarbonate relieve the underlying cause of some arrhythmias. Other agents, such as digitalis, propranolol, phenylephrine, edrophonium, and neostigmine, act

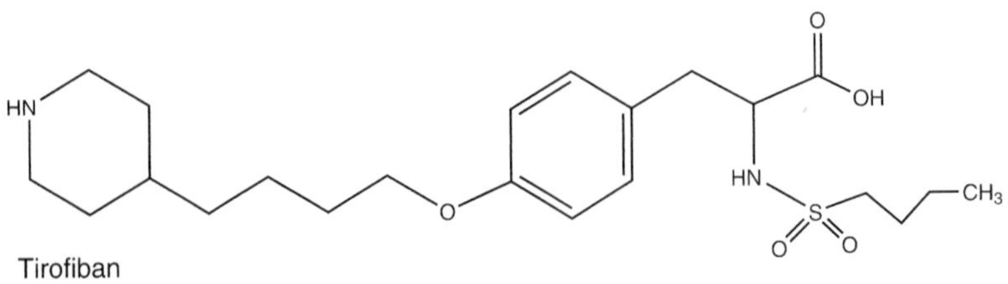

Tirofiban
(Aggrastat)

on the cardiovascular system by affecting heart muscle or on the autonomic nerves to the heart. Finally, there are drugs that alter the electrophysiological mechanisms causing arrhythmias. The latter group of drugs is discussed in this chapter.

Within the past five decades, research on normal cardiac tissues and, in the clinical setting, on patients with disturbances of rhythm and conduction has brought to light information on the genesis of cardiac arrhythmias and the mode of action of antiarrhythmic agents. In addition, laboratory tests have been developed to measure blood levels of antiarrhythmic drugs such as phenytoin, disopyramide, lidocaine, procainamide, and quinidine, to help evaluate the pharmacokinetics of these agents. As a result, it is possible to maintain steady-state plasma levels of these drugs, which allows the clinician to use these and other agents more effectively and with greater safety. No other clinical intervention has been more effective at reducing mortality and morbidity in coronary care units.

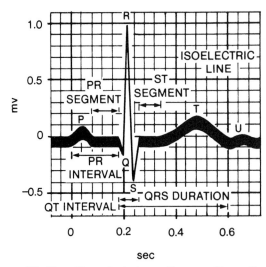

Figure 19-10 ■ Normal electrocardiogram. (From Ganong, W. F.: Review of Medical Physiology, 9th ed. San Francisco, Lange Medical Publications, 1985.)

Cardiac Electrophysiology

The heart depends on the synchronous integration of electrical impulse transmission and myocardial tissue response to carry out its function as a pump. When the impulse is released from the SA node, excitation of the heart tissue takes place in an orderly manner by a spread of the impulse throughout the specialized automatic fibers in the atria, the AV node, and the Purkinje fiber network in the ventricles. This spreading of impulses produces a characteristic electrocardiographic pattern that can be equated to predictable myocardial cell membrane potentials and Na^+ and K^+ fluxes in and out of the cell.

A single fiber in the ventricle of an intact heart during the diastolic phase (see phase 4, Fig. 19-4) has a membrane potential (resting potential) of 90 mV. This potential is created by differential concentrations of K^+ and Na^+ in the intracellular and extracellular fluid. An active transport system (pump) on the membrane is responsible for concentrating the K^+ inside the cell and maintaining higher concentrations of Na^+ in the extracellular fluid. Diastolic depolarization is caused by a decreased K^+ ionic current into the extracellular tissue and a slow inward leakage of Na^+ until the threshold potential (60 to 55 mV) is reached. At this time the inward sodium current suddenly increases, and a self-propagated wave occurs to complete the membrane depolarization process. Pacemaker cells possess this property, which is termed *automaticity*. This maximal rate of depolarization (MRD) is represented by phase 0 or the spike action potential (Fig. 19-4).

The form, duration, resting potential level, and amplitude of the action potential are characteristic for different types of myocardial cells. The rate of rise of the response (phase 0) is related to the level of the membrane potential at the time of stimulation and has been termed *membrane responsiveness*. Less negative potentials produce smaller slopes of phase 0 and are characterized by slower conduction times. The phase 0 spike of the SA node corresponds to the inscription of the P wave on the electrocardiogram (Fig. 19-10). Repolarization is divided into three phases. The greatest amount of repolarization is represented by phase 3, in which there is a passive flux of K^+ ions out of the cell. Phase 1

repolarization is caused by an influx of Cl^- ions. During phase 2, a small inward movement of Ca^{2+} ions occurs through a slow channel mechanism that is believed to be important in the process of coupling excitation with contraction. The process of repolarization determines the duration of the action potential and is represented by the QT interval. The action potential duration is directly related to the refractory period of cardiac muscle.

Mechanisms of Arrhythmias

The current understanding of the electrophysiological mechanisms responsible for the origin and perpetuation of cardiac arrhythmias is that they are due to altered impulse formation (i.e., change in automaticity), altered conduction, or both, acting simultaneously from different locations of the heart. The generation of cardiac impulses in the normal heart is usually confined to specialized tissues that spontaneously depolarize and initiate the action potential. These cells are located in the right atrium and are referred to as the *SA node* or the *pacemaker cells*. Although the spontaneous electrical depolarization of the SA pacemaker cells is independent of the nervous system, these cells are innervated by both sympathetic and parasympathetic fibers, which may cause an increase or decrease of the heart rate, respectively. Other special cells in the normal heart that possess the property of automaticity may influence cardiac rhythm when the normal pacemaker is suppressed or when pathological changes occur in the myocardium to make these cells the dominant source of cardiac rhythm (i.e., ectopic pacemakers). Automaticity of subsidiary pacemakers may develop when myocardial cell damage occurs because of infarction or from digitalis toxicity, excessive vagal tone, excessive catecholamine release from sympathomimetic nerve fibers to the heart, or even high catecholamine levels in plasma. The development of automaticity in specialized cells, such as that found in special atrial cells, certain AV node cells, bundle of His, and Purkinje fibers, may lead to cardiac arrhythmias. Because production of ectopic impulses is often due to a

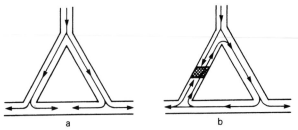

Figure 19–11 ■ Reentry mechanism of Purkinje fibers. **a.** Normal conduction of impulses through triangular arrangement of cardiac fibers. **b.** Unidirectional block on left arm of triangular section allows impulse to reenter the regional conducting system and recycle.

defect in the spontaneous phase 4 diastolic depolarization ("T wave"), drugs that can suppress this portion of the cardiac stimulation cycle are effective agents for these types of arrhythmia.

Arrhythmias are also caused by disorders in the conduction of impulses and changes in the refractory period of the myocardial tissue. Pharmacological intervention is based on these two properties. The Purkinje fibers branch into a network of interlacing fibers, particularly at their most distant positions. This creates several pathways in which a unidirectional block in a localized area may establish circular (circus) microcellular or macrocellular impulse movements that reenter the myocardial fibers and create an arrhythmia (Fig. 19-11). Unidirectional block results from localized myocardial disease *(infarcts)* or from a change in dependence of the tissue to Na^+ fluxes that causes a longer conduction time and allows the tissue to repolarize to propagate the retrograde impulse.

Classes of Antiarrhythmic Drugs

Antiarrhythmic drugs can be placed into four separate classes, based on their mechanism of action or pattern of electrophysiological effects produced on heart tissue. Table 19-4 summarizes the four-part classification of antiarrhythmic drugs as first proposed by Vaughan Williams in 1970[19] and expanded in 1984.[20] Note that drugs within the same

TABLE 19–4 Classes of Antiarrhythmic Drugs

Class	Drugs	Mechanism of Action
IA	Quinidine, procainamide, disopyramide	Lengthens refractory period
IB	Lidocaine, phenytoin, tocainide, mexiletine	Shortens duration of action potential
IC	Encainide, flecainide, lorcainide, moricizine, propafenone	Slows conduction
II	β-Adrenergic blockers (e.g., propranolol)	Slows AV conduction time, suppresses automaticity
III	Amiodarone, bretylium, sotalol	Prolongs refractoriness
IV	Calcium channel blockers (e.g., verapamil, diltiazem)	Blocks slow inward Ca^{2+} channel

category are placed there because they demonstrate similar clinical actions. That patients do not respond to a drug in this class, however, should not rule out use of other drugs in the same class.[21] Despite the well-intentioned use of these agents, most antiarrhythmic drugs have the potential to aggravate the arrhythmia they treat *(proarrhythmia)*. Proarrhythmia develops from an increase in the density of single ectopic beats and is more likely to occur in patients who have a dysfunction in the left ventricle or sustained ventricular tachycardia. Class I antiarrhythmic agents (see below) are especially proarrhythmic in myocardial infarction patients.

CLASS I. MEMBRANE-DEPRESSANT DRUGS

Class I antiarrhythmic agents are drugs that have membrane-stabilizing properties (i.e., they shift membranes to more negative potentials). Drugs in this class act on the fast Na^+ channels and interfere with the process by which the depolarizing charge is transferred across the membrane. It is assumed that these drugs bind to the Na^+ channel and block its function, preventing Na^+ conductance as long as the drug is bound. The prototypical drugs in this class are quinidine and procainamide. During the 1970s, several drugs were studied for their antiarrhythmic effects. Most of them were local anesthetics that affected Na^+ membrane channels, and they were grouped in a single class (class I). Studies on the antiarrhythmic properties of these chemicals have shown that there are sufficient differences to place them into separate subgroups.[21]

Class I antiarrhythmic drugs can be subdivided on the basis of the relative ease with which they dissociate from the Na^+ ion channel. Drugs in class IC, such as encainide, lorcainide and moricizine, are the most potent sodium channel–blocking agents of the class I antiarrhythmic drugs. They slowly dissociate from the Na^+ channel, causing a slowing of the conduction time of the impulse through the heart. Class IB drugs, which include lidocaine, tocainide, and mexiletine, dissociate rapidly from the Na^+ channels and thus have the lowest potency as sodium channel blockers. They produce little, if any, change in action potential duration. Quinidine, procainamide, and disopyramide are drugs that have an intermediate rate of dissociation from Na^+ channels. These are categorized as class IA antiarrhythmic agents, and they lengthen the refractory period of cardiac tissue to cause cessation of arrhythmias.[22]

Studies have shown that Na^+ channels on the membranes of Purkinje fiber cells normally exist in at least three states: *R,* rested, closed near the resting potential but able to be opened by stimulation and depolarization; *A,* activated, allowing Na^+ ions to pass selectively through the membrane; and *I,* inactivated and unable to be opened (i.e., inactive).[23] The affinity of the antiarrhythmic drug for the receptor on the ion channel varies with the state of the channel or with the membrane potential. Because of this, *R, A,* and *I* ion channels can have different kinetics of interaction with antiarrhythmic drugs. A review of the recent literature shows that the antiarrhythmic drugs have low affinity for *R* channels but relatively high affinity for the *A* or *I* channels or both. Regardless of which channel state is blocked by class I antiarrhythmic drugs, the unblocking rate directly determines the amount of depression present at normal heart rates.

CLASS II. β-ADRENERGIC BLOCKING AGENTS

β-Adrenergic blocking drugs cause membrane-stabilizing or depressant effects on myocardial tissue. Their antiarrhythmic properties, however, are considered to be principally the result of inhibition of adrenergic stimulation to the heart. The principal electrophysiological property of these β-blocking agents is reduction of the phase 4 slope of potential sinus or ectopic pacemaker cells such that the heart rate decreases and ectopic tachycardias are either slowed or converted to sinus rhythm.

CLASS III. REPOLARIZATION PROLONGATORS

Drugs in this class (e.g., amiodarone, bretylium, sotalol, ibutilide, dofetilide) cause several different electrophysiological changes on myocardial tissue but share one common effect, prolonging the action potential, which increases the effective refractory period of the membrane action potential without altering the phase of depolarization or the resting membrane potential. Drugs in this class produce their effects by more than one mechanism. Sotalol is a K^+ channel blocker and has some β-adrenergic blocking properties.[24] Amiodarone and bretylium, drugs that also prolong the action potential by means that are unclear, also have Na^+ channel–blocking properties.

CLASS IV. CALCIUM CHANNEL BLOCKERS

Although not all Ca^{2+} channel blockers possess antiarrhythmic activity, some members of this class of antiarrhythmic drugs (verapamil, diltiazem) block the slow inward current of Ca^{2+} ions during phase 2 of the membrane action potential in cardiac cells. For example, the prototypical drug in this group, verapamil, selectively blocks entry of Ca^{2+} into the myocardial cell. It acts on the slow-response fibers found in the sinus node and the AV node, slowing conduction velocity and increasing refractoriness in the AV node.

pH and Activity

The action of class I local anesthetic-type antiarrhythmic drugs is pH dependent and may vary with each drug.[25] Antiarrhythmic drugs are weak bases, with most having pK_a values ranging from 7.5 to 9.5. At physiological pH of 7.40, these bases exist in an equilibrium mixture consisting of both the free base and the cationic form. Ionizable drugs, such as lidocaine (pK_a 7.86), have stronger electrophysiological effects in ischemic rather than normal myocardial cells. This potentiation has been attributed in part to the increase in H^+ concentration within the ischemic areas of the heart. Acidosis increases the proportion of Na^+ ion channels occupied by the protonated form of the antiarrhythmic agent. Nevertheless, the effect of pH on the antiarrhythmic activity of drugs can be complex, as both the free base and cationic species have been proposed as the active form of some drugs. The uncharged form of the Na^+ channel blocker can penetrate directly from the lipid phase of the surrounding cell membrane to block the channel.

Small changes in pH can alter these drugs' effectiveness by changing the charged-to-uncharged molecular ratio in the myocardial cells. Acidosis external to the myocardial cell promotes the cationic form. Because this species does not partition in the membrane as readily, onset of these drugs' action would be delayed. Furthermore, concentration of these drugs in the membrane would be reduced. Therefore, drugs that act on the channel only in the inactivated (closed) state would have a reduced effect in acidotic conditions. Acidosis may also prolong the effect of these drugs. External acidosis facilitates protonation of receptor-bound drugs. Because only neutral drugs can dissociate from closed channels, recovery is prolonged by acidosis.

Alkalosis tends to hyperpolarize the cell membrane and, thereby, reduces the effect of antiarrhythmic drugs. Because of this, alkalosis promotes the formation of more of the free-base antiarrhythmic agent, increasing the rate of recovery from the block. Alkalosis-inducing salts such as sodium lactate have been used to counteract toxicity caused by the antiarrhythmic quinidine.

CLASS I ANTIARRHYTHMICS

Quinidine Sulfate, USP. Quinidine sulfate is the sulfate of an alkaloid obtained from various species of *Cinchona* and their hybrids. It is a dextrorotatory diastereoisomer of quinine. The salt crystallizes from water as the dihydrate, in the form of fine, needle-like, white crystals. Quinidine sulfate contains a hydroxymethyl group that serves as a link between a quinoline ring and a quinuclidine moiety. The structure contains two basic nitrogens, of which the quinuclidine nitrogen is the stronger base (pK_a 10). Quinidine sulfate is bitter and light sensitive. Aqueous solutions are nearly neutral or slightly alkaline. It is soluble to the extent of 1% in water and more highly soluble in alcohol or chloroform.

Quinidine
(Cardioquin)
(Quinora)
(Auinidex)

Quinidine sulfate is the prototype of antiarrhythmic drugs and a class IA antiarrhythmic agent according to the Vaughan Williams classification. It reduces Na^+ current by binding the open ion channels (i.e., state A). The decreased Na^+ entry into the myocardial cell depresses phase 4 diastolic depolarization and shifts the intracellular threshold potential toward zero. These combined actions diminish the spontaneous frequency of pacemaker tissues, depress the automaticity of ectopic foci, and, to a lesser extent, reduce impulse formation in the SA node. This last action results in bradycardia. During the spike action potential, quinidine sulfate decreases transmembrane permeability to passive influx of Na^+, thus slowing the process of phase 0 depolarization, which decreases conduction velocity. This is shown as a prolongation of the QRS complex of electrocardiograms. Quinidine sulfate also prolongs action potential duration, which results in a proportionate increase in the QT interval. It is used to treat supraventricular and ventricular ectopic arrhythmias, such as atrial and ventricular premature beats, atrial and ventricular tachycardia, atrial flutter, and atrial fibrillation.

Quinidine sulfate is used most frequently as an oral preparation and is occasionally given intramuscularly. Quinidine sulfate that has been absorbed from the gastrointestinal tract or from the site of intramuscular injection is bound 80% to serum albumin.[18] The drug is taken up quickly from the bloodstream by body tissues; consequently, a substantial concentration gradient is established within a few minutes. Onset of action begins within 30 minutes, with the peak effect attained in 1 to 3 hours. Quinidine is metabolized primarily in the liver by hydroxylation, and a small amount is excreted by the liver.[25] Because of serious side effects and the advent of more effective oral antiarrhythmic agents, quinidine is now used less, except in selected patients for long-term oral antiarrhythmic therapy.

Quinidine Gluconate, USP.

Quinidinium gluconate (Duraquin, Quinaglute) occurs as an odorless, very bitter, white powder. In contrast with the sulfate salt, it is freely soluble in water. This is important because there are emergencies when the condition of the patient and the need for a rapid response make the oral route of administration inappropriate. The high water solubility of the gluconate salt along with a low irritant potential makes it valuable when an injectable form is needed in these emergencies. Quinidine gluconate forms a stable aqueous solution. When used for injection, it usually contains 80 mg/mL, equivalent to 50 mg of quinidine or 60 mg of quinidine sulfate.

Quinidine Polygalacturonate.

Quinidine polygalacturonate (Cardioquin) is formed by reacting quinidine and polygalacturonic acid in a hydroalcoholic medium. It contains the equivalent of approximately 60% quinidine. This salt is only slightly ionized and slightly soluble in water, but studies have shown that although equivalent doses of quinidine sulfate give higher peak blood levels earlier, a more uniform and sustained blood level is achieved with the polygalacturonate salt.

In many patients, the local irritant action of quinidine sulfate in the gastrointestinal tract causes pain, nausea, vomiting, and especially diarrhea, often precluding oral use in adequate doses. Studies with the polygalacturonate salt yielded no evidence of gastrointestinal distress. It is available as 275-mg tablets. Each tablet is the equivalent of 200 mg of quinidine sulfate or 166 mg of free alkaloid.

Procainamide Hydrochloride, USP.

Procainamide hydrochloride, *p*-amino-*N*-[2-(diethylamino)ethyl]benzamide monohydrochloride, procainamidium chloride (Pronestyl, Procan SR), has emerged as a major antiarrhythmic drug. It was developed in the course of research for compounds structurally similar to procaine, which had limited effect as an antiarrhythmic agent because of its central nervous system (CNS) side effects and short-lived action due to rapid hydrolysis of its ester linkage by plasma esterases. Because of its amide structure, procainamide hydrochloride is also

more stable in water than is procaine. Aqueous solutions of procainamide hydrochloride have a pH of about 5.5. A kinetic study of the acid-catalyzed hydrolysis of procainamide hydrochloride showed it to be unusually stable to hydrolysis in the pH range 2 to 7, even at elevated temperatures.[26]

Procainamide
(Pronestyl)
(Procan SR)

Procainamide hydrochloride is metabolized through the action of *N*-acetyltransferase. The product of enzymatic metabolism of procainamide hydrochloride is *N*-acetylprocainamide (NAPA), which possesses only 25% of the activity of the parent compound.[25] A study of the disposition of procainamide hydrochloride showed that 50% of the drug was excreted unchanged in the urine, with 7 to 24% recovered as NAPA.[27,28] Unlike quinidine, procainamide hydrochloride is bound only minimally to plasma proteins. Between 75 and 95% of the drug is absorbed from the gastrointestinal tract. Plasma levels appear 20 to 30 minutes after administration and peak in about 1 hour.[29]

Procainamide hydrochloride appears to have all of the electrophysiological effects of quinidine. It diminishes automaticity, decreases conduction velocity, and increases action potential duration and, thereby, the refractory period of myocardial tissue. Clinicians have favored the use of procainamide hydrochloride for ventricular tachycardias and quinidine for atrial arrhythmias, even though the two drugs are effective in either type of disorder.

Disopyramide Phosphate, USP.

Disopyramide phosphate, α-[2(diisopropylamino)ethyl]-α-phenyl-2-pyridineacetamide phosphate (Norpace), is an oral and intravenous class IA antiarrhythmic agent. It is quite similar to quinidine and procainamide in its electrophysiological properties, in that it decreases phase 4 diastolic depolarization, decreases conduction velocity, and has vagolytic properties.[30] It is used clinically in the treatment of refractory, life-threatening ventricular tachyarrhythmias. Oral administration of the drug produces peak plasma levels within 2 hours. The drug is bound approximately 50% to plasma protein and has a half-life of 6.7 hours in humans. More than 50% is excreted unchanged in the urine. Therefore, patients with renal insufficiency should be monitored carefully for evidence of overdose. Disopyramide phosphate commonly exhibits side effects of dry mouth, constipation, urinary retention, and other cholinergic blocking actions because of its structural similarity to anticholinergic drugs.

Disopyramide
(Norpace)

Lidocaine Hydrochloride, USP. Lidocaine hydrochloride, 2-(diethylamino)-2',6'-acetoxylidide monohydrochloride (Xylocaine), was conceived as a derivative of gramine (3-dimethylaminomethylindole) and introduced as a local anesthetic. It is now being used intravenously as a standard parenteral agent for suppression of arrhythmias associated with acute myocardial infarction and cardiac surgery. It is the drug of choice for the parenteral treatment of premature ventricular contractions.

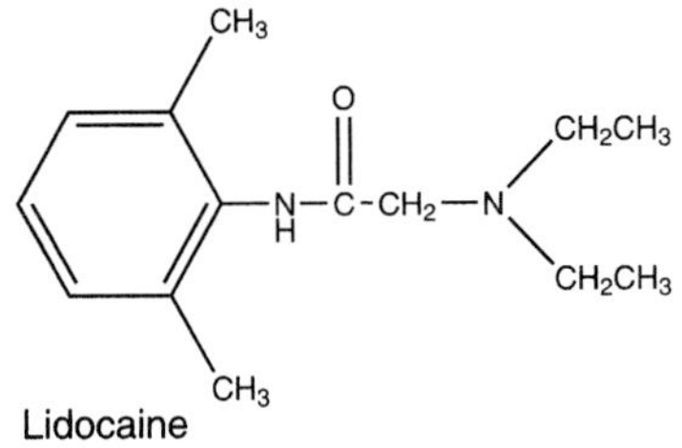

Lidocaine
(Xylocaine)

Lidocaine hydrochloride is a class IB antiarrhythmic agent with a different effect on the electrophysiological properties of myocardial cells from that of procainamide and quinidine. It binds with equal affinity to the active (A) and inactive (I) Na^+ ion channels. It depresses diastolic depolarization and automaticity in the Purkinje fiber network and increases the functional refractory period relative to action potential duration, as do procainamide and quinidine. It differs from the latter two drugs, however, in that it does not decrease, and may even enhance, conduction velocity and increases membrane responsiveness to stimulation. There are fewer data available on the subcellular mechanisms responsible for the antiarrhythmic actions of lidocaine than on the more established drug quinidine. It has been proposed that lidocaine has little effect on membrane cation exchange of the atria. Sodium ion entrance into ventricular cells during excitation is not influenced by lidocaine because it does not alter conduction velocity in this area. Lidocaine hydrochloride does depress Na^+ influx during diastole, as do all other antiarrhythmic drugs, to diminish automaticity in myocardial tissue. It also alters membrane responsiveness in Purkinje fibers, allowing increased conduction velocity and ample membrane potential at the time of excitation.[31]

Lidocaine hydrochloride administration is limited to the parenteral route and is usually given intravenously, though adequate plasma levels are achieved after intramuscular in-jections. Lidocaine hydrochloride is not bound to any extent to plasma proteins and is concentrated in the tissues. It is metabolized rapidly by the liver (Fig. 19-12). The first step is deethylation with the formation of monoethylglycinexylidide, followed by hydrolysis of the amide.[32] Metabolism is rapid, the half-life of a single injection ranging from 15 to 30 minutes. Lidocaine hydrochloride is a popular drug because of its rapid action and its relative freedom from toxic effects on the heart, especially in the absence of hepatic disease. Monoethylglycinexylidide, the initial metabolite of lidocaine, is an effective antiarrhythmic agent; its rapid hydrolysis by microsomal amidases, however, prevents its use in humans.

Precautions must be taken so that lidocaine hydrochloride solutions containing epinephrine salts are not used as cardiac depressants. Such solutions are intended only for local anesthesia and are not used intravenously. The aqueous solutions without epinephrine may be autoclaved several times, if necessary.

Phenytoin Sodium, USP. Phenytoin sodium, 5,5-diphenyl-2,4-imidazolidinedione, 5,5-diphenylhydantoin, diphenyl-hydantoin sodium (Dilantin), has been used for decades in the control of grand mal types of epileptic seizure. It is structurally analogous to the barbiturates but does not possess their extensive sedative properties. The compound is available as the sodium salt. Solutions for parenteral administration contain 40% propylene glycol and 10% alcohol to dissolve the sodium salt.

Phenytoin sodium's cardiovascular effects were uncovered during observation of toxic manifestations of the drug in patients being treated for seizure disorders. Phenytoin sodium was found to cause bradycardia, prolong the PR interval, and produce T-wave abnormalities on electrocardiograms. It is a class IB antiarrhythmic agent. Today, phenytoin sodium's greatest clinical use as an antiarrhythmic drug is in the treatment of digitalis-induced arrhythmias.[33] Its action is similar to that of lidocaine. It depresses ventricular automaticity produced by digitalis, without adverse intraventricular conduction. Because it also reverses the prolongation of AV conduction by digitalis, phenytoin sodium is useful in supraventricular tachycardias caused by digitalis intoxication.

Phenytoin sodium is located in high amounts in the body tissues, especially fat and liver, leading to large gradients

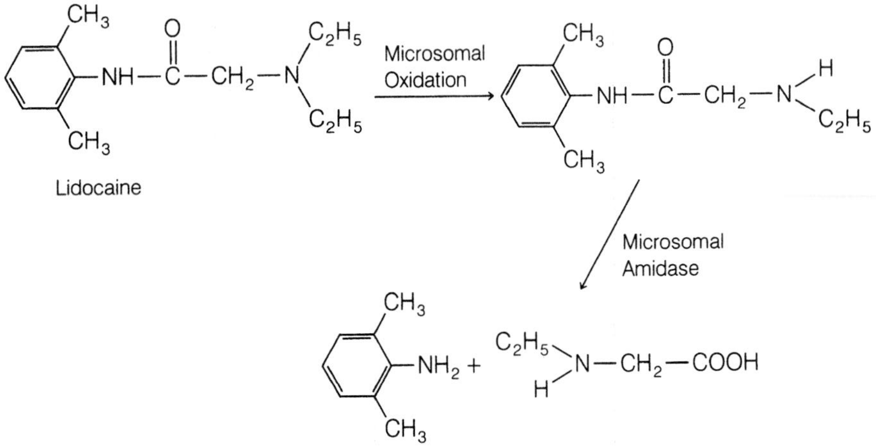

Figure 19–12 ■ Metabolism of lidocaine.

between the drug in tissues and the plasma concentrations. It is metabolized in the liver.

Mexiletine Hydrochloride.   Mexiletine hydrochloride, 1-methyl-2-(2,6-xylyloxy)ethylamine hydrochloride (Mexitil) (pK_a 8.4), is a class IB antiarrhythmic agent that is effective when given either intravenously or orally. It resembles lidocaine in possessing a xylyl moiety but otherwise is different chemically. Mexiletine hydrochloride is an ether and is not subject to the hydrolysis common to the amides lidocaine and tocainide. Its mean half-life on oral administration is approximately 10 hours.

Mexiletine
(Mexitil)

Although not subject to hydrolysis, mexiletine hydrochloride is metabolized by oxidative and reductive processes in the liver. Its metabolites, *p*-hydroxymexiletine and hydroxymethylmexiletine, are not pharmacologically active as antiarrhythmic agents.[34]

Mexiletine hydrochloride, like class I antiarrhythmic agents, blocks the fast Na^+ channel in cardiac cells. It is especially effective on the Purkinje fibers in the heart. The drug increases the threshold of excitability of myocardial cells by reducing the rate of rise and amplitude of the action potential and decreases automaticity.

Mexiletine hydrochloride is used for long-term oral prophylaxis of ventricular tachycardia. The drug is given in 200- to 400-mg doses every 8 hours.

Tocainide Hydrochloride.   Tocainide hydrochloride, 2-amino-2',6'-propionoxyxylidide hydrochloride (Tonocard) (pK_a 7.7), is an analogue of lidocaine. It is orally active and has electrophysiological properties like those of lidocaine.[35] Total body clearance of tocainide hydrochloride is only 166 mL/min, suggesting that hepatic clearance is not large. Because of low hepatic clearance, the hepatic extraction ratio must be small; therefore, tocainide hydrochloride is unlikely to be subject to a substantial first-pass effect. The drug differs from lidocaine, in that it lacks two ethyl groups, which provides tocainide hydrochloride some protection from first-pass hepatic elimination after oral ingestion. Tocainide hydrochloride is hydrolyzed in a manner similar to that of lidocaine. None of its metabolites is active.

Tocainide
(Tonocard)

Tocainide hydrochloride is classed as a IB antiarrhythmic agent and used orally to prevent or treat ventricular ectopy and tachycardia. The drug is given in 400- to 600-mg doses every 8 hours.

Flecainide Acetate.   Flecainide acetate, *N*-(2-piperidinylmethyl)-2,5-bis (2,2,2-trifluoroethoxy)benzamide monoacetate (Tambocor), is a class IC antiarrhythmic drug with local anesthetic activity; it is a chemical derivative of benzamide. The drug undergoes biotransformation, forming a meta-O-dealkylated compound, whose antiarrhythmic properties are half as potent as those of the parent drug, and a meta-O-dealkylated lactam of flecainide with little pharmacological activity.[36] Flecainide acetate is given orally to suppress chronic ventricular ectopy and ventricular tachycardia. It has some limitations because of CNS side effects.

Flecainide
(Tambocor)

Moricizine.   Moricizine, ethyl 10-(3-morpholinopropionyl)phenothiazine-2-carbamate (Ethmozine), is a phenothiazine derivative used for the treatment of malignant ventricular arrhythmias. It is categorized as a class IC antiarrhythmic agent, blocking the Na^+ channel with 1:1 stochiometry. The drug has higher affinity for the inactivated state than the activated or resting states. It appears to bind to a site on the external side of the Na^+ channel membrane.[37] It has been used to suppress life-threatening ventricular arrhythmias.

Moricizine
(Ethmozine)

Propafenone.   Propafenone, 2-[2'-hydroxy-3-(propylamino)propoxy]-3-phenylpropiophenone (Rythmol), a class IC antiarrhythmic drug, contains a chiral center and is marketed as the racemic mixture. Therapy with the racemic mixture of propafenone produces effects that can be attributed to both (*S*) and (*R*) enantiomers. Although (*R*) and (*S*) enantiomers exert similar Na^+ channel–blocking effects, the (*S*) enantiomer also produces a β-adrenergic blockade. As a result, the (*S*) enantiomer is reported to be 40-fold more potent than the (*R*) enantiomer as an antiarrhythmic agent.[38] The enantiomers also display stereoselective disposition characteristics. The (*R*) enantiomer is cleared more quickly. Hepatic metabolism is polymorphic and determined genetically. Ten percent of Caucasians have a reduced capacity to hydroxylate the drug to form 5-hydroxypropafenone. This polymorphic metabolism accounts for the interindividual variability in the relationships between dose and concentration and, thus, variability in the pharmacodynamic effects of the drug. The 5-hydroxy metabolites of both enantiomers are as potent as the parent compound in blocking Na^+ channels. Propafenone also depresses the slow inward current of Ca^{2+} ions. This drug has been used for acute termination or long-term suppression of ventricular arrhythmias. It is bound in excess of 95% to α_1-acid glycoprotein in the plasma. It is absorbed effectively, but bioavailability is estimated to be less than 20% because of first-pass metabolism. Less than 1% is eliminated as unchanged drug. Therapy with propafenone may produce effects that can be attributed to both (S) and (R) enantiomers. Thus, the effects may be modulated because of an enantiomer–enantiomer interaction when patients are treated with the racemate.[39]

Propafenone
(Rythmol)

CLASS II ANTIARRHYTHMICS

Class II antiarrhythmics are discussed under the heading, Adrenergic System Inhibitors.

CLASS III ANTIARRHYTHMICS

Amiodarone. Amiodarone, 2-butyl-3-benzofuranyl-4-[2-(diethylamino)ethoxy]-3,5-diiodophenyl ketone (Cordarone), was introduced as an antianginal agent. It has very pronounced class III action and is especially effective in maintaining sinus rhythm in patients who have been treated by direct current shock for atrial fibrillation.[40] Like class III antiarrhythmic drugs, amiodarone lengthens the effective refractory period by prolonging the action potential duration in all myocardial tissues. Amiodarone is eliminated very slowly from the body, with a half-life of about 25 to 30 days after oral doses.[41] Although the drug has a broad spectrum of antiarrhythmic activity, its main limitation is a slow onset of action. Drug action may not be initiated for several days, and the peak effect may not be obtained for several weeks.

Amiodarone has adverse effects involving many different organ systems. It also inhibits metabolism of drugs cleared by oxidative microsomal enzymes. It contains iodine in its molecular structure and, as a result, has an effect on thyroid hormones. Hypothyroidism occurs in up to 11% of patients receiving amiodarone.[42] The principal effect is the inhibition of peripheral conversion of T_4 to T_3. Serum reverse T_3 (rT_3) is increased as a function of the dose as well as the length of amiodarone therapy. As a result, rT_3 levels have been used as a guide for judging adequacy of amiodarone therapy and predicting toxicity.[43]

Amiodarone
(Cordarone)

Bretylium Tosylate. Bretylium tosylate, (o-bromobenzyl)ethyl dimethylammonium p-toluenesulfonate (Bretylol), is an extremely bitter, white, crystalline powder. The chemical is freely soluble in water and alcohol. Bretylium tosylate is an adrenergic neuronal blocking agent that accumulates selectively in the neurons and displaces norepinephrine. Because of this property, bretylium was used initially, under the trade name of Darenthin, as an antihypertensive agent. It caused postural decrease in arterial pressure.[43] This use was discontinued because of the rapid development of tolerance, erratic oral absorption of the quaternary ammonium compound, and persistent pain in the parotid gland on prolonged therapy. Currently, bretylium is reserved for use in ventricular arrhythmias that are resistant to other therapy. Bretylium does not suppress phase 4 depolarization, a common action of other antiarrhythmic agents. It prolongs the effective refractory period relative to the action potential duration but does not affect conduction time and is categorized as a class III antiarrhythmic agent. Because bretylium does not have properties similar to those of the other antiarrhythmic agents, it has been suggested that its action is due to its adrenergic neuronal blocking properties; the antiarrhythmic properties of the drug, however, are not affected by administration of reserpine. Bretylium is also a local anesthetic, but it has not been possible to demonstrate such an effect on atria of experimental animals, except at very high concentrations.[44] Therefore, the precise mechanism of the antiarrhythmic action of bretylium remains to be resolved.

Bretylium
(Bretylol)

Dofetilide. Dofetilide, N-[4-(3-{[2-(4-methanesulfonyl-aminophenyl)ethyl]methylamino}propoxy)phenyl]methanesulfonamide (Tikosyn), acts by blocking the cardiac ion channel carrying the rapid component of the delayed rectifier potassium currents (Ikr) and is used to terminate supraventricular arrhythmias, prevent the recurrence of atrial fibrillation, and treat life-threatening ventricular arrhythmias. Unlike sotalol and ibutilide, which are also methanesulfonanilides, it has no effect on adrenergic receptors or sodium channels, respectively. Dofetilide has high specificity for the delayed rectifier potassium currents.[45]

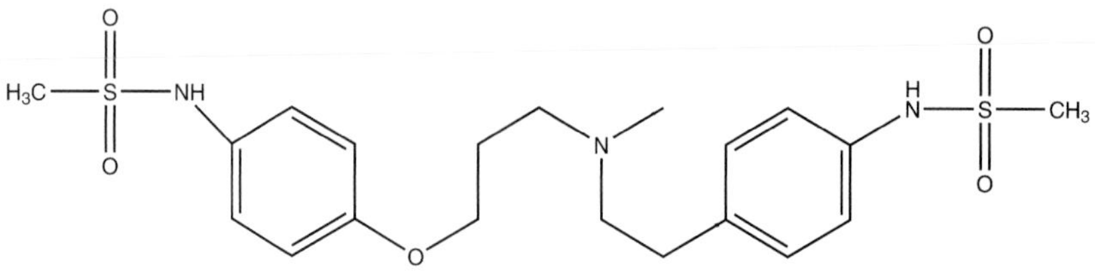

Dofetilide
(Tikosyn)

Ibutilide. Ibutilide, *N*-{4-[4-(ethylheptylamino)-1-hydroxybutyl]phenyl}methanesulfonamide (Corvert), a class III antiarrhythmic belonging to the methanesulfonanilide class of agents, is indicated for rapid conversion of atrial fibrillation or atrial flutter to normal sinus rhythm. Unlike dofetilide, it is not highly specific for the delayed rectifier potassium currents (Ikr) and does have some affinity for sodium channels.

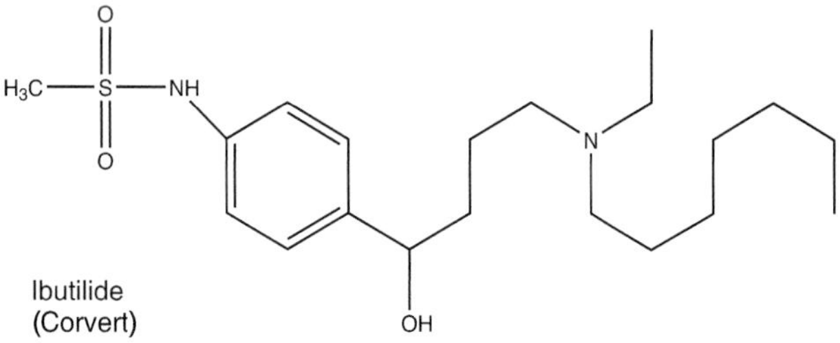

Ibutilide
(Corvert)

Sotalol. Sotalol, 4'[1-hydroxy-2-(isopropylamino)ethyl]methylsulfonanilide (Betapace), is a relatively new antiarrhythmic drug, characterized most often as a class III agent, and although it has effects that are related to the class II agents, it is not therapeutically considered a class II antiarrhythmic. It contains a chiral center and is marketed as the racemic mixture. Because of its enantiomers, its mechanism of action spans two of the antiarrhythmic drug classes. The *l*(−) enantiomer has both β-blocking (class II) and potassium channel–blocking (class III) activity. The d(+) enantiomer has class III properties similar to those of the (−) isomer, but its affinity for the β-adrenergic receptor is 30 to 60 times lower. The sotalol enantiomers produce different effects on the heart. Class III action of *d*-sotalol in the sinus node is associated with slowing of sinus heart rate, whereas β-adrenergic blockade contributes to the decrease in heart rate observed with *l*- or *d,l*-sotalol. Sotalol is not metabolized, nor is it bound significantly to proteins. Elimination occurs by renal excretion, with more than 80% of the drug eliminated unchanged. Sotalol is characteristic of class III antiarrhythmic drugs, in that it prolongs the duration of the action potential and, thus, increases the effective refractory period of myocardial tissue. It is distinguished from the other class III drugs (amiodarone and bretylium) because of its β-adrenergic receptor–blocking action.

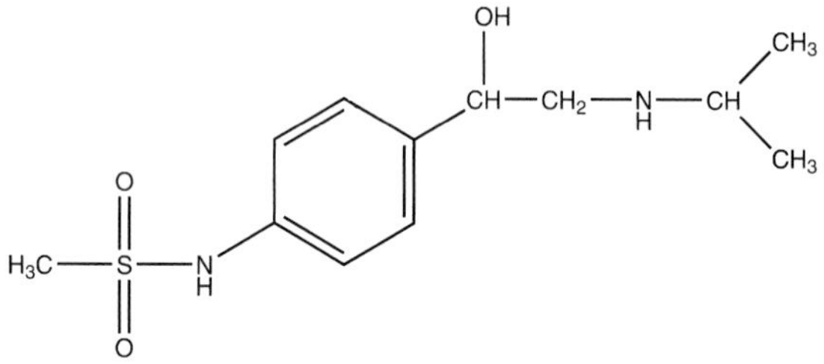

Sotalol
(Betapace)

Azimilide. Azimilide, *E*-1-[[[5-(4-chlorophenyl)-2-furanyl]methylene]amino]-3-[4-(4-methyl-1-piperazinyl)butyl]-2,4-imidazolidinedione, is a class III agent that significantly blocks the delayed rectifier potassium current, Iks, including the Ikr component. Its ability to block multichannels may be due to a lack of the methane sulfonamide group that is common to other class III agents, which selectively block the Ikr potassium current. It is believed that blocking both Ikr and Iks potassium currents yields consistent class III antiarrhythmic effects at any heart rate.[46]

CLASS IV ANTIARRHYTHMICS

Verapamil and Diltiazem. Both verapamil and diltiazem block the slow inward Ca^{2+} currents (voltage-sensitive channel) in cardiac fibers. This slows down AV conduction and the sinus rate. These drugs are used in controlling atrial and paroxysmal tachycardias and are categorized as class IV antiarrhythmic agents according to the Vaughan Williams classification.[20] (A more detailed description of calcium channel blockers is given above.)

ANTIHYPERTENSIVE AGENTS

Hypertension is a consequence of many diseases. Hemodynamically, blood pressure is a function of the amount of

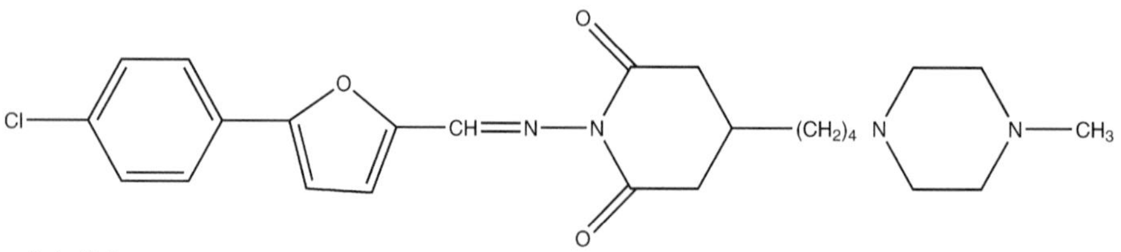

Azimilide

blood pumped by the heart and the ease with which the blood flows through the peripheral vasculature (i.e., resistance to blood flow by peripheral blood vessels). Diseases of components of the central and peripheral nervous systems, which regulate blood pressure and abnormalities of the hormonal system, and diseases of the kidney and peripheral vascular network, which affect blood volume, can create a hypertensive state in humans. Hypertension is generally defined as mild when the diastolic pressure is between 90 and 104 mm Hg, moderate when it is 105 to 114 mm Hg, and severe when it is above 115 mm Hg. It is estimated that about 15% of the adult population in the United States (about 40 million) are hypertensive.

Primary (essential) hypertension is the most common form of hypertension. Although advances have been made in the identification and control of primary hypertension, the etiology of this form of hypertension has not yet been resolved. *Renal hypertension* can be created by experimentally causing renal artery stenosis in animals. Renal artery stenosis also may occur in pathological conditions of the kidney, such as nephritis, renal artery thrombosis, renal artery infarctions, or other conditions that restrict blood flow through the renal artery. Hypertension also may originate from pathological states in the CNS, such as malignancies. Tumors in the adrenal medulla that cause release of large amounts of catecholamines create a hypertensive condition known as *pheochromocytoma.* Excessive secretion of aldosterone by the adrenal cortex, often because of adenomas, also produces hypertensive disorders.

Arterial blood pressure is regulated by several physiological factors, such as heart rate, stroke volume, peripheral vascular network resistance, blood vessel elasticity, blood volume, and viscosity of blood. Endogenous chemicals also play an important part in the regulation of arterial blood pressure. The peripheral vascular system is influenced greatly by the sympathetic–parasympathetic balance of the autonomic nervous system, the control of which originates in the CNS. Enhanced adrenergic activity is a principal contributor to primary (essential) hypertension.

Therapy using antihypertensive agents evolved rapidly between 1950 and 1960. During that time, a number of drugs for the treatment and control of hypertensive disease were discovered. Despite the many years of experience, treatment remains empiric because the etiology of the principal form of hypertension, primary hypertension, is unknown. The first drugs used to produce symptomatic relief of hypertension were α-adrenergic blocking agents. These drugs had limitations because their duration of action was far too short and side effects precluded long-term therapy. Contemporary therapy of primary hypertension uses one of several drug classes as the first course. These drugs may be diuretics to reduce blood volume, inhibitors of the renin–angiotensin system (ACE inhibitors), and agents that reduce peripheral vascular resistance (e.g., calcium channel blockers, vasodilators, and sympathetic nervous system depressants). The antihypertensive drug classes discussed in this section include ACE inhibitors, sympathetic nervous system depressants, and vasodilators acting on smooth muscle. Calcium channel blockers and other vasodilators are included in previous discussions in this chapter. Diuretics are discussed in Chapter 18.

The Renin–Angiotensin System and Hypertension

The renin–angiotensin system is a hormonal system that plays a central role in the control of sodium excretion and body fluid volume. It interacts closely with the sympathetic nervous system and aldosterone secretion in the regulation of blood pressure. Figure 19-13 shows the relationship of the component parts of the renin–angiotensin system and their main physiological effects.

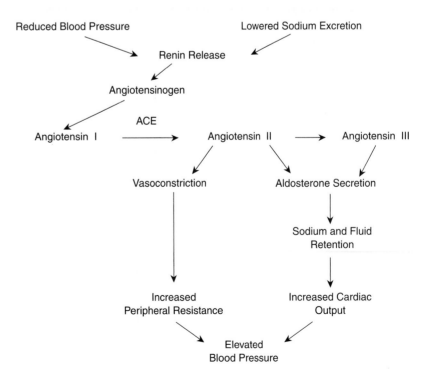

Figure 19-13 ■ Renin–angiotensin system of blood pressure control.

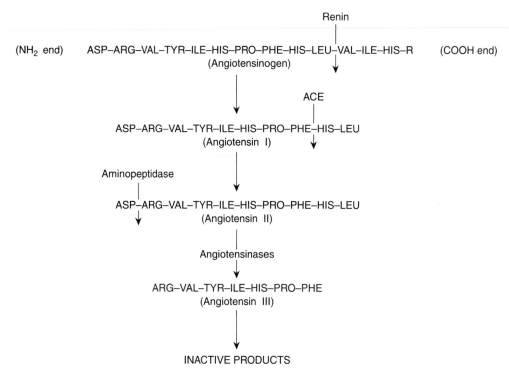

Figure 19–14 ■ Biochemistry of the renin–angiotensin system: formation of angiotensins from angiotensinogen.

The relationship between the renin–angiotensin system and blood pressure in humans has been known since before the beginning of the 20th century. Tigerstedt and Bergman[47] demonstrated in 1898 that when injected in a host, kidney extract produced a potent vasopressor response. The substance was named *renin*. Many years later, this substance was shown to require a cofactor to produce vasoconstriction.[48] Eventually, in 1939, this hypertensive substance was isolated, identified as a decapeptide, and later called *angiotensin*. This cofactor existed as an inactive precursor, angiotensinogen. Later studies revealed that angiotensin existed in two forms, the biologically inactive decapeptide angiotensin I and the active octapeptide angiotensin II.[49]

The precursor of angiotensin, angiotensinogen, is a glycoprotein of molecular weight (MW) 58,000 to 61,000, synthesized primarily in the liver and brought into the circulatory system. Renin, an aspartyl protease (MW 35,000 to 40,000), whose primary source is the kidney, cleaves the Leu-Val bond from the aspartic acid end of the angiotensinogen polypeptide molecule to release the decapeptide angiotensin I (Fig. 19-14). The biochemical conversion continues with the cleavage of a dipeptide (His-Leu) from the carboxyl terminal of angiotensin I by ACE to form the octapeptide angiotensin II, a potent vasoconstrictor. Angiotensin III is formed by removal of the N-terminal aspartate residue of angiotensin II, a reaction catalyzed by glutamyl aminopeptidase. In contrast to angiotensin II, angiotensin III has a less potent but significant regulatory effect on sodium excretion by the renal tubules.

The regulatory action of the renin–angiotensin system in controlling sodium and potassium balance and arterial blood pressure is modified by vasodilators called *kinins*. Proteolytic enzymes that circulate in the plasma form kinins. Kallikrein is activated in plasma by noxious influences to act on a kinin, callidin, which is converted to bradykinin by tissue enzymes. Bradykinin enhances release of the prostaglandins PGE_2 and PGI_2 within certain tissues to produce a vasodilatory effect (Fig. 19-15). Bradykinin is converted to inactive products by ACE and other carboxypeptidases. Although ACE causes activation of angiotensin and inactivation of bradykinin, actions that appear to be opposite, the balance of the system seems to favor vasoconstriction.

ACE is a membrane-bound enzyme anchored to the cell membrane through a single transmembrane domain located near the carboxy-terminal extremity. The enzyme is a zinc-containing glycoprotein with a MW about 130,000. It is a nonspecific peptidyldipeptide hydrolase, widely distributed in mammalian tissues, that cleaves dipeptides from the carboxy terminus of a number of endogenous peptides. The minimum structural requirement for binding and cleavage of a substrate by ACE is that it be a tripeptide with a free carboxylate group. A general exception is that this enzyme does not cleave peptides with a penultimate prolyl residue. This accounts for the biological stability of angiotensin II.[50] The important binding points at the active site of ACE are a cationic site to attract a carboxylate ion and a zinc ion that can polarize a carbonyl group of an amide function to make it more susceptible to hydrolysis. In the active site, there is a nucleophilic attack of the amide carbonyl by the γ-carbonyl

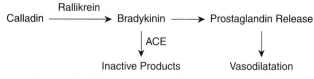

Figure 19–15 ■ Bradykinin formation and action.

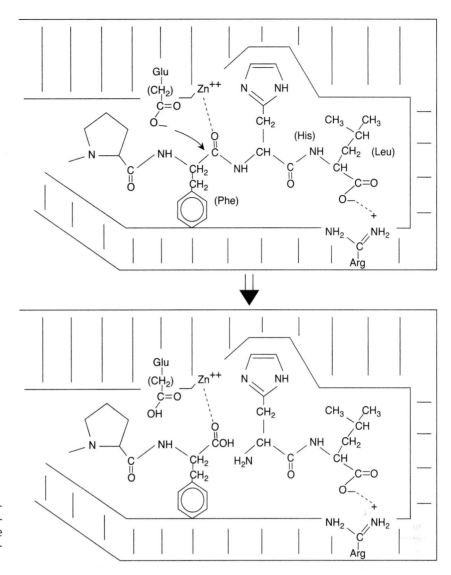

Figure 19–16 ■ Model showing cleavage of the histidine–phenylalanine residue of angiotensin I by ACE to form the octapeptide antiotensin II and the dipeptide residue of histidine and leucine.

group of a glutamic acid residue to cause hydrolysis of the peptide. Figure 19-16 shows a hypothetical model of the hydrolysis of angiotensin I by the active site of ACE. ACE exists in more than one form. Somatic ACE that regulates blood pressure, found in most tissues, differs from the isoenzyme ACE found in the testis. Somatic ACE, in contrast to testicular ACE, contains two binding domains. The principal active site for hydrolysis is the domain located in the C-terminal half of somatic ACE.[51]

RENIN–ANGIOTENSIN SYSTEM INHIBITORS

Captopril. Captopril, 1-[(2S)-3-mercapto-2-methyl-1-oxopropionyl]proline (Capoten), blocks the conversion of angiotensin I to angiotensin II by inhibiting the converting enzyme. The rational development of captopril as an inhibitor of ACE was based on the hypothesis that ACE and carboxypeptidase A functioned by similar mechanisms. It was noted that *d*-2-benzylsuccinic acid[50] was a potent inhibitor of carboxypeptidase A but not ACE. By use of this small molecule as a prototype, captopril was designed with a carboxyl group on a proline and a thiol group was introduced to enhance the binding to the zinc ion of ACE. The important

binding points at the active site of ACE are thought to be an arginine residue, which provides a cationic site that attracts a carboxylate ion, and a zinc ion, which can polarize a carbonyl group of an amide function to make it more susceptible to hydrolysis. Hydrophobic pockets lie between these groups in the active site, as does a functional group that forms a hydrogen bond with an amide carbonyl. Figure 19-17 shows the hypothetical binding of captopril in the active site of ACE.

Captopril
(Capoten)

Lisinopril. Lisinopril, 1-[N^2-[*S*-1-carboxy-3-phenylpropyl]-L-lysyl]-L-proline dihydrate (Prinivil, Zestril), is a ly-

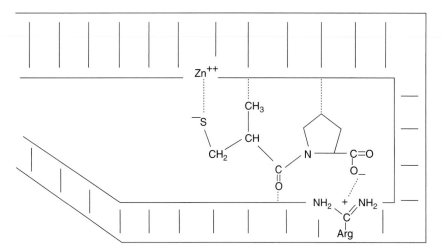

Figure 19–17 ■ Accommodation of captopril to the active site of ACE.

sine derivative of enalaprilat, the active metabolite of enalapril. Like all ACE inhibitors, it is an active site-directed inhibitor of the enzyme, with the zinc ion used in an effective binding interaction at a stoichiometric ratio of 1:1. The pharmacological effects of lisinopril are similar to those of captopril and enalapril.

Lisinopril
(Prinivil)
(Zestril)

ACE INHIBITOR PRODRUGS

Many new ACE inhibitors became available for the treatment of hypertension following the clinical effectiveness of enalapril. Enalapril is a non–thiol-containing ACE inhibitor devoid of the side effects of rash and loss of the sense of taste characteristic of the thiol-containing compound captopril. With the exception of the phosphorus-containing fosinopril, these antihypertensive agents have a 2-(S)-amino-phenylbutyric acid ethyl ester moiety differing only in the substituents on the amino group. They have the common property of acting as prodrugs, being converted to the active enzyme inhibitor following absorption and metabolism by liver and intestinal enzymes. These drugs (Fig. 19-18), like the prototypical drug captopril, are used in the treatment of mild-to-moderate hypertension, either alone or in conjunction with diuretics or calcium channel blockers. Table 19-5 compares some of their properties.

Enalapril Maleate. Enalapril maleate, 1-[*N*[(*S*)-1-carboxy-3-phenylpropyl]-L-alanyl]-L-proline 1′-ethyl ester maleate (Vasotec), is a long-acting ACE inhibitor. It requires activation by hydrolysis of its ethyl ester to form the diacid enalaprilat. Enalapril is devoid of the side effects of rash

and loss of taste seen with captopril. These side effects are similar to those of the mercapto-containing drug penicillamine. The absence of the thiol group in enalapril maleate may free it from these side effects. The half-life is 11 hours.

Enalapril
(Vasotec)

Benazepril Hydrochloride. Benazepril hydrochloride, (3*S*)-3-[[(1*S*)-1-carbethoxy-3-phenylpropyl]amino]-2,3,4,5-tetrahydro-2-oxo-1*H*-1-benzazepine-1-acetic acid 3-ethyl ester hydrochloride (Lotensin), is metabolized rapidly to the active diacid benazaprilat. As with the ACE prodrugs, no mutagenicity has been found, even though these drugs cross the placenta.

Benazepril
(Lotensin)

Quinapril Hydrochloride. Quinapril hydrochloride, (*S*)-[(*S*)-*N*-[(*S*)21-carboxy3-phenylpropyl]alanyl]-1,2,3,4-tetrahydro-3-isoquinolinecarboxylic acid 1-ethyl ester hydrochloride (Acuretic), forms the diacid quinaprilate in the body. It is more potent than captopril and equipotent to the active form of enalapril.

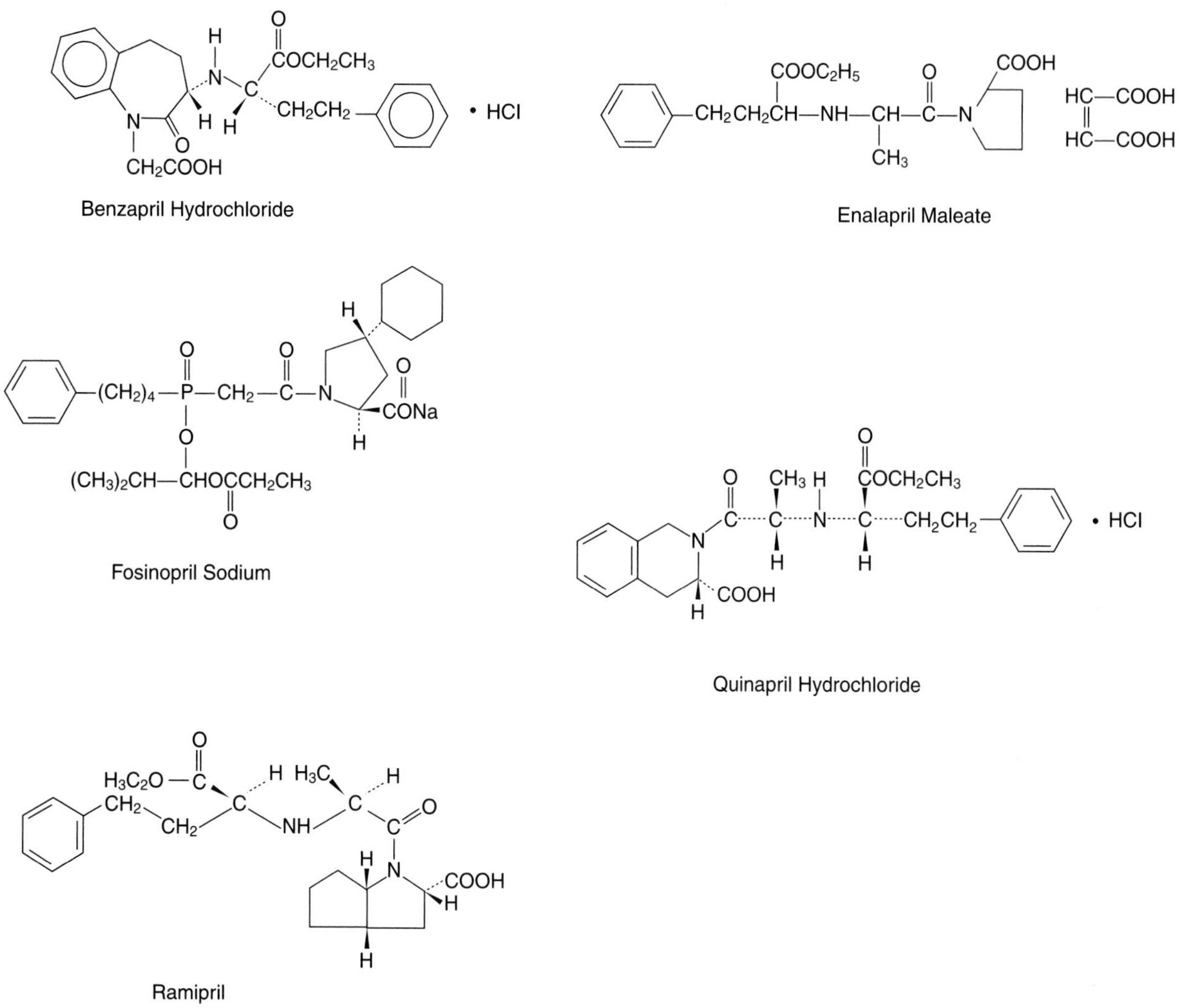

Benzapril Hydrochloride

Enalapril Maleate

Fosinopril Sodium

Quinapril Hydrochloride

Ramipril

Figure 19–18 ■ ACE inhibitor prodrugs.

TABLE 19–5   ACE-Inhibitor Prodrugs

Prodrug	Metabolite	Metabolite Protein Binding (%)	Metabolite Plasma $t_{1/2}$ (hours)	Mode of Excretion
Benazepril	Benazeprilat	95	10–11	Renal
Enalapril	Enalaprilat	50–60	11.0	Renal
Fosinopril	Fosinoprilat	97	11.5	Renal/fecal
Quinapril	Quinaprilat	97	3.0	Renal/fecal
Ramipril	Ramiprilat	56	13–17	Renal/fecal

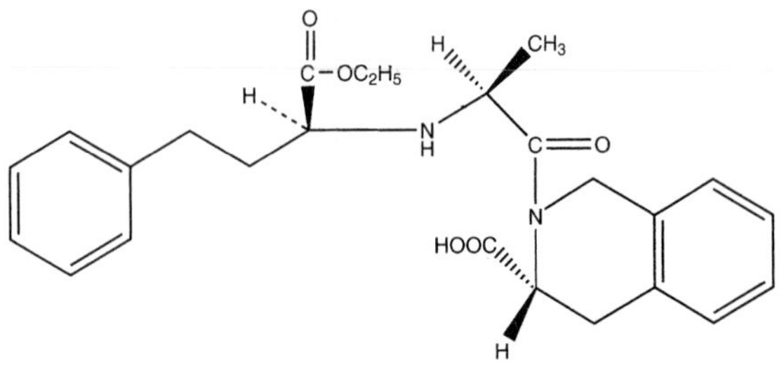

Quinapril
(Accupril)

Ramipril. Ramipril, (2S, 3aS, 6aS)-1-[(S)-N-[(S)-1-carboxy-3-phenylpropyl]alanyl]octahydrocyclopenta[b]pyrrole-2-carboxylic acid 1-ethyl ester (Altace), is hydrolyzed to ramiprilat, its active diacid form, faster than enalapril is hydrolyzed to its active diacid form. Peak serum concentrations from a single oral dose are achieved between 1.5 and 3.0 hours. The ramiprilate formed completely suppresses ACE activity for up to 12 hours, with 80% inhibition of the enzyme still observed after 24 hours.

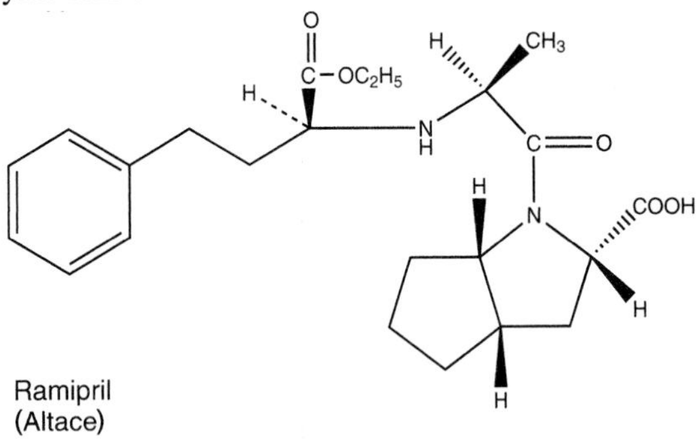

Ramipril
(Altace)

Fosinopril Sodium. Fosinopril sodium, (4S)-4-cyclohexyl-1-[[[(RS)-1-hydroxy-2-methylpropoxy](4-phenyl-butyl)phosphinyl]acetyl]-L-proline sodium salt (Monopril), is a phosphorus-containing ACE inhibitor. It is inactive but serves as a prodrug, being completely hydrolyzed by intestinal and liver enzymes to the active diacid fosinoprilat.

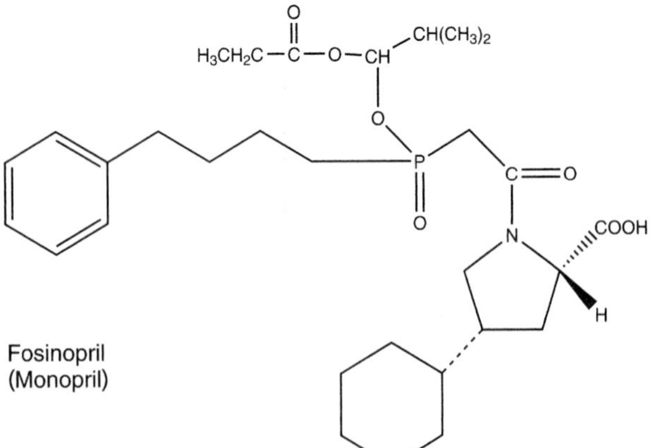

Fosinopril
(Monopril)

Trandolapril. Trandolapril, 1-[2-(1-ethoxycarbonyl-3-phenylpropylamino)propionyl]octahydroindole-2-carboxylic acid (Mavik), is an indole-containing ACE inhibitor that is structurally related to most of the agents discussed above. Enalapril is very similar to trandolapril, with the primary difference occurring in the heterocyclic systems. The

pyrrolidine of enalapril has been replaced with an octahydroindole system. Much like enalaprilate, trandolapril must be hydrolyzed to tranolaprilate, which is the bioactive species.

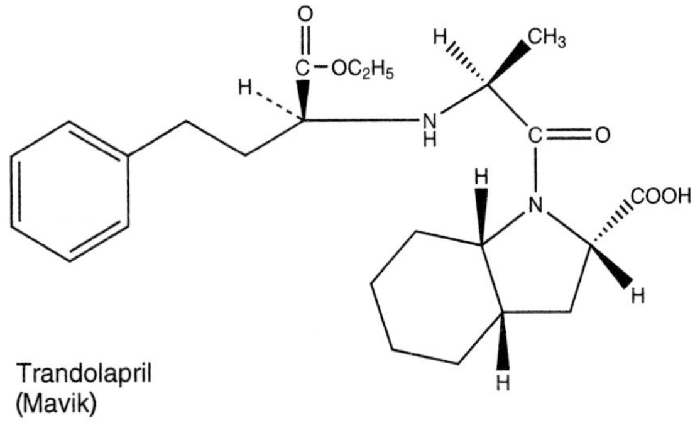

Trandolapril
(Mavik)

ANGIOTENSIN ANTAGONISTS

Administration of a competitive antagonist can inhibit angiotensin II to produce a vasodilatory effect. Since the substrate for this receptor is an octapeptide, much of the earlier work was performed by using various peptide systems. One such agent, saralasin, is an octapeptide that differs from angiotensin by two amino acids. This agent's use was limited because it had some partial agonistic properties. Nevertheless, it served as a lead in the development of other agents that are useful in antagonizing the angiotensin II receptor. The most significant lead in the development of this class came from a series of imidazole-5-acetic acid derivatives that attenuated pressor response to angiotensin II in test animals. Molecular modeling revealed that the imidazole-5-acetic acid could be exploited to more closely mimic the pharmacophore of angiotensin II. The first successful agent to be developed through this method is losartan. Later, four other agents were introduced into the U.S. market. These tend to be biphenylmethyl derivatives that possess certain acidic moieties, which can interact with various positions on the receptor, much like the substrate, angiotensin II. Since the late 1980s, this particular class has received a great deal of attention. In the early 1990s, the receptor for angiotensin II was found to exist as four isozymes, AT_1, AT_2, AT_3, and AT_4, with AT_1 being responsible for smooth muscle contraction, sympathetic pressor mechanisms, and aldosterone release.

ANGIOTENSIN II BLOCKERS

Losartan. Losartan, 2-butyl-4-chloro-1-[p-(o-1H-tetrazol-5-yl-phenyl)benzyl]imidazole-5-methanol monopotassium salt (Cozarr), was the first nonpeptide imidazole to be introduced as an orally active angiotensin II antagonist with high specificity for AT_1. When administered to patients, it undergoes extensive first-pass metabolism, with the 5-methanol being oxidized to a carboxylic acid. This metabolism is mediated by CYP 2C9 and 3A4 isozymes. The 5-methanol metabolite is approximately 15 times more potent than the parent hydroxyl compound. Since the parent hydroxyl compound has affinity for the AT_1 receptor, strictly speaking, it is not a prodrug.

Candesartan. Candesartan, (+)-1-[[(cyclohexyloxy)carbonyl]-oxy]ethyl 2-ethoxy-1-[[2'-(1H-tetrazol-5-yl)[1,1'-biphenyl]-4-yl]methyl]-1H-benzimidazole-7-carboxyl-

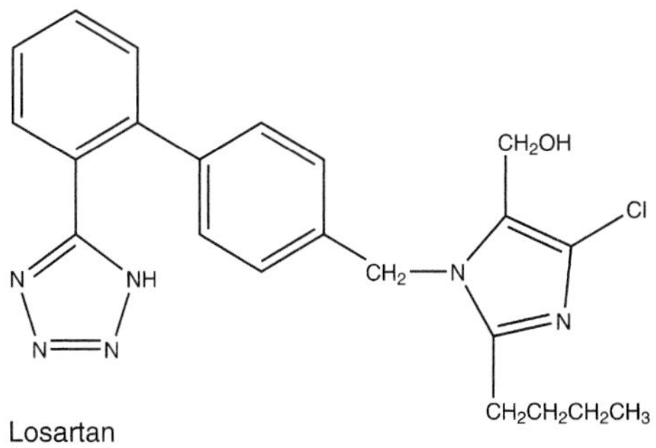

Losartan
(Cozaar)

ate (Atacand), like losartan, possesses the acidic tetrazole system, which most likely plays a role in binding to the angiotensin II receptor similarly to the acidic groups of angiotensin II. Also, the imidazole system has been replaced with a benzimidazole possessing an ester at position 7. This ester must be hydrolyzed to the free acid. Fortunately, this conversion takes place fairly easily because of the carbonate in the ester side chain. This facilitates hydrolysis of the ester so much that conversion to the free acid takes place during absorption from the gastrointestinal tract.

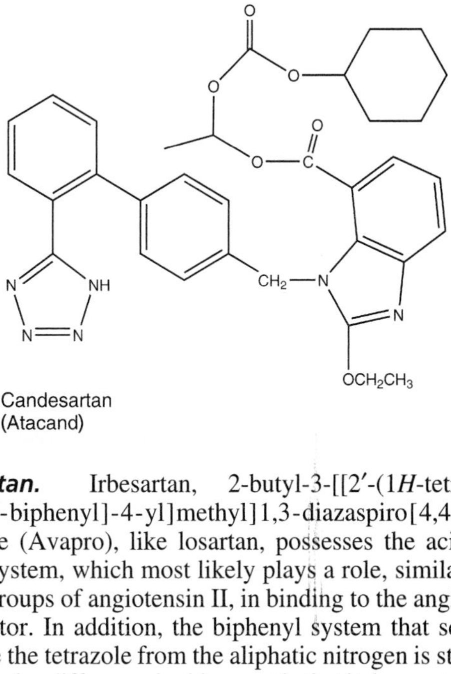

Candesartan
(Atacand)

Irbesartan. Irbesartan, 2-butyl-3-[[2′-(1*H*-tetrazol-5-yl)[1,1′-biphenyl]-4-yl]methyl]1,3-diazaspiro[4,4]non-1-en-4-one (Avapro), like losartan, possesses the acidic tetrazole system, which most likely plays a role, similar to the acidic groups of angiotensin II, in binding to the angiotensin II receptor. In addition, the biphenyl system that serves to separate the tetrazole from the aliphatic nitrogen is still present. A major difference in this agent is that it does not possess the acidic side chain. Even so, irbesartan has good affinity for the angiotensin II receptor because of hydrogen bonding with the carbonyl moiety of the amide system. Also, this particular agent does not require metabolic activation as candesartan does.

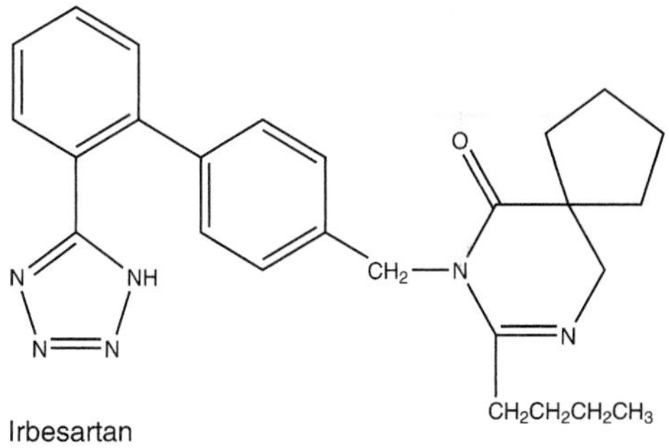

Irbesartan
(Avapro)

Telmisartan. Telmisartan, 4′-[(1,4′-dimethyl-2′-propyl[2,6′-bi-1*H*-benzimidazol]-1′-yl)methyl]-[1,1′-biphenyl]-2-carboxylic acid (Micardis), does not appear to bear any structural relationship to this class, but there is actually a great deal of overlap in the chemical architecture with other agents. The first, and most significant, difference is the replacement of the acidic tetrazole system with a simple carboxylic acid. This acid, like the tetrazole, plays a role in receptor binding. The second difference is the lack of a carboxylic acid near the imidazole nitrogen that also contributes to receptor binding. As with irbesartan, however, there is not a need for this group to be acidic but, rather, to be one that participates in receptor binding. The second imidazole ring, much like a purine base in DNA, can hydrogen bond with the angiotensin II receptor.

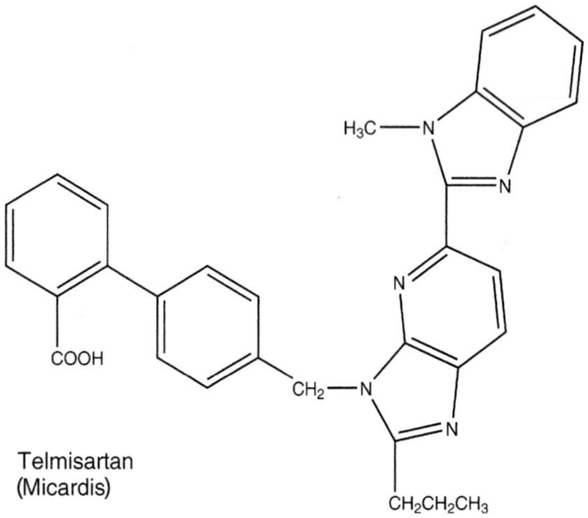

Telmisartan
(Micardis)

Valsartan. Valsartan, *N*-(1-oxopentyl)-*N*-[[2′-(1*H*-tetrazol-5-yl)[1,1′-biphenyl]-4-yl]methyl]-L-valine (Diovan), like losartan, possesses the acidic tetrazole system, which most likely plays a role, similar to that of the acidic groups of angiotensin II, in binding to the angiotensin II receptor. In addition, the biphenyl system that serves to separate the tetrazole from the aliphatic nitrogen is still present. In addition, there is a carboxylic acid side chain in the valine moiety that also serves to bind to the angiotensin II receptor.

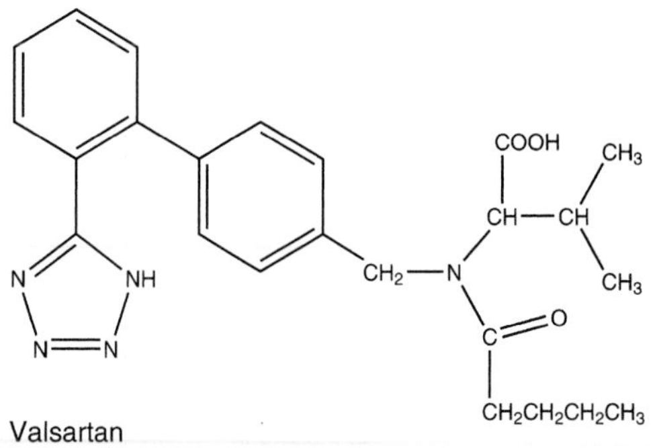

Valsartan
(Diovan)

ADRENERGIC SYSTEM INHIBITORS

Drugs that reduce blood pressure by depressing the activity of the sympathetic nervous system have been used as effective agents in the treatment of hypertension. This can be accomplished in several ways: *(a)* depleting the stores of neurotransmitter, *(b)* reducing the number of impulses traveling in sympathetic nerves, *(c)* antagonizing the actions of the neurotransmitter on the effector cells, and *(d)* inhibiting neurotransmitter release.

AGENTS DEPLETING NEUROTRANSMITTER STORES

Folk remedies prepared from species of *Rauwolfia,* a plant genus belonging to the Apocynaceae family, were reported as early as 1563. The root of the species *R. serpentina* has been used for centuries as an antidote to stings and bites of insects, to reduce fever, as a stimulant to uterine contractions, for insomnia, and particularly for the treatment of insanity. Its use in hypertension was recorded in the Indian literature in 1918, but not until 1949 did hypotensive properties of *Rauwolfia* spp. appear in the Western literature.[52] *Rauwolfia* preparations were introduced in psychiatry for the treatment of schizophrenia in the early 1950s, following confirmation of the folk remedy reports on their use in mentally deranged patients. By the end of the 1960s, however, the drug had been replaced by more efficacious neurotropic agents. Reserpine and its preparations remain useful in the control of mild essential hypertension.

The effects of reserpine do not correlate well with tissue levels of the drug. The pharmacological effects of reserpine were still present in animals when it could no longer be detected in the brain.[53] Reserpine depletes catecholamines and serotonin from central and peripheral neurons by interfering with the uptake of these amines from the cytosol into the vesicles and granules.[54,55] As a consequence, norepinephrine cannot be stored intraneuronally in adrenergic neurons, and much of the norepinephrine in the cytosol is metabolized by monoamine oxidase (Fig. 19-19). The binding of reserpine to the storage vesicle membrane is firm, and as a result, the storage granule is destroyed, reducing the ability of the nerve to concentrate and store norepinephrine. Since reserpine acts on both central and peripheral adrenergic neurons, its antihypertensive effects may result from neurotransmitter depletion from both of these sites.

Chemical investigations of the active components of *R. serpentina* roots have yielded several alkaloids (e.g., ajmaline, ajmalicine, ajmalinine, serpentine, and serpentinine).

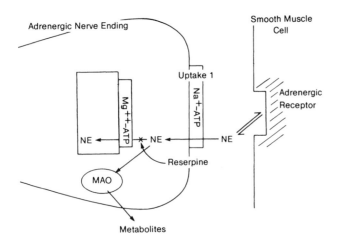

Figure 19-19 ■ Action of reserpine at adrenergic nerve ending.

Reserpine, which is the major active constituent of *Rauwolfia,*[56] was isolated in 1952 and is a much weaker base than the alkaloids just mentioned. Reserpinoid alkaloids are yohimbine-like bases that have an additional functional group on C-18. Only three naturally occurring alkaloids possess reserpine-like activity strong enough for use in treating hypertension: reserpine, deserpidine, and rescinnamine.

Reserpine is absorbed rapidly after oral administration. Fat tissue accumulates reserpine slowly, with a maximal level reached between 4 and 6 hours. After 24 hours, small amounts of reserpine are found in the liver and fat, but none is found in the brain or other tissues. Reserpine is metabolized by the liver and intestine to methyl reserpate and 3,4,5-trimethoxybenzoic acid.

Powdered Rauwolfia Serpentina, USP. Rauwolfia (Raudixin, Rauserpal, Rauval) is the powdered whole root of *R. serpentina* (Benth). It is a light tan to light brown powder, sparingly soluble in alcohol and only slightly soluble in water. It contains the total alkaloids, of which reserpine accounts for about 50% of the total activity. Orally, a dosage of 200 to 300 mg is roughly equivalent to 500 μg of reserpine. It is used in the treatment of mild or moderate hypertension or in combination with other hypotensive agents in severe hypertension.

Reserpine, USP. Reserpine (Serpasil, Reserpoid, Rau-Sed, Sandril) is a white to light yellow, crystalline alkaloid, practically insoluble in water, obtained from various species of *Rauwolfia.* In common with other compounds with an indole nucleus, it is susceptible to decomposition by light and oxidation, especially when in solution. In the dry state, discoloration occurs rapidly when reserpine is exposed to light, but the loss in potency is usually small. In solution, reserpine may break down with no appreciable color change when exposed to light, especially in clear glass containers; thus, color change cannot be used as an index of the amount of decomposition.

Reserpine is effective orally and parenterally for the treatment of hypertension. After a single intravenous dose, the onset of antihypertensive action usually begins in about 1 hour. After intramuscular injection, the maximum effect occurs within approximately 4 hours and lasts about 10 hours. When it is given orally, the maximum effect occurs within about 2 weeks and may persist up to 4 weeks after the final dose. When used in conjunction with other hypotensive drugs in the treatment of severe hypertension, the daily dose varies from 100 to 250 μg.

Guanethidine and Related Compounds. Guanethidine has been classified traditionally as an adrenergic blocking agent because it can prevent the release of norepinephrine from postganglionic neurons in response to adrenergic stimulation. Guanethidine and other compounds discussed in this section have other actions on catecholamine metabolism and can cause significant depletion of these amines in adrenergic neurons. They do not interfere with release of epinephrine from the adrenal medulla.

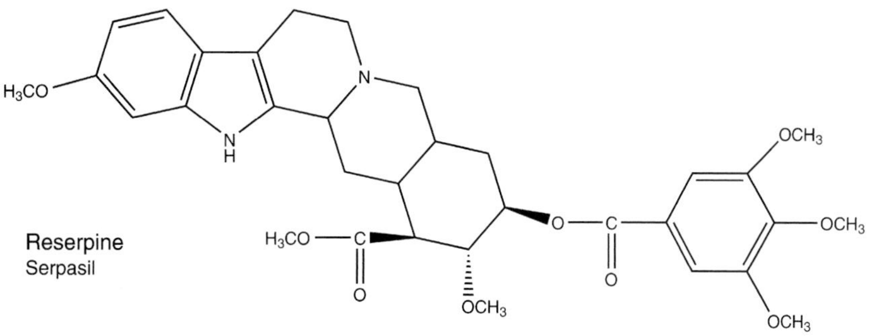

Reserpine
Serpasil

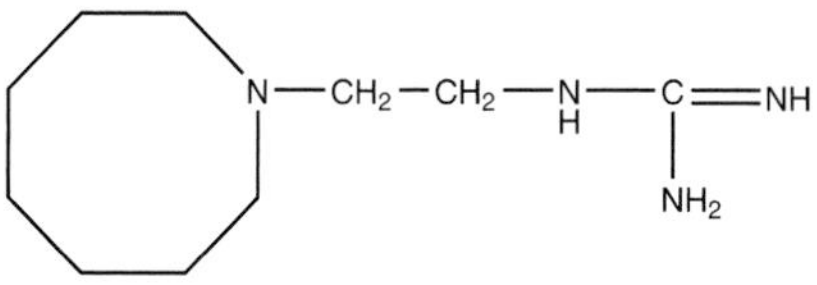

Guanethidine
(Ismelin)

Guanethidine Monosulfate, USP.

Guanethidine monosulfate, [2-(hexahydro-1 (2*H*)-azocinyl)ethyl]guanidine sulfate (Ismelin sulfate), is a white, crystalline material that is very soluble in water. It was one of a series of guanidine compounds prepared in the search for potent antitrypanosomal agents. There is an absence of CNS effects, such as depression, because the drug is highly polar and does not easily cross the blood–brain barrier. Guanethidine monosulfate produces a gradual, prolonged fall in blood pressure. Usually, 2 to 7 days of therapy are required before the peak effect is reached, and usually, this peak effect is maintained for 3 or 4 days. Then, if the drug is discontinued, the blood pressure returns to pretreatment levels over a period of 1 to 3 weeks. Because of this slow onset and prolonged duration of action, only a single daily dose is needed.

Guanethidine monosulfate is metabolized by microsomal enzymes to 2-(6-carboxyhexylamino)ethylguanidine and guanethidine *N*-oxide (Fig. 19-20). Both metabolites have very weak antihypertensive properties. Guanethidine mono-

sulfate is taken up by the amine pump located on the neuronal membrane and retained in the nerve, displacing norepinephrine from its storage sites in the neuronal granules. The displaced norepinephrine is metabolized to homovanillic acid by mitochondrial monoamine oxidase, depleting the nerve ending of the neurotransmitter. The usefulness of guanethidine monosulfate also resides in the fact that once it is taken up by the nerve, it produces a sympathetic blockade by inhibiting release of nonepinephrine that would occur on neuronal membrane response to stimulation[28] by the nerve action potential. Guanethidine monosulfate stored in the granules is released by the nerve action potential but has very low intrinsic activity for the adrenergic receptors on the postjunctional membrane. Moderate doses for a prolonged period or large doses may produce undesirable side effects by causing neuromuscular blockade and adrenergic nerve conduction blockade.

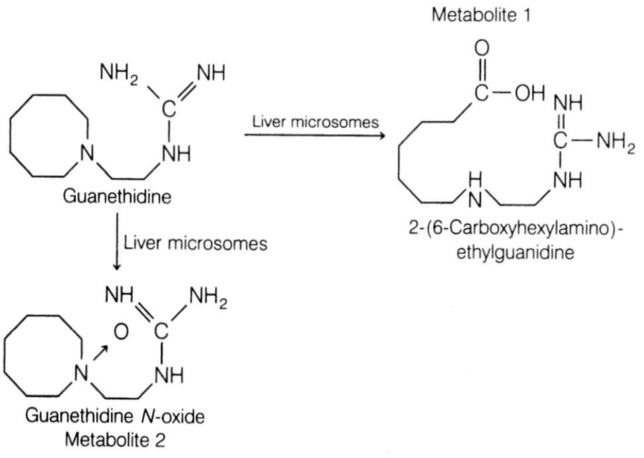

Guanadrel Sulfate.

Guanadrel sulfate, (1,4-dioxaspiro[4.5]dec-2-ylmethyl)guanadine sulfate (Hylorel), is similar to guanethidine monosulfate in the manner in which it reduces elevated blood pressure. It acts as a postganglionic adrenergic blocking agent by displacing norepinephrine in adrenergic neuron storage granules, thereby preventing release of the endogenous neurotransmitter on nerve stimulation. Guanadrel sulfate has a much shorter half-life (10 hours) than guanethidine monosulfate, whose half-life is measured in days. In the stepped-care approach to hypertension, guanadrel sulfate is usually a step 2 agent.

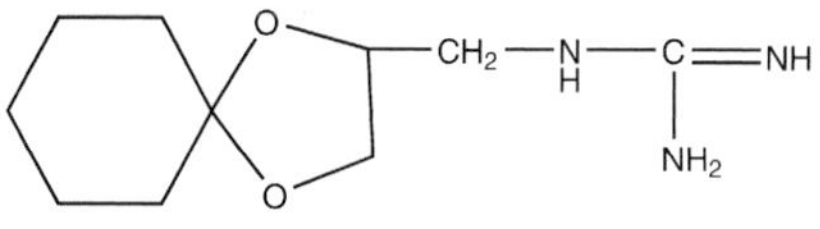

Guanadrel
(Hylorel)

Metabolite 1

Guanethidine

2-(6-Carboxyhexylamino)-
ethylguanidine

Guanethidine *N*-oxide
Metabolite 2

Figure 19–20 ■ Metabolism of guanethidine monosulfate.

SELECTIVE α-ADRENERGIC ANTAGONISTS

The principal clinical use of α-adrenergic antagonists is in the treatment of catecholamine-dependent hypertension. Classic drugs such as phentolamine and phenoxybenzamine are nonspecific blocking agents of both α_1 and α_2 receptors on the presynaptic membrane of the adrenergic neuron. Specific antagonists of α_1 receptors are effective antihypertensive agents by blocking the vasocontricting effect on smooth muscle and not interfering with the activation of α_2 receptors on the adrenergic neuron, which when activated inhibit further release of norepinephrine.

Prazosin Hydrochloride. The antihypertensive effects of prazosin hydrochloride, 1-(4-amino-6,7-dimethoxy-2-quinazolinyl)-4-(2-furoyl)piperazine monohydrochloride (Minipress), are due to peripheral vasodilation as a result of its blockade of α_1-adrenergic receptors. In ligand-binding studies, prazosin hydrochloride has 5,000-fold greater affinity for α_1 receptors than for some α_2-adrenergic receptors.[57]

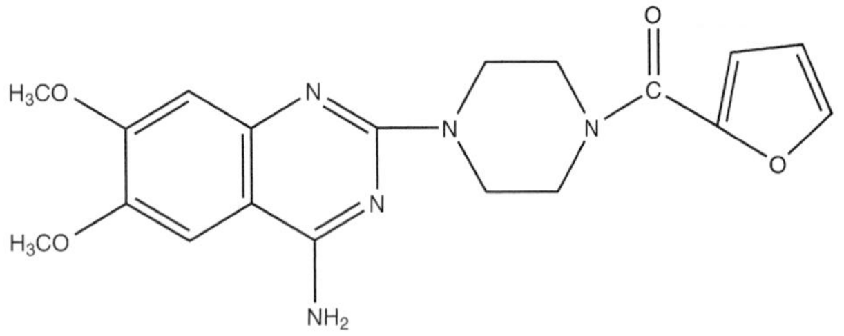

Prazosin
(Minipress)

Prazosin hydrochloride is readily absorbed, and plasma concentrations reach a peak about 3 hours after administration. Plasma half-life is between 2 and 3 hours. Prazosin hydrochloride is highly bound to plasma protein; it does not cause adverse reactions, however, with drugs that might be displaced from their protein-binding sites (e.g., cardiac glycosides). It may cause severe orthostatic hypertension because of its α-adrenergic blocking action, which prevents the reflex venous constriction that is activated when an individual sits up from a prone position.

Terazosin Hydrochloride. Terazosin hydrochloride, 1-(4-amino-6,7-dimethoxy-2-quinazolinyl)-4-(tetrahydro-2-furoyl)piperazine monohydrochloride (Hytrin), is a structural congener of prazosin hydrochloride. It possesses similar selective properties of specifically inhibiting α_1-adrenergic receptors. The drug is slightly less potent than prazosin hydrochloride. Terazosin hydrochloride has a half-life of approximately 12 hours, which is much longer than that of prazosin. This lends itself to a once-daily dose to control hypertension in many patients.

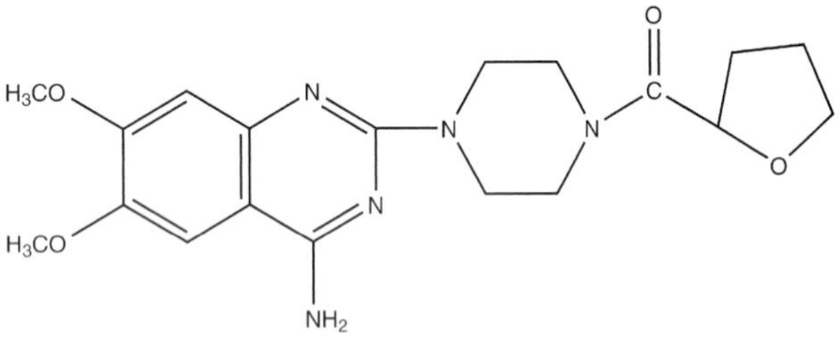

Terazosin
(Hytrin)

Doxazosin. Doxazosin, 1-(4-amino-6,7-dimethoxy-2-quinazolinyl)-4-(1,4-benzodioxan-2-ylcarbonyl)piperazine (Cardura), is a quinazoline compound that selectively inhibits the α_1 subtype of α-adrenergic receptors. This agent is very useful in the management of hypertension associated with pheochromocytoma.

CENTRALLY ACTING ADRENERGIC DRUGS

The use of agents that directly affect the peripheral component of the sympathetic nervous system represents an important approach to the treatment of hypertension. A second approach to modifying sympathetic influence on the cardiovascular system is through inhibition or reduction of CNS control of blood pressure. Several widely used medications act by stimulating α_2 receptors, which in the CNS reduces sympathetic outflow to the cardiovascular system and produces a hypotensive effect.

Methyldopate Hydrochloride, USP. Methyldopate hydrochloride, L-3-(3,4-dihydroxyphenyl)-2-methylalanine ethyl ester hydrochloride (Aldomet ester hydrochloride), α-methyldopa, lowers blood pressure by inhibiting the outflow of sympathetic vasoconstrictor impulses from the brain. Early studies had suggested that the hypotensive action of α-methyldopa was due to the peripheral properties of the drug as a decarboxylase inhibitor or a false transmitter.

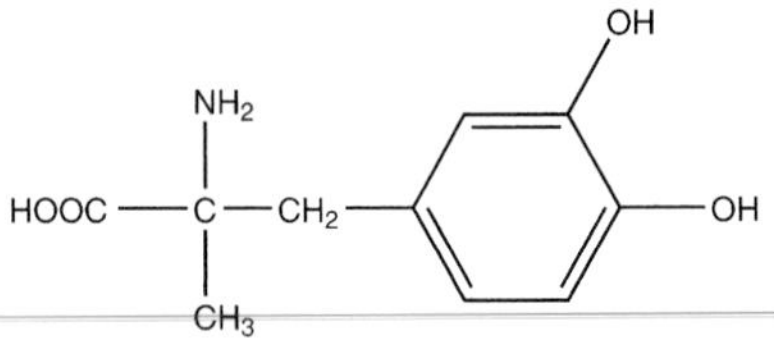

Methyldopa
(Aldomet)

The current hypothesis concerning the hypotensive activity of methyldopa involves the CNS as the site of action.[58] Methyldopa, on conversion to α-methylnorepinephrine, acts on α_2-adrenergic receptors to inhibit the release of norepinephrine, resulting in decreased sympathetic outflow from the CNS and activation of parasympathetic outflow.

Methyldopa is used as a step 2 agent and is recommended for patients with high blood pressure who are not responsive to diuretic therapy alone. Methyldopa, suitable for oral use, is a zwitterion and is not soluble enough for parenteral use. The problem was solved by making the ester, leaving the amine free to form the water-soluble hydrochloride salt. It is supplied as a stable, buffered solution, protected with antioxidants and chelating agents.

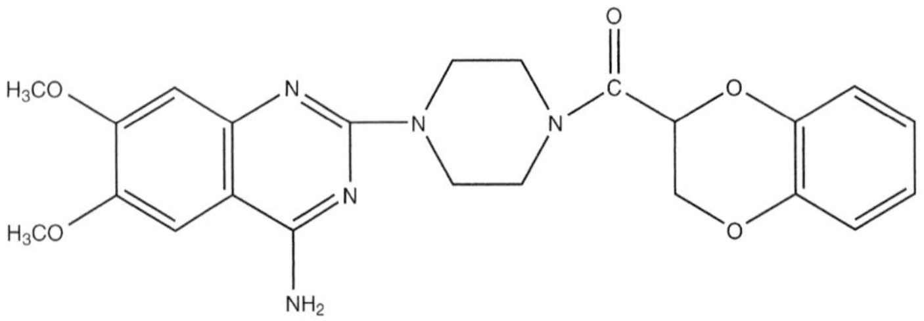

Doxazosin
(Cardura)

Clonidine Hydrochloride. Clonidine hydrochloride, 2-[(2,6-dichlorophenyl)imino]imidazolidine monohydrochloride (Catapres), was the first antihypertensive known to act on the CNS. It was synthesized in 1962 as a derivative of the known α-sympathomimetic drugs naphazoline and tolazoline, potential nasal vasoconstrictors, but instead it proved to be effective in the treatment of mild-to-severe hypertension.

Clonidine hydrochloride acts by both peripheral and central mechanisms in the body to affect blood pressure. It stimulates the peripheral α-adrenergic receptors to produce vasoconstriction, resulting in a brief period of hypertension. Clonidine hydrochloride acts centrally to inhibit the sympathetic tone and cause hypotension that is of much longer duration than the initial hypertensive effect. Administration of clonidine hydrochloride thus produces a biphasic change in blood pressure, beginning with a brief hypertensive effect and followed by a hypotensive effect that persists for about 4 hours. This biphasic response is altered by dose only: Larger doses produce a greater hypertensive effect and delay the onset of the hypotensive properties of the drug. Clonidine hydrochloride acts on α_2 adrenoreceptors located in the hindbrain to produce its hypotensive action. Clonidine hydrochloride also acts centrally to cause bradycardia and to reduce plasma levels of renin. Sensitization of baroreceptor pathways in the CNS appears to be responsible for the bradycardia transmitted by way of the vagus nerve. The central mechanism that results in decreased plasma renin is not known, however. The hypotensive properties of clonidine in animals can be blocked by applying α-adrenergic blocking agents directly to the brain.[59]

Clonidine hydrochloride has advantages over antihypertensive drugs such as guanethidine monosulfate and prazosin hydrochloride, in that it seldom produces orthostatic hypotensive side effects. It does, however, have some sedative properties that are undesirable; it also may cause constipation and dryness of the mouth.

Clonidine hydrochloride is distributed throughout the body, with the highest concentrations found in the organs of elimination: kidney, gut, and liver. Brain concentrations are low but higher than plasma concentrations. The high concentration in the gut is due to an enterohepatic cycle in which clonidine hydrochloride is secreted into the bile in rather high concentrations. The half-life in humans is about 20 hours. Clonidine hydrochloride is metabolized by the body to form two major metabolites, *p*-hydroxyclonidine and its glucuronide. *p*-Hydroxyclonidine does not cross the blood–brain barrier and has no hypotensive effect in humans.

Clonidine
(Catapres)

Guanabenz Acetate. Guanabenz acetate, [(2,6-dichlorobenzylidene)amino]guanidine monoacetate (Wytensin), is a central α_2-adrenergic agonist that reduces the release of

norepinephrine from the neuron when stimulated. The effect of the drug results in decreased sympathetic tone in the heart, kidneys, and peripheral blood vessels. The drug does not produce orthostatic hypotension.

Guanabenz
(Wytensin)

Guanfacine Hydrochloride. Guanfacine hydrochloride, *N*-(aminoiminomethyl)-2,6-dichlorobenzeneacetamide (Tenex), is structurally related to clonidine hydrochloride and guanabenz acetate and shares many of their pharmacological properties. The drug has a longer duration of action than either clonidine hydrochloride or guanabenz acetate. It lasts up to 24 hours. It also requires much longer (8 to 12 hours) for a peak effect to occur after the drug is administered.

Guanfacine
(Tenex)

VASODILATORY DRUGS ACTING ON SMOOTH MUSCLE

Reduction of arterial smooth muscle tone may occur by many mechanisms, such as reduction in sympathetic tone, stimulation of β-adrenergic receptors, or even direct action on the vasculature without interference from the autonomic innervation. Drugs acting on the arteriolar smooth muscle also increase sympathetic reflex activity, causing an increase in heart rate and cardiac output and stimulating renin release, which increases sodium retention and plasma volume. As a result, it is common to coadminister saluretics and β-adrenergic blocking drugs with these agents.

Antihypertensive agents that produce vasodilation of smooth muscle can be divided into two categories: direct-acting and indirect-acting vasodilators. Indirect-acting vasodilators may be distinguished from direct-acting vasodilators, in that they produce their effect by interfering with the vasoconstrictor stimuli and their primary site of action is not necessarily the vascular smooth muscle itself. Indirect-acting vasodilators include sympatholytic drugs, such as reserpine; α-adrenergic antagonists, such as prazosin hydrochloride; ACE inhibitors; and angiotensin II receptor antagonists, such as saralysin. Direct-acting vasodilators include hydralazine hydrochloride, sodium nitroprusside, potassium channel openers, and calcium channel–blocking agents.[59]

Hydralazine Hydrochloride, USP. Hydralazine hydrochloride, 1-hydrazinophthalazine monohydrochloride (Apresoline hydrochloride), originated from the work of a chemist[60] attempting to produce some unusual chemical

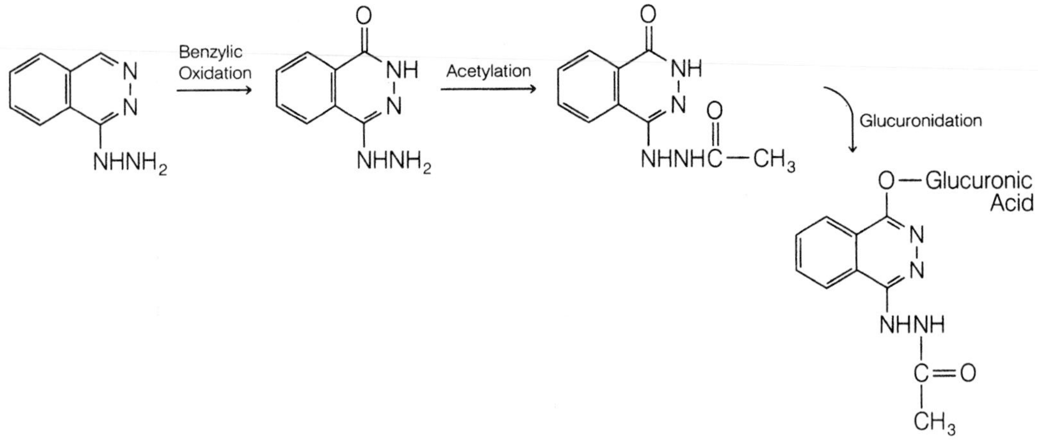

Figure 19-21 ■ Metabolism of hydralazine hydrochloride.

compounds and from the observation[61] that this compound had antihypertensive properties. It occurs as yellow crystals and is soluble in water to the extent of about 3%. A 2% aqueous solution has a pH of 3.5 to 4.5.

Hydralazine hydrochloride is useful in the treatment of moderate-to-severe hypertension. It is often used in conjunction with less potent antihypertensive agents because side effects occur frequently when it is used alone in adequate doses. In combinations, it can be used in lower and safer doses. Its action appears to be centered on the smooth muscle of the vascular walls, with a decrease in peripheral resistance to blood flow. This results in increased blood flow through the peripheral blood vessels. It also has the unique property of increasing renal blood flow, an important consideration in patients with renal insufficiency.

Hydralazine hydrochloride acts on vascular smooth muscle to cause relaxation. Its mechanism of action is unclear. It interferes with Ca^{2+} entry and Ca^{2+} release from intracellular stores and reportedly causes activation of guanylate cyclase, resulting in increased levels of cGMP. All of these biochemical events can cause vasodilation.

Absorption of hydralazine hydrochloride taken orally is rapid and nearly complete. The maximal hypotensive effect is demonstrable within 1 hour. The drug is excreted rapidly by the kidneys, and within 24 hours, 75% of the total amount administered appears in the urine as metabolites or unchanged drug. Hydralazine hydrochloride undergoes benzylic oxidation, glucuronide formation, and N-acetylation by the microsomal enzymes in the tissues (Fig. 19-21). Acetylation appears to be a major determinant of the rate of hepatic removal of the drug from the blood and, therefore, of systemic availability.[62] Rapid acetylation results in a highly hepatic extraction ratio from blood and greater first-pass elimination.

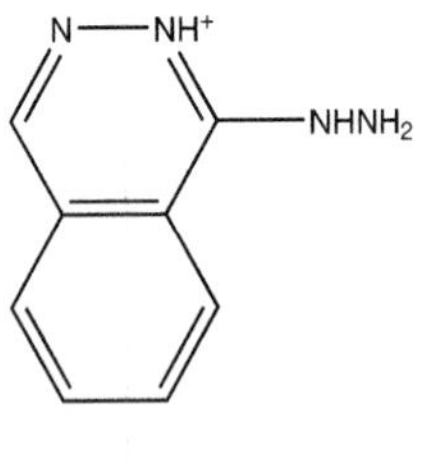

Hydralazine
(Apresoline)

Hydralazine hydrochloride is more effective clinically when coadministered with drugs that antagonize adrenergic transmission (e.g., β-adrenergic antagonists, reserpine, guanethidine monosulfate, methyldopa, and clonidine hydrochloride). When given with diuretics, it is useful in the treatment of CHF.

Sodium Nitroprusside, USP. Sodium nitroprusside, sodium nitroferricyanide, disodium pentacyanonitrosylferrate(2) $Na_2[Fe(CN)_5NO]$ (Nipride, Nitropress), is one of the most potent blood pressure–lowering drugs. Its use is limited to hypertensive emergencies because of its short duration of action. The effectiveness of sodium nitroprusside as an antihypertensive has been known since 1928, but not until 1955 was its efficacy as a drug established.[63] The drug differs from other vasodilators, in that vasodilation occurs in both venous and arterial vascular beds. Sodium nitroprusside is a reddish-brown water-soluble powder that is decomposed by light when in solution. The hypotensive effect of the chemical is due to the formation of NO in situ (look under the heading, Nitrovasodilators), elevating cellular levels of cGMP. Sodium nitroprusside is metabolized by the liver, yielding thiocyanate. Because thiocyanate is excreted by the kidneys, patients with impaired renal function may suffer thiocyanate toxicity.

$$Na_2[Fe(CN)_5NO] \cdot 2H_2O$$

Sodium Nitroprusside
(Nipride)
(Nitropress)

POTASSIUM CHANNEL AGONISTS

The two agents that can be classified in this category are diazoxide and minoxidil. These drugs are also called *potassium channel openers*. These agents activate ATP-sensitive potassium channels, which leads to a decrease of intracellular Ca^{2+} and reduces the excitability of smooth muscle. The primary action of these drugs is to open potassium channels in the plasma membrane of vascular smooth muscle. An efflux of potassium from the cell follows, resulting in hyperpolarization of the membrane, which produces an inhibitory influence on membrane excitation and subsequent vasodilation.

Diazoxide, USP. Diazoxide is used as the sodium salt of 7-chloro-3-methyl-2*H*-1,2,4-benzothiadiazine 1,1-dioxide (Hyperstat IV). Diazoxide lowers peripheral vascular resistance, increases cardiac output, and does not compromise renal blood flow.

This is a des-sulfamoyl analogue of the benzothiazine diuretics and has a close structural similarity to chlorothiazide. It was developed intentionally to increase the antihypertensive action of the thiazides and to minimize the diuretic effect.

It is used by intravenous injection as a rapidly acting antihypertensive agent for emergency reduction of blood pressure in hospitalized patients with accelerated or malignant hypertension. Over 90% is bound to serum protein, and caution is needed when it is used in conjunction with other protein-bound drugs that may be displaced by diazoxide. The injection is given rapidly by the intravenous route to ensure maximal effect. The initial dose is usually 1 mg/kg of body weight, with a second dose given if the first injection does not lower blood pressure satisfactorily within 30 minutes. Further doses may be given at 4- to 24-hour intervals if needed. Oral antihypertensive therapy is begun as soon as possible.

The injection has a pH of about 11.5, which is necessary to convert the drug to its soluble sodium salt. There is no significant chemical decomposition after storage at room temperature for 2 years. When the solution is exposed to light, it darkens.

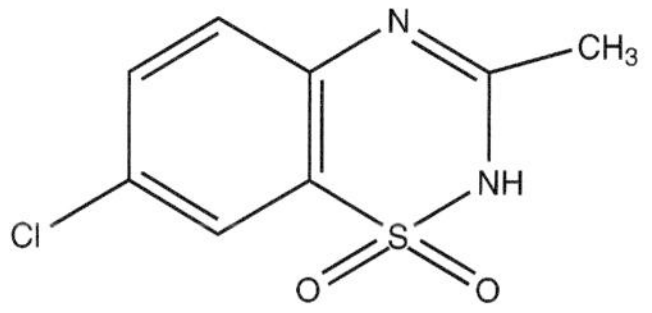

Diazoxide
(Hyperstat)

Minoxidil, USP. Minoxidil, 2,4-diamino-6-piperidinopyrimidine-3-oxide (Loniten), was developed as a result of isosteric replacement of a triaminotriazine moiety by triaminopyrimidine. The triaminotriazines were initially observed to be potent vasodilators in cats and dogs following their formation of *N*-oxides in these animals. The triazines were inactive in humans because of their inability to form *N*-oxide metabolites; this led to the discovery of minoxidil. Minoxidil is the only direct-acting vasodilator that requires metabolic activation to produce its antihypertensive effect (Fig. 19-22). It is converted to minoxidil sulfate in the liver by a sulfotransferase enzyme.[64]

The antihypertensive properties of minoxidil are similar to those of hydralazine hydrochloride, in that minoxidil can decrease arteriolar vascular resistance. Minoxidil exerts its vasodilatory action by a direct effect on arteriolar smooth muscle and appears to have no effect on the CNS or on the adrenergic nervous system in animals.[65] The serum half-life is 4.5 hours, and the antihypertensive effect may last up to 24 hours.

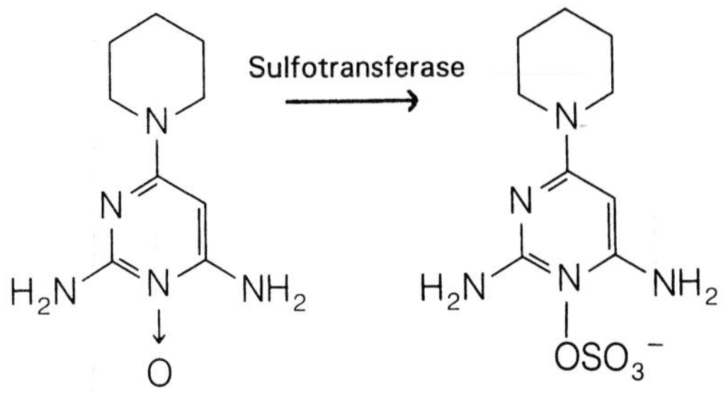

Figure 19–22 ■ Activation of minoxidil.

Minoxidil is used for severe hypertension that is difficult to control with other antihypertensive agents. The drug has some of the characteristic side effects of direct vasodilatory drugs. It causes sodium and water retention and may require coadministration of a diuretic. Minoxidil also causes reflex tachycardia, which can be controlled by use of a β-adrenergic blocking agent.

Minoxidil topical solution is used to treat alopecia androgenitica (male pattern baldness). Although the mechanism is not clearly understood, topical minoxidil is believed to increase cutaneous blood flow, which may stimulate hair growth. The stimulation of hair growth is attributed to vasodilation in the vicinity of application of the drug, resulting in better nourishment of the local hair follicles.

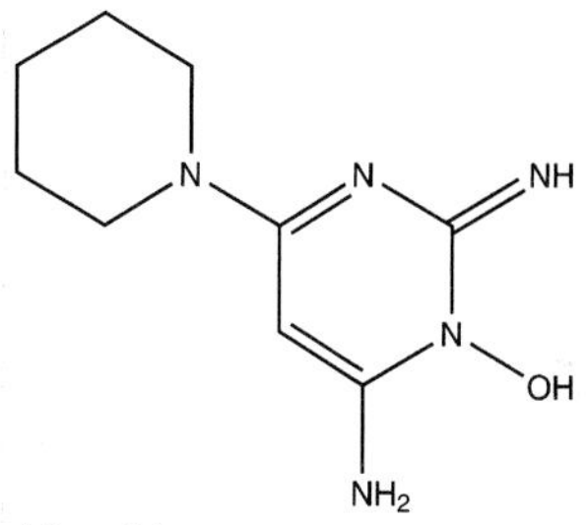

Minoxidil
(Loniten)

POSITIVE INOTROPIC AGENTS

Agents that successfully increase the force of contraction of the heart may be particularly useful in the treatment of CHF. In CHF, the heart cannot maintain sufficient blood flow to various organs to provide oxygen-rich blood. Agents that increase the force of contraction allow greater amounts of blood to be distributed throughout the body and, in turn, reduce the symptoms associated with CHF. Most of the positive inotropic agents exhibit their effects on the force of contraction by modifying the coupling mechanism involved in the myocardial contractile process.

Digitalis glycosides, a mixture of products isolated from foxglove, *Digitalis* spp., were first used as a heart medication as early as 1500 BC when in the *Ebers Papyrus* the ancient Egyptians reported their success in using these products. Throughout history these plant extracts have also been used as arrow poisons, emetics, and diuretics. The dichotomy of the poisonous effects and the beneficial heart properties is still evident today. Cardiac glycosides are still used today in the treatment of CHF and atrial fibrillation, with careful attention paid to monitoring the toxicity these agents possess.

The cardiac glycosides include two distinct classes of compounds—the cardenolides and the bufadienolides. These differ in the substitutions at the C-17 position, where the cardenolides possess an unsaturated butyrolactone ring, while the bufadienolides have an α-pyrone ring. Pharmacologically, both have similar properties and are found in many of the same natural sources, including plant and toad species. By far, the most important sources include *Digitalis purpurea* and *D. lanata*. In 1785, William Withering published "An Account of the Foxglove and Its Medical Uses: With Practical Remarks on Dropsy and Other Diseases," in which he describes the beneficial use of foxglove in dropsy (edema), which often exists in CHF.

Even with recent advances in synthetic organic chemistry coupled with the use of combinatorial chemistry, no new therapeutics have displaced the cardiac glycosides. Furthermore, the perennial use of these agents over many centuries is even more remarkable when one considers the useful life of a "block buster" drug in today's marketplace. This remarkable fact is based, quite simply, on the unique ability of nature to produce extraordinarily bioactive substances, which characteristically possess both a lipophilic portion in the steroidal ring and a hydrophilic moiety in the glycosidic rings. The therapeutic use of these agents depends largely on a balance between the different solubility characteristics of the steroid structure, and the type and number of sugar units attached to it. Although the fundamental pharmacological properties reside with the steroidal nucleus, the sugars play a critical role in the biological effects elicited, since they increase the water solubility of the lipid system, making them more available for translocation in an aqueous environment and, at the same time, allowing transportation across fatty sites. These properties uniquely balance each other and allow successful translocation to the receptive sites in the body. Ultimately, the lipophilic steroid also plays a specific role in the agent's onset and duration of action. As the steroidal rings are modified with polar groups (e.g., hydroxyls), the onset increases and the duration of action decreases. The sugar residues are substituted on C-3 of the steroid and generally are digitoxose, glucose, rhamnose, or cymarose.

The cardiac glycosides elicit their effects through inhibition of the Na^+/K^+-ATPase pump. Inhibition of this pump increases the intracellular Na^+ concentration, which affects Na^+/Ca^{2+} exchange. This increases intracellular concentrations of Ca^{2+}, which is available to activate the contractile proteins actin and myosin, thereby enhancing the force of contraction. Also, it is suggested that these agents have other compensatory mechanisms including baroreceptor sensitivity, which result in improved conditions for patients suffering from CHF.

Digoxin. Digoxin (Lanoxin) is a purified digitalis preparation from *Digitalis lanata* and represents the most widely used digitalis glycoside. This wide use is primarily due to its fast onset and short half-life. Position 3 of the steroid is substituted with three digitoxose residues that, when removed, provide a genin or aglycone steroid that is still capable of receptor binding but with altered pharmacokinetics.

Digitalis. Digitalis (Crystodigin) is isolated from *D. lanata* and *D. purpurea*, among other *Digitalis* spp. and is the chief active glycoside in digitalis leaf, with 1 mg digitoxin equal to 1 g of digitalis leaf therapy. In patients who miss doses, digitalis is very useful for maintenance therapy because of the longer half-life it provides. The longer duration and increased half-life are due to the lack of the C-12 hydroxy that is present in digoxin. In digoxin, this hydroxy plays two roles: *(a)* it serves as a site for metabolism, which reduces the compound's half-life; and *(b)* it gives more hydrophilic character, which results in greater water solubility and ease in renal elimination.

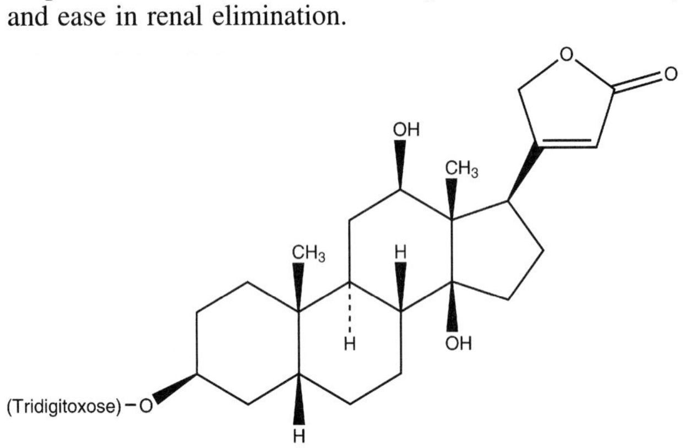

Digoxin
(Lanoxin)

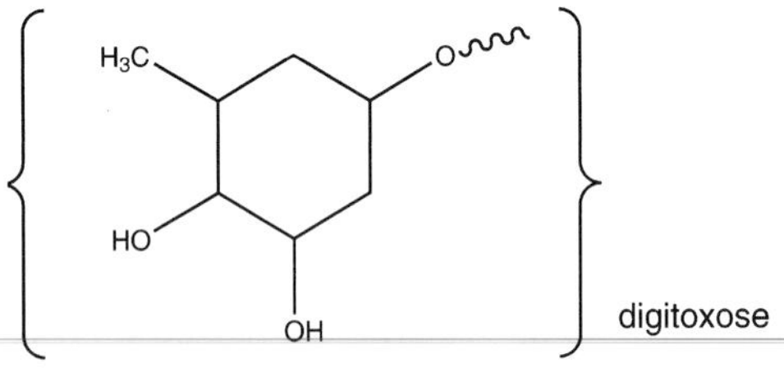

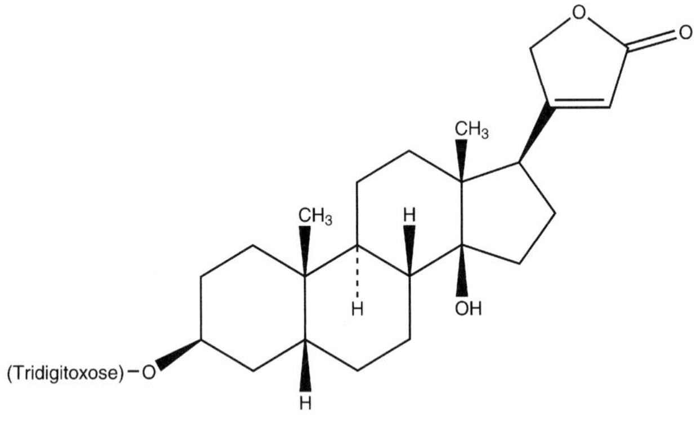

digitoxose

Digitalis
(Crystodigin)

digitoxose

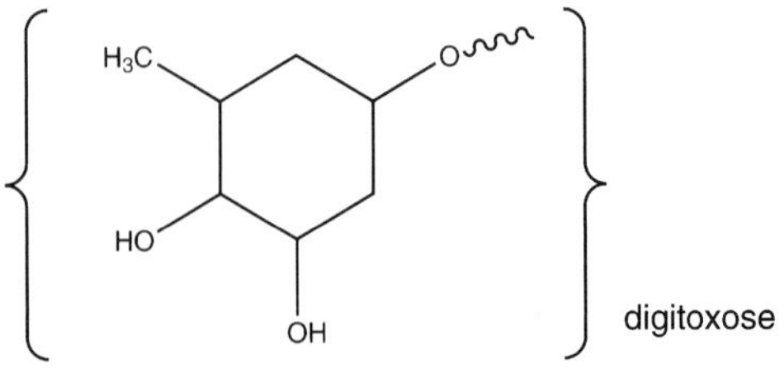

Amrinone. During normal heart function, cAMP performs important roles in regulating intracellular calcium levels. That is, certain calcium channels and storage sites for calcium must be activated by cAMP-dependant protein kinases. Since cAMP plays an indirect role in the contractility process, agents that inhibit its degradation will provide more calcium for cardiac contraction. One phosphodiesterase enzyme that is involved in the hydrolysis of myocardium cAMP is F-III. Amrinone, 5-amino (3,4′-dipyridin)-6 1(*H*)-one (Inocor), possesses positive isotropic effects as a result of its ability to inhibit this phosphodiesterase. In 1999, the U. S. Pharmacopoeia (USP) Nomenclature Committee and the United States Adopted Names (USAN) Council approved changing the nonproprietary name and the current official monograph title of amrinone to inamrinone. This change in nomenclature was a result of amrinone being confused with amiodarone because of the similarity of the names. This was reported to cause confusion between the products that led to medication errors, some of which resulted in serious injury or death.

Amrinone
(Inocor)

Milrinone. Milrinone, 1,6-dihydro-2-methyl-6-oxo-3,4′-bipyridine-5-carbonitrile (Primacor), is another dipyridine phosphodiesterase F-III inhibitor that possesses pharmacological properties similar to those of amrinone. The inhibition of the degradation of cAMP results in an increase in the cardiac muscle's force of contraction.

Milrinone
(Primacor)

ANTIHYPERLIPIDEMIC AGENTS

The major cause of death in the Western world today is vascular disease, of which the most prevalent form is atherosclerotic heart disease. Although many causative factors of this disease are recognized (e.g., smoking, stress, diet), atherosclerotic disease can be treated through medication or surgery.

Hyperlipidemia is the most prevalent indicator for susceptibility to atherosclerotic heart disease; it is a term used to describe elevated plasma levels of lipids that are usually in the form of lipoproteins. Hyperlipidemia may be caused by

an underlying disease involving the liver, kidney, pancreas, or thyroid, or it may not be attributable to any recognizable disease. In recent years, lipids have been implicated in the development of atherosclerosis in humans. *Atherosclerosis* may be defined as degenerative changes in the intima of medium and large arteries. This degeneration includes the accumulation of lipids, complex carbohydrates, blood, and blood products and is accompanied by the formation of fibrous tissue and calcium deposition on the intima of the blood vessels. These deposits or *plaques* decrease the lumen of the artery, reduce its elasticity, and may create foci for thrombi and subsequent occlusion of the blood vessel.

Lipoprotein Classes

Lipoproteins are macromolecules consisting of lipid substances (cholesterol, triglycerides) noncovalently bound with protein and carbohydrate. These combinations solubilize the lipids and prevent them from forming insoluble aggregates in the plasma. They have a spherical shape and consist of a nonpolar core surrounded by a monolayer of phospholipids whose polar groups are oriented toward the lipid phase of the plasma. Included in the phospholipid monolayer are a small number of cholesterol molecules and proteins termed *apolipoproteins*. The apolipoproteins appear to be able to solubilize lipids for transport in an aqueous surrounding such as plasma (Fig. 19-23).

The various lipoproteins found in plasma can be separated by ultracentrifugal techniques into chylomicrons, very-low-density lipoprotein (VLDL), intermediate-density lipoprotein (IDL), low-density lipoprotein (LDL), and high-density lipoprotein (HDL). These correlate with the electrophoretic separations of the lipoproteins as follows: chylomicrons, pre-β-lipoprotein (VLDL), broad β-lipoprotein (IDL), β-lipoprotein (LDL), and α-lipoprotein (HDL).

Chylomicrons contain 90% triglycerides by weight and originate from exogenous fat from the diet. They are the least dense of the lipoproteins and migrate the least under the

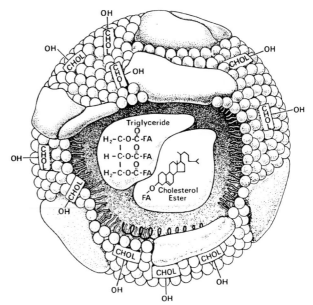

Figure 19–23 ▪ Hypothetical model of lipoprotein particle.

influence of an electric current. Chylomicrons are normally absent in plasma after 12 to 24 hours of fasting. The VLDL is composed of about 60% triglycerides, 12% cholesterol, and 18% phospholipids. It originates in the liver from FFAs. Although VLDL can be isolated from plasma, it is catabolized rapidly into IDL, which is degraded further into LDL. Normally, IDL also is catabolized rapidly to LDL, but it is usually not isolated from plasma. The LDL consists of 50% cholesterol and 10% triglycerides. This is the major cholesterol-carrying protein. In normal persons, this lipoprotein accounts for about 65% of the plasma cholesterol and is of major concern in hyperlipidemic disease states. The LDL is formed from the intravascular catabolism of VLDL. The HDL is composed of 25% cholesterol and 50% protein and accounts for about 17% of the total cholesterol in plasma.

Lipoprotein Metabolism

The rate at which cholesterol and triglycerides enter the circulation from the liver and small intestine depends on the supply of the lipid and proteins necessary to form the lipoprotein complexes. Although the protein component must be synthesized, the lipids can be obtained either from de novo biosynthesis in the tissues or from the diet. Reduction of plasma lipids by diet can delay the development of atherosclerosis. Furthermore, the use of drugs that decrease assimilation of lipids into the body plus diet decreases mortality from cardiovascular disease.[66]

Lipid transport mechanisms exist that shuttle cholesterol and triglycerides among the liver, intestine, and other tissues. Normally, plasma lipids, including lipoprotein cholesterol, are cycled into and out of plasma and do not cause extensive accumulation of deposits in the walls of arteries. Genetic factors and changes in hormone levels affect lipid transport by altering enzyme concentrations and apoprotein content, as well as the number and activity of lipoprotein receptors. This complex relationship makes the treatment of all hyperlipoproteinemias by a singular approach difficult, if not impractical.

Lipids are transported by both *exogenous* and *endogenous* pathways. In the exogenous pathway, dietary fat (triglycerides and cholesterol) is incorporated into large lipoprotein particles (chylomicrons), which enter the lymphatic system and are then passed into the plasma. The chylomicrons are acted on by lipoprotein lipase in the adipose tissue capillaries, forming triglycerides and monoglycerides. The FFAs cross the endothelial membrane of the capillary and are incorporated into triglycerides in the tissue for storage as fat or are used for energy by oxidative metabolism. The chylomicron remnant in the capillary reaches the liver and is cleared from the circulation by binding to a receptor that recognizes the apoprotein E and B-48 protein components of the chylomicron remnant.

In the endogenous pathway of lipid transport, lipids are secreted from the liver. These are triglycerides and cholesterol combined with apoprotein B-100 and apoprotein E to form VLDL. The VLDL is acted on by lipoprotein lipase in the capillaries of adipose tissue to generate FFAs and an IDL. Some IDL binds to LDL receptors in the liver and is cleared from plasma by endocytosis. Approximately half of the circulating IDL is converted to LDL in the plasma by additional loss of triglycerides. This LDL has a half-life in

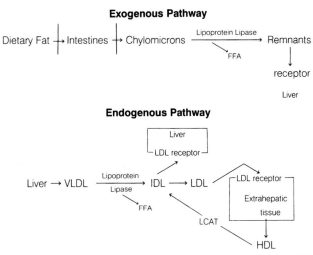

Figure 19–24 ■ Exogenous and endogenous pathways of lipoprotein metabolism.

plasma of about 1.5 days and represents 60 to 70% of the cholesterol in plasma. These LDL particles bind to LDL receptors in extrahepatic tissues and are removed from the plasma. Levels of LDL receptors vary depending on the need of extrahepatic tissues to bind LDL to use cholesterol. The extrahepatic tissue subsequently releases HDL. Free plasma cholesterol can be adsorbed onto HDL and the cholesterol esters formed by the enzyme lecithin–cholesterol acyltransferase (LCAT). These esters are transferred from HDL to VLDL or LDL in plasma to complete the cycle. The pathways for plasma lipoprotein metabolism by the exogenous and endogenous routes are shown in Figure 19-24.

Hyperlipoproteinemias

Lipid disorders are related to problems of lipoprotein metabolism[67] that create conditions of hyperlipoproteinemia. The hyperlipoproteinemias have been classified into six types, each of which is treated differently (Table 19-6).

The abnormal lipoprotein pattern characteristic of type I is caused by a decrease in the activity of lipoprotein lipase, an enzyme that normally hydrolyzes the triglycerides present in chylomicrons and clears the plasma of this lipoprotein fraction. Because the triglycerides found in chylomicrons come primarily from exogenous sources, this type of hyperlipoproteinemia may be treated by decreasing the intake of dietary fat. There are no drugs at present that can be used to counteract type I hyperlipidemia effectively.

Type II hyperlipoproteinemia has been divided into types IIa and IIb. Type IIa is characterized by elevated levels of LDL (β-lipoproteins) and normal levels of triglycerides. This subtype disorder is very common and may be caused by disturbed catabolism of LDL. Type IIb differs from type IIa, in that this hyperlipidemia has elevated VLDL levels in addition to LDL levels. Type II hyperlipoproteinemia is often clearly familial and frequently inherited as an autosomal dominant abnormality with complete penetrance and expression in infancy. Patients have been treated by use of dietary restrictions on cholesterol and saturated fats. This type of hyperlipoproteinemia responds to some form of

TABLE 19–6 Characterization of Hyperlipoproteinemia Types

Hyperlipo-proteinemia	Abnormality		Appearance of Plasma[a]	Triglycerides	Total Cholesterol
	Electrophoresis	**Ultracentrifuge**			
I	Massive chylomicronemia	Clear; creamy layer of chylomicronemia on top	Massively elevated	Slightly to moderately elevated	
IIa	β-Lipoproteins elevated	LDL increased	Clear	Normal	Heavily elevated
IIb	Pre-β-lipoproteins elevated	LDL + VLDL increased	Slightly turbid	Slightly elevated	Heavily elevated
III	Broad β-lipoprotein band	VLDL/LDL of abnormal composition	Slightly turbid to turbid	Elevated	Elevated
IV	Pre-β-lipoproteins elevated	VLDL increased	Turbid	Moderately to heavily elevated	Normal to elevated
V	Pre-β-lipoproteins elevated; chylomicronemia	VLDL increased; chylomicronemia	Turbid; on top, chylomicronemia	Massively elevated	Slightly elevated

Adapted from Witte, E. C.: Prog. Med. Chem. 11:199, 1975.
[a]After having been kept standing at 4°C for 25 hours.

chemotherapy. The combined therapy may bring LDL levels back to normal.

Type III is a rare disorder characterized by a broad band of β-lipoprotein. Like type II, it is also familial. Patients respond favorably to diet and drug therapy.

In type IV hyperlipoproteinemia, levels of VLDL are elevated. Because this type of lipoprotein is rich in triglycerides, plasma triglyceride levels are elevated. The metabolic defect that causes type IV is still unknown; this form of hyperlipidemia, however, responds to diet and drug therapy.

Type V hyperlipoproteinemia has high levels of chylomicrons and VLDL, resulting in high levels of plasma triglycerides. The biochemical defect of type V hyperlipoproteinemia is not understood. Clearance of dietary fat is impaired, and reduction of dietary fat is indicated along with drug therapy.

Clofibrate, USP. Clofibrate, ethyl 2-(*p*-chlorophenoxy)-2-methylpropionate (Atromid-S), is a stable, colorless to pale yellow liquid with a faint odor and a characteristic taste. It is soluble in organic solvents but insoluble in water.

Clofibrate is prepared by a Williamson synthesis, condensing *p*-chlorophenol with ethyl α-bromoisobutyrate, or by the interaction of a mixture of acetone, *p*-chlorophenol, and chloroform in the presence of excess potassium hydroxide. The acid obtained by either of these methods is esterified to give clofibrate. Both acid and ester are active; the latter, however, is preferred for medicinal use. Clofibrate is hydrolyzed rapidly to 2-*p*-chlorophenoxy-2-methylpropionic acid by esterases in vivo and, bound to serum albumin, circulates in blood. The acid has been investigated as a hypolipidemic agent. It is absorbed more slowly and to a smaller extent than is the ester. The aluminum salt of the acid gives even lower blood levels than *p*-chlorophenoxy-2-methylpropionic acid.[68]

Clofibrate is the drug of choice in the treatment of type III hyperlipoproteinemias and may also be useful, to a lesser extent, in types IIb and IV hyperlipoproteinemias. The drug is not effective in types I and IIa.

Clofibrate can lower plasma concentrations of both triglycerides and cholesterol, but it has a more consistent clinical effect on triglycerides. It also affects lipoprotein plasma levels by enhancing removal of triglycerides from the circulation and causes reduction of VLDL by stimulating lipoprotein lipase to increase the catabolism of this lipoprotein to LDL.[69] Clofibrate lowers triglyceride levels in the serum much more than cholesterol levels and decreases levels of FFAs and phospholipids. The lowering of cholesterol levels may result from more than one mechanism. Clofibrate inhibits the incorporation of acetate into the synthesis of cholesterol, between the acetate and mevalonate step, by inhibiting *sn*-glyceryl-3-phosphate acyltransferase. Clofibrate also regulates cholesterol synthesis in the liver by inhibiting microsomal reduction of 3-hydroxy-3-methylglutaryl-CoA (HMG-CoA), catalyzed by HMG-CoA reductase. Clofibrate may lower plasma lipids by means other than impairment of cholesterol biosynthesis, such as increasing excretion through the biliary tract.

Clofibrate is tolerated well by most patients; the most common side effects are nausea and, to a smaller extent, other gastrointestinal distress. The dosage of anticoagulants, if used in conjunction with this drug, should be reduced by one third to one half, depending on the individual response, so that the prothrombin time may be kept within the desired limits.

Clofibrate
(Atromid)

Gemfibrozil. Gemfibrozil, 5-(2,5-dimethylphenoxy)-2,2-dimethylpentanoic acid (Lopid), is a congener of clofibrate that was used first in the treatment of hyperlipoproteinemia in the mid-1970s. Its mechanism of action and use are similar to those of clofibrate. Gemfibrozil reduces plasma levels of VLDL triglycerides and stimulates clearance of VLDL from plasma. The drug has little effect on cholesterol plasma levels but does cause an increase of HDL.

Gemfibrozil is absorbed quickly from the gut and excreted

unchanged in the urine. The drug has a plasma half-life of 1.5 hours, but reduction of plasma VLDL concentration takes between 2 and 5 days to become evident. The peak effect of its hypolipidemic action may take up to 4 weeks to become manifest.

Gemfibrozil
(Lopid)

Fenofibrate. Fenofibrate, 2-[4-(4-chlorobenzoyl)phenoxy]-2-methylpropanoic acid 1-methylethyl ester (Tricor), has structural features represented in clofibrate. The primary difference involves the second aromatic ring. This imparts a greater lipophilic character than exists in clofibrate, resulting in a much more potent hypocholesterolemic and triglyceride-lowering agent. Also, this structural modification results in a lower dose requirement than with clofibrate or gemfibrozil.

Fenofibrate
(Tricor)

Dextrothyroxine Sodium, USP. Dextrothyroxine sodium, *O*-(4-hydroxy-3,5-diiodophenyl)-3,5-diiodo-D-tyrosine monosodium salt hydrate, sodium D-3,3′,5,5′-tetraiodothyronine (Choloxin), occurs as a light yellow to buff powder. It is stable in dry air but discolors on exposure to light; hence, it should be stored in light-resistant containers. It is very slightly soluble in water, slightly soluble in alcohol, and insoluble in acetone, chloroform, and ether.

The hormones secreted by the thyroid gland have marked hypocholesterolemic activity along with their other well-known actions. The finding that not all active thyroid principles possessed the same degree of physiological actions led to a search for congeners that would cause a decrease in serum cholesterol levels without other effects such as angina pectoris, palpitation, and congestive failure. D-Thyroxine resulted from this search. At the dosage required, however, L-thyroxine contamination must be minimal; otherwise, it will exert its characteristic actions. One route to optically pure (at least 99% pure) D-thyroxine is the use of an L-amino acid oxidase from snake venom, which acts only on the L isomer and makes separation possible.

The mechanism of action of D-thyroxine appears to be stimulation of oxidative catabolism of cholesterol in the liver through stimulation of 7-α-cholesterol hydroxylase, the rate-limiting enzyme in the conversion of cholesterol to bile acids. The bile acids are conjugated with glycine or taurine and excreted by the biliary route into the feces. Although thyroxine does not inhibit cholesterol biosynthesis, it increases the number of LDL receptors, enhancing removal of LDL from plasma.

Dextrothyroxine
(Choloxin)

Use of thyroxine in the treatment of hyperlipidemias is not without adverse effects. The drug increases the frequency and severity of anginal attacks and may cause cardiac arrhythmias.

D-Thyroxine potentiates the action of anticoagulants such as warfarin or dicumarol; thus, the dosage of the anticoagulants used concurrently should be reduced by one third and then, if necessary, further modified to maintain the prothrombin time within the desired limits. Also, it may increase the dosage requirements for insulin or oral hypoglycemic agents if used concurrently with them.

Cholestyramine Resin, USP. Cholestyramine (Cuemid, Questran) is the chloride form of a strongly basic anion-exchange resin. It is a styrene copolymer with divinylbenzene with quaternary ammonium functional groups. After oral ingestion, cholestyramine resin remains in the gastrointestinal tract, where it readily exchanges chloride ions for bile acids in the small intestine, to be excreted as bile salts in the feces. Cholestyramine resin is also useful in lowering plasma lipids. The reduction in the amounts of reabsorbed bile acids results in increased catabolism of cholesterol in bile acids in the liver. The decreased concentration of bile acids returning to the liver lowers the feedback inhibition by bile acids of 7-α-hydroxylase, the rate-limiting enzyme in the conversion of cholesterol to bile acids, increasing the breakdown of hepatic cholesterol. Although biosynthesis of cholesterol is increased, it appears that the rate of catabolism is greater, resulting in a net decrease in plasma cholesterol levels by affecting LDL clearance. The increase of LDL receptors in the liver that occurs when its content of cholesterol is lowered augments this biochemical event.

Cholestyramine resin does not bind with drugs that are neutral or with amine salts; acidic drugs (in the anion form) could be bound, however. For example, in animal tests, absorption of aspirin given concurrently with the resin was depressed only moderately during the first 30 minutes.

Cholestyramine Resin
(Cholybar)
(Questran)

Cholestyramine resin is the drug of choice for type IIa hyperlipoproteinemia. When used in conjunction with a controlled diet, it reduces β-lipoproteins. The drug is an insoluble polymer and, thus, probably one of the safest because it is not absorbed from the gastrointestinal tract to cause systemic toxic effects.

Colestipol Hydrochloride. Colestipol (Colestid) is a high-molecular-weight, insoluble, granular copolymer of tetraethylenepentamine and epichlorohydrin. It functions as an anion-exchange, resin-sequestering agent in a manner similar to that of cholestyramine resin. Colestipol hydrochloride reduces cholesterol levels without affecting triglycerides and seems to be especially effective in the treatment of type II hyperlipoproteinemias.

Colestipol
(Colestid)

Colesevelam. Colesevelam (Welchol) is one of the more recent additions to the class of bile acid-sequestering agents. Its structure is rather novel, and at first glance, it appears to look like the previous examples of cholestyramine and colestipol. It does not possess the chloride ions, however, and, strictly speaking, is not an anion-exchange resin. This compound has good selectivity for both the trihydroxy and dihydroxy bile acids. The selectivity for these hydroxylated derivatives lends some insight into the reduced side effects colesevelam possesses, compared with cholestyramine and colestipol. Unlike the older agents, colesevelam does not have a high incidence of causing constipation. This results from the compound's ability to "pick up" water because of its affinity for hydroxyl system (i.e., hydrogen bonding with either the bile acid or water). In turn, this yields softer, gel-like materials that are easier to excrete.

Colesevelam
(Welchol)

Nicotinic Acid. Nicotinic acid, 3-pyridinecarboxylic acid (Niacin), is effective in the treatment of all types of hyperlipoproteinemia except type I, at doses above those given as a vitamin supplement. The drug reduces VLDL synthesis and, subsequently, its plasma products, IDL and LDL. Plasma triglyceride levels are reduced because of the decreased VLDL production. Cholesterol levels are lowered, in turn, because of the decreased rate of LDL formation from VLDL. Although niacin is the drug of choice for type II hyperlipoproteinemias, its use is limited because of the vasodilating side effects. Flushing occurs in practically all patients but generally subsides when the drug is discontinued.

The hypolipidemic effects of niacin may be due to its ability to inhibit lipolysis (i.e., prevent the release of FFAs and glycerol from fatty tissues). As a consequence, there is a reduced reserve of FFA in the liver and diminution of lipoprotein biosynthesis, which reduces the production of VLDL. The decreased formation of lipoproteins leads to a pool of unused cholesterol normally incorporated in VLDL. This excess cholesterol is then excreted through the biliary tract.

Niacin (nicotinic acid) may be administered as aluminum nicotinate (Nicalex). This is a complex of aluminum hydroxy nicotinate and niacin. The aluminum salt is hydrolyzed to aluminum hydroxide and niacin in the stomach. The aluminum salt seems to have no advantage over the free acid. Hepatic reaction appears more prevalent than with niacin.

Nicotinic acid has been esterified to prolong its hypolipidemic effect. Pentaerythritol tetranicotinate has been more effective experimentally than niacin in reducing cholesterol levels in rabbits. Sorbitol and *myo*-inositol hexanicotinate polyesters have been used in the treatment of patients with atherosclerosis obliterans.

The usual maintenance dose of niacin is 3 to 6 g/day given in three divided doses. The drug is usually given at mealtimes to reduce the gastric irritation that often accompanies large doses.

Nicotinic Acid
(Niacin)

β-Sitosterol. Sitosterol is a plant sterol, whose structure is identical with that of cholesterol, except for the substituted ethyl group on C-24 of its side chain. Although the mechanism of its hypolipidemic effect is not clearly understood, it is suspected that the drug inhibits the absorption of dietary cholesterol from the gastrointestinal tract. Sitosterols are absorbed poorly from the mucosal lining and appear to compete with cholesterol for absorption sites in the intestine.

β-Sitosterol

Probucol, USP. Probucol, 4,4'-[(1-methylethylidene)-bis(thio)]bis[2,6-bis(1,1-dimethylethyl)phenol], DH-581 (Lorelco), is a chemical agent that was developed for the plastics and rubber industry in the 1960s. The probucol molecule has two tertiary butylphenol groups linked by a dithio-propylidene bridge, giving it a high lipophilic character with strong antioxidant properties. In humans, it causes reduction of both liver and serum cholesterol levels, but it does not alter plasma triglycerides. It reduces LDL and (to a lesser extent) HDL levels by a unique mechanism that is still not clearly delineated. The reduction of HDL may be due to the ability of probucol to inhibit the synthesis of apoprotein A-1, a major protein component of HDL.[70] It is effective at reducing levels of LDL and is used in hyperlipoproteinemias characterized by elevated LDL levels.

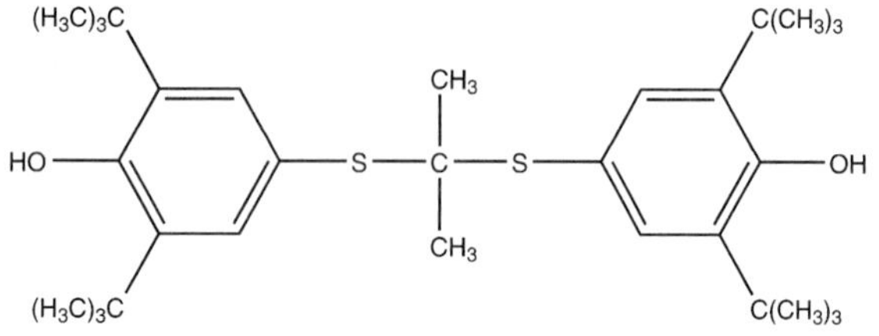

Probucol
(Lorelco)

HMG-CoA Reductase Inhibitors

Drugs in this class of hypolipidemic agents inhibit the enzyme HMG-CoA reductase, responsible for the conversion of HMG-CoA to mevalonate in the synthetic pathway for the synthesis of cholesterol (Fig. 19-25). HMG-CoA reductase is the rate-limiting catalyst for the irreversible conversion of HMG-CoA to mevalonic acid in the synthesis of cholesterol. The activity of HMG-CoA reductase is also under feedback regulation. When cholesterol is available in sufficient amounts for body needs, the enzyme activity of HMG-CoA reductase is suppressed.

Elevated plasma cholesterol levels have been correlated with an increase in cardiovascular disease. Of the plasma lipoproteins, the LDL fraction contains the most cholesterol. The source of cholesterol in humans is either the diet or de novo synthesis with the reduction of HMG-CoA by HMG-CoA reductase as the rate-limiting step. Ingested cholesterol as the free alcohol or ester is taken up after intestinal absorption and transported to the liver and other body organs through the exogenous pathway (Fig. 19-25). The LDL delivers cholesterol to peripheral cells. This process occurs after binding of LDL to specific LDL receptors located on the surface of cell membranes. After binding and endocytosis of the receptor and LDL, lysosomal degradation of this complex in the cell makes cholesterol available for use in cellular membrane synthesis. It is generally accepted that total plasma cholesterol is lowered most effectively by reducing LDL levels. Therefore, the population of LDL receptors is an important component of clearing the plasma of cholesterol. HMG-CoA reductase inhibitors contribute to this by directly blocking the active site of the enzyme. This action has a twofold effect on cholesterol plasma levels; it causes a decrease in de novo cholesterol synthesis and an increase in hepatic LDL receptors. These HMG-CoA reductase inhibitors are effective hypocholesteremic agents in patients with familial hypercholesteremia.

Three drugs, lovastatin, simvastatin, and pravastatin, compose the list of approved HMG-CoA reductase inhibitors for the treatment of hyperlipidemia in patients. The three drugs have structures similar to the substrate, HMG-CoA, of the enzyme HMG-CoA reductase. Lovastatin and simvastatin are lactones and prodrugs, activated by hydrolysis in the liver to their respective β-hydroxy acids. Pravastatin, in contrast, is administered as the sodium salt of the β-hydroxy acid.

Lovastatin. Lovastatin, 2-methylbutanoic acid 1,2,3,7,8,8a-hexahydro-3,7-dimethyl-8-[2-(tetrahydro-4-hydroxy-6-oxo-2*H*-pyran-2-yl)ethyl]-1-naphthalenyl ester, mevinolin, MK-803 (Mevacor) (formerly called mevinolin), is a potent inhibitor of HMG-CoA. The drug was obtained originally from the fermentation products of the fungi *Aspergillus terreus* and *Monascus ruber*. Lovastatin was one of two original HMG-CoA reductase inhibitors. The other drug, mevastatin (formerly called compactin), was isolated from cultures of *Penicillium cillium citrum*. Mevastatin was withdrawn from clinical trials because it altered intestinal morphology in dogs. This effect was not observed with lovastatin. For inhibitory effects on HMG-CoA reductase, the lactone ring must be hydrolyzed to the open-ring heptanoic acid.

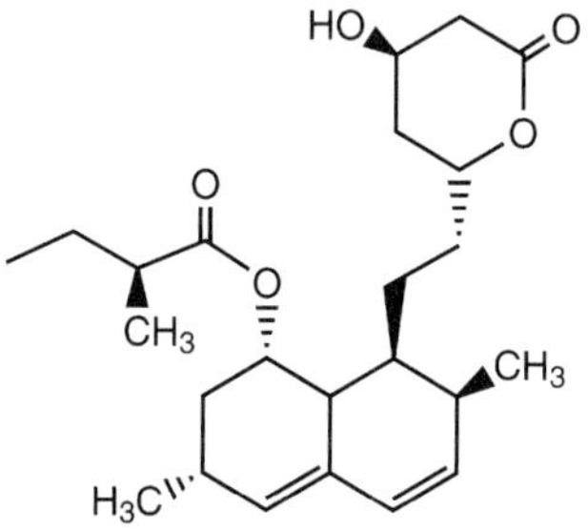

Lovastatin
(Mevacor)

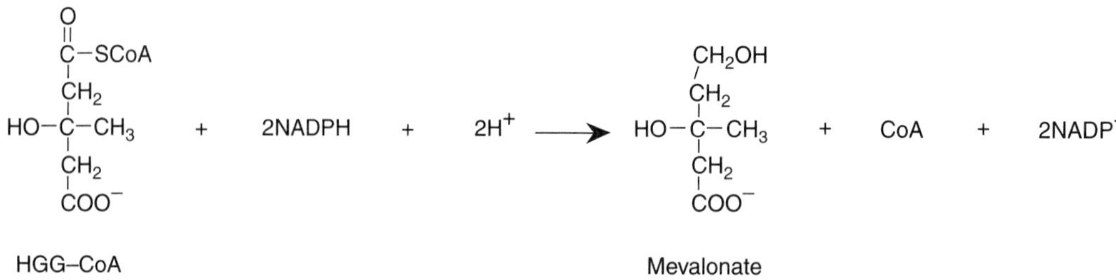

Figure 19-25 ■ HMG-CoA reductase reaction.

Simvastatin. Simvastatin, 2,2-dimethyl butanoic acid, 1,2,3,7,8,8a-hexahydro-3,7-dimethyl-8-[2-(tetrahydro-4-hydroxy-6-oxo-2-pyran-2-yl)ethyl]-1-naphthalenyl ester (Zocor), is an analogue of lovastatin. These two drugs have many similar properties. Both drugs, in the prodrug form, reach the liver unchanged after oral administration, where they undergo extensive metabolism to a number of open-ring hydroxy acids, including the active β-hydroxy acids. They are also highly bound to plasma proteins. These actions make the bioavailability of simvastatin rather poor but better than that of lovastatin, which has been estimated to be 5%.

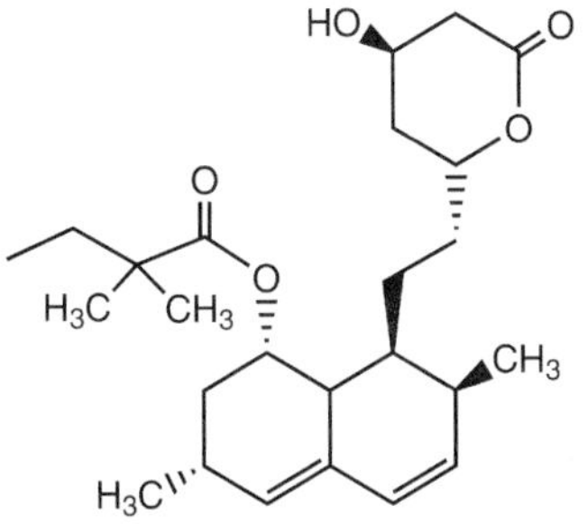

Simvastatin
(Zocor)

Pravastatin. Pravastatin, sodium 1,2,6,7,8,8a-hexahydro-β,δ,6-trihydroxy-2-methyl-8-(2-methyl-1-oxobutoxy)-1-naphthaleneheptanoate (Pravachol), is the most rapid-acting of the three HMG-CoA reductase inhibitor drugs, reaching a peak concentration in about 1 hour. The sodium salt of the β-hydroxy acid is more hydrophilic than the lactone forms of the other two agents, which may explain this property. In addition, the open form of the lactone ring contributes to a more hydrophilic agent, which, in turn, results in less CNS penetration. This explains, in part, why pravastatin has fewer CNS side effects than the more lipophilic lactone ester of this class of agents. Absorption of pravastatin following oral administration can be inhibited by resins such as cholestyramine because of the presence of the carboxylic acid function on the drug. The lactone forms of lovastatin and simvastatin are less affected by cholestyramine.

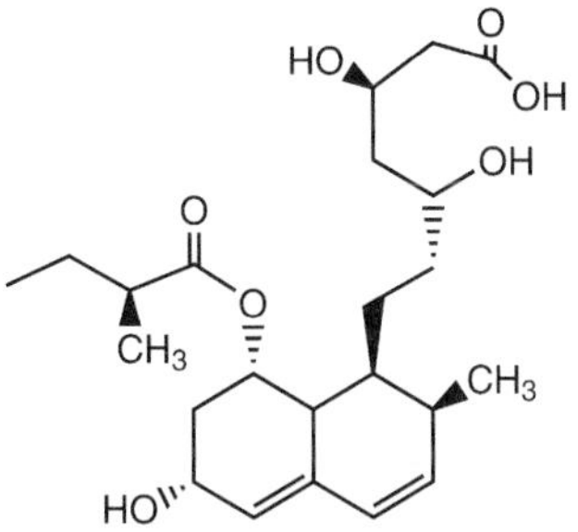

Pravastatin
(Pravachol)

Fluvastatin. Fluvastatin, [R*,S*-(E)]-(±)-7-[3-(4-fluorophenyl)-1-(1-methylethyl)-1H-indol-2-yl]-3,5-dihydroxy-6-heptenoic acid monosodium salt (Lescol), is very similar to pravastatin. It possesses a heptanoic acid side chain that is superimposable over the lactone ring found in lovastatin and simvastatin. It is this side chain that is recognized by HMG-CoA reductase. Also, much like pravastatin, the CNS side effects of this lipid-lowering agent are much

lower than those of the agents that possess a lactone ring as part of their architectural design.

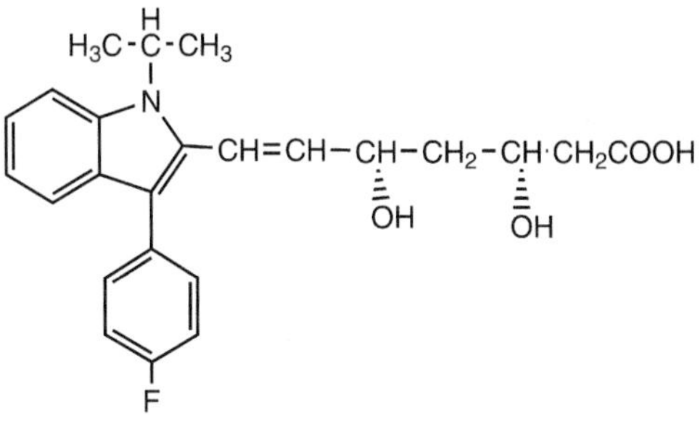

Fluvastatin
(Lescol)

Atorvastatin. Atorvastatin, [R-(R*,R*)]-2-(4-fluorophenyl)-b,d-dihydroxy-5-(1-methylethyl)-3-phenyl-4 [(phenylamino)carbonyl]-1H-pyrrole-1-heptanoic acid (Lipitor), also possesses the heptanoic acid side chain, which is critical for inhibition of HMG-CoA reductase. Although the side chain is less lipophilic than the lactone form, the high amount of lipophilic substitution causes this agent to have a slightly higher level of CNS penetration than pravastatin, resulting in a slight increase in CNS side effects. Even so, its CNS profile is much lower than that of lovastatin.

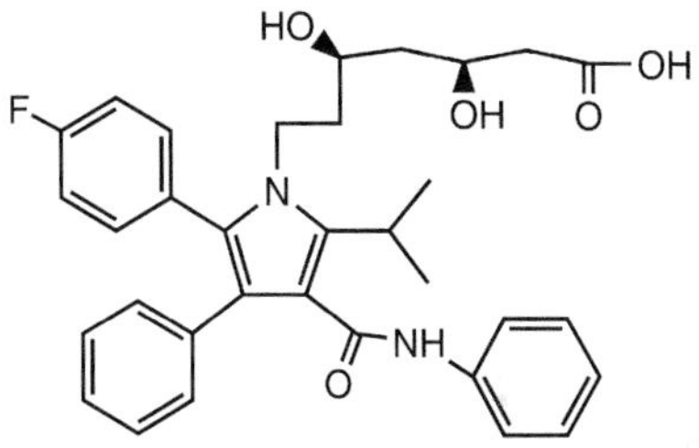

Atorvastatin
(Lipitor)

Cerivastatin. Cerivastatin (Baycol) is one of the newer agents in this class of cholesterol-lowering agents. It carries, however, a higher incidence of rhabdomyolysis and, as a result, was voluntarily withdrawn from the market by its manufacturer in 2001.

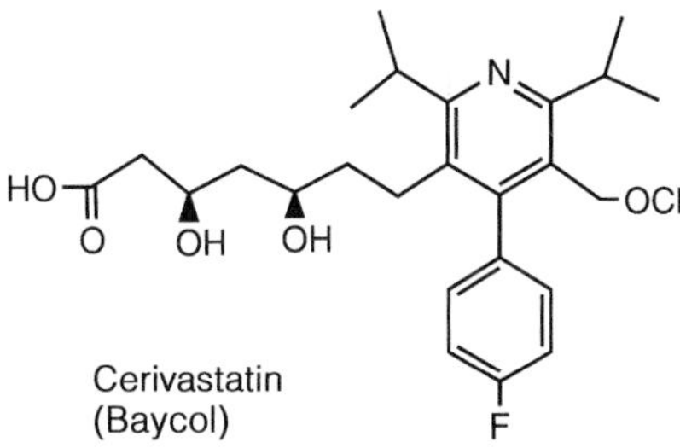

Cerivastatin
(Baycol)

ANTICOAGULANTS

A theory of blood clotting introduced in 1905 was based on the existence of four factors: thromboplastin (thrombokinase), prothrombin, fibrinogen, and ionized calcium. The clotting sequence proposed was that when tissue damage occurred, thromboplastin entered the blood from the platelets

TABLE 19–7 Roman Numerical Nomenclature of Blood-Clotting Factors and Some Common Synonyms

Factor	Synonyms
I	Fibrinogen
II	Prothrombin
III	Thromboplastin, tissue factor
IV	Calcium
V	Proaccelerin, accelerator globulin, labile factor
VI	(This number is not now used)
VII	Proconvertin, stable factor, autoprothrombin I, SPCA
VIII	Antihemophilic factor, antihemophilic globulin, platelet cofactor I, antihemophilic factor A
IX	Plasma thromboplastin component (PTC), Christmas factor, platelet cofactor II, autoprothrombin II, antihemophilic factor B
X	Stuart-Power factor, Stuart factor, autoprothrombin III
XI	Plasma thromboplastin antecedent (PTA), antihemophilic factor C
XII	Hageman factor
XIII	Fibrin-stabilizing factor, fibrinase, Laki-Lorand factor

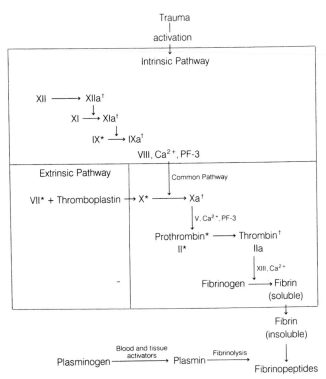

Figure 19–26 ■ Scheme of blood coagulation and fibrinolysis. *, a vitamin K–dependent factor; †, inhibition by heparin and antithrombin III.

and reacted with prothrombin in the presence of calcium to form thrombin. Thrombin then reacted with fibrinogen to form insoluble fibrin, which enmeshed red blood cells to create a clot. The concept remained unchallenged for almost 50 years, but it has now been modified to accommodate the discovery of numerous additional factors that enter into the clotting mechanism (Table 19-7).

Mechanism of Blood Coagulation

The fluid nature of blood can be attributed to the flat cells (endothelial) that maintain a nonthrombogenic environment in the blood vessels. This is a result of at least four phenomena: *(a)* the maintenance of a transmural negative electric charge that prevents adhesion between platelets; *(b)* the release of a plasmalogen activator, which activates the fibrinolytic pathway; *(c)* the release of thrombomodulin, a cofactor that activates protein C, a coagulation factor inhibitor; and *(d)* the release of PGI_2, a potent inhibitor of platelet aggregation.

The process of blood coagulation (Fig. 19-26) involves a series of steps that occur in a cascade and terminate in the formation of a fibrin clot. Blood coagulation occurs by activation of either an intrinsic pathway, a relatively slow process of clot formation, or an extrinsic pathway, which has a much faster rate of fibrin formation. Both pathways merge into a common pathway for the conversion of prothrombin to thrombin and subsequent transformation of fibrinogen to the insoluble strands of fibrin. Lysis of intravascular clots occurs through a plasminogen–plasmin system, which consists of plasminogen, plasmin, urokinase, kallikrein, plasminogen activators, and some undefined inhibitors.

The *intrinsic* pathway refers to the system for coagulation that occurs from the interaction of factors circulating in the blood. It is activated when blood comes into contact with a damaged vessel wall or a foreign substance. Each of the plasma coagulation factors (Table 19-7), with the exception of factor III (tissue thromboplastin), circulates as an inactive proenzyme. Except for fibrinogen, which precipitates as fibrin, these factors are usually activated by enzymatic removal of a small peptide in the cascade of reactions that make up the clotting sequence (Fig. 19-26). The *extrinsic* clotting system refers to the mechanism by which thrombin is generated in plasma after the addition of tissue extracts. When various tissues, such as brain or lung (containing thromboplastin), are added to blood, a complex between thromboplastin and factor VII in the presence of calcium ions activates factor X, bypassing the time-consuming steps of the intrinsic pathway that form factor X.

The intrinsic and extrinsic pathways interact in vivo. Small amounts of thrombin formed early after stimulation of the extrinsic pathway accelerate clotting by the intrinsic pathway by activating factor VIII. Thrombin also speeds up the clotting rate by activating factor V, located in the common pathway. Thrombin then converts the soluble protein fibrinogen into a soluble fibrin gel by acting on Gly–Arg bonds to remove small fibrinopeptides from the N terminus, enabling the remaining fibrinogen molecule to polymerize. It also activates factor XIII, which stabilizes the fibrin gel in the presence of calcium by cross-linking between the chains of the fibrin monomer through intermolecular γ-glutamyl–lysine bridges to form an insoluble mass.

Anticoagulant Mechanisms

In the milieu of biochemicals being formed to facilitate the clotting of blood, the coagulation cascade in vivo is controlled by a balance of inhibitors in the plasma to prevent all of the blood in the body from solidifying. Thrombin plays a pivotal role in blood coagulation. It cleaves fibrinogen, a reaction that initiates formation of the fibrin gel, which constitutes the framework of the blood clot. As mentioned above, it activates the cofactors factor V and factor VIII to accelerate the coagulation process. Intact endothelial cells express a receptor, thrombomodulin, for thrombin. When thrombin is bound to thrombomodulin, it does not have coagulant activity, which thus prevents clot formation beyond damaged areas and onto intact endothelium. In this bound state, however, thrombin does activate protein C, which then inactivates two cofactors and impedes blood clotting. Thrombin also activates factor XIII, leading to cross-linking of the fibrin gel. The activity of thrombin is regulated by its inactivation by plasma protein inhibitors: α_1-proteinase inhibitor, α_2-macroglobulin, antithrombin (antithrombin III), and heparin cofactor II. These belong to a family of proteins called *serpins,* an acronym for *serine protease inhibitors.*

Antithrombin III, an α_2-globin, neutralizes thrombin and the serine proteases in the coagulation cascade—Xa, IXa, XIa, and XIIa. Although antithrombin III is a slow-acting inhibitor, it becomes a rapid-acting inhibitor of thrombin in the presence of heparin. Heparin is a naturally occurring anticoagulant that requires antithrombin III (see above) for its biological property of preventing blood clot formation. It binds at the lysine site of the antithrombin III molecule, causing a change in the conformation of antithrombin III and increasing its anticoagulant properties. Heparin can then dissociate from antithrombin III to bind to another antithrombin III molecule. An additional system, which controls unwanted coagulation, involves protein C, a vitamin K–dependent zymogen in the plasma. Protein C is converted to a serine protease when thrombin and factor Xa, formed in the blood in the coagulation cascade, interact with thrombomodulin. The now-activated protein C inhibits factors V and VIII and, in so doing, blocks further production of thrombin. Protein C also enhances fibrinolysis by causing release of the tissue plasminogen activator.

The biosynthesis of prothrombin (factor II) depends on an adequate supply of vitamin K. A deficiency of vitamin K results in the formation of a defective prothrombin molecule. The defective prothrombin is antigenically similar to normal prothrombin but has reduced calcium-binding ability and no biological activity. In the presence of calcium ions, normal prothrombin adheres to the surface of phospholipid vesicles and greatly increases the activity of the clotting mechanism. The defect in the abnormal prothrombin is in the NH_2-terminal portion, in which the second carboxyl residue has not been added to the γ-carbon atom of some glutamic acid residues on the prothrombin molecule to form γ-carboxyglutamic acid.[71] Administration of vitamin K antagonists decreases synthesis of a biologically active prothrombin molecule and increases the clotting time of blood in humans.[72]

Vitamin K is critical to the formation of clotting factors VII, IX, and X. These factors are glycoproteins that have γ-carboxyglutamic acid residues at the N-terminal end of the peptide chain. The enzyme involved in forming an active prothrombin is a vitamin K–dependent carboxylase located in the microsomal fraction of liver cells. It has been suggested that vitamin K drives the carboxylase reaction by abstracting a proton from the relatively unreactive methylene carbon of the glutamyl residue, forming a 2,3-epoxide. Oral anticoagulants interfere with the γ-carboxylation of glutamic acid residues by preventing the reduction of vitamin K to its hydroquinone form (Fig. 19-27).

Hemophilia A, a blood disease characterized by a deficiency of coagulation factor VIII, is the most common inherited blood coagulation disorder. Treatment of this disease over the past 25 years has depended on the concentration of the antihemophilic factor (factor VIII) by cryoprecipitation and immunoaffinity chromatography separation technology. The impact of this therapy has been diminished by the presence of viruses that cause the acquired immunodeficiency syndrome (AIDS) and other less tragic viral diseases in humans. Recombinant antihemophilic factor preparations have been produced since 1989 with use of mammalian cells genetically altered to secrete human factor VIII. Kogenate and Helixate are recombinant preparations, obtained from genetically altering baby hamster kidney cells that contain high concentrations of factor VIII. Recombinant factor VIIa, an active factor in the extrinsic pathway, now in phase III clinical trials (Novo Seven), has been used to treat patients with hemophilia A factor VII deficiency. Hemophilia B, another genetic blood disorder, which constitutes about 20% of hemophilia cases, is caused by a deficiency of factor IX and has been treated from cryoprecipitated fractions obtained from plasma. Monoclonal antibody technology has produced an essentially pure, carrier-free preparation of native factor IX (Mononine). Recombinant technology has solved the problem of limited supply and viral contamination of these critical blood factors.

Platelet Aggregation and Inhibitors

Blood platelets play a pivotal role in hemostasis and thrombus formation. Actually, they have two roles in the cessation of bleeding: a hemostatic function, in which platelets, through their mass, cause physical occlusion of openings in blood vessels, and a thromboplastic function, in which the chemical constituents of the platelets take part in the blood coagulation mechanism. The circulatory system is self-sealing because of the clotting properties of blood. The pathological formation of clots within the circulatory system, however, creates a potentially serious clinical situation that must be dealt with through the use of anticoagulants.

Platelets do not adhere to intact endothelial cells. They do become affixed to subendothelial tissues, which have been exposed by injury, to cause hemostasis. Platelets bind to collagen in the vessel wall and trigger other platelets to adhere to them. This adhesiveness is accompanied by a change in shape of the platelets and may be caused by mobilization of calcium bound to the platelet membrane. The growth of the platelet mass depends on the adenosine diphosphate (ADP) released by the first few adhering cells and enhances the aggregation process. A secondary phase (phase II) immediately follows, with additional platelet aggregation. In this secondary phase, the platelets undergo a secretory process during which enzymes such as cathepsin and acid hydrolases, along with fibrinogen, are released from α granules in the platelets and ADP, ATP, serotonin, and calcium are released from dense bodies in the platelets. The dense bodies

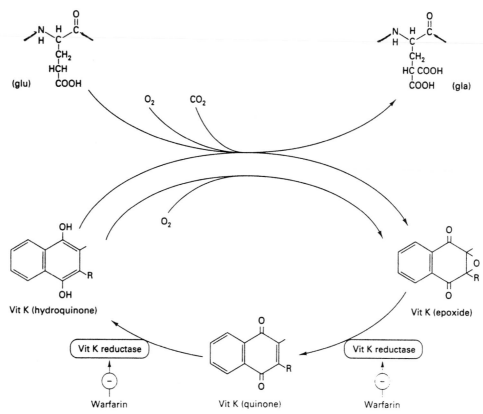

Figure 19–27 ■ Mechanism of action of vitamin K and sites of action of warfarin.

are likened to the storage granules associated with adrenergic neurons. Increased levels of cAMP inhibit platelet aggregation. cAMP activates specific dependent kinases, which form protein–phosphate complexes that chelate calcium ions. The reduced levels of calcium inhibit aggregation (Fig. 19-28). Inhibitors of platelet aggregation can increase cAMP levels by either stimulating adenylate cyclase or inhibiting phosphodiesterase.[72] Substances such as glucagon, adenosine, and isoproterenol increase cAMP levels and inhibit platelet aggregation. Drugs such as theophylline, aminophylline, dipyridamole, papaverine, and adenosine inhibit phosphodiesterase and aggregation of platelets. Epinephrine, collagen, and serotonin inhibit adenylate cyclase and stimulate platelet aggregation.[73] The role of platelets in arterial thrombosis is

similar to that in hemostasis. The factors contributing to venous thrombosis are circulatory stasis, excessive generation of thrombin formation of fibrin, and, to a lesser extent than in the artery, platelet aggregation.

Aspirin, sulfinpyrazone, and indomethacin have an inhibitory effect on platelet aggregation. They inhibit cyclooxygenase, the enzyme that controls the formation of prostaglandin endoperoxides and increases the tendency for platelets to aggregate.[74] Aspirin also inhibits the platelet-release reaction. Dipyridamole inhibits adenosine deaminase and adenosine uptake by platelets. As a result, the increased plasma concentrations of adenosine inhibit ADP-induced aggregation of platelets.

Among the many pharmacological actions of prostaglandins is the ability of some to stimulate or inhibit the aggregation of platelets and alter the clotting time of blood. Prostaglandins are synthesized from 20-carbon polyunsaturated fatty acids containing from three to five double bonds. These fatty acids are present in the phospholipids of cell membranes of all mammalian tissues. The main precursor of prostaglandins is arachidonic acid. Arachidonic acid is released from membrane phospholipids by the enzyme phospholipase A_2. Once released, arachidonic acid is metabolized by cyclooxygenase synthetase to form unstable cyclic endoperoxides, PGG_2 and PGH_2, which subsequently are transformed into PGI_2 and thromboxane A_2 (TXA_2). The conversion to TXA_2 is aided by the enzyme thromboxane synthetase. The formation of PGI_2 can occur nonenzymatically. Blood platelets convert arachidonic acid to TXA_2, whereas PGI_2 is formed mainly by the vascular endothelium.

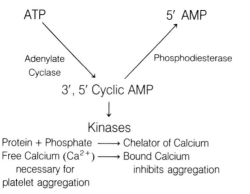

Figure 19–28 ■ Role of adenosine 3′,5′-cyclic monophosphate (cAMP) in inhibition of platelet aggregation.

Both PGI$_2$ and TXA$_2$ are unstable at physiological pH and temperatures. Their half-lives are 2 to 3 minutes.

PGI$_2$ inhibits platelet aggregation by stimulating adenylate cyclase to increase cAMP levels in the platelets. PGI$_2$ is also a vasodilator and, as a result, has potent hypotensive properties when given intravenously or by intra-arterial administration. TXA$_2$ induces platelet aggregation. Together with PGI$_2$, TXA$_2$ plays a role in the maintenance of vascular homeostasis. In addition to being a platelet aggregator, TXA$_2$ is a potent vasoconstrictor.

Retardation of clotting is important in blood transfusions, to avoid thrombosis after surgery or from other causes, to prevent recurrent thrombosis in phlebitis and pulmonary embolism, and to lessen the propagation of clots in the coronary arteries. This retardation may be accomplished by agents that inactivate thrombin (heparin) or substances that prevent the formation of prothrombin in the liver (the coumarin derivatives and the phenylindanedione derivatives).

Although heparin is a useful anticoagulant, it has limited applications. Many of the anticoagulants in use today were developed following the discovery of dicumarol, an anticoagulant present in spoiled sweet clover. These compounds are orally effective, but there is a lag period of 18 to 36 hours before they increase the clotting time significantly. Heparin, in contrast, produces an immediate anticoagulant effect after intravenous injection. A major disadvantage of heparin is that the only effective therapeutic route is parenteral.

Dicumarol and related compounds are not vitamin K antagonists in the classic sense. They appear to act by interfering with the function of vitamin K in the liver cells, which are the sites of synthesis of the clotting factors, including prothrombin. This lengthens the clotting time by decreasing the amount of biologically active prothrombin in the blood.

The discovery that dicumarol and related compounds were potent reversible competitors of vitamin K coagulant-promoting properties (although at high levels dicumarol is not reversed by vitamin K) led to the development of anti–vitamin K compounds such as phenindione, which was designed in part according to metabolite–antimetabolite concepts. The active compounds of the phenylindanedione series are characterized by a phenyl, a substituted phenyl, or a diphenylacetyl group in the 2 position. Another requirement for activity is a keto group in the 1 and 3 positions, one of which may form the enol tautomer. A second substituent, other than hydrogen, at the 2 position prevents this keto–enol tautomerism, and the resulting compounds are ineffective as anticoagulants.

PRODUCTS

Protamine Sulfate, USP. Protamine sulfate has an anticoagulant effect, but if used in the proper amount, it counteracts the action of heparin and is used as an antidote for the latter in cases of overdosage. It is administered intravenously in a dose that depends on the circumstances.

Dicumarol, USP. Dicumarol, 3,3′-methylenebis[4-hydroxycoumarin], is a white or creamy white crystalline powder with a faint, pleasant odor and a slightly bitter taste. It is practically insoluble in water or alcohol, slightly soluble in chloroform, and dissolved readily by solutions of fixed

alkalies. The effects after administration require 12 to 72 hours to develop and persist for 24 to 96 hours after discontinuance.

Dicumarol

Dicumarol is used alone or as an adjunct to heparin in the prophylaxis and treatment of intravascular clotting. It is used in postoperative thrombophlebitis, pulmonary embolus, acute embolic and thrombotic occlusion of peripheral arteries, and recurrent idiopathic thrombophlebitis. It has no effect on an already-formed embolus but may prevent further intravascular clotting. Because the outcome of acute coronary thrombosis depends largely on extension of the clot and formation of mural thrombi in the heart chambers, with subsequent embolization, dicumarol has been used in this condition. It has also been administered to arrest impending gangrene after frostbite. The dose, after determination of the prothrombin clotting time, is 25 to 200 mg, depending on the size and the condition of the patient. The drug is given orally in the form of capsules or tablets. On the second day and thereafter, it may be given in amounts sufficient to maintain the prothrombin clotting time at about 30 seconds. If hemorrhages should occur, a dosage of 50 to 100 mg of menadione sodium bisulfite is injected, supplemented by a blood transfusion.

Warfarin Sodium, USP. Warfarin sodium, 3-(α-acetonylbenzyl)-4-hydroxycoumarin sodium salt (Coumadin, Panwarfin), is a white, odorless, crystalline powder, with a slightly bitter taste; it is slightly soluble in chloroform and soluble in alcohol or water. A 1% solution has a pH of 7.2 to 8.5.

By virtue of its great potency, warfarin sodium at first was considered unsafe for use in humans and was used very effectively as a rodenticide, especially against rats. At the proper dosage level, however, it can be used in humans, especially by the intravenous route.

Wafarin Sodium
(Coumadin)

Warfarin Potassium, USP. Warfarin potassium, 3-(α-acetonylbenzyl)-4-hydroxycoumarin potassium salt (Athrombin-K), is readily absorbed after oral administration, and a therapeutic hypoprothrombinemia is produced within 12 to 24 hours after administration of 40 to 60 mg. This salt is therapeutically interchangeable with warfarin sodium.

Anisindione, USP.   Anisindione, 2-(*p*-methoxyphenyl)-1,3-indandione, 2-(*p*-anisyl)-1,3-indandione (Miradon), is a *p*-methoxy congener of phenindione. It is a white, crystalline powder, slightly soluble in water, tasteless, and absorbed well after oral administration.

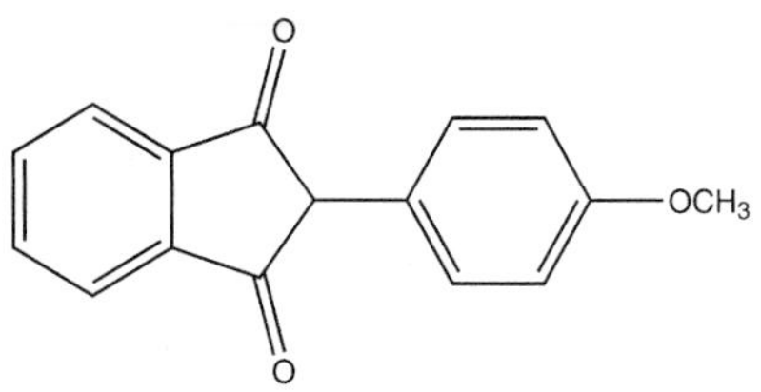

Anisindione
(Miradon)

In instances when the urine may be alkaline, an orange color may be detected. This is due to metabolic products of anisindione and is not hematuria.

SYNTHETIC HYPOGLYCEMIC AGENTS

The discovery that certain organic compounds will lower the blood sugar level is not recent. In 1918, guanidine was shown to lower the blood sugar level. The discovery that certain trypanosomes need much glucose and will die in its absence was followed by the discovery that galegine lowered the blood sugar level and was weakly trypanocidal. This led to the development of several very active trypanocidal agents, such as the bisamidines, diisothioureas, bisguanidines, and others. Synthalin (trypanocidal at 1:250 million) and pentamidine are outstanding examples of very active trypanocidal agents. Synthalin lowers the blood sugar level in normal, depancreatized, and completely alloxanized animals. This may be due to reduced oxidative activity of mitochondria, resulting from inhibition of the mechanisms that simultaneously promote phosphorylation of ADP and stimulate oxidation by nicotinamide adenine dinucleotide (NAD) in the citric acid cycle. Hydroxystilbamidine isethionate, USP, is used as an antiprotozoan agent.

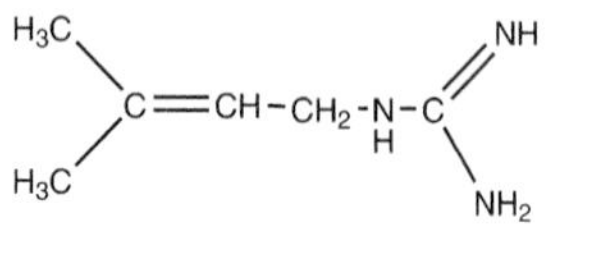

Galegine

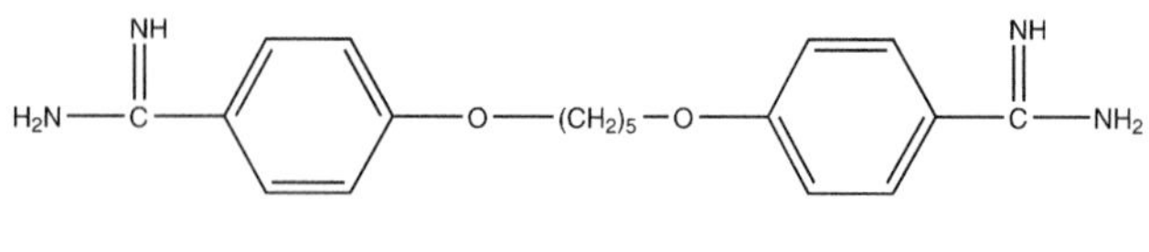

Pentamidine

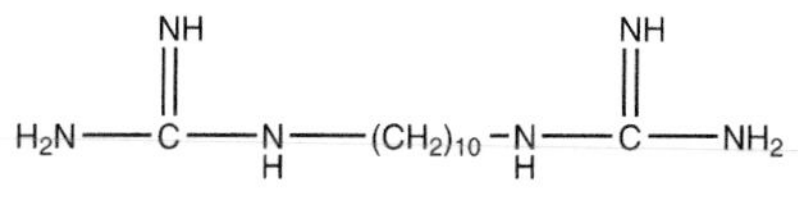

Synthalin

In 1942, *p*-aminobenzenesulfonamidoisopropylthiadiazole (an antibacterial sulfonamide) was found to produce hypoglycemia. These results stimulated research for the development of synthetic hypoglycemic agents, several of which are in use today.

Sulfonylureas became widely available in 1955 for the treatment of non–ketosis-prone mild diabetes and are still the drugs of choice. A second class of compounds, the biguanides, in the form of a single drug, phenformin, has been used since 1957. Phenformin was withdrawn from the U. S. market, however, because it causes lactic acidosis, from which fatalities have been reported.

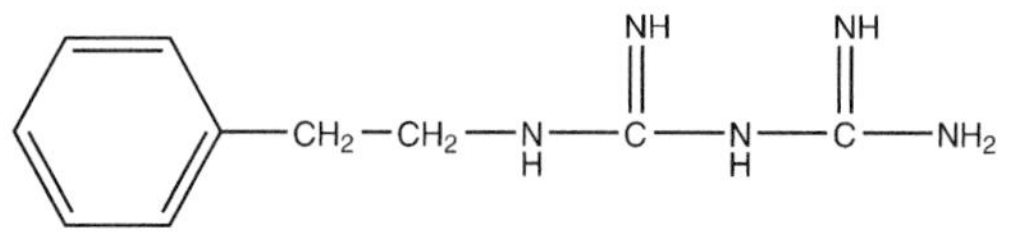

Phenformin

Sulfonylureas

The sulfonylureas may be represented by the following general structure:

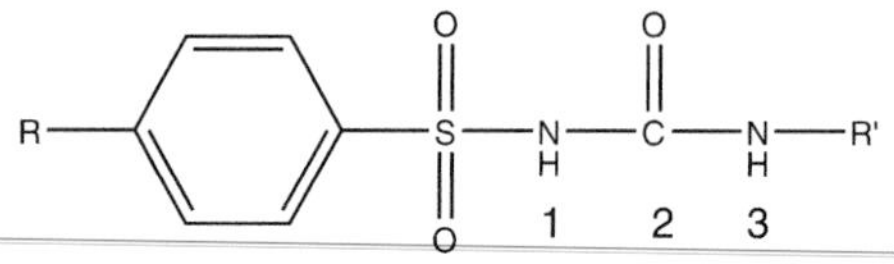

These are urea derivatives with an arylsulfonyl group in the 1 position and an aliphatic group at the 3 position. The aliphatic group, R′, confers lipophilic properties to the molecule. Maximal activity results when R′ consists of three to six carbon atoms, as in chlorpropamide, tolbutamide, and acetohexamide. Aryl groups at R′ generally give toxic compounds. The R group on the aromatic ring primarily influences the duration of action of the compound. Tolbutamide disappears quite rapidly from the bloodstream by being metabolized to the inactive carboxy compound, which is excreted rapidly. Chlorpropamide, however, is metabolized more slowly and persists in the blood much longer.

The mechanism of action of the sulfonylureas is to stimulate the release of insulin from the functioning β cells of the intact pancreas. In the absence of the pancreas, they have no significant effect on blood glucose. The sulfonylureas may have other actions, such as inhibition of secretion of glucagon and action at postreceptor intracellular sites to increase insulin activity.

For a time, tolbutamide, chlorpropamide, and acetohexamide were the only oral hypoglycemic agents. Subsequently, a second generation of these drugs became available. Although they did not present a new method of lowering blood glucose levels, they were more potent than the existing drugs. Glipizide and glyburide are the second-generation oral hypoglycemic agents.

Whether they are first- or second-generation oral hypoglycemic drugs, this group of agents remains a valuable adjunct to therapy in adult-onset diabetes patients. Accordingly, the sulfonylureas are not indicated in juvenile-onset diabetes.

Tolbutamide, USP. Tolbutamide, 1-butyl-3-(*p*-tolyl-sulfonyl)urea (Orinase), occurs as a white, crystalline powder that is insoluble in water and soluble in alcohol or aqueous alkali. It is stable in air.

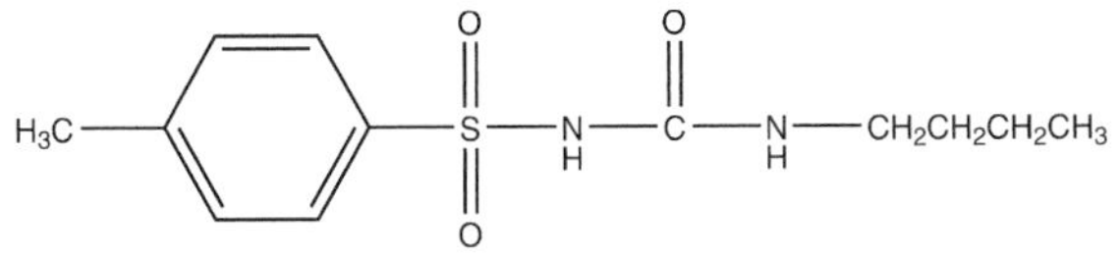

Tolbutamide
(Orinase)

Tolbutamide is absorbed rapidly in responsive diabetic patients. The blood sugar level reaches a minimum after 5 to 8 hours. It is oxidized rapidly in vivo to 1-butyl-3-(*p*-carboxyphenyl)sulfonylurea, which is inactive. The metabolite is freely soluble at urinary pH; if the urine is strongly acidified, however, as in the use of sulfosalicylic acid as a protein precipitant, a white precipitate of the free acid may be formed.

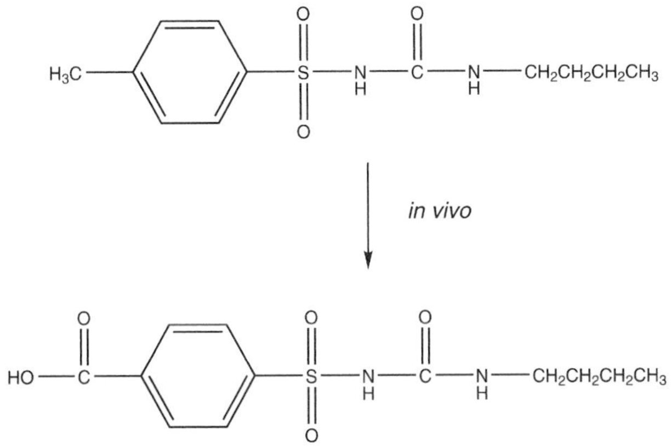

Tolbutamide should be used only when the diabetic patient is an adult or shows adult-onset diabetes, and the patient should adhere to dietary restrictions.

Tolbutamide Sodium, USP. Tolbutamide sodium, 1-butyl-3-(*p*-tolylsulfonyl)urea monosodium salt (Orinase Diagnostic), is a white, crystalline powder, freely soluble in water, soluble in alcohol and chloroform, and very slightly soluble in ether.

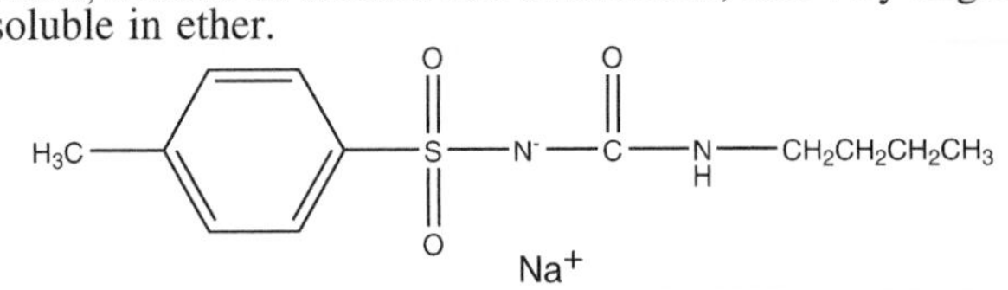

Tolbutamide Sodium

This water-soluble salt of tolbutamide is used intravenously for the diagnosis of mild diabetes mellitus and of functioning pancreatic islet cell adenomas. The sterile dry powder is dissolved in sterile water for injection to make a clear solution, which then should be administered within 1

hour. The main route of breakdown is to butylamine and sodium *p*-toluene sulfonamide.

Chlorpropamide, USP. Chlorpropamide, 1-[(*p*-chlorophenyl)-sulfonyl]-3-propylurea (Diabinese), is a white, crystalline powder, practically insoluble in water, soluble in alcohol, and sparingly soluble in chloroform. It will form water-soluble salts in basic solutions. This drug is more resistant to conversion to inactive metabolites than is tolbutamide and, as a result, has a much longer duration of action. One study showed that about half of the drug is excreted as metabolites, with the principal one being hydroxylated in the 2 position of the propyl side chain.[75] After control of the blood sugar level, the maintenance dose is usually on a once-a-day schedule.

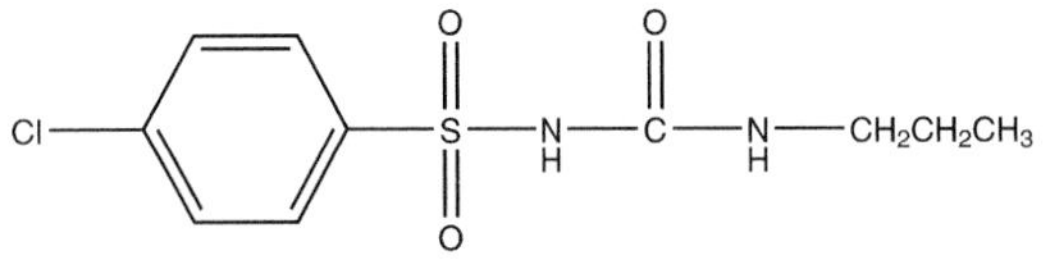

Chlorpropamide
(Diabinese)

Tolazamide, USP. Tolazamide, 1-(hexahydro-1*H*-azepin-1-yl)-3-(*p*-tolylsulfonyl)urea (Tolinase), is an analogue of tolbutamide and is reported to be effective, in general, under the same circumstances in which tolbutamide is useful. Tolazamide, however, appears to be more potent than tolbutamide and is nearly equal in potency to chlorpropamide. In studies with radioactive tolazamide, investigators found that 85% of an oral dose appeared in the urine as metabolites that were more soluble than tolazamide itself.

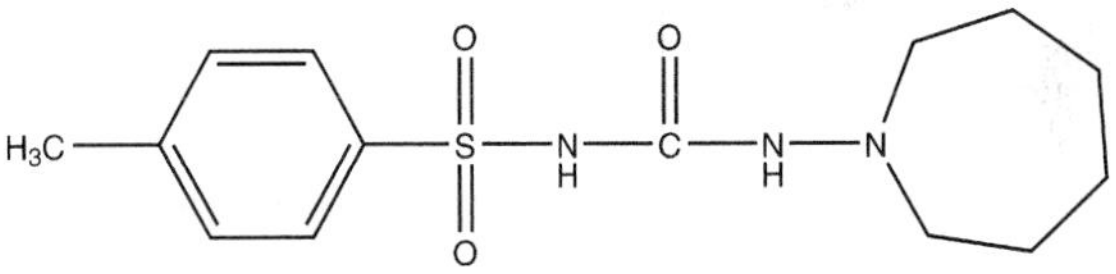

Tolazamide
(Tolinase)

Acetohexamide, USP. Acetohexamide, 1-[(*p*-acetylphenyl)sulfonyl]-3-cyclohexylurea (Dymelor), is related chemically and pharmacologically to tolbutamide and chlorpropamide. Like the other sulfonylureas, acetohexamide lowers the blood sugar level, primarily by stimulating the release of endogenous insulin.

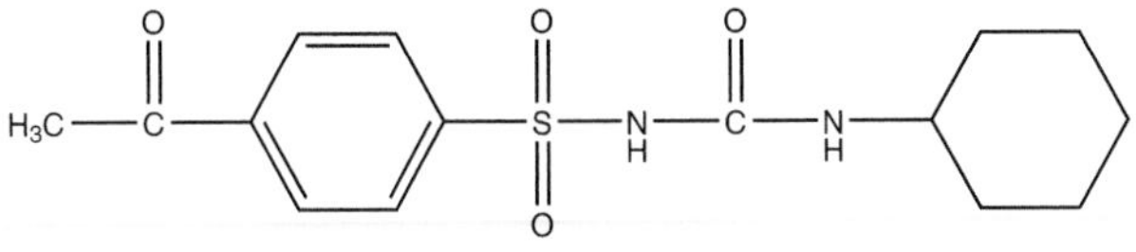

Acetohexamide
(Dymelor)

Acetohexamide is metabolized in the liver to a reduced form, the α-hydroxyethyl derivative. This metabolite, the main one in humans, possesses hypoglycemic activity. Acetohexamide is intermediate between tolbutamide and chlor-

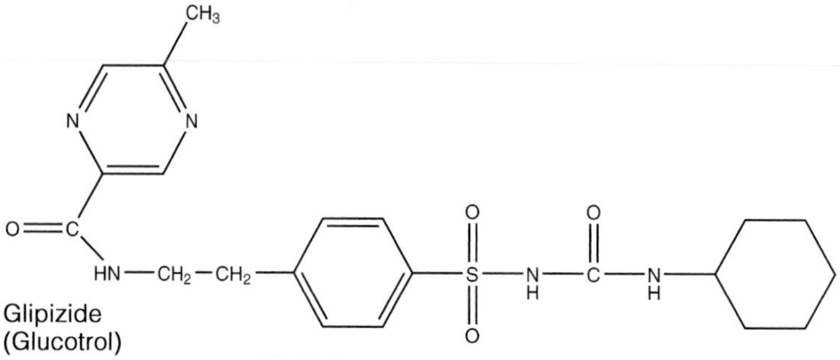

Glipizide
(Glucotrol)

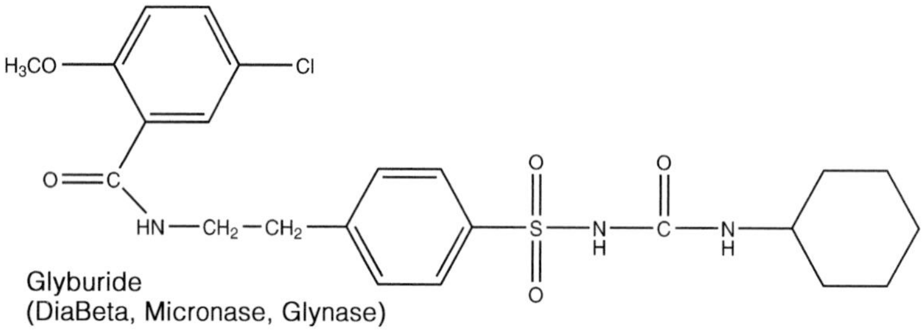

Glyburide
(DiaBeta, Micronase, Glynase)

propamide in potency and duration of effect on blood sugar levels.

Glipizide. Structurally, glipizide, 1-cyclohexyl-3-[[*p*-[2-(methylpyrazinecarboxamido)ethyl]phenyl]sulfonyl]urea (Glucotrol), is a cyclohexylsulfonylurea analogue similar to acetohexamide and glyburide. The drug is absorbed rapidly on oral administration. Its serum half-life is 2 to 4 hours, and it has a hypoglycemic effect that ranges from 12 to 24 hours.

Glyburide. Similar to glipizide, glyburide, 1-[[*p*-[2-(5-chloro-*o*-anisamido)ethyl]-phenyl]sulfonyl]-3-cyclohexyl-urea (DiaBeta, Micronase, Glynase), is a second-generation oral hypoglycemic agent. The drug has a half-life elimination of 10 hours, but its hypoglycemic effect remains for up to 24 hours.

Glipizide. Glipizide, 1-cyclohexyl-3-[[*p*-(2-(5-methyl-pyrazinecarboxamido)ethyl]phenyl]sulfonyl]urea (Glucotrol), is an off-white, odorless powder with a pKa of 5.9. It is insoluble in water and alcohols, but soluble in 0.1 N NaOH. Even though on a weight basis it is approximately 100 times more potent than tolbutamide, the maximal hypoglycemic effects of these two agents are similar. It is rapidly absorbed on oral administration, with a serum half-life of 2

to 4 hours, while the hypoglycemic effects range from 12 to 24 hours. Metabolism of glipizide is generally through oxidation of the cyclohexane ring to the *p*-hydroxy and *m*-hydroxy metabolites. A minor metabolite that occurs involves the *N*-acetyl derivative, which results from the acetylation of the primary amine following hydrolysis of the amide system by amidase enzymes.

Glimepiride. Glimepiride, 1-[[*p*-[2-(3-ethyl-4-methyl-2-oxo-3-pyrroline-1-carboxamido)ethyl]phenyl]sulfonyl]-3-(*trans*-4-methylcyclohexyl)urea (Amaryl), is very similar to glipizide with the exception of their heterocyclic rings. Instead of the pyrazine ring found in glipizide, glimepiride contains a pyrrolidine system. It is metabolized primarily through oxidation of the alkyl side chain of the pyrrolidine, with a minor metabolic route involving acetylation of the amine.

Gliclazide. Chemically, gliclazide, 1-(3-azabicyclo [3.3.0]oct-3-yl)-3-*p*-tolylsulfonylurea (Diamicron), is very similar to tolbutamide, with the exception of the bicyclic heterocyclic ring found in gliclazide. The pyrrolidine increases its lipophilicity over that of tolbutamide, which increases its half-life. Even so, the *p*-methyl is susceptible to the same oxidative metabolic fate as observed for tolbutamide, namely, it will be metabolized to a carboxylic acid.

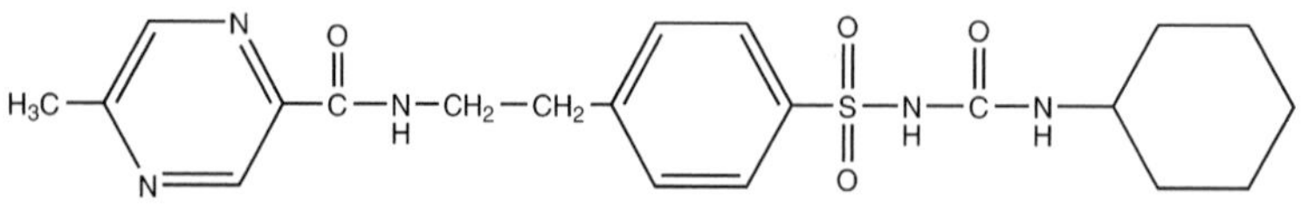

Glipizide
(Glucotrol)

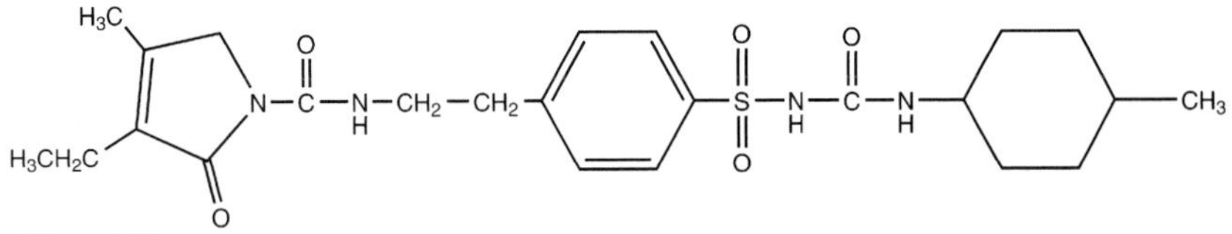

Glimepiride
(Amaryl)

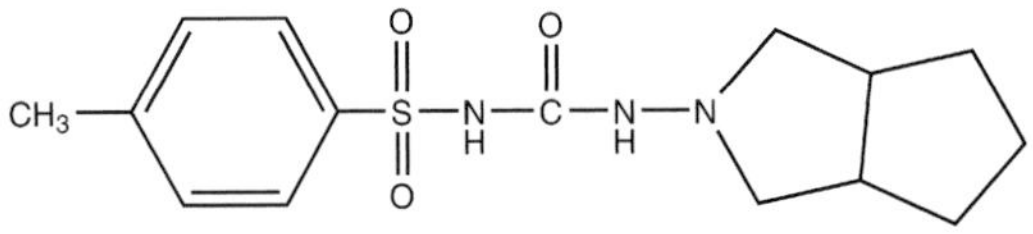

Gliclazide
(Diamicron)

Nonsulfonylureas—Metaglinides

The metaglinides are nonsulfonylurea oral hypoglycemic agents used in the management of type 2 diabetes (non–insulin-dependent diabetes mellitus, NIDDM). These agents tend to have a rapid onset and a short duration of action. Much like the sulfonylureas, these induce insulin release from functioning pancreatic β cells. The mechanism of action for the metaglinides, however, differs from that of the sulfonylureas. The mechanism of action is through binding to specific receptors in the β-cell membrane, leading to the closure of ATP-dependent K^+ channels. The K^+ channel blockade depolarizes the β-cell membrane, which in turn leads to Ca^{2+} influx, increased intracellular Ca^{2+}, and stimulation of insulin secretion. Because of this different mechanism of action from the sulfonylureas, there are two major differences between these seemingly similar classes of agents. The first is that the metaglinides cause much faster insulin production than the sulfonylureas. As a result, the metaglinides should be taken during meals, as the pancreas will produce insulin in a much shorter period. The second difference is that the effects of the metaglinides do not last as long as the effects of the sulfonylureas. The effects of this class appear to last less than 1 hour, while sulfonylureas continue to stimulate insulin production for several hours. One advantage of a short duration of action is that there is less risk of hypoglycemia.

Repaglinide. Repaglinide, (+)-2-ethoxy-4-[N-[3-methyl-1(S)-[2-(1-piperidinyl)phenyl]butyl]carbamoyl-methyl]benzoic acid (Prandin), represents a new class of nonsulfonylurea oral hypoglycemic agents. With a fast onset and a short duration of action, the medication should be taken with meals. It is oxidized by CYP 3A4, and the carboxylic acid may be conjugated to inactive compounds. Less than 0.2% is excreted unchanged by the kidney, which may be an advantage for elderly patients who are renally impaired. The most common side effect involves hypoglyce-

mia, resulting in shakiness, headache, cold sweats, anxiety, and changes in mental state.

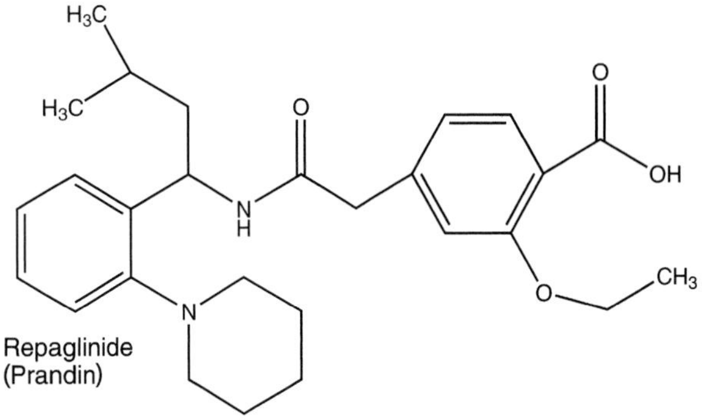

Repaglinide
(Prandin)

Nateglinide. Although nateglinide, N-(4-isopropyl-cyclohexanecarbonyl)-D-phenylalanine (Starlix), belongs to the metaglinides, it is a phenylalanine derivative and represents a novel drug in the management of type 2 diabetes.

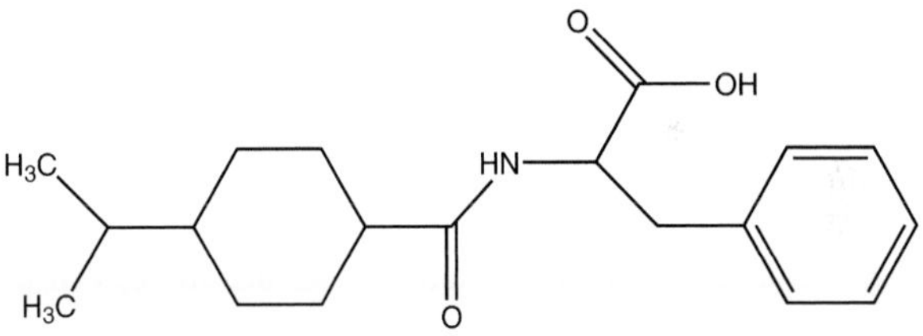

Nateglinide
(Starlix)

Thiazolindiones

The thiazolindiones represent a novel nonsulfonylurea class of hypoglycemic agents for the treatment of NIDDM. Much like the sulfonylureas, the use of these agents requires a functioning pancreas that can successfully secrete insulin from β cells. Although insulin may be released in normal levels from the cells, peripheral sensitivity to this hormone may be reduced or lacking. The thiazolidinediones are highly selective agonists for the peroxisome proliferator-activated receptor-γ (PPARγ), which is responsible for improving glycemic control, primarily through the improvement of insulin sensitivity in muscles and adipose tissue. In addition, they inhibit hepatic gluconeogenesis. These agents normalize glucose metabolism and reduce the amount of insulin needed to achieve glycemic control. They are only effective in the presence of insulin.

Rosiglitazone. Rosiglitazone, (±)-5-[[4-[2-(methyl-2-pyridinylamino)ethoxy]phenyl]methyl]-2,4-thiazolidinedione

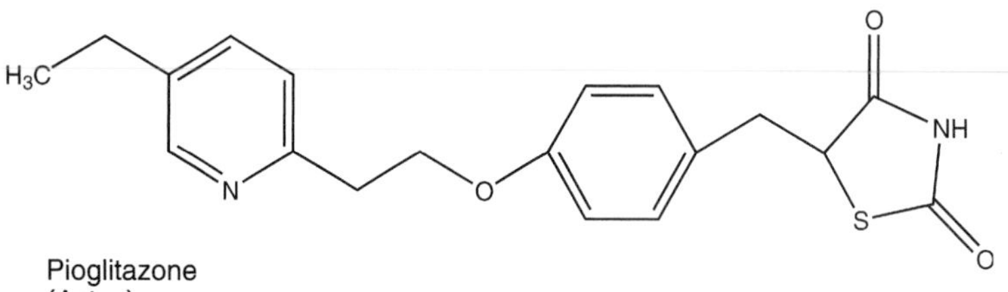

Pioglitazone
(Actos)

(Avandia), is a white to off-white solid with pK_a values of 6.8 and 6.1. Rosiglitazone is readily soluble in ethanol and a buffered aqueous solution with pH of 2.3; solubility decreases with increasing pH in the physiological range. The molecule has a single chiral center and is present as a racemate. Even so, the enantiomers are functionally indistinguishable because of rapid interconversion.

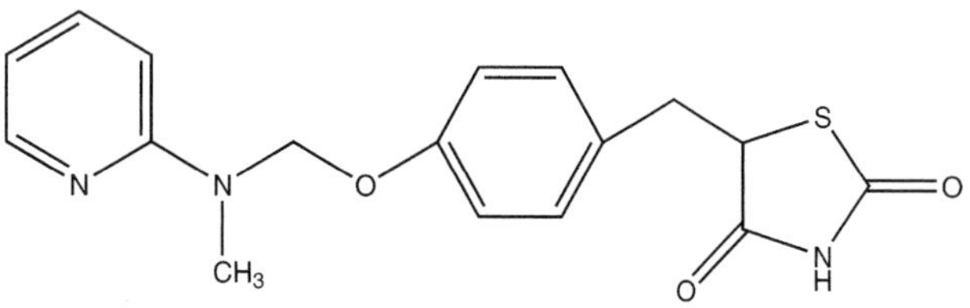

Rosiglitazone
(Avandia)

Pioglitazone. Pioglitazone, (±)-5-[[4-[2-(5-ethyl-2-pyridinyl)ethoxy]phenyl]methyl]-2,4-thiazolidinedione (Actos), is an odorless, white, crystalline powder that must be converted to a salt such as its hydrochloride before it will have any water solubility. Although the molecule contains one chiral center, the compound is used as the racemic mixture. This is primarily due to the in vivo interconversion of the two enantiomers. Thus, there are no differences in the pharmacological activity of the two enantiomers.

Bisguanidines

Metformin. Metformin, *N,N*-dimethylimidodicarbonimidic diamide hydrochloride (Glucophage), is a bisguanidine. This class of agents is capable of reducing sugar absorption from the gastrointestinal tract. Also, they can decrease gluconeogenesis while increasing glucose uptake by muscles and fat cells. These effects, in turn, lead to lower blood glucose levels. Unlike the sulfonylureas, these are not hypoglycemic agents but rather can act as antihyperglycemics. This difference in nomenclature is due to the inability of these agents to stimulate the release of insulin from the pancreas. Often, metformin is coadministered with the nonsulfonylureas to improve the efficacy of those agents.

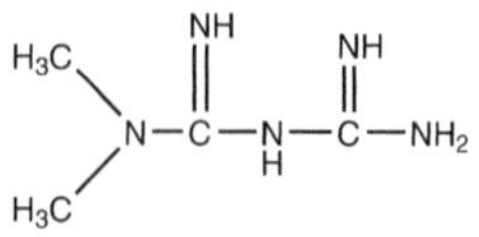

Metformin
(Glucophage)

α-Glucosidase Inhibitors

The enzyme α-glucosidase is present in the brush border of the small intestine and is responsible for cleaving dietary carbohydrates and facilitating their absorption into the body. Inhibition of this enzyme allows less dietary carbohydrate to be available for absorption and, in turn, less available in the blood following a meal. The inhibitory properties of these agents are greatest for glycoamylase, followed by sucrose, maltase, and dextranase, respectively. Since these do not enhance insulin secretion when used as monotherapy, hypoglycemia is generally not a concern when using these agents.

Acarbose. Acarbose, *O*-4,6-dideoxy-4-[[(1*S*,4*R*,5*S*,6*S*)-4,5,6-trihydroxy-3-(hydroxymethyl)-2-cyclohexen-1-yl]amino]α-D-glucopyranosyl-(1,4)-*O*-α-D-glucopyranosyl-(1,4)-D-glucose (Precose), is a naturally occurring oligosaccharide, which is obtained from the microorganism *Actinoplanes utahensis*. It is a white to off-white powder that is soluble in water and has a pK_a of 5.1. As one might expect, its affinity for α-glucosidase is based on it being a polysaccharide that the enzyme attempts to hydrolyze. This allows acarbose to act as a competitive inhibitor, which in turn reduces the intestinal absorption of starch, dextrin, and dissacharides.

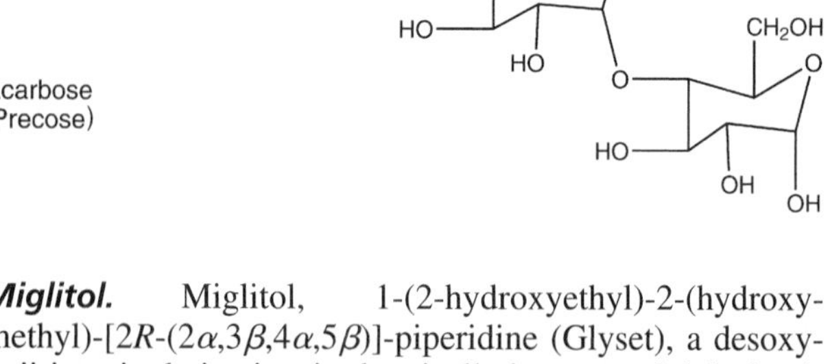

Acarbose
(Precose)

Miglitol. Miglitol, 1-(2-hydroxyethyl)-2-(hydroxymethyl)-[2*R*-(2α,3β,4α,5β)]-piperidine (Glyset), a desoxynojirimycin derivative, is chemically known as 3,4,5-piperidinetriol. It is a white to pale-yellow powder that is soluble in water, with a pK_a of 5.9. In chemical structure, this agent is very similar to a sugar, with the heterocyclic nitrogen serving as an isosteric replacement of the sugar oxygen. This feature allows recognition by the α-glucosidase as a substrate. This results in competitive inhibition of the enzyme and delays complex carbohydrate absorption from the gastrointestinal tract.

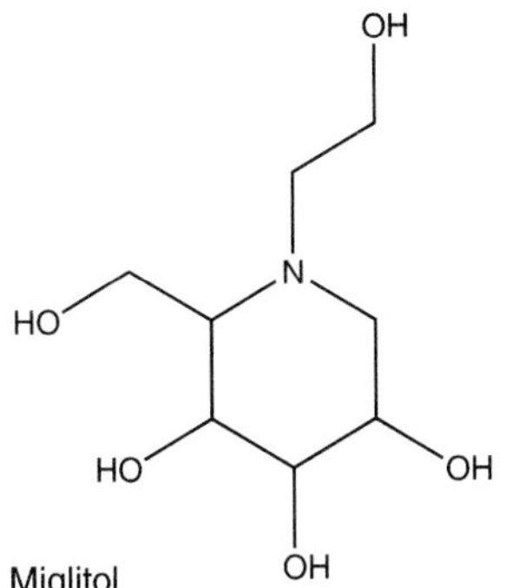

Miglitol
(Glyset)

THYROID HORMONES

Desiccated, defatted thyroid substance has been used for many years as replacement therapy in thyroid gland deficiencies. The efficacy of the whole gland is now known to depend on its thyroglobulin content. This is an iodine-containing globulin. Thyroxine was obtained as a crystalline derivative by Kendall[76] of the Mayo Clinic in 1915. It showed much the same action as the whole thyroid substance. Later, thyroxine was synthesized by Harington and Barger in England.[77] Later studies showed that an even more potent iodine-containing hormone existed, which is now known as triiodothyronine. Evidence now indicates that thyroxine may be the storage form of the hormone, whereas triiodothyronine is the circulating form. Another point of view is that in the blood, thyroxine is bound more firmly to the globulin fraction than is triiodothyronine, which can then enter the tissue cells.

Levothyroxine Sodium, USP. Levothyroxine sodium, *O*-(4-hydroxy-3,5-diiodophenyl)-3,5-diiodo-2-tyrosine monosodium salt, hydrate (Synthroid, Letter, Levoxine, Levoid), is the sodium salt of the *levo* isomer of thyroxine, which is an active physiological principle obtained from the thyroid gland of domesticated animals used for food by humans. It is also prepared synthetically. The salt is a light yellow, tasteless, odorless powder. It is hygroscopic but stable in dry air at room temperature. It is soluble in alkali hydroxides, 1:275 in alcohol, and 1:500 in water, to give a pH of about 8.9.

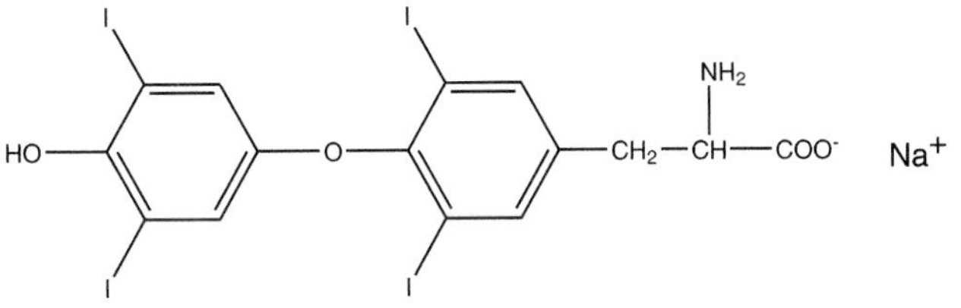

Levothyroxine Sodium
(Synthroid, Letter, Levoxine, Levoid)

Levothyroxine sodium is used in replacement therapy of decreased thyroid function (hypothyroidism). In general, a dosage of 100 μg of levothyroxine sodium is clinically equivalent to 30 to 60 mg of Thyroid USP.

Liothyronine Sodium, USP. Liothyronine sodium, *O*-(4-hydroxy-3-iodophenyl)-3,5-diiodo-L-thyroxine monosodium salt (Cytomel), is the sodium salt of L-3,3′,5-triiodothyronine. It occurs as a light-tan, odorless, crystalline powder, which is slightly soluble in water or alcohol and has a specific rotation of +18 to 22° in a mixture of diluted HCl and alcohol.

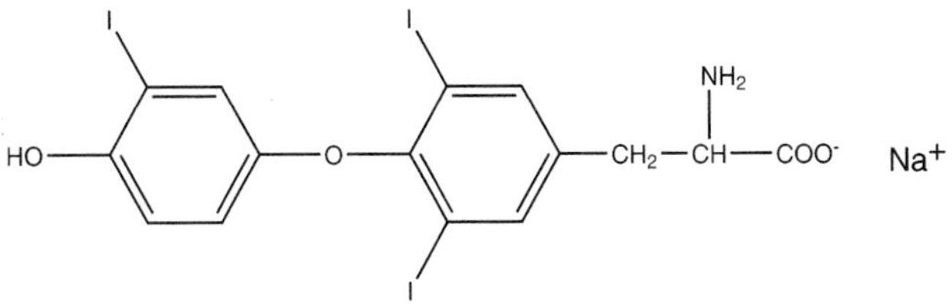

Liothyronine Sodium
(Cytomel)

Liothyronine sodium occurs in vivo together with levothyroxine sodium; it has the same qualitative activities as thyroxine but is more active. It is absorbed readily from the gastrointestinal tract, is cleared rapidly from the bloodstream, and is bound more loosely to plasma proteins than is thyroxine, probably because of the less acidic phenolic hydroxyl group.

Its uses are the same as those of levothyroxine sodium, including treatment of metabolic insufficiency, male infertility, and certain gynecological disorders.

ANTITHYROID DRUGS

Hyperthyroidism (excessive production of thyroid hormones) usually requires surgery, but before surgery the patient must be prepared by preliminary abolition of the hyperthyroidism through the use of antithyroid drugs. Thiourea and related compounds show an antithyroid activity, but they are too toxic for clinical use. The more useful drugs are 2-thiouracil derivatives and a closely related 2-thioimidazole derivative. All of these appear to have a similar mechanism of action (i.e., prevention of the iodination of the precursors of thyroxine and triiodothyronine). The main difference in the compounds lies in their relative toxicities.

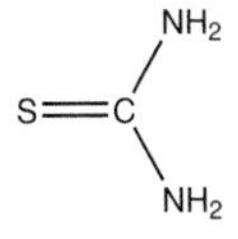

Thiourea

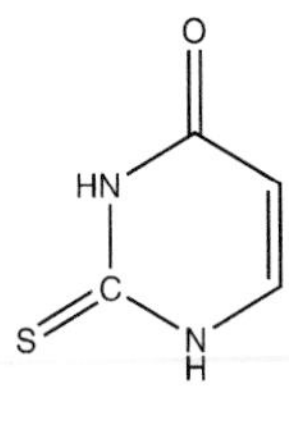

2-Thiouracil

These compounds are absorbed well after oral administration and excreted in the urine.

The 2-thiouracils, 4-keto-2-thiopyrimidines, are undoubtedly tautomeric compounds and can be represented as follows:

Some 300 related structures have been evaluated for antithyroid activity, but of these, only the 6-alkyl-2-thiouracils and closely related structures possess useful clinical activity. The most serious adverse effect of thiouracil therapy is agranulocytosis.

Propylthiouracil, USP. Propylthiouracil, 6-propyl-2-thiouracil (Propacil), is a stable, white, crystalline powder with a bitter taste. It is slightly soluble in water but readily soluble in alkaline solutions (salt formation).

Propylthiouracil
(Propacil)

This drug is useful in the treatment of hyperthyroidism. There is a delay in appearance of its effects because propylthiouracil does not interfere with the activity of thyroid hormones already formed and stored in the thyroid gland. This lag period may vary from several days to weeks, depending on the condition of the patient. The need for three equally spaced doses during a 24-hour period is often stressed, but evidence now indicates that a single daily dose is as effective as multiple daily doses in the treatment of most hyperthyroid patients.[78]

Methimazole, USP. Methimazole, 1-methylimidazole-2-thiol (Tapazole), occurs as a white to off-white, crystalline powder with a characteristic odor and is freely soluble in water. A 2% aqueous solution has a pH of 6.7 to 6.9. It should be packaged in well-closed, light-resistant containers.

Methimazole
(Tapazole)

Methimazole is indicated in the treatment of hyperthyroidism. It is more potent than propylthiouracil. The side effects are similar to those of propylthiouracil. As with other antithyroid drugs, patients using this drug should be under medical supervision. Also, like the other antithyroid drugs, methimazole is most effective if the total daily dose is subdivided and given at 8-hour intervals.

REFERENCES

1. Robinson, B. F.: Adv. Drug. Res. 10:93, 1975.
2. Aronow, W. S.: Am. Heart J. 84:273, 1972.
3. Sonnenblick, E., Ross, J., Jr., and Braunwald, E.: Am. J. Cardiol. 22: 328, 1968.
4. Ignarro, L. J., et al.: J. Pharmacol. Exp. Ther. 218:739, 1981.
5. Feelisch, M.: Eur. Heart J. 14(Suppl. I):123, 1993.
6. Needleman, P.: Annu. Rev. Pharmacol. Toxicol. 16:81, 1976.
7. Chung, S. J., and Fung, H. L.: J. Pharmacol. Exp. Ther. 253:614, 1990.
8. Fusari, S. A.: J. Pharm. Sci. 62:123, 1973.
9. Fusari, S. A.: J. Pharm. Sci. 62:2012, 1973.
10. McCall, D., et al.: Curr. Probl. Cardiol. 10:1, 1985.
11. Heschler, J., et al.: Eur. J. Biochem. 165:261, 1987.
12. Beridge, M. J.: Annu. Rev. Biochem. 56:159, 1987.
13. van Zweiten, P. A., and van Meel, J. C.: Prog. Pharmacol. 5:1, 1982.
14. Atkinson, J., et al.: Naunyn Schmeidbergs Arch. Pharmacol. 337:471, 1988.
15. Smith, H. J., and Briscoe, M. G.: J. Mol. Cell Cardiol. 17:709, 1985.
16. Sanguinetti, M. C., and Kass, R. S.: Circ. Res. 55:336, 1984.
17. Rosenkirchen, R., et al.: Naunyn Schmiedebergs Arch. Pharmacol. 310: 69, 1979.
18. Triggle, D. J., Calcium antagonists. In: Antonoccio, P. N. (ed.). Cardiovascular Pharmacology, 3rd ed. New York, Raven Press, 1990.
19. Vaughan Williams, E. M.: In Sandoe E., Flensted-Jansen, E., and Olesen, K. H. (eds.). Symposium on Cardiac Arrhythmias. Sodertalje, Sweden, B. Astra, 1970, pp. 449–472.
20. Vaughan Williams, E. M.: J. Clin. Pharmacol. 24:129, 1984.
21. CAPS Investigators: Am. J. Cardiol. 61:501, 1988.
22. Woosley, R. L.: Annu. Rev. Pharmacol. Toxicol. 31:427, 1991.
23. Campbell, T. J.: Cardiovasc. Res. 17:344, 1983.
24. Yool, A. J.: Mol. Pharmacol. 46:970, 1994.
25. Hondeghem, L. M., and Katzung, B. G.: Annu. Rev. Pharmacol. Toxicol. 24:387, 1984.
26. Nies, A. S., and Shang, D. G.: Clin. Pharmacol. Exp. Ther. 14:823, 1973.
27. Koch-Wester, J.: Ann. N. Y. Acad. Sci. 179:370, 1971.
28. Giardinia, E. V., et al.: Clin. Pharmacol. Ther. 19:339, 1976.
29. Elson, J., et al.: Clin. Pharmacol. Ther. 17:134, 1975.
30. Belfer, B., et al.: Am. J. Cardiol. 35:282, 1975.
31. Bigger, T. J., and Jaffe, C. C.: Am. J. Cardiol. 27:82, 1971.
32. Hollunger, G.: Acta Pharmacol. Toxicol. 17:356, 1960.
33. Helfant, R. H., et al.: Am. Heart J. 77:315, 1969.
34. Beckett, A. H., and Chiodomere, E. C.: Postgrad. Med. J. 53(Suppl. 1):60, 1977.
35. Anderson, J. L., Mason, J. W., and Roger, M. D.: Circulation 57:685, 1978.
36. Guehler, J., et al.: Am. J. Cardiol. 55:807, 1985.
37. Saeki, T., et al.: Eur. J. Pharmacol. 261:249, 1994.
38. Groshner, K., et al.: Br. J. Pharmacol. 102:669, 1991.
39. Hii, J. T., Duff, H. J., and Burgess, E. D.: Clin. Pharmacokinet. 21:1, 1991.
40. Olsson, S. B., Brorson, L., and Varnauskas, E.: Br. Heart J. 35:1255, 1973.
41. Kannan, R., et al.: Clin. Pharmacol. 31:438, 1982.
42. Witt, D. M., Ellsworth, A. J., and Leversee, J. H.: Ann. Pharmacother. 27:1463, 1993.
43. Nademanee, K., et al.: Circulation 66:202, 1982.
44. Papp, J. G., and Vaughan Williams, E. M.: Br. J. Pharmacol. 37:380, 1969.
45. Boyer, E. W., Stork, C., and Wang, R. Y.: Int. J. Med. Toxicol. 2001; 4: 16.
46. Salata, J. J., and Brooks, R. R.: Cardiol. Drug Rev. 15:137–156, 1997.
47. Tigerstedt, R., and Bergman, P. G.: Scand. Arch. Physiol. 8:223, 1898.
48. Page, F., and Helmer, O. A.: J. Exp. Med. 71:29, 1940.

49. Skeggs, L., et al.: J. Exp. Med. 99:275, 1954.
50. Shapiro, R., and Riordan, J. F.: Biochemistry 23:5225, 1984.
51. Ehlers, M. R., and Riordan, J. F.: Biochemistry 30:7118, 1991.
52. Vakil, R.: Br. Heart J. 11:350, 1949.
53. Hess, S. M., Shore, P. A., and Brodie, P. P.: Br. J. Pharmacol. Exp. Ther. 118:84, 1956.
54. Kirshner, N.: J. Biol. Chem. 237:2311, 1962.
55. von Euler, U. S., and Lishajko, F.: Int. J. Neuropharmacol. 2:127, 1963.
56. Muller, J. M., Schlittler, E., and Brin, H. J.: Experientia 8:338, 1952.
57. U'Prichard, D., et al.: Eur. J. Pharmacol. 50:87, 1978.
58. Langer, S. Z., and Cavero, I.: Hypertension 2:372, 1980.
59. Starke, K., and Montel, H.: Neuropharmacology 12:1073, 1973.
60. Meisheri, K. D.: Direct-acting vasodilators. In Singh, B. J., et al. (eds.). Cardiovascular Pharmacology. New York, Churchill Livingstone, 1994, p. 173..
61. Gross, F., Druey, J., and Meier, R.: Experientia 6:19, 1950.
62. Zacest, R., Koch-Wesesr, J.: Clin. Pharmacol. 13:4420, 1972.
63. Page, I. H., et al.: Circulation 11:188, 1955.
64. Cook, N. S.: Potassium Channels: Structure, Classification, Function and Therapeutic Potential. New York, John Wiley & Sons, 1990, p. 181.
65. DuCharme, D. W., et al.: Pharmacol. Exp. Ther. 184:662, 1973.
66. Levy, R. I., et al.: Circulation 69:325, 1984.
67. Levy, R. I.: Annu. Rev. Pharmacol. Toxicol. 47:499, 1977.
68. Mannisto, P. T., et al.: Acta Pharmacol. Toxicol. 36:353, 1975.
69. Kesaniemi, Y. A., and Grundy, S. M.: JAMA 251:2241, 1984.
70. Atmeh, R. F., et al.: J. Lipid Res. 24:588, 1983.
71. Stenflo, J., et al.: Proc. Natl. Acad. Sci. U. S. A. 71:2730, 1974.
72. Jackson, C. M., and Suttie, J. W.: Prog. Hematol. 10:333, 1978.
73. Triplett, D. A. (ed.): Platelet Function. Chicago, American Society of Clinical Pathology, 1978.
74. Hamberg, M., et al.: Proc. Natl. Acad. Sci. U. S. A. 71:345, 1974.
75. Thomas, R. C., and Ruby, R. W.: J. Med. Chem. 15:964, 1972.
76. Kendall, E. C.: JAMA 64:2042, 1915.
77. Harrington, C. R., and Barger, C.: Biochem. J. 21:169, 1927.
78. Greer, M. A., and Meihoff, W. C.: N. Engl. J. Med. 272:888, 1965.

Local Anesthetic Agents

GARETH THOMAS

Local anesthetics are blocking drugs that, when administered locally in the correct concentration, "block" the nerves that carry nerve impulses in local areas of the body. They do not block coarse touch or movement, and the action is reversible. Their method of administration is governed by such properties as toxicity, stability, duration of action, water solubility, membrane permeability, and point of application, while their modes of action (see under heading, Mechanism of Action) depend on their lipid solubility, pK$_a$, vasodilation, and protein-binding characteristics.

Although given locally, the drug may exert a systemic effect because of transport in the blood from the site of administration to other areas, such as the heart and central nervous system (CNS). These systemic effects, which depend on the concentration of the local anesthetic in the blood, are usually sedation and lightheadedness, but restlessness, nausea, and anxiety may also occur. High plasma concentrations can result in convulsions, chiropidy, and coma with respiratory and cardiac depression.

Local anesthetics are used to alleviate the pain caused by a wide variety of situations. They are used in dentistry, in ophthalmology, in minor surgical operations including endoscopy, and in relieving pain in intractable medical conditions, such as tumors growing in the spine. Local anesthetics are also used topically for the temporary relief of pain from insect bites, burns, and other types of surface wounds. They are particularly effective when they are used on mucous membranes, such as the mouth, vagina, or rectum

HISTORICAL DEVELOPMENT

The start of the search for ways to relieve pain is lost in the past. People have used religious exorcism, hypnotism, acupuncture, hypothermia, nerve compression, and drugs. Each of these methods has had its periods of popularity, and most are still used in one form or another. The modern development of the use of drugs to induce local anesthesia probably started in the mid-19th century. The earliest recorded use of hypothermia as a local anesthetic, however, is believed to be by Larrey, Napoleon's chief army surgeon during the retreat from Moscow. He recorded that amputations were carried out in subzero temperatures had a higher patient survival rate than those carried out in warmer conditions. Later in the century, Thompson reported that ether acted as a refrigerant when poured onto the skin. These observations lay dormant until 1848 when Arnott reported that he had used a pig's bladder filled with crushed ice to alleviate the pain caused by incisions made in the skin. This was followed by Snow's unsuccessful attempts to find a viable way of using refrigeration as a local anesthetic. Success was

achieved eventually by his protégé Richardson, who replaced the cologne in the then recently introduced Eau-de-Cologne spray with ether. This achieved temperatures that allowed minor surgery to be carried out. Richardson and other workers improved the efficiency of the procedure by using a petroleum distillate, then ethyl bromide, and ultimately ethyl chloride. The success of the Richardson spray inspired Koller to search for a local anesthetic that could be safely applied to the eye.

Koller qualified in medicine in 1882 and went on to specialize in ophthalmology in Vienna. His experience as an eye surgeon made him increasingly aware of the need for a local anesthetic that could be used in the eye. In 1884, while he was collaborating with Freud to study the effect of cocaine on fatigue, a colleague remarked that the drug numbed his tongue. Koller and Gaertner investigated this claim and found that a dilute aqueous solution of cocaine hydrochloride caused local anesthesia of the cornea. Brettauer presented Koller's results on his behalf at an ophthalmology meeting in Heidelberg in September 1884, since Koller could not afford the train fare from Vienna to Heidelberg. Koller's paper resulted in the immediate widespread use of cocaine in Europe and the United States. Koller also recommended the use of cocaine as a local anesthetic in ear, nose, and throat operations. At the time, however, little was known about its addictive properties.

In 1885, degradation studies by Camels and Gossin suggested that there were some structural similarities between cocaine and atropine. This led Filehne at the University of Breslau (now Wroclaw) in Poland to determine whether atropine had any local anesthetic activity in the eye. Atropine had been isolated from the roots of belladonna in 1831 by Mein, a German apothecary. Filehne found that atropine had little local anesthetic activity and was toxic, causing eye irritation at the doses required for any activity. Earlier, Lossen showed that atropine could be split into tropic acid and a nitrogenous base called *tropine*. Later, in 1880, Ladenburg synthesized a series of physiologically active compounds, which he called *tropeines,* by esterifying tropine with a variety of aromatic acids. Filehne investigated these semisynthetic analogues of atropine for local anesthetic activity and found that homatropine (Fig. 20-1a) was less irritating to

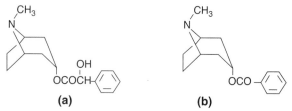

Figure 20–1 ■ **a.** Homatropine. **b.** Benzoyltropine.

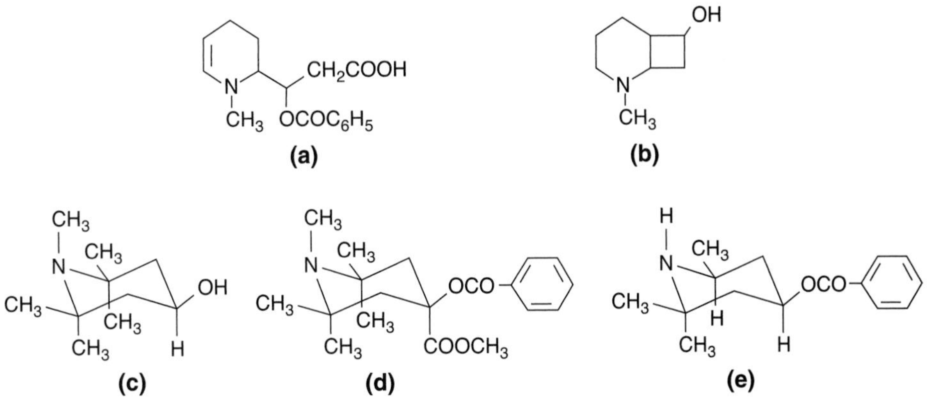

Figure 20–2 ■ The incorrect structures proposed for cocaine **(a)** and tropine **(b)** by Albert Einhorn and Georg Merling. Structures of methyltriacetone alkamine **(c)**, *alpha-Eucaine* **(d)**, and *beta-Eucaine* **(e)**.

the eyes and a better local anesthetic than atropine, whereas benzoyltropine (Fig. 20-1b) was a strong local anesthetic but caused too much irritation to be of any clinical use. The identification of a benzoyl group in the structures of the most active atropine analogues and also in cocaine, however, led Filehne to test the activity of the benzoyl derivatives of quinine, cinchonine, hydrocotarnine, and morphine. His results, which were published in 1887, showed that these benzoate esters acted as local anesthetics, but many had unwanted side effects.

By 1888 the toxic and addictive effects of cocaine were beginning to concern the medical world, and many workers were seeking a safe substitute. In 1892, Einhorn,[1] professor of chemistry at the University of Munich, suggested a structure for cocaine (Fig. 20-2a) based on the structure of tropine proposed in 1883 by Merling[2] at the University of Berlin (Fig. 20-2b). Merling decided, on the basis of these incorrect structures, to synthesize a benzoyl analogue containing only a piperidine ring. He produced a compound whose structure was similar to that of the weakly active methyltriacetone alkamine analogue of atropine (Fig. 20-2c). It was marketed under the name alpha-Eucaine (Fig. 20-2d) but was not popular, as it caused a burning sensation when applied to the eyes. It was rapidly replaced by beta-Eucaine (Fig. 20-2e), but this also caused eye irritation.

Einhorn, on realizing Merling's success with the benzoate

derivatives of piperidine, attempted to synthesize active benzoate compounds based on the simpler hexane ring. His syntheses, which were based on the reduction of aromatic benzoate esters, failed, so he decided to have a number of unrelated aromatic benzoate esters tested for local anesthetic activity. Some were found to be active, but more importantly, several of the phenols formed by the hydrolysis of the esters were also found to be active, and in 1896, Einhorn introduced Orthoform (orthocaine) into clinical use. Problems with its production and its side effects led him to introduce Orthoform New in 1897. Einhorn's work was important in that it gave the first indication that a benzoate ester was not essential for local anesthesia.

Although the Orthoforms were relatively successful as topical anesthetics, their poor water solubility made them unsuitable for other medicinal uses. Consequently, Einhorn attempted to improve their water solubility by introducing amine-containing aliphatic side chains. He reasoned that the formation of their amine hydrochlorides would improve water solubility without making the preparation too acidic. One of Einhorn's compounds, Nirvanin, was introduced in 1898. Its activity was low, and it had to be used in high doses, which caused toxic effects.

In 1898, Willstatter determined the correct structures of both atropine and cocaine. He followed this by synthesizing cocaine in 1901.

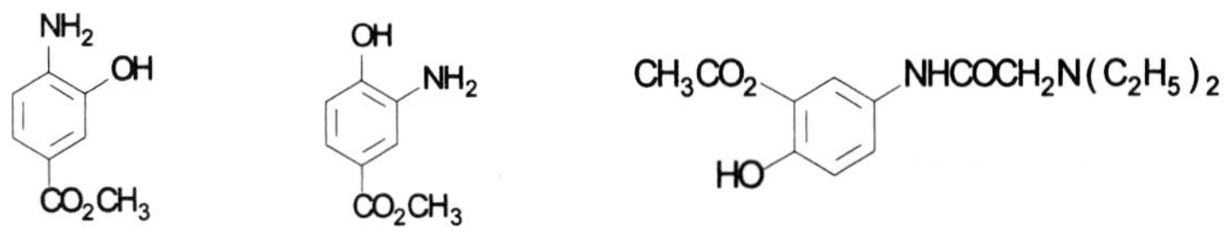

Orthoform *Orthoform New* *Nirvanin*

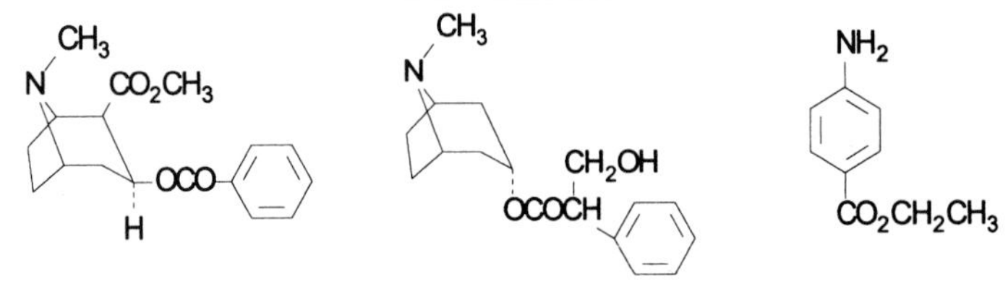

Cocaine *Atropine* *Benzocaine*

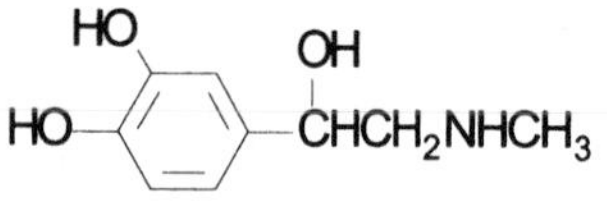

Adrenaline

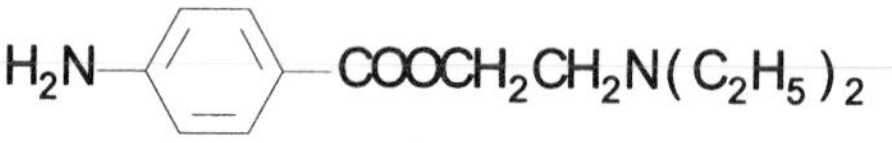

Procaine

Einhorn's clinical success with the poorly water soluble Orthoforms resulted in the introduction of ethyl 4-aminobenzoate into clinical use in 1902 under the name Anesthesine. It was later given the approved name of benzocaine. Ritsert had noticed in 1890 that this water-insoluble compound had numbed his tongue and so to improve its water solubility, it had been formulated as the hydrochloride. As aromatic amines are weak bases, however, the resulting solution had proved too acidic, and he had discounted its clinical use.

In 1902, Fourneau in France designed a drug whose structure incorporated functional groups similar to those found in the structure of the cocaine molecule. He did not include the piperidine ring, however, which he considered to be responsible for the toxicity of cocaine. His compound, which he marketed under the name Stovaine, was the first nonirritant local anesthetic that could be given by injection and used as a safe substitute for cocaine. Stovaine was later given the approved name of amylocaine.

Amylocaine

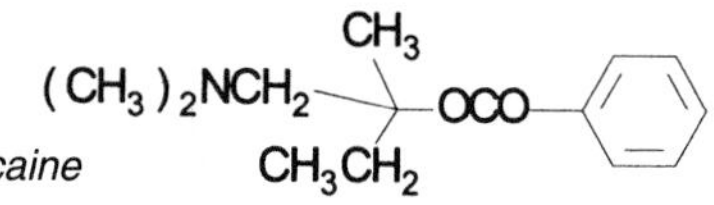

Earlier work in 1885 by Corning in the United States had shown that the anesthetic effect of cocaine could be enhanced by the use of tourniquets to keep the drug from being carried away from the site of application. This increased the effectiveness of the drug and allowed lower doses to be used. Applications of the tourniquet technique were limited, however. In 1900, the publication of the observation that adrenal extracts caused blood vessels to contract resulted in Braun demonstrating that mixtures of cocaine and adrenal extracts were more effective than cocaine alone. The isolation of adrenaline, the active component of adrenal extracts, and its subsequent structure determination led Braun in 1904 to design a drug based on the structure of both adrenaline and Einhorn's local anesthetics. It was marketed as Novocaine and was later given the approved name of procaine. Procaine dominated the local anesthetic market for half a century and is still in use today.

In the next 30 or so years after the synthesis of procaine, large numbers of compounds were tested for local anesthetic activity, but none of importance emerged. Miescher, working for Ciba in Switzerland, found, however, that some of

the acetanilide analogues he had synthesized as potential antipyretic agents also exhibited local anesthetic activity. In 1931, his synthetic work led to the production of cinchocaine (Nupercaine), a long-acting local anesthetic that was particularly useful in spinal anesthesia.

Cinchocaine

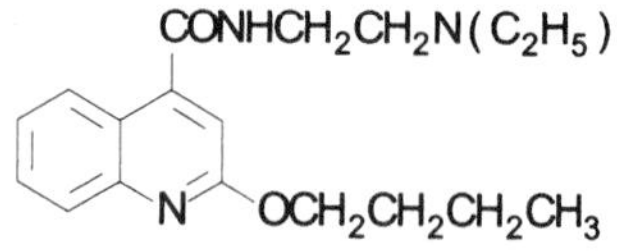

At about the same time that cinchocaine was developed, an investigation of the chemical structure of the alkaloid gramine at Stockholm University resulted in Erdtman synthesizing its isomer, isogramine. As luck would have it, Erdtman tasted isogramine and found that his tongue went numb. Realizing its potential, he tested its open-chain precursor and found that it also exhibited local anesthetic activity. For the next 7 years, Erdtman and his student Lofregen synthesized and tested compounds with similar structural characteristics. Their search was rewarded 57 compounds later, by the discovery of lignocaine (Lidocaine, Xylocaine). This drug was marketed in 1948 by Astra in Sweden, and because of its rapidity of action, nonirritant and relatively safe nature, it has become the leading local anesthetic.

In 1957, scientists at AB Bofors replaced the acyclic tertiary amino side chain of lignocaine with a cyclic tertiary amine for no reason other than it produced novel compounds. This irrational approach led to two useful local anesthetics, mepivacaine (Carbocaine) and bupivacaine (Marcain). Bupivacaine was long acting, producing nerve blocks for up to 8 hours.

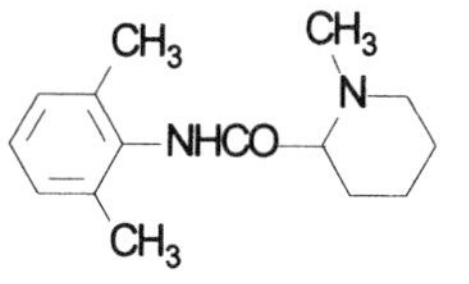

Mepivacaine

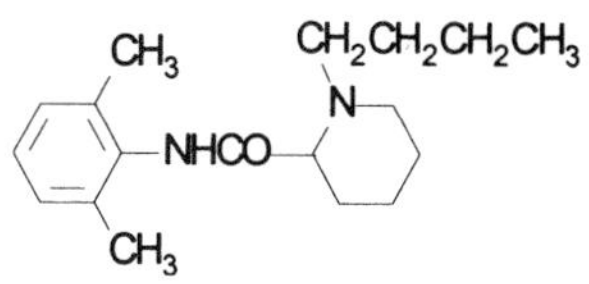

Bupivacaine

A large number of active compounds have now been synthesized, but lignocaine, procaine, and many of the pre-1957 compounds are still in current use. In 1974, Hughes isolated and, in 1975,[3] determined the structures of the natural pain-

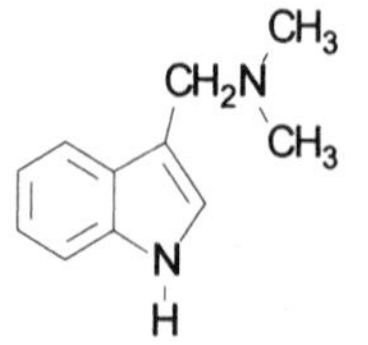

*Gramine 3-
(dimethylaminomethyl)indole*

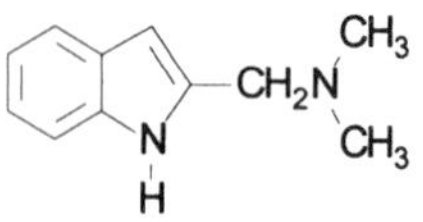

*Isogramine 2-
(dimethylaminomethyl)indole*

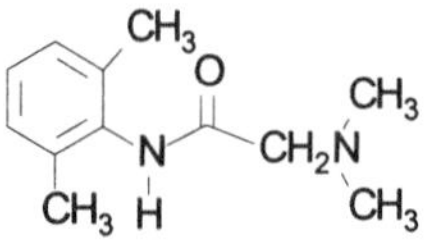

Lignocaine

control agents, methionine-enkephalin (met-enkephalin) and leucine-enkephalin (leu-enkephalin). The isolation of these and other peptides with similar activity opened up a possible new structural route to the synthesis of local anesthetic agents that has yet to be fully exploited.

H-Try-Gly-Gly-Phe-Met(OH)   H-Try-Gly-Gly-Phe-Leu(OH)

    Met-enkephalin   Leu-enkephalin

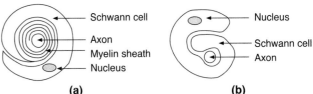

Figure 20–4 ■ Representations of myelinated **(a)** and unmyelinated **(b)** axons.

THE NERVOUS SYSTEM

The nervous system consists of sensory and motor components. The sensory component responds to various external stimulations, which it transmits in the form of a nerve impulse to the CNS for interpretation. The motor component of the nervous system carries a signal from the CNS to the appropriate part of the body to elicit the response to the stimulation. One of these responses is the sensation known as pain. Nerve impulses are now known to take the form of an electrical impulse. Experimental evidence suggests that both stimulation and the transmission of a nerve impulse may be blocked by the action of local anesthetic agents.[4] Consequently, understanding this action requires a knowledge of the structure and action of the nervous system.

The basic building blocks of the nervous system are the *nerve cells* or *neurons.* Associated with the neurons are the *glial cells.* In humans, the complete system contains over 10 billion neurons and about 10 to 15 times that number of glial cells. Extending from the brain, the *command center* of the nervous system, is the cluster of neurons and glial cells that form the spinal cord. The brain together with the spinal cord forms the CNS. Extending outward from the CNS is the peripheral nervous system *(PNS).* The motor and sensory components of the PNS are subdivided into somatic and vegetative systems. Somatic systems control conscious functions, such as physical movements, while the vegetative systems control unconscious functions. The motor vegetative system is referred to as the *autonomic* or *involuntary nervous system*[5] and controls body functions such as breathing, digestion, and heart beat.

Neurons receive, conduct, and transmit electrical signals in the form of ionic currents. A typical neuron usually consists of a central cell body from which radiate out a number of thin, branch-like protuberances (Fig. 20-3). These branches are of two types, a single branch known as the

axon, which acts as a conductor of signals from the cell body, and a number of other separate branches known as the *dendrites,* which act as antennae, receiving signals from the axon of other neurons. Both the axons and dendrites of neurons can exhibit an astonishing variety of branching, but axon branching is usually simpler. The terminal branches of the axon end in *synaptic knobs,* which are also known as *terminal buttons* or *axon telondria.*

The axon arises from a thickened area of the cell body called the *axon hillock.* Its membrane is mainly composed of lipids and proteins and is known as the *axolemma.* Many of the axons of the CNS and PNS are partly covered from near the axon hillock to the synaptic knob by a sheath of *myelin* (myelinated axons), but some axons do not have this type of covering (unmyelinated axons). The myelin sheath of PNS myelinated axons is not continuous but is broken at about 1-mm intervals to expose the axolemma to the extracellular fluid. These exposed areas, which are about 1 μm long, are known as the *nodes of Ranvier.* The distance between the nodes is often referred to as the *internodal distance.*

A segment of the PNS myelin sheath consists of a single glial cell known as a *Schwann cell,* tightly wrapped around the axon so as to form several tightly bound layers of the same cell (Fig. 20-4a). In unmyelinated axons, the Schwann cells simply surround the axon and are not tightly wrapped around it (Fig. 20-4b). The CNS myelinated sheath is a much more complicated structure. In all cases, however, the main function of myelin is to act as an insulating material, electrically insulating the axon from the extracellular fluid.

A nerve consists of myelinated or unmyelinated nerve fibers (Fig. 20-5a). These nerve fibers consist of "chains" of neurons. The junction between adjacent neurons in the chain consists of the synaptic knob of the transmitting neuron separated by a gap of about 30 to 50 nm from either the dendrite, axon hillock, or cell body of the other neuron. This

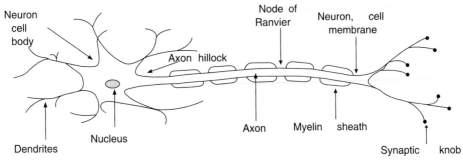

Figure 20–3 ■ Schematic diagram of a neuron. Representation of the variety of branching found in dendrites.

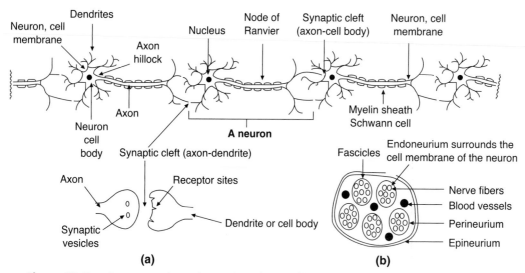

Figure 20–5 ■ Representations of a section of nerve fiber **(a)** (reproduced from Thomas, G.: Medicinal Chemistry, An Introduction. Chichester, U. K., John Wiley & Sons, 2000, by permission of John Wiley & Sons, Ltd.) and a cross section of a nerve **(b)**.

gap is known as the *synaptic cleft,* and the whole area where transmission and reception of the impulse from one neuron to the other occur is known as a *synapse.* The nerve fibers are enclosed in different layers of protective tissues (Fig. 20-5b). For example, in a spinal nerve the individual nerve fibers, whether myelinated or unmyelinated, are wrapped in a layer of protective connective tissue known as the *endoneurium.* These endoneurium-coated fibers are grouped in bundles known as *fascicles.* Each fascicle is coated with a layer of connective tissue called the *perineurium.* The complete nerve consists of a number of fascicles embedded in tissue through which run various blood vessels, the whole structure being covered by a layer of connective tissue known as the *epineurium.*

Neurons are excited by electrical, chemical, and mechanical stimuli. They convey the information provided by this stimulation in the form of electrical signals. The precise nature of the information carried depends on the type of neuron, however. For example, a *motor neuron* will convey electrical signals that cause a particular muscle to contract. In all cases, the signals take the form of changes in the electrical potential across the neuronal membranes. In myelinated neurons, a change in the membrane potential in one node of Ranvier will stimulate further changes in an adjacent node and so on; that is, a change in electrical potential at A stimulates a change in electrical potential at B, which in turn initiates a change in the electrical potential at C and so on (Fig. 20-6). The process whereby the change in potential jumps from one node to another is known as *saltatory conduction.* It results in the movement of an electrical impulse that is referred to as either the *nerve impulse* or *action potential* along

the axon. In unmyelinated nerves, the change in potential of one section of the membrane stimulates a change in potential of an immediately adjacent section of the membrane. These nerve impulses are transmitted or conducted along an axon sheathed with myelin at speeds up to 120 m/sec or more, but only up to 10 m/sec in unmyelinated axons. In large neurons, the strength of the nerve impulse is maintained by an automatic amplification system, but many smaller neurons have no such systems.

If the center of an axon is stimulated, the nerve impulse will be transmitted in both directions along that axon (Fig. 20-7). The synapse allows, however, only the transmission of the impulse from the axon to the next neuron, i.e., in only one direction. Consequently, an impulse will only travel in one direction along a nerve fiber.

In most cells, the electrical potential difference between the inner and outer surfaces of the cell membrane is due to the movement of ions across that membrane.[5] In all axons, the interior face of the membrane is the negative side of the potential difference, largely because of the excess of anions, such as chloride ions, found in the interior of the neuron. For a cell at rest (i.e., a cell that is not subject to any outside stimulation), this electrical potential is known as the *resting potential* and can vary from −20 to −200 mV, where by convention the extracellular side of the membrane is taken to be 0 volts. The resting potential of neurons is about −70 mV. The *action potential* of the axon is the series of potential changes that occurs when the axon is stimulated. Microelectrodes implanted in the axon *(intracellular recording)* show that stimulation causes an initial depolarization of the membrane by about 20 mV. This is followed by the rapid rise of the membrane's potential to a maximum value of about +35 mV. The membrane is then said to be *depolarized.* This is immediately followed by the potential dropping back toward the resting potential *(repolarization).* The repolarization overshoots the resting potential *(hyperpolarization)* before slowly recovering to the resting potential (Fig. 20-8). The rapid rise and fall of the potential is termed the *spike poten-*

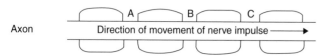

Figure 20–6 ■ Representation of the transmission of a nerve impulse along a neuron fiber by saltatory conduction.

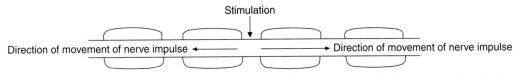

Figure 20–7 ■ Stimulation at the center of an axon results in a nerve impulse being transmitted in both directions.

tial, and the point at which it starts, the *firing level* or *threshold* of the axon. No action potential is produced if the stimulus is below the threshold potential. Once the threshold level is reached, however, the action potential will occur regardless of the strength of the stimulus. Furthermore, the amplitude of this action potential is independent of the intensity of the stimulant. The action potential is said to obey the *"all-or-nothing"* law.

The peripheral nerves of mammals consist of bundles of neurons held together in a fibrous envelope called the *epineurium.* The change in potential for these systems is the sum of the action potentials of all the axons in the system if extracellular recording is attempted. Each axon in the system has a different threshold potential, and so the number of axons firing will initially increase with increased intensity of the stimulus. Eventually, all the axons in the nerve will fire, and at this point, further increases in the intensity of the stimulus will cause no further increase in the size of the action potential. In bundles of mixed nerves, there will be multiple peaks in the action potential profile, however, because the differing types of nerve fiber will have different conduction speeds.

The electrical potential across the lipid membrane of an axon is mainly due to the transport of small inorganic ions, such as Ca^{2+}, Na^+, K^+, and Cl^-, across the membrane by active or passive transport. Active transport usually involves the intervention of a carrier protein that physically carries the ion to the other side of the membrane. It can occur against the electrochemical and concentration gradients across the membrane *(uphill).* Passive transport occurs by the diffusion of the ions through water-filled channels (ion channels) formed by the integral proteins of the membrane. The ions move from high concentration to low concentration *(downhill)* at rates on the order of 10^6 or more ions per second, which is 100 times faster than the active transport of ions. Passive transport of the ions is usually in the opposite direction to active transport. For example, Na^+ ions are transported into an axon by passive transport but out of an axon by active transport. Similarly, K^+ ions may be transported

out of an axon by passive transport but into an axon by active transport. A small movement of ions across a membrane can lead to the generation of electric fields that are enormous by macroscopic standards. For example, the transfer of one ion pair per million, the cation leaving and the anion entering the neuron across a membrane, results in an electrical potential of about $150,000$ V cm^{-1}.

The highest density of Na^+ ion channels occurs at the nodes of Ranvier.[6] The myelinated internodal sections of the neuron contain far fewer Na^+ channels. In addition, these internodal regions are electrically insulated and so do not contribute to the action potential. Consequently, the potential produced at the nodes of Ranvier must be strong enough to produce an effect up to 1 mm away.

Ion channels are formed by groups of integral proteins that run from one side of the membrane to the other. The channels are selective, allowing the passage of certain ions but preventing the passage of others. This suggests that parts of the channel must act as a selective filter. Furthermore, some of the channels are not permanently open; changes in the conformation of the proteins that form the channel effectively open and close the channel as though it contained a gate. These *gates* usually open briefly in response to various membrane changes, such as a change in voltage across the membrane *(voltage-gated channels)* or the binding of a ligand to a receptor *(ligand-gated channels).* Over 50 types of gated channel have been discovered.[7]

The axolemma is more permeable to K^+ ions than to Na^+ ions. These ions diffuse out of the neuron through the so-called *potassium leak channels,* whose opening does not appear to require a specific membrane change. The movement of K^+ ions is concentration driven; K^+ ions move from inside the neuron, where the concentration is high, to the extracellular fluid, where the concentration is lower (Fig. 20-9a). This tendency of K^+ ions to leak out of the neuron *(driven by the concentration gradient)* is balanced to some extent by a limited movement of K^+ ions back into the neuron, both by diffusion through K^+ channels and by active transport mechanisms such as the sodium pump. These

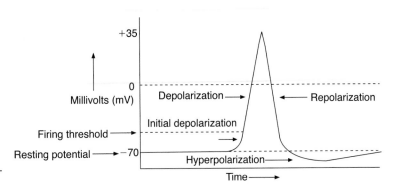

Figure 20–8 ■ Changes in electrical potential observed during a nerve impulse.

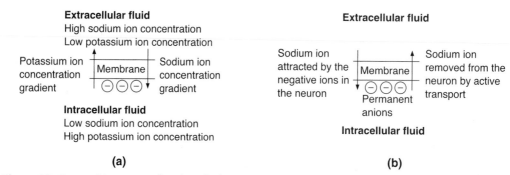

(a)   **(b)**

Figure 20–9 ■ **a.** Movement of Na$^+$ and K$^+$ ions across a membrane because of differences in concentration. **b.** Attraction of positive ions into a cell by electrostatic attraction and their removal by active transport.

movements of K$^+$ result in a potential difference across the membrane, which is a major contributor to the *equilibrium potential* that exists between the opposite faces of a biological membrane in a normal cell at rest with a switched-on sodium pump. Its value for a particular ion when the system is in equilibrium and the cell is at rest may be calculated by using the Nernst equation:

$$V = V_i - V_o = \frac{RT}{zF} \ln \frac{C_o}{C_i} \qquad \text{(Eq. 20-1)}$$

where V is the equilibrium potential, V_i is the internal potential, V_o is the external potential, C_i is the internal concentration of the ion (mol dm^{-3}), C_o is the external concentration of the ion (mol dm^{-3}), R is the ideal gas constant, and T is the temperature (°K). F is Faraday's constant (96,487 coulombs), and z is the charge on the ion.

The axolemma of a neuron at rest with a switched-on sodium pump does not allow the free movement of Na$^+$ ions, even though it contains channels that are specific for them. If the sodium pump is switched off, however, the concentration of Na$^+$ starts to build up in the cell, as the membrane is not completely impermeable to Na$^+$. The Na$^+$ ions pass into the cell down the concentration gradient through the so-called *sodium ion channels,* aided by an attraction for the anions in the cell. This inward movement of Na$^+$ neutralizes the negative charges of some of these anions and so reduces *(depolarizes)* the membrane potential, which allows a greater concentration of K$^+$ ions to leave the cell (Fig. 20-9b).

Ca^{2+} ions will also move into a cell, attracted by the anions permanently present inside and will also leak out of cells via *calcium channels.* Similarly, under the appropriate conditions, Cl$^-$ ions move in and out of cells. The movement of both of these ions also contributes to the membrane potential of the cell, which for a cell at rest can vary from −20 to −200 mV. The more permeable a membrane is to a particular ion, the more closely the membrane potential approaches the equilibrium potential for that ion.

The initial depolarization of the neuron (Fig. 20-8) was shown by Hodgkin and Huxley in 1953 to be due to increased movement of Na$^+$ into the neuron, which is followed almost immediately by increased movement of K$^+$ ions out of the neuron. Consequently, the gated ion channels of neurons are believed to be responsible for the transmittance of the action potentials that carry information to and from the body of the nerve cell. It is thought that the action potential is triggered by a stimulation that causes momentary shift of the membrane potential of a small section of the membrane to a less negative value *(depolarization of the membrane).* This causes the gated Na$^+$ channels in this section of the membrane to open, which allows Na$^+$ to enter the cell. This process depolarizes the membrane still further, until the action potential reaches a critical value (the *firing threshold*), when it triggers the opening of large numbers of adjacent Na$^+$ channels so that Na$^+$ ions flood into the axon. This process continues until the membrane potential of this section of membrane reaches about +60 mV, which is the equilibrium potential (V_{Na}) for Na$^+$ ions when the cell is at rest (calculated using Eq. 20-1). At this point, all the Na$^+$ channels of the membrane should be permanently open. This situation is not reached, however, because each channel has an automatic closing mechanism that operates even though the cell membrane is still depolarized (Fig. 20-10). Once

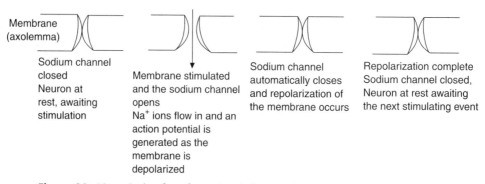

Figure 20–10 ■ Cycle of conformational changes that occur in a sodium channel.

closed, the ion channel cannot open again until the membrane potential in its vicinity returns to its original negative value, which is brought about by the leakage of K^+ ions out of the neuron through K^+ channels. Hodgkin and Huxley showed that a membrane becomes more permeable to K^+ ions a fraction of a millisecond after the Na^+ channels have started to open. As a result, K^+ ions flow out of the neuron, which reduces the electrical potential of the membrane, and so at the peak of the action potential, the membrane potential has a value of about $+40$ mV relative to the exterior of the axon. The movement of the K^+ ions out of the axon, coupled with the automatic closing of the sodium channel gates and the action of the sodium pump transporting Na^+ ions out of the neuron, results in a net flow of positive ions out of the neuron. This repolarizes the membrane and causes its membrane potential to drop below its resting potential to almost the K^+ ion equilibrium value. As the sodium channels close and K^+ ions flow back into the axon, the membrane potential returns to its resting value. The entire process of depolarization and repolarization is normally accomplished within 1 millisecond. The action of the sodium pump is very slow, however, compared with that of the Na^+ and K^+ ion channels.

An action potential originating from the cell body will trigger the depolarization of an adjacent section of the axon membrane, which in turn will produce an action potential in this area through the same process. These new areas, in turn, will affect further adjacent sections of the membrane and so on. In this way the initial electrical impulse will move along the neuron. The impulse will flow in one direction, since the channels will automatically close and will not open until the next stimulus reaches them down the neuron. Furthermore, since each action potential requires the same membrane trigger potential of about -20 mV, the amplitude of the impulse remains the same as it proceeds along the axon. Moreover, since only a small change in the Na^+ and K^+ ion concentrations is required to form the action potential, the axon is able to transmit a nerve impulse every few milliseconds.

Neurons contain many thousands of sodium ion channels. Experimental work by Catterall in 1984 using radioactive neurotoxins and antibodies showed that their distribution in the plasma membranes of electrically excitable cells is nonuniform. Sodium channels appear to occupy at least 15% of the surface area of the nodes of Ranvier, but very few have been detected in the internodal regions of myelinated axons. Experimental work by Moczydlowski and coworkers in 1986[8] indicated that the nature of sodium channels varied with the type of membrane. Their results demonstrated the existence of three different Na-channel subtypes or "isochannels" and that each of these individual isochannels is the predominant Na-channel types in mammalian brain, skeletal muscle, and cardiac muscle, respectively. Further work by Schneider and Dubois in1986 attributed the action of benzocaine on the voltage clamped frog nodes of Ranvier to two different types of channel with different rates of inactivation and affinities for the drug.[9] Since then, numerous different types of ion channel have been identified, and it is likely that these different types of ion channels respond differently to local anesthetic agents.

Patch clamp recording has shown that a sodium channel either opens completely to allow the passage of a Na^+ ion or remains shut. Sodium channels appear to open on a random basis, but when open, a channel always has the same conductance. In other words, the rate of ion transfer from one side of the membrane to the other is always the same. Since a membrane is about 5 nm thick, the voltage gradient across a membrane is of the order of 150,000 V cm^{-1}. Consequently, the proteins forming the channels are subjected to very strong electrical fields. Changes in this electrical field are believed to be responsible for the changes in the conformations of the proteins that form the gated channels; that is, changes in the electrical field of the membrane cause the opening and closing of the so-called gates in the ion channels.

Neurons communicate with each other and with muscle cells and glands at sites known as *synapses*. A nerve impulse arriving at the synapse *(presynaptic site or cell)* of a neuron *(A)* triggers the release, by exocytosis, of a chemical known as a *neurotransmitter,* which is stored in the synaptic vesicles (Fig. 20-11). The neurotransmitter diffuses across the synaptic cleft to a receptor *(postsynaptic cell or site)* on either a dendrite of a neuron cell body *(B)* and/or another suitable cell. This initiates a process that either promotes or inhibits the transmission of the action potential. Promotion causes a change in the electrical potential of the postsynaptic site that exceeds the neuron's firing potential. The receiving neuron will subsequently transmit this action potential along its length to the next synapse, where a similar process of neurotransmission will be repeated. Synapses usually permit conduction of impulses in one direction only.

The chemical structures of neurotransmitters are very varied and include acetylcholine, simple amino acids, small peptides, and miscellaneous amines, such as the catecholamines (Table 20-1). The mechanism of their release is not fully understood but is known to be triggered by a change in the membrane potential at the presynaptic site. For example, the process that stimulates the contraction of a muscle cell is initiated by the opening of a calcium ion channels, caused by the arrival of an action potential at the presynaptic site. Since the concentration of Ca^{2+} ions is far higher in the extracellular fluid, Ca^{2+} flow into the neuron. This increase in intracellular Ca^{2+} concentration initiates the release of acetylcholine into the synaptic cleft by exocytosis of the synaptic vesicles. The mechanism of this Ca^{2+}-stimulated release of acetylcholine is not known. However, the quantity of neurotransmitter released is proportional to the concentration of Ca^{2+} flowing into the neuron.

The arrival of the neurotransmitter at the postsynaptic receptor activates the relevant *transmitter-gated ion channel,* which changes the membrane's permeability to ions, which produces a change in the membrane potential.[5] However, transmitter-gated ion channels are not sensitive to changes in the membrane potential and so cannot transmit an action potential. Consequently, the opening of transmitter-gated channels must stimulate the opening of voltage-gated channels that can transmit an action potential through the neuron in the manner described above. The neurotransmitter will continue to act unless it is removed from the site of action by blood circulation, is metabolized, or is reabsorbed into the presynaptic neuron. Metabolism is usually rapid. However, some toxins prevent the metabolism of the neurotransmitter and, in effect, leave the action potential system switched on, with potentially fatal results. Reabsorption into the presynap-

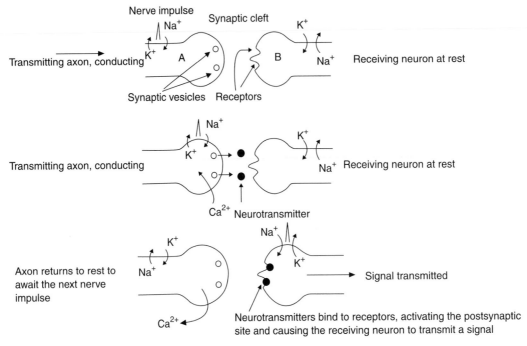

Figure 20–11 ■ Representation of the action of a neurotransmitter.

tic neuron may result in either vesicle formation or the neurotransmitter being transported to, and metabolized in, the mitochondria of the cell.

Many drugs act by interfering with either the synthesis and/or action and/or metabolism of the neurotransmitter. For example, the enkephalins are believed to act as endogenous painkillers by inhibiting substance P, a neurotransmitter that transmits pain signals across the synaptic cleft. It is thought that the activation of a pain-transmitting neuron causes both the presynaptic and postsynaptic neurons to release enkephalins. The enkephalins produced at the presynaptic site inhibit the release of substance P, while those produced at the postsynaptic site hypopolarize the postsynaptic membrane, which makes it more difficult to generate the postsynaptic action potential in the receiving neuron. Other drugs act by replacing the neurotransmitter.

Some neurotransmitters, such as glycine and γ-aminobutanoic acid (GABA), act as inhibitors by opening Cl⁻ ion channels and allowing Cl⁻ ions to flow into the neuron causing hyperpolarization. This makes the internal face of the membrane relatively more electronegative, and so the neuron requires more intense depolarization if it is to transmit a signal. Ethanol is believed to act by inducing GABA receptors to open their Cl⁻ channels in the brain. This inhibits the excitability of the affected neurons and so reduces their ability to transmit nerve impulses. However, the ability of a neurotransmitter to either excite or inhibit a neuron appears to depend on the nature of its receptor rather than its structure.

Transmitter-gated channels are ion selective, and their receptor sites are highly selective for a particular neurotransmitter.[5] The first to be characterized was the acetylcholine

TABLE 20–1   Examples of Neurotransmitters

Amino Acids	Small Peptides	Miscellaneous Amines and Their Derivatives
$H_3\overset{+}{N}CH_2COO^-$ Glycine	H-Try-Gly-Gly-Phe-Met(OH) Met-enkephalin	HO—, HO—⟨ ⟩—$CH_2CH_2NH_2$ Dopamine
$H_3\overset{+}{N}CH_2CH_2CH_2COO^-$ γ-Aminobutanoic acid (GABA)	H-Try-Gly-Gly-Phe-Leu(OH) Leu-enkephalin	HO—, HO—⟨ ⟩—$\overset{OH}{C}HCH_2NH_2$ Noradrenaline
$H_3\overset{+}{N}CH\overset{\displaystyle COO^-}{\underset{\displaystyle CH_2CH_2COOH}{}}$ Glutamic acid		$(CH_3)_3\overset{+}{N}CH_2CH_2OCOCH_3$ Acetylcholine

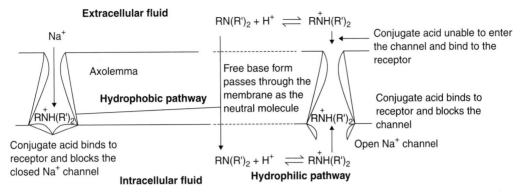

Figure 20–12 ■ Representation of the mechanism of action of local anesthetics in blocking closed and open sodium channels.

receptor. This is a glycoprotein that consists of five integral proteins. There are about 20,000 per mm^2 of these receptors in the synapse sites of muscle cells. When two acetylcholine molecules bind to the receptor, they cause a change in conformation of the proteins that opens the channel. The channel has a cluster of negatively charged amino acid residues at its entrance, which is thought to prevent the passage of negative ions. Its diameter is about 0.65 nm, so it will allow the passage of positive ions such as Na^+, K^+, and Ca^{2+}. In muscle cells, Na^+ ions are the main contributors to the change in membrane potential (~30,000 ions per channel per millisecond). Ca^+ ions make a small contribution because their extracellular concentration is much lower than that of Na^+ ions, while for K^+ ions, the leakage out almost balances the voltage gradient-driven inward movement.

MECHANISM OF ACTION

Experimental work has shown that the main site of local anesthetic action is on the cell membrane. Local anesthetics do not appear to have any appreciable effect on the intracellular fluid *(axoplasm)*. Various theories have been put forward to explain the mechanism of the action.[10] Many of these postulate prevention of conduction and formation of an action potential by either fully or partially blocking the Na^+ ion channels. Blocking is believed to be achieved either by the drug molecule causing a physical block in the channel, like a cork in a bottle, or by the drug molecule distorting the channel. If enough sodium channels are blocked, there would be no significant changes in membrane potential, the firing potential would not be reached, and conduction of an action potential along the neuron would be prevented. Blocking of conduction would automatically prevent the release of neurotransmitter at the presynaptic site. Increasing the Ca^+ ion concentration of the extracellular fluid may either enhance or reduce the activity of a local anesthetic by affecting the opening of sodium channels.

Shanes[11] suggested in 1958 that local anesthetics acted by increasing the surface pressure of the cell membrane, which would result in the closure of ion channels. In 1968, Metcalfe and Burgen[12] proposed that the nerve impulse was blocked by the drug increasing disorder of the membrane, which caused distortion of the ion channels. However, based on the work of several research groups (Ritchie[10] in 1975, Hille[14] in 1980, Strichartz[15] in 1980, and Strichartz and Ritchie[13] in 1985), it is now believed that the main mechanism of local anesthetic action is associated with the blocking of sodium channels (Fig. 20-12). Strichartz[15] also showed, in 1981, that the receptor for the blocking action appears to be about halfway down the sodium channel. Work by Schneider and Dubois[9] in 1986 indicated that benzocaine blocks two different types of sodium channel. Their work suggested that these channels have different affinities for the drug and so differing rates of inactivation. Other investigations in 1986 by Moczydlowski et al.[8] of the blocks imposed by local anesthetic agents indicated that there are at least two sites of action of local anesthetic agents and not one in the interior entrance of the channel, as previously proposed by Hille. Their work also supported the idea of a wide internal entryway into the channel but a constricted external entry. This internal entry was large enough to allow the passage of organic molecules, but the external entry was small enough to prevent the ingress of organic molecules with a single methyl group. It was, however, large enough to permit the entry of divalent cations such as Ca^{2+} and Co^{2+}. The observations made by Moczydlowski et al. were supported by the work of MacIver and Roth[16] (1987) on a single isolated neuron (crayfish stretch receptor), which also suggested the existence of receptor sites that can discriminate between the structures of different anesthetics. These deductions were supported by those of Elliot et al.[17] in 1987, who concluded from their investigation of the inhibition of sodium current in giant squid axon by benzocaine that there were at least two sites for the action of the drug.

It is an important feature of the local anesthetics in clinical use that their structures include tertiary amine groups that coexist in equilibrium with the conjugate acid at physiological pH:

$$RN(R')_2 \ + \ H^+ \ \rightleftharpoons \ R\overset{+}{N}H(R')_2$$

Local anesthetic (neutral molecule)   Conjugate acid

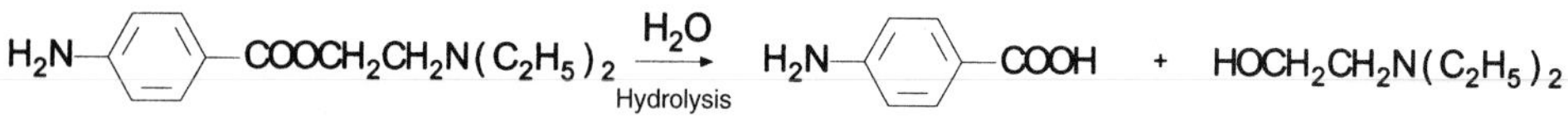

$$H_2N-\!\!\!\langle\ \rangle\!\!\!-COOCH_2CH_2N(C_2H_5)_2 \xrightarrow[\text{Hydrolysis}]{H_2O} H_2N-\!\!\!\langle\ \rangle\!\!\!-COOH \ + \ HOCH_2CH_2N(C_2H_5)_2$$

Procaine   4-Aminobenzoic acid   Diethylaminoethanol

Experimental studies carried out by Narahashi and Frazier[18] in 1971 and Strichartz and Ritchie[13] in 1985 indicated that the site of action of local anesthetics is only accessible from the interior of the neuron. Consequently, as neutral molecules cross membranes more easily than charged molecules, the drug must cross the membrane in its uncharged form before it can enter and block the ion channel. Once inside the neuron, experimental evidence suggests that the action of the drug is mainly due to its charged form and that its binding to the receptor is voltage dependent.[18, 19]

Analysis of the work of Strichartz, Hille, and Ritchie has shown that the block caused by many local anesthetic agents depends on the number of channels open; the greater the number open, the greater the block. This suggests that the activity of the local anesthetic agent depends on it entering the channel from inside the neuron ("the hydrophilic pathway"). However, blocks can arise even if the channel is not open. This is explained by the local anesthetic agent entering the channel directly from the membrane ("the hydrophobic pathway"). The relative effects of these two pathways appear to depend on the lipid solubility of the drug, but both appear to contribute to the blocking effect.

Local anesthetic agents are removed from the site of application by the blood flowing through the tissues and membranes in the area of application. Metabolism occurs through a variety of routes in both the plasma and the liver. Ester-type agents such as procaine are either eliminated by hydrolysis in the plasma, catalyzed by plasma esterases, or in the liver, catalyzed by specific liver esterases.

The 4-aminobenzoic acid (PABA) produced in this hydrolysis inhibits the action of sulfonamides. However, the PABA is excreted in the urine, partly in the form of conjugates. The diethylaminoethanol is also excreted in the urine but about 70% is metabolized by the liver. Amide-based local anesthetics may also be hydrolyzed by plasma esterases, but the rate of hydrolysis is usually slower than that for the corresponding ester agents. Consequently, amide local anesthetic agents are more likely to be hydrolyzed in the liver. Amide local anesthetic agents are also metabolized by oxidation and N-alkylation in the liver. For example lignocaine is metabolized by both hydrolysis and N-dealkylation (Fig. 20-13). The importance of the liver in the metabolism of amide-based local anesthetics means that use of these agents in patients with severe liver damage should be avoided, as any toxic effects of the local anesthetic agent will be increased because of a reduced rate of metabolism.

The delivery of local anesthetic agents to the liver for metabolism appears to be related to their degree of binding to

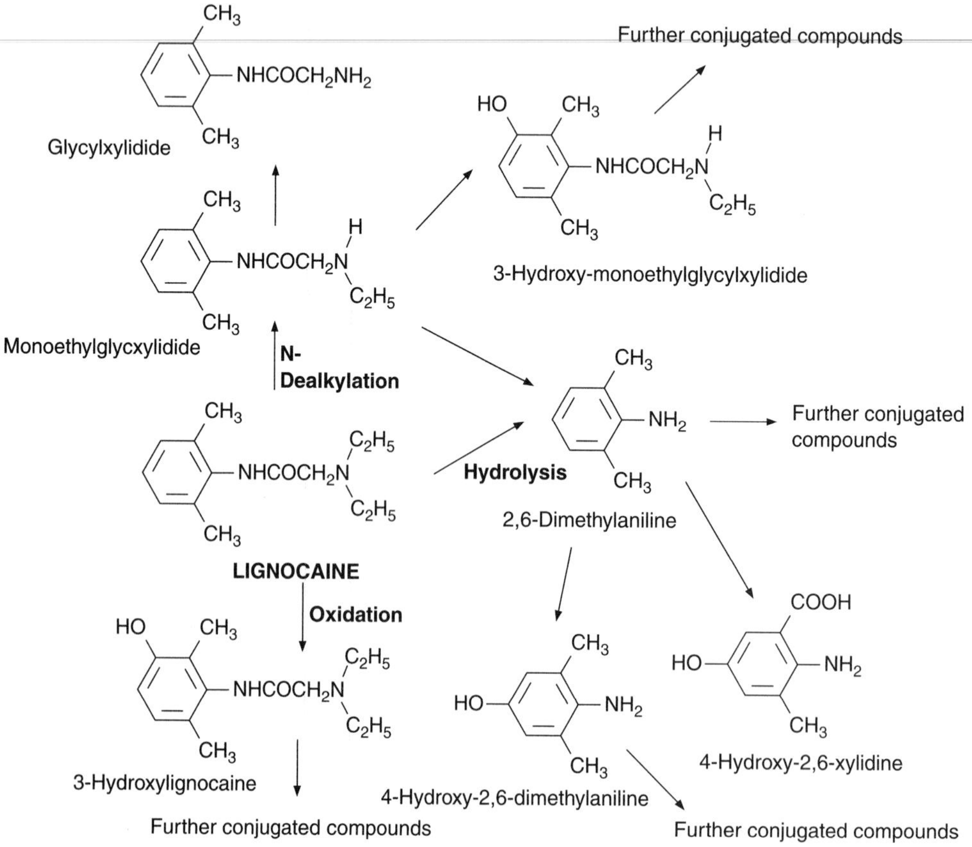

Figure 20-13 ■ Metabolism of lignocaine.

plasma proteins. Experimental work by Tucker et al. (1970) showed that amide-based local anesthetic agents bind more readily to plasma and tissue proteins than do ester-based agents. The binding of amide-based agents often involves the anesthetic binding to α_1-acid glycoprotein. This binding is usually significant, ranging from 55 to 95% of the drug. However, many factors influence the concentration of plasma proteins; for example, cancer, smoking and trauma decrease the concentration of plasma proteins, while oral contraceptives increase their concentration. Plasma protein concentration may also be altered in many diseases. Obviously these changes will influence the quantity and rate of delivery of the local anesthetic to the liver, with subsequent changes in the systemic toxicity of the drug.

The elimination of local anesthetics and their metabolites from the liver depends on hepatic blood flow. If this flow is reduced, it can result in an increase in concentration of agents and their metabolites in the body when large doses are administered over long periods. This buildup may result in an increase in the systemic toxicity of the local anesthetic agent.[20]

ADMINISTRATION

Topical or Surface Anesthesia[10, 21]

Direct application of a local anesthetic agent to the skin or a mucous membrane blocks the sensory nerve endings. The local anesthetic may be applied in the form of a liquid, spray, cream, ointment, or gel. It appears that the form used is often selected subjectively. For example, in the use of local anesthetic agents as premedication in gastrointestinal endoscopy, the patients preferred sprays, even though the degree of anesthesia was the same for sprays and gargles.

Anesthesia of the mucous membranes of the ear, nose, and throat is usually brought about by use of aqueous solutions of the salts of tetracaine, lignocaine, or cocaine. The vasodilator effect of cocaine reduces bleeding in surgical procedures. However, all local anesthetics are rapidly absorbed through mucous membranes, and so their use may be accompanied by an increased risk of toxic systemic reactions. As a result, dosage must be carefully controlled.

Infiltration Anesthesia

A set dose of the local anesthetic in a suitable solvent system is injected directly into the area of the body that is to be anesthetized. These areas range from the skin to deeper tissues. The most frequently used local anesthetics for infiltration are lignocaine, bupivacaine, and procaine.

The technique produces a good degree of anesthesia in a localized area without disrupting general bodily functions. However, the use of this technique may require large concentrations of anesthetic to bring about the desired degree of anesthesia, with an attendant increase in the risk of toxic systemic reactions.

Field Block Anesthesia

A solution of the local anesthetic is injected subcutaneously at a point adjacent to the area that is to be anesthetized, so that it blocks the nerve transmissions to that region. Field block anesthesia is brought about by the same drugs used for infiltration anesthesia. However, the technique produces a larger region of anesthesia with a lower dose of the local anesthetic than is required by the infiltration technique.

Regional Nerve Block Anesthesia

Regional nerve block anesthesia is usually brought about by either injection of the anesthetic in a suitable solvent system into the nerve or infiltration of the anesthetic into the tissue surrounding a nerve or plexus supplying the region to be anesthetized. For example, spinal anesthesia may be brought about by injection into the cerebrospinal fluid in the subarachnoid space. Dental anesthesia is brought about by flooding the area around the nerve by injecting the anesthetic into the adjacent tissue. The local anesthetic agent used for a nerve block depends on which nerve is to be blocked, the length of time the anesthesia is required, and the medical condition and physique of the patient. Duration of action is usually prolonged by the use of vasoconstrictors rather than by increasing the dose. This approach reduces the chances of the drug spreading to regions that do not require anesthesia.

Intravenous Regional Anesthesia

Intravenous regional anesthesia is used to anesthetize a large region, such as a limb. The anesthetic is injected into a suitable vein in a limb that has had its blood flow restricted by a tourniquet. The efficiency and safety of the technique depends on preventing arterial flow for the duration of the anesthesia. Lignocaine is frequently used to produce intravenous regional anesthesia, but bupivacaine is not approved for this purpose because of its long duration of action.

Spinal Anesthesia

Spinal anesthesia is carried out by injecting the anesthetic agent into the subarachnoid space in the spinal cord. The anesthetic acts mainly on the nerve fibers and blocks the pain regions of the body served by the sections of the spinal cord affected.

Epidural Anesthesia

The drug is injected into the epidural space between the vertebrae and spinal cord. This numbs the nerves leading to the uterus and the pelvic area and leads to pain relief during labor. Epidural anesthesia may sometimes cause headaches.

FACTORS INFLUENCING THE EFFECTIVENESS OF THE ANESTHETIC ACTION

Susceptibility of the Neuron to Anesthesia

Pain information is carried by the largely unmyelinated C fibers, while sharp pain is transmitted by myelinated Aδ fibers. The sensitivity of nerve fibers to local anesthetic appears to vary according to the size, anatomical type, and degree of conductance of the nerve fiber. In general, the order of onset of local anesthesia with increasing concentration of agent is often small nonmyelinated fibers > small myelinated fibers > large fibers. However, this order is not strictly followed in practice. Some myelinated fibers are blocked with lower concentrations of local anesthetics than some nonmyelinated fibers, while large fibers are often blocked before smaller fibers. Furthermore, in experimental work, the outer fibers in the nerve are affected first, regardless of their nature.

Experimental work by Franz and Perry[22] in 1974 supported by the work of Chiu and Ritchie[23] in 1984 suggests that the differential blocking of nerve fibers depends on the length of axon that has to be exposed to the local anesthetic to bring about anesthesia. Shorter nerve fibers have shorter internodal distances and in the early stages of anesthesia are fully exposed to the local anesthetic, with the result that they are more readily blocked than longer fibers. In most patients, the sensation of pain is the first to be lost, followed by temperature and touch.

pH of the Extracellular and Intracellular Fluids

Local anesthetics are normally weak bases (pK$_a$ ~8.5), which are only slightly soluble in water. Consequently, they are usually marketed as aqueous solutions of their more soluble salts. These solutions are often quite acidic, which makes them less prone to bacterial and fungal contamination. However, an aqueous solution of the salt of a local anesthetic will normally contain between 2 and 15% of the free base in equilibrium with the salt.

Although the drug is mainly transferred through the cell membrane in its free base form, administration of the drug in alkaline solution does not enhance its activity. This is because the structure of the drug is controlled by the pH of the extracellular fluid and not the pH of the dosage form. Once inside the neuron, equilibrium is reestablished. Both the free base and its protonated form are known to be active, but it is not known whether they bind to the same receptor site. However, it does appear that the protonated base plays the major part in anesthetic activity.[12, 24, 25]

Vasoconstrictors

The anesthetic action of local anesthetics is proportional to the time that the agent is in contact with nerve tissue. As early as 1903, Braun discovered that the addition of adrenaline to solutions of local anesthetics increased and prolonged their action. It is now accepted that the addition of vasoconstrictors such as adrenaline to local anesthetic solutions prolongs and intensifies their action. The agent is confined to its site of action by reducing the rate at which the blood carries it away. Vasoconstrictors such as adrenaline also reduce the rate of absorption of a drug by allowing the metabolic rate of the local anesthetic to keep pace with the rate at which it is absorbed into the bloodstream. This also reduces systemic toxicity. However, prolonged use of a vasoconstrictor on major arteries may cause irreversible tissue damage and can lead to gangrene.

The main vasoconstrictors in current use with local anesthetics are adrenaline (epinephrine), noradrenaline (norepinephrine), and felypressin. Solutions of local anesthetics often contain either adrenaline or a synthetic analogue such as phenylephrine. The effect of vasoconstrictors depends on the local anesthetic agent used; for example, adrenaline significantly prolongs the action of lignocaine but has less effect with prilocaine. The concentrations of vasoconstrictors are kept as low as possible to reduce the risk of unwanted side effects, such as chest pains, palpitations, and increased heart rate. Local anesthetic preparations containing vasoconstrictors should never be used on digits, since they have no alternative blood supply. Consequently, restriction of blood supply can cause necrosis, a form of enforced cell death. Additionally, preparations containing adrenaline should not normally be used on patients with diseases including poorly controlled diabetes, cardiovascular disease, and thyrotoxicosis. Cocaine is a vasoconstrictor and so probably owes some of its effectiveness to this property.

Neuron Stimulation

The effectiveness of the blocking action of a given concentration of a local anesthetic agent depends on the frequency and extent to which a neuron has been recently stimulated. The greater the frequency of this stimulation, the more effective the local anesthetic agent is in blocking a response.[14, 26]

RATE OF ONSET AND DURATION OF ANESTHESIA

The time for the onset of action appears to be related to the type of tissue being anesthetized, the method of administration, and the percentage of the local anesthetic agent in its unprotonated form at physiological pH. Since the degree of protonation is indicated by the pK$_a$ value of the drug, local anesthetic agents with a low pK$_a$ value and high lipid solubility usually have a more rapid onset of action than those with higher pK$_a$ values and lower lipid solubility. For example, lignocaine, which is about 35% unprotonated at pH 7.4, usually has a more rapid onset of action than bupivacaine, which is about 8% unprotonated at this pH. The time taken for the

Adrenaline
(Epinephrine)

Noradrenaline (Norepinephrine)

Phenylephrine

Cys-Phe-Phe-Gln-Asn-Cys-Pro-Lys-GlyNH$_2$

Felypressin

drug to diffuse from its site of application to its site of action will also affect the rate of onset of anesthesia.[10]

Reportedly,[27, 28] the time taken for the onset of anesthesia can be reduced by the use of the hydrogen carbonate form of the drug. This does not increase the toxicity of the local anesthetic agent, but it has been reported to reduce the pain associated with injection and improve the effectiveness of the block in some cases.

The duration of action appears to be related to the lipid solubility of the local anesthetic agent and its ability to bind to protein. As a general rule, the more lipid soluble the drug, the longer the duration of its action. It is difficult, to classify local anesthetics in terms of the duration of anesthesia, however, because although the period of action depends on the dose, the relationship between dose and duration of anesthesia is not clear. In most cases, increasing the dose increases the duration of the anesthesia, but the relationship is not linear. For example, doubling a dose does not necessarily double the time of action.

The dose used clinically is usually determined by factors such as systemic toxicity, potency, and the time for which the anesthesia is required. When long periods of anesthesia are required, it is better to repeat applications rather than use large doses. This keeps dose levels to a minimum, which reduces the level of any possible systemic toxicity.

SECONDARY PHARMACOLOGICAL ACTION

Local anesthetics do not rely on blood circulation to reach their site of action, as they are usually administered at, or close to, their site of action. Systemic side effects arise because the local anesthetic agent is carried away in the blood before it can be fully metabolized. Consequently, the chemical and pharmacological properties of local anesthetics are of major importance in determining not only the effectiveness of the drug but also its systemic side effects.

Local anesthetic agents can affect the function of any organs in which electrical impulse transmission occurs. The nature and the extent of these unwanted side effects depend on the drug used, the concentration of the drug in circulation, the site of application, and the technique used. The secondary effects of local anesthetic agents in these situations are discussed in this section.

Cardiovascular System

Local anesthetic agents usually affect the cardiovascular system by decreasing the force of contraction, electrical excitability, and conduction of the myocardium. A high systemic concentration of local anesthetic is usually necessary, however, before any of these effects are observed. Occasionally, low concentrations administered by infiltration cause cardiovascular collapse and death. The reason for cardiovascular collapse is not known,[29] it appears, however, that local anesthetic agents may act as antiarrhythmic agents by blocking the Na^+, K^+, and Ca^{2+} channels responsible for the excitation of heart muscle. For example, many workers believe that lignocaine may reduce the possibility of Na^+ channels opening during depolarization. Recovery from this type of block, however, is usually rapid.

Central Nervous System

All amide-based local anesthetics can stimulate the CNS, causing symptoms ranging from restlessness to clonic convulsions. Stimulation may be followed by depression of the CNS and death, usually from respiratory failure. These unwanted side effects appear to be related to the potency of the anesthetic. It is therefore possible to predict these side effects from a knowledge of the drug and its concentration in the bloodstream. Unfortunately, convulsions can occur with little or no warning but can be prevented or stopped by the use of sedatives, such as diazepam or barbiturates, although near-anesthetic doses of the latter are required.

Other types of local anesthetic can stimulate the CNS system but often lead to drowsiness. Individual compounds may cause other unwanted side effects, however. For example, at blood concentrations of 5 $\mu g\ cm^{-3}$, lignocaine may produce muscle twitching, dysphoria, and euphoria. Both lignocaine and procaine can produce symptoms of sedation, followed by unconsciousness. Cocaine, in common with some other local anesthetic agents, has an effect on mood and behavior.

Blood[30–32]

Amethocaine (tetracaine), benzocaine, lignocaine, and prilocaine have been reported to induce methemoglobinemia. This is a condition in which the level of methemoglobin in erythrocytes exceeds the normal 1 to 2%. Methemoglobin is hemoglobin that contains iron III instead of iron II and so cannot transport oxygen. Concentrations of about 15% result in the appearance of cyanosis in which the lips take on a purple-blue coloration. High concentrations are rare but are associated with a high mortality rate. It has been suggested that methemoglobinemia may be due to either the presence of an aromatic amine in the local anesthetic or the metabolism of the local anesthetic to an aromatic amine.

Wound Healing

Local anesthetics may interfere with wound healing. This is particularly important in surgery carried out on the hands and feet.

Hypersensitivity

Hypersensitivity to local anesthetics appears to be related to both chemical structure and the method of administration. Allergic reactions occur most frequently with ester-based local anesthetic agents (benzoic acid derivatives). Adverse effects include allergic dermatitis, asthmatic attack, or, in extreme cases, death due to anaphylactic shock. Individuals suffering a hypersensitive reaction from one local anesthetic agent are often sensitive to compounds with a similar structure. For example, patients sensitive to procaine are often also sensitive to amethocaine

Amide-based local anesthetic agents do not usually produce hypersensitivity reactions, although they may be responsible for other unwanted effects and have been implicated in malignant hyperpyrexia. Families with a history of this disease should only be treated with ester-based local anesthetics.

Patch testing frequently provides adequate warning of hypersensitivity. When Ruzicka et al. (1987) conducted allergy

TABLE 20–4   Miscellaneous Compounds With Local Anesthetic Activity

Dimethisoquin	
Diperodon	
Dyclonine hydrochloride	
Euprocin	
Fomocaine	
Myrtecaine	
Phenacaine hydrochloride	
Pramoxine hydrochloride	

weak bases with distinct hydrophilic and lipophilic regions. In addition, a wide variety of compounds, including benzyl alcohol, phenol, and some antihistamines, also show some local anesthetic activity.

REFERENCES

1. Einhorn, A.: Justus Leibigs Ann. Chem. 216:236–237, 1891.
2. Merling, G.: Justus Leibigs Ann. Chem. 265:329–356, 1883.
3. Hughes, J.: Brain Res. 88:295, 1975.
4. Smith, T. (ed.): British Medical Association: Guide to Medicines and Drugs. Godalming, U. K., Colour Library Books, 1992.
5. Alberts, B., Bray, D., Lewis, J., et al.: Molecular Biology of the Cell, 3rd ed. New York, Garland Publishing, 1994, pp. 523–546.
6. Catterall, W. A.: Science 223:653–661, 1984.
7. Watson, S., and Girdlestone, D. (eds.): Reference Receptor and Ion Channel Nomenclature Supplement. Trends Pharmacol. Sci. 1994.
8. Moczydlowski, E., Uehara, A., Guo, X., and Heiny J.: Ann. N. Y. Acad. Sci. 479:269–292, 1986.
9. Schneider, M. F., and Dubois, J. M.: Biophys. J. 50:523–530, 1986.
10. Ritchie, J. M., and Greene, N. M.: Local anesthetics. In Goodman, L. S., and Gilman, A. (eds.). Goodman and Gilman's The Pharmacological Basis of Therapeutics, 7th ed. New York, Macmillan, 1985, pp. 302–321.
11. Shanes, A. M.: Pharmacol. Rev. 10:59–273, 1958.
12. Metcalfe, J. C., and Burgen, A. S. V.: Nature 220:587–588, 1968.
13. Strichartz, G. R., and Ritchie, J. M.: Action of local anesthetics on ion channels of excitable tissues. In Strichartz, G. R. (ed.). Local Anesthetics; Handbook of Experimental Pharmacology. Berlin, Springer-Verlag, 1985.
14. Hille, B.: Theories of anesthesia: General perturbations versus specific receptors. In Fink, B. R. (ed.). Mechanisms of Anesthesia, vol. 2: Progress in Anesthesiology. New York, Raven Press, 1980, pp. 1–5.
15. Strichartz, G. R.: J. Dent. Res. 60:1460–1467, 1981.
16. MacIver, M. B., and Roth, S. H.: Eur. J. Pharmacol. 139:43–52, 1987.
17. Elliot, J. R., Haydon, D. A., and Hendry, B. M.: Pflueugers Arch. 409:596–600, 1987.
18. Narahashi, T., and Frazier, D. T.: Neurosci. Res. 4:65–99, 1971.
19. Ritchie, J. M., and Greengard, P.: Annu. Rev. Pharmacol. 6:405–430, 1966.
20. Tucker, G. T., and Mather, L. E.: Br. J. Anesth. 47:213, 1975.
21. Neal, M. J.: Medical Pharmacology at a Glance. Oxford, Blackwell Scientific Publications, 1987, pp. 16–17.

22. Franz, D. N., and Perry, R. S.: J. Physiol. (Lond.) 236:193–210, 1974.
23. Chiu, S. Y., and Ritchie, J. M.: Proc. R. Soc. Lond. (Biol.) 220: 415–422, 1984.
24. Hille, B.: J. Gen. Physiol. 69:497–515, 1977.
25. Mrose, H., and Ritchie, J. M.: J. Gen. Physiol. 71: 223–225, 1978.
26. Courtney, K. R.: J. Pharmacol. Exp. Ther. 213:114–119, 1980.
27. Bromage, P. R.: Acta Anesthesiol. Scand. Suppl. 16:55–69, 1965.
28. Bromage, P. R.: Can. Med. Assoc. J. 97:1377–1384, 1967.
29. Grant, A. O., Jr.: Am. Heart J. 123:1130–1136, 1992.
30. Ferraro, L., Zeichner, S., Greenblott, G., and Groeger, J. S.: Anesthesiology 69:614–615, 1988.
31. Anderson, S. T., Hajduczek, J., and Barker, S. J.: Anesth. Analg. 67: 1099–1101, 1988.
32. Hall, A. H., Kulig, K. W., and Rumack, B. H.: Med. Toxicol. 1(4): 253–260, 1986.
33. Martindale, W. (ed.): Martindale: The Extra Pharmacopoeia, 30th ed. London, Pharmaceutical Press, 1993, pp. 995–1018.
34. Muhtadi, F. J., and Al-Badr, A. A.: Anal. Profiles Drug Subst. 15: 151–231, 1986.
35. Buchi, J., and Perlia, X.: Structure-activity relations and physiochemical properties of local anesthetics. In Lachat, P. (ed.). Local Anesthetics, Encyclopedia of Pharmacology and Therapeutics, sect. 8, vol. 1. New York, Pergamon, 1971, p. 39.
36. Buchi, J., and Perlia, X.: Design of local anesthetics. In Ariens, E. J. (ed.). Drug Design, vol. III. New York, Academic Press, 1972, p. 243.

SELECTED READING

Neal, M. J.: Medical Pharmacology at a Glance, 3rd ed. Blackwell Scientific Publications, 1997.
Rang, H. P., Dale, M. M., and Ritter, J. M.: Pharmacology, 4th ed. Edinburgh, Churchill Livingstone, 1999.
Reynolds, J. E. F., and Prasad, A. B. (eds): The Merck Index, 12th ed. Rahway, NJ, Merck & Co., 1996.
Sneader, W.: Drug Discovery: the Evolution of Modern Medicines. Chichester, U. K., John Wiley & Sons, 1985.
Speight, T. M., and Holford, P. (eds.): Avery's Drug Treatment, Principles and Practice of Clinical Pharmacology and Therapeutics, 4th. ed. Auckland, ADIS Press, 1997.
Tortora, G. J., Anagnostakos, N. P., and Marieb, E. N.: Principles of Anatomy and Physiology. San Francisco, Canfield Press, 2000.
Thomas, G.: Medicinal Chemistry, An Introduction. Chichester, U. K., John Wiley & Sons, 2000.
Voet, D., Voet, J. G., and Pratt, C.: Fundamentals of Biochemistry. New York, John Wiley & Sons, 1999.

Histamine and Antihistaminic Agents

THOMAS N. RILEY AND JACK DERUITER

Histamine is a β-imidazolylethylamine derivative that is present in essentially all mammalian tissues. The major physiological actions of histamine are centered on the cardiovascular system, nonvascular smooth muscle, exocrine glands, and the adrenal medulla.[1] In a general sense, histamine plays an important role as a "chemical messenger" component of a variety of pathways that have evolved in multicellular organisms, allowing them to communicate efficiently and effectively. The involvement of histamine in the mediation of allergic and hypersensitivity reactions and the regulation of gastric acid secretion has led to the development of important drug classes useful in the treatment of symptoms associated with allergic and gastric hypersecretory disorders.

HISTAMINE

Nomenclature

Histamine, known trivially as 4(5-)(2-aminoethyl)imidazole, structurally is composed of an imidazole heterocycle and ethylamine side chain. The methylene groups of the aminoethyl side chain are designated α and β. The side chain is attached, via the β-CH_2 group, to the 4 position of an imidazole ring. The imidazole N at position 3 is designated the *pros* (π) N, whereas the N at position 1 is termed the *tele* (τ) N. The side chain N is distinguished as N^α.

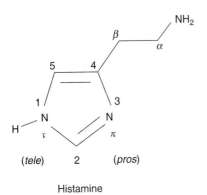

Histamine

Ionization and Tautomerism

Histamine is a basic organic compound (N^π, $pK_{a1} = 5.80$; N^α, $pK_{a2} = 9.40$; N^τ, $pK_{a3} = 14.0$) capable of existing as a mixture of different ionic and uncharged tautomeric species (Fig. 21-1).[2,3] Histamine exists almost exclusively (96.6%)

as the monocationic conjugate species (αNH_3^+) at physiological pH (7.4). The ratio of the concentrations of the tautomers N^τ-H/N^π-H has been calculated to be 4.2, indicating that in aqueous solution, 80% of the histamine monocation exists as N^τ-H and 20% exists as N^π-H.

Structure–activity relationship studies suggest that the α-NH_3^+ monocation is important for agonist activity at histamine receptors and that transient existence of the more lipophilic uncharged histamine species may contribute to translocation of cell membranes. Other studies support the proposal that the N^τ-H tautomer of the histamine monocation is the pharmacophoric species at the H_1 receptor, while a 1,3-tautomeric system is important for selective H_2-receptor agonism.

Stereochemistry

Histamine is an achiral molecule; histamine receptors, however, are known to exert high stereoselectivity toward chiral ligands.[4] Molecular modeling and steric-activity relationship studies of the influence of conformational isomerism on the activity of histamine suggest the importance of *trans-gauche* rotameric structures (Fig. 21-2) in the receptor activities of this substance. Studies with conformationally restricted histamine analogues suggest that while the *trans* rotamer of histamine possesses affinity for both H_1 and H_2 histamine receptors, the *gauche* conformer does not act at H_2 sites.

HISTAMINE LIFE CYCLE

Knowledge of the biodisposition of histamine is important to understanding the involvement of this substance in various pathophysiologies as well as the actions of various ligands that either enhance or block its actions. Each of the steps in the "life cycle" of histamine represents a potential site for pharmacological intervention.

Biosynthesis and Distribution

Histamine is synthesized in cytoplasmic granules of its principal storage cells, mast cells and basophils.[5] Histamine is formed from the naturally occurring amino acid, *S*-histidine, via the catalysis of either the pyridoxal phosphate–dependent enzyme histidine decarboxylase (HDC, EC 4.1.1.22) or aromatic amino acid decarboxylase (Fig. 21-3). Substrate specificity is higher for HDC. HDC inhibitors (HDCIs) in-

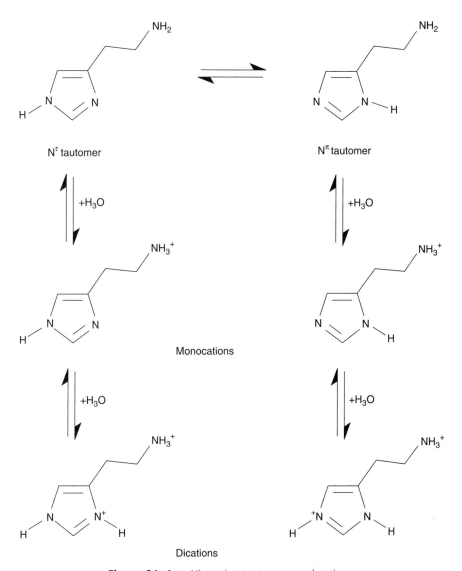

Figure 21–1 ■ Histamine tautomers and cations.

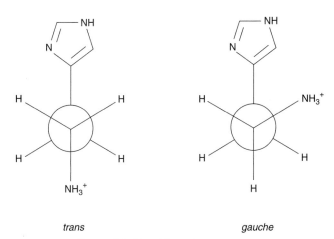

Figure 21–2 ■ Histamine rotamers.

clude α-fluoromethyl histidine (FMH) and certain flavonoids, although no HDCIs have proved useful clinically.

Histamine is found in almost all mammalian tissues in concentrations ranging from 1 to more than 100 μg/g. This substance is in particularly high concentration in skin, bronchial mucosa, and intestinal mucosa. It is found in higher concentrations in mammalian cerebrospinal fluid than in plasma and other body fluids.

Storage and Release

Most histamine is synthesized and stored in mast cells and basophilic granulocytes.[6] Protein-complexed histamine is then stored in secretory granules and released by exocytosis in response to a wide variety of immune (antigen and antibody) and nonimmune (bacterial products, xenobiotics, physical effects, and cholinergic effects) stimuli. The release of histamine as one of the mediators of hypersensitivity reactions is initiated by the interaction of an antigen–IgE complex with the membrane of a histamine storage cell. This interaction triggers activation of intracellular phosphokinase C (PKC), leading to accumulation of inositol phosphates, diacylglycerols, and Ca^{2+}. Exocytotic release of histamine follows the degranulation of histamine storage cells. Histamine is released from mast cells in the gastric mucosa by gastrin and acetylcholine. Neurochemical studies also suggest that histamine is stored in selected neuronal tracts in the central nervous system (CNS).

Receptors

Once released, the physiological effects of histamine are mediated by specific cell-surface receptors.[7] Extensive pharmacological analysis suggests the existence of at least three different histamine receptor subtypes, H_1, H_2, and H_3.

Histamine H_1 receptors have been detected in a wide variety of tissues including mammalian brain; smooth muscle from airways, gastrointestinal (GI) tract, genitourinary system, and the cardiovascular system; adrenal medulla; and endothelial cells and lymphocytes. The structure of the H_1 receptor has been determined and shown to possess several important features that distinguish it from the H_2 receptor.[8] The H_1-receptor protein has a molecular mass of 56 kDa. The deduced sequence of the bovine H_1-receptor protein represents 491 amino acid residues. Structurally, this receptor contains seven hydrophobic transmembrane domains (TMs) characteristic of most G-protein receptors. The third intracellular loop of the receptor is very large (212 amino acids), and the intracellular C-terminal tail is relatively short (17 amino acids). Site-directed mutagenesis studies have provided evidence for the binding domains of H_1 agonists and antagonists. The third (TM3) and fifth (TM5) transmembrane domains of the receptor protein are responsible for binding histamine. Aspartate (107) of the human H_1 receptor is essential for the binding of histamine and H_1 antagonists to the receptor, perhaps by being involved in an Asp-$COO^-\cdots H_3N^+$–R interaction. Asparagine (207) of the TM5 domain is known to interact with the N^τ-nitrogen of the imidazole ring of histamine, while lysine (200) has been shown to interact with the nucleophilic N^π-nitrogen of the natural ligand. Signal transduction of the H_1 receptor involves the activation of phospholipase C (PLC), resulting in inositol phosphate accumulation and calcium mobilization in most tissues.

H_2 receptors have been detected in a wide variety of tissues (most notably for therapeutic consideration, myocardial cells and cell membranes of acid-secreting cells [parietal] of the gastric mucosa) and mediate the gastric acid secretory actions of histamine. The H_2 receptor has the general characteristics of a G-protein–coupled receptor, with a molecular mass of 59 kDa and nonessential N-glycosylation sites in the N-terminal region.[9] The most notable difference between structures of cloned H_1 and H_2 receptors is the much shorter third intracellular loop and longer C-terminal loop of the H_2-receptor protein. A TM3 aspartate along with an aspartate and threonine residue in TM5 is apparently responsible for binding histamine. The physiological and pharmacological effects of H_2-receptor ligands are mediated by a stimulatory G_s-protein–coupled receptor, which in turn activates the adenylate cyclase/cyclic adenosine monophosphate (cAMP) intracellular second-messenger system.

The cloning of the human histamine H_3 receptor in 1999 evoked considerable renewed interest in the field of histamine receptors.[10] The H_3 receptor is proposed to function as a neural autoreceptor (presynaptic) serving to modulate histamine synthesis and release in the CNS. Subsequent studies have also located H_3 sites in peripheral tissue, including the gastric mucosa where this receptor may negatively control gastric acid secretion and on the cardiac sympathetic terminals in the myocardium. Although signal transduction mechanisms of the H_3 receptor have not been fully elucidated, increasing evidence suggests that this receptor belongs to the superfamily of G-protein–coupled receptors.[10]

A new histamine receptor, the H_4 subtype, was first reported in 2000 and characterized as a 390-amino acid, G_i-coupled protein with 40% identity to the H_3 receptor.[10] This new receptor exhibits a very restricted localization; expression is primarily found in intestinal tissue, spleen, thymus, and immune active cells, such as T cells, neutrophils, and eosinophils, which suggests an important role for H_4 receptors in the regulation of immune function.

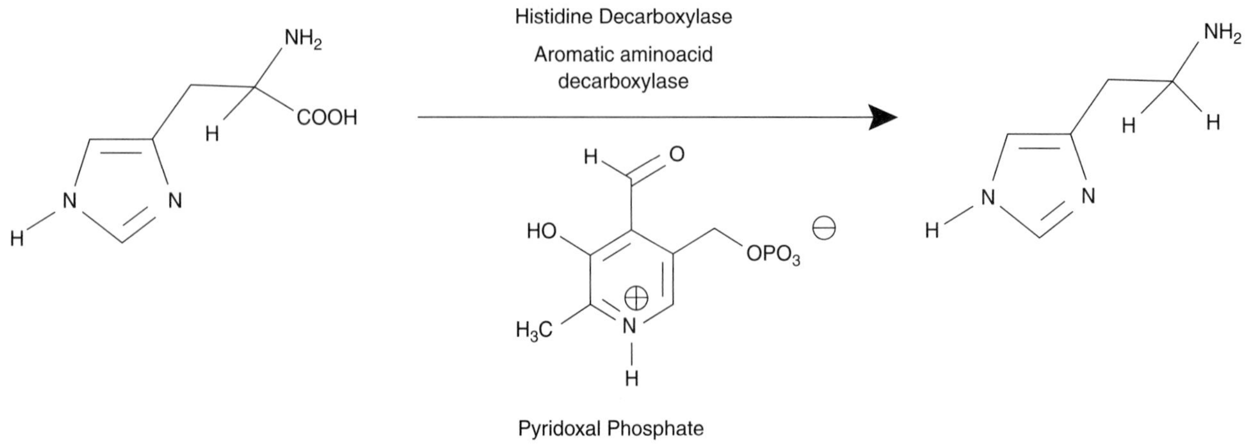

Figure 21–3 ■ Histamine biosynthesis.

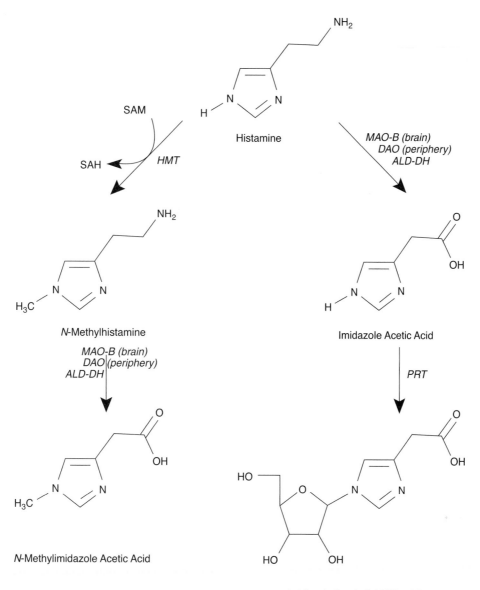

Figure 21–4 ▪ Metabolism of histamine. *ALD-DH,* aldehyde dehydrogenase; *PRT* phosphoribosyltransferase.

Termination of Histamine Action

Three principal ways exist to terminate the physiological effects of histamine[3]:

- *Cellular uptake.* Animal studies have documented the uptake of histamine by many cells. In particular, uptake is a temperature- and, partially, Na^+-dependent process in rabbit gastric glands, and the histamine is metabolized once in the cell.
- *Desensitization of cells.* Some H_1 receptor–containing tissues exhibit a homogeneous loss of sensitivity to the actions of histamine, perhaps as a result of receptor modification.
- *Metabolism* (Fig. 21.4).[11] The most common pathway for terminating histamine action involves enzymatic inactivation.

The enzyme histamine *N*-methyltransferase (HMT; EC 2.1.1.8) is widely distributed among mammalian tissues and catalyzes the transfer of a methyl group from *S*-adenosyl-L-methionine (SAM) to the ring *tele*-nitrogen of histamine, producing N^τ-methylhistamine and *S*-adenosyl-L-homocysteine. Histamine is also subject to oxidative deamination by diamine oxidase (DAO; EC 1.4.3.6), yielding imidazole acetic acid, a physiologically inactive product excreted in the urine. Similarly, N^τ-methylhistamine is converted by both DAO and monoamine oxidase (MAO) to *N*-methyl imidazole acetic acid.

Functions of Endogenous Histamine as Related to Pharmacological Intervention

Histamine exhibits a wide variety of both physiological and pathological functions in different tissues and cells. The actions of histamine that are of interest from both a pharmacological and therapeutic point of view include *(a)* its important but limited role as a chemical mediator of hypersensitivity reactions, *(b)* a major role in the regulation of gastric acid secretion, and *(c)* an emerging role as a neurotransmitter in the CNS.

HISTAMINE H₁ ANTAGONISTS (ANTIHISTAMINIC AGENTS)

The term *antihistamine* historically has referred to drugs that antagonize the actions of histamine at H_1 receptors rather than H_2 receptors. The development of antihistamine drugs began more than five decades ago with the discovery that piperoxan could protect animals from the bronchial spasm induced by histamine.[12] This finding was followed by the synthesis of a number of *N*-phenylethylenediamines with antihistaminic activities superior to those of piperoxan.[13] Further traditional structure–activity studies in this series, based largely on the principles of isosterism and functional group modification, led to the introduction in the 1940s to 1970s of a variety of H_1 antagonists containing the diarylalkylamine framework.[14, 15] These H_1 antagonists, referred to now as the *first-generation* or *classical* antihistamines, are related structurally and include a number of aminoalkyl ethers, ethylenediamines, piperazines, propylamines, phenothiazines, and dibenzocycloheptenes. In addition to H_1-receptor antagonism, these compounds display an array of other pharmacological activities that contribute toward therapeutic applications and adverse reactions. More recently, a number of second-generation or "nonsedating" antihistamines have been developed and introduced.[16] The second-generation agents bear some structural resemblance to the first-generation agents but have been modified to be more specific in action and limited in their distribution profiles.

Mechanism of Action

H_1 antagonists may be defined as drugs that competitively inhibit the action of histamine on tissues containing H_1 receptors. Traditionally, H_1 antagonists have been evaluated in vitro in terms of their ability to inhibit histamine-induced spasms in an isolated strip of guinea pig ileum. Antihistamines may be evaluated in vivo in terms of their ability to protect animals against the lethal effects of histamine administered intravenously or by aerosol.

To distinguish competitive antagonism of histamine from other modes of action, the index pA is applied to in vitro assays. The index pA_2 is defined as the inverse of the logarithm of the molar concentration of the antagonist that reduces the response of a double dose of the agonist to that of a single one. The more potent H_1 antagonists exhibit a pA_2 value significantly higher than 6. Although there are many pitfalls[17] to be avoided in the interpretation of structure–activity relationship (SAR) studies using pA_2 values, the following example illustrates distinguishing competitive antagonism. pA_2 values for pyrilamine (mepyramine) antagonism range from 9.1 to 9.4 with human bronchi and guinea

pig ileum.[15] By contrast, the pA_2 value in guinea pig atria (H_2 receptor) is 5.3. Thus, one may conclude that pyrilamine is a weak, noncompetitive inhibitor of histamine at the atrial receptors and a competitive inhibitor at H_1 receptors. The structural features required for effective interaction with these receptors are discussed below. Some H_1 antagonists also block histamine release. The concentrations required, however, are considerably higher than those required to produce significant histamine receptor blockade. The H_1 antagonists do not block antibody production or antigen–antibody interactions.[18]

Structure–Activity Relationships

The H_1 antagonists are now commonly subdivided into two broad groups—the first- generation, or classical, antihistamines and the second-generation, or "nonsedating," antihistamines—based primarily on their general pharmacological profiles.[16, 19] The differences between these two series are discussed in more detail in the sections that follow. The most detailed published SAR analyses for H_1 antagonists, however, focus on the structural requirements for the first-generation agents.[14, 15] From these studies, the basic structural requirements for H_1-receptor antagonism have been identified as those shown in Figure 21-5. In this structure, *Ar* is aryl (including phenyl, substituted phenyl, and heteroaryl groups such as 2-pyridyl); *Ar'* is a second aryl or arylmethyl group; *X* is a connecting atom of O, C, or N; *(CH₂)ₙ* represents a carbon chain, usually ethyl; and *NRR'* represents a basic, terminal amine function. The nature of the connecting atom, as well as the diaryl substitution pattern and amine moiety, has been used to subclassify the first-generation antihistamines as indicated in the sections below.

This diaryl substitution pattern is present in both the first- and second-generation antihistamines and is essential for significant H_1-receptor affinity. Furthermore, several SAR studies suggest that the two aryl moieties must be able to adopt a noncoplanar conformation relative to each other for optimal interaction with the H_1 receptor.[20] The two aromatic systems may be linked, as in the tricyclic antihistamines (phenothiazines, dibenzocycloheptanes, and heptenes, etc.), but again they must be noncoplanar for effective receptor interaction. Most H_1 antagonists contain substituents in one of the aryl rings (usually benzene), and these influence antihistamine potency as well as biodisposition, as discussed for individual classes of compounds in the sections below.

In many of the first-generation, or classical, antihistamines, the terminal nitrogen atom is a simple dimethylamino moiety. The amine may also be part of a heterocyclic structure, however, as illustrated by the piperazines, some propylamines (pyrrolidines and piperidines), some phenothiazines, the dibenzocycloheptenes, and the second-generation

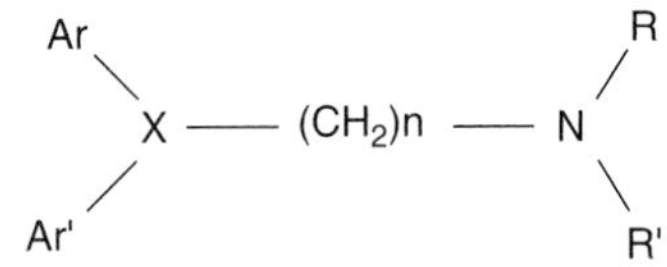

Figure 21–5 ■ General antihistamine structure.

antihistamines. In all cases, the amino moiety is basic, with pK$_a$s ranging from 8.5 to 10, and thus is presumed to be protonated when bound on the receptor. The moiety is also important in the development of stable, solid dosage forms through salt formation.

The carbon chain of typical H$_1$ antagonists consists of two or three atoms. As a result, the distance between the central point of the diaryl ring system and the terminal nitrogen atom in the extended conformation of these compounds ranges from 5 to 6 angstroms (Å). A similar distance between these key moieties is observed for those antihistamines with less conformational freedom. In some series, branching of the carbon chain results in reduced antihistaminic activity. There are exceptions, however, as evidenced by promethazine, which has greater activity than its nonbranched counterpart. When the carbon adjacent to the terminal nitrogen atom is branched, the possibility of asymmetry exists. Stereoselective H$_1$-receptor antagonism is typically not observed, however, when chirality exists at this site.[21] Also, in compounds with an asymmetrically substituted unsaturated carbon chain (pyrrobutamine and triprolidine), one geometric isomer typically displays higher receptor affinity than the other.

The X connecting moiety of typical H$_1$ antagonists may be a saturated carbon–oxygen moiety or simply a carbon or nitrogen atom. This group, along with the carbon chain, appears to serve primarily as a spacer group for the key pharmacophoric moieties. Many antihistamines containing a carbon atom in the connecting moiety are chiral and exhibit stereoselective receptor binding. For example, in the pheniramine series and carbinoxamine, this atom is chiral, and in vitro analyses indicate that enantiomers with the *S* configuration have higher H$_1$-receptor affinity.[22]

Generally, the first- and second-generation antihistamines are substantially more lipophilic than the endogenous agonist histamine (or the H$_2$ antagonists).[23] This lipophilicity difference results primarily from the presence of the two aryl rings and the substituted amino moieties and thus may simply reflect the different structural requirements for antagonist versus agonist action at H$_1$ receptors.

The nature of this connecting moiety and the structural nature of the aryl moieties have been used to classify the antihistamines as indicated in the sections below. Furthermore, variations in the diaryl groups, X connecting moieties, and the nature of substitution in the alkyl side chain or terminal nitrogen among the various drugs account for differences observed in antagonist potency as well as pharmacological, biodisposition, and adverse reaction profiles. The ability of these drugs to display an array of pharmacological activities is largely because they contain the basic pharmacophore required for binding to muscarinic as well as adrenergic and serotonergic receptors. The relationships of antihistamine structure to these overlapping actions (H$_1$ antagonist, anticholinergic, and local anesthetic) have been analyzed.

General Pharmacological Considerations

The classical antihistamines have been used extensively for the symptomatic treatment (sneezing, rhinorrhea, and itching of eyes, nose, and throat) of allergic rhinitis (hay fever, polli-

nosis), chronic idiopathic urticaria, and a number of other histamine-related diseases. These uses are clearly attributable to their antagonism of the action of histamine at peripheral H$_1$ receptors. The drugs best relieve the symptoms of allergic diseases at the beginning of the season when pollen counts are low. Although the symptoms of the common cold might be modified by antihistamines, these agents do not prevent or cure colds, nor do they shorten the course of the disease.[19] The antihistamines also are of little or no value in diseases such as systemic anaphylaxis and bronchial asthma, in which autocoids other than histamine are important.[18]

A number of the antihistamines, particularly the phenothiazines and aminoalkyl ethers, have antiemetic actions and thus may be useful in the treatment of nausea, vomiting, and motion sickness.[18, 19] Also, those agents that produce pronounced sedation have application as nonprescription sleeping aids.[18, 19] Several of the phenothiazines have limited use in Parkinson-like syndromes as a result of their ability to block central muscarinic receptors.[18, 19] And, a number of antihistamines, including promethazine, pyrilamine, tripelennamine and diphenhydramine, display local anesthetic activity that may be therapeutically useful.[24]

As the general pharmacological profiles above suggest, most antihistamines can interact with a variety of neurotransmitter receptors and other biomacromolecular targets. This is most evident among the first-generation agents, many of which function as antagonists at muscarinic receptors and, to a lesser extent, adrenergic, serotonergic, and dopamine receptors.[16, 18, 19] Although some of these non–target-receptor interactions may have some therapeutic value (as discussed above), more frequently they are manifested as adverse reactions that limit drug use. This is particularly true of the peripheral anticholinergic effects produced by these drugs and of interactions with a number of neurotransmitter systems in the CNS that result in sedation, fatigue, and dizziness.[16, 18, 19]

The primary objective of antihistamine research over the past 10 to 15 years has centered on developing new drugs with higher selectivity for H$_1$ receptors and lacking undesirable CNS actions. The pronounced sedative effects of some of the first-generation agents were attributed to the ability of these drugs to penetrate the blood–brain barrier (BBB) because of their lipophilic nature and then block cerebral H$_1$ receptors and possibly other receptors.[16] Thus research efforts were initiated to design novel antihistamines with reduced ability to penetrate the CNS and decreased affinity for central histamine receptors. These efforts led to the introduction of the second-generation antihistamines, which are nonsedating and have little antagonist activity at other neurotransmitter receptors at therapeutic concentrations. The pharmacological properties of these agents are discussed in more detail below.

Surprisingly little information is available concerning the pharmacokinetic and biodisposition profiles of the first-generation antihistamines.[23] Generally, the compounds are orally active and well absorbed, but oral bioavailability may be limited by first-pass metabolism. The metabolites formed depend on drug structure to a large extent but commonly involve the tertiary amino moiety. This functionality may be subject to successive oxidative N-dealkylation, deamination, and amino acid conjugation of the resultant acid. The amine group may also undergo N-oxidation, which may be reversible, or direct glucuronide conjugation. First-generation agents with unsubstituted and activated aromatic rings (phenothiazines) may undergo aromatic hydroxylation to yield phenols, which may be eliminated as conjugates.[23] More detailed pharmacokinetic data are available for the second-generation agents and are included in the monographs that follow.

The H_1 antagonists display a variety of significant drug interactions when coadministered with other therapeutic agents. For example, MAO inhibitors prolong and intensify the anticholinergic actions of the antihistamines.[16, 18, 19, 23] Also, the sedative effects of these agents may potentiate the depressant activity of barbiturates, alcohol, narcotic analgesics, and other depressants. Recently, it was discovered that several of the second-generation antihistamines may produce life-threatening arrhythmias when coadministered with drugs that inhibit their metabolism.[16, 18] These interactions are discussed in more detail in the sections below.

First-Generation H₁-Antagonist Drug Classes

AMINOALKYL ETHERS (ETHANOLAMINES)

The aminoalkyl ether antihistamines are characterized by the presence of a CHO connecting moiety (X) and a two- or three-carbon atom chain as the linking moiety between the key diaryl and tertiary amino groups (Fig. 21-6). Most compounds in this series are simple *N,N*-dimethylethanolamine derivatives and are so classified in a number of texts. Clemastine and diphenylpyraline differ from this basic structural pattern, in that the basic nitrogen moiety and at least part of the carbon chain are part of a heterocyclic ring system and there are three carbon atoms between the oxygen and nitrogen atoms.

The simple diphenyl derivative diphenhydramine was the first clinically useful member of the ethanolamine series and serves as the prototype. Other therapeutically useful derivatives of diphenhydramine have been obtained by *para* substitution of methyl (methyldiphenhydramine), methoxy (medrylamine), chloro (chlorodiphenhydramine), or bromo (bromodiphenhydramine) on one of the phenyl rings. These derivatives reportedly have better therapeutic profiles than diphenhydramine because of reduced adverse effects.[23]

Replacement of one of the phenyl rings of the diphenhydramine with a 2-pyridyl group, as in doxylamine and carbi-noxamine, enhances antihistaminic activity. These compounds display oral antihistaminic activities 40 and 2 times greater, respectively, than diphenhydramine in animals.[23]

As a result of an asymmetrically substituted benzylic carbon, most of the aminoalkyl ethers are optically active. Most studies indicate that the individual enantiomers differ significantly in antihistaminic activity, with activity residing predominantly in the *S* enantiomer.[22]

The diaryl tertiary aminoalkyl ether structure that characterizes these compounds also serves as a pharmacophore for muscarinic receptors. As a result, the drugs in this group possess significant anticholinergic activity, which may enhance the H_1-blocking action on exocrine secretions. Drowsiness is a side effect common to the tertiary aminoalkyl ethers, presumably as a result of the ability of these compounds to penetrate the BBB and occupy central H_1 receptors. Although this side effect is exploited in over-the-counter (OTC) sleeping aids, it may interfere with the performance of tasks requiring mental alertness.[18, 19] The frequency of GI side effects in this series of antihistamines is relatively low, compared with the ethylenediamine antihistamines.[18, 19]

In spite of their extensive use, pharmacokinetic data on this series of compounds are relatively limited. Most members of this series apparently are extensively metabolized by pathways including N-oxidation and successive oxidative N-dealkylation followed by amino acid conjugation of the resultant acid metabolites.[23]

The structures of the aminoalkyl ether derivatives, along with physicochemical properties, basic therapeutic activity data, and dosage form information are provided in the monographs that follow.

Diphenhydramine Hydrochloride, USP. Diphenhydramine hydrochloride, 2-(diphenylmethoxy)-*N,N*-dimethylethanamine hydrochloride (Benadryl), has an oily, lipid-soluble free base available as the bitter-tasting hydrochloride salt, which is a stable, white crystalline powder soluble in water (1:1), alcohol (1:2), and chloroform (1:2). The salt has a pK_a value of 9, and a 1% aqueous solution has a pH of about 5.

In addition to antihistaminic action, diphenhydramine exhibits antidyskinetic, antiemetic, antitussive, and sedative properties. It is used in OTC sleep-aid products. In the usual dose range of 25 to 400 mg, diphenhydramine is not a highly active H_1 antagonist; it has anticholinergic and sedative properties. Conversion to a quaternary ammonium salt does not alter the antihistaminic action greatly but does increase the anticholinergic action.

As an antihistaminic agent, diphenhydramine is recommended in various allergic conditions and, to a lesser extent, as an antispasmodic. It is administered either orally or parenterally in the treatment of urticaria, seasonal rhinitis (hay fever), and some dermatoses. The most common side effect is drowsiness, and the concurrent use of alcoholic beverages and other CNS depressants should be avoided.

Usual adult dose: Oral, 25–50 mg; IM or IV, 10–50 mg
Dosage forms: Capsules, elixir, syrup, tablets, injection

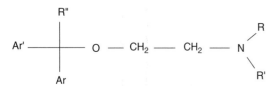

Figure 21–6 ▪ General structure of the aminoalkyl ethers.

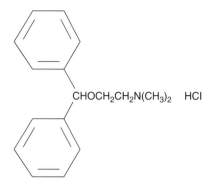

Diphenhydramine Hydrochloride

Bromodiphenhydramine Hydrochloride

Dimenhydrinate, USP. The 8-chlorotheophyllinate (theoclate) salt of diphenhydramine, 8-chlorotheophylline 2-(diphenylmethoxy)-*N,N*-dimethylethylamine compound (Dramamine), is a white crystalline, odorless powder that is slightly soluble in water and freely soluble in alcohol and chloroform.

Dimenhydrinate (see structure below) is recommended for the nausea of motion sickness and for hyperemesis gravidarum (nausea of pregnancy). For the prevention of motion sickness, the dose should be taken at least one-half hour before beginning the trip. The cautions listed for diphenhydramine should be observed.

Usual adult dose: Oral, 50–100 mg/4 hours; IM or IV, 50 mg/ 4 hours; rectal, 100 mg q.d. or b.i.d.
Dosage forms: Elixir, syrup, tablets, injection, suppositories

Bromodiphenhydramine Hydrochloride, USP. Bromodiphenhydramine hydrochloride, 2-[(4-bromophenyl)-phenylmethoxy]-*N,N*-dimethylethanamine hydrochloride (Ambodryl Hydrochloride), is a white to pale-buff crystalline powder that is freely soluble in water and in alcohol. Relative to diphenhydramine, bromodiphenhydramine is more lipid soluble and was twice as effective in protecting guinea pigs against the lethal effects of histamine aerosols.

Usual adult dose: Oral, 25 mg/4–6 hours
Dosage forms: Capsules and elixir

Doxylamine Succinate, USP. The acid succinate salt (bisuccinate) of doxylamine, 2-[α-[2-(dimethylamino)ethoxy]-α-methylbenzyl]pyridine bisuccinate (Decapryn Succinate), is a white to creamy-white powder with a characteristic odor. It is soluble in water (1:1), alcohol (1:2), and chloroform (1:2). A 1% solution has a pH of about 5.

Doxylamine succinate is comparable in potency to diphenhydramine. It is a good nighttime hypnotic, compared with secobarbital.[25] Concurrent use of alcohol and other CNS depressants should be avoided.

Usual adult dose: Oral, 12.5–25 mg/4–6 hours
Dosage forms: Syrup and tablets

Doxylamine Succinate

Carbinoxamine Maleate, USP. The oily, lipid-soluble free base of carbinoxamine is available as the bitter bimaleate salt, (*d,l*)-2-[*p*-chloro-α-[2-(dimethylamino)ethoxy]-

Dimenhydrinate

benzyl]pyridine bimaleate (Clistin), a white crystalline powder that is very soluble in water and freely soluble in alcohol and in chloroform. The pH of a 1% solution is between 4.6 and 5.1.

Carbinoxamine is a potent antihistaminic and is available as the racemic mixture. Carbinoxamine differs structurally from chlorpheniramine only in having an oxygen atom separate the asymmetric carbon atom from the aminoethyl side chain. The more active *levo* isomer of carbinoxamine has the (*S*) absolute configuration[26] and can be superimposed on the more active *dextro* isomer (*S* configuration[22]) of chlorpheniramine.

Usual adult dose: Oral, 4–8 mg t.i.d. or q.i.d.
Dosage forms: Elixir and tablets

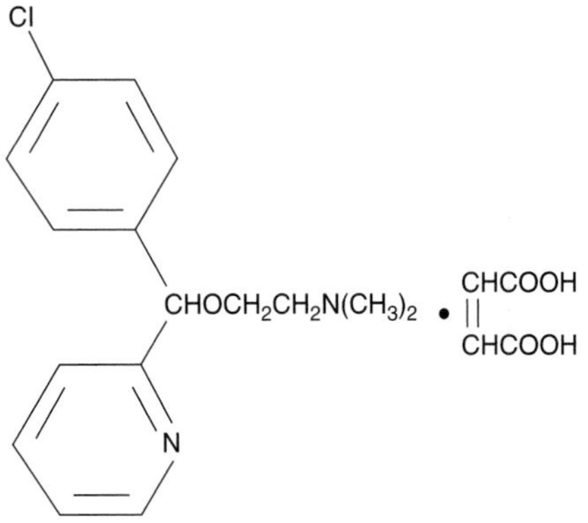

Carbinoxamine Maleate

Clemastine Fumarate, USP.

Dextrorotatory clemastine, 2-[2-[1-(4-chlorophenyl)-1-phenylethoxy]ethyl]-1-methylpyrrolidine hydrogen fumarate (1:1) (Tavist), has two chiral centers, each of which is of the (*R*) absolute configuration. A comparison of the activities of the antipodes indicates that the asymmetric center close to the side chain nitrogen is of lesser importance to antihistaminic activity.[15]

This member of the ethanolamine series is characterized by a long duration of action, with an activity that reaches a maximum in 5 to 7 hours and persists for 10 to 12 hours. It is well absorbed when administered orally, and it is excreted primarily in the urine. The side effects are those usually encountered with this series of antihistamines. Clemastine is closely related to chlorphenoxamine, which is used for its central cholinergic-blocking activity. Therefore, it is not surprising that clemastine has significant antimuscarinic activity.

Usual adult dose: Oral, 1.34 mg b.i.d. or 2.68 mg q.d. to t.i.d.
Dosage forms: Syrup and tablets

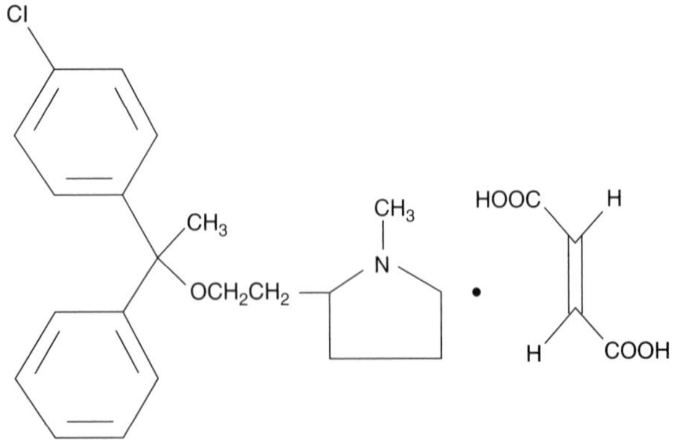

Clemastine Fumarate

Diphenylpyraline Hydrochloride, USP.

Diphenylpyraline hydrochloride, 4-(diphenylmethoxy)-1-methylpiperidine hydrochloride (Hispril, Diafen) occurs as a white or slightly off-white crystalline powder that is soluble in water or alcohol. Diphenylpyraline is structurally related to diphenhydramine with the aminoalkyl side chain incorporated in a piperidine ring. It is a potent antihistaminic, and the usual dose is 2 mg 3 or 4 times daily. The hydrochloride is available as 5-mg sustained-release capsules.

Usual adult dose: Oral, 5 mg/12 hours
Dosage forms: Extended-release capsules

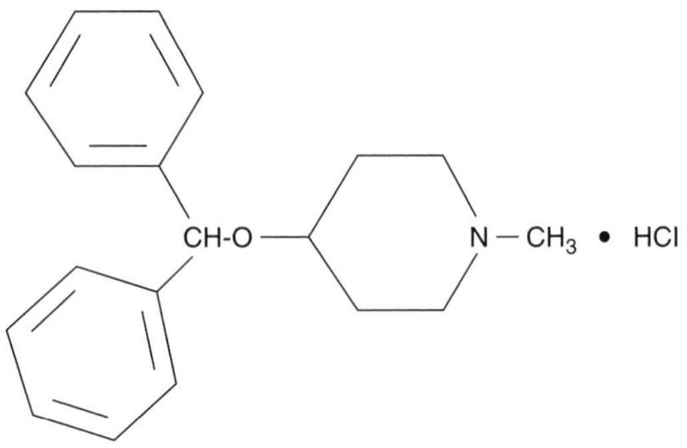

Diphenylpyraline Hydrochloride

ETHYLENEDIAMINES

The ethylenediamine antihistamines are characterized by the presence of a nitrogen connecting atom (X) and a two-carbon atom chain as the linking moiety between the key diaryl and tertiary amino moieties (Fig. 21-7). All compounds in this series are simple diarylethylenediamines except antazoline, in which the terminal amine and a portion of the carbon chain are included as part of an imidazoline ring system. Because it differs significantly in its pharmacological profile, antazoline is not always classified as an ethylenediamine derivative.

Phenbenzamine was the first clinically useful member of this class and served as the prototype for the development of more effective derivatives. Replacement of the phenyl moiety of phenbenzamine with a 2-pyridyl system yielded tripelennamine, a significantly more effective histamine receptor blocker.[23] Substitution of a *para* methoxy (pyrilamine or mepyramine), chloro (chloropyramine), or bromo (bromtripelennamine) further enhances activity.[23] Replacement of the benzyl group of tripelennamine with a 2-thienylmethyl group provided methapyrilene, and replacement of tripelennamine's 2-pyridyl group with a pyrimidinyl moiety (along with *p*-methoxy substitution) yielded thonzylamine, both which function as potent H_1-receptor antagonists.[23]

In all of these compounds the aliphatic or terminal amino group is significantly more basic than the nitrogen atom bonded to the diaryl moiety; the nonbonded electrons on the diaryl nitrogen are delocalized by the aromatic ring, and the

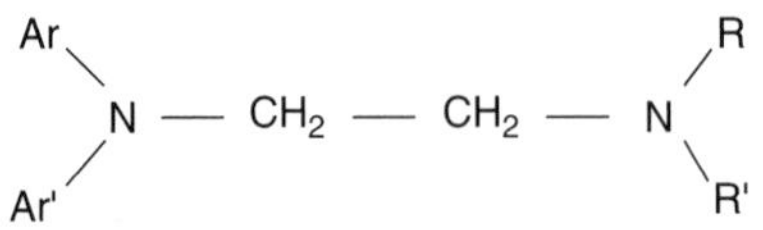

Figure 21–7 ■ General structure of the ethylenediamines.

resultant reduction in electron density on nitrogen decreases basicity. Thus the aliphatic amino group in the ethylenediamines is sufficiently basic for the formation of pharmaceutically useful salts.

The ethylenediamines were among the first useful antihistamines.[23] They are highly effective H_1 antagonists, but they also display a relatively high frequency of CNS depressant and GI side effects.[19] The anticholinergic and antiemetic actions of these compounds are relatively low, compared with those of most other classical antihistamines. The piperazine- and phenothiazine-type antihistamines also contain the ethylenediamine moiety, but these agents are discussed separately because they exhibit significantly different pharmacological properties.

Relatively little information is available concerning the pharmacokinetics of this series of compounds. Tripelennamine is metabolized in humans by N-glucuronidation, N-oxidation, and pyridyl oxidation followed by phenol glucuronidation. It is anticipated that other members of this series are similarly metabolized.[23]

The structures of the salt forms of the marketed ethylenediamine antihistamines, along with physicochemical properties, basic therapeutic activity profiles, and dosage form information, are provided in the monographs below.

Tripelennamine Citrate, USP. The oily free base of tripelennamine citrate, 2-[benzyl[2-(dimethylamino)ethyl]amino]pyridine citrate (1:1), PBZ (Pyribenzamine Citrate), is available as the less bitter monocitrate salt, which is a white crystalline powder freely soluble in water and in alcohol. A 1% solution has a pH of 4.25. For oral administration in liquid dose forms, the citrate salt is less bitter and thus more palatable than the hydrochloride. Because of the difference in molecular weights, the doses of the two salts must be equated—30 mg of the citrate salt is equivalent to 20 mg of the hydrochloride salt.

Usual adult dose: Oral, 25–50 mg/4–6 hours
Dosage forms: Elixir

Tripelennamine Citrate or HCl

Tripelennamine Hydrochloride, USP. Tripelennamine hydrochloride is a white crystalline powder that darkens slowly on exposure to light. The salt is soluble in water (1:0.77) and in alcohol (1:6). It has a pK_a of about 9, and a 0.1% solution has a pH of about 5.5.

Tripelennamine, the first ethylenediamine developed in American laboratories, is well absorbed when given orally. On the basis of clinical experience, it appears to be as effective as diphenhydramine and may have the advantage of fewer and less severe side reactions. Drowsiness may occur,

however, and may impair the ability to perform tasks requiring alertness. The concurrent use of alcoholic beverages should be avoided.

Usual adult dose: Oral tablets, 25–50 mg/4–6 hours; extended-release, 100 mg/8–12 hours
Dosage forms: Tablets, extended-release tablets

Pyrilamine Maleate, USP. The oily free base of pyrilamine is available as the acid maleate salt, pyrilamine maleate, 2-[[2-(dimethylamino)ethyl](p-methoxybenzyl)amino]pyridine maleate (1:1), mepyramine, which is a white crystalline powder with a faint odor and a bitter, saline taste. The salt is soluble in water (1:0.4) and freely soluble in alcohol. A 10% solution has a pH of approximately 5. At a pH of 7.5 or above, the oily free base begins to precipitate.

Pyrilamine differs structurally from tripelennamine by having a methoxy group in the *para* position of the benzyl radical. It differs from its more toxic and less potent precursor phenbenzamine (Antergan) by having a 2-pyridyl group on the nitrogen atom in place of a phenyl group.

Clinically, pyrilamine and tripelennamine are considered among the less potent antihistaminics. They are highly potent, however, in antagonizing histamine-induced contractions of guinea pig ileum.[14] Because of the pronounced local anesthetic action, the drug should not be chewed, but taken with food.

Usual adult dose: Oral, 25–50 mg/6–8 hours
Dosage forms: Tablets

Pyrilamine Maleate

Methapyrilene Hydrochloride. The oily free base is available as the bitter-tasting monohydrochloride salt, methapyrilene hydrochloride, 2-[[2-(dimethylamino)ethyl]-2-thienylamino]pyridine monohydrochloride (Histadyl). It is a white crystalline powder that is soluble in water (1:0.5), in alcohol (1:5), and in chloroform (1:3). Its solutions have a pH of about 5.5. It differs structurally from tripelennamine in having a 2-thenyl (thiophene-2-methylene) group in place of the benzyl group. The thiophene ring is considered isosteric with the benzene ring, and the isosteres exhibit similar activity. A study of the solid-state conformation of methapyrilene hydrochloride showed that the *trans* conformation is preferred for the two ethylenediamine nitrogen atoms. The Food and Drug Administration declared methapyrilene a potential carcinogen in 1979, and all products containing it have been recalled.

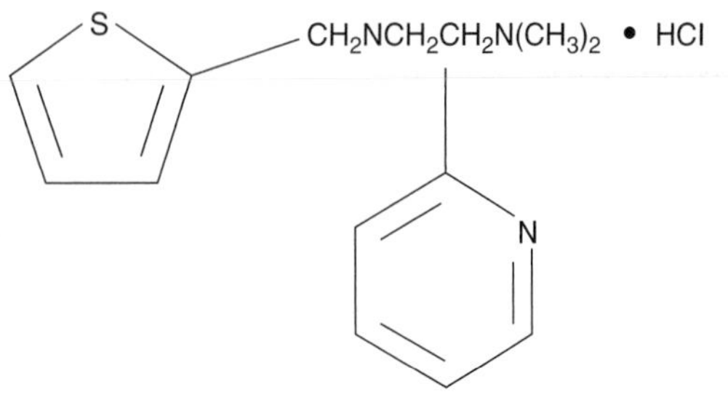

CH$_2$NCH$_2$CH$_2$N(CH$_3$)$_2$ • HCl

Methapyrilene Hydrochloride

Thonzylamine Hydrochloride. Thonzylamine hydrochloride, 2-[[2-(dimethylamino)ethyl](p-methoxybenzyl) amino]pyrimidine hydrochloride, is a white crystalline powder soluble in water (1:1), in alcohol (1:6), and in chloroform (1:4). A 2% aqueous solution has a pH of 5.5. It is similar in activity to tripelennamine but is claimed to be less toxic. The usual dose is 50 mg up to 4 times daily. It is available in certain combination products.

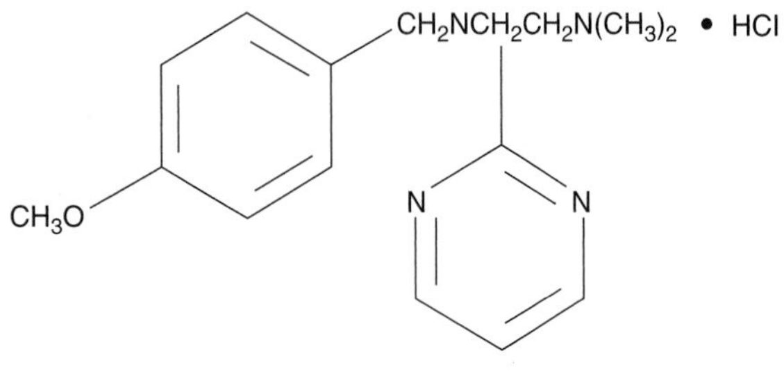

CH$_2$NCH$_2$CH$_2$N(CH$_3$)$_2$ • HCl

Thonzylamine Hydrochloride

Antazoline Phosphate. Antazoline phosphate, 2-[(N-benzylanilino)methyl]-2-imidazoline dihydrogen phosphate, occurs as a bitter, white to off-white crystalline powder that is soluble in water. It has a pK$_a$ of 10.0, and a 2% solution has a pH of about 4.5. Antazoline, like the ethylenediamines, contains an N-benzylanilino group linked to a basic nitrogen through a two-carbon chain.

Antazoline is less active than most of the other antihistaminic drugs, but it is characterized by the lack of local irritation. The more soluble phosphate salt is applied topically to the eye in a 0.5% solution. The less soluble hydrochloride is given orally. In addition to its use as an antihistamine, antazoline has more than twice[27] the local anesthetic potency of procaine and also exhibits anticholinergic actions.

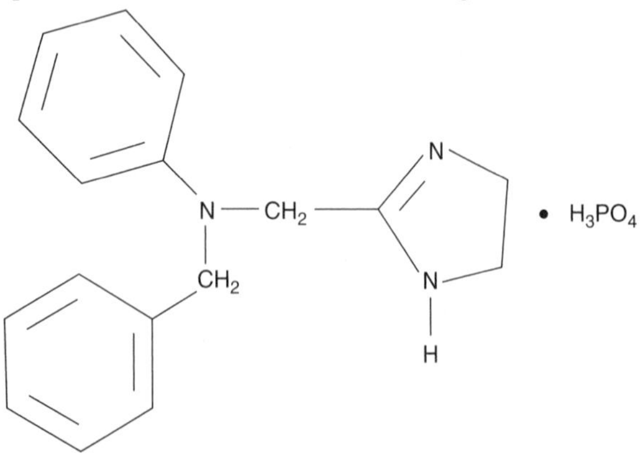

• H$_3$PO$_4$

Antazoline Phosphate

PIPERAZINES (CYCLIZINES)

The piperazines or cyclizines can also be considered ethylenediamine derivatives or cyclic ethylenediamines (cyclizines); in this series, however, the connecting moiety (X) is a CHN group, and the carbon chain, terminal amine functionality, and the nitrogen atom of the connecting group are all part of a piperazine moiety (Fig. 21-8). Both nitrogen atoms in these compounds are aliphatic and thus display comparable basicities. The primary structural differences within this series involve the nature of the *para* aromatic ring substituent (H or Cl) and, more importantly, the nature of the terminal piperazine nitrogen substituent.

The piperazines are moderately potent antihistaminics with a low incidence of drowsiness.[18, 19, 23] A warning of the possibility of some dulling of mental alertness is advised, however. The activity of the piperazine-type antihistaminics is characterized by a slow onset and long duration of action. These agents exhibit peripheral and central antimuscarinic activity, which may be responsible for the antiemetic and antivertigo effects.[18, 19] The agents diminish vestibular stimulation and may act on the medullary chemoreceptor trigger zone. Thus as a group, these agents are probably more useful as antiemetics and antinauseants and in the treatment of motion sickness.

Some members of this series have exhibited a strong teratogenic potential, inducing a number of malformations in rats. Norchlorcyclizine, a metabolite of these piperazines, was proposed as responsible for the teratogenic effects of the parent drugs.[28]

Metabolic studies in this series of compounds have focused primarily on cyclizine and chlorcyclizine, and these compounds undergo similar biotransformation. The primary pathways involve N-oxidation and N-demethylation, and both of these metabolites are devoid of antihistaminic activity.[23]

The structures of the marketed salt forms of the piperazine antihistamines, along with physicochemical properties, basic therapeutic activity profiles, and dosage form information, are provided in the monographs below.

Cyclizine Hydrochloride, USP. Cyclizine hydrochloride, 1-(diphenylmethyl)-4-methylpiperazine monohydrochloride (Marezine), occurs as a light-sensitive, white crystalline powder with a bitter taste. It is slightly soluble

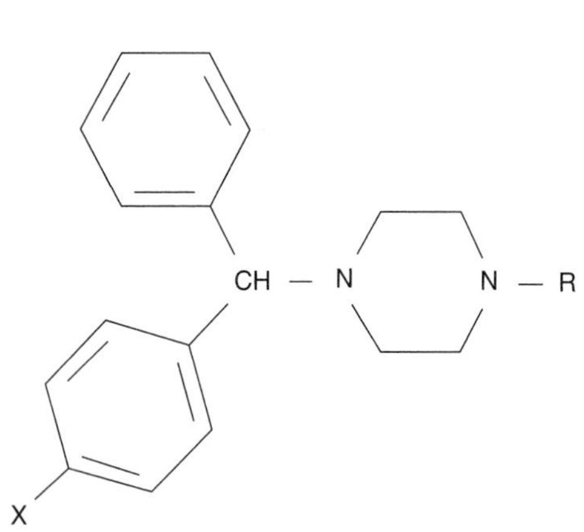

CH — N ⟩ N — R

X

Figure 21–8 ■ General structure of the piperazines.

in water (1:115), in alcohol (1:115), and in chloroform (1:75). It is used primarily in the prophylaxis and treatment of motion sickness. The lactate salt (Cyclizine Lactate Injection, USP) is used for intramuscular injection because of the limited water solubility of the hydrochloride. The injection should be stored in a cold place because if it is stored at room temperature for several months, a slight yellow tint may develop. This does not indicate a loss in biologic potency.

Usual adult dose: Oral, 50 mg/4–6 hours; IM, 50 mg/4–6 hours
Dosage forms: Tablets (HCl) and injection (lactate)

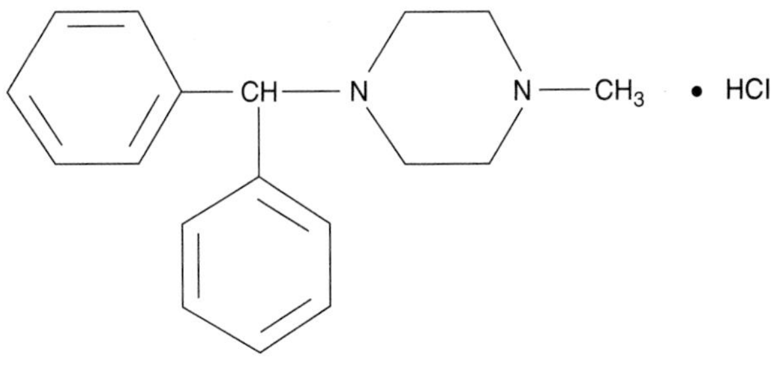

Cyclizine Hydrochloride or Lactate

Chlorcyclizine Hydrochloride, USP.

Chlorcyclizine hydrochloride, 1-(p-chloro-α-phenylbenzyl)-4-methylpiperazine monohydrochloride, a light-sensitive, white crystalline powder, is soluble in water (1:2), in alcohol (1:11), and in chloroform (1:4). A 1% solution has a pH between 4.8 and 5.5.

Disubstitution or substitution of halogen in the 2 or 3 position of either of the benzhydryl rings results in a much less potent compound. Chlorcyclizine is indicated in the symptomatic relief of urticaria, hay fever, and certain other allergic conditions.

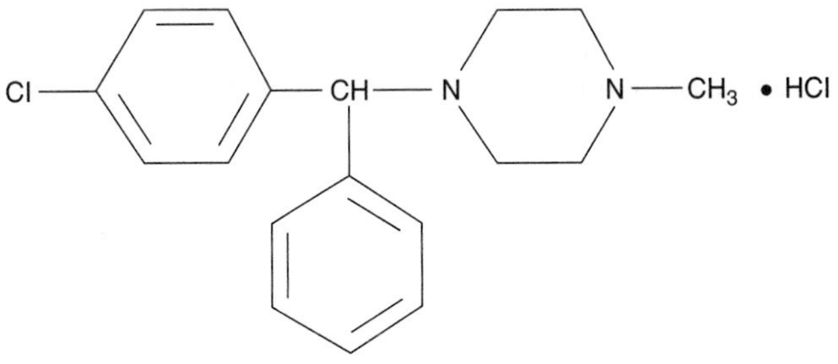

Chlorcyclizine Hydrochloride

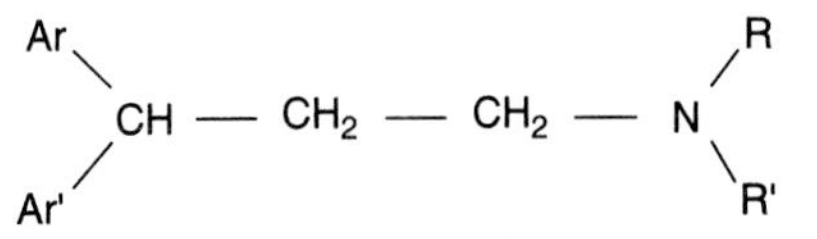

Figure 21–9 ■ General structure of the propylamines.

Meclizine Hydrochloride, USP.

Meclizine hydrochloride, 1-(p-chloro-α-phenylbenzyl)-4-(m-methylbenzyl)piperazine dihydrochloride monohydrate (Bonine, Antivert), is a tasteless, white or slightly yellowish crystalline powder that is practically insoluble in water (1:1,000). It differs from chlorcyclizine in having an N-m-methylbenzyl group in place of the N-methyl group. Although it is a moderately potent antihistaminic, meclizine is used primarily as an antinauseant in the prevention and treatment of motion sickness and in the treatment of nausea and vomiting associated with vertigo and radiation sickness.

Usual adult dose: Oral, 25–50 mg
Dosage forms: Tablets and chewable tablets

Buclizine Hydrochloride, USP.

Buclizine hydrochloride, 1-(p-tertbutylbenzyl)-4-(p-chloro-α-phenylbenzyl)piperazine dihydrochloride (Bucladin-S), occurs as a white to slightly yellow crystalline powder that is insoluble in water. The highly lipid-soluble buclizine has CNS depressant, antiemetic, and antihistaminic properties. The salt is available in 50-mg tablets for oral administration. The usual dose is 50 mg 30 minutes before travel and is repeated in 4 to 6 hours as needed.

Usual adult dose: Oral, 50 mg/4–6 hours
Dosage forms: Tablets

PROPYLAMINES (MONOAMINOPROPYL DERIVATIVES)

The propylamine antihistamines are characterized structurally by an sp^3 or sp^2 carbon connecting atom with a carbon chain of two additional carbons linking the key tertiary amino and diaryl pharmacophore moieties (Fig. 21-9). Those propylamines with a saturated carbon connecting moiety are commonly referred to as the *pheniramines*. All of the pheniramines consist of a phenyl and a 2-pyridyl aryl group and a terminal dimethylamino moiety. These compounds differ only in the phenyl substituent at the *para* position—H (phe-

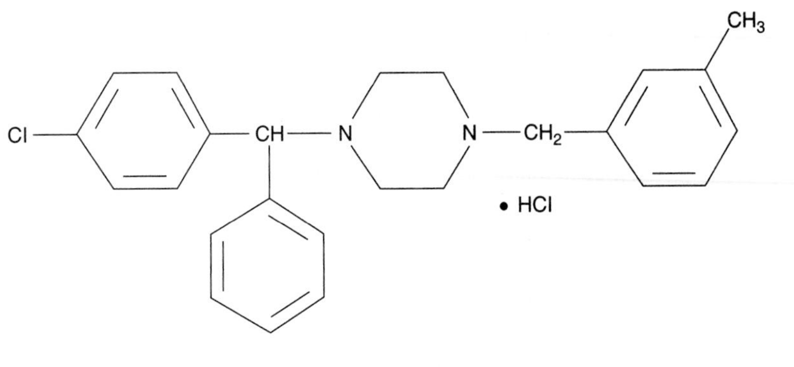

Meclizine Hydrochloride

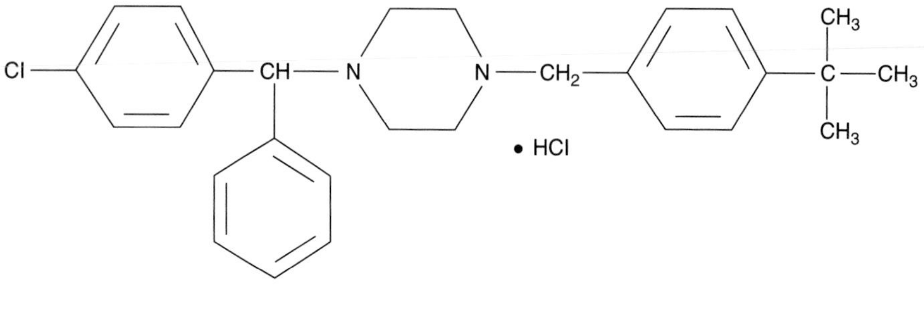

Buclizine Hydrochloride

niramine), Cl (chlorpheniramine), and Br (brompheniramine). The halogenated pheniramines are significantly more potent (20 to 50 times) and have a longer duration of action.[23]

All pheniramines are chiral molecules, and the halogen-substituted derivatives have been resolved by crystallization of salts formed with *d*-tartaric acid. Antihistaminic activity resides almost exclusively in the *S* stereoisomers.[22]

The propylamines with an unsaturated connecting moiety include the open derivatives pyrrobutamine and triprolidine and the cyclic analogues dimethindene and phenindamine. In the open-chain propylamines, a coplanar aromatic double-bond system appears to be an important factor for antihistaminic activity. The pyrrolidino group of these compounds is the side chain tertiary amine that imparts greatest antihistaminic activity. The conformational rigidity of the unsaturated propylamines has provided a useful model to determine distances between the key diaryl and tertiary pharmacophoric moieties in H_1-receptor antagonists, a distance of 5 to 6 Å.

The antihistamines in this group are among the most active H_1 antagonists. The agents in this class also produce less sedation than the other classical antihistamines (yet a significant proportion of patients do experience this effect) and have little antiemetic action. They do, however, exhibit significant anticholinergic activity, albeit less than the aminoalkyl ethers and phenothiazines.[18, 19, 23]

In the propylamine series, the pharmacokinetics of chlorpheniramine have been studied most extensively in humans.[23] Oral bioavailability is relatively low (30 to 50%) and may be limited by first-pass metabolism. The primary metabolites for this compound and other members of this series are the mono- and di-N-dealkylation products. Complete oxidation of the terminal amino moiety followed by glycine conjugation has also been reported for brompheniramine. Chlorpheniramine plasma half-lives range from about 12 hours to 28 hours, depending on the route of administration (oral versus IV).[23]

The structures of the marketed salt forms of the propylamine antihistamines, along with physicochemical properties, basic therapeutic activity profiles, and dosage form information, are provided in the monographs below.

Pheniramine Maleate. Pheniramine maleate, 2-[α-[2-dimethylaminoethyl]benzyl]pyridine bimaleate (Trimeton, Inhiston), is a white crystalline powder, with a faint amine-like odor, that is soluble in water (1:5) and very soluble in alcohol.

This drug is the least potent member of the series and is marketed as the racemate. The usual adult dose is 20 to

40 mg 3 times daily. It is available in certain combination products.

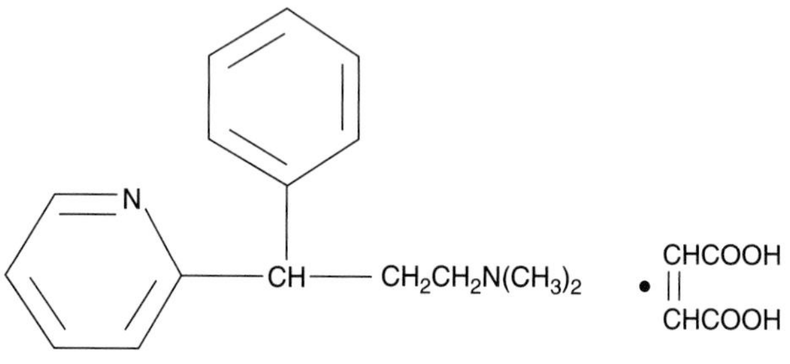

Pheniramine Maleate

Chlorpheniramine Maleate, USP. Chlorpheniramine maleate, ($\pm$)2-[*p*-chloro-α-[2-dimethylamino)ethyl]benzyl]-pyridine bimaleate (Chlor-Trimeton), is a white crystalline powder that is soluble in water (1:3.4), in alcohol (1:10), and in chloroform (1:10). It has a pK_a of 9.2, and an aqueous solution has a pH between 4 and 5. Chlorination of pheniramine in the *para* position of the phenyl ring increases potency 10-fold with no appreciable change in toxicity. Most of the antihistaminic activity resides with the *dextro* isomer (see dexchlorpheniramine below). The usual dose is 2 to 4 mg 3 or 4 times a day. It has a half-life of 12 to 15 hours.

Usual adult dose: Oral, 4 mg/4–6 hours; extended release, 8–12 mg/8–12 hours; IM, IV, or SC, 5–40 mg
Dosage forms: Extended-release capsules, syrup, tablets, chewable tablets, extended release tablets, injection

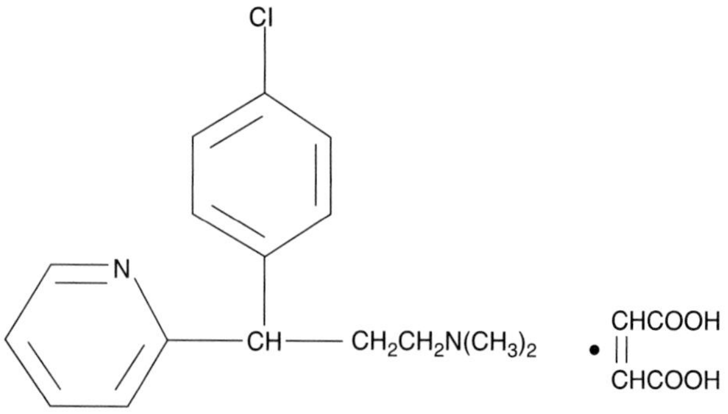

Chlorpheniramine Maleate
Dexchlorpheniramine Maleate

Dexchlorpheniramine Maleate, USP. Dexchlorpheniramine (Polaramine) is the dextrorotatory enantiomer of chlorpheniramine. In vitro and in vivo studies of the enantio-morphs of chlorpheniramine showed that the antihistaminic activity exists predominantly in the *dextro* isomer. As mentioned above, the *dextro* isomer has the (S) configuration,[22] which is superimposable on the (S) configuration of the more active levorotatory enantiomorph of carbinoxamine.

Usual adult dose: Oral, 2 mg t.i.d. or q.i.d.
Dosage forms: Syrup, tablets, extended-release tablets

Brompheniramine Maleate, USP. Brompheniramine maleate, (+)2-[*p*-bromo-*α*-[2-(dimethylamino)ethyl]benzyl]pyridine bimaleate (Dimetane), differs from chlorpheniramine by the substitution of a bromine atom for the chlorine atom. Its actions and uses are like those of chlorpheniramine. It has a half-life of 25 hours, which is almost twice that of chlorpheniramine.

Usual adult dose: Oral, 4 mg t.i.d. or q.i.d.; extended-release, 8–12 mg/8–12 hours; IM, IV, or SC, 10 mg/8–12 hours
Dosage forms: Elixir, tablets, extended-release tablets, injection

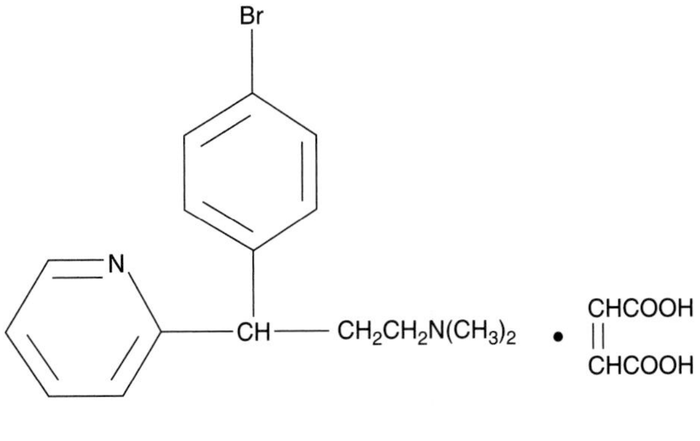

Brompheniramine Maleate

Dexbrompheniramine Maleate, USP. Like the chlorine congener, the antihistaminic activity of brompheniramine exists predominantly in the *dextro* isomer, dexbrompheniramine maleate (Disomer), and is of comparable potency.

Pyrrobutamine Phosphate. Pyrrobutamine phosphate, (E)-1-[4-(4-chlorophenyl)-3-phenyl-2-butenyl]pyrrolidine diphosphate (Pyronil), occurs as a white crystalline

powder that is soluble to the extent of 10% in warm water. Pyrrobutamine was investigated originally as the hydrochloride salt, but the diphosphate was absorbed more readily and completely. Clinical studies indicate that it is long acting, with a comparatively slow onset of action. The feeble antihistaminic properties of several analogues point to the importance of having a planar ArC = CH-CH$_2$N unit and a pyrrolidino group as the side chain tertiary amine.[14]

Triprolidine Hydrochloride, USP. Triprolidine hydrochloride, (E)-2-[3(1-pyrrolidinyl)-1-*p*-tolylpropenyl]pyridine monohydrochloride monohydrate (Actidil), occurs as a white crystalline powder with no more than a slight, but unpleasant, odor. It is soluble in water and in alcohol, and its solutions are alkaline to litmus.

The activity is confined mainly to the geometric isomer in which the pyrrolidinomethyl group is *trans* to the 2-pyridyl group. Pharmacological studies[29] confirm the high activity of triprolidine and the superiority of (E) over corresponding (Z) isomers as H$_1$ antagonists. At guinea pig ileum sites, the affinity of triprolidine for H$_1$ receptors was more than 1,000 times the affinity of its (Z) partner.

The relative potency of triprolidine is of the same order as that of dexchlorpheniramine. The peak effect occurs about 3.5 hours after oral administration, and the duration of effect is about 12 hours.

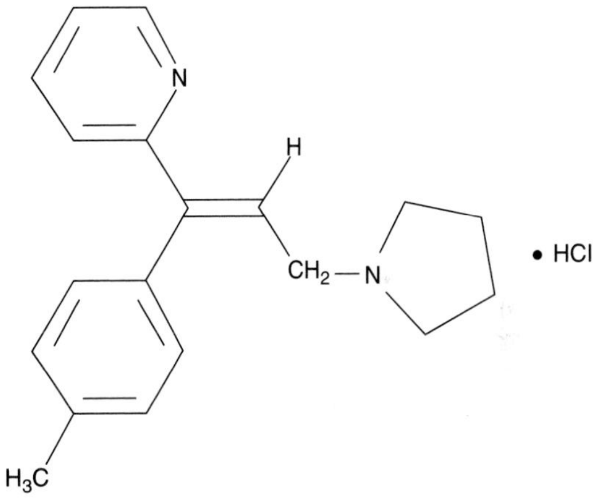

Triprolidine Hydrochloride

Phenindamine Tartrate, USP. Phenindamine tartrate, 2,3,4,9-tetrahydro-2-methyl-9-phenyl-1*H*-indeno[2,1-c]pyr-

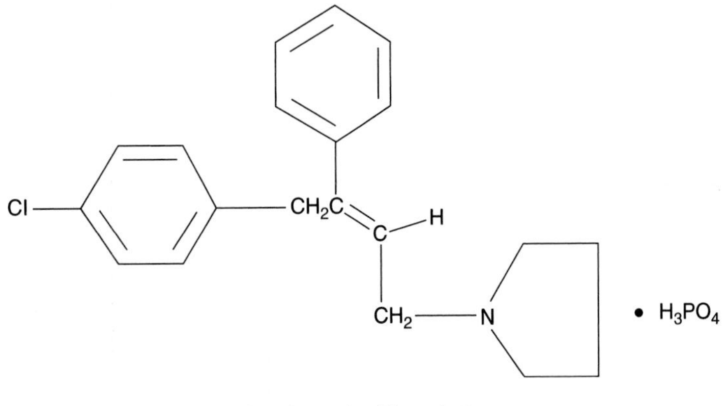

Pyrrobutamine Phosphate

idine bitartrate, occurs as a creamy-white powder, usually with a faint odor and sparingly soluble in water (1:40). A 2% aqueous solution has a pH of about 3.5. It is most stable in the pH range of 3.5 to 5.0 and is unstable in solutions of pH 7 or higher. Oxidizing substances or heat may cause isomerization to an inactive form.

Structurally, phenindamine can be regarded as an unsaturated propylamine derivative, in that the rigid ring system contains a distorted, *trans* alkene. Like the other commonly used antihistamines, it may produce drowsiness and sleepiness; it may also cause a mildly stimulating action in some patients and insomnia when taken just before bedtime.[30]

Usual adult dose: Oral, 25 mg/4–6 hours
Dosage forms: Tablets

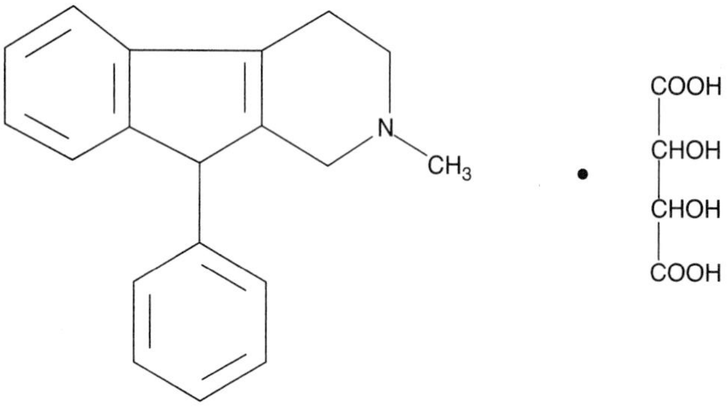

Phenindamine Tartrate

Dimethindene Maleate.

Dimethindene maleate, (±)2-[1-[2-[2-dimethylamino)ethyl]inden-3-yl]ethyl]pyridine bimaleate (1:1) (Forhistal Maleate), occurs as a white to off-white crystalline powder that has a characteristic odor and is sparingly soluble in water. This potent antihistaminic agent may be considered a derivative of the unsaturated propylamines. The principal side effect is some sedation or drowsiness. The antihistaminic activity resides mainly in the levorotatory isomer.[14]

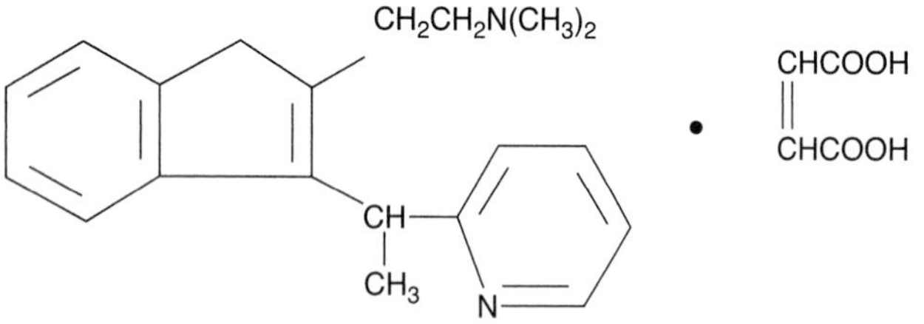

Dimethindene Maleate

PHENOTHIAZINES

Beginning in the mid-1940s, several antihistaminic drugs have been discovered as a result of bridging the aryl units of agents related to the ethylenediamines. The search for effective antimalarials led to the investigation of phenothiazine derivatives in which the bridging entity is sulfur. Subsequent testing found that the phenothiazine class of drugs had not only antihistaminic activity but also a pharmacologi-

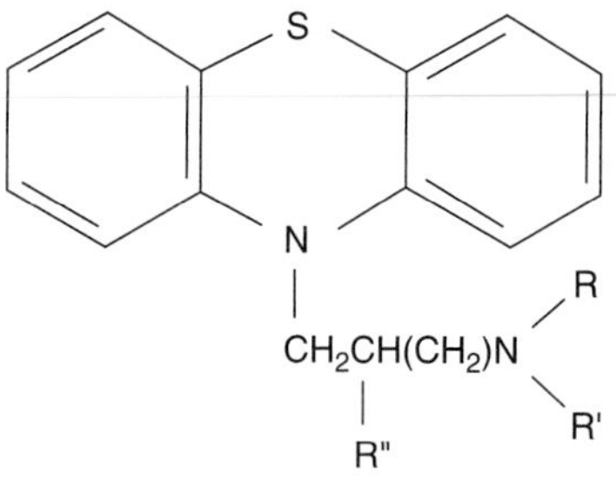

Figure 21–10 ■ General structure of the phenothiazines.

cal profile of its own, considerably different from that of the ethylenediamines (Fig. 21-10). Thus began the era of the useful psychotherapeutic agent.[19, 31]

The phenothiazine derivatives that display therapeutically useful antihistaminic actions contain a two- or three-carbon, branched alkyl chain between the ring system and terminal nitrogen atom. This differs significantly from the phenothiazine antipsychotic series in which an unbranched propyl chain is required. The phenothiazines with a three-carbon bridge between nitrogen atoms are more potent in vitro. Also, unlike the phenothiazine antipsychotics, the heterocyclic ring of the antihistamines is unsubstituted.[23]

The enantiomers of promethazine have been resolved and have similar antihistaminic and other pharmacological properties as described below.[32] This is in contrast with results of studies of the pheniramines and carbinoxamine compounds in which the chiral center is closer to the aromatic feature of the molecule. Asymmetry appears to have less influence on antihistaminic activity when the chiral center lies near the positively charged side-chain nitrogen.

Promethazine, the parent member of this series, is moderately potent by present standards, with prolonged action and pronounced sedative side effects. In addition to its antihistaminic action, it is a potent antiemetic, anticholinergic, and sedating agent and significantly potentiates the action of analgesic and sedative drugs.[19] The other members of this series display a similar pharmacological profile and thus may cause drowsiness and impair the ability to perform tasks requiring alertness. Also, concurrent administration of alcoholic beverages and other CNS depressants with the phenothiazines should be avoided.[19] In general, the combination of lengthening of the side chain and substitution of lipophilic groups in the 2 position of the aromatic ring results in compounds with decreased antihistaminic activity and increased psychotherapeutic properties.

Although few pharmacokinetic data are available for the phenothiazine antihistamines, the metabolism of the close structural analogue promethazine has been studied in detail.[23] This compound undergoes mono- and di-N-dealkylation, sulfur oxidation, aromatic oxidation at the 3 position to yield the phenol, and N-oxidation. A number of these metabolites, particularly the phenol, may yield glucuronide conjugates. It is expected that the phenothiazine antihistamines would display similar metabolic profiles.

Promethazine Hydrochloride, USP.

Promethazine hydrochloride, (±)10-[2-(dimethylamino)propyl]phenothiazine monohydrochloride (Phenergan), occurs as a white to faint-yellow crystalline powder that is very soluble in water, in hot absolute alcohol, and in chloroform. Its aqueous solutions are slightly acid to litmus.

Usual adult dose: Oral, 12.5 mg/4–6 hours or 25 mg q.d.; IM or IV, 12.5–25 mg/4–6 hours

Dosage forms: Syrup, tablets, injection, suppositories

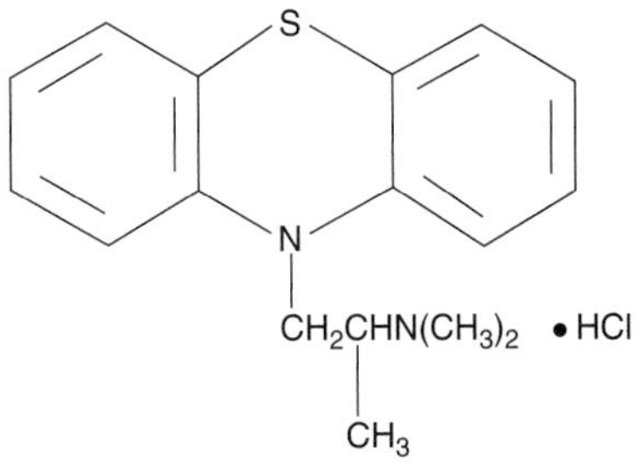

Promethazine Hydrochloride

Trimeprazine Tartrate, USP. Trimeprazine tartrate, (±)10-[3-(dimethylamino)-2-methylpropyl]phenothiazine tartrate (Temaril), occurs as a white to off-white crystalline powder that is freely soluble in water and soluble in alcohol. Its antihistaminic action is reported to be from 1.5 to 5 times that of promethazine. Clinical studies have shown it has a pronounced antipruritic action. This action may be unrelated to its histamine-antagonizing properties.

Usual adult dose: Oral, 2.5 mg q.i.d.
Dosage forms: Syrup and tablets

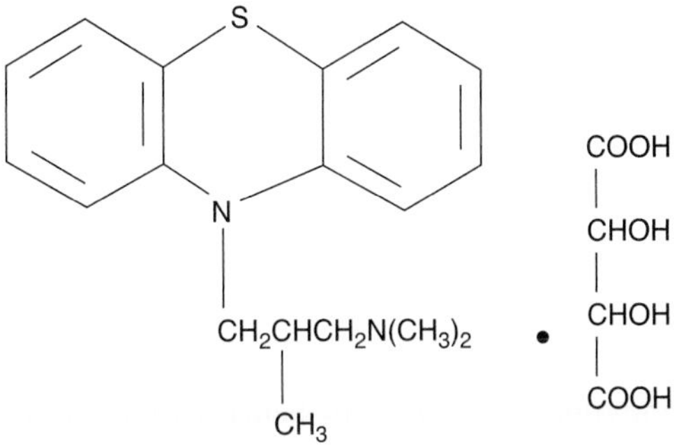

Trimeprazine Tartrate

Methdilazine, USP. Methdilazine, 10-[(1-methyl-3-pyrrolidinyl)methyl]phenothiazine (Tacaryl), occurs as a light-tan crystalline powder that has a characteristic odor and is practically insoluble in water. Methdilazine, as the free base, is used in chewable tablets because its low solubility in water contributes to its tastelessness. Some local anesthesia of the buccal mucosa may be experienced if the tablet is chewed and not swallowed promptly.

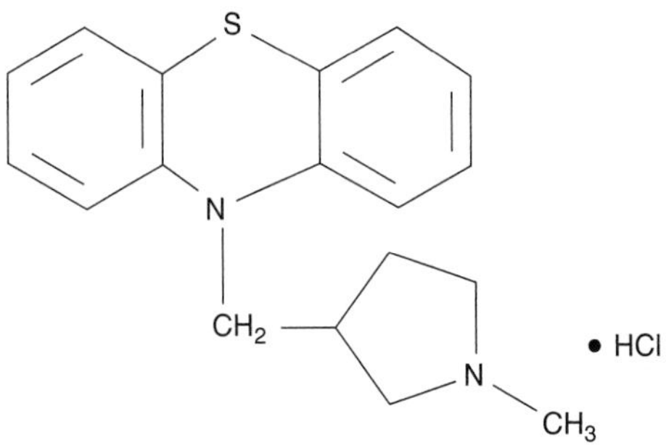

Methdilazine Hydrochloride

Methdilazine Hydrochloride, USP. Methdilazine hydrochloride, 10-[(1-methyl-3-pyrrolidinyl)methyl]phenothiazine monohydrochloride (Tacaryl Hydrochloride), also occurs as a light-tan crystalline powder with a slight characteristic odor. The salt is freely soluble in water and in alcohol, however. The activity is like that of methdilazine, and it is administered orally for its antipruritic effect.

DIBENZOCYCLOHEPTENES AND DIBENZOCYCLOHEPTANES

The dibenzocycloheptene and dibenzocycloheptane antihistamines may be regarded as phenothiazine analogues in which the sulfur atom has been replaced by an isosteric vinyl group (cyproheptadine) or a saturated ethyl bridge (azatadine), and the ring nitrogen has been replaced by an sp^2 carbon atom (Fig. 21-11). The two members of this series are closely related in structure; azatadine is an aza (pyridyl) isostere of cyproheptadine in which the 10,11-double bond is reduced. The properties of each agent are detailed in the monographs below.

Cyproheptadine Hydrochloride, USP. Cyproheptadine hydrochloride, 4-(5*H*-dibenzo-[a,d]-cyclohepten-5-ylidene)-1-methylpiperidine hydrochloride sesquihydrate (Periactin), is slightly soluble in water and sparingly soluble in alcohol.

Cyproheptadine possesses both antihistamine and antiserotonin activity and is used as an antipruritic agent. Sedation is the most prominent side effect, and this is usually brief, disappearing after 3 or 4 days of treatment.

Usual adult dose: Oral, 4 mg t.i.d or q.i.d.
Dosage forms: Syrup and tablets

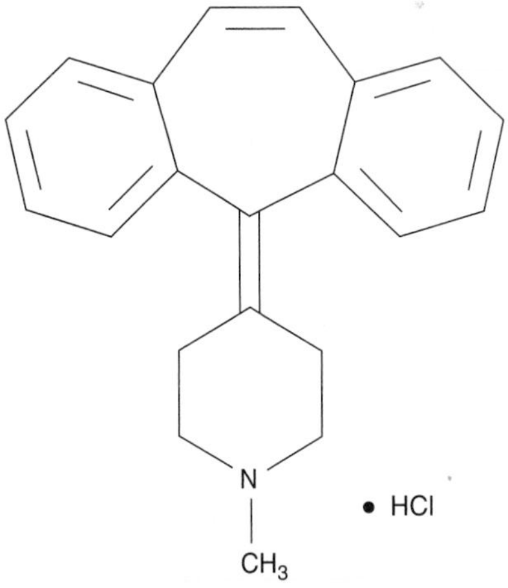

Cyproheptadine Hydrochloride

Azatadine Maleate, USP. Azatadine maleate, 6,11-dihydro-11-(1-methyl-4-piperidylidene)-5*H*-benzo-[5,6]cyclohepta[1,2-b]pyridine maleate (1:2) (Optimine), is a potent, long-acting antihistaminic with antiserotonin activity. In early testing, azatadine exhibited more than 3 times the potency of chlorpheniramine in the isolated guinea pig ileum screen and more than 7 times the oral potency of chlorpheniramine in protection of guinea pigs against a double lethal dose of intravenously administered histamine.[33] The

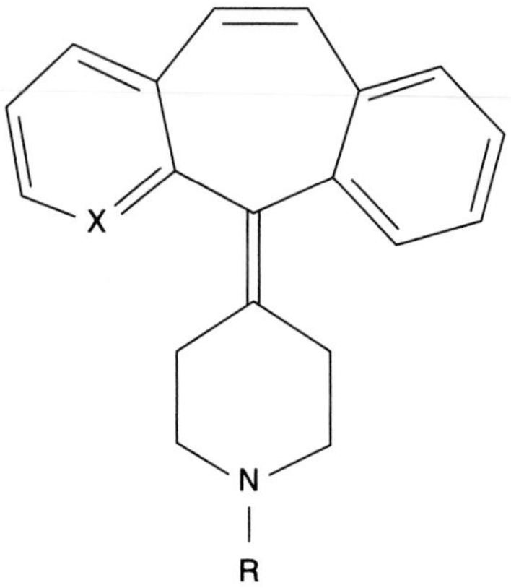

Figure 21–11 ■ General structure of the dibenzocycloheptenes and dibenzocycloheptanes.

usual dosage is 1 to 2 mg twice daily. Azatadine is available in 1-mg tablets.

Usual adult dose: Oral, 1–2 mg b.i.d.
Dosage forms: Tablets

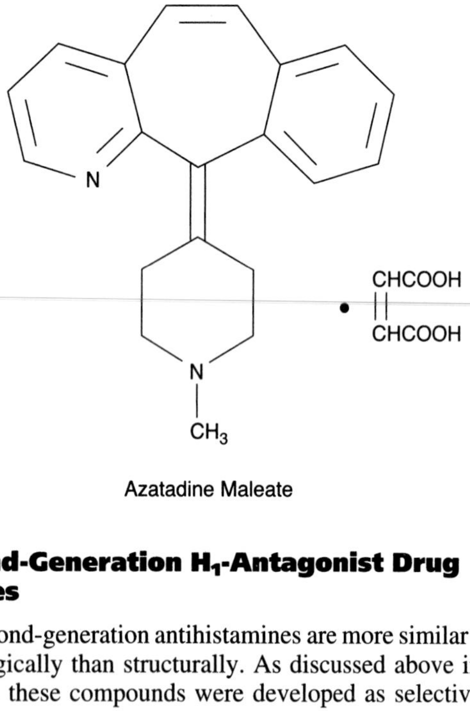

Azatadine Maleate

Second-Generation H₁-Antagonist Drug Classes

The second-generation antihistamines are more similar pharmacologically than structurally. As discussed above in this chapter, these compounds were developed as selective H₁-

receptor antagonists with relatively high potency. Most of these compounds also produce prolonged antihistaminic effects as a result of slow dissociation from H₁ receptors and the formation of active metabolites with similar receptor-binding profiles.[16] The second-generation agents have little affinity for muscarinic, adrenergic, or serotonergic receptors and, therefore, display a lower incidence of side effects associated with antagonism at these receptors. Their affinities for these receptors vary somewhat, as indicated in the monographs below. Perhaps most importantly, all of these compounds lack sedating effects at therapeutic concentrations because of poor CNS penetration and, possibly, lowered affinities for central histaminic,[16] cholinergic, and adrenergic receptors. The first members of this antihistamine subclass introduced in the United States included terfenadine (Seldane) and astemizole (Hismanal) (Fig. 21-12). Although these compounds offered several advantages over the classical antihistamines, widespread use revealed a number of therapeutic limitations, most notably the ability to produce life-threatening arrhythmias when used concurrently with drugs that inhibit their metabolism. This drug interaction has been most evident with the imidazole antifungals (ketoconazole, itraconazole, and fluconazole) and the macrolides (erythromycin, clarithromycin), which inhibit the metabolism of terfenadine and astemizole and thus elevate levels of the parent drugs, which are proarrhythmic.[18] As a result of these concerns, both astemizole and terfenadine have been withdrawn from the U. S. market. Subsequent research efforts focused on the development of second-generation antihistamines that maintained the desired receptor-binding profiles of astemizole and terfenadine but were devoid of proarrhythmic toxicity. These efforts led to the introduction of fexofenadine, loratadine, cetirizine, and acrivastine, as described in the monographs below.

Fexofenadine Hydrochloride.   Fexofenadine hydrochloride, (±)-4-[1-hydroxy-4-[4-(hydroxydiphenylmethyl)-1-piperinyl]butyl-α,α-dimethylbenzeneacetic acid (Allegra), occurs as a white to off-white crystalline powder that is freely soluble in methanol and ethanol, slightly soluble in chloroform and water, and insoluble in hexane. This compound is marketed as a racemate and exists as a zwitterion in aqueous media at physiological pH.

Fexofenadine is a primary oxidative metabolite of terfenadine. Terfenadine was developed during a search for new butyrophenone antipsychotic drugs as evidenced by the presence of the *N*-phenylbutanol substituent. It also contains a

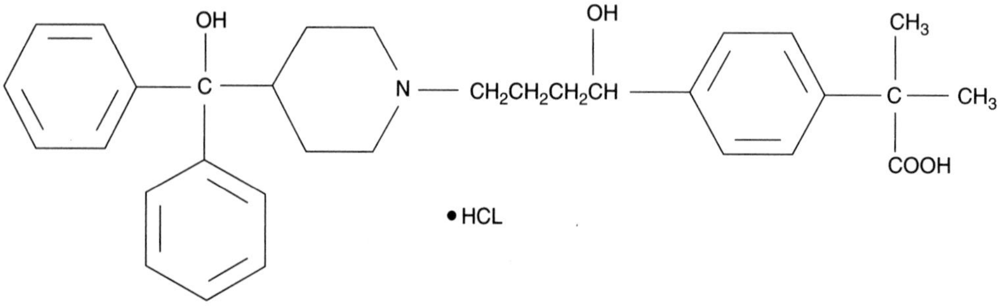

Fexofenadine Hydrochloride

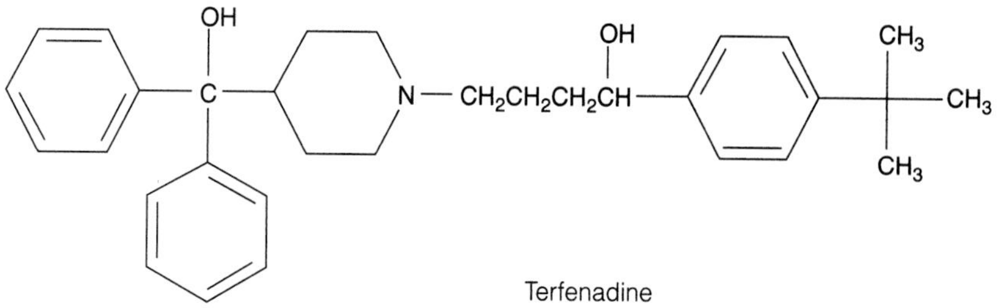

Figure 21–12 ■ Structures of terfenadine and astemizole.

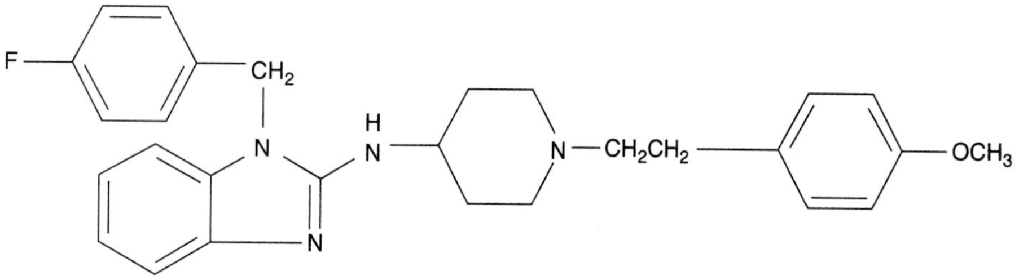

diphenylmethylpiperidine moiety analogous to that found in the piperazine antihistamines. Terfenadine is a selective, long-acting (>12 hours) H_1 antagonist with little affinity for muscarinic, serotonergic, or adrenergic receptors. The histamine receptor affinity of this compound is believed to be related primarily to the presence of the diphenylmethylpiperidine moiety. The prolonged action results from very slow dissociation from these receptors.[18] The lack of anticholinergic, adrenergic, or serotonergic actions appears to be linked to the presence of the *N*-phenylbutanol substituent. This substituent also limits distribution of terfenadine to the CNS.[34, 35] Terfenadine undergoes significant first-pass metabolism, with the predominant metabolite being fexofenadine, an active metabolite resulting from methyl group oxidation. When drugs that inhibit this transformation, such as the imidazole antifungals and macrolides, are used concurrently, terfenadine levels may rise to toxic levels, resulting in potentially fatal heart rhythm problems. The observation that fexofenadine displays antihistaminic activity comparable with that of terfenadine but is less cardiotoxic led to its development as an alternative to terfenadine for the relief of the symptoms of seasonal allergies.[36]

Fexofenadine is a selective peripheral H_1-receptor blocker that, like terfenadine, produces no clinically significant anticholinergic effects or α_1-adrenergic receptor blockade at therapeutic doses. No sedative or other CNS effects have been reported for this drug, and animal studies indicate that fexofenadine does not cross the BBB. In vitro studies also suggest that unlike terfenadine, fexofenadine does not block potassium channels in cardiocytes. Furthermore, in drug interaction studies no prolongation of the QTc interval or related heart rhythm abnormalities were detected when fexofenadine was administered concurrently with erythromycin or ketoconazole.[16, 37]

Fexofenadine is rapidly absorbed after oral administration, producing peak serum concentrations in about 2.5 hours. Fexofenadine is 60 to 70% plasma protein bound.

Unlike its parent drug, only 5% of the total dose of fexofenadine is metabolized. The remainder is excreted in the bile and urine; the mean elimination half-life is about 14 hours.[16, 37]

Usual adult dose: Oral, 60 mg b.i.d.
Dosage form: Capsules

Loratadine, USP. Loratadine, 4-(8-chloro-5,6-dihydro-11*H*-benzo[5,6]-cyclohepta[1,2-b]pyridin-11-ylidene-1-carboxylic acid ethyl ester, is a white to off-white powder not soluble in water but very soluble in acetone, alcohols, and chloroform.

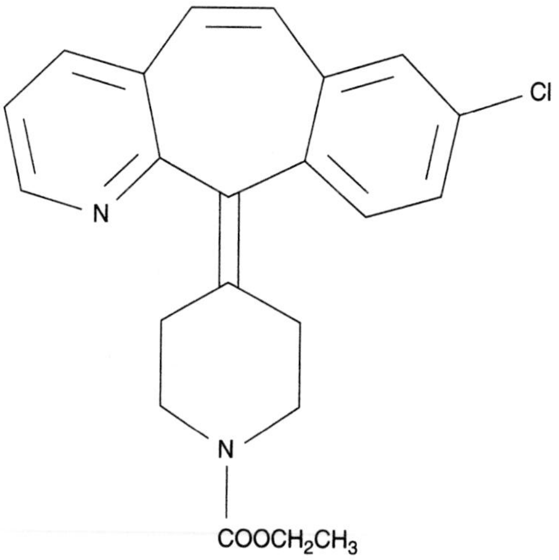

Loratadine

Loratadine is structurally related to the antihistamines azatadine and cyproheptadine. It differs from azatadine, in that a neutral carbamate group has replaced the basic tertiary amino moiety, and a phenyl ring has been substituted with a chlorine atom. The replacement of the basic group with a neutral functionality is believed to preserve antihistaminic action while reducing CNS effects. Loratadine is also structurally related to a number of tricyclic antidepressants.[16, 38]

Loratadine is a selective peripheral H_1 antagonist with a receptor-binding profile like that of the other members of this series, except that it has more antiserotonergic activity. Thus it produces no substantial CNS or autonomic side effects. Loratadine displays potency comparable with that of astemizole and greater than that of terfenadine.[16, 39]

Loratadine is rapidly absorbed after oral administration, producing peak plasma levels in about 1.5 hours. This drug is extensively metabolized, primarily to the descarboethoxy metabolite, which retains some antihistaminic activity. Both parent drug and metabolite have elimination half-lives ranging from 8 to 15 hours. The metabolite is excreted renally as a conjugate.

Usual adult dose: Oral, 10–40 mg daily

Cetirizine, USP.

Cetirizine, USP. Cetirizine, [2-[4-[(4-chlorophenyl) phenylmethyl]-1-piperazinyl]ethoxy]acetic acid (Zyrtec), is a racemic compound available as a white crystalline powder that is water soluble.

Cetirizine is the primary acid metabolite of hydroxyzine, resulting from complete oxidation of the primary alcohol moiety. This compound is zwitterionic and relatively polar and thus does not penetrate the BBB readily. Before its introduction in the United States, cetirizine was one of the most widely prescribed H_1 antihistamines in Europe. It is highly selective in its interaction with various hormonal binding sites and highly potent (>> terfenadine) as well.[40, 41]

The advantages of this compound appear to be once-daily dosing, rapid onset of activity, minimal CNS effects, and a lack of clinically significant effects on cardiac rhythm when administered with imidazole antifungals and macrolide antibiotics. The onset of action is within 20 to 60 minutes in most patients. Cetirizine produces qualitatively different effects on psychomotor and psychophysical functions from the first-generation antihistamines. The most common adverse reaction associated with cetirizine is dose-related somnolence, however, so patients should be advised that cetirizine may interfere with the performance of certain psychomotor and psychophysical activities Other effects of this drug include fatigue, dry mouth, pharyngitis, and dizziness. Be-

cause the drug is primarily eliminated by a renal route, its adverse reactions may be more pronounced in individuals suffering from renal insufficiency. No cardiotoxic effects, such as QT prolongation, are observed with the new drug when used at its recommended or higher doses or when co-administered with imidazole antifungals and macrolide antibiotics. Other typical drug interactions of H_1 antihistamines, however, apply to cetirizine. Concurrent use of this drug with alcohol and other CNS depressants should be avoided.[41–43]

Dose-proportional C_{max} values are achieved within 1 hour of oral administration of cetirizine. Food slows the rate of cetirizine absorption but does not affect the overall extent. Consistent with the polar nature of this carboxylic acid drug, less than 10% of peak plasma levels have been measured in the brain. Cetirizine is not extensively metabolized, and more than 70% of a 10-mg oral dose is excreted in the urine (>80% as unchanged drug) and 10% is recovered in the feces. The drug is highly protein bound (93%) and has a terminal half-life of 8.3 hours. The clearance of cetirizine is reduced in elderly subjects and in renally and hepatically impaired patients.[44]

Usual adult dose: Oral, 5–10 mg q.d.
Dosage form: Tablets

Acrivastine, USP.

Acrivastine, USP. Acrivastine, USP, (E,E)-3-[6-[1-(4-methylphenyl)-3-(1-pyrrolidinyl)-1-propenyl-2-pyridinyl]-2-propenoic acid (Semprex), is a fixed-combination product of the antihistamine acrivastine (8 mg) with the decongestant pseudoephedrine (60 mg). Acrivastine is an odorless, white to pale-cream crystalline powder that is soluble in chloroform and alcohol and slightly soluble in water.

Acrivastine is an analogue of triprolidine containing a carboxyethenyl moiety at the 6 position of the pyridyl ring. Acrivastine shows antihistaminic potency and duration of action comparable to those of triprolidine. Unlike triprolidine, acrivastine does not display significant anticholinergic activity at therapeutic concentrations. Also, the enhanced polarity of this compound resulting from carboxyethenyl substitution limits BBB penetration, and thus, this compound produces less sedation than triprolidine.[38, 43]

Limited pharmacokinetic data are available for this compound. Orally administered drug has a half-life of about 1.7 hours and a total body clearance of 4.4 mL/min per kg. The mean peak plasma concentrations are reported to vary

Cetirizine

widely, and the drug appears to penetrate the CNS poorly. The metabolic fate of acrivastine has not been reported.

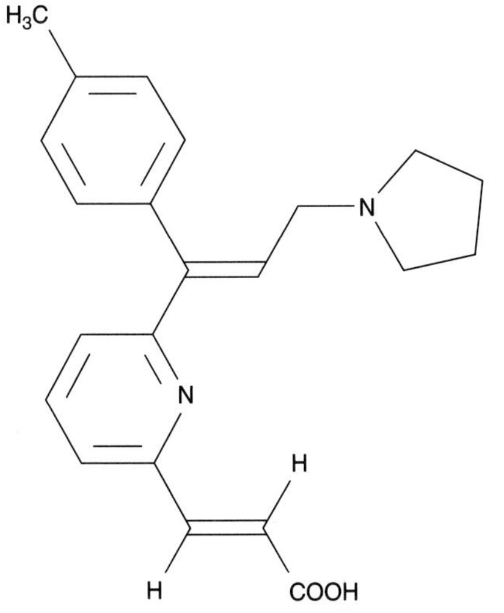

Acrivastine

Usual adult dose: Oral, 8 or 60 mg t.i.d. to q.i.d.
Dosage form: Tablets

INHIBITION OF HISTAMINE RELEASE: MAST CELL STABILIZERS

The discovery of the bronchodilating activity of the natural product khellin led to the development of the bis(chromones) as compounds that stabilize mast cells and inhibit the release of histamine and other mediators of inflammation. The first therapeutically significant member of this class was cromolyn sodium.[30, 44] Further research targeting more effective agents resulted in the introduction of nedocromil, followed more recently by pemirolast and lodoxamide. Generally, the mast cell stabilizers inhibit activation of, and mediator release from, a variety of inflammatory cell types associated with allergy and asthma, including eosinophils, neutrophils, macrophages, mast cells, monocytes, and platelets. In addition to histamine, these drugs inhibit the release of leukotrienes (C4, D4, E4) and prostaglandins. In vitro studies suggest that these drugs indirectly inhibit calcium ion entry into the mast cell and that this action prevents mediator release. In addition to their mediator release, some of these drugs also inhibit the chemotaxis of eosinophils at the site of application (i.e., ocular tissue). In lung tissue, pretreatment with the mast cell stabilizers cromolyn and nedocromil blocks the immediate and delayed bronchoconstrictive reactions induced by the inhalation of antigens. These drugs also attenuate the bronchospasm associated with exercise, cold air, environmental pollutants, and certain drugs (aspirin). The mast cell stabilizers do not have intrinsic bronchodilator, antihistamine, anticholinergic, vasoconstrictor, or glucocorticoid activity and, when delivered by inhalation at the recommended dose, have no known therapeutic systemic activity. The structures, chemical properties, pharmacological profiles, and dosage data for these agents are provided in the monographs below.

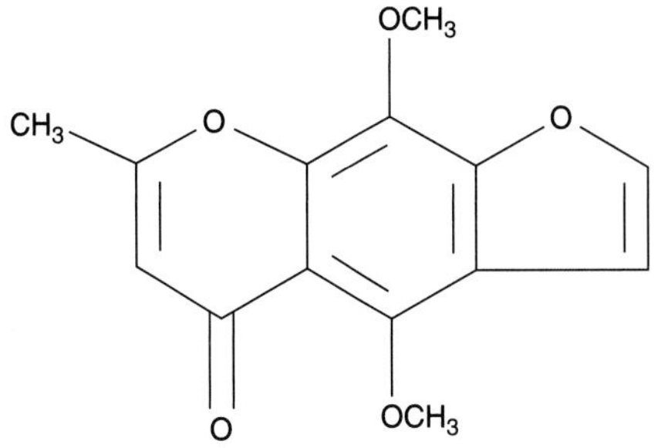

Khellin

Cromolyn Sodium, USP. Cromolyn sodium, disodium 1,3-bis(2-carboxychromon-5-yloxy)-2-hydroxypropane (Intal), is a hygroscopic, white, hydrated crystalline powder that is soluble in water (1:10). It is tasteless at first but leaves a very slightly bitter aftertaste. The pK$_a$ of cromolyn is 2.0. It is available as a solution for a nebulizer, an aerosol spray, a nasal solution, an ophthalmic solution, and an oral concentrate.

Nebulized and aerosol cromolyn is used for prophylactic management of bronchial asthma and prevention of exercise-induced bronchospasm. Cromolyn nasal solution is used for the prevention and treatment of allergic rhinitis, and oral concentrate is used to treat the histaminic symptoms of mastocytosis (diarrhea, flushing, headaches, vomiting, urticaria, abdominal pain, nausea, and itching). In the treatment of asthma, cromolyn efficacy is manifested by decreased severity of clinical symptoms, or need for concomitant therapy, or both. Long-term use is justified if the drug significantly reduces the severity of asthma symptoms; permits a significant reduction in, or elimination of, steroid dosage; or im-

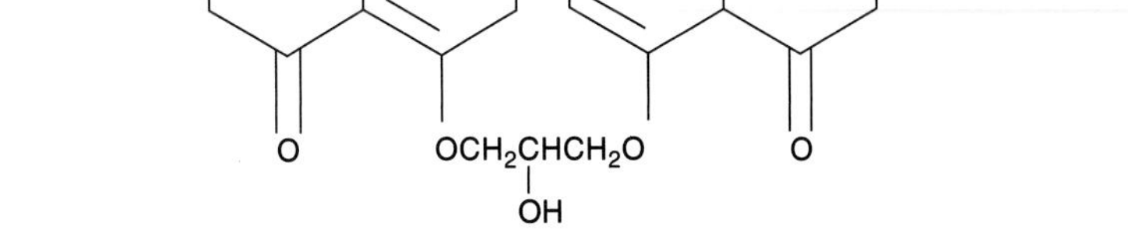

Cromolyn Sodium

proves management of those who have intolerable side effects to sympathomimetic agents or methylxanthines. For cromolyn to be effective, it must be administered at least 30 minutes prior to antigen challenge and administered at regular intervals (see dosing information below). Overuse of cromolyn results in tolerance.

Usual adult dose:
Nebulizer solution, 20 mg inhaled q.i.d.
Aerosol, 2 metered sprays inhaled q.i.d.
Intranasal, 5.2 mg (one metered spray) in each nostril t.i.d. or q.i.d. at regular intervals
Ophthalmic, 1 drop of a 2–4% solution q.i.d. to 6 times daily
Oral, 2 ampules q.i.d. 30 minutes before meals and at bedtime

Nedocromil Sodium, USP.
Nedocromil sodium, disodium 9-ethyl-6,9-dihydro-4,6-dioxo-10-propyl-4*H*-pyrano [3,2-g]quinoline-2,8-dicarboxylate (Tilade), is available as an aerosol in a metered-dose inhaler.

Nedocromil is structurally related to cromolyn and displays similar, but broader, pharmacological actions. Nedocromil is indicated for maintenance therapy in the management of patients with mild-to-moderate bronchial asthma. It was developed in a search for a compound with a better biological profile than cromolyn, which has limitations in the treatment of certain patients, such as the elderly asthmatic patient and patients with intrinsic asthma. Cromolyn is more effective in stabilizing connective tissue mast cells than mucosal mast cells, and since release of mediators from mast cells in the lung is an important component of inflammation and bronchial hyperreactivity in asthmatic patients, an agent with greater effects on mucosal mast cells was desirable. Available data suggest that nedocromil, although having profile of activity like that of cromolyn, is more effective in stabilizing mucosal mast cells.[45]

Nedocromil Disodium

The antiasthmatic effects of nedocromil may also involve inhibition of axon reflexes. Axon reflexes may be produced by bradykinin in the presence of damage to the airway epithelium, resulting in release of sensory neuropeptides (substance P, neurokinin A), which can produce bronchoconstriction and edema. Nedocromil is more effective than cromolyn in reversing bradykinin-induced and neurokinin A–induced bronchoconstriction in humans.

Usual adult dose: Intranasal, 14 mg (two inhalations) q.i.d. at regular intervals

Lodoxamide Tromethamine.
The only significant structurally similarity between lodoxamide and cromolyn and nedocromil is the presence of two acidic groups. Lodoxamide tromethamine, *N,N*′-(2-chloro-5-cyano-*m*-phenylene)-dioxamic acid (Alomide), is a white crystalline, water-soluble powder. It is available as a 0.1% solution, with each milliliter containing 1.78 mg of lodoxamide tromethamine equivalent to 1 mg of lodoxamide. The solution contains the preservative benzalkonium chloride (0.007%) as well as mannitol, hydroxypropyl methylcellulose, sodium citrate, citric acid, edetate disodium, tyloxapol, hydrochloric acid and/or sodium hydroxide (to adjust pH), and purified water.

Lodoxamide is indicated in the treatment of the ocular disorders including vernal keratoconjunctivitis, vernal conjunctivitis, and vernal keratitis.[46] The dose for adults and children older than 2 years of age is 1 to 2 drops in each affected eye 4 times daily for up to 3 months. The most frequently reported ocular adverse experiences were transient burning, stinging, or discomfort on instillation.

Pemirolast Potassium Ophthalmic Solution.
Pemirolast can be considered an analogue of one portion of the cromolyn structure in which the carboxyl group has been replaced with an isosteric tetrazole moiety. Pemirolast potassium, 9-methyl-3-(1*H*-tetrazol-5-yl)-4*H*-pyrido[1,2-*α*]-pyrimidin-4-one potassium (Alamast), is a yellow, water-soluble powder. The commercial preparation is available as a 0.1% sterile ophthalmic solution for topical administration to the eyes. Each milliliter of this solution contains 1.0 mg of pemirolast potassium, as well as the preservative lauralkonium chloride (0.005%), and glycerin, phosphate buffers, and sodium hydroxide to maintain a solution pH of 8.0. The solution has an osmolality of approximately 240 mOsm/L. The recommended dose is one to two drops instilled into each affected eye 4 times a day. This drug product is for ocular administration only and not for injection or oral use. Pemiro-

Lodoxamide Tromethamine

last solution should be used with caution during pregnancy or while nursing, since its safety has not been studied under these circumstances.[47]

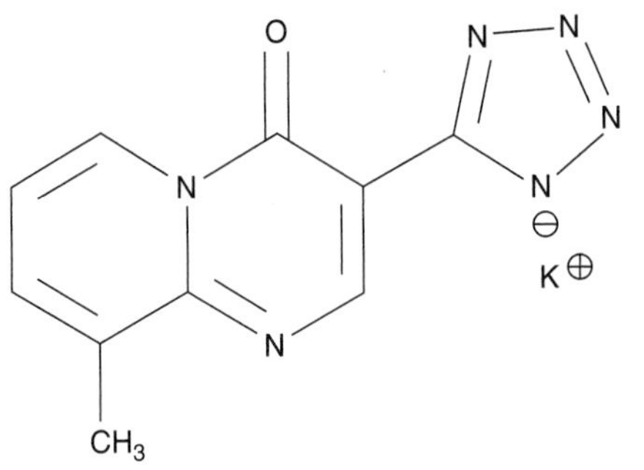

Pemirolast Potassium

RECENT ANTIHISTAMINE DEVELOPMENTS: THE "DUAL-ACTING" ANTIHISTAMINES

Over the past decade there has been considerable interest in the development of novel antihistaminic compounds with dual mechanisms of action including H_1-receptor antagonism and mast cell stabilization. Currently available drugs that exhibit such dual antihistaminic actions include azelastine and ketotifen. These compounds contain the basic pharmacophore to produce relatively selective histamine H_1 antagonism (diarylalkylamines) as well as inhibition of the release of histamine and other mediators (e.g., leukotrienes and PAF) from mast cells involved in the allergic response. In vitro studies suggest that these compounds also decrease chemotaxis and activation of eosinophils. Azelastine and ketotifen currently are indicated for the treatment of itching of the eye associated with allergic conjunctivitis. Their antiallergy actions occur within minutes after administration and may persist for up to 8 hours. The structures, chemical properties, pharmacological profiles, and dosage data for these agents are provided in the monographs below.

Azelastine Hydrochloride Ophthalmic Solution.
Azelastine hydrochloride, (±)-1-(2*H*)-phthalazinone, 4-[(4-chlorophenyl)methyl]-2-(hexahydro-1-methyl-1*H*-azepin-4-yl)-1-(2*H*)-phthalazinone monohydrochloride (Optivar), is a white crystalline powder that is sparingly soluble in water, methanol, and propylene glycol and slightly soluble in ethanol, octanol, and glycerine. The commercial preparation is available as a 0.05% sterile ophthalmic solution for topical administration to the eyes. Each milliliter of azelastine solution contains 0.5 mg azelastine hydrochloride equivalent to 0.457 mg of azelastine base, the preservative benzalkonium chloride (0.125 mg), and inactive ingredients including disodium edetate dihydrate, hydroxypropylmethylcellulose, sorbitol solution, sodium hydroxide, and water for injection. The solution has a pH of approximately 5.0 to 6.5 and an osmolality of approximately 271 to 312 mOsm/L.

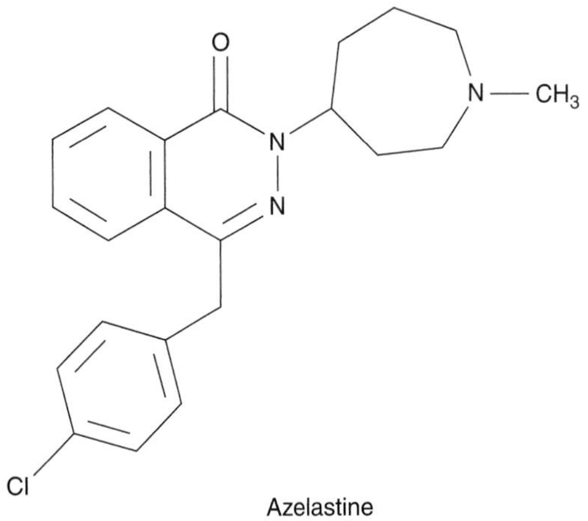

Azelastine

The recommended dose of azelastine solution is one drop instilled into each affected eye twice a day. This drug product is for ocular administration only and not for injection or oral use. Absorption of azelastine following ocular administration is relatively low (less than 1 ng/mL). Absorbed drug undergoes extensive oxidative N-demethylation by cytochrome P-450, and the parent drug and metabolite are eliminated primarily in the feces. The most frequently reported adverse reactions are transient eye burning or stinging, headaches, and bitter taste. Azelastine solution should be used with caution during pregnancy or while nursing, since its safety has not been studied under these circumstances.[48]

Ketotifen Fumarate Ophthalmic Solution.　Ketotifen fumarate, 4-(1-methyl-4-piperidylidene)-4*H*-benzo[4,5]cyclohepta[1,2-b]thiophen-10(9*H*)-one hydrogen fumarate (Zaditor), is a fine crystalline powder. Ketotifen is a ketothiophene isostere analogue of the dibenzocycloheptane antihistamines. The solution contains 0.345 mg of ketotifen fumarate, which is equivalent to 0.25 mg of ketotifen. The solution also contains the preservative benzalkonium chloride (0.01%) as well as glycerol, sodium hydroxide and/or hydrochloric acid (to adjust pH), and purified water. It has a pH of 4.4 to 5.8 and an osmolality of 210 to 300 mOsm/kg.

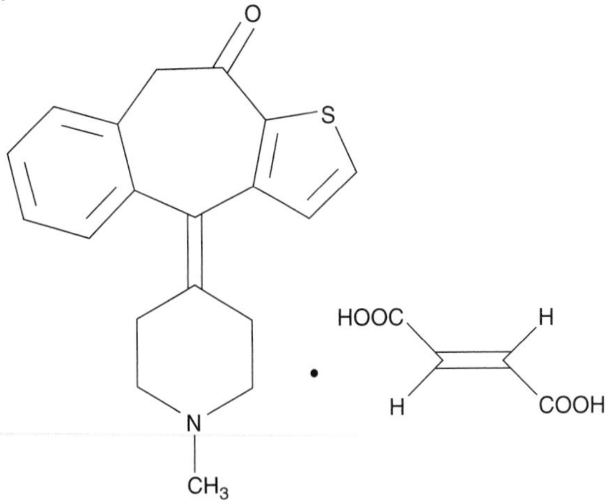

Ketotifen Fumarate

The recommended dose of ketotifen solution is one drop instilled into each affected eye every 8 to 12 hours. The most frequently reported adverse reactions are conjunctival injection, headaches, and rhinitis. This drug product is for ocular administration only and not for injection or oral use. Ketotifen solution should be used with caution during pregnancy or while nursing, since its safety has not been studied under these circumstances.[49]

HISTAMINE H₂ ANTAGONISTS

Drugs whose pharmacological action primarily involves antagonism of the action of histamine at its H_2 receptors find therapeutic application in the treatment of acid-peptic disorders ranging from heartburn to peptic ulcer disease, Zollinger-Ellison syndrome, gastroesophageal reflux disease (GERD), acute stress ulcers, and erosions.[50, 51]

Peptic Acid Secretion

A characteristic feature of the mammalian stomach is its ability to secrete acid as part of its involvement in digesting food for absorption later in the intestine. The presence of acid and proteolytic pepsin enzymes, whose formation is facilitated by the low gastric pH, is generally assumed to be required for the hydrolysis of proteins and other foods.

The acid secretory unit of the gastric mucosa is the parietal (oxyntic) cell. Parietal cells contain a hydrogen ion pump, a unique H_3O^+/K^+-ATPase system that secretes H_3O^+ in exchange for the uptake of K^+ ion. Secretion of acid by gastric parietal (oxyntic) cells is regulated by the actions of various mediators at receptors located on the basolateral membrane, including histamine agonism of H_2 receptors (cellular), gastrin activity at G receptors (blood), and acetylcholine (ACh) at M_2 muscarinic receptors (neuronal) (Fig. 21.13).

Peptic Ulcer Disease[52]

Peptide ulcer disease (PUD) is a group of upper GI tract disorders that result from the erosive action of acid and pepsin. Duodenal ulcer (DU) and gastric ulcer (GU) are the most common forms, although PUD may occur in the esophagus or small intestine. Factors involved in the pathogenesis and

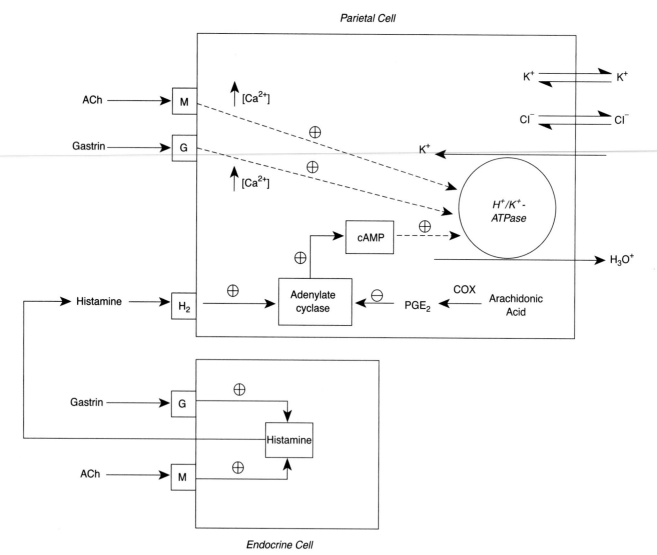

Figure 21–13 ▪ Hormonal regulation of acid secretion by parietal cells.

recurrence of PUD include hypersecretion of acid and pepsin and GI infection by *Helicobacter pylori,* a Gram-negative spiral bacterium. *H. pylori* has been found in virtually all patients with DU and approximately 75% of patients with GU. Some risk factors associated with recurrence of PUD include cigarette smoking, chronic use of ulcerogenic drugs (e.g., nonsteroidal anti-inflammatory drugs [NSAIDs]), male gender, age, alcohol consumption, emotional stress, and family history.

The goals of PUD therapy are to promote healing, relieve pain, and prevent ulcer complications and recurrences. Medications used to heal or reduce ulcer recurrence include antacids, histamine H_2-receptor antagonists, protective mucosal barriers, proton pump inhibitors, prostaglandins, and bismuth salt and antibiotic combinations.

Structural Derivation

A review of the characterization and development of histamine H_2-receptor antagonists reveals a classic medicinal chemistry approach to problem solving.[53] Structural evolution of the first discovered, clinically useful H_2 antagonist, cimetidine, is depicted in Figure 21-14. Methylation of the 5 position of the imidazole heterocycle of histamine produces a selective agonist at atrial histamine receptors (H_2). The guanidino analogue of histamine possesses weak antagonist activity to the acid-secretory actions of histamine. Increasing the length of the side chain from two to four carbons, coupled with replacement of the strongly basic guanidino group by the neutral methyl thiourea function, leads to burimamide, the first antagonist to be developed lacking detectable agonist activity in laboratory assays. The

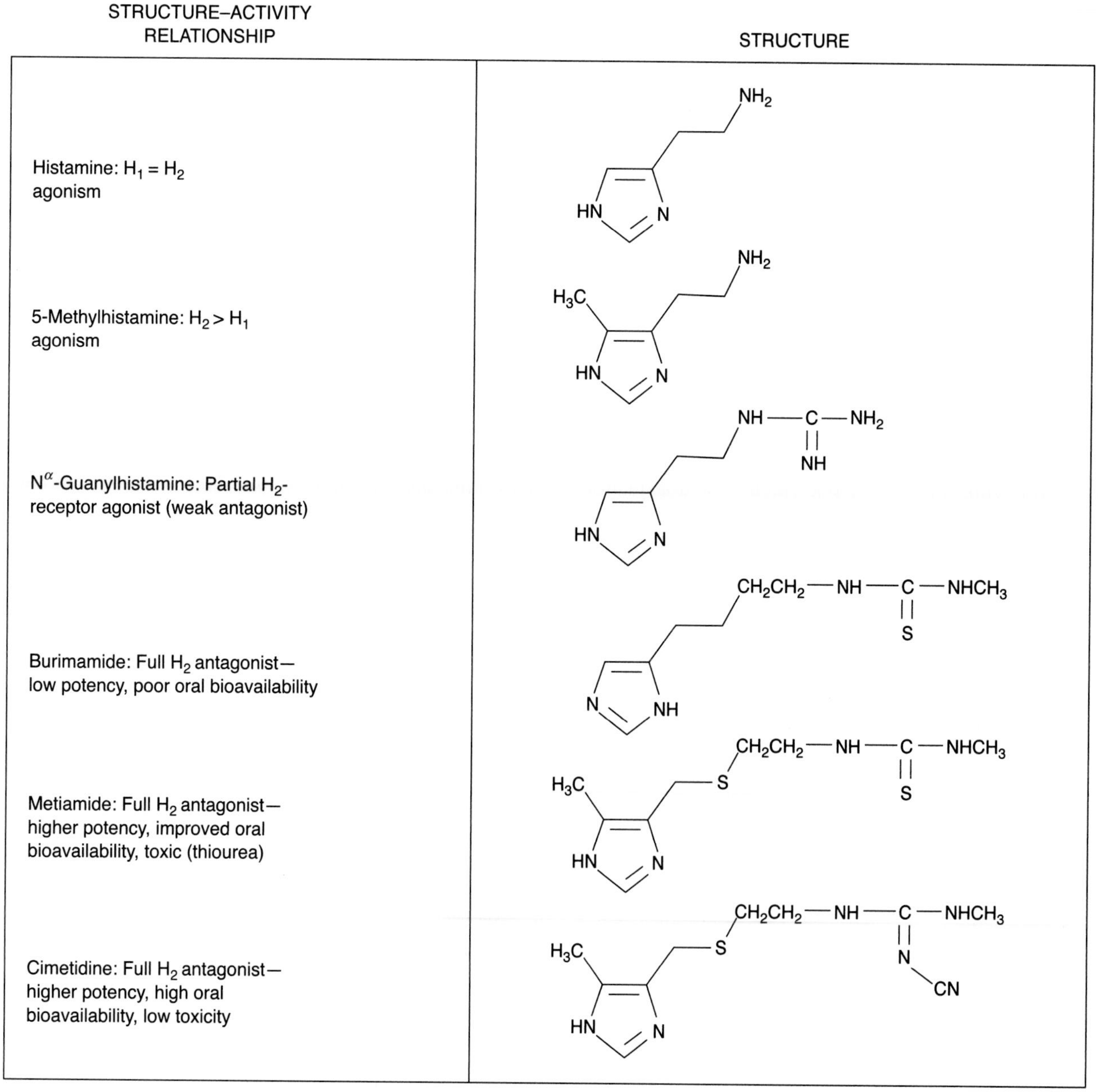

STRUCTURE–ACTIVITY RELATIONSHIP

STRUCTURE

Histamine: $H_1 = H_2$ agonism

5-Methylhistamine: $H_2 > H_1$ agonism

N^α-Guanylhistamine: Partial H_2-receptor agonist (weak antagonist)

Burimamide: Full H_2 antagonist— low potency, poor oral bioavailability

Metiamide: Full H_2 antagonist— higher potency, improved oral bioavailability, toxic (thiourea)

Cimetidine: Full H_2 antagonist— higher potency, high oral bioavailability, low toxicity

Figure 21–14 ■ Structural derivation of histamine H_2 antagonists.

low potency of burimamide is postulated to be related to its nonbasic, electron-releasing side chain, which favors the nonpharmacophoric N^π-H imidazole tautomer over the basic, electron-withdrawing side chain in histamine, which predominantly presents the higher-affinity N^τ-H imidazole tautomer to the receptor. Insertion of an electronegative thioether function in the side chain in place of a methylene group favors the N^τ tautomer, and introduction of the 5-methyl group favors H_2-receptor selectivity and leads to metiamide, a H_2 blocker of higher potency and oral bioavailability than burimamide. Toxicity associated with the thiourea structural feature is eliminated by replacing the thiourea sulfur with a cyano-imino function to produce cimetidine.

Introduction of cimetidine into human medicine revealed an effective gastric antisecretory agent that promotes the healing of duodenal ulcers. Cimetidine is not without a number of limitations, however. Because it is short acting, it requires a frequent-dosing schedule in humans, and in addition, its selectivity is poor. Cimetidine has antiandrogenic activity, which can lead to gynecomastia, and it inhibits the cytochrome P-450 mixed-function oxygenase-metabolizing enzyme system in the liver, an action that potentiates the effects of drugs whose clearance also depends on biotransformation by this system. Cimetidine also causes confusional states in some elderly patients. Subsequent development of additional drugs of this class indicates that a great deal of structural latitude is available in the design of H_2 antagonists (Table 21.1).[54]

Examination of the structural features of H_2 antagonists that came after cimetidine confirms that the imidazole ring of histamine is not required for competitive antagonism of histamine at H_2 receptors. Other heterocycles may be used and may, in fact, enhance both potency and selectivity of H_2-receptor antagonism. If the imidazole ring is used, however, the N^τ-H tautomer should be the predominant species for maximal H_2-antagonist activity. The electronic effects of the ring substituents and side-chain structural features determine the tautomerism. Separation of the ring and the nitrogen group with the equivalent of a four-carbon chain appears to be necessary for optimal antagonist activity. The isosteric thioether link is present in the four agents currently marketed in the United States. The terminal nitrogen–containing functionality should be a polar, nonbasic substituent for maximal antagonist activity. Groups that are positively charged at physiological pH appear to confer agonist activity. In general, antagonist activity varies inversely with the hydrophilic character of the nitrogen group. The hydrophilic group, 1,1-diaminonitroethene, found in ranitidine and nizatidine is an exception, however; it is much more active than is predicted by relative solubility effects.

Cimetidine, USP. Cimetidine, N^π-cyano-N-methyl-N'-[2-[[5-methylimidazol-4-yl)methyl]-thio]ethyl]guanidine (Tagamet), is a colorless crystalline solid that is slightly soluble in water (1.14% at 37°C). The solubility is greatly increased by the addition of dilute acid to protonate the imidazole ring (apparent pK_a of 6.8). At pH 7, aqueous solutions are stable for at least 7 days. Cimetidine is a relatively hydrophilic molecule with an octanol/water partition coefficient of 2.5.

Cimetidine

Cimetidine reduces the hepatic metabolism of drugs biotransformed by the cytochrome P-450 mixed-oxidase system, delaying elimination and increasing serum levels of these drugs. Concomitant therapy of patients with cimetidine and drugs metabolized by hepatic microsomal enzymes, particularly those of low therapeutic ratio or in patients with renal or hepatic impairment, may require dosage adjustment. Table 21.2 provides a compilation of drugs whose combination therapy with cimetidine may increase their pharmacological effects or toxicity. Antacids interfere with cimetidine absorption and should be administered at least 1 hour before or after a cimetidine dose.

Cimetidine has a weak antiandrogenic effect. Gynecomastia may occur in patients treated for 1 month or more.

Cimetidine exhibits high oral bioavailability (60 to 70%) and a plasma half-life of about 2 hours, which is increased

TABLE 21–1 Currently Available H₂ Antagonists

	Relative Potency	Oral Bioavailability (%)	Metabolism, Enzyme	Metabolites	Dose Metabolized (%)	Route of Elimination	Renal Clearance (L/hour)
Cimetidine	1	63–78	FMO3	Sulfoxide, hydroxymethyl	~25	Renal	24–36
Famotidine	40	37–45	?	S-Oxide	~30	Renal	14–26
Nizatidine	10	98	?	N₂-monodesmethyl, N₂-oxide	~37	Renal	27–36
Ranitidine	6	52	FMO3; P-450	N-Oxide, N-desmethyl sulfoxide	~30	Renal, biliary	24–32

From Laethem, R.M., and Serabjit-Singh, C.J.: H₂-antagonists, proton-pump inhibitors, and antiemetics. In Levy, R.H., Thummel, K.E., Trager, W.F., Hansten, P.D., and Eichelbaum, M. (eds). Metabolic Drug Interactions. Philadelphia, Lippincott Williams & Wilkins, 2000, chap. 36.

TABLE 21–2   Cimetidine Drug Interactions

Benzodiazepines	Metronidazole	Sulfonylurea
Caffeine	Moricizine	Tacrine
Calcium channel blockers	Pentoxifylline	Theophylline
Carbamazepine	Phenytoin	Triamterene
Chloroquine	Propafenone	Tricyclic antidepressants
Labetalol	Propranolol	Valproic acid
Lidocaine	Quinidine	Warfarin
Metoprolol	Quinine	

From Histamine H2-antagonists. In Olinm, B. R. (ed.). Drug Facts and Comparisons. St. Louis, MO, Facts and Comparisons, 1995, pp. 304–305.

in renal and hepatic impairment and in the elderly. Approximately 30 to 40% of a cimetidine dose is metabolized (S-oxidation, 5-CH_3 hydroxylation), and the parent drug and metabolites are eliminated primarily by renal excretion.

Usual adult oral dose:
Duodenal ulcer: Treatment dose, 800–1,200 mg q.d. to q.i.d. with meals and at bedtime; maintenance dose, 400 mg q.d.
Benign gastric ulcer: 800–1,200 mg q.d. to q.i.d.
Hypersecretory condition: 1,200–2,400 mg q.i.d.
Heartburn: 200 mg (2 OTC tablets) up to twice daily
Usual pediatric dose: Oral, 20–40 mg (base) per kilogram of body weight q.i.d. with meals and at bedtime
Dosage forms: Tablet (200, 300, 400, 800 mg), liquid (300 mg/5 mL), injection (300 mg/2 and 50 mL)

Famotidine, USP.   Famotidine, N'-(aminosulfonyl)-3-[[[2[(diaminomethylene)-amino]-4-thiazolyl]methyl]thio]propanimidamide (Pepcid), which uses a thiazole bioisostere of the imidazole heterocycle, is a white to pale-yellow crystalline compound that is very slightly soluble in water and practically insoluble in ethanol.

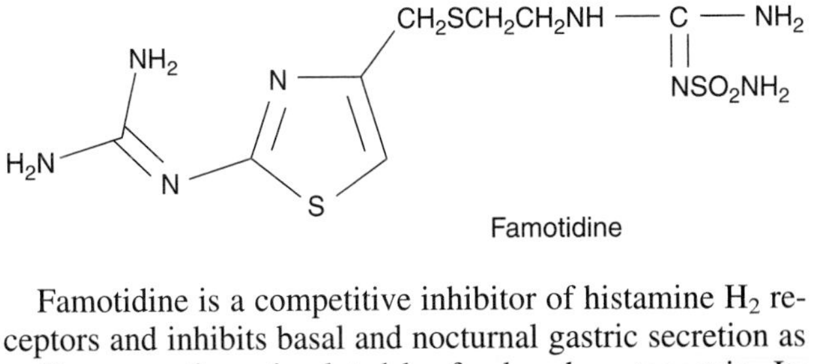

Famotidine

Famotidine is a competitive inhibitor of histamine H_2 receptors and inhibits basal and nocturnal gastric secretion as well as secretion stimulated by food and pentagastrin. Its current labeling indications are for the short-term treatment of duodenal and benign gastric ulcers, GERD, pathological hypersecretory conditions (e.g., Zollinger-Ellison syndrome), and heartburn (OTC only).

No cases of gynecomastia, increased prolactin levels, or impotence have been reported, even at the higher dosage levels used in patients with pathological hypersecretory conditions. Studies with famotidine in humans, in animal models, and in vitro have shown no significant interference with the disposition of compounds metabolized by the hepatic microsomal enzymes (e.g., cytochrome P-450 system).

Famotidine is incompletely absorbed (40 to 45% bioavail

ability). The drug is eliminated by renal (65 to 70%) and metabolic (30 to 35%) routes. Famotidine sulfoxide is the only metabolite identified in humans. The effects of food or antacid on the bioavailability of famotidine are not clinically significant.

Usual adult oral dose:
Duodenal ulcer: Treatment dose, 40 mg q.d. to b.i.d. at bedtime; maintenance dose, 20 mg q.d. at bedtime
Benign gastric ulcer: 40 mg q.d.
Hypersecretory condition: 80–640 mg q.i.d.
Heartburn: 10 mg (1 OTC tablet) for relief or 1 hour before a meal for prevention
Dosage forms: Tablet (20 and 40 mg), oral suspension (40 mg/5 mL), injection (10 mg/mL)

Ranitidine, USP.   Ranitidine, N-[2-[[[5-[dimethylamino)methyl]-2-furanyl]methyl]thio]ethyl]-N'-methyl-2-nitro-1,1-ethenediamine (Zantac), is an aminoalkyl furan derivative with pK_a values of 2.7 (side chain) and 8.2 (dimethylamino). It is a white solid. The hydrochloride salt is highly soluble in water.

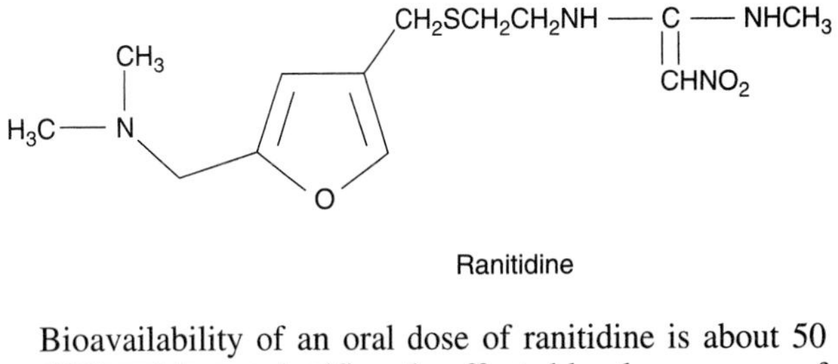

Ranitidine

Bioavailability of an oral dose of ranitidine is about 50 to 60% and is not significantly affected by the presence of food. Some antacids may reduce ranitidine absorption and should not be taken within 1 hour of administration of the H_2-blocker. The plasma half-life of the drug is 2 to 3 hours, and it is excreted along with its metabolites in the urine. Three metabolites, ranitidine N-oxide, ranitidine S-oxide, and desmethyl ranitidine, have been identified. Ranitidine is only a weak inhibitor of the hepatic cytochrome P-450 mixed-function oxidase system

In addition to being available in a variety of dosage forms as the hydrochloride salt, ranitidine is also available as a bismuth citrate salt for use with the macrolide antibiotic clarithromycin in treating patients with an active duodenal ulcer associated with *H. pylori* infection. Eradication of *H. pylori* reduces the risk of duodenal ulcer recurrence.

> Usual adult oral dose:
> Duodenal ulcer: Treatment dose, 200–3,000 mg q.d. to b.i.d.; maintenance dose, 150 mg q.d.
> Benign gastric ulcer: 300 mg q.d.
> Hypersecretory condition: 300–6,000 mg 2 or more times daily
> Dosage forms: Tablets (150 and 300 mg of HCl salt), syrup (15 mg/mL as HCl salt), injection (0.5 and 25 mg/mL as HCl salt)

Nizatidine. Nizatidine, *N*-[2-[[[2-[(dimethylamino)methyl]-4-thiazolyl]methyl]thio]ethyl]-*N*′-methyl-2-nitro-1,1-ethenediamine (Axid), is an off-white to buff crystalline solid that is soluble in water, alcohol, and chloroform. The pK_as of the drug in water are 2.1 (side chain) and 6.8 (dimethylamino).

Nizatidine

Nizatidine has excellent oral bioavailability (>90%). The effects of antacids or food on its bioavailability are not clinically significant. The elimination half-life is 1 to 2 hours. It is excreted primarily in the urine (90%) and mostly as unchanged drug (60%). Metabolites include nizatidine sulfoxide (6%), *N*-desmethylnizatidine (7%), and nizatidine N_2-oxide (dimethylaminomethyl function). Nizatidine has no demonstrable antiandrogenic action or inhibitory effects on cytochrome P-450-linked drug-metabolizing enzyme system.

> Usual adult oral dose:
> Duodenal ulcer: Treatment dose, 300 mg q.d. to b.i.d.; maintenance dose, 150 mg q.d.
> Hypersecretory condition: 150 mg b.i.d.
> Dosage forms: Capsules (150 and 300 mg)

Other Antiulcer Therapies

PROTON PUMP INHIBITORS

The final step in acid secretion in the parietal cell is the extrusion ("pumping") of protons. The membrane pump, an H^+/K^+-ATPase, catalyzes the exchange of hydrogen ions for potassium ions. Inhibition of this proton pump acts beyond the site of action of second messengers (e.g., Ca^{2+} and cAMP) and is independent of the action of secretogogues histamine, gastrin, and acetylcholine. Thus, acid pump inhibitors block basal and stimulated secretion.

In 1972, a group of Swedish medicinal chemists discovered that certain pyridylmethyl benzimidazole sulfides were active proton pump H^+/K^+-ATPase inhibitors (PPIs).[55]

These compounds were subsequently converted to sulfoxide derivatives, which exhibited highly potent, irreversible inhibition of the proton pump. The benzimidazole PPIs are prodrugs that are rapidly converted to a sulfenamide intermediate in the highly acidic environment of gastric parietal cells. The weakly basic benzimidazole PPIs accumulate in these acidic compartments on the luminal side of the tubuvesicular and canalicular structures of the parietal cells. The benzimidazole PPIs are chemically converted by acid to a sulfenamide intermediate that inhibits the proton pump via covalent interaction with cysteine residues (813 or 822) of the pump H^+/K^+-ATPase (Fig. 21-15).[56] The acid lability of the benzimidazole PPIs dictates that these drugs must be formulated as delayed-release, enteric-coated granular dosage forms.

The PPIs are more effective in the short term than the H_2-blockers in healing duodenal ulcers and erosive esophagitis and can heal esophagitis resistant to treatment with the H_2-blockers.[57] In addition, the benzimidazole PPIs have antimicrobial activity against *H. pylori* and thus possess efficacy in treating gastric ulcers or with one or more antimicrobials, in eradicating infection by this organism. Four benzimidazole PPIs are currently approved for marketing in the United States (Table 21-3). Adverse effect profiles of the various PPIs are difficult to compare because comparative clinical trials do not usually include sufficient individuals to allow reliable conclusions. Relatively early in its marketing, the use of omeprazole was associated with the occurrence of diarrhea, headache, and rashes; longer-term experience suggests, however, that these adverse responses are rare. Similarly, characterization of adverse reaction profiles of other PPIs must await more extensive use in patients.

The PPIs are eliminated almost entirely by rapid metabolism to inactive or less active metabolites (Fig. 21-16).[58] Virtually no unchanged drug is excreted in the urine and feces. The cytochrome P-450 enzyme system is primarily involved in PPI metabolism and can be the source of drug–drug interactions for the PPIs. Inhibition of oxidative metabolism by omeprazole (but not esomeprazole) is responsible for prolonging the clearance of benzodiazepines, phenytoin, and warfarin. Lansoprazole decreases theophylline concentration slightly and may decrease the efficacy of oral contraceptives. Pantoprazole and rabeprazole appear to be free of these interactions. Further, the profound and long-lasting inhibition of gastric acid secretion by the PPIs may interfere with the bioavailability of drugs when gastric pH is an important determinant, such as the azole antifungals (e.g., ketoconazole), ampicillin, iron salts, digoxin, and cyanocobalamin.

Omeprazole. Omeprazole, 5-methoxy-2-(((4-methoxy-3,5-dimethyl-2-pyridinyl)methyl)sulfinyl)-1*H*-benzimidazole (Losec), is a white to off-white crystalline powder with very slight solubility in water. Omeprazole is an amphoteric compound (pyridine N, pK_a 4.13; benzimidazole N-H, pK_a 1.68), and consistent with the proposed mechanism of action of the substituted benzimidazoles, it is acid labile. Hence, the omeprazole product is formulated as delayed-release capsules containing enteric-coated granules. The absolute bioavailability of orally administered omeprazole is 30 to 40% related to substantial first-pass biotransformation. The drug has a plasma half-life of about 1 hour. Most (77%) of an oral dose of omeprazole is excreted in the urine as metabolites with insignificant antisecretory activity. The pri-

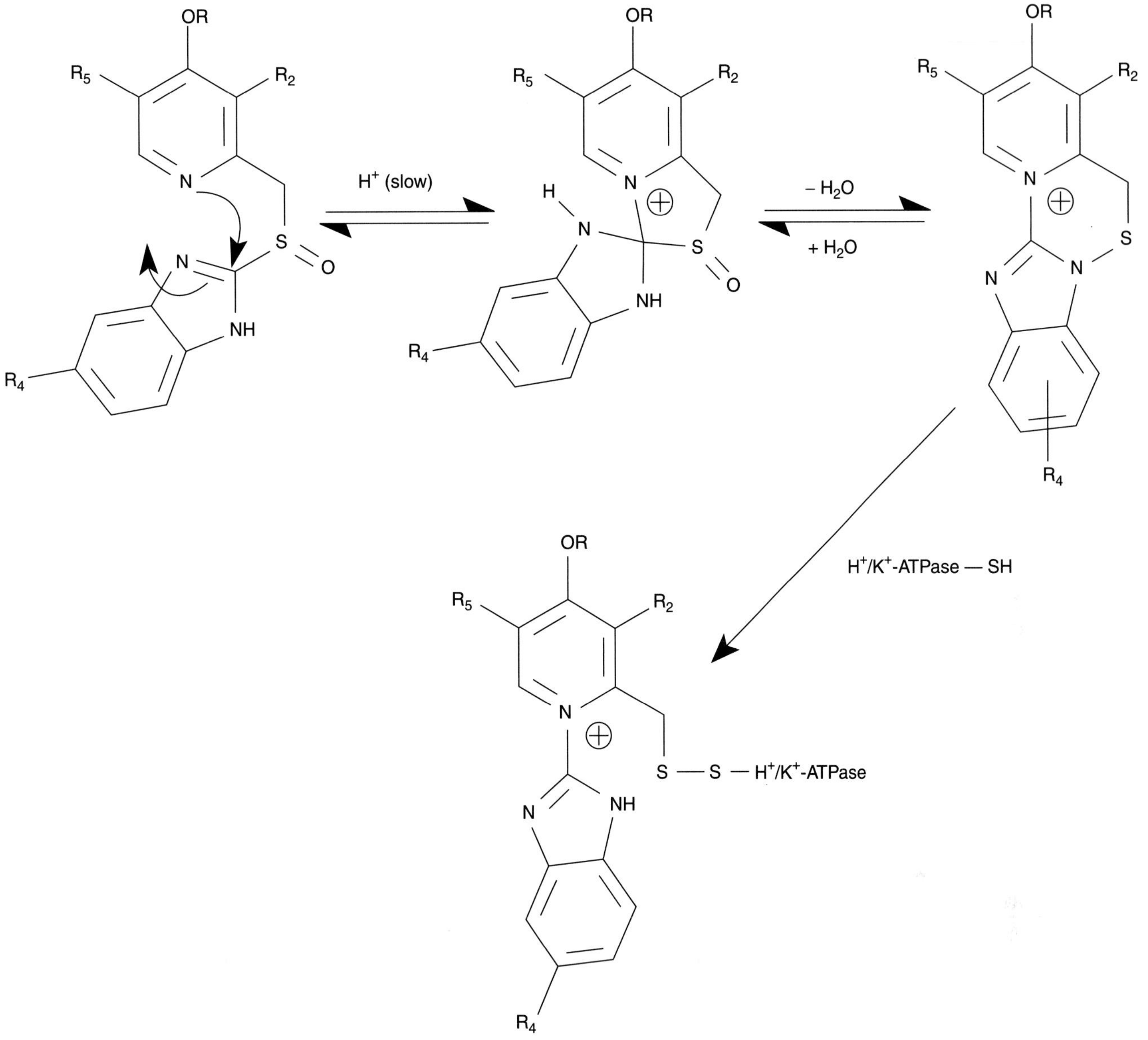

Figure 21–15 ■ Mechanism of action of PPIs.

TABLE 21–3   Proton Pump Inhibitors Marketed in the United States

Indication	Omeprazole	Lansoprazole	Pantoprazole Sodium	Rabeprazole Sodium	Esomeprazole Magnesium
Duodenal ulcer	✓	✓		✓	
Duodenal ulcer/*H. pylori*	✓	✓			✓
Erosive esophagitis	✓	✓	✓	✓	✓
Gastric ulcer	✓	✓			
GERD	✓	✓	✓	✓	✓
Hypersecretory conditions	✓	✓		✓	

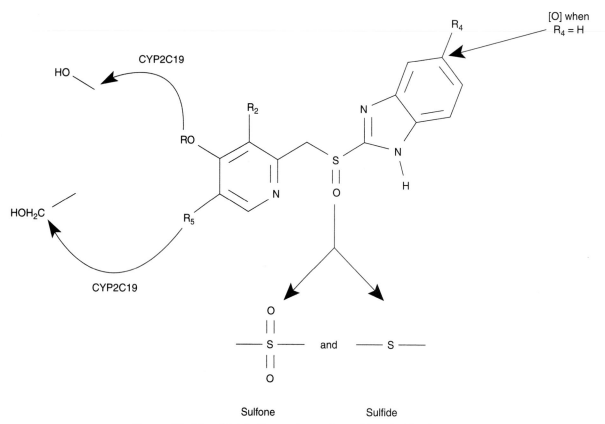

Figure 21–16 ■ Metabolic transformations of benzimidazole PPIs.

mary metabolites of omeprazole are 5-hydroxymeprazole (cytochrome P-450 [CYP] isozyme 2C19) and omeprazole sulfone (CYP 3A4). The antisecretory actions of omeprazole persist for 24 to 72 hours, long after the drug has disappeared from plasma, which is consistent with its suggested mechanism of action involving irreversible inhibition of the proton pump H+/K+-ATPase.[59]

Omeprazole is approved for the treatment and reduction of risk of recurrence of duodenal ulcer, GERD, gastric ulcer, and pathological hypersecretory conditions.

Usual adult dose: Oral, 20 mg q.d.
Dosage form: Delayed-release capsules containing 20 mg of omeprazole in enteric-coated granules

Esomeprazole Magnesium. Esomeprazole magnesium, *S*-bis(5-methoxy-2-[(*S*)-[(4-methoxy-3,5-dimethyl-2-pyridinyl)methyl]sulfinyl]-1*H*-benzimidazole-1-yl) magne-

sium trihydrate (Nexium), is the *S* enantiomer of omeprazole. The benzimidazole PPIs contain a chiral sulfur atom that forms an enantiomeric pair that is stable and insoluble under standard conditions. The *S* isomer of omeprazole has slightly greater PPI activity, and its intrinsic clearance is approximately 3 times lower than that of *R* omeprazole (15 versus 43 μL/min). The lower clearance of *S*-omeprazole is related to slower metabolic clearance by the CYP 2C19 isozyme. Although *R*-omeprazole is primarily transformed to the 5-hydroxy metabolite, the *S* isomer is metabolized by O-demethylation and sulfoxidation, which contribute little to intrinsic clearance.

Usual adult dose:
  Erosive esophagitis: Healing dose: 20 or 40 mg q.d. for 4–8 weeks; maintenance dose: 20 mg q.d.
  Treatment of GERD: 20 mg q.d. for 4 weeks;
  H. pylori eradication: 40 mg q.d. for 10 days in combination with amoxicillin (1 g b.i.d. for 10 days) and clarithromycin (500 mg b.i.d. for 10 days)
Dosage form:
  Oral: Delayed-release capsules, 20 or 40 mg of esomeprazole (present as 22.3 mg or 44.5 mg esomeprazole magnesium trihydrate) as enteric-coated pellets

Lansoprazole. Lansoprazole, 2-[[[3-methyl-4-(2,2,2-trifluoroethoxy)-2-pyridyl]methyl]sulfinyl]benzimidazole (Prevacid), is a white to brownish-white, odorless crystalline powder that is practically insoluble in water. Lansoprazole is a weak base (pyridine N, pK$_a$ 4.01) and a weak acid (benzimidazole N-H, pK$_a$ 1.48). Like omeprazole, lansoprazole is

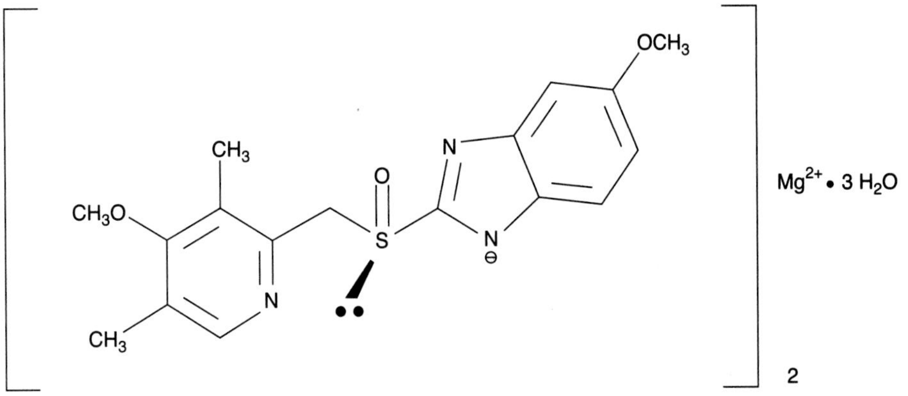

Esomeprazole Magnesium

essentially a prodrug that, in the acidic biophase of the parietal cell, forms an active metabolite that irreversibly interacts with the target ATPase of the pump. Lansoprazole must be formulated as encapsulated enteric-coated granules for oral administration to protect the drug from the acidic environment of the stomach.

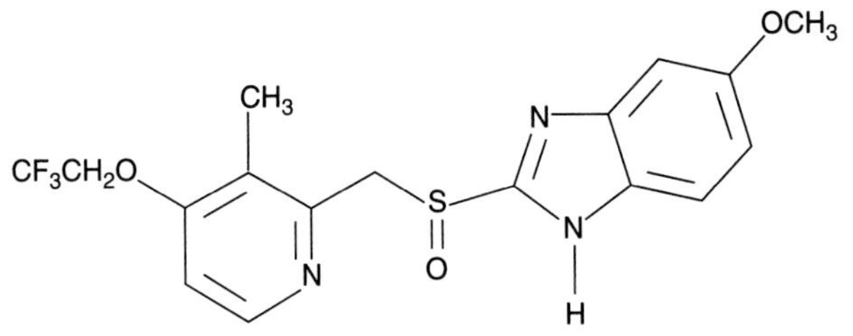

Lansoprazole

In the fasting state, about 80% of a dose of lansoprazole (versus ~50% of omeprazole) reaches the systemic circulation, where it is 97% bound to plasma proteins. The drug is metabolized in the liver (sulfone and hydroxy metabolites) and excreted in bile and urine, with a plasma half-life of about 1.5 hours.[60]

Usual adult dose: Daily oral dose administered before breakfast
    Duodenal ulcer: 15 mg once daily

Erosive esophagitis: 30 mg
Zollinger-Ellison syndrome: 60 mg
NSAID-induced gastric ulcers: treatment and prevention
Dosage form: Delayed-release capsules containing 15 and 30 mg of lansoprazole in enteric-coated granules

Pantoprazole Sodium. The active ingredient in Protonix (pantoprazole sodium) is a substituted benzimidazole, sodium 5-(difluoromethoxy)-2-[[(3,4-dimethoxy-2-pyridinyl)methyl]sulfinyl]-1*H*-benzimidazole sesquihydrate (1.5 H_2O), a compound with a molecular weight of 432.4. The benzimidazoles have weakly basic (pyridine N, pK_a 3.96) and acidic (benzimidazole N-H, pK_a 0.89) properties, which facilitate their formulation as salts of alkaline materials (Fig. 21-17). Pantoprazole sodium sesquihydrate is a white to off-white crystalline powder and is racemic. Pantoprazole sodium sesquihydrate is freely soluble in water, very slightly soluble in phosphate buffer at pH 7.4, and practically insoluble in *n*-hexane. The stability of the compound in aqueous solution is pH dependent; the rate of degradation increases with decreasing pH. At ambient temperature, the degradation half-life is approximately 2.8 hours at pH 5.0 and approximately 220 hours at pH 7.8.

The absorption of pantoprazole is rapid (C_{max} of 2.5 μg/mL, T_{max} ~2.5 hours) after single or multiple oral 40-mg doses. Pantoprazole is well absorbed (~77% bioavailability). Administration of pantoprazole with food may delay its absorption but does not alter its bioavailability. Pantoprazole

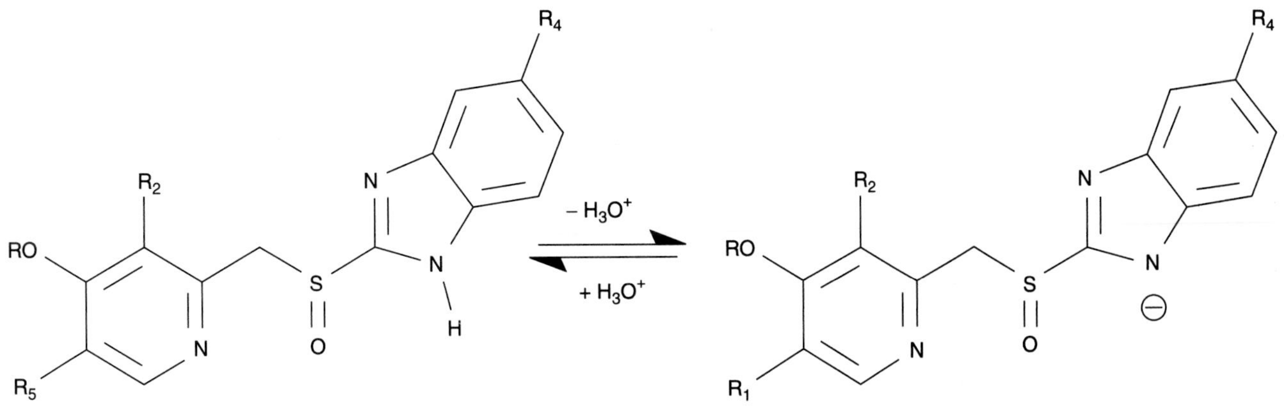

Figure 21-17 ■ Ionization of benzimidazole PPIs.

is distributed mainly in extracellular fluid. The serum protein binding of pantoprazole is about 98%, primarily to albumin. Pantoprazole is extensively metabolized in the liver through the CYP system, including O-demethylation (CYP 2C19), with subsequent sulfation. Other metabolic pathways include sulfur oxidation by CYP 3A4. There is no evidence that any of the pantoprazole metabolites have significant pharmacological activity. Approximately 71% of a dose of pantoprazole is excreted in the urine, with 18% excreted in the feces through biliary excretion.

Pantoprazole Sodium

Usual adult dose:
Erosive esophagitis associated with GERD: 40 mg q.d. for ≤8 weeks; if not healed after 8 weeks of treatment, an additional 8-week course may be considered
Long-term treatment of erosive esophagitis and GERD: IV treatment of erosive esophagitis as an alternative to continued oral therapy, 40 mg q.d. by infusion for 7–10 days
Short-term treatment (7 to 10 days) of GERD
Treatment of pathological hypersecretory conditions associated with Zollinger-Ellison syndrome
Dosage form:
Protonix: Delayed-release tablet for oral administration; each tablet contains 45.1 mg of pantoprazole sodium sesquihydrate (equivalent to 40 mg pantoprazole)
Protonix I.V.: Freeze-dried powder for injection equivalent to 40 mg pantoprazole/vial

Rabeprazole Sodium. Rabeprazole sodium, 2-[[[4-(3-methoxypropoxy)-3-methyl-2-pyridinyl]methyl]sulfinyl]-1 *H*-benzimidazole sodium salt (Aciphex), is a substituted benzimidazole with a molecular weight of 381.43. Rabeprazole sodium is a white to slightly yellowish-white solid. It is very soluble in water and methanol, freely soluble in ethanol, chloroform, and ethyl acetate, and insoluble in ether and *n*-hexane. Rabeprazole is a weak base (pyridine N, pK_a 4.90) and a weak acid (benzimidazole N-H, pK_a 1.60).

Rabeprazole Sodium

Rabeprazole sodium is formulated as enteric-coated, delayed-release tablets to allow the drug to pass through the stomach relatively intact. After oral administration of 20 mg, peak plasma concentrations (C_{max}) occur over a range of 2.0 to 5.0 hours (T_{max}). Absolute bioavailability for a 20-mg oral tablet of rabeprazole (versus IV administration) is approximately 52%. The plasma half-life of rabeprazole ranges from 1 to 2 hours. The effects of food on the absorption of rabeprazole have not been evaluated. Rabeprazole is 96.3% bound to human plasma proteins. Rabeprazole is extensively metabolized in the liver. The thioether and sulfone are the primary metabolites measured in human plasma resulting from CYP 3A oxidation. Additionally, desmethyl rabeprazole is formed via the action of CYP 2C19. Approximately 90% of the drug is eliminated in the urine, primarily as thioether carboxylic acid and its glucuronide and mercapturic acid metabolites. The remainder of the dose is recovered in the feces. Total recovery of radioactivity was 99.8%. No unchanged rabeprazole was recovered in the urine or feces.

Usual adult dose: Oral, 20 mg once daily (duodenal ulcer for 4 weeks; erosive or ulcerative GERD for 4–8 weeks); gastric hypersecretory disorders, 60 mg once daily titrated to a maximum of 120 mg/day
Dosage form: 20-mg delayed release tablets of the sodium salt

CHEMICAL COMPLEXATION

The sulfate esters and sulfonate derivatives of polysaccharides and lignin form chemical complexes with the enzyme pepsin. These complexes have no proteolytic activity. Because polysulfates and polysulfonates are poorly absorbed from the GI tract, specific chemical complexation appears to be a desirable mechanism of pepsin inhibition. Unfortunately, these polymers are also potent anticoagulants.

The properties of chemical complexation and anticoagulant action are separable by structural variation. In a comparison of selected sulfated saccharides of increasing number of monosaccharide units, from disaccharides through starch-derived polysaccharides of differing molecular size, three conclusions are supported by the data: (a) the anticoagulant activity of sulfated saccharide is positively related to molecular size, (b) anticoagulant activity is absent in the disaccharides, and (c) the inhibition of pepsin activity and the protection against experimentally induced ulceration depend on the degree of sulfation and not on molecular size.

The readily available disaccharide sucrose has been used to develop a useful antiulcer agent, sucralfate.

Sucralfate. Sucralfate, 3,4,5,6-tetra-(polyhydroxyaluminum)-α-D-glucopyranosyl sulfate-2,3,4,5-tetra-(polyhydroxyaluminum)-β-D-fructofuranoside sulfate (Carafate), is the aluminum hydroxide complex of the octasulfate ester of sucrose. It is practically insoluble in water and soluble in strong acids and bases. It has a pK_a value between 0.43 and 1.19.

Sucralfate is minimally absorbed from the GI tract and thus exerts its antiulcer effect through local rather than systemic action. It has negligible acid-neutralizing or buffering capacity in therapeutic doses.

Its mechanism of action has not been established. Studies suggest that sucralfate binds preferentially to the ulcer site to form a protective barrier that prevents exposure of the lesion to acid and pepsin. In addition, it adsorbs pepsin and bile salts. Either would be very desirable modes of action.

R = SO$_3$Al(OH)$_2$

[Al(OH)$_3$]$_x$ [H$_2$O]$_y$
(x = 8 to 10 and y = 22 to 31)

The product labeling states that the simultaneous administration of sucralfate may reduce the bioavailability of certain agents (e.g., tetracycline, phenytoin, digoxin, or cimetidine). It further recommends restoration of bioavailability by separating administration of these agents from that of sucralfate by 2 hours. Presumably, sucralfate binds these agents in the GI tract.

The most frequently reported adverse reaction to sucralfate is constipation (2.2%). Antacids may be prescribed as needed but should not be taken within one-half hour before or after sucralfate.

Usual adult dose: Oral, 1 g q.i.d. on an empty stomach
Dosage form: 1-g sucralfate tablets

PROSTAGLANDINS

The prostaglandins are endogenous 20-carbon unsaturated fatty acids biosynthetically derived from arachidonic acid. These bioactive substances and their synthetic derivatives have been of considerable research and development interest as potential therapeutic agents because of their widespread physiological and pharmacological actions on the cardiovascular system, GI smooth muscle, the reproductive system, the nervous system, platelets, kidney, the eye, etc.[61] Prostaglandins of the E, F, and I series are found in significant concentrations throughout the GI tract. The GI actions of the prostaglandins include inhibition of basal and stimulated gastric acid and pepsin secretion in addition to prevention of ulcerogen or irritant-induced gross mucosal lesions of the stomach and intestine (termed *cytoprotection*). The prostaglandins can both stimulate (PGFs) and inhibit (PGEs and PGIs) intestinal smooth muscle contractility and accumulation of fluid and electrolytes in the gut lumen (PGEs). Therapeutic application of the natural prostaglandins in the treatment of GI disorders is hindered by their lack of pharmacological selectivity coupled with a less-than-optimal biodisposition profile.

Misoprostol. Misoprostol, (±)-methyl 11α,16-dihydroxy-16-methyl-9-oxoprost-13*E*-en-1-oate, is a semisynthetic derivative of PGE$_1$ that derives some pharmacological selectivity as well as enhanced biostability from its 16-methyl, 16-hydroxy structural features. Misoprostol exhibits both antisecretory and cytoprotectant effects characteristic of the natural prostaglandins and has a therapeutically acceptable biodisposition profile. Although the antisecretory effects of misoprostol are thought to be related to its agonistic actions at parietal cell prostaglandin receptors, its cyto-

protective actions are proposed to be related to increases in GI mucus and bicarbonate secretion, increases in mucosal blood flow, and/or prevention of back diffusion of H$_3$O$^+$ into the gastric mucosa.[62]

Misoprostol

Misoprostol is rapidly absorbed following oral administration and undergoes rapid deesterification to the pharmacologically active free acid with a terminal half-life of 20 to 40 minutes.[62] Misoprostol is commonly used to prevent NSAID-induced gastric ulcers in patients at high risk of complications from a gastric ulcer, such as elderly patients and patients with a history of ulcer. Misoprostol has also been used in treating duodenal ulcers unresponsive to histamine H$_2$ antagonists; the drug does not prevent duodenal ulcers, however, in patients taking NSAIDS. Misoprostol can cause miscarriage, often associated with potentially dangerous bleeding.

Usual adult dose: Oral, 200 μg q.i.d. with food
Dosage form: 100- and 200-μg tablets

HISTAMINE H$_3$-RECEPTOR LIGANDS[63, 64]

Histamine H$_3$ receptors are members of the G-protein–coupled receptor family involved in the regulation of neurotransmitter release in both central and peripheral neurons. The cDNA for the human histamine H$_3$ receptor encodes a 445-amino acid protein that, when recombinantly expressed, couples to inhibition of adenylate cyclase, presumably through Gαi. The histamine H$_3$-receptor mRNA is highly expressed in central nervous tissues. Histamine H$_3$ heteroreceptors have been identified in stomach, lung, and cardiac tissues of animals. Presynaptic H$_3$ receptors have been implicated in regulating neurotransmitter release from histaminergic, noradrenergic, dopaminergic, cholinergic, serotoninergic, and peptidergic neurons. The potential therapeutic roles of histamine H$_3$-receptor antagonists in the CNS have been evaluated in models of learning and memory impairment, attention-deficit hyperactivity disorder, obesity, and epilepsy. Studies of the regulation of inflammatory processes, gastroprotection, and cardiovascular function suggest several therapeutic possibilities for peripherally acting histamine H$_3$-receptor agonists. As yet, no histamine H$_3$-receptor ligands have been approved for marketing in the United States.

Potent H$_3$ agonists (Fig. 21-18) are obtained by simple modifications of the histamine molecule. The imidazole ring is a common structural feature in almost all H$_3$ agonists. Methylation of the aminoethyl side chain of histamine favors

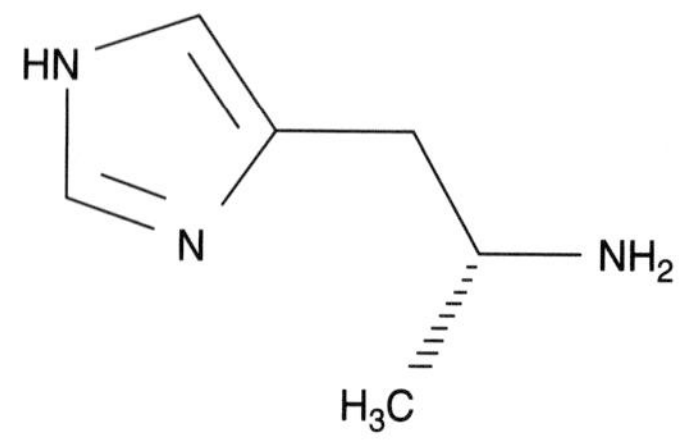

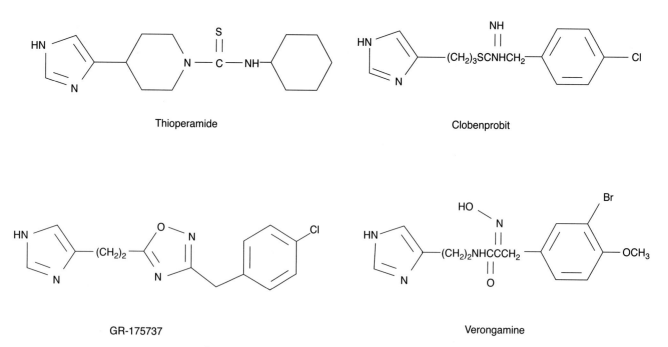

R-α-Methylhistamine

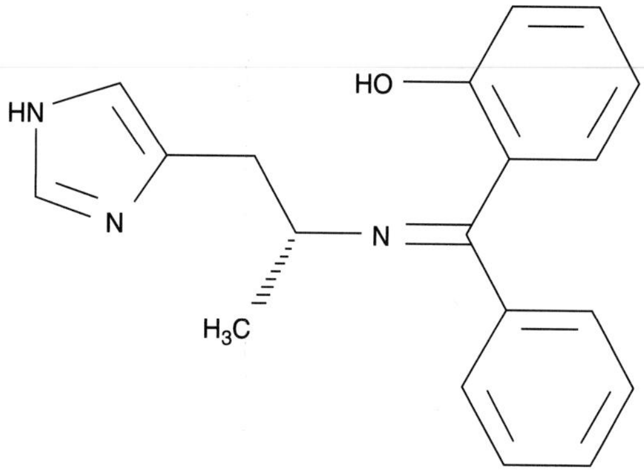

Azomethine derivative of
R-α-Methylhistamine

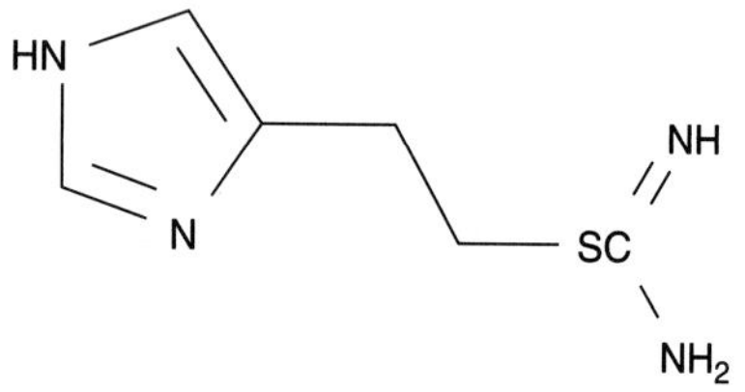

Imetit

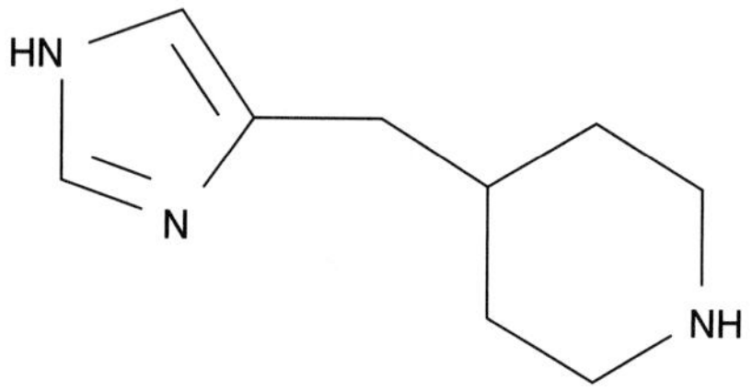

Immepip

Figure 21–18 ■ Histamine H₃-receptor agonists.

Thioperamide

Clobenprobit

GR-175737

Verongamine

Figure 21–19 ■ Histamine H₃-receptor antagonists.

H_3 activity. Introduction of one or two methyl groups to give α-methylhistamine and α,α-dimethylhistamine yields potent H_3 agonists that show little selectivity among the three histamine receptors. The increased potency of α-methyl-histamine is ascribed almost completely to its R isomer (H_3/H_1 ratio = 17). The clinical use of R-α-methylhistamine is compromised by rapid catabolism by histamine-N-methyltransferase. Azomethine derivatives of R-α-methylhistamine have been developed and shown to possess anti-inflammatory and antinociceptive properties. Other H_3 agonists include the isothiourea derivative, imetit, a highly selective, full agonist that is more potent than R-α-methylhistamine. A third type of H_3 agonist is immepip, which may be considered as a histamine analogue with an elongated and cyclized side chain. Immepip is both a highly selective and potent H_3 agonist.

A large number of H_3 antagonists have been described. Antagonist studies have suggested the presence of H_3-receptor subtypes. In general, antagonist structures conform to the following general representation:[65]

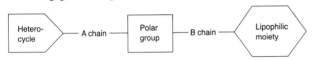

The heterocycle component of this general structure is most commonly a 4-monosubstituted imidazole or bioisosteric equivalent. Chains A and B can be of various structures and lengths, and there is also wide latitude in the structural requirements for the polar group. Halogenated phenyl, cycloalkyl, and heteroaryl structures are usually found for the lipophilic moiety (Fig. 21-19).

Thioperamide was the first potent H_3 antagonist to be described. This agent enhances arousal and/or vigilant patterns in a dose-dependent fashion in animals, suggesting possible use of CNS-acting H_3 antagonists in treating sleep disorders characterized by excessive daytime sleep, such as narcolepsy. Other H_3-antagonist structures are shown below, including the natural product verongamine, isolated from a sea sponge.

REFERENCES

1. Garrison, J. C.: Histamine, bradykinin, 5-hydroxytryptamine, and their antagonists. In Gilman, A. G., Rall, T. W., Nies, A. S., and Taylor, P. (eds.). Goodman and Gilman's The Pharmacological Basis of Therapeutics, 8th ed. New York, Pergamon, 1990, p. 575.
2. Saxena, A. K., and Saxena, M.: Prog. Drug Res. 39:35, 1992.
3. Durant, G. J., Ganellin, C. R., and Parsons, M. E.: J. Med. Chem. 18: 905–909, 1975.
4. Casy, A. F.: The Steric Factor in Medicinal Chemistry. Dissymmetric Probes of Pharmacological Receptors. New York, Plenum Press, 1993, Chap. 11.
5. Falus, A.: Histamine and Inflammation. Austin, TX, R. G. Landes, 1994, Chap. 1.1, p. 2.
6. Falus, A.: Histamine and Inflammation. Austin, TX, R. G. Landes, 1994, Chap. 1.3, p. 33.
7. Hill, S. J., Ganellin, C. R., Timmerman, H., et al. Pharmacol. Rev. 49: 253–278, 1997.
8. Timmerman, H.: Trends Pharmacol. Sci. 13:6–7, 1992.
9. Birdsall, N. J. M.: Trends Pharmacol. Sci., 12:9–10, 1991.
10. Leurs, R., Timmerman, H., and Watanabe T.: Trends Pharmacol. Sci. 22:337–339, 2001.
11. Maslinski, C., and Fogel, W. A.: Catabolism of Histamine. In Uvnäs, B. (ed.). Histamine and Histamine Antagonists, Handbook of Experimental Pharmacology, vol. 97. New York, Springer-Verlag, 1991, Chap. 5.
12. Pelletier, G.: Naturally occurring antihistaminics in body tissues. In Rocha e Silva, M. (ed.). Handbook of Experimental Pharmacology, vol. 18/2. New York, Springer-Verlag, 1978, p. 369.
13. Best, C. H., et al.: J. Physiol. (Lond.) 62:397, 1927.
14. Fourneau, E., and Bovet, D.: Arch. Int. Pharmacodyn. 46:178, 1933.
15. Casy, A. F.: Chemistry of anti-H1 histamine antagonists. In Rocha e Silva, M. (ed.). Handbook of Experimental Pharmacology, vol. 18/2. New York, Springer-Verlag, 1978, p. 175.
16. Witiak, D. T.: Antiallergenic agents. In Burger, A. (ed.). Medicinal Chemistry, 3rd ed. New York, Wiley Interscience, 1970, p. 1643.
17. Paton, D. M.: Receptors for histamine. In Schachter, M. (ed.). Histamine and Antihistamines, New York, Pergamon Press, 1973, p. 3.
18. Rocha e Silva, M., and Antonio, A.: Bioassay of antihistaminic action. In Rocha e Silva, M. (ed.). Handbook of Experimental Pharmacology, vol. 18/2. New York, Springer-Verlag, 1978, p. 381.
19. Biel, J. H., and Martin, Y. C.: Organic synthesis as a source of new drugs. In Gould, R. F. (ed.). Drug Discovery, Advances in Chemistry Series no. 108. Washington, DC, American Chemical Society, 1971, p. 81.
20. Ahlquist, R. P.: Am. J. Physiol. 153:586, 1948.
21. Lin, T. M., et al.: Ann. N. Y. Acad. Sci. 99:30, 1962.
22. Ash, A. S. F., and Schild, H. O.: Br. J. Pharmacol. Chemother. 27:427, 1966.
23. Black, J. W., et al.: Nature 236:385, 1972.
24. Metzler, D. E., Ikawa, M., and Snell, E. E.: J. Am. Chem. Soc. 76: 648, 1954.
25. Schayer, R. W., and Cooper, J. A. D.: J. Appl. Physiol. 9:481, 1956.
26. Schayer, R. W.: Biogenesis of histamine. In Rocha e Silva, M. (ed.). Handbook of Experimental Pharmacology, vol. 18/2. New York, Springer-Verlag, 1978, p. 109.
27. Wetterqvist, H.: Histamine metabolism and excretion. In Rocha e Silva, M. (ed.). Handbook of Experimental Pharmacology, vol. 18/2. New York, Springer-Verlag, 1978, p. 131.
28. Ganellin, C. R., and Parsons, M. E. (eds.): Pharmacology of Histamine Receptors. Bristol, U. K., Wright, 1982.
29. Fordtran, J. S., and Grossman, M. I. (eds.): Third Symposium on Histamine H2-Receptor Antagonists: Clinical Results with Cimetidine. Gastroenterology 74(2):339, 1978.
30. Douglas, W. W.: Histamine and 5-hydroxytryptamine (serotonin) and their antagonists.. In Gilman, A. G., Goodman, L. S., Rall, T. W., and Murad, F. (eds.). Goodman and Gilman's The Pharmacological Basis of Therapeutics, 7th ed. New York, Macmillan, 1985, p. 605.
31. van den Brink, F. G., and Lien, E. J.: Competitive and noncompetitive antagonism. In Rocha e Silva, M. (ed.). Handbook of Experimental Pharmacology, vol. 18/2. New York, Springer-Verlag, 1978, p. 333.
32. Nauta, W. T., and Rekker, R. F.: Structure-activity relationships of Hl-receptor antagonists. In Rocha e Silva, M. (ed.). Handbook of Experimental Pharmacology, vol. 18/2. New York, Springer-Verlag, 1978, p. 215.
33. Ganellin, C. R.: Annu. Rep. Med. Chem. 14:91, 1979.
34. Sjoquist, F., and Lasagna, L.: Clin. Pharmacol. Ther. 8:48, 1967.
35. Barouh, V., et al.: J. Med. Chem. 14:834, 1971.
36. Shafi'ee, A., and Hite, G.: J. Med. Chem. 12:266, 1969.
37. Nobles, W. L., and Blanton, C. D.: J. Pharm. Sci. 53:115, 1964.
38. Toldy, L., et al.: Acta Chim. Acad. Sci. Hung. 19:273, 1959.
39. Ison, R. R., Franks, F. M., and Soh, K. S.: J. Pharm. Pharmacol. 25: 887, 1973.
40. King, C. T. G., Weaver, S. R., and Narrod, S. A.: J. Pharmacol. Exp. Ther. 147:391, 1965.
41. Criep, L. H.: Lancet 68:55, 1948.
42. Landau, S. W., Nelson, W. A., and Gay. L. N.: J. Allergy 22:19, 1951.
43. Villani, F. J., et al.: J. Med. Chem. 15:750, 1972.
44. Intal 0, Cromolyn Sodium, A Monograph. Bedford, MA, Fisons Corporation, 1973.
45. Johnson, P. C., Gillespie, E., and Temple, D. L.: Annu. Rep. Med. Chem. 17:55, 1982.
46. Caldwell, D. R., Verin, P., Hartwich-Young, R., et al. Am. J. Ophthalmol. 113:632–637, 1992.
47. Tanaka, M.: Drugs Today 28:29–31, 1992.
48. McTavish, D., and Sorkin, E. M.: Drugs 38:778–800, 1989.
49. Martin, U., and Romer, D.: Arzneimittelforschung 28:770–782, 1978.
50. Feldman, M., and Burton, M. E.: N. Engl. J. Med. 323:1672–1680, 1990.
51. Feldman, M., and Burton, M. E.: N. Engl. J. Med. 323:1749–1755, 1990.

52. Soll, A. H.: N. Engl. J. Med. 322:909–916, 1990.
53. Black, J.: Science 245:486–493, 1989.
54. Brittain, R. T., Jack, D., and Price, B. J.: Trends Pharmacol. Sci. 2: 310–313, 1981.
55. Brändström, A., Lindberg, P., and Junggren, U.: Scand. J. Gastroenterol. 20(Suppl. 108):15–22, 1985.
56. Bauer, R. F., Collins, P. W., and Jones, P. H.: Annu. Rep. Med. Chem. 22:191, 1987.
57. Langman, M. J. S.: Gut 49:309–310, 2001.
58. Meyer, U. A.: Yale J. Biol. Med. 69:203–209, 1996.
59. Lampkin, T. A., Ouellet, D., Hak, L. J., and Dukes, G. E.: DICP 24: 393–402, 1990.
60. Spencer, C. M., and Faulds, D.: Drugs 48:405–431, 1992.
61. Konturek, S. J., and Pawlik, W.: Dig. Dis. Sci. 31:6–19, 1986.
62. Monk, J. P., and Clissold, S. P.: Drugs 33:1–30, 1987.
63. Leurs, R., and Timmerman, H.: Prog. Drug Res. 39:127, 1992.
64. Phillips, J. G., Ali, S. M., Yates, S. L., and Tedford, C. E.: Annu. Rep. Med. Chem. 33:31–40, 1998.
65. Stark, H., Ligneau, X., Arrang, J.-M., et al.: Bioorg. Med. Chem. Lett. 8:2011–2016, 1998.

SELECTED READING

Bass, P.: Gastric antisecretory and antiulcer agents. Adv. Drug Res. 8:206, 1974.
Beaven, M. A.: Histamine, Its Role in Physiological and Pathological Processes. Monogr. Allergy, vol. 13. New York, S. Karger, 1978.
Burland, W. L., and Simkins, M. A. (eds.): Cimetidine, Proceedings of the Second International Symposium on Histamine H2-Receptor Antagonists. New York, Excerpta Medica/Elsevier, 1977.
Fordtran, J. S., and Grossman, M. I. (eds.): Third Symposium on Histamine H2-Receptor Antagonists, Clinical Results with Cimetidine. Gastroenterology 74(2, Part 2):339, 1978.
GERD Information Resource Center: http://www.gerd.com/
Leurs, R., Smit, M. J., and Timmerman, H.: Molecular pharmacological aspects of histamine receptors. Pharmacol. Ther. 66:413–463, 1995.
Nelson, W. L.: Antihistamines and related antiallergic and antiulcer agents. In Williams, D.A., and Lemke, T. L. (ed.). Foye's Principles of Medicinal Chemistry, 5th ed. Baltimore, Lippincott Williams & Wilkins, 2002, pp. 794–818.
Rocha e Silva, M. (ed.): Histamine and antihistaminics. In Handbook of Experimental Pharmacology, vol. 18/1. New York, Springer-Verlag, 1966.
Rocha e Silva, M. (ed.): Histamine II and antihistaminics. In Handbook of Experimental Pharmacology, vol. 18/2. New York, Springer-Verlag, 1978.
Schachter, M. (ed.): Histamine and antihistamines. In International Encyclopedia of Pharmacology and Therapeutics, sect. 74, vol. 1. New York, Pergamon, 1973.
Sippy, B. W.: JAMA 250:2192, 1983.
Thompson, J. H.: Gastrointestinal disorders—peptic ulcer disease. In Rubin, A. A. (ed.). Search for New Drugs, Medicinal Research Series, vol. 6. New York, Marcel Dekker, 1972, p. 115.
van der Goot, H., and Timmerman, H.: Selective ligands as tools to study histamine receptors. Eur. J. Med. Chem. 35:5–20, 2000.

Analgesic Agents

ROBERT E. WILLETTE

The struggle to relieve pain began with the origin of humanity. Ancient writings, both serious and fanciful, dealt with secret remedies, religious rituals, and other methods of pain relief. Slowly, the present modern era of synthetic analgesics evolved. An *analgesic* may be defined as a drug bringing about insensibility to pain without loss of consciousness. (The etymologically correct term *analgetic* may be used in place of the incorrect but popular *analgesic*, but the latter is used almost universally.)

Tainter[1] has divided the history of analgesic drugs into four major eras, namely:

1. The period of discovery and use of naturally occurring plant drugs
2. Isolation of pure plant principles (e.g., alkaloids) from the natural sources and their identification with analgesic action
3. Development of organic chemistry and the first synthetic analgesics
4. Development of modern pharmacological techniques, making it possible to undertake a systematic testing of new analgesics

A new era has emerged with the discovery of opioid receptors and endogenous chemicals that have analgesic activity.

The isolation of morphine from opium by Sertürner, in 1803, and the discovery of its analgesic activity (he named it *morphine* after the Greek god of dreams, Morpheus) ushered in the second era. It continues today only on a small scale. Wöhler introduced the third era indirectly with his synthesis of urea in 1828. He showed that chemical synthesis could be used to make and produce drugs. In the third era, the first synthetic analgesics used in medicine were the salicylates, originally found in nature (methyl salicylate, salicin) and then synthesized by chemists. Other early synthesized drugs were acetanilid (1886), phenacetin (1887), and aspirin (1899).

These early discoveries were the principal contributions in this field until modern methods of pharmacological testing initiated the fourth era. The effects of small structural modifications of synthetic molecules then could be assessed accurately by pharmacological means. This permitted systematic study of the relationship of structure to activity during this era. The development of these pharmacological testing procedures, coupled with the fortuitous discovery of meperidine by Eisleb and Schaumann,[2] made possible a period of rapid strides in the development of potent analgesics.

PAIN

The primary use of the drugs covered in this chapter is to relieve pain of a wide array of causes and mechanisms. Pain is the most common complaint for which patients seek treatment. For various reasons, however, including politics and lack of training and ignorance, pain is not well managed; less than half of those with pain are adequately treated. This is primarily due to a fear of addiction, which often limits the proper use of the narcotic or opioid class of analgesics, and lack of training of health care professionals. To understand how and when this broad class of drugs is and should be used in the management of pain requires a brief review of pain.

Pain has been classified into the following types: physiological, inflammatory, and neuropathic. The first is the most common, for example, touching a hot object or getting a cut. Inflammatory pain can be initiated in a wide variety of ways, such as infection and tissue injury. The last type is due to injury to the peripheral or central nervous system (CNS). Within these classes of pain there are different levels of pain or categories of pain. These include acute, chronic, cancer, arthropathy (e.g., arthritis), visceral, neuropathic, and diabetic pain. A separate category is recognized for acquired immunodeficiency syndrome (AIDS) because of its disseminated nature. Clearly, these all require different approaches to pain management.

In the following sections of this chapter, several classes of pain-relieving drugs are described. The three major classes of drugs used to manage pain are opioids, nonsteroidal anti-inflammatory agents, and acetaminophen. A newly emerging class, known as *analgesic adjuvants,* is not covered here.

Of these drug classes, the historically important group of drugs in the opioid class has been the most problematic for use in the proper management of pain. The term *opiophobia* was coined to describe the reluctance of physicians to prescribe opioid drugs in adequate amounts or for long enough periods. As early as the 1970s, the National Institutes of Health formed a committee, at the request of the president, to investigate therapies for rare diseases, but the initial focus was on pain management. There was political pressure to approve the use of heroin for pain, under the mistaken impression that a more potent drug was needed, after several studies showed poor pain management. The committee found that the problem was a lack of training of physicians in pain management and misconceptions about the use of opioids and addiction.[3]

Unfortunately, the problem continued through the end of the 20th century and into the 21st. Over the past few years, major national medical groups, state medical boards, and pharmaceutical groups have formulated guidelines directed at improving pain therapy. Pharmacists and other health professionals must clearly recognize the advances in pain management and the advantages and limitations of the various drugs. For further information on pain and its management, refer to a number of articles and American Pharmaceutical Association continuing education programs.[4–7]

The consideration of naturally occurring and synthetic analgesics is facilitated greatly by dividing them into two groups: *(a)* morphine and related compounds and *(b)* the antipyretic and anti-inflammatory analgesics. Also, numerous drugs that possess distinctive pharmacological activities in other areas also possess analgesic properties and are used as analgesic adjuvants. The analgesic property exerted may be a direct effect or may be indirect, but it is subsidiary to some other, more pronounced effect. Some examples of these, which are discussed elsewhere in this text, are sedatives (e.g., barbiturates), muscle relaxants (e.g., mephenesin, methocarbamol), and tranquilizers (e.g., meprobamate). These drugs are not considered in this chapter.

MORPHINE AND RELATED COMPOUNDS

Historical Perspective

The discovery of morphine early in the 19th century and the demonstration of its potent analgesic properties led directly to the search for similar drugs from plant sources. In tribute to the remarkable potency and action of morphine, it and codeine have remained alone as outstanding and indispensable analgesics from a plant source. Only since 1938 have synthetic compounds rivaling morphine in its action been found, although many earlier synthetic changes made on morphine itself gave more effective agents.

Modifications of the morphine molecule are considered under the following headings:

1. Early changes on morphine before the work of Small, Eddy, and their coworkers
2. Changes on morphine initiated in 1929 by Small, Eddy, and coworkers[8] under the auspices of the Committee on Drug Addiction of the National Research Council and extending to the present time
3. Research initiated by Eisleb and Schaumann[2] in 1938, with their discovery of the potent analgesic action of meperidine, a compound that departs radically from the typical morphine molecule
4. Research initiated by Grewe, in 1946, leading to the successful synthesis of the morphinan group of analgesics

EARLY MORPHINE MODIFICATIONS

Morphine is obtained from opium, which is the partly dried latex from incised unripe capsules of *Papaver somniferum*. Opium contains numerous alkaloids (as meconates and sulfates), of which morphine, codeine, noscapine (narcotine), and papaverine are therapeutically the most important. Thebaine, which has convulsant properties, is an important starting material for many other drugs. Other opium alkaloids, such as narceine, have been tested medicinally but are not of great importance. The action of opium is principally due to its morphine content. As an analgesic, opium is not as effective as morphine because of its slower absorption, but it has a greater constipating action and, thus, is better suited for antidiarrheal preparations (e.g., paregoric). Opium, as a constituent of Dover's powders and Brown Mixture, also

exerts a valuable expectorant action that is superior to that of morphine.

Two basic types of structures are recognized among the opium alkaloids, the *phenanthrene* (morphine) type and the *benzylisoquinoline* (papaverine) type (see structures).

Phenanthrene Type
(Morphine, R & R' = H)

Benzylisoquinoline Type
(Papaverine)

The pharmacological actions of the two types of alkaloids are dissimilar. The morphine group acts principally on the CNS as a depressant and stimulant; the papaverine group has little effect on the nervous system but a marked antispasmodic action on smooth muscle. Clinically, the depressant action of the morphine group is the most useful property, resulting in increased tolerance to pain, a sleepy feeling, a lower perception of external stimuli, and a feeling of well-being (euphoria). Respiratory depression, central in origin, is perhaps the most serious objection to this type of alkaloid, aside from its tendency to cause addiction. The stimulant action is well illustrated by the convulsions produced by certain members of this group (e.g., thebaine).

Before 1929, the derivatives of morphine that were made primarily resulted from simple changes on the molecule, such as esterification of the phenolic and/or alcoholic hydroxyl groups, etherification of the phenolic hydroxyl group, and similar minor changes. The net result was the discovery of some compounds with greater activity than morphine but also with greater toxicity and addiction potential. No compounds were found that completely lacked the addiction liabilities of morphine. (The term *addiction liability* or the preferred term *dependence liability*, as used in this text, indicates the ability of a substance to induce true addictive tolerance and physical dependence and/or to suppress the morphine abstinence syndrome after withdrawal of morphine from addicts.)

Some of the compounds in common use before 1929 are listed in Table 22-1 together with some more recently introduced. All have the common morphine skeleton. Among the earlier compounds is codeine, the phenolic methyl ether of morphine, which also had been obtained from opium. It has survived as a good analgesic and cough depressant, together

TABLE 22–1 Synthetic Derivatives of Morphine

Compound Proprietary Name	R	R'	R"	Principal Use
Morphine	H	H	(with H, OH)	Analgesic
Codeine	CH₃	H	Same as above	Analgesic and to depress cough reflex
Ethylmorphine *Dionin*	C₂H₅	H	Same as above	Ophthalmology
Diacetylmorphine (heroin)	CH₃CO	H	(—O—C(=O)—CH₃)	Analgesic (prohibited in US)
Hydromorphone (dihydromorphinone) *Dilaudid*	H	H	(=O)	Analgesic
Hydrocodone (dihydrocodeinone) *Dicodid*	CH₃	H	Same as above	Analgesic and to depress cough reflex
Oxymorphone (dihydrohydroxymorphinone)	H	OH	Same as above	Analgesic
Oxycodone (dihydrohydroxycodeinone)	CH₃	OH	Same as above	Analgesic and to depress cough reflex
Dihydrocodeine *Paracodin*	CH₃	H	(—OH)	Depress cough reflex
Dihydromorphine	H	H	Same as above	Analgesic
Methyldihydromorphinone *Metopon*	H	H	(OCH₃, O)	

with the corresponding ethyl ether, which has found its principal application in ophthalmology. The diacetyl derivative of morphine, heroin, has been known for a long time; it has been banished for years from the United States and is being used less in other countries. It is the most widely used illicit drug among narcotic addicts. Among the reduced compounds are dihydromorphine and dihydrocodeine and their C-6 oxidized congeners, dihydromorphinone (hydromorphone) and dihydrocodeinone (hydrocodone). Derivatives of the last two compounds that possess a hydroxyl group in position 14 are dihydrohydroxymorphinone, or oxymorphone, and dihydrohydroxycodeinone, or oxycodone. These are the principal compounds that either had been on the market or had been prepared before the studies of Small, Eddy, and coworkers. To this time, no really systematic effort had been made to investigate the structure–activity relationships in the molecule, and only the easily changed peripheral groups had been modified. The only exception is oxymorphone, introduced in the United States in 1959 but mentioned here because it obviously is closely related to oxycodone.

MORPHINE MODIFICATIONS INITIATED BY THE RESEARCH OF SMALL AND EDDY

The avowed purpose of Small, Eddy, and coworkers[8] in 1929 was to approach the morphine problem from the standpoint that it might be possible to separate chemically the addictive property of morphine from its other, more salutary attributes, or if that was not possible, it might be possible to find other synthetic molecules without this undesirable property. Proceeding on these assumptions, these workers first examined the morphine molecule exhaustively. As a starting point, morphine offered the advantages of ready availability, proven potency, and ease of alteration. In addition to its addictive tendency, they hoped that other liabilities (e.g., respiratory depression, emetic properties, and gastrointestinal tract and circulatory disturbances) could be minimized or abolished as well. Because early modifications of morphine (e.g., acetylation or alkylation of hydroxyls and quaternization of the nitrogen) caused variations in the addictive potency, they felt that the physiological effects of morphine could be related, at least in part, to the peripheral groups.

It was not known if the actions of morphine were primarily a function of the peripheral groups or of the structural skeleton. This did not matter, however, because modification of the groups would alter activity in either case. These groups and the effects on activity by modifying them are listed in Table 22-2. The results of these and earlier studies[9] have not always shown the effects of simple modifications on the analgesic action of morphine quantitatively, but they do indicate the direction in which the activity is likely to go. The studies are far more comprehensive than Table 22-2 indicates, and the conclusions usually depend on more than one pair of compounds. Unfortunately, these studies on morphine did not eliminate the addiction potential from these compounds. In fact, the studies suggested that any modification that increased the analgesic activity caused a concomitant increase in addiction liability.

The second phase of the studies[8] dealt with the attempted synthesis of substances with central narcotic and, especially, analgesic action. The morphine molecule contains certain well-defined types of chemical structures. Among these are the phenanthrene nucleus, the dibenzofuran nucleus, and, as a variant of the latter, carbazole. These synthetic studies, although extensive and interesting, provided no significant findings and are not discussed further in this text.

One of the more useful results of the investigations was the synthesis of 5-methyldihydromorphinone (Table 22-1), whose methyl substituent was originally assigned to position

TABLE 22–2   Some Structural Relationships in the Morphine Molecule

Peripheral Groups of Morphine	Modification (On Morphine Unless Otherwise Indicated)	Effects on Analgesic Activity (Morphine or Another Compound as Indicated = 100)
Phenolic hydroxyl	—OH → —OCH$_3$ (codeine)	15
	—OH → —OC$_2$H$_5$ (ethylmorphine)	10
	—OH → —OCH$_2$CH$_2$—N◯O (pholcodine)	1
Alcoholic hydroxyl	—OH → —OCH$_3$ (heterocodeine)	500
	—OH → —OC$_2$H$_5$	240
	—OH → —OCOCH$_3$	420
	—OH → =O (morphinone)	37
	—OH → =O (dihydromorphine to dihydromorphinone)	600 (Dihydromorphine vs. dihydromorphinone)
	—OH → =O (dihydrocodeine to dihydrocodeinone)	390 (Dihydrocodeine vs. dihydrocodeinone)
	—OH → —H (dihydromorphine to dihydrodesoxymorphine-D)	1,000 (Dihydromorphine vs. dihydrodesoxymorphine-D)
Ether bridge	=C—O—CH— → =C—OH HCH— (dihydrodesoxymorphine-D to tetrahydrodesoxymorphine)	13 (Dihydrodesoxymorphine-D vs. tetrahydrodesoxymorphine)
Alicyclic unsaturated linkage	—CH=CH— → —CH$_2$CH$_2$— (dihydromorphine)	120
	—CH=CH— → —CH$_2$CH$_2$— (codeine to dihydrocodeine)	115 (Codeine vs. dihydrocodeine)
Tertiary nitrogen	N—CH$_3$ → N—H (normorphine)	5
	N—CH$_3$ → N—CH$_2$CH$_2$—C$_6$H$_5$	1,400
	N—CH$_3$ → N—R	Reversal of activity (morphine antagonism); R = propyl, isobutyl, allyl, methallyl
	N—CH$_3$ → N$^+$(CH$_3$)$_2$ Cl—	1 (Strong curare action)
	Opening of nitrogen ring (morphimethine)	Marked decrease in action

(Continued)

TABLE 22–2—*Continued*

Peripheral Groups of Morphine	Modification (On Morphine Unless Otherwise Indicated)	Effects on Analgesic Activity (Morphine or Another Compound as Indicated = 100)	
Nuclear substitution	Substitution of:		
	—NH_2 (most likely at position 2)		Marked decrease in action
	—Cl or —Br (at position 1)	50	
	—OH (at position 14 in dihydromorphinone)	250	(Dihydromorphinone vs. oxymorphone)
	—OH (at position 14 in dihydrocodeinone)	530	(Dihydrocodeinone vs. oxycodone)
	—CH_3 (at position 6)	280	
	—CH_3 (at position 6 in dihydromorphine)	33	(Dihydromorphine vs. 6-methyldihydromorphine)
	—CH_3 (at position 6 in dihydrodesoxymorphine-D)	490	(Dihydrodesoxymorphine-D vs. 6-methyldihydrodesoxymorphine)
	=CH_2 (at position 6 in dihydrodesoxymorphine-D)	600	(Dihydrodesoxymorphine-D vs. 6-methylenedihydrodesoxymorphine)

7.[10] Although it possessed addiction liabilities, it was a very potent analgesic with a minimum of the undesirable side effects of morphine, such as emetic action and mental dullness. Later, the high analgesic activity demonstrated by morphine congeners in which the alicyclic ring is either reduced or methylated (or both) and the alcoholic hydroxyl at position 6 is absent prompted the synthesis of related compounds possessing these features. These include 6-methyldihydromorphine and its dehydrated analogue 6-methyl-Δ^6-desoxymorphine or methyldesorphine,[11] both of which have high potency. Also of interest were the compounds morphinone; 6-methylmorphine; and 6-methyl-7-hydroxy-, 6-methyl-, and 6-methylenedihydrodesoxymorphine.[12, 13] In analgesic activity in mice, the last-named compound was 82 times more potent, milligram for milligram, than morphine. Its therapeutic index (TI_{50}) was 22 times that of morphine.[14]

The structure–activity relationships of 14-hydroxymorphine derivatives have been reviewed,[8] and several related compounds were synthesized.[15] Of these, the dihydrodesoxy compounds possessed the most analgesic activity. Also, esters of 14-hydroxycodeine derivatives have shown very high activity.[16] For example, in rats, 14-cinnamyloxycodeinone was 177 times more active than morphine.

In 1963, Bentley and Hardy[17] reported the synthesis of a novel series of potent analgesics derived from the opium alkaloid thebaine. In rats, the most active members of the series (I, R_1 = H, R_2 = CH_3, R_3 = isoamyl; and I, R_1 = $COCH_3$, R_2 = CH_3, R_3 = n-C_3H_7) were several thousand times stronger than morphine.[18] These compounds exhibited marked differences in activity of optical isomers, as well as other interesting structural effects. It was postulated that the more rigid molecular structure might allow them to fit the receptor surface better. Extensive structural and pharmacological studies have been reported.[19] Some of the N-cyclopropylmethyl compounds are the most potent antagonists yet discovered and have been studied very intensively.

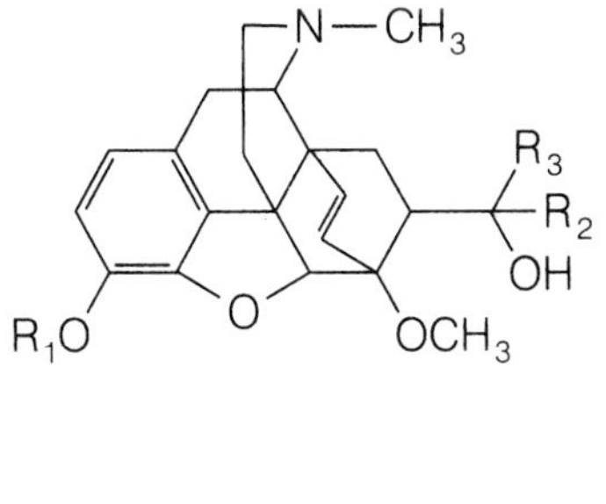

As indicated in Table 22-2, replacement of the N-methyl group in morphine by larger alkyl groups not only lowers analgesic activity, but also confers morphine-antagonistic properties on the molecule (discussed below). In direct contrast to this effect, the N-phenethyl derivative has 14 times the analgesic activity of morphine. This enhancement of activity by N-aralkyl groups has wide application, as is shown below.

Some of the morphine antagonists, such as nalorphine, are also strong analgesics.[20] The similarity of the ethylenic double bond and the cyclopropyl group has prompted the synthesis of N-cyclopropylmethyl derivatives of morphine and its derivatives.[21] This substituent usually confers strong narcotic antagonistic activity, with variable effects on analgesic potency. The dihydronormorphinone derivative has only moderate analgesic activity.

MORPHINE MODIFICATIONS INITIATED BY THE RESEARCH OF EISLEB AND SCHAUMANN

In 1938, Eisleb and Schaumann[2] reported the fortuitous discovery that a simple piperidine derivative, now known as meperidine, possessed analgesic activity. It was prepared as an antispasmodic, a property it also possesses. As the story is told, during the pharmacological testing of meperidine in mice, it was observed to cause the peculiar erection of the tail known as the Straub reaction. Because this reaction is characteristic of morphine and its derivatives, the compound then was tested for analgesic properties and found to be about one fifth as active as morphine. This finding led not only to the discovery of an active analgesic, but far more important, it stimulated research. The status of research on analgesic compounds with an activity comparable to that of morphine was at a low ebb in 1938. Many felt that potent compounds could not be prepared, unless they were very closely related structurally to morphine. The demonstration of high potency in a synthetic compound that was related only distantly to morphine, however, spurred the efforts of various research groups.[22, 23]

The first efforts, naturally, were made on the meperidine-type molecule in an attempt to enhance its activity further. It was found that replacement of the 4-phenyl group by hydrogen, alkyl, other aryl, aralkyl, and heterocyclic groups reduced analgesic activity. Placement of the phenyl and ester groups at the 4 position of 1-methylpiperidine also gave optimum activity. Several modifications of this fundamental structure are listed in Table 22-3.

Among the simplest changes shown to increase activity is the insertion of an *m*-hydroxyl group on the phenyl ring.

It is in the same relative position as in morphine. The effect is more pronounced on the keto compound (Table 22-3, A-4) than on meperidine (A-1). Ketobemidone is equivalent to morphine in activity and was once widely used.

More significantly, Jensen et al.[24] discovered that replace-

TABLE 22–3 Compounds Related to Meperidine

(R$_5$ = H except in trimeperidine, where it is CH$_3$)

Com-pound	Structure				Name (If Any)	Analgesic Activity (Meperidine = 1)
	R$_1$	R$_2$	R$_3$	R$_4$		
A-1	—C$_6$H$_5$	—COOC$_2$H$_5$	—CH$_2$CH$_2$—	—CH$_3$	Meperidine	1.0
A-2	(phenyl with OH)	—COOC$_2$H$_5$	—CH$_2$CH$_2$	—CH$_3$	Bemidone	1.5
A-3	—C$_6$H$_5$	—COOCH(CH$_3$)$_2$	—CH$_2$CH$_2$—	—CH$_3$	Properidine	15
A-4	—C$_6$H$_5$	—C(=O)—C$_2$H$_5$	—CH$_2$CH$_2$—	—CH$_3$		0.5
A-5	(phenyl with OH)	—C(=O)—C$_2$H$_5$	—CH$_2$CH$_2$—	—CH$_3$	Ketobemidone	6.2
A-6	—C$_6$H$_5$	—O—C(=O)—C$_2$H$_5$	—CH$_2$CH$_2$—	—CH$_3$		5
A-7	—C$_6$H$_5$	—O—C(=O)—C$_2$H$_5$	—CH$_2$CH(CH$_3$)—	—CH$_3$	Alphaprodine / Betaprodine	5 / 14
A-8	—C$_6$H$_5$	—O—C(=O)—C$_2$H$_5$	—CH$_2$CH(CH$_3$)—	—CH$_3$ (R$_5$ = CH$_3$)	Trimeperidine	7.5
A-9	—C$_6$H$_5$	—COOC$_2$H$_5$	—CH$_2$CH$_2$—	—CH$_2$CH$_2$C$_6$H$_5$	Pheneridine	2.6
A-10	—C$_6$H$_5$	—COOC$_2$H$_5$	—CH$_2$CH$_2$—	—CH$_2$CH$_2$—(C$_6$H$_4$)—NH$_2$	Anileridine	3.5
A-11	—C$_6$H$_5$	—COOC$_2$H$_5$	—CH$_2$CH$_2$—	—(CH$_2$)$_3$—NH—C$_6$H$_5$	Piminodine	55
A-12	—C$_6$H$_5$	—O—C(=O)—C$_2$H$_5$	—CH$_2$CH$_2$—	—CH$_2$CH$_2$CHC$_6$H$_5$ (O—C(=O)—C$_2$H$_5$)		1,880
A-13	—C$_6$H$_5$	—COOC$_2$H$_5$	—CH$_2$CH$_2$—	—CH$_2$CH$_2$C(C$_6$H$_5$)$_2$ (CN)	Diphenoxylate	None

(Continued)

TABLE 22–3—*Continued*

Com-pound	Structure				Name (If Any)	Analgesic Activity (Meperidine = 1)
	R_1	R_2	R_3	R_4		
A-14	$-C_6H_4$-*p*-Cl	$-OH$	$-CH_2CH_2-$	$-CH_2CH_2C(C_6H_5)_2$ $\overset{\mid}{\underset{\overset{\parallel}{O}}{C}}N(CH_3)_2$	Loperamide	None
A-15	$-C_6H_5$	$-COOC_2H_5$	$-CH_2CH_2CH_2-$	$-CH_3$	Ethoheptazine	1
A-16	$-C_6H_5$	$-O-\overset{\overset{\parallel}{O}}{C}C_2H_5$	$-\overset{\underset{\mid}{CH_3}}{C}H-$	$-CH_3$	Prodilidine	0.3
A-17	$-H$	$-\overset{\overset{\displaystyle O}{\parallel}}{\underset{\underset{\mid}{C_6H_5}}{N}}-\overset{}{C}C_2H_5$	$-CH_2CH_2-$	$-CH_2CH_2C_6H_5$	Fentanyl	940
A-18	$-COOCH_3$	$-\overset{\overset{\displaystyle O}{\parallel}}{\underset{\underset{\mid}{C_6H_5}}{N}}-\overset{}{C}C_2H_5$	$-CH_2\overset{\underset{\mid}{CH_3}}{C}H-$	$-CH_2CH_2C_6H_5$	Lofentanil (R 34,995)	8,400

ment of the carbethoxyl group in meperidine by acyloxyl groups gave better analgesic, as well as spasmolytic, activity. The ''reversed'' ester of meperidine, the propionoxy compound (A-6), was the most active, being 5 times as active as meperidine. These findings were validated and expanded on by Lee et al.[25–28] In an extensive study of structural modifications of meperidine, Janssen and Eddy[29] concluded that the propionoxy compounds were always more active, usually about twofold, regardless of what group was attached to the nitrogen.

Lee[30] had postulated that the configuration of the propionoxy derivative (A-6) more closely resembled that of morphine, with the ester chain taking a position similar to that occupied by C-6 and C-7 in morphine. His speculations were based on space models and certainly did not reflect the actual conformation of the nonrigid meperidine. He did arrive at the correct assumption, however, that introduction of a methyl group into position 3 of the piperidine ring in the propionoxy compound would yield two isomers, one with activity approximating that of desomorphine and the other with less activity. One of the two diastereoisomers (A-7), betaprodine, has an activity in mice about 9 times that of morphine and 3 times that of A-6. Beckett et al.[31] have established that it is the *cis* (methyl/phenyl) form. The *trans* form, alphaprodine, is twice as active as morphine. Resolution of the racemates shows that one enantiomer has the predominant activity. In humans, however, the sharp differences in analgesic potency are not so marked. The *trans* form is marketed as the racemate. The significance of the 3-methyl has been attributed to discrimination of the enantiotropic edges of these molecules by the receptor. This is even more dramatic in the 3-allyl and 3-propyl isomers, for which the *α-trans* forms are considerably more potent than the *β* isomers, indicating that three-carbon substituents are not tolerated in the axial orientation. The 3-ethyl isomers are nearly equal in activity,

further indicating that two or fewer carbons are more acceptable in the drug–receptor interaction.[32, 33]

A small substituent, such as methyl, attached to the nitrogen had seemed to be optimal for analgesic activity. This was believed to be true not only for the meperidine series of compounds but also for all the other types. It is now well established that replacement of the methyl group by various aralkyl groups can increase activity markedly.[29] A few examples of this type of compound in the meperidine series are shown in Table 22-3. The phenethyl derivative (A-9) is about 3 times as active as meperidine (A-1). The *p*-amino congener, anileridine (A-10), is about 4 times more active. Piminodine, the phenylaminopropyl derivative (A-11), has 55 times the activity of meperidine in rats and is about 5 times as effective in humans as an analgesic.[34] The most active meperidine-type compounds, to date, are the propionoxy derivative (A-12), which is nearly 2,000 times as active as meperidine, and the *N*-phenethyl analogue of betaprodine, which is over 2,000 times as active as morphine.[31] Diphenoxylate (A-13), a structural hybrid of meperidine and methadone types, lacks analgesic activity, although it reportedly suppresses the morphine abstinence syndrome in morphine addicts.[35, 36] It is quite effective as an intestinal spasmolytic and is used for the treatment of diarrhea (Lomotil). Several other derivatives of it have been studied.[37] The related *p*-chloro analogue, loperamide (A-14), binds to opiate receptors in the brain but does not penetrate the blood–brain barrier enough to produce analgesia.[38]

Another way to modify the structure of meperidine with favorable results was to enlarge the piperidine ring to the seven-membered hexahydroazepine (or hexamethylenamine) ring. As was true in the piperidine series, the most active compound is the one containing a methyl group on position 3 of the ring adjacent to the quaternary carbon atom in the propionoxy derivative, that is, 1,3-dimethyl-4-phenyl-

4-propionoxyhexahydroazepine, to which the name *proheptazine* was given. In the study by Eddy and coworkers, cited above, proheptazine was one of the more active analgesics included and had one of the highest addiction liabilities. The higher ring homologue of meperidine, ethoheptazine, was on the market. Although originally thought to be inactive,[39] it is less active than codeine as an analgesic in humans but is free of addiction liability and has a low incidence of side effects.[40] It is no longer available.

Contraction of the piperidine ring to the five-membered pyrrolidine ring was also successful. The lower ring homologue of alphaprodine, prodilidine (A-16), is an effective analgesic; a dose of 100 mg is equivalent to 30 mg of codeine, but because of its potential abuse liability, it was never marketed.[41]

A more unusual modification of the meperidine structure is found in fentanyl (A-17), in which the phenyl and the acyl groups are separated from the ring by a nitrogen. It is a powerful analgesic, 50 times stronger than morphine in humans, with minimal side effects.[42] Its short duration of action makes it well suited for use in anesthesia.[43] It is marketed for this purpose in combination with a neuroleptic, droperidol. The *cis*-(−)-3-methyl analogue with an ester group at the 4 position, like meperidine (A-18), was 8,400 times more potent than morphine as an analgesic. In addition, it has the highest binding affinity to isolated opiate receptors of all compounds tested.[38] Fentanyl and its 3-methyl and *α*-methyl analogues have found their way into the illicit drug market and are sold as substitutes for heroin. Because of their extreme potency, they have caused many deaths.

When the nitrogen ring of morphine is opened, as in the formation of morphimethines, the analgesic activity is virtually abolished. On this basis, predicting whether a compound would or would not have activity without the nitrogen in a ring would favor a lack of activity or, at best, low activity. The first report indicating that this was a false assumption was based on the initial work of Bockmuehl and Ehrhart,[44] in which they claimed that the type of compound represented by B-1 in Table 22-4 possessed both analgesic and spasmolytic properties. The Hoechst laboratories in Germany followed up this lead during World War II by preparing the ketones corresponding to these esters. Some of the compounds they prepared with high activity are represented by formulas B-2 through B-7. Compound B-2 is the well-known methadone. In the meperidine and bemidone types, the introduction of a *m*-hydroxyl group in the phenyl ring brought about slightly to markedly increased activity, whereas the same operation with the methadone-type compound markedly decreased action. Phenadoxone (B-8), the morpholine analogue of methadone, was marketed in England. The piperidine analogue, dipanone, was once under study in this country after successful results in England.

Methadone was first brought to the attention of American pharmacists, chemists, and allied workers by the Kleiderer report[45] and by the early reports of Scott and Chen.[46, 47] Since then, much work has been done on this compound, its isomer isomethadone, and related compounds. The report by Eddy, Touchberry, and Lieberman[48] covers most of the points concerning the structure–activity relationships of methadone. The *levo* isomer (B-3) of methadone (B-2) and the *levo* isomer of isomethadone (B-4) are twice as effective as their racemic mixtures. Also, all structural derivatives of

methadone demonstrate greater activity than the corresponding structural derivatives of isomethadone. In other words, the superiority of methadone over isomethadone seems to hold, even through the derivatives. Conversely, the methadone series of compounds was always more toxic than the isomethadone group.

More extensive permutations, such as replacing the propionyl group (R_3 in B-2) by hydrogen, hydroxyl, or acetoxyl, decreased activity. In a series of amide analogues of methadone, Janssen and Jageneau[49–51] synthesized racemoramide (B-12), which is more active than methadone. The (6) isomer, dextromoramide (B-13), is the active isomer and has been marketed. A few of the other modifications that have been carried out and their effect on analgesic activity relative to methadone are described in Table 22-4, which includes most of the methadone congeners that are or were on the market. Much deviation in structure from these examples will result in varying degrees of loss of activity.

Particular attention should be paid to the two phenyl groups in methadone and the sharply decreased action resulting from removal of one of them. It is believed that the second phenyl residue helps to lock the —COC_2H_5 group of methadone in a position to simulate the alicyclic ring of morphine, even though the propionyl group is not particularly rigid. In this connection, however, the compound with a propionoxy group in place of the propionyl group (R_3 in B-2) lacks significant analgesic action.[23] In direct contrast with this is (6)-propoxyphene (B-14), which is a propionoxy derivative with one of the phenyl groups replaced by a benzyl group. In addition, it is an analogue of isomethadone (B-4), making it an exception to the rule. This compound is lower than codeine in analgesic activity, possesses few side effects, and has a limited addiction liability.[52] Replacement of the dimethylamino group in (6)-propoxyphene with a pyrrolidyl group gives a compound that is nearly three-fourths as active as methadone and possesses morphine-like properties. The *levo* isomer of alphacetylmethadol (B-9), known as LAAM, has been marketed as a long-acting substitute for methadone in the treatment of addicts.[53]

MORPHINE MODIFICATIONS INITIATED BY GREWE

Grewe, in 1946, approached the problem of synthetic analgesics from another direction when he synthesized the tetracyclic compound that he first named morphan and then revised to *N*-methylmorphinan. The relationship of this compound to morphine is obvious.

N-Methylmorphinan

N-Methylmorphinan differs from the morphine nucleus in lacking the ether bridge between C-4 and C-5. This compound possesses a high degree of analgesic activity, which suggests that the ether bridge is not essential. The 3-hydroxyl derivative of *N*-methylmorphinan (racemorphan) was on the market and had an intensity and duration of action that exceeded that of morphine. The original racemorphan was in-

TABLE 22–4 Compounds Related to Methadone

$$R_1 \underset{R_2}{\overset{R_3}{\underset{|}{\overset{|}{C}}}} R_4$$

Com-pound	Structure				Name	Isomer, Salt	Analgesic Activity (Methadone = 1)
	R_1	R_2	R_3	R_4			
B-1	$-C_6H_5$	$-C_6H_5$	$-COO-Alkyl$	$-CH_2CH_2N(CH_5)_2$		—	0.17
B-2	$-C_6H_5$	$-C_6H_5$	$-\overset{\|}{\underset{O}{C}}-C_2H_5$	$-CH_2\overset{\|}{\underset{CH_3}{C}}HN(CH_3)_2$	Methadone	$(\pm)$-HCl	1.0
B-3	Same as in B-2				Levanone	$(-)$-Bitartrate	1.9
B-4	$-C_6H_5$	$-C_6H_5$	$-\overset{\|}{\underset{O}{C}}-C_2H_5$	$-CH\overset{\|}{\underset{CH_3}{C}}H_2N(CH_3)_2$	Isomethadone	$(\pm)$-HCl	0.65
B-5	$-C_6H_5$	$-C_6H_5$	$-\overset{\|}{\underset{O}{C}}-C_2H_5$	$-CH_2CH_2N(CH_3)_2$	Normethadone	HCl	0.44
B-6	$-C_6H_5$	$-C_6H_5$	$-\overset{\|}{\underset{O}{C}}-C_2H_5$	$-CH_2\overset{\|}{\underset{CH_3}{C}}HN\langle$piperidine$\rangle$	Dipanone	$(\pm)$-HCl	0.80
B-7	$-C_6H_5$	$-C_6H_5$	$-\overset{\|}{\underset{O}{C}}-C_2H_5$	$-CH_2CH_2N\langle$piperidine$\rangle$	Hexalgon	HBr	0.50
B-8	$-C_6H_5$	$-C_6H_5$	$-\overset{\|}{\underset{O}{C}}-C_2H_5$	$-CH_2\overset{\|}{\underset{CH_3}{C}}HN\langle$morpholine$\rangle$	Phenadoxone	$(\pm)$-HCl	1.4
B-9	$-C_6H_5$	$-C_6H_5$	$-\underset{O-\overset{\|}{\underset{O}{C}}CH_3}{CHC_2H_5}$	$-CH_2\overset{\|}{\underset{CH_3}{C}}HN(CH_3)_2$	Alphacetylmethadol	$\alpha,(\pm)$-HCl	1.3
B-10	Same as in B-9				Betacetylmethadol	$\beta,(\pm)$-HCl	2.3
B-11	$-C_6H_5$	$-C_6H_5$	$-COOC_2H_5$	$-CH_2CH_2N\langle$morpholine$\rangle$	Dioxaphetyl buty-rate	HCl	0.25
B-12	$-C_6H_5$	$-C_6H_5$	$-\overset{\|}{\underset{O}{C}}-N\langle$pyrrolidine$\rangle$	$-CH\overset{\|}{\underset{CH_3}{C}}H_2N\langle$morpholine$\rangle$	Racemoramide	$(+)$-Base	3.6
B-13	Same as in B-12				Dextromoramide	$(+)$-Base	13
B-14	$-C_6H_5$	$-CH_2C_6H_5$	$O-\overset{\|}{\underset{O}{C}}-C_2H_5$	$-CH\overset{\|}{\underset{CH_3}{C}}H_2N(CH_3)_2$	Propoxyphene	$(+)$-HCl	0.21

troduced as the hydrobromide and was the (*dl*), or racemic, form as obtained by synthesis. Realizing that the levorotatory form of racemorphan was the analgesically active portion of the racemate, the manufacturer resolved the (*dl*) form and marketed the *levo* form as the tartrate salt (levorphanol). The *dextro* form has found use as a cough suppressant (see dextromethorphan). The ethers and acylated derivatives of the 3-hydroxyl form also exhibit considerable activity. The 2- and 4-hydroxyl isomers are, not unexpectedly, without value as analgesics. Likewise, the *N*-ethyl derivative lacks activity, and the *N*-allyl compound, levallorphan, is a potent morphine antagonist.

Eddy et al.[54] reported on an extensive series of *N*-aralkylmorphinan derivatives. The effect of the *N*-aralkyl substitution was more dramatic in this series than it was for morphine or meperidine. The *N*-phenethyl and *N*-*p*-aminophenethyl analogues of levorphanol are about 3 and 18 times more active, respectively, than the parent compound in analgesic activity in mice. The most potent member of the series was the *N*-β-furylethyl analogue, which was nearly 30 times as active as levorphanol or 160 times as active as morphine. The *N*-acetophenone analogue, levophenacylmorphan, was once under clinical investigation. In mice, it is about 30 times more active than morphine, and in humans a 2-mg dose is equivalent to 10 mg of morphine in its analgesic response.[55] It has a much lower physical-dependence liability than morphine.

The *N*-cyclopropylmethyl derivative of 3-hydroxymorphinan (cyclorphan) was reported to be a potent morphine antagonist, capable of precipitating morphine withdrawal symptoms in addicted monkeys, indicating that it is nonaddicting.[21] Clinical studies have indicated that it is about 20 times stronger than morphine as an analgesic, but it has some undesirable side effects, primarily hallucinatory. The *N*-cyclobutyl derivative, butorphanol, possesses mixed agonist–antagonist properties, however, and has been marketed as a potent analgesic.

Since removal of the ether bridge and all the peripheral groups in the alicyclic ring in morphine did not destroy its analgesic action, May et al.[56] synthesized a series of compounds in which the alicyclic ring was replaced by one or two methyl groups. These are known as *benzomorphan derivatives* or, more correctly, *benzazocines*. They may be represented by the following formula:

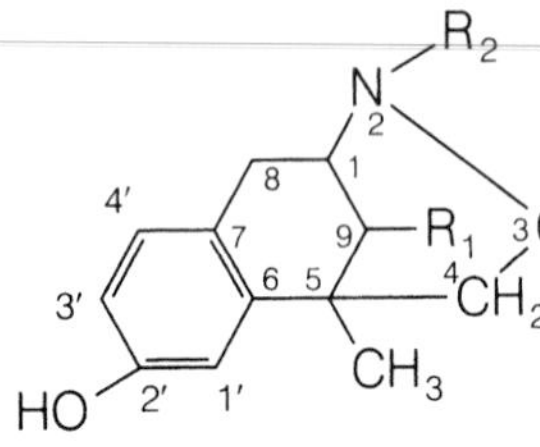

The trimethyl compound (II, $R_1 = R_2 = CH_3$) is about 3 times more potent than the dimethyl (II, $R_1 = H$, $R_2 = CH_3$). The *N*-phenethyl derivatives have almost 20 times the analgesic activity of the corresponding *N*-methyl compounds. Again, the more potent was the one containing two ring methyls (II, $R_1 = CH_3$, $R_2 = CH_2CH_2C_6H_5$). Deracemization proved the *levo* isomer of this compound to be more active, being about 20 times as potent as morphine in mice. The ($\pm$) form, phenazocine, was on the market but was removed in favor of pentazocine.

May et al.[57] demonstrated an extremely significant difference between the two isomeric *N*-methyl benzomorphans in which the alkyl in the 5 position is *n*-propyl (R_1) and the alkyl in the 9 position is methyl (R_2). These have been termed the α and the β isomer and have the groups oriented as indicated. The isomer with the alkyl *cis* to the phenyl possesses analgesic activity (in mice) equal to that of morphine but has little or no capacity to suppress withdrawal symptoms in addicted monkeys. On the other hand, the *trans* isomer has one of the highest analgesic potencies among the benzomorphans, but it is quite able to suppress morphine

withdrawal symptoms. Further differences in properties are found between the enantiomers of the *cis* isomer. The (+) isomer has weak analgesic activity, but a high physical-dependence capacity. The (−) isomer is a stronger analgesic, without the dependence capacity, and possesses antagonistic activity.[58] The same is true of the 5,9-diethyl and 9-ethyl-5-phenyl derivatives. The (−) *trans*-5,9-diethyl isomer is similar, except it has no antagonistic properties. This demonstrates that it is possible to divorce analgesic activity comparable to that of morphine from addiction potential. That *N*-methyl compounds have shown antagonistic properties is of great interest as well. The most potent of these is the benzomorphan with an α-methyl and β-3-oxoheptyl group at position 9. The (−) isomer shows greater antagonistic activity than naloxone and is still 3 times more potent than morphine as an analgesic.[59]

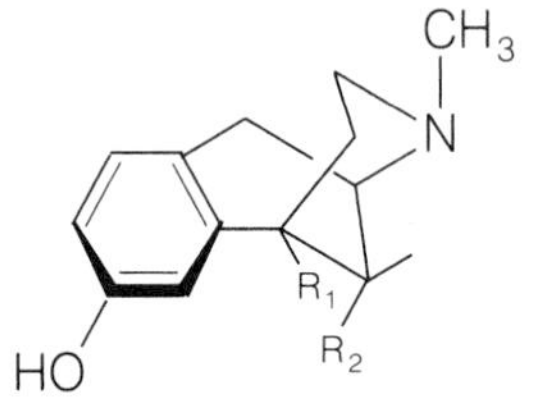

α isomer (*cis*)   β isomer (*trans*)

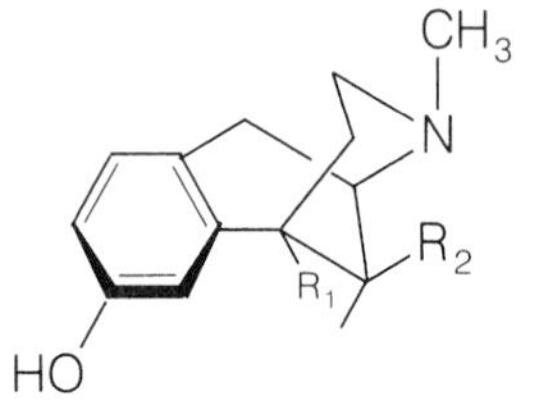

An extensive series of the antagonist-type analgesics in the benzomorphans was reported.[60] Of these, pentazocine (II, $R_1 = CH_3$, $R_2 = CH_2CH = C(CH_3)_2$) and cyclazocine (II, $R_1 = CH_3$, $R_2 = CH_2$–cyclopropyl) have been the most interesting. Pentazocine has about half the analgesic activity of morphine, with a lower incidence of side effects.[61] Its addiction liability is much lower, approximating that of propoxyphene.[62] It is currently available in parenteral and tablet form. Cyclazocine is a strong morphine antagonist, showing about 10 times the analgesic activity of morphine.[63] It was investigated as an analgesic and for the treatment of heroin addiction, but it was never marketed because of hallucinatory side effects.

As mentioned above, replacement of the *N*-methyl group in morphine by larger alkyl groups lowered analgesic activity. In addition, these compounds counteracted the effect of morphine and other morphine-like analgesics and are thus known as *narcotic antagonists*. The reversal of activity increases from ethyl, to propyl, to allyl, with the cyclopropylmethyl usually being maximal. This property was true not only for morphine but also for other analgesics. *N*-Allylnormorphine (nalorphine) was the first of these but because of side effects was taken off the market. Levallorphan, the corresponding allyl analogue of levorphanol, naloxone (*N*-allylnoroxymorphone), and naltrexone (*N*-cyclopropyl-noroxymorphone) are the three narcotic antagonists now on the market. Naloxone and naltrexone appear to be pure antagonists with no morphine- or nalorphine-like effects. They also block the effects of other antagonists. These drugs are used to prevent, diminish, or abolish many of the actions or the side effects encountered with the narcotic analgesics. Some of these are respiratory and circulatory depression, euphoria, nausea, drowsiness, analgesia, and hyperglycemia. They are thought to act by competing with the analgesic molecule for attachment at its, or a closely related, receptor site. The observation that some narcotic antagonists that lack addiction liability are also strong analgesics spurred considerable interest in them.[20] The *N*-cyclopropylmethyl compounds mentioned are the most potent antagonists but appear to produce psychotomimetic effects and may not be useful as analgesics. One of these, buprenorphine, has shown an interesting study profile, however, and has been introduced in Europe and in the United States as a potent analgesic.[64] It is being introduced as a treatment for narcotic addicts in a novel treatment program, Office Based Opioid Treatment (OBOT), provided by private physicians rather than formal treatment clinics.[65]

Other efforts have been under way to develop narcotic antagonists that can be used to treat narcotic addiction.[66] The continuous administration of an antagonist will block the euphoric effects of heroin, thereby aiding rehabilitation of an addict. The cyclopropylmethyl derivative of naloxone, naltrexone, has been marketed for this purpose. The oral dose of 100 to 150 mg 3 times a week suffices to block several usual doses of heroin.[67] Long-acting preparations were once also under study.[68]

Much research, other than that described above, has been carried out by the systematic dissection of morphine to give several interesting fragments. These approaches have not yet produced important analgesics and so are not discussed in this chapter. The interested reader may find a key to this literature, however, in the excellent reviews of Eddy,[9] Bergel and Morrison,[23] and Lee.[30]

Structure–Activity Relationships

Several reviews on the relationship between chemical structure and analgesic action have been published.[9, 35, 69–77] Only the major conclusions are considered here, and the reader is urged to consult these reviews for more complete discussion of the subject.

From the time Small et al. started their studies on the morphine nucleus to the present, there has been much light shed on the structural features connected with morphine-like analgesic action. In a very thorough study made for the United Nations Commission on Narcotics in 1955, Braenden et al.[70] found that the features possessed by all known morphine-like analgesics were as follows:

1. A tertiary nitrogen, with the group on the nitrogen being relatively small
2. A central carbon atom, of which none of the valences is connected with hydrogen
3. A phenyl group or a group isosteric with phenyl, which is connected to the central carbon atom
4. A two-carbon chain separating the central carbon atom from the nitrogen for maximal activity

The above discussion shows that several exceptions to these generalizations exist in the structures of compounds that have been synthesized in the past several years. Eddy[35] has discussed the more significant exceptions. Relative to the first feature mentioned, extensive studies of the action of normorphine have shown that it possesses analgesic activity that approximates that of morphine. In humans, it is about one fourth as active as morphine when administered intramuscularly, but it was slightly superior to morphine when administered intracisternally. On the basis of the last-mentioned effect, Beckett et al.[78] postulated that N-dealkylation was a step in the mechanism of analgesic action. This has

been questioned.[79] Additional studies indicate that dealkylation does occur in the brain, although its exact role is not clear.[80] It is clear, from the *N*-aralkyl derivatives discussed above, that a small group is not necessary.

Several exceptions to the second feature have been synthesized. In these series, the central carbon atom has been replaced by a tertiary nitrogen. They are related to methadone and have the following structures:

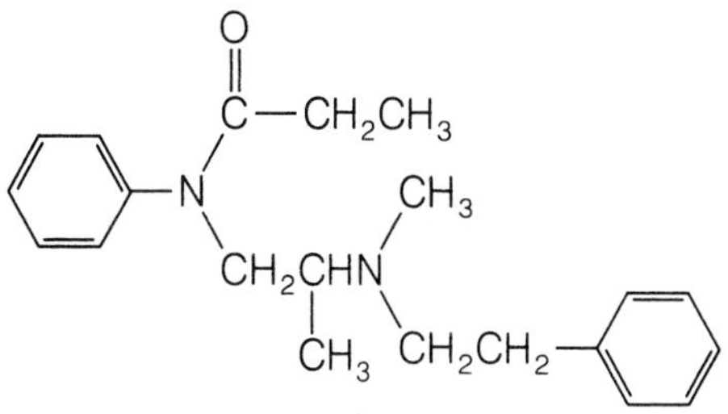

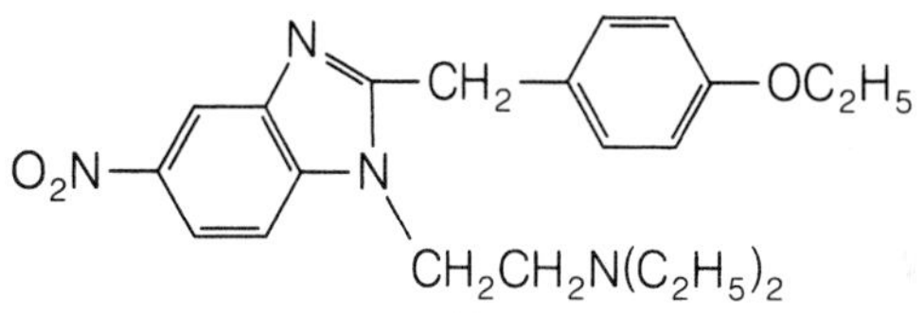

Diampromide (III) and its related anilides have potencies that are comparable with those of morphine;[81] they have shown addiction liability, however, and have not appeared on the market. The closely related cyclic derivative fentanyl (Table 22-3, A-17) is used in surgery. The benzimidazoles, such as etonitazene (IV), are very potent analgesics but show the highest addiction liabilities yet encountered.[82, 83]

Possibly an exception to feature 3, and the only one that has been encountered, may be the cyclohexyl analogue of A-6 (Table 22-3), which has significant activity. Eddy[35] mentions two possible exceptions to feature 4 in addition to fentanyl.

The many studies on molecules of varying types that possess analgesic activity revealed that activity was associated not only with certain structural features but also with the size and the shape of the molecule. The hypothesis of Beckett and Casy[84] has dominated thinking for several years in the area of stereochemical specificity of these molecules. They initially noted that the more active enantiomers of the methadone- and thiambutene-type analgesics were related configurationally to (*R*)-alanine. This suggested to them that a stereoselective fit at a receptor could be involved in analgesic activity. To depict the dimensions of an analgesic receptor, they selected morphine (because of its semirigidity and high activity) to provide them with information on a complementary receptor. The features thought to be essential for proper receptor fit were

1. A basic center able to associate with an anionic site on the receptor surface
2. A flat aromatic structure, coplanar with the basic center, allowing van der Waals bonding to a flat surface on the receptor site to reinforce the ionic bond
3. A suitably positioned projecting hydrocarbon moiety forming a three-dimensional geometric pattern with the basic center and the flat aromatic structure

These features were selected, among other reasons, because they are present in *N*-methylmorphinan, which may be looked on as a "stripped down" morphine (i.e., morphine without the characteristic peripheral groups [except for the basic center]). Since *N*-methylmorphinan possessed substantial activity of the morphine type, these three features were considered the fundamental ones determining activity, and the peripheral groups of morphine were considered to essentially modulate the activity.

In accord with the foregoing postulates, Beckett and Casy[84] proposed a complementary receptor site (Fig. 22-1) and suggested ways[85, 86] in which the known active molecules could be adapted to it. After their initial postulates, natural (−)-morphine was shown to be related configurationally to methadone and thiambutene, which lent weight to the hypothesis. Fundamental to their proposal was that such a receptor was essentially inflexible and that a lock-and-key-type situation existed. Subsequently, the unnatural (+)-morphine was synthesized and shown to be inactive.[87]

Although the foregoing hypothesis appeared to fit the facts quite well and was a useful hypothesis for several years, it now appears that certain anomalies exist that cannot be accommodated by it. For example, the more active enantiomer of *α*-methadol is not related configurationally to (*R*)-alanine, in contrast with the methadone and thiambutene series. This is also true for the carbethoxy analogue of methadone (V) and for diampromide (III) and its analogues. Another factor that was implicit in considering a proper receptor fit for the morphine molecule and its congeners was that the phenyl ring at the 4 position of the piperidine moiety should be in the axial orientation for maximum activity. The fact that structure VI has only an equatorial phenyl group, yet possesses activity equal to that of morphine, would seem to cast doubt on the necessity for axial orientation as a receptor-fit requirement.

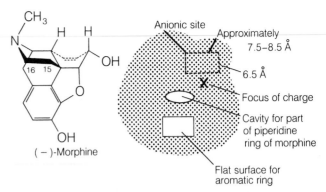

(−)-Morphine

Figure 22–1 ■ Diagram of the surface of the analgesic receptor site with the corresponding lower surface of the drug molecule. The three-dimensional features of the molecule are shown by the bonds: —, - - -, and – –, which represent in front of, behind, and in the plane of the paper, respectively. (From Gourley, D. R. H.: Prog. Drug Res. 7:36, 1964.]

V

VI

In view of the difficulty of accepting Beckett and Casy's hypothesis as a complete picture of analgesic–receptor interaction, Portoghese[88–90] has offered an alternative hypothesis. This hypothesis is based, in part, on the established ability of enzymes and other types of macromolecules to undergo conformational changes[91, 92] on interaction with small molecules (substrates or drugs). The fact that configurationally unrelated analgesics can bind and exert activity is interpreted as meaning that more than one mode of binding may be possible at the same receptor. Such different modes of binding may be due to differences in positional or conformational interactions with the receptor. The manner in which

the hypothesis can be applied to the methadol anomaly is illustrated in Figure 22-2.

After considering activity changes in various structural types (i.e., methadones, meperidines, prodines) as related to the identity of the N-substituent, Portoghese noted that in certain series, when identical changes in N-substituents were made, there was parallelism in the direction of activity, whereas in others there appeared to be nonparallelism. He has interpreted parallelism and nonparallelism, respectively, as being due to similar and dissimilar modes of binding. Viewed by this hypothesis, although analgesic molecules must still be bound in a fairly precise manner, the concept of binding is liberalized, in that a response may be obtained by two different molecules binding stereoselectively in two different precise modes at the same receptor. A schematic representation of such different possible binding modes is shown in Figure 22-3. This representation will aid in visualizing the meaning of *similar* and *dissimilar* binding modes. If two different analgesiophores (the analgesic molecule

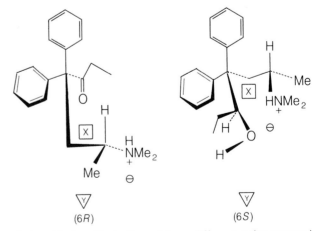

(6*R*)   (6*S*)

Figure 22–2 ■ Illustration of how different polar groups in analgesic molecules may cause inversion in the configurational selectivity of an analgesic receptor. A hydrogen-bonding moiety, denoted by *X* and *Y*, represents a site that is capable of being hydrogen bonded.

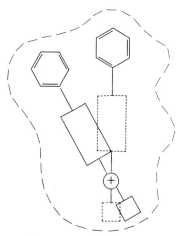

Figure 22–3 ■ Schematic illustration of two different molecular modes of binding to a receptor. ⊕, protonated nitrogen; □, an N-substituent. The anionic sites lie directly beneath the pronated nitrogen.

minus the N-substituent, i.e., that portion of the molecule that gives the characteristic analgesic response) bearing identical N-substituents are positioned on the receptor surface such that the N-substituent occupies essentially the same position, a similar pharmacological response may be anticipated. Thus, as one proceeds from one N-substituent to another, the response should likewise change, resulting in parallelism of effect. On the other hand, if two different analgesiophores are bound to the receptor such that the N-substituents are not arranged identically, one may anticipate nonidentical responses to changing the N-substituent (i.e., a nonparallel response). The preceding statements, as well as the diagram, do not imply that the analgesiophore necessarily will be bound in the identical position within a series. They do suggest, however, that in series with parallel activities, the pairs being compared will be bound identically to produce the parallel effect. Interestingly, when binding modes are similar, Portoghese has been able to demonstrate the existence of a linear free-energy relationship. There is also the possibility that more than one receptor is involved.

Considerable evidence now demonstrates that multiple receptors exist. Martin has characterized and named these by responses to probe molecules: μ (mu) receptors for morphine-specific effects, δ (delta) for cyclazocine, and κ (kappa) for ketocyclazocine.[93] A different designation for these receptors, based on pharmacological criteria, is OP3, OP1, and OP2, respectively. Various combinations of these in different tissues could be responsible for the varying effects observed.[94, 95]

This discovery has stimulated much research into the search for drugs that have selectivity for single receptors. The natural opiates and related synthetic opioids have predominantly μ receptor agonist activity, with morphine and minor analogues showing 10 to 20 times the selectivity over the other receptors. Other analgesic drugs have shown even higher ratios. The antagonists show lower selectivity. Drugs with high κ receptor affinity have high analgesic activity, lack many of the opioid side effects, but have not been useful because of dysphoric and hallucinogenic effects. There are

also no useful drugs developed to date that are selective for δ receptors.

Another highly important development in structure–activity correlations is the development of highly active analgesics from the N-allyl-type derivatives that were once thought to be only morphine antagonists and devoid of analgesic properties. Serendipity played a major role in this discovery: Lasagna and Beecher,[96] in attempting to find some "ideal" ratio of antagonist (N-allylnormorphine, nalorphine) to analgesic (morphine) to maintain the desirable effects of morphine while minimizing the undesirable ones, discovered that nalorphine was, milligram for milligram, as potent an analgesic as morphine. Unfortunately, nalorphine has depersonalizing and psychotomimetic properties that preclude its use clinically as a pain reliever. The discovery led, however, to the development of related derivatives such as pentazocine and cyclazocine. Pentazocine has achieved some success in providing an analgesic with low addiction potential, although it is not totally free of some of the other side effects of morphine. The pattern of activity in these and other N-allyl and N-cyclopropylmethyl derivatives indicates that most potent antagonists possess psychotomimetic activity, whereas the weak antagonists do not. It is from this latter group that useful analgesics, such as pentazocine, butorphanol, and nalbuphine, have been found. The latter two possess N-cyclobutylmethyl groups.

What structural features are associated with antagonist-like activity is uncertain. The N-allyl and dimethylallyl substituent does not always confer antagonist properties. This is true in the meperidine and thevinol series. Demonstration of antagonist-like properties by specific isomers of N-methyl benzomorphans has raised still further speculation. The exact mechanisms by which morphine and the narcotic antagonists act are not clear, and much research is presently being carried on. Published reviews and symposia may be consulted for further discussions of these topics.[66, 97–99]

A further problem also is demonstrated in the testing for analgesic activity. The analgesic activity of the antagonists was not apparent from animal testing; it was observed only in humans. Screening in animals can be used to assess the antagonistic action, which indirectly indicates possible analgesic properties in humans.[100]

It has been customary in the area of analgesic agents to attribute differences in their activities to structurally related differences in their receptor interactions. This rather universal practice continues in spite of early warnings and recent findings. It now appears clear that much of the difference in relative analgesic potencies can be accounted for on the basis of pharmacokinetic or distribution properties.[98] For example, a definite correlation was found between the partition coefficients and the intravenous analgesic data for 17 agents of widely varying structures.[101] Usual test methods do not help distinguish which structural features are related to receptors and which to distribution phenomena. Studies directed toward distinction have used the measurement of actual brain and plasma levels[102, 103] or direct injection into the ventricular area,[101] the measurement of ionization potentials and partition coefficients,[104] and the application of molecular orbital theories and quantum mechanics.[99, 105–107] These are providing valuable insight into designing of new and more successful agents.

All of the foregoing work had strongly suggested the existence of specific binding sites or *receptors* in brain and other tissue. The demonstration of the high steric and structural specificity in the action of the opiates and their antagonists led many investigators to search for such receptors.[108, 109] Thus in 1971, Goldstein and coworkers demonstrated stereospecific binding in brain homogenates.[110] This was quickly followed by refinements and further discoveries by Simon, Terenius, and Pert and Snyder.[111–113] These receptor-binding studies have now become a routine assay for examining structure–activity relationships.

In addition to the binding studies, considerable attention continued on the use of in vitro models, in particular the isolated guinea pig ileum, rat jejunum, and mouse vas deferens.[114] While working with these preparations, Hughes was the first to discover the existence of an endogenous factor from pig brains that possessed opiate-like properties.[115, 116] This factor, given the name *enkephalin,* consisted of two pentapeptides, called *methonine-*, or *metenkephalin,* and *leucine-*, or *leuenkephalin.* These two enkephalins have subsequently been shown to exist in all animals, including humans, and to possess all morphine-like properties.[117–119] They exist as segments of a pituitary hormone, the 91-amino acid β-lipotropin, which is cleaved selectively to release specific segments that have now been found to have functions within the body. Thus, segment 61 to 65 is metenkephalin, 61 to 76 is α-endorphin, 61 to 77 is γ-endorphin, and, probably the most important, 61 to 91 is β-endorphin.

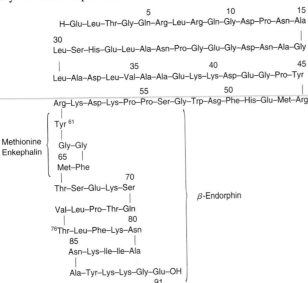

β-Lipotropin, β-Endorphin, Methionine–Enkephalin Relationships

The last of these endorphins (short for *end*ogenous mor*phine*) has 20 times the analgesic potency of morphine when injected into rat brain. These substances can also produce tolerance and dependence.

Clearly, all of these techniques will lead to new concepts and understanding of the processes of analgesia, tolerance, and dependence. It is hoped that learning how these mechanisms operate will aid in the design and development of better analgesics.

Products

In General Circular No. 253, March 10, 1960, the Treasury Department, Bureau of Narcotics, Washington, DC, pub-

lished an extensive listing of narcotics of current interest in the drug trade. This listing is much more extensive than the following monographs covering compounds primarily of interest to American pharmacists.

Morphine. Morphine was isolated first in 1803 by Derosne, but the credit for isolation generally goes to Sertürner (1803), who first called attention to the basic properties of this alkaloid. Morphine, incidentally, was the first plant base isolated and recognized as such. Although intensive research was carried out on the structure of morphine, it was in 1925 that Gulland and Robinson[120] postulated the currently accepted formula. The total synthesis of morphine finally was effected by Gates and Tschudi[121, 122] in 1952, confirming the Gulland and Robinson formula.

Morphine is obtained only from the opium poppy, *Papaver somniferum,* either from opium, the resin obtained by lancing the unripe pod, or from poppy straw. The latter process is favored, as it helps to eliminate illicit opium from which heroin is readily produced. Morphine occurs in opium in amounts varying from 5 to 20% (*USP* requires not less than 9.5%). It is isolated by various methods, but the final step is usually the precipitation of morphine from an acid solution by use of excess ammonia. The precipitated morphine then is recrystallized from boiling alcohol.

The free alkaloid occurs as levorotatory, odorless, white, needle-like crystals possessing a bitter taste. It is almost insoluble in water (1:5,000, 1:1,100 at the boiling point), ether (1:6,250), or chloroform (1:1,220). It is somewhat more soluble in ethyl alcohol (1:210, 1:98 at boiling point). (Note that in this chapter, a solubility of 1:5,000 indicates that 1 g is soluble in 5,000 mL of the solvent at 25°C. Solubilities at other temperatures are so indicated.) Because of the phenolic hydroxyl group, it is readily soluble in solutions of alkali or alkaline earth metal hydroxides.

Morphine is a monoacidic base and readily forms water-soluble salts with most acids. Thus, because morphine itself is so poorly soluble in water, the salts are the preferred form for most uses. Numerous salts have been marketed, but the ones in use are principally the sulfate and, to a lesser extent, the hydrochloride.

Many writers have pointed out the "indispensable" nature of morphine, based on its potent analgesic properties toward all types of pain. It is properly termed a *narcotic analgesic.* Because it causes addiction so readily, however, it should be used only when other pain-relieving drugs prove inadequate. It controls pain caused by serious injury, neoplasms, migraine, pleurisy, biliary and renal colic, and numerous other conditions. It is often administered as a preoperative sedative, together with atropine to control secretions. With scopolamine, it is given to obtain the so-called twilight sleep. This effect is used in obstetrics, but care is needed to prevent respiratory depression in the fetus. The toxic properties of morphine are much more evident in young and old people.

Morphine Hydrochloride. Morphine hydrochloride may be prepared by neutralizing a hot aqueous suspension of morphine with diluted hydrochloric acid and then concentrating the resultant solution to crystallization. It is no longer commercially available. It occurs as silky, white, glistening needles, as cubical masses, or as a white crystalline powder. The hydrochloride is soluble in water (1:17.5, 1:0.5 at boiling point), alcohol (1:52, 1:46 at 60°), or glycerin, but it is practically insoluble in ether or chloroform. Solutions have a pH of approximately 4.7 and may be sterilized by boiling. Its uses are the same as those of morphine. The usual oral and subcutaneous dose is 15 mg every 4 hours as needed, with a suggested range of 8 to 20 mg.

Morphine Sulfate, USP. Morphine sulfate is prepared in the same manner as the hydrochloride (i.e., by neutralizing morphine with diluted sulfuric acid). It occurs as feathery, silky, white crystals, as cubical masses of crystals, or as a white crystalline powder. Although it is a fairly stable salt, it loses water of hydration and darkens on exposure to air and light. It is soluble in water (1:16, 1:1 at 80°), poorly soluble in alcohol (1:570, 1:240 at 60°), and insoluble in chloroform or ether. Aqueous solutions have a pH of about 4.8 and may be sterilized by heating in an autoclave.

This common morphine salt is used widely in England, and now in the United States, by oral administration for the management of pain in cancer patients. It has largely replaced Brompton's mixture or cocktail, a combination of heroin and cocaine in chloroform water. In the United States, this preparation has become mistakenly popular, substituting morphine sulfate for the heroin. Moreover, Twycross has advised that the stimulant cocaine is contraindicated because it interferes with sleep,[123] and its original use was for cough in tuberculosis patients. Morphine sulfate is available in a variety of dosage forms: tablets, oral solution, parenteral, suppositories, and controlled-release tablets (MS Contin) and capsules (Kadian).

Codeine, USP. Codeine is an alkaloid that occurs naturally in opium, but the amount present is usually too small to be of commercial importance. Consequently, most commercial codeine is prepared from morphine by methylating the phenolic hydroxyl group. The methylation methods make use of reagents such as diazomethane, dimethyl sulfate, and methyl iodide. Newer methods are based on its synthesis from thebaine, which makes it possible to use *Papaver bracteatum* as a natural source (see above).

It occurs as levorotatory, colorless, efflorescent crystals or as a white crystalline powder. It is light sensitive. Codeine is slightly soluble in water (1:120) and sparingly soluble in ether (1:50). It is freely soluble in alcohol (1:2) and very soluble in chloroform (1:0.5). Codeine is a monoacidic base and readily forms salts with acids, with the most important being the sulfate and the phosphate. The acetate and methylbromide derivatives have been used to a limited extent in cough preparations.

The general pharmacological action of codeine is similar to that of morphine, but as indicated above, it does not possess the same analgesic potency. Studies indicate that a dose of 30 to 120 mg of codeine is considerably less efficient parenterally than 10 mg of morphine, and the usual side effects of morphine—respiratory depression, constipation, nausea, and such—occur. Codeine is less effective orally than parenterally, and Houde and Wallenstein[124] stated that a dose of 32 mg of codeine is about as effective as 650 mg of aspirin in relieving terminal cancer pain. Combinations

of aspirin and codeine act additively as analgesics, however, thus giving some support to the common practice of combining the two drugs.

Codeine has a reputation as an antitussive, depressing the cough reflex, and is used in many cough preparations. It is one of the most widely used morphine-like analgesics. It is considerably less addicting than morphine, and in the usual doses, respiratory depression is negligible, although an oral dose of 60 mg causes such depression in a normal person. Much of codeine's reputation as an antitussive probably rests on subjective impressions rather than on objective studies. The average 5-mL dose contains 10 mg of codeine. Several cough preparations containing codeine are available, with some that may be sold over-the-counter as exempt narcotic preparations. Abuse or misuse of these preparations, however, has led many states to place them on prescription-only status.

Codeine Phosphate, USP. Codeine phosphate may be prepared by neutralizing codeine with phosphoric acid and precipitating the salt from aqueous solution with alcohol. Codeine phosphate occurs as fine, needle-shaped, white crystals or as a white crystalline powder. It is efflorescent and is sensitive to light. It is freely soluble in water (1:2.5, 1:0.5 at 80°) but less soluble in alcohol (1:325, 1:125 at boiling point). Solutions may be sterilized by boiling. Because of its high solubility in water, compared with the sulfate, this salt is used widely. It is often the only salt of codeine stocked by pharmacies and is dispensed, rightly or wrongly, on all prescriptions calling for either the sulfate or the phosphate.

Codeine Sulfate, USP. Codeine sulfate is prepared by neutralizing an aqueous suspension of codeine with diluted sulfuric acid and then effecting crystallization. It occurs as white crystals, usually needle-like, or as a white crystalline powder. The salt is efflorescent and light sensitive. It is soluble in water (1:30, 1:6.5 at 80°), much less soluble in alcohol (1:1,280), and insoluble in ether or chloroform. This salt of codeine is prescribed frequently but is not as suitable as the phosphate for liquid preparations. Solutions of the sulfate and the phosphate are incompatible with alkaloidal reagents and alkaline substances.

Diacetylmorphine Hydrochloride. Although diacetylmorphine hydrochloride, heroin hydrochloride, diamorphine hydrochloride, heroin, is 2 to 3 times more potent than morphine as an analgesic, its sale and use are prohibited in the United States because of its intense addiction liability. It is available in some European countries, where it has a limited use as an antitussive and as an analgesic in terminal cancer patients. Because of its superior solubility over morphine sulfate, arguments have been raised for its availability. The other more potent analgesics described here have, however, significant advantages in being more stable and longer acting. It remains one of the most widely used narcotics for illicit purposes and places major economic burdens on society.

Hydromorphone. Hydromorphone, dihydromorphinone, a synthetic derivative of morphine, is prepared by the catalytic hydrogenation and dehydrogenation of morphine under acidic conditions, using a large excess of platinum or palladium. The free base is similar in properties to morphine, being slightly soluble in water, freely soluble in alcohol, and very soluble in chloroform.

This compound, of German origin, was introduced in 1926. It is a substitute for morphine (5 times as potent) but has approximately equal addicting properties and a shorter duration of action. It possesses the advantage over morphine of giving less daytime sedation or drowsiness. It is a potent antitussive and is often used for coughs that are difficult to control.

Hydromorphone Hydrochloride, USP.

Hydromorphone hydrochloride, dihydromorphinone hydrochloride (Dilaudid), occurs as a light-sensitive, white crystalline powder that is freely soluble in water (1:3), sparingly soluble in alcohol, and practically insoluble in ether. It is used in about one-fifth the dose of morphine for any of the indications of morphine. It is available in tablet, liquid, parenteral, and suppository dosage forms. The dose is 1 to 8 mg.

Hydrocodone Bitartrate, USP.

Hydrocodone bitartrate, dihydrocodeinone bitartrate (Dicodid, Codone), is prepared by the catalytic rearrangement of codeine or by hydrolyzing dihydrothebaine. It occurs as fine, white crystals or as a white crystalline powder. It is soluble in water (1:16), slightly soluble in alcohol, and insoluble in ether. It forms acidic solutions and is affected by light. The hydrochloride is also available.

Hydrocodone has a pharmacological action midway between those of codeine and morphine, with 15 mg being equivalent to 10 mg of morphine in analgesic power. Although it possesses more addiction liability than codeine, it reportedly gives no evidence of dependence or addiction with long-term use. Its principal advantage is in the lower frequency of side effects encountered with its use. It is more effective than codeine as an antitussive and is used primarily for this purpose. It is on the market in many cough preparations, as well as in tablet and parenteral forms. It has also been marketed in an ion-exchange resin complex form under the trade name of Tussionex. The complex releases the drug at a sustained rate and is said to produce effective cough suppression over a 10- to 12-hour period. Hydrocodone is also marketed in combination with acetaminophen (e.g., Hydrocet, Vicodin, Lortab, and Zydone) and with homatropine as Hycodan. Although this drug found extensive use in antitussive formulations for many years, it has been placed under more stringent narcotic regulations.

Oxymorphone Hydrochloride, USP.

Oxymorphone hydrochloride, (−)-14-hydroxydihydromorphinone hydrochloride (Numorphan), introduced in 1959, is prepared by cleavage of the corresponding codeine derivative. It is used as the hydrochloride salt, which occurs as a white crystalline powder freely soluble in water and sparingly soluble in alcohol. In humans, oxymorphone is as effective as morphine in one-eighth to one-tenth the dosage, with good duration and a slightly lower frequency of side effects.[125] It has high addiction liability. It is used for the same purposes as morphine, such as control of postoperative pain, pain of advanced neoplastic diseases, and other types of pain that respond to morphine. Because of the risk of addiction, it should not be used for relief of minor pains that can be controlled with codeine. It has poor antitussive activity and is not used as a cough suppressant. It may be administered orally, parenterally (intravenously, intramuscularly, or subcutaneously), or rectally, and for these purposes is supplied as a solution for injection (1.0 and 1.5 mg/mL) and in suppositories (5 mg).

Nalbuphine Hydrochloride.

Nalbuphine hydrochloride, N-cyclobutylmethyl-14-hydroxy-N-nordihydromorphinone hydrochloride (Nubain), N-cyclobutylmethylnoroxymorphone hydrochloride, was introduced in 1979 as a potent analgesic of the agonist–antagonist type, with little to no abuse liability. It is a somewhat less potent analgesic than its parent oxymorphone but shares some of the antagonist properties of the closely related, but pure, antagonists naloxone and naltrexone. Nalbuphine hydrochloride occurs as a white to off-white powder that is soluble in water and sparingly soluble in alcohol. It is prepared from cyclobutylmethyl bromide and noroxycodone followed by cleavage of the O-methyl group.

This analgesic shows a very rapid onset with a duration of action of up to 6 hours. It has relatively low abuse liability, judged to be less than that of codeine and propoxyphene. The injection is, therefore, available without narcotic controls, although caution is urged for long-term administration or use in emotionally disturbed patients. Abrupt discontinuation after prolonged use has given rise to withdrawal signs. Usual doses cause respiratory depression comparable to that of morphine, but no further decrease is seen with higher doses. It has fewer cardiac effects than pentazocine and butorphanol. The most frequent adverse effect is sedation, and as with most other CNS depressants and analgesics, caution should be urged when it is administered to ambulatory patients who may need to drive a car or operate machinery.

Nalbuphine is marketed as an injectable (10 and 20 mg/mL). The usual dose is 10 mg administered subcutaneously, intramuscularly, or intravenously at 3- to 6-hour intervals, with a maximal daily dose of 160 mg.

Oxycodone Hydrochloride.

Oxycodone hydrochloride, dihydrohydroxycodeinone hydrochloride, is prepared by the catalytic reduction of hydroxycodeinone prepared by hydrogen peroxide (in acetic acid) oxidation of thebaine. This derivative of morphine occurs as a white crystalline powder that is soluble in water (1:10) or alcohol. Aqueous solutions may be sterilized by boiling. Although this drug is almost as likely to cause addiction as morphine, it is sold in the United States in Percodan and several other products in combination with aspirin or acetaminophen.

It is used as a sedative, an analgesic, and a narcotic. To depress the cough reflex, it is used in 3- to 5-mg doses and as an analgesic in 5- to 10-mg doses. For severe pain, a dose of 20 mg is given subcutaneously. Oxycodone is also marketed as controlled-release tablets (OxyContin, 10 to 160 mg) for use in managing chronic pain. Unfortunately, these high-dose preparations have become popular with drug users and addicts, who crush the tablets, dissolve the contents, and inject the mixture. Several overdose deaths have resulted from this practice, leading to tighter controls over their availability.

Dihydrocodeine Bitartrate. Dihydrocodeine is obtained by the reduction of codeine. The bitartrate salt occurs as white crystals that are soluble in water (1:4.5) and only slightly soluble in alcohol. Subcutaneously, a dose of 30 mg of this drug is almost equivalent to 10 mg of morphine as an analgesic, with faster onset and negligible side effects. It has addiction liability. It is available in combination with aspirin or acetaminophen for pain.

Normorphine. Normorphine may be prepared by N-demethylation of morphine.[126] In humans, by normal routes of administration, it is about one fourth as active as morphine in producing analgesia but has a much lower physical dependence capacity. Its analgesic effects are nearly equal by the intraventricular route. It does not show the sedative effects of morphine in single doses but does so cumulatively. Normorphine suppresses the morphine abstinence syndrome in addicts, but after its withdrawal, it gives a slow onset and a mild form of the abstinence syndrome.[127, 128] It was once considered for possible use in the treatment of narcotic addiction, but it has no current use.

Opium. An extract of opium, containing a mixture of the total alkaloids of opium, is available as an alcoholic aqueous solution. It is available as Deodorized Opium Tincture (15 mg/mL of morphine base) and Paregoric (2 mg/mL of morphine base). These are used primarily for the treatment of diarrhea.

Tramadol Hydrochloride. Tramadol hydrochloride, (±)-*cis*-2-[(dimethylamino)methyl]-1-(*m*-methoxyphenyl) cyclohexanol hydrochloride (Ultram), represents a fragment of codeine's structure, consisting of the phenyl and cyclohexane rings. The drug possesses opioid activity but has other analgesic activity that is not reversed by naloxone. The principal effect is attributed to the O-demethylated metabolite, which is 6 times more potent than the parent compound, an observation consistent with the differences between codeine and morphine. It produces significantly lower morphine-like side effects. It is available in tablet form for use in moderate-to-severe pain in a dose of 50 to 100 mg every 4 to 6 hours and in combination (37.5 mg) with acetaminophen (Ultracet) for short-term management of acute pain.

Apomorphine Hydrochloride, USP. When morphine or morphine hydrochloride is heated at 140° under pressure with strong (35%) hydrochloric acid, it loses a molecule of water and yields a compound known as apomorphine.

The hydrochloride is odorless and occurs as minute, glistening, white or grayish white crystals or as a white powder.

It is light sensitive and turns green on exposure to air and light. It is sparingly soluble in water (1:50, 1:20 at 80°) and in alcohol (1:50) and is very slightly soluble in ether or chloroform. Solutions are neutral to litmus.

The change in structure from morphine to apomorphine profoundly changes its physiological action. The central depressant effects of morphine are much less pronounced, and the stimulant effects are enhanced greatly, thereby producing emesis by a purely central mechanism. It is administered subcutaneously to obtain emesis. It is ineffective orally. Apomorphine is one of the most effective, prompt (10 to 15 minutes), and safe emetics in use today. Care should be exercised in its use, however, because it may be depressant in already-depressed patients. It is currently classified as an "orphan drug" for use in Parkinson's disease.

Meperidine Hydrochloride, USP. Meperidine hydrochloride, ethyl 1-methyl-4-phenylisonipecotate hydrochloride, ethyl 1-methyl-4-phenyl-4-piperidinecarboxylate hydrochloride (Demerol Hydrochloride), is a fine, white, odorless crystalline powder that is very soluble in water, soluble in alcohol, and sparingly soluble in ether. It is stable in the air at ordinary temperature, and its aqueous solution is not decomposed by a short period of boiling. The free base may be made by heating benzyl cyanide with bis(β-chloroethyl)methylamine, hydrolyzing to the corresponding acid and esterifying the latter with ethyl alcohol.[2]

Meperidine first was synthesized to study its spasmolytic character, but it was found to have far greater analgesic properties. The spasmolysis is primarily due to a direct papaverine-like depression of smooth muscle and, also, to some action on parasympathetic nerve endings. In therapeutic doses, it exerts an analgesic effect that lies between those of morphine and codeine, but it shows little tendency toward hypnosis. It is indicated for the relief of pain in most patients for whom morphine and other alkaloids of opium generally are used, but it is especially valuable when the pain is due to spastic conditions of intestine, uterus, bladder, bronchi, and so on. Its most important use seems to be in lessening the severity of labor pains in obstetrics and, with barbiturates or tranquilizers, producing amnesia in labor. In labor, a dose of 100 mg is injected intramuscularly as soon as contractions occur regularly, and a second dose may be given after 30 minutes if labor is rapid or if the cervix is thin and dilated (≥2 to 3 cm). A third dose may be necessary an hour or two later, and at this stage a barbiturate may be administered in a small dose to ensure adequate amnesia for several hours. Meperidine possesses addiction liability. Psychic dependence develops in individuals who experience euphoria lasting for an hour or more. The development of tolerance has been observed, and meperidine can be substituted successfully for morphine in addicts who are being treated by gradual withdrawal. Furthermore, mild withdrawal symptoms have been noted in certain persons who have become purposely addicted to meperidine. The possibility of dependence is great enough to put it under the federal narcotic laws. It is available in oral liquid, tablet, and parenteral dosage forms.

Alphaprodine Hydrochloride, USP. Alphaprodine hydrochloride, (±)-1,3-dimethyl-4-phenyl-4-piperidinol propanoate hydrochloride, is prepared by the method of Ziering and Lee.[129] It occurs as a white crystalline powder that is freely soluble in water, alcohol, and chloroform but insoluble in ether. The compound is an effective analgesic, similar to meperidine, and of special value in obstetric analgesia. It appears to be quite safe for use in this capacity, causing little or no respiratory depression in either mother or fetus. It is currently not marketed in the United States.

Anileridine, USP. Anileridine, ethyl 1-(*p*-aminophenethyl)-4-phenylisonipecotate (Leritine), is prepared by the method of Weijlard et al.[130] It occurs as a white to yellowish-white crystalline powder that is freely soluble in alcohol but only very slightly soluble in water. It is oxidized on exposure to air and light. The injection is prepared by dissolving the free base in phosphoric acid solution. Anileridine is more active than meperidine and has the same usefulness and limitations. Its dependence capacity is less, and it is considered a suitable substitute for meperidine. It is currently not marketed in the United States.

Anileridine Hydrochloride, USP. Anileridine hydrochloride, ethyl 1-(*p*-aminophenethyl)-4-phenylisonipecotate dihydrochloride (Leritine Hydrochloride), is prepared as cited for anileridine, except that it is converted to the dihydrochloride by conventional procedures. It occurs as a white or nearly white, crystalline odorless powder that is stable in air. It is freely soluble in water, sparingly soluble in alcohol, and practically insoluble in ether and chloroform. This salt has the same activity as anileridine. It is currently not marketed in the United States.

Diphenoxylate Hydrochloride, USP. Diphenoxylate hydrochloride, ethyl 1-(3-cyano-3,3-diphenylpropyl)-4-phenylisonipecotate monohydrochloride (Lomotil, Lonox, Logen, Lomanate), occurs as a white, odorless, slightly water-soluble powder with no distinguishing taste. Although this drug has a strong structural relationship to the meperidine-type analgesics, it has very little, if any, such activity itself. Its most pronounced activity is its ability to inhibit excessive gastrointestinal motility, an activity reminiscent of the constipating side effect of morphine itself. Investigators have demonstrated the possibility of addiction,[35, 36] particularly with large doses, but virtually all studies using ordinary dosage levels show nonaddiction. Its safety is reflected in its classification as an exempt narcotic, with the warning, however, that it may be habit forming. To discourage possible abuse of the drug, the commercial product (Lomotil) once contained a subtherapeutic dose (25 μg) of atropine sulfate in each 2.5-mg tablet and in each 5 mL of the liquid, which contains a like amount of the drug.

It is indicated in the oral treatment of diarrhea resulting from a variety of causes. The usual initial adult dose is 5 mg 3 or 4 times a day, with the maintenance dose usually substantially lower and individually determined. Appropriate dosage schedules for children are available in the manufacturer's literature.

The incidence of side effects is low, but the drug should be used with caution, if at all, in patients with impaired hepatic function. Similarly, patients taking barbiturates concurrently with the drug should be observed carefully, in view of reports of barbiturate toxicity under these circumstances.

Loperamide Hydrochloride, USP. Loperamide hydrochloride, 4-(4-chlorophenyl)-4-hydroxy-*N,N*-dimethyl-α,α-diphenyl-1-piperidinebutanamide, 4-(4-*p*-chlorophenyl-4-hydroxypiperidino)-*N,N*-dimethyl-2,2-diphenylbutyramide hydrochloride (Imodium), a hybrid of a methadone-like and meperidine molecule, is closely related to diphenoxylate but is more specific, more potent, and longer acting. It acts as an antidiarrheal by a direct effect on the circular and longitudinal intestinal muscles. After oral administration it reaches peak blood levels within 4 hours and has a very long plasma half-life (40 hours). Tolerance to its effects has not been observed.[131] Although it has shown minimal CNS effects, it has been controlled under Schedule V. Loperamide is available as 2-mg capsules (Loperamide hydrochloride capsules, USP) for treatment of acute and chronic diarrhea. Recommended dosage is 4 mg initially, with 2 mg after each loose stool for a maximum of 16 mg/day.

Ethoheptazine Citrate. Ethoheptazine citrate, ethyl hexahydro-1-methyl-4-phenyl-1*H*-azepine-4-carboxylate citrate, 1-methyl-4-carbethoxy-4-phenylhexamethylenimine citrate (Zactane Citrate), is effective orally against moderate pain in doses of 50 to 100 mg, with minimal side effects. Parenteral administration is limited because of central stimulating effects. It appears to have no addiction liability, but toxic reactions have occurred with large doses. A double-blind study in humans rated 100 mg of the hydrochloride salt equivalent to 30 mg of codeine and found that the addition of 600 mg of aspirin increased analgesic effectiveness.[39] In another study, a dose of 150 mg was found equal to 65 mg of propoxyphene, with both better than placebo.[132] It was once available as a 75-mg tablet and in combination with 600 mg of aspirin (Zactirin).

Fentanyl Citrate, USP. Fentanyl citrate, *N*-(1-phenethyl-4-piperidyl)propionanilide citrate (Sublimaze), occurs as a crystalline powder soluble in water (1:40) and methanol and sparingly soluble in chloroform. This novel anilide derivative has analgesic activity 50 times that of morphine in humans.[42] It has a very rapid onset (4 min) and short duration of action. Side effects similar to those of other potent analgesics are common, particularly respiratory depression and bradycardia. It is used primarily as an adjunct to anesthesia. For use as a neuroleptanalgesic in surgery, it is available in combination with the neuroleptic droperidol (Innovar). It is also available as a transdermal release system (Duragesic, at total dose levels ranging from 20 to 100 mg) for management of chronic pain. It has dependence liability.

Alfentanil Hydrochloride. Alfentanil hydrochloride, *N*-[1-[2-(4-ethyl-5-oxo-2-tetrazolin-1-yl)-ethyl]-4-(methoxymethyl)-4-piperidyl]propionanilide hydrochloride monohydrate (Alfenta), is closely related to fentanyl. It is a potent analgesic used as a primary anesthetic or as an adjunct in the maintenance of anesthesia. It has the same properties and side effects as fentanyl. It is available as an injection (0.5 mg/mL).

Remifentanil Hydrochloride. Remifentanil hydrochloride, 4-carboxy-4-(*N*-phenylpropionamido)-1-piperidineproprionic acid methyl ester hydrochloride (Ultiva), a structural analogue of fentanyl, has similar properties and is also used in anesthesia. It is available as an injection (1 mg/mL).

Sufentanil Citrate.

Sufentanil citrate, *N*-[4-(methoxymethyl)-1-[2-(2-thienyl)ethyl]-4-piperidyl]propionanilide citrate (Sufenta), a structural analogue of fentanyl, has similar properties and is also used in anesthesia. It is available as an injection (0.05 mg/mL).

Methadone Hydrochloride, USP.

Methadone hydrochloride, 6-(Dimethylamino)-4,4-diphenyl-3-heptanone hydrochloride (Dolophine Hydrochloride), occurs as a bitter, white crystalline powder. It is soluble in water, freely soluble in alcohol and chloroform, and insoluble in ether. Methadone is synthesized in several ways. The method of Easton et al.[133] is noteworthy, in that it avoids the formation of the troublesome isomeric intermediate aminonitriles.[44, 133] The analgesic effect and other morphine-like properties are exhibited chiefly by the (−) form. Aqueous solutions are stable and may be sterilized by heat for intramuscular and intravenous use. Like all amine salts, it is incompatible with alkali and salts of heavy metals. It is somewhat irritating when injected subcutaneously.

The toxicity of methadone is 3 to 10 times that of morphine, but its analgesic effect is twice that of morphine and 10 times that of meperidine. It has been placed under federal narcotic control because of its high addiction liability. Methadone is a most effective analgesic, used to alleviate many types of pain. It can replace morphine for the relief of withdrawal symptoms. It produces less sedation and narcosis than morphine and appears to have fewer side reactions in bedridden patients. Methadone is especially valuable in spasm of the urinary bladder and in the suppression of the cough reflex,.

The *levo* isomer, levanone, reportedly does not produce euphoria or other morphine-like sensations and has been advocated for the treatment of addicts.[134] Methadone itself is used quite extensively in addict treatment, although not without some controversy.[135] It suppresses withdrawal effects and is widely used to maintain former heroin addicts during this rehabilitation. Large doses are often used to "block" the effects of heroin during treatment. The use of methadone in treating addicts is subject to Food and Drug Administration (FDA) regulations that require special registration of physicians and dispensers. Methadone is available for use as an analgesic, however, under the usual narcotic requirements.

Levomethadyl Acetate Hydrochloride.

Levomethadyl acetate hydrochloride, *l*-*α*-acetylmethadol, (-)-*α*-6-(dimethylamino)-4,4-diphenyl-3-heptyl acetate hydrochloride, methadyl acetate, LAAM, occurs as a white crystalline powder that is soluble in water but dissolves with some difficulty. It is prepared by hydride reduction of (+)-methadone followed by acetylation. Of the four possible methadol isomers, the (3*S*,6*S*) isomer LAAM has the unique characteristic of producing long-lasting narcotic effects. Extensive metabolism studies have shown that this is due to its N-demethylation to give (−)-*α*-acetylnormethadol, which is more potent than its parent, LAAM, and possesses a long half-life.[136]

This is further accentuated by its demethylation to the dinor metabolite, which has similar properties.[136, 137]

Because of the need to administer methadone daily, which inconveniences the maintenance patient and leads to illicit diversion, the long-acting LAAM was actively investigated as an addict-maintenance drug to replace methadone. Generally, an 80- to 100-mg dose 3 times a week suffices for routine maintenance.[53, 138] The FDA has approved the drug for use, and it is marketed as ORLAAM in solution form (10 mg/mL). By law, it can be dispensed only by treatment programs certified by the Department of Health and Human Services' Substance Abuse and Mental Health Services Administration and registered with the Drug Enforcement Administration. It also carries a warning about possible serious cardiac arrhythmia. The racemate of the normetabolite, noracylmethadol, was once studied in the clinic as a potential analgesic.[139]

Propoxyphene Hydrochloride, USP.

Propoxyphene hydrochloride, (2*S*,3*R*)-(+)-4(dimethylamino)-3-methyl-1,2-diphenyl-2-butanol propanoate hydrochloride (Darvon, Dolene, Doxaphene), was introduced into therapy in 1957. It may be prepared by the method of Pohland and Sullivan.[140] It occurs as a bitter, white crystalline powder that is freely soluble in water, soluble in alcohol, chloroform, and acetone, but practically insoluble in benzene and ether. It is the *α*-(+) isomer; the *α*-(−) isomer and *β* diastereoisomers are far less potent in analgesic activity. The *α*-(−) isomer, *levo*-propoxyphene, is an effective antitussive (see below).

In analgesic potency, propoxyphene is approximately equal to codeine phosphate and has a lower frequency of side effects. It has no antidiarrheal, antitussive, or antipyretic effect, thus differing from most analgesic agents. It can suppress the morphine abstinence syndrome in addicts but has shown a low level of abuse because of its toxicity. It is not very effective in deep pain and appears to be no more effective in minor pain than aspirin. Its widespread use in dental pain seems justified, since aspirin is reported to be relatively ineffective. It has been classified as a narcotic and controlled under federal law. It does give some euphoria in high doses and has been abused. It has been responsible for numerous overdosage deaths. Refilling the prescription should be avoided if misuse is suspected. It is available in several combination products with aspirin or acetaminophen (e.g., Wygesic).

Propoxyphene Napsylate, USP.

Propoxyphene napsylate, (+)-*α*-4-dimethylamino-3-methyl-1,2-diphenyl-2-butanol propanoate (ester) 2-naphthylenesulfonate (salt) (Darvon-N), is very slightly soluble in water, but soluble in alcohol, chloroform, and acetone. The napsylate salt of propoxyphene was introduced shortly before the patent on Darvon expired. The insoluble salt form is claimed to be less prone to abuse because it cannot be readily dissolved for injection and, on oral administration, gives a slower, less pronounced peak blood level.

Because of its mild narcotic-like properties, it was once investigated as an addict-maintenance drug to be used in place of methadone. It was hoped that it would provide easier withdrawal and serve as an addict-detoxification drug. Unfortunately, toxicity at higher doses has limited this application. It is available in combination with acetaminophen (Propacet, Darvocet-N).

Levorphanol Tartrate, USP.
Grewe made the basic studies in the synthesis of compounds of the type of levorphanol tartrate, (−)-3-hydroxy-*N*-methylmorphman bitartrate (Levo-Dromoran), as mentioned above. Schnider and Gräussner synthesized the hydroxymorphinans, including the 3-hydroxyl derivative, by similar methods. The racemic 3-hydroxy-*N*-methylmorphinan hydrobromide (racemorphan, (±)-Dromoran) was the original form in which this potent analgesic was introduced. This drug is prepared by resolution of racemorphan. The *levo* compound is available in Europe under the original name, Dromoran. As the tartrate, it occurs in the form of colorless crystals. The salt is sparingly soluble in water (1:60) and is insoluble in ether.

The drug is used for the relief of severe pain and is in many respects similar in its actions to morphine, except that it is 6 to 8 times as potent. The addiction liability of levorphanol is as great as that of morphine and, for that reason, caution should be observed in its use. It is claimed that the gastrointestinal effects of this compound are significantly lower than those experienced with morphine. Naloxone is an effective antidote for overdosage. Levorphanol is useful for relieving severe pain originating from a multiplicity of causes (e.g., inoperable tumors, severe trauma, renal colic, biliary colic). In other words, it has the same range of usefulness as morphine and is considered an excellent substitute. It is supplied in ampuls, in multidose vials, and as oral tablets (2 mg). The drug requires a narcotic form.

Butorphanol Tartrate, USP.
Butorphanol tartrate, 17-(cyclobutyl-methyl)morphinan-3,14-diol D-(−)-tartrate, (−)-*N*-cyclobutylmethyl-3,14-dihydroxymorphinan bitartrate (Stadol), a potent analgesic, occurs as a white crystalline powder soluble in water and sparingly soluble in alcohol. It is prepared from the dihydroxy-*N*-normorphinan obtained by a modification of the Grewe synthesis. It is the cyclobutyl analogue of levorphanol and levallorphan, and is as potent an analgesic as the former and a somewhat less active antagonist than the latter.

Butorphanol

The onset and duration of action of the drug are comparable to those of morphine, but it has the advantages of showing a maximal ceiling effect on respiratory depression and a greatly reduced abuse liability. The injectable form was marketed without narcotic controls; this product was considered for placement in Schedule IV, however, because of reported misuse and lack of recognition of its potential abuse liability. The drug has also been used illegally for doping racehorses.

Butorphanol shares the adverse hemodynamic effects of pentazocine, causing increased pressure in specific arteries and on the heart workload. It should thus be used with caution and only with patients hypersensitive to morphine for the treatment of myocardial infarction or other cardiac problems. Other adverse effects include a high incidence of sedation and, less frequently, nausea, headache, vertigo, and dizziness.[141]

It is available as a parenteral for intramuscular and intravenous administration in a dose of 1 or 2 mg every 3 to 4 hours, with a maximal single dose of 4 mg. It is also available as a nasal spray (Stadol NS).

Buprenorphine Hydrochloride.
Buprenorphine hydrochloride, 21-cyclopropyl-7α-[(*S*)-1-hydroxy-1,2,2-trimethylpropyl]-6,14-*endo*-ethano-6,7,8,14-tetrahydrooripavine hydrochloride (Buprenex), is a rapidly acting, centrally acting analgesic in the agonist–antagonists class. It is about 30 times more potent than morphine. It is available for treating moderate-to-severe pain as a parenteral for intramuscular or intravenous administration in a dose of 0.3 mg every 6 hours.

After several years of investigation for use in treating opioid addiction, buprenorphine, alone or in combination with naloxone, has been approved for use in a highly regulated treatment program called *Office Based Opioid Treatment* (OBOT). Under federal legislation, the Substance Abuse and Mental Health Administration's Center for Drug Abuse Treatment has established criteria and training programs for private physicians to administer these special dosage forms to opioid addicts. The intent of the program is to make treatment available to persons who are not likely to seek treatment in traditional treatment clinics, such as adolescents, executives, and the like.

Dezocine.
Dezocine, (−)-13β-amino-5,6,7,8,9,10,11α, 12-octahydro-5α-methyl-5,11-methanobenzocyclodecen-3-ol (Dalgan), is a synthetic agonist–antagonist analgesic, with an unusual structure. It is similar to morphine in analgesic potency and duration. It produces fewer side effects, due to its antagonist activity, with reported minimal dependence capacity. It is available for treating moderate-to-severe pain as a parenteral for intramuscular or intravenous administration in a dose of 5 to 20 mg every 3 to 6 hours.

Nalbuphine Hydrochloride.
Nalbuphine hydrochloride, 17-(cyclobutylmethyl)-4,5α-epoxymorphinan-3,6α, 14-triol hydrochloride (Nubain), is a combination of the oxymorphine nucleus and the nitrogen substituent of butorphanol. It is a potent analgesic of the agonist–antagonist class, similar to morphine in potency but with an abuse potential rated less than that of codeine. It is useful in treating moderate-to-severe pain and is available for parenteral use with a usual dose of 10 mg/70 kg every 3 to 6 hours.

Pentazocine, USP.
Pentazocine, 1,2,3,4,5,6-hexahydro-*cis*-6,11-dimethyl-3-(3-methyl-2-butenyl)-2,6-methano3-benzazocin-8-ol, *cis*-2-dimethylallyl-5,9-dimethyl-2'-hydroxy-6,7-benzomorphan (Talwin), occurs as a white crystalline powder that is insoluble in water and sparingly soluble in alcohol. It forms a poorly soluble hydrochloride salt, but is readily soluble as the lactate.

Pentazocine in a parenteral dose of 30 mg or an oral dose of 50 mg is about as effective as 10 mg of morphine in most patients. There is some evidence that the analgesic action resides principally in the (–) isomer, and a dose of 25 mg is approximately equivalent to 10 mg of morphine sulfate.[142] Occasionally, doses of 40 to 60 mg may be required. Pentazocine's plasma half-life is about 3.5 hours.[143] At the lower dosage levels, it appears to be well tolerated, although some sedation occurs in about one third of persons receiving it. The incidence of other morphine-like side effects is as high as with morphine and other narcotic analgesics. In patients who have been receiving other narcotic analgesics, large doses of pentazocine may precipitate withdrawal symptoms. It shows an equivalent or greater respiratory depressant activity. Pentazocine has given rise to a few cases of possible dependence. It has been placed under control, and its abuse potential should be recognized and close supervision of its use maintained. Levallorphan cannot reverse its effects, although naloxone can, and methylphenidate is recommended as an antidote for overdosage or excessive respiratory depression.

Pentazocine as the lactate is available in injection form containing the base equivalent of 30 mg/mL, buffered to pH 4 to 5. It should not be mixed with barbiturates. Tablets of 50 mg (as the hydrochloride in combination with nalorone to prevent abuse) are available for oral administration. It is also available in combination with aspirin (Talwin Compound) and with acetaminophen (Talacen).

Methotrimeprazine, USP. Methotrimeprazine, (–)-10-[3-(dimethylamino)-2-methylpropyl]-2-methoxyphenothiazine (Levoprome), a phenothiazine derivative closely related to chlorpromazine, possesses strong analgesic activity. An intramuscular dose of 15 to 20 mg is equal to 10 mg of morphine in humans. It has not shown any dependence liability and appears not to produce respiratory depression. The most frequent side effects are similar to those of phenothiazine tranquilizers, namely, sedation and orthostatic hypotension. These often result in dizziness and fainting, limiting the use of methotrimeprazine to nonambulatory patients. It should be used with caution along with antihypertensives, atropine, and other sedatives. It shows some advantage in patients for whom addiction and respiratory depression are problems.[144]

Narcotic Antagonists

Nalorphine Hydrochloride, USP. Nalorphine hydrochloride, *N*-allylnormorphine hydrochloride, may be prepared according to the method of Weijlard and Erickson.[126] It occurs in the form of white or practically white crystals that slowly darken on exposure to air and light. It is freely soluble in water (1:8), sparingly soluble in alcohol (1:35), and almost insoluble in chloroform and ether. The phenolic hydroxyl group confers water solubility in the presence of fixed alkali. Aqueous solutions of the salt are acid, with a pH of about 5.

Nalorphine has a direct antagonistic effect against morphine, meperidine, methadone, and levorphanol. It has little antagonistic effect toward barbiturate or general anesthetic depression, however. It has strong analgesic properties, but it is not acceptable for such use owing to the high incidence of undesirable psychotic effects. Because of these properties and the availability of alternate antagonists, it was withdrawn from the market.

Levallorphan Tartrate, USP. Levallorphan tartrate, 17-(2-propenyl)-morphinan-3-ol tartrate, (–)-*N*-allyl-3-hydroxymorphinan bitartrate (Lorfan), occurs as a white or practically white, odorless crystalline powder. It is soluble in water (1:20), sparingly soluble in alcohol (1:60), and practically insoluble in chloroform and ether. Levallorphan resembles nalorphine in its pharmacological action and is about 5 times more effective as a narcotic antagonist. It was useful in combination with analgesics such as meperidine, alphaprodine, and levorphanol to prevent the respiratory depression usually associated with these drugs. It is no longer marketed.

Narcotic Antagonists

Naloxone Hydrochloride, USP. Naloxone hydrochloride, 4,5-epoxy-3,14-dihydroxy-17-(2-propenyl)morphinan-6-one hydrochloride, *N*-allyl-14-hydroxynordihydromorphinone hydrochloride (Narcan), *N*-allylnoroxymorphone hydrochloride, is presently on the market as the agent of choice for treating narcotic overdosage. It lacks not only the analgesic activity shown by other antagonists, but also all of the other agonist effects. It is almost 7 times more active than nalorphine in antagonizing the effects of morphine. It shows no withdrawal effects after long-term administration. The duration of action is about 4 hours. It was briefly investigated for the treatment of heroin addiction. With adequate doses of naloxone, the addict does not receive any effect from heroin. It is given to an addict only after a detoxification period. Its long-term usefulness is currently limited because its short duration of action requires large oral doses. Long-acting, alternative antagonists are available (Table 22-5).

Cyclazocine. Cyclazocine, 3-(cyclopropylmethyl)-1,2,3,4,5,6-hexahydro-6,11-dimethyl-2,6-methano-3-benzazocin-8-ol, *cis*-2-cyclopropylmethyl-5,9-dimethyl-2'-hydroxy-6,7-benzomorphan, is a potent narcotic antagonist that has shown analgesic activity in humans in 1-mg doses. It once was investigated as a clinical analgesic. It does possess hallucinogenic side effects at higher doses, which limited its usefulness as an analgesic. It was studied like naloxone in the treatment of narcotic addiction. Voluntary treatment with cyclazocine deprives addicts of the euphorogenic effects of heroin. Its dependence liability is lower, and the effects of withdrawal develop more slowly and are milder. Tolerance develops to the side effects of cyclazocine, but not to its antagonist effects.[147] The effects are long lasting and are not reversed by other antagonists such as nalorphine. It has not been marketed.

Naltrexone. Naltrexone, 17-(cyclopropylmethyl)-4,5 α-epoxy-3,14-dihydroxymorphinan-6-one, *N*-cyclopropylmethyl-14-hydroxynordihydromorphinone, *N*-cyclopropylmethylnoroxymorphone (ReVia, Depade), a naloxone analogue, has been marketed as the preferred agent for treating former opiate addicts. Oral doses of 50 mg daily or 100 mg 3 times weekly suffice to "block" or protect a patient from

TABLE 22–5 Narcotic Antagonists

Name *Proprietary Name*	Preparations	Usual Adult Dose	Usual Dose Range	Usual Pediatric Dose
Levallorphan tartrate, NF *Lorfan*	Levallorphan tartrate injection, NF	IV, 1 mg, repeated twice at 10- to 15-minute intervals, if necessary	500 μg–2 mg, repeated, if necessary	0.05–0.1 mg in neonates to decrease respiratory depression
Naloxone hydrochloride, USP *Narcan*	Naloxone hydrochloride injection, USP	Parenteral, 400 μg, repeated at 2- to 3-minute intervals, as necessary		0.01 mg as above

the effects of heroin. Its metabolism,[148, 149] pharmacokinetics,[150] and pharmacology[151] have been studied intensely because of the tremendous governmental interest in developing new agents for the treatment of addiction.[67]

It is available as 50-mg tablets (ReVia) for use in treating narcotic addiction. It has also shown promise for suppressing craving in the treatment of alcoholism and is available for that use. Sustained-release or depot dosage forms of naltrexone were once investigated to avoid the recurrent decision on the part of the former addict of whether a protecting dose of antagonist is needed.[68, 152]

Nalmefene Hydrochloride.   Nalmefene hydrochloride, 17-(cyclopropylmethyl)-4,5 α-epoxy-6-methylenemorphinan-3,14-diol hydrochloride (Revex), is the 6-methylene analogue of naloxone. It is the latest pure antagonist to be introduced for use in reversing the effects of opioid agonists. It is longer acting than naltrexone and is used for the same indications. It is available as an injection (0.1 and 1.0 mg/mL).

Others.   Several other narcotic antagonists have been investigated (e.g., diprenorphine[153] and oxilorphan).[154]

ANTITUSSIVE AGENTS

Cough is a protective, physiological reflex that occurs in health as well as in disease. It is very widespread and commonly ignored as a mild symptom. In many conditions, however, it is desirable to take measures to reduce excessive coughing. Many etiological factors cause this reflex, and when a cough has been present for an extended period or accompanies any unusual symptoms, the person should be referred to a physician. Cough preparations are widely advertised and often sold indiscriminately; the pharmacist must warn the public of the inherent dangers.

Among the agents used in the symptomatic control of cough are those that act by depressing the cough center located in the medulla. These have been termed *anodynes, cough suppressants,* and *centrally acting antitussives.* Until recently, the only effective drugs in this area were narcotic analgesic agents. The more important and widely used ones are morphine, hydromorphone, codeine, hydrocodone, methadone, and levorphanol, which are discussed above.

In recent years, several compounds have been synthesized that possess antitussive activity without the addiction liabili-

ties of the narcotic agents. Some of these act in a similar manner through a central effect. In a hypothesis for the initiation of the cough reflex, Salem and Aviado[155] proposed that bronchodilatation is an important mechanism for the relief of cough. Their hypothesis suggests that irritation of the mucosa initially causes bronchoconstriction that in turn excites the cough receptors.

Chappel and von Seemann[156] have pointed out that most antitussives of this type fall into two structural groups. The larger group has structures that bear a resemblance to methadone. The other group has large, bulky substituents on the acid portion of an ester, usually connected by means of a long, ether-containing chain to a *tertiary* amino group. The notable exceptions are benzonatate and sodium dibunate. Noscapine could be considered as belonging to the first group.

Many of the cough preparations sold contain various other ingredients in addition to the primary antitussive agent. The more important ones include antihistamines, useful when the cause of the cough is allergic, although some antihistaminic drugs (e.g., diphenhydramine) have a central antitussive action as well; sympathomimetics, which are quite effective owing to their bronchodilatory activity, the most useful being ephedrine, methamphetamine, phenylpropanolamine, homarylamine, isoproterenol, and isooctylamine; parasympatholytics, which help to dry secretions in the upper respiratory passages; and expectorants. It is not known if these drugs potentiate the antitussive action, but they usually are considered adjuvant therapy. The more important drugs in this class are discussed in the following section. For more exhaustive coverage of the field, the reader is urged to consult the excellent review of Chappel and von Seemann.[156]

Products

Some of the narcotic antitussive products are discussed above with the narcotic analgesics. Others are discussed below (Table 22-6).

Noscapine, USP.   Noscapine, (−)-narcotine (Tusscapine), an opium alkaloid, was isolated in 1817 by Robiquet. It is isolated rather easily from the drug by ether extraction. It makes up 0.75 to 9% of opium. With the discovery of its unique antitussive properties, the name of this alkaloid was changed from narcotine to noscapine. It was realized that it would not meet with widespread acceptance as long as its name was associated with the narcotic opium alkaloids. The name *noscapine* was probably selected because a precedent

TABLE 22–6   Antitussive Agents

Name *Proprietary Name*	Preparations	Usual Adult Dose	Usual Dose Range
Dextromethorphan hydrobromide, USP *Romilar*	Dextromethorphan hydrobromide syrup, USP	15–30 mg qd to qid	
Levopropoxyphene napsylate, USP *Novrad*	Levopropoxyphene napsylate capsules, USP Levopropoxyphene napsylate oral suspension, USP	50–100 mg of levopropoxyphene, as the napsylate, every 4 hours	
Benzonatate, USP *Tessalon*	Benzonatate capsules, USP	100 mg tid	100–200 mg

existed in the name of (±)-narcotine, namely, *gnoscopine*. It was once available in various cough preparations.

Dextromethorphan Hydrobromide, USP.

Dextromethorphan hydrobromide, (+)-3-methoxy-17-methyl-$9\alpha,13\alpha,14\alpha$-morphinan hydrobromide (Romilar), is the O-methylated (+)-form of racemorphan left after the resolution necessary in the preparation of levorphanol. It occurs as practically white crystals or as a crystalline powder, with a faint odor. It is sparingly soluble in water (1:65), freely soluble in alcohol and chloroform, and insoluble in ether.

It possesses the antitussive properties of codeine, without the analgesic, addictive, central depressant, and constipating features. Ten milligrams is suggested as equivalent to a 15-mg dose of codeine in antitussive effect. It affords an opportunity to note the specificity exhibited by very closely related molecules. Here, the (+) and (−) forms both must attach to receptors responsible for the suppression of the cough reflex, but the (+) form is apparently in a steric relationship that precludes attaching to the receptors involved in analgesic, constipative, addictive, and other actions exhibited by the (−) form. It has largely replaced many older antitussives, including codeine, in prescription and nonprescription cough preparations.

Benzonatate, USP.

Benzonatate, 2,5,8,11,14,17,20,23,26-nonaoxaoctacosan-28-yl *p*-(butylamino)benzoate (Tessalon), introduced in 1956, is a pale-yellow, viscous liquid insoluble in water and soluble in most organic solvents. It is chemically related to *p*-aminobenzoate local anesthetics, except that the aminoalcohol group has been replaced by a methylated polyethylene glycol group.

Benzonatate reportedly possesses both peripheral and central activity in producing its antitussive effect. It somehow blocks the stretch receptors thought to be responsible for cough. Clinically, it is not as effective as codeine, but it produces far fewer side effects and has very low toxicity. It is available in 100-mg capsules ("perles").

Carbetapentane Citrate.

Carbetapentane citrate, 2-[2-(diethylamino)-ethoxy]ethyl 1-phenylcyclopentanecarboxylate citrate, is a white, odorless crystalline powder that is freely soluble in water (1:1), slightly soluble in alcohol, and insoluble in ether. It is reportedly equivalent to codeine as an antitussive. Introduced in 1956, it is well tolerated and has a low frequency of side effects. It is available as a pediatric suspension (2.5 mg/5 mL) or as capsules (20 mg, Cophene-X), and in various combinations with antihistamines and decongestants. The tannate is also available (Rynatuss) as a 60-mg tablet and is said to give a more sustained action.

ANTI-INFLAMMATORY ANALGESICS

The early growth of the anti-inflammatory analgesic group was related closely to the belief that lowering or "curing" fever was an end in itself. Drugs that induced a drop in temperature in feverish conditions were considered quite valuable and were sought eagerly. The decline of interest in these drugs coincided more or less with the realization that fever was an outward symptom of some other, more fundamental ailment. During the use of the several antipyretics, however, some were noted to be excellent analgesics for the relief of minor aches and pains. These drugs have survived to the present time on the basis of the analgesic, rather than the antipyretic, effect. Although these drugs are still widely used for the alleviation of minor aches and pains, they are also used extensively in the symptomatic treatment of rheumatic fever, rheumatoid arthritis (RA), and osteoarthritis (OA). The dramatic effect of salicylates in reducing the inflammatory effects of rheumatic fever is time honored, and even with the development of the corticosteroids, these drugs are still of great value in this respect. The steroids are reportedly no more effective than the salicylates in preventing the cardiac complications of rheumatic fever.[157]

The analgesic drugs that fall into this category have been disclaimed by some as not deserving the term *analgesic* because of their low activity in comparison with the morphine-type compounds. Indeed, Fourneau has suggested the name *antalgics* to designate this general category and, in this way, to emphasize the distinction from the narcotic or so-called true analgesics. Two of the principal features distinguishing these analgesics from the narcotic analgesics are the low activity for a given dose (which is not increased significantly at a higher dosage) and the lack of addiction potential.

Research has intensified in an effort to find new nonsteroidal anti-inflammatory drugs (NSAIDs). Long-term therapy with the corticosteroids is often accompanied by various side effects. Efforts to discover new agents have been limited, for the most part, to structural analogues of active compounds owing to a lack of knowledge about the causes and mechanisms of inflammatory diseases.[158] Although several new agents have been introduced for use in RA, aspirin remains one of the most widely used drugs for this purpose. It also protects against myocardial infarctions.

A significant stimulus to this search was the observation that prostaglandins play a major role in the inflammatory processes.[159] Drugs such as aspirin and indomethacin inhibit prostaglandin synthesis in several tissues.[160] Furthermore, almost all classes of NSAIDs strongly inhibit the conversion of arachidonic acid into prostaglandin E_2 (PGE_2).[161, 162] This occurs at the stage of conversion of arachidonic acid, released by the action of phospholipase A on damaged tissues, by prostaglandin H_2 synthetase, now called *cyclooxygenase*, to the cyclic endoperoxides PGG_2 and PGH_2. These are known to cause vasoconstriction and pain. They, in turn, are converted in part to PGE_2 and $PGF_{2\alpha}$, which can cause pain and vasodilatation. This effect of the NSAIDs parallels their relative potency in various tests and is stereospecific.[161]

The search for specific inhibitors of cyclooxygenase has opened a new area of research in this field. This enzyme occurs in two forms, cyclooxygenase 1 (COX-1) and cyclooxygenase 2 (COX-2). COX-1 is a constitutive enzyme and plays a role in the production of essential prostaglandins. Inhibition of this enzyme by all the older, nonselective NSAIDs is primarily responsible for a number of their side effects. The COX-2 enzyme is induced in response to the release of several proinflammatory mediators, leading to the inflammatory response and pain. Thus, there was an active search for specific inhibitors of the COX-2 enzyme. This has been successful with the approval of three COX-2 inhibitors, discussed below.

Even with the significant advances achieved in the discovery of new and more specific NSAIDs, they all have a ceiling effect on their ability to relieve all pain. It is becoming common practice to use combinations of the opioid drugs with NSAIDs to treat severe and intractable pain. These drugs are considered below in their various chemical categories.

Salicylic Acid Derivatives

Historically, the salicylates were among the first of this group to achieve recognition as analgesics. Leroux, in 1827, isolated salicin, and Piria, in 1838, prepared salicylic acid. After these discoveries, Cahours (1844) obtained salicylic acid from oil of wintergreen (methyl salicylate), and Kolbe and Lautermann (1860) prepared it synthetically from phenol. Sodium salicylate was introduced in 1875 by Buss, followed by the introduction of phenyl salicylate by Nencki in 1886. Aspirin, or acetylsalicylic acid, was first prepared in 1853 by Gerhardt but remained obscure until Felix Hoffmann discovered its pharmacological activities in 1899. It was tested and introduced into medicine by Dreser, who named it *aspirin* by taking the *a* from acetyl and adding it to *spirin*, an old name for salicylic or spiric acid, derived from its natural source of spirea plants.

The pharmacology of the salicylates and related compounds has been reviewed extensively by Smith.[163, 164] Salicylates, in general, exert their antipyretic action in febrile patients by increasing heat elimination of the body via the mobilization of water and consequent dilution of the blood. This brings about perspiration, causing cutaneous dilatation.

This does not occur with normal temperatures. The antipyretic and analgesic actions are believed to occur in the hypothalamic area of the brain. Some think that the salicylates exert their analgesia by their effect on water balance, reducing the edema usually associated with arthralgias. Aspirin is particularly effective for this. For an interesting account of the history of aspirin and a discussion of its mechanisms of action, the reader should consult an article by Collier,[165] as well as the reviews by Smith[163, 164] and by Nickander et al.[162]

The possibility of hypoprothrombinemia and concomitant capillary bleeding in conjunction with salicylate administration accounts for the inclusion of menadione in some salicylate formulations. There is some doubt, however, about the necessity for this measure. A more serious aspect of salicylate medication is the possibility of inducing hemorrhage from direct irritative contact with the mucosa. Alvarez and Summerskill have pointed out a definite relationship between salicylate consumption and massive gastrointestinal hemorrhage from peptic ulcer.[166] Barager and Duthie[167] in an extensive study found, however, no danger of increased anemia or development of peptic ulcer. Leonards and Levy[168] used radiolabeled iron and demonstrated that bleeding does occur following administration of aspirin. The effects varied with the formulation. Davenport[169] suggests that back diffusion of acid from the stomach is responsible for capillary damage.

Because of these characteristics of aspirin, it has been extensively studied as an antithrombotic agent in the treatment and prevention of clinical thrombosis.[170, 171] It is thought to act by its selective action on the synthesis of the prostaglandin-related thromboxane A_2 and prostacyclin, which are the counterbalancing factors involved in platelet aggregation and are released when tissue is injured. It is unique from the other NSAIDs, in that it irreversibly inhibits the cyclooxygenase enzymes by acetylation. Aspirin has now been approved for the prevention of transient ischemic attacks, indicators of an impending stroke.[172]

The salicylates are readily absorbed from the stomach and the small intestine and depend strongly on the pH of the media. Absorption slows considerably as the pH rises (more alkaline) because of the acidic nature of these compounds and the necessity for the presence of undissociated molecules for absorption through the lipoidal membrane of the stomach and the intestines. Therefore, buffering agents administered at the same time in *excessive* amounts decrease the rate of absorption. In small quantities, their principal effect may be to aid in the dispersion of the salicylate into fine particles. This would help to increase absorption and decrease the possibility of gastric irritation by the accumulation of large particles of the undissolved acid and their adhesion to the gastric mucosa. Levy and Hayes[173] have shown that the absorption rate of aspirin and the incidence of gastric distress were a function of the dissolution rate of its particular dosage form. A more rapid dissolution rate of calcium and buffered aspirin was believed to account for faster absorption. They also demonstrated significant variations in dissolution rates of different nationally distributed brands of plain aspirin tablets. This may account for some of the conflicting reports and opinions concerning the relative advantages of plain and buffered aspirin tablets. Lieberman et al.[174] have also shown that buffering is effective in raising the blood levels of aspirin. A measure of the antianxiety effect of aspirin by means of electroencephalograms (EEGs) found differences between buffered, brand name, and generic aspirin preparations.[175]

Potentiation of salicylate activity by simultaneous administration of *p*-aminobenzoic acid or its salts has been the basis for the introduction of numerous products of this kind. Salassa and coworkers have shown that this effect is due to the inhibition of both salicylate metabolism and excretion in the urine.[176] This effect has been proved amply, provided that the ratio of 24 g of *p*-aminobenzoic acid to 3 g of salicylate per day is observed. There is no strong evidence, however, to substantiate any significant elevation of plasma salicylate levels when less *p*-aminobenzoic acid is used.

The derivatives of salicylic acid are of two types [I and II (a and b)]:

I

IIa   IIb

Type I represents those that are formed by modifying the carboxyl group (e.g., salts, esters, or amides). Type II (a and b) represents those that are derived by substitution on the hydroxyl group of salicylic acid. The derivatives of salicylic acid were introduced in an attempt to prevent the gastric symptoms and the undesirable taste inherent in the common salts of salicylic acid. Most hydrolysis of type I takes place in the intestine, and most of the type II compounds are absorbed unchanged into the bloodstream (see aspirin).

COMPOUNDS OF TYPE I

The alkyl and aryl esters of salicylic acid (type I) are used externally, primarily as counterirritants, where most of them are well absorbed through the skin. This type of compound is of little value as an analgesic. A few inorganic salicylates are used internally when the effect of the salicylate ion is intended. These compounds vary in their irritation of the stomach. To prevent the development of pink or red coloration in the product, contact with iron should be avoided in their manufacture.

Sodium Salicylate, USP.

Sodium salicylate may be prepared by the reaction, in aqueous solution, between 1 mole each of salicylic acid and sodium bicarbonate; evaporating to dryness yields the white salt. Generally, the salt has a pinkish tinge or is a white microcrystalline powder. It is odorless or has a faint, characteristic odor, and it has a sweet, saline taste. It is affected by light. The compound is soluble in water (1:1), alcohol (1:10), and glycerin (1:4).

In solution, particularly in the presence of sodium bicarbonate, the salt will darken on standing (see salicylic acid). This darkening may be lessened by the addition of sodium sulfite or sodium bisulfite. Also, use of recently boiled distilled water and dispensing in amber-colored bottles lessens color change. Sodium salicylate forms a eutectic mixture with antipyrine and produces a violet coloration with iron or its salts. Solutions of the compound must be neutral or slightly basic to prevent precipitation of free salicylic acid. The USP salt forms neutral or acid solutions, however.

This salt is the one of choice for salicylate medication and usually is administered with sodium bicarbonate to lessen gastric distress, or it is administered in enteric-coated tablets. The use of sodium bicarbonate[177] is ill advised because it decreases the plasma levels of salicylate and increases the excretion of free salicylate in the urine.

Sodium Thiosalicylate.

Sodium thiosalicylate (Rexolate) is the sulfur or thio analogue of sodium salicylate. It is more soluble and better absorbed, thus allowing lower dosages. It is recommended for gout, rheumatic fever, and muscular pains in doses of 100 to 150 mg every 3 to 6 hours for 2 days, and then 100 mg once or twice daily. It is available only for injection.

Magnesium Salicylate, USP.

Magnesium salicylate (Mobidin, Magan) is a sodium-free salicylate preparation for use when sodium intake is restricted. It is claimed to produce less gastrointestinal upset. The dosage and indications are the same as those for sodium salicylate.

Choline Salicylate.

Choline salicylate (Arthropan) is extremely soluble in water and is available as a flavored liquid. It is claimed to be absorbed more rapidly than aspirin, giving faster peak blood levels. It is used when salicylates are indicated in a recommended dose of 870 mg to 1.74 g 4 times daily. It is also available in combination with magnesium salicylate (Trilisate, Tricosal).

Others.

Ammonium, lithium, and strontium salts of salicylic acid have also found use. They offer no distinct advantage over sodium salicylate.

SALOL PRINCIPLE

Nencki introduced salol in 1886 and so presented to the science of therapy the "salol principle." In salol, two toxic substances (phenol and salicylic acid) were combined into an ester that taken internally slowly hydrolyzes in the intestine to give the antiseptic action of its components. This type of ester is referred to as a *full salol* or *true salol* when both components of the ester are active compounds. Examples are guaiacol benzoate, *β*-naphthol benzoate, and salol. The salol principle can be applied to esters in which only the alcohol or the acid is the toxic, active or corrosive portion; this type is called a *partial salol*. Examples of partial salols that contain an active acid are ethyl salicylate and methyl salicylate. Examples of partial salols that contain an active phenol are creosote carbonate, thymol carbonate, and guaiacol carbonate. Although many salol-type compounds have been prepared and used to some extent, none is presently valuable in therapeutics, and all are surpassed by other agents.

Phenyl Salicylate.

Phenyl salicylate, salol, occurs as fine white crystals or a white crystalline powder with a characteristic taste and a faint, aromatic odor. It is insoluble in water (1:6,700), slightly soluble in glycerin, and soluble in alcohol (1:6), ether, chloroform, acetone, or fixed and volatile oils. Damp or eutectic mixtures form readily with many organic materials, such as thymol, menthol, camphor, chloral hydrate, and phenol.

Salol is sold in combination with methenamine and atropine alkaloids as a urinary tract antiseptic and analgesic (e.g., Prosed/OS, Trac Tabs, Urised and others). Salol is insoluble in gastric juice but is slowly hydrolyzed in the intestine into phenol and salicylic acid. Because of this property, coupled with its low melting point (41 to 43°C), it has been used in the past as an enteric coating for tablets and capsules. It is not efficient as an enteric-coating material, however, and its use has been superseded by more effective materials. It has also been used externally as a sun filter (10% ointment) for sunburn prevention (Rayderm).

Salicylamide.

Salicylamide, *o*-hydroxybenzamide, is a derivative of salicylic acid that has been known for almost a century. It is readily prepared from salicyl chloride and ammonia. The compound occurs as a nearly odorless, white crystalline powder. It is fairly stable to heat, light, and moisture. It is slightly soluble in water (1:500); soluble in hot water, alcohol (1:15), and propylene glycol; and sparingly soluble in chloroform and ether. It is freely soluble in solutions of alkalies. In alkaline solution with sodium carbonate or triethanolamine, decomposition takes place, resulting in a yellow to red precipitate.

Salicylamide

Salicylamide reportedly exerts a moderately quicker and deeper analgesic effect than aspirin. Long-term studies on rats revealed no untoward symptomatic or physiological reactions. Its metabolism differs from that of other salicylic compounds, and it is not hydrolyzed to salicylic acid.[163] Its analgesic and antipyretic activity is probably no greater than that of aspirin, and possibly less. It can be used in place of salicylates, however, and is particularly useful for patients with a demonstrated sensitivity to salicylates. It is excreted much more rapidly than other salicylates, which probably accounts for its lower toxicity and, thus, does not permit high blood levels.

The dose for simple analgesic effect may vary from 300 mg to 1 g administered 3 times daily; but for rheumatic conditions, the dose may be increased to 2 to 4 g 3 times a day. Gastric intolerance may limit the dosage, however. The usual period of the higher dosage should not exceed 3 to 6 days. It is available in several combination products (e.g., Saleto, BC Powder).

Aspirin, USP.

Aspirin, acetylsalicylic acid (Aspro, Empirin), was introduced into medicine by Dreser in 1899. It is prepared by treating salicylic acid, which was first prepared by Kolbe in 1874, with acetic anhydride. The hydrogen atom of the hydroxyl group in salicylic acid is replaced by the acetyl group; this also may be accomplished by using acetyl chloride with salicylic acid or ketene with salicylic acid.

Aspirin

Aspirin occurs as white crystals or as a white crystalline powder. It is slightly soluble in water (1:300) and soluble in alcohol (1:5), chloroform (1:17), and ether (1:15). Also, it dissolves easily in glycerin. Aqueous solubility may be increased by using acetates or citrates of alkali metals, although these are said to decompose it slowly. It is stable in dry air, but in the presence of moisture, it slowly hydrolyzes into acetic and salicylic acids. Salicylic acid will crystallize out when an aqueous solution of aspirin and sodium hydroxide is boiled and then acidified.

Aspirin itself is acidic enough to produce effervescence with carbonates and, in the presence of iodides, to cause the slow liberation of iodine. In the presence of alkaline hydroxides and carbonates, it decomposes, although it does form salts with alkaline metals and alkaline earth metals. The presence of salicylic acid, formed on hydrolysis, may be confirmed by the formation of a violet color on the addition of ferric chloride solution.

Aspirin is not hydrolyzed appreciably on contact with weakly acid digestive fluids of the stomach but, on passage into the intestine, is subjected to some hydrolysis. Most of it is absorbed unchanged, however. Garrett[178] has ascribed the gastric mucosal irritation of aspirin to salicylic acid formation, the natural acidity of aspirin, or the adhesion of undissolved aspirin to the mucosa. He has also proposed that the nonacidic anhydride of aspirin is superior for oral administration. Davenport[169] concludes that aspirin alters mucosal cell permeability, allowing back diffusion of stomach acid, which damages the capillaries. A number of proprietaries (e.g., Bufferin) use compounds such as sodium bicarbonate, aluminum glycinate, sodium citrate, aluminum hydroxide, or magnesium trisilicate to counteract this acidic property. One of the better antacids is dihydroxyaluminum aminoacetate, USP. Aspirin is unusually effective when prescribed with calcium glutamate. The more stable, nonirritant calcium acetylsalicylate is formed, and the glutamate portion (glutamic acid) maintains a pH of 3.5 to 5.

Preferably, dry dosage forms (i.e., tablets, capsules, or powders) should be used, since aspirin is somewhat unstable in aqueous media. In tablet preparations, the use of acid-washed talc improves the stability of aspirin.[179] Also, aspirin has been found to break down in the presence of phenylephrine hydrochloride.[180] Aspirin in aqueous media will hydrolyze almost completely in less than 1 week; solutions made with alcohol or glycerin do not decompose as quickly. Citrates retard hydrolysis only slightly. Some studies have indicated that sucrose tends to inhibit hydrolysis. A study of aqueous aspirin suspensions indicated that sorbitol exerts a pronounced stabilizing effect.[181] Stable liquid preparations are available that use triacetin, propylene glycol, or a polyethylene glycol. Aspirin lends itself readily to combination with many other substances but tends to soften and become damp with methenamine, aminopyrine, salol, antipyrine, phenol, or acetanilid.

Aspirin is one of the most widely used compounds in therapy and, for many years, was not associated with untoward effects. Allergic reactions to aspirin are now observed commonly. Asthma and urticaria are the most common manifestations and, when they occur, are extremely acute and difficult to relieve. Like sodium salicylate, aspirin caused congenital malformations when administered to mice.[182] Pretreatment with sodium pentobarbital or chlorpromazine significantly lowered these effects.[183] Similar effects have been attributed to the consumption of aspirin by women, and its use during pregnancy should be avoided. Other studies, however, found no untoward effects. The reader is urged to consult the excellent review by Smith for an account of the pharmacological aspects of aspirin.[163, 164]

Practically all salts of aspirin, except those of aluminum and calcium, are unstable for pharmaceutical use. These salts appear to have fewer undesirable side effects and to induce analgesia faster than aspirin. A timed-release preparation of aspirin is available. It does not appear to offer any advantages over aspirin, except for bedtime dosage.

Aspirin is used as an antipyretic, analgesic, and antirheumatic, usually in powder, capsule, suppository, or tablet form. Its use in rheumatism has been reviewed, and it is reportedly the drug of choice over all other salicylate derivatives.[184, 185] There is some anesthetic action when applied locally, especially in powder form in tonsillitis or pharyngitis, and in ointment form for skin itching and certain skin diseases. In the usual dose, 52 to 75% is excreted in the urine, in various forms, in a period of 15 to 30 hours. Analgesia is believed to be due to the unhydrolyzed acetylsalicylic acid molecule.[163–165]

A low-dosage form of aspirin, 81 mg, equivalent to the dose recommended for infants (the ''baby aspirin''), is recommended as a daily dose for individuals who are at even a low cardiovascular risk. Several large studies found that this low dose of aspirin reduces the number of heart attacks and thrombotic strokes. Other salicylates and NSAIDs have not shown similar effects. In fact, the NSAIDs can interfere with aspirin's cardiovascular benefits, and they should not be taken within 12 hours of each other.

Salsalate. Salsalate, salicylsalicylic acid (Amigesic, Disalcid, etc.), is the ester formed between two salicylic acid molecules to which it is hydrolyzed following absorption. It reportedly causes less gastric upset than aspirin because it is relatively insoluble in the stomach and is not absorbed until it reaches the small intestine. Limited clinical trials[186–188] suggest that it is as effective as aspirin and that it may have fewer side effects.[189] The recommended dose is 325 to 1,000 mg 2 or 3 times a day. It is available only on prescription.

Diflunisal. Over the years, several hundred analogues of aspirin have been made and tested to produce a compound that was more potent, was longer acting, and had less gastric irritation. By the introduction of a hydrophobic group in the 5 position, diflunisal, 5-(2,4-difluorophenyl)salicylic acid, 2',4'-difluoro-4-hydroxy-3-biphenylcarboxylic acid (Dolobid), appears to meet these criteria. In animal tests, it is at least 4 times more potent. In humans, it appears to be about twice as effective, with twice the duration.[190] Like other aryl acids, it is highly bound to plasma protein as its deacylated metabolite. It is marketed in tablets (250 and 500 mg) for treating mild-to-moderate pain and RA and OA.

N-Arylanthranilic Acids

One of the early advances in the search for nonnarcotic analgesics was centered in the *N*-arylanthranilic acids. Their outstanding characteristic is that they are primarily NSAIDs, and secondarily, some possess analgesic properties.

Mefenamic Acid. Mefenamic acid, *N*-2,3-xylylanthranilic acid (Ponstel), occurs as an off-white crystalline powder that is insoluble in water and slightly soluble in alcohol. It appears to be the first genuine antiphlogistic analgesic discovered since aminopyrine. Because it is believed that aspirin and aminopyrine owe their general purpose analgesic efficacy to a combination of peripheral and central effects,[191] a wide variety of arylanthranilic acids were screened for antinociceptive (analgesic) activity if they showed significant anti-inflammatory action. The combination of both effects is a rarity among these compounds. The mechanism of analgesic action is believed to be related to the ability to block prostaglandin synthetase. No relationship to lipid-plasma distribution, partition coefficient, or pK_a has been noted. The interested reader, however, will find additional information on antibradykinin and anti-UV erythema activities of these compounds, together with speculations on a receptor site, in the literature.[192]

(a) $R_1 = CH_3$, X = CH, R_2 = H
(b) R_1 = H, $R_2 = CF_3$, X = CH

Mefenamic acid in a dose of 250 mg is superior to 600 mg of aspirin as an analgesic, and doubling the dose sharply increases its efficacy.[193] A study examining this drug relative to gastrointestinal bleeding indicated a lower incidence of this side effect than exhibited by aspirin.[194] Diarrhea, drowsiness, and headache have accompanied its use. The possibility of blood disorders has prompted limitation of its administration to 7 days. It is not recommended for children or during pregnancy. It has been approved for use in the management of primary dysmenorrhea (PD), which is thought to be caused by excessive concentrations of prostaglandins and endoperoxides.

Meclofenamate Sodium. Meclofenamate sodium, sodium *N*-(2,6-dichloro-*m*-tolyl)anthranilate, Meclomen, is available in 50- and 100-mg capsules for use in the treatment of acute and chronic RA. The most significant side effects are gastrointestinal, including diarrhea.

Meclofenamate Sodium

Arylacetic Acid Derivatives

The arylacetic acid derivative group of agents has received the most intensive attention for new clinical candidates. As a group, they show high analgesic potency in addition to their anti-inflammatory activity.

Indomethacin, USP. Indomethacin, 1-(p-chlorobenzoyl)-5-methoxy-2-methylindole-3-acetic acid (Indocin), occurs as a pale-yellow to yellow-tan crystalline powder that is soluble in ethanol and acetone and practically insoluble in water. It is unstable in alkaline solution and sunlight. It shows polymorphism; one form melts at about 155°C, and the other at about 162°C. It may occur as a mixture of both forms with a melting range between these melting points.

Indomethacin

Since its introduction in 1965, it has been widely used as an anti-inflammatory analgesic in RA, spondylitis, and OA, and to a lesser extent in gout. Although both its analgesic and anti-inflammatory activities are well established, it appears to be no more effective than aspirin.[195]

The most frequent side effects are gastric distress and headache. It has also been associated with peptic ulceration, blood disorders, and possible deaths. The side effects appear to be dose related and sometimes can be minimized by reducing the dose. It is not recommended for use in children because of possible interference with resistance to infection. Like many other acidic compounds, it circulates bound to blood protein, thus requiring caution in the concurrent use of other protein-binding drugs. Indomethacin is recommended only for patients who cannot tolerate aspirin and in place of phenylbutazone in long-term therapy, for which it appears to be less hazardous than corticosteroids or phenylbutazone.

Sulindac, USP. Sulindac, (Z)-5-fluoro-2-methyl-1-[[p-(methylsulfinyl)phenyl]methylene]-1H-indene-3-acetic acid (Clinoril), occurs as yellow crystals soluble in alkaline but insoluble in acidic solutions. The drug reaches peak blood levels within 2 to 4 hours and undergoes a complicated, reversible metabolism as follows:

inactive   parent   active

The parent sulfinyl has a plasma half-life of 8 hours, and that of the active sulfide metabolite is 16.4 hours. The more polar and inactive sulfoxide is virtually the only form excreted. The long half-life is due to extensive enterohepatic recirculation.[196] Only the sulfide species inhibits prostaglandin synthetase in vitro. Although these forms are highly protein bound, the drug does not appear to affect binding of anticoagulants or hypoglycemics. Coadministration of aspirin is contraindicated because it considerably reduces the sulfide blood levels.

Sulindac

Careful monitoring of patients with a history of ulcers is recommended. Gastric bleeding, nausea, diarrhea, dizziness, and other adverse effects have been noted, but with a lower frequency than with aspirin. Sulindac is recommended for RA, OA, and ankylosing spondylitis in a 150- to 200-mg dose, twice daily.[197, 198] It is available as tablets (150 and 200 mg).

Tolmetin Sodium, USP. Tolmetin sodium, 1-methyl-5-(p-toluoyl)pyrrole-2-acetate dihydrate sodium, McN-2559 (Tolectin), is an arylacetic acid derivative with a pyrrole as the aryl group. This drug is absorbed rapidly, with a relatively short plasma half-life (1 hour). It is recommended for use in the management of acute and chronic RA. It shares similar, but less frequent, adverse effects with aspirin. It does not potentiate coumarin-like drugs nor alter the blood levels of sulfonylureas or insulin. Like other drugs in this class, it inhibits prostaglandin synthetase and lowers PGE blood levels.

Tolmetin: $R_1 = CH_3$, $R_2 = H$
Zomepirac: $R_1 = Cl$, $R_2 = CH_3$

Available as tablets (200 and 600 mg) and a capsule (400 mg), a dose of 400 mg 3 times daily, with a maximum of 2,000 mg, is recommended. Clinical trials indicate a usual daily dose of 1,200 mg is comparable in relief to 3.9 g of aspirin and 150 mg of indomethacin per day.[199]

Ibuprofen, USP. Ibuprofen, 2-(4-isobutylphenyl)propionic acid (Motrin, Advil, Nuprin), was introduced into clinical practice following extensive clinical trials. It appears to be comparable to aspirin in the treatment of RA, with a lower incidence of side effects.[202] It has also been approved for use in PD.

Ibufenac R = H
Ibuprofen R = CH₃

In this series of compounds, potency was enhanced by introduction of the α-methyl group on the acetic acid moiety. The precursor ibufenac (R = H), which was abandoned owing to hepatotoxicity, was less potent. Moreover, the activity resides in the (*S*)-(+) isomer, not only in ibuprofen but throughout the arylacetic acid series. Furthermore, these isomers are the more potent inhibitors of prostaglandin synthetase.[161] The recommended dosage is 400 mg. Ibuprofen is also available over-the-counter as 200-mg tablets.

Naproxen, USP. Naproxen, (+)-6-methoxy-α-methyl-2-naphthaleneacetic acid (Anaprox, Naprosyn), occurs as white to off-white crystals that are sparingly soluble in acidic solutions, freely soluble in alkaline solutions, and highly soluble in organic or lipid-like solutions. After oral administration, it is well absorbed, giving peak blood levels in 2 to 4 hours and a half-life of 13 hours. A steady-state blood level is usually achieved after four to five doses. Naproxen is very highly protein bound and displaces most protein-bound drugs. Dosages of these must be adjusted accordingly.

Naproxen

Naproxen is recommended for use in rheumatoid and gouty arthritis. It shows good analgesic activity—400 mg is comparable to 75 to 150 mg of oral meperidine and superior to 65 mg of propoxyphene and 325 mg of aspirin plus 30 mg of codeine. A 220- to 330-mg dose is comparable to 600 mg of aspirin alone. It reportedly produces dizziness, drowsiness, and nausea, with infrequent mention of gastrointestinal tract irritation. Like aspirin, it inhibits prostaglandin synthetase and prolongs blood-clotting time. It is not recommended for pregnant or lactating women or children under 16.[204] It is also available over-the-counter as 200-mg tablets (Aleve).

Fenoprofen Calcium, USP. Fenoprofen calcium, α-methyl-3-phenoxybenzeneacetic acid dihydrate calcium (Nalfon), occurs as a white crystalline powder that is slightly soluble in water, soluble in alcohol, and insoluble in benzene. It is rapidly absorbed orally, reaches peak blood levels within 2 hours, and has a short plasma half-life (3 hours). It is highly protein bound like the other acylacetic acids, and caution is needed when it is used concurrently with hydantoins, sulfonamides, and sulfonylureas. It shares many of the adverse effects common to this group of drugs, with

gastrointestinal bleeding, ulcers, dyspepsia, nausea, sleepiness, and dizziness reported at a lower incidence than with aspirin. It inhibits prostaglandin synthetase.[205]

Fenoprofen

Available as capsules (200 and 300 mg) and tablets (600 mg), it is recommended for RA and OA in divided doses 4 times a day for a maximum of 3,200 mg/day. It should be taken at least 30 minutes before or 2 hours after meals. It is not yet recommended for the management of acute flare-ups. Doses of 2.4 g per day are comparable to 3.9 g per day of aspirin in arthritis. For pain relief, 400 mg gave results similar to 650 mg of aspirin.[206]

Ketoprofen. Ketoprofen, 3-benzoyl-α-methylbenzeneacetic acid, *m*-benzoylhydratropic acid (Orudis), is closely related to fenoprofen in structure, properties, and indications. It has a low incidence of side effects and has been approved for over-the-counter sale (Orudis KT, Actron). It is available as capsules and tablets (25 and 50 mg), with a recommended daily dose of 150 to 300 mg divided into three or four doses. It is also available as extended-release capsules (100, 150, and 200 mg).

Flurbiprofen, USP. Flurbiprofen, (±)-2-(2-fluoro-4-biphenylyl)propionic acid (Ansaid, Ocufen), is another hydrotropic acid analogue that is used in the acute or long-term management of RA and OA. It is available as tablets (50 and 100 mg), with a recommended dose of 200 to 300 mg divided into 2, 3, or 4 times daily.

Diclofenac Potassium and Sodium. Diclofenac sodium, sodium [*o*-(2,6-dichloroanilino)phenyl]acetate (Voltaren), is indicated for short- and long-term treatment of RA, OA, and ankylosing spondylitis. The potassium salt (Cataflam), which is faster acting, is indicated for the management of acute pain and PD. The sodium salt is available as delayed-release tablets (25, 50, 75, and 100 mg), with a recommended daily dose of 100 to 200 mg in divided doses. The potassium salt is available as a tablet (50 mg), with a recommended dose of 50 mg 3 times daily.

Nabumetone. Nabumetone, 4-(6-methoxy-2-naphthyl)-2-butanone (Relafen), serves as a prodrug to its active metabolite, 6-methoxy-2-naphthylacetic acid. Like the other arylacetic acid drugs, it is used in short- or long-term management of RA and OA. It is available as tablets (500 and 750 mg), with a recommended single daily dose of 1,000 mg.

Ketorolac Tromethamine. Ketorolac tromethamine, (±)-benzoyl-2,3-dihydro-1*H*-pyrrolizine-1-carboxylic acid compound with 2-amino-2-(hydroxymethyl)-1,3-propanediol (Toradol), is a potent NSAID analgesic indicated for the treatment of moderately severe, acute pain. Because of a number of potential side effects, its administration should not exceed 5 days. Treatment is usually initiated by intravenous (30 mg) or intramuscular (60 mg) administration, with analgesia maintained by initial oral doses of 20 or 30 mg, followed by 10 mg every 4 to 6 hours.

Etodolac. Etodolac, 1,8-diethyl-1,3,4,9-tetrahydropyrano[3,4-*b*]indole-1-acetic acid (Lodine), possesses an indole ring as the aryl portion of this group of NSAID drugs. It shares many of the properties of this group and is indicated for short- and long-term management of pain and OA. It is available as capsules (200 and 300 mg), tablets (400 and 500 mg) and extended-release tablets (400, 500, and 600 mg), with a recommended daily dose of 800- to 1,200-mg in divided doses.

Oxaprozin. Oxaprozin, 4,5-diphenyl-2-oxazolepropionic acid (Daypro), differs from the other members of this group in being an arylpropionic acid derivative. It shares the same properties and side effects of other members in this group. It is indicated for the short- and long-term management of OA and RA, administered as a single 1,200-mg dose. It is available as 600-mg caplets.

Piroxicam, USP. Piroxicam, 4-hydroxy-2-methyl-*N*-2-pyridyl-2*H*-1,2-benzothiazine-3-carboximide 1,1-dioxide (Feldene), represents a class of acidic inhibitors of prostaglandin synthetase, although it does not antagonize PGE_2 directly.[207] This drug is very long acting, with a plasma half-life of 50 hours, thus requiring a dose of only 20 to 30 mg once daily. It is reported to give results similar to those from 25 mg of indomethacin or 400 mg of ibuprofen 3 times a day.[208, 209]

Piroxicam

Meloxicam. Like piroxicam in structure, meloxicam, 4-hydroxy-2-methyl-*N*-(5-methyl-2-thiazoyl)-2*H*-1,2-benzothiazine-3-carboxamide 1,1-dioxide (Mobic), is also indicated for use in OA. It also has a relatively long half-life of 15 to 20 hours. Available as a 7.5-mg tablet, the recommended dose is 7.5 mg/day, with a maximum of 15 mg/day.

Celecoxib. The first of the COX-2 inhibitor drugs to be marketed, celecoxib, 4-[5-(4-methylphenyl)-3-(trifluorophenyl)-1*H*-pyrazol-1-yl]benzenesulfonamide (Celebrex), has been approved for use in RA and OA, with a dose of 100 or 200 mg twice a day for RA and 200 mg/day for OA in a single dose of 200 mg or 100 mg twice a day. It has also been approved for reducing the number of adenomatous colorectal polyps in familial adenomatous polyposis (FAP). It is available as 100- and 200-mg tablets.

Rofecoxib. Rofecoxib, 4-[4-(methylsulfinyl)phenyl]-3-phenyl-2(5*H*)-furanone (Vioxx), is a COX-2 inhibitor with greater potency and a longer half-life than celecoxib (17 versus 11 hours). It is approved for use in OA, acute pain, and PD, with a dose of 12.5 mg/day and a maximum of 25 mg/day for OA, and a single dose of 50 mg daily recommended for a maximum of 5 days for acute pain and PD. It is available as tablets (12.5, 25, and 50 mg) and suspensions (12.5 and 25 mg/mL).

Valdecoxib. Introduced in late 2001, the COX-2 inhibitor valdecoxib, 4-[5-methyl-3-phenylisoxazol-4-yl]-benzenesulfonamide (Bextra), had the same approved uses as celecoxib and rofecoxib, with a recommended dose of 10 mg/day for RA and OA and 40 mg for PD. It is available as 10- and 20-mg tablets. Several other COX-2 enzyme inhibitors are under investigation and clinical trials, including the highly specific etoricoxib and the parenteral parecoxib.

Aniline and *p*-Aminophenol Derivatives

The introduction of aniline derivatives as analgesics is based on the discovery by Cahn and Hepp, in 1886, that aniline (C-1) and acetanilid (C-2) (Table 22-7) both have powerful antipyretic properties. The origin of this group from aniline has led to their being called "coal tar analgesics." Acetanilid was introduced by these workers because of the known toxicity of aniline itself. Aniline brings about the formation of methemoglobin, a form of hemoglobin that cannot function as an oxygen carrier. The acyl derivatives of aniline were thought to exert their analgesic and antipyretic effects by first being hydrolyzed to aniline and the corresponding acid, after which the aniline was oxidized to *p*-aminophenol (C-3). This is then excreted in combination with glucuronic or sulfuric acid.

The aniline derivatives do not appear to act on the brain cortex; the pain impulse appears to be intercepted at the hypothalamus, wherein also lies the thermoregulatory center of the body. It is not clear if this is the site of their activity because most evidence suggests that they act at peripheral thermoceptors. They are effective in returning feverish individuals to normal temperature. Normal body temperatures are not affected by the administration of these drugs. Of the antipyretic analgesic group, the aniline derivatives show little if any anti-inflammatory activity.

Table 22-7 shows some of the types of aniline derivatives that have been made and tested in the past. In general, any type of substitution on the amino group that reduces its basicity also lowers its physiological activity. Acylation is one type of substitution that accomplishes this effect. Acetanilid (C-2) itself, although the best of the acylated derivatives, is toxic in large doses, but when administered in analgesic doses, it is probably without significant harm. Formanilid (C-4) is readily hydrolyzed and too irritant. The higher homologues of acetanilid are less soluble and, therefore, less active and less toxic. Those derived from aromatic acids (e.g., C-5) are virtually without analgesic and antipyretic effects. One of these, salicylanilide (C-6), is used as a fungicide and antimildew agent. Exalgin (C-7) is too toxic.

The hydroxylated anilines *(o, m, p)*, better known as the aminophenols, are considerably less toxic than aniline. The *para* compound (C-3) is of particular interest from two

TABLE 22–7   Some Analgesics Related to Aniline

Compound	Structure R₁	R₂	R₃	Name
C-1	—H	—H	—H	Aniline
C-2	—H	—H	$-\overset{O}{\underset{\|}{C}}-CH_3$	Acetanilid
C-3	—OH	—H	—H	p-Aminophenol
C-4	—H	—H	$-\overset{\|}{\underset{O}{C}}-H$	Formanilid
C-5	—H	—H	$-\overset{\|}{\underset{O}{C}}-C_6H_5$	Benzanilid
C-6	—H	—H	$-\overset{\|}{\underset{O}{C}}-$ (salicyl) HO	Salicylanilide (not an analgesic, but is an antifungal agent)
C-7	—H	—CH₃	$-\overset{\|}{\underset{O}{C}}-CH_3$	Exalgin
C-8	—OH	—H	$-\overset{\|}{\underset{O}{C}}-CH_3$	Acetaminophen
C-9	—OCH₃	—H	—H	Anisidine
C-10	—OC₂H₅	—H	—H	Phenetidine
C-11	—OC₂H₅	—H	$-\overset{\|}{\underset{O}{C}}-CH_3$	Phenacetin
C-12	—OC₂H₅	—H	$-\overset{\|}{\underset{O}{C}}-\underset{OH}{CHCH_3}$	Lactylphenetidin
C-13	—OC₂H₅	—H	$-\overset{\|}{\underset{O}{C}}-CH_2NH_2$	Phenocoll
C-14	—OC₂H₅	—H	$-\overset{\|}{\underset{O}{C}}-CH_2OCH_3$	Kryofine
C-15	$-O\overset{\|}{\underset{O}{C}}-CH_3$	—H	$-\overset{\|}{\underset{O}{C}}-CH_3$	p-Acetoxyacetanilid
C-16	$-O\overset{\|}{\underset{O}{C}}-$ (salicyl) OH	—H	$-\overset{\|}{\underset{O}{C}}-CH_3$	Phenetsal
C-17	—OCH₂CH₂OH	—H	$-\overset{\|}{\underset{O}{C}}-CH_3$	Pertonal

standpoints: namely, it is the metabolic product of aniline, and it is the least toxic of the three possible aminophenols. It also possesses a strong antipyretic and analgesic action. It is too toxic to serve as a drug, however, and therefore, numerous modifications were attempted. One of the first was the acetylation of the amine group to provide N-acetyl-*p*-aminophenol (acetaminophen) (C-8), a product that retained a good measure of the desired activities. Another approach to the detoxification of *p*-aminophenol was the etherification of the phenolic group. The best known of these are anisidine (C-9) and phenetidine (C-10), which are the methyl and ethyl ethers, respectively. A free amino group in these compounds however, although promoting a strong antipyretic action, was also conducive to methemoglobin formation. The only exceptions to this were compounds in which a carboxyl group or sulfonic acid group had been substituted on the benzene nucleus. In these compounds, however, the antipyretic effect also had disappeared. These considerations led to the preparation of the alkyl ethers of N-acetyl-*p*-aminophenol, of which the ethyl ether was the best and is known as phenacetin (C-11). The methyl and propyl homologues were undesirable from the standpoint of causing emesis, salivation, diuresis, and other reactions. Alkylation of the nitrogen with a methyl group potentiates the analgesic action but, unfortunately, has a highly irritant action on mucous membranes.

The phenacetin molecule has been modified by changing the acyl group on the nitrogen, with sometimes beneficial results. Among these are lactylphenetidin (C-12), phenocoll (C-13), and kryofine (C-14). None of these, however, is in current use.

Changing the ether group of phenacetin to an acyl type of derivative has not always been successful. *p*-Acetoxyacetanilid (C-15) has about the same activity and disadvantages as the free phenol. The salicyl ester (C-16), however, exhibits diminished toxicity and increased antipyretic activity. Pertonal (C-17) is a somewhat different type in which glycol has been used to etherify the phenolic hydroxyl group. It is very similar to phenacetin. None of these is currently on the market.

Relative to the fate in humans of the types of compounds just discussed, Brodie and Axelrod[210–212] point out that acetanilid and phenacetin are metabolized by two different routes. Acetanilid is metabolized primarily to N-acetyl-*p*-aminophenol and acetaminophen and only a small amount to aniline, which they showed to be the precursor of phenylhydroxylamine, the compound responsible for methemoglobin formation. Phenacetin is mostly deethylated to acetaminophen, whereas a small amount is converted by deacetylation to *p*-phenetidine, also responsible for methemoglobin formation. With both acetanilid and phenacetin, the metabolite acetaminophen is believed to be responsible for the analgesic activity. Because of the toxicity described above, both are no longer available, replaced primarily by acetaminophen.

Acetaminophen, USP. Acetaminophen, N-Acetyl-*p*-aminophenol, 4-hydroxyacetanilide, APAP (Panado, Tempra, Tylenol, etc.), may be prepared by reduction of *p*-nitrophenol in glacial acetic acid, acetylation of *p*-aminophenol with acetic anhydride or ketene, or from *p*-hydroxy-acetophenone hydrazone. It occurs as a white, odorless, slightly bitter crystalline powder. It is slightly soluble in water and ether and is soluble in boiling water (1:20), alcohol (1:10), and sodium hydroxide T.S.

Acetaminophen has analgesic and antipyretic activities comparable to those of acetanilid and is used in the same conditions. It exerts its effects by inhibiting the cyclooxygenase enzyme centrally but has very little effect peripherally. Although it possesses the same toxic effects as acetanilid, they occur less frequently and are less severe; therefore, it is considered safer. Several precautions should be recognized, however, including not to exceed the recommended dosages and the risk of liver toxicity in chronic alcoholics.

It is available in several nonprescription forms and, also, is marketed in combination with aspirin and caffeine (Excedrin, Vanquish).

Pyrazolone and Pyrazolidinedione Derivatives

The simple doubly unsaturated compound containing two nitrogen and three carbon atoms in the ring, with the nitrogen atoms neighboring, is known as *pyrazole*. The reduction products, named as are other rings of five atoms, are pyrazoline and pyrazolidine. Several pyrazoline substitution products are used in medicine. Many of these are derivatives of 5-pyrazolone. Some can be related to 3,5-pyrazolidinedione.

Ludwig Knorr, a pupil of Emil Fischer, while searching for antipyretics of the quinoline type, in 1884, discovered the 5-pyrazolone now known as *antipyrine*. This discovery initiated the beginnings of the great German drug industry that dominated the field for about 40 years. Knorr, although at first mistakenly believing that he had a quinoline-type compound, soon recognized his error, and the compound was interpreted correctly as a pyrazolone. Within 2 years, the analgesic properties of this compound became apparent when favorable reports began to appear in the literature, particularly with reference to its use in headaches and neuralgias. Since then, it has retained some of its popularity as an analgesic, although its use as an antipyretic has declined steadily. Since its introduction into medicine, there have been more than 1,000 compounds made in an effort to find others with more potent analgesic action combined with less toxicity. Many modifications of the basic compound have been made. The few derivatives and modifications on the market are listed in Tables 22-8 and 22-9. Phenylbutazone, although analgesic itself, was originally developed as a solubilizer for the insoluble aminopyrine. It is now being used for the relief of many forms of arthritis, in which capacity it also reduces swelling and spasm by an anti-inflammatory action.

TABLE 22–8 Derivatives of 5-Pyrazole

Compound *Proprietary Name*	Structure			
	R₁	**R₂**	**R₃**	**R₄**
Antipyrine *Phenazone*	—C_6H_5	—CH_3	—CH_3	—H
Aminopyrine *Amidopyrine*	—C_6H_5	—CH_3	—CH_3	—$N(CH_3)_2$
Dipyrone *Methampyrone*	—C_6H_5	—CH_3	—CH_3	—NCH_2SO_3Na | CH_3

Antipyrine, USP. Antipyrine, 2,3-dimethyl-1-phenyl-3-pyrazolin-5-one, phenazone, was one of the first important drugs to be made (1887) synthetically. Antipyrine and many related compounds are prepared by the condensation of hydrazine derivatives with various esters. Antipyrine itself is prepared by the action of ethyl acetoacetate on phenylhydrazine and subsequent methylation.

It consists of colorless, odorless crystals or a white powder, with a slightly bitter taste. It is very soluble in water, alcohol, or chloroform and less so in ether. Its aqueous solution is neutral to litmus paper. It is basic in nature, however, which is due primarily to the nitrogen at position 2.

Locally, antipyrine exerts a paralytic action on the sensory and the motor nerves, resulting in some anesthesia and vasoconstriction, and it also exerts a feeble antiseptic effect. Systemically, it causes results that are very similar to those of acetanilid, although they are usually more rapid. It is readily absorbed after oral administration, circulates freely, and is excreted chiefly by the kidneys without having been changed chemically. Any abnormal temperature is reduced rapidly by an unknown mechanism, usually attributed to an effect on the serotonin-mediated thermal regulatory center of the nervous system. It has greater anti-inflammatory activity than aspirin, phenylbutazone, and indomethacin. It also lessens perception to pain of certain types, without any alteration in central or motor functions, which differs from the effects of morphine. Very often it produces unpleasant and possibly alarming symptoms, even in small or moderate doses. These are giddiness, drowsiness, cyanosis, great reduction in temperature, coldness in the extremities, tremor, sweating, and morbilliform or erythematous eruptions; very large doses produce asphyxia, epileptic convulsions, and collapse. Treatment for such untoward reactions must be symptomatic. It is probably less likely to produce collapse than acetanilid and is not known to cause the granulocytopenia that sometimes follows aminopyrine.

The great success of antipyrine in its early years led to the introduction of a great many derivatives, especially salts with a variety of acids, but none of these has any advantage over the parent compound. Its use is limited to a combination with benzocaine as an ear drop. Other drugs in this group, which once included aminopyrine, phenylbutazone, and oxyphenbutazone, are no longer marketed. The pharmacology of these and other analogues has been reviewed extensively.[213, 214]

TABLE 22–9 Derivatives of 3,5-Pyrazolidinedione

Compound *Proprietary Name*	Structure	
	R₁	**R₂**
Phenylbutazone *Azolid, Butazolidin*	—C_6H_5	—C_4H_9 (n)
Oxyphenbutazone *Oxalid, Tandearil*	—$C_6H_4(OH)$ (p)	—C_4H_9 (n)

REFERENCES

1. Tainter, M. L.: Ann. N. Y. Acad. Sci. 51:3, 1948.
2. Eisleb, O., and Schaumann, O.: Dtsch. Med. Wochenschr. 65:967, 1938.
3. U. S. Department of Health, Education and Welfare. The Interagency Committee on New Therapies for Pain and Discomfort: Report to the White House, 1979.
4. Williams, M., Kowalik, E. A., and Anuric, S. P.: J. Med. Chem. 42:1401, 1999.
5. Bonomi, A. E., et al.: J. Am. Pharm. Assoc. 39:558, 1999.
6. American Pharmaceutical Association: Pharmacists' Responsibilities in Managing Opioids: A Resource. Washington, DC, American Pharmaceutical Association, 2002.
7. American Pharmaceutical Association: Achieving Optimal Therapeutic Outcomes with Nonprescription Analgesics. Washington, DC, American Pharmaceutical Association, 1996.
8. Small, L. F., Eddy, N. B., Mosettig, E., and Himmelsbach, C. K.: Studies on Drug Addiction. Suppl. 138 to the Public Health Reports. Washington, DC, Superintendent of Documents, U. S. Government Printing Office, 1938.
9. Eddy, N. B., Halbach, H., and Braenden, O. J.: Bull. WHO 14:353, 1956.
10. Stork, G., and Bauer, L.: J. Am. Chem. Soc. 75:4373, 1953.
11. U. S. Patent 2,831,531. Chem. Abstr. 52:13808, 1958.
12. Rapoport, H., Baker, D. R., and Reist, H. N.: J. Org. Chem. 22:1489, 1957.
13. Chadha, M. S., Rapoport, H.: J. Am. Chem. Soc. 79:5730, 1957.
14. Okun, R., and Elliott, H. W.: J. Pharmacol. Exp. Ther. 124:255, 1958.
15. Seki, I., Takagi, H., and Kobayashi, S.: J. Pharm. Soc. Jpn. 84:280, 1964.
16. Buckett, W. R., Farquharson, M. E., and Haining, C. G.: J. Pharm. Pharmacol. 16:174, 1964.
17. Bentley, K. W., and Hardy, D. G.: Proc. Chem. Soc. 220, 1963.
18. Lister, R. E.: J. Pharm. Pharmacol. 16:364, 1964.
19. Bentley, K. W., and Hardy, D. G.: J. Am. Chem. Soc. 89:3267, 1967.
20. Telford, J., Papadopoulos, C. N., and Keats, A. S.: J. Pharmacol. Exp. Ther. 133:106, 1961.
21. Gates, M., and Montzka, T. A.: J. Med. Chem. 7:127, 1964.
22. Schaumann, O.: Arch. Exp. Pathol. Pharmakol. 196:109, 1940.
23. Bergel, F., and Morrison, A. L.: Q. Rev. (Lond.) 2:349, 1948.
24. Jensen, K. A., Lindquist, F., Rekling, E., and Wolffbrandt, C. G.: Dan. Tidsskr. Farm. 17:173, 1943; through Chem. Abstr. 39:2506, 1945.

25. Lee, J., Ziering, A., Berger, L., and Heineman, S. D.: Jubilee Volume–Emil Barell. Basel, Reinhardt, 1946, p. 267.
26. Lee, J., Ziering, A., Berger, L., and Heineman, S. D.: J. Org. Chem. 12:885, 894, 1947.
27. Berger, L., Ziering, A., Lee, J.: J. Org. Chem. 12:904, 1947.
28. Ziering, A., and Lee, J.: J. Org. Chem. 12:911, 1947.
29. Janssen, P. A. J., and Eddy, N. B.: J. Med. Pharm. Chem. 2:31, 1960.
30. Lee, J.: Analgesics: B. Partial structures related to morphine. In American Chemical Society: Medicinal Chemistry, vol. 1. New York, John Wiley & Sons, 1951, pp. 438–466.
31. Beckett, A. H., Casy, A. F., and Kirk, G.: J. Med. Pharm. Chem. 1: 37, 1959.
32. Bell, K. H., and Portoghese, P. S.: J. Med. Chem. 16:203, 589, 1973.
33. Bell, K. H., and Portoghese, P. S.: J. Med. Chem. 17:129, 1974.
34. Groeber, W. R., et al.: Obstet. Gynecol. 14:743, 1959.
35. Eddy, N. B.: Chem. Ind. (Lond.) Nov. 21:1462, 1959.
36. Fraser, H. F., and Isbell, H.: Bull. Narc. 13:29, 1961.
37. Janssen, P. A. J., et al.: J. Med. Pharm. Chem. 2:271, 1960.
38. Stahl, K. D., et al.: Eur. J. Pharmacol. 46:199, 1977.
39. Blicke, F. F., and Tsao, E.: J. Am. Chem. Soc. 75:3999, 1953.
40. Cass, L. J., et al.: JAMA 166:1829, 1958.
41. Batterham, R. C., Mouratoff, G. J., and Kaufman, J. E.: Am. J. Med. Sci. 247:62, 1964.
42. Finch, J. S., and DeKornfeld, T. J.: J. Clin. Pharmacol. 7:46, 1967.
43. Yelnosky, J., and Gardocki, J. F.: Toxicol. Appl. Pharmacol. 6:593, 1964.
44. Bockmuehl, M., and Ehrhart, G.: German Patent 711,069.
45. Kleiderer, E. C., Rice, J. B., and Conquest, V.: Pharmaceutical Activities at the I. G. Farbenindustrie Plant, Höchstam-Main, Germany. Report 981. Washington, DC, Office of the Publication Board, Department of Commerce, 1945.
46. Scott, C. C., and Chen, K. K.: Fed. Proc. 5:201, 1946.
47. Scott, C. C., and Chen, K. K.: J. Pharmacol. Exp. Ther. 87:63, 1946.
48. Eddy, N. B., Touchberry, C., and Lieberman, J.: J. Pharmacol. Exp. Ther. 98:121, 1950.
49. Janssen, P. A. J., and Jageneau, A. H.: J. Pharm. Pharmacol. 9:381, 1957.
50. Janssen, P. A. J., and Jageneau, A. H.: J. Pharm. Pharmacol. 10:14, 1958.
51. Janssen, P. A. J.: J. Am. Chem. Soc. 78:3862, 1956.
52. Cass, L. J., and Frederik, W. S.: Antibiot. Med. 6:362, 1959.
53. Blaine, J., and Renault, P. (eds.): Rx 3 Times/Wk LAAM–Methadone Alternative. NIDA Research Monograph 8. Washington, DC, DHEW, 1976.
54. Eddy, N. B., Besendorf, H., and Pellmont, B.: Bull. Narc. 10:23, 1958.
55. DeKornfeld, T. J.: Curr. Res. Anesth. 39:430, 1960.
56. Murphy, J. G., Ager, J. H., and May, E. L.: J. Org. Chem. 25:1386, 1960.
57. Chignell, C. F., Ager, J. H., and May, E. L.: J. Med. Chem. 8:235, 1965.
58. May, E. L., and Eddy, N. B.: J. Med. Chem. 9:851, 1966.
59. Michne, W. F., et al.: J. Med. Chem. 22:1158, 1979.
60. Archer, S., et al.: J. Med. Chem. 7:123, 1964.
61. Cass, L. J., Frederik, W. S., and Teodoro, J. V.: JAMA 188:112, 1964.
62. Fraser, H. F., and Rosenberg, D. E.: J. Pharmacol. Exp. Ther. 143: 149, 1964.
63. Lasagna, L., DeKornfeld, T. J., and Pearson, J. W.: J. Pharmacol. Exp. Ther. 144:12, 1964.
64. Houde, R. W.: Br. J. Clin. Pharmacol. 7:297, 1979.
65. Harris, D. S., et al.: Drug Alcohol Depend. 61:85, 2000.
66. Martin, W. R.: Pharmacol. Rev. 19:463, 1967.
67. Julius, D., and Renault, P. (eds.): Narcotic Antagonists: Naltrexone, Progress Report. NIDA Research Monograph 9. Washington, DC, DHEW, 1976.
68. Willette, R. E. (ed.): Narcotic Antagonists: The Search for Long-Acting Preparations. NIDA Research Monograph 4. Washington, DC, DHEW, 1975.
69. deStevens, G. (ed.): Analgetics. New York, Academic Press, 1965.
70. Braenden, O. J., Eddy, N. B., and Halbach, H.: Bull. WHO 13:937, 1955.
71. Leutner, V.: Arzneimittelforschung 10:505, 1960.
72. Janssen, P. A. J.: Br. J. Anaesth. 34:260, 1962.
73. Beckett, A. H., and Casy, A. F.: Prog. Med. Chem. 2:43–87, 1962.
74. Mellet, L. B., and Woods, L. A.: Prog. Drug Res. 5:156, 1963.
75. Casy, A. F.: Prog. Med. Chem. 7:229–284, 1970.

76. Lewis, J., Bentley, K. W., and Cowan, A.: Annu. Rev. Pharmacol. 11:241, 1970.
77. Eddy, N. B., and May, E. L.: Science 181:407, 1973.
78. Beckett, A. H., Casy, A. F., and Harper, N. J.: Pharm. Pharmacol. 8: 874, 1956.
79. Lasagna, L., and DeKornfeld, T. J.: J. Pharmacol. Exp. Ther. 124: 260, 1958.
80. Fishman, J., Hahn, E. F., and Norton, B. I.: Nature 261:64, 1976.
81. Wright, W. B., Jr., Brabander, H. J., and Hardy, R. A., Jr.: J. Am. Chem. Soc. 81:1518, 1959.
82. Gross, F., and Turrian, H.: Experientia 13:401, 1957.
83. Gross, F., and Turrian, H.: Fed. Proc. 19:22, 1960.
84. Beckett, A. H., and Casy, A. F.: J. Pharm. Pharmacol. 6:986, 1954.
85. Beckett, A. H.: J. Pharm. Pharmacol. 8:848, 860, 1958.
86. Beckett, A. H.: Pharm. J. 256, 1959.
87. Jacquet, Y. F., et al.: Science 198:842, 1977.
88. Portoghese, P. S.: J. Med. Chem. 8:609, 1965.
89. Portoghese, P. S.: J. Pharm. Sci. 55:865, 1966.
90. Portoghese, P. S.: Acc. Chem. Res. 11:21, 1978.
91. Koshland, D. E., Jr.: Proc. First Int. Pharmacol. Meet. 7:161, 1963.
92. Belleau, B.: J. Med. Chem. 7:776, 1964.
93. Martin, W. R., et al.: J. Pharmacol. Exp. Ther. 197:517, 1976.
94. Gilbert, P. E., and Martin, W. R.: J. Pharmacol. Exp. Ther. 198:66, 1976.
95. Beaumont, A., and Hughes, J.: Annu. Rev. Pharmacol. Toxicol. 19: 245, 1979.
96. Lasagna, L., and Beecher, H. K.: J. Pharmacol. Exp. Ther. 112:356, 1954.
97. Soulairac, A., Cahn, J., and Charpentier, J. (eds.): Pain. New York, Academic Press, 1968.
98. Willette, R. E.: Am. J. Pharm. Ed. 34:662, 1970.
99. Barnett, G., Trsic, M., and Willette, R. E. (eds.): Quantitative Structure-Activity Relationships of Analgesics, Narcotic Antagonists, and Hallucinogens. NIDA Research Monograph 22. Washington, DC, DHEW, 1978.
100. Archer, S., and Harris, L. S.: Prog. Drug Res. 8:262, 1965.
101. Kutter, E., et al.: J. Med. Chem. 13:801, 1970.
102. Portoghese, P. S., et al.: J. Med. Chem. 14:144, 1971.
103. Portoghese, P. S., et al.: J. Med. Chem. 11:219, 1968.
104. Kaufman, J. J., Semo, N. M., and Koski, W. S.: J. Med. Chem. 18: 647, 1975.
105. Kaufman, J. J., Kerman, E., and Koski, W. S.: Int. J. Quantum Chem. 289, 1974.
106. Loew, G. H., and Berkowitz, D. S.: J. Med. Chem. 21:101, 1978.
107. Loew, G. H., and Berkowitz, D. S.: J. Med. Chem. 22:603, 1979.
108. Simon, E. J., and Hiller, J. B.: Annu. Rev. Pharmacol. Toxicol. 18: 371, 1978.
109. Goldstein, A.: Life Sci. 14:615, 1974.
110. Goldstein, A., Lowney, L. I., and Pal, B. K.: Proc. Natl. Acad. Sci. U. S. A. 68:1742, 1971.
111. Simon, E. J., Hiller, J. M., and Edelman, I.: Proc. Natl. Acad. Sci. U. S. A. 70:1947, 1973.
112. Terenius, L.: Acta Pharmacol. Toxicol. 32:317, 1973.
113. Pert, C. B., and Snyder, S. H.: Science 179:1011, 1973.
114. Kosterlitz, H. W., and Watt, A. J.: Br. J. Pharmacol. Chemother. 33: 266, 1968.
115. Hughes, J.: Brain Res. 88:295, 1975.
116. Hughes, J.: Neurosci. Res. Program Bull. 13:55, 1975.
117. Terenius, L.: Annu. Rev. Pharmacol. Toxicol. 18:189, 1978.
118. Goldstein, A.: Science 193:1081, 1976.
119. Kolanta, G. B.: Science 205:774, 1979.
120. Gulland and Robinson: Proc. Manchester Lit. Phil. Soc. 69–79, 1925.
121. Gates, M., and Tschudi, G.: J. Am. Chem. Soc. 74:1109, 1952.
122. Gates, M., and Tschudi, G.: J. Am. Chem. Soc. 78:1380, 1956.
123. Twycross, R. G.: Int. J. Clin. Pharmacol. 9:184, 1974.
124. Houde, R. W., and Wallenstein, S. L.: Minutes of the 11th meeting, Committee on Drug Addiction and Narcotics, National Research Council, 1953.
125. Eddy, N. B., and Lee, L. E.: J. Pharmacol. Exp. Ther. 125:116, 1959.
126. Weijlard, J., and Erickson, A. E.: J. Am. Chem. Soc. 64:869, 1942.
127. Fraser, H. F., et al.: J. Pharmacol. Exp. Ther. 122:359, 1958.
128. Cochin, J., Axelrod, J.: J. Pharmacol. Exp. Ther. 125:105, 1959.
129. Ziering, A., and Lee, J.: J. Org. Chem. 12:911, 1947.
130. Weijlard, J., et al.: J. Am. Chem. Soc. 78:2342, 1956.
131. Med. Lett. 19:73, 1977.

132. Wang, R. I. H.: Eur. J. Clin. Pharmacol. 7:183, 1974.
133. Easton, N. R., Gardner, J. H., and Stevens, J. R.: J. Am. Chem. Soc. 69:2941, 1947.
134. Freedman, A. M.: JAMA 197:878, 1966.
135. Med. Lett. 11:97, 1969.
136. Smits, S. E.: Res. Commun. Chem. Pathol. Pharmacol. 8:575, 1974.
137. Billings, R. E., Booher, R., and Smits, S. E., et al.: J. Med. Chem. 16:305, 1973.
138. Jaffe, J. H., Senay, E. C., and Schuster, C. R., et al.: JAMA 222:437, 1972.
139. Gruber, C. M., and Babtisti, A.: Clin. Pharmacol. Ther. 4:172, 1962.
140. Pohland, A., and Sullivan, H. R.: J. Am. Chem. Soc. 75:4458, 1953.
141. Med. Lett. 20:111, 1978.
142. Forrest, W. H., et al.: Clin. Pharmacol. Ther. 10:468, 1969.
143. Ehrnebo, M., Boreus, L. O., and Lönroth, V.: Clin. Pharmacol. Ther. 22:888, 1977.
144. Med. Lett. 9:49, 1967.
145. Deleted in proof.
146. Deleted in proof.
147. Jasinski, D. R., Martin, W. R., and Sapira, J. D.: Clin. Pharmacol. Ther. 9:215, 1968.
148. Cone, E. J.: Tetrahedron Lett. 28:2607, 1973
149. Chatterjie, N., et al.: Drug Metab. Dispos. 2:401, 1974.
150. Batra, V. K., Sams, R. A., Reuning, R. H., and Malspeis, L.: Acad. Pharm. Sci. 4:122, 1974.
151. Blumberg, H., and Dayton, H. B.: In Kosterlitz, H., Villarreal, J. E. (eds.). Agonist and Antagonist Actions of Narcotic Analgesic Drugs. London, Macmillan, 1972.
152. Woodland, J. H. R., et al.: J. Med. Chem. 16:897, 1973.
153. Takemori, A. E. A., Hayashi, G., and Smits, S. E.: Eur. J. Pharmacol. 20:85, 1972.
154. Nutt, J. G., and Jasinsky, D. R.: Pharmacologist 15:240, 1973.
155. Salem, H., and Aviado, D. M.: Am. J. Med. Sci. 247:585, 1964.
156. Chappel, C. I., and von Seemann, C.: Prog. Med. Chem. 3:133–136, 1963.
157. Five-Year Report. Br. Med. J. 2:1033, 1960.
158. Wong, S.: Annu. Rep. Med. Chem. 10:172–181, 1975.
159. Collier, H. O. J.: Nature 232:17, 1971.
160. Vane, J. R.: Nature 231:232, 1971.
161. Shen, T. Y.: Angew. Chem. Int. Ed. 11:460, 1972.
162. Nickander, R., McMahon, F. G., and Ridolfo, A. S.: Annu. Rev. Pharmacol. Toxicol. 19:469, 1979.
163. Smith, P. K.: Ann. N. Y. Acad. Sci. 86:38, 1960.
164. Smith, M. J. H., and Smith, P. K. (eds.): The Salicylates. A. Critical Bibliographic Review. New York, John Wiley & Sons, 1966.
165. Collier, H. O. J.: Sci. Am. 209:97, 1963.
166. Alvarez, A. S., and Summerskill, W. H. J.: Lancet 2:920, 1958.
167. Barager, F. D., and Duthie, J. J. R.: Br. Med. J. 1:1106, 1960.
168. Leonards, J. R., and Levy, G.: Abstr. of the 116th meeting. Am. Pharm. Assoc., Montreal, May 17–22, 1969, p. 67.
169. Davenport, H. W.: N. Engl. J. Med. 276:1307, 1967.
170. Weiss, H. J.: Schweiz. Med. Wochenschr. 104:114, 1974
171. Elwood, P. C., et al.: Br. Med. J. 1:436, 1974.
172. Aspirin Myocardial Infarction Study Research Group: JAMA 243:661, 1980.
173. Levy, G., and Hayes, B. A.: N. Engl. J. Med. 262:1053, 1960.
174. Lieberman, S. V., et al.: J. Pharm. Sci. 53:1486, 1492, 1964.
175. Pfeiffer, C. C.: Arch. Biol. Med. Exp. 4:10, 1967.
176. Salassa, R. M., Bollman, J. M., and Dry, T. J.: J. Lab. Clin. Med. 33:1393, 1948.
177. Smith, P. K., et al.: J. Pharmacol. Exp. Ther. 87:237, 1946.
178. Garrett, E. R.: J. Am. Pharm. Assoc. Sci. Ed. 48:676, 1959.
179. Gold, G., and Campbell, J. A.: J. Pharm. Sci. 53:52, 1964.
180. Troup, A. E., and Mitchner, H.: J. Pharm. Sci. 53:375, 1964.
181. Blaug, S. M., and Wesolowski, J. W.: J. Am. Pharm. Assoc. Sci. Ed. 48:691, 1959.
182. Obbink, H. J. K.: Lancet 1:565, 1964.
183. Goldman, A. S., and Yakovac, W. C.: Proc. Soc. Exp. Biol. Med. 115:693, 1964.
184. Br. Med. J. 2:131T, 1963.
185. Med. Lett. 8:7, 1966.
186. Liyanage, S. P., and Tambar, P. K.: Curr. Med. Res. Opin. 5:450, 1978.
187. Deodhar, S. D., et al.: Curr. Med. Res. Opin. 5:185, 1978.
188. Regaldo, R. G.: Curr. Med. Res. Opin. 5:454, 1978.
189. Leonards, J. R.: J. Lab. Clin. Med. 74:911, 1969.
190. Bloomfield, S. S., Barden, T. P., and Hille, R.: Clin. Pharmacol. Ther. 11:747, 1970.
191. Winder, C. V.: Nature 184:494, 1959.
192. Scherrer, R. A.: Analgesics. In Scherrer, R. A., and Whitehouse, M. W. (eds.). Anti-inflammatory Agents. New York, Academic Press, 1974, p. 191.
193. Cass, L. J., and Frederik, W. S.: J. Pharmacol. Exp. Ther. 139:172, 1963.
194. Lane, A. Z., Holmes, E. L., and Moyer, C. E.: J. New Drugs 4:333, 1964.
195. Med. Lett. 10:37, 1968.
196. Walker, R. W., et al.: Anal. Biochem. 95:579, 1979.
197. Brogden, R. N., et al.: Drugs 16:97, 1978.
198. Brogden, R. N., et al.: Med. Lett. 21:1, 1979.
199. Brogden, R. N., et al.: Drugs 15:429, 1978.
200. Deleted in proof.
201. Deleted in proof.
202. Dornan, J., and Reynolds, W.: Can. Med. Assoc. J. 110:1370, 1974.
203. Deleted in proof.
204. Brogden, R. N., et al.: Drugs 18:241, 1979.
205. Brogden, R. N., et al.: Drugs 13:241, 1977.
206. Chernish, S. M., et al.: Arthritis Rheum. 22:376, 1979.
207. Wiseman, E. H.: R. Soc. Med. Int. Congr. Ser. 1:11, 1978.
208. Weintraub, M., et al.: J. Rheumatol. 4:393, 1979.
209. Balogh, Z., et al.: Curr. Med. Res. Opin. 6:148, 1979.
210. Brodie, B. B., and Axelrod, J.: J. Pharmacol. Exp. Ther. 94:29, 1948.
211. Brodie, B. B., and Axelrod, J.: J. Pharmacol. Exp. Ther. 97:58, 1949.
212. Axelrod, J.: Postgrad. Med. 34:328, 1963.
213. Burns, J. J., et al.: Ann. N. Y. Acad. Sci. 86:253, 1960.
214. Domenjoz, R.: Ann. N. Y. Acad. Sci. 86:263, 1960.

SELECTED READING

American Chemical Society: First National Medicinal Chemistry Symposium. Columbus, OH, American Chemical Society, 1948, pp. 15–49.
Anonymous: Codeine and Certain Other Analgesic and Antitussive Agents: A Review. Rahway, NJ, Merck & Co., 1970.
Archer, S., and Harris, L. S.: Narcotic antagonists. Prog. Drug Res. 8:262, 1965.
Arrigoni-Martelli, E.: Inflammation and Anti-inflammatories. New York, Spectrum, 1977.
Barlow, R. B.: Morphine-like analgesics. In Introduction to Chemical Pharmacology. New York, John Wiley & Sons, 1955, pp. 39–56.
Beckett, A. H., and Casy, A. F.: The testing and development of analgesic drugs. Prog. Med. Chem. 2:43–87, 1963.
Bengsston, V., Johansson, S., and Angervall, L.: Kidney Int. 13:107, 1978.
Bengsston, V., Johansson, S., and Angervall, L.: Science 240:129, 1979.
Bergel, F., and Morrison, A. L.: Q. Rev. (Lond.) 2:349, 1948.
Berger, F. M., et al.: Ann. N. Y. Acad. Sci. 86:310, 1960.
Bonica, J. J., and Allen, G. D.: In Modell, W. (ed.). Drugs of Choice 1970–1971. St. Louis, C. V. Mosby, 1970, p. 210.
Braenden, O. J., Eddy, N. B., and Hallbach, H.: Bull. WHO 13:937, 1955.
Braude, M. C., et al. (eds.): Narcotic Antagonists. New York, Raven Press, 1973.
Brümmer, T.: Fortschr. Ther. 12:24, 1936.
Brown, D. M., and Hardy, T. L.: Br. J. Pharmacol. Chemother. 32:17, 1968.
Casy, A. F.: Prog. Med. Chem. 7:229–284, 1970.
Chappel, C. I., and von Seemann, C.: Prog. Med. Chem. 3:89–145, 1963.
Chen, K. K.: Physiological and pharmacological background, including methods of evaluation of analgesic agents. J. Am. Pharm. Assoc. Sci. Ed. 38:51, 1949.
Clouet, D. H.: Narcotic Drugs: Biochemical Pharmacology. New York, Plenum Press, 1971.
Collins, P. W.: Antitussives. In Burger, A. (ed.). Medicinal Chemistry, 3rd ed. New York, Wiley-Interscience, 1970, pp. 1351–1364.
Coyne, W. E.: Nonsteroidal anti-inflammatory agents and antipyretics. In Burger, A. (ed.). Medicinal Chemistry, 3rd ed. New York, Wiley-Interscience, 1970, pp. 953–975.
deStevens, G. (ed.): Analgetics. New York, Academic Press. 1965.
Eddy, N. B.: Chemical structure and action of morphine-like analgesics and related substances. Chem. Ind. (Lond.) 1462, 1959.
Eddy, N. B., Halbach, H., and Braenden, O. J.: Bull. WHO 14:353–402, 1956.

Eddy, N. B., Halbach, H., and Braenden, O. J.: Bull. WHO 17:569–863, 1957.

Evens, R. P.: Drug therapy reviews: Antirheumatic agents. Am. J. Hosp. Pharm. 36:622, 1979.

Fellows, E. J., and Ullyot, G. E.: Analgesics: A. Aralkylamines. In American Chemical Society, Medicinal Chemistry, vol. 1. New York, John Wiley & Sons, 1951, pp. 390–437.

Gold, H., and Cattell, M.: Am. J. Med. Sci. 246:590, 1963.

Greenberg, L.: Antipyrine: A Critical Bibliographic Review. New Haven, CT, Hillhouse, 1950.

Gross, M.: Acetanilid: A Critical Bibliographic Review. New Haven, CT, Hillhouse, 1946.

Hellerbach, J., Schnider, O., Besendorf, H., et al.: Synthetic Analgesics: Part II. Morphinans and 6,7-Benzomorphans. New York, Pergamon Press, 1966.

Jacobson, A. E., May, E. L., and Sargent, L. J.: Analgetics. In Burger, A. (ed.). Medicinal Chemistry, 3rd ed. New York, Wiley-Interscience, 1970, pp. 1327–1350.

Janssen, P. A. J.: Synthetic Analgesics: Part I. Diphenylpropylamines. New York, Pergamon Press, 1960.

Janssen, P. A. J., and van der Eycken, C. A. M.: In Burger, A. (ed.). Drugs Affecting the Central Nervous System. New York, Marcel Dekker, 1968, pp. 25–85.

Lasagna, L.: The clinical evaluation of morphine and its substitutes as analgesics: Pharmacol. Rev. 16:47–83, 1964.

Lee, J.: Analgesics: B. Partial structures related to morphine. In American Chemical Society. Medicinal Chemistry, vol. 1. New York, John Wiley & Sons, 1951, pp. 438–466.

Martin, W. R.: Opioid antagonists. Pharmacol. Rev. 19:463–521, 1967.

Mellet, L. B., and Woods, L. A.: Analgesia and addiction. Prog. Drug Res. 5:156–267, 1963.

Med. Lett. 6:78, 1964.

Portoghese, P. S.: Stereochemical factors and receptor interactions associated with narcotic analgesics. J. Pharm. Sci. 55:865, 1966.

Portoghese, P. S.: Selective nonpeptide opioid antagonists. In Hertz, A. (ed.). Handbook of Experimental Pharmacology: Opioids I, vol. 104/I. Berlin, Springer-Verlag, 1993.

Reynolds, A. K., and Randall, L. O.: Morphine and Allied Drugs. Toronto, University of Toronto Press, 1957.

Salem, H., and Aviado, D. M.: Antitussive Agents, vols. 1–3 (Sect. 27 of International Encyclopedia of Pharmacology and Therapeutics). Oxford, Pergamon Press, 1970.

Scherrer, R. A., and Whitehouse, M. W.: Anti-inflammatory Agents. New York, Academic Press, 1974.

Shen, T. Y.: Perspectives in nonsteroidal anti-inflammatory agents. Angew. Chem. Int. Ed. 11:460, 1972.

Simon, E. J., and Gioannini, T. L.: Opioid receptor multiplicity: Isolation, purification, and chemical characterization of binding sites. In Hertz, A. (ed.). Handbook of Experimental Pharmacology: Opioids I, vol. 104/I. Berlin, Springer-Verlag, 1993.

Snyder, S. H.: Opiate receptors and internal opiates. Sci. Am. 237:236–244, 1977.

Tomatis, L., et al.: Cancer Res. 38:877, 1978.

Winder, C. A.: Nonsteroid anti-inflammatory agents. Prog. Drug Res. 10: 139–203, 1966.

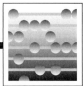

Steroid Hormones and Therapeutically Related Compounds

PHILIP J. PROTEAU

Steroid hormones and related products represent one of the most widely used classes of therapeutic agents. These drugs are used primarily in birth control, hormone-replacement therapy (HRT), inflammatory conditions, and cancer treatment. Most of these agents are chemically based on a common structural backbone, the steroid backbone. Although they share a common structural foundation, the variations in the structures provide specificity for the unique molecular targets. Five general groups of steroid hormones are discussed: estrogens, progestins, androgens, glucocorticoids, and mineralocorticoids. The structural bases for the differences in actions and the various therapeutic uses for these compounds are explored. Several review articles and texts provide excellent coverage of the pharmacology and chemistry of steroid hormones.[1-3]

STEROID NOMENCLATURE, STEREOCHEMISTRY, AND NUMBERING

As shown in Figure 23-1, nearly all steroids are named as derivatives of cholestane, androstane, pregnane, or estrane. The standard system of numbering is illustrated with 5α-cholestane.

The absolute stereochemistry of the molecule and any substituents is shown with solid (β) and dashed (α) bonds. Most carbons have one β bond and one α bond, with the β bond lying closer to the "top" or C18 and C19 methyl side of the molecule. Both α and β substituents may be axial or equatorial. This system of designating stereochemistry can best be illustrated by use of 5α-androstane (Fig. 23-2).

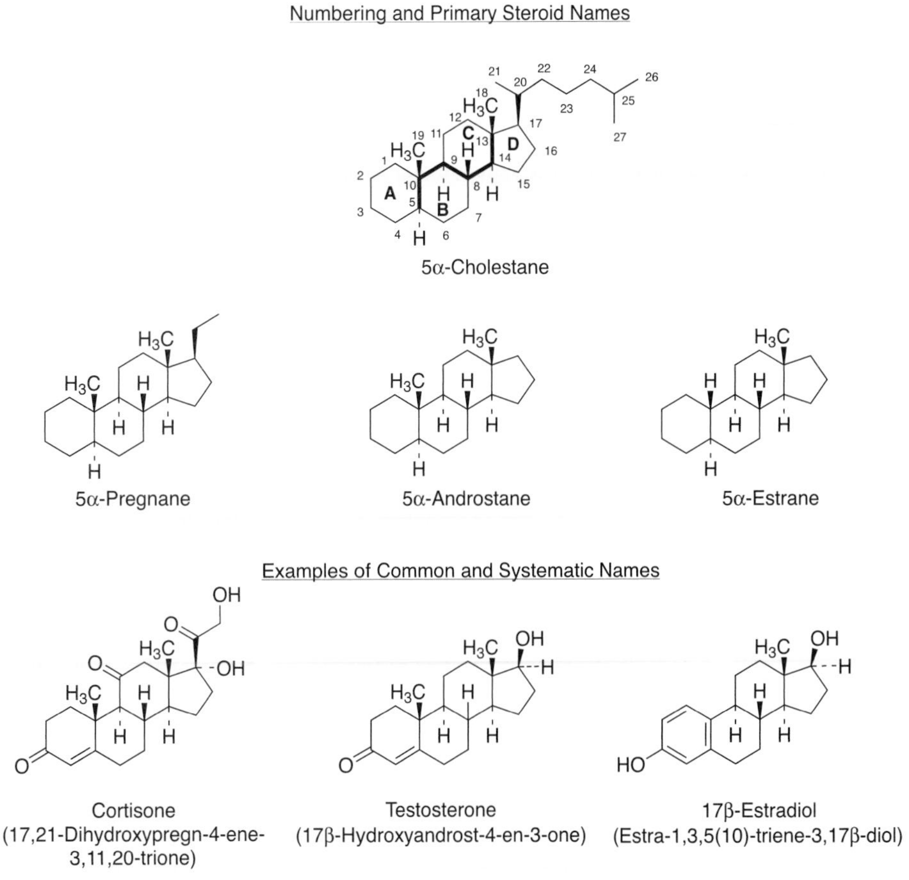

Numbering and Primary Steroid Names

5α-Cholestane

5α-Pregnane

5α-Androstane

5α-Estrane

Examples of Common and Systematic Names

Cortisone
(17,21-Dihydroxypregn-4-ene-3,11,20-trione)

Testosterone
(17β-Hydroxyandrost-4-en-3-one)

17β-Estradiol
(Estra-1,3,5(10)-triene-3,17β-diol)

Figure 23–1 ■ Steroid nomenclature and numbering.

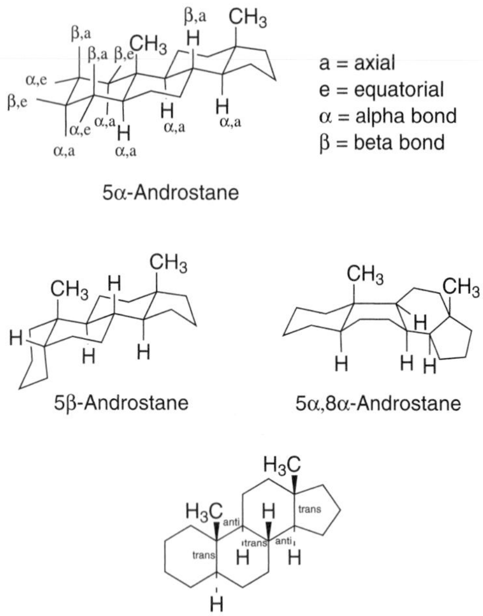

a = axial
e = equatorial
α = alpha bond
β = beta bond

5α-Androstane

Figure 23–2 ■ Steroid nomenclature—stereochemistry.

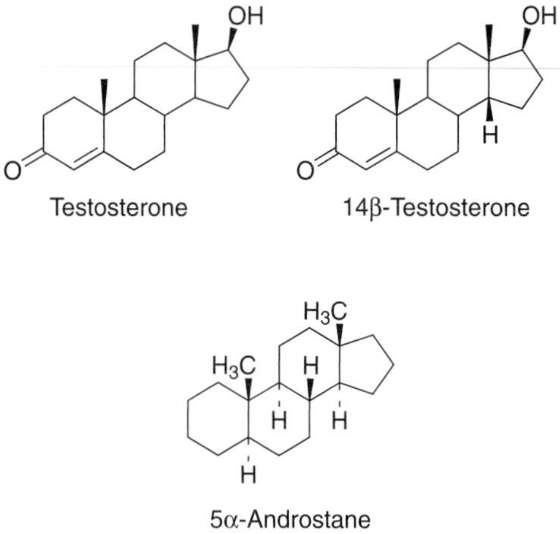

The stereochemistry of the H at C5 is always indicated in the name. The stereochemistry of the other H atoms is not indicated unless it differs from 5α-cholestane. Changing the stereochemistry of any of the ring juncture or backbone carbons (shown in Fig. 23-1 with a heavy line on 5α-cholestane) greatly changes the shape of the steroid, as seen in the examples of 5α,8α-androstane and 5β-androstane (Fig. 23-2).

Because of the immense effect that "backbone" stereochemistry has on the shape of the molecule, the International Union of Pure and Applied Chemistry (IUPAC) rules[4] strongly recommend that the stereochemistry at all backbone carbons be clearly shown. That is, all hydrogens along the backbone should be drawn. When the stereochemistry is not known, a wavy line is used in the drawing, and the Greek letter xi (ζ) is used in the name instead of α or β. Methyls are explicitly indicated as CH3.

The terms *cis* and *trans* are occasionally used in steroid

5-Androstene or
Δ^5-Androstene or
Androst-5-ene

5α-Androst-8-ene or
5α-Δ^8-Androstene

5α-Androst-8(14)-ene or
5α-$\Delta^{8(14)}$-Androstene

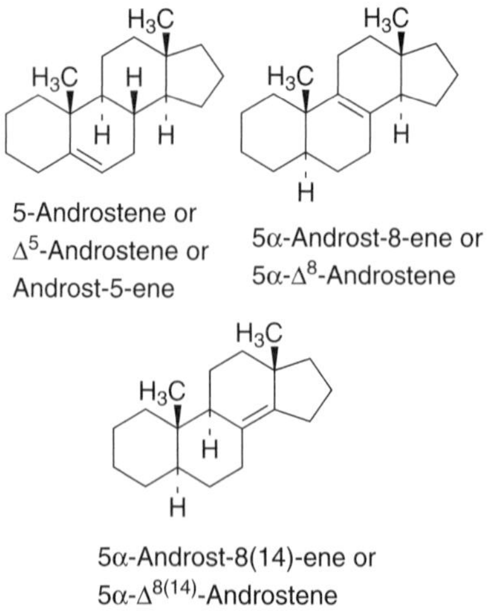

Figure 23–3 ■ Steroid nomenclature—double bonds.

Testosterone

14β-Testosterone

5α-Androstane

Figure 23–4 ■ Alternative representations of steroids.

nomenclature to indicate the backbone stereochemistry between rings. For example, 5α steroids are A/B *trans*, and 5β steroids are A/B *cis*. The terms *syn* and *anti* are used analogously to *trans* and *cis* for indicating stereochemistry in bonds connecting rings (e.g., the C9:C10 bond that connects rings A and C). The use of these terms is indicated in Figure 23-2.

The position of double bonds can be designated in any of the various ways shown below. Double bonds from C8 may go toward C9 or C14, and those from C20 may go toward C21 or C22. In such cases, both carbons are indicated in the name if the double bond is not between sequentially numbered carbons (e.g., 5α-androst-8(14)-ene or 5α-$\Delta^{8(14)}$-androstene; see Fig. 23-3). These principles of modern steroid nomenclature are applied to naming several common steroid drugs shown in Figure 23-1.

Such common names as *testosterone* and *cortisone* are obviously much easier to use than the long systematic names. Substituents must always have their position and stereochemistry clearly indicated, however, when common names are used (e.g., 17α-methyltestosterone, 9α-fluorocortisone).

Steroid drawings sometimes appear with lines drawn instead of methyls (CH3), and backbone stereochemistry is not indicated unless it differs from that of 5α-androstane (Fig. 23-4). This manner of representation should only be used when there is no ambiguity in the implied stereochemistry.

STEROID BIOSYNTHESIS

Steroid hormones in mammals are biosynthesized from cholesterol, which in turn is made in vivo from acetyl-coenzyme A (acetyl-CoA) via the mevalonate pathway. Although humans do obtain approximately 300 mg of cholesterol per day in their diets, a greater amount (about 1 g) is biosynthesized per day. A schematic outline of these biosynthetic pathways is shown in Figure 23-5.

Conversion of cholesterol to pregnenolone is the rate-limiting step in steroid hormone biosynthesis. It is not the enzymatic transformation itself that is rate limiting, however; the translocation of cholesterol to the inner mitochondrial membrane of steroid-synthesizing cells is rate limiting.[5] A key protein involved in the translocation is the *S*teroidogenic

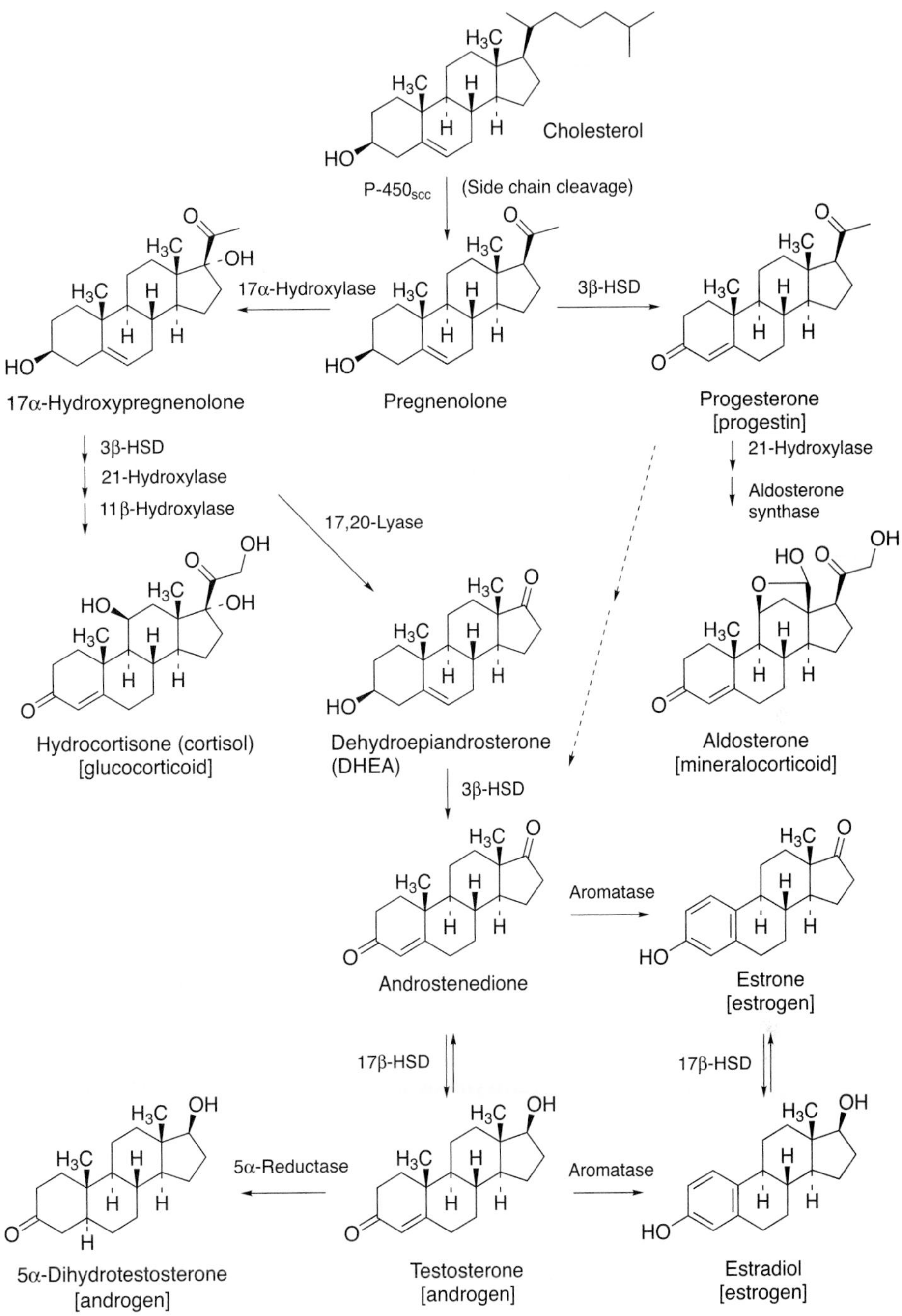

Figure 23–5 ■ Outline of the biosynthesis of steroid hormones. *3β-HSD*, 3β-hydroxysteroid dehydrogenase/Δ^{5-4} isomerase; *17β-HSD*, 17β-hydroxysteroid dehydrogenase.

Acute *R*egulatory protein (StAR). Defects in the StAR gene lead to congenital lipoid adrenal hyperplasia, a rare condition marked by a deficiency of adrenal and gonadal steroid hormones.[6] The enzymes involved in the transformation of cholesterol to the hormones are mainly cytochromes P-450 and dehydrogenases. The main routes of biosynthesis of the hormones are depicted in Figure 23-5. Estradiol, testosterone, progesterone, aldosterone, and hydrocortisone are representatives of the distinct steroid receptor ligands that are shown. Further metabolic fates of these compounds are presented under the specific structural class.

An enzyme denoted cytochrome P-450$_{\text{scc}}$ (SCC for side chain cleavage) mediates the cleavage of the C17 side chain on the D ring of the sterol to provide pregnenolone, the C21

precursor of the steroids. This enzyme mediates a three-step process involved in the oxidative metabolism of the side chain. Successive hydroxylations at C20 and C22 are followed by oxidative cleavage of the C20–C22 bond, providing pregnenolone. Pregnenolone can be either directly converted into progesterone or modified for synthesis of glucocorticoids, estrogens, and androgens. Introduction of unsaturation into the A ring leads to the formation of progesterone. Specifically, oxidation of the alcohol at C3 to the ketone provides a substrate in which isomerization of the $\Delta^{5,6}$ double bond to the $\Delta^{4,5}$ double bond is facilitated. This transformation is mediated by a bifunctional enzyme, 3β-hydroxysteroid dehydrogenase/Δ^{5-4} isomerase (3β-HSD). This enzyme can act on several 3-ol-5-ene steroids in addition to pregnenolone. Hydroxylation at C17 provides the precursor for both sex steroid hormones and glucocorticoids. Cytochrome P-450c17 hydroxylates pregnenolone and progesterone to provide the corresponding 17α-hydroxylated compounds. 17α-Hydroxypregnenolone can be converted to 17α-hydroxyprogesterone by 3β-HSD. Cytochrome P-450c17 is also a bifunctional enzyme, with lyase activity in addition to the hydroxylase action. The C17,20 lyase activity is crucial for the formation of the sex hormones. The lyase oxidatively removes the two carbons at C17, providing the C17 ketone. In the case of 17α-hydroxypregnenolone, the product is dehydroepiandrosterone (DHEA). If 17α-hydroxyprogesterone is the substrate for the lyase, androstenedione results. The conversion of 17α-hydroxyprogesterone to androstenedione is limited in humans, although in other species this is an important pathway. DHEA is converted to androstenedione by the action of 3β-HSD. Androstenedione can either be converted to testosterone by the action of 17β-hydroxysteroid dehydrogenase (17β-HSD) or be transformed into estrone by aromatase, a unique cytochrome P-450 that aromatizes the A ring of certain steroid precursors. Testosterone is aromatized to 17β-estradiol by the same enzyme. 17β-HSD acts on estrone to form 17β-estradiol. If testosterone is acted on by 5α-reductase, 5α-dihydrotestosterone (DHT), an androgen important in the prostate is produced.

The major route to glucocorticoids diverges at 17α-hydroxypregnenolone. Instead of oxidative cleavage at C17, 3β-HSD acts on this substrate to provide 17α-hydroxyprogesterone. Small amounts of 17α-hydroxyprogesterone can be produced directly from progesterone, although this is not a major pathway in humans. Sequential action of 21-hydroxylase (Cyp21) and 11β-hydroxylase (Cyp11B1) provide hydrocortisone, the key glucocorticoid in humans.

If progesterone is directly acted on by 21-hydroxylase (Cyp21), 11-deoxycorticosterone is produced, a precursor to the mineralocorticoid aldosterone. In tissues where aldosterone is synthesized, the multifunctional enzyme aldosterone synthase (Cyp11B2) mediates the hydroxylation at C11 as well as the two-step oxidation of C18 to an aldehyde, providing aldosterone, which exists predominantly in the cyclic hemiacetal form.

CHEMICAL AND PHYSICAL PROPERTIES OF STEROIDS

With few exceptions, the steroids are white crystalline solids. They may be in the form of needles, leaflets, platelets, or amorphous particles, depending on the particular compound, the solvent used in crystallization, and the skill and luck of the chemist. As the steroids have 17 or more carbon atoms, it is not surprising that they tend to be water insoluble. Addition of hydroxyl or other polar groups (or decreasing carbons) increases water solubility slightly, as expected. Salts are the most water soluble. Examples are shown in Table 23-1.

CHANGES TO MODIFY PHARMACOKINETIC PROPERTIES OF STEROIDS

As with many other compounds described in previous chapters, the steroids can be made more lipid soluble or more

TABLE 23–1 Solubilities of Steroids

	Solubility (g/100 mL)		
	CHCl$_3$	EtOH	H$_2$O
Cholesterol	22	1.2	Insoluble
Testosterone	50	15	Insoluble
Testosterone propionate	45	25	Insoluble
Dehydrocholic acid	90	0.33	0.02
Estradiol	1.0	10	Insoluble
Estradiol benzoate	0.8	8	Insoluble
Betamethasone	0.1	2	Insoluble
Betamethasone acetate	10	3	Insoluble
Betamethasone NaPO$_4$ salt	Insoluble	15	50
Hydrocortisone	0.5	2.5	0.01
Hydrocortisone acetate	1.0	0.4	Insoluble
Hydrocortisone NaPO$_4$ salt	Insoluble	1.0	75
Prednisolone	0.4	3	0.01
Prednisolone acetate	1.0	0.7	Insoluble
Prednisolone NaPO$_4$ salt	0.8	13	25

water soluble by making suitable ester derivatives of hydroxyl groups. Derivatives with increased lipid solubility are often made to decrease the rate of release of the drug from intramuscular injection sites (i.e., in depot preparations). More lipid-soluble derivatives also have improved skin absorption properties and thus are preferred for dermatological preparations. Derivatives with increased water solubility are needed for intravenous preparations. Since hydrolyzing enzymes are found throughout mammalian cells, especially in the liver, converting hydroxyl groups to esters does not significantly modify the activity of most compounds.

Some steroids (e.g., estradiol, progesterone, and testosterone) are particularly susceptible to rapid metabolism after absorption or rapid inactivation in the gastrointestinal tract before absorption. These inactivation processes limit the effectiveness of these hormones as orally available drugs, although micronized forms of estradiol and progesterone are available for oral administration. Sometimes, a simple chemical modification can decrease the rate of inactivation and, thereby, increase the drug's half-life or make it possible to be taken orally.

Examples of common chemical modifications are illustrated in Figure 23-6. Drugs such as testosterone *cyclopentylpropionate* (cypionate) and methylprednisolone sodium succinate are *prodrugs* that require hydrolysis to release the active hormone in the body.

STEROID HORMONE RECEPTORS

Steroid hormones regulate tissue-specific gene expression. The individual hormones exhibit remarkable tissue selectivity, even though their structural differences are relatively minor. Estrogens such as estradiol increase uterine cell proliferation, for example, but not prostate cell proliferation.

1. Increase Lipid Solubility (Slower rate of release for depot preparation; increase skin absorption)

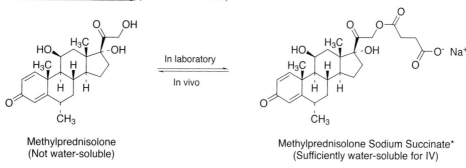

(IM dose: 10–25 mg
2–3 times/week)

Testosterone Cyclopentylpropionate*
(Testosterone cypionate; IM dose: 200–
400 mg every 4 weeks)

Triamcinolone

Triamcinolone Acetonide
(Increased topical activity)

2. Increase Water Solubility (Suitable for IV use)

Methylprednisolone
(Not water-soluble)

Methylprednisolone Sodium Succinate*
(Sufficiently water-soluble for IV)

3. Decrease Inactivation

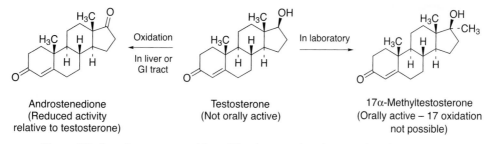

Androstenedione
(Reduced activity
relative to testosterone)

Testosterone
(Not orally active)

17α-Methyltestosterone
(Orally active – 17 oxidation
not possible)

Figure 23–6 ▪ Common steroid modifications to alter therapeutic utility. *, prodrug.

Androgens such as testosterone do the reverse, but neither androgens nor estrogens affect stomach epithelium. The basis for this selectivity is the presence of selective steroid hormone receptors in individual tissues. This section provides an overview of steroid hormone receptors and their mode of action.[1, 2]

The steroid receptors themselves are key players in gene expression, but many other proteins are involved in this process. Chaperone proteins, for example, help fold the receptor proteins into the proper three-dimensional shape for binding the steroid ligand. Together, the steroid hormone receptor and associated proteins (Fig. 23-7) make up the mature receptor complex. Once the ligand is bound to the receptor, the chaperone proteins dissociate, and the receptors dimerize and are posttranslationally modified, typically by phosphorylation. Some of the steroid receptor–ligand complexes must be transported into the nucleus prior to interaction with DNA. The activated receptor–ligand complex binds to target DNA, and various coactivators or corepressors are recruited to the DNA–receptor complex. Transcription (or repression

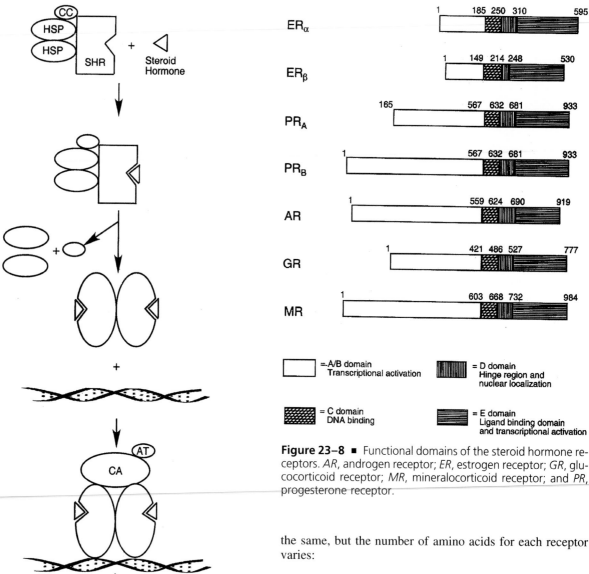

Figure 23–7 ■ Generic structural model of a steroid hormone–receptor complex and its activation for gene transcription. *AT,* histone acetyltransferase; *CA,* coactivator; *CC,* cochaperone; *HSP,* heat shock protein; *SHR,* steroid hormone receptor.

Figure 23–8 ■ Functional domains of the steroid hormone receptors. *AR,* androgen receptor; *ER,* estrogen receptor; *GR,* glucocorticoid receptor; *MR,* mineralocorticoid receptor; and *PR,* progesterone receptor.

of transcription) occurs when all of the necessary associated proteins have been recruited to the DNA–receptor complex.

Structure of Steroid Hormone Receptors

The complementary DNAs (cDNAs) of all the major steroid hormone receptors have been cloned, giving the complete amino acid sequence of each. Although the whole three-dimensional structure of a steroid hormone receptor has not been solved (structures of the ligand-binding domains of the estrogen, androgen, and progesterone receptors have been elucidated; see below in this section), the functional role of each part is well known (see Fig. 23-8).[7] The organization of the domains for all types of steroid hormone receptors is the same, but the number of amino acids for each receptor varies:

1. *N-terminal (''A/B'') domain.* Once the steroid receptor complex has bound to the target gene(s), this domain (also called the *A/B modulator domain*) activates the hormone response elements adjacent to the genes. The hormone response elements are on the DNA adjacent to the target gene. They contain about 12 to 18 base-pair DNA sequences and consist of two ''half sites'' that are separated by a variable spacer. In the nucleus, steroid hormone receptor complexes exist as dimers; the dimeric structure allows access to both half sites. The nucleotide sequence and spacing between the half sites are essential for the specificity of the various steroid hormone complexes. After the dimer binds and all accessory proteins have been recruited to the receptor–DNA complex, transcription is initiated.
2. *DNA-binding (''C'') domain.* This short section is made up of about 65 amino acids, organized into two zinc finger motifs that are important for recognition and binding to the DNA response elements. The zinc fingers are also responsible for dimerization of the receptor.
3. *Hinge (''D'') domain.* This variable linker region appears to be involved with nuclear localization and transport (translocation) of the steroid–receptor complex into the nucleus.
4. *C-terminal ''ligand-binding'' (''E'') domain (LBD).* The C-terminal domain includes about 250 amino acids. This section has the steroid hormone-binding site and is also involved with ligand-dependent transcriptional activation, receptor dimeriza-

tion, binding to chaperone proteins (discussed below), and, in some cases, repressing ("silencing") particular genes.

Structure of Steroid Hormone Receptor Complexes

Steroid hormone receptor complexes include the steroid hormone receptor as well as other proteins, predominantly chaperone (heat shock) proteins, cochaperones, and immunophilins (Fig. 23-7).[8, 9] Their role is to "chaperone" the correct conformation and folding of complex proteins, which is otherwise much more difficult as temperatures increase. At normal physiological temperatures, the chaperone proteins assist the proper folding of large proteins such as steroid hormone receptors. The individual components vary depending on the type of steroid hormone receptor. Without the chaperones, the steroid hormone-binding site on the receptor does not have the proper folding and conformation for optimal steroid binding.

Once the steroid hormone binds to the receptor, a conformational change of the receptor occurs, and the mature receptor complex dissociates (Fig. 23-7). The receptor is dimerized, phosphorylated, and transported into the nucleus, if necessary. There, the zinc fingers on the steroid hormone receptor bind to the target gene(s) in the DNA. Additional proteins are recruited to the receptor–DNA complex prior to initiation or repression of transcription.[10] These additional proteins include coactivators or corepressors and histone acetyltransferases. Typically, the receptor–DNA–coactivator complex displays histone acetyltransferase action, which relaxes the chromatin structure, allowing binding of RNA polymerase II and the subsequent initiation of transcription. If corepressors are recruited to the complex, deacetylation of the histone complex is facilitated, preventing transcription.

X-RAY CRYSTALLOGRAPHY AND STEROID FIT AT THE RECEPTOR

As mentioned above, x-ray structures have been solved for the ligand-binding domains of several of the steroid hormone receptors. The structures for the ligand-binding domains for the estrogen receptors α and β,[11–13] the progesterone receptor,[14] and the androgen receptor[15] have all been determined. Homology modeling structures for the glucocorticoid and mineralocorticoid receptors have been created based on the progesterone structure.[16, 17]

The x-ray crystal structures of the estrogen, progesterone, and androgen receptors have revealed a key difference that leads to the unique ligand specificity of the estrogen receptors.[12, 18] In the region of the ligand-binding domain, where the A ring of steroids binds, are key residues that bind to either the phenolic A ring of estrogens or the enone A ring of progesterone or testosterone. In the case of the estrogen receptor, glutamate and arginine residues are important in a hydrogen-bonding network that involves the phenolic hydroxyl. In contrast to this structural arrangement, the progesterone and androgen receptors have glutamine and arginine residues that hydrogen bond to the A-ring enones of progesterone and testosterone. The change from glutamate, a hydrogen-bond acceptor, to glutamine, a hydrogen-bond donor, is critical for the discrimination between estrogens and other steroid hormones.

The x-ray crystal structures of the steroid hormones themselves have also provided important information. Although the conformations of rigid molecules in crystals and their preferred conformations in solution with receptors can differ, it is now clear from x-ray crystallography studies of steroids, prostaglandins, thyroid compounds, and many other drug classes that this technique can be a powerful tool in understanding drug action and in designing new drugs.[19–21] The relationship is straightforward: Steroid drugs usually do not have a charge and, as a result, are held to their receptors by relatively weak forces of attraction. The same is true for steroid molecules as they "pack" into crystals. In both events, the binding energy is too small to hold any but low-energy conformations. In short, the steroid conformation observed in steroid crystals often is the same or very similar to that at the receptor.

ESTROGEN RECEPTORS

There are two distinct estrogen receptors (ERs), estrogen receptor α (ER$_\alpha$) and estrogen receptor β (ER$_\beta$), which are encoded by different genes.[22] The ERs have distinct tissue distributions and can have distinct actions on the target genes. ER$_\alpha$ can be found in high abundance in the uterus, vagina, and ovaries, as well as in the breast, the hypothalamus, endothelial cells, and vascular smooth muscle. ER$_\beta$ is found in greatest abundance in the ovaries and the prostate, with reduced occurrence in the lungs, brain, and vasculature.[23] Although many ligands bind with similar affinities to both receptor subtypes, some ligands are selective for one or the other receptor.[24–26] ERs have received extensive investigation, to date, and although much has been learned about how the ERs function when bound to agonists or antagonists, new insights are continually being gained.[26–30]

PROGESTERONE RECEPTORS

The progesterone receptor can also be found in two forms, but these are derived from a single gene. PR$_A$ has had 164 amino acids truncated from the N terminus of PR$_B$, providing a receptor that has different interactions with target genes and associated proteins. PR$_B$ mainly mediates the stimulatory actions of progesterone. PR$_A$ acts as a transcriptional inhibitor of estrogen, androgen, glucocorticoid, mineralocorticoid, and PR$_B$ receptors.[23] These differential actions are believed to be due to interactions with different coactivators and corepressors. The DNA- and ligand-binding domains for the two receptors are identical.

ANDROGEN, GLUCOCORTICOID, AND MINERALOCORTICOID RECEPTORS

The androgen, glucocorticoid, and mineralocorticoid receptors are present in only a single form. Only one gene and one protein are known for each receptor. Mutant forms of the androgen[31] and glucocorticoid[32] receptors are known, and evidence is mounting that some of these mutant receptors are associated with disease states.

GnRH AND GONADOTROPINS

The gonadotropins are peptides that have a close functional relationship to the estrogens, progesterone, and testosterone.

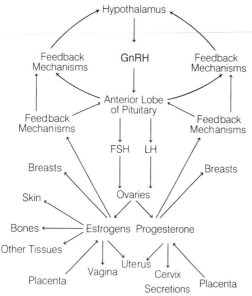

Figure 23–9 ■ Regulation of ovulation by GnRH.

They are called *gonadotropins* because of their actions on the gonads. As shown in Figures 23-9 through 23-11, they control ovulation, spermatogenesis, and development of sex organs, and they maintain pregnancy. An additional peptide, gonadotropin-releasing hormone (GnRH), regulates release of the gonadotropins. Included in this group are the following:

- Gonadotropin-releasing hormone (GnRH)
- Luteinizing hormone (LH)
- Follicle-stimulating hormone (FSH)
- Chorionic gonadotropin (CG; hCG is human gonadotropin), a glycopeptide produced by the placenta; its pharmacological actions are essentially the same as those of LH

GnRH

The hypothalamus releases GnRH, a peptide that stimulates the anterior pituitary to secrete LH and FSH in males and females. This peptide controls and regulates both male and female reproduction (Figs. 23-9 and 23-10). GnRH is a mod-

ified decapeptide (10 amino acids): PyroGlu-His-Trp-Ser-Tyr-Gly-Leu-Arg-Pro-Gly-NH$_2$. The pyroglutamate at the N terminus and the C-terminal amide distinguish this peptide from unmodified decapeptides. Analogues of GnRH that are used therapeutically are covered in Chapter 25.

Pituitary Gonadotropins: LH and FSH

The pituitary gonadotropins LH and FSH, their structures, genes, receptors, biological roles, and their regulation (including by negative feedback actions of steroid hormones) have been studied intensively.[33, 34] FSH, LH, and CG are all glycopeptide dimers with the same α subunit but different β subunits.

In females, LH and FSH regulate the menstrual cycle (see Figs. 23-9 and 23-11). At the start of the cycle, plasma concentrations of estradiol and other estrogens (Fig. 23-11) and progesterone are low. FSH and LH stimulate several ovarian follicles to enlarge and begin developing more rapidly than others. After a few days, only one follicle continues developing to the release of a mature ovum. The granulosa cells of the maturing follicles begin secreting estrogens, which then cause the uterine endometrium to thicken. Vaginal and cervical secretions increase. Gonadotropins and estrogen reach their maximum plasma concentrations at about day 14 of the cycle. The release in LH causes the follicle to break open, releasing a mature ovum. Under the stimulation of LH, the follicle changes into the corpus luteum, which begins secreting progesterone as well as estrogen.

The increased concentrations of estrogens and progesterone regulate the hypothalamus and the anterior pituitary by a feedback inhibition process that decreases GnRH, LH, and FSH production. The result is that further ovulation is inhibited. As described below in this chapter, this is the primary mechanism by which steroid birth control products inhibit ovulation.

If fertilization does not occur by about day 25, the corpus luteum begins to degenerate, slowing down its production of

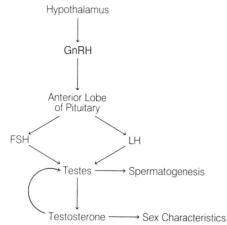

Figure 23–10 ■ Regulation of spermatogenesis.

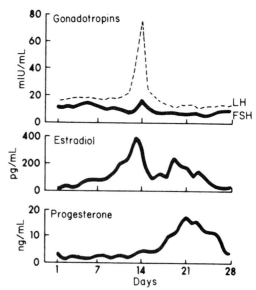

Figure 23–11 ■ Hormone changes in the normal menstrual cycle.

hormones. The concentrations of estrogens and progesterone become too low to maintain the vascularization of the endometrium, and menstruation results.

The pharmacological actions of hCG are essentially the same as those of LH. In females during pregnancy, the hCG secreted by the placenta maintains the corpus luteum to continue secretion of estrogen and progesterone, thus inhibiting ovulation and menstruation.

In males (Fig. 23-10), LH stimulates testosterone synthesis by the testes, and together, testosterone and LH promote spermatogenesis (sperm production) and development of the testes. Testosterone is also essential for development of secondary sex characteristics in males. FSH stimulates production of proteins and nutrients required for sperm maturation.

SEX HORMONES

Although the estrogens and progesterone are usually called female sex hormones and testosterone is called a male sex hormone, all of these steroids are biosynthesized in both males and females. For example, examination of the biosynthetic pathway in Figure 23-5 reveals that progesterone serves as a biosynthetic precursor to hydrocortisone and aldosterone and, to a lesser extent, to testosterone and the estrogens. Testosterone is one of the precursors of the estrogens. The estrogens and progesterone are produced in much larger amounts in females, however, as is testosterone in males. These hormones play profound roles in reproduction, in the menstrual cycle, and in giving women and men their characteristic physical differences.

Several modified steroidal compounds, as well as some nonsteroidal compounds, have estrogenic activity. A large number of synthetic or semisynthetic steroids with biological activities similar to those of progesterone have been made, and these are commonly called *progestins*. Although the estrogens and progestins have had their most extensive use as chemical contraceptive agents for women and in HRT, their wide spectrum of activity has given them a diversity of therapeutic uses in women as well as a few uses in men.

Testosterone has two primary kinds of activities—androgenic (promoting male physical characteristics) and anabolic (muscle building). Many synthetic and semisynthetic androgenic and anabolic steroids have been prepared. Despite efforts to prepare selective anabolic agents (e.g., for use in aiding recovery from debilitating illness or surgery), all "anabolic" steroids have androgenic effects. The androgenic agents are mainly used in males, but they do have some therapeutic usefulness in women (e.g., in the palliation of certain sex organ cancers).

In summary, although many sex hormone products have their greatest therapeutic uses in either women or men, nearly all have some uses in both sexes. Nevertheless, the higher concentrations of estrogens and progesterone in women and of testosterone in men cause the development of the complementary reproductive systems and characteristic physical differences of women and men.

Estrogens[35]

ENDOGENOUS ESTROGENS

The active endogenous estrogens are estradiol, estrone, and estriol. Estradiol provides the greatest estrogenic activity, with less activity for estrone, and the least activity with estriol. This range of activity parallels the affinity of these estrogens for the ER,[36] but the in vivo activities of these compounds are also affected by interconversions between active and inactive metabolites.

BIOSYNTHESIS

The estrogens are synthesized by the action of the enzyme aromatase on androstenedione or testosterone (Fig. 23-5). They are normally produced in relatively large quantities in the ovaries and placenta, in lower amounts in the adrenal glands, and in trace quantities in the testes. In postmenopausal women, most estrogens are synthesized in adipose tissue and other nonovarian sites. About 50 to 350 μg/day of estradiol are produced by the ovaries (especially the corpus luteum) during the menstrual cycle. During the first months of pregnancy, the corpus luteum produces larger amounts of estradiol and other estrogens; the placenta produces most of the circulating hormone in late pregnancy. During pregnancy, the estrogen blood levels are up to 1,000 times higher than during the menstrual cycle.

METABOLISM OF ESTROGENS

The metabolism of natural estrogens has been reviewed in detail.[37] The three primary estrogens in women are 17β-estradiol, estrone, and estriol (16α,17β-estriol). Although 17β-estradiol is produced in the greatest amounts, it is quickly oxidized (see Fig. 23-12) to estrone, the estrogen found in highest concentration in the plasma. Estrone, in turn, is converted to estriol, the major estrogen found in human urine, by hydroxylation at C16 (to provide the 16α-hydroxyl) and reduction of the C17 ketone (17β-hydroxyl). Estradiol can also be directly converted to estriol. In the human placenta, the most abundant estrogen synthesized is estriol. In both pregnant and nonpregnant women, however, the three primary estrogens are also metabolized to small amounts of other derivatives (e.g., 2-hydroxyestrone, 2-methoxyestrone, 4-hydroxyestrone, and 16β-hydroxy-17β-estradiol). Only about 50% of therapeutically administered estrogens (and their various metabolites) are excreted in the urine during the first 24 hours. The remainder are excreted into the bile and reabsorbed; consequently, several days are required for complete excretion of a given dose.

Conjugation appears to be very important in estrogen transport and metabolism. Although the estrogens are unconjugated in the ovaries, significant amounts of conjugated estrogens may predominate in the plasma and other tissues. Most of the conjugation takes place in the liver. The primary estrogen conjugates found in plasma and urine are glucuronides and sulfates. As sodium salts, they are quite water soluble. The sodium glucuronide of estriol and the sodium sulfate ester of estrone are shown in Figure 23-12.

BIOLOGICAL ACTIVITIES OF ESTROGENS

In addition to having important roles in the menstrual cycle (described above), the estrogens and, to a lesser extent, progesterone are largely responsible for the development of secondary sex characteristics in women at puberty. The estrogens cause a proliferation of the breast ductile system, and progesterone stimulates development of the alveolar system.

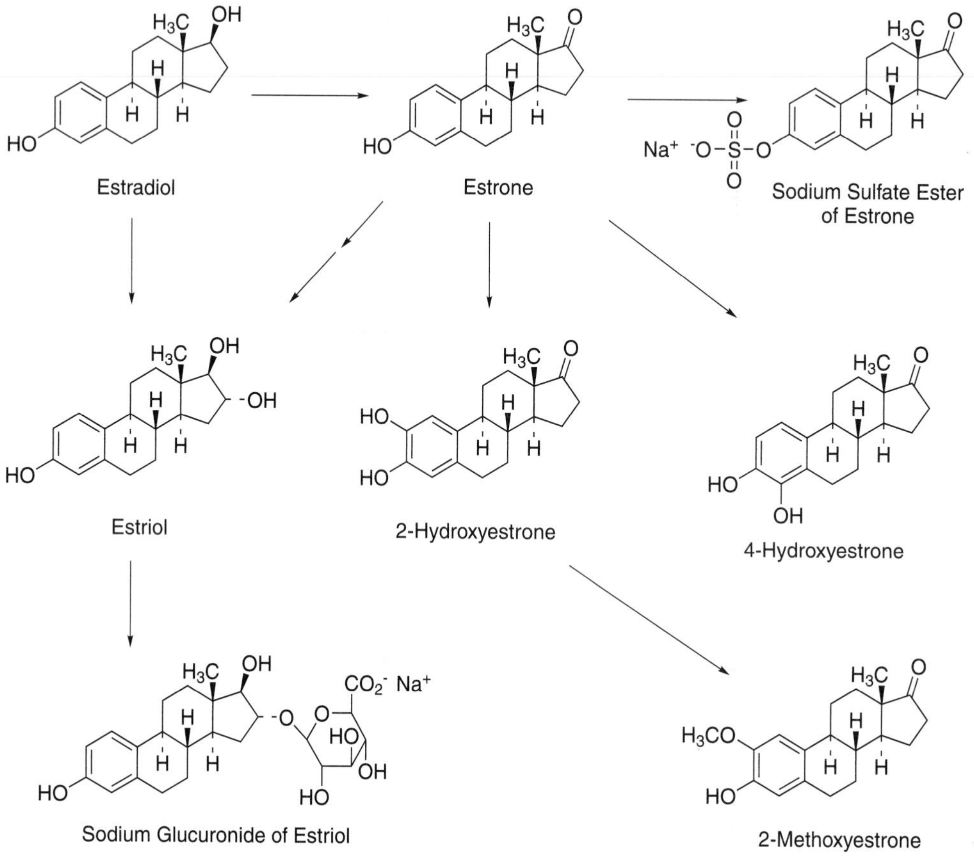

Figure 23–12 ■ Metabolites of 17β-estradiol and estrone.

The estrogens also stimulate the development of lipid and other tissues that contribute to breast shape and function. Pituitary hormones and other hormones are also involved. Fluid retention in the breasts during the later stages of the menstrual cycle is a common effect of the estrogens.

The estrogens directly stimulate the growth and development of the vagina, uterus, and fallopian tubes and, in combination with other hormones, play a primary role in sexual arousal and in producing the body contours of the mature woman. Pigmentation of the nipples and genital tissues and growth stimulation of pubic and underarm hair (possibly with the help of small amounts of testosterone) are other results of estrogen action.

The physiological changes at menopause emphasize the important roles of estrogens in the young woman. Breast and reproductive tissues atrophy, the skin loses some of its suppleness, coronary atherosclerosis and gout become potential health problems for the first time, and the bones begin to lose density because of decreased mineral content.

STRUCTURAL CLASSES—ESTROGENS

As shown in Figure 23-13, there are three structural classes of estrogens: steroidal estrogens, diethylstilbestrol and derivatives, and phytoestrogens. (Each class is summarized in the sections that follow.) The steroidal estrogens include the naturally occurring estrogens found in humans and other mammals, as well as semisynthetic derivatives of these compounds. Because of rapid metabolism, estradiol itself has poor oral bioavailability. The addition of a 17α-alkyl group to the estradiol structure blocks oxidation to estrone. Ethinyl estradiol is therefore very effective orally, whereas estradiol itself is not. Most of the therapeutically useful steroidal estrogens are produced semisynthetically from natural precursors such as diosgenin, a plant sterol.

Steroidal Estrogens—Conjugated Estrogens, Esterified Estrogens.
Conjugated estrogens (sometimes called equine estrogens) are estradiol-related metabolites originally obtained from the urine of horses, especially pregnant mares. Premarin, the major conjugated estrogen product on the market, is a mixture of numerous components that is still obtained from mare urine. Equine estrogens are largely mixtures of estrone sodium sulfate and equilin sodium sulfate. Little or no equilin and equilenin are produced in humans. The sulfate groups must be removed metabolically to release the active estrogens. Conjugated estrogens that derive exclusively from plant precursors are also on the market. Esterified estrogens are also mainly a combination of estrone sodium sulfate and equilin sodium sulfate, but in a different ratio than in conjugated estrogens. The esterified estrogens are now prepared exclusively from plant sterols.

Diethylstilbestrol Derivatives.
At first glance, it might be surprising that nonsteroidal molecules such as diethylstil-

bestrol (DES) could have the same activity as estradiol or other estrogens. DES can be viewed, however, as a form of estradiol with rings B and C open and a six-carbon ring D. The activity of DES analogues was explained in 1946.[38] It was proposed that the distance between the two DES phenol OH groups was the same as the 3-OH to 17-OH distance of estradiol; therefore, they could both fit the same receptor. Modern medicinal chemists have shown the OH-to-OH distance to be actually 12.1 Å in DES and 10.9 Å in estradiol. In aqueous solution, however, estradiol has two water molecules hydrogen-bonded to the 17-OH. If one of the two water molecules is included in the distance measurement, there is a perfect fit with the two OH groups of DES (Fig. 23-14). This suggests that water may have an important role for estradiol in its receptor site. It is now generally accepted that the estrogens must have a phenolic moiety for binding,

but some investigators propose that the receptor may be flexible enough to accommodate varying distances between the two key hydroxyls. This point about estrogens needing a phenolic ring for high-affinity binding to the ER is critical. Steroids with a phenolic A ring and related phenolic compounds lack high-affinity binding to the other steroid hormone receptors.

Thousands of DES analogues were synthesized, and from them emerged many products, including dienestrol and benzestrol. As long as the OH-to-OH distance relationship is maintained, significant estrogenic activity is usually found in the DES derivative. Without the central double bond and two ethyl or other alkyl groups, the molecule loses all its rigidity and shape, the OH-to-OH distance is not fixed, and activity is abolished. Reduction of the double bond of DES results in two diastereomers of hexestrol. The *meso* form is

1. <u>Steroidal Estrogens and Derivatives</u>

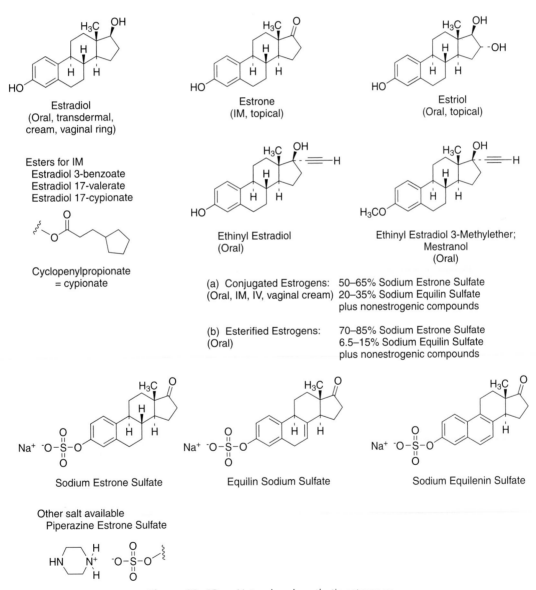

Figure 23–13 ■ Natural and synthetic estrogens.

1. Steroidal Estrogens and Derivatives (continued)

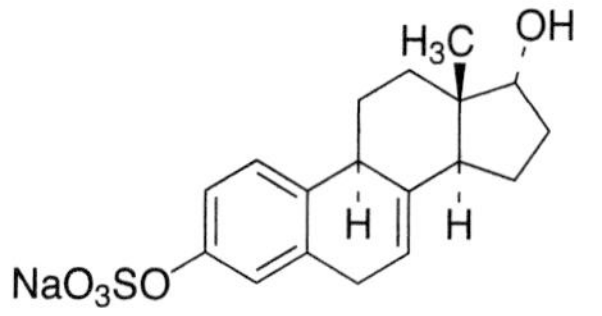

Sodium 17α-Dihydroequilin Sulfate

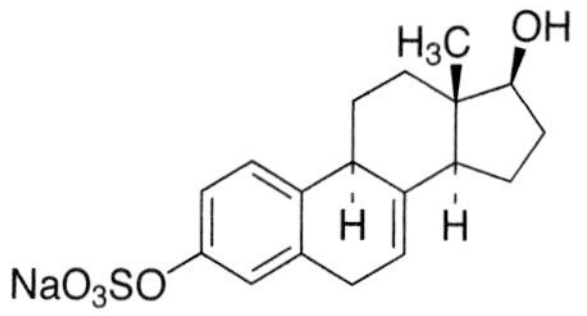

Sodium 17β-Dihydroequilin Sulfate

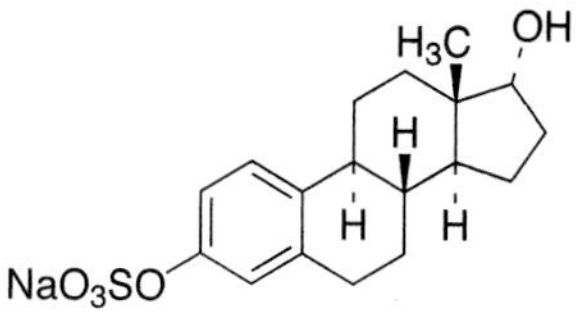

Sodium 17α-Estradiol Sulfate

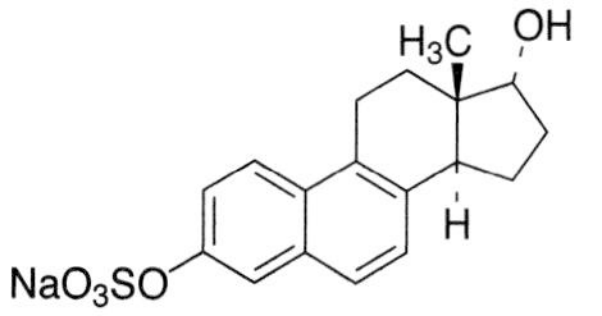

Sodium 17α-Dihydroequilenin Sulfate

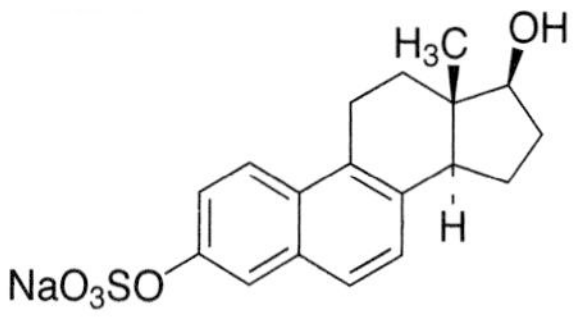

Sodium 17β-Dihydroequilenin Sulfate

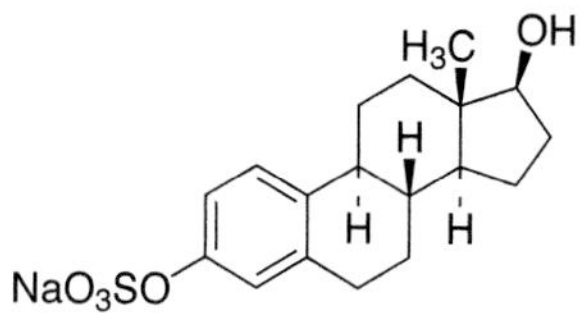

Sodium 17β-Estradiol Sulfate

2. Diethylstilbestrol and Derivatives (Oral, vaginal cream)

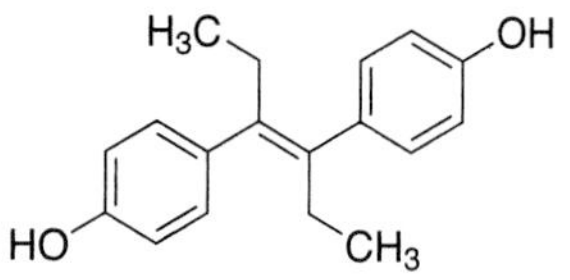

Diethylstilbestrol (available as the diphosphate for IV injection)

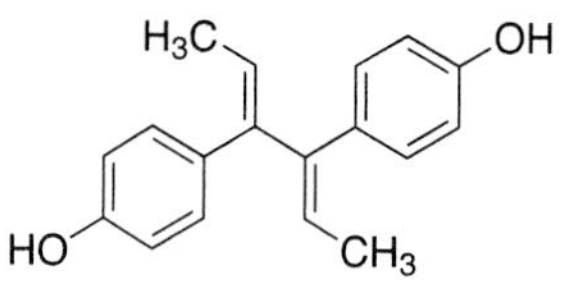

Dienestrol

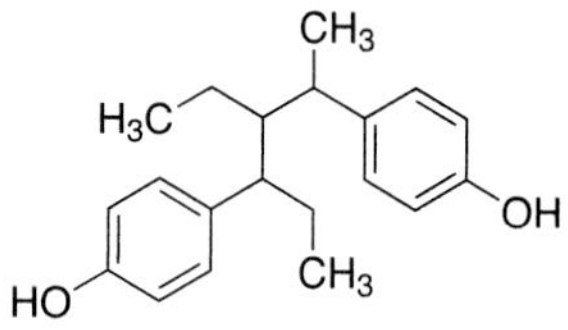

Benzestrol

3. Estrogens From Plants (Phytoestrogens)

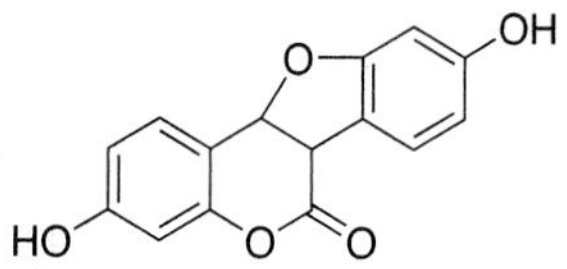

Coumestrol

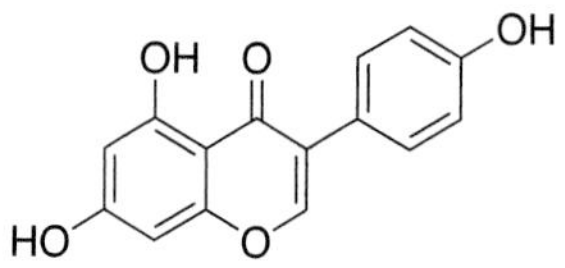

Genistein

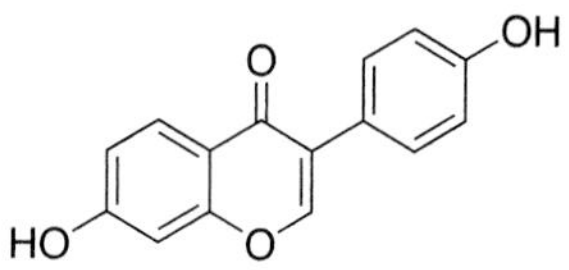

Daidzein

Figure 23–13 ■ *Continued.*

active because the OH-to-OH distance is maintained. In the *threo* isomer, however, there is steric repulsion of the two ethyl groups. The two phenol groups rotate to relieve the repulsion, the OH-to-OH distance is changed, and consequently, the *threo* isomer is inactive (Fig. 23-15).

Phytoestrogens. Several natural plant substances that have general structural features similar to those of DES and estradiol also have estrogenic effects and have been termed *phytoestrogens.*[39] These include genistein, from soybeans and a species of clover; daidzein, from soybeans; and coumestrol, found in certain legumes. Genistein and daidzein are

examples of isoflavones. These and others have antifertility activity in animals.[40] Many claims have been made about the beneficial effects of consuming products containing these phytoestrogens, including preventing and treating cardiovascular disease, reducing postmenopausal symptoms, and preventing osteoporosis. Because of the numerous other components present in many of the commercial products as well as a lack of well-designed studies to test the effects of the phytoestrogens themselves, however, positive health effects specifically due to direct hormonal action of the phytoestrogens are uncertain. Questions have also been raised about a possible contribution of phytoestrogens to an increased

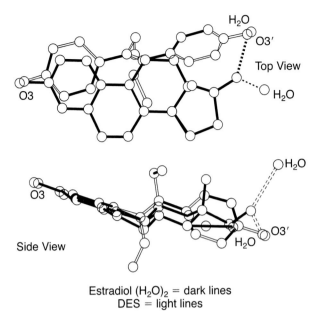

Estradiol $(H_2O)_2$ = dark lines
DES = light lines

Figure 23–14 ■ Computer graphics. Superposition of estradiol $(H_2O)_2$ *(dark lines)* with DES *(light lines)*. (Courtesy of Medical Foundation of Buffalo, Inc.)

incidence of breast cancer. These concerns, however, are contradicted by studies that suggest a chemoprotective role for soy products containing phytoestrogens (this could well be due to other components of the mixture). The long history of use of soy products in the world and no global correlations with increased breast cancer risks suggest that any connection between phytoestrogens in general and breast cancer is quite small.[41]

Recent studies have demonstrated that genistein (and likely other phytoestrogens) binds preferentially to ER_β over ER_α.[42] The clinical relevance of this difference in binding is unclear, but it suggests differences between the phytoestrogens and classical estrogens that should be explored.

THERAPEUTIC USES OF ESTROGENS

Birth Control. A major use of estrogens is for inhibition of ovulation, in combination with progestins. Steroidal birth control agents containing estrogens are discussed in the section on chemical contraception later in this chapter.

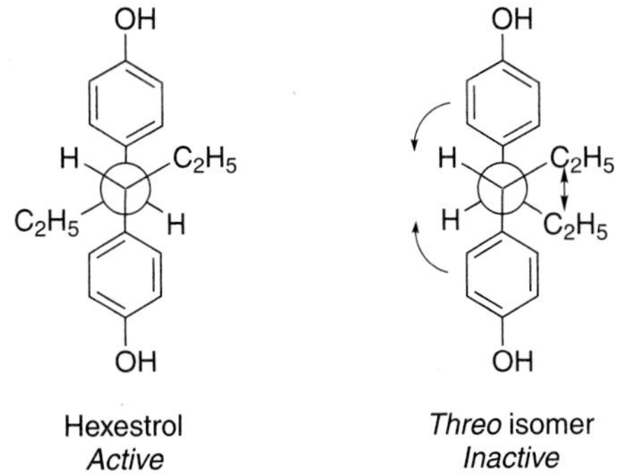

![Figure showing Hexestrol (Active) and Threo isomer (Inactive) chemical structures with OH, H, C2H5 groups]

Hexestrol
Active

Threo isomer
Inactive

Figure 23–15 ■ Importance of conformation and rigidity in estrogen activity.

Hormone Replacement Therapy. Another major use of estrogens is in HRT for postmenopausal women. For this use, a progestin is often included to oppose the effects of estrogens on endometrial tissue. HRT is covered in more depth later in the chapter.

Treatment of Estrogen Deficiency From Ovarian Failure or After Oophorectomy. Estrogen therapy, usually with a progestin, is common in cases of ovarian failure and after an oophorectomy.

Treatment of Advanced, Inoperable Breast Cancer in Men and Postmenopausal Women and of Advanced, Inoperable Prostate Cancer in Men. Estrogens are used to treat inoperable breast cancer in men and in postmenopausal women, but estrogen therapy can actually stimulate existing breast cancers in premenopausal women. The selective ER modulator tamoxifen is reported to have fewer side effects; hence, it is usually preferred. Estrogens have also been used to treat inoperable prostate cancer, but GnRH analogues are now generally preferred because of fewer unwanted side effects.

Estrogens and Cancer. Many years of study have firmly established an association between estrogen use and increased risk of breast cancer. The risk is associated, however, with the timing of estrogen exposure, the estrogen dose, the length of use, and the type of estrogen used.[43] A patient should discuss the potential risks of breast cancer with her doctor carefully before starting estrogen therapy. Unopposed estrogens in HRT for postmenopausal women are also linked to an increased risk of endometrial carcinoma, which is the basis for inclusion of a progestin in many forms of HRT.[44]

DES Babies. During the late 1930s through the early 1950s, it was believed that DES treatment could help pregnant women who tended to miscarry to have full-term pregnancies. Not only was the belief incorrect, it was subsequently reported that daughters of women who had taken DES during pregnancy (''DES babies'') had a high risk of vaginal, cervical, and uterine abnormalities, along with a low risk of vaginal clear cell adenocarcinoma.[45] Women exposed to DES in utero who developed genital tract problems have a much higher risk of infertility than unexposed women.[46] A long-term effect on women who were treated with DES during their pregnancies is a slightly higher risk of breast cancer than for women who were not exposed, although no increased risk of ovarian, endometrial, or other cancers was observed.[47]

ESTROGEN PRODUCTS

Estrogens are commercially available in a wide variety of dosage forms: oral tablets, vaginal creams and foams, transdermal patches, and intramuscular dosage preparations.

Estradiol, USP. Estradiol, estra-1,3,5(10)-triene-3,17β-diol, is the most active of the natural steroid estrogens. Although its 17β-OH group is vulnerable to bacterial and enzymatic oxidation to estrone (Fig. 23-12), it can be temporarily protected as an ester or permanently protected by adding a 17α-alkyl group (giving 17α-ethinyl estradiol and the 3-methyl ether, mestranol, the most commonly used estrogens in oral contraceptives). The increased oil solubility of the 3- and 17β-esters (relative to estradiol) permits the esters to remain in oil at the injection site for extended periods. These derivatives illustrate the principles of steroid modification shown in Figure 23-6. Transdermal estradiol products avoid first-pass metabolism, allowing estradiol to be as effective as oral estrogens for treating menopausal symptoms. Estradiol itself is typically not very effective orally because of rapid metabolism, but an oral formulation of micronized estradiol that allows more rapid absorption of the drug is available (Estrace). The commercially available estradiol esters are the following:

Estradiol 3-benzoate, USP
Estradiol 17-valerate, USP
Estradiol 17-cypionate, USP

Estrone, USP.

Estrone, 3-hydroxyestra-1,3,5(10)-trien-17-one, is less active than estradiol but more active than its metabolite, estriol. As the salt of its 3-sulfate ester, estrone is the primary ingredient in conjugated estrogens, USP, and esterified estrogens, USP. Although originally obtained from the urine of pregnant mares (about 10 mg/L), estrone is now prepared synthetically.

PIPERAZINE ESTRONE SULFATE (3-SULFOXY-ESTRA-1,3,5(10)-TRIEN-17-ONE PIPERAZINE SALT), USP. All the estrone 3-sulfate salts have the obvious pharmaceutical advantage of increased water solubility and better oral absorption. Acids convert the salts to the free 3-sulfate esters and cause some hydrolysis of the ester. This does not seem to affect absorption adversely, but precipitation of the free sulfate esters in acidic pharmaceutical preparations should be avoided. The dibasic piperazine molecule acts as a buffer, giving it somewhat greater stability.

CONJUGATED ESTROGENS, USP. The term *conjugated estrogens* refers to the mix of sulfate conjugates of estrogenic components isolated from *pregnant mare urine* (Premarin). These compounds are also referred to as *CEE* (conjugated equine estrogens). Conjugated estrogens contain 50 to 65% sodium estrone sulfate and 20 to 35% sodium equilin sulfate (based on the total estrogen content of the product). Premarin also contains the sulfate esters of 17α-estradiol, 17α-dihydroequilin, and 17β-dihydroequilin, in addition to other minor components. Although most commonly used in HRT to treat postmenopausal symptoms, the conjugated estrogens are used for the entire range of indications described above, except birth control.

SYNTHETIC CONJUGATED ESTROGENS, A. Cenestin is a mixture of nine estrogenic substances (Fig. 23-13): sodium estrone sulfate, sodium equilin sulfate, sodium equilenin sulfate, sodium 17α-estradiol sulfate, sodium 17β-estradiol sulfate, sodium 17α-dihydroequilin sulfate, sodium 17β-dihydroequilin sulfate, sodium 17α-dihydroequilenin sulfate, and sodium 17β-dihydroequilenin sulfate. These estrogenic substances are synthesized from soy sterols. The term *synthetic* has been added before conjugated estrogens to indicate that

this product is distinct from (not equivalent to) the conjugated estrogens derived from mare urine. The "A" following the name indicates that this is the first approved mixture of synthetic conjugated estrogens. Subsequent synthetic conjugated estrogen products will be named in order, with the final descriptors "B, C, D," etc. Cenestin is approved for the treatment of moderate-to-severe vasomotor symptoms and vulvar and vaginal atrophy associated with menopause.

ESTERIFIED ESTROGENS, USP. Esterified estrogens (Estratab, Menest) contain some of the same sulfate conjugates of estrogens present in conjugated estrogens, but the ratios of these components and the composition of minor components of the products differ. These products contain 75 to 85% sodium estrone sulfate and 6 to 15% sodium equilin sulfate, in such proportion that the total of these 2 components is 90% of the total esterified estrogens content. The esterified estrogens find the same uses as the conjugated estrogens.

Estriol, USP.

Estriol, estra-1,3,5(10)-triene-3,16α,17β-triol, is available for compounding into a number of different formulations for use in HRT. It can be used alone or in combinations with estradiol (Bi-Est) or with estradiol and estrone (Tri-Est).

Ethinyl Estradiol, USP.

17α-Ethinyl estradiol has the great advantage over other estradiol products of being orally active. It is equal to estradiol in potency by injection but is 15 to 20 times more active orally. The primary metabolic path for ethinyl estradiol is 2-hydroxylation by cytochrome P-450 isozyme 3A4 (CYP 3A4), followed by conversion to the 2- and 3-methyl ethers by catechol-*O*-methyltransferase. The 3-methyl ether of ethinyl estradiol is mestranol, USP, used in oral contraceptives. Mestranol is a prodrug that is 3-*O*-demethylated to the active ethinyl estradiol. An oral dose of about 50 μg of mestranol has an estrogenic action approximately equivalent to 35 μg of oral ethinyl estradiol. The demethylation is mainly mediated by CYP 2C9.[48]

Diethylstilbestrol, USP.

Diethylstilbestrol, α,α-diethyl-(*E*)-4,4/-stilbenediol, DES, is the most active of the nonsteroidal estrogens (see under the heading, Structural Classes—Estrogens, above), having about the same activity as estrone when given intramuscularly. The *cis* isomer has only one-tenth the activity of the *trans*. This is mainly due to the improper positioning and distance (~7Å) between the hydroxyls in the *cis* isomer. The *trans* isomer is well absorbed orally and metabolized slowly and, consequently, was a popular estrogen for many medical purposes, but undesirable side effects have severely limited its use. The diphosphate ester, *diethylstilbestrol diphosphate, USP*, available for intravenous use, is used only for cancer of the prostate. Cardiovascular toxicity including deep vein thrombosis and myocardial infarction limit its use, however.[49] The diphosphate salt has great water solubility, as one would predict from Table 23-1. Prior to the 1970s, DES was used extensively in low doses as an aid to fatten cattle, but due to a potential link to cancer, it was banned as an additive in animal feed.

Note: All stilbene derivatives, such as DES and dienestrol, are light sensitive and must be kept in light-resistant containers.

Dienestrol, USP. Dienestrol, 4,4'-(1,2-diethylidene-1,2-ethanediyl)bisphenol, is orally active but is only currently available as a topical cream. The cream is used to treat atrophic vaginitis.

SELECTIVE ESTROGEN RECEPTOR MODULATORS AND ANTIESTROGENS

Whereas estrogens have been very important in chemical contraception and HRT, compounds that can antagonize the ER have been of great interest for the treatment of estrogen-dependent breast cancers. Tumor biopsies have shown ER to be present in about 60% of primary breast cancers, and most are responsive to estrogen blockade. Unfortunately, most of these ER-related breast cancers also develop resistance to antiestrogen therapy within 5 years. In contrast, only about 6% of nonmalignant breast tissues have significant ER present. Three compounds that are used clinically for estrogen antagonist action in the treatment of breast cancer are tamoxifen, toremifene, and fulvestrant (Fig. 23-16). Two

additional agents that can antagonize ERs are clomiphene, which is used as an ovulation stimulant, and raloxifene, which is used for the prevention and treatment of osteoporosis.

Tamoxifen and clomiphene were traditionally called *estrogen receptor (ER) antagonists* or *antiestrogens*. Referring to these compounds as ER antagonists, however, does not accurately portray how these compounds work in vivo. While tamoxifen is an ER antagonist in breast tissue, it has agonist actions on the endometrium, liver, bone, and cardiovascular system. Because of the differential agonist and antagonist effects of these types of compounds on the ER, depending on the specific tissue, a new term was coined: *selective estrogen receptor modulators* (SERMs). A SERM is a drug that has tissue-specific estrogenic activity. Although many compounds exhibit SERM activity, a few agents are antagonists in all tissues. These compounds are termed *antiestrogens,* and fulvestrant is one example (Fig. 23-16). Tamoxifen and clomiphene are often referred to in older literature as *antiestrogens.*

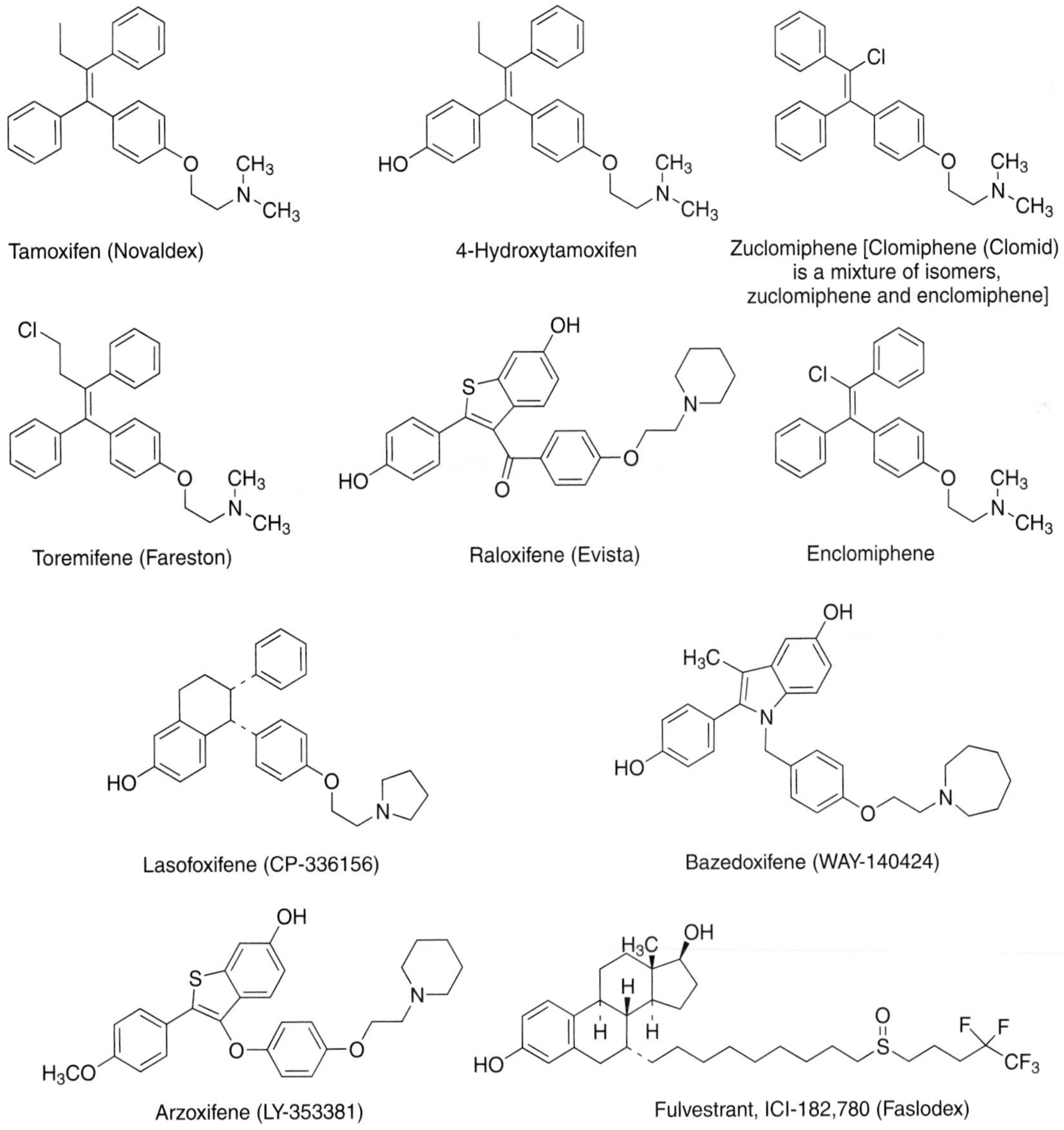

Figure 23–16 ■ Selective estrogen receptor modulators (SERMs) and antiestrogens.

Tamoxifen has seen extensive use in treating primary breast cancers that are ER dependent.[50, 51] For premenopausal women with metastatic disease, tamoxifen is an alternative and adjuvant with oophorectomy, ovarian irradiation, and mastectomy. Tamoxifen use, however, is not problem free. Tamoxifen increases the incidence of endometrial polyps, hyperplasia, and carcinoma and uterine sarcomas. The risk of endometrial cancer resulting from tamoxifen is, however, much lower than the ''modest but highly significant reductions in morbidity and mortality of breast cancer.''[52] Because of the increased risk of endometrial cancer with tamoxifen therapy, tamoxifen should be used to prevent breast cancer only in women at high risk. Women without a family history of breast cancer or other risks should not use tamoxifen in this manner.

Raloxifene is another SERM, but its profile of activity differs from that of tamoxifen. Raloxifene is an ER antagonist in both breast and endometrial tissue, but has agonist action on bone and acts as an estrogen agonist in lowering total cholesterol and low-density lipoprotein (LDL). The subtle structural differences between the two drugs underlie the distinct activity profiles.[53] The agonist action on bone tissue is the basis for the use of this drug for treating osteoporosis.

A key question is why do compounds like tamoxifen and raloxifene exhibit antagonist action in some tissues, but agonist action in other tissues? Major developments in the past few years are beginning to provide the answer to this question.[11, 26, 27, 54] Tamoxifen,[55] raloxifene, and estradiol[11] all bind to the ER at the same site, but their binding modes are different. In addition, each induces a distinct conformation in the transactivation region of the ligand-binding domain.[11] These unique conformations dictate how the receptor–ligand complex will interact with coregulator proteins (coactivators or corepressors).[27] In all tissues, the estradiol–ER complex recruits coactivators, so gene transcription is stimulated. In breast tissue, both raloxifene- and tamoxifen-bound receptors prevent the association with coactivators, but rather recruit corepressors, so antagonist action is observed. In uterine tissue, however, the raloxifene–ER complex recruits corepressors, whereas the tamoxifen–ER complex recruits a coactivator, SRC-1, which leads to agonist action.[54] An additional factor involved in this agonist action of tamoxifen is the context in which the liganded receptor interacts with the target gene. The liganded ER can interact directly with DNA or can interact indirectly by being tethered to other transcription factors. When the tamoxifen-bound receptor interacts in a tethered manner with the target genes in uterine tissue, the SRC-1 coactivator is recruited, and gene transcription is promoted.[27, 54] A deeper understanding of how the liganded receptors interact with target genes and the mechanisms for recruitment of coregulators may help to explain the phenomenon of tamoxifen resistance, which results from increased tamoxifen agonism in breast tissue.[27]

Lasofoxifene, bazedoxifene, and arzoxifene are several of the newer SERMs that are in late-stage clinical trials (Fig. 23-16). Lasofoxifene and bazedoxifene are being studied for use in the treatment of osteoporosis, while arzoxifene is being investigated for breast cancer treatment. Structurally, arzoxifene is most similar to raloxifene, with an ether bridge, rather than a carbonyl bridge, attached to the benzothiophene core. Bazedoxifene uses an indole ring system in place of the benzothiophene of raloxifene. Bazedoxifene was the result of a screening program that selected for compounds that did not stimulate breast or uterine tissue.[56] Lasofoxifene can be viewed as a constrained, saturated analogue of 4-hydroxytamoxifen.

Clomiphene is another drug that exhibits antiestrogen actions, but it is not used for treating breast cancer or osteoporosis; rather, it is used for increasing the odds of a successful pregnancy. Clomiphene's therapeutic application as an ovulation stimulant results from its ability to increase GnRH production by the hypothalamus. The mechanism is presumably a blocking of feedback inhibition of ovary-produced estrogens (via ER antagonism). The hypothalamus and pituitary interpret the false signal that estrogen levels are low and respond by increasing the production of GnRH. The increased GnRH, in turn, leads to increased secretion of LH and FSH, maturation of the ovarian follicle, and ovulation (as described above in this chapter; see Fig. 23-9). Support for the feedback inhibition mechanism is provided by tests with experimental animals in which clomiphene has no effect in the absence of a functioning pituitary gland.

Multiple births occur about 10% of the time with patients taking clomiphene, and birth defects in 2 to 3% of live newborns. Vasomotor ''hot flashes'' occur about 10% of the time, and abnormal enlargement of the ovaries about 14%. Abdominal discomfort should be discussed immediately with the physician.

SERM AND ANTIESTROGEN PRODUCTS

Tamoxifen Citrate, USP. Tamoxifen, 2-[4-(1,2-diphenyl-1-butenyl)phenoxy]-*N,N*-dimethylethanamine (Nolvadex), is a triphenylethylene SERM used to treat early and advanced breast carcinoma in postmenopausal women. Tamoxifen is used as adjuvant treatment for breast cancer in women following mastectomy and breast irradiation. It reduces the occurrence of contralateral breast cancer in patients receiving adjuvant tamoxifen therapy. It is also effective in the treatment of metastatic breast cancer in both women and men. In premenopausal women with metastatic breast cancer, tamoxifen is an alternative to oophorectomy or ovarian irradiation. Tamoxifen can be used preventatively to reduce the incidence of breast cancer in women at high risk. Antiestrogenic and estrogenic side effects can include hot flashes, nausea, vomiting, platelet reduction, and (in patients with bone metastases) hypercalcemia. Like all triphenylethylene derivatives, it should be protected from light.

The major metabolite of tamoxifen is *N*-desmethyltamoxifen, which reaches steady-state levels higher than tamoxifen itself. It is believed that *N*-desmethyltamoxifen contributes significantly to the overall antiestrogenic effect. Another metabolite, 4-hydroxytamoxifen, is a more potent antiestrogen than tamoxifen, but because it is only a minor metabolite of tamoxifen, it probably does not contribute significantly to the therapeutic effects. 4-Hydroxytamoxifen, with its greater affinity for the ERs, however, has been used extensively in pharmacological studies of these receptors. Tamoxifen concentrations are reduced if coadministered with rifampin, a cytochrome P-450 inducer.

Toremifene Citrate, USP. Toremifene, 2-[4-[(1*Z*)-4-chloro-1,2-diphenyl-1-butenyl]phenoxy]-*N,N*-dimethylethanamine (Fareston), differs structurally from tamoxifen only by having a chloroethyl group (rather than an ethyl group) attached to the triphenylethylene structure. As might be expected, the pharmacological actions of toremifene and tamoxifen are quite similar. Toremifene is also a SERM, with estrogen antagonist action in breast tissue but agonist action in the endometrium, on bone tissue, and on serum lipid profiles. Although toremifene appears to carry less risk of causing endometrial cancer than tamoxifen, its limited use in comparison with tamoxifen requires the use of caution in evaluating the safety profile for toremifene.[57] Toremifene is used in the treatment of metastatic breast cancer in postmenopausal women.

Raloxifene, USP.

Raloxifene, [6-hydroxy-2-(4-hydroxyphenyl)benzo[*b*]thien-3-yl][4-[2-(1 - piperidinyl)ethoxy]phenyl]methanone (Evista), is a benzothiophene derivative that differs slightly from the triphenylethylene SERMs. A key structural difference is the carbonyl "hinge" that connects the modified phenolic side chain to the benzothiophene ring system. This hinge is the key structural element that leads to the differing actions at the ERs.[53] Raloxifene, unlike tamoxifen and toremifene, has antagonist properties on the endometrium and breast tissue and agonist properties on bone and the cardiovascular system. The lack of agonist action on endometrial tissue has been suggested as a reason for the lack of endometrial cancer associated with raloxifene use. Raloxifene is approved for the prevention and treatment of osteoporosis in postmenopausal women and is being studied for the prevention of breast cancer in women at high risk.

Fulvestrant, USP.

Fulvestrant, 7α-[9-[(4,4,5,5,5-pentafluoropentyl)sulfinyl]nonyl]estra-1,3,5(10)-triene-3, 17β-diol (Faslodex), is an antagonist structurally based on the estradiol structure, with a long, substituted alkyl chain attached at the 7α position of the steroid skeleton. When bound to the ERs, this alkyl chain induces a conformation of the receptor distinctive from that formed upon estradiol or tamoxifen binding, preventing agonist action. Fulvestrant is a pure antagonist at both ER_α and ER_β and an ER downregulator (stimulates degradation of the ER), completely lacking the agonist activity that is seen with tamoxifen or raloxifene. The different pharmacological profile of fulvestrant allows the use of this agent in women who have had disease progression after prior antiestrogen therapy (typically tamoxifen), providing an alternative to aromatase inhibitors.[58]

Clomiphene Citrate, USP.

Clomiphene citrate, 2-[4-(2-chloro-1,2-diphenylethenyl)phenoxy]-*N*,*N*-diethylethanamine (Clomid), is used as an ovulation stimulant in women desiring pregnancy. Although early literature refers to clomiphene as an estrogen antagonist, it is more accurately a SERM.[59] Clomiphene is chemically a mixture of two geometric isomers, zuclomiphene, the *cis* isomer, and enclomiphene, the *trans* isomer. In animal studies, these isomers have different estrogenic actions in different tissues. Zuclomiphene appears to have weak agonist actions on all tissues studied, whereas enclomiphene has antagonist actions on uterine tissue, but agonist action on bone tissue.[60] The actions of clomiphene in humans are likely a composite of the actions of the two isomers.

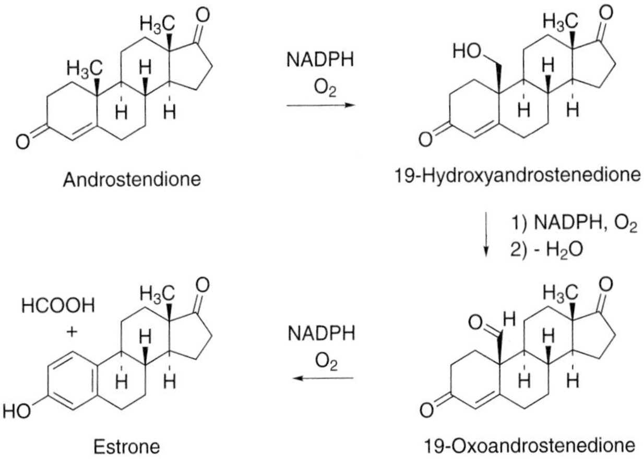

Figure 23-17 ■ Conversion of androstenedione to estrone by aromatase.

AROMATASE INHIBITORS

Aromatase is a cytochrome P-450 enzyme complex that catalyzes the conversion of androstenedione to estrone and testosterone to estradiol (Figs. 23-5 and 23-17).[61–63] The complex is made up of reduced nicotinamide adenine dinucleotide phosphate (NADPH)-cytochrome P-450 reductase, and cytochrome P-450 hemoprotein. In the first two steps, the C19 methyl is hydroxylated to CH_2OH, and then to an aldehyde hydrate form that dehydrates to provide the C19 aldehyde. In the final aromatization step, the C19 carbon is oxidatively cleaved to formate. A hydride shift, proton transfer, and free radical pathways have been proposed, with *cis* elimination of the 1β and 2β hydrogens.[64] In premenopausal women, aromatase is primarily found in ovaries, but in postmenopausal women, aromatase is largely in muscle and adipose tissue.

As discussed above with SERMs, some types of breast cancer are estrogen dependent. Because the aromatase reaction is unique in steroid biosynthetic pathways, it would be anticipated that aromatase inhibitors would be very specific in their estrogen biosynthesis blockade. This has proved to be true, and aromatase inhibitors offer a useful approach to decreasing estrogen levels in the treatment of estrogen-dependent breast cancer. Initially, aromatase inhibitors were used as second-line therapy in postmenopausal women who failed on tamoxifen therapy. Recent studies have indicated, however, that the newer aromatase inhibitors can be used as first-line therapy and possibly for cancer prevention in patients at high risk.[65]

Aromatase inhibitors include both steroidal and nonsteroidal compounds. Examples of aromatase inhibitors are shown in Fig. 23-18. The first- generation aromatase inhibitors were aminoglutethimide, a nonsteroidal compound, and the steroid-based testolactone, two compounds that were developed before it was recognized that their effectiveness in breast cancer treatment was due to aromatase inhibition.[66] Aminoglutethimide also inhibits other P-450s involved in steroid hormone biosynthesis, which limits its use in breast cancer treatment. The newer drugs are more potent and more specific inhibitors of aromatase than the earlier compounds.

In addition to testolactone, two other steroid analogues have been used. A well-studied steroid analogue is 4-hydroxy-

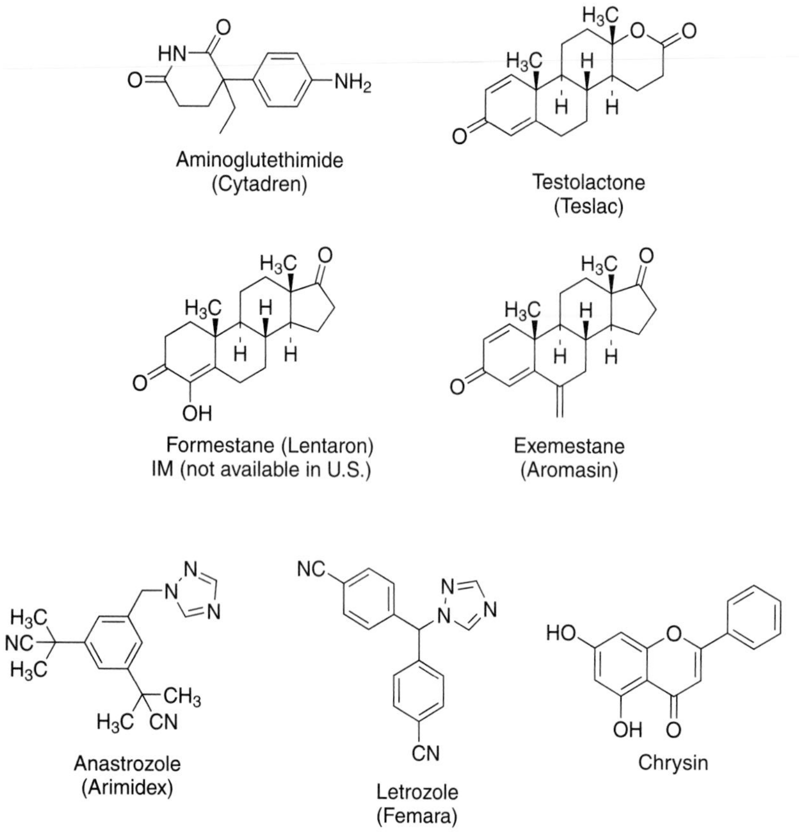

Figure 23–18 ■ Aromatase inhibitors.

androstenedione (4-OHA; formestane; Lentaron), which has been marketed in the United Kingdom since the early 1990s for treatment of breast cancer. Although initially thought to be a completely reversible inhibitor, it is now known that formestane is an enzyme activated irreversible (''suicide'') inhibitor of aromatase. A limitation for formestane is lack of oral availability. Exemestane is the latest steroidal aromatase inhibitor. It is another mechanism-based inactivator of aromatase, but it is orally available and is highly selective for aromatase. Both compounds reflect minor structural modifications to the natural substrate, androstenedione.

The nonsteroidal aromatase inhibitors are competitive inhibitors that bind to the enzyme active site by coordinating the iron atom present in the heme group of the P-450 protein. Aside from aminoglutethimide, the first selective aromatase inhibitor to be marketed in the United States was anastrozole (Arimidex). Anastrozole incorporates a triazole ring into its structure that can coordinate to the heme iron. Letrozole is another triazole-containing inhibitor that is also effective in the treatment of breast cancer.

Currently available inhibitors suppress plasma estrogen levels (estradiol, estrone, and estrone sulfate) by 80 to 95%. Earlier aromatase inhibitors, such as aminoglutethimide and testolactone, suppressed plasma estrogens to a lesser extent. The side effects often seen with aminoglutethimide because of additional inhibition of other biosynthetic enzymes are avoided with the newest agents. The selectivity of these drugs for aromatase is quite high.

As with the SERMs, these drugs are only effective when the breast cancer cells are ''estrogen receptor (ER) posi-tive,'' meaning that they respond and proliferate in the presence of estrogen. Aromatase inhibitors can cause fetal harm in pregnant women and are therefore contraindicated.

Additional nonsteroidal inhibitors are based on the flavone structure. Chrysin is a flavonoid natural product that has aromatase inhibitory action in vitro similar to that of aminoglutethimide.[67] It is isolated from *Passiflora coerulea* and other plants. While this compound is not used therapeutically as an aromatase inhibitor, it has found questionable use as a nutritional supplement in combination with anabolic steroids to enhance muscle building and athletic performance. The theory for use is that an aromatase inhibitor reduces the estrogenic side effects of androgenic compounds. Although a variety of nutritional supplement products containing chrysin are available, it is unlikely that significant aromatase inhibition is being achieved in vivo. The oral bioavailability of chrysin is very low, mainly because of efficient conversion to the corresponding glucuronide and sulfate conjugates, so the plasma concentration of free chrysin is minimal.[68]

AROMATASE INHIBITOR PRODUCTS

Anastrozole, USP.   Anastrozole, $\alpha,\alpha,\alpha',\alpha'$-tetramethyl-5-(1$H$-1,2,4-triazol-1-ylmethyl)-1,3-benzenediacetonitrile, was the first specific aromatase inhibitor approved in the United States. It is indicated for first-line treatment of post-menopausal women with advanced or metastatic breast cancer and for second-line treatment of postmenopausal patients with advanced breast cancer who have had disease progression following tamoxifen therapy. An additional indication for adjuvant treatment of women with early breast cancer was added in 2002. Patients who did not respond to tamoxifen therapy rarely respond to anastrozole.

Anastrozole reduces serum estradiol approximately 80% after 14 days of daily dosing. Due to an elimination half-life of 50 hours, anastrozole is effective with once-daily dosing (1 mg). Metabolism of anastrozole includes hydroxylation and glucuronidation, as well as N-dealkylation to produce triazole. The metabolites of anastrozole are inactive. Although anastrozole can inhibit CYPs 1A2, 2C9, and 3A4 with K_i values in the low micromolar range, the concentrations of anastrozole reached under standard therapeutic dosing are much lower, so anastrozole should lack significant P-450 interactions.[69]

Letrozole, USP. Letrozole, 4,4′-(1*H*-1,2,4-triazol-1-ylmethylene)dibenzonitrile (Femara), is used for most of the same indications as anastrozole. It reduces concentrations of estrogens by 75 to 95%, with maximal suppression achieved within 2 to 3 days. Letrozole is specific for aromatase inhibition, with no additional effects on adrenal corticoid biosynthesis. CYPs 3A4 and 2A6 are involved in the metabolism of letrozole to the major carbinol metabolite, which is inactive. The loss of the triazole ring, which is involved in coordination of the heme iron, would explain the loss of activity. Letrozole strongly inhibits CYP 2A6 in vitro, with moderate inhibition of CYP 2C19. The effect of this in vitro inhibition on the pharmacokinetics of coadministered drugs is unknown. Tamoxifen reduces the levels of letrozole significantly if they are used together, so combination treatment with these agents is not recommended.[70]

Exemestane, USP. Exemestane, 6-methylenandrosta-1,4-diene-3,17-dione (Aromasin), is the first steroid-based aromatase inhibitor approved for the treatment of breast cancer in the United States. It is a mechanism-based inactivator that irreversibly inhibits the enzyme. Plasma estrogen levels are reduced by 85 to 95% within 2 to 3 days, and effects last 4 to 5 days. Exemestane does not inhibit any of the major cytochromes P-450 and has essentially no interaction with steroid receptors, with only a very weak affinity for the androgen receptor. The 17β-hydroxyexemestane reduction product, however, has much higher affinity for the androgen receptor than the parent (still several fold less than DHT, 0.28% for parent versus ~30% for metabolite). The clinical significance of the affinity is likely minimal because of the low levels of the metabolite produced.

Aminoglutethimide, USP. Aminoglutethimide, 3-(4-aminophenyl)-3-ethyl-2,6-piperidinedione, is mainly used to treat Cushing's syndrome, a condition of adrenal steroid excess, a use in which the P-450$_{scc}$ inhibition of this compound is exploited rather than its aromatase inhibition. Aminoglutethimide is a weak inhibitor of aromatase and has been used successfully in the treatment of estrogen-dependent breast cancer. Because of the development of more selective aromatase inhibitors, the use of aminoglutethimide for its ability to inhibit aromatase is not supported.

Testolactone, USP. Testolactone, 13-hydroxy-3-oxo-13,17-secoandrosta-1,4-dien-17-oic acid δ-lactone, was originally synthesized as a possible anabolic steroid, considering its structural similarity to testosterone. The key structural difference from anabolic steroids is the D-ring lactone instead of the typical cyclopentyl ring. Although considered in many texts an androgen or anabolic steroid (it is a Schedule III drug because of its classification as an anabolic steroid), testolactone lacks androgenic effects in vivo. Its action is believed to be due to irreversible inhibition of aromatase. It is a relatively weak inhibitor of aromatase, but the irreversible nature of the inhibition can lead to prolonged effects. Its relatively weak inhibition of aromatase and its undesirable dosage schedule (5 × 50-mg tablets q.i.d.) give this older agent only limited use in breast cancer treatment because of better available options.

Formestane. Formestane, 4-hydroxyandrost-4-ene-3,17-dione (Lentaron), was originally believed to be a competitive inhibitor of aromatase, but later studies determined it to be a mechanism-based irreversible inactivator of aromatase. Formestane was the first aromatase inhibitor approved for use in treating breast cancer in Europe, but it is not available in the United States. It lacks oral activity and is used as a once-every-2-weeks injection.

Progestins

ENDOGENOUS PROGESTINS

The key endogenous steroid hormone that acts at the progesterone receptors is progesterone. All other endogenous steroids lack significant progestational action.

BIOSYNTHESIS

Progesterone is produced in the ovaries, testes, and adrenal glands. Much of the progesterone that is synthesized from pregnenolone is immediately converted to other hormonal intermediates and is not secreted. See the biosynthetic pathway (Fig. 23-5). The corpus luteum secretes the most progesterone, 20 to 30 mg/day during the last or "luteal" stage of the menstrual cycle. Normal men secrete about 1 to 5 mg of progesterone daily.

METABOLISM OF PROGESTERONE

Progesterone has a half-life of only about 5 minutes when taken orally, because of rapid metabolism. Progesterone can be transformed to many other steroid hormones (Fig. 23-5) and, in that sense, has numerous metabolic products. The principal excretory product of progesterone metabolism, however, is 5β-pregnane-3α,20α-diol and its conjugates (Fig. 23-19). The steps that are involved in the formation of this metabolite are reduction of the C4-5 double bond, reduction of the C3 ketone providing the 3α-ol, and reduction of the C20 ketone. The reduction at C5 must precede the reduction of the C3 ketone, but the timing of the C20 can vary, depending on the tissue.[71, 72] Structural features that can block reduction at C5 or C20 have greatly increased the half-lives of progesterone derivatives.

BIOLOGICAL ACTIVITIES OF THE PROGESTINS[1]

Like the estrogens, progesterone has a variety of pharmacological actions, with the main target tissues being the uterus,

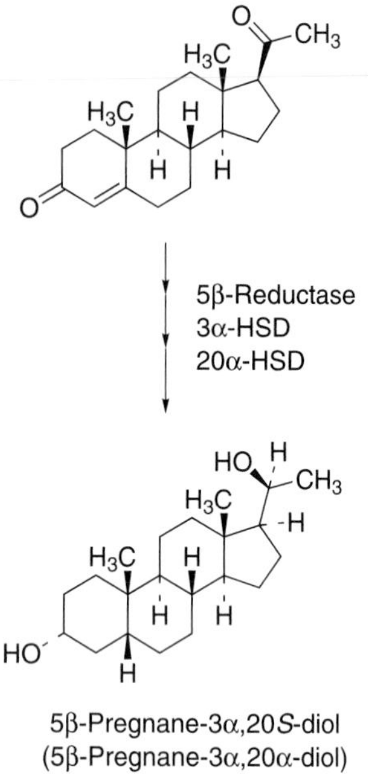

Figure 23–19 ■ Progesterone metabolism (timing of the reduction steps can vary). *HSD,* hydroxysteroid dehydrogenase.

breast, and brain. Progesterone decreases the frequency of the hypothalamic pulse generator and increases the amplitude of LH pulses released from the pituitary. The actions of progesterone in the uterus include development of the secretory endometrium. When release of progesterone from the corpus luteum at the end of the menstrual cycle declines, menstruation begins. Progesterone also acts to thicken cervical secretions, decreasing cervical penetration by sperm. Progesterone is critical for the maintenance of pregnancy by suppressing menstruation and decreasing uterine contractility. Progesterone has important actions in the breast during pregnancy, acting in conjunction with estrogens to prepare for lactation.

A thermogenic action is also associated with progesterone. During the menstrual cycle, progesterone mediates a slight temperature increase near midcycle and maintains the increased temperature until the onset of menstruation. The exact mechanism for this temperature increase is not known. Progesterone and its metabolites have additional central effects, which are being actively explored.[73]

STRUCTURAL CLASSES—PROGESTINS

Progestins are compounds with biological activities similar to those of progesterone. They include three structural classes: *(a)* progesterone and derivatives, *(b)* testosterone and 19-nortestosterone derivatives, and *(c)* miscellaneous synthetic progestins (Fig. 23-20). Progesterone itself has low oral bioavailability because of poor absorption and almost complete metabolism in one passage through the liver. A recently available oral formulation is micronized progesterone in gelatin capsules. The micronized drug is much more readily absorbed, allowing oral delivery of progesterone, even though the dose must be much higher than a parenteral dose to compensate for extensive liver metabolism. Adding 17α-acyl groups slows metabolism of the 20-one, whereas

a 6-methyl group enhances activity and reduces metabolism. Medroxyprogesterone acetate is a particularly potent example (Table 23-2).

Duax and coworkers[19, 20] have studied the structural requirements of the progesterone receptor in detail. They conclude that the progesterone 4-en-3-one ring A is a key to binding but only when it is in a conformation quite different from that of testosterone or the glucocorticoids. Their reviews contain stereo drawings that show the required conformations in three dimensions. Structural features modifying the steroid D ring are also important for optimal interactions with the progesterone receptor.

Two important discoveries led to the development of the nortestosterone derivatives. One was the discovery that 19-norprogesterone still maintained significant progestational activity. The second was that 17α-alkynyl testosterone (ethisterone) had greater progestational than androgenic activity. Although the 19-nortestosterones do have androgenic side effects, their primary activity, nevertheless, is progestational. In addition to causing a marked increase in progestational activity, the 17α-alkynyl group also blocks metabolic or bacterial oxidation to the corresponding 17-ones. Thus, by adding a 17α-ethinyl group to testosterone, one can simultaneously decrease androgenic activity, promote good progestational activity, and have an orally active compound as well. Table 23-2 illustrates the relative progestational activity of a number of progestins. A further modification to the nortestosterones yields progestins with minimal androgenic activities. Changing the alkyl group at C13 from a methyl to an ethyl group, as in levonorgestrel, reduces the androgenic effects, while maintaining the progestational effects.

THERAPEUTIC USES OF PROGESTINS

Progestin therapy may cause menstrual irregularities, such as spotting or amenorrhea. Weight gain and acne have been associated with testosterone and 19-nortestosterone analogues, in part because of their slight androgenic effects.

TABLE 23–2 Comparative Progestational Activity of Selected Progestins

	Relative Oral Activity	Activity SC
Progesterone	(nil)	1
17 α-Ethinyltestosterone (ethisterone)	1	0.1
17 α-Ethinyl-19-nortestosterone (norethindrone)	5–10	0.5–1
Norethynodrel	0.5–1	0.05–1
17 α-Hydroxyprogesterone caproate	2–10	4–10
Medroxyprogesterone acetate	12–25	50
19-Norprogesterone		5–10
Norgestrel		3
Dimethisterone	12	

Data from Salhanick, H. A., et al.: Metabolic Effects of Gonadal Hormones and Contraceptive Steroids. New York, Plenum Press, 1969.

Birth Control. A significant use of the progestins, as of the estrogens, is inhibition of ovulation. Steroidal birth control agents are discussed in the following section on chemical contraception.

Reduction of the Risk of Endometrial Cancer From Postmenopausal Estrogens. As discussed in the section on therapeutic uses of estrogens, several studies have suggested that the combination of a progestin with an estrogen may significantly reduce the risk of endometrial cancer in women taking postmenopausal estrogens. Because of this, a progestin is often included in HRT.

Primary and Secondary Amenorrhea and Functional Uterine Bleeding Caused by Insufficient Progesterone Production or Estrogen–Progesterone Imbalance. Progestins have been used very effectively to treat primary and secondary amenorrhea, functional uterine bleeding, and related menstrual disorders caused by hormonal deficiency or imbalance.

Breast or Endometrial Carcinoma. Progestins can be used for palliative treatment of advanced carcinoma of the breast or endometrium. These agents should not be used in place of surgery, radiation, or chemotherapy.

Progestins for Premenstrual Syndrome (PMS). There have been claims that progesterone may reduce the effects of PMS. Continued analyses of various studies indicate, however, that progestins are not effective for this use.[74]

PROGESTIN PRODUCTS

The progestins are primarily used in oral contraceptive products and in hormone replacement regimens for women. They are also used to treat several gynecological disorders: dys-

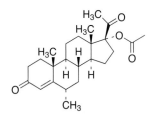

1. Progesterone and Derivatives

Progesterone

Hydroxyprogesterone Caproate
(Hy-gestrone, Hylutin)

Medroxyprogesterone Acetate
(Provera, Cycrin)

Megestrol Acetate
(Megace)

2. Synthetic Progestins – Testosterone and Nortestosterone Derivatives

Ethisterone

Dimethisterone

Norethindrone

Norethynodrel

Ethynodiol Diacetate

Figure 23–20 ▪ Natural and synthetic progestins.

2. Synthetic Progestins (continued)

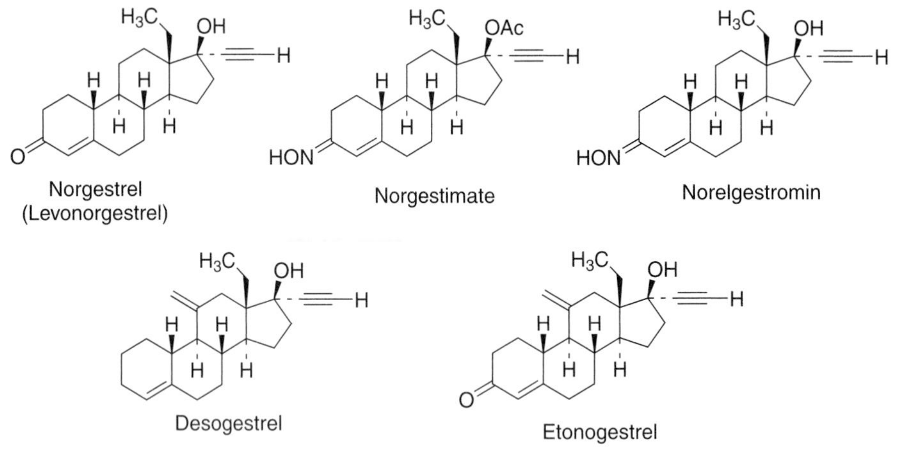

Norgestrel
(Levonorgestrel)

Norgestimate

Norelgestromin

Desogestrel

Etonogestrel

3. Miscellaneous Synthetic Progestins

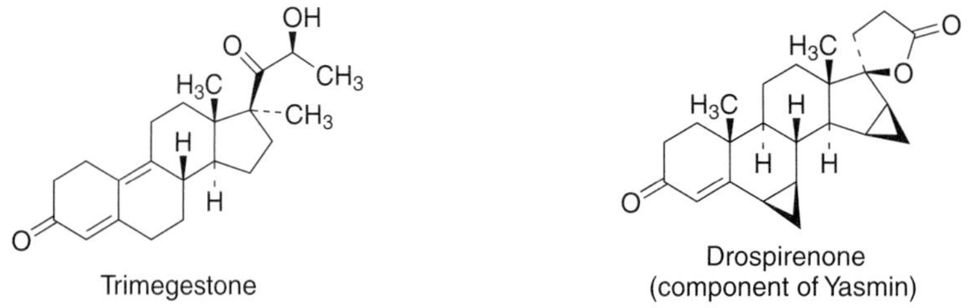

Trimegestone

Drospirenone
(component of Yasmin)

Figure 23–20 ▪ *Continued.*

menorrhea, endometriosis, amenorrhea, and dysfunctional uterine bleeding. Estrogens are given simultaneously in most of these situations.

Progesterone, USP. Progesterone, pregn-4-en-3,20-dione is so rapidly metabolized that it is not particularly effective orally, being only one-twelfth as active as intramuscularly. An oral formulation of micronized progesterone (Prometrium) is available. Progesterone given intramuscularly can be very irritating. A vaginal gel containing 4 or 8% progesterone offers an alternative dosage form. Progesterone was originally obtained from animal ovaries but is now prepared synthetically from plant sterol precursors. The discovery of 19-nortestosterones with progesterone activity made synthetically modified progestins of tremendous therapeutic importance.

Progesterone (and all other steroid 4-ene-3-ones) is light sensitive and should be protected from light.

Hydroxyprogesterone Caproate, USP. Hydroxyprogesterone caproate, 17-hydroxypregn-4-ene-3,20-dione hexanoate, is much more active and longer acting than progesterone (see Table 23-2), probably because the 17α ester hinders reduction to the 20-ol. In contrast, hydroxyprogesterone itself lacks progestational activity. The caproate ester is given only intramuscularly. The ester greatly increases oil

solubility, allowing it to be slowly released from depot preparations, as one would predict from Figure 23-6.

Medroxyprogesterone Acetate, USP. Medroxyprogesterone acetate, 17-acetyloxy-6α-methylpregn-4-ene-3,20-dione (Provera), adds a 6α-methyl group to the basic 17α-hydroxyprogesterone structure to greatly decrease the rate of reduction of the 4-ene-3-one system. The 17α-acetate group also decreases reduction of the 20-one, similar to the 17α-caproate. Medroxyprogesterone acetate (MPA) is very active orally (see Table 23-2) and has such a long duration of action intramuscularly that it cannot be routinely used intramuscularly for treating many menstrual disorders. The intramuscular formulation is useful in the palliative treatment of advanced endometrial, breast, and renal carcinomas. MPA also has an important role in several birth control products (Depo-Provera, Lunelle).

Megestrol Acetate, USP. Megestrol acetate, 17-hydroxy-6-methylpregna-4,6-diene-3,20-dione acetate (Megace), is a progestin used primarily for the palliative management of recurrent, inoperable, or metastatic endometrial or breast carcinoma. Megestrol acetate has also been indicated for appetite enhancement in AIDS patients. The biochemical basis for this use of megestrol is unclear.

Norethindrone, USP, and Norethynodrel, USP. Norethindrone, 17α-ethinyl-19-nortestosterone, and its $\Delta^{5(10)}$ isomer, norethynodrel, might appear at first glance to be subtle copies of each other. One would predict that the $\Delta^{5(10)}$ double bond would isomerize in the stomach's acid to the Δ^4 position. In fact, however, the two drugs were developed simultaneously and independently; hence, neither can be considered a copy of the other. Furthermore, norethindrone is about 10 times more active than norethynodrel (see Table 23-2), indicating that isomerization is not as facile in vivo as one might predict. Although they are less active than progesterone when given subcutaneously, they have the important advantage of being orally active. The discovery of the potent progestin activity of 17α-ethinyltestosterone (ethisterone) and 19-norprogesterone preceded the development of these potent progestins. Both are orally active, with the 17α-ethinyl group blocking oxidation to the less active 17-one. The rich electron density of the ethinyl group and the absence of the 19-methyl group greatly enhance progestin activity. Both compounds were of great importance as progestin components of oral contraceptives, although currently, use of norethynodrel is minimal. Norethindrone, USP, and norethindrone acetate, USP, are widely used for all the usual indications of the progestins, as well as being components of oral contraceptives. Because these compounds retain key features of the testosterone structure, including the 17β-OH, it is not surprising that they possess some androgenic side effects.

Ethynodiol Diacetate, USP. Ethynodiol diacetate, 19-norpregn-4-en-20-yne-$3\beta,17\alpha$-diol diacetate, is a prodrug of norethindrone. A combination of hydrolysis of both esters and oxidation of the C3 alcohol to the ketone is necessary to provide the fully active progestin.[75]

Norgestrel, USP, and Levonorgestrel, USP. Norgestrel, (17α)-$(\pm)$-13-ethyl-17-hydroxy-18,19-dinorpregn-4-en-20-yn-3-one, and levonorgestrel, (17α)-$(-)$-13-ethyl-17-hydroxy-18,19-dinorpregn-4-en-20-yn-3-one, have a C13 ethyl group instead of the C13 methyl but have progestational properties similar to those of norethindrone, with decreased androgenic effects. The ethyl group apparently provides unfavorable steric interactions with the androgen receptor that reduce the affinity compared with that with the progesterone receptors. Norgestrel is a racemic mixture, while levonorgestrel is the single active levorotatory enantiomer. Norgestrel is used only in oral contraceptives. Levonorgestrel is used in both oral combination birth control products and polymeric implants that provide contraception for up to 5 years.

Desogestrel, USP. Desogestrel, (17α)-13-ethyl-11-methylene-18,19-dinorpregn-4-en-20-yn-17-ol (Desogen), is a 19-nortestosterone analogue with good progestin activity. Like the other progestins, it is orally active and used in combination with an estrogen in oral contraceptives. Desogestrel is a prodrug that must be oxidized to the 3-one in vivo to have progestational action. CYPs 2C9 and 2C19 have been implicated in the initial hydroxylation of desogestrel at C3.[76]

Norgestimate, USP. Norgestimate, (17α)-17-acetyloxy-13-ethyl-18,19-dinor-pregn-4-en-20yn-3-one oxime (Cyclen, Tri-Cyclen), is a 19-nortestosterone, 3-oxime prodrug that is orally active and used with an estrogen in oral contraceptive products. It has minimal androgenic action. Norgestimate is metabolized to 17-deacetylnorgestimate (norelgestromin) and norgestrel, which provide the progestational action.[77]

Norelgestromin, USP. Norelgestromin, (17α)-13-ethyl-17-hydroxy-18,19-dinor-pregn-4-en-20-yn-3-one, oxime, is the progestin component in the contraceptive patch (Ortho-Evra). First-pass metabolism in the liver is avoided by the transdermal application. Hepatic metabolism does occur, however, and norgestrel, an active metabolite, and other hydroxylated and conjugated metabolites are formed.

Etonogestrel, USP. Etonogestrel, 17α-13-ethyl-17-hydroxy-11-methylene-18,19-dinorpregn-4-en-20-yn-3-one, 3-ketodesogestrel, is the active metabolite of desogestrel. It is the progestin component in a newer implantable contraceptive (Implanon) and in the vaginal contraceptive ring (NuvaRing).

Drospirenone, USP. Drospirenone, 3-oxo-$6\beta,7\beta$:15β, 16β-dimethylene-17α-pregn-4-en-21,17-carbolactone, differs structurally from all of the other commercially available progestins. Its structure is similar to that of spironolactone, a mineralocorticoid receptor antagonist, and drospirenone does have antimineralocorticoid activity as well as progestational activity. It is also reported to have some antiandrogenic effects. The spirolactone at C17 and the two cyclopropyl groups at C6-C7 and C15-C16 contribute to these unique actions. Drospirenone is the progestin component in a new oral contraceptive, Yasmin.

Trimegestone. Trimegestone, 17β-(S)-lactoyl-17-methyl-estra-4,9-dien-3-one, is a highly modified norprogesterone derivative that is being investigated for its use in HRT and as a component of oral contraceptives. The key structural differences are a 17β-lactoyl group in place of the typical acetyl group, a 17α-methyl, and a C9-C10 double bond. Trimegestone lacks androgenic action and has little to no affinity for the estrogen and glucocorticoid receptors.[78]

CHEMICAL CONTRACEPTIVE AGENTS

Political, cultural, and research-cost barriers have enormously complicated the development of contraceptive agents in modern times. The reviews by Djerassi,[79] inventor of norethindrone, and by Lednicer[80] are important reading. (Their "insider's viewpoint" of the research competition during the 1950s and 1960s to develop steroid products is especially interesting.) More recent reviews provide a slightly different perspective on the overall development of oral contraceptives.[81, 82]

The most notable achievement in chemical contraception came in the late 1950s and early 1960s with the development of oral contraceptive agents—"the pill." Since then, a variety of contraceptive products have been introduced, including hormone-releasing intrauterine devices, polymer implants, injectable formulations, and a transdermal patch. Additionally, postcoital contraceptives and abortifacients have been developed. Despite the advances in chemical contraceptive agents for women, no hormonal male contraceptives are currently available, although limited research in this area has been conducted. In the following pages, each of these approaches to chemical contraception is discussed. Individual compounds are discussed above with the estrogens and progestins.

Ovulation Inhibitors and Related Hormonal Contraceptives

HISTORY[79, 80, 83]

In the 1930s, several research groups found that injections of progesterone inhibited ovulation in rats, rabbits, and guinea pigs.[84–86] Kurzrok, Albright, and Sturgis, in the early 1940s, are generally credited with the concept that estrogens, progesterone, or both could be used to prevent ovulation in women.[87, 88] In 1965, Pincus[89] reported that progesterone given from day 5 to day 25 of the menstrual cycle would inhibit ovulation in women. During this time, Djerassi et al.[90] of Syntex, and Colton[91] of G. D. Searle and Co. reported the synthesis of norethindrone and norethynodrel. These progestins possessed very high progestational and ovulation-inhibiting activity.

Extensive animal and clinical trials conducted by Pincus, Rock, and Garcia confirmed, in 1956, that Searle's norethynodrel and Syntex's norethindrone were effective ovulation inhibitors in women. In 1960, Searle marketed Enovid (a mixture of norethynodrel and mestranol), and in 1962, Ortho marketed Ortho Novum (a mixture of norethindrone and mestranol) under contract with Syntex. Norethindrone has remained the most extensively used progestin in oral contraceptives, but several other useful agents have been developed. These are discussed in the sections below.

THERAPEUTIC CLASSES AND MECHANISM OF ACTION

The modern hormonal contraceptives fall into several major categories (Table 23-3), each with its own mechanism of contraceptive action. Individual compounds are discussed with the estrogens and progestins in the section above.

Combination Tablets: Mechanism of Action.

Although, as noted above, Sturgis and Albright recognized in the early 1940s that either estrogens or progestins could inhibit ovulation, it was subsequently found that combinations were highly effective. Some problems, such as breakthrough (midcycle) bleeding, were also reduced by the use of a combination of progestin and estrogen.

Although all the details of the process are still not completely understood, it is now believed that the combination tablets suppress the production of LH, FSH, or both by a feedback-inhibition process (see Fig. 23-9). Without FSH or LH, ovulation is prevented. The process is similar to the natural inhibition of ovulation during pregnancy, caused by the release of estrogens and progesterone from the placenta and ovaries. An additional effect comes from the progestin causing the cervical mucus to become very thick, providing a

barrier for the passage of sperm through the cervix. Because pregnancy is impossible without ovulation, however, the contraceptive effects of thick cervical mucus or alterations in the lining of the uterus (to decrease the probability of implantation of a fertilized ovum) would appear to be quite secondary. Nevertheless, occasional ovulation may occur, and thus the alterations of the cervical mucus and the endometrium may actually serve an important contraceptive function (especially, perhaps, when the patient forgets to take one of the tablets). During combination drug treatment, the endometrial lining develops enough for withdrawal bleeding to occur about 4 or 5 days after taking the last active tablet of the series (see Table 23-3).

MONOPHASIC (FIXED) COMBINATIONS. The monophasic combinations of a progestin and estrogen contain the same amount of drug in each active tablet (see Table 23-3). As discussed below in this chapter, the trend in prescribing has been toward lower doses of estrogen. As estrogen levels are reduced, however, breakthrough bleeding (or ''spotting'') becomes an annoying side effect for some patients at early to midcycle. Spotting after midcycle or amenorrhea appears to be related to too little progestin relative to the estrogen. The biphasic and triphasic combinations were developed to solve these breakthrough-bleeding problems in some patients.

BIPHASIC AND TRIPHASIC (VARIABLE) COMBINATIONS. In the natural menstrual cycle, progesterone plasma concentrations peak late in the cycle. The higher estrogen/progesterone ratio early in the cycle is believed to assist in development of the endometrium. The higher progesterone concentration later contributes to proliferation of the endometrium and a resultant ''normal'' volume of menstrual flow. The biphasic and triphasic combinations attempt to mimic this variation in estrogen/progestin levels, and thereby to reduce the incidence of spotting associated with low-dose monophasic combinations. With proper selection of patients, the goal has been achieved; but in other patients, the incidence of spotting has not decreased appreciably.

EXTENDED ORAL CONTRACEPTIVE THERAPY. Clinical trials are currently in progress that use a 91-day cycle as opposed to the current 28-day cycles typically used for oral contraceptives. The monophasic combinations in testing have levonorgestrel and ethinyl estradiol as the progestin and estrogen, respectively. Instead of 21 days of hormones, followed by a week of inert tablets, these regimens have 84 days of hormones, followed by a week of inert tablets. The key difference with this approach is that the number of menstrual cycles during the year would be reduced from 12 to 4. If shown to be effective and safe, this type of product could allow women to reduce the frequency of cramps and anemia associated with menstruation.

HOW SAFE?

The safety of the ''pill'' has been investigated extensively because of the widespread use of these drugs in healthy young women. Overall, oral contraceptives have an excellent safety profile in healthy, nonsmoking women of child-bearing age.[92] Early studies, based largely on the earlier products that contained high doses of estrogen, showed an alarming

TABLE 23–3 Comparison of Steroid Contraceptive Regimens

1. Combination—Monophasic

Products are available in 21- or 28-day dispensers and refills. The 28-day dispensers contain several inert (or Fe^{2+}-containing) tablets of a different color, taken daily after the 21 days of active tablets. Doses of active tablets are shown.

Brand	Progestin	Estrogen
Necon 1/50	Norethindrone, 1 mg	Mestranol, 50 μg
Norinyl 1 + 50	Norethindrone, 1 mg	Mestranol, 50 μg
Ortho-Novum 1/50	Norethindrone, 1 mg	Mestranol, 50 μg
Ovcon 50	Norethindrone, 1 mg	Ethinyl estradiol, 50 μg
Demulen 1/50	Ethynodiol diacetate, 1 mg	Ethinyl estradiol, 50 μg
Zovia 1/50E	Ethynodiol diacetate, 1 mg	Ethinyl estradiol, 50 μg
Ovral-28	Norgestrel, 0.5 mg	Ethinyl estradiol, 50 μg
Ogestrel	Norgestrel, 0.5 mg	Ethinyl estradiol, 50 μg
Necon 1/35	Norethindrone, 1 mg	Ethinyl estradiol, 35 μg
Norinyl 1 + 35	Norethindrone, 1 mg	Ethinyl estradiol, 35 μg
Nortrel 1/35	Norethindrone, 1 mg	Ethinyl estradiol, 35 μg
Ortho-Novum 1/35	Norethindrone, 1 mg	Ethinyl estradiol, 35 μg
Modicon	Norethindrone, 0.5 mg	Ethinyl estradiol, 35 μg
Necon 0.5/35	Norethindrone, 0.5 mg	Ethinyl estradiol, 35 μg
Nortrel 0.5/35	Norethindrone, 0.5 mg	Ethinyl estradiol, 35 μg
Ovcon-35	Norethindrone, 0.4 mg	Ethinyl estradiol, 35 μg
Ortho-Cyclen	Norgestimate, 0.25 mg	Ethinyl estradiol, 35 μg
Demulen 1/35	Ethynodiol diacetate, 1 mg	Ethinyl estradiol, 35 μg
Zovia 1/35E	Ethynodiol diacetate, 1 mg	Ethinyl estradiol, 35 μg
Yasmin	Drospirenone, 3 mg	Ethinyl estradiol, 30 μg
Loestrin 21 1.5/30	Norethindrone acetate, 1.5 mg	Ethinyl estradiol, 30 μg
Loestrin Fe 1.5/30	Norethindrone acetate, 1.5 mg	Ethinyl estradiol, 30 μg
Microgestin Fe 1.5/30	Norethindrone acetate, 1.5 mg	Ethinyl estradiol, 30 μg
Lo/Ovral	Norgestrel, 0.3 mg	Ethinyl estradiol, 30 μg
Low-Ogestrel	Norgestrel, 0.3 mg	Ethinyl estradiol, 30 μg
Desogen	Desogestrel, 0.15 mg	Ethinyl estradiol, 30 μg
Ortho-Cept	Desogestrel, 0.15 mg	Ethinyl estradiol, 30 μg
Apri	Desogestrel, 0.15 mg	Ethinyl estradiol, 30 μg
Levlen	Levonorgestrel, 0.15 mg	Ethinyl estradiol, 30 μg
Levora	Levonorgestrel, 0.15 mg	Ethinyl estradiol, 30 μg
Nordette	Levonorgestrel, 0.15 mg	Ethinyl estradiol, 30 μg
Alesse	Levonorgestrel, 0.1 mg	Ethinyl estradiol, 20 μg
Aviane	Levonorgestrel, 0.1 mg	Ethinyl estradiol, 20 μg
Levlite	Levonorgestrel, 0.1 mg	Ethinyl estradiol, 20 μg
Loestrin 21 1/20	Norethindrone acetate, 1 mg	Ethinyl estradiol, 20 μg
Loestrin Fe 1/20	Norethindrone acetate, 1 mg	Ethinyl estradiol, 20 μg
Microgestin Fe 1/20	Norethindrone acetate, 1 mg	Ethinyl estradiol, 20 μg

2. Combination—Biphasic

Products are available in 21- or 28-day dispensers and refills. They are taken on the same schedule of 21 days plus 7 days of no (or inert) tablets as the monophasics above, except Mircette. Doses of active tablets are shown.

Brand	Progestin and Estrogen
Jenest-28	7 days: Norethindrone, 0.5 mg, and ethinyl estradiol, 35 μg
	14 days: Norethindrone, 1 mg, and ethinyl estradiol, 35 μg
Necon 10/11	10 days: Norethindrone, 0.5 mg, and ethinyl estradiol, 35 μg
	11 days: Norethindrone, 1 mg, and ethinyl estradiol, 35 μg
Ortho-Novum	10 days: Norethindrone, 0.5 mg, and ethinyl estradiol, 35 μg

(Continued)

TABLE 23–3   Comparison of Steroid Contraceptive Regimens—*Continued*

Brand	Progestin and Estrogen
10/11 21	11 days: Norethindrone, 1 mg, and ethinyl estradiol, 35 μg
Mircette	21 days: Desogestrel, 0.15 mg, and ethinyl estradiol, 20 μg
	5 days: Ethinyl estradiol, 10 μg
	2 days: Inert

3. Combination—Triphasic

Products are available in 21- or 28-day dispensers and refills. They are taken on the same schedule of 21 days plus 7 days of no (or inert) tablets as the monophasics above. Doses of active tablets are shown.

Brand	Progestin and Estrogen
Ortho-Novum 7/7/7	7 days: Norethindrone, 0.5 mg, and ethinyl estradiol, 35 μg
	7 days: Norethindrone, 0.75 mg, and ethinyl estradiol, 35 μg
	7 days: Norethindrone, 1 mg, and ethinyl estradiol, 35 μg
Ortho-Tri-Cyclen	7 days: Norgestimate, 0.18 mg, and ethinyl estradiol, 35 μg
	7 days: Norgestimate, 0.215 mg, and ethinyl estradiol, 35 μg
	7 days: Norgestimate, 0.25 mg, and ethinyl estradiol, 35 μg
Trinorinyl	7 days: Norethindrone, 0.5 mg, and ethinyl estradiol, 35 μg
	9 days: Norethindrone, 1 mg, and ethinyl estradiol, 35 μg
	5 days: Norethindrone, 0.5 mg, and ethinyl estradiol, 35 μg
Tri-Levlen	6 days: Levonorgestrel, 0.05 mg, and ethinyl estradiol, 30 μg
	5 days: Levonorgestrel, 0.075 mg, and ethinyl estradiol, 40 μg
	10 days: Levonorgestrel, 0.125 mg, and ethinyl estradiol, 30 μg
Tri-Phasil	6 days: Levonorgestrel, 0.05 mg, and ethinyl estradiol, 30 μg
	5 days: Levonorgestrel, 0.075 mg, and ethinyl estradiol, 40 μg
	10 days: Levonorgestrel, 0.125 mg, and ethinyl estradiol, 30 μg
Trivora	6 days: Levonorgestrel, 0.05 mg, and ethinyl estradiol, 30 μg
	5 days: Levonorgestrel, 0.075 mg, and ethinyl estradiol, 40 μg
	10 days: Levonorgestrel, 0.125 mg, and ethinyl estradiol, 30 μg
Estrostep	5 days: Norethindrone acetate, 1 mg, and ethinyl estradiol, 20 μg
	7 days: Norethindrone acetate, 1 mg, and ethinyl estradiol, 30 μg
	9 days: Norethindrone acetate, 1 mg, and ethinyl estradiol, 35 μg

4. Progestin Only

An active tablet is taken each day of the year.

Brand	Progestin	Dose
Micronor	Norethindrone	0.35 mg
Nor-Q.D.	Norethindrone	0.35 mg
Ovrette	Norgestrel	0.075 mg

5. Injectable Depot Hormonal Contraceptives

Brand	Drug	Dosage Cycle
Depo-Provera	Medroxyprogesterone acetate alone	150 mg/month
		150 mg every 3 months
Lunelle	Medroxyprogesterone acetate (MPA), 25 mg, and estradiol cypionate (E2C), 5 mg/0.5 mL	0.5-mL IM injection once in deltoid, gluteus maximus, or anterior thigh every 28 to 30 days

6. Transdermal Contraceptive Patch

Brand	Release Rate	Total Hormone Content	Dosage Cycle
Ortho-Evra	0.15 mg norelgestromin, 0.02 mg, ethinyl estradiol/24 hours	6 mg norelgestromin, 0.075 mg, ethinyl estradiol	One patch each week for 3 weeks, 1 week no patch.

TABLE 23–3—*Continued*

7. Hormone-Releasing Implants, IUDs, and Vaginal Rings

Brand	Drug	Dosage Cycle
Progestasert	Progesterone-releasing IUD	38-mg dose in IUD lasts 1 year
Mirena	Levonorgestrel-releasing intrauterine system (LRIS)	52-mg dose in LRIS provides contraception for up to 5 years
Norplant	6 Silastic capsules with 36 mg levonorgestrel; all 6 capsules are inserted subdermally in the middle upper arm	Contraceptive efficacy lasts for 5 years if the implants are not removed
Implanon	One polymeric rod with 68 mg etonorgestrel, released at a rate of ~40 μg/day.	Contraceptive efficacy lasts up to 3 years if the implant is not removed
NuvaRing	11.7 mg etonogestrel, 2.7 mg ethinyl estradiol in a flexible, polymeric vaginal ring	Vaginal ring is inserted for 3 weeks duration, then 1 week off before insertion of a new ring

8. Emergency Contraceptives

Brand	Drug	Dosage
Plan B	0.75 mg levonorgestrel	The first dose (1 tablet) should be taken as soon as possible within 72 hours of intercourse; the second dose (1 tablet) must be taken 12 hours later
Preven	0.25 mg levonorgestrel, 0.05 mg ethinyl estradiol	The first dose (2 tablets) should be taken as soon as possible within 72 hours of intercourse; the second dose (2 tablets) must be taken 12 hours later

incidence of thromboembolic disease (blood clots). More recent studies have shown a greatly reduced risk of cardiovascular effects with lower estrogen doses. Another concern has been an association between estrogens and increased cancer risk. Recent reanalysis of clinical data supports a slightly increased risk of breast cancer in women taking oral contraceptives, but the risk subsides within 10 years of discontinuation of use.[93] This small increase in incidence of breast cancer is not greatly affected by duration of use, dose, age at first use, or progestin component. Additionally, use of oral contraceptives has shown a decreased risk for endometrial and ovarian cancers.[93]

The overall results of these studies have been that (*a*) the sequential contraceptive products with their high doses of estrogen have been removed from American markets; (*b*) most combination contraceptives now marketed contain less than 0.050 mg of estrogen per dose (see Table 23-3); (*c*) progestin-only or minipill products are available (see Table 23-3); and (*d*) a few groups of women have been identified who should definitely not take oral contraceptives (e.g., women with a history of thromboembolic disease or other cardiovascular disease, women who are heavy smokers over the age of 35, and women with a history of breast cancer in their immediate family). The actual incidence of "pill-induced" cardiovascular death for nonsmoking young women is quite small, and there is not a widespread link between oral contraceptive use and cancer. Cigarette smoking increases the risk of thromboembolic disorders associated with oral contraceptive use, so women should be counseled to abstain from smoking while using oral contraceptives.

Progestin Only (Minipill). The estrogen component of sequential and combination oral contraceptive agents has been related to some side effects, with thromboembolism being a concern. One solution to this problem has been to develop new products with decreased estrogen content. The minipill contains no estrogen at all.

Although higher doses of progestin are known to suppress ovulation, minipill doses of progestin do not suffice to suppress ovulation in all women. Some studies have indicated that increased viscosity of the cervical mucus (or sperm barrier) could account for much of the contraceptive effect. Low doses of progestin have also been found to increase the rate of ovum transport and to disrupt implantation. There is a good probability that most, or all, of these factors contribute to the overall contraceptive effect of the minipill. The incidence of pregnancy with the minipill is slightly higher than with combination products, although still very low when the minipill is used as directed.

Depo-Provera. Medroxyprogesterone acetate intramuscular (IM) injection (Depo-Provera) provides contraception for 3 months after a single 150-mg IM dose. Most women experience some irregular bleeding or spotting and often experience small weight gain. Fertility returns for most women within the first 12 months after discontinuance of Depo-Provera. Contraception typically continues for a few weeks beyond the 3-month term, giving patients a short grace period if the subsequent IM dose is delayed.

Lunelle. Lunelle is a newer injectable contraceptive formulation that combines the effects of a progestin, medroxyprogesterone acetate (MPA), and an estrogen, estradiol cypionate (E2C). This product is also referred to as MPA/E2C. The cypionate ester at C17 provides a lipophilic prodrug that is slowly released from the injection site, providing sustained action of the estrogen component. The progestin is also slowly released from the injection site. The MPA/E2C injection is given once a month in the deltoid, gluteus maximus, or anterior thigh.

Transdermal Contraceptives. In 2001, the Food and Drug Administration (FDA) approved the first transdermal contraceptive patch, Ortho-Evra. The product contains norelgestromin and ethinyl estradiol. A patch is applied once a week for 3 weeks, followed by a week with no patch. The pregnancy rate for this product is 1 in 100, a rate similar to that often observed with oral contraceptives.

Progesterone IUD. The low progestin doses of the mini-pill seem to have a direct effect on the uterus and associated reproductive tract. Therefore, it would seem possible to lower the progestin dose even more if the drug were released in the reproductive tract itself.

The Progestasert IUD (Progesterone Intrauterine Contraceptive System, USP) has 38 mg of microcrystalline progesterone dispersed in silicone oil. The dispersion is contained in a flexible polymer in the approximate shape of a T. The polymer acts as a membrane to permit 65 μg of progesterone to be released slowly into the uterus each day for 1 year. The progesterone-containing IUD has had some of the therapeutic problems of other IUDs, including a relatively low patient continuation rate, some septic abortions, and some perforations of uterus and cervix.

Levonorgestrel-Releasing Intrauterine System (LRIS). Because the Progestasert system provided evidence that a progestin-releasing intrauterine device was an effective contraceptive, another intrauterine system has been developed with use of a different progestin. Mirena is a plastic T-shaped frame, with the stem of the "T" containing 52 mg of levonorgestrel. The levonorgestrel is released slowly, at a dose lower than in a pill (approximately one-seventh strength), directly to the lining of the uterus. This local release and absorption of the hormone helps to reduce systemic progesterone-type side effects. The contraceptive effectiveness of this device lasts up to 5 years.

Mirena acts as a contraceptive in two ways: it thickens the mucus at the cervix, preventing sperm from getting through, and it also thins the lining of the uterus, preventing implantation. In some women it also prevents ovulation. An additional feature of the LRIS is that menstrual periods are typically lighter than usual. The LRIS may be useful to alleviate the difficulties associated with heavy periods, even in patients who do not need contraception.

There is a small chance that the device may dislodge in the early months of use. Although the LRIS releases a reduced amount of progestin, it does slightly increase progesterone levels in the bloodstream. This increased progesterone can cause side effects including headache, water retention, breast tenderness, or acne, although these are typically mild. Bleeding problems are the most common side effect, but this effect usually ceases after 3 to 6 months of use.

Intrauterine Ring. A new entry into the contraceptive market is a flexible polymeric ring, approximately 2.1 inches in diameter, that contains etonogestrel and ethinyl estradiol (NuvaRing). The ring is inserted into the vagina by the woman herself and remains inserted for 3 weeks. The spent ring is removed for 1 week to allow the menstrual period. A new ring is inserted 1 week after removal of the prior ring. The ring contains 11.7 mg of etonogestrel and 2.7 mg of ethinyl estradiol, with a release rate of 0.12 mg etonogestrel/day and 0.015 mg of ethinyl estradiol/day. Unlike a diaphragm, the placement of the vaginal ring contraceptive device is not critical. Clinical trials suggest a 1 to 2% pregnancy rate for women using the ring as indicated. Like other hormone-based contraceptives, the ring should not be used by women who have cardiovascular disease, blood clots, or hormone-dependent breast cancer. Women should also abstain from smoking while using the ring.

CONTRACEPTIVE IMPLANTS

Norplant. The first implantable contraceptive was Norplant, a set of six flexible Silastic (dimethylsiloxane/methylvinylsiloxane copolymer) capsules that contain levonorgestrel. The capsules implanted in the midportion of the upper arm provided contraception for up to 5 years. Contraceptive efficacy was very high. Most women experienced changes in menstrual bleeding, ranging from irregular cycles to prolonged bleeding or amenorrhea. A problem that arose with Norplant was that removal of the product, either at the end of 5 years, or earlier in patients who wished to stop using contraception, often entailed a sometimes painful surgical procedure. The insertion and removal procedures required extra training of physicians, another feature that reduced the desirability of this product. Although Norplant was extremely effective as a contraceptive, a variety of legal issues, public concerns, and production issues led the manufacturers to discontinue production of Norplant. Norplant II, a two-rod implantable system that had reduced problems with insertion and removal, was approved by the FDA but was never marketed in the United States.

A new implantable system may be available soon in the United States. Implanon is a single-rod system (40 × 2 mm) that releases etonogestrel (3-ketodesogestrel) rather than the levonorgestrel in Norplant. The contraceptive efficacy is up to 3 years. With a single rod and a specially designed applicator system, the insertion/removal difficulties with Norplant should be avoided. The Implanon system has been used successfully in Europe for several years.

Other Methods of Chemical Contraception

POSTCOITAL CONTRACEPTIVES

Two products specifically designated for postcoital or emergency contraception have been approved. Plan B uses a high-dose progestin-only approach, whereas Preven combines a progestin and an estrogen. Both must be taken within 72 hours of unprotected intercourse, followed by another dose 12 hours later. Some monophasic oral contraceptives must also be used in a similar fashion. A specific drug that has been used in this manner is Ovral, which combines norgestrel (0.5 mg) and ethinyl estradiol (50 μg). Two Ovral tablets are taken within 72 hours of unprotected intercourse or failure of other method, followed by another two tablets 12 hours later. Some patients experience nausea, which is usually mild. The treatment successfully prevents pregnancy with about 90% of patients. This treatment is intended, however, only for use in short-term emergency situations.

ABORTIFACIENTS

History records many different compounds that have been tried as abortifacients, but many of these compounds also are toxic or mutagenic or cause severe hemorrhaging along with the abortion. Several therapeutically acceptable abortifacients, however, are currently available. Two prostaglandins have been approved by the FDA to induce second-trimester abortions, and mifepristone (Mifeprex), a progesterone receptor antagonist, is available for use in the first 49 days of pregnancy (Fig. 23-21).

Prostaglandins $F_{2\alpha}$ ($PGF_{2\alpha}$) and E_2 (PGE_2) concentrations increase significantly in amniotic fluid before normal labor and childbirth and are involved in stimulating uterine contractions. In a similar fashion, the prostaglandin drugs stimulate the uterus to contract. These contractions usually suffice to expel the fetus from the uterus. Good surgical support is essential with carboprost and dinoprostone because some clinicians report a high incidence of incomplete abortions that require additional treatment. Carboprost is approved only for intramuscular injection, while dinoprostone (prostaglandin E_2) is available as a vaginal suppository. Both products are used for second-trimester abortions. Carboprost is a $PGF_{2\alpha}$ analogue.

Mifepristone acts directly by antagonizing the effects of progesterone at progesterone receptors, as well as indirectly by causing a decrease in progesterone secretion from the corpus luteum. These combined effects lead to an increase in the level of prostaglandins, which stimulates uterine contractions. Mifepristone also causes a softening of the cervix, which aids in expulsion of the fertilized ovum. Mifepristone treatment is followed by the use of misoprostol, a prostaglandin E_2 analogue, to ensure a complete abortion. Mifepristone also has antagonist action at glucocorticoid receptors.

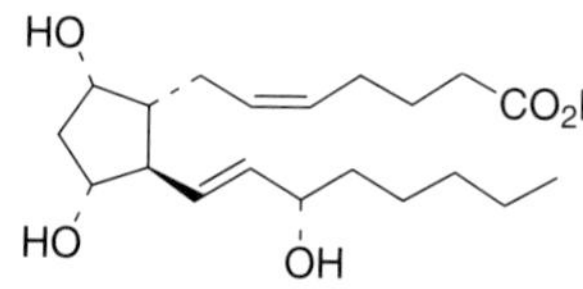

Relative Contraceptive Effectiveness of Various Methods

Some caution is required in interpreting data on the effectiveness of contraceptive methods. Even the "best" method can lead to pregnancy if not used consistently and correctly. Even the generally least effective method is better than no contraceptive at all. Table 23-4 presents some data on numbers of pregnancies per method.

Prostaglandin $F_{2\alpha}$

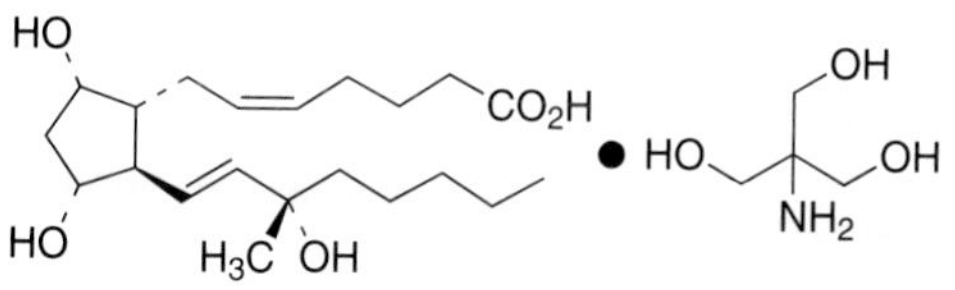

Carboprost Tromethamine (Hemabate)
15S-Methyl-prostaglandin $F_{2\alpha}$

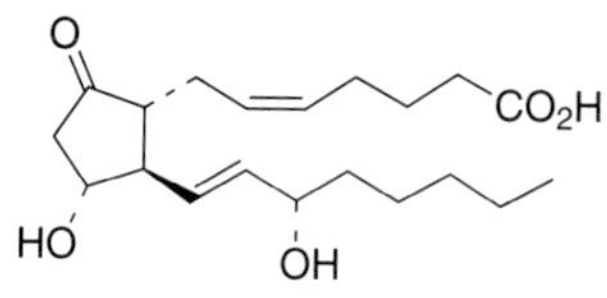

Prostaglandin E_2
Dinoprostone (Prostin E_2)

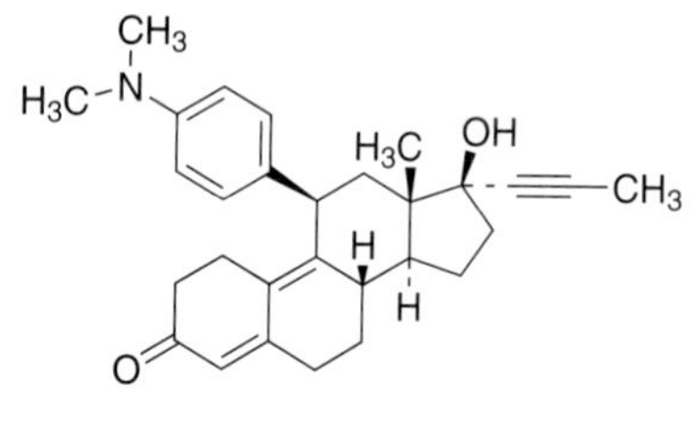

Mifepristone (Mifeprex; RU-486)

Figure 23–21 ■ Abortifacients.

TABLE 23–4   Failure Rate of Contraceptive Methods

Method	Pregnancies/100 Woman Years
Tubal ligation	0.5
Vasectomy	0.15
Norplant	0.05
Implanon	(0.05)[a]
Depo-Provera injection	0.3
MPA/E2C injection	<1
Combination oral contraceptives	0.1–3
Progestin only minipill (oral)	0.5–3
Progestasert IUD	1.5–2
Copper T IUD	0.6–0.8
Levonorgestrel-releasing intrauterine system	0.1
NuvaRing	1–2
Transdermal combination contraceptive	1
Diaphragm (with spermicide)	6–20
Condom (female)	5–21
Condom (male)	3–14
Withdrawal	4–19
Spermicides	6–26
Periodic abstinence	9–25
No contraceptive method	85

Modified from Trussel, J.: Contraceptive Efficacy. In Hatcher, R. A, Trussel, J., Stewart, F., et al. Contraceptive Technology, 17th rev. ed. New York, Irvington Publishers, 1998.

[a]The failure rate for Implanon is estimated to be similar to that of Norplant. Several thousand women have used Implanon, and as of the end of 2001, no pregnancies were reported with proper use.

Combined Estrogen/Progestin Hormone Replacement Therapy

Similar to the combined estrogen and progestin oral contraceptives, combination estrogen/progestin products are available for use in HRT in women. In contrast to the oral contraceptives, in which the estrogen component is almost always ethinyl estradiol, the estrogen component of HRT products is typically conjugated estrogens or estradiol. The progestin component for HRT is often medroxyprogesterone acetate or norethindrone acetate. Table 23-5 lists the currently available combination products. Both oral tablets and a transdermal patch are used.

TREATMENT OF VASOMOTOR SYMPTOMS OF MENOPAUSE AND ATROPHIC VAGINITIS

Estrogens have been very useful in treating the "hot flashes" associated with early menopause, as well as atrophic vaginitis and other vaginal symptoms of inadequate estrogen production. The evidence that they result in enhanced mood and improved cognitive function in postmenopausal women is less clear, however, and more studies are needed to sort out the competing claims in these areas.[94–96]

OSTEOPOROSIS PREVENTION AND TREATMENT[97–99]

Osteoporosis is an enormous public health problem, responsible for approximately 1.5 million fractures in the United States each year. Because of the prevalence of osteoporosis, especially in older women, the prevention and treatment of this condition have received much attention. Prior to menopause, a good diet and exercise are essential for young women, to decrease the risk of osteoporosis later in life. After menopause, supplemental estrogens can have a positive effect relative to osteoporosis. Estrogens mainly act by decreasing bone resorption, so estrogens are better at preventing bone loss than restoring bone mass. Estrogens taken after menopause (often with a supplemental progestin) have been unequivocally shown to greatly decrease the incidence and severity of osteoporosis, especially when combined with good nutrition and exercise. The long-term use of estrogens plus a progestin for preventing osteoporosis should be carefully considered in light of the recent results of a study examining HRT for lowering the risk of heart disease (see below). Alternatives to estrogens for the prevention of osteoporosis, such as raloxifene, should also be considered.

POSTMENOPAUSAL ESTROGENS IN LOWERING RISK OF HEART DISEASE[100]

After years of general recommendations for the beneficial use of estrogens after menopause for lowering the risk of heart disease, the results of a long-term study with conjugated estrogens supplemented with a progestin have indicated that the risks of this approach outweigh the benefits. The Women's Health Initiative (WHI) trial, which enrolled over 16,000 postmenopausal women between 1993 and 1998, was terminated early in 2002 because of an unacceptably high level of adverse effects relative to the benefits gained. With long-term use (average follow-up of 5.2 years), there was a slight increase in the incidence of coronary heart disease, as well as an increase in breast cancer risk. Although there was a slight decrease in the risk of colorectal cancer and fewer hip fractures, the effects on the heart and breast argue against the use of estrogens plus a progestin for the prevention of coronary heart disease in postmenopausal women. Another WHI trial with estrogen alone in postmenopausal women without a uterus is still in progress. The estrogen-plus-progestin trial used, however, only one drug regimen (0.625 mg of conjugated equine estrogens and 2.5 mg of medroxyprogesterone acetate), so care should be taken in extending these results to other regimens and products. Also, the short-term use in the management of hot flashes and other postmenopausal symptoms is still appropriate.

An alternative to a combination estrogen/progestin drug for HRT would be a single compound that has both estrogenic and progestogenic actions. Tibolone (17α-hydroxy-7α-methyl-19-norpregn-5(10)-en-20-yn-3-one) is such a compound. It is a synthetic steroid that has diverse actions and is used alone in HRT in Europe as an alternative to standard estrogen or estrogen-plus-progestin therapy. Tibolone is awaiting FDA approval for use in HRT and for treating osteoporosis. It has been described as a tissue-specific compound with beneficial actions on bone, vagina, climacteric symptoms, mood, and sexual well-being but without stimulation of breast and endometrial tissue.[101, 102] Tibolone has estrogenic, progestogenic, and weak androgenic actions. This range of actions has been attributed to metabolites of tibolone (Fig. 23-22). Tibolone is rapidly converted to 3α- and 3β-hydroxy metabolites as well as a Δ^4 metabolite.[102] Despite the lack of an A-ring phenol, the hydroxy metabolites bind to the ER, while the Δ^4 metabolite binds to the progesterone and androgen receptors. The absence of stimu-

TABLE 23–5 Combined Progestin/Estrogen Hormone Replacement Therapy Products (Available in Tablets or a Transdermal Patch)

Brand	Progestin	Estrogen
Prempro	Medroxyprogesterone acetate, 2.5 or 5 mg	Conjugated estrogens, 0.625 mg
Premphase[a]	Medroxyprogesterone acetate, 5 mg	Conjugated estrogens, 0.625 mg
Femhrt	Norethindrone acetate, 1 mg	Ethinyl estradiol, 5 μg
Activella	Norethindrone acetate, 0.5 mg	Estradiol, 1 mg
Ortho-Prefest[b]	Norgestimate, 0.09 mg	Estradiol, 1 mg
CombiPatch	Norethindrone acetate, 0.14 or 0.25 mg	Estradiol, 50 μg

[a]Premphase is dosed 14 days of estrogen-only tablets (0.625 mg conjugated estrogens), followed by 14 days of combined progestin/estrogen.
[b]Ortho-Prefest is dosed 15 days of estradiol (1 mg) alone, then 15 days of the combined progestin/estrogen.

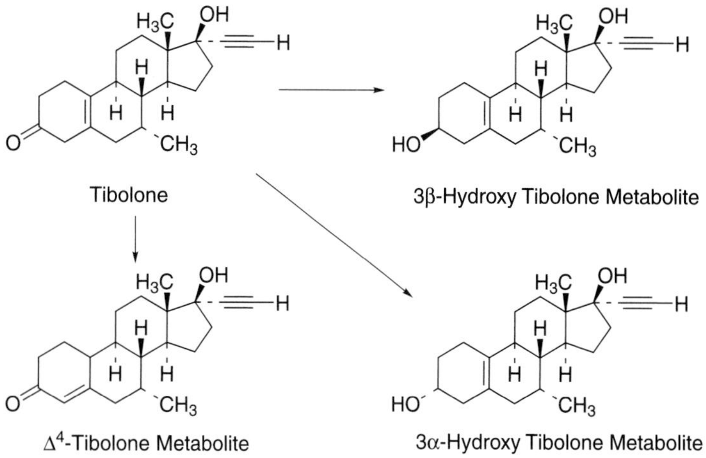

Figure 23–22 ■ Tibolone and its active metabolites.

lation of endometrial tissue has been attributed to progestational action of the Δ^4 metabolite. Tibolone and the 3β-hydroxy metabolite inhibit estrone sulfatase, which may partly explain the lack of breast tissue stimulation (the decreased amount of estrone that would be available for conversion to estradiol).[103] Although tibolone reduces high-density lipoprotein (HDL) levels, it has other positive effects on the cardiovascular system that may be beneficial.[104]

ANDROGENS[105]

Endogenous Androgens

Testosterone and its more potent reduction product 5α-DHT are produced in significantly greater amounts in males than in females, but females also produce low amounts of these "male" sex hormones. These endogenous compounds have two important activities: androgenic activity (promoting male sex characteristics) and anabolic activity (muscle-building).

DHEA and androstenedione are referred to as *adrenal androgens,* although this nomenclature is somewhat misleading. DHEA and androstenedione are biosynthetic precursors to the androgens but have only low affinity for the androgen receptors themselves.[106, 107] Therefore, DHEA or androstenedione can have androgenic actions, but only after in vivo conversion to testosterone and DHT. DHEA and androstenedione are, however, also precursors to the estrogens, so estrogenic actions may also occur.

Biosynthesis

As shown in Figure 23-5, testosterone can be synthesized through pregnenolone, DHEA, and androstenedione. About 7 mg/day is synthesized by young human adult males. Labeling experiments have also shown that it can be biosynthesized from androst-5-ene-3β,17β-diol, a reduction product of DHEA.

Testosterone is primarily produced by the interstitial cells of the testes, synthesized largely from cholesterol made in Sertoli cells. DHT is also secreted by the testes, as well as being produced in other tissues. The ovaries and adrenal cortex synthesize androstenedione and DHEA, which can be rapidly converted to testosterone in many tissues. Testosterone levels in the plasma of men are 5 to 100 times higher than those in the plasma of women.

Testosterone is produced in the testes in response to LH release by the anterior pituitary, as shown in Figure 23-10. Testosterone and DHT inhibit the production of LH and FSH by a feedback-inhibition process. This is quite similar to the feedback inhibition by estrogens and progestins in FSH and LH production.

Metabolism of Androgens

Testosterone is rapidly converted to 5α-DHT in many tissues by the action of 5 α-reductase. Depending on the tissue, this is either to activate testosterone to the more potent androgen, DHT (e.g., in the prostate), or a step in the metabolic inactivation of this androgen. The primary route for metabolic inactivation of testosterone and DHT is oxidation to the 17-one. The 3-one group is also reduced to the 3α- (major) and 3β-ols (minor). The metabolites are shown in Figure 23-23. Androsterone is the major urinary metabolite and was the first "androgenic" steroid isolated. These metabolites are excreted mainly as the corresponding glucuronides. Other minor metabolites have also been detected.[105]

Biological Activities of Androgens

Testosterone and DHT cause pronounced masculinizing effects, even in the male fetus. They induce the development of the prostate, penis, and related sexual tissues. At puberty, the secretion of testosterone by the testes increases greatly, leading to an increase in facial and body hair, deepening of the voice, increased protein anabolic activity and muscle mass, rapid growth of long bones, and loss of some subcutaneous fat. Spermatogenesis begins, and the prostate and seminal vesicles increase in activity. Sexual organs increase in size. The skin becomes thicker, and sebaceous glands increase in number, leading to acne in many young people. The androgens also play important roles in male psychology and behavior. In women, testosterone plays a role in libido, mood, muscle mass and strength, as well as bone density.[108, 109]

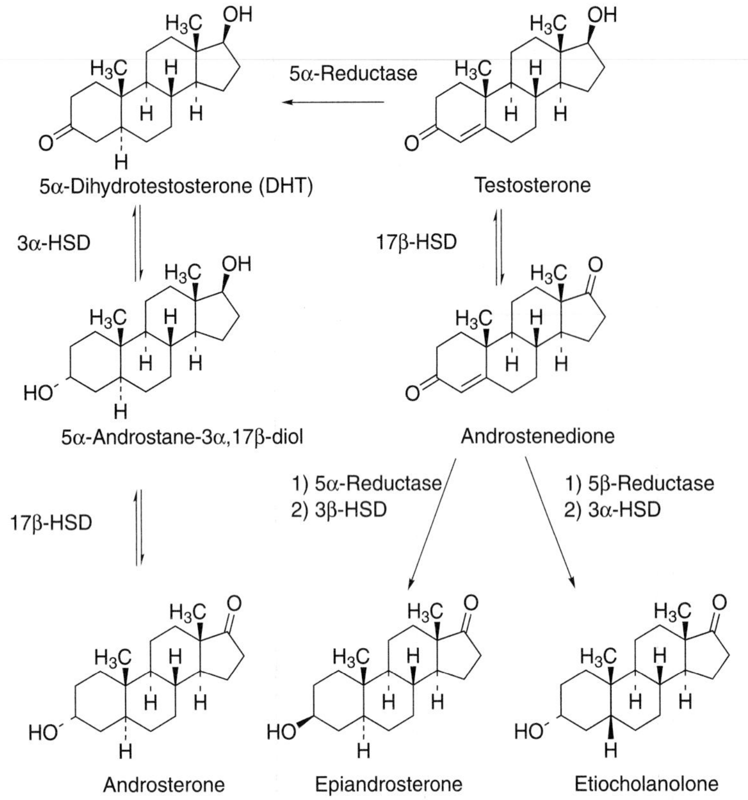

Figure 23–23 ■ Metabolism of testosterone and 5α-DHT (conjugates of the metabolites are also formed). *HSD*, hydroxysteroid dehydrogenase.

Structural Classes—Anabolic Androgenic Steroids

The androgens, also known as anabolic androgenic steroids (AAS), include all of the therapeutic agents whose main actions are mediated by the androgen receptors. The inclusion of both *anabolic* and *androgenic* in referring to these compounds reflects the fact that no products are available in which the anabolic properties of androgens can be separated from the androgenic properties. The commonly used AAS are shown in Figure 23-24. Several recent reviews on AAS have been published.[105, 110]

SEMISYNTHETIC ANALOGUES

Because bacterial and hepatic oxidation of the 17β-hydroxyl to the 17-one is a key component of metabolic inactivation, 17α-alkyl groups have been added to prevent oxidation of the alcohol. Even though 17α-methyltestosterone is only about half as active as testosterone, it can be taken orally because its half-life is longer than that of testosterone. 17α-Ethyltestosterone has greatly reduced activity, as shown in Table 23-6.[111] As mentioned above, addition of an α-alkynyl group provides more progestogenic action than androgenic action, although some activity at androgen receptors is retained. A disadvantage of the 17α-methyl testosterones is hepatotoxicity. Hepatic disturbances, jaundice (occasionally), and death (in rare cases) may occur, particularly in the high doses often used by athletes (see next section).

Table 23-6 illustrates some structure–activity effects of the androgens, such as the greatly decreased activity of the 17α-ol isomer of testosterone (epitestosterone). Hundreds

TABLE 23–6 Androgenic Activities of Some Androgens

Compound	μg Equivalent to an International Unit
Testosterone (17 β-ol)	15
Epitestosterone (17 α-ol)	400
17 α-Methyltestosterone	25–30
17 α-Ethyltestosterone	70–100
17 α-Methylandrostane-3α, 17 β-diol	35
17 α-Methylandrostane-3-one-17 β-ol	15
Androsterone	100
Epiandrosterone	700
Androstane-3α, 17 β-diol	20–25
Androstane-3α, 17 α-diol	350
Androstane-3β, 17 β-diol	500
Androstane-17β-ol-3-one	20
Androstane-17α-ol-3-one	300
Δ^5-Androstene-3α, 17β-diol	35
Δ^5-Androstene-3β, 17β-diol	500
Androstanedione-3, 17	120–130
Δ^4-Androstenedione	120

Data are from Djerassi, C.: J. Chem. Soc. 76:4092, 1954.

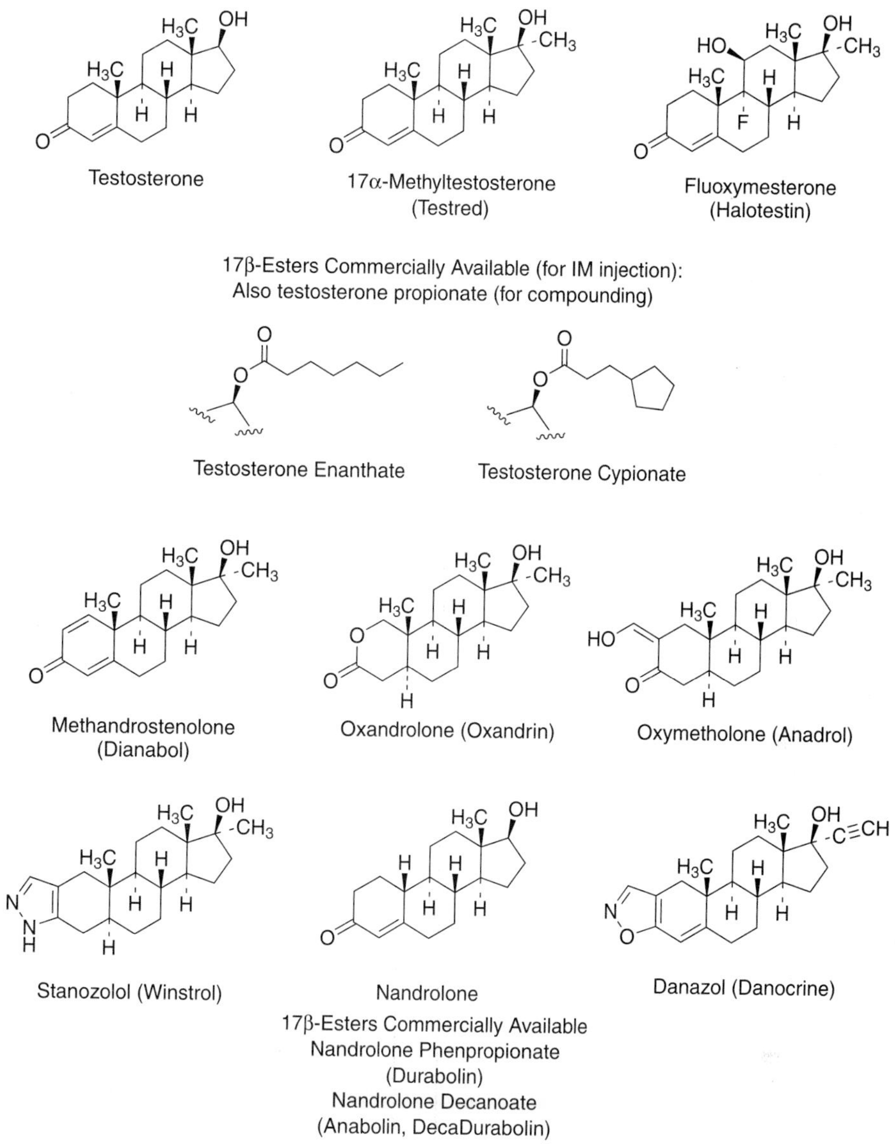

Testosterone

17α-Methyltestosterone
(Testred)

Fluoxymesterone
(Halotestin)

17β-Esters Commercially Available (for IM injection):
Also testosterone propionate (for compounding)

Testosterone Enanthate

Testosterone Cypionate

Methandrostenolone
(Dianabol)

Oxandrolone (Oxandrin)

Oxymetholone (Anadrol)

Stanozolol (Winstrol)

Nandrolone
17β-Esters Commercially Available
Nandrolone Phenpropionate
(Durabolin)
Nandrolone Decanoate
(Anabolin, DecaDurabolin)

Danazol (Danocrine)

Figure 23–24 ■ Testosterone and synthetic anabolic androgenic steroids.

of different AAS have been synthesized and studied. The goal of many synthetic programs was to make a compound that possessed the anabolic properties of testosterone but lacked its androgenic actions. While numerous compounds were prepared that did display improved anabolic/androgenic ratios in vitro, no compounds completely lacked androgenic action.[110] Also, the high anabolic/androgenic ratios did not appear to be maintained when these drugs were used in humans. Despite the many compounds that have been examined, the structure–activity relationships of these drugs are not well delineated. Many hypotheses have been made in an attempt to summarize the structure–activity relationships of all the known androgens.[105] As with other compounds that have been discussed, hydroxyl groups in the testosterones are often converted to the corresponding esters to prolong activity or to provide some protection from oxidation.

Therapeutic Uses of Anabolic Androgenic Steroids

The primary use of AAS is in androgen replacement therapy in men, either at maturity or in adolescence. The cause of

testosterone deficiency may be either hypogonadism or hypopituitarism.

The use of the AAS for their anabolic activity or for uses other than androgen replacement has been limited because of their masculinizing actions. This has greatly limited their use in women and children. Although anabolic activity is often needed clinically, none of the products presently available is free of significant androgenic side effects.

The masculinizing (androgenic) side effects in females include hirsutism, acne, deepening of the voice, clitoral enlargement, and depression of the menstrual cycle. Furthermore, AAS generally alter serum lipid levels and increase the probability of atherosclerosis, characteristically a disease of men and postmenopausal women.

The masculinizing effects of the AAS preclude their use in most circumstances in women. Secondary treatment of advanced or metastatic breast carcinoma in selected patients is generally considered to be the only indication for large-dose, long-term androgen therapy in women. In lower doses, androgen replacement therapy is more often being considered for use in menopausal and postmenopausal women for the positive effects on libido, mood, vasomotor symptoms, and muscle mass, all areas negatively affected by decreased testosterone levels in aging women.[112]

Androgens are also used to relieve bone pain associated with osteoporosis and to treat certain anemias, although this use has greatly decreased because of the availability of erythropoietin. In all cases, use of these agents requires caution.

Androgens and Sports

The use of androgens for their anabolic effects (hence the term *anabolic steroids*) by athletes began in the late 1940s and has, at times, been widespread.[113] Prior to urine testing requirements, it was estimated that up to 80% of competitive weight lifters and about 75% of professional football players used these drugs, along with a variety of other athletes. International awareness of the abuse of steroids by athletes, however, was limited until the 1988 Olympics when Canada's Ben Johnson was disqualified as the winner of the gold medal in the 100-yard dash for having traces of stanozolol in his urine. The shocking disqualification brought the international misuse of AAS to headlines worldwide. Unfortunately, abuse of steroids is still a problem at all levels of competitive sports.

Although numerous "anabolic" steroids have been synthesized and used/abused by athletes, most likely all of the androgens have been used by athletes in an attempt to improve strength and increase muscle mass. In the early years, the 17α-alkylated steroids with high anabolic/androgenic ratios in vitro were used with the belief that the anabolic properties of these drugs were greater than those of other androgens such as testosterone. With the ban on the use of steroids in most sports and the prevalence of drug testing, however, the 17α-alkylated steroids have fallen out of favor because of the ease of detecting these compounds by mass spectrometry. This has led to a greater use of testosterone and its esters, as well as the androgen precursors androstenedione ("andro"), androstenediol, androstanediol, and DHEA. The belief is that because these steroids all occur naturally, detecting them will be much more difficult. While it is true that assays for the endogenous steroids must now discriminate deviations from normal ratios, it is possible to detect the abuse of these compounds. Externally supplied testosterone, for example, can be detected by a urine test examining the ratio of testosterone glucuronide to epitestosterone glucuronide. A ratio greater than 6:1 usually indicates abuse.[114]

Many studies have attempted to determine if taking anabolic steroids improves athletic performance.[110, 115] Some failed to use controls (athletes who trained in an identical manner but did not take anabolic steroids). Others failed to use placebos in at least a single-blind research design (neither the treated nor control groups knowing which they were taking). An additional problem with many of the studies has been that typical therapeutic doses have been tested for their anabolic properties in clinical settings, whereas athletes typically use much higher doses.[110, 116] Of the studies using at least a single-blind protocol, some have reported that anabolic steroids did increase athletic performance, whereas others found they did not. It would be fair to say, therefore, that the benefit of anabolic steroids to athletic performance is uncertain. The risks of using these drugs appear to outweigh their uncertain benefits.

As summarized by the FDA,[117] the side effects include

In both sexes
  Increased risk of coronary heart disease, stroke, or obstructed blood vessels
  Increased aggression and antisocial behavior (known as "steroid rage")
  Liver tumors, peliosis hepatis (blood-filled cysts), and jaundice (for 17α-alkylated androgens only)
In men
  Testicular atrophy with consequent sterility or decreased sperm count and abnormal motility and morphology
  Impotence
  Enlarged prostate
  Breast enlargement
In women
  Clitoral enlargement
  Beard growth
  Baldness
  Deepened voice
  Breast diminution

Because of these risks, the International Olympic Committee, numerous professional sports organizations, and the National Collegiate Athletic Association (NCAA) banned all anabolic drugs. Testing of elite athletes for performance-enhancing drugs of all types is commonplace. Despite the known problems with the use of AAS, however, some professional sports have been slow to enact testing for performance-enhancing drugs. As of the summer of 2002, Major League Baseball was finalizing a testing policy for its athletes, while the National Hockey League still lacked a policy on the use of anabolic steroids.

An additional risk is associated with self-injection of long-lasting anabolic steroid preparations. The risk of contracting hepatitis A, hepatitis C, and human immunodeficiency virus (HIV) is increased if needles used for injecting steroids are shared.[118]

Anabolic Androgenic Steroid Products

Therapeutic uses of the androgens are discussed above. 17β-Esters and 17α-alkyl products are available for a complete range of therapeutic uses. These drugs are contraindicated in men with prostatic cancer; in men or women with heart, kidney, or liver disease; and in pregnancy. Diabetics using the androgens should be carefully monitored. Androgens potentiate the action of oral anticoagulants, causing bleeding in some patients, and they may also interfere with some laboratory tests. Female patients may develop virilization side effects, and doctors should be warned that some of these effects may be irreversible (e.g., voice changes). All of the "anabolic" agents currently commercially available (methandrostenolone, oxymetholone, oxandrolone, stanozolol, nandrolone) have significant androgenic activity; hence, virilization is a potential problem for all women patients. Many of the anabolic agents are orally active, as one would predict by noting a 17α-alkyl group in many of them (see Fig. 23-24). Those without the 17α-alkyl (nandrolone decanoate and nandrolone phenpropionate) are active only intramuscularly. The 17α-alkyl products may induce liver toxicity in some patients.

All steroid 4-en-3-ones are light sensitive and should be kept in light-resistant containers.

Testosterone, USP.   Testosterone, 17β-hydroxyandrost-4-en-3-one, is a naturally occurring androgen in men.

In women, it mainly serves as a biosynthetic precursor to estradiol but also has other hormonal effects. It is rapidly metabolized to relatively inactive 17-ones (see Fig. 23-23), however, preventing significant oral activity. Testosterone is available in a transdermal delivery system (patch), a gel formulation, and as implantable pellets. Testosterone 17β-esters are available in long-acting intramuscular depot preparations illustrated in Figure 23-24, including the following:

- Testosterone cypionate, USP: Testosterone 17β-cyclopentylpropionate
- Testosterone enanthate, USP: Testosterone 17β-heptanoate
- Testosterone propionate, USP: Testosterone 17β-propionate

Methyltestosterone, USP. Methyltestosterone, 17β-hydroxy-17-methylandrost-4-en-3-one, is only about half as active as testosterone (intramuscularly), but it has the great advantage of being orally active.

Fluoxymesterone, USP. Fluoxymesterone, 9α-fluoro-11β,17β-dihydroxy-17-methylandrost-4-en-3-one, is a highly potent, orally active androgen, about 5 to 10 times more potent than testosterone. It can be used for all the indications discussed above, but its great androgenic activity has made it useful primarily for treatment of the androgen-deficient male.

Methandrostenolone, USP. Methandrostenolone, 17β-hydroxy-17-methylandrosta-1,4-dien-3-one, is orally active and about equal in potency to testosterone.

Oxymetholone, USP. Oxymetholone, 17β-hydroxy-2-(hydroxymethylene)-17-methylandrostan-3-one, is approved for the treatment of a variety of anemias.

Oxandrolone, USP. Oxandrolone, 17β-hydroxy-17-methyl-2-oxaandrostan-3-one, is approved to aid in the promotion of weight gain after weight loss following surgery, chronic infections, or severe trauma and to offset protein catabolism associated with long-term corticosteroid use. Oxandrolone is also used to relieve bone pain accompanying osteoporosis. It has been used to treat alcoholic hepatitis and HIV wasting syndrome.

Stanozolol, USP. Stanozolol, 17-methyl-2′/H-5α-androst-2-eno[3,2,c]-pyrazol-17β-ol, is used prophylactically in the management of hereditary angioedema to reduce the frequency and severity of attacks.

Nandrolone Decanoate, USP, and Nandrolone Phenpropionate, USP. Nandrolone decanoate, 17β-hydroxyestr-4-en-3-one 17-decanoate, has been used in the management of certain anemias, but the availability of erythropoietin has greatly reduced this use. Nandrolone phenpropionate is 17β-hydroxyestr-4-en-3-one 17-(3′-phenyl)propionate.

Danazol and Endometriosis

Danazol, USP. Danazol, 17α-pregna-2,4-dien-20-yno[2,3-d]isoxazol-17-ol (Danocrine), is a weak androgen that, in spite of the 17α-ethinyl group, has little estrogenic or progestogenic activity. Danazol has been called a synthetic steroid with diverse biological effects.[119] Danazol binds to sex-hormone-binding globulin (SHBG) and decreases the hepatic synthesis of this estradiol and testosterone carrier. Free testosterone thus increases. Danazol inhibits FSH and LH production by the hypothalamus and pituitary. It binds to progesterone receptors, glucocorticoid receptors, androgen receptors, and ERs. Although the exact mechanism of action is unclear, danazol alters endometrial tissue so that it becomes inactive and atrophic, which allows danazol to be an effective treatment for endometriosis. Danazol is also used to treat hereditary angioedema and fibrocystic breast disease.

Antiandrogens

A variety of compounds (Fig. 23-25) have been intensively studied as androgen receptor antagonists, or antiandrogens.[120, 121] Antiandrogens are of therapeutic use in treating conditions of hyperandrogenism (e.g., hirsutism, acute acne, and premature baldness) or androgen-stimulated cancers (e.g., prostatic carcinoma). The ideal antiandrogen would be nontoxic, highly active, and devoid of any hormonal activity. Both steroidal and nonsteroidal antiandrogens have been investigated, but only nonsteroidal antiandrogens have been approved for use in the United States. Cyproterone acetate, a steroidal antiandrogen, is used in Europe. The steroidal antiandrogens typically have actions at other steroid receptors that limit their use. The nonsteroidal antiandrogens, while lacking hormonal activity, bind with lower affinity to the androgen receptor than the endogenous hormones.

FLUTAMIDE, BICALUTAMIDE, AND NILUTAMIDE

Three nonsteroidal antiandrogens are in clinical use in the United States—flutamide, bicalutamide, and nilutamide (Fig. 23-25). They are mainly used in the management of prostate cancer. Flutamide was the first of these compounds approved for use by the FDA, but liver toxicity and thrice-daily dosing offered room for improvement. It was also determined that a metabolite of flutamide, hydroxyflutamide, had greater antiandrogen action than the parent. Bicalutamide, which has greater potency than flutamide, incorporates a hydroxyl into its structure at the same relative position as in hydroxyflutamide. Bicalutamide is dosed once a day and has less toxicity than flutamide and nilutamide, making it a preferred choice when initiating therapy.

Prostate cancer is strongly androgen sensitive, so by blocking androgen receptors, the cancer can be inhibited or slowed. Studies have shown that these drugs completely inhibit the action of testosterone and other androgens by binding to androgen receptors. In clinical trials when given as a single agent for prostate cancer, serum testosterone and estradiol increase. But when given in combination with a GnRH agonist, such as goserelin or leuprolide, bicalutamide and flutamide do not affect testosterone suppression, which is the result of GnRH. GnRH agonists greatly decrease gonadal function—the medical equivalent of castration in men. Thus, the combination of GnRH with bicalutamide or flutamide blocks the production of testosterone in the testes and androgen receptors in the prostate.

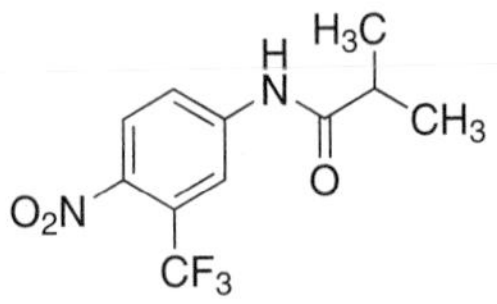

Flutamide (Eulexin)

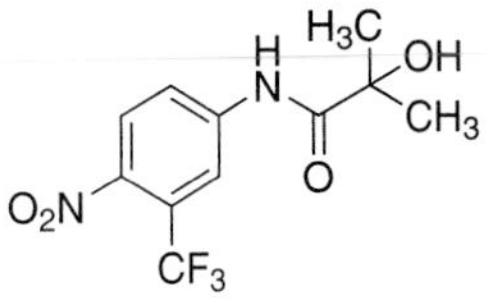

Hydroxyflutamide

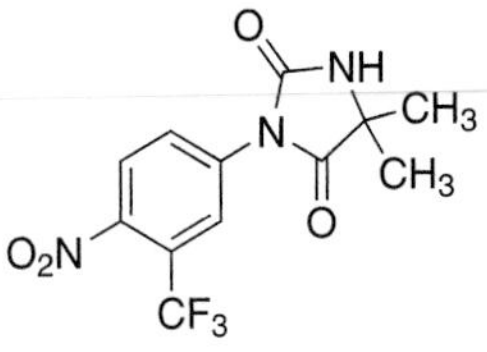

Nilutamide (Nilandron)

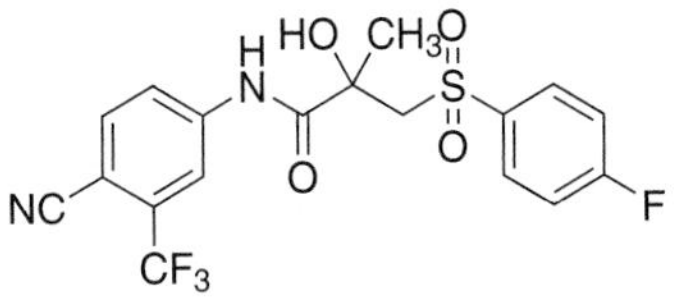

Bicalutamide (Casodex)

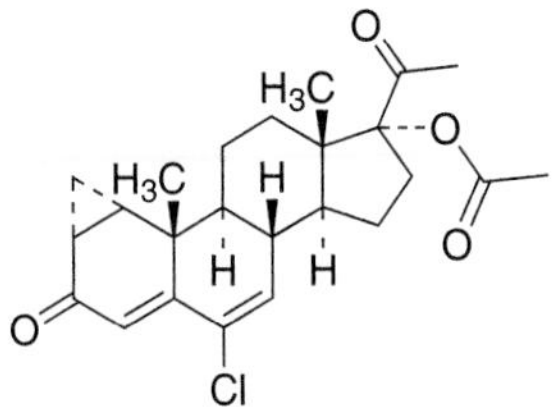

Cyproterone Acetate

Figure 23–25 ■ Antiandrogens.

Antiandrogen Products

Flutamide, USP. Flutamide, 2-methyl-*N*-[4-nitro-3-(trifluoromethyl)phenyl]propanamide (Eulexin), is dosed 3 times daily (250-mg dose; 750-mg total daily dose). A major metabolite of flutamide, hydroxyflutamide, is a more potent androgen receptor antagonist than the parent compound. This metabolite, which is present at a much higher steady-state concentration than is flutamide, contributes a significant amount of the antiandrogen action of this drug. A limiting factor in the use of flutamide is hepatotoxicity in from 1 to 5% of patients. Although the hepatotoxicity usually is reversible following cessation of treatment, rare cases of death associated with hepatic failure have been reported to be associated with flutamide therapy. Diarrhea is also a limiting side effect with flutamide therapy for some patients.

Bicalutamide, USP. Bicalutamide, *N*-4-cyano-3-(trifluoromethyl)phenyl-3-[(4-fluorophenyl)sulfonyl]-2-hydroxy-2-methyl-propanamide (Casodex), is more potent than flutamide and has a much longer half-life (5.9 days versus 6 hours for hydroxyflutamide). Because of the longer half-life, bicalutamide is used for once-a-day (50 mg) treatment of advanced prostate cancer. Bicalutamide is available as a racemic mixture, but both animal and human studies with the androgen receptor show that the *R* enantiomer has higher affinity for the androgen receptor than the *S* enantiomer.[122]

Nilutamide, USP. Nilutamide, 5,5-dimethyl-3-[4-nitro-3-(trifluoromethyl)phenyl]-2,4-imidazolidinedione, is used in combination with surgical castration for the treatment of metastatic prostate cancer. Nilutamide, which has an elimination half-life of approximately 40 hours, can also be used in once-daily dosing, but it has side effects that limit its use—visual disturbances, alcohol intolerance, and allergic pneumonitis.

Inhibition of 5α-Reductase

5α-DHT is important for maintaining prostate function in men. The formation of DHT is mediated by 5α-reductase, an enzyme that has two distinct forms, type I and type II.[123, 124] The type I enzyme is located in the liver and some peripheral tissues and is involved mainly in the metabolism of testosterone and other A-ring enones. The type II enzyme is located in the prostate gland and testes and is responsible for the conversion of testosterone to DHT for androgenic action. Blocking this enzyme is one approach for controlling androgen action. The 1997 review by Harris and Kozarich provides an excellent background and details the development of finasteride, the first 5α-reductase inhibitor approved for use in the United States (Fig. 23-26).[125]

DHT also plays a major role in the pathogenesis of benign prostatic hyperplasia (BPH). Finasteride, (5α,17β)-*N*-(1,1-dimethylethyl)-3-oxo-4-azaandrost-1-ene-17-carboxamide (Proscar, Propecia), is a potent, slow, tight-binding inhibitor of 5α-reductase that functions by a unique mechanism. Finasteride is activated by the enzyme and irreversibly binds to the NADP cofactor, yielding a finasteride–NADP complex that is only slowly released from the enzyme active site, producing essentially irreversible inhibition of the enzyme (Fig. 23-27).[126] The turnover from the finasteride–5α-reductase complex is very slow ($t_{1/2}$ ~30 days).

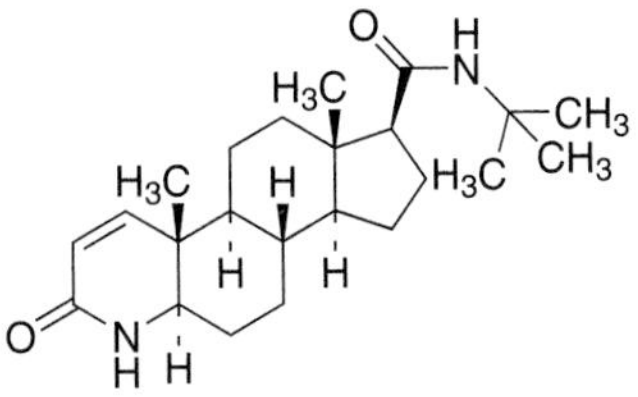

Finasteride
(Proscar, Propecia)

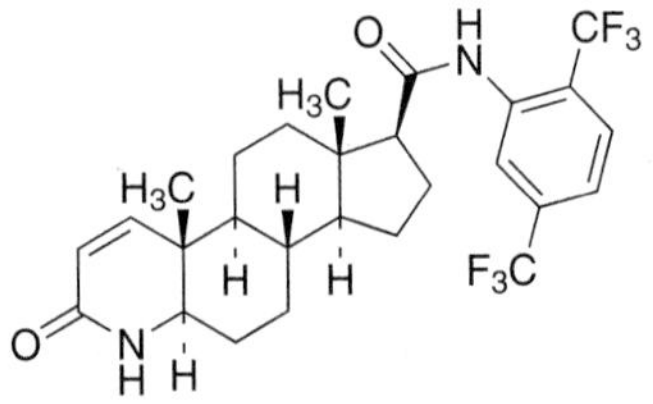

Dutasteride

Figure 23–26 ■ Steroid 5α-reductase inhibitors.

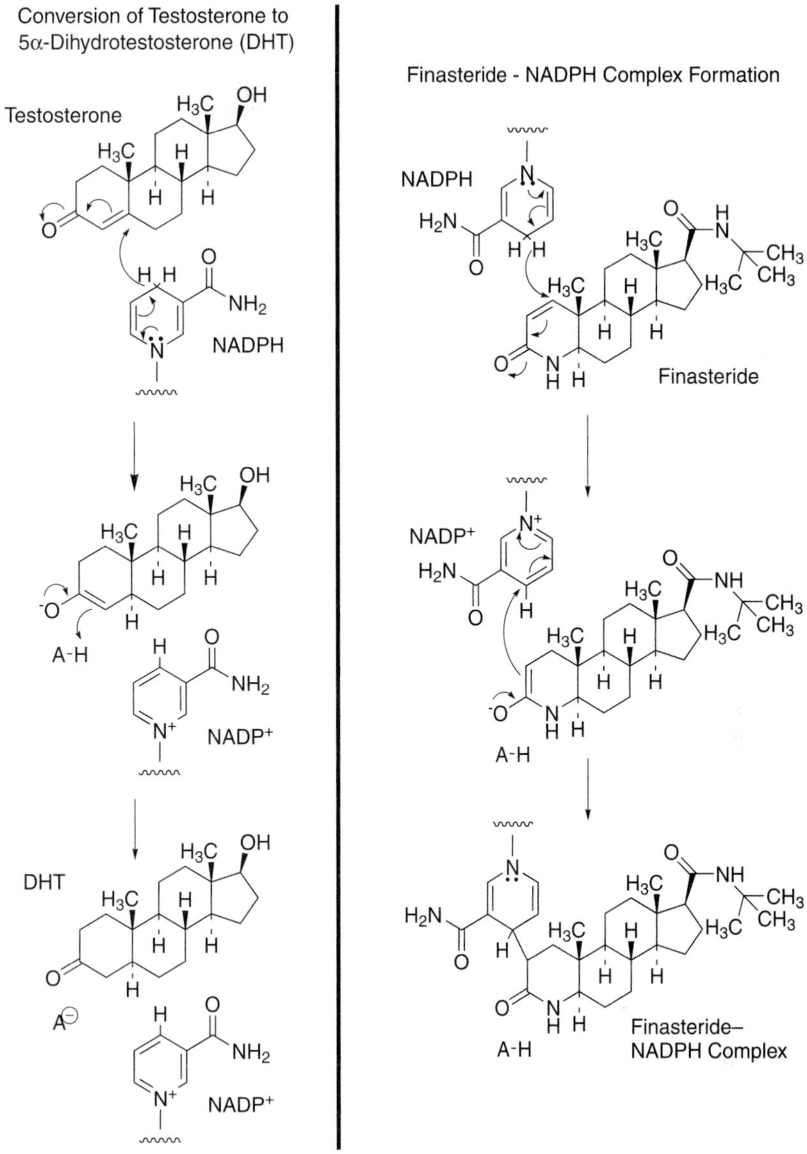

Figure 23–27 ■ Comparison of 5α-reductase action on testosterone and finasteride. This scheme is an oversimplification of the exact mechanisms, but it indicates that when finasteride is bound at the active site of 5α-reductase, NADPH is positioned closer to C1 of finasteride than to the normal C5 of testosterone, leading to essentially irreversible inhibition.

Finasteride is a relatively selective inhibitor of type II 5α-reductase. This enzyme is present in high levels in the prostate and at lower levels in other tissues. Because of the strong connection to the formation of DHT in the prostate, it was theorized that specific inhibition of this isoform would yield the greatest therapeutic effect. More recent studies suggest, however, that the type I isoform may also play a role in the progression of hormone-dependent prostate cancer.[127] Because of this, dual 5α-reductase inhibitors have been developed. Dutasteride, a compound recently approved for treating BPH, inhibits both isoforms of the enzyme and may be found to have superior therapeutic effects once it is broadly used (Fig. 23-26). Dutasteride bears an aromatic amide at C17, rather than the *t*-butyl amide seen in finasteride.

A second use of finasteride is in the treatment of male pattern baldness. The conversion of testosterone to DHT in advancing years leads to thinning of hair in men. Inhibition of this conversion was envisioned as a possible baldness treatment. After finasteride was shown to be safe and effective in the treatment of BPH, a lower dose formulation was studied for treating male pattern baldness. The trials were a success, and Propecia (1 mg/day) was the result. Although finasteride preferentially inhibits the type II enzyme, it is believed to be the peripheral type-I 5α-reductase that is being targeted for the baldness treatment. Dutasteride is also being investigated for use as a baldness treatment.

Saw palmetto *(Serenoa repens)* extract is an herbal product used to treat BPH, and it has been suggested that the effects can be attributed to a constituent of the extract with 5α-reductase inhibition, but other mechanisms have also been proposed.[128] Further studies and identification of a specific component that inhibits 5α-reductase are necessary.

ADRENAL CORTEX HORMONES

Endogenous Corticosteroids

The adrenal glands (which lie just above the kidneys) secrete over 50 different steroids, including precursors for other steroid hormones. The most important hormonal steroids produced by the adrenal cortex, however, are aldosterone and hydrocortisone. Aldosterone is the primary *mineralocorticoid* in humans (i.e., it causes significant salt retention). Hydrocortisone is the primary *glucocorticoid* in humans (i.e., it has its primary effects on intermediary metabolism). The glucocorticoids have become very important in modern medicine, especially for their anti-inflammatory effects.

Aldosterone and, to a lesser extent, other mineralocorticoids maintain a constant electrolyte balance and blood vol-ume. The glucocorticoids have key roles in controlling carbohydrate, protein, and lipid metabolism.

Biosynthesis

As shown in the scheme in Figure 23-28, aldosterone and hydrocortisone are biosynthesized from pregnenolone through a series of steps involving hydroxylations at C17, C11, and C21 that convert pregnenolone to hydrocortisone. Deficiencies in any of the enzymes cause congenital adrenal

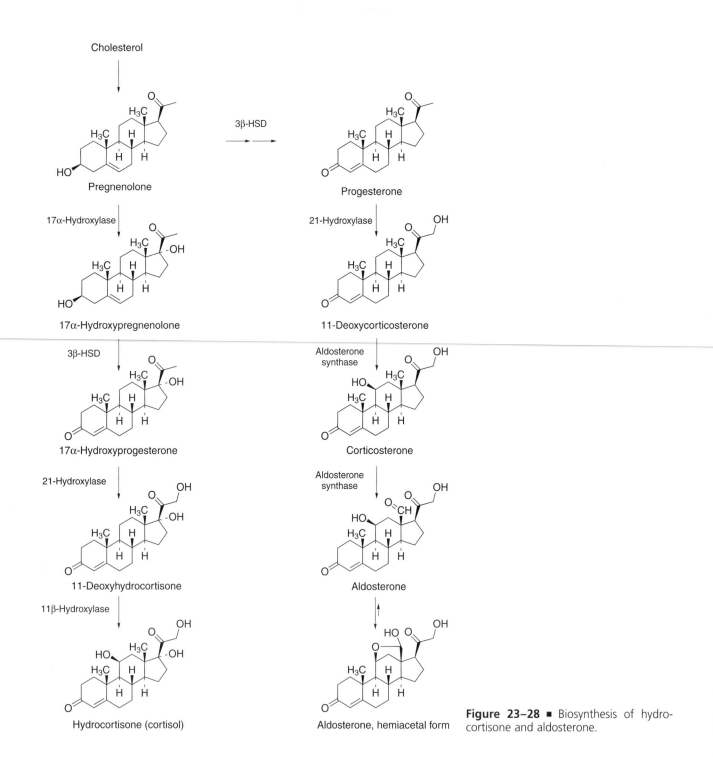

Figure 23–28 ■ Biosynthesis of hydrocortisone and aldosterone.

hyperplasia. Defects in the gene regulation, as well as the enzymes that catalyze the hydroxylation have been studied intensively.[129–131] Investigators have linked defects in particular genes or steroid-binding sites to the pathophysiology of patients with the corresponding metabolic diseases.[131]

These disorders are usually caused by an inability of the adrenal glands to carry out 11β-, 17α-, or 21-hydroxylations. The most common is a lack of 21-hydroxylase activity, which will result in decreased production of hydrocortisone and a compensatory increase in adrenocorticotropic hormone (ACTH) production. Furthermore, the resultant buildup of 17α-hydroxyprogesterone will lead to an increase of testosterone. The 21-hydroxylase is important for the synthesis of both mineralocorticoids and glucocorticoids. When 11β-hydroxylase activity is low, large amounts of 11-deoxycorticosterone will be produced. Because 11-deoxycorticosterone is a potent mineralocorticoid, there will be symptoms of mineralocorticoid excess, including hypertension. When 17α-hydroxylase activity is low, there will be decreased production of testosterone and estrogens as well as hydrocortisone.

Although the details are not completely known, the 39-amino acid peptide ACTH (corticotropin) produced by the anterior pituitary is necessary for the conversion of cholesterol to pregnenolone. ACTH acts at the ACTH receptor, a G-protein–coupled receptor that activates adenylyl cyclase, leading to increased cAMP levels. Activation of the ACTH receptors has short- and long-term effects on steroidogenesis. The short-term phase involves an increase in the supply of cholesterol for use by cytochrome P-450$_{scc}$ in the formation of pregnenolone. The long-term effects are due to increased transcription of steroidogenic enzymes.[132] An overall result of ACTH action is increased synthesis and release of hydrocortisone. Hydrocortisone then acts by feedback inhibition to suppress the formation of additional ACTH. (ACTH is discussed in more detail in Chapter 25.)

The release of the primary mineralocorticoid aldosterone depends only slightly on ACTH. Aldosterone is an active part of the angiotensin–renin–blood pressure cycle that controls blood volume. A decrease in blood volume stimulates the kidneys to secrete the enzyme renin. Renin, in turn, converts angiotensinogen to angiotensin, which stimulates the adrenal cortex to release aldosterone. Aldosterone then causes the kidneys to retain sodium, and blood volume increases. When the blood volume has increased sufficiently, renin production decreases, until blood volume drops again.

Metabolism of Hydrocortisone

Hydrocortisone and cortisone are enzymatically interconvertible, and thus one finds metabolites with both the 11-keto and the 11β-hydroxy functionality. Most of the metabolic processes occur in the liver, with the metabolites excreted primarily in the urine. Although many metabolites have been isolated, the primary routes of catabolism are (a) reduction of the C4,5 double bond to yield 5β-pregnanes, (b) reduction of the 3-one to give 3α-ols, and (c) reduction of the 20-one to the corresponding 20α- and 20β-ols. These are the same steps that are involved in progesterone metabolism. The two primary metabolites are tetrahydrocortisol and tetrahydrocortisone and their conjugates. The cortols (20α and 20β),

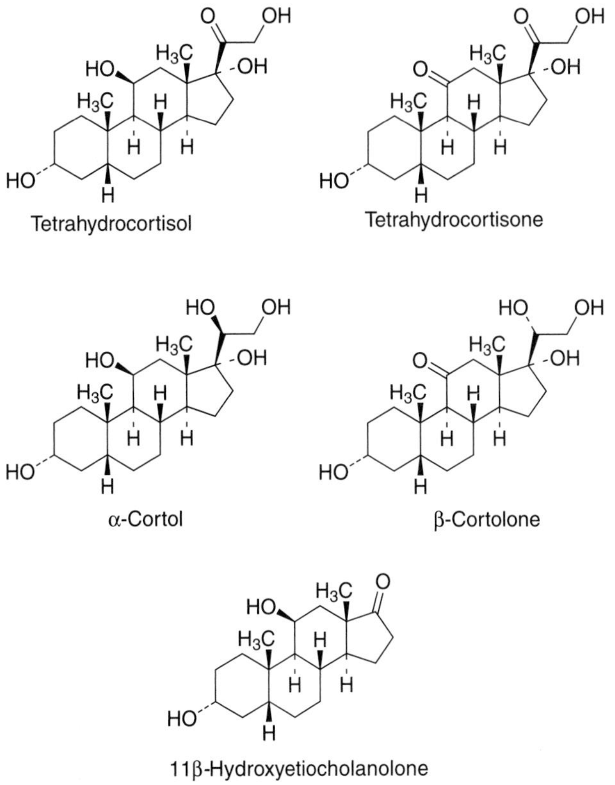

Figure 23–29 ▪ Metabolites of cortisone and hydrocortisone.

cortolones (20α and 20β), and 11β-hydroxyetiocholanolone are some of the minor metabolites of hydrocortisone (Fig. 23-29).

Biological Activities of Mineralocorticoids and Glucocorticoids

The adrenocortical steroids permit the body to adjust to environmental changes, to stress, and to changes in the diet. Aldosterone and, to a lesser extent, other mineralocorticoids maintain a constant electrolyte balance and blood volume, and the glucocorticoids have key roles in controlling carbohydrate, protein, and lipid metabolism.

Aldosterone increases sodium reabsorption in the kidneys. An increase in plasma sodium concentration, in turn, will lead to increased blood volume, because blood volume and urinary excretion of water are directly related to the plasma sodium concentration. Simultaneously, aldosterone increases potassium ion excretion. 11-Deoxycorticosterone also is quite active as a mineralocorticoid. Similar actions are exhibited with hydrocortisone and corticosterone, but to a much smaller degree.

Aldosterone controls the movement of sodium ions in most epithelial structures involved in active sodium transport. Although aldosterone acts primarily on the distal convoluted tubules of the kidneys, it also acts on the proximal convoluted tubules and collecting ducts. Aldosterone controls the transport of sodium in sweat glands, small intestine, salivary glands, and the colon. In all of these tissues, aldosterone enhances the inward flow of sodium ions and promotes the outward flow of potassium ions.

The glucocorticoids have many physiological and pharmacological actions. They control or influence carbohydrate, protein, lipid, and purine metabolism. They also affect the cardiovascular and nervous systems and skeletal muscle. They regulate growth hormone gene expression. In addition, glucocorticoids have anti-inflammatory and immunosuppressive actions that arise through complex mechanisms.

Glucocorticoids stimulate glycogen storage synthesis by inducing the synthesis of glycogen synthase and stimulate gluconeogenesis in the liver. They have a catabolic effect on muscle tissue, stimulating the formation and transamination of amino acids into glucose precursors in the liver. The catabolic actions in Cushing's syndrome are demonstrated by wasting of the tissues, osteoporosis, and reduced muscle mass. Lipid metabolism and synthesis increase significantly in the presence of glucocorticoids, but the actions usually seem to depend on the presence of other hormones or cofactors. A lack of adrenal cortex steroids also causes depression, irritability, and even psychoses, reflecting significant effects on the central nervous system.

ANTI-INFLAMMATORY/IMMUNOSUPPRESSIVE ACTIONS OF GLUCOCORTICOIDS[133–137]

Glucocorticoid-receptor complexes (see Fig. 23-7) may activate or repress the genes to which they associate. Repression in particular may have an important role in glucocorticoid anti-inflammatory actions. Glucocorticoids inhibit the transcription of genes encoding cytokines such as interferon-γ, tumor necrosis factor-α (TNF-α), the interleukins, and granulocyte/monocyte colony-stimulating factor, all factors involved in the immune system and inflammatory responses.[132] Glucocorticoids inhibit the production and release of other mediators of inflammation, including prostaglandins, leukotrienes, and histamine. In addition, glucocorticoids inhibit the expression of the gene encoding collagenase, an important enzyme involved with inflammation.

RESISTANCE TO GLUCOCORTICOIDS[138–140]

A few patients with chronic inflammatory illnesses such as asthma, rheumatoid arthritis, and lupus develop resistance to the anti-inflammatory effects of the glucocorticoids. The mechanism is not fully understood but appears to be a decrease in the binding or activation ability of glucocorticoid receptor complexes and their target or "activator" genes. Disruption of the translocation of the glucocorticoid receptor to the nucleus has also been implicated in glucocorticoid resistance.[141]

Structural Classes: Mineralocorticoids and Glucocorticoids

Medically important adrenal cortex hormones and synthetic mineralocorticoids and glucocorticoids are shown in Figure 23-30. Because salt retention activity is usually undesirable, the drugs are classified by their salt retention activities. As illustrated in Figure 23-30, the adrenal cortex hormones are classified by their biological activities into three major groups.

MINERALOCORTICOIDS

The mineralocorticoids are adrenal cortex steroids and analogues with high salt-retaining activity. They are used mainly for treatment of Addison's disease, or primary adrenal insufficiency. The naturally occurring hormone aldosterone has an 11β-OH and an 18-CHO that naturally bridge to form a hemiacetal (as drawn in Fig. 23-28). Aldosterone is too expensive to produce commercially; therefore other semisynthetic analogues have taken its place for treatment of Addison's disease. Adding a 9α-fluoro group to hydrocortisone greatly increases both salt retention and anti-inflammatory activity. Deoxycorticosterone (11-deoxy), an intermediate in the biosynthesis of aldosterone, has lower mineralocorticoid activity than aldosterone (~20-fold) but may play a role if the 11β-hydroxylase is deficient. Deoxycorticosterone is not available for therapeutic uses.

Extensive modifications have been made to the basic hydrocortisone structure to alter the properties of glucocorticoids. Modifications at all sites of the steroid backbone have been tried. Aside from addition of a double bond at C1–C2, the most beneficial changes are made to rings B and D of the steroid skeleton and modification of the C17 side chain. Table 23-7 summarizes the relative effects of various substituents seen in commercially available products on salt retention and glucocorticoid activity. The salt-retaining actions

TABLE 23–7 Effects of Substituents on Glucocorticoid/Mineralocorticoid Activity

Functional Group	Glycogen Deposition	Anti-inflammatory Activity	Effects on Urinary Sodium[a]
9α-Fluoro	10	7–10	+++
9α-Chloro	3–5	3–4	++
1-Dehydro	3–4	3–4	−
6α-Methyl	2–3	1–2	−−−
16α-Hydroxy	0.4–0.5	0.1–0.2	−−−−
17α-Hydroxy	1–2	4	−
21-Hydroxy	4–7	25	++

Adapted from Rodig, O.R.: In Burger, A. (ed.). Medicinal Chemistry, Part 2, 3rd ed. New York, Wiley-Interscience, 1970. Used with permission.
[a] +, retention; −, excretion.

are approximately additive. For example, the $3+$ increase in salt retention of a 9α-fluoro group can be eliminated by the $3-$ decrease of a 6α-methyl.

GLUCOCORTICOIDS WITH MODERATE-TO-LOW SALT RETENTION

The glucocorticoids with moderate-to-low salt retention include cortisone, hydrocortisone, and their 1-enes predniso-lone and prednisone. As shown in Table 23-8, an 11β-OH maintains good topical anti-inflammatory activity, but 11-ones have little or none. The 11β-hydroxysteroid dehydrogenase in the skin oxidizes an 11β-hydroxyl to an 11-ketone.[142] For activation of an 11-one glucocorticoid for topical action, reduction at C11 would be necessary. The 1-ene of prednisolone and prednisone increases anti-inflammatory activity about fourfold and somewhat decreases salt retention. Duax and coworkers[20] have shown that the increase in

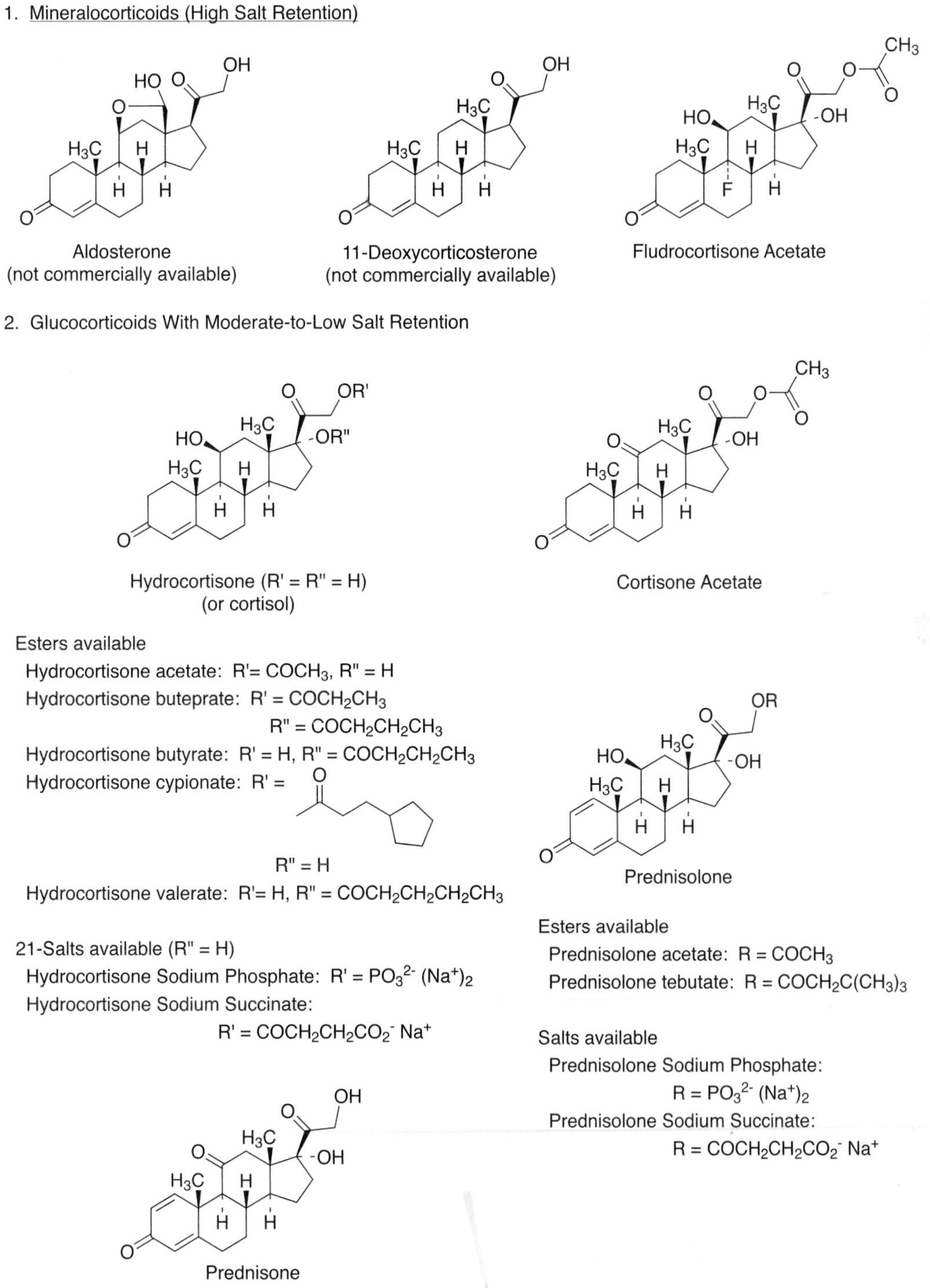

1. Mineralocorticoids (High Salt Retention)

Aldosterone
(not commercially available)

11-Deoxycorticosterone
(not commercially available)

Fludrocortisone Acetate

2. Glucocorticoids With Moderate-to-Low Salt Retention

Hydrocortisone (R' = R" = H)
(or cortisol)

Cortisone Acetate

Esters available
  Hydrocortisone acetate: R'= COCH$_3$, R" = H
  Hydrocortisone buteprate: R' = COCH$_2$CH$_3$
                             R" = COCH$_2$CH$_2$CH$_3$
  Hydrocortisone butyrate: R' = H, R" = COCH$_2$CH$_2$CH$_3$
  Hydrocortisone cypionate: R' =
  R" = H
  Hydrocortisone valerate: R'= H, R" = COCH$_2$CH$_2$CH$_2$CH$_3$

21-Salts available (R" = H)
  Hydrocortisone Sodium Phosphate: R' = PO$_3^{2-}$ (Na$^+$)$_2$
  Hydrocortisone Sodium Succinate:
       R' = COCH$_2$CH$_2$CO$_2^-$ Na$^+$

Prednisolone

Esters available
  Prednisolone acetate: R = COCH$_3$
  Prednisolone tebutate: R = COCH$_2$C(CH$_3$)$_3$

Salts available
  Prednisolone Sodium Phosphate:
       R = PO$_3^{2-}$ (Na$^+$)$_2$
  Prednisolone Sodium Succinate:
       R = COCH$_2$CH$_2$CO$_2^-$ Na$^+$

Prednisone

Figure 23–30 ■ Natural and synthetic corticosteroids.

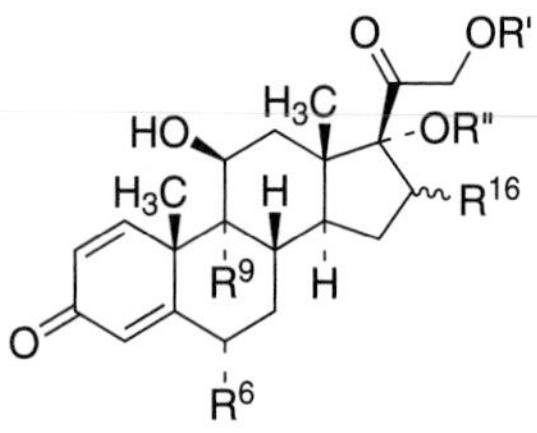

Betamethasone
R^6 = H
R^9 = F
R^{16} = —CH_3
R' = R" = H

Dexamethasone
R^6 = H
R^9 = F
R^{16} = - -CH_3
R' = R" = H

Diflorasone Diacetate
R^6 = R^9 = F
R^{16} = —CH_3
R' = R" = $COCH_3$

Methylprednisolone
R^6 = CH_3
R^9 = R^{16} = H
R' = R" = H

Prednicarbate
R^6 = R^9 = R^{16} = H
R' = R" = $COCH_2CH_3$

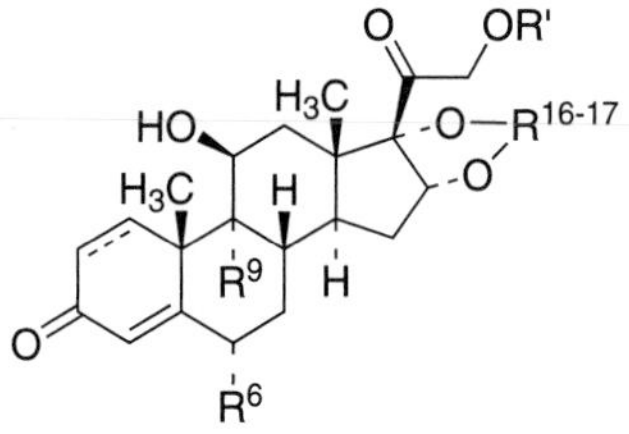

R^{16-17} = I =

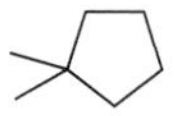

= II =
CH_3
CH_3

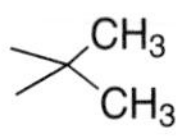

Amcinonide
1-ene
R^6 = H
R^9 = F
R^{16-17} = I
R' = $COCCH_3$

Desonide
1-ene
R^6 = R^9 = H
R^{16-17} = II
R' = H

Fluocinolone Acetonide
1-ene
R^6 = R^9 = F
R^{16-17} = II
R' = H (fluocinonide is
the C21 acetate)

Flurandrenolide
R^6 = F
R^9 = H
R^{16-17} = II
R' = H

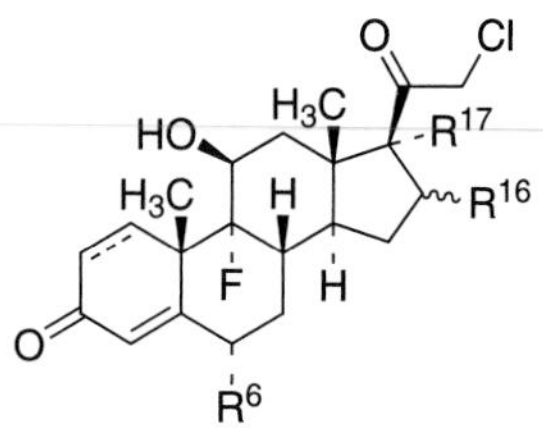

Clobetasol Propionate
1-ene
R^6 = H
R^{16} = —CH_3
R^{17} = $OCOCH_2CH_3$

Halobetasol Propionate
1-ene
R^6 = F
R^{16} = —CH_3
R^{17} = $OCOCH_2CH_3$

Halcinonide
R^6 = H
$R^{16,17}$ = acetonide

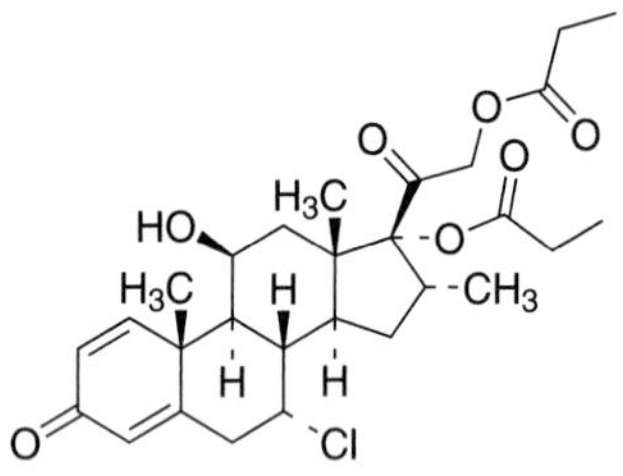

Alclometasone Dipropionate

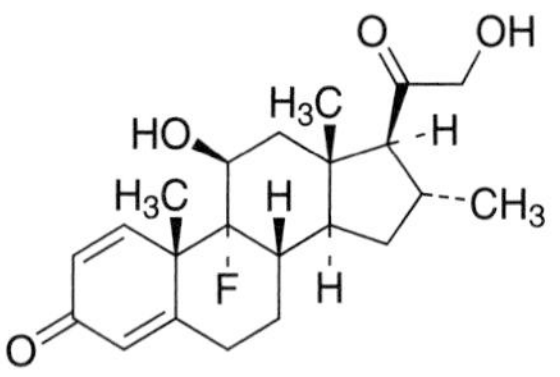

Desoximetasone

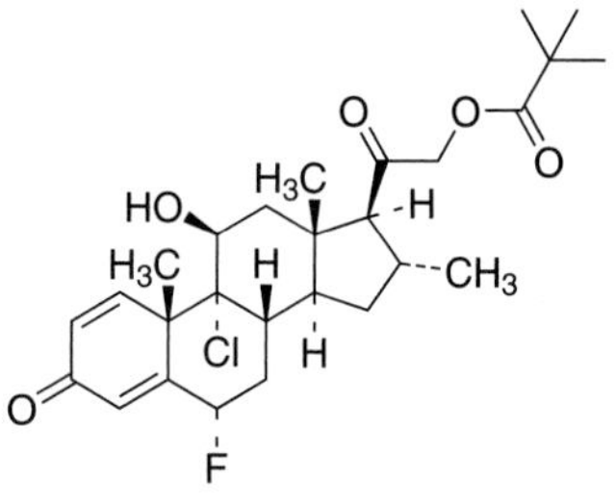

Clocortolone Pivalate

Figure 23–30 ■ *Continued.*

activity may be due to a change in shape of ring A. Specifically, analogues more active than hydrocortisone appear to have their ring A bent underneath the molecule to a much greater extent than hydrocortisone.

The 11β-OH of hydrocortisone is of major importance in binding to the receptors. Cortisone is reduced in vivo to yield hydrocortisone as the active agent. The increased activity of 9α-halo derivatives may be due to the electron-withdrawing inductive effect on the 11β-OH, making it more acidic and, therefore, better able to form hydrogen bonds with the recep-

tor. A 9α-halo substituent also reduces oxidation of the 11β-OH to the inactive 11-one.

GLUCOCORTICOIDS WITH VERY LITTLE OR NO SALT RETENTION

Cortisone and hydrocortisone, and even prednisone and prednisolone, have too much salt-retaining activity in the doses needed for some therapeutic purposes. Over the past several decades, a number of substituents have been discov-

TABLE 23–8 Approximate Relative Activities of Corticosteroids[a]

	Anti-inflammatory Activity	Topical Activity	Salt-Retaining Activity	Equivalent Dose (mg)
Mineralocorticoids				
Aldosterone	0.2	0.2	800	
Deoxycorticosterone	0	0	40	
Fludrocortisone	10	5–40	800	2
Glucocorticoids				
Hydrocortisone	1	1	1	20
Cortisone	0.8	0	0.8	25
Prednisolone	4	4	0.6	5
Prednisone	3.5	0	0.6	5
Methylprednisolone	5	5	0	4
Triamcinolone acetonide	5	5–100	0	4
Triamcinolone		1–5		
Fluocinolone acetonide		Over 40		
Flurandrenolide		Over 20		
Fluocinolone		Over 40		
Fluocinonide		40–100		
Betamethasone	35	5–100	0	0.6
Dexamethasone	30	10–35	0	0.75

[a] The data in this table are only approximate. Blanks indicate that comparative data are not available to the author or that the product has only one use (e.g., topical). Data were taken from several sources, and there is an inherent risk in comparing such data. The table should, however, serve as a guide to relative activities.

ered that greatly decrease salt retention. They include 16α-hydroxy; 16α,17α-ketal; 6α-methyl; and 16α- and 16β-methyl. Other substituents have been found to increase both glucocorticoid and mineralocorticoid activities: 1-ene, 9α-fluoro, 9α-chloro, and 21-hydroxy.

As a result of the great economic benefit of having a potent anti-inflammatory product on the market, pharmaceutical manufacturers have made numerous combinations of these various substituents. In almost every case a 16-methyl or a modified 16-hydroxy (to eliminate salt retention) has been combined with another substituent to increase glucocorticoid or anti-inflammatory activity. The number of permutations and combinations has resulted in a redundant array of analogues with very low salt retention and high anti-inflammatory activity.

A primary goal of these highly anti-inflammatory drugs has been to increase topical potency. As shown in Table 23-8, some are as much as 100 times more active topically than hydrocortisone. Relative potency is as follows:

Very high potency
  Augmented betamethasone dipropionate ointment, 0.05%
  Clobetasol propionate, 0.05%
  Diflorasone diacetate ointment, 0.05%
High potency
  Amcinonide, 0.1%
  Betamethasone dipropionate ointment, 0.05%
  Desoximetasone, 0.25%
  Diflorasone diacetate cream, 0.05%
  Fluocinonide, 0.05%
  Halcinonide, 0.1%
  Halobetasol propionate, 0.05%
  Triamcinolone acetonide, 0.5%

Medium potency
  Betamethasone valerate, 0.1%
  Clocortolone pivalate, 0.1%
  Desoximetasone, 0.05%
  Fluocinolone acetonide, 0.025%
  Fluticasone propionate, 0.005%
  Hydrocortisone butyrate, 0.1%
  Hydrocortisone valerate, 0.2%
  Mometasone furoate, 0.1%
  Prednicarbate, 0.1%
  Triamcinolone acetonide, 0.1%
Low potency
  Alclometasone dipropionate, 0.05%
  Desonide, 0.05%
  Fluocinolone acetonide, 0.01%
  Triamcinolone acetonide cream, 0.1%
Lowest potency
  Hydrocortisone, 1.0%
  Hydrocortisone, 2.5%

Although, as shown in Table 23-8, cortisone and prednisone are not active topically, most other glucocorticoids are active. Some compounds, such as clobetasol and betamethasone dipropionate, have striking activity topically. Skin absorption is favored by increased lipid solubility of the drug.

Absorption of topical glucocorticoids can also be greatly affected by the extent of skin damage, concentration of the glucocorticoid, cream or ointment base used, and similar factors. One must not assume, therefore, from a study of Table 23-8 that, for example, a 0.25% cream of prednisolone is necessarily exactly equivalent in anti-inflammatory potency to 1% hydrocortisone. Nevertheless, the table can serve as a preliminary guide. Furthermore, particular patients may seem to respond better to one topical anti-inflammatory glucocorticoid than to another, irrespective of the relative potencies shown in Table 23-8.

RISK OF SYSTEMIC ABSORPTION

The topical corticosteroids do not typically cause significant absorption effects when used on small areas of intact skin. When these compounds are used on large areas of the body, however, systemic absorption may occur, especially if the skin is damaged or if occlusive dressings are used. Up to 20 to 40% of hydrocortisone given rectally may also be absorbed.

Therapeutic Uses of Adrenal Cortex Hormones

The adrenocortical steroids are used primarily for their glucocorticoid effects, including immunosuppression, anti-inflammatory activity, and antiallergic activity. The mineralocorticoids are used only for treatment of Addison's disease. Addison's disease is caused by chronic adrenocortical insufficiency and may be due to either adrenal or anterior pituitary failure. The glucocorticoids are also used in the treatment of congenital adrenal hyperplasias.

The symptoms of Addison's disease illustrate the great importance of the adrenocortical steroids in the body and, especially, the importance of aldosterone. These symptoms include increased loss of body sodium, decreased loss of potassium, hypoglycemia, weight loss, hypotension, weakness, increased sensitivity to insulin, and decreased lipolysis.

Hydrocortisone is also used during postoperative recovery after surgery for Cushing's syndrome—excessive adrenal secretion of glucocorticoids. Cushing's syndrome can be caused by bilateral adrenal hyperplasia or adrenal tumors and is treated by surgical removal of the tumors or resection of hyperplastic adrenal gland(s).

The use of glucocorticoids during recovery from surgery for Cushing's syndrome illustrates a most important principle of glucocorticoid therapy: abrupt withdrawal of glucocorticoids may result in adrenal insufficiency, showing clinical symptoms similar to those of Addison's disease. For that reason, patients who have been on long-term glucocorticoid therapy must have the dose reduced gradually. Furthermore, prolonged treatment with glucocorticoids can cause adrenal suppression, especially during times of stress. The symptoms are similar to those of Cushing's syndrome, such as rounding of the face, hypertension, edema, hypokalemia, thinning of the skin, osteoporosis, diabetes, and even subcapsular cataracts.

The glucocorticoids are used in the treatment of collagen vascular diseases, including rheumatoid arthritis and disseminated lupus erythematosus. Although there is usually prompt remission of redness, swelling, and tenderness by the glucocorticoids in rheumatoid arthritis, continued long-term use may lead to serious systemic forms of collagen disease. As a result, the glucocorticoids should be used infrequently in rheumatoid arthritis.

The glucocorticoids are used extensively topically, orally, and parenterally to treat inflammatory conditions. They also usually relieve the discomforting symptoms of many allergic conditions—intractable hay fever, exfoliative dermatitis, generalized eczema, and others. The glucocorticoids are also used to treat asthmatic symptoms unresponsive to bronchodilators. They are especially useful in inhaled formulations (see section below). The glucocorticoids' lymphocytopenic actions make them particularly useful for treatment of chronic lymphocytic leukemia in combination with other antineoplastic drugs.

The adrenocortical steroids are contraindicated or should be used with great caution in patients who have (a) peptic ulcer (in which the steroids may cause hemorrhage), (b) heart disease, (c) infections (the glucocorticoids suppress the body's normal infection-fighting processes), (d) psychoses (since behavioral disturbances may occur during steroid therapy), (e) diabetes (the glucocorticoids increase glucose production, so more insulin may be needed), (f) glaucoma, (g) osteoporosis, or (h) herpes simplex involving the cornea.

When administered topically, the glucocorticoids present relatively infrequent therapeutic problems, but their anti-inflammatory action can mask symptoms of infection. Many physicians prefer not giving a topical anti-inflammatory steroid until after an infection is controlled with topical antibiotics. The immunosuppressive activity of the topical glucocorticoids can also prevent natural processes from curing the infection. Topical steroids actually may also cause dermatoses in some patients.

Finally, as discussed above with the oral contraceptives, steroid hormones should not be used during pregnancy. If it is absolutely necessary to use glucocorticoids topically during pregnancy, they should be limited to small areas of intact skin and used for a limited time.

Mineralocorticoid and Glucocorticoid Products

The corticosteroids used in commercial products are shown in Figures 23-30, 23-31, and 23-32. The structures illustrate the usual changes (see Fig. 23-6) made to modify solubility of the products and, therefore, their therapeutic uses. In particular, the 21-hydroxyl can be converted to an ester to make it less water soluble to modify absorption or to a phosphate ester salt or hemisuccinate ester salt to make it more water soluble and appropriate for intravenous use. The products also reflect the structure–activity relationship changes discussed above to increase anti-inflammatory activity or potency or decrease salt retention.

Again, patients who have been on long-term glucocorticoid therapy must have the dose reduced gradually. This "critical rule" and indications are discussed above under the heading, Therapeutic Uses of Adrenal Cortex Hormones. Dosage schedules and gradual dosage reduction can be quite complex and specific for each indication.

Many of the glucocorticoids are available in topical dosage forms, including creams, ointments, aerosols, lotions, and solutions. They are usually applied 3 to 4 times a day to well-cleaned areas of affected skin. Ointments are usually prescribed for dry, scaly dermatoses. Lotions are well suited for weeping dermatoses. Creams are of general use for many other dermatoses. When applied to very large areas of skin or to damaged areas of skin, significant systemic absorption can occur. The use of an occlusive dressing can also greatly increase systemic absorption.

The glucocorticoids that are mainly used for inflammation of the eye are shown in Figure 23-31. These compounds differ structurally from other glucocorticoids, in that the 21-

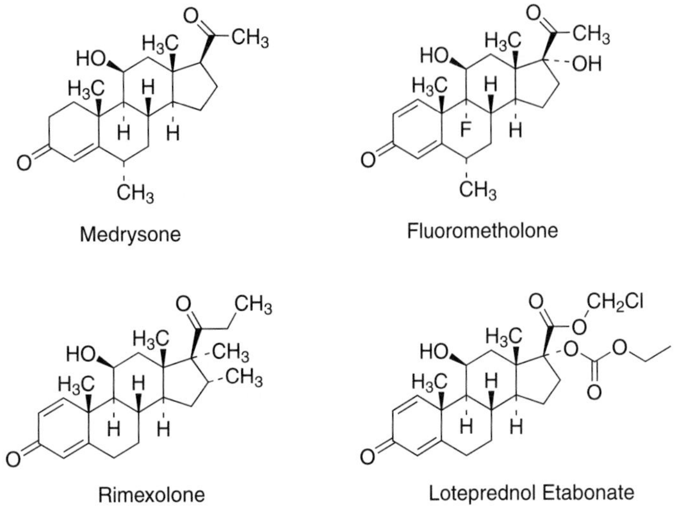

Figure 23–31 ■ Ophthalmic glucocorticoids.

hydroxyl is missing from medrysone, fluorometholone, and rimexolone, while loteprednol etabonate has a modified ester at C17 that leads to rapid degradation upon systemic absorption.

MINERALOCORTICOIDS

Fludrocortisone Acetate, USP.   Fludrocortisone acetate, 21-acetyloxy-9-fluoro-11β,17-dihydroxypregn-4-ene-3,20-dione, 9α -fluorohydrocortisone (Florinef Acetate), is used only for the treatment of Addison's disease and for inhibition of endogenous adrenocortical secretions. As shown in Table 23-8, it has up to about 800 times the mineralocorticoid activity of hydrocortisone and about 11 times the glucocorticoid activity. Its potent activity stimulated the synthesis and study of the many fluorinated steroids shown in Figure 23-30. Although its great salt-retaining activity limits its use to Addison's disease, it has sufficient glucocorticoid activity that in some cases of the disease, additional glucocorticoids need not be prescribed.

GLUCOCORTICOIDS WITH MODERATE-TO-LOW SALT RETENTION

Hydrocortisone, USP.   Hydrocortisone, 11β,17,21-trihydroxypregn-4-ene-3,20-dione, is the primary natural glucocorticoid in humans. Despite the large number of synthetic glucocorticoids, hydrocortisone, its esters, and its salts remain a mainstay of modern adrenocortical steroid therapy and the standard for comparison of all other glucocorticoids and mineralocorticoids (see Table 23-8). It is used for all the indications mentioned above. Its esters and salts illustrate the principles of chemical modification to modify pharmacokinetic use shown in Figure 23-6. The commercially available salts and esters (see Fig. 23-30) include

Hydrocortisone acetate, USP (21-acetate)
Hydrocortisone buteprate, USP (17-butyrate, 21-propionate)
Hydrocortisone butyrate, USP (17-butyrate)
Hydrocortisone cypionate, USP (21-cypionate)
Hydrocortisone sodium phosphate, USP (21-sodium phosphate)
Hydrocortisone sodium succinate, USP (21-sodium succinate)
Hydrocortisone valerate, USP (17-valerate)

Cortisone Acetate, USP.   Cortisone acetate, 21-(acetyloxy)-17-hydroxypregn-4-ene-3,11,20-trione, is the 21-acetate of naturally occurring cortisone with good systemic anti-inflammatory activity and low-to-moderate salt-retention activity after its in vivo conversion to hydrocortisone acetate. This conversion is mediated by 11β-hydroxysteroid dehydrogenase. It is used for the entire spectrum of uses discussed above under the heading, Therapeutic Uses of Adrenal Cortex Hormones—collagen diseases, Addison's disease, severe shock, allergic conditions, chronic lymphocytic leukemia, and many other indications. Cortisone acetate is relatively ineffective topically, mainly because it must be reduced in vivo to hydrocortisone. Its plasma half-life is only about 30 minutes, compared with 90 minutes to 3 hours for hydrocortisone.

Prednisolone, USP.   Prednisolone, Δ^1-hydrocortisone, 11β,17,21-trihydroxypregna-1,4-diene-3,20-dione, has less salt-retention activity than hydrocortisone (see Table 23-8), but some patients have more frequently experienced complications such as gastric irritation and peptic ulcers. Because of low mineralocorticoid activity, it cannot be used alone for adrenal insufficiency. Prednisolone is available in a variety of salts and esters to maximize its therapeutic utility (see Fig. 23-30):

Prednisolone acetate, USP (21-acetate)
Prednisolone sodium phosphate, USP (21-sodium phosphate)
Prednisolone sodium succinate, USP (21-sodium succinate)
Prednisolone tebutate, USP (21-tebutate)

Prednisone, USP.   Prednisone, Δ^1-cortisone, 17,21-dihydroxypregna-1,4-diene-3,11,20-trione, has systemic activity very similar to that of prednisolone, and because of its lower salt-retention activity, it is often preferred over cortisone or hydrocortisone. Prednisone must be reduced in vivo to prednisolone to provide the active glucocorticoid.

GLUCOCORTICOIDS WITH VERY LITTLE OR NO SALT RETENTION

Most of the key differences between the many glucocorticoids with minimal salt retention (see Fig. 23-30) have been summarized in Tables 23-7 and 23-8. The tremendous therapeutic and, therefore, commercial importance of these drugs has stimulated the proliferation of new compounds and their products. Many compounds also are available as salts or esters to give the complete range of therapeutic flexibility illustrated in Figure 23-30. When additional pertinent information is available, it is given below. The systemic name for each drug is provided after the common name.

Alclometasone Dipropionate, USP. Alclometasone dipropionate, 7α-chloro-11β-hydroxy-16α-methyl-17,21-bis(1-oxopropoxy)-pregna-1,4-diene-3,20-dione (Aclovate), is one of the few commercially used glucocorticoids that bears a halogen substituent in the 7α position.

Amcinonide, USP. Amcinonide, 21-(acetyloxy)-16α, 17-[cyclopentylidenebis(oxy)]-9-fluoro-11β-hydroxypregna-1,4-diene-3,20-dione (Cyclocort).

Beclomethasone Dipropionate, USP. Beclomethasone dipropionate, 9-chloro-11β-hydroxy-16β-methyl-17,21-bis(1-oxopropoxy)-pregna-1,4-diene-3,20-dione (Beconase, Vancenase, Vanceril, QVAR), is used in nasal sprays and aerosol formulations to treat allergic rhinitis and asthma (see section below).

Betamethasone, USP. Betamethasone, 9-fluoro-11β, 17,21-trihydroxy-16β-methylpregna-1,4-diene-3,20-dione, is available as a variety of ester derivatives.

 Betamethasone valerate, USP (17-valerate)
 Betamethasone acetate, USP (21-acetate)
 Betamethasone sodium phosphate, USP (21-sodium phosphate)
 Betamethasone dipropionate, USP (17-propionate, 21-propionate)

Budesonide, USP. Budesonide, 16α,17-[butylidenebis(oxy)]-11β,21-dihydroxypregna-1,4-diene-3,20-dione (Entocort), in oral capsules is used to treat Crohn's disease. The affinity for the GR is approximately 200-fold greater than that of hydrocortisone and 15-fold greater than that of prednisolone. Budesonide is a mixture of epimers, with the 22R form having twice the affinity for the GR of the S epimer. This glucocorticoid is metabolized by CYP 3A4, and its levels can be increased in the presence of potent CYP 3A4 inhibitors. Budesonide is also used in an inhaled formulation for the treatment of asthma (see below).

Clobetasol Propionate, USP. Clobetasol propionate, 21-chloro-9-fluoro-11β-hydroxy-16β-methyl-17-(1-oxopropoxy)-pregna-1,4-diene-3,20-dione (Temovate).

Clocortolone Pivalate, USP. Clocortolone pivalate, 9-chloro-21-(2,2-dimethyl-1-oxopropoxy)-6α-fluoro-11β-hydroxy-16α-methylpregna-1,4-diene-3,20-dione (Cloderm), along with desoximetasone, lacks the C17α oxygen functionality that is present in other glucocorticoids but still retains good glucocorticoid activity.

Desonide, USP. Desonide, 11β,21-dihydroxy-16α,17-[(1-methylethylidene)bis(oxy)]pregna-1,4-diene-3,20-dione (DesOwen, Tridesiol).

Desoximetasone, USP. Desoximetasone, 9-fluoro-11β, 21-dihydroxy-16α-methylpregna-1,4-diene-3,20-dione, like clocortolone pivalate, lacks a C17α hydroxyl group in its structure.

Dexamethasone, USP. Dexamethasone, 9-fluoro-11β, 17,21-trihydroxy-16α-methylpregna-1,4-diene-3,20-dione, is the 16α isomer of betamethasone.

 Dexamethasone acetate, USP (21-acetate)
 Dexamethasone sodium phosphate, USP (21-sodium phosphate)

Diflorasone Diacetate, USP. Diflorasone diacetate, 17,21-bis(acetyloxy)-6α,9-difluoro-11β-hydroxy-16α-methylpregna-1,4-diene-3,20-dione.

Flunisolide, USP. Flunisolide, 6α-fluoro-11β,21-dihydroxy-16α,17-[(1-methylethylidene)bis(oxy)]pregna-1,4-diene-3,20-dione. (See following section for use of flunisolide in the treatment of asthma.)

Fluocinolone Acetonide, USP. Fluocinolone acetonide, 6α,9-difluoro-11β,21-dihydroxy-16α,17-[(1-methylethylidene)bis(oxy)]pregna-1,4-diene-3,20-dione, also known as 6α-fluorotriamcinolone acetonide, is the 21-acetate derivative of fluocinolone acetonide and is about 5 times more potent than fluocinolone acetonide in at least one topical activity assay.

Fluorometholone, USP. Fluorometholone, 9-fluoro-11β,17-dihydroxy-6α-methylpregn-4-ene-3,20-dione(FluorOp, FML), lacks the typical C21 hydroxyl group of glucocorticoids and is used exclusively in ophthalmic products. The 17-acetate of fluorometholone is also used as an ophthalmic suspension (Flarex).

Flurandrenolide, USP. Flurandrenolide, 6α-fluoro-11β,21-dihydroxy-16 α,17-[(1-methylethylidene)bis(oxy)]-pregn-4-ene-3,20-dione, although available as a tape product, can stick to and remove damaged skin, so it should be avoided with vesicular or weeping dermatoses.

Fluticasone Propionate, USP. Fluticasone propionate, S-(fluoromethyl) 6α,9-difluoro-11β-hydroxy-16α-methyl-3-oxo-17α-(1-oxopropoxy)androsta-1,4-diene-17-carbothioate (Cutivate), is 3- to 5-fold more potent than dexamethasone in receptor binding assays. (See also the following section on inhaled corticosteroids.)

Halcinonide. Halcinonide, 21-chloro-9-fluoro-11β-hydroxy-16α,17-[(1-methylethylidene)bis(oxy)]pregn-4-ene-3,20-dione, was the first chloroglucocorticoid marketed. Like many of the other potent glucocorticoids, it is used only topically.

Halobetasol Propionate, USP. Halobetasol propionate, 21-chloro-6α,9-difluoro-11β-hydroxy-16β-methyl -17-(1-oxopropoxy)pregna-1,4-diene-3,20-dione.

Loteprednol Etabonate, USP. Loteprednol etabonate, chloromethyl 17α-[(ethoxycarbonyl)oxy]-11β-hydroxy-3-oxoandrosta-1,4-diene-17-carboxylate (Alrex, Lotemax), has a modified carboxylate at the C17 position rather than the typical ketone functionality. This modification maintains affinity for the glucocorticoid receptor but allows facile metabolism to inactive metabolites. This limits the systemic action of the drug. Loteprednol etabonate is used as an ophthalmic suspension that has greatly reduced systemic action due to rapid metabolism to the inactive carboxylate (Fig. 23-31).

Medrysone, USP. Medrysone, 11β-hydroxy-6α-methylpregn-4-ene-3,20-dione, is unique among the corticosteroids, in that it lacks the usual 17α,21-diol system of the others (Fig. 23-31). Currently, it is used only for treatment of inflammation of the eyes.

Methylprednisolone, USP. Methylprednisolone, 11β,17,21-trihydroxy-6α-methyl-1,4-pregnadiene-3,20-dione, is available unmodified or as ester derivatives.

Methylprednisolone acetate, USP
Methylprednisolone sodium succinate, USP

Mometasone Furoate, USP. Mometasone furoate, 9,21-dichloro-17α-[(2-furanylcarbonyl)oxy]-11β-hydroxy-16α-methylpregna-1,4-diene-3,20-dione (Elocon), is a high-potency glucocorticoid available in cream, lotion, or ointment formulations for topical use. In addition, mometasone furoate monohydrate is formulated in a nasal spray for treating allergic rhinitis (see following section).

Prednicarbate, USP. Prednicarbate, 17-[(ethoxycarbonyl)oxy]-11β-hydroxy-21-(1-oxopropoxy)pregna-1,4-diene-3,20-dione, is a prednisolone derivative with a C21 propionate ester and a C17 ethyl carbonate group. It is available for use only in a 0.1% topical cream. Prednicarbate is a medium-potency glucocorticoid.

Rimexolone, USP. Rimexolone, 11β-hydroxy-16α,17α-dimethyl-17-(1-oxopropyl)androsta-1,4-diene-3-one, like medrysone and fluorometholone, lacks the C21 hydroxyl group. In addition, rimexolone has an additional methyl group in the 17α position, a site where a hydroxyl group is typically found. Rimexolone is available as a suspension for ophthalmic use (Fig. 23-31).

Triamcinolone, USP. Triamcinolone, 9-fluoro-11β,16α,17,21-tetrahydroxypregna-1,4-diene-3,20-dione.

Triamcinolone acetonide, USP: Triamcinolone-16α,17-acetonide
Triamcinolone hexacetonide, USP: Triamcinolone acetonide 21-[3-(3,3-dimethyl)butyrate]
Triamcinolone diacetate, USP: 16,21-Diacetate

Triamcinolone acetonide is approximately 8 times more potent than prednisone in animal inflammation models. Topically applied triamcinolone acetonide is a potent anti-inflammatory agent (see Table 23-8), about 10 times more so

than triamcinolone. The plasma half-life is approximately 90 minutes, although the plasma half-life and biological half-lives for glucocorticoids do not correlate well. The hexacetonide is slowly converted to the acetonide in vivo and is given only by intra-articular injection. Only triamcinolone and the diacetate are given orally. The acetonide and diacetate may be given by intra-articular or intrasynovial injection; additionally, the acetonide may be given by intrabursal or, sometimes, intramuscular or subcutaneous injection. A single intramuscular dose of the diacetate or acetonide may last up to 3 or 4 weeks. Plasma levels with intramuscular doses of the acetonide are significantly higher than with triamcinolone itself. The acetonide is also used to treat asthma and allergic rhinitis (see following section).

INHALED CORTICOSTEROIDS FOR ASTHMA AND ALLERGIC RHINITIS

The National Asthma Education and Prevention Program has provided recent recommendations on the treatment of asthma, including a strong recommendation for the first-line use of inhaled corticosteroids for severe and moderate persistent asthma in all age groups. The corticosteroids currently used in inhaled formulations are all relatively potent topical corticosteroids that have the advantage of rapid deactivation/inactivation for the portion of the dose that is swallowed. The development of glucocorticoids that are efficiently inactivated metabolically when swallowed has greatly reduced the systemic side effects associated with the use of steroids in asthma treatment. The older corticosteroids that are used orally (e.g., methylprednisolone, prednisolone, and prednisone) have much greater systemic side effects, and their use should be limited, if possible. Although systemic side effects are reduced, they are not completely eliminated. The side effects can vary with the steroid used and the frequency of administration.

The five glucocorticoids that are currently approved for use in the United States for asthma as inhaled formulations are beclomethasone dipropionate, budesonide, flunisolide, fluticasone propionate, and triamcinolone acetonide (Fig. 23-32). Mometasone furoate will likely be added soon for an asthma indication. Ciclesonide is the newest glucocorticoid being pursued for use in the treatment of asthma. Ciclesonide is in phase III clinical trials and may be available in the United States within a few years. Clinical trials suggest that it may have better tolerability than some of the currently available inhaled steroids.

The following agents are also available in nasal inhalers for the treatment of allergic rhinitis. Details are provided below for the mode of metabolic inactivation involved for each of these products. Although all of these agents have much lower systemic effects than the oral steroids, some systemic effects, as measured by suppression of the hypothalamic–pituitary–adrenal (HPA) axis, have been observed for these products.

GLUCOCORTICOIDS FOR ASTHMA AND ALLERGIC RHINITIS

Beclomethasone Dipropionate. Beclomethasone dipropionate (Beclovent, Beconase, Vanceril, Vancenase) (BDP) is rapidly converted in the lungs to beclomethasone

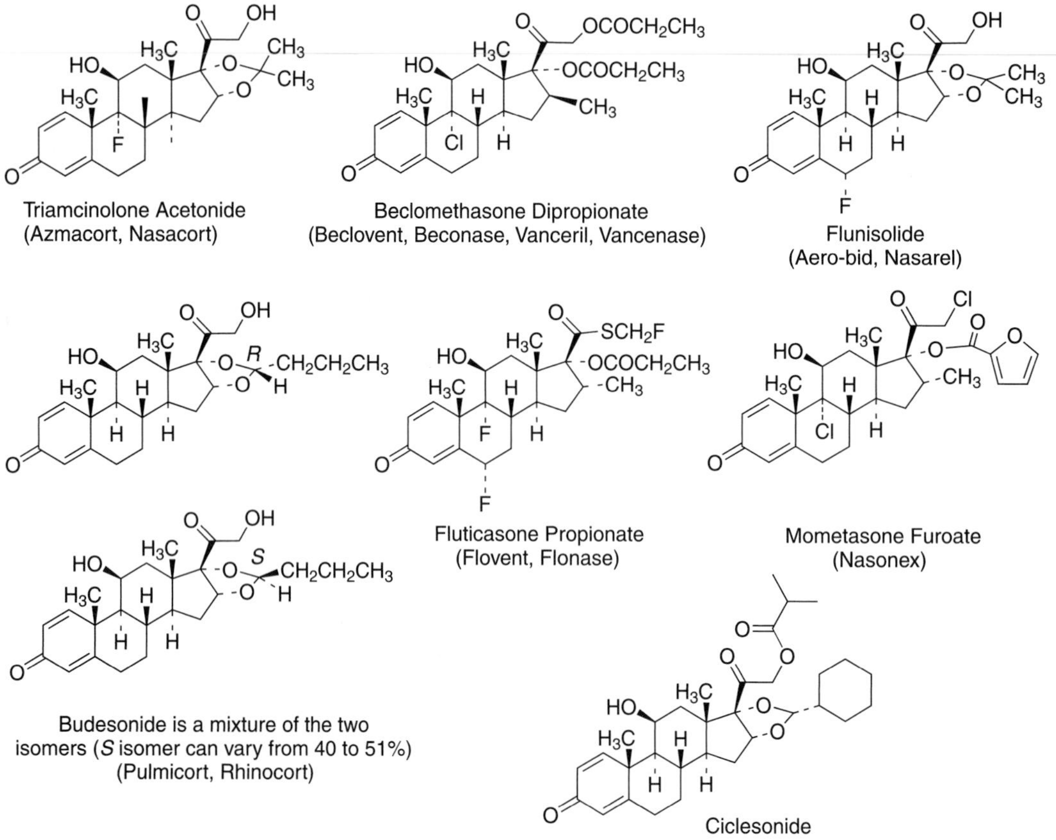

Figure 23–32 ■ Glucocorticoids used to treat asthma and allergic rhinitis (some are also used topically).

17-monopropionate (17-BMP), the metabolite that provides the bulk of the anti-inflammatory activity. The monopropionate also has higher affinity for the GR than either the dipropionate or beclomethasone. The portion of BDP that is swallowed is rapidly hydrolyzed to 17-BMP, 21-BMP (which arises by a transesterification reaction from 17-BMP), and beclomethasone itself.[143] Beclomethasone has much less glucocorticoid activity than the monopropionate.[144]

Budesonide. Budesonide (Pulmicort Turbuhaler, Rhinocort) is extensively metabolized in the liver, with 85 to 95% of the orally absorbed drug metabolized by the first-pass effect. The major metabolites are 6β-hydroxybudesonide and 16α-hydroxyprednisolone, both with less than 1% of the activity of the parent compound. Metabolism involves the CYP 3A4 enzyme, so coadministration of budesonide with a known CYP 3A4 inhibitor should be monitored carefully.

Flunisolide. The portion of a flunisolide (AeroBid, Nasarel) dose that is swallowed is rapidly converted to the 6β-hydroxy metabolite after first-pass metabolism in the liver. The 6β-hydroxy metabolite is approximately as active as hydrocortisone itself, but the small amount produced usually has limited systemic effects. Water-soluble conjugates are inactive.

Fluticasone Propionate. The main metabolite of fluticasone propionate (Flovent, Flonase) found in circulation in

humans is the 17β-carboxylate derivative. As expected, a charged carboxylate in place of the normal acetol functionality at C17 greatly reduces affinity for the glucocorticoid receptor (2,000-fold less than the parent), and this metabolite is essentially inactive. The metabolite is formed via the CYP 3A4 system, so care should be taken if fluticasone propionate is coadministered with a CYP 3A4 inhibitor such as ketoconazole or ritonavir. Clinically induced Cushing's syndrome has been observed when inhaled fluticasone propionate was administered concurrently with ritonavir.[145]

Fluticasone is also available in an inhaled formulation in combination with the long-acting β_2-agonist salmeterol (Advair Diskus).

Mometasone Furoate. Mometasone furoate (Nasonex) undergoes extensive metabolism to multiple metabolites. No major metabolites are detectable in human plasma after oral administration, but the 6β-hydroxy metabolite is detectable by use of human liver microsomes. This metabolite is formed via the CYP 3A4 pathway.

Triamcinolone Acetonide. The three main metabolites of triamcinolone acetonide (Azmacort, Nasacort) are 6β-hydroxytriamcinolone acetonide, 21-carboxytriamcinolone acetonide, and 6β-hydroxy-21-carboxytriamcinolone acetonide. All are much less active than the parent compound. The 6β-hydroxyl group and the 21-carboxy group are both structural features that greatly reduce glucocorticoid action. The increased water solubility of these metabolites also facilitates more rapid excretion.

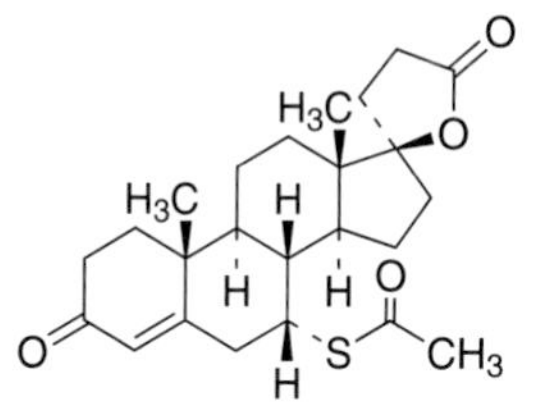

Spironolactone (Aldolactone)

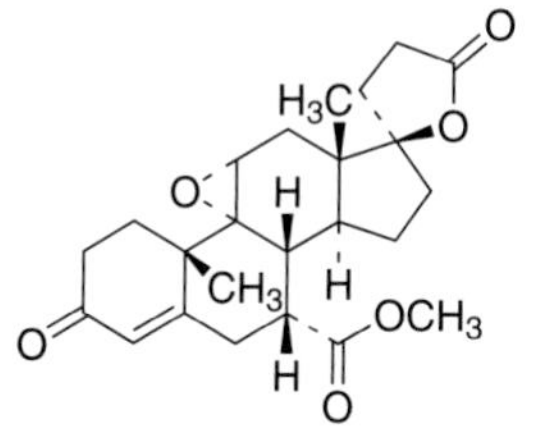

Eplerenone (Inspra)

Figure 23–33 ■ Aldosterone receptor antagonists.

Mineralocorticoid Receptor Antagonists (Aldosterone Antagonists)

Antagonism of the mineralocorticoid receptor can have profound effects on the renin–angiotensin system, thus having significant cardiac effects. Structurally, these compounds have an A-ring enone, essential for recognition by the receptor, but the 7α substituent and the D-ring spirolactone provide structural elements that lead to antagonism (Fig. 23-33).

Spironolactone, USP. Spironolactone, 7α-(acetylthio)-17α-hydroxy-3-oxopregn-4-ene-3-one-21-carboxylic acid γ-lactone (Aldactone), is an aldosterone antagonist of great medical importance because of its diuretic activity. Spironolactone is discussed in Chapter 18.

Eplerenone, USP. Eplerenone, $9,11\alpha$-epoxy-17α-hydroxy-3-oxopregn-4-ene-7α,21-dicarboxylic acid, γ-lactone, methyl ester (Inspra), is a new aldosterone antagonist that was approved by the FDA in 2002 for the treatment of hypertension.

Acknowledgment

I would like to thank Debra Peters for assistance with the illustration of several figures. I would also like to express my appreciation to the authors of various review articles on the steroids. Without the dedication and hard work of these individuals, the assembly of this chapter would have been a much more challenging task.

REFERENCES

1. Hardman, J. G., and Limbird, L. E. (eds.): Goodman & Gilman's The Pharmacological Basis of Therapeutics, 10th ed. New York, McGraw-Hill, 2001.
2. Norman, A. W., and Litwack, G.: Hormones, 2nd ed. San Diego, Academic Press, 1997.
3. Williams, D. A., and Lemke, T. L. (eds.): Foye's Principles of Medicinal Chemistry, 5th ed. Philadelphia, Lippincott Williams & Wilkins, 2002.
4. Moss, G. P.: Eur. J. Biochem. 186:429–458, 1989.
5. Stocco, D. M.: Annu. Rev. Physiol. 63:193–213, 2001.
6. Lin, D., Sugawara, T., Strauss, J. F., III, et al.: Science 267: 1828–1831, 1995.
7. Aranda, A., and Pascual, A.: Physiol. Rev. 81:1269–1304, 2001.
8. Cheung, J., and Smith, D. F.: Mol. Endocrinol. 14:939–946, 2000.
9. Pratt, W. B., and Toft, D. O.: Endocr. Rev. 18:306–360, 1997.
10. DeFranco, D. B.: Mol. Endocrinol. 16:1449–1455, 2002.
11. Brzozowski, A. M., Pike, A. C., Dauter, Z., et al.: Nature 389: 753–758, 1997.
12. Tanenbaum, D. M., Wang, Y., Williams, S. P., and Sigler, P. B.: Proc. Natl. Acad. Sci. U. S. A. 95:5998–6003, 1998.
13. Pike, A. C., Brzozowski, A. M., Hubbard, R. E., et al.: Embo J. 18: 4608–4618, 1998.
14. Williams, S. P., and Sigler, P. B.: Nature 393:392–396, 1998.
15. Sack, J. S., Kish, K. F., Wang, C., et al.: Proc. Natl. Acad. Sci. U. S. A. 98:4904–4909, 2001.
16. Dey, R., Roychowdhury, P., and Mukherjee, C.: Protein Eng. 14: 565–571, 2001.
17. Dey, R., and Roychowdhury, P.: J. Biomol. Struct. Dyn. 20:21–29, 2002.
18. Ekena, K., Katzenellenbogen, J. A., and Katzenellenbogen, B. S.: J. Biol. Chem. 273:693–699, 1998.
19. Duax, W. L., et al.: Biochemical Actions of Hormones, vol 11. New York, Academic Press, 1984.
20. Duax, W. L., Griffin, J. F., Weeks, C. M., and Wawrzak, Z.: J. Steroid Biochem. 31:481–492, 1988.
21. Hanson, J. R.: Nat. Prod. Rep. 19:381–389, 2002.
22. Mosselman, S., Polman, J., and Dijkema, R.: FEBS Lett. 392:49–53, 1996.
23. Loose-Mitchell, D. S., and Stancel, G. M.: Estrogens and progestins. In Hardman, J. G., and Limbird, L. E. (eds.). Goodman & Gilman's The Pharmacological Basis of Therapeutics, 10th ed. New York, McGraw-Hill, 2001, pp. 1597–1634.
24. Harris, H. A., Katzenellenbogen, J. A., and Katzenellenbogen, B. S.: Endocrinology 143:4172–4177, 2002.
25. Harris, H. A., Bapat, A. R., Gonder, D. S., and Frail, D. E.: Steroids 67:379–384, 2002.
26. Katzenellenbogen, B. S., Sun, J., Harrington, W. R., et al.: Ann. N. Y. Acad. Sci. 949:6–15, 2001.
27. Katzenellenbogen, B. S., and Katzenellenbogen, J. A.: Science 295: 2380–2381, 2002.
28. McDonnell, D. P., Connor, C. E., Wijayaratne, A., et al.: Recent Prog. Horm. Res. 57:295–316, 2002.
29. McDonnell, D. P., and Norris, J. D.: Science 296:1642–1644, 2002.
30. Sanchez, R., Nguyen, D., Rocha, W., et al.: Bioessays 24:244–254, 2002.
31. Gelmann, E. P.: J. Clin. Oncol. 20:3001–3015, 2002.
32. DeRijk, R. H., Schaaf, M., and de Kloet, E. R.: J. Steroid Biochem. Mol. Biol. 81:103–122, 2002.
33. Burns, K. H., and Matzuk, M. M.: Endocrinology 143:2823–2835, 2002.
34. Themmen, A. P. N., and Huhtaniemi, I. T.: Endocr. Rev. 21:551–583, 2000.
35. Ruenitz, P. C.: Female sex hormones and analogs. In Wolff, M. E. (ed.). Burger's Medicinal Chemistry and Drug Discovery, 5th ed. New York, John Wiley & Sons, vol. 4. 1996, pp. 553–587.
36. Rich, R. L., Hoth, L. R., Geoghegan, K. F., et al.: Proc. Natl. Acad. Sci. U. S. A. 99:8562–8567, 2002.
37. Martin, C. R.: Endocrine Physiology. New York, Oxford University Press, 1985.
38. Schuler, F. S.: Science 103:221, 1946.
39. Jordan, V. C., Mittal, S., Gosden, B., et al.: Environ. Health Perspect. 61:97–110, 1985.
40. Adams, N. R.: J. Anim. Sci. 73:1509–1515, 1995.
41. Setchell, K. D.: J. Am. Coll. Nutr. 20:354S–362S, 2001; discussion 381S–383S.
42. An, J., Tzagarakis-Foster, C., Scharschmidt, T. C., et al.: J. Biol. Chem. 276:17808–17814, 2001.

43. Hilakivi-Clarke, L., Cabanes, A., Olivo, S., et al.: J. Steroid Biochem. Mol. Biol. 80:163–174, 2002.
44. Shapiro, S., Kelly, J. P., Rosenberg, L., et al.: N. Engl. J. Med. 313:969–972, 1985.
45. Mittendorf, R.: Teratology 51:435–445, 1995.
46. Palmer, J. R., Hatch, E. E., Rao, R. S., et al.: Am. J. Epidemiol. 154:316–321, 2001.
47. Titus-Ernstoff, L., Hatch, E. E., Hoover, R. N., et al.: Br. J. Cancer 84:126–333, 2001.
48. Schmider, J., Greenblatt, D. J., von Moltke, L. L., et al.: J. Clin. Pharmacol. 37:193–200, 1997.
49. Malkowicz, S. B.: Urology 58:108–113, 2001.
50. Cummings, F. J.: Clin. Ther. 24(Suppl C):C3–25, 2002.
51. Carlson, R. W.: Breast Cancer Res. Treat. 75(Suppl 1):S27–32, 2002; discussion S33–35.
52. Ross, D., and Whitehead, M.: Curr. Opin. Obstet. Gynecol. 7:63–68, 1995.
53. Grese, T. A., Sluka, J. P., Bryant, H. U., et al.: Proc. Natl. Acad. Sci. U. S. A. 94:14105–14110, 1997.
54. Shang, Y., and Brown, M.: Science 295:2465–2468, 2002.
55. Shiau, A. K., Barstad, D., Loria, P. M., et al.: Cell 95:927–937, 1998.
56. Komm, B. S., and Lyttle, C. R.: Ann. N. Y. Acad. Sci. 949:317–326, 2001.
57. Buzdar, A. U., and Hortobagyi, G. N.: J. Clin. Oncol. 16:348–353, 1998.
58. Wardley, A. M.: Int. J. Clin. Pract. 56:305–309, 2002.
59. Goldstein, S. R., Siddhanti, S., Ciaccia, A. V., and Plouffe, L., Jr.: Hum. Reprod. Update 6:212–224, 2000.
60. Turner, R. T., Evans, G. L., Sluka, J. P., et al.: Endocrinology 139:3712–3720, 1998.
61. Brueggemeier, R. W.: Am. J. Ther. 8:333–344, 2001.
62. Recanatini, M., Cavalli, A., and Valenti, P.: Med. Res. Rev. 22:282–304, 2002.
63. Simpson, E. R., Clyne, C., Rubin, G., et al.: Annu. Rev. Physiol. 64:93–127, 2002.
64. Osawa, Y., Higashiyama, T., Fronckowiak, M., et al.: J. Steroid Biochem. 27:781–789, 1987.
65. Simpson, E. R., and Dowsett, M.: Recent Prog. Horm. Res. 57:317–338, 2002.
66. Cocconi, G.: Breast Cancer Res. Treat. 30:57–80, 1994.
67. Campbell, D. R., and Kurzer, M. S.: J. Steroid Biochem. Mol. Biol. 46:381–388, 1993.
68. Walle, T., Otake, Y., Brubaker, J. A., et al.: Br. J. Clin. Pharmacol. 51:143–146, 2001.
69. Grimm, S. W., and Dyroff, M. C.: Drug Metab. Dispos. 25:598–602, 1997.
70. Dowsett, M., Pfister, C., Johnston, S. R., et al.: Clin. Cancer Res. 5:2338–2343, 1999.
71. Charbonneau, A., and The, V. L.: Biochim. Biophys. Acta 1517:228–235, 2001.
72. Blom, T., Ojanotko-Harri, A., Laine, M., and Huhtaniemi, I.: J. Steroid Biochem. Mol. Biol. 44:69–76, 1993.
73. Mellon, S. H., and Griffin, L. D. Trends Endocrinol. Metab. 13:35–43, 2002.
74. Wyatt, K., Dimmock, P., Jones, P., et al.: Br. Med. J. 323:776–780, 2001.
75. Briggs, M. H.: Curr. Med. Res. Opin. 3:95–98, 1975.
76. Gentile, D. M., Verhoeven, C. H., Shimada, T., and Back, D. J.: J. Pharmacol. Exp. Ther. 287:975–982, 1998.
77. Kuhnz, W., Fritzemeier, K. H., Hegele-Hartung, C., and Krattenmacher, R.: Contraception 51:131–139, 1995.
78. Zhang, Z., Lundeen, S. G., Zhu, Y., et al.: Steroids 65:637–643, 2000.
79. Djerassi, C.: The Politics of Contraception. New York, W. W. Norton, 1979.
80. Lednicer, D. (ed.): Contraception, The Chemical Control of Fertility. New York, Marcel Dekker, 1969.
81. Marks, L. V.: Sexual Chemistry. New Haven, Yale University Press, 2001.
82. Asbell, B.: The Pill. New York, Random House, 1995.
83. Chester, E.: Woman of Valor, Margaret Sanger. New York, Simon & Schuster, 1992.
84. Makepeace, A. W., et al.: Am. J. Physiol. 119:512, 1937.
85. Selye, H., Tache, Y., and Szabo, S.: Fertil. Steril. 22:735–740, 1971.
86. Dempsey, E. W.: Am. J. Physiol. 120:926, 1937.
87. Kurzrok, R.: J. Contracept. 2:27, 1937.
88. Sturgis, S. H., and Albright, F.: Endocrinology 26:68, 1940.
89. Pincus, G.: The Control of Fertility. New York, Academic Press, 1965.
90. Djerassi, C., et al.: J. Chem. Soc. 76:4092, 1954.
91. Colton, F. B.: U. S. Patent 2,691,028, 1954.
92. Borgelt-Hansen, L.: J. Am. Pharm. Assoc. (Wash) 41:875–886, 2001; quiz 925–926.
93. La Vecchia, C., Altieri, A., Franceschi, S., and Tavani, A. Drug Safety 24:741–754, 2001.
94. Schleifer, L. A., Justice, A. J., and de Wit, H.: Pharmacol. Biochem. Behav. 71:71–77, 2002.
95. Shepherd, J. E.: J. Am. Pharm. Assoc. (Wash) 41:221–228, 2001.
96. Lawrence, D. M.: Lancet 359:1493, 2002.
97. Gennari, L., Becherini, L., Falchetti, A., et al.: J. Steroid Biochem. Mol. Biol. 81:1–24, 2002.
98. Riggs, B. L., Khosla, S., and Melton, L. J., 3rd: Endocr. Rev. 23:279–302, 2002.
99. Notelovitz, M.: J. Reprod. Med. 47:71–81, 2002.
100. JAMA 288:321–333, 2002.
101. Kloosterboer, H. J.: J. Steroid Biochem. Mol. Biol. 76:231–238, 2001.
102. Vos, R. M. E., Krebbers, S. F. M., Verhoeven, C. H. J., and Delbressine, L. P. C.: Drug Metab. Dispos. 30:106–112, 2002.
103. Purohit, A., Malini, B., Hooymans, C., and Newman, S. P.: Horm. Metab. Res. 34: 1–6, 2002.
104. Barnes, J. F., Farish, E., Rankin, M., and Hart, D. M.: Atherosclerosis 160:185–193, 2002.
105. Brueggemeier, R.: Male sex hormones and analogs. In Wolff, M. E. (ed.). Burger's Medicinal Chemistry and Drug Discovery, vol. 3, 5th ed. New York, John Wiley & Sons, 1996, pp. 445–510.
106. George, F. W.: Endocrinology 138:871–877, 1997.
107. Williams, M. R., Ling, S., Dawood, T., et al.: J. Clin. Endocrinol. Metab. 87:176–181, 2002.
108. Davis, S. R., and Tran, J.: Trends Endocrinol. Metab. 12:33–37, 2001.
109. Padero, M. C., Bhasin, S., and Friedman, T. C.: J. Am. Geriatr. Soc. 50:1131–1140, 2002.
110. Kuhn, C. M.: Recent Prog. Horm. Res. 57:411–434, 2002.
111. Djerassi, C.: J. Chem. Soc. 76:4092, 1954.
112. Burd, I. D., and Bachmann, G. A.: Curr. Womens Health Rep. 1:202–205, 2001.
113. Hoberman, J. M., and Yesalis, C. E.: Sci. Am. 272:76–81, 1995.
114. van de Kerkhof, D. H., de Boer, D., Thijssen, J. H., and Maes, R. A.: J. Anal. Toxicol. 24:102–115, 2000.
115. Yesalis, C. E., and Bahrke, M. S.: Sports Med. 19:326–340, 1995.
116. Wu, F. C.: Clin. Chem. 43:1289–1292, 1997.
117. FDA Drug Bull. 17:27, 1987.
118. Rich, J. D., Dickinson, B. P., Feller, A., et al.: Int. J. Sports Med. 20:563–566, 1999.
119. Dmowski, W. P.: J. Reprod. Med. 35:69–74, 1990; discussion 74–75.
120. Reid, P., Kantoff, P., and Oh, W.: Invest. New Drugs 17:271–284, 1999.
121. Singh, S. M., Gauthier, S., and Labrie, F.: Curr. Med. Chem. 7:211–247, 2000.
122. Mukherjee, A., Kirkovsky, L., Yao, X. T., et al.: Xenobiotica 26:117–122, 1996.
123. Li, X., Chen, C., Singh, S. M., et al.: Steroids 60:430–441, 1995.
124. Jin, Y., and Penning, T. M.: Best Pract. Res. Clin. Endocrinol. Metab. 15:79–94, 2001.
125. Harris, G. S., and Kozarich, J. W. Curr. Opin. Chem. Biol. 1:254–259, 2001.
126. Bull, H. G., Garcia-Calvo, M., Andersson, S., et al.: J. Am. Chem. Soc. 118:2359–2365, 1996.
127. Steers, W. D.: Urology 58:17–24, 2001; discussion 24.
128. Gerber, G. S.: J. Urol. 163:1408–1412, 2000.
129. Stowasser, M., and Gordon, R. D.: J. Steroid Biochem. Mol. Biol. 78:215–229, 2001.
130. Peter, M., Dubuis, J. M., and Sippell, W. G.: Horm. Res. 51:211–222, 1999.
131. Dacou-Voutetakis, C., Maniati-Christidi, M., and Dracopoulou-Vabouli, M.: J. Pediatr. Endocrinol. Metab. 14(Suppl. 5):1303–1308, 2001; discussion 1317.
132. Schimmer, B. P., and Parker, K. L.: Adrenocorticotropic hormone; adrenocortical steroids and their synthetic analogs; inhibitors of the synthesis and actions of adrenocortical hormones. In Hardman, J. G., and Limbird, L. E. (eds). Goodman & Gilman's The Pharmacological Basis of Therapeutics, vol. 1, 10th ed. New York, McGraw-Hill, 2001, pp. 1679–1714.

133. Amsterdam, A., Tajima, K., and Sasson, R.: Biochem. Pharmacol. 64:843–850, 2002.
134. Van Laethem, F., Baus, E., Andris, F.: Cell Mol. Life Sci. 58: 1599–1606, 2001.
135. Karin, M., and Chang, L.: J. Endocrinol. 169:447–451, 2001.
136. Sternberg, E. M.: J. Endocrinol. 169:429–435, 2001.
137. De Bosscher, K., Vanden Berghe, W., and Haegeman, G.: J. Neuroimmunol. 109: 16–22, 2000.
138. Chikanza, I. C.: Ann. N. Y. Acad. Sci. 966:39–48, 2002.
139. Loke, T. K., Sousa, A. R., Corrigan, C. J., and Lee, T. H.: Curr. Allergy Asthma Rep. 2:144–150, 2002.
140. Kino, T., and Chrousos, G. P.: J. Endocrinol. 169:437–445, 2001.
141. Goleva, E., Kisich, K. O., and Leung, D. Y.: J. Immunol. 169: 5934–5940, 2002.
142. Hennebold, J. D., and Daynes, R. A.: Arch. Dermatol. Res. 290: 413–419, 1998.
143. Foe, K., Cheung, H. T., Tattam, B. N., et al.: Drug Metab. Dispos. 26:132–137, 1998.
144. Daley-Yates, P. T., Price, A. C., Sisson, J. R., et al.: Br. J. Clin. Pharmacol. 51:400–409, 2001.
145. Clevenbergh, P., Corcostegui, M., Gerard, D., et al.: J. Infect. 44: 194–195, 2002.

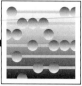

Prostaglandins, Leukotrienes, and Other Eicosanoids

THOMAS J. HOLMES, JR.

The prostaglandins (PGA through PGJ) are one group of naturally occurring 20-carbon fatty acid derivatives produced by the oxidative metabolism of 5,8,11,14-eicosatetraenoic acid, also called *arachidonic acid*. Other so-called eicosanoids produced in the complex biological oxidation scheme called the arachidonic acid cascade (Figs. 24-1 and 24-2) are thromboxane A_2 (TXA$_2$), the leukotrienes (LKTs A to F), and the highly potent antithrombotic agent prostacyclin (PGI$_2$). The naming and the numbering of these 20-carbon acids are included in Figures 24-1 to 24-3. Although eicosanoid-derived agents in current human clinical therapy are few, the promise of future contributions from this area is presumed to be very great. This promise stems from the fact that intermediates of arachidonic acid metabolism play an essential modulatory role in many normal and disease-related cellular processes. In fact, much of the pain, fever, swelling, nausea, and vomiting associated with "illness," in general, probably results from excessive prostaglandin production in damaged tissues.

HISTORY OF DISCOVERY

Early in the past century (1931), Kurzrok and Lieb noted that human seminal fluid could increase or decrease spontaneous muscle contractions of uterine tissue under controlled conditions.[1] This observed effect on uterine musculature was believed to be induced by an acidic vasoactive substance formed in the prostate gland, which was later (1936) termed *prostaglandin* by von Euler.[2] Much later (1950s), it was found that the acidic extract contained not one but several structurally related prostaglandin substances.[3] These materials subsequently were separated, purified, and characterized as the prostaglandins (PGA through PGJ), varying somewhat in degree of oxygenation and dehydrogenation and markedly in biological activity (Table 24-1). Specific stereochemical syntheses of the prostaglandins provided access to sufficient purified material for wide-scale biological evaluation and confirmed the structural characterization of these complex substances.[4]

Although many scientists have contributed to refined characterization of the eicosanoid biosynthetic pathways and the biological consequences of this cascade, the discerning and persistent pioneering efforts of Sune Bergstrom, Bengt Samuellson, and John R. Vane were recognized by the award of a shared Nobel Prize in Medicine in 1982. These scientists not only dedicated themselves to the chemical and biological characterization of the eicosanoid substances but also were the first to realize the profound significance of the arachidonic acid cascade in disease processes, particularly inflammation. These individuals first proved that the mechanism of the anti-inflammatory action of aspirin and related nonsteroidal anti-inflammatory drugs (NSAIDs) was directly due to their inhibitory effect on prostaglandin formation. It was shown subsequently that the analgesic and antipyretic effects of these NSAIDs, as well as their proulcerative and anticoagulant side effects, also result from their effect on eicosanoid metabolism (e.g., inhibition of cyclooxygenases 1 and 2 [COX-1 and COX-2]).

Many books have been published describing the role of eicosanoids in the inflammatory process, the immune system, carcinogenesis, the cardiovascular system, reproductive processes, gastric ulceration, and the central nervous system (see Selected Reading). An annual update of research results in this area has been published since 1975, *Advances in Prostaglandins, Thromboxanes, and Leukotriene Research*. Recent research findings in this area may appear in a variety of biochemical and clinical journals but are the primary concern of two specific journals: *Prostaglandins and Other Lipid Mediators* and *Prostaglandins, Leukotrienes, and Essential Fatty Acids*.

EICOSANOID BIOSYNTHESIS

Prostaglandins and other eicosanoids are produced by the oxidative metabolism of free arachidonic acid. Under normal circumstances, arachidonic acid is not available for metabolism as it is present as a conjugated component of the phospholipid matrix of most cellular membranes. Release of free arachidonic acid, which subsequently may be oxidatively metabolized, occurs by stimulation of phospholipase (PLA$_2$) enzyme activity in response to some traumatic event (e.g., tissue damage, toxin exposure, or hormonal stimulation). It is believed that the clinical anti-inflammatory effect of glucocortical steroids (i.e., hydrocortisone) is due to their ability to suppress PLA$_2$ activity via lipocortins and thus prevent the release of free arachidonic acid.[5] Modulation of PLA$_2$ activity by alkali metal ions, toxins, and various therapeutic agents has become a major focus of biological research because of the changes in eicosanoid production and the dramatic biological effects accompanying PLA$_2$ stimulation or suppression. Although initially it was believed that the inflammatory response (swelling, redness, pain) was princi-

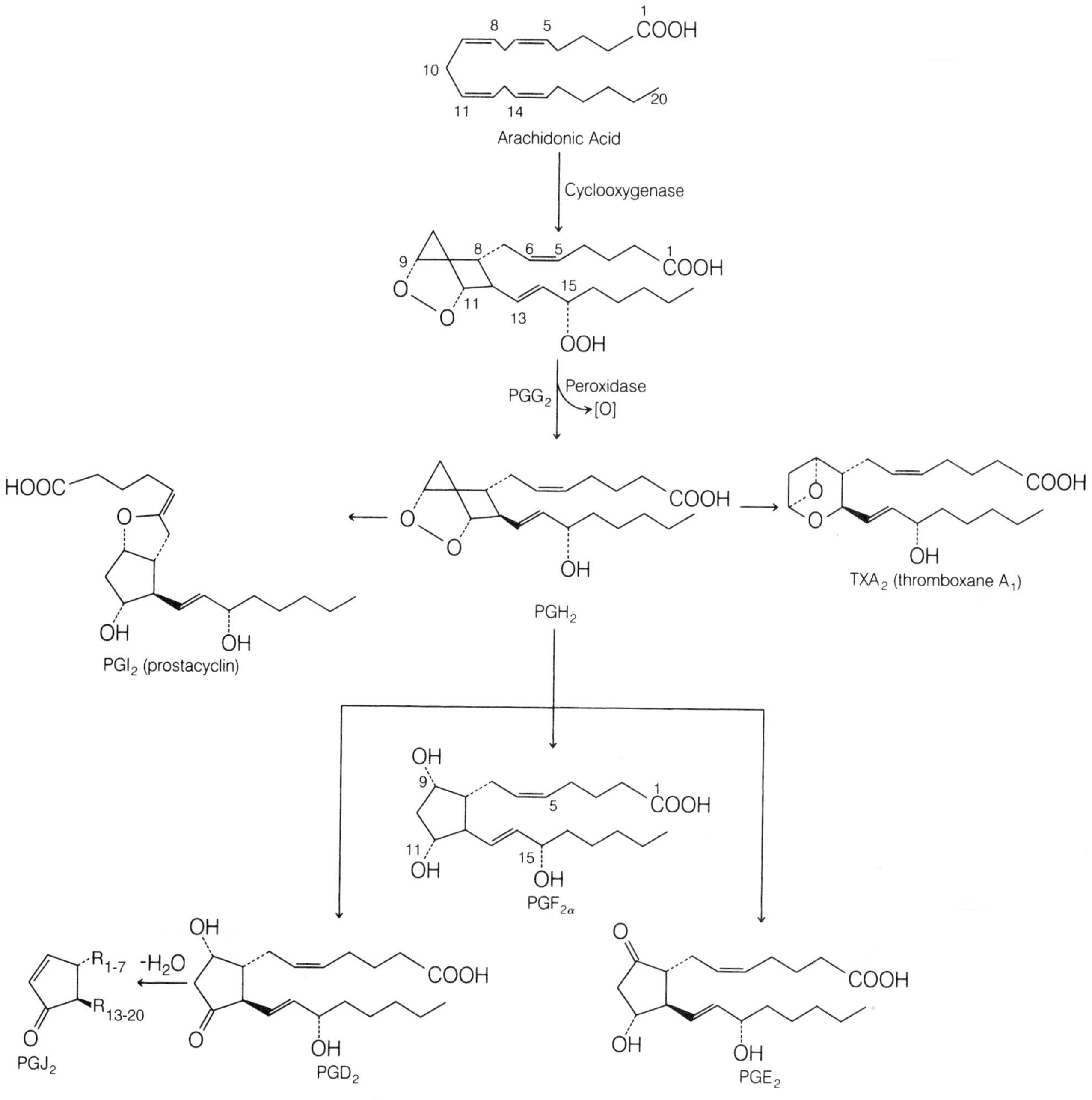

Figure 24–1 ■ Cyclooxygenase pathway.

pally due to PGE$_2$, recent interest has focused on the interrelationships of PGE-type eicosanoids with PGI$_2$ and cytokines, such as interleukin-1 and interleukin-2, in the modulation of inflammatory reactions.[6]

Two different routes for oxygenation of arachidonic acid have been defined: the cyclooxygenase pathway (Fig. 24-1) and the lipoxygenase pathway (Fig. 24-2). The relative significance of each of these pathways may vary in a particular tissue or disease state. The cyclooxygenase pathway, so named because of the unusual bicyclic endoperoxide (PGG$_2$) produced in the first step of the sequence, involves the highly stereospecific addition of two molecules of oxygen to the arachidonic acid substrate, followed by subsequent enzyme-

controlled rearrangements to produce an array of oxygenated eicosanoids with diverse biological activities (see Table 24-1). The first enzyme in this pathway, PGH synthase, is a hemoprotein that catalyzes both the addition of oxygen (to form PGG$_2$) and the subsequent reduction (peroxidase activity) of the 15-position hydroperoxide to the 15-(S)-configuration alcohol (PGH$_2$).[7] PGH synthase (also called *cyclooxygenase-1 [COX-1]* or *cyclooxygenase-2 [COX-2]*, and formerly *PG synthetase*) has been the focus of intense investigation because of its key role as the first enzyme in the arachidonic acid cascade.[8] It is this enzyme in constitutive (COX-1) or inducible (COX-2) form that is susceptible to inhibition by NSAIDs, leading to relief of pain, fever, and

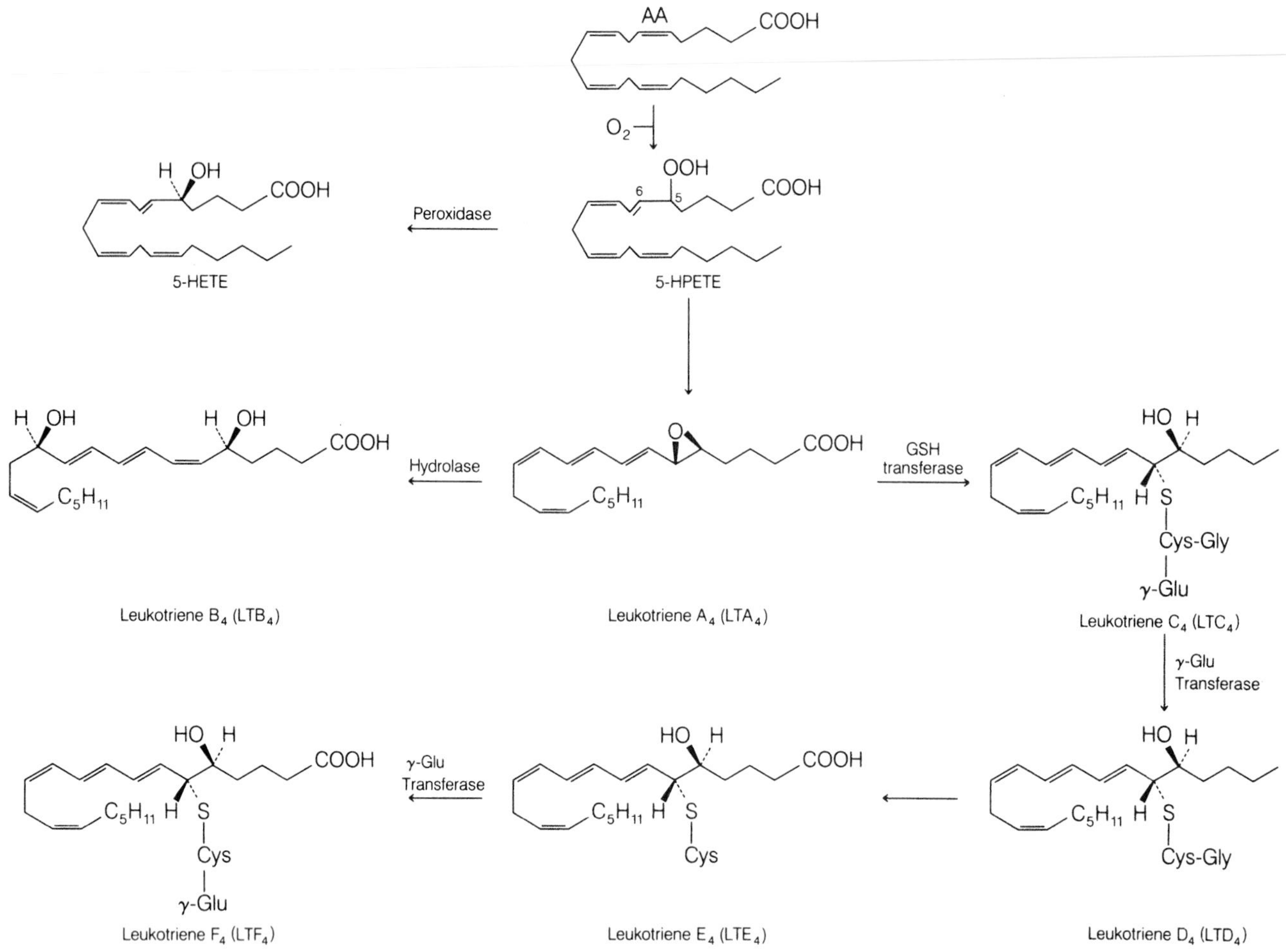

Figure 24–2 ■ Lipoxygenase pathway.

inflammation.[6, 9] This enzyme is also inhibited by the ω-3 (omega-3) fatty acids (eicosapentaenoic acid [EPA] and docosahexaenoic acid [DHA]) found in certain cold-water fish and provided commercially as nutritional supplements, leading to beneficial cardiovascular effects.[10] This enzyme will metabolize 20-carbon fatty acids with one more or one less double bond than arachidonic acid, leading to prostaglandins of varied degrees of unsaturation (e.g., PGE_1 or PGE_3, for which the subscript number indicates the number of double bonds in the molecule).

Prostaglandin H_2 serves as a branch-point substrate for specific enzymes, leading to the production of the various prostaglandins, TXA_2, and PGI_2. Even though most tissues can produce PGH_2, the relative production of each of these derived eicosanoids is highly tissue specific and may be subject to secondary modulation by a variety of cofactors. The complete characterization of enzymes involved in branches of the cyclooxygenase pathway is currently under way.

Specific cellular or tissue responses to the eicosanoids are apparently a function of available surface receptor recognition sites.[11] The variety of tissue responses observed on eicosanoid exposure is outlined in Table 24-1. Non–tissue-selective inhibitors of the cyclooxygenase pathway, such as aspirin, thus may exert a diversity of therapeutic effects or side effects (e.g., decreased uterine muscle contraction and platelet aggregation, gastric ulceration, lowering of elevated body temperature, central and peripheral pain relief, and decreased vascular perfusion) based on their tissue distributions.

The lipoxygenase pathway of arachidonic acid metabolism (Fig. 24-2) produces a variety of acyclic lipid peroxides (hydroperoxyeicosatetraenoic acids [HPETEs]) and derived alcohols (hydroxyeicosatetraenoic acids [HETEs]).[12] Although the specific biological function of each of these lipoxygenase-derived products is not completely known, they are believed to play a major role as chemotactic factors that promote cellular mobilization toward sites of tissue injury. In addition, the glutathione (GSH) conjugates LKT-C_4 and LKT-D_4 are potent, long-acting bronchoconstrictors that are released in the lungs during severe hypersensitivity episodes (leading to their initial designation as the "slow-reacting substances of anaphylaxis" [SRSAs]). Because of the presumed benefit of preventing formation of LKTs in asthmatic patients, much research effort is being dedicated to the design and discovery of drugs that might selectively inhibit the lipoxygenase pathway of arachidonic acid metabolism without affecting the cyclooxygenase pathway.[13] Zileuton (Zyflo by Abbott Laboratories) specifically inhibits the lipoxygenase pathway. It has been proposed that aspirin hypersensitivity in susceptible individuals may result from effectively "shutting down" the cyclooxygenase metabolic route, allowing only the biosynthesis of lipoxygenase path-

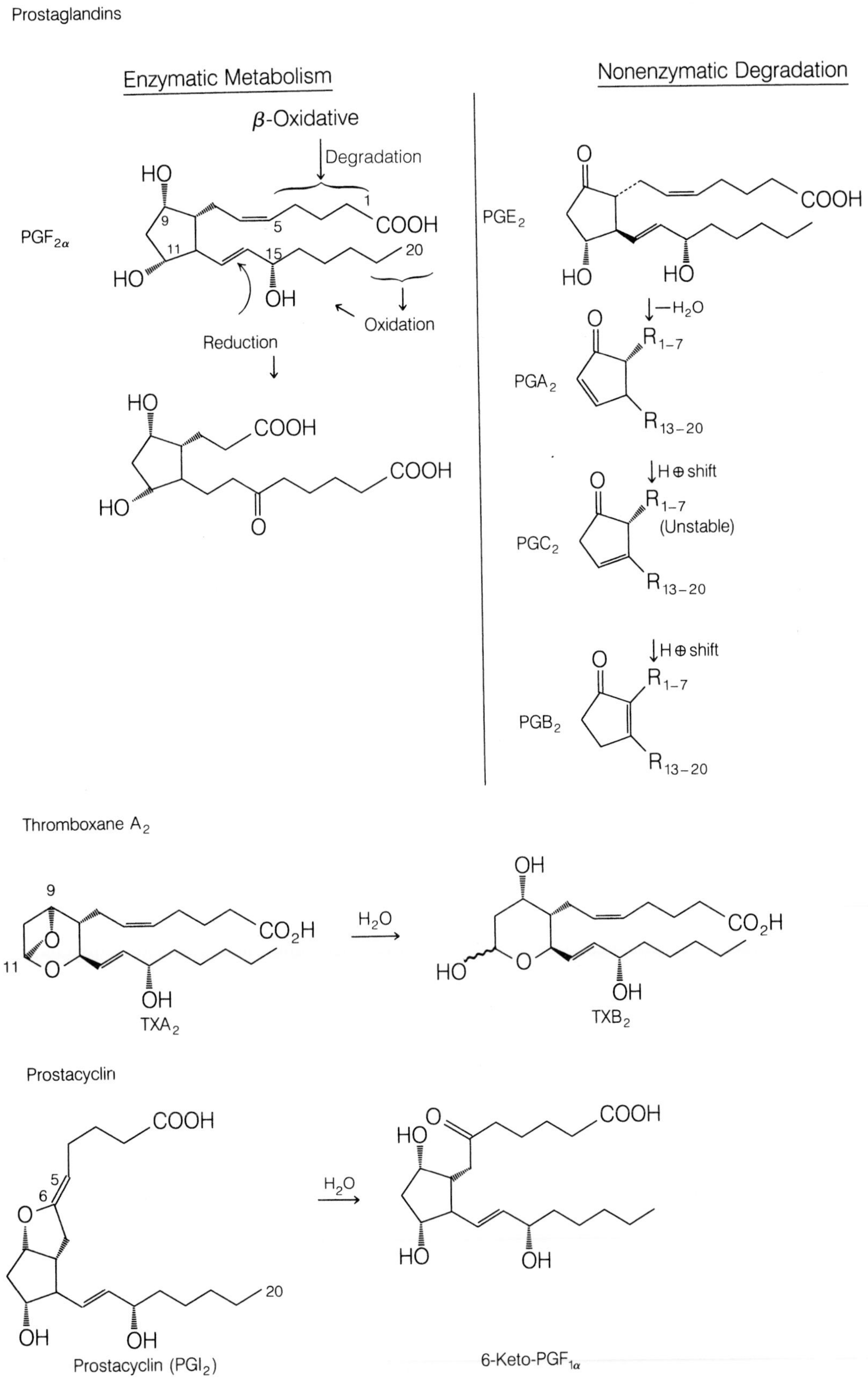

Prostaglandins

Enzymatic Metabolism

Nonenzymatic Degradation

Figure 24–3 ■ Eicosanoid degradation.

TABLE 24–1 Biological Activities Observed with the Eicosanoids

Substance	Observed Biological Activity
PGD_2	Weak inhibitor of platelet aggregation
PGE_1	Vasodilation
	Inhibitor of lipolysis
	Inhibitor of platelet aggregation
	Bronchodilatation
	Stimulates contraction of gastrointestinal smooth muscle
PGE_2	Stimulates hyperalgesic response
	Renal vasodilatation
	Stimulates uterine smooth muscle contraction
	Protects gastrointestinal epithelia from acid degradation
	Reduces secretion of stomach acid
PGF_2	Elevates thermoregulatory set point in anterior hypothalamus
	Stimulates breakdown of corpus luteum (luteolysis) in animals
	Stimulates uterine smooth muscle contraction
PGI_2	Potent inhibitor of platelet aggregation
	Potent vasodilator
	Increases cAMP levels in platelets
PGJ_2	Stimulates osteogenesis
	Inhibits cell proliferation
TXA_2	Potent inducer of platelet aggregation
	Potent vasoconstrictor
	Decreases cAMP levels in platelets
	Stimulates release of ADP and serotonin from platelets
LTB_4	Increases leukocyte chemotaxis and aggregation
LTC/D_4	Slow-reacting substances of anaphylaxis
	Potent and prolonged contraction of guinea pig ileum smooth muscle
	Contracts guinea pig lung parenchymal strips
	Bronchoconstrictive in humans
	Increased vascular permeability in guinea pig skin (augmented by PGEs)
5- or 12-HPETE	Vasodilatation of rat and rabbit gastric circulation
	Inhibits induced platelet aggregation
5- or 12-HETE	Aggregates human leukocytes
	Promotes leukocyte chemotaxis

way intermediates, including the bronchoconstrictive LKTs.[14]

DRUG ACTION MEDIATED BY EICOSANOIDS

The ubiquitous nature of the eicosanoid-producing enzymes implies their significance in a variety of essential cellular processes. Additionally, the sensitivity of these enzymes to structurally varied hydrophobic materials, particularly car-

boxylic acids and phenolic antioxidants, implies their susceptibility to influence by a variety of exogenously administered agents. Because most aromatic drug molecules undergo hepatic hydroxylation, phenolic derivatives of administered drugs become readily available in vivo. Even more directly, aromatic molecules on in vitro incubation with microsomal PGH synthase will become hydroxylated directly during arachidonic acid metabolism, in a process labeled *cooxidation*.[15] This cooxidative process presumably occurs during the peroxidase conversion of PGG_2 to PGH_2, which effectively makes available a nonspecific oxidizing equivalent. The cooxidation process has been implicated in the activation of polycyclic aromatic hydrocarbons to form proximate carcinogens.[16]

The only group of drugs that has been thoroughly characterized for its effect on arachidonic acid metabolism is the NSAIDs. This large group of acidic, aromatic molecules exerts a diverse spectrum of activities (mentioned above) by inhibition of the first enzyme in the arachidonic acid cascade, PGH synthase (also called *COX-1* and *COX-2*). Such agents as salicylic acid, phenylbutazone, naproxen, sulindac, and ibuprofen presumably act by a competitive, reversible inhibition of arachidonic acid oxygenation.[17] Aspirin and certain halogenated aromatics (including indomethacin, flurbiprofen, and Meclomen) appear to inhibit PGH synthase in a time-dependent, irreversible manner.[18] Since this irreversible inhibition appears critical for aspirin's significant effect on platelet aggregation and, therefore, prolongation of bleeding time,[19] this discovery has led clinicians to recommend the daily consumption of low doses of aspirin (81 mg) by patients at risk for myocardial infarction (MI, heart attack), particularly a second MI.

Interestingly, aspirin's primary competitor in the commercial analgesic marketplace, acetaminophen, is a rather weak inhibitor of arachidonic acid oxygenation in vitro.[20] This, in fact, is a characteristic of reversible, noncompetitive, phenolic antioxidant inhibitors in general.[21] This determination, in concert with its lack of in vitro anti-inflammatory activity (while maintaining analgesic and antipyretic activity equivalent to that of the salicylates) has led to the proposal that acetaminophen is more active as an inhibitor of cyclooxygenases in the brain, where peroxide levels (which stimulate cyclooxygenase activity) are lower than in inflamed peripheral joints, where lipid peroxide levels are high.[17] In fact, when in vitro experimental conditions are modified to reduce the so-called peroxide tone, acetaminophen becomes as effective as aspirin in reducing arachidonic acid metabolism.[20]

COX-2 INHIBITORS

The newer anti-inflammatory COX-2 inhibitors (e.g., celecoxib, rofecoxib, and valdecoxib) are claimed to show greater inhibitory selectivity for the inducible form of cyclooxygenase.[22] Although not absolute, this selectivity provides a potential therapeutic advantage by reducing side effects, particularly gastric irritation and ulceration.[23] Unfortunately, this altered profile of activity is not totally risk free. The manufacturer of rofecoxib (Vioxx) has recently (April 2002) issued a warning regarding the use of this product in patients with a medical history of ischemic heart disease.

COX-2 inhibitors do not share the beneficial effects of aspirin in preventing cardiovascular thrombotic events.

DESIGN OF EICOSANOID DRUGS

The ability to capitalize successfully on the highly potent biological effects of the various eicosanoids to develop new therapeutic agents currently seems an unfulfilled promise to medicinal chemists. Although these natural substances are highly potent effectors of various biological functions, their use as drugs has been hampered by several factors: (a) their chemical complexity and relative instability, which have limited, to some extent, their large-scale production and formulation for clinical testing; (b) their susceptibility to rapid degradation (Fig. 24-3), which limits their effective bioactive half-life; and (c) their ability to affect diverse tissues (particularly the gastrointestinal tract, which may lead to severe nausea and vomiting) if they enter the systemic circulation, even in small amounts. Caution is always recommended with the use of prostaglandin analogues in females of childbearing age because of their potential for inducing dramatic contraction of uterine muscles, possibly leading to miscarriage.

Several approaches have been used to overcome these difficulties. First, structural analogues of particular eicosanoids have been synthesized that are more resistant to chemical and metabolic degradation but maintain, to a large extent, a desirable biological activity. Although commercial production and formulation may be facilitated by this approach, biological potency of these analogues is usually reduced by several orders of magnitude. Also, systemic side effects may become troublesome because of broader tissue distribution as a result of the increased biological half-life.

Structural alterations of the eicosanoids have been aimed primarily at reducing or eliminating the very rapid metabolism of these potent substances to relatively inactive metabolites (see Fig. 24-3). Several analogues are presented in Table 24-2 to illustrate approaches that have led to potentially useful eicosanoid drugs. Methylation at the 15 or 16 position will eliminate or reduce oxidation of the essential 15-(S)-alcohol moiety. Esterification of the carboxylic acid function may affect formulation or absorption characteristics of the eicosanoid, whereas esterase enzymes in the bloodstream or tissues would be expected to regenerate the active therapeutic agent quickly. Somewhat surprisingly, considering the restrictive configurational requirements at the naturally asymmetric centers, a variety of hydrophobic substituents (including phenyl rings) may replace the saturated alkyl chains, with retention of bioactivity.

A second major approach has been aimed at delivering the desired agent, either a natural eicosanoid or a modified analogue, to a localized site of action by a controlled delivery method. The exact method of delivery may vary according to the desired site of action (e.g., uterus, stomach, lung) but has included aerosols and locally applied suppository, gel formulations, or cyclodextrin complexes. The recent commercial development of PGF-type derivatives for use in the eye to lower intraocular pressure (IOP) in glaucoma (discussed below under the heading, Prostaglandins for Ophthalmic Use) relies on their potent therapeutic effects coupled with their limited distribution from this site of administration.[24]

DEVELOPMENT OF PROSTACYCLIN-DERIVED PRODUCTS

The ongoing development of potent, effective, and long-acting forms of naturally occurring PGI_2 is an excellent illustration of strategies that capitalize on the beneficial but short-lived biological effects of eicosanoid derivatives. PGI_2 itself is currently marketed as the sodium salt (epoprostenol; Flolan by GlaxoSmithKline) for continuous intravenous infusion in patients suffering from primary pulmonary hypertension (PPH). The solution for infusion is prepared within 48 hours of expected use because of its limited chemical stability. The potent vasodilatory, platelet antiaggregatory effect and vascular smooth muscle antiproliferative effect of this naturally occurring eicosanoid produce a dramatic but short-lived (half-life less than 6 minutes) therapeutic effect in PPH patients. Continuous, uninterrupted administration of the drug by portable infusion pump is necessary, however, to prevent symptoms of rebound pulmonary hypertension. To ensure proper use of this therapy, its distribution is relatively restricted.[25]

Three more-stable derivatives of PGI_2 are being developed to extend the duration of action of this drug to improve the safety and convenience of PPH therapy and, perhaps, broaden the therapeutic indications for its use. Treprostinil (Remodulin) with an extended half-life has been developed for continuous subcutaneous injection for PPH patients. This

TABLE 24–2 Prostaglandin Analogues under Investigation as Receptor Ligands and Future Drug Candidates

Structure	Name	Activity
	Butaprost	EP$_2$-receptor ligand
	BW245C: R=H BWA 868C: R = CH$_2$	DP-receptor ligands
	Cicaprost	IP-receptor ligand
	Enprostil (Roche)	EP$_3$-receptor ligand antiulcer therapy
	Enisoprost (Searle)	Orphan status: cyclosporine toxicity
	Gemeprost (Cervagem by Ono Pharmaceuticals)	Abortifacient
	S-145	TP-receptor ligand

(Continued)

TABLE 24–2—*Continued*

Structure	Name	Activity
	SQ-29548	TP-receptor ligand
	Sulprostone (Glofil Banca Dati Sanitaria Farmaceutical)	EP-receptor ligand Oxytoxic
	U-46619	TP-receptor ligand

method of administration and longer half-life would markedly improve the convenience and safety of "prostacyclin" therapy in PPH patients. Localized intermittent subcutaneous administration of Uniprost is proposed for the treatment of critical limb ischemia.

Another stable derivative of PGI_2, iloprost, is intended for nasal inhalation to provide a direct vasodilatory effect on pulmonary blood vessels and thus decrease vascular resistance. Currently available in Europe, patients inhale 6 to 8 puffs of aerosolized iloprost every 2 to 3 hours. Side effects such as coughing, headaches, and jaw pain have been reported.

An even more chemically and biologically stable derivative of PGI_2 is beraprost, which is being evaluated in an oral formulation for the treatment of early-stage pulmonary arterial hypertension[26,27] and peripheral vascular disease.[28] This prostacyclin has been approved for use in Japan but not yet in the United States.

EICOSANOID RECEPTORS

Another approach to developing new therapies based on the known biological activities of the prostaglandins and leukotrienes requires characterization of the naturally occurring tissue receptors for these agents. A thorough knowledge of the tissue distribution (localization) of such receptors and their binding characteristics would allow the design of receptor-specific agonists or antagonists that might not possess the same limitations as the natural eicosanoids but could affect tissue function nonetheless.

An excellent historical description of prostanoid receptor isolation and characterization has been published,[29] and a more recent review of developments in this field is available.[11] Basically, prostanoid receptors are identified by their primary eicosanoid agonist (e.g., DP, EP, IP, and TP), although subclassification of PGE receptors has been necessary (e.g., EP_1, EP_2, EP_3, and EP_4). In fact, the existence of subtypes of the EP_3 receptor (EP_{3A}, EP_{3B}, EP_{3C}, EP_{3D}) and TP receptor (TP_α, TP_β) has been proposed. Complete characterization of receptors (and subtypes) includes tissue localization, biological effect produced, cellular signal transduction mechanism, inhibitor sensitivity, protein structure, and genetic origin. Not all receptors or subtypes have been completely characterized in this way, but significant progress toward this goal has occurred recently. Table 24-3 indicates characteristics of the prostanoid receptors identified thus far.

Although receptor studies have required the use of nonhuman species (principally the mouse but also the rat, cow, sheep, and rabbit), a high correlation of structural homology of receptor subtypes between species (~80 to 90%) has been observed, while structural homology among receptor subtypes is relatively low (30 to 50%). All prostanoid receptors, however, are believed belong to a "rhodopsin-type" superfamily of receptors that function via G-protein–coupled transduction mechanisms. Three general classes of prostanoid receptors are proposed[11]: *(a)* relaxant, including DP, EP_2, EP_4, and IP, which promote smooth muscle relaxation by raising intracellular cyclic adenosine monophosphate (cAMP) levels; *(b)* contractile, including EP_1, FP, and TP, which promote smooth muscle contraction via calcium ion mobilization; and *(c)* inhibitory, such as EP_3, which prevents smooth muscle contraction by lowering intracellular cAMP levels. Although structural and functional characterization of prostanoid receptors has permitted the identification and differentiation of selective receptor ligands (Table 24-3, both agonists and antagonists), overlapping tissue distributions

---

TABLE 24–3 Prostanoid Receptor Characteristics

Receptor	Principle Ligands	Tissue/Action	Transduction	Gene Knockout Effect
DP	PGD_2 BW245C BWA868C	Ileum/muscle relaxation Brain (leptomeninges)/ sleep induction	↑cAMP/Gs	Not available
EP_1	PGE_2 17-phenyl-PGE_2 Sulprostone Iloprost Bimatoprost	Kidney/papillary ducts Lung/bronchoconstriction Stomach/smooth muscle contraction	↑Ca^{2+}	Not available
EP_2 (inducible)	PGE_2; PGE_1 Butaprost (misoprostol)	Lung/bronchodilation Uterus/implantation	↑cAMP/G_s	↓Ovulation ↓Fertilization ↑Na^+ hypertension
EP_3	PGE_2; PGE_1 Sulprostone Misoprostol Enprostil Gemeprost	Gastric/antisecretory Gastric/cytoprotective Uterus/inhibits contraction Brain/fever response	EP_{3A} ↓ cAMP/G_i EP_{3B} ↑ cAMP/G_s EP_{3C} ↑ cAMP/G_s EP_{3D} ↑PI turnover/G_q	Pyrogen response
EP_4	PGE_2; PGE_1 Misoprostol	Ductus arteriosus/relaxant Kidney/glomerulus Gastric antrum/mucous secretion Uterus/endometrium	↑cAMP/G_s	Patent ductus arteriosus ↓Bone resorption
FP	$PGF_{2\alpha}$ Fluprostenol Carboprost Latanoprost Unoprostone Travoprost Bimatoprost	Eye/decreases intraocular pressure Corpus luteum/luteolysis Lung/bronchoconstriction	↑PI turnover/G_q	Lost parturition
IP	PGI_2 Iloprost Cicaprost Beraprost	Platelets/aggregation Arteries/dilation DRG neurons/pain Kidney/afferent arterioles (↑GFR)	↑cAMP/Gs	↑Thrombosis ↓Inflammatory edema
TP	TXA_2 S-145 SQ-29548 U-46619	Lung/bronchoconstriction Kidney/↓ GFR Arteries/constriction Thymus/↓ immature thymocytes	TP_α ↓ cAMP TP_β ↑ cAMP	↑Bleeding

From Narumiya, S., Sugimoto, Y., and Ushikubi, F.: Physiol. Rev. 79: 1193–1226, 1999.

and common signal transduction mechanisms present formidable obstacles to the development of specific pharmacological therapies.

EICOSANOIDS APPROVED FOR HUMAN CLINICAL USE

Prostaglandin F$_{2\alpha}$. PGF$_{2\alpha}$, dinoprost (Prostin F2 Alpha), is a naturally occurring prostaglandin that was administered intra-amniotically to induce labor or abortion within the first trimester.

This product, which was supplied as a solution of the tromethamine salt (5 mg/mL) for direct administration, is no longer available in the United States for human use but is still formulated for veterinary use as described elsewhere in this chapter.

Prostaglandin E$_2$. PGE$_2$, dinoprostone (Prostin E$_2$, Cervidil), is a naturally occurring prostaglandin that is administered in a single dose of 20 mg by vaginal suppository to induce labor or abortion.

Carboprost Tromethamine. Carboprost tromethamine, 15-(S)-methyl-PGF$_{2\alpha}$ (Hemabate), is a prostaglandin derivative that has been modified to prevent metabolic oxidation of the 15-position alcohol function.

This derivative is administered in a dose of 250 μg by deep intramuscular injection to induce abortion or to ameliorate severe postpartum hemorrhage.

Prostaglandin E$_1$, USP. PGE$_1$, alprostadil (Prostin VR Pediatric), is a naturally occurring prostaglandin that has found particular use in maintaining a patent (opened) ductus arteriosus in infants with congenital defects that restrict pulmonary or systemic blood flow.

Alprostadil must be administered intravenously continually at a rate of approximately 0.1 μg/kg per minute to temporarily maintain the patency of the ductus arteriosus until corrective surgery can be performed. Up to 80% of circulating alprostadil may be metabolized in a single pass through the lungs. Because apnea occurs in 10 to 12% of neonates with congenital heart defects, this product should be administered only when ventilatory assistance is immediately available. Other commonly observed side effects include decreased arterial blood pressure (which should be monitored during infusion), inhibited platelet aggregation (which might aggravate bleeding tendencies), and diarrhea. Prostin VR Pediatric is provided as a sterile solution in absolute alcohol (0.5 mg/mL) that must be diluted in saline or dextrose solution before intravenous administration. A liposomal preparation is available (Liposome Company) to extend the biological half-life of the active prostaglandin.

Alprostadil (Caverject) is also available in glass vials for reconstitution to provide 1.0 mL of solution containing either 10 or 20 μg/mL for intercavernosal penile injection to diagnose or correct erectile dysfunction in certain cases of impotence. A urethral suppository is also available; this therapeutic use has been all but eliminated, however, by the availability of orally administered Viagra.

Prostaglandin E$_1$ Cyclodextrin. The cyclic polysaccharide complex of PGE$_1$ (Vasoprost) is available as an orphan drug for the treatment of severe peripheral arterial occlusive disease when grafts or angioplasty are not indicated. Cyclodextrin complexation is used to enhance water solubility and reduce rapid metabolic inactivation.

Misoprostol. Misoprostol, 16-(R,S)-methyl-16-hydroxy-PGE$_1$ methyl ester (Cytotec), is a modified prostaglandin analogue that shows potent gastric antisecretory and gastroprotective effects when administered orally.

Misoprostol is administered orally in tablet form in a dose

of 100 to 200 μg 4 times a day to prevent gastric ulceration in susceptible individuals who are taking NSAIDs. Misoprostol is combined with the NSAID diclofenac in an analgesic product (Arthrotec by Pharmacia) that is potentially safe for long-term antiarthritic therapy. This prostaglandin derivative should be avoided by pregnant women because of its potential to induce abortion. In fact, the combined use of intramuscular methotrexate and intravaginal misoprostol has been claimed to be a safe and effective, noninvasive method for the termination of early pregnancy.[30]

PROSTAGLANDINS FOR OPHTHALMIC USE

Several prostaglandin analogues have recently come to market for the treatment of open-angle glaucoma or ocular hypertension in patients who have not benefited from other available therapies. These products are marketed as sterile solutions for use in the eye (as indicated below). Each of these agents is presumed to lower IOP by stimulation of FP receptors to open the uveoscleral pathway, thus increasing aqueous humor outflow. Commonly occurring side effects reported for this product group include conjunctival hyperemia, increased pigmentation and growth of eyelashes, ocular pruritus, and increased pigmentation of the iris and eyelid. Contact lenses should be removed during and after (15 minutes) administration of these products.

Bimatoprost. Bimatoprost (Lumigan) is supplied as a sterile 0.03% ophthalmic solution in 2.5- and 5.0-mL sizes. The recommended dosage of bimatoprost is limited to one drop into the affected eye once daily in the evening. Increased use may decrease its beneficial effect. If used concurrently with other IOP-lowering drugs, a waiting period of 5 minutes should separate administrations.

Latanoprost. Latanoprost (Xalatan) is available as a 0.005% sterile ophthalmic solution in a 2.5-mL dispenser bottle. Latanoprost is also marketed as a combination ophthalmic product with the β-adrenergic blocking agent timolol, which apparently enhances IOP-lowering by decreasing the production of aqueous humor. Cautions and side effects are similar to those for other ophthalmic prostanoids.

Travoprost. Travoprost (Travatan) is supplied as a 2.5-mL sterile 0.004% ophthalmic solution in a 3.5-mL container. Travoprost is claimed to be the most potent and FP-specific analogue in this product category.[31] Cautions and side effects are similar to those given above.

Unoprostone. Unoprostone (Rescula) is supplied as a 0.15% sterile ophthalmic solution. Unoprostone is somewhat unusual, in that it is a docosanoid (22-carbon atom) $PGF_{2\alpha}$ analogue marketed as the isopropyl ester. The natural 15-position alcohol is oxidized to the ketone, as would be expected to occur in vivo. Cautions and side effects are similar to those given above.

VETERINARY USES OF PROSTANOIDS

Since McCracken and coworkers demonstrated that $PGF_{2\alpha}$ acts as a hormone in sheep to induce disintegration of the corpus luteum (luteolysis),[32] salts of this prostaglandin and a variety of analogues have been marketed to induce or synchronize estrus in breed animals. This procedure allows artificial insemination of many animals during one insemination period. The following two products are currently available for this purpose.

Cloprostenol Sodium. Cloprostenol sodium (Estrumate) is available as the sodium salt from Bayer Agricultural Division or Bayvet Division of Miles Laboratory as an aqueous solution containing 250 mg/mL.

Dinoprost Trimethamine. Dinoprost trimethamine (Lutalyse) marketed by Upjohn (veterinary) is a pH-balanced aqueous solution of the trimethylammonium salt of $PGF_{2\alpha}$ (5.0 mg/mL).

EICOSANOIDS IN CLINICAL DEVELOPMENT FOR HUMAN TREATMENT

Numerous prostaglandin analogues are under investigation for the treatment of human diseases (see Table 24-2). Efforts are being focused on the areas of gastroprotection for antiulcer therapy, fertility control, the development of thrombolytics (e.g., prostacyclin or thromboxane synthetase inhibitors) to treat cerebrovascular or coronary artery diseases, and the development of antiasthmatics through modulation of the lipoxygenase pathway. Future application of eicosanoids to the treatment of cancer, hypertension, or immune system disorders cannot be ruled out, however. Thus, although progress has been slow, the expanded use of eicosanoids or eicosanoid analogues as therapeutic agents in the future is almost ensured.

REFERENCES

1. Kurzrok, R., and Lieb, C.: Proc. Soc. Exp. Biol. 28:268, 1931.
2. von Euler, U. S.: J. Physiol. (Lond.) 88:213, 1937.
3. Bergstrom, S., et al.: Acta Chem. Scand. 16:501, 1962.
4. Nicolaou, K. C., and Petasis, N. A.: In Willis, A. L. (ed.). Handbook of Eicosanoids: Prostaglandins and Related Lipids, vol. I, part B. Boca Raton, FL, CRC Press, 1987, pp. 1–18.
5. Flower, R. J., Blackwell, G. J., and Smith, D. L.: In Willis, A. L. (ed.). Handbook of Eicosanoids: Prostaglandins and Related Lipids, vol. II. Boca Raton, FL, CRC Press, 1989, pp. 35–46.
6. Parnham, M. J., Day, R. O., and Van den Berg, W. B.: Agents Actions 41:C145–C149, 1994.
7. Tsai, A.-L., and Kulmacz, R. J.: Prostaglandins Other Lipid Mediators 62:231-254, 2000.
8. Smith, W. L., and Dewitt, D. L.: Adv. Immunol. 62:167–215, 1996.
9. Vane, J. R., Bakhle, Y. S., and Botting, R. M.: Annu. Rev. Pharmacol. Toxicol. 38:97–120, 1998.
10. Lands, W. E. M.: Prostaglandins Leukot. Essent. Fatty Acids 63:125–126, 2000.
11. Narumiya, S., Sugimoto, Y., and Ushikubi, F.: Physiol. Rev. 79:1193–1226, 1999.
12. Kuhn, H.: Prostaglandins Other Lipid Mediators 62:255–270, 2000.
13. Bell, R. L., Summers, J. B., and Harris, R. R.: Annu. Rep. Med. Chem. 32:91–100, 1997.
14. Szczeklik, A.: Adv. Prostaglandin Thromboxane Leukot. Res. 22:185–198, 1994.
15. Marnett, L. J., and Eling, T. E.: Rev. Biochem. Toxicol. 5:135, 1984.
16. Robertson, I. G. C., et al.: Cancer Res. 43:476, 1983.
17. Lands, W. E. M., Jr.: Trends Pharmacol. Sci. 1:78, 1981.
18. Rome, L. H., and Lands, W. E. M.: Proc. Natl. Acad. Sci. U. S. A. 72:4863, 1975.
19. Higgs, G. A., et al.: Proc. Natl. Acad. Sci. U. S. A. 84:1417, 1987.
20. Hanel, A. M., and Lands, W. E. M.: Biochem. Pharmacol. 31:3307, 1982.
21. Kuehl, F. A., et al.: In Ramwell, P. (ed.). Prostaglandin Synthetase Inhibitors: New Clinical Applications. New York, Alan R. Liss, 1980, pp. 73-86.
22. Cryer, B., and Feldman, M.: Am. J. Med. 104:413-421, 1998.
23. Warner, T. D., Giuliano, F., Vojnovic, I., et al.: Proc. Natl. Acad. Sci. U. S. A. 96:7563–7568, 1999.
24. Susanna, R., Giampani, J., Borges, A. S., et al.: Ophthalmology 108:259–263, 2001.
25. Am. J. Health-Syst. Pharm. 53:976 and 982, 1996.
26. Vizza, C. D., Sciomer, S., Morelli, S., et al.: Heart 86:661–665, 2001.
27. Nagaya, N., Shimizu, Y., Satoh, T., et al.: Heart 87:340–345, 2002.
28. Lievre, M., Morand, S., Besse, B., et al.: Circulation 102:426–431, 2000.
29. Coleman, R. A., Smith, W. L., and Narumiya, S.: Pharmacol. Rev. 46:205–229, 1994.
30. Hausknecht, R. V.: N. Engl. J. Med. 333:537–540, 1995.
31. Sharif, N. A., Davis, T. L., and Williams, G. W.: J. Pharm. Pharmacol. 51:685–694, 1999.
32. McCracken, J. A., et al.: Nature 238:129, 1972.

SELECTED READING

Bailey, J. M. (ed.): Prostaglandins, Leukotrienes, and Lipoxins. New York, Plenum Press, 1985.
Batt, D. G.: 5-Lipoxygenase inhibitors and their anti-inflammatory activities. Prog. Med. Chem. 29:1–63, 1992.
Chandra, R. K. (ed.): Health Effects of Fish and Fish Oils. St. John's, Newfoundland, ARTS Biomedical Publishers and Distributors, 1989.
Cohen, M. M. (ed.): Biological Protection with Prostaglandins, vols. 1 and 2. Boca Raton, FL, CRC Press, 1985, 1986.
Dunn, M. J., Patrono, C., and Cinotti, G. A. (eds.): Renal eicosanoids. Adv. Exp. Med. Biol. 259:1–421, 1989.
Edqvist, L. E., and Kindahl, H. (eds.): Prostaglandins in Animal Reproduction. New York, Elsevier, 1984.
Fukushima, M.: Biological activities and mechanisms of action of PGJ_2 and related compounds: an update. Prostaglandins Leukot. Essent. Fatty Acids 47:1–12, 1992.
Gryglewski, R. J., and Stock, G. (eds.): Prostacyclin and Its Stable Analogue Iloprost. New York, Springer-Verlag, 1987.
Gryglewski, R. J., Szczeklik, A., and McGiff, J. C. (eds.): Prostacyclin Clinical Trials. New York, Raven Press, 1985.
Hillier, K. (ed.): Advances in Eicosanoid Research, vols. 1–4. Boston, MTP Press, 1987–1988.
Lands, W. E. M., and Smith, W. L. (eds.): Prostaglandins and arachidonate metabolites. Methods Enzymol. 86:1–705, 1982.
Lefer, A. M., and Gee, M. H. (eds.): Leukotrienes in cardiovascular and pulmonary function. Prog. Clin. Biol. Res. 199:1–270, 1985.
Pace-Asciak, C. R.: Mass spectra of prostaglandins and related products. In Samuelsson, B., and Paoletti, R. (ed.): Adv. Prostaglandin Thromboxane Leukot. Res. 18:1–565, 1989.
Rainsford, K. D.: Anti-Inflammatory and Anti-Rheumatic Drugs, vols. 1–3. Boca Raton, FL, CRC Press, 1985.
Robinson, H. J., and Vane, J. R. (eds.): Prostaglandin Synthetase Inhibitors. New York, Raven Press, 1974.
Rokach, J. (ed.): Leukotrienes and Lipoxygenases. Amsterdam, Elsevier, 1989.
Ruzicka, T.: Eicosanoids and the Skin. Boca Raton, FL, CRC Press, 1990.
Schror, K., and Sinzinger, H. (eds.): Prostaglandins in Clinical Research: Cardiovascular System, vol. 301. New York, Alan R. Liss, 1989.
Simopoulos, A. P., Kifer, R. R., and Martin, R. E.: Health Effects of Polyunsaturated Fatty Acids in Seafoods. New York, Academic Press, 1986.
Stansby, M. E. (ed.): Fish Oils in Nutrition. New York, Van Nostrand Reinhold, 1990.
Thaler-Dao, H., dePaulet, A. C., and Paoletti, R.: Icosanoids and Cancer. New York, Raven Press, 1984.
Vane, J. R., and O'Grady, J. (eds.): Therapeutic Applications of Prostaglandins. Boston, Edward Arnold, 1993.
Watkins, W. D., Peterson, M. B., and Fletcher, J. R. (eds.): Prostaglandins in Clinical Practice. New York, Raven Press, 1989.
Willis, A. L. (ed.): Handbook of Eicosanoids: Prostaglandins and Related Lipids, vol. II. Boca Raton, FL, CRC Press, 1989.
Zor, U., Naor, Z., and Danon, A. (eds.): In Braquet, P. (ed.). Leukotrienes and Prostanoids in Health and Disease, New Trends in Lipid Mediators Research, vol. 3. Basel, S. Karger, 1989.

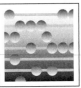

Proteins, Enzymes, and Peptide Hormones

STEPHEN J. CUTLER AND HORACE G. CUTLER

Proteins are essential to all living matter and perform numerous functions as cellular components. Fundamental cellular events are catalyzed by proteins called enzymes, while other proteins serve as architectural constituents of protoplasm and cell membranes. Most important are the classes of hormones that are characterized as proteins or protein-like compounds because of their polypeptidic structure.

Protein chemistry, essential in understanding the mechanisms of molecular biology and how cellular components participate in physiology, is also key to certain aspects of medicinal chemistry. An examination of the chemical nature of proteins explains the action of those medicinal agents that are proteins or protein-like compounds and elucidates their physicochemical and biochemical properties. This, in turn, relates to their mechanisms of action. Furthermore, in medicinal chemistry, drug–receptor interactions are directly related to structure–activity relationships (SARs) and aid in the process of rational drug design. Drug receptors are considered to be macromolecules, some of which appear to be proteins or protein-like.

Recombinant DNA (rDNA) technology[1] has had a dramatic impact on our ability to produce complex proteins and polypeptides structurally identical with those found in vivo. Many of the endogenous proteins or polypeptides have exhibited neurotransmitter and hormonal properties that regulate a variety of important physiological processes. rDNA-derived technology products currently being used are discussed below in this chapter.

Although this chapter reviews the medicinal chemistry of proteins, it includes some enzymology, not only because many drugs affect enzyme systems and vice versa but also because basic discoveries in enzymology have been practically applied to the study of drug–receptor interactions. Hence, a basic introduction to enzymes is included.

PROTEIN HYDROLYSATES

In therapeutics, agents affecting volume and composition of body fluids include various classes of parenteral products. Ideally, it would be desirable to have available parenteral fluids that provide adequate calories and important proteins and lipids to mimic, as closely as possible, an appropriate diet. Unfortunately, this is not the case. Usually, sufficient carbohydrate is administered intravenously to prevent ketosis, and in some cases, it is necessary to give further sources of carbohydrate by vein to reduce protein waste. Sources of protein are made available in the form of protein hydrolysates, and these can be administered to induce a favorable balance.

Protein deficiencies in human nutrition are sometimes treated with protein hydrolysates. The lack of adequate protein may result from several conditions, but the problem is not always easy to diagnose. The deficiency may be due to insufficient dietary intake, temporarily increased demands (as in pregnancy), impaired digestion or absorption, liver malfunction, increased catabolism, or loss of proteins and amino acids (e.g., in fevers, leukemia, hemorrhage, surgery, burns, fractures, or shock).

Protein Hydrolysate. Protein hydrolysate is a solution of amino acids and short-chain oligopeptides that represent the approximate nutritive equivalent of the casein, lactalbumin, plasma, fibrin, or other suitable protein from which it is derived by acid, enzymatic, or other hydrolytic methods. It may be modified by partial removal, and restoration or addition of one or more amino acids. It may contain dextrose or another carbohydrate suitable for intravenous infusion. Not less than 50% of the total nitrogen present is in the form of α-amino nitrogen. It is a yellowish to red-amber transparent liquid with a pH of 4 to 7.

Parenteral preparations are used to maintain a positive nitrogen balance in patients who exhibit interference with ingestion, digestion, or absorption of food. For such patients, the material to be injected must be nonantigenic and must not contain pyrogens or peptides of high molecular weight. Injection may result in untoward effects such as nausea, vomiting, fever, vasodilatation, abdominal pain, twitching and convulsions, edema at the site of injection, phlebitis, and thrombosis. Sometimes, these reactions are due to inadequate cleanliness or too-rapid administration.

AMINO ACID SOLUTIONS

Amino acid solutions contain a mixture of essential and nonessential crystalline amino acids, with or without electrolytes (e.g., Aminosyn, ProCalamine, Travasol, Novamine). Although oral studies have shown a comparison between protein hydrolysates and free amino acid diets,[2] protein hydrolysates are being replaced by crystalline amino acid solutions for parenteral administration because the free amino acids are used more efficiently than the peptides produced by the enzymatic cleavage of protein hydrolysates.[3]

PROTEINS AND PROTEIN-LIKE COMPOUNDS

The chemistry of proteins is complex, with many facets not completely understood. Protein structure is usually studied in basic organic chemistry and, to a greater extent, in biochemistry, but for the purposes of this chapter some of the more important topics are summarized, with emphasis on relationships to medicinal chemistry. Much progress has been made in understanding the more sophisticated features of protein structure[4] and its correlation with physicochemical and biological properties. With the total synthesis of ribonuclease in 1969, new approaches to the study of SARs among proteins have involved the synthesis of modified proteins.

Many types of compounds important in medicinal chemistry are classified structurally as proteins, including enzymes, antigens, and antibodies. Numerous hormones are low relative-molecular-mass proteins and so are called *simple proteins*. Fundamentally, all proteins are composed of one or more polypeptide chains; that is, the primary organizational level of protein structure is the polypeptide (polyamide) chain composed of naturally occurring amino acids bonded to one another by amide linkages (Fig. 25-1). The specific physicochemical and biological properties of proteins depend not only on the nature of the specific amino acids and their sequence within the polypeptide chain but also on conformational characteristics.

Conformational Features of Protein Structure

As stated, the polypeptide chain is considered to be the primary level of protein structure, and the folding of the polypeptide chains into a specific coiled structure is maintained through hydrogen-bonding interactions (intramolecular) (Fig. 25-2). The folding pattern is the secondary level of protein structure. The intramolecular hydrogen bonds involve the partially negative oxygens of amide carbonyl groups and the partially positive hydrogens of the amide –NH. Additional factors, such as ionic bonding between positively and negatively charged groups and disulfide bonds, help stabilize such folded structures.

The arrangement and interfolding of the coiled chains into layers determine the tertiary and higher levels of protein structure. Such final conformational character is determined by various types of interaction, primarily hydrophobic forces and, to some extent, hydrogen bonding and ion pairing.[4, 5] Hydrophobic forces are implicated in many biological phenomena associated with protein structure and interactions.[6] The side chains (R groups) of various amino acids have hydrocarbon moieties that are hydrophobic, and they have minimal tendency to associate with water molecules, whereas water molecules are strongly associated through hydrogen bonding. Such hydrophobic R groups tend to get close to one another, with exclusion of water molecules, to form ''bonds'' between different segments of the chain or

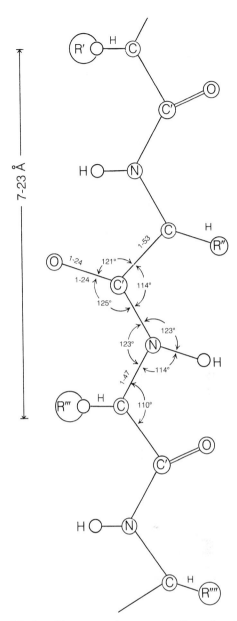

Figure 25–1 ■ Diagrammatic representation of a fully extended polypeptide chain with the bond lengths and the bond angles derived from crystal structures and other experimental evidence. (From Corey, R. B., and Pauling, L.: Proc. R. Soc. Lond. Ser. B 141:10, 1953.)

between different chains. These are often termed *hydrophobic bonds, hydrophobic forces,* or *hydrophobic interactions.*

The study of protein structure has required several physicochemical methods of analysis.[4] Ultraviolet spectrophotometry has been applied to the assessment of conformational changes that proteins undergo. Conformational changes can be investigated by the direct plotting of the difference in absorption of the protein under various sets of conditions. X-ray analysis has been most useful in the elucidation of the structures of several proteins (e.g., myoglobulin and lysozyme). Absolute determinations of conformation and helical content can be made by x-ray diffraction analysis. Optical rotation of proteins has also been studied

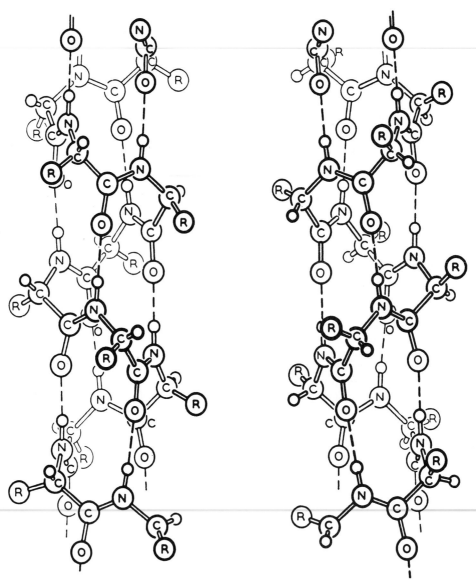

Figure 25–2 ■ Left-handed and right-handed α helices. The R and H groups on the α-carbon atom are in the correct position corresponding to the known configuration of the L-amino acids in proteins. (From Pauling, L., and Corey, R. B.: unpublished drawings.)

fruitfully. The specific rotations of proteins are always negative, and extreme changes in pH (when the protein is in solution) and conditions that promote denaturation (urea solutions, increased temperatures) tend to augment the negative optical rotation. Accordingly, it is thought that the changes in rotation are due to conformational changes (i.e., changes in protein structure at the secondary and higher levels of organization). Optical rotatory dispersion has also been used to study conformational alterations and differences among globular proteins. Additionally, circular dichroism methodology has been involved in structural studies. The shape and the magnitude of rotatory dispersion curves and circular dichroism spectra are very sensitive to conformational alterations; thus, the effects of enzyme inhibitors on conformation can be analyzed. Structural studies have included the investigation of the tertiary structures of proteins in high-frequency nuclear magnetic resonance

(NMR).[7, 8] NMR spectroscopy has been of some use in the study of interactions between drug molecules and proteins such as enzymes, proteolipids, and others. NMR has been applied to the study of binding of atropine analogues to acetylcholinesterase[9] and interactions involving cholinergic ligands and housefly brain and torpedo electroplax.[10] NMR was also used in the determination of the tertiary structure of the capsid protein of the human immunodeficiency virus (HIV).[11]

Factors Affecting Protein Structure

Conditions that promote the hydrolysis of amide linkages affect protein structure (see under the heading, Protein Hydrolysates, above). The highly ordered conformation of a protein can be disorganized (without hydrolysis of the amide linkages), and in the process, the protein's biological activity is lost. This process, customarily called *denaturation,* involves unfolding of the polypeptide chains, loss of the native conformation of the protein, and disorganization of the uniquely ordered structure, without the cleavage of covalent bonds (e.g., cooked egg albumin). The rupture of native disulfide bonds is usually considered a more extensive and drastic change than denaturation. Criteria for the detection of denaturation involve detection of previously masked –SH, imidazole, and –NH_2 groups; decreased solubility; increased susceptibility to the action of proteolytic enzymes; decreased diffusion constant and increased viscosity of protein solution; loss of enzymatic activity if the protein is an enzyme; and modification of antigenic properties.

Purification and Classification

It might be said that it is old-fashioned to classify proteins according to the following system, since so much progress has been made in understanding protein structure. Nevertheless, an outline of this system of classification is given because the terms used are still found in the pharmaceutical and medical literature. Table 25-1 includes the classification and characterization of simple proteins. Before classification, the protein material must be purified as much as possible, which is a very challenging task. Several criteria are used to determine homomolecularity, including crystallinity, constant solubility at a given temperature, osmotic pressure in different solvents, diffusion rate, electrophoretic mobility, dielectric constant, chemical assay, spectrophotometry, and quantification of antigenicity. The methodology of purification is complex; procedures can involve various techniques of chromatography (column), electrophoresis, ultracentrifugation, and others. High-performance liquid chromatography (HPLC) has been applied to the separation of peptides (e.g., the purification of some hypothalamic peptides by a combination of chromatographic methods including HPLC).[12, 13]

Conjugated proteins contain a nonprotein structural component in addition to the protein moiety, whereas simple proteins contain only the polypeptide chain of amino acid units. Nucleoproteins are conjugated proteins containing nucleic acids as structural components. Glycoproteins are carbohydrate-containing conjugated proteins (e.g., thyroglobulin). Phosphoproteins contain phosphate moieties (e.g., casein). Lipoproteins are lipid bearing. Metalloproteins have some bound metal. Chromoproteins, such as hemoglobin or cytochrome, have some chromophoric moiety.

Properties of Proteins

The classification in Table 25-1 is based on solubility properties. Fibrous proteins are water insoluble and highly resistant to hydrolysis by proteolytic enzymes; the collagens, elastins, and keratins are in this class. Globular proteins (albumins, globulins, histones, and protamines) are relatively water soluble; they are also soluble in aqueous solutions containing salts, acids, bases, or ethanol. Enzymes, oxygen-carrying proteins, and protein hormones are globular proteins.

Another important characteristic of proteins is their amphoteric behavior. In solution, proteins migrate in an electric field, and the direction and rate of migration are a function of the net electrical charge of the protein molecule, which in turn depends on the pH of the solution. The isoelectric point is the pH value at which a given protein does not migrate in an electric field; it is a constant for any given protein and can be used as an index of characterization. Proteins differ in rate of migration and in their isoelectric points. Electrophoretic analysis is used to determine purity and for quantitative estimation because proteins differ in electrophoretic mobility at any given pH.[4]

Because they are ionic in solution, proteins bind with cations and anions depending on the pH of the environment. Sometimes, complex salts are formed, and precipitation takes place (e.g., trichloroacetic acid is a precipitating agent for proteins and is used for deproteinizing solutions).

Proteins possess chemical properties characteristic of their component functional groups, but in the native state, some of these groups are "buried" within the tertiary protein structure and may not react readily. Certain denaturation procedures can expose these functions and allow them to respond to the usual chemical reagents (e.g., an exposed –NH_2 group can be acetylated by ketene; –CO_2H can be esterified with diazomethane).

TABLE 25–1 Simple (True) Proteins

Class	Characteristics	Occurrence
Albumins	Soluble in water, coagulable by heat and reagents	Egg albumin, lactalbumin, serum albumin, leucosin of wheat, legumelin of legumes
Globulins	Insoluble in water, soluble in dilute salt solution, coagulable	Edestin of plants, vitelline of egg, serum globulin, lactoglobulin, amandin of almonds, myosin of muscles
Prolamines	Insoluble in water or alcohol, soluble in 60–80% alcohol, not coagulable	Found only in plants (e.g., gliadin of wheat, hordein of barley, zein of corn, and secalin of rye)
Glutelins	Soluble only in dilute acids or bases, coagulable	Found only in plants (e.g., glutenin of wheat and oryzenin of rice)
Protamines	Soluble in water or ammonia, strongly alkaline, not coagulable	Found only in the sperm of fish (e.g., salmine from salmon)
Histones	Soluble in water, but not in ammonia, predominantly basic, not coagulable	Globin of hemoglobin, nucleohistone from nucleoprotein
Albuminoids	Insoluble in all solvents	In keratin of hair, nails, and feathers; collagen of connective tissue; chondrin of cartilage; fibroin of silk; and spongin of sponges

Color Tests and Miscellaneous Separation and Identification Methods

Proteins respond to the following color tests: *(a)* biuret, pink to purple with an excess of alkali and a small amount of copper sulfate; *(b)* ninhydrin, a blue color when boiled with ninhydrin (triketohydrindene hydrate), which is intensified by the presence of pyridine; *(c)* Millon's test for tyrosine, a brick-red color or precipitate when boiled with mercuric nitrate in an excess of nitric acid; *(d)* Hopkins-Cole test for tryptophan, a violet zone with a salt of glyoxylic acid and stratified over sulfuric acid; and *(e)* xanthoproteic test, a brilliant orange zone when a solution in concentrated nitric acid is stratified under ammonia. Almost all so-called alkaloidal reagents will precipitate proteins in slightly acid solution.

The qualitative identification of the amino acids found in proteins and other substances has been simplified greatly by the application of paper chromatographic techniques to the proper hydrolysate of proteins and related substances. End-member degradation techniques for the detection of the sequential arrangements of the amino acid residues in polypeptides (proteins, hormones, enzymes, etc.) have been developed to such a high degree with the aid of paper chromatography that very small samples of the polypeptides can be used. These techniques, together with statistical methods, have led to the elucidation of the amino acid sequences in oxytocin, vasopressin, insulin, hypertensin, glucagon, corticotropins, and others.

Ion exchange chromatography has been applied to protein analysis and to the separation of amino acids. The principles of ion exchange chromatography can be applied to the design of automatic amino acid analyzers with appropriate recording instrumentation.[4] One- or two-dimensional thin-layer chromatography has been used to accomplish separations not possible with paper chromatography. Another method for separating amino acids and proteins involves a two-dimensional analytical procedure that uses electrophoresis in one dimension and partition chromatography in the other. The applicability of HPLC was noted above.[12, 13]

Products

Gelatin, NF. Gelatin, NF, is a protein obtained by the partial hydrolysis of collagen, an albuminoid found in bones, skin, tendons, cartilage, hoofs, and other animal tissues. The products seem to be of great variety, and from a technical standpoint, the raw material must be selected according to the purpose intended (Table 25-2). This is because collagen is usually accompanied in nature by elastin and, especially, mucoids such as chondromucoid, which enter into the product in a small amount. The raw materials for official gelatin, and that used generally for food, are skins of calf or swine and bones. The bones are first treated with hydrochloric acid to remove the calcium compounds and then are digested with lime for a prolonged period, which solubilizes most other impurities. The fairly pure collagen is extracted with hot water at a pH of about 5.5, and the aqueous solution of gelatin is concentrated, filtered, and cooled to a stiff gel. Calf skins are treated in about the same way, but those from hogs are not given any lime treatment. The product derived from an acid-treated precursor is known as type A and exhibits an isoelectric point between pH 7 and 9; that for which alkali is used is known as type B and exhibits an isoelectric point between pH 4.7 and 5. The minimum gel strength officially is that a 1% solution kept at 0°C for 6 hours must show no perceptible flow when the container is inverted.

Gelatin occurs in sheets, shreds, flakes, or coarse powder. It is white or yellowish, has a slight but characteristic odor and taste, and is stable in dry air but subject to microbial decomposition when moist or in solution. It is insoluble in cold water but swells and softens when immersed and gradually absorbs 5 to 10 times its own weight of water. It dissolves in hot water to form a colloidal solution; it also dissolves in acetic acid and in hot dilute glycerin. Gelatin commonly is bleached with sulfur dioxide, but the medicinal product must not have over 40 parts per million of sulfur dioxide. A proviso is made, however, for the manufacture of capsules or pills, which may have certified colors added, may contain as much as 0.15% sulfur dioxide, and may have a lower gel strength.

Gelatin is used in the preparation of capsules, in the coating of tablets, and, with glycerin, as a vehicle for suppositories. It has also been used as a vehicle when slow absorption is desired for drugs. When dissolved in water, the solution becomes somewhat viscous, and in cases of shock, these solutions may be used to replace the loss in blood volume. Presently, this replacement is accomplished more efficiently with blood plasma, which is safer to use. In hemorrhagic conditions, it is sometimes administered intravenously to increase the clotting of blood or is applied locally for the treatment of wounds.

The most important value in therapy is as an easily digested and adjuvant food. Notably, it fails to provide any tryptophan and is lacking in adequate amounts of other essential amino acids; approximately 60% of the total amino acids consist of glycine and the prolines. Nevertheless, when supplemented, it is very useful in various forms of malnutrition, gastric hyperacidity or ulcer, convalescence, and general diets of the sick. It is especially useful in the preparation of modified milk formulas for feeding infants.

Gelatin Film, Absorbable, USP. Gelatin film, absorbable (Gelfilm), is a sterile, nonantigenic, absorbable, water-insoluble gelatin film. The gelatin films are prepared from a solution of specially prepared gelatin–formaldehyde combination, by spreading on plates and drying under controlled humidity and temperature. The film is available as light yellow, transparent, brittle sheets 0.076 to 0.228 mm thick. Although insoluble in water, they become rubbery after being in water for a few minutes.

TABLE 25–2 Pharmaceutically Important Protein Products

Name Proprietary Name	Category
Gelatin, NF	Pharmaceutical acid (encapsulating agent; suspending agent; tablet binder and coating agent)
Gelatin film, absorbable, USP *Gelfilm*	Local hemostatic
Gelatin sponge, absorbable, USP *Gelfoam, Surgiform*	Local hemostatic

Gelatin Sponge, Absorbable, USP. Gelatin sponge absorbable (Gelfoam, Surgifoam) is a sterile, absorbable, water-insoluble, gelatin-based sponge that is a light, nearly white, nonelastic, tough, porous matrix. It is stable to dry heat at 150°C for 4 hours. It absorbs 50 times its own weight of water or 45 times oxalated whole blood.

It is absorbed in 4 to 6 weeks when used as a surgical sponge. When applied topically to control capillary bleeding, it should be moistened with sterile isotonic sodium chloride solution or thrombin solution.

Venoms. Cobra (Naja) venom solution, from which the hemotoxic and proteolytic principles have been removed, has been credited with virtues because of its toxins and has been injected intramuscularly as a nonnarcotic analgesic in doses of 1 mL/day. Snake venom solution of the water moccasin is used subcutaneously in doses of 0.4 to 1.0 mL as a hemostatic in recurrent epistaxis and thrombocytopenic purpura and as a prophylactic before tooth extraction and minor surgical procedures. Stypven, from the Russell viper, is used topically as a hemostatic and as a thromboplastic agent in Quick's modified clotting-time test. Ven-Apis, the purified and standardized venom from bees, is furnished in graduated strengths of 32, 50, and 100 bee-sting units. It is administered topically in acute and chronic arthritis, myositis, and neuritis.

The frog venom, caerulein, isolated from the red-eyed tree frog *Agalychnis callidryas* mimics the effects of cholecystokinin and has been used in radiography procedures to contract the gallbladder. In addition, sauvagine, an anxiolytic, has been isolated from *A. callidryas*. Finally, bombesin, a 14-amino acid peptide that also possesses anxiolytic properties, has been isolated from the European fire-bellied frog. Although not a complete list of the peptides isolated from frogs, these provide an insight into the ancient defense mechanisms these reptiles possess and the possibility of exploitation for such uses as analgetics, antimicrobials (especially against resistant organisms), and cardiovascular agents.

Nucleoproteins. The nucleoproteins mentioned above are found in the nuclei and cytoplasm of all cells. They can be deproteinized by several methods. The compounds that occur in yeast are usually treated by grinding with a very dilute solution of potassium hydroxide, adding picric acid in excess, and precipitating the nucleic acids with hydrochloric acid, leaving the protein in solution. The nucleic acids are purified by dissolving in dilute potassium hydroxide, filtering, acidifying with acetic acid, and finally precipitating with a large excess of ethanol.

The nucleoproteins found in the nucleus of eukaryotic cells include a variety of enzymes, such as DNA and RNA polymerases (involved in nucleic acid synthesis), nucleases (involved in the hydrolytic cleavage of nucleotide bonds), isomerases, and others. The nucleus of eukaryotic cells also contains specialized proteins, such as tubulin (involved in the formation of mitotic spindle before mitosis) and histones. Histones are proteins rich in the basic amino acids arginine and lysine, which together make up one fourth of the amino acid residues. Histones combine with negatively charged double-helical DNA to form complexes that are held together by electrostatic interactions. Histones package and order the DNA into structural units called *nucleosomes*. Because of the enormous amount of research on histones, the reader is encouraged to evaluate the Selected Reading list provided at the end of this chapter.

ENZYMES

Proteins that have catalytic properties are called *enzymes* (i.e., enzymes are biological catalysts of protein nature). Some enzymes have full catalytic reactivity per se; these are considered to be simple proteins because they do not have a nonprotein moiety. Other enzymes are conjugated proteins, and the nonprotein structural components are necessary for reactivity. Occasionally, enzymes require metallic ions. Because enzymes are proteins or conjugated proteins, the general review of protein structural studies presented above in this chapter (e.g., protein conformation and denaturation) is fundamental to the following topics. Conditions that affect denaturation of proteins usually have an adverse effect on the activity of the enzyme.

General enzymology is discussed effectively in numerous standard treatises, and one of the most concise discussions appears in the classic work by Ferdinand,[14] who includes reviews of enzyme structure and function, bioenergetics, and kinetics and appropriate illustrations with a total of 37 enzymes selected from the six major classes. For additional basic studies of enzymology, the reader should refer to this classic monograph and to a comprehensive review of this topic.[15]

Relation of Structure and Function

Koshland[16] has reviewed concepts concerning correlations of protein conformation and conformational flexibility of enzymes with enzyme catalysis. Enzymes do not exist initially in a conformation complementary to that of the substrate. The substrate induces the enzyme to assume a complementary conformation. This is the so-called induced-fit theory. There is proof that proteins do possess conformational flexibility and undergo conformational changes under the influence of small molecules. This does not mean that all proteins must be flexible; nor does it mean that conformationally flexible enzymes must undergo conformational changes when interacting with all compounds. Furthermore, a regulatory compound that is not directly involved in the reaction can exert control on the reactivity of the enzyme by inducing conformational changes (i.e., by inducing the enzyme to assume the specific conformation complementary to the substrate). (Conceivably, hormones as regulators function according to the foregoing mechanism of affecting protein structure.) So-called flexible enzymes can be distorted conformationally by molecules classically called *inhibitors*. Such inhibitors can induce the protein to undergo conformational changes, disrupting the catalytic functions or the binding function of the enzyme. In this connection, it is noteworthy how the work of Belleau[17] and the molecular perturbation theory of drug action relate to Koshland's studies presented above in this textbook.

Evidence continues to support the explanation of enzyme catalysis on the basis of the active site (reactive center) of amino acid residues, which is considered to be that relatively small region of the enzyme's macromolecular surface involved in catalysis. Within this site, the enzyme has strategically positioned functional groups (from the side chains of amino acid units) that participate cooperatively in the catalytic action.[18]

Some enzymes have absolute specificity for a single substrate; others catalyze a particular type of reaction that various compounds undergo. In the latter, the enzyme is said to have *relative specificity*. Nevertheless, compared with other catalysts, enzymes are outstanding in their specificity for certain substrates.[19] The physical, chemical, conformational, and configurational properties of the substrate determine its complementarity to the enzyme's reactive center. These factors, therefore, determine whether a given compound satisfies the specificity of a particular enzyme. Enzyme specificity must be a function of the nature, including conformational and chemical reactivity, of the reactive center, but when the enzyme is a conjugated protein with a coenzyme moiety, the nature of the coenzyme also contributes to specificity characteristics.

In some instances, the active center of the enzyme is apparently complementary to the substrate molecule in a strained configuration, corresponding to the "activated" complex for the reaction catalyzed by the enzyme. The substrate molecule is attracted to the enzyme, and the forces of attraction cause it to assume the strained state, with conformational changes that favor the chemical reaction; that is, the enzyme decreases the activation energy requirement of the reaction to such an extent that the reaction proceeds ap-

preciably faster than it would in the absence of the enzyme. If enzymes were always completely complementary in structure to the substrates, then no other molecule would be expected to compete successfully with the substrate in combination with the enzyme, which in this respect would be similar in behavior to antibodies. Occasionally, however, an enzyme complementary to a strained substrate molecule attracts a molecule resembling the strained substrate molecule more strongly; for example, the hydrolysis of benzoyl-L-tyrosylglycineamide is practically inhibited by an equal amount of benzoyl-D-tyrosylglycineamide. This example illustrates a type of antimetabolite activity.

Several types of interaction contribute to the formation of enzyme–substrate complexes: attractions between charged (ionic) groups on the protein and the substrate, hydrogen bonding, hydrophobic forces (the tendency of hydrocarbon moieties of side chains of amino acid residues to associate with the nonpolar groups of the substrate in a water environment), and London forces (induced dipole interactions).

Many studies of enzyme specificity have involved proteolytic enzymes (proteases). Configurational specificity can be exemplified by the aminopeptidase that cleaves L-leucylglycylglycine but does not affect D-leucylglycylglycine. D-Alanylglycylglycine is cleaved slowly by this enzyme. These phenomena illustrate the significance of steric factors; at the active center of aminopeptidase, the closeness of approach affects the kinetics of the reaction.

One can easily imagine how difficult it is to study the reactivity of enzymes on a functional group basis because the mechanism of enzyme action is so complex.[16] Nevertheless, the –SH group probably is found in more enzymes as a functional group than are the other polar groups. In some

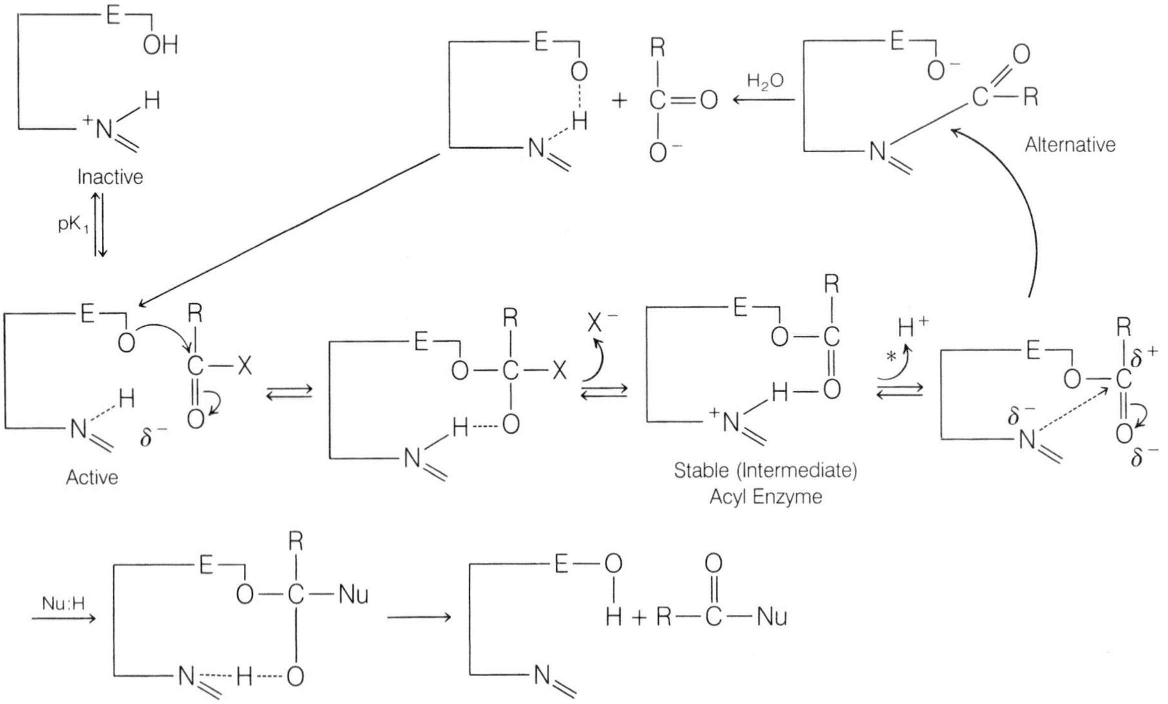

Figure 25–3 ■ Proposed generalized mechanism for enzyme-catalyzed hydrolysis of R—C(=O)—X.

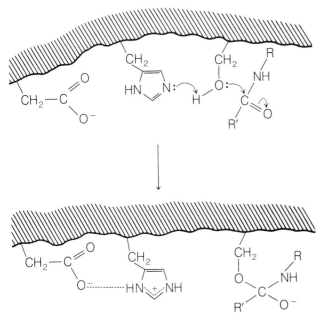

Figure 25–4 ▪ Generalized mechanism of protease catalysis. (Adapted from Chem. Eng. News, Apr. 16, 1979, p. 23.)

enzymes (e.g., urease), the less readily available SH groups are necessary for biological activity and cannot be detected by the nitroprusside test, which is used to detect freely reactive SH groups.

A free –OH group of the tyrosyl residue is necessary for the activity of pepsin. Both the –OH of serine and the imidazole portion of histidine appear to be necessary parts of the active center of certain hydrolytic enzymes, such as trypsin and chymotrypsin, and furnish the electrostatic forces involved in a proposed mechanism (Fig. 25-3), in which E denotes enzyme and the other symbols are self-evident. (Alternative mechanisms have been proposed;[15] esterification and hydrolysis were studied extensively by M. L. Bender [see *Journal of the American Chemical Society* 79:1258, 1957; 80:5338, 1958; 82:1900, 1960; 86:3704, 5330, 1964]. D. M. Blow reviewed studies concerning the structure and mechanism of chymotrypsin [see *Accounts of Chemical Research* 9:145, 1976].)

These two groups (i.e., –OH and =NH) could be located on separate peptide chains in the enzyme as long as the specific three-dimensional structure formed during activation of the zymogen brought them near enough to form a hydrogen bond. The polarization of the resulting structure would cause the serine oxygen to be the nucleophilic agent that attacks the carbonyl function of the substrate. The com-

plex is stabilized by the simultaneous "exchange" of the hydrogen bond from the serine oxygen to the carbonyl oxygen of the substrate.

The intermediate acylated enzyme is written with the proton on the imidazole nitrogen. The deacylation reaction involves the loss of this positive charge simultaneously with the attack of the nucleophilic reagent (abbreviated Nu:H).

Roberts[20] used nitrogen-15 (^{15}N) NMR to study the mechanism of protease catalysis. A schematic summary of the generalized mechanism is represented in Figure 25-4. It is concluded that the tertiary N-1 nitrogen of the histidine unit within the reactive center of the enzyme deprotonates the hydroxyl of the neighboring serine unit and simultaneously the hydroxyl oxygen exerts a nucleophilic attack on the carbonyl carbon of the amide substrate, as depicted in the scheme. A tetrahedral intermediate is implicated, and the carboxylate group of the aspartate unit (the third functional group within the reactive center) stabilizes the developing imidazolium ion by hydrogen bonding to the N-3 hydrogen. Finally, decomposition of the anionic tetrahedral intermediate toward product formation (amine and acylated serine) is promoted by prior protonation of the amide nitrogen by the imidazolium group.

A possible alternative route to deacylation would involve the nucleophilic attack of the imidazole nitrogen on the newly formed ester linkage of the postulated acyl intermediate, leading to the formation of the acyl imidazole. The latter is unstable in water, hydrolyzing rapidly to give the product and regenerated active enzyme.

The reaction of an alkyl phosphate in such a scheme may be written in an entirely analogous fashion, except that the resulting phosphorylated enzyme would be less susceptible to deacylation through nucleophilic attack. The diagrammatic scheme in Figure 25-5 has been proposed to explain the function of the active thiol ester site of papain. This ester site is formed and maintained by the folding energy of the enzyme (protein) molecule.

Zymogens (Proenzymes)

Zymogens, also called *proenzymes,* are enzyme precursors. These proenzymes are said to be activated when they are transformed to the enzyme. Activation usually involves catalytic action by some proteolytic enzyme. Occasionally, the activators merely effect a reorganization of the tertiary structure (conformation) of the protein so that the groups involved within the reactive center become functional (i.e., unmasked).

Synthesis and Secretion of Enzymes

Exportable proteins (enzymes), such as amylase, ribonuclease, chymotrypsin(ogen), trypsin(ogen), and insulin,

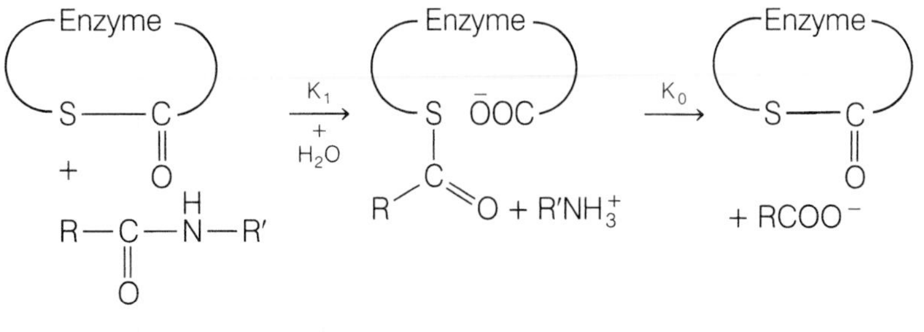

Figure 25–5 ▪ Proposed scheme for the action of papain.

are synthesized on the ribosomes. They pass across the membrane of the endoplasmic reticulum into the cisternae and directly into a smooth vesicular structure, which effects further transportation. They are finally stored in highly concentrated form within membrane-bound granules called *zymogen granules*. The exportable protein content of zymogen granules may reach a value of 40% of the total protein of the gland cell. In the enzyme sequences above, the newly synthesized exportable protein (enzyme) is not free in the cell sap. The stored exportable digestive enzymes are released into the extracellular milieu and the hormones into adjacent capillaries. Release of these proteins is initiated by specific inducers. For example, cholinergic agents (but not epinephrine) and Ca^{2+} effect a discharge of amylase, lipase, or others into the medium, increased glucose levels stimulate the secretion of insulin, and so on. This release of the reserve enzymes and hormones is completely independent of the synthetic process, as long as the stores in the granules are not depleted. Energy oxidative phosphorylation does not play an important role in these releases. Electron microscope studies indicate a fusion of the zymogen granule membrane with the cell membrane so that the granule opens directly into the extracellular lumen of the gland.

Classification

There are various systems for the classification of enzymes. The International Union of Biochemistry system includes some of the terminology used in the literature of medicinal chemistry, and in many instances the terms are self-explanatory. For example, transferases catalyze transfer of a group (e.g., methyltransferase); hydrolases catalyze hydrolysis reactions (e.g., esterases and amidases); and lyases catalyze nonhydrolytic removal of groups, leaving double bonds. There are also oxidoreductases, isomerases, and ligases. Other systems are sometimes used to classify and characterize enzymes, and the following terms are frequently encountered: *lipase, peptidase, protease, phosphatase, kinase, synthetase, dehydrogenase, oxidase,* and *reductase.*

Products

Pharmaceutically important enzyme products are listed in Table 25-3.

Pancreatin, USP. Pancreatin (Panteric) is a substance obtained from the fresh pancreas of the hog or the ox and contains a mixture of enzymes, principally pancreatic amylase (amylopsin), protease, and pancreatic lipase (steapsin). It converts not less than 25 times its weight of USP Potato Starch Reference Standard into soluble carbohydrates and not less than 25 times its weight of casein into proteoses. Pancreatin of higher digestive power may be brought to this standard by admixture with lactose, sucrose containing not more than 3.25% of starch, or pancreatin of lower digestive power. Pancreatin is a cream-colored amorphous powder with a faint, characteristic, but not offensive, odor. It dissolves slowly but incompletely in water and is insoluble in alcohol. It acts best in neutral or faintly alkaline media, and excessive acid or alkali renders it inert. Pancreatin can be prepared by extracting the fresh gland with 25% alcohol or with water and subsequently precipitating with alcohol.

Besides the enzymes mentioned, it contains some trypsinogen, which can be activated by intestinal enterokinase; chymotrypsinogen, which is converted by trypsin to chymotrypsin; and carboxypeptidase.

Pancreatin is used largely for predigestion of food and for the preparation of hydrolysates. The value of its enzymes orally must be very small because they are digested by pepsin and acid in the stomach, although some of them may escape into the intestines without change. Even if they are protected by enteric coatings, it is doubtful they could be of great assistance in digestion.

Trypsin Crystallized, USP. Trypsin crystallized is a proteolytic enzyme crystallized from an extract of the pancreas gland of the ox, *Bos taurus*. It occurs as a white to yellowish white, odorless, crystalline or amorphous powder, and 500,000 USP trypsin units are soluble in 10 mL of water or saline TS.

Trypsin has been used for several conditions in which its proteolytic activities relieve certain inflammatory states, liquefy tenacious sputum, and so forth. Many side reactions are encountered, however, particularly when it is used parenterally, which mitigate against its use.

Pancrelipase, USP. Pancrelipase (Cotazym) has a greater lipolytic action than other pancreatic enzyme preparations. Hence, it is used to help control steatorrhea and in other conditions in which pancreatic insufficiency impairs the digestion of fats in the diet.

Chymotrypsin, USP. Chymotrypsin (Chymar) is extracted from mammalian pancreas and is used in cataract surgery. A dilute solution is used to irrigate the posterior chamber of the eye to dissolve the fine filaments that hold the lens.

Dornase Alpha, USP. Dornase alpha (Pulmozyme) is a highly purified solution of recombinant human deoxyribonuclease I (rhDNAse). It is indicated for use in cystic fibrosis because of its ability to liquefy secretions from the lung effectively. It accomplishes this by cleaving the extracellular DNA in purulent sputum and reducing the viscosity and elasticity of the secretion.

Hyaluronidase for Injection, USP. Hyaluronidase for injection (Alidase, Wydase) is a sterile, dry, soluble enzyme product prepared from mammalian testes and capable of hydrolyzing the mucopolysaccharide hyaluronic acid. It contains not more than 0.25 μg of tyrosine for each USP hyaluronidase unit. Hyaluronidase in solution must be stored in a refrigerator. Hyaluronic acid, an essential component of tissues, limits the spread of fluids and other extracellular material, and because the enzyme destroys this acid, injected fluids and other substances tend to spread farther and faster than normal when administered with this enzyme. Hyaluronidase may be used to increase the spread and consequent absorption of hypodermoclytic solutions; to diffuse local anesthetics, especially in nerve blocking; and to increase diffusion and absorption of other injected materials, such as penicillin. It also enhances local anesthesia in surgery of the eye

TABLE 25–3 Pharmaceutically Important Enzyme Products

Name *Proprietary Name*	Preparations	Category	Application	Usual Adult Dose[a]	Usual Dose Range[a]
Pancreatin, USP *Panteric*	Pancreatin capsules, USP Pancreatin tablets, USP	Digestive aid		325 mg–1 g	
Trypsin crystallized, USP	Trypsin crystallized for aerosol, USP	Proteolytic enzyme		Aerosol, 125,000 USP units in 3 mL of saline daily	
Pancrelipase, USP *Cotazym*	Pancrelipase capsules, USP Pancrelipase tablets, USP	Digestive aid			An amount of pancrelipase equivalent to 8,000–24,000 USP units of lipolytic activity before each meal or snack, or to be determined by the practitioner according to the needs of the patient
Chymotrypsin, USP *Chymar*	Chymotrypsin for ophthalmic solution, USP	Proteolytic enzyme (for zonule lysis)	1–2 mL by irrigation to the posterior chamber of the eye, under the iris, as a solution containing 75–150 U/mL		
Dornase Alfa *Pulmozyme*	Aerosol	Proteolytic enzyme	Nebulizer		
Hyaluronidase for injection, USP *Alidase, Wydase*	Hyaluronidase injection, USP	Spreading agent		Hypodermoclysis, 150 USP hyaluronidase units	
Imiglucerase *Cerezyme*	Injection	Proteolytic enzyme			Dose based on body weight; range is 15–60 U/kg IV over 1–2 hours
Sutilains, USP *Travase*	Sutilains ointment, USP	Proteolytic enzyme	Topical, ointment, b.i.d. to q.i.d.		

[a]See USP DI for complete dosage information.

and is useful in glaucoma because it causes a temporary drop in intraocular pressure.

Hyaluronidase is practically nontoxic, but caution must be exercised in the presence of infection because the enzyme may cause a local infection to spread, through the same mechanism. It should never be injected in an infected area. Sensitivity to the drug is rare.

The activity of hyaluronidase is determined by measuring the reduction in turbidity of a substrate of native hyaluronidate and certain proteins or by measuring the reduction in viscosity of a buffered solution of sodium or potassium hyaluronidate. Each manufacturer defines its product in turbidity or viscosity units, but values are not the same because they measure different properties of the enzyme.

Imiglucerase Injection.   Imiglucerase injection (Cerezyme) is a form of human placental glucocerebrosidase from which the terminal mannose residues have been removed. This product is produced through recombinant technology

and is used to treat type-1 Gaucher's disease because its ability to hydrolyze glucocerebroside prevents the accumulation of this lipid in organs and tissues.

Sutilains, USP.   Sutilains (Travase) is a proteolytic enzyme obtained from cultures of *Bacillus subtilis* and used to dissolve necrotic tissue occurring in second- and third-degree burns as well as bed sores and ulcerated wounds.

Many substances are contraindicated during the topical use of sutilains. These include detergents and anti-infectives that denature the enzyme preparation. The antibiotics penicillin, streptomycin, and neomycin do not inactivate sutilains. Mafenide acetate is also compatible with the enzyme.

Streptokinase.   Streptokinase (Kabikinase, Streptase) is a catabolic 47,000-Da protein secreted by group C β-hemolytic streptococci. It is a protein with no intrinsic enzymatic activity. Streptokinase activates plasminogen to plasmin, a proteolytic enzyme that hydrolyzes fibrin and promotes the dissolution of thrombi. Plasminogen is activated when streptokinase forms a 1:1 stoichiometric complex with it. Allergic reactions to streptokinase occur commonly because of antibody formation in individuals treated with it. Furthermore, the antibodies inactivate streptokinase and reduce its ability to prolong thrombin time. Streptokinase is indicated for acute myocardial infarction, for local perfusion of an occluded vessel, and before angiography, by intravenous, intra-arterial, and intracoronary administration, respectively.

Urokinase. Urokinase (Abbokinase) is a glycosylated serine protease consisting of 411 amino acid residues, which exists as two polypeptide chains connected by a single disulfide bond. It is isolated from human urine or tissue culture of human kidneys. The only known substrate of urokinase is plasminogen, which is activated to plasmin, a fibrinolytic enzyme. Unlike streptokinase, urokinase is a direct activator of plasminogen. Urokinase is nonantigenic because it is an endogenous enzyme and, therefore, may be used when streptokinase use is impossible because of antibody formation. It is administered intravenously or by the intracoronary route. Its indications are similar to those of streptokinase.

Alteplase. Alteplase (Activase) is a tissue plasminogen activator (t-PA) produced by rDNA technology. It is a single-chain glycoprotein protease consisting of 527 amino acid residues. Native t-PA is isolated from a melanoma cell line. The single-chain molecule is susceptible to enzymatic digestion to a two-chain molecule, in which the two chains remain linked with a disulfide bond. Both forms of the native t-PA are equipotent in fibrinolytic (and plasminogen-activating) properties. It is an extrinsic plasminogen activator associated with vascular endothelial tissue, which preferentially activates plasminogen bound to fibrin. The fibrinolytic action of alteplase (t-PA) is confined to thrombi, with minimal systemic activation of plasminogen. It is produced commercially by rDNA methods by inserting the alteplase gene (acquired from human melanoma cells) into ovarian cells of the Chinese hamster, serving as host cells. The melanoma-derived alteplase is immunologically and chemically identical with the uterine form. Alteplase is indicated for the intravenous management of acute myocardial infarction.

Papain, USP. Papain (Papase), the dried and purified latex of the fruit of *Carica papaya* L. (Caricaceae), can digest protein in either acidic or alkaline media; it is best at a pH between 4 and 7 and at 65 to 90°C. It occurs as light brownish gray to weakly reddish brown granules or as a yellowish gray to weakly yellow powder. It has a characteristic odor and taste and is incompletely soluble in water to form an opalescent solution. The commercial material is prepared by evaporating the juice, but the pure enzyme has also been prepared and crystallized. In medicine, it has been used locally in various conditions similar to those for which pepsin is used. It has the advantage of activity over a wider range of conditions, but it is often much less reliable. Intraperitoneal instillation of a weak solution has been recommended to counteract a tendency to develop adhesions after abdominal surgery, and several enthusiastic reports have been made about its value under these conditions. Papain has been reported to cause allergies in persons who handle it, especially those who are exposed to inhalation of the powder.

Bromelains. Bromelains (Ananase) is a mixture of proteolytic enzymes obtained from the pineapple plant. It is proposed for use in the treatment of soft tissue inflammation and edema associated with traumatic injury, localized inflammation, and postoperative tissue reactions. The swelling that accompanies inflammation may be caused by occlusion of the tissue spaces with fibrin. If this is true, enough Ananase would have to be absorbed and reach the target area after oral administration to act selectively on the fibrin. This is yet to be established, and its efficacy as an anti-inflammatory agent is inconclusive. An apparent inhibition of inflammation, however, has been demonstrated with irritants such as turpentine and croton oil (granuloma pouch technique). Ananase is available in 50,000-unit tablets for oral use.

Diastase. Diastase (Taka-Diastase) is derived from the action of a fungus, *Aspergillus oryzae* Cohn (Ahlburg), on rice hulls or wheat bran. It is a yellow, hygroscopic, almost tasteless powder that is freely soluble in water and can solubilize 300 times its weight of starch in 10 minutes. It is used in doses of 0.3 to 1.0 g in the same conditions as malt diastase. Taka-Diastase is combined with alkalies as an antacid in Takazyme, with vitamins in Taka-Combex, and in other preparations.

HORMONES

The hormones discussed in this chapter may be classified structurally as polypeptides, proteins, or glycoproteins. These hormones include metabolites elaborated by the hypothalamus, pituitary gland, pancreas, gastrointestinal tract, parathyroid gland, liver, and kidneys. A comprehensive review of the biochemistry of these polypeptides and other related hormones is beyond the scope of this chapter. For a detailed discussion, the reader should refer to the review by Wallis et al.[21] and other literature cited throughout this chapter.

Hormones From the Hypothalamus

Spatola provides an excellent, although somewhat dated, review on the physiological and clinical aspects of hypothalamic-releasing hormones.[22] Through use of these hormones, the central nervous system regulates other essential endocrine systems, including the pituitary, which in turn controls still other systems (e.g., the thyroid).

Thyroliberin (thyrotropin-releasing hormone [TRH]) is the hypothalamic hormone responsible for the release of the pituitary's thyrotropin. Thyrotropin stimulates the production of thyroxine and liothyronine by the thyroid. The latter thyroid hormones, by feedback regulation, inhibit the action of TRH on the pituitary. TRH is a relatively simple tripeptide that has been characterized as pyroglutamyl-histidyl-prolinamide. TRH possesses interesting biological properties. In addition to stimulating the release of thyrotropin, it promotes the release of prolactin. It has also some central nervous system effects that have been evaluated for antidepressant therapeutic potential, but the results of clinical studies are not yet considered conclusive.

Gonadoliberin, as the name implies, is the gonadotropin-releasing hormone (Gn-RH), also known as luteinizing hormone–releasing hormone (LH-RH). This hypothalamic decapeptide stimulates the release of luteinizing hormone (LH) and follicle-stimulating hormone (FSH) by the pituitary. LH-RH is considered to be of potential therapeutic importance in the treatment of hypogonadotropic infertility in both males and females.[23]

$$\begin{array}{cc} & 10 \\ \text{(pyro)}^1\text{Glu} & \text{Gly-NH}_2 \\ | & | \\ \text{His} & \text{Pro} \\ | & | \\ \text{Trp} & \text{Arg} \\ | & | \\ \text{Ser} & \text{Leu} \\ | & | \\ {}^5\text{Tyr} — \text{Gly} \end{array}$$

Luteinizing Hormone-Releasing Hormone
(LH-RH)

A hypothalamic growth-releasing factor (GRF), also called somatoliberin, continues to be under intensive investigation. Its identification and biological characterization remain to be completed, but physiological and clinical data support the existence of hypothalamic control of pituitary release of somatotropin.

Somatostatin is another very interesting hypothalamic hormone.[22] It is a tetradecapeptide possessing a disulfide bond linking two cysteine residues, 3 and 14, in the form of a 38-member ring. Somatostatin suppresses several endocrine systems. It inhibits the release of somatotropin and thyrotropin by the pituitary. It also inhibits the secretion of insulin and glucagon by the pancreas. Gastrin, pepsin, and secretin are intestinal hormones that are likewise affected by somatostatin. The therapeutic potential of somatostatin is discussed below in relation to the role of glucagon in the pathology of human diabetes.

Other hypothalamic hormones include the luteinizing hormone release-inhibiting factor (LHRIF), prolactin-releasing factor (PRF), corticotropin-releasing factor (CRF), melanocyte-stimulating hormone-releasing factor (MRF), and melanocyte-stimulating hormone release-inhibiting factor (MIF).

As the foregoing discussion illustrates, the hypothalamic endocrine system performs many essential functions affecting other endocrine systems. In turn, the thalamus and cortex exert control on the secretion of these (hypothalamic) factors. A complete review of this field is beyond the scope of this chapter; the interested reader should refer to the literature cited.[21–23]

Pituitary Hormones

The pituitary gland, or the hypophysis, is located at the base of the skull and is attached to the hypothalamus by a stalk. The pituitary gland plays a major role[21] in regulating activity of the endocrine organs, including the adrenal cortex, the gonads, and the thyroid. The neurohypophysis (posterior pi-

tuitary), which originates from the brain, and the adenohypophysis (anterior pituitary), which is derived from epithelial tissue, are the two embryologically and functionally different parts of the pituitary gland. The adenohypophysis is under the control of hypothalamic regulatory hormones, and it secretes adrenocorticotropic hormone (ACTH), growth hormone (GH), LH, FSH, prolactin, and others. The neurohypophysis is responsible for the storage and secretion of the hormones vasopressin and oxytocin, controlled by nerve impulses traveling from the hypothalamus.

ADRENOCORTICOTROPIC HORMONE

ACTH (adrenocorticotropin, corticotropin) is a medicinal agent that has been the center of much research. In the late 1950s, its structure was elucidated, and the total synthesis was accomplished in the 1960s. Related peptides also have been synthesized, and some of these possess similar physiological action. Human ACTH has 39 amino acid units within the polypeptide chain.

SAR studies of ACTH[24] showed that the COOH-terminal sequence is not particularly important for biological activity. Removal of the NH$_2$-terminal amino acid results in complete loss of steroidogenic activity. Full activity has been reported for synthetic peptides containing the first 20 amino acids. A peptide containing 24 amino acids has full steroidogenic activity, without allergenic reactions. This is of practical importance because natural ACTH preparations sometimes produce clinically dangerous allergic reactions.

Corticotropin exerts its major action on the adrenal cortex, promoting steroid synthesis by stimulating the formation of pregnenolone from cholesterol.[25] An interaction between ACTH and specific receptors is implicated in the mechanism leading to stimulation of adenylate cyclase and acceleration of steroid production. The rate-limiting step in the biosynthesis of steroids from cholesterol is the oxidative cleavage of the side chain of cholesterol, which results in the formation of pregnenolone. This rate-limiting step is regulated by cyclic adenosine monophosphate (cAMP). Corticotropin, through cAMP, stimulates the biosynthesis of steroids from cholesterol by increasing the availability of free cholesterol. This involves activation of cholesterol esterase by phosphorylation. Corticotropin also stimulates the uptake of cholesterol from plasma lipoproteins. Other biochemical effects exerted by ACTH include stimulation of phosphorylase and hydroxylase activities. Glycolysis also is increased by this hormone. Enzyme systems that catalyze processes involving the production of reduced nicotinamide adenine dinucleotide phosphate (NADPH) are also stimulated. (NADPH is required by the steroid hydroxylations that take place in the overall transformation of cholesterol to hydrocortisone, the major glucocorticoid hormone.) Pharmaceutically important ACTH products are listed in Table 25-4.

cAMP

TABLE 25–4   Pharmaceutically Important ACTH Products

Preparation Proprietary Name	Category	Usual Adult Dose[a]	Usual Dose Range[a]	Usual Pediatric Dose[a]
Corticotropin injection, USP Corticotropin for injection, USP *Acthar*	Adrenocorticotropic hormone; adrenocortical steroid (anti-inflammatory): diagnostic aid (adrenocortical insufficiency)	Adrenocorticotropic hormone: parenteral, 20 USP units, q.i.d. Adrenocortical steroid (anti-inflammatory): parenteral, 20 USP units q.i.d. Diagnostic aid (adrenocortical insufficiency): rapid test—IM or IV, 25 USP units, with blood sampling in 1 hour; adrenocortical steroid output—IV infusion, 25 U in 500–1,000 mL of 5% dextrose injection over a period of 8 hours on each of 2 successive days, with 24-hour urine collection each day	Adrenocorticotropic hormone: 40–80 U/day; adrenocortical steroid (anti-inflammatory): 40–80 U/day	Parenteral, 0.4 U/kg of body weight or 12.5 U/m^2 of body surface, q.i.d.
Repository corticotropin injection, USP *Acthar Gel, Cortrophin Gel*	Adrenocorticotropic hormone; adrenocortical steroid (anti-inflammatory); diagnostic aid (adrenocortical insufficiency)	Adrenocorticotropic hormone: IM or SC, 40–80 U every 24–72 hours; IV infusion, 40–80 U in 500 mL of 5% dextrose injection given over an 8-hour period, q.d. Adrenocortical steroid (anti-inflammatory): IM or SC, 40–80 U every 24–72 hours; IV infusion, 40–80 U in 500 mL of 5% dextrose injection given over an 8-hour period, q.d. Diagnostic aid (adrenocortical insufficiency): IM, 40 U b.i.d. on each of 2 successive days, with 24-hour urine collection each day		Adrenocorticotropic hormone: parenteral, 0.8 U/kg of body weight or 25 U/m^2 of body surface per dose
Sterile corticotropin zinc hydroxide suspension, USP *Cortrophin-Zinc*	Adrenocorticotropic hormone; adrenocortical steroid (anti-inflammatory); diagnostic aid (adrenocortical insufficiency)	Adrenocorticotropic hormone: IM, initial, 40–60 U/day, increasing interval to 48, then 72 hours: reduce dose per injection thereafter; maintenance, 20 U/day to twice weekly Adrenocortical steroid (anti-inflammatory): IM, initial, 40–60 U/day, increasing interval to 48, then 72 hours; reduce dose per injection thereafter; maintenance, 20 U/day to twice weekly Diagnostic aid (adrenocortical insufficiency): IM, 40 U on each of 2 successive 24-hour periods		
Cosyntropin *Cortrosyn*	Diagnostic aid (adrenocortical insufficiency)	IM or IV, 250 μg		Children 2 years of age or less, 0.125 mg

[a]See USP DI for complete dosage information.

Corticotropin Injection, USP.   Adrenocorticotropin injection (ACTH injection, Acthar) is a sterile preparation of the principle or principles derived from the anterior lobe of the pituitary of mammals used for food by humans. It occurs as a colorless or light straw-colored liquid or a soluble, amorphous solid by drying such liquid from the frozen state. It exerts a tropic influence on the adrenal cortex. The solution has a pH range of 3.0 to 7.0 and is used for its adrenocorticotropic activity.

Repository Corticotropin Injection, USP.   ACTH purified (ACTH-80, corticotropin gel, purified corticotropin) is corticotropin in a solution of partially hydrolyzed gelatin to be used intramuscularly for a more uniform and prolonged maintenance of activity.

Sterile Corticotropin Zinc Hydroxide Suspension, USP.   Sterile corticotropin zinc hydroxide suspension is a sterile suspension of corticotropin, adsorbed on zinc hydroxide, which contains no less than 45 and no more than 55 μg of zinc for each 20 USP corticotropin units. Because of its prolonged activity due to slow release of corticotropin, an initial dose of 40 USP units can be administered intramuscularly, followed by a maintenance dose of 20 units 2 or 3 times a week.

```
¹Ser    Val²⁰ — Lys
 |       |       |
Tyr     Pro     Val     Phe
 |       |       |       |
Ser     Arg     Tyr     Glu
 |       |       |       |
Met     Arg     Pro     Leu
 |       |       |       |
⁵Glu    Lys     Asn²⁵   Pro
 |       |       |       |
His     Lys¹⁵   Gly     Phe³⁵
 |       |       |       |
Phe     Gly     Ala     Ala
 |       |       |       |
Arg     Val     Glu     Glu
 |       |       |       |
Tyr     Pro     Asp     Ala
 |       |       |       |
¹⁰Gly — Lys     Gln³⁰ — Ser
```

Corticotropin

Cosyntropin. Cosyntropin (Cortrosyn) is a synthetic peptide containing the first 24 amino acids of natural corticotropin. Cosyntropin is used as a diagnostic agent to test for adrenal cortical deficiency. Plasma hydrocortisone concentration is determined before and 30 minutes after the administration of 250 μg of cosyntropin. Most normal responses result in an approximate doubling of the basal hydrocortisone concentration in 30 to 60 minutes. If the response is not normal, adrenal insufficiency is indicated. Such adrenal insufficiency could be due to either adrenal or pituitary malfunction, and further testing is required to distinguish between the two. Cosyntropin (250 μg infused within 4 to 8 hours) or corticotropin (80 to 120 U/day for 3 to 4 days) is administered. Patients with functional adrenal tissue should respond to this dosage. Patients who respond accordingly are suspected of hypopituitarism, and the diagnosis can be confirmed by other tests for pituitary function. Patients who have Addison's disease, however, show little or no response.

Corticorelin. Corticorelin (Acthrel) is a synthetic peptide that may be used as an injectable in the determination of pituitary responsiveness. It possesses the amino acid sequence found in corticotropin-releasing hormone that is responsible for stimulating the release of ACTH.

MELANOTROPINS (MELANOCYTE-STIMULATING HORMONE)

Melanocyte-stimulating hormone (MSH) is elaborated by the intermediate lobe of the pituitary gland and regulates pigmentation of skin in fish, amphibians, and, to a lesser extent, humans. Altered secretion of MSH has been implicated in causing changes in skin pigmentation during the menstrual cycle and pregnancy. The two major types of melanotropin, α-MSH and β-MSH, are derived from ACTH and β-lipotropin, respectively. α-MSH contains the same amino acid sequence as the first 13 amino acids of ACTH; β-MSH has 18 amino acid residues. A third melanotropin, γ-melano-

tropin, is derived from a larger peptide precursor, proopiomelanocortin (POMC). Some important endocrinological correlations include inhibitory actions of hydrocortisone on the secretion of MSH and the inhibitory effects of epinephrine and norepinephrine on MSH action.

LIPOTROPINS (ENKEPHALINS AND ENDORPHINS)

Opiates, such as opium and morphine, have been known for centuries as substances that relieve pain and suffering. Neuropharmacologists have theorized that opiates interact with receptors in the brain that are affected by endogenous substances that function as regulators of pain perception. The important breakthrough came in 1975, with the isolation of two peptides with opiate-like activity[26] from pig brains. These related pentapeptides, called methionine-enkephalin (metenkephalin) and leucine-enkephalin (leuenkephalin), are abundant in certain nerve terminals and have been found in the pituitary gland.

```
¹Tyr            ¹Tyr
 |               |
Gly             Gly
 |               |
Gly             Gly
 |               |
Phe             Phe
 |               |
⁵Met            ⁵Leu
```
[Met]Enkephalin   [Leu]Enkephalin

```
¹Tyr    Asn²⁰ — Ala
 |       |       |
Gly     Lys     Ile
 |       |       |
Gly     Phe     Ile
 |       |       |
Phe     Leu     Lys
 |       |       |
⁵Met    Thr     Asn²⁵
 |       |       |
Thr     Val¹⁵   Ala
 |       |       |
Ser     Leu     His
 |       |       |
Gly     Pro     Lys
 |       |       |
Lys     Thr     Lys
 |       |       |
¹⁰Ser — Gln     Gly³⁰
                 |
                Gln
```
β-Endorphin (sheep)

An examination of the structures of enkephalins revealed that the amino acid sequence of metenkephalin was identical with the sequence of residues 61 to 65 of β-lipotropin (β-LPH), a larger peptide found in the pituitary gland. This discovery suggested that β-LPH might be a precursor for other larger peptides containing the metenkephalin sequence. Soon after the structural relationship between β-LPH and metenkephalin was established, longer peptides, called *endorphins,* were isolated from the intermediate lobe of the pituitary gland. The endorphins (α, β, and γ) contained the metenkephalin amino acid sequence and possessed morphine-like activity.[27] The longest of these peptides, β-endorphin, a 31-residue peptide (residues 61 to 91 of β-LPH), is about 20 to 50 times more potent than morphine as an analgesic and has a considerably longer duration of action than enkephalins. Numerous enkephalin analogues and derivatives have been prepared, and their biological activity has been evaluated. Like morphine, β-endorphin and the enkephalins can induce tolerance and dependence.

In addition to the enkephalins and endorphins, several other opioid peptides have been extracted from pituitary, adrenal, and nervous tissue, including dynorphins and neo-endorphins. The peptides β-LPH, ACTH, and γ-MSH are derived from the same precursor, POMC.

The endorphins and enkephalins have a wide range of biological effects, and most of their actions are in the central nervous system. Their actions include inhibition of release of dopamine in brain tissue and inhibition of release of acetylcholine from neuromuscular junctions. The role of endorphins and enkephalins as inhibitory neurotransmitters agrees well with the observed biological effects of these peptides in lowering response to pain and other stimuli. The role of endorphins and enkephalins as neurotransmitters and neuromodulators, with emphasis on receptor interactions, has been reviewed.[28] Also, see Chapter 22, Analgesic Agents, in this textbook.

GROWTH HORMONE (SOMATOTROPIN)

GH is a 191-residue polypeptide elaborated by the anterior pituitary. The amino acid sequence of GH has been determined, and comparison with growth hormones of different species has revealed considerable structural variation.[29] In addition, the structure and properties of human GH have been reviewed.[30]

The major biological action of GH is to promote overall somatic growth. Deficiency in the secretion of this hormone can cause dwarfism, and an overproduction of this hormone can cause acromegaly and giantism. Secretion of this hormone is stimulated by growth hormone–releasing hormone (GH-RH), a 44-residue polypeptide secreted by the hypothalamus. Secretion of GH is inhibited by somatostatin.

GH stimulates protein synthesis, both in the skeletal muscles and in the liver. In the liver, GH stimulates uptake of amino acids and promotes the synthesis of all forms of RNA. It stimulates glucagon secretion by the pancreas, increases synthesis of glycogen in muscles, augments the release of fatty acids from adipose tissue, and increases osteogenesis. It also causes acute hypoglycemia followed by elevated blood glucose concentration and, perhaps, glycosuria.

GH has been recognized as an effective replacement therapy for GH-deficient children. The supply of GH, however, was very limited because its source was the pituitary glands of human cadavers, and several reports of deaths in children with Creutzfeldt-Jakob disease (caused by viral contamination of GH) halted the distribution of GH in 1977. Both of these problems were solved with the application of rDNA technology in the commercial production of somatrem and somatropin.

Somatrem (Systemic). Somatrem (Protropin) is a biosynthetic form of human GH that differs from the pituitary-derived GH and recombinant somatotropin by addition of an extra amino acid, methionine. Because of its structural difference from the natural GH, patients receiving somatrem may develop antibodies, which may result in a decreased response to it. Somatrem is administered intramuscularly or subcutaneously, and the therapy is continued as long as the patient responds, until the patient reaches mature adult height, or until the epiphyses close. The dosage range is 0.05 to 0.1 IU.

Somatropin (rDNA Origin). Somatropin for injection (Humatrope) is a natural-sequence human GH of rDNA origin. Its composition and sequence of amino acids are identical with those of human GH of pituitary origin. It is administered intramuscularly or subcutaneously. The dosage range is 0.05 to 0.1 IU.

PROLACTIN

Prolactin (PRL), a hormone secreted by the anterior pituitary, was discovered in 1928. It is a 198-residue polypeptide with general structural features similar to those of GH. PRL stimulates lactation of parturition.

Gonadotropic Hormones

The two principal gonadotropins elaborated by the adenohypophysis are FSH and LH. LH is also known as *interstitial cell–stimulating hormone*. The gonadotropins along with thyrotropin form the incomplete glycoprotein group of hormones. FSH and LH may be produced by a single cell, the gonadotroph. The secretion of FSH and LH is controlled by the hypothalamus, which produces LH-RH. LH-RH stimulates the secretion of both FSH and LH, although its effects on the secretion of LH are more pronounced.

FOLLICLE-STIMULATING HORMONE

FSH promotes the development of ovarian follicles to maturity as well as spermatogenesis in testicular tissue. It is a glycoprotein, and the carbohydrate component is considered to be associated with its activity.

LUTEINIZING HORMONE

LH is another glycoprotein. It acts after the maturing action of FSH on ovarian follicles, stimulates production of estrogens, and transforms the follicles into corpora lutea. LH also acts in the male to stimulate the Leydig cells that produce testosterone.

MENOTROPINS

Pituitary hormones prepared from the urine of postmenopausal women whose ovarian tissue does not respond to gonadotropin are available for medicinal use as the product menotropins (Pergonal). The latter has FSH and LH gonadotropin activity in a 1:1 ratio. Menotropins are useful in the treatment of anovular women whose ovaries respond to pituitary gonadotropins but who have a gonadotropin deficiency caused by either pituitary or hypothalamus malfunction. Usually, menotropins are administered intramuscularly in an initial dose of 75 IU of FSH and 75 IU of LH daily for 9 to 12 days, followed by 10,000 IU of chorionic gonadotropin 1 day after the last dose of menotropins.

Thyrotropin

The thyrotropic hormone, also called *thyrotropin* and *thyroid-stimulating hormone* (TSH), is a glycoprotein consisting of two polypeptide chains. This hormone promotes production of thyroid hormones by affecting the kinetics of the mechanism by which the thyroid concentrates iodide ions from the bloodstream, thereby promoting incorporation of the halogen into the thyroid hormones and release of hormones by the thyroid.

TSH (Thyropar) appears to be a glycoprotein (relative molecular mass [M_r] 26,000 to 30,000) containing glucosamine, galactosamine, mannose, and fucose, whose homogeneity is yet to be established. It is produced by the basophil cells of the anterior lobe of the pituitary gland. TSH enters the circulation from the pituitary, presumably traversing cell membranes in the process. After exogenous administration, it is widely distributed and disappears very rapidly from circulation. Some evidence suggests that the thyroid may directly inactivate some of the TSH by an oxidation mechanism that may involve iodine. TSH thus inactivated can be reactivated by certain reducing agents. TSH regulates the production by the thyroid gland of thyroxine, which stimulates the metabolic rate. Thyroxine feedback mechanisms regulate the production of TSH by the pituitary gland.

The decreased secretion of TSH from the pituitary is a part of a generalized hypopituitarism that leads to hypothyroidism. This type of hypothyroidism can be distinguished from primary hypothyroidism by the administration of TSH in doses sufficient to increase the uptake of radioiodine or to elevate the blood or plasma protein-bound iodine (PBI) as a consequence of enhanced secretion of hormonal iodine (thyroxine). Interestingly, massive doses of vitamin A inhibit the secretion of TSH. Thyrotropin is used as a diagnostic agent to differentiate between primary and secondary hypothyroidism. Its use in hypothyroidism caused by pituitary deficiency has limited application; other forms of treatment are preferable.

Somatostatin

Somatostatin was discovered in the hypothalamus. It is elaborated by the δ cells of the pancreas and elsewhere in the body. Somatostatin is an oligopeptide (14 amino acid residues) and is referred to as *somatotropin release–inhibiting factor* (SRIF).

Its primary action is inhibiting the release of GH from the pituitary gland. Somatostatin also suppresses the release of both insulin and glucagon. It causes a decrease in both cAMP levels and adenylate cyclase activity. It also inhibits calcium ion influx into the pituitary cells and suppresses glucose-induced pancreatic insulin secretion by activating and deactivating potassium ion and calcium ion permeability, respectively. The chemistry, SARs, and potential clinical applications have been reviewed.[22, 31]

```
¹Ala
 |
Gly
 |
Cys-S-S-Cys
 |         |
Lys       Ser
 |         |
⁵Asn      Thr
 |         |
Phe       Phe
 |         |
Phe       Thr¹⁰
 |         |
Trp———————Lys
```
Somatostatin

A powerful new synthetic peptide that mimics the action of somatostatin, octreotide acetate (Sandostatin), is approved by the Food and Drug Administration (FDA) for the treatment of certain rare forms of intestinal endocrine cancers, such as malignant carcinoid tumors and vasoactive intestinal peptide-secreting tumors (VIPomas). Octreotide acetate is indicated for long-term treatment of severe diarrhea associated with these carcinomas.

Placental Hormones

HUMAN CHORIONIC GONADOTROPIN

Human chorionic gonadotropin (hCG) is a glycoprotein synthesized by the placenta. Estrogens stimulate the anterior pituitary to produce placentotropin, which in turn stimulates hCG synthesis and secretion. hCG is produced primarily during the first trimester of pregnancy. It exerts effects that are similar to those of pituitary LH.

hCG is used therapeutically in the management of cryptorchidism in prepubertal boys. It also is used in women in conjunction with menotropins to induce ovulation when the endogenous availability of gonadotropin is not normal.

HUMAN PLACENTAL LACTOGEN

Human placental lactogen (hPL) also is called *human choriomammotropin* and *chorionic growth-hormone prolactin*. This hormone exerts numerous actions. In addition to mammotropic and lactotropic effects, it exerts somatotropic and luteotropic actions. It is a protein composed of 191 amino acid units in a single-peptide chain with two disulfide bridges.[23] hPL resembles human somatotropin.

Neurohypophyseal Hormones (Oxytocin, Vasopressin)

The posterior pituitary (neurohypophysis) is the source of vasopressin, oxytocin, α- and β-MSH, and coherin. The synthesis, transport, and release of these hormones have been reviewed by Brownstein.[32] Vasopressin and oxytocin are synthesized and released by neurons of the hypothalamic–neurohypophyseal system. These peptide hormones, and their respective neurophysin carrier proteins, are synthesized as structural components of separate precursor proteins, and these proteins appear to be partially degraded into smaller bioactive peptides in the course of transport along the axon.

Oxytocin

Vasopressin

The structures of vasopressin and oxytocin have been elucidated, and these peptides have been synthesized. Actually, three closely related nonapeptides have been isolated from mammalian posterior pituitary: oxytocin and arginine vasopressin from most mammals and lysine vasopressin from pigs. The vasopressins differ from one another in the nature of the eighth amino acid residue: arginine and lysine, respectively. Oxytocin has leucine at position 8 and its third amino acid is isoleucine instead of phenylalanine. Several analogues of vasopressin have been synthesized and their antidiuretic activity evaluated. Desmopressin, 1-desamino-8-arginine-vasopressin, is a synthetic derivative of vasopressin. It is a longer-acting and more potent antidiuretic than vasopressin, with much less pressor activity. Desmopressin is much more resistant to the actions of peptidases because of the deamination at position 1, which accounts for its longer duration of action. The substitution of D- for L-arginine in position 8 accounts for its sharply lower vasoconstrictive effects.

Vasopressin also is known as the *pituitary antidiuretic hormone* (ADH). This hormone can effect graded changes in the permeability of the distal portion of the mammalian nephron to water, resulting in either conservation or excretion of water; thus, it modulates the renal tubular reabsorption of water. ADH has been shown to increase cAMP production in several tissues. Theophylline, which promotes cAMP by inhibiting the enzyme (phosphodiesterase) that catalyzes its hydrolysis, causes permeability changes similar to those caused by ADH. Cyclic AMP also effects similar permeability changes; hence, it is suggested that cAMP is involved in the mechanism of action of ADH.

The nonrenal actions of vasopressin include its vasoconstrictor effects and neurotransmitter actions in the central nervous system, such as regulation of ACTH secretion, circulation, and body temperature.

ADH is therapeutically useful in the treatment of diabetes insipidus of pituitary origin. It also has been used to relieve intestinal paresis and distention.

Oxytocin is appropriately named on the basis of its oxytocic action. Oxytocin exerts stimulant effects on the smooth muscle of the uterus and mammary gland and has a relaxing effect on vascular smooth muscle when administered in high doses. It is considered the drug of choice to induce labor, particularly in cases of intrapartum hypotonic inertia. Oxytocin also is used in inevitable or incomplete abortion after the 20th week of gestation. It also may be used to prevent or control hemorrhage and to correct uterine hypotonicity. In some cases, oxytocin is used to promote milk ejection; it acts by contracting the myoepithelium of the mammary glands. Oxytocin is usually administered parenterally by intravenous infusion, intravenous injection, or intramuscular injection. Oxytocin citrate buccal tablets are also available, but the rate of absorption is unpredictable, and buccal administration is less precise. Topical administration (nasal spray)

TABLE 25–5   Neurohypophyseal Hormones: Pharmaceutical Products

Preparation *Proprietary Name*	Category	Usual Adult Dose[a]	Usual Pediatric Dose[a]
Oxytocin injection, USP *Pitocin, Syntocinon*	Oxytocic	IM, 3–10 U after delivery of placenta; IV, initially no more than 1–2 mU/minute, increased every 15–30 minutes in increments of 1–2 mU	
Oxytocin nasal solution, USP *Syntocinon*	Oxytocic	1 spray or 3 drops in 1 or both nostrils 2–3 minutes before nursing or pumping of breasts	
Vasopressin injection, USP *Pitressin*	Antidiuretic posterior pituitary hormone	IM or SC, 2.5–10 U t.i.d. or q.i.d. as necessary	IM or SC, 2.5–10 U t.i.d. or q.i.d. as necessary
Sterile vasopressin tannate oil suspension *Pitressin*	Antidiuretic posterior pituitary hormone	IM, 1.5–5 U every 1–3 days	IM, 1.25–2.5 U every 1–3 days
Desmopressin acetate nasal solution *DDAVP*	Antidiuretic posterior pituitary hormone	Maintenance: intranasal, 2–4 μg/day, as a single dose or in 2–3 divided doses	Maintenance: intranasal, 2–4 μg/kg of body weight per day or 5–30 mg/day or in 2–3 divided doses
Desmopressin acetate injection *DDAVP, Stimate*	Antidiuretic posterior pituitary hormone	IV or SC, 2–4 μg/day usually in 2 divided doses in the morning or evening	IV, 3 μg/kg of body weight diluted in 0.9% sodium chloride injection USP

[a]See USP DI for complete dosage information.

2 or 3 minutes before nursing to promote milk ejection is sometimes recommended.[33] See Table 25-5 for product listing.

Oxytocin Injection, USP. Oxytocin injection is a sterile solution in water for injection of oxytocic principle prepared by synthesis or obtained from the posterior lobe of the pituitary of healthy, domestic animals used for food by humans. The pH is 2.5 to 4.5; expiration date, 3 years.

Oxytocin preparations are widely used with or without amniotomy to induce and stimulate labor. Although injection is the usual route of administration, the sublingual route is extremely effective. Sublingual and intranasal spray (Oxytocin Nasal Solution, USP) routes of administration also will stimulate milk letdown.

Vasopressin Injection, USP. Vasopressin injection (Pitressin) is a sterile solution of the water-soluble pressor principle of the posterior lobe of the pituitary of healthy, domestic animals used for food by humans; it also may be prepared by synthesis. Each milliliter possesses a pressor activity equal to 20 USP posterior pituitary units; expiration date, 3 years.

Vasopressin Tannate. Vasopressin tannate (Pitressin Tannate) is a water-insoluble tannate of vasopressin administered intramuscularly (1.5 to 5 pressor units daily) for its prolonged duration of action by the slow release of vasopressin. It is particularly useful for patients who have diabetes insipidus, but it should never be used intravenously.

Felypressin. Felypressin, 2-L-phenylalanine-8-L-lysine vasopressin, has relatively low antidiuretic activity and little oxytocic activity. It has considerable pressor (i.e., vasoconstrictor) activity, which differs from that of epinephrine (i.e., following capillary constriction in the intestine it lowers the pressure in the vena portae, whereas epinephrine raises the portal pressure). Felypressin also causes increased renal blood flow in the cat, whereas epinephrine brings about a fall in renal blood flow. Felypressin is 5 times more effective as a vasopressor than is lysine vasopressin and is recommended in surgery to minimize blood flow, especially in obstetrics and gynecology.

Lypressin. Lypressin is synthetic 8-L-lysine vasopressin, a polypeptide similar to ADH. The lysine analogue is considered more stable, and it is absorbed rapidly from the nasal mucosa. Lypressin (Diapid) is pharmaceutically available as a topical solution, spray, 50 pressor units (185 μg)/mL in 5-mL containers. Usual dosage, topical (intranasal), one or more sprays applied to one or both nostrils one or more times daily.

Desmopressin Acetate. Desmopressin acetate (DDAVP, Stimate) is synthetic 1-desamino-8-D-arginine vasopressin. Its efficacy, ease of administration (intranasal), long duration of action, and lack of side effects make it the drug of choice for the treatment of central diabetes insipidus. It may also be administered intramuscularly or intravenously. It is preferred to vasopressin injection and oral anti-diuretics for use in children. It is indicated in the management of temporary polydipsia and polyuria associated with trauma to, or surgery in, the pituitary region.

Pancreatic Hormones

Relationships between lipid and glucose levels in the blood and the general disorders of lipid metabolism found in diabetic subjects have received the attention of many chemists and clinicians. To understand diabetes mellitus, its complications, and its treatment, one has to begin with the basic biochemistry of the pancreas and the ways carbohydrates are correlated with lipid and protein metabolism. The pancreas produces insulin, as well as glucagon; β-cells secrete insulin and α-cells secrete glucagon. Insulin is considered first.

INSULIN

One of the major triumphs of the 20th century occurred in 1922, when Banting and Best extracted insulin from dog pancreas.[34] Advances in the biochemistry of insulin have been reviewed with emphasis on proinsulin biosynthesis, conversion of proinsulin to insulin, insulin secretion, insulin receptors, metabolism, effects by sulfonylureas, and so on.[35–38]

Insulin is synthesized by the islet β-cells from a single-chain, 86-amino-acid polypeptide precursor, proinsulin.[39] Proinsulin itself is synthesized in the polyribosomes of the rough endoplasmic reticulum of the β-cells from an even larger polypeptide precursor, preproinsulin. The B chain of preproinsulin is extended at the NH_2-terminus by at least 23 amino acids. Proinsulin then traverses the Golgi apparatus and enters the storage granules, where the conversion to insulin occurs.

The subsequent proteolytic conversion of proinsulin to insulin is accomplished by the removal of the Arg-Arg residue at positions 31 and 32 and the Arg-Lys residue at positions 64 and 65 by an endopeptidase that resembles trypsin in its specificity and a thiol-activated carboxypeptidase B-like enzyme.[40]

The actions of these proteolytic enzymes on proinsulin result in the formation of equimolar quantities of insulin and the connecting C-peptide. The resulting insulin molecule consists of chains A and B, with 21 and 31 amino acid residues, respectively. The chains are connected by two disulfide linkages, with an additional disulfide linkage within chain A (Fig. 25-6).

The three-dimensional structure of insulin was determined by x-ray analysis of single crystals. These studies demonstrated that the high bioactivity of insulin depends on the integrity of the overall conformation. The biologically active form of the hormone is thought to be the monomer. The receptor-binding region consists of A-1 Gly, A-4 Glu, A-5 Gln, A-19 Tyr, A-21 Asn, B-12 Val, B-16 Tyr, B-24 Phe, and B-26 Tyr. The three-dimensional crystal structure appears to be conserved in solution and during its receptor interaction.

The amino acid sequence of insulins from various animal species has been examined.[35] Details of these are shown in Table 25-6. It is apparent from the analysis that frequent changes in sequence occur within the interchain disulfide ring (positions 8, 9, and 10). The hormonal sequence for porcine insulin is the closest to that of humans, differing

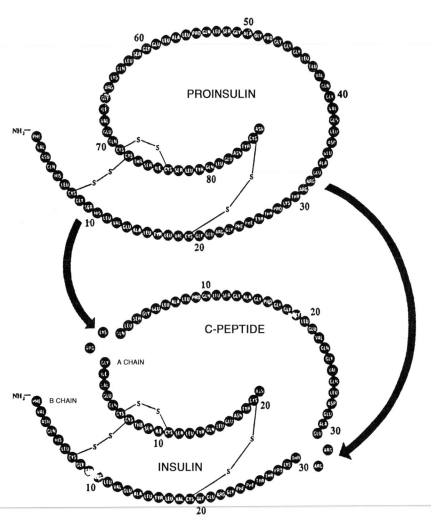

Figure 25–6 ■ Conversion of proinsulin to insulin.

TABLE 25–6 Some Sequence Differences in Insulins of Various Species

Species	A Chain				B Chain			
	1	8	9	10	−1	1	29	30
Human	Gly.	Thr.	Ser.	Ile.		Phe.	Lys.	Thr.
Pork	Gly.	Thr.	Ser.	Ile.		Phe.	Lys.	Ala.
Beef	Gly.	Ala.	Ser.	Val.		Phe.	Lys.	Ala.
Sheep	Gly.	Ala.	Gly.	Val.		Phe.	Lys.	Ala.
Horse	Gly.	Thr.	Gly.	Ile.		Phe.	Lys.	Ala.
Rabbit	Gly.	Thr.	Ser.	Ile.		Phe.	Lys.	Ser.
Chicken	Gly.	His.	Asn.	Thr.		Ala.	Lys.	Ala.
Cod	Gly.	His.	Arg.	Pro.	Met.	Ala.	Lys.	—
Rat I[a]	Gly.	Thr.	Ser.	Ile.		Phe.	Lys.	Ser.
Rat II[a]	Gly.	Thr.	Ser.	Ile.		Phe.	Met.	Ser.

See Reference 55 for details.
[a]Asp substitution for Glu at position 4 on A chain.

only by the substitution of an alanine residue at the COOH-terminus of the B chain. Porcine insulin, therefore, is a good starting material for the synthesis of human insulin.

Insulin composes 1% of pancreatic tissue, and secretory protein granules contain about 10% insulin. These granules fuse with the cell membrane with simultaneous liberation of equimolar amounts of insulin and the C-peptide. Insulin enters the portal vein, and about 50% is removed in its first passage through the liver. The plasma half-life of insulin is approximately 4 minutes, compared with 30 minutes for the C-peptide.

Usually, exogenous insulin is weakly antigenic. Insulin antibodies have been observed to neutralize the hypoglycemic effect of injected insulin. The antibody-binding sites on insulin are quite different from the sites involved in binding of insulin with its receptors.[41]

Regulation of insulin secretion is affected by numerous factors, such as food, hormonal and neuronal stimuli, and ionic mechanisms.[42] In humans, the principal substrate that stimulates the release of insulin from the islet β-cells is glucose. In addition to glucose, other substrates (e.g., amino acids, free fatty acids, and ketone bodies) also can stimulate insulin secretion directly. Secretin and ACTH can directly stimulate insulin secretion. Glucagon and other related peptides can increase the secretion of insulin, whereas somatostatin inhibits its secretion.

Autonomic neuronal mechanisms also play an important role in regulating insulin release. In the sympathetic nervous system, α-adrenergic agonists inhibit insulin release, whereas β-adrenergic agonists stimulate the release of insulin. In the parasympathetic nervous system, cholinomimetic drugs stimulate insulin release.

''Clinical'' insulin that has been crystallized 5 times and then subjected to countercurrent distribution (2-butanol:1% dichloroacetic acid in water) yields about 90% insulin A, with varying amounts of insulin B together with other minor components. A and B differ by an amide group and have the same activity. End-member analysis, sedimentation, and diffusion studies indicate an M_r of about 6,000. The value of 12,000 M_r for insulin containing trace amounts of zinc (obtained by physical methods) is probably a bimolecular association product through the aid of zinc. Insulin was the first protein for which a complete amino acid sequence was determined. The extensive studies of Sanger[43] and others elucidated the amino acid sequence and structure of insulin. Katsoyannis[44] and others followed with the synthesis of A and B chains of human, bovine, and sheep insulin. The A and B chains were combined to form insulin in 60 to 80% yields, with a specific activity comparable to that of the natural hormone.

The total synthesis of human insulin was reported by Rittel et al.[45] These workers selectively synthesized the final molecule appropriately cross-linked by disulfide (-S-S-) groups in yields ranging between 40 and 50%, whereas earlier synthetic methods involved random combination of separately prepared A and B chains of the molecule.

rDNA technology has been applied successfully in the production of human insulin on a commercial scale. Human insulin is produced in genetically engineered *Escherichia coli*.[46] Eli Lilly and Co., in cooperation with Genentech, began marketing rDNA-derived human insulin (Humulin) in 1982. There are two available methods of applying rDNA technology in the production of human insulin. The earlier method involved insertion of genes, for production of either the A or the B chain of the insulin molecule, into a special strain of *E. coli* (KI2) and subsequently combining the two chains chemically to produce an insulin that is structurally and chemically identical with pancreatic human insulin. The second, and more recent, method involves the insertion of genes for the entire proinsulin molecule into special *E. coli* cells that are then grown in fermentation process. The connecting C-peptide is then enzymatically cleaved from proinsulin to produce human insulin.[47] Human insulin produced by rDNA technology is less antigenic than that from animal sources.

Although insulin is readily available from natural sources (e.g., porcine and bovine pancreatic tissue), partial syntheses and molecular modifications have been developed as the basis for SAR studies. Such studies have shown that amino acid units cannot be removed from the insulin peptide chain A without significant loss of hormonal activity. Several amino acids of chain B, however, are not considered essential for activity. Up to the first six and the last three amino acid units can be removed without significant decrease in activity.[23]

Two insulin analogues, which differ from the parent hormone in that the NH_2-terminus of chain A (A^1) glycine has been replaced by L- and D-alanine, respectively, have been synthesized by Cosmatos et al.[48] for SAR studies. The relative potencies of the L and D analogues reveal interesting SARs. The L- and D-alanine analogues are 9.4 and 95%, respectively, as potent as insulin in glucose oxidation. The relative binding affinity to isolated fat cells is reported to be approximately 10% for the L- and 100% for the D analogue. Apparently, substitution on the α carbon of A^1 glycine of insulin with a methyl in a particular configuration interferes with the binding; hence, the resulting analogue (that of L-alanine) is much less active. Methyl substitution in the opposite configuration affects neither the binding nor the bioactivity.

Molecular modifications of insulin on the amino groups appear to reduce bioactivity, but modifications of the ε-amino group of lysine number 29 on chain B (B-29) may yield active analogues. Accordingly, May et al.[49] synthesized N-ε-(+)-biotinyl insulin, which was equipotent with natural insulin. Complexes of this biotinyl-insulin derivative with avidin also were prepared and evaluated biologically; these complexes showed a potency decrease to 5% of that of insulin. Such complexes conjugated with ferritin are expected to be useful in the development of electron microscope stains of insulin receptors.

Alteration in the tertiary structure of insulin appears to drastically reduce biological activity as well as receptor binding. The three-dimensional structure provided by x-ray crystallography of the insulin monomer has revealed an exposed hydrophobic face that is thought to be involved directly in interacting with the receptor.[50] Thus, loss of biological activity in insulin derivatives, produced by chemical modification, can be interpreted in terms of adversely affecting this hydrophobic region. Also, species variation in this hydrophobic region is very unusual.

Insulin is inactivated in vivo by *(a)* an immunochemical system in the blood of insulin-treated patients, *(b)* reduction of disulfide bonds (probably by glutathione), and *(c)* insulinase (a proteolytic enzyme) that occurs in liver. Pepsin and chymotrypsin hydrolyze some peptide bonds that lead to inactivation. Insulin is inactivated by reducing agents such as sodium bisulfite, sulfurous acid, and hydrogen.

Advances in the area of insulin's molecular mechanisms have been reviewed[36–38, 51] with emphasis on receptor interactions, effect on membrane structure and functions, effects on enzymes, and the role of second messengers. The insulin receptor is believed to be a glycoprotein complex with a high M_r. The receptor is thought to consist of four subunits: two identical α units with an M_r of about 130,000 Da and two identical β units with an M_r of 95,000 Da, joined together by disulfide bonds. The α subunits are primarily responsible for binding insulin to its receptor, and the β subunits are thought to possess intrinsic protein kinase activity that is stimulated by insulin. The primary effect of insulin may be a kinase stimulation leading to phosphorylation of the receptor as well as other intracellular proteins.[52, 53] Additionally, insulin binding to its receptors may result in the generation of a soluble intracellular second messenger (possibly a peptide) that may mediate some insulin activity relating to activation of enzymes such as pyruvate dehydrogenase and glycogen synthetase. The insulin–receptor complex becomes internalized and may serve as a vehicle for translocating insulin to the lysosomes, in which it may be broken down and recycled back to the plasma membrane. The half-life of insulin is about 10 hours.

The binding of insulin to its target tissue is determined by several factors. The number of receptors in the target tissue and their affinity for insulin are two important determinants. These factors vary substantially from tissue to tissue. Another important consideration is the concentration of insulin itself. Elevated levels of circulating insulin decrease the number of insulin receptors on target cell surfaces and vice versa. Other factors that affect insulin binding to its receptors include pH, temperature, membrane lipid composition, and ionic strength.[53] It is conceivable, therefore, that conditions associated with insulin resistance, such as obesity and type I and type II diabetes mellitus, could be caused by altered receptor kinase activity or impaired generation of second messengers (low-M_r peptides), increased degradation of the messenger, or fewer substrates (enzymes involved in metabolic activity) for the messenger or receptor kinase.[54]

Metabolic Effects of Insulin.   Insulin has pronounced effects on the metabolism of carbohydrates, lipids, and proteins.[55] The major tissues affected by insulin are muscle (cardiac and skeletal), adipose tissue, and liver. The kidney is much less responsive, and others (e.g., brain tissue and red blood cells) do not respond at all. The actions of insulin are highly complex and diverse. Because many of the actions of insulin are mediated by second messengers, it is difficult to distinguish between its primary and secondary actions.

In muscle and adipose tissue, insulin promotes transport of glucose and other monosaccharides across cell membranes; it also facilitates transport of amino acids, potassium ions, nucleosides, and ionic phosphate. Insulin also activates certain enzymes—kinases and glycogen synthetase in muscle and adipose tissue. In adipose tissue, insulin decreases the release of fatty acids induced by epinephrine or glucagon. cAMP promotes fatty acid release from adipose tissue; therefore, it is possible that insulin decreases fatty acid release by reducing tissue levels of cAMP. Insulin also facilitates the incorporation of intracellular amino acids into protein.

Insulin is believed to influence protein synthesis at the ribosomal level in various tissues.[56] In skeletal muscles, insulin predominantly stimulates translation by increasing the rate of initiation of protein synthesis and the number of ribosomes. In the liver, the predominant effect is on transcription. In cardiac muscles, insulin is believed to decrease the rate of protein degradation.

In the liver, there is no barrier to the transport of glucose into cells; nevertheless, insulin influences liver metabolism, decreasing glucose output, decreasing urea production, lowering cAMP levels, and increasing potassium and phosphate uptake. The lower cAMP levels result in decreased activity of glycogen phosphorylase, leading to diminished glycogen breakdown and increased activity of glycogen synthetase. It appears that insulin induces specific hepatic enzymes involved in glycolysis, while inhibiting gluconeogenic enzymes. Thus, insulin promotes glucose use through glycolysis by increasing the synthesis of glucokinase, phosphofructokinase, and pyruvate kinase. Insulin decreases the availability of glucose from gluconeogenesis by suppressing pyruvate carboxylase, phosphoenolpyruvate carboxykinase, fructose-1,6-diphosphatase, and glucose-6-phosphatase.

Insulin's effects on lipid metabolism also are important. In adipose tissue, it has an antilipolytic action (i.e., an effect opposing the breakdown of fatty acid triglycerides). It also decreases the supply of glycerol to the liver. Thus, at these two sites, insulin decreases the availability of precursors for the formation of triglycerides. Insulin is necessary for the activation and synthesis of lipoprotein lipases, enzymes responsible for lowering very low-density lipoprotein (VLDL) and chylomicrons in peripheral tissue. Other effects include stimulation of the synthesis of fatty acids (lipogenesis) in the liver.

Diabetes mellitus is a systemic disease caused by a decrease in the secretion of insulin or reduced sensitivity or responsiveness to insulin by target tissue (insulin receptor activity). The disease is characterized by hyperglycemia, hyperlipidemia, and hyperaminoacidemia. Diabetes mellitus frequently is associated with the development of micro- and macrovascular diseases, neuropathy, and atherosclerosis. Various types of diabetes have been recognized and classified and their pathophysiology discussed.[57]

The two major types of diabetes are type I, insulin-dependent diabetes mellitus (IDDM), and type II, non-insulin-dependent diabetes mellitus (NIDDM). Type I diabetes (also known as juvenile-onset diabetes) is characterized by a destruction of pancreatic β-cells, resulting in a deficiency of insulin secretion. Autoimmune complexes and viruses have been mentioned as two possible causes of β-cell destruction. Generally, in type I diabetes, receptor sensitivity to insulin is not decreased. Type II diabetes, also known as adult-onset diabetes, is characterized primarily by insulin receptor defects or postinsulin receptor defects. There is no destruction of β-cells, and insulin secretion is relatively normal. In reality, however, the two types of diabetes show a considerable overlap of clinical features.[57]

Diabetes mellitus is associated with both microangiopathy (damage to smaller vessels, e.g., the eyes and kidney) and macroangiopathy (damage to larger vessels, e.g., atherosclerosis). Hyperlipidemia (characterized by an increase in the concentration of lipoproteins such as VLDL, intermediate density lipoprotein [IDL], and LDL) has been implicated in the development of atherosclerosis and is known to occur in diabetes. Severe hyperlipidemia may lead to life-threatening attacks of acute pancreatitis. It also seems that severe hyperlipidemia causes xanthoma. Considering the effects of insulin on lipid metabolism, as summarized above, one can rationalize that in type II diabetes, in which the patient may actually have an absolute excess of insulin, in spite of the evidence of glucose tolerance tests, the effect of the excessive insulin on lipogenesis in the liver may suffice to increase the levels of circulating triglycerides and VLDL. In type I diabetes, with a deficiency of insulin, the circulating level of lipids may rise because too much precursor is available, with fatty acids and carbohydrates going to the liver.

The relationship between the carbohydrate metabolic manifestations of diabetes and the development of micro- and macrovascular diseases has been studied extensively.[58, 59] It is becoming increasingly clear that hyperglycemia plays a major role in the development of vascular complications of diabetes, including intercapillary glomerulosclerosis, premature atherosclerosis, retinopathy with its specific microaneurysms and retinitis proliferans, leg ulcers, and limb gangrene. First, hyperglycemia causes an increase in the activity of lysine hydroxylase and galactosyl transferase, two important enzymes involved in glycoprotein synthesis. Increased glycoprotein synthesis in the collagen of kidney basement membrane may lead to the development of diabetic glomerulosclerosis. Second, increased uptake of glucose by non-insulin-sensitive tissues (e.g., nerve Schwann cells and ocular lens cells) occurs during hyperglycemia. Intracellular glucose is converted enzymatically first to sorbitol and then to fructose. The buildup of these sugars inside the cells increases the osmotic pressure in ocular lens cells and Schwann cells, resulting in increased water uptake and impairing cell functions. Some forms of diabetic cataracts and diabetic neuropathy are believed to be caused by this pathway. Third, hyperglycemia may precipitate nonenzymatic glycosylation of a variety of proteins in the body, including hemoglobin, serum albumin, lipoprotein, fibrinogen, and basement membrane protein. Glycosylation is believed to alter the tertiary structures of proteins and possibly their rate of metabolism. The rate of glycosylation is a function of plasma glucose concentration and the duration of hyperglycemia. Needless to say, this mechanism might play an important role in both macro- and microvascular lesions. Finally, hyperglycemia increases the rate of aggregation and agglutinization of circulating platelets. Platelets play an important role in promoting atherogenesis. The increase in the rate of platelet aggregation and agglutinization leads to the development of microemboli, which can cause transient cerebral ischemic attacks, strokes, and heart attacks.[57]

Concepts of the therapeutics of diabetes mellitus have been reviewed by Maurer.[60] This review emphasizes that insulin therapy does not always prevent serious complications. Even diabetic patients considered under insulin therapeutic control experience wide fluctuations in blood glucose concentration, and it is hypothesized that these fluctuations eventually cause the serious complications of diabetes (e.g., kidney damage, retinal degeneration, premature atherosclerosis, cataracts, neurological dysfunction, and a predisposition to gangrene).

Insulin Preparations. The various commercially available insulin preparations are listed in Table 25-7. Amorphous insulin was the first form made available for clinical use. Further purification afforded crystalline insulin, which is now commonly called "regular insulin." Insulin injection, USP, is made from zinc insulin crystals. For some time, regular insulin solutions have been prepared at a pH of 2.8 to 3.5; if the pH were increased above the acidic range, particles would be formed. More highly purified insulin, however, can be maintained in solution over a wider pH range, even when unbuffered. Neutral insulin solutions have

TABLE 25–7 Insulin Preparations

Name	Particle Size (μm)	Action	Composition	pH	Duration (hours)
Insulin injection,[a] USP		Prompt	Insulin + $ZnCl_2$	2.5–3.5	5–7
Prompt insulin zinc suspension,[a] USP	2[b]	Rapid	Insulin + $ZnCl_2$ + buffer	7.2–7.5	12
Insulin zinc suspension,[a] USP	10–40 (70%) 2 (30%)[b]	Intermediate	Insulin + $ZnCl_2$ + buffer	7.2–7.5	18–24
Extended insulin zinc suspension,[a] USP	10–40	Long-acting	Insulin + $ZnCl_2$ + buffer	7.2–7.5	24–36
Globin zinc insulin injection[a] USP		Intermediate	Globin[c] + $ZnCl_2$ + insulin	3.4–3.8	12–18
Protamine zinc insulin suspension,[d] USP		Long-acting	Protamine[e] + insulin + Zn	7.1–7.4	24–36
Isophane insulin suspension,[a] USP	30	Intermediate	Protamine[f] $ZnCl_2$ insulin buffer	7.1–7.4	18–24

[a]Clear or almost clear.
[b]Amorphous.
[c]Globin (3.6–4.0 mg/100 USP units of insulin) prepared from beef blood.
[d]Turbid.
[e]Protamine (1.0–1.5 mg/100 USP units of insulin) from the sperm or the mature testes of fish belonging to the genus *Oncorhynchus* or *Salmo*.
[f]Protamine (0.3–0.6 mg/100 USP units of insulin).

greater stability than acidic solutions; neutral insulin solutions maintain nearly full potency when stored up to 18 months at 5 and 25°C. As noted in Table 25-7, the various preparations differ in onset and duration of action. A major disadvantage of regular insulin is its short duration of action (5 to 7 hours), which necessitates its administration several times daily.

Many attempts have been made to prolong the duration of action of insulin, for example, development of insulin forms less water soluble than the highly soluble (in body fluids) regular insulin. Protamine insulin preparations proved to be less soluble and less readily absorbed from body tissue. Protamine zinc insulin (PZI) suspensions were even longer acting (36 hours) than protamine insulin; these are prepared by mixing insulin, protamine, and zinc chloride with a buffered solution. The regular insulin/PZI ratios in clinically useful preparations range from 2:1 to 4:1.

Isophane insulin suspension incorporates some of the qualities of regular insulin injection and is usually long acting enough (although not as much as PZI) to protect the patient from one day to the next (the term *isophane* is derived from the Greek *iso* and *phane,* meaning equal and appearance, respectively). Isophane insulin is prepared by careful control of the protamine/insulin ratio and the formation of a crystalline entity containing stoichiometric amounts of insulin and protamine. (Isophane insulin also is known as *NPH;* the *N* indicates neutral pH, the *P* stands for protamine, and the *H* for Hegedorn, the developer of the product.) NPH insulin has a quicker onset and a shorter duration of action (28 hours) than PZI. NPH is given in single morning doses and normally exhibits greater activity during the day than at night. NPH and regular insulin can be combined conveniently and effectively for many patients with diabetes.

The posology of various insulin preparations is summarized in Table 25-7.

A major concern with PZI and NPH insulins is the potential antigenicity of protamine (obtained from fish). This concern led to the development of lente insulins. By varying the amounts of excess zinc, by using an acetate buffer (instead of phosphate), and by adjusting the pH, two types of lente insulin were prepared. At high concentrations of zinc, a microcrystalline form precipitates and is called *ultralente.* Ultralente insulin is relatively insoluble and has a slower onset and a longer duration of action than PZI. At a relatively low zinc concentration, an amorphous form precipitates and is called *semilente insulin.* The latter is more soluble and has a quicker onset and a shorter duration of action than regular insulins. A third type of insulin suspension, lente insulin, is a 70:30 mixture of ultralente and semilente insulins. Lente insulin has a rapid onset and an intermediate duration of action (comparable to that of NPH insulin). Lente insulins are chemically incompatible with the PZI and NPH insulins because of the different buffer system used in the preparation of these insulins (an acetate buffer is used in lente insulins and a phosphate buffer is used in PZI and NPH insulins). Dosage and sources are summarized in Table 25-8.

Additionally, regular insulin will remain fast acting when combined with NPH but not when added to lente. The rapid action of regular insulin is neutralized by the excess zinc present in lente insulin.[54] Similar products[61] containing rDNA-derived human insulin (instead of the bovine- and porcine-derived insulin) are available.

TABLE 25–8   Dosage and Source of Insulin Preparations

USP Insulin Type	Strengths and Sources	Usual Adult Dose[a]
Insulin injection (regular insulin, crystalline zinc insulin, Cispro)	U-40 mixed, U-100 mixed: purified beef, pork; purified pork; biosynthetic human; semisynthetic human U-500: purified pork	Diabetic hyperglycemia: SC, as directed by physician 15–30 minutes before meals up to t.i.d. or q.i.d.
Isophane insulin suspension (NPH insulin)	U-40 mixed, U-400 mixed: beef; purified beef, pork; purified pork; biosynthetic human; semisynthetic human	SC, as directed by physician, q.d. 30–60 minutes before breakfast; an additional dose before breakfast may be necessary for some patients about 30 minutes before a meal or at bedtime
Isophane insulin suspension (70%) and insulin injection (30%)	U-100: purified pork; semisynthetic human	SC, as directed by physician, q.d. 15–30 minutes before breakfast, or as directed
Insulin zinc suspension (Lente insulin)	U-40 mixed, U-100 mixed: beef; purified beef; purified pork; biosynthetic human; semisynthetic human	SC, as directed by physician, q.d. 30–60 minutes before breakfast; an additional dose may be necessary for some patients about 30 minutes before a meal or at bedtime
Extended insulin zinc suspension (Ultralente insulin)	U-40 mixed, U-100 mixed: beef; purified beef	SC, as directed by physician, q.d. 30–60 minutes before breakfast
Prompt insulin zinc suspension (Semilente insulin)	U-40 mixed, U-100 mixed: beef; purified pork	SC, as directed by physician, q.d. 30–60 minutes before breakfast; an additional dose may be necessary for some patients about 30 minutes before a meal or at bedtime
Protamine zinc insulin suspension (PZI Insulin)	U-40 mixed, U-100 mixed: purified pork	SC, as directed by physician, q.d. 30–60 minutes before breakfast

SC, subcutaneously.
[a]See USP DI for complete dosage information.

Progress in alternative routes of delivery of insulin has been prompted by problems associated with conventional insulin therapy, mentioned above. First, various types of electromechanical devices (infusion pumps) have been developed with the aim of reducing fluctuations in blood glucose levels associated with conventional insulin therapy (subcutaneous injections). These continuous-infusion pumps are either close-loop or open-loop systems. The ultimate goal of research in this area is to develop a reliable implantable (miniature) device for long-term use that would eliminate the need for daily administration and monitoring of blood glucose levels. The second area of research studies alternative routes of administration such as oral, nasal, and rectal. Preliminary results indicate that absorption of insulin at these sites is not uniform and is unpredictable. The third approach to correcting the problems of conventional insulin therapy is to supplement the defective pancreas by transplantation with a normally functioning pancreas from an appropriate donor. The major problem with this approach is rejection of the donor pancreas by the recipient, as well as problems associated with the draining of exocrine enzymes. A modified procedure transplants only viable pancreatic islet cells or fetal or neonatal pancreas. The possibility remains, however, that in type I diabetes, the newly transplanted pancreatic β-cells could be destroyed by the same autoimmune process that caused the disease in the first place.

GLUCAGON

Glucagon, USP. The hyperglycemic–glycogenolytic hormone elaborated by the α cells of the pancreas is known as glucagon. It contains 29 amino acid residues in the sequence shown. Glucagon has been isolated from the amorphous fraction of a commercial insulin sample (4% glucagon).

Glucagon

Attention has been focused on glucagon as a factor in the pathology of human diabetes. According to Unger et al.,[62] the following observations support this implication of glucagon: elevated glucagon blood levels (hyperglucagonemia) have been observed in association with every type of hyperglycemia; when secretion of both glucagon and insulin is suppressed, hyperglycemia is not observed unless the glucagon levels are restored to normal by the administration of glucagon; the somatostatin-induced suppression of glucagon release in diabetic animals and humans restores blood sugar levels to normal and alleviates certain other symptoms of diabetes.

Unger et al.[62] propose that although the major role of insulin is regulation of the transfer of glucose from the blood to storage in insulin-responsive tissues (e.g., liver, fat, and muscle), the role of glucagon is regulation of the liver-mediated mobilization of stored glucose. The principal consequence of high concentrations of glucagon is liver-mediated release into the blood of abnormally high concentrations of glucose, thereby causing persistent hyperglycemia. This indicates that a relative excess of glucagon is an essential factor in the development of diabetes.

Glucagon's solubility is 50 $\mu g/mL$ in most buffers between pH 3.5 and 8.5. It is soluble, 1 to 10 mg/mL, in the pH ranges 2.5 to 3.0 and 9.0 to 9.5. Solutions of 200 $\mu g/mL$ at pH 2.5 to 3.0 are stable for at least several months at 4°C if sterile. Loss of activity by fibril formation occurs readily at high concentrations of glucagon at room temperature or above at pH 2.5. The isoelectric point appears to be at pH 7.5 to 8.5. Because it has been isolated from commercial insulin, its stability properties should be comparable to those of insulin.

As with insulin and some of the other polypeptide hormones, glucagon-sensitive receptor sites in target cells bind glucagon. This hormone–receptor interaction leads to activation of membrane adenylate cyclase, which catalyzes cAMP formation. Thus, intracellular cAMP levels are elevated. The mode of action of glucagon in glycogenolysis is basically the same as the mechanism of epinephrine (i.e., stimulation of adenylate cyclase). Subsequently, the increase in cAMP activates the protein kinase that catalyzes phosphorylation of phosphorylase kinase to phosphophosphorylase kinase. The latter is necessary for the activation of phosphorylase to form phosphorylase *a*. Finally, phosphorylase *a* catalyzes glycogenolysis, which is the basis for the hyperglycemic action of glucagon. Although both glucagon and epinephrine exert hyperglycemic action through cAMP, glucagon affects liver cells and epinephrine affects both muscle and liver cells.

Fain[63] reviewed the many phenomena associated with hormones, membranes, and cyclic nucleotides, including several factors that activate glycogen phosphorylase in rat liver. These factors involve not only glucagon but also vasopressin and the catecholamines. Glucagon and β-catecholamines mediate their effects on glycogen phosphorylase through cAMP but may involve other factors as well.

Glucagon exerts other biochemical effects. Gluconeogenesis in the liver is stimulated by glucagon, and this is accompanied by enhanced urea formation. Glucagon inhibits the incorporation of amino acids into liver proteins. Fatty acid synthesis is decreased by glucagon. Cholesterol formation is also reduced. Glucagon activates liver lipases, however, and stimulates ketogenesis. Ultimately, the availability of fatty acids from liver triglycerides is elevated, fatty acid oxidation increases acetyl-CoA and other acyl-CoAs, and ketogenesis is promoted. As glucagon effects elevation of cAMP levels, release of glycerol and free fatty acids from adipose tissue also is increased.

Glucagon, whose regulatory effect on carbohydrate and fatty acid metabolism is well understood, is therapeutically important. It is recommended for the treatment of severe hypoglycemic reactions caused by the administration of insulin to diabetic or psychiatric patients. Of course, this treatment is effective only when hepatic glycogen is available. Nausea and vomiting are the most frequently encountered reactions to glucagon.

Usual dose: parenteral, adults, 500 μg to 1 mg (0.5 to 1 unit), repeated in 20 minutes if necessary; pediatric, 25 μg/kg of body weight, repeated in 20 minutes if necessary.

Gastrointestinal Hormones

There is a formidable array of polypeptide hormones of the gastrointestinal tract that includes secretin, pancreozymin–cholecystokinin, gastrin, motilin, neurotensin, vasoactive intestinal peptide, somatostatin, and others. The biosynthesis, chemistry, secretion, and actions of these hormones have been reviewed.[64]

GASTRIN

Gastrin is a 17-residue polypeptide isolated from the antral mucosa. It was isolated originally in two different forms. In one of the forms, the tyrosine residue in position 12 is sulfated. Both forms are biologically active. Cholinergic response to the presence of food in the gastrointestinal tract provides the stimulus for gastrin secretion. The lowering of pH in the stomach inhibits the secretion of gastrin. The effects of structural modification of gastrin on gastric acid secretion have been reviewed.[65] These studies revealed that the four residues at the COOH terminus retain significant biological activity and that the aspartate residue is the most critical for activity. The most important action of gastrin is to stimulate the secretion of gastric acid and pepsin. Other actions of gastrin include increased secretion of pancreatic enzymes; contraction of smooth muscles; water and electrolyte secretion by the stomach and pancreas; water and electrolyte absorption by the small intestine; and secretion of insulin, glucagon, and somatostatin. A synthetic pentapeptide derivative, pentagastrin, is currently used as a gastric acid secretagogue.

Gastrin

Pentagastrin. Pentagastrin (Peptavlon), a physiological gastric acid secretagogue, is the synthetic pentapeptide derivative *N-t*-butyloxycarbonyl-β-alanyl-L-tryptophyl-L-methionyl-L-aspartyl-L-phenylalanyl amide. It contains the COOH-terminal tetrapeptide amide (H · Try · Met · Asp · Phe · NH$_2$), which is considered to be the active center of the natural gastrins. Accordingly, pentagastrin appears to

have the physiological and pharmacological properties of the gastrins, including stimulation of gastric secretion, pepsin secretion, gastric motility, pancreatic secretion of water and bicarbonate, pancreatic enzyme secretion, biliary flow and bicarbonate output, intrinsic factor secretion, and contraction of the gallbladder.

Pentagastrin is indicated as a diagnostic agent to evaluate gastric acid secretory function, and it is useful in testing for anacidity in patients with suspected pernicious anemia, atrophic gastritis or gastric carcinoma, hypersecretion in suspected duodenal ulcer or postoperative stomal ulcers, and Zollinger-Ellison tumor.

Pentagastrin is usually administered subcutaneously; the optimal dose is 6 μg/kg. Gastric acid secretion begins approximately 10 minutes after administration, and peak responses usually occur within 20 to 30 minutes. The usual duration of action is from 60 to 80 minutes. Pentagastrin has a relatively short plasma half-life, perhaps less than 10 minutes. The available data from metabolic studies indicate that pentagastrin is inactivated by the liver, kidney, and tissues of the upper intestine.

Contraindications include hypersensitivity or idiosyncrasy to pentagastrin. It should be used with caution in patients with pancreatic, hepatic, or biliary disease.

SECRETIN

Secretin is a 27-amino-acid polypeptide that is structurally similar to glucagon. The presence of acid in the small intestine is the most important physiological stimulus for the secretion of secretin. The primary action of secretin is on pancreatic acinar cells that regulate the secretion of water and bicarbonate. Secretin also promotes the secretion of pancreatic enzymes, to a lesser extent. Secretin inhibits the release of gastrin and, therefore, gastric acid. It also increases stomach-emptying time by reducing the contraction of the pyloric sphincter.[64]

Secretin

CHOLECYSTOKININ–PANCREOZYMIN

It was thought originally that cholecystokinin and pancreozymin were two different hormones. Cholecystokinin was thought to be responsible for contraction of the gallbladder, whereas pancreozymin was believed to induce secretion of pancreatic enzymes. It is now clear that both actions are caused by a single 33-residue polypeptide, referred to as *cholecystokinin–pancreozymin* (CCK-PZ). CCK-PZ is secreted in the blood in response to the presence of food in the duodenum, especially long-chain fatty acids. The five COOH-terminal amino acid residues are identical with those in gastrin. The COOH-terminal octapeptide retains full activity of the parent hormone.

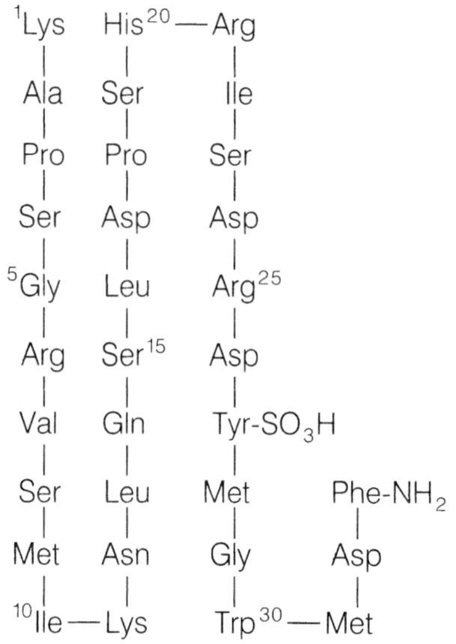

Cholecystokinin

The octapeptide is found in the gut as well as the central nervous system. SARs of cholecystokinin have been reviewed.[64] The COOH-terminal octapeptide is present in significant concentrations in the central nervous system. Its possible actions here, the therapeutic implications in the treatment of Parkinson's disease and schizophrenia, and its SAR have been reviewed.[65]

VASOACTIVE INTESTINAL PEPTIDE

Vasoactive intestinal peptide (VIP) is widely distributed in the body and is believed to occur throughout the gastrointestinal tract. It is a 28-residue polypeptide with structural similarities to secretin and glucagon. It causes vasodilatation and increases cardiac contractibility. VIP stimulates bicarbonate secretion, relaxes gastrointestinal and other smooth muscles, stimulates glycogenesis, inhibits gastric acid secretion, and stimulates insulin secretion. Its hormonal and neurotransmitter role has been investigated.[66]

GASTRIC INHIBITORY PEPTIDE

Gastric inhibitory peptide (GIP) is a 43-amino-acid polypeptide isolated from the duodenum. Secretion of GIP into the blood is stimulated by food. The primary action of GIP is inhibition of gastric acid secretion. Other actions include stimulation of insulin and glucagon secretion and stimulation of intestinal secretion.[64]

MOTILIN

Motilin is a 22-residue polypeptide isolated from the duodenum. Its secretion is stimulated by the presence of acid in

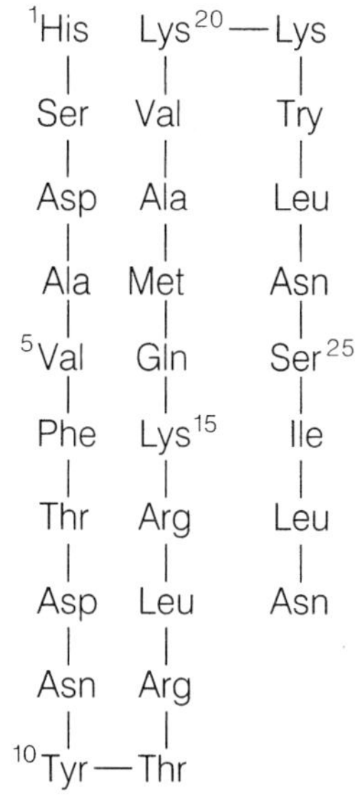

Vasoactive Intestinal Peptide

the duodenum. Motilin inhibits gastric motor activity and delays gastric emptying.

NEUROTENSIN

Neurotensin is a 13-amino-acid peptide, first isolated from bovine hypothalamus. It has now been identified in the intestinal tract. The ileal mucosa contains 90% of the total neurotensin of the body. It is implicated as a releasing factor for several adenohypophyseal hormones. It causes vasodilatation, increases vascular permeability, and increases gastrin secretion. It decreases secretion of gastric acid and secretin.

Parathyroid Hormone

This hormone is a linear polypeptide containing 84 amino acid residues. SAR studies[67] of bovine parathyroid hormone revealed that the biological activity is retained by an NH2-terminal fragment consisting of 8 amino acid residues. It regulates the concentration of calcium ion in the plasma within the normal range, in spite of variations in calcium intake, excretion, and anabolism into bone. Also, for this hormone, cAMP is implicated as a second messenger. Parathyroid hormone activates adenylate cyclase in renal and skeletal cells, and this effect promotes formation of cAMP from ATP. The cAMP increases the synthesis and release of the lysosomal enzymes necessary for the mobilization of calcium from bone.

Parathyroid Injection, USP. Parathyroid injection has been used therapeutically as an antihypocalcemic agent for the temporary control of tetany in acute hypoparathyroidism.

CALCITONIN

Calcitonin (thyrocalcitonin) is a 32-amino-acid polypeptide hormone secreted by parafollicular cells of the thyroid glands in response to hypocalcemia. The entire 32-residue peptide appears to be required for activity, because smaller fragments are totally inactive. Common structural features of calcitonin isolated from different species are a COOH-terminal prolinamide, a disulfide bond between residues 1

salts that dissolve the lecithin, by soaps or alkalies, by saponins, by immune hemolysins, and by hemolytic sera, such as those from snake venom and numerous bacterial products.

Hemoglobin (Hb) is a conjugated protein; the prosthetic group heme (hematin) and the protein (globin), which is composed of four polypeptide chains, are usually in identical pairs. The total M_r is about 66,000, including four heme molecules. The molecule has an axis of symmetry and, therefore, is composed of identical halves with an overall ellipsoid shape of the dimensions $55 \times 55 \times 70$ Å.

Iron in the heme of hemoglobin (ferrohemoglobin), is in the ferrous state and can combine reversibly with oxygen to function as a transporter of oxygen.

$$Hb + O_2 \leftrightarrow \text{Oxyhemoglobin (HbO}_2)$$

In this process, the formation of a stable oxygen complex, the iron remains in the ferrous form because the heme moiety lies within a cover of hydrophobic groups of the globin. Both Hb and O_2 are magnetic, whereas HbO_2 is diamagnetic because the unpaired electrons in both molecules have become paired. When oxidized to the ferric state (methemoglobin or ferrihemoglobin), this function is lost. Carbon monoxide combines with hemoglobin to form carboxyhemoglobin (carbonmonoxyhemoglobin) to inactivate it.

The stereochemistry of the oxygenation of hemoglobin is very complex, and it has been investigated to some extent. Some evidence from x-ray crystallographic studies reveals that the conformations of the α and β chains are altered when their heme moieties complex with oxygen, thus promoting complexation with oxygen. It is assumed that hemoglobin can exist in two forms, the relative position of the subunits in each form being different. In the deoxy form, α and β subunits are bound to each other by ionic bonds in a compact structure that is less reactive toward oxygen than is the oxy form. Some ionic bonds are cleaved in the oxy form, relaxing the conformation. The latter conformation is more reactive to oxygen.

IMPACT OF BIOTECHNOLOGY ON THE DEVELOPMENT AND COMMERCIAL PRODUCTION OF PROTEINS AND PEPTIDES AS PHARMACEUTICAL PRODUCTS

Over the past decade and a half, far-reaching and revolutionary breakthroughs in molecular biology, especially research involving gene manipulations (i.e., genetic engineering), have led the way in the development of new biotechnology-derived products for the treatment of diseases. The term *biotherapy* has been coined to describe the clinical and diagnostic use of biotechnology-derived products. Generally, these products are proteins, peptides, or nucleic acids that are structurally and/or functionally similar to naturally occurring biomolecules. The large-scale production of these complex biomolecules was beyond the capabilities of traditional pharmaceutical technologies. According to the 1995 survey[74] conducted by the Pharmaceutical Research and Manufacturers of America, there are currently more than 230 biotechnology-derived products in various stages of development and 24 approved biotechnology-derived products available in the market. The currently approved biotechnology products are listed in Table 25-9. There are 14 approval applications pending at the FDA and 49 in the third and final stage of clinical testing. A detailed discussion of the various processes and methodologies involved in biotechnology and the wide array of biotechnology-derived pharmaceutical products is beyond the scope of this chapter and is covered in Chapter 6. There are a number of reference sources[72, 75-77] available.

Since the emphasis in this chapter is on proteins, peptides, and enzymes, the discussion of biotechnology processes and products is limited to these topics. The various biotechnology-derived products[74] include enzymes, receptors, hormones and growth factors, cytokines, vaccines, monoclonal antibodies, and nucleic acids (genes and antisense RNA).

Biotechnology techniques are constantly changing and expanding; however, the two primary techniques responsible for the development of most of the products are rDNA technology and monoclonal antibody technology. The emphasis in this chapter is on rDNA technology and products derived from this technology. The monoclonal antibody technology and resulting products are discussed elsewhere in this book. Excellent references[78, 79] are available for review. The following discussion of rDNA technology assumes that the reader has thorough comprehension of the normal process of genetic expression in human cells (i.e., replication, transcription, and translation). A number of biochemistry textbooks are available for review.

rDNA Technology

rDNA technology frequently has been referred to as *genetic engineering* or *gene cloning*. A comprehensive discussion of the process and application of rDNA technology is available in several good reviews.[72, 75-77] The concept of genetic engineering is based on the fact that the genetic material (DNA) in all living organisms is made of the same four building blocks, that is, four different deoxymononucleotides. Therefore, genetic material from one organism or cell may be combined with the genetic material of another organism or cell. Since every single protein, regardless of its source, is produced as a result of expression of a specific gene coding for it, the application of this technology in the mass production of desired human proteins is obvious. A number of human diseases are caused by deficiencies of desired proteins or peptides. For example, insulin deficiency is a major cause of diabetes, and human growth hormone deficiency causes dwarfism. If a human gene coding for a deficient protein is identified and isolated, then it may be combined with fast-replicating, nonchromosomal bacterial DNA (i.e., plasmids). The recombined DNA is placed back into the bacteria, which then are grown in ideal media. The plasmids replicate and the genes within the plasmid are expressed, including the human gene, resulting in large quantities of the desired human protein.

The major steps in a typical rDNA process used in commercial-scale synthesis of human proteins are discussed below and summarized in Fig. 25-7.

1. Identification and isolation of the desired gene: The possible nucleotide sequence of a desired gene can be ascertained by *(a)* isolating and determining the amino acid sequence of the protein expressed by the gene and then determining the possible nucleotide sequences for the corresponding mRNA and the DNA

TABLE 25–9 Approved Biotechnology of Drugs and Vaccines

Product Name	Company	Indication (Date of U. S. Approval)
Actimmune Interferon gamma-1b	Genentech[a] (San Francisco, CA)	Management of chronic granulomatous disease (December 1990)
Activase Alteplase, recombinant	Genentech[a] (San Francisco, CA)	Acute myocardial infarction (November 1987); acute massive pulmonary embolism (June 1990)
Alferon N Interferon alfa-n3 (injection)	Interferon Sciences (New Brunswick, NJ)	Genital warts (October 1989)
Betaseron Interferon beta-1b, recombinant	Berlex Laboratories[a] (Wayne, NJ) Chiron[a] (Emeryville, CA)	Relapsing, remitting multiple sclerosis (July 1993)
Cerezyme Imiglucerase for injection (recombinant glucocerebrosidase)	Genzyme (Cambridge, MA)	Treatment of Gaucher's disease (May 1994)
Engerix-B Hepatitis B vaccine (recombinant)	SmithKline Beecham[a] (Philadelphia, PA)	Hepatitis B (September 1989)
Epogen Epoetin alfa (rEPO)	Amgen[a] (Thousand Oaks, CA)	Treatment of anemia associated with chronic renal failure, including patients on dialysis and not on dialysis, and anemia in Retrovir-treated, HIV-infected patients (June 1989); treatment of anemia caused by chemotherapy in patients with nonmyeloid malignancies (April 1993)
Procrit[c] Epoetin alfa (rEPO)	Ortho Biotech[a] (Raritan, NJ)	Treatment of anemia associated with chronic renal failure, including patients on dialysis and not on dialysis, and anemia in Retrovir-treated, HIV-infected patients (December 1990); treatment of anemia caused by chemotherapy in patients with nonmyeloid malignancies (April 1993)
Humatrope Somatropin (rDNA origin) for injection	Eli Lilly[a] (Indianapolis, IN)	Human growth hormone deficiency in children (March 1987)
Humulin Human insulin (rDNA origin)	Eli Lilly[a] (Indianapolis, IN)	Diabetes (October 1982)
Intron A Interferon alfa-2b (recombinant)	Schering-Plough[a] (Madison, NJ)	Hairy cell leukemia (June 1986); genital warts (June 1988); AIDS-related Kaposi's sarcoma (November 1988); hepatitis C (February 1991); hepatitis B (July 1992)
KoGENate Antihemophiliac factor (recombinant)	Miles[a] (West Haven, CT)	Treatment of hemophilia A (February 1993)
Leukine Sargramostim (yeast-derived GM-CSF)	Immunex[a] (Seattle, WA)	Autologous bone marrow transplantation (March 1991)
Neupogen Filgrastim (rG-CSF)	Amgen[a] (Thousand Oaks, CA)	Chemotherapy-induced neutropenia (February 1991); autologous or allogeneic bone marrow transplantation (June 1994); chronic severe neutropenia (December 1994)
Nutropin Somatropin for injection	Genentech[a] (San Francisco, CA)	Growth failure in children due to chronic renal insufficiency, growth hormone inadequacy in children (March 1994)
OncoScint CR/OV Satumomab pendetide	CYTOGEN[a] (Princeton, NJ)	Detection, staging, and follow-up of colorectal and ovarian cancers (December 1992)
ORTHOCLONE OKT 3 Muromonab-CD3	Ortho Biotech[a] (Raritan, NJ)	Reversal of acute kidney transplant rejection (June 1986); reversal of heart and liver transplant rejection (June 1993)
Proleukin Aldesleukin (interleukin-2)	Chiron[a] (Emeryville, CA)	Renal cell carcinoma (May 1992)
Protropin Somatrem for injection	Genentech[a] (San Francisco, CA)	Human growth hormone deficiency in children (October 1985)
Pulmozyme DNAse (dornase alpha)	Genentech[a] (San Francisco, CA)	Cystic fibrosis (December 1993)
RECOMBINATE Antihemophilic factor recombinant (rAHF)	Baxter Healthcare/Hyland Division (Glendale, CA) Genetics Institute[b] (Cambridge, MA)	Hemophilia A (December 1992)

(Continued)

TABLE 25–9   Approved Biotechnology of Drugs and Vaccines—*Continued*

Product Name	Company	Indication (Date of U. S. Approval)
RECOMBIVAX HB Hepatitis B vaccine (recombinant), MSD	Merck[a] (Whitehouse Station, NJ)	Hepatitis B prevention (July 1986)
ReoPro	Centocor (Malvern, PA)	
Abciximab	Eli Lilly[a] (Indianapolis, IN)	Antiplatelet prevention of blood clots (December 1994)
Roferon-A Interferon alfa-2a, recombinant	Hoffmann-La Roche[a] (Nutley, NJ)	Hairy cell leukemia (June 1986); AIDS-related Kaposi's sarcoma (November 1988)

Adapted from Biotechnology Medicines in Development: Approved Biotechnology Drugs and Vaccines [survey]. Pharmaceutical Research and Manufacturers of America, 1995, p. 20.
[a]PhRMA member company.
[b]PhRMA research affiliate.
[c]Procrit was approved for marketing under Amgen's epoetin alfa PLA. Amgen manufactures the product for Ortho Biotech. Under an agreement between the two companies, Amgen licensed to Ortho Pharmaceuticals the U.S. rights to epoetin for indications in human use excluding dialysis and diagnostics.

(gene), *(b)* isolating the mRNA and determining its nucleotide sequence, and *(c)* using DNA probes to "fish out" the desired gene from the genomic library (cellular DNA chopped up into segments 10,000 to 20,000 nucleotides long).

2. Constructing rDNA: Once the desired human gene is identified and isolated, it is recombined with genes of microbial cells that are known to have rapid rates of cell division. To accomplish this task, bacterial enzymes known as *restriction endonucleases* are used. Over 100 different variations of these hydrolytic enzymes, which act like scissors in hydrolyzing the phosphodiester bonds of DNA at specific sites (i.e., nucleotide sequences), are available. The use of a specific restriction endonuclease both to obtain the human gene and to open a site on the microbial gene allows easy formation of the hybrid (recombined) DNA molecule because of the "sticky" ends on both genes. The ends of the human gene and the microbial DNA vector are "glued" together by enzymes known as *DNA ligases*. The human genes are placed in specific locations on the microbial DNA vectors to ensure expression of the human gene when the microbial cells divide. Plasmids are the most commonly used microbial DNA. These extrachromosomal circular DNAs replicate independently of the chromosomes and are much smaller than chromosomal DNA. Plasmids are easy to manipulate and are considered excellent vectors to carry human genes. Other microbial cells used as hosts are yeast cells. Mammalian cells, such as Chinese hamster ovary cells, are used when glycosylation of the rDNA-derived protein is essential for biological activity (e.g., erythropoietin). Nonmammalian cells cannot glycosylate proteins.

3. Cloning: The cells carrying the recombined human gene are then allowed to grow in appropriate media. As the cells divide, the rDNA replicates and expresses its products, including the desired human protein as well as the normal bacterial proteins.

4. Isolation and purification of rDNA-derived protein: From this complex mixture containing bacterial proteins, cell components, chemicals used in preparing the media, etc., isolating and purifying the desired human protein is a daunting task indeed. This task requires sophisticated isolation techniques, such as complex filtrations, precipitations, and HPLC. The primary goal of the purification process is to ensure that the protein isolated will retain the biological activity of the native protein in the body. The rDNA-derived protein is then formulated into a pharmaceutical product that is stable during transportation, storage, and administration to a patient.

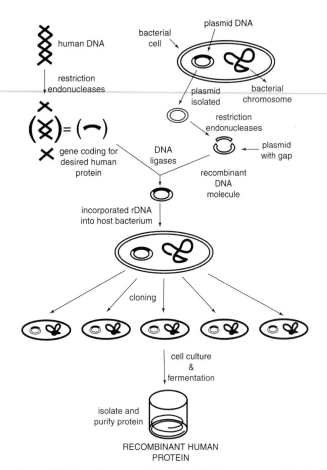

Figure 25–7 ■ Summary of a typical rDNA process used in the commercial-scale production of human proteins.

BIOTECHNOLOGY-DERIVED PHARMACEUTICAL PRODUCTS

The two dozen FDA-approved biotechnology-derived pharmaceutical products are listed in Table 25-9. There are more than 200 other products in various stages of development.[74] The FDA-approved products fall loosely into five major categories: enzymes, hormones, lymphokines, hematopoietic factors, and biologicals. A detailed discussion of all of these products is beyond the scope of this chapter. Since most of these products are proteins or peptides, a cursory evaluation of them and their uses[80] follows.

rDNA-DERIVED ENZYMES

Alteplase, Recombinant. Alteplase (Activase) was discussed above in this chapter.

Dornase Alpha. Dornase alpha, rhDNAse (Pulmozyme), is a mucolytic enzyme identical with the natural human DNAse and is used in the treatment of cystic fibrosis. Patients with cystic fibrosis suffer from decreased pulmonary function and infections caused by the secretion of thick mucus. Proteins contained in the mucus are bound to extracellular DNA, produced as a result of disintegration of bacteria in the lungs. This enzyme is involved in cleaving extracellular DNA and separates DNA from proteins, allowing proteolytic enzymes to break down proteins and thus decrease the viscosity of mucus in the lungs.[81] Proteins bound to extracellular DNA are not susceptible to proteolytic enzymes.[82] Dornase alpha is a glycoprotein containing 260 amino acids that is commercially produced in genetically engineered Chinese hamster ovary cells.

Dornase alpha is indicated for the treatment of cystic fibrosis in conjunction with other available therapies, such as antibiotics, bronchodilators, and corticosteroids. Adult dosage is 2.5 mg inhaled once daily, administered via a recommended nebulizer. Dornase alpha should not be mixed or diluted with other agents in the nebulizer because of the possibility of adverse physicochemical changes that may affect activity. Common adverse effects include sore throat, hoarseness, and facial edema.

Imiglucerase. Imiglucerase (Cerezyme)[80] is a glycoprotein containing 497 amino acid residues and is N-glycosylated at four different positions. It is an analogue of the natural human enzyme β-glucocerebrosidase and contains arginine at position 495 instead of the histidine in the natural enzyme. It is commercially produced in genetically engineered Chinese hamster ovary cells.

Like the natural enzyme, imiglucerase catalyzes the hydrolysis of glucocerebroside, a glycolipid, to glucose and ceramide within the lysosomes of phagocytic cells. Gaucher's disease is caused by a deficiency of this enzyme, which results in the accumulation of glucocerebroside within tissue macrophages. The glycolipid-engorged macrophages are known as *Gaucher cells* and are responsible for the numerous clinical manifestations of Gaucher's disease. The common clinical manifestations of Gaucher's disease are severe anemia, thrombocytopenia, and skeletal complications that include osteonecrosis and osteopenia.

Imiglucerase is indicated for the long-term replacement therapy of Gaucher's disease. It is administered intravenously at an initial dose of 2.5 to 60 U/kg, infused over 1 to 2 hours. This dose is usually repeated every 2 weeks. Both the dose and the frequency of administration may be varied, however, depending on the response.[83] Common adverse effects include dizziness, headache, abdominal discomfort, nausea, and rash.

rDNA-DERIVED HORMONES

The rDNA-derived hormones include insulin human injection USP (Humulin R, Novolin R, Velosulin Human), growth hormone (somatotropin; Humatrope), and somatrem (Protropin). All of these products, as well as other products containing human insulin, are discussed above in this chapter.

rDNA-DERIVED CYTOKINES

Interferons.[80] Interferons are natural glycoproteins produced by virtually all eukaryotic cells; they possess immunomodulating, antiviral, and cytotoxic activities. This family of glycoproteins is produced by cells in response to a wide range of stimuli.[84] In humans, interferons bind to cellular receptors, which leads to the synthesis of over a dozen proteins that contribute to viral resistance. The antiviral effects of interferons may be caused by inhibition of the synthesis of viral mRNA or proteins or prevention of viral penetration or uncoating.[85, 86] Based on their antigenic subtypes, the interferons are classified into three major groups: α, β, and γ. α-Interferon and β-interferon are produced by virtually all cells in response to a viral infection and various other stimuli. γ-Interferon is produced specifically by the T lymphocytes and the natural killer cells. γ-Interferons have greater immunoregulatory, but lower antiviral, effects than α- or β-interferons.[86] More than 12 subspecies of α-interferons, 1 β-interferon, and 2 γ-interferons are known to exist. In general, the interferons are glycoproteins consisting of 165 to 166 amino acid residues. There are four rDNA-derived α-interferons available for clinical use around the world and three available in the United States (described below). All α-interferons exhibit antiviral and antiproliferative activity, enhance phagocytic activity, and augment specific cytotoxicity of lymphocytes for certain target cells.[87] The most common adverse effects of α- and β-interferons include flu-like symptoms, bone marrow suppression, neurotoxic effects, hypocalcemia, anorexia and other gastrointestinal symptoms, and weight loss.

Interferon Alfa-2a, Recombinant. Interferon alfa-2a, recombinant (Roferon), is produced from genetically engineered *E. coli* and contains 165 amino acid residues. At position 23, interferon alfa-2a has a lysine residue. The pharmaceutical product contains a single α-interferon subtype. A murine monoclonal antibody is used during purification by affinity chromatography. Interferon alfa-2a is used in the treatment of hairy cell leukemia and acquired immunodeficiency syndrome (AIDS)-related Kaposi's sarcoma. It is absorbed well after intramuscular or intravenous administration and has a half-life of 5 to 7 hours when administered by the intramuscular route. The solution should be stored in the refrigerator at 36 to 46°F and should not be frozen or shaken.

Interferon Alfa-2b, Recombinant. Interferon alfa-2b, recombinant (Intron A), also contains a single subtype of α-interferon. It is a glycoprotein containing 165 amino acid residues and is commercially produced from genetically engineered *E. coli*. It differs from interferon alfa-2b in possessing an arginine residue at position 23. It is used in the treatment of hairy cell leukemia, condyloma acuminata (genital warts), AIDS-related Kaposi's sarcoma, hepatitis C, and hepatitis B. It is administered intramuscularly or subcutaneously with a half-life of 2 to 3 hours and via intravenous infusion with a half-life of 8 hours. The reconstituted solution is stable for 1 month when stored at a temperature of 36 to 46°F.

Interferon Alfa-n3 (injection). Interferon alfa-n3 (Alferon N) is a polyclonal mixture of up to 14 natural *α*-interferon subtypes and contains 166 amino acid residues. Its commercial production involves induction of pooled units of human leukocytes with an avian virus (Sendai virus). The purification process involves immunoaffinity and filtration chromatography. It is indicated primarily by intralesional injection for the treatment of genital warts. The solution should be stored at a temperature of 36 to 46°F and should not be shaken.

Interferon Beta-1b, recombinant. Interferon beta-1b, recombinant (Betaseron), has biological effects similar to those of natural *β*-interferon and *α*-interferons. The natural *β*-interferon is a glycoprotein containing 166 amino acid residues. The rDNA product differs from the natural form, in that it is not glycosylated, it lacks the amino-terminal methionine, and it has serine in the place of methionine at position 17.[88] It is used for a wide variety of indications via intravenous, intramuscular, subcutaneous, intrathecal, and intralesional routes. Its primary indication is for the prevention of exacerbations in patients suffering from relapsing/remitting multiple sclerosis. Recommended dosage is 8 million units, administered subcutaneously, every other day. It also is indicated in the treatment of malignant glioma and malignant melanoma. Recommended temperature for storage is 36 to 46 °F, and unused reconstituted solution should be discarded.

Aldesleukin. Aldesleukin, interleukin-2 (Proleukin),[80] is an rDNA-derived lymphokine that differs structurally from native interleukin-2 (IL-2) but has biological activity similar to that of the natural lymphokine.[89] Natural IL-2 is produced primarily by the peripheral blood lymphocytes and contains 133 amino acid residues. The immunoregulatory effects of aldesleukin include enhancing mitogenesis of lymphocytes, stimulating the growth of IL-2–dependent cell lines, enhancing cytotoxicity of lymphocytes, inducing lymphokine-activated killer (LAK) cells and natural killer (NK) cells, and inducing interferon-*γ* production. The exact mechanism of the antitumor activity of aldesleukin in humans is unknown.

The rDNA process involves genetically engineered *E. coli* (pBR 322 plasmids). The gene for IL-2 was synthesized after first isolating and identifying the mRNA from the human Jurkat cell line and then preparing the complementary DNA (cDNA). The IL-2 gene was genetically engineered before it was hybridized into pBR 322 plasmid. Further manipulation of the hybridized plasmid resulted in the production of a modified IL-2, aldesleukin.[90] Aldesleukin differs structur-

ally from the native IL-2 in that the former is not glycosylated, it lacks the N-terminal alanine residue, and it has serine in the place of cysteine at position 125. Noncovalent, molecular aggregation of aldesleukin is different from IL-2, and the former exists as a microaggregate of 27 molecules.

The primary indication for aldesleukin is in the treatment of adult metastatic renal carcinoma. It is administered via intravenous infusion in doses of 10,000 to 50,000 U/kg every 8 hours for 12 days. It is primarily metabolized by the kidneys, with no active form found in the urine. Aldesleukin causes serious adverse effects in patients, including fever, hypotension, pulmonary congestion and dyspnea, coma, gastrointestinal bleeding, respiratory failure, renal failure, arrhythmias, seizures, and death.

rDNA-DERIVED HEMATOPOIETIC FACTORS

Hematopoietic growth factors are glycoproteins produced by a number of peripheral and marrow cells. More than 200 billion blood cells are produced each day; and the hematopoietic factors, along with other lymphopoietic factors such as the stem cell factor and the interleukins, are involved in the proliferation, differentiation, and maturation of various types of blood cells derived from the pluripotent stem cells.

Erythropoietin.[80] Erythropoietin is a heavily glycosylated protein containing 166 amino acid residues. It is produced primarily by the peritubular cells in the cortex of the kidney, and up to 15% is produced in the liver. It is the principal hormone responsible for stimulating the production of red blood cells from erythroid progenitor cells, erythrocyte burst-forming units, and erythrocyte colony-forming units.[91] Small amounts of erythropoietin are detectable in the plasma; however, most of the hormone is secreted by the kidneys in response to hypoxia or anemia, when levels of the hormone can rise more than 100-fold.

Decreased erythropoietin production is one of several potential causes of anemia of chronic renal disease. Other causes of anemia of chronic renal disease include infection or inflammatory condition in the kidneys, iron deficiency, marrow damage, and vitamin or mineral deficiency. Regardless of the underlying disease causing renal failure, erythropoietin levels decrease in patients with renal failure. Until rDNA technology was used to produce commercial quantities of erythropoietin, it was obtained from the urine of patients suffering from severe aplastic anemia. This process of obtaining natural hormone was costly and time-consuming and produced only small quantities of the hormone.

Epoetin Alfa. Epoetin alfa, rEPO (Epogen, Procrit), is the recombinant human erythropoietin produced in Chinese hamster ovary cells into which the human erythropoietin gene has been inserted. These mammalian cells glycosylate the protein in a manner similar to that observed in human cells.[92]

Epoetin alfa is indicated in anemic patients with chronic renal failure, including both those who require regular dialysis and those who do not. Epoetin alfa is also indicated in anemia associated with AIDS, treatment of AIDS with zidovudine, frequent blood donations, and neoplastic diseases. It is indicated to prevent anemia in patients who donate blood prior to surgery for future autologous transfusions and to reduce the need for repeated maintenance transfusions.[93] The hormone is available as an isotonic buffered solution, which is administered by the intravenous route. The solution should not be frozen or shaken and is stored at 36 to 46°F.

Colony-Stimulating Factors.[80]

Colony-stimulating factors are natural glycoproteins produced in lymphocytes and monocytes. These factors bind to cell-surface receptors of hematopoietic progenitor cells and stimulate proliferation, differentiation, and maturation of these cells into recognizable mature blood cells.[93] Colony-stimulating factors produced by rDNA technology have the same biological activity as the natural hormones. Currently, there are two colony-stimulating factors commercially produced by rDNA technology. These products are discussed below.

Filgrastim.

Filgrastim, rG-CSF (Neupogen), is a 175-amino-acid polypeptide produced in genetically engineered *E. coli* cells containing the human granulocyte colony-stimulating factor (G-CSF) gene. Filgrastim differs from the natural hormone in that the former is not glycosylated and contains an additional methionine group at the N terminus, which is deemed necessary for expression of the gene in *E. coli*.

Filgrastim specifically stimulates the proliferation and maturation of neutrophil granulocytes and, hence, is considered lineage specific. Accepted indications for filgrastim include the following: *(a)* to decrease the incidence of febrile neutropenia in patients with nonmyeloid malignancies who receive myelosuppressive chemotherapeutic agents, thus lowering the incidence of infections in these patients; *(b)* to accelerate myeloid recovery in patients undergoing autologous bone marrow transplantation; and *(c)* in AIDS patients, to decrease the incidence of neutropenia caused by the disease itself or by drugs used to treat the disease. The usual starting dose for filgrastim is 5 μg/kg per day in patients with nonmyeloid cancer who receive myelosuppressive chemotherapy.

Filgrastim solution should be stored at 36 to 46°F and used within 24 hours of preparation. The solution should not be shaken or allowed to freeze. Any solution left at room temperature for more than 6 hours should be discarded. The most frequent adverse effects of filgrastim are medullary bone pain, arthralgia, and myalgia.

Sargramostim.

Sargramostim, rGM-CSF (Leukine), is a glycoprotein commercially produced in genetically engineered yeast cells. Its polypeptide chain contains 127 amino acids. It differs from the natural hormone by substitution of leucine at position 23 and variations in the glycosylation.[94] Sargramostim is a lineage-nonspecific hematopoietic factor because it promotes the proliferation and maturation of granulocytes (neutrophils and eosinophils) and monocytes (macrophages and megakaryocytes).

The primary indication for sargramostim is in myeloid engraftment following autologous bone marrow transplantation and hematopoietic stem cell transplantation. Handling, storage precautions, and adverse effects are similar to those for filgrastim.

rDNA-DERIVED MISCELLANEOUS PRODUCTS

Antihemophilic Factor.

Antihemophilic factor (factor VIII) (Humate-P, Hemophil M, Koate HP, Monoclate-P) is a glycoprotein found in human plasma and a necessary cofactor in the blood-clotting mechanism. This high-molecular-weight glycoprotein has a complex structure with several components (subcofactors).[95] The commercially available concentrates derived from blood collected from volunteer donors by the American Red Cross Blood Services are used primarily for the treatment of patients with hemophilia A. Since the commercially available products are purified concentrates derived from blood pooled from millions of donors, the major precautions in using the products relate to transmission of viruses, such as hepatitis virus, herpesvirus, and HIV. This major problem has been alleviated, mostly because of the development and marketing of rDNA-derived antihemophilic factors.

Antihemophilic Factor (Recombinant).

Antihemophilic factor (recombinant), rAHF (KoGENate, Helixate), is an rDNA-derived factor VIII expressed in genetically engineered baby hamster kidney cells.[96] KoGENate has the same biological activity as the human plasma-derived antihemophilic factor (pdAHF). The purification process for rAHF includes monoclonal antibody immunoaffinity chromatography to remove any protein contaminants.

rAHF is indicated for the treatment of hemophilia A and is administered by the intravenous route. Patients suffering from hemophilia A exhibit a decrease in the activity of plasma clotting factor VIII. This product temporarily prevents bleeding episodes in hemophiliacs and may be used to prevent excessive bleeding during surgical procedures in these patients. A major advantage of the rAHF over the natural factor VIII is the lack of virus in the product. rAHF does not contain von Willebrand's factor; therefore, it is not indicated in the treatment of von Willebrand's disease. Patients receiving rAHF should be monitored carefully for the development of antibodies.

Bioclate is an rDNA-derived factor VIII expressed in genetically engineered Chinese hamster ovary cells. It has the same biological activity as pdAHF and is structurally similar. Its indications and adverse effects are similar to those for KoGENate.

REFERENCES

1. Ahmad, F., et al. (eds.): From Gene to Protein: Translation into Biotechnology, vol. 19. New York, Academic Press, 1982.
2. Boza, J. J., Moennoz, D., Vuichoud, J., et al.: Eur. J. Nutr. 39(6):237, 2000.
3. American Medical Association Department of Drugs: Drug Evaluations, 6th ed. New York, John Wiley & Sons, 1986, pp. 867–870.
4. Stryer, L.: Biochemistry, 5th ed. New York, W. H. Freeman & Co., 2002, Chap. 3.
5. Corey, R. B., and Pauling, L.: Proc. R. Soc. Lond. Ser. B 141:10, 1953 (see also Adv. Protein Chem. 8:147, 1957).
6. Tanford, C.: The Hydrophobic Effect: Formation of Micelles and Biological Membranes, 2nd ed. New York, John Wiley & Sons, 1979.
7. McDonald, C. C., and Phillips, W. D.: J. Am. Chem. Soc. 89:6332, 1967.
8. Rienstra, C. M., Tucker-Kellogg, L., Jaroniec, C. P., et al.: Proc. Natl. Acad. Sci. U. S. A. 99(16):10260, 2002.
9. Kato, G., and Yung, J.: Mol. Pharmacol. 7:33, 1971.
10. Elefrawi, M. E., et al.: Mol. Pharmacol. 7:104, 1971.
11. Tang, C., Ndassa, Y., Summers, M. F.: Nat. Strict. Biol. 9(7):537, 2002.

12. Kodak, A., Kenna, K., Tarnish, H., et al.: Endocrinology 143(2):411, 2002.
13. Catrina, S. B., Cocilescu, M., and Andersson, M.: J. Cell Mol. Med. 5(2):195, 2001.
14. Ferdinand, W.: The Enzyme Molecule. New York, John Wiley & Sons, 1976.
15. Stryer, L.: Biochemistry, 5th ed. New York, W. H. Freeman & Co., 2002, Chap. 4.
16. Koshland, D. E.: Sci. Am. 229:52, 1973 (see also Annu. Rev. Biochem. 37:359, 1968).
17. Belleau, B.: J. Med. Chem. 7:776, 1964.
18. Lowe, J. N., and Ingraham, L. L.: An Introduction to Biochemical Reaction Mechanisms. Englewood Cliffs, NJ, Prentice-Hall, 1974.
19. Hanson, K. R., and Rose, I. A.: Acc. Chem. Res. 8:1, 1975 (see also Science 193:121, 1976).
20. Roberts, J. D.: Chem. Eng. News, 57:23, 1979.
21. Wallis, M., Howell, S. L., and Taylor, K. W.: The Biochemistry of the Peptide Hormone. Chichester, U. K., John Wiley & Sons, 1986.
22. Spatola, A. F.: Annu. Rep. Med. Chem. 16:199, 1981.
23. Brueggemeier, R. W.: Peptide and protein hormones. In Wolff, M. E. (ed.). Burger's Medicinal Chemistry, vol. 3, 5th ed. New York, John Wiley & Sons, 1996, pp. 464–465.
24. Otsuka, H., and Inouye, L. K.: Pharmacol. Ther. [B] 1:501, 1975.
25. Schimmer, B. P., and Parker, K. L.: In Hardman, J. G., and Limbird, L. E. (eds.). Goodman and Gilman's The Pharmacological Basis of Therapeutics, 10th ed. New York, Macmillan, 2001, pp. 1650–1655.
26. Hughes, J., et al.: Nature 258:577, 1975.
27. Gutstein, H. B., and Akil, H.: In Hardman, J. G., and Limbird, L. E. (eds.). Goodman and Gilman's The Pharmacological Basis of Therapeutics, 10th ed. New York, Macmillan, 2001, pp. 569–579.
28. Snyder, S. H.: Science 224:22, 1984.
29. Wallis, M.: J. Mol. Evol. 17:10, 1981.
30. Lewis, U. J., Sinha, Y. N., and Lewis, G. P.: Endocr. J. 47(Suppl.): S1–8, 2000.
31. Janecka, A., Zubrzycka, M., and Janecki, T.: J. Pept. Res. 58(2):91, 2001.
32. Brownstein, M. J.: Science 207:373, 1980.
33. Drug Information for the Health Care Professional, vol. 1, 22nd ed. Rockville, MD, U. S. Pharmacopeial Convention, 2002, p. 2275.
34. Banting, F. G., and Best, C. H.: J. Lab. Clin. Med. 7:251, 1922.
35. Wallis, M., Howell, S. L., and Taylor, K. W.: The Biochemistry of Peptide Hormones. Chichester, U. K., John Wiley & Sons, 1985, pp. 257–297.
36. Alrefai, H., Allababidi, H., Levy, S., and Levy, J: Endocrine 18(2): 105, 2002.
37. Newgard, C. B.: Diabetes 51(11):3141, 2002.
38. De Meyts, P., and Whittaker, J.: Nat. Rev. Drug Discov. 1(10):769, 2002.
39. Steiner, D. F., et al.: Recent Prog. Horm. Res. 25:207–282, 1969.
40. Docherty, K., et al.: Proc. Natl. Acad. Sci. U. S. A. 79:4613, 1982.
41. Arquilla, E. R., et al.: In Steiner, D. F., and Freinkel, N. (eds.). Handbook of Physiology, Sect. 7: Endocrinology, vol. 1. Washington, DC, American Physiological Society, 1972, pp. 159–173.
42. Gerich, J., et al.: Annu. Rev. Physiol. 38:353, 1976.
43. Sanger, F.: Annu. Rev. Biochem. 27:58, 1958.
44. Katsoyannis, P. G.: Science 154:1509, 1966.
45. Rittel, W., et al. Helv. Chim. Acta 67:2617, 1974.
46. Chance, R. E., et al.: Diabetes Care 4:147, 1981.
47. Johnson, I. S.: Diabetes Care 5(Suppl. 2):4, 1982.
48. Cosmatos, A., et al.: J. Biol. Chem. 253:6586, 1978.
49. May, J. M., et al.: J. Biol. Chem. 253:686, 1978.
50. Blundell, T. L., et al.: Crit. Rev. Biochem. 13:141, 1982.
51. Larner, J.: Diabetes 37:262, 1988.
52. Kasuga, M., et al.: Science 215:185, 1982.
53. Gerich, J. E.: In Diabetes Mellitus, 9th ed. Indianapolis, Eli Lilly & Co., 1988, p. 53.
54. Galloway, J. A.: In Diabetes Mellitus, 9th ed. Indianapolis, Eli Lilly & Co., 1988, pp. 109–122.
55. Wallis, M., et al.: The Biochemistry of the Polypeptide Hormones. Chichester, U. K., John Wiley & Sons, 1985, p. 280.
56. Jefferson, L. S.: Diabetes 29:487, 1980.
57. Feldman, J. M.: In Diabetes Mellitus, 9th ed. Indianapolis, Eli Lilly & Co., 1988, pp. 28–42.
58. Pirat, J.: Diabetes Care 1(part 1):168–188, (part 2):252–263, 1978.
59. Raskin, P., and Rosenstock, J.: Ann. Intern. Med. 105:254, 1986.
60. Maurer, A. C.: Am. Sci. 67:422, 1979.
61. USP DI: Drug Information for the Health Care Professional, vol. I, 22nd ed. Rockville, MD, U. S. Pharmacopeial Convention, 2002, pp. 1701–1730.
62. Unger, R. J., et al.: Science 188:923, 1975.
63. Fain, J. N.: Recept. Recogn. Ser. A 6:3, 1978.
64. Wallis, M., Howell, S. L., and Taylor, K. W.: The Biochemistry of the Polypeptide Hormones. Chichester, U. K., John Wiley & Sons, 1985, pp. 318–335.
65. Emson, P. C., and Sandberg, B. E.: Annu. Rep. Med. Chem. 18:31, 1983.
66. Miller, R. J.: J. Med. Chem. 27:1239, 1984.
67. Adams, A. E., Bisello, A., Chorev, M., et al.: Mol. Endocrinol. 12(11): 1673, 1998.
68. Bumpus, F. M.: Fed. Proc. 36:2128, 1977.
69. Ondetti, M. A., and Cushman, J.: J. Med. Chem. 24:355, 1981.
70. Ogonowski, A. A., May, S. W., Moore, A. B., et al.: J. Pharm. Exp. Ther. 280:846–853, 1997.
71. May, S. W., and Pollock, S. H.: U. S. Patent #6,495,514. Issued December 2002.
72. Pezzuto, J. M., Johnson, M. E., and Manasse, H. R. (eds.): Biotechnology and Pharmacy. New York, Chapman & Hall, 1993.
73. Richards, F. F., et al.: Science 187:130, 1975.
74. Biotechnology Medicines in Development [survey], Pharmaceutical Research and Manufacturers of America, Washington, DC, 1995.
75. Zito, S. W. (ed.): Pharmaceutical Biotechnology: A Programmed Text. Lancaster, PA, Technomic Publishing, 1992.
76. Hudson, R. A., and Black, C. D.: Biotechnology—The New Dimension in Pharmacy Practice: A Working Pharmacists' Guide. Columbus, OH, Council of Ohio Colleges of Pharmacy, 1992, p. 1.
77. Primrose, S. B.: Modern Biotechnology. Boston, Blackwell Scientific Publications, 1987.
78. Hudson, R. A., and Black, C. D.: Biotechnology—The New Dimension in Pharmacy Practice: A Working Pharmacists' Guide, Council of Ohio Colleges of Pharmacy, 1992, p. 2.
79. Birch, J. R., and Lennox, E. S. (eds.): Monoclonal Antibodies: Principles and Applications. New York, John Wiley & Sons, 1995.
80. Gelman, C. R., Rumack, B. H., and Hess, A. J. (eds.): DRUGDEX (R) System. Englewood, CO, MICROMEDEX, Inc. (expired 11/30/95).
81. Shak, S., et al.: Recombinant human DNAse I reduces viscosity of cystic fibrosis sputum. Proc. Natl. Acad. Sci. U. S. A. 87:9188, 1990.
82. Lieberman, J., and Kurnick, N. B.: Nature 196:988, 1962.
83. Brady, R. O., et al.: Efficacy of enzyme replacement therapy in Gaucher disease. Prog. Clin. Biol. Res. 95:669, 1982.
84. Kirkwood, J. M., and Ernstoff, M. S.: J. Clin. Oncol. 2:336, 1984.
85. Houglum, J. E.: Clin. Pharm. 2:202, 1983.
86. Hayden, F. G.: Antiviral agents. In Hardman, J. G., and Limbird, L. E. (eds.). Goodman and Gilman's The Pharmacological Basis of Therapeutics, 10th ed. New York, Macmillan, 2001, pp. 1332–1335.
87. USP DI: Drug Information for the Health Care Professional, vol. I, 22nd ed. Rockville, MD, U. S. Pharmacopeial Convention, 2002, pp. 1730–1733.
88. Von Hoff, D. D., and Huong, A. M.: Effect of recombinant interferon beta-ser on primary human tumor colony-forming units. J. Interferon Res. 8:813, 1988.
89. Doyle, M. V., Lee, M. T., and Fong, S.: Comparison of the biological activities of human recombinant interleukin-2125 and native interleukin-2. J. Biol. Response Mod. 4:96, 1985.
90. Kato, K., et al.: Purification and characterization of recombinant human interleukin-2 produced in *Escherichia coli*. Biochem. Biophys. Res. Commun. 130:692, 1985.
91. Erslev, A. J.: Erythropoietin coming of age. N. Engl. J. Med. 316:101, 1981.
92. Lin, F. K., et al.: Cloning and expression of the human erythropoietin gene. Proc. Natl. Acad. Sci. U. S. A. 82:7580, 1985.
93. USP DI: Drug Information for the Health Care Professional, vol. I, 22nd ed. Rockville, MD, U. S. Pharmacopeial Convention, 2002, pp. 941–947.
94. Lee, F., et al.: Isolation of c-DNA for human granulocyte-macrophage colony stimulating factor by functional expression in mammalian cells. Proc. Natl. Acad. Sci. U. S. A. 82:4360, 1985.
95. Fulcher, C., and Zimmerman, T.: Proc. Natl. Acad. Sci. U. S. A. 79: 1648, 1982.
96. Lawn, R. M., and Vehar, G. A.: The molecular genetics of hemophilia. Sci. Am. 254:48, 1986.

SELECTED READING

Birch, J. R., and Lennox, E. S. (eds.): Monoclonal Antibodies: Principles and Applications. New York, John Wiley & Sons, 1995.

Boyer, P. D. (ed.): The Enzymes, 3rd ed. New York, Academic Press, 1970.

Brockerhoff, H., and Jensen, R. G.: Lipolytic Enzymes. New York, Academic Press, 1974.

Ferdinand, W.: The Enzyme Molecule. New York, John Wiley & Sons, 1976.

Galloway, J. A., Potvin, J. H., and Shuman, C. R. (eds.): Diabetes Mellitus, 9th ed. Indianapolis, Eli Lilly & Co., 1988.

Grollman, A. P.: Inhibition of protein biosynthesis. In Brockerhoff, H., and Jensen, R. G. (eds.). Lipolytic Enzymes. New York, Academic Press, 1974, pp. 231–247.

Hardman, J. G., and Limbird, L. E. (eds.). Goodman and Gilman's The Pharmacological Basis of Therapeutics, 10th ed. New York, Macmillan, 2001.

Haschemeyer, R. H., and de Harven, E.: Electron microscopy of enzymes. Annu. Rev. Biochem. 43:279, 1974.

Hruby, V. J., de Chavez, C. G., and Kavarana, M.: Peptide and protein hormones, peptide neurotransmitters, and therapeutic agents. In Abraham, D. J. (ed). Burger's Medicinal Chemistry and Drug Discovery, vol. 4, 6th ed. New York, John Wiley & Sons, 2003.

Jenks, W. P.: Catalysis in Chemistry and Enzymology. New York, McGraw-Hill, 1969.

Lowe, J. N., and Ingraham, L. L.: An Introduction to Biochemical Reaction Mechanisms. Englewood Cliffs, NJ, Prentice-Hall, 1974. (This book includes elementary enzymology including mechanisms of coenzyme function.)

Mildvan, A. S.: Mechanism of enzyme action. Annu. Rev. Biochem. 43: 357, 1974.

Pezzuto, J. M., Johnson, M. E., and Manasse, H. R. (eds.): Biotechnology and Pharmacy. New York, Chapman & Hall, 1993.

Pikes, S. J., and Parks, C. R.: The mode of action of insulin. Annu. Rev. Pharmacol. 14:365, 1974.

Schaeffer, H. J.: Factors in the design of reversible and irreversible enzyme inhibitors. In Ariens, E. J. (ed). Drug Design, vol. 2. New York, Academic Press, 1971, pp. 129–159.

Stryer, L. S.: Biochemistry, 5th ed. New York, W. H. Freeman & Co., 2002.

Tager, H. S., and Steiner, D. F.: Peptide hormones. Annu. Rev. Biochem. 43:509, 1974.

Waife, S. O. (ed.): Diabetes Mellitus, 8th ed. Indianapolis, Eli Lilly & Co., 1980.

Wallis, M., Howell, S. L., and Taylor, K. W.: The Biochemistry of the Peptide Hormones. Chichester, U. K., John Wiley & Sons, 1985.

Wilson, C. A.: Hypothalamic amines and the release of gonadotrophins and other anterior pituitary hormones. Adv. Drug Res. 8:119–204, 1974.

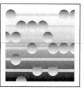

Vitamins and Related Compounds

GUSTAVO R. ORTEGA, MICHAEL J. DEIMLING, JAIME N. DELGADO[*]

Vitamins traditionally have been considered to be "accessory food factors." Generally, vitamins are among those nutrients that the human organism cannot synthesize from other dietary components. Together with certain amino acids (i.e., essential amino acids), the vitamins constitute a total of 24 organic compounds that have been characterized as dietarily essential.[1] Many vitamins function biochemically as precursors in the synthesis of coenzymes necessary in human metabolism; thus, vitamins perform essential functions. When they are not available in appropriate amounts, the consequences may lead to serious disease states.

Although there are relatively few therapeutic indications for vitamin pharmaceutical preparations, diseases caused by certain vitamin deficiencies do respond favorably to vitamin therapy. Additionally, there are products indicated for prophylactic use as dietary supplements. An optimal diet provides all of the necessary nutrients; in some cases of increased demands, however, vitamin and mineral supplementation is recommended.[2]

Two organizations provide guidelines for daily vitamin intake in the United States. The first, the Food and Drug Administration (FDA), regulates the labeling of foods with respect to their nutritional content, including vitamins. The current labeling requirements for vitamins, established following the Dietary Supplement Health and Education Act (DSHEA) of 1994 and published in the Code of Federal Regulations (CFR),[3] requires that the vitamin content of food be listed as a percentage of the daily value (DV). The daily value for nutrients is determined by using the daily reference value (DRV) if the nutrient is a source of energy, such as protein, carbohydrates, and fats, or by using the reference daily intake (RDI) for vitamins and minerals. The RDI replaces the previously used term, U. S. RDA (recommended daily allowance), to prevent confusion with the RDAs published by the National Academy of Sciences. The RDIs for each of the vitamins as published in the CFR are the same as the values used under the older term, RDAs. The DV for each of the vitamins (Table 26-1) is based on a 2,000-calorie diet, and the %DV that is placed on the food label is determined by dividing the content of one serving of the food by the DV and expressing the result as a percentage.

The second organization that provides nutritional guidelines is the Nutrition Board of the National Academy of Sciences, Institute of Medicine. Their guidelines are published in the form of dietary reference intakes (DRIs), which include several ways of evaluating the proper intake of vitamins and minerals, such as the estimated average requirement (EAR), recommended dietary allowance (RDA), adequate intake (AI), and tolerable upper intake level (UL). Generally, the RDA is the most specific recommendation of the recommended daily intake, with the AI used if not enough data exist to support determination of a RDA. Table 26-2 contains the current dietary DRIs, in terms of the RDA (when available) or the AI (when the RDA is not available) for the vitamins covered in this chapter.

The medicinal chemistry of vitamins is fundamental not only to the therapeutics of nutritional problems but also to the understanding of the biochemical actions of other medicinal agents that directly or indirectly affect the metabolic functions of vitamins and coenzymes. Accordingly, this chapter includes a brief summary of the basic biochemistry of vitamins, structure–activity relationships, physicochemical properties and some stability considerations, nutritional and therapeutic applications, and brief characterizations of representative pharmaceutical products.

In 1912, Funk[4] described a substance, present in rice polishings and in foods, that cured polyneuritis in birds and beriberi in humans. This substance was referred to as *vitamine* because it was characterized as an amine and as a vital nutritional component. After other food factors were noted to be vital nutritional components that were not amines and did not even contain nitrogen,[5] Drummond suggested the modification that led to the term *vitamin*. McCollum and

[*]Deceased.

TABLE 26-1 Daily Values of the Vitamins Used in Food Labeling

Vitamin	Daily Value[a]
Vitamin A	5,000 IU[b]
Vitamin C	60 mg
Vitamin D	400 IU
Vitamin E	30 IU
Vitamin K	80 μg
Thiamin	1.5 mg
Riboflavin	1.7 mg
Niacin	20 mg
Vitamin B_6	2 mg
Folate	400 μg
Vitamin B_{12}	6 μg
Biotin	300 μg
Pantothenic acid	10 mg

From Code of Federal Regulations. Section 101.9. 1977.
[a]Based on a 2,000-calorie diet.
[b]International units.

TABLE 26-2 Dietary Reference Intakes of the Vitamins for Individuals[a]

Life Stage Group	Biotin (mg/d)	Choline (mg/d)	Folate (mg/d)	Niacin (mg/d)	Pantothenic Acid (mg/d)	Riboflavin (mg/d)	Thiamin (mg/d)	Vitamin A (mg/d)	Vitamin B$_6$ (mg/d)	Vitamin B$_{12}$ (mg/d)	Vitamin C (mg/d)	Vitamin D (mg/d)	Vitamin E (mg/d)	Vitamin K (mg/d)
Infants														
0–6 mo	5*	125*	65*	2*	1.7*	0.3*	0.2*	400*	0.1*	0.4*	40*	5*	4*	2.0*
7–12 mo	6*	150*	80*	4*	1.8*	0.4*	0.3*	500*	0.3*	0.5*	50*	5*	5*	2.5*
Children														
1–3 y	8*	200*	150	6	2*	0.5	0.5	300	0.5	0.9	15	5*	6	30*
4–8 y	12*	250*	200	8	3*	0.6	0.6	400	0.6	1.2	25	5*	7	55*
Males														
9–13 y	20*	375*	300	12	4*	0.9	0.9	600	1.0	1.8	45	5*	11	60*
14–18 y	25*	550*	400	16	5*	1.3	1.2	900	1.3	2.4	75	5*	15	75*
19–30 y	30*	550*	400	16	5*	1.3	1.2	900	1.3	2.4	90	5*	15	120*
31–50 y	30*	550*	400	16	5*	1.3	1.2	900	1.3	2.4	90	5*	15	120*
51–70 y	30*	550*	400	16	5*	1.3	1.2	900	1.7	2.4	90	10*	15	120*
>70 y	30*	550*	400	16	5*	1.3	1.2	900	1.7	2.4	90	15*	15	120*
Females														
9–13 y	20*	375*	300	12	4*	0.9	0.9	600	1.0	1.8	45	5*	11	60*
14–18 y	25*	400*	400	14	5*	1.0	1.0	700	1.2	2.4	65	5*	15	75*
19–30 y	30*	425*	400	14	5*	1.1	1.1	700	1.3	2.4	75	5*	15	90*
31–50 y	30*	425*	400	14	5*	1.1	1.1	700	1.3	2.4	75	5*	15	90*
51–70 y	30*	425*	400	14	5*	1.1	1.1	700	1.5	2.4	75	10*	15	90*
>70 y	30*	425*	400	14	5*	1.1	1.1	700	1.5	2.4	75	15*	15	90*
Pregnancy														
≤18 y	30*	450*	600	18	6*	1.4	1.4	750	1.9	2.6	80	5*	15	75*
19–30 y	30*	450*	600	18	6*	1.4	1.4	770	1.9	2.6	85	5*	15	90*
31–50 y	30*	450*	600	18	6*	1.4	1.4	770	1.9	2.6	85	5*	15	90*
Lactation														
≤18 y	35*	550*	500	17	7*	1.6	1.4	1,200	2.0	2.8	115	5*	19	75*
19–30 y	35*	550*	500	17	7*	1.6	1.4	1,300	2.0	2.8	120	5*	19	90*
31–50 y	35*	550*	500	17	7*	1.6	1.4	1,300	2.0	2.8	120	5*	19	90*

Dietary Reference Intakes: Applications in Dietary Assessment. 2001 Food and Nutrition Board, National Academy of Sciences, Institute of Medicine. Washington, DC, National Academy Press, 2001; and Dietary Reference Intakes for Vitamin A, Vitamin K, Arsenic, Boron, Chromium, Copper, Iodine, Iron, Manganese, Molybdenum, Nickel, Silicon, Vanadium, and Zinc. 2001 Food and Nutrition Board, National Academy of Sciences, Institute of Medicine. Washington, DC, National Academy Press, 2001.

Abbreviations: d, day; y, year.

[a]Numbers in this table represent the current Recommended Daily Allowance (RDA) as determined by the Food and Nutrition Board of the Institute of the National Academy of Sciences, Institute of Medicine unless marked by an asterisk (*), in which case they represent the Adequate Intake (IA)

Davis[6, 7] described a lipid-soluble essential food factor in butterfat and egg yolk, and 2 years later, reference was made to a water-soluble factor in wheat germ. Thus, the terms *fat-soluble A* and *water-soluble B,* respectively, were applied to these food factors. Since then, many other dietary components have been discovered to be essential nutritional components (i.e., vitamins). It is traditional to classify these compounds as either lipid-soluble or water-soluble vitamins. This classification is convenient because members of each category possess important properties in common.

LIPID-SOLUBLE VITAMINS

The lipid-soluble vitamins include vitamins A, D, E, and K. These compounds possess other characteristics in common besides solubility. They are usually associated with the lipids in foods and are absorbed from the intestine with these dietary lipids. The lipid-soluble vitamins are stored in the liver and, thus, conserved by the organism, whereas storage of the water-soluble vitamins is usually not significant.

Vitamin As

Vitamin A was first recognized as a vitamin by McCollum and Davis[6, 7] in 1913 to 1915, but studies of the molecular mechanism of action of retinol in the visual process were not significantly productive until 1968 to 1972. The mechanism of action of vitamin A in physiological processes other than vision has been very difficult to study. Advances in molecular biology have, however, started to identify the role of retinoids in bone growth, reproduction, embryonic development, protein synthesis, sperm production, and control and differentiation of epithelial tissues. This has led to the suggestion that vitamin A has hormone-like properties. There is convincing evidence that vitamin A performs an important function in the biosynthesis of glycoproteins and in sugar-transfer reactions in mammalian membranes.[8] Investigations on the mechanism of this action were stymied by difficulties in clearly defining the biochemically active form of the vitamins, whether it is all-*trans*-retinol or retinoic acid. This question was reviewed comprehensively by Chytil and Ong.[9] Most, if not all, vitamin A actions in development, differentiation, and metabolism are mediated through nuclear receptors that bind to retinoic acid.[10]

TABLE 26-3   Weight Equal to 1 IU

Retinoid	µg
All-*trans*-retinol	0.3
All-*trans*-retinol acetate	0.334
All-*trans*-retinol propionate	0.359
All-*trans*-retinol palmitate	0.55
β-Carotene	0.6

TABLE 26-4   USP Units per Gram of Selected Retinoids

Retinoid	U/g
All-*trans*-retinol	2,907,000
Neovitamin A	2,190,000
9-*cis*-Retinol	634,000
9,13-Di-*cis*-retinol	688,000
9,11-Di-*cis*-retinol	679,000
All-*trans*-retinal	3,050,000
11-*cis*-Retinal	3,120,000
9-*cis*-Retinal	637,000
9,13-Di-*cis*-retinal	581,000
9,11-Di-*cis*-retinal	11,610,000

The term *vitamin A* currently is applied to compounds possessing biological activity like that of retinol. The term *vitamin A₁* refers to all-*trans*-retinol. The term *retinoid* is applied to retinol and its naturally occurring derivatives plus synthetic analogues, which need not have vitamin A activity.

Vitamin A activity is expressed as USP units, international units (IU), retinol equivalents (RE), and β-carotene equivalents. The USP units and IU are equivalent. Each unit expresses the activity of 0.3 µg of all-*trans*-retinol. Thus, 1 mg of all-*trans*-retinol has the activity of 3,333 units. Other equivalents are listed in Table 26-3. One RE represents the biological activity of 1 µg of all-*trans*-retinol, 6 µg of β-carotene, and 12 µg of mixed dietary carotenoids. The RE is used to convert all dietary sources of vitamin A into a single unit for easy comparison.[11]

The stereochemistry of vitamin A and related compounds is complex, and a complete stereochemical analysis is beyond the scope of this chapter. A brief summary of some stereochemical features is presented here as the basis for the characterization of the biochemical actions exerted by this vitamin. The study of the structural relationships among vitamin A and its stereoisomers has been complicated by the common use of several numbering systems, as shown below. The first numbering system (A) is the one currently recommended by the International Union of Pure and Applied Chemistry (IUPAC). The second system (B) places emphasis on the conjugated π system, while the third (C) is used by the *USP Dictionary of USAN and International Drug Names.*

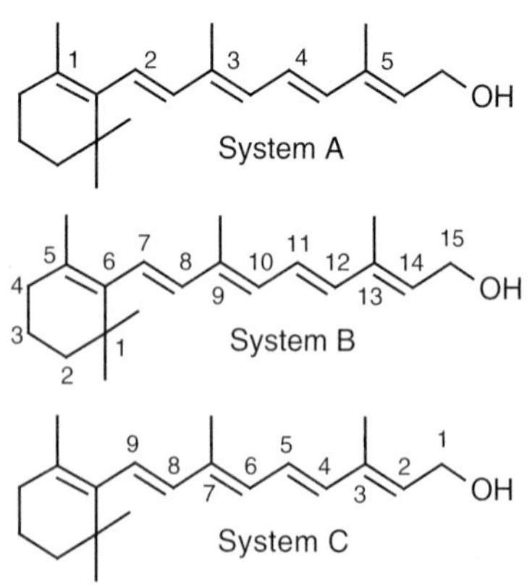

System A

System B

System C

For steric reasons, the number of isomers of vitamin A most likely to occur is limited. These are all-*trans*, 9-*cis*, 13-*cis*, and the 9,13-di-*cis*. A *cis* linkage at double bond 7 or 11 encounters steric hindrance. The 11-*cis* isomer is twisted as well as bent at this linkage; nevertheless, this is the only isomer that is active in vision. The biological activity[12] of the isomers of vitamin A acetate, in terms of USP units per gram, are listed in Table 26-4. Disregarding stereochemical variations, several compounds with structures corresponding to vitamin A, its ethers, and its esters have been prepared.[13–16] These compounds as well as synthetic vitamin A acid possess biological activity.

Dietary vitamin A is obtained exclusively from foods of animal origin as retinyl esters. The provitamin carotenoids are obtained from plant and dairy sources. The highest sources of natural vitamin A are fish liver oils, which vary greatly in the content of this vitamin (Table 26-5). Most liver oils contain vitamin A and neovitamin A in the ratio of 2:1. Vitamin A occurs free and combined as the biologically active esters, chiefly of palmitic and some myristic and dodecanoic acids. It is also found in the livers of animals, especially those that are herbivorous. Milk and eggs are fair sources of this vitamin.

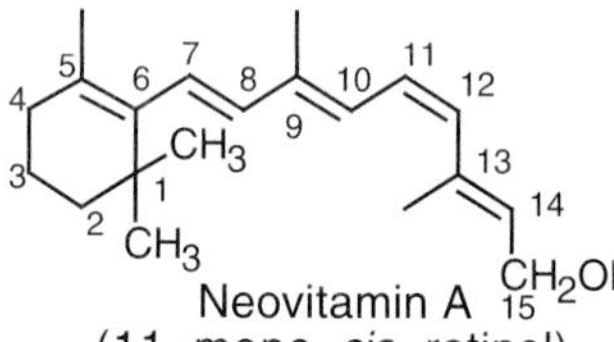

Neovitamin A
(11–mono–*cis*–retinol)

The livers of freshwater fish contain vitamin A₂ (3,4-dehydroretinol).

TABLE 26-5   Vitamin A Content of Some Fish Liver Oils

Source	Animal Species	Potency (IU/g)
Halibut, liver	*Hippoglossus hippoglossus*	60,000
Percomorph, liver	*Percomorph* fishes (mixed oils)	60,000
Shark, liver	*Galeus zygopterus*	25,500
Shark, liver	*Hypoprion brevirostris* and other varieties	16,500
Burbot, liver	*Lota maculosa*	4,880
Cod, liver	*Gadus morrhua*	850

Vitamin A₂ (all–*trans*)
3,4–Dehydroretinol or Dehydroretinol

Dietary retinyl esters are hydrolyzed in the intestinal lumen by various hydrolases. The retinol is absorbed into the enterocytes by facilitated diffusion in normal concentrations. At pharmacological doses, however, retinol can be absorbed by passive diffusion.[17] Within the enterocytes, the retinol is esterified by two enzymes, acylcoenzyme A (CoA): retinol acyltransferase (ARAT) and lecithin:retinal acyltransferase (LRAT). LRAT esterifies retinol bound to an intracellular protein, cellular retinol-binding protein type II (CRBP [II]), while ARAT can esterify unbound retinol. It has been proposed that LRAT esterifies retinol at normal doses, while ARAT esterifies excess retinol.[18]

The retinyl esters are incorporated into chylomicrons, which in turn enter the lymph. Once in the general circulation, chylomicrons are converted into chylomicron remnants, which are cleared primarily by the liver. As the esters enter the hepatocytes, they are hydrolyzed. In the endoplasmic reticulum, the retinol is bound to retinol-binding protein (RBP). This complex is released into the blood or transferred to liver stellate cells for storage. Within the stellate cells, the retinol is bound to CRBP(I) and esterified for storage by ARAT and LRAT. Stellate cells contain up to 95% of the liver vitamin A stores. The RBP–retinol complex released into the general circulation from hepatocytes or stellate cells, in turn, is bound to transthyretin (TTR), which protects retinol from metabolism and renal excretion.[19]

The cellular uptake of plasma retinol remains to be fully understood. This is further complicated because chylomicron remnants also contribute retinol to the target cells. The fate of retinol after absorption is just beginning to be understood. RBP and TTR do not enter the cell. On entering the cell, the retinol is bound to CRBP(I) in the cytoplasm. Most tissues contain CRBP(I) and CRBP(II). These intracellular proteins function in the transport and metabolism of retinol and retinoic acid by solubilizing them in aqueous media and presenting them to the appropriate enzymes while protecting them from catabolizing enzymes.[20] These proteins also limit the concentration of free retinoids within the cell. CRBP(I) regulates the esterification of retinol and its oxidation to retinoic acid from retinal, while CRBP(II) controls the reduction of retinal to retinol and its subsequent esterification.[21]

Retinol is susceptible to glucuronide conjugation, followed by enterohepatic recycling. It may be oxidized to retinoic acid by two enzymes, retinol dehydrogenase and retinal dehydrogenase, with the former being rate-limiting.[22] Unlike retinol, retinoic acid has no specific carrier in the blood. Retinoic acid undergoes decarboxylation, followed by glucuronide conjugation. Normally, no unchanged retinol is excreted. Retinal, retinoic acid, and other metabolites are, however, found in the urine and feces.

Although fish liver oils are used for their vitamin A content, purified or concentrated forms of vitamin A are of great commercial significance. These are prepared in three ways: *(a)* saponification of the oil and concentration of the vitamin A in the nonsaponifiable matter by solvent extraction, with the product marketed as such; *(b)* molecular distillation of the nonsaponifiable matter, from which the sterols have been removed by freezing, giving a distillate of vitamin A containing 1 to 2 million IU/g; and *(c)* subjecting the fish oil to direct molecular distillation to recover the free vitamin A, vitamin A palmitate, and myristate.

Pure crystalline vitamin A occurs as pale yellow plates or crystals. It melts at 63 to 64°C and is insoluble in water but soluble in alcohol, the usual organic solvents, and the fixed oils. It is unstable in the presence of light and oxygen and in oxidized or readily oxidized fats and oils. It can be protected by the exclusion of air and light and by the presence of antioxidants.

Like all substances that have a polyene structure, vitamin A gives color reactions with many reagents, most of which are either strong acids or chlorides of polyvalent metals. An intense blue is obtained with vitamin A in dry chloroform solution on the addition of a chloroform solution of antimony trichloride. This color reaction (Carr-Price reaction) has been studied extensively and is the basis of a colorimetric assay for vitamin A.[23]

Vitamin A (all–*trans*-retinol) is biosynthesized in animals from plant pigments called *carotenoids,* which are terpenes composed of isoprenoid units. These pigments protect plant cells from photochemical damage and transfer radiant energy to the pigments responsible for photosynthesis. Although hundreds of carotenoids have been identified, only a few function as provitamins.[24]

α–Carotene

β–Carotene

γ–Carotene

δ–Carotene

Cryptoxanthin

The provitamin As (e.g., α-, β-, and γ-carotenes and cryptoxanthin) are found in deep green, yellow, and orange fruits and vegetables, such as carrots, spinach, broccoli, kale, collard and turnip greens, mangoes, apricots, nectarines, pumpkins, and sweet potatoes. The carotenoid pigments are used poorly by humans, whereas animals differ in their ability to use these compounds. These carotenoid pigments are provitamins A because they are converted to the active vitamin A. For example, β-carotene is absorbed intact by the intestinal mucosa, then cleaved to retinal by β-carotene-15,15′-dioxygenase, which requires molecular oxygen.[25] β-Carotene can give rise to two molecules of retinal, whereas with the other three carotenoids, only one molecule is possible by this transformation. These carotenoids have only one ring (see formula for β-carotene) at the end of the polyene chain, which is identical with that found in β-carotene and is necessary for vitamin A activity. This accounts for the low activity of β-carotene.

The conjugated double-bond systems found in vitamin A and β-carotene are necessary for activity; when these compounds are partially or completely reduced, activity is lost. The β-ionone ring of retinol or the dehydro-β-ionone ring found in dehydroretinol (vitamin A_2) is essential for activity. Saturation results in loss of activity. The ester and methyl ethers of vitamin A have a biological activity on a molar basis equal to that of vitamin A. Retinoic acid (vitamin A acid) is biologically active but is not stored in the liver.

Carotenoid absorption is by passive diffusion and depends on absorbable fats and bile. It is assumed that one sixth of normal dietary β-carotene but only one twelfth of the other provitamin A carotenoids is absorbed. The enterocytes convert the carotenes into retinol, but up to 20 to 30% are absorbed unchanged.

The intestinal mucosa is the main site of β-carotene transformation[25] to retinal, but the enzymes that catalyze the transformation also occur in hepatic tissue. Two mechanisms for the conversion to retinal have been proposed. Originally, it was proposed that cleavage occurred centrally by β-carotene-15,15′-dioxygenase.[26] Evidence exists, however, for peripheral cleavage to yield apo-carotinals, which can be converted further to retinal.[27] The retinal thus formed is reduced to retinol and esterified before entering the chylomicrons for transport from the liver.

β–Carotene

β–Apo–8′–carotenal

β–Cyclocitral

β–Apo–10′–carotenal

β–Apo–12′–carotenal

β–Apo–8′–carotenal

β–Apo–14′–carotenal

11–Mono–*cis*–retinal

Retinoic acid, the corresponding carboxylic acid, promotes development of bone and soft tissues and sperm production, but it does not participate in the visual process. Retinoic acid is found in the bile in the glucuronide form.

Vitamin A is often called the *growth vitamin* because a deficiency of it in the diet causes cessation of growth in young rats. A deficiency of vitamin A is manifested chiefly by degeneration of the mucous membranes throughout the body. This degeneration is more pronounced in the eye than in any other part of the body and gives rise to a condition known as xerophthalmia. In the earlier stages of vitamin A deficiency, night blindness (*nyctalopia*) may develop, which can be cured by vitamin A. *Night blindness* can be defined as the inability to see in dim light.

Dark adaptation or *visual threshold* is a more suitable description than *night blindness* in many subclinical cases of vitamin A deficiency. The *visual threshold* at any moment is just that light intensity required to elicit a visual sensation. *Dark adaptation* is the change that the visual threshold undergoes during a stay in the dark after an exposure to light. This change may be very great. After exposure of the eye to daylight, a stay of 30 minutes in the dark decreases the threshold by a factor of 1 million. This phenomenon is used as the basis for detecting subclinical cases of vitamin A deficiency. These tests vary in their technique, but essentially they measure visual dark adaptation after exposure to bright light and compare it with the normal.[28, 29]

Advanced deficiency of vitamin A gives rise to dryness and scaliness of the skin, accompanied by a tendency to infection. Characteristic lesions of the human skin caused by vitamin A deficiency usually occur in sexually mature persons between the ages of 16 and 30 and not in infants. These lesions appear first on the anterolateral surface of the thigh and the posterolateral portion of the upper forearms and later spread to adjacent areas of the skin. The lesions consist of pigmented papules, up to 5 mm in diameter, at the site of the hair follicles.

Vitamin A regulates the activities of osteoblasts and osteoclasts, influencing the shape of the bones in the growing animal. The teeth also are affected. In vitamin A deficiency states, a long overgrowth occurs. Overdoses of vitamin A in infants for prolonged periods lead to irreversible changes in the bones, including retardation of growth, premature closure of the epiphyses, and differences in the lengths of the lower extremities. Thus, a close relationship exists between the functions of vitamins A and D relative to cartilage, bones, and teeth.[30] The tocopherols exert a sparing and what appears to be a synergistic action[31] with vitamin A.

Blood levels of vitamin A decrease very slowly, and decreased dark adaptation was observed in only 2 of 27 volunteers (maintained on a vitamin A–free diet) after 14 months, at which time blood levels had decreased from 88 to 60 IU/100 mL of blood.

Vitamin A performs numerous biochemical functions. It promotes the production of mucus by the basal cells of the epithelium, whereas in its absence keratin can be formed. Vitamin A performs a function in the biosynthesis of glycogen and some steroids, and increased quantities of coenzyme Q are found in the livers of vitamin-deficient rats. Significantly, the best-known action of vitamin A is its function in the chemistry of vision.

Hypervitaminosis A can lead to both short- and long-term effects.[32] Short-term doses of 0.5 to 4 million IU can lead, within hours to several days, to central nervous system effects including increased intracranial pressure, headache, irritability, and seizures; gastrointestinal effects including nausea, vomiting, and pain; dermatological effects such as desquamation; ophthalmic effects such as papilledema, scotoma, and photophobia; and liver damage. Most of these reactions have been reported in infants following treatment with large doses of vitamin A, but some have resulted from ingestion of food rich in vitamin A, such as liver, especially from polar bears.

Long-term intake of doses of vitamin A lower than the intake required for short-term toxicity but still above that required by the body can lead to long-term effects, including effects on the skin, liver, central nervous system, and bone. Although the amount required varies, doses as low as 15,000 IU/day have led to some adverse effects, although higher doses, generally above 100,000 IU/day, are required to see all the reported adverse effects. In patients with low body weight, malnutrition, or liver or renal disease, the doses required for long-term adverse effects may be lower still.

Dermatological adverse effects include drying of the skin and mucosa, dermatitis, pruritus, swelling and fissuring of the lips, and (sometimes) loss of body hair. Hepatic effects include hypertrophy and hyperplasia of the Ito cells (which store vitamin A), hepatomegaly, fibrosis, and cirrhosis, which can lead to portal hypertension, ascites, and jaundice. Splenomegaly is also seen. Central nervous system effects include increased intracranial pressure (pseudotumor cerebri) leading to headache, visual disturbances (e.g., diplopia), drowsiness, vomiting, seizures, and a bulging fontanel in infants. Finally, pain in the bone and joints, with accompanying tenderness, and reduced bone mineralization[33] have also been reported.

The teratogenic effects of vitamin A are also well known.[32, 34] Intake of as little as 10,000 IU/day during pregnancy may increase the risk of birth defects, and the risk increases with increasing intake of vitamin A.[35] Birth defects include craniofacial, neural tube, and urogenital and musculoskeletal abnormalities.

β-Carotene, in contrast, is relatively nontoxic. After long-term exposure to high levels of β-carotene (30 to 180 mg/day for 15 years), which is equivalent to 50,000 to 300,000 IU of vitamin A, patients have not developed any problems other than skin discoloration and asymptomatic hypercarotenemia. Furthermore, β-carotene is not teratogenic. The most likely mechanism is the slow rate of conversion of β-carotene to retinol.

The molecular mechanism of action of vitamin A in the visual process has been under investigation for many years. Wald in 1968[36] and Morton in 1972[37] characterized this mechanism of action. The chemistry of vision was reviewed comprehensively in *Accounts of Chemical Research* (1975) by numerous investigators. These reviews include theoretical studies of the visual chromophore, characterization of rhodopsin in synthetic systems, dynamic processes in vertebrate rod visual pigments and their membranes, and the dynamics of the visual protein opsin.[38–43]

Vitamin A (all-*trans*-retinol) undergoes isomerization to the 11-*cis* form in the liver. This transformation is catalyzed by a retinol isomerase. Subsequently, 11-*cis*-retinol interacts with RBP to form a complex that is transported to the retinal photoreceptor cells, which contain specific receptors for the RBP–retinol complex.

The retina has been considered[41, 43] to be a double-sense organ in which the rods are concerned with colorless vision at low light intensities and the cones are concerned with color vision at high light intensities. A dark-adapted, excised retina is rose red; when it is exposed to light, its color changes to chamois, to orange, to pale yellow; finally, on prolonged irradiation, it becomes colorless. The rods contain photosensitive visual purple (rhodopsin), which, when acted on by light of a definite wavelength, is converted to visual yellow and initiates a series of chemical steps necessary to vision. Visual purple is a conjugated carotenoid protein with a relative molecular mass (M_r) of about 40,000 and one prosthetic group per molecule. It contains seven hydrophobic α-helices, which are embedded in the membrane. Short hydrophilic loops interconnect the helices and are exposed to the aqueous environment on either side of the membrane. It has an absorption maximum of about 510 nm. The prosthetic group is retinene (neoretinene b or retinal), which is joined to the protein through a protonated Schiff base linkage.

The function of retinene in visual purple is to increase the absorption coefficient in visible light and, thereby, sensitize the protein, which is denatured. This process initiates a series of physical and chemical steps necessary to vision. The protein itself differs from other proteins in having a lower energy of activation, which permits it to be denatured by a quantum of visible light. Other proteins require a quantum of ultraviolet (UV) light to be denatured. The bond between the pigment and the protein is much weaker when the protein is denatured than when it is native. The denaturation of the protein is reversible and takes place more readily in the dark to give rise, when combined with retinene, to visual purple. The effectiveness of the spectrum in bleaching visual purple runs fairly parallel with its absorption spectrum (510 nm) and with the sensibility distribution of the eye in the spectrum at low illuminations. It has been calculated that for a human to see a barely perceptible flash of light, only one molecule of visual purple in each 5 to 14 rod cells needs to be photochemically transformed in a dark-adapted eye. The system possesses such sensitivity because of biological amplification. In vivo, visual purple is re-formed constantly as it is bleached by light, and under continuous illumination, an equilibrium is maintained between visual purple, visual yellow, and visual white. If an animal is placed in the dark, the regeneration of visual purple continues until a maximum concentration is obtained. Visual purple in the eyes of an intact animal may be bleached by light and regenerated in the dark an enormous number of times.

In the resting state (dark), rod and cone membranes exhibit a steady electrical current. The membrane allows sodium ions to enter freely through specific channels. A Na^+/K^+-ATPase pump maintains the ion gradient. The closing of the pores hyperpolarizes the membrane and initiates the neuronal response.

The pores are kept open by binding to cyclic guanosine monophosphate (cGMP). The light-induced isomerization of retinal causes a conformational change in the protein part of rhodopsin, activating the molecule. One active rhodopsin activates several hundred G-protein molecules, called *transducin*. (G proteins can bind with guanosine nucleotides.) Activation of transducin consists of an exchange of bound guanosine diphosphate (GDP) for guanosine triphosphate (GTP). Activated transducin, in turn, activates a phosphodiesterase, which hydrolyzes thousands of cGMP molecules. The decreased concentration of cGMP results in closing of the sodium channels.

Hydrolysis of transducin-bound GTP to GDP inactivates the phosphodiesterases. The activated rhodopsin must also be deactivated, however. This is accomplished by phosphorylation of opsin by opsin kinase. Guanylate cyclase replenishes the cGMP concentration, which reopens the channels.

Visual purple occurs in all vertebrates. It is not distributed evenly over the retina. It is missing in the fovea, and in the regions outside the fovea, its concentration undoubtedly increases to a maximum in the region about 20° off center, corresponding to the high density of rods in this region. Therefore, to see an object best in the dark, one should not look directly at it.

The diagrams represent some of the changes that take place in the visual cycle involving the rhodopsin system in which the 11-mono-*cis* isomer of vitamin A is functional in the aldehyde form.[44]

After the light-catalyzed reaction, all-*trans*-retinal is released, which in turn is reduced to all-*trans*-retinol. To be used again by opsin, the all-*trans*-retinol must be converted to 11-*cis*-retinol. Isomerization occurs in the pigment epithelium of the retina.[45] Oxidation of 11-*cis*-retinol to 11-*cis*-retinaldehyde occurs while retinol is bound to the protein cellular retinaldehyde-binding protein (CRALBP) by a microsomal enzyme in the pigment epithelium.[46]

The isomerization of *trans*-retinal may take place in the presence of blue light. Vision continues very well, however, in yellow, orange, and red light, in which no isomerization takes place. The 11-mono-*cis*-retinal under these circumstances is replaced by an active form of vitamin A from the bloodstream, which came from stores in the liver. The isomerization of *trans*-vitamin A in the body to *cis-trans*-vitamin A seems to keep pace with long-term processes such as growth, since vitamin A, neovitamin A, and 11-mono-*cis*-retinal are equally active in growth tests in rats. The sulfhydryl groups (two for each 11-mono-*cis*-retinal molecule isomerized) exposed on the opsin initiate the transmission of impulses in the phenomenon of vision.

Research since the mid-1980s has taken vast strides in determining the molecular mechanism of action of vitamin A. It appears that the vitamin exerts its biological function with respect to development, differentiation, and metabolism like a steroid hormone.[47–49] The biologically active species is believed to be retinoic acid. Two intracellular retinoic acid–binding proteins have been isolated, CRABP(I) and CRABP(II). These appear to have functions similar to those of the CRBPs.

More importantly, several retinoic acid receptors (RARs) have been identified: RARα, RARβ, and RARγ.[48] These differ in their tissue distribution and the level of expression during cell development and differentiation. After binding with retinoic acid, the complex binds to specific recognition sequences on DNA (RAREs), thus influencing the transcription of specific genes. The ultimate biological effects of retinoic acid are mediated through various proteins that remain to be identified. Retinoids influence embryonic development by inhibiting cell proliferation and inducing cell differentiation and apoptosis.[50] A new family of retinoic acid receptors has been identified.[51] These are called *retinoid X receptors,* RXRα, RXRβ, and RXRγ. They have a different tissue distribution from the RARs. The ligand for RXR has been identified as 9-*cis*-retinoic acid.[52]

These retinoid receptors must form dimers before they interact with RAREs. RARs must form heterodimers with RXRs, whereas RXRs may also form homodimers. It appears that the RAREs for the homodimers differ from those for the heterodimers. This implies that they may activate different sets of genes.[53, 54] RXRs also form heterodimers with thyroid hormone receptors and vitamin D receptors, increasing their affinity for DNA.[55] Several enzymes whose expression depends on RXR have been found.[52] The available experimental data provide convincing evidence that these proteins are, in fact, nuclear receptors belonging to the steroid/thyroid hormone superfamily. They mediate important aspects of vitamin A function. The existence of proteins that specifically bind retinoic acid substantiates the implication of retinoic acid as a physiological form of vitamin A.

Studies have shown a correlation between a diet high in β-carotene and a reduced risk of certain cancers. Several reviews of these studies are available.[56, 57]

PRODUCTS

Vitamin A, USP. Vitamin A (Aquasol A) contains retinol (vitamin A alcohol) or its esters from edible fatty acids (chiefly acetic and palmitic acids), whose activity is not less than 95% of the labeled amount; a dosage of 0.3 μg of vitamin A alcohol (retinol) equals 1 USP unit.

Vitamin A is indicated only for treatment of vitamin A deficiencies. Because the vitamin is prevalent in the diet, especially with supplementation of milk, this disorder is not common. It is associated with conditions that result in the malabsorption of fats (e.g., biliary or pancreatic diseases, sprue, hepatic cirrhosis).

Pure vitamin A has an activity of 3.5 million IU/g. Moderate-to-massive doses of vitamin A have been used in pregnancy, lactation, acne, termination of colds, removal of persistent follicular hyperkeratosis of the arms, persistent and abnormal warts, corns, and calluses, and similar conditions. Phosphatides or the tocopherols enhance the absorption of vitamin A. Vitamin A applied topically appears to reverse the impairment of wound healing by corticoids.

Vitamin A occurs as a yellow to red, oily liquid. It is nearly odorless or has a fishy odor and is unstable to air and light. It is insoluble in water or glycerin and is soluble in absolute alcohol, vegetable oils, ether, and chloroform.

Tretinoin, USP.

Tretinoin, retinoic acid (Retin-A), is a yellow to light-orange, crystalline powder. It is insoluble in water and slightly soluble in alcohol.

Tretinoin

Tretinoin, indicated for topical treatment of acne vulgaris, was initially used systemically. Therapeutic doses frequently resulted in hypervitaminosis A, however. It appears to exert its action by decreasing the adhesion of corneocytes and by increasing the proliferation of the follicular epithelium.[58]

Tretinoin is usually applied as a 0.05% polyethylene glycol (PEG)-400/ethanol liquid or a 0.05% hydrophilic cream. Daily application results in inflammation, erythema, and peeling of the skin. After 3 to 4 weeks, pustular eruptions may be seen, causing the expulsion of microcomedones. Treatment may then be changed to applications every 2 or 3 days. Because the horny layer is thinned, the skin is more susceptible to irritation by chemical or physical abuse. Thus, it is recommended that other kerolytic agents (salicylic, sulfur, resorcinol, benzoyl peroxide) be discontinued before beginning treatment with tretinoin.

Sunscreens labeled SPF-15 or higher are recommended. Unlabeled uses of tretinoin include the treatment of some forms of skin cancer, lamellar ichthyosis, Darier's disease, and photoaging. Photoaging of the skin is mainly the result of excessive exposure to sunlight and is manifested by lax, yellow, mottled, wrinkled, leathery, rough skin. Once-daily application has been reported to aid in the early stages of photoaging.[59] Tretinoin is believed to exert this action by its function in regulating epithelial differentiation, cell division, and protein synthesis.[60] Termination of treatment, however, results in reversal within 1 year. Tretinoin is believed to exert its antineoplastic effect by promoting cellular differentiation toward normal cells.[61]

Isotretinoin, USP.

Isotretinoin, 13-*cis*-retinoic acid (Accutane), is a yellow-orange to orange, crystalline powder. It is insoluble in water and sparingly soluble in alcohol.

Isotretinoin

Isotretinoin is indicated for the treatment of severe recalcitrant cystic acne. Because of the risks of adverse effects, its use should be reserved for patients who are unresponsive to conventional acne therapies. Treatment should be individualized and modified depending on the course of the disease. The mechanism is believed to involve inhibition of sebaceous gland function and follicular keratinization. Isotretinoin reduces sebum production, the size of the glands, and gland differentiation.

The initial dose is 0.5 to 1 mg/kg daily in two divided doses. Absorption is rapid, but bioavailability is low (~25%) because of degradation in the lumen and metabolism by the gastrointestinal mucosa and the liver on the first pass. The chief metabolite is 4-oxoisotretinoin. Both isotretinoin and its metabolite are conjugated to the glucuronide and excreted in the urine and feces. The usual course of therapy is 15 to 20 weeks.

The adverse effects of isotretinoin are typical of chronic hypervitaminosis A. Because of the high potential to cause teratogenic effects, isotretinoin should be used with extreme caution in females of childbearing age. The manufacturer of the drug strongly recommends that patients have pregnancy tests performed before starting therapy and use a form of birth control during therapy.

Etretinate.

Etretinate (Tegison) is indicated for the treatment of severe recalcitrant psoriasis. Because of its potential adverse effects, therapy should be limited to diseases that do not respond to standard therapies. The exact mechanism of etretinate's action is unknown but is believed to result from some of the actions common to the retinoids.

Etretinate

Oral bioavailability of etretinate is approximately 40%. Milk and lipids increase the absorption. Etretinate is converted significantly to the free acid on the first pass through the liver. The free acid (acitretin) is also active. After a single dose, the half-life of etretinate is 6 to 13 hours, but after long-term therapy, the half-life is 120 days. Etretinate's high lipid character results in storage in adipose tissue, from which it is released slowly. After discontinuation of therapy, etretinate can be detected for up to 1 year.

Acitretin has the advantage of a shorter half-life, 2 hours after a single dose and 50 hours after multiple doses. It is, however, more susceptible to conversion to 13-*cis*-etretin. Thus, it appears that the ester provides metabolic stability.

The initial dosage of etretinate is 0.75 to 1 mg/kg in divided doses. After 8 to 16 weeks, a maintenance dosage of 0.5 to 0.75 mg/kg may be started. As with isotretinoin, extreme caution is needed in the administration of etretinate. The manufacturer discontinued this product in 1998.

Acitretin. Acitretin (Soriatane) is a yellow to greenish-yellow powder. It is the active species of etretinate. After absorption, acitretin is extensively metabolized and also undergoes isomerization to its 13-*cis* isomer. Acitretin is less lipid soluble than etretinate and thus is eliminated faster by the body. The elimination half-life is 50 hours.

Acitretin is indicated for the treatment of severe psoriasis. The initial dose is 25 to 50 mg in a single dose with food. Because of significant variation in pharmacokinetics and efficacy, however, the maintenance dose should be individualized. Initial response may occur in 2 weeks, but maximal response requires 2 to 3 months. Because of significant adverse effects associated with its use, acitretin should be reserved for patients who do not respond to other therapies or whose clinical condition contraindicates the use of other treatments.

Concurrent administration with ethanol is contraindicated because etretinate is formed. Because the half-life of etretinate is much longer, the teterogenic risk to women is significantly increased.[61]

Alitretinoin. Alitretinoin, 9-*cis*-retinoic acid (Panretin), is a yellow powder that is slightly soluble in ethanol and insoluble in water. Alitretinoin is a naturally occurring endogenous retinoid.

Alitretinoin is indicated for the treatment of cutaneous lesions in patients with AIDS-related Kaposi's sarcoma. It is not indicated when systemic anti–Kaposi's sarcoma therapy is required. It is not indicated as a systemic drug.

Alitretinoin is applied as a 0.1% gel. Initial application is twice daily but may be increased gradually to 4 times daily. Application, however, must be limited to the lesion. Application to normal skin and mucosal tissue should be avoided. The gel should be allowed to dry before dressing. Occlusive dressings should not be used.

Unlike its geometric isomer all *trans*-retinoid acid, which binds only RAR receptors, alitretinoin is a ligand for both RAR and RXR. It has been called a "pan-agonist," since it binds all retinoid receptors. Because of this ability it has been proposed that alitretinoin may be more potent and thus more effective than other retinoids.[62]

Adapalene. Adapalene (Differin) is a white to off-white powder that is soluble in tetrahydrofuran, sparingly soluble in ethanol, and practically insoluble in water. Adapalene is applied as a 0.1% solution or gel for the treatment of acne vulgaris. The eyes, lips, and mucous membranes should be avoided.

Adapalene is a naphthoic acid derivative, thus differing markedly from the endogenous retinoids. This results in different ability to bind the many retinoic acid–binding proteins. It binds with RARs but not RXRs or CRABPs.[63]

Bexarotene. Bexarotene (Targretin) is a white to off-white powder that is insoluble in water and slightly soluble in ethanol and vegetable oil. It is available in 75-mg soft capsules. Bexarotene has FDA approval for use in the treatment of cutaneous T-cell lymphoma (CTCL) refractory to at least one prior systemic therapy. The recommended initial dose is 300 mg/m^2 daily with a meal. Depending on toxicity, the dose may be adjusted up to 400 mg/m^2 or down by 100 mg/m^2 or be temporarily suspended.

Bexarotene binds selectively with retinoid X receptors.[64] Activation of the RXR pathway leads to apoptosis and other cellular activities mediated by proteins resulting from gene expression. The exact mechanism in the treatment of cutaneous T-cell lymphoma is not known.

Absorption of bexarotene is enhanced by fatty meals, thus the recommendation that it be taken with a meal. It is oxidized by P-450 isozyme 3A4 (CYP 3A4), but its interactions with CYP 3A4 inhibitors or inducers have not been studied. Because this drug is administered orally, it must not be given to pregnant women or those expecting to get pregnant.

Tazarotene. Tazarotene (Tazorac) is indicated for the treatment of stable plaque psoriasis. It is applied topically as a 0.05% or 0.1% emollient cream. It has been used on up to 20% of the skin. As with other topical retinoids, care must be taken to protect eye, mouth, and mucous membranes, and occlusive dressings should be avoided.

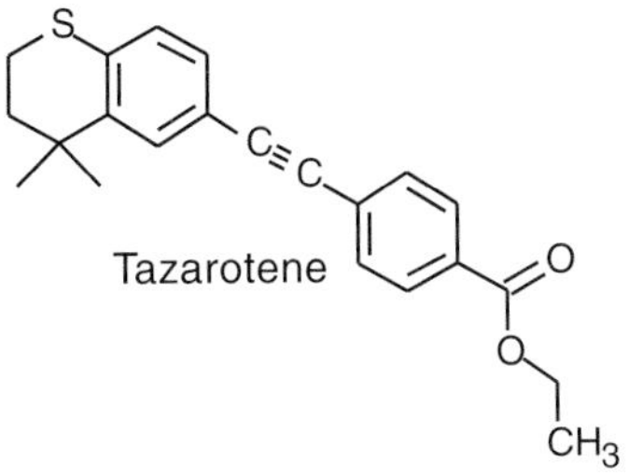

Tazarotene

Tazarotene is an acetylenic prodrug. On application, it is rapidly converted to the active form, tazarotenic acid.[65] Although tazarotenic acid can bind all three RARs, it shows selectivity for RARβ and RARγ. The latter is the primary receptor found in the epidermis.[66] Gene expression then normalizes keratinocyte differentiation, producing less inflammation and decreasing hyperproliferation.[67] Tazarotenic acid is retained in the skin for up to 3 months, and its therapeutic effect continues after cessation of therapy.[65]

β-Carotene, USP.

β-Carotene (Soletene) is a red or reddish-brown to violet-brown powder. It is insoluble in water and alcohol and sparingly soluble in vegetable oils. It is a naturally occurring carotenoid pigment found in green and yellow vegetables.

β-Carotene is indicated for the treatment of erythropoietic protoporphyria. It does not provide total protection against the sun, but patients who respond to its treatment can remain in the sun the same as normal individuals. Discontinuance of the drug results in a return of hypersensitivity. β-Carotene does not function as a sunscreen in normal patients and should not be used as such.

The dosage range is 30 to 300 mg/day in a single or divided dose, usually administered with food because its absorption depends on the presence of bile and absorbable fat.

Most β-carotene is converted to retinol during absorption, but the fraction that is absorbed is distributed widely and accumulates in the skin. The metabolic pathway of β-carotene is similar to that of retinol. Several weeks of therapy are required before enough accumulates in the skin to exert protective effects. Carotenodermia, a result of accumulation in the skin, is the major side effect. A "tanning" capsule containing β-carotene and canthaxanthin, however, uses this effect.

VITAMIN A₂

Vitamin A_2 is found in vertebrates that live or, at least, begin their lives in freshwater. Vitamin A_2 exhibits chemical, physical, and biological properties very similar to those of vitamin A. It has the structural formula depicted above (see page 869). Vitamin A_2 has a biological potency of 1.3 million USP U/g, which is approximately 40% of the activity of crystalline vitamin A acetate.

Vitamin Ds

The recognition in 1919 that rickets was the result of a nutritional deficiency led to the isolation of antirachitic compounds from food products.[68] The role of sunlight in the prevention of rickets was noted at the same time.[69] The term *vitamin D* was applied to all agents with antirachitic activity. Several compounds were isolated, designated D_1, D_2, or D_3. D_1 was the material obtained by irradiation of yeast ergosterol. This material later was found to be a 1:1 mixture of ergocalciferol and lumisterol. On purification and further characterization, ergocalciferol (calciferol) proved to possess the antirachitic properties and became known as *vitamin D_2*. Cholecalciferol was designated *vitamin D_3*.

In a classical sense, vitamin D_3, the form produced in animals, is not a true "vitamin" because it is produced in the skin from 7-dehydrocholesterol by UV radiation in the range of 290 to 300 nm.[70] 7-Dehydrocholesterol is produced from cholesterol metabolism. Only when exposure to sunlight is inadequate does vitamin D_3 become a vitamin in the historical sense. Further, vitamin D_3 is now termed a *provitamin* because it requires hydroxylation by the liver and the kidney to be fully active.

On UV irradiation, 7-dehydrocholesterol is converted rapidly to previtamin D_3. Previtamin D_3 undergoes slow thermal conversion to vitamin D_3 and the biologically inactive lumisterol₃ and tachysterol₃. Excess exposure increases production of the inactive compounds. The slow conversion of previtamin D_3 to vitamin D_3 ensures adequate supplies when the exposure is brief. Further, lumisterol and tachysterol can be converted back to previtamin D_3 and thus serve as a reservoir.[70] It has been estimated that a 10-minute exposure of just the uncovered hands and face will produce sufficient vitamin D_3.[71]

The mechanism responsible for the movement of vitamin D_3 from the skin to the blood is not known. In the blood, vitamin D_3 is bound primarily to an α protein known as vitamin D–binding protein (VDBP). This protein selectively removes vitamin D_3 from the skin because it has low affinity for 7-dehydrocholesterol, previtamin D_3, lumisterol, and tachysterol.

Cholecalciferol (vitamin D_3) does not perform its function directly. It must be transformed by the liver and the kidney. The first step occurs in the liver by the enzyme vitamin D_3 25-hydroxylase. This enzyme converts the provitamin to 25-hydroxyvitamin D_3 (25-OHD₃). This enzyme, which requires both molecular oxygen and reduced nicotinamide adenine dinucleotide phosphate (NADPH), appears to be a cytochrome P-450 monooxygenase and is found in the endoplasmic reticulum and the mitochondria.[72] The rate of this hydroxylation correlates with substrate concentration.[70] The 25-OHD₃ thus formed is the major circulating form of the vitamin bound to VDBP. The circulating levels of 25-OHD₃ are proportional to vitamin D intake. Thus plasma levels of 25-OHD₃ are used to indicate vitamin D status.[73]

The epithelial cells of the proximal convoluted tubules convert 25-OHD₃ to 1α,25-OHD₃ by the enzyme 25-OHD 1α-hydroxylase. The activity of this mitochondrial cytochrome P-450 enzyme is controlled by 1α,25-OHD₃ and parathyroid hormone as well as high concentrations of calcium and phosphate.[70]

Catabolism of vitamin D is initiated by the enzyme vitamin D 24-hydroxylase, whose expression is stimulated by 1α,25-OHD₃ itself. 24-Hydroxylation is followed by oxidation to the ketone. Subsequent hydroxylation at C-23 leads to cleavage of the side chain, resulting in the biologically inactive product calcitronic acid.[73, 74]

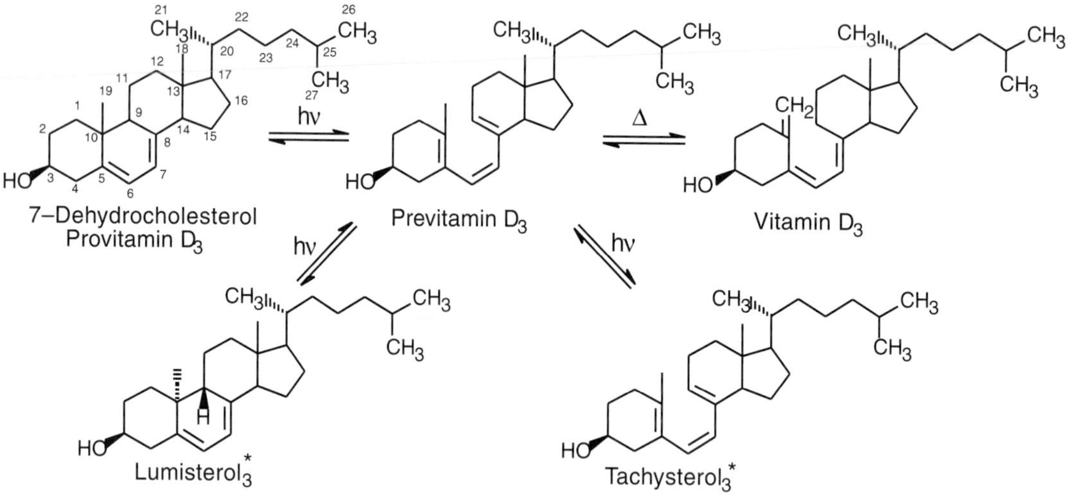

7–Dehydrocholesterol
Provitamin D$_3$

Previtamin D$_3$

Vitamin D$_3$

Lumisterol$_3$*

Tachysterol$_3$*

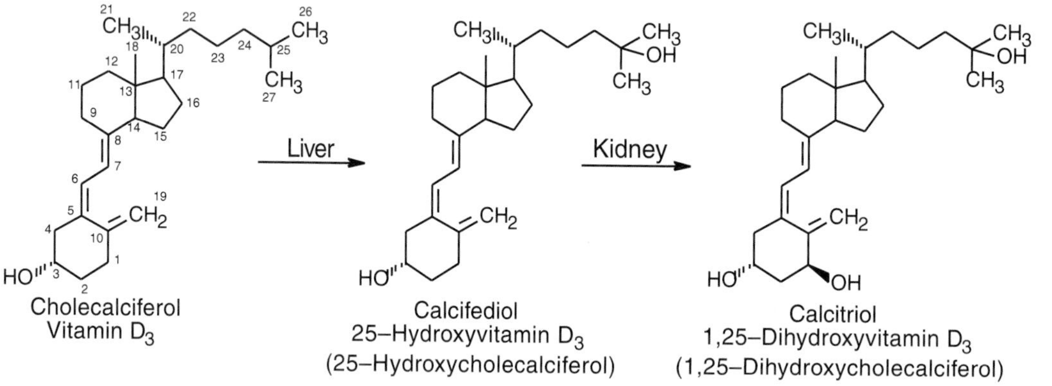

Cholecalciferol
Vitamin D$_3$

Calcifediol
25–Hydroxyvitamin D$_3$
(25–Hydroxycholecalciferol)

Calcitriol
1,25–Dihydroxyvitamin D$_3$
(1,25–Dihydroxycholecalciferol)

The need for calcium stimulates parathyroid hormone secretion. Parathyroid hormone, in turn, suppresses the 24-hydroxylase and stimulates the 1α-hydroxylase system. When phosphate availability is below normal, the 1α-hydroxylase is stimulated and the 24-hydroxylase is suppressed.

As with vitamin A, most of the effects of vitamin D involve a nuclear receptor. The vitamin D receptor is a member of the steroid/thyroid hormone superfamily of receptors. When 1α,25-OHD$_3$ binds to its receptor, the complex forms a heterodimer with an unoccupied RXR. This heterodimer subsequently binds to the regulatory regions on specific genes in target tissue. These regions are called *vitamin D response elements* (VDREs). The binding to VDREs can increase or decrease expression of genes.[70] The proteins thus made carry out the functions of vitamin D.

The physiological role of vitamin D is to maintain calcium homeostasis. Phosphate metabolism is also affected. Vitamin D accomplishes its role by enhancing the absorption of calcium and phosphate from the small intestines, promoting their mobilization from bone, and decreasing their excretion by the kidney. Also involved are parathyroid hormone and calcitonin.

1α,25-OHD$_3$ promotes Ca^{2+} intestinal absorption and increases Ca^{2+} renal reabsorption in the distal tubules and mobilization of Ca^{2+} from bone. The mechanism of action promoting Ca^{2+} transport in the intestine involves formation of a calcium-binding protein. 1α,25-OHD$_3$ promotes availability of this protein. A calcium-dependent ATPase, Na$^+$, and the calcium-binding protein are necessary for intestinal Ca^{2+} transport. 1α,25-OHD$_3$ also promotes intestinal phosphate absorption, mobilization of Ca^{2+} and phosphate from bone, and renal reabsorption of Ca^{2+} and phosphate. 1α,25-OHD$_3$ induces the synthesis of a Na–Pi cotransport.[75]

Vitamin D deficiency results in rickets in infants and children as a result of inadequate calcification of bones. In adults, osteomalacia most often occurs during pregnancy and lactation. Rickets is rare in the United States because of fortification of foods. Deficiencies in the elderly, however, result from underexposure to sunlight.

Hypervitaminosis D apparently cannot arise from excessive exposure to sunlight[76] but only occurs following ingestion of large quantities of synthetic vitamin D for months. The amount necessary has been estimated at 50,000 units or more in a person with normal parathyroid function.[77] The mechanism may involve formation of excessive amounts of the vitamin D metabolite 25-OHD. Toxicity involves derangements of calcium metabolism, resulting in hypercalcemia and metastatic calcification of soft tissue. Most problems result from the hypercalcemia, which typically causes muscular weakness, anorexia, nausea, vomiting, and depression of the central nervous system (which can result in coma and death). In addition, deposition of calcium salts in the kidneys (nephrocalcinosis) and the tubules (nephrolithiasis)

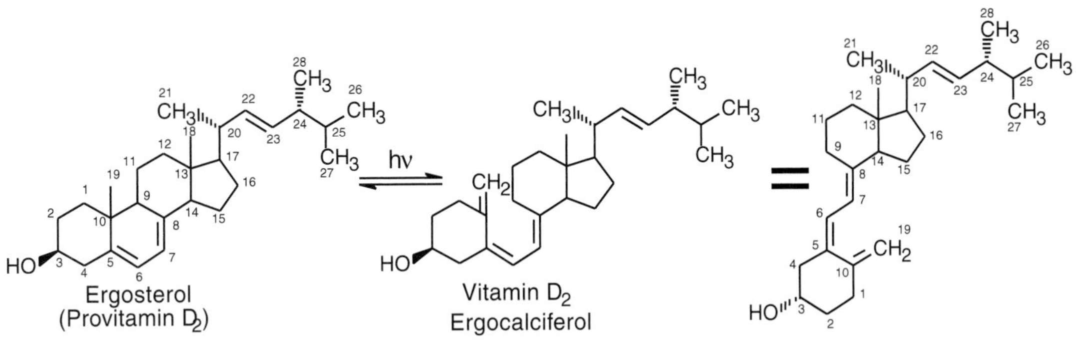

Ergosterol
(Provitamin D₂)

Vitamin D₂
Ergocalciferol

can lead to potentially irreversible renal damage. Early signs are polyuria and nocturia due to damage to the renal concentrating mechanism.

Ergosterol (precursor of D₂) occurs naturally in fungi and yeast. Eggs and butter contain vitamin D₂ (ergocalciferol) or D₃ (cholecalciferol). Milk and bread are fortified with vitamin D₂. Cholecalciferol is found in fish liver oils.

Ergocalciferol (vitamin D₂) is produced in plants from ergosterol on UV irradiation. Vitamin D₂ is the form most often used in commercial products and to fortify foods. Although different in structure, its biological activity is comparable to that of vitamin D₃ and must be bioactivated in a similar fashion.

The gastrointestinal absorption of the vitamin Ds requires bile. Vitamin D₃ may be absorbed better than vitamin D₂. The vitamin Ds enter the circulation through lymph chylomicrons. In the blood they are associated with vitamin D–binding protein (VDBP). The 25-hydroxylated compounds are the major circulating metabolites and may be stored in fats and muscle for prolonged periods. The 24-hydroxy metabolites are excreted primarily in the bile. Because the vitamin D metabolites are very lipophilic, protein binding helps in their transport in plasma. Protein binding also prolongs the circulatory half-lives by making them less susceptible to hepatic metabolism and biliary excretion.[78] Albumin and lipoproteins also bind vitamin D but with lower affinity than VDBP.

The vitamin Ds are important in the therapeutics of hypoparathyroidism and of vitamin D deficiency.[2] Ergocalciferol, cholecalciferol, and dihydrotachysterol are recognized by

the USP. Although dihydrotachysterol has relatively weak antirachitic activity, it is effective and faster acting in increasing serum Ca^{2+} concentrations in parathyroid deficiency. Dihydrotachysterol has a shorter duration of action; hence, it has less potential for toxicity from hypercalcemia.

Vitamin D receptors have been identified in tissue not normally associated with bone mineral homeostasis. Besides the intestines, kidneys, and osteoblasts, vitamin D receptors have been located in the parathyroid gland, the pancreatic islet cells, the mammary epithelium, and the skin keratinocytes. This has resulted in many investigational uses for vitamin D, including suppression of parathyroid hormone and treatment of colon and breast cancers and psoriasis.[70] These investigational treatments require high doses of vitamin D, and the resultant hypercalcemia and hypercalciuria limit the use of vitamin D natural metabolites. Vitamin D analogues with a decreased tendency to cause hypercalcemia and hypercalciuria are being developed and investigated. These analogues have low affinity for VDBP but retain high affinity for the vitamin D receptors.[70] The only approved use of a vitamin D analogue is in the treatment of psoriasis with calcipotriene.

PRODUCTS

Ergocalciferol, USP. One USP or IU of ergocalciferol, (3β,5Z,7E,22E)-9,10-secoergosta-5,7,10(19),22-tetraen-3-ol, vitamin D₂, calciferol, activated ergosterol, is 0.025 µg of vitamin D₃. Thus, 1 µg equals 40 USP units. Because ergocalciferol is the least expensive of the vitamin D analogues, it is preferred, unless the patient cannot activate it.

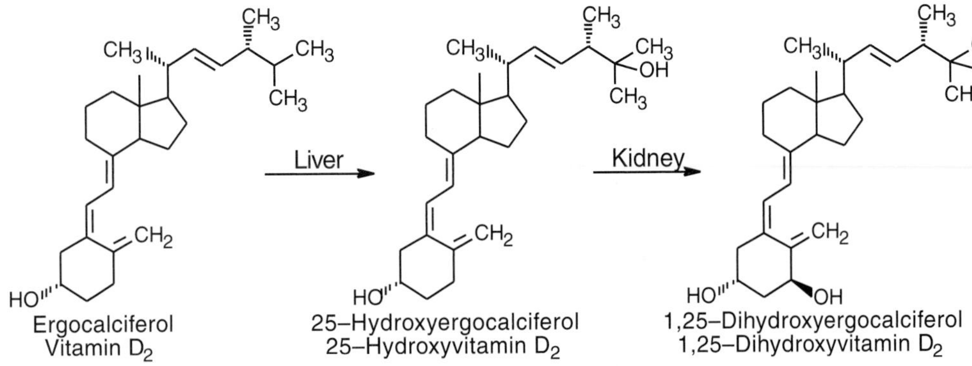

Ergocalciferol
Vitamin D₂

25–Hydroxyergocalciferol
25–Hydroxyvitamin D₂

1,25–Dihydroxyergocalciferol
1,25–Dihydroxyvitamin D₂

Ergocalciferol has a half-life of 24 hours (19 to 48 hours) and a duration of action of up to 6 months. After oral or intramuscular administration, the onset of action (hypercalcemia) is 10 to 24 hours, with maximal effects seen 4 weeks after daily administration.

After irradiation, the steroid undergoes fission of ring B; therefore, it is known as a secosteroid. This is indicated in the name by the "9,10-seco" portion. The "ergosta" portion indicates the presence of 28 atoms in the carbon skeleton.

The history and preparation of this vitamin are described above. Vitamin D_2 is a white, odorless crystalline compound that is soluble in fats and in the usual organic solvents, including alcohol. It is insoluble in water. Vitamin D_2 is oxidized slowly in oils by oxygen from the air, probably through the fat peroxides that are formed. Vitamin A is much less stable under the same conditions.

Cholecalciferol, USP.

Cholecalciferol, (3β,5Z,7E)-9,10-secocholesta-5,7,10(19)-trien-3-ol, vitamin D_3, activated 7-dehydrocholesterol, occurs as white odorless crystals that are soluble in fatty oils, alcohol, and many organic solvents. It is insoluble in water. Vitamin D_3 also occurs in tuna and halibut liver oils. It has the same activity as vitamin D_2 in rats but is more effective in the chick; both vitamins, however, have equal activity in humans. Vitamin D_3 exhibits stability comparable to that of vitamin D_2.

Epimerization of the hydroxyl at C-3 in vitamin D_2 or D_3 or conversion of the hydroxyl at C-3 to a ketone group greatly diminishes the activity but does not completely destroy it. Ethers and esters that cannot be cleaved in the body have no vitamin D activity. Inversion of the hydrogen at C-9 in ergosterol and other 7-dehydrosterols prevents the normal course of irradiation.

Dihydrotachysterol, USP.

Tachysterol (represented below) is a by-product of ergosterol irradiation. Reduction of tachysterol led to dihydrotachysterol, (3β,5E,7E,10α,22E)-9,10-ergosta-5,7,22-trien-3ol, dihydrotachysterol$_2$, dichysterol, DHT.

Dihydrotachysterol occurs as colorless or white crystals or a white, crystalline odorless powder. It is soluble in alcohol, freely soluble in chloroform, sparingly soluble in vegetable oils, and practically insoluble in water.

Dihydrotachysterol has slight antirachitic activity. It increases the calcium concentration in the blood, an effect for which tachysterol is only one tenth as active. In high doses, dihydrotachysterol is more effective than the other analogues in mobilizing calcium. Thus, it is used in hypoparathyroidism.

After oral administration, the onset of action is seen within hours. This fast onset of action is an advantage of this drug. Maximal activity is seen in 2 weeks after daily administration. Its duration of action is 2 weeks.

Dihydrotachysterol is activated by hepatic enzymes to its 25-hydroxylated metabolite. It does not require renal activation, for the hydroxy on ring A occupies the same position as that of the 1-hydroxyl in the activated forms of the vitamin Ds. 25-Hydroxydihydrotachysterol$_3$ has weak antirachitic activity, but it is a more important bone-mobilizing agent and is more effective than dihydrotachysterol$_3$. Also, it is more effective in increasing intestinal calcium transport and bone mobilization in thyroparathyroidectomized rats. Its activity suggests that it may be the drug of choice in the treatment of hypoparathyroidism and similar bone diseases.[79]

Calcifediol, USP.

Calcifediol, (3β,5Z,7E)-9,10-secocholesta-5,7,10(19)-trien-3,25-diol, 25-hydroxycholecalciferol, 25-hydroxyvitamin D_3, occurs as a white powder. It is practically insoluble in water and sensitive to light and heat. The half-life of calcifediol is 16 days (10 to 22 days). Its onset of action occurs within 2 to 6 hours, and its duration of action is 15 to 20 days.

Calcifediol is indicated for patients receiving long-term renal dialysis.

Calcitriol.

Calcitriol, (1α,3β,5Z,7E)-9,10-secocholesta-5,7,10(19)-trien-1,3,25-triol, 1,25-dihydroxycholecalciferol, 1,25-dihydroxyvitamin D_3, occurs as colorless crystals that are insoluble in water. Because calcitriol does not require activation, increased calcium absorption is seen within 2 hours of administration. Its half-life is 3 to 8 hours, and its duration of action is 1 to 2 days.

Calcitriol is the most active form of vitamin D_3. It is indicated in patients who are receiving long-term renal dialysis or who cannot properly metabolize ergocalciferol.

Calcipotriene.

Calcipotriene, (1α,3β,5Z,7E,22E,24S)-24-cyclopropyl-9,10-secochola-5,7,10(19),22-tetraene-1,3,24-triol, calcipotriol (Dovonex), is a synthetic vitamin D_3 analogue indicated for topical application in the treatment of moderate plaque psoriasis. It has the same affinity for the vitamin D receptor as calcitriol, but its effect on calcium metabolism is 100 to 200 times less. Calcipotriene inhibits epidermal cell proliferation and enhances cell differentia-

Tachysterol$_2$ $\longrightarrow$ Dihydrotachysterol $\xrightarrow{\text{Liver}}$ 25–Hydroxydihydrotachysterol

tion. It reduces cell numbers and total DNA content.[80] Antiproliferative effects are caused by a reduction in the mRNA levels of a cellular oncogene associated with proliferation, c-*myc*. The mechanism resulting in differentiation changes is not completely known but involves the secondary messengers inositol triphosphate (IP_3) and diacylglycerol (DAG).[70]

Calcipotriene

Doxercalciferol. Doxercalciferol, ($1\alpha,3\beta,5Z,7E,22E$)-9, 10-secoergosta-5,7,10(19),22-tetraene-1,3-diol, 1α-hydroxyergocalciferol, 1α-hydroxyvitamin D_3 (Hectorol), is a colorless crystalline compound soluble in oils and organic solvents but relatively insoluble in water. Doxercalciferol is indicated for the reduction of elevated intact parathyroid hormone (iPTH) in the management of secondary hyperparathyroidism in patients undergoing chronic renal dialysis.

Doxercalciferol

Following gastrointestinal absorption after oral administration, doxercalciferol is activated in the liver to $1\alpha,25(OH)_2D_2$. The activation does not require involvement of the kidney. Being a prodrug, doxercalciferol does not stimulate the absorption of dietary calcium and phosphorus.[81] The mean half-life in healthy volunteers is approximately 32 to 37 hours, which is similar to the half-life in patients with end-stage renal disease.[82]

The dose must be individualized for each patient. The goal is to lower blood iPTH into the 150 to 300 pg/mL range. The recommended initial dose is 10 μg 3 times weekly, administered at dialysis. If the iPTH levels are not lowered by 50% and fail to reach the indicated range, the dose may be increased by 2.5 μg every 8 weeks. The maximal recommended dose is 60 μg/week.

Paricalcitol. Paricalcitol, ($1\alpha,3\beta,5Z,7E,22E$)-19-nor-9,10-secoergosta-5,7,22-triene-1,3,25-triol (Zemplar), is a white powder. Paricalcitol is indicated for the prevention and treatment of secondary hyperparathyroidism in patients undergoing chronic renal dialysis. It has a lower incidence of hypercalcemia and hyperphosphatemia than calcitriol.[83]

Paricalcitol

Paricalcitol is a calcitriol analogue intended for intravenous use. The recommended initial dose is 0.04 to 0.1 μg/kg as a bolus dose during dialysis. The dose may be given no more often than every other day. The goal of therapy is to lower iPTH levels to no more than 1.5 to 3 times the nonuremic upper normal limit. The dose may be increased by 2 to 4 μg at 2- to 4-week intervals.

Vitamin E

Since the early 1920s, it has been known that rats fed only cow's milk cannot produce offspring. The principle from wheat germ that can rectify this deficiency in both male and female rats was named *vitamin E*. When the compound known as vitamin E was isolated in 1936, it was named *tocopherol*. Since then, several other closely related compounds have been discovered from natural sources, and this family of natural products took the generic name *tocopherols*.

The tocopherols are especially abundant in wheat germ, rice germ, corn germ, other seed germs, lettuce, soya, and cottonseed oil. All green plants contain some tocopherols, and there is evidence that some green leafy vegetables and rose hips contain more than wheat germ. It is probably synthesized by leaves and translocated to the seeds. All four tocopherols have been found in wheat germ oil; α-, β-, and γ-tocopherols have been found in cottonseed oil. Corn oil contains predominantly γ-tocopherol and thus furnishes a convenient source for the isolation of this difficult member of the tocopherols to prepare. δ-Tocopherol is 30% of the mixed tocopherols of soya bean oil.

Several tocopherols have been isolated. Some have the 4',8',12'-trimethyltridecyl-saturated side chain; others have unsaturation in the side chain. It has been suggested that these polyunsaturated tocols be named "tocotrienols." The best known is α-tocopherol (vitamin E), which has the greatest biological activity. The base structure, represented below, shows that the tocopherols are methyl-substituted tocol derivatives: α-tocopherol is 5,7,8-trimethyltocol; β-tocopherol is 5,8-dimethyltocol; the γ-compound is 7,8-dimethyltocol; and δ-tocopherol is 8-methyltocol. The tocotrienols have similar substituents. Natural α-(+)-tocopherol has the configuration 2R,4'R,8'R. The natural tocotrienols have a 2R,3'E,7'E configuration. The tocopherols are diterpenoid natural products biosynthesized from a combination of four isoprenoid units; geranylgeranyl pyrophosphate is the key intermediate that leads to these compounds.[84]

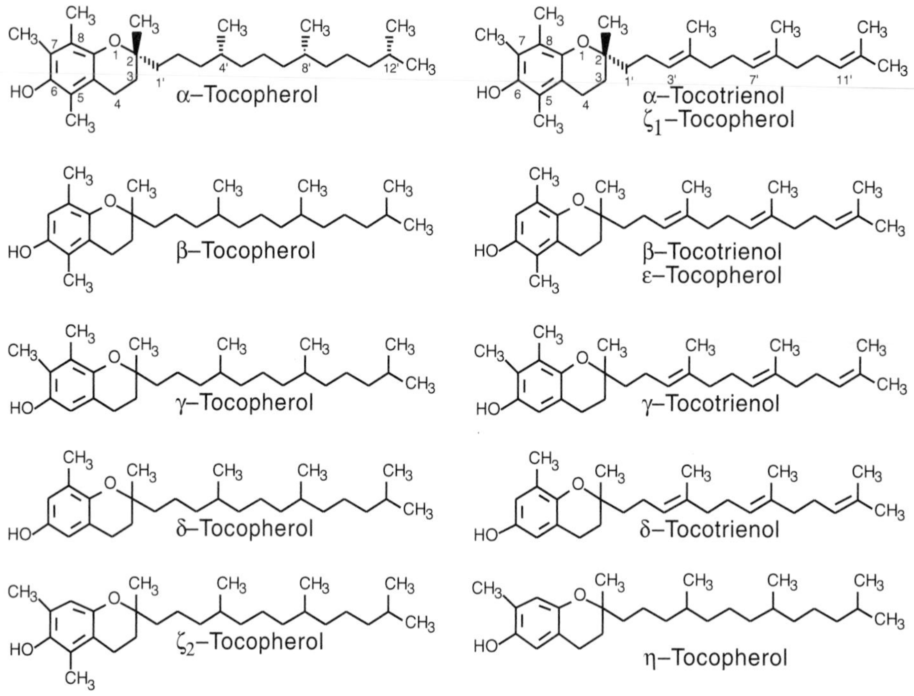

α–Tocopherol

α–Tocotrienol
ζ₁–Tocopherol

β–Tocopherol

β–Tocotrienol
ε–Tocopherol

γ–Tocopherol

γ–Tocotrienol

δ–Tocopherol

δ–Tocotrienol

ζ₂–Tocopherol

η–Tocopherol

The tocopherols and their acetates are light yellow, viscous, odorless oils that have an insipid taste. They are insoluble in water and soluble in alcohol, organic solvents, and fixed oils. The acid succinate esters are white powders insoluble in water and soluble in ethanol and vegetable oils. Tocopherols are stable in air for reasonable periods but are oxidized slowly by air. They are oxidized readily by ferric salts, mild oxidizing agents, and air in the presence of alkali. They are inactivated rapidly by exposure to UV light; not all samples behave alike in this respect, however, because traces of impurities apparently greatly affect the rate of oxidation. Tocopherols have antioxidant properties for fixed oils in the following decreasing order of effectiveness: δ, γ, β, and α.[85] In the process of acting as antioxidants, tocopherols are destroyed by the accumulating fat peroxides that they decompose. They are added to Light Mineral Oil NF and Mineral Oil USP because of their antioxidant property. Tocopherols can be converted to acetates and benzoates, which are oils as active as the parent compounds but more stable toward oxidation.

(+)-α-Tocopherol is about 1.36 times as effective as (±)-α-tocopherol in rat antisterility bioassays. β-Tocopherol is about half as active as α-tocopherol, and the γ- and δ-tocopherols are only 1/100 times as active as α-tocopherol. The esters of tocopherol (e.g., acetate, propionate, and butyrate) are more active than the parent compound.[86] This is also true of the phosphoric acid ester of (±)-δ-tocopherol when it is administered parenterally.[87] The ethers of the tocopherols are inactive. Oxidation of the tocopherols to their corresponding quinones also leads to inactive compounds. Replacement of the methyl groups by ethyl groups decreases activity. The introduction of a double bond in the 3,4 position of α-tocopherol reduces its activity by about two thirds. Reduction of the size of the long alkyl side chain or the introduction of double bonds in this side chain markedly reduces activity. Vitamin E activity currently is expressed in terms

of the α-(+)-tocopherol equivalents based on the former USP units and mass listed in Table 26-6. One former USP unit is equal to one former IU. Vitamin E, USP, may consist of (+)- or (±)-α-tocopherols or their acetates or succinates, 96.0 to 102.0% pure.

(−)-α-Tocopherol is absorbed from the gut more rapidly than the (+)-form; absorption of the mixture of (+)- and (−)-α-tocopherol, however, was considerably higher (about 55%) than that expected from the data obtained after administration of the single compounds. As doses increase, the fraction absorbed decreases. No marked differences were noted in the distribution in various tissues and the metabolic degradation of (+)- and (−)-α-tocopherols.[88] The liver is

TABLE 26-6 Relative Potencies of Various Commercial Forms of Vitamin E

Form of Vitamin E	Potency
Potency (in former USP units) of 1 mg	
(±)-α-Tocopherol	1.1
(±)-α-Tocopherol acetate	1.0
(±)-α-Tocopherol acid succinate	0.89
(+)-α-Tocopherol	1.49
(+)-α-Tocopherol acetate	1.36
(+)-α-Tocopherol acid succinate	1.21
Potency (in terms of (+)-tocopherol equivalents) of 1 mg	
(+)-α-Tocopherol acetate	0.91
(+)-α-Tocopherol acid succinate	0.81
(±)-α-Tocopherol	0.74
(±)-α-Tocopherol acetate	0.67
(±)-α-Tocopherol acid succinate	0.60

an important storage site. Most of the gastrointestinal absorption of vitamin E occurs through the mucosa and the lymphatic system. Bile performs an important function in promoting tocopherol absorption. The ester derivatives are hydrolyzed by pancreatic enzymes before absorption. Although hydrolysis of the ester is not required, it does improve absorption. Vitamin E preparations are absorbed better from aqueous solutions than from oily solutions. α-Tocopherol and γ-tocopherol are absorbed from the intestines and distributed to the liver equally well. γ-Tocopherol is secreted primarily into the bile, however, while α-tocopherol enters the circulation, where it is found in much higher levels than γ-tocopherol, even though the latter predominates in the diet. This difference is attributed to a liver cytosolic binding protein that is selective for α-tocopherol.

The tocopherols in lymph are associated with chylomicrons and very-low-density lipoproteins (VLDLs). Circulating tocopherols are also associated mainly with the blood low-density lipoproteins (LDLs). The tocopherols are readily and reversibly bound to most tissues, including adipose tissue, and the vitamin is thus stored. The vitamin is concentrated in membrane structures, such as mitochondria, endoplasmic reticulum, and nuclear and plasma membranes.

Vitamin E is metabolized primarily to tocopheronic acid and its γ-lactone, followed by glucuronide conjugation. The terminal methyl group is oxidized to a carboxylic acid and shortened by β-oxidation to produce tocopheronic acid. The chroman ring is hydrolyzed to a quinone, which subsequently is reduced to a hydroquinone. Nucleophilic attack by a hydroxyl on the carbonyl side chain produces tocopheronolactone. These metabolites are excreted in the bile. Vitamin E may undergo some enterohepatic circulation.

Tocopheronic acid

Tocopheronolactone

For decades, there has been significant interest in investigating the biochemical functions of vitamin E, but it is still difficult to explain many of the biochemical derangements caused by vitamin E deficiency in animals. There seems to be general agreement that one of the primary metabolic functions of the vitamin is preventing the oxidation of lipids, particularly unsaturated fatty acids. This antioxidant function does not, however, explain all of the biochemical abnormalities caused by vitamin E deficiency. Moreover, vitamin E is not the only in vivo antioxidant. Two enzyme systems, glutathione reductase and *o*-phenylenediamine peroxidase, also function in this capacity.[89]

It has been postulated that vitamin E has a role in the regulation of protein synthesis. Other actions of this vitamin have also been investigated, for example, effects on muscle creatine kinase and liver xanthine oxidase. Vitamin E deficiency leads to an increase in the turnover of creatine kinase. Vitamin E–deficient animals also exhibit increased liver xanthine oxidase activity, which is due to increased de novo synthesis.[89]

Although it has been difficult to establish clinical correlates of vitamin E deficiency in humans, Bieri and Farrell[89] have summarized some useful generalizations and conclusions. These workers noted that the infant, especially the premature infant, is susceptible to tocopherol deficiency because of ineffective transfer of the vitamin from placenta to fetus and that growth in infants requires greater availability of the vitamin. In adults, the tocopherol storage depots provide adequate availability that is not readily depleted, but intestinal malabsorption syndromes, when persistent, can lead to depletion of the storage depots. Children with cystic fibrosis suffer from severe vitamin E deficiency caused by malabsorption. Tropical sprue, celiac disease, gastrointestinal resections, hepatic cirrhosis, biliary obstruction, and excessive ingestion of mineral oil may also cause long-term malabsorption.

Vitamin E therapeutic indications include the clinical conditions characterized by low serum tocopherol levels and increased fragility of red blood cells to hydrogen peroxide or conditions that require additional amounts. The latter can be exemplified by individuals who consume excessive amounts of polyunsaturated fatty acids (more than 20 g/day over normal diet).[90]

It has been claimed that vitamin E could be of therapeutic benefit in ischemic heart disease, but evidence against this claim continues to accumulate. It has also been suggested that megadoses of tocopherol be used in the treatment of peripheral vascular disease with intermittent claudication. Although some studies support this proposal, experts in the field state that further clinical studies are necessary to make a definitive recommendation. Nevertheless, it continues to be popular and controversial to consider the beneficial effects of vitamin E and other vitamins in large (mega) dietary supplements, and investigations of megavitamin E therapy for cardiovascular disease continue to appear in the literature.[89]

The eminent vitamin biochemist R. J. Williams has emphasized that

> [l]ipid peroxidation, the formation of harmful peroxides, from the interaction between oxygen and highly unsaturated fats (polyunsaturates) needs to be controlled in the body. Both oxygen and the polyunsaturated lipids are essential to our existence, but if the protection against peroxidation is inadequate, serious damage to various body proteins may result. Vitamin E is thought to be the leading agent for the prevention of peroxidation and the free radical production that is associated both with it and with radiation.[91–93]

Williams also noted that although exact mechanisms of action of these antioxidants are not yet known,

> [p]roviding plenty of vitamin E and ascorbic acid (both harmless antioxidants) is indicated as a possible means of preventing premature aging, especially if one's diet is rich in polyunsaturated acids.

Considering the foregoing implication of unnecessary peroxidation of unsaturated lipids, it is interesting that atherosclerosis appears to be due to a deficiency of prostacyclin, which is caused by inhibition of prostacyclin synthetase by lipid peroxides or by free radicals that are likely to be generated during hyperlipidemia. Although no direct evidence indicates that in experimental or human atherosclerosis, lipid peroxidation is the earliest sign of the disease state, lipid peroxides have been found in arteries from atherosclerotic patients and in ceroid atheromatic plaques, and at the same time, hardly any prostacyclin is generated in human atheromatic plaques.[94]

Vitamin E used in high doses, as high as 3,200 mg/day, has a proven record of safety.[32] A variety of reports, many single case reports or uncontrolled studies, have suggested adverse effects such as interference with clotting, weakness, decreased thyroid hormone levels, and gastrointestinal upset. The importance of these is unknown. The only notable adverse effects have occurred in premature infants given large doses of this vitamin. Hepatotoxicities have been seen in premature infants of less than 1,500 g birth weight given vitamin E intravenously, and the incidence of necrotizing enterocolitis and sepsis increased under similar conditions following oral or intravenous dosing.

Vitamin Ks

Lipid-free diet research by Henrik Dam starting in 1929 resulted in the discovery of an antihemorrhagic factor that was named *vitamin K* (from the German word *Koagulation*). Along with the work of Edward A. Doisy, the structure of vitamin K was determined in 1931 as shown below. For their work, Dam and Doisy shared the 1943 Nobel Prize in medicine. The term *vitamin K* was applied to the vitamin isolated from alfalfa, and a similar principle from fish meal was named *vitamin K₂*. *Vitamin K₂* refers to a series of compounds called the *menaquinones*. These have a longer side chain with more unsaturation. This side chain may be composed of 1 to 13 isoprenyl units. The most common are depicted below.

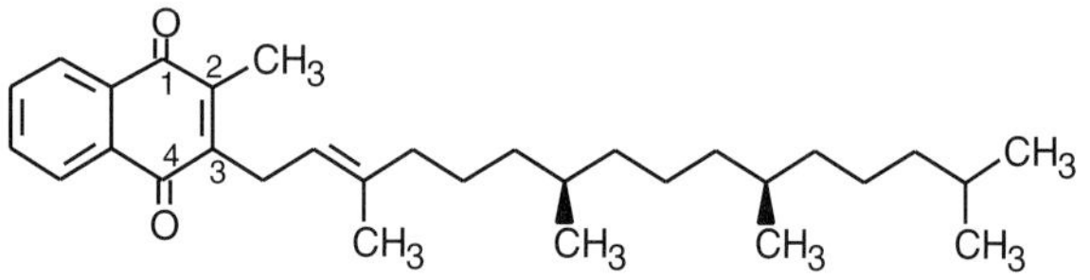

Vitamin K$_1$
Phytonadione
(2–Methyl–3–phytyl–1,4–naphthoquinone)

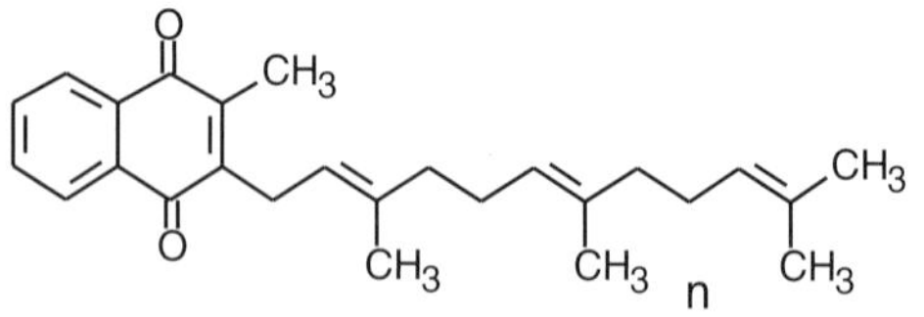

n = 4 = Vitamin K$_{2(30)}$ Menaquinone–6
n = 5 = Vitamin K$_{2(35)}$ Menaquinone–7

Many other closely related compounds possess vitamin K activity (e.g., menadione [2-methyl-1,4-naphthoquinone] is as active as vitamin K on a molar basis). The synthetic compounds menadione and menadiol are referred to as *vitamins K₃* and *K₄*, respectively. Vitamin K is a naphthoquinone derivative containing diterpenoid units biosynthesized by the intermediate geranylpyrophosphate.[95]

TABLE 26-7 Vitamin K Content of Selected Foods

Food	µg/100 g
Broccoli	200
Brussels sprouts	220
Cabbage, Chinese	175
Cabbage, red	50
Cabbage, white	80
Green onions	60
Kale	750
Lettuce	120
Parsley	700
Spinach	350
Turnip greens	300
Watercress	200

Animals depend on two sources for their intake of this vitamin, dietary and bacterial synthesis. Table 26-7 lists excellent sources of vitamin K$_1$.

Natural K$_1$ occurs as a *trans* isomer and has an *R,R,E* configuration. The synthetic, commercially available form is a mixture of *cis* and *trans* isomers, with no more than 20% *cis*. Vitamin K$_2$ is synthesized by the intestinal flora, especially by Gram-positive bacteria. It is not available commercially.

Numerous compounds have been tested for their antihemorrhagic activity, and significant biological activity is manifested in compounds with the following structure

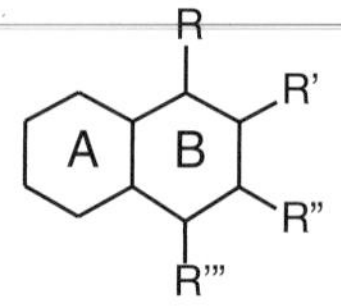

when

1. Ring A is aromatic or hydroaromatic.
2. Ring A is not substituted.
3. Ring B is aromatic or hydroaromatic.
4. R is OH, CO, OR, OAc (the R in OR is methyl or ethyl).
5. R′ is methyl.
6. R″ is H, sulfonic acid, dimethylamino, or an alkyl group containing 10 or more carbon atoms. A double bond in the β,γ position of this alkyl group enhances potency; if the double bond is further removed, it exerts no effect. Isoprenoid groups are more effective than straight chains. In the vitamin K$_{2(30)}$-type compounds, the 6′,7′-mono-*cis*- isomer is significantly less active than the all-*trans*- or the 18′,19′-mono-*cis*- isomer. This was also true of the vitamin K$_{2(30)}$-isoprenologue. A vitamin K$_{2(25)}$ isoprenologue was 20% more active than vitamin K$_{1(37)}$.
7. R‴ is H, OH, NH$_2$, CO, OR, Ac (the R in OR is methyl or ethyl).

Decreased antihemorrhagic activity is obtained when

1. Ring A is substituted.
2. R′ is an alkyl group larger than a methyl.
3. R″ is a hydroxyl group.
4. R″ contains a hydroxyl group in a side chain.

If ring A is benzenoid, the introduction of sulfur in place of a —CH=CH— in this ring in 2-methylnaphthoquinone permits the retention of some antihemorrhagic activity. This might indicate that in the process of exerting vitamin K activity, the benzenoid end of the molecule must fit into a pocket carefully tailored to it. That the other end is not so closely surrounded is shown by the retention of activity on changing the alkyl group in the 2 position.

Although marked antihemorrhagic activity is found in many naphthoquinone compounds, these compounds may be converted in the body to a vitamin K_1-type compound. The esters of the hydroquinones may be hydrolyzed, and the resulting hydroquinone may be oxidized to the quinone. The methyl tetralones, which are very active, could be dehydrogenated to the methylnaphthols, which are hydroxylated, and the latter product converted to the biologically equivalent quinone. Compounds with a dihydrobenzenoid ring (e.g., 5,8-dihydrovitamin K_1) appear to be moderately easily dehydrogenated, whereas the corresponding tetrahydrides are resistant to such change.

Vitamins K_1 and K_2 are absorbed by an active process in the proximal small intestines. Bile of normal composition is necessary to facilitate the absorption. The bile component principally concerned in the absorption and transport of fat-soluble vitamin K from the digestive tract is thought to be deoxycholic acid. The molecular compound of vitamin K with deoxycholic acid was effective on oral administration to rats with biliary fistula. Vitamin K is absorbed through the lymph in chylomicrons. It is transported to the liver, where it is concentrated, but no significant storage occurs.

The entire metabolic pathway of vitamin K has not been elucidated. The major urinary metabolites, however, are glucuronide conjugates of carboxylic acids derived from shortening of the side chain. High fecal concentrations are probably due to bacterial synthesis.

The accepted mechanism for vitamin K is to function as a cofactor in the posttranslational synthesis of γ-carboxyl–glutamic acid (Gla) from glutamic acid residues.[96] The discovery of Gla in 1974[97, 98] clarified the mechanism of vitamin K and led to the identification of additional vitamin K–dependent proteins. The only known function of vitamin K in mammals is to maintain adequate levels of vitamin K–dependent proteins involved in coagulation. These include prothrombin (factor II), factor VII (proconvertin), factor IX (autoprothrombin II), factor X (Stuart-Prower factor), and proteins C, S, and Z. Prothrombin and factors VII, IX, and X promote coagulation, while proteins C and S have anticoagulant activity. The function of protein Z is not known.

It follows that any condition that does not permit full use of the antihemorrhagic agents or the production of prothrombin would lead to increased clotting time or hemorrhagic disorders. Some of these conditions are *(a)* faulty absorption caused by several disorders (e.g., obstructive jaundice, biliary fistulas, intestinal polyposis, chronic ulcerative colitis, intestinal fistula, intestinal obstruction, and sprue); *(b)* damaged livers or primary hepatic diseases (e.g., atrophy, cirrhosis, or chronic hepatitis); *(c)* insufficient amounts of bile or abnormal bile in the intestinal tract; and *(d)* insufficient amounts of vitamin K.

Prothrombin and factors VII, IX, and X participate in the cascade of reactions leading to fibrin clot formation. Protein C exerts its anticoagulant effect by inactivating activated factors V_a and VIII_a.[99] Protein C is first activated by prothrombin. This activation requires a cell surface receptor, thrombomodulin, calcium, and protein S. Protein C also increases fibrinolysis by inactivating the major inhibitor of tissue plasminogen activator.[100] Protein S functions as a cofactor in the protein C inactivation of activated factor V_a and VIII_a. Protein S is found in the plasma and is bound to C4b-binding protein, an inhibitor in the complement system.[101] Protein S is also a cofactor in protein C fibrinolysis.

All of these proteins are synthesized in the liver, and they have considerable structural homology. All contain 10 to 12 Gla residues.[102, 103] The coagulation activity is proportional to the number of Gla residues present. For example, prothrombin has 10 Gla residues. Loss of just two residues decreases activity by 80%.[103]

This system requires reduced vitamin K (a hydroquinone, KH_2), carbon dioxide, and molecular oxygen. Although the reaction does not require ATP, it uses the energy from the oxidation of KH_2 to execute the carboxylation of glutamic acid.[104] The carboxylase must create a carbanion by extracting a proton from the glutamate γ-carbon. This requires a base with a pK_a of 26 to 28. The anion of the hydroquinone, however, has a pK_a of only about 9.

A proposed mechanism for the above carboxylation creates such a base from vitamin K.[105, 106] Vitamin K is reduced to its hydroquinone form (vitamin KH_2). Molecular oxygen is incorporated into the conjugate acid form of vitamin KH_2 to form a peroxy anion, which subsequently forms a dioxetane intermediate. The peroxy bond is cleaved by the adjacent enolate anion to produce an intermediate sufficiently basic to deprotonate the α-carbon.

Extraction of the proton allows the carboxylase to carboxylate the glutamate residue. The vitamin K intermediate is converted to vitamin K oxide, which must be reduced back to vitamin K. Vitamin K oxide is recycled back to vitamin K by vitamin K epoxide reductase and vitamin K quinone reductase. Both of these enzymes are dithiol dependent and are inhibited by the 4-hydroxycoumarin anticoagulants.

All vitamin K–dependent proteins contain Gla residues. Vitamin K thus participates in the formation of specific γ-carboxylglutamic acid Ca^{+2}-binding sites on the vitamin K–dependent proteins. Further, the Gla residues are found in essentially the same region, near the amino terminus, and this region is called the *Gla domain*.[107] These Gla residues function as ion bridges linking the blood-clotting protein to phospholipids on endothelial cells and platelets.[108] The vitamin K–dependent carboxylase system is located on the endoplasmic reticulum.[109] Binding to membrane surfaces is critical in the activation of these proteins.[108]

The discovery of Gla not only clarified the biochemical mechanism of vitamin K but also resulted in the isolation of several nonhepatic vitamin K–dependent proteins: osteocalcin, matrix Gla protein, Gas6, PRGP 1 and PRGP 2. Osteocalcin is synthesized in the osteoplast and odontoblasts. Its expression is regulated by 1α,25-dihydroxyvitamin D[109] and retinoic acid.[110] Studies on osteocalcin-deficient mice indicate that osteocalcin is a negative regulator of bone formation via an unknown mechanism but does not alter bone resorption or mineralization.[111] Matrix Gla protein is found in bone, cartilage, and soft tissue. Its synthesis is regulated by 1α,25-dihydroxyvitamin D_3 and retinoic acid, and it inhibits soft tissue calcification.[112] Gas6 is encoded by growth arrest–specific gene 6, and it contains 10 to 11 Gla residues.[113] It is involved in cell proliferation regulation through an unknown mechanism. The physiological roles of three other Gla-containing proteins remain unknown. Nephrocalcin has been isolated from renal tissue,[114] while plaque Gla protein has been isolated from atherosclerotic plaque.[115] The latest Gla-containing proteins have wide tissue distribution and are rich in proline residues; thus they have been named proline-rich Gla proteins (PRGP 1 and PRGP 2).[116]

Phytonadione is considered relatively nontoxic even at high doses. Rare cases of hemolytic anemia have been reported, and the manufacturer has reported anaphylactic reactions following use of the injectable product. Menadione, in contrast, can produce hemolytic anemia, hyperbilirubinemia, and kernicterus in newborns, especially premature infants. In addition, menadione can cause hemolytic anemia in patients with glucose-6-phosphate dehydrogenase deficiency.[117–119]

PRODUCTS

Phytonadione, USP. Phytonadione, 2-methyl-3-phytyl-1,4-naphthoquinone, vitamin K_1 (Mephyton, Aqua-MEPHYTON), is a clear, yellow, very viscous, odorless or nearly odorless liquid. Pure vitamin K_1 is a yellow crystalline solid that melts at 69°C. It is insoluble in water, slightly soluble in alcohol, and soluble in vegetable oils and in the usual fat solvents. It is unstable toward light, oxidation, strong acids, and halogens. It can be reduced easily to the corresponding hydroquinone, which in turn can be esterified.

The therapeutic use of vitamin K as a systemic hemostatic agent is based on the critical function that the vitamin performs in blood coagulation. Vitamin K_1 (phytonadione) is effective both in the treatment of hypoprothrombinemia caused by dietary deficiency of the vitamin or malabsorption and in the bleeding caused by oral anticoagulants (e.g., coumadin derivatives). Phytonadione exerts prompt and prolonged action. It can be administered orally, subcutaneously, or intramuscularly; in emergencies it can be given by slow intravenous injection.

Vitamin K is administered in conjunction with bile salts or their derivatives in preoperative and postoperative jaundiced patients to bring about and maintain a normal prothrombin level in the blood. In the average infant, the birth values of prothrombin content are adequate, but during the first few days of life, they appear to fall rapidly, even dangerously low, and then slowly recover spontaneously. This transition period was and is critical because of the numerous sites of hemorrhagic manifestations, traumatic or spontaneous, that may prove serious if not fatal. This condition is now considered a type of alimentary vitamin K deficiency. The spontaneous recovery is perhaps due to establishment of an intestinal flora that can synthesize vitamin K after ingestion of food. Oral administration of vitamin K, however, effects a prompt recovery.

Vitamin K_1 acts more rapidly (effect on prothrombin time) than menadione, within 2 hours after intravenous administration. No difference, however, could be detected after 2 hours.[120] The menadiones are much less active than vitamin K_1 in normalizing the prolonged blood-clotting times caused by dicumarol and related drugs.[120] Vitamin K_1 is the drug of choice for humans because of its low toxicity. Its duration of action is longer than that of menadione and its derivatives. Vitamin K should not be administered to patients receiving warfarin or coumarin anticoagulants.

Vitamin K can be used to diagnose liver function accurately. Intramuscular injection of 2 mg of 2-methyl-1,4-naphthoquinone elicits a response in prothrombin index in patients with jaundice of extrahepatic origin but not in those with jaundice of intrahepatic origin (e.g., cirrhosis).

Menadione, USP. Menadione, 2-methyl-1,4-naphthoquinone, menaphthone, vitamin K_3, can be prepared readily by the oxidation of 2-methylnaphthalene with chromic acid. It is a bright yellow, crystalline powder and is nearly odorless. It is affected by sunlight. Menadione is practically insoluble in water; it is soluble in vegetable oils, and 1 g of it is soluble in about 60 mL of alcohol. The USP/NF cautions that menadione powder is irritating to the respiratory tract and the skin and that an alcoholic solution has vesicant properties.

On a mole-for-mole basis, menadione is equal to vitamin K_1 in activity and can be used as a complete substitute for this vitamin. It is effective orally, intravenously, and intramuscularly. Oral absorption occurs in the distal small intestines and the colon. If given orally to patients with biliary obstruction, bile salts or their equivalent should be administered simultaneously to facilitate absorption. It can be administered intramuscularly in oil when the patient cannot tolerate an oral product or has a biliary obstruction or when a prolonged effect is desired.

Carbon-14–labeled menadiol diacetate in small physiological doses is converted in vivo to vitamin $K_{2(20)}$, and the side chain probably originates from mevalonic acid. This suggests that menadione may be an intermediate or a provitamin K.[120]

Menadione in oil is 3 times more effective than a menadione suspension in water. More of menadione than of vitamin K_1 is absorbed orally, but 38% of menadione is excreted by the kidney in 24 hours, whereas only very small amounts of vitamin K_1 are excreted by this route in 24 hours. In rats, menadione in part is reduced to the hydroquinone and excreted as the glucuronide (19%) and the sulfate (9.3%).

Menadione Sodium Bisulfate. Menadione sodium bisulfate, 2-methyl-1,4-naphthoquinone sodium bisulfite, is prepared by adding a solution of sodium bisulfite to menadione.

Menadione   Menadione Sodium Bisulfate

Menadione sodium bisulfate occurs as a white, crystalline, odorless powder. One gram of it dissolves in about 2 mL of water, and it is slightly soluble in alcohol. It decomposes in the presence of alkali to liberate the free quinone.

Menadiol Sodium Diphosphate, USP. Menadiol sodium diphosphate, tetrasodium 2-methyl-1,4-naphthalenediol bis(dihydrogen phosphate), tetrasodium 2-methylnaphthohydroquinone diphosphate, vitamin K_4, is a white hygroscopic powder, very soluble in water, giving solutions with a pH of 7 to 9. It is available in ampuls for use subcutaneously, intramuscularly, or intravenously and in tablets for oral administration. Unlike the other vitamin K analogues, menadiol[59] oral absorption does not depend on the presence of bile. Once absorbed, it is converted to menadione.

Menadiol Sodium Diphosphate

Menadione bisulfite and menadiol diphosphate produce hemolytic symptoms (reticulocytosis, increase in Heinz bodies) in newborn, premature infants when given in excessive doses (more than 5 to 10 mg/kg). In severe cases, overt hemolytic anemia with hemoglobinuria may occur. The increased red cell breakdown may lead to hyperbilirubinemia and kernicterus.

These compounds may also interfere with bile pigment secretion. Newborns with a congenital defect of glucose-6-phosphate dehydrogenase can react with severe hemolysis, even to small doses of menadione derivatives. Small nonhemolyzing doses, however, can be used in the newborn, and a combination with vitamin E is not considered essential.[121]

WATER-SOLUBLE VITAMINS

Although the water-soluble vitamins are structurally diverse, they are put in a general class to distinguish them from the lipid-soluble vitamins. This class includes the B-complex vitamins and ascorbic acid (vitamin C). The term *B-complex vitamins* usually refers to thiamine, riboflavin, pyridoxine, nicotinic acid, pantothenic acid, biotin, cyanocobalamin, and folic acid. Dietary deficiencies of any of the B vitamins commonly are complicated by deficiencies of another member(s) of the group, so treatment with B-complex preparations is usually indicated.

Thiamine (Vitamin B₁)

Thiamine was the first water-soluble vitamin to be discovered (1926), but the complete determination of its structure and synthesis was not accomplished until 1936.

Thiamine Hydrochloride

Many natural foods provide adequate amounts of this vitamin. The germ of cereals, brans, egg yolks, yeast extracts, peas, beans, and nuts usually provide enough thiamine to satisfy adult requirements. The requirement for thiamine is related directly to caloric intake, 0.2 to 0.3 mg/1,000 calories. It is not economically practical to isolate the crystalline vitamin from natural sources on a commercial scale, so commercially available thiamine is prepared synthetically.

Thiamine is synthesized biologically from the pyrimidine derivative 4-amino-5-hydroxymethyl-2-methyl pyrimidine methylpyrimidine and 5-(β-hydroxyethyl)-4-methylthiazole. These two precursors are converted to phosphate derivatives under kinase catalysis, which requires ATP. The respective phosphate derivatives then interact to form thiamine phosphate in a reaction catalyzed by thiamine phosphate pyrophosphorylase.

In higher mammalian organisms, thiamine is transformed to the coenzyme thiamine pyrophosphate by direct pyrophosphate transfer from ATP. This coenzyme performs important metabolic functions, for example, as cocarboxylase in the decarboxylation of α-keto acids (such as pyruvate to form acetyl-CoA) and in transketolases (such as use of pentoses in the hexose monophosphate shunt).

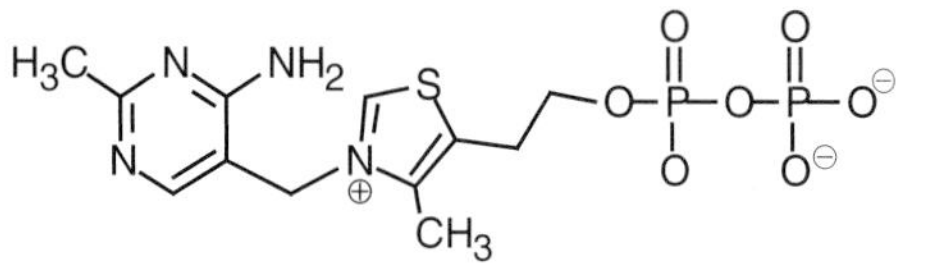

Thiamine Pyrophosphate

In the decarboxylation of pyruvate, the coenzyme interacts with pyruvic acid to form so-called active aldehyde, as shown below.

The active aldehyde intermediate then interacts with thioctic acid to form acetyl-thioctate, which is responsible for acetylating CoA-SH to form acetyl-CoA. In deficiency states, the oxidation of α-keto acids is decreased, resulting in increased pyruvate levels in the blood.

Thiamine hydrochloride is stable in acid but unstable in aqueous solutions with a pH above 5. Under these conditions, it undergoes decomposition and inactivation. Exposure of thiamine to the atmosphere or to oxidizing reagents such as hydrogen peroxide, permanganate, or alkaline potassium ferricyanide oxidizes it readily to thiochrome, shown below. Thiochrome exhibits a vivid blue fluorescence; hence, this reaction is the basis for the quantitative fluorometric assay of thiamine in the USP.

Oxythiamine and neopyrithiamine are antivitamins used in the study of the deficiency state. Oxythiamine is a competitive inhibitor of thiamine pyrophosphate. Neopyrithiamine inhibits the pyrophosphorylation of thiamine.

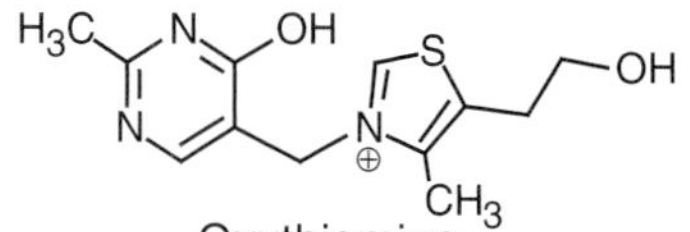

Oxythiamine

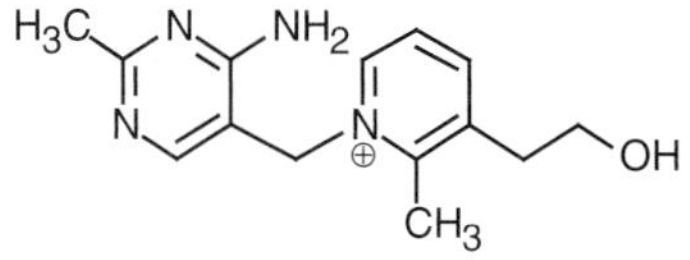

Neopyrithiamine

PRODUCTS

Thiamine Hydrochloride, USP. Thiamine hydrochloride, thiamine monohydrochloride, thiamine chloride, vitamin B_1 hydrochloride, vitamin B_1, aneurine hydrochloride, occurs as small white crystals or as a crystalline powder. It has a slight, characteristic yeast-like odor. The anhydrous product, when exposed to air, rapidly absorbs about 4% of water. One gram is soluble in 1 mL of water and in about 100 mL of alcohol. It is soluble in glycerin. An aqueous solution, 1:20, has a pH of 3. Aqueous solutions 1:100 have a pH of 2.7 to 3.4. Thiamine has pK_a values of 4.8 and 9.0. Thiamine hydrochloride is sensitive to alkali. The addition of 3 moles of sodium hydroxide per mole of thiamine hydrochloride gives the reaction shown on page 887.

Thiamine hydrochloride absorption is sodium dependent; thus, saturation limits absorption to 8 to 15 mg daily. Absorption is decreased in alcoholism and cirrhosis. Food affects the rate, but not the amount, absorbed. After absorption, thiamine hydrochloride is distributed to all tissues. There is limited storage of the vitamin in the body (about 30 mg). Normally, little or no thiamine is excreted in the urine. If doses exceed physiological needs after body stores are saturated, however, thiamine can be found in the urine as pyrimidine or as the unchanged compound.

Severe thiamine deficiency is called *beriberi*. The major organs affected are the nervous system (in dry beriberi), the cardiovascular system (in wet beriberi), and the gastrointestinal tract. Thiamine administration reverses the gastrointestinal and cardiovascular symptoms. The neurological damage may be permanent, however, if the deficiency has been severe or of long duration. Thiamine hydrochloride is indicated

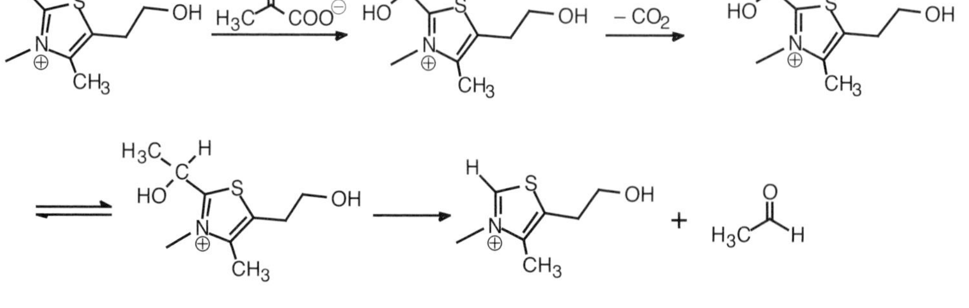

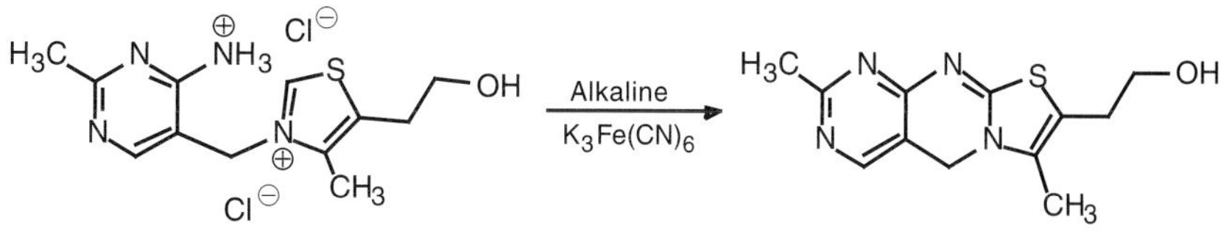

Thiamine Hydrochloride

Alkaline
K₃Fe(CN)₆

Thiochrome

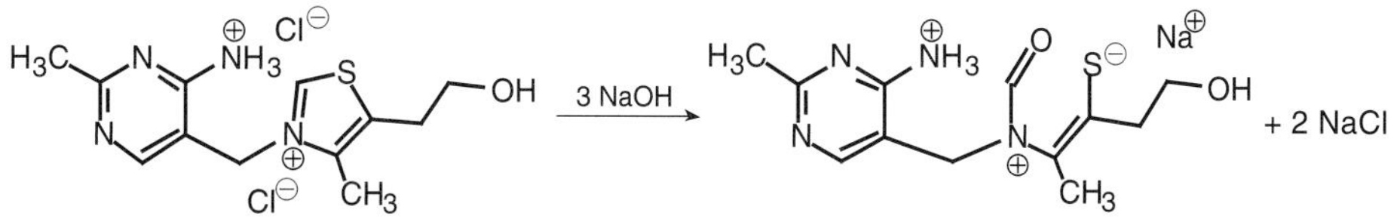

Thiamine Hydrochloride

3 NaOH

+ 2 NaCl

in the treatment or prophylaxis of thiamine deficiencies. Dietary deficiencies are rare in the United States; alcoholism is the most common cause of the disease. Alcoholics have poor dietary habits (deficient diet), and alcohol interferes with absorption of the vitamin.

Thiamine dosage of 5 mg/day for 4 to 5 weeks has resulted in headache, insomnia, irritability, increased heart rate, and weakness. In addition, thiamine can cause anaphylactic reactions following parenteral use.[122]

Thiamine Mononitrate, USP.
Thiamine mononitrate, thiamine nitrate, vitamin B_1 mononitrate, is a colorless compound. It is soluble in water (1:35) and slightly soluble in alcohol; 2% aqueous solutions have a pH of 6.0 to 7.1. This salt is more stable than the chloride hydrochloride in the dry state, less hygroscopic, and recommended for multivitamin preparations and enrichment of flour mixes.

Pantothenic Acids

During the 1930s, R. J. Williams and his collaborators recognized, isolated, and synthesized pantothenic acid. Because its occurrence is so widespread, it was called *pantothenic acid* from the Greek, meaning "from everywhere."

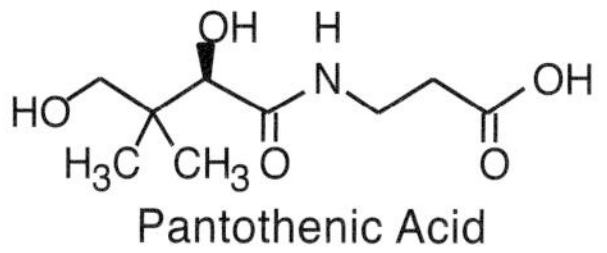

Pantothenic Acid

Pantothenic acid has also been called *vitamin B_5*. Excellent sources of the vitamin are liver, eggs, and cereals. It is found, however, in the form of CoA. This coenzyme cannot be absorbed directly from the gut. Although no experiments have been conducted in humans, studies on animals indicate that the coenzyme must be hydrolyzed to panthenene and pantothenate,[40] which are absorbed by passive diffusion. Human intestinal cells contain enzymes that can hydrolyze the coenzyme. Pantothenate is the major form circulating in the blood and is absorbed by individual cells. Once inside the cell, CoA is synthesized.

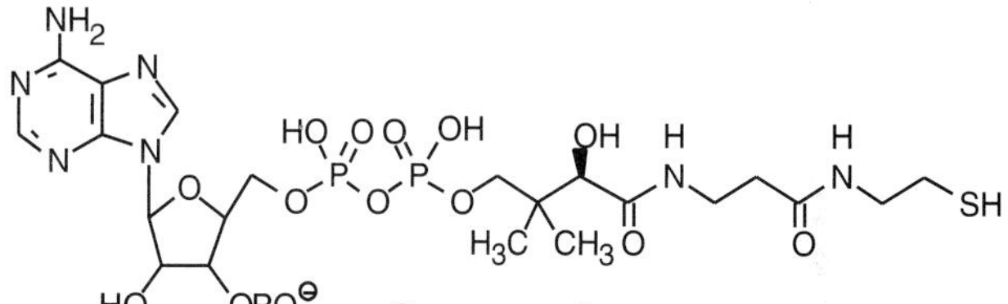

Coenzyme A

This vitamin is synthesized by most green plants and microorganisms. The precursors are γ-ketoisovaleric acid and β-alanine.[1] The latter originates from the decarboxylation of aspartic acid. γ-Ketoisovaleric acid is converted to ketopantoic acid by N^5,N^{10}-methylenetetrahydrofolic acid; then, on reduction, pantoic acid is formed. Finally, pantoic acid and β-alanine react by amide formation to form pantothenic acid.

The metabolic functions of pantothenic acid in human biochemistry are mediated through the synthesis of CoA. Pantothenic acid is a structural component of CoA, which is necessary for many important metabolic processes. Pantothenic acid is incorporated into CoA by a series of five enzyme-catalyzed reactions. CoA is involved in the activation of fatty acids before β-oxidation, which requires ATP to form the respective fatty acyl-CoA derivatives. Pantothenic acid also participates in fatty acid β-oxidation in the final step, forming acetyl-CoA. Acetyl-CoA is also formed from pyruvate decarboxylation, in which CoA participates with thiamine pyrophosphate and lipoic acid, two other important coenzymes. Thiamine pyrophosphate is the actual decarboxylating coenzyme that functions with lipoic acid to form acetyldihydrolipoic acid from pyruvate decarboxylation. CoA then accepts the acetyl group from acetyldihydrolipoic acid to form acetyl-CoA. Acetyl-CoA is an acetyl donor in many processes and is the precursor in important biosyntheses (e.g., those of fatty acids, steroids, porphyrins, and acetylcholine).

Clinical cases of pantothenic acid deficiency develop rarely, unless they arise in combination with deficiencies of the other B vitamins.[2] Accordingly, pantothenic acid is usually included in multivitamin preparations. The calcium salt is commonly used in pharmaceutical preparations. Panthenol, the alcohol derivative, is also commonly used.

PRODUCTS

Pantothenic Acid.

Pantothenic acid, vitamin B_5, occurs as a viscous hygroscopic oil, freely soluble in water but unstable to heat, acid, and alkali. Because of this instability, the calcium salt is used commercially.

Pantothenic acid and its derivatives have essentially no pharmacological actions per se. Because of the ubiquitous nature of the vitamin, deficiency states usually do not develop. They have been produced by use of synthetic diets devoid of the vitamin or by use of a vitamin antagonist. ω-Methylpantothenic acid has produced fatigue, headache, paresthesia of the hands and feet, cardiovascular instability, and gastrointestinal problems.

ω–Methylpantothenic Acid

Pantothenic acid and its derivatives are readily absorbed and widely distributed. The highest concentrations are found in the liver, adrenal glands, heart, and kidneys. Pantothenic acid apparently undergoes little if any metabolism; the amount eliminated approximates the amount consumed. About 70% of a dose is eliminated unchanged in the urine, and the remainder is eliminated in the feces.

The only official indication for pantothenic acid is in the prevention or treatment of vitamin B deficiencies. Because a deficiency of a single B vitamin is rare, it is commonly formulated in multivitamin preparations or B-complex preparations.

Calcium Pantothenate, USP.

Calcium pantothenate, calcium D-pantothenate, is a slightly hygroscopic, white, odorless, bitter powder that is stable in air. It is insoluble in alcohol and soluble 1:3 in water; aqueous solutions have a pH of about 9 and $[\alpha]_D = +25$ to $+27.5°$. Autoclaving calcium pantothenate at 120°C for 20 minutes may cause 10 to 30% decomposition. Some of the phosphates of pantothenic acid that occur naturally in coenzymes are quite stable to both acid and alkali, even on heating.[123]

Calcium Pantothenate

Racemic Calcium Pantothenate, USP.

Racemic calcium pantothenate provides a more economical source of this vitamin. Other than containing not less than 45% of the dextrorotatory biologically active form, its properties are very similar to those of calcium pantothenate, USP.

Panthenol, USP.

Panthenol, the racemic alcohol analogue of pantothenic acid, exhibits both qualitatively and quantitatively the vitamin activity of pantothenic acid. It is considerably more stable than pantothenic acid in solutions with pH values of 3 to 5 but of about equal stability at pH 6 to 8. It appears to be absorbed more readily from the gut, particularly in the presence of food.

Dexpanthenol, USP.

Dexpanthenol occurs as a slightly hygroscopic, viscous oil freely soluble in water and alcohol. It is the dextrorotatory alcohol derivative of pantothenic acid and is converted readily in vivo to the acid form.

Dexpanthenol

Dexpanthenol and the racemic mixture are used in the treatment of paralytic ileus and postoperative distention. Dexpanthenol in combination with choline is used to relieve gas retention.

Nicotinic Acid

Nicotinic acid (niacin) was prepared first by oxidation of the alkaloid nicotine, but not until 1913 was it isolated from yeast and recognized as an essential food factor (see the structures). In 1934–1935, nicotinamide was obtained from the hydrolysis of a coenzyme isolated from horse red blood cells. This coenzyme was later named *coenzyme II* and is now more commonly called *nicotinamide adenine dinucleotide phosphate* (NADP).

Nicotine → Niacin

Generous sources of this vitamin include pork, lamb, and beef livers; hog kidneys; yeasts; pork; beef tongue; hearts; lean meats; wheat germ; peanut meal; and green peas. Nicotinic acid can be synthesized by almost all plants and animals. Tryptophan can be metabolized to a nicotinic acid nucleotide in animals, but the efficiency of this multistep process varies from species to species. Plants and many microorganisms synthesize this vitamin through alternative routes by use of aspartic acid.

In the human, nicotinic acid reacts with 5-phosphoribosyl-1-pyrophosphate to form nicotinic acid mononucleotide, which then reacts with ATP to produce desamido-NAD (the intermediate dinucleotide with the nicotinic acid moiety). Finally, the latter intermediate is converted to NAD (originally called *coenzyme I*) by transformation of the carboxyl of the nicotinic acid moiety to the amide by glutamine. This final step is catalyzed by NAD synthetase; NADP is produced from NAD by ATP under kinase catalysis.[1]

R = H = Nicotinamide adenine dinucleotide
R = PO_3^{-2} = Nicotinamide adenine dinucleotide phosphate

NAD and NADP are oxidizing coenzymes for many (more than 200) dehydrogenases. Some dehydrogenases require

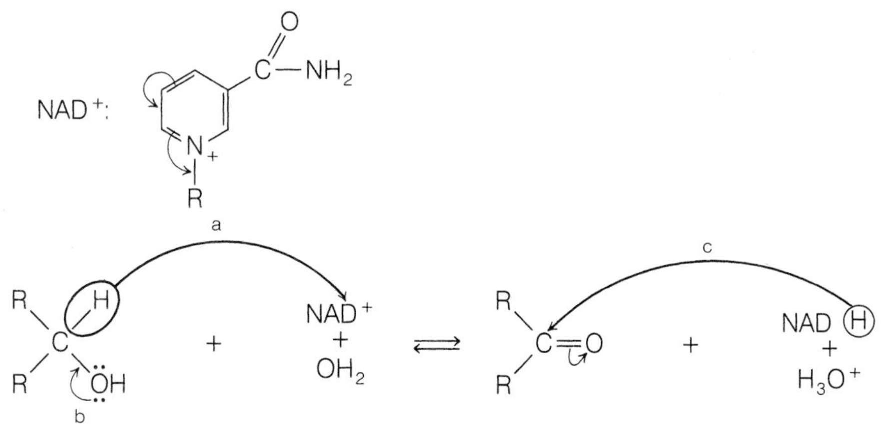

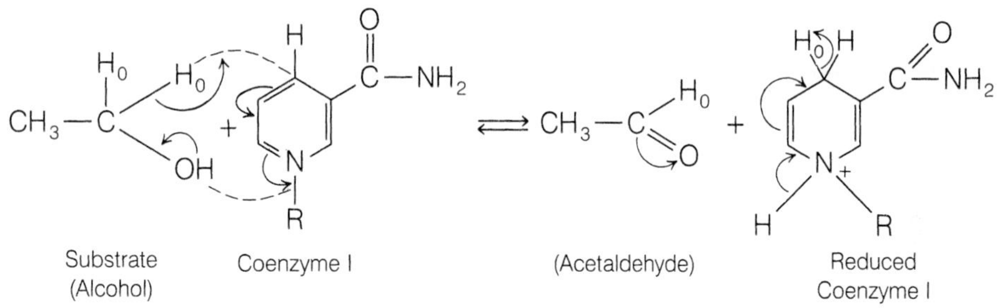

Figure 26–1 ■ Generalized representation of the hydride transfer reaction.

Substrate (Alcohol)   Coenzyme I   (Acetaldehyde)   Reduced Coenzyme I

Ethanol oxidation is schematically illustrated below:

NAD, others require NADP, and some function with either. The generalized representation in Figure 26-1 illustrates the function of these coenzymes in metabolic oxidations and reductions. The abbreviation [NAD^+] emphasizes the electrophilicity of the pyridine C_4 moiety (which is the center of reactivity) and the substrate designated

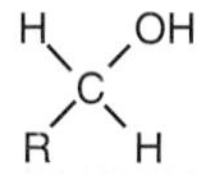

could be a primary or secondary alcohol. *Arrow a* in Figure 26-1 symbolizes the function of NAD as oxidant in the hydride transfer from the substrate to the coenzyme, forming NADH, reduced coenzyme. The hydroxyl of the substrate is visualized as undergoing deprotonation concertedly by either water or the pyridine nitrogen of NADH. *Arrow b* shows concerted formation of the carbonyl π-bond of the oxidation product. *Arrow c* symbolizes the reverse hydride transfer from reduced coenzyme, NADH, to the carbonyl carbon; and concertedly, as the carbonyl oxygen undergoes protonation, the reduction of the carbonyl group forms the corresponding alcohol. Thus, NAD and NADP are hydride

acceptors, and NADH and NADPH are hydride donors. Although this is a simplistic representation, it shows the dynamism of the oxidation–reduction reactions effected by these coenzymes under appropriate dehydrogenase catalysis. Alternatively, the reduced coenzymes may be used in ATP production through the electron-transport system.

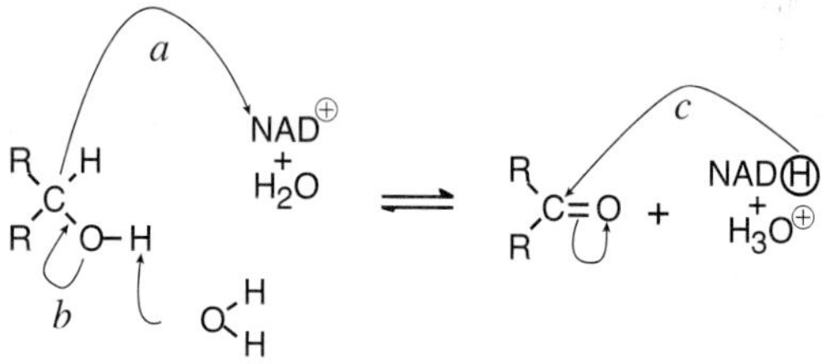

Ethanol Oxidation Is Schematically Illustrated Below

As noted above, nicotinic acid (also known as *niacin* to avoid confusion with nicotine) can be made available in nucleotide form from the amino acid tryptophan. It has been estimated that a dosage of 60 mg of tryptophan equals that of 1 mg of nicotinic acid. Consequently, humans and other mammals can synthesize the vitamin, provided there is appropriate dietary availability of tryptophan. (Thus, nicotinic

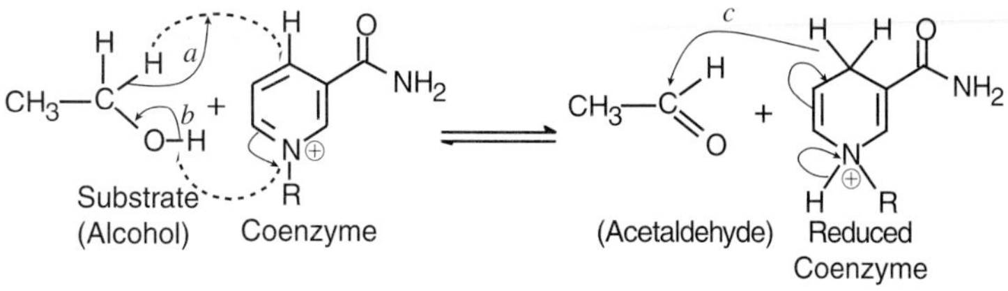

Substrate (Alcohol)   Coenzyme   (Acetaldehyde)   Reduced Coenzyme

acid is not a true vitamin by the classic definition of the term.)

PRODUCTS

Niacin, USP. Niacin, nicotinic acid, 3-pyridine carboxylic acid, vitamin B$_3$, occurs as white crystals or as a crystalline powder. It is odorless or may have a slight odor. One gram of nicotinic acid dissolves in 60 mL of water. It is freely soluble in boiling water, boiling alcohol, and solutions of alkali hydroxides and carbonates but is almost insoluble in ether. A 1% aqueous solution has a pH of 6. Nicotinic acid has a pK$_a$ of 4.85. Nicotinic acid is stable under normal storage conditions. It sublimes without decomposition.

Serious deficiency of niacin or tryptophan may lead to pellagra (from the Italian, *pelle agra,* for "rough skin"). The major systems affected are the gastrointestinal tract (diarrhea, enteritis, stomatitis), the skin (dermatitis), and the central nervous system (headache, dizziness, depression). Severe cases may result in delusions, hallucinations, and dementia. In the United States, pellagra has become rare because flour is supplemented with nicotinic acid. Chronic alcoholism is the chief cause of pellagra and is associated with multiple vitamin deficiency. The symptoms of pellagra are completely reversed by niacin; therefore, it is indicated for the treatment and prevention of the deficiency.

Adverse effects of niacin are most commonly seen when this vitamin is used at pharmacological doses above 1 g/day in the treatment of dyslipidemia. Notable adverse effects include flushing due to vasodilatation; dermatological effects including dry skin pruritus and hyperkeratosis; gastrointestinal effects including peptic ulcer, stomach pain, nausea, and diarrhea; elevations in serum uric acid and glucose; and hepatotoxicity.[122, 124]

Niacin (but not niacinamide) is also indicated in hyperlipidemia to lower triglycerides and cholesterol. Triglycerides, VLDLs, and LDLs are reduced; HDLs are increased. The exact mechanism is not known. Because niacin at high doses has a direct vasodilatory effect believed to be mediated through the prostaglandins, the dose required (1 to 3 g 3 times daily) often limits the usefulness.

Niacin is absorbed readily from the gastrointestinal tract and distributed widely. At physiological doses, little niacin is excreted unchanged. Most is excreted as *N*-methylniacin or the glycine conjugate (nicotinuric acid). After administration of large doses, niacin can be found in the urine unchanged.

Niacinamide, USP. Niacinamide, nicotinamide, nicotinic acid amide, is prepared by the amidation of esters of nicotinic acid or by passing ammonia gas into nicotinic acid at 320°C. Nicotinamide is a white crystalline powder that is odorless, or nearly so, and bitter. One gram is soluble in about 1 mL of water, 1.5 mL of alcohol, and about 10 mL of glycerin. Aqueous solutions are neutral to litmus. For occurrence, action, and uses, see nicotinic acid. Niacinamide has pK$_a$ values of 0.5 and 3.35.

Ethyl Nicotinate   Niacinamide
                          Nicotinamide

Like niacin, niacinamide is indicated in the treatment and prevention of deficiency states. Unlike niacin, niacinamide has no vasodilatory effect, which may be of therapeutic importance for compliance reasons. Niacinamide has no effect on triglycerides and lipoproteins. This product is formulated with potassium iodide and used as an iodine supplement.

Niacinamide hydrochloride is also available. It is more stable in solution and more compatible with thiamine chloride in solution.

Riboflavin (Vitamin B$_2$)

Although crystalline riboflavin was not isolated until 1932, interest in this compound as a pigment dates back to 1881 in connection with the color in the whey of milk. In 1932, riboflavin was isolated as a coenzyme–enzyme complex from yeast by Warburg and Christian and was designated *yellow oxidation ferment.*

Riboflavin

Riboflavin is synthesized by all green plants and by most bacteria and fungi. Although yeast is the richest source, eggs, dairy products, legumes, and meats are the major sources in the diet. The precursor is a guanosine phosphate derivative, but the exact synthetic steps leading to the vitamin are not understood completely.

In higher mammals, riboflavin is absorbed readily from the intestines and distributed to all tissues. It is the precursor in the biosynthesis of the coenzymes flavin mononucleotide (FMN) and flavin adenine dinucleotide (FAD). The metabolic functions of this vitamin involve these two coenzymes, which participate in numerous vital oxidation–reduction processes. FMN (riboflavin 5′-phosphate) is produced from the vitamin and ATP by flavokinase catalysis. This step can be inhibited by phenothiazines and the tricyclic antidepressants. FAD originates from an FMN and ATP reaction that involves reversible dinucleotide formation catalyzed by flavin nucleotide pyrophosphorylase. These coenzymes function in combination with several enzymes as coenzyme–enzyme complexes, often characterized as *flavoproteins.*

Flavin Mononucleotide

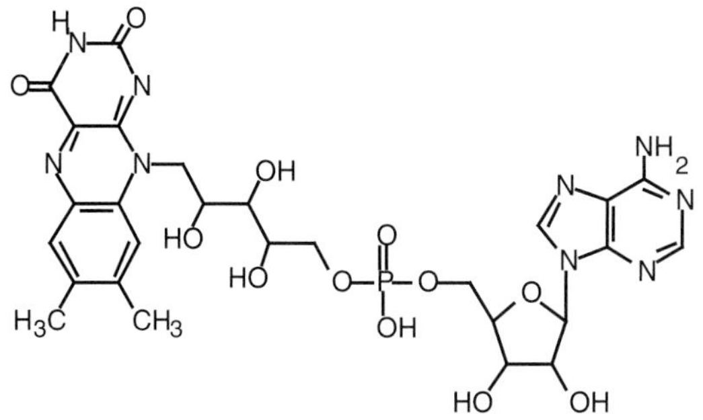

Flavin Adenine Dinucleotide

These flavoproteins function in aerobic or anaerobic conditions as oxidases and dehydrogenases. Examples include glucose oxidase, xanthine oxidase, cytochrome reductase, and acyl-CoA dehydrogenase. The riboflavin moiety of the complex is considered a hydrogen-transporting agent (carrier) functioning as a hydrogen acceptor; the hydrogen donors may be NADH, NADPH, or some suitable substrate. The isoalloxazine rings accept two hydrides stepwise to form the dihydroriboflavin derivative.

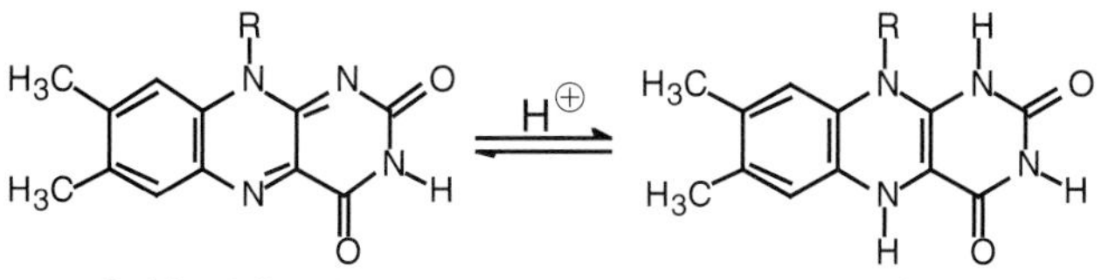

Oxidized Species   Reduced Species

PRODUCTS

Riboflavin, USP.   Riboflavin, lactoflavin, vitamin B₂, vitamin G, is a yellow to orange-yellow, crystalline powder with a slight odor. It is soluble in water 1:3,000 to 1:20,000 mL, with the variation in solubility being due to differences in internal crystalline structure, but it is more soluble in an isotonic solution of sodium chloride. A saturated aqueous solution has a pH of 6. Riboflavin has a pK_a of 10.5. It is less soluble in alcohol and insoluble in ether or chloroform. Benzyl alcohol (3%), gentisic acid (3%), urea in varying amounts, and niacinamide are used to solubilize riboflavin when relatively high concentrations of it are needed for parenteral solutions. Gentisic ethanol amide and sodium 3-hydroxy-2-naphthoate also solubilize riboflavin effectively.

When dry, riboflavin is not affected appreciably by diffused light; it deteriorates, however, in solution in the presence of light. This deterioration is very rapid in the presence of alkalies, producing lumiflavine. This deterioration may be retarded by buffering on the acid side, but under acid conditions, light can produce lumichrome. Neither of these decomposition products possesses biological activity.

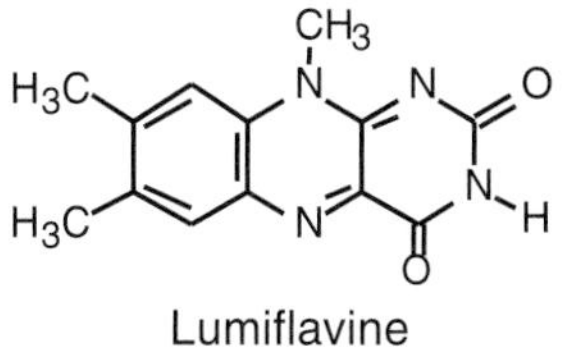

Lumiflavine

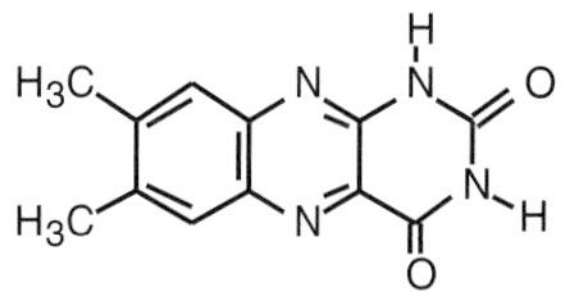

Lumichrome

The vitamin is commercially available as riboflavin, riboflavin 5-phosphate, and riboflavin 5-phosphate sodium. The phosphate esters are used commercially only in multivitamin preparations, and they are hydrolyzed before absorption occurs. Absorption occurs through an active transport system in which riboflavin is phosphorylated by the intestinal mucosa during absorption. Food and bile enhance absorption. Riboflavin is distributed widely in the body, with limited stores in the liver, spleen, heart, and kidneys. Conversion to FAD occurs primarily in the liver. FMN and FAD circulate primarily protein bound. Only small amounts (~9%) are excreted in the urine unchanged. Larger amounts can be found after administration of large doses.

Severe riboflavin deficiency is known as *ariboflavinosis*. Its major symptoms include cheilosis, seborrheic dermatitis, and vascularization of the cornea. Ariboflavinosis occurs in chronic alcoholism in combination with other vitamin deficiencies. It has also resulted from phenothiazine, tricyclic antidepressant, and probenecid therapy. Riboflavin has no pharmacological action and is relatively nontoxic. The only approved indication is in the treatment and prevention of ariboflavinosis.

Pyridoxine

In 1935, the term *vitamin B₆* was applied to the principle that cured dermatitis in rats fed a vitamin-free diet supplemented with thiamine and riboflavin. Three years later, vitamin B₆ was isolated from rice paste and yeast. In 1935, P. Gyorgy showed that rat pellagra was not the same as human pellagra but that it resembled a particular disease of infancy known as ''pink disease'' or acrodynia. This rat acrodynia is characterized by a symmetric dermatosis affecting first the paws and the tips of the ears and the nose. These areas become swollen, red, and edematous, with ulcers developing frequently around the snout and on the tongue. Thickening and scaling of the ears are noted, and there is weight loss; fatalities occur 1 to 3 weeks after the appearance of the symptoms. Gyorgy was able to cure these conditions with a supplement obtained from yeast, which he called *vitamin B₆*. In 1938, this factor was isolated from rice paste and yeast in a crystalline form in a number of laboratories. A single dose of about 100 μg produced healing in 14 days in a rat with severe vitamin B₆–deficiency symptoms.

Chemical tests, electrometric titration determinations, and absorption spectrum studies gave clues to its composition. These were substantiated by the synthesis of vitamin B₆ (1938 and 1939). Two additional chemical forms, pyridoxal (an aldehyde) and pyridoxamine (a primary amine), have been isolated from natural sources. These three compounds are interrelated metabolically and functionally. The interconversion between the different forms is shown below.

Gyorgy proposed the term *pyridoxine* for the original compound isolated. Soon it became synonymous with *vitamin B₆*. In 1960, IUPAC recommended using the term *pyri-*

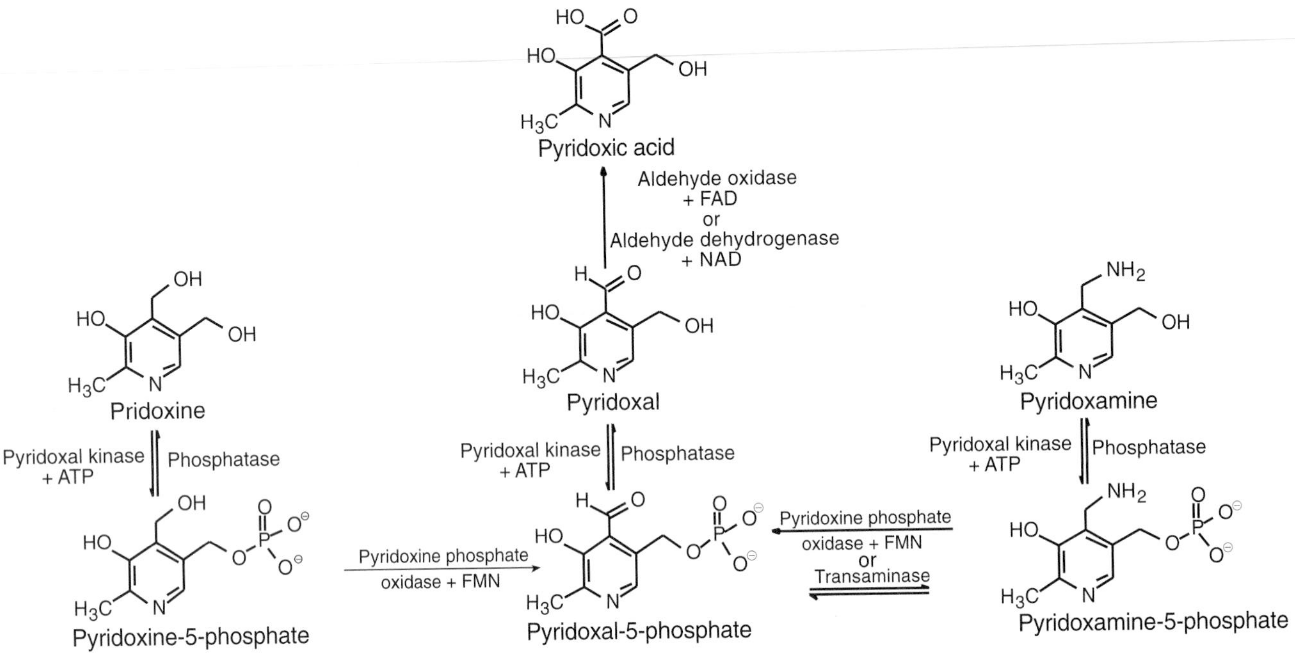

Pyridoxic acid

Aldehyde oxidase
+ FAD
or
Aldehyde dehydrogenase
+ NAD

Pridoxine

Pyridoxal

Pyridoxamine

Pyridoxal kinase
+ ATP   Phosphatase

Pyridoxal kinase
+ ATP   Phosphatase

Pyridoxal kinase
+ ATP   Phosphatase

Pyridoxine-5-phosphate

Pyridoxine phosphate
oxidase + FMN

Pyridoxine phosphate
oxidase + FMN
or
Transaminase

Pyridoxal-5-phosphate

Pyridoxamine-5-phosphate

doxine as a generic descriptor for all forms of the vitamin and *pyridoxol* as the trivial name for the alcohol form of the vitamin. In 1973, IUPAC revised its recommendations. Presently, the term *vitamin B_6* is the approved descriptor for all forms of the vitamin, and the term *pyridoxine* refers to the alcohol form. The term *pyridoxol* is no longer recommended. IUPAC further recommends that the phosphate esters be called *pyridoxine 5'-phosphate, pyridoxal 5'-phosphate,* and *pyridoxamine 5'-phosphate.* These may be abbreviated to *pyridoxine 5'-P, pyridoxine-P,* etc. when no ambiguity arises.

Pyridoxine is available from whole-grain cereals, peanuts, corn, meat, poultry, and fish. Up to 40% of the vitamin may be destroyed, however, during cooking. Food sources contain all three forms, either in their free form or phosphorylated. Plants contain primarily pyridoxol and pyridoxamine, while animal sources provide chiefly pyridoxal. Many plants also contain a glycoside of pyridoxol, which is included in vitamin content determinations. Although this conjugate is absorbed, it is not used well.[5] This may explain the lower bioavailability of the vitamin from plant sources than from animal sources.

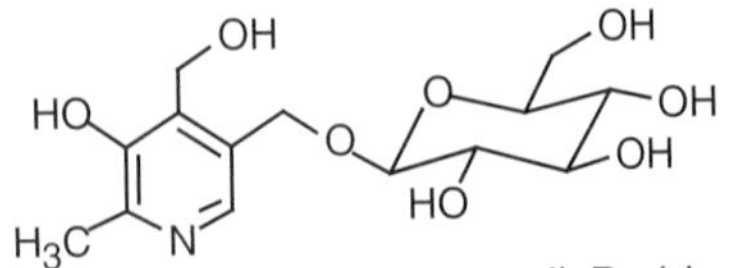

5–O–(β–D–Glycospyranosyl) Pyridoxol

Vitamin B_6 is absorbed via passive diffusion, chiefly in the jejunum, and transported to the liver. The liver is a major organ of storage (16 to 27 mg), metabolism, and interconversion between the three forms. Excess B_6 is oxidized to 4-pyridoxic acid. This acid is the primary form found in the urine, accounting for up to 60% of ingested vitamin B_6.

In the liver, all three forms are converted to pyridoxal 5-phosphate, which circulates in the blood bound to albumin.

Before entry into cells, the phosphate must be dephosphorylated. Inside the cells, pyridoxal kinase rephosphorylates the vitamin. This kinase is found in many cell types, although other enzymes involved in the interconversions are not expressed in all cells.[125] Although large amounts of the vitamin are found in the liver, the muscles contain higher amounts in the form of glycogen phosphorylase.[126] This vitamin B_6 is not readily available, however, during deficiency states.[127]

Pyridoxal 5-phosphate is a coenzyme[128, 129] that performs many vital functions in human metabolism. It functions in the transaminations and decarboxylations that amino acids generally undergo. For example, it functions as a cotransaminase in the transamination of alanine to form pyruvic acid and as a codecarboxylase in the decarboxylation of dopa to form dopamine. Other biological transformations[123, 128] of amino acids in which pyridoxal can function are racemization, elimination of the α-hydrogen together with a β-substituent (i.e., OH or SH) or a γ-substituent, and probably the reversible cleavage of β-hydroxyamino acids to glycine and carbonyl compounds.

An electromeric displacement of electrons from bonds *a, b,* or *c* (see diagram below) would result in the release of a cation (H, R', or COOH) and, subsequently, lead to the variety of reactions observed with pyridoxal. The extent to which one of these displacements predominates over others depends on the structure of the amino acid and the environment (pH, solvent, catalysts, enzymes, and such). When this mechanism applies in vivo, the pyridoxal component is linked to the enzyme through the phosphate of the hydroxymethyl group.

Metals such as iron and aluminum, which markedly catalyze nonenzymatic transaminations in vitro, probably do so by promoting formation of the Schiff base and maintaining planarity of the conjugated system through chelate ring formation, which requires the presence of the phenolic group. This chelated metal ion also provides an additional electron-

heterocyclic nitrogen atom (or nitro group), thereby increasing the electron displacements from the α-carbon atom as shown above.

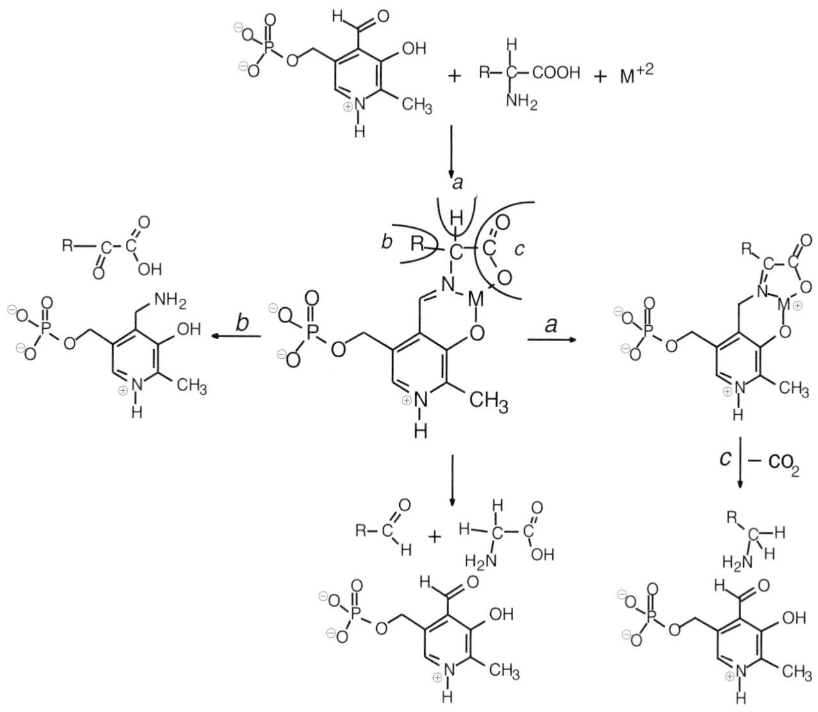

Certain hydrazine derivatives, when administered therapeutically (e.g., isoniazid), can induce a deficiency of the coenzyme (pyridoxal 5-phosphate) by inactivation through the mechanism of hydrazone formation with the aldehyde functional group. Another hydrazine derivative, hydralazine, when administered in high doses to control hypertension, can cause similar B_6 deficiency, conceivably through a similar mechanism involving hydrazone formation.

Hypochromic anemias caused by familiar-type pyridoxine dependency respond to pyridoxine therapy. Similarly, this vitamin has been useful in the treatment of hypochromic or megaloblastic anemias that are not due to iron deficiency and do not respond to other hematopoietic agents.[2]

A review by Rose[130] summarizes studies on the effects of certain hormones on vitamin B_6 nutrition in humans, on the biochemical interrelationship between steroid hormones and pyridoxal phosphate-dependent enzymes, and on the role of vitamin B_6 in regulating hypothalamus–pituitary functions. Some of these studies have important clinical implications. The use of estrogen-containing oral contraceptives has been investigated as a factor leading to an abnormality of tryptophan metabolism. This abnormality resembles dietary vitamin B_6 deficiency and responds favorably to treatment with the vitamin. For some time, there has been clinical interest in the relationship between certain hormones and vitamin B_6 function because abnormal urinary excretion of tryptophan metabolites was observed during pregnancy and in patients with hyperthyroidism.

Estrogens and tryptophan metabolism have been studied because estrogen administration occasionally leads to the excretion of abnormally large amounts of xanthurenic acid, a metabolic product of tryptophan. This metabolic malfunc-tion has been related to the inhibitory effect of estrogen sulfate conjugates on another pathway of tryptophan metabolism—the transamination of kynurenine from tryptophan. Consequently, xanthurenic acid formation appears to be abnormally high because of this estrogen effect or B_6 deficiency.

In vitro studies have been conducted to determine the effect of estrogens on kynurenine aminotransferase, which catalyzes the B_6-dependent transamination of kynurenine to kynurenic acid. Some estrogen conjugates (e.g., estradiol disulfate and diethylstilbestrol sulfate) interfere with this transamination, apparently by reversible inhibition of the aminotransferase apoenzyme. Apparently, the estrogen sulfate competes with pyridoxal 5-phosphate for interaction with the apoenzyme. In contrast, free estradiol and estrone do not possess this inhibitory property.

Some women suffer from mental depression when taking estrogen-containing oral contraceptives, and this depression could be due to another malfunction in tryptophan metabolism, leading to 5-hydroxytryptamine (serotonin). Some evidence indicates that the decarboxylation of 5-hydroxytryptophan is inhibited (in vitro) by estrogen conjugates competing with pyridoxal phosphate for the decarboxylase apoenzyme.

Other endocrine systems are interrelated. Both corticosteroids and thyroid hormones may increase the requirement for pyridoxine and affect pyridoxal 5-phosphate–dependent metabolic processes. Moreover, there appear to be associations between vitamin B_6 and anterior pituitary hormones that seem to involve the hypothalamus, 5-hydroxytryptamine, and dopamine. The latter two neurotransmitters are synthesized by metabolic processes that require pyridoxal 5-phosphate.

Interestingly, studies have shown that vitamin B_6, in turn, influences the function of steroid hormones.[25] Pyridoxal 5-phosphate binds to lysine residues on the steroid receptors.

It has been proposed that the lysine residues are found at the site where the steroid binds to the receptor and where the receptor binds DNA.[125] Thus, pyridoxal 5-phosphate decreases the number of receptors able to bind with the steroids and the number of steroid–receptor complexes binding to DNA. The overall result is decreased expression of DNA.

PRODUCTS

Pyridoxine Hydrochloride, USP.

Pyridoxine hydrochloride, 5-hydroxy-6-methyl-3,4-pyridinedimethanol hydrochloride, vitamin B_6 hydrochloride, rat antidermatitis factor, is a white, odorless, crystalline substance that is soluble 1:5 in water and 1:100 in alcohol and insoluble in ether. It is relatively stable to light and air in the solid form and in acid solutions at a pH no greater than 5, at which pH it can be autoclaved at 15 pounds at 120°C for 20 to 30 minutes. Pyridoxine is unstable when irradiated in aqueous solutions at pH 6.8 or above. It is oxidized readily by hydrogen peroxide and other oxidizing agents. Pyridoxine is as stable in mixed vitamin preparations as riboflavin and nicotinic acid. A 1% aqueous solution has a pH of 3. The pK_{a1} values for pyridoxine, pyridoxal, and pyridoxamine are 5.00, 4.22, and 3.40, respectively, and their pK_{a2} values are 8.96, 8.68, and 8.05, respectively.

Pyridoxine deficiencies have been studied by the use of antivitamins such as 4-desoxypyridoxal. As with the other B vitamins, dietary deficiencies are rare and are associated mainly with alcoholism. The symptoms involve the skin, nervous system, and erythropoiesis.

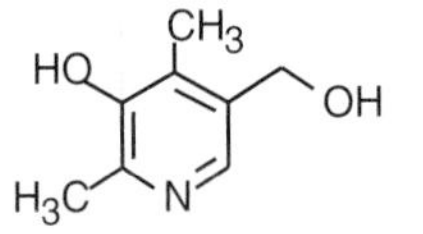

4–Desoxypyridoxal

Because of inadequate diets, some infants suffer from severe vitamin B_6 deficiencies that can lead to epilepsy-like convulsive seizures, and the convulsions can be controlled by treatment with pyridoxine.[1] The convulsions are believed to be due to below-normal availability of the central nervous

system neurohormone γ-aminobutyric acid (GABA), from glutamic acid decarboxylation, which is effected by the coenzyme pyridoxal 5-phosphate.

Pyridoxine hydrochloride is indicated in the treatment and prevention of vitamin deficiency. It is also approved for concurrent administration with isoniazid and cycloserine to decrease their toxicity. Concurrent administration of pyridoxine hydrochloride and levodopa is not recommended. The decarboxylation of levodopa to dopamine in the periphery is increased by pyridoxine, so that less levodopa reaches the central nervous system.

Peripheral neuropathy can occur following ingestion of high doses of pyridoxine. Doses of 2 g/day can produce paresthesia and alter proprioception.[131] Some studies suggest the dose required may be as low as 50 to 500 mg/day. Symptoms may actually increase for several weeks after discontinuing pyridoxine, a phenomenon called *coasting*.[132]

Cobalamins

Vitamin B_{12}, cyanocobalamin, occurs in nature as a cofactor that originally was isolated as cyanocobalamin and vitamin B_{12b} (hydroxocobalamin). In April 1948, Rickes et al.[133–135] isolated from clinically active liver fractions, minute amounts of a red crystalline compound that was also highly effective in promoting the growth of *Lactobacillus lactis*. This compound was called *vitamin B_{12}*, and in single doses as small as 3 to 6 μg, it produced positive hematological activity in patients with addisonian pernicious anemia. Evidence indicates that its activity is comparable with that of Castle's extrinsic factor and that it can be stored in the liver.

Vitamin B_{12} is found in commercial fermentation processes of antibiotics, such as those of *Streptomyces griseus, S. olivaceus, S. aureofaciens*, sewage, milorganite, and others. Some of these fermentations furnish a commercial source of vitamin B_{12}. Excellent dietary sources are meats, eggs, seafood, dairy, and fermented products. De novo synthesis of vitamin B_{12}, however, is restricted to microorganisms. Animals depend on intestinal flora synthesis or, as in humans, consumption of products from animal that have already obtained vitamin B_{12}. The only dietary plant prod-

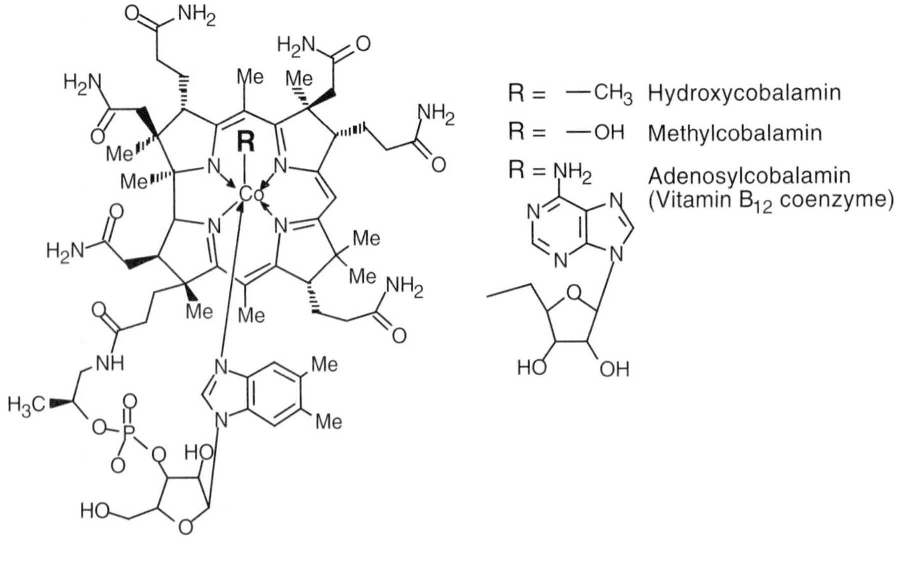

R = —CH₃ Hydroxycobalamin

R = —OH Methylcobalamin

R = NH₂ Adenosylcobalamin (Vitamin B_{12} coenzyme)

ucts containing the vitamin are legumes, because of their symbiosis with microorganisms.

Because dietary vitamin B_{12} is protein bound, the first step in absorption is its release in the stomach. Release is enhanced by gastric pH and pancreatic proteases. The freed vitamin is bound immediately to a glycoprotein, the *intrinsic factor,* secreted by parietal cells of the gastric mucosa. The vitamin B_{12}–intrinsic factor complex is carried to the intestines, where it binds with receptors in the ileum. Absorption is mainly by an active process, which can be saturated by 1.5 to 3 μg of vitamin B_{12}. Excess amounts may be absorbed passively.

In the intestinal cells, the complex is broken and vitamin B_{12} is absorbed into the blood, where it binds to transcobalamin II, a β-globulin, for distribution. In the liver, the vitamin is converted to the active form and stored as such. Up to 90% of the vitamin (5 to 11 mg) is stored in the liver. Vitamin B_{12} is excreted through the bile and undergoes extensive reabsorption.

In the biosynthesis of the coenzymes[136] derived from vitamin B_{12}, cobalt is reduced from a trivalent to a monovalent state before the organic anionic ligands are attached to the structure. The two types of cobamide that participate as coenzymes in human metabolism are the adenosylcobamides and the methylcobamides. These coenzymes perform vital functions in methylmalonate–succinate isomerization and in methylation of homocysteine to methionine.

Methylcobalamin is the major form of the coenzyme in the plasma, and 5-deoxyadenosylcobalamine is the major form in the liver and other tissues. The enzyme system methylmalonyl-CoA mutase requires 5′-deoxyadenosylcobamide; this enzyme system catalyzes the methylmalonyl-CoA transformation to succinyl-CoA, which is the major pathway of propionyl-CoA metabolism. Propionyl-CoA from lipid metabolism must be processed through this pathway by succinyl-CoA to enter the Krebs citric acid cycle to be either converted to γ-oxaloacetate, leading to gluconeogenesis, or oxidized aerobically to CO_2, with production of ATP. The methylation of homocysteine to form methionine requires methylcobalamin and is catalyzed by a transmethylase that also requires 5-methyltetrahydrofolic acid and reduced FAD.[136]

A deficiency of vitamin B_{12} leads to anemia. Pernicious anemia is due to a lack of the intrinsic factor. The symptoms involve systems that have rapidly dividing cells and the nervous system. Herbert and Das[136] reviewed the biochemical roles of vitamin B_{12} and folic acid in hematopoiesis and other cellular development. They emphasize that vitamin B_{12} and folic acid are essential for normal growth and proliferation of all human cells. Vitamin B_{12} also functions to maintain myelin throughout the nervous system. Deficiency of either vitamin leads to megaloblastic anemia involving below-normal DNA synthesis. Interference with DNA synthesis results in the inability of cells to mature properly. These symptoms are readily reversed by vitamin B_{12} supplementation; the nerve damage, however, is irreversible. It has been postulated that the myelin damage results from low levels of *S*-adenosylmethionine caused by a methionine synthetase deficiency.[137] Most vitamin B_{12} deficiencies are due to malabsorption (lack of intrinsic factor, alcoholism) or increased need (pregnancy). It has been postulated that vitamin B_{12} deficiency is largely a conditioned folic acid deficiency

caused by below-normal transformation of 5-methyltetrahydrofolic acid to tetrahydrofolic acid (THFA) by the B_{12}-dependent homocysteine methyl transferase reaction and defective cellular uptake of 5-methyl-THFA in vitamin B_{12} deficiency. This so-called methyl-THFA trap hypothesis seems to rationalize a mechanism for the pathogenesis of megaloblastic anemia in vitamin B_{12} deficiency, and investigations continue to provide evidence that supports this rationalization.

High doses of vitamin B_{12} are not associated with toxicity. Rare anaphylactic reactions and mild diarrhea have occurred, although vitamin B_{12} therapy has involved adverse events that result more from problems with resolution of the disease being treated (usually megaloblastic anemia) than from the high doses of B_{12} used. For example, after B_{12} therapy for megaloblastic anemia, serious hypokalemia has resulted from increased potassium requirements for erythropoiesis.[138]

PRODUCTS

Cyanocobalamin, USP. Cyanocobalamin, vitamin B_{12}, is a cobalt-containing substance usually produced by the growth of suitable organisms or obtained from liver. It occurs as dark red crystals or an amorphous or crystalline powder. The anhydrous form is very hygroscopic and may absorb about 12% water. One gram is soluble in about 80 mL of water. It is soluble in alcohol but insoluble in chloroform and in ether.

Vitamin B_{12} loses about 1.5% of its activity per day when stored at room temperature in the presence of ascorbic acid; vitamin B_{12b} (hydroxocobalamin) is very unstable (completely inactivated in 1 day). This loss in activity is accompanied by release of cobalt and a loss of color. The greater stability of vitamin B_{12} is attributed to the increased strength of the bond between cobalt and the benzimidazole nitrogen by cyanide. Unusual resonance energy is imputed to the cobalt–cyanide complex, giving a positive charge to the cobalt atom and, thereby, strengthening the Co—N bond. The protective action of certain liver extracts of vitamin B_{12b} toward ascorbic acid and its sodium salt is, no doubt, due to the presence of copper and iron. Iron salts protect vitamin B_{12b} in 0.001% concentration. Catalysis of the oxidative destruction of ascorbate by iron is well known. On exposure to air, liver extracts containing B_{12} lose most of the B_{12} activity in 3 months. The most favorable pH for a mixture of cyanocobalamin and ascorbic acid appears to be 6 to 7. Niacinamide can stabilize aqueous parenteral solutions of cyanocobalamin and folic acid at a pH of 6 to 6.5; it is, however, unstable in B-complex solution. Cyanocobalamin is stable in solutions of sorbitol and glycerin but not in dextrose or sucrose.

Aqueous solutions of vitamin B_{12} are stable to autoclaving for 15 minutes at 121°C. It is almost completely inactivated in 95 hours by 0.015 N sodium hydroxide or 0.01 N hydrochloric acid. Cyanocobalamin is most stable at pH 4.5 to 5.0 and is stable in a wide variety of solvents.

Hydroxocobalamin, USP. Hydroxocobalamin, cobinamide dihydroxide, dihydrogen phosphate (ester) mono(inner salt), 3′-ester with 5,6-dimethyl-1-α-D-ribofuranosylbenzimidazole, vitamin B_{12b}, is cyanocobalamin in which the CN group is replaced by an OH group. It occurs as dark red crystals or a red crystalline powder that is sparingly soluble in water or alcohol and practically insoluble in the usual organic solvents. Under the usual conditions, in the absence of cyanide ions, only the hydroxo form of cobalamin is isolated from natural sources. It has good depot properties but is less stable than cyanocobalamin.

Cyanocobalamin Radioactive Cobalt (^{57}Co) Capsules, USP.
Cyanocobalamin ^{57}Co capsules contain cyanocobalamin in which some of the molecules contain radioactive cobalt (^{57}Co). Each microgram of this cyanocobalamin preparation has a specific activity of not less than 0.02 MBq (0.5 μCi). The USP cautions that in making dosage calculations one should correct for radioactive decay. The radioactive half-life of ^{57}Co is 270 days.

Cyanocobalamin ^{57}Co Solution, USP.
Cyanocobalamin ^{57}Co solution has the same potency, dosage, and use as described under Cyanocobalamin Radioactive Cobalt (^{57}Co) Capsules, USP. It is a clear, colorless to pink solution that has a pH range of 4.0 to 5.5.

Cyanocobalamin Radioactive Cobalt (^{60}Co) Capsules, USP.
Cyanocobalamin ^{60}Co capsules are the counterpart of cyanocobalamin ^{57}Co capsules in potency, dosage, and use. They differ only in radioactive half-life, which is 5.27 years.

Cyanocobalamin Radioactive Cobalt (^{60}Co) Solution, USP.
Cyanocobalamin ^{60}Co solution has the same potency, dosage, and use as cyanocobalamin ^{60}Co capsules. It is a clear, colorless to pink solution with a pH range of 4.0 to 5.5.

These four preparations must be labeled ''Caution—Radioactive Material'' and ''Do not use after 6 months from date of standardization.''

Cobalamin Concentrate, USP.
Cobalamin concentrate, derived from cultures of *Streptomyces* spp. or of other cobalamin-producing microorganisms, contains 500 μg of cobalamin per gram of concentrate. A cyanocobalamin–zinc tannate complex can be used as a repository form for the slow release of cyanocobalamin when it is administered by injection.

Commercial products containing liver extract for oral and parenteral use are available. Liver extract is assayed to contain 10 to 20 μg of cyanocobalamin activity per mL. Crude liver extract contains 2 μg of activity per mL.

Vitamin B$_{12}$ with intrinsic factor is a mixture whose potency is expressed in terms of oral units of hematopoietic activity. One unit has no more than 15 μg of cyanocobalamin activity. The intrinsic factor is obtained from dried hog stomach, pylorus, or duodenum. One unit contains not more than 300 mg of dried product.

Folic Acid

In the early 1940s, R. J. Williams et al.[139, 140] used the term *folic acid* in referring to a vitamin occurring in leaves and foliage of spinach, from the Latin for leaf *(folium)*. Previously, it was called *vitamin M* and *vitamin B$_9$*. Since then, folic acid has been found in whey, mushrooms, liver, yeast, bone marrow, soybeans, and fish meal, all of which are excellent dietary sources. The structure (see diagram) has been proved by synthesis in many laboratories (e.g., see Waller et al.[141, 142]).

Folic Acid

Folic acid is a pteridine derivative (rings A and B constitute the pteridine heterocyclic system) synthesized by bacteria from GTP, *p*-aminobenzoic acid, and glutamic acid. Accordingly, the structure of folic acid is composed of three moieties: the pteridine moiety derived from GTP, the *p*-aminobenzoic acid moiety, and the glutamic acid moiety. (Antibacterial sulfonamides [see Chapter 8] compete with *p*-aminobenzoic acid and, thereby, interfere with bacterial folic acid synthesis.) Humans cannot synthesize folic acid.

In the human, dietary folic acid must be reduced metabolically to THFA to exert its vital biochemical actions. This reaction, which proceeds through the intermediate dihydrofolic acid, is catalyzed by a reductase. This reductase enzyme system has been implicated as the catalyst in both reaction steps—folic acid reduction and dihydrofolic acid reduction. The coenzyme THFA is converted to other cofactors by formulation of the N-10 and/or N-5 nitrogen.

Folic Acid   Dihydrofolic Acid   Tetrahydrofolic Acid

These coenzymes derived from folic acid participate in many important reactions, including conversion of homocysteine to methionine, synthesis of glycine from serine, purine synthesis (C-2 and C-8), and histidine metabolism.

N^5	$-CH_3$	N^5-Methyltetrahydrofolic acid
N^5	$-CHO$	N^5-Formyltetrahydrofolic acid (folinic acid)
N^{10}	$-CHO$	N^{10}-Formyltetrahydrofolic acid
N^{5-10}	$=CH-$	N^{5-10}-Methenyltetrahydrofolic acid
N^{5-10}	$-CH_2-$	N^{5-10}-Methylenetetrahydrofolic acid
N^5	$-CH=NH$	N^5-Formiminotetrahydrofolic acid
N^5	$-CH_2-OH$	N^5-Hydroxytetrahydrofolic acid

The most critical "one-carbon" transfer involved in DNA synthesis requires N^5,N^{10}-methylene-THFA as the methylating coenzyme responsible for converting uridylic acid to thymidylic acid. Interestingly, some folic acid antagonists useful in cancer chemotherapy (e.g., methotrexate [see Chapter 12]) interfere with DNA synthesis by inhibiting this methylation step.[143]

There is a fundamental relationship between folic acid metabolism and vitamin B_{12}. The reduction of methylene-THFA to 5-methyl-THFA is essentially irreversible; hence, there is only one pathway for the regeneration of THFA from 5-methyl-THFA. THFA is regenerated by the B_{12}-dependent methyl group transfer from 5-methyl-THFA to homocysteine. This biochemical interrelationship has been implicated in the etiology of megaloblastic anemia (see corresponding discussion under vitamin B_{12}[136]).

PRODUCTS

Folic Acid, USP. Folic acid, *N*-[[[(2-amino-4-hydroxy-6-pteridinyl)methyl]amino]benzoyl]glutamic acid, pteroylglutamic acid (Folacine, Folvite), occurs as a yellow or yellowish-orange powder that is only slightly soluble in water (1 mg/100 mL). It is insoluble in the common organic solvents. The sodium salt is soluble (1:66) in water. Aqueous solutions of folic acid or its sodium salt are stable to oxygen of the air, even on prolonged standing. These solutions can be sterilized by autoclaving at a pressure of 15 pounds in the usual manner. Folic acid in the dry state and in very dilute solutions is decomposed readily by sunlight or UV light. Although folic acid is unstable in acid solutions, particularly below a pH of 6, the presence of liver extracts has a stabilizing effect at lower pH levels than are otherwise possible. Iron salts do not materially affect the stability of folic acid solutions. The water-soluble vitamins that have a deleterious effect on folic acid are (in descending order of effectiveness) as follows: riboflavin, thiamine hydrochloride, ascorbic acid, niacinamide, pantothenic acid, and pyridox-

ine. This deleterious effect may be largely overcome by inclusion of approximately 70% sugar in the mixture.

Folic acid in foods is destroyed more readily by cooking than are the other water-soluble vitamins. These losses range from 46% in halibut to 95% in pork chops and from 69% in cauliflower to 97% in carrots.

Folic acid occurs in the diet as pteroylpolyglutamates that must be hydrolyzed to the monoglutamates before absorption. The hydrolysis is catalyzed by pteroyl-γ-glutamyl carboxy-peptidase, found in the membrane of the intestinal mucosa. The monoglutamates are absorbed actively in the jejunum and upper duodenum. This absorption is pH sensitive and is facilitated by the slightly acidic conditions found in these regions. The vitamin is transported as monoglutamates bound to albumin.

n = 1 = Pteroylglutamic acid
n = 6 = Pteroylpolyglutamic acid

Although the mucosa in these regions possesses dihydrofolate reductase, most reduction and methylation occur in the liver. THFA is distributed to all tissues, where it is stored as polyglutamates. The N^5-methyl derivative is the main transport and storage form in the body. The body stores 5 to 10 mg, approximately 50% in the liver. The major elimination pathway for the vitamin is biliary excretion as the N^5-methyl derivative. Extensive reabsorption occurs. Only trace amounts are found in the urine. Large doses that exceed the tubular reabsorption limit, however, result in substantial amounts in the urine.

As with vitamin B_{12}, folic acid deficiencies mainly result from malabsorption or alcoholism. No neurological abnormalities are associated with folic acid deficiency. The resulting megaloblastic anemia is indistinguishable from that caused by vitamin B_{12} because both vitamins are involved in the critical biochemical step. Folic acid can correct the anemia caused by vitamin B_{12} deficiency, but it has no effect on the neurological damage. Thus, only small amounts are found in over-the-counter preparations.

Folic acid administered to healthy adults in a daily dose of 15 mg for 1 month resulted in gastrointestinal disturbances (including anorexia, nausea and pain) and central nervous system effects (including sleep disturbances, vivid dreams, malaise, irritability and increased excitability).[144]

Leucovorin Calcium, USP. Leucovorin calcium, *N*[4-[[(2-amino-5-formyl1,4,5,6,7,8-hexahydro-4-oxo-6-pteridinyl)methyl]amino]benzoyl]-L-glutamic acid, calcium salt, calcium 5-formyl-5,6,7,8-tetrahydrofolate, calcium folinate, occurs as a yellowish-white or yellow, odorless, microcrystalline powder that is insoluble in alcohol and very soluble in water.

Leucovorin Calcium

This product is used in chemotherapy concurrently with dihydrofolate reductase inhibitors to prevent damage to normal cells. It is not indicated for use in folic acid deficiencies.

Ascorbic Acid

The historical significance of vitamin C was summarized eloquently by the eminent medicinal chemist and pharmacist Professor Ole Gisvold, and the following direct quotation from the 7th edition of this textbook is an appropriate introduction to the significance of ascorbic acid in medicinal chemistry and basic biochemistry:

> The disease scurvy, which now is known as a condition due to a deficiency of ascorbic acid in the diet, has considerable historical significance.[145] For example, in the war between Sweden and Russia (most likely the march of Charles XII into the Ukraine in the winter of 1708–1709) almost all of the soldiers of the Swedish army became incapacitated by scurvy. But further progress of the disease was stopped by a tea prepared from pine needles. The Iroquois Indians cured Jacques Cartier's men in the winter of 1535–1536 in Quebec by giving them a tea brewed from an evergreen tree. Many of Champlain's men died of scurvy when they wintered near the same place in 1608–1609. During the long siege of Leningrad, lack of vitamin C made itself particularly felt, and a decoction made from pine needles played an important role in the prevention of scurvy. It is somewhat common knowledge that sailors on long voyages at sea were subject to the ravages of scurvy. The British used supplies of limes to prevent this, and the sailors often were referred to as "limeys."
>
> Holst and Frolich,[146] in 1907, first demonstrated that scurvy could be produced in guinea pigs. A comparable condition cannot be produced in rats.
>
> Although Waugh and King[147–152] (1932) isolated crystalline vitamin C from lemon juice and showed it to be the antiscorbutic factor of lemon juice, Szent-Gyorgyi[153] had isolated the same substance from peppers in 1928, in connection with his biological oxidation–reduction studies. At the time, he failed to recognize its vitamin properties and reported it as a hexuronic acid because some of its properties resembled those of sugar acids. Hirst et al.[154] suggested that the correct formula should be one of a series of possible tautomeric isomers and offered basic proof that the formula now generally accepted is correct. The first synthesis of L-ascorbic acid (vitamin C) was announced almost simultaneously by Haworth et al.[155] and Reichstein[156] in 1933. Since that time, ascorbic acid has been synthesized in a number of different ways.

This vitamin is now better known as ascorbic acid because of its acidic character and its effectiveness in the treatment and prevention of scurvy. The acidic character is due to the two enolic hydroxyls; the C-3 hydroxyl has a pK_a value of 4.1, and the C-2 hydroxyl has a pK_a of 11.6. The monobasic sodium salt is the usual salt form (e.g., Sodium Ascorbate, USP).

Ascorbic Acid

Ascorbic acid can be synthesized by nearly all living organisms, plants, and animals; but primates, guinea pigs, bats, and some other species cannot produce this vitamin. The consensus is that organisms that cannot synthesize ascorbic acid lack the liver microsomal enzyme L-gulonolactone oxidase, which catalyzes the terminal step of the biosynthetic process. Sato and Udenfriend[157] summarized studies of the biosynthesis of ascorbic acid in mammals and the biochemical and genetic basis for the incapability of some species to synthesize the vitamin. Because humans are one of the few animal species that cannot synthesize ascorbic acid, the vitamin has to be available as a dietary component.

Ascorbic acid performs important metabolic functions, as evidenced by the severe manifestations of its deficiency in humans. This vitamin is involved in metabolic hydroxylations in numerous important metabolic processes (e.g., the synthesis of steroids and of neurotransmitters and in collagen and drug metabolism). Ascorbic acid has also been implicated as important in other critical oxidation–reduction processes in human metabolism.[1]

Although ascorbic acid is an effective reducing agent and antioxidant, the biochemical functions of this vitamin are not well understood. It is controversial to consider ascorbic acid an antiviral agent, but some scientists argue that ascorbic acid is an effective cure or preventative of "common colds."[158, 159] One study provides some evidence that ascorbic acid appears to help the organism recover from viral infections through an indirect mechanism on the body's immune system.[160] Ascorbic acid has also received attention as a possible anticancer agent. In cell culture studies, ascorbic acid, both alone and in combination with copper ions, is selectively toxic to melanoma cancer cells.[161]

PRODUCTS

Ascorbic Acid, USP. Ascorbic acid, vitamin C, L-ascorbic acid (Cevitamic Acid, Cebione), occurs as white or slightly yellow crystals or powder. It is odorless and, on exposure to light, gradually darkens. One gram dissolves in about 3 mL of water and in about 30 mL of alcohol. A 1% aqueous solution has a pH of 2.7. Aqueous solutions are not very stable. The ascorbic acid in such preparations undergoes oxidation, particularly under aerobic conditions. Oxidation to dehydroascorbic acid is followed by hydrolytic cleavage of the lactone. The effect of pH on the aerobic degradation of ascorbic acid aqueous solutions has been studied by various investigators. Rogers and Yacomeni[162] found that the degradation rate shows a maximum near pH 4 and a minimum near pH 5.6. Further, if a preparation of ascorbic acid with an initial pH between 5 and 5.6 develops acidity on storage, the rate of degradation will increase as the pH decreases; hence, an initial pH in the range of 5.6 to 6 is recommended.

Ascorbic Acid   Dehydroascorbic Acid   2,3–Diketo–L– gulonic Acid

Dietary sources of ascorbic acid include citrus fruits, tomatoes, and potatoes. Although the sources of some commercial products are rose hips and citrus fruits, most ascorbic acid is prepared synthetically.

Ascorbic acid is readily absorbed by an active process. Large doses can saturate this system, limiting the amounts absorbed. Once absorbed, it is distributed to all tissue. The vitamin is metabolized to oxalic acid before excretion. Ascorbic acid-2-sulfate is also a metabolite found in the urine. Large doses result in the excretion of substantial amounts of unchanged ascorbic acid. The resultant acidification of the urine is the basis for most of the vitamin's adverse effects.

High doses of vitamin C (ascorbic acid) can lead to renal, bone, hematological and gastrointestinal effects.[32] Renal calculi due to oxalate or urate result from enhanced renal excretion of these compounds in the presence of high doses of vitamin C. Increased release of calcium and phosphorus from bone have been observed. Hematological effects include increased absorption of nonheme iron without significant increases in total body iron stores. Diarrhea, likely resulting from an osmotic effect, has been reported following large doses, and ascorbic acid tablets that lodge in the esophagus can cause local erosion. Finally, ascorbic acid has been shown to interfere with a number of laboratory tests because of its ability to act as a reducing agent and interfere with colorimetric redox assays.

The vitamin is indicated for the treatment and prevention of ascorbic acid deficiency. Although scurvy occurs infrequently, it is seen in the elderly, infants, alcoholics, and drug users. Ascorbic acid (but not the sodium salt) frequently is administered with methenamine to improve the effectiveness of this antibacterial agent. Because ascorbic acid increases iron chelation by deferoxamine, it is used in the treatment of chronic iron toxicity. It is also a useful adjunct in the treatment of methemoglobinemia.

Ascorbic Acid Injection, USP.   Ascorbic acid injection is a sterile solution of sodium ascorbate that has a pH of 5.5 to 7.0. It is prepared from ascorbic acid with the aid of sodium hydroxide, sodium carbonate, or sodium bicarbonate. It may be used for intravenous injection; ascorbic acid is too acidic for this purpose.

Sodium Ascorbate, USP.   Sodium ascorbate is a white crystalline powder that is soluble 1:1.3 in water and insoluble in alcohol.

Sodium Ascorbate   Ascorbyl Palmitate

Ascorbyl Palmitate, NF.   Ascorbyl palmitate, ascorbic acid palmitate (ester), is the C-6 palmitic acid ester of ascorbic acid. It occurs as a white to yellowish-white powder that is very slightly soluble in water and in vegetable oils. It is freely soluble in alcohol. Ascorbic acid has antioxidant properties and is a very effective synergist for the phenolic antioxidants such as propylgallate, hydroquinone, catechol, and nordihydroguaiaretic acid, when they are used to inhibit oxidative rancidity in fats, oils, and other lipids. Long-chain, fatty acid esters of ascorbic acid are more soluble and more suitable for use with lipids than is ascorbic acid.

Biotin

Biotin was discovered, isolated, and identified structurally in the 1930s. Previously, it was known also as vitamin H. Since then, it has been noted that small amounts of biotin can be detected in almost all higher animals. The D isomer possesses all of the activity. The highest concentrations have been found in liver, kidney, eggs, and yeast, as a water-insoluble complex. Considerable quantities are found both free and in the complex form in vegetables, grains, and nuts. Alfalfa, string beans, spinach, and grass are fair sources of this vitamin.

Biotin

Microorganisms synthesize biotin from the fatty acid oleic acid. The biosynthetic process involves numerous complex reactions that remain to be better understood. The final reaction step requires formation of the sulfur heterocycle, but the source of the sulfur is not yet known.

Although this vitamin is known to perform essential metabolic functions in the human, the minimal nutritional requirement has not been established because it has been difficult to quantify the amounts of the vitamin made available by intestinal microorganisms. Nevertheless, deficiency states may develop as a result of prolonged feeding of large quantities of raw egg white. Raw egg white contains avidin, a protein that complexes biotin and minimizes its absorption from the gastrointestinal tract. The symptoms of biotin deficiency include dermatitis, hyperesthesia, and glossitis.

Biotin performs vital metabolic functions in important carboxylation processes in the form of carboxybiotin, which is in combination with a carboxylase, as represented below.

$$Biotin-enzyme + HCO_3 \xrightleftharpoons{Mg^{2+}}$$
$$CO_2-biotin-enzyme + ADP + Pi$$

The oxygen for ATP cleavage is derived from bicarbonate and appears in the Pi.

CO₂–Biotin Enzyme

Purified preparations of acetyl-CoA carboxylase contain biotin (1 mole of biotin per 350,000 g of protein [enzyme]). It catalyzes the first step in palmitate synthesis as follows:

$$CH_3COSCoA + HCO_3 + ATP \xrightleftharpoons{Mg^{2+}} {}^-OOCCH_2COSCoA + ADP + Pi$$

Biotin also appears to be associated intimately in carboxylation by β-methylerotonyl-CoA carboxylase, propionyl-CoA carboxylase, pyruvate carboxylase, and methylmalonyloxalacetic transcarboxylase.

Biotin is also joined in an amide linkage to the ε-amino group of a lysine residue of carbamyl phosphate synthetase (CPS) to form biotin–CPS, which participates with two ATPs, HCO_3^-, and glutamine in the synthesis of carbamyl phosphate. This takes place stepwise as follows:

1. Biotin CPS + ATP + HCO_3^- ↔ carbonic phosphoric anhydride biotin–CPS (CPA biotin–CPS) + ADP
2. CPA biotin–CPS ↔ $^-$OOC–biotin–CPS + Pi
3. $^-$OOC–biotin–CPS + glutamine ↔ H_2NOC–biotin–CPS + ATP ↔ biotin–CPS + carbamyl phosphate + ADP

Carbamyl phosphate can participate in amino acid metabolism and some nucleic acid syntheses.

Biotin is absorbed readily from the gastrointestinal tract. The body appears unable to break the fused imidazolidine and tetrahydrothiophene ring system. Biotin appears in the urine, predominantly as the unchanged molecule. Only small amounts of the metabolites biotin sulfoxide and bisnorbiotin appear in the urine.

MISCELLANEOUS CONSIDERATIONS

Some dietary components are difficult to characterize as essential nutritional factors in human metabolism because the organism can produce these compounds from other dietary components. (Consider vitamin D and nicotinic acid, which are discussed above.) Vitamin D and nicotinic acid, however, generally are considered among the classic vitamins. Moreover, there is no clear consensus on the necessity for inositol, choline, and *p*-aminobenzoic acid. Nevertheless, such dietary components do perform important metabolic functions; hence, a brief characterization of these follows.

Inositol. Inositol, 1,2,3,5-*trans*-4,6-cyclohexanehexol, *i*-inositol, *meso*-inositol (*myo*-inositol, mouse antialopecia factor), is prepared from natural sources such as corn steep liquors and is available in limited commercial quantities. It is a white crystalline powder that is soluble in water 1:6 and in dilute alcohol. It is slightly soluble in alcohol, the usual organic solvents, and fixed oils. It is stable under normal storage conditions.

Inositol is one of nine different *cis–trans* isomers of hexahydroxycyclohexane and is usually assigned the following configuration:

Inositol

Inositol has been found in most plant and animal tissues. It has been isolated from cereal grains, other plant parts, eggs, blood, milk, liver, brain, kidney, heart muscle, and other sources. The concentration of inositol in leaves reaches a maximum shortly before the fruit ripens. Good sources of this factor are fruits, especially citrus fruits,[163] and cereal grains. Inositol occurs free and combined in nature. In plants, it is present chiefly as the well-known phytic acid, which is inositol hexaphosphate. It is also present in the phosphatide fraction of soybean as a glycoside. In animals, much of it occurs free.[164] Inositol in the form of phosphoinositides is almost as widely distributed as inositol, and some of these forms are more active metabolically. Phosphatidylinositol (monophosphoinositide) is the most widely distributed of the inositides, and the chief fatty acid residue is stearic acid.

Phosphoinositides serve as storage forms for secondary messengers. Phosphoinositides compose only a minor fraction (2-8%) of the lipids in cell membranes, yet they can be converted to at least three intracellular messenger molecules: arachidonic acid, inositol 1,4,5-trisphosphate (IP_3), and 1,2-diacylglycerol (DAG). The functions of arachidonic acid derivatives are discussed in Chapter 24. IP_3 releases intracellular calcium, and DAG is an essential cofactor in the activation of protein kinase C.[165]

The binding of many different hormones, neurotransmitters, and growth factors to the cell surface results in activation of the polyphosphoinositide receptor system.[166] Binding to the specific receptor activates the enzyme phospholipase C through the intermediacy of a G protein. Phospholipase C converts phosphatidylinositol 4,5-bisphosphate (PIP_2) into IP_3 and DAG. IP_3 releases calcium ion, which in turn affects many cellular responses in the target cells.

IP_3 is also converted to inositol 1,3,4,5-tetrakisphosphate (IP_4). IP_4 also acts as an intracellular messenger, resulting in an influx of extracellular calcium. IP_4 is converted to IP_3(1,3,4), which is dephosphorylated stepwise to inositol 1,4-diphosphate, inositol 1-phosphate, then inositol. The inositol is then incorporated into DAG to form phosphatidylinositol (PI). PI is sequentially phosphorylated to form phosphatidylinositol 4-phosphate (PIP) and PIP_2.

The DAG released has several possible fates. It can be converted to PI, as mentioned, or it can be hydrolyzed further to release the arachidonic acid component. DAG in conjunction with calcium ion stimulates protein kinase C. By phosphorylating proteins, kinases regulate many cellular activities. The cycle is completed by the phosphorylation of DAG to phosphatidic acid, which in turn is converted to PI. The complete system remains to be fully understood. Cyclic phosphoinositol derivatives appear also to be secondary messengers.

Inositol is a growth factor for a wide variety of human cell lines in tissue culture. It is considered a characteristic

Phosphatidylinositol PIP₂

Inositol Trisphosphate IP₃

Diacylglycerol DAG

component of seminal fluid, and the content is an index of the secretory activity of the seminal vesicles.

Evidence is accumulating that inositol will reduce elevated blood cholesterol levels. This in turn may prevent or mitigate cholesterol depositions in the intima of blood vessels in humans and animals and, therefore, be of value in atherosclerosis. Inositol has also been considered a lipotropic agent. Because humans can synthesize inositol, the need for it as a nutritional requirement has not been proved.[2]

Methionine, USP. An adequate diet should provide the methionine necessary for normal metabolism in the human. Methionine is considered an essential amino acid in humans. It is the precursor in the biosynthesis of *S*-adenosylmethionine, which is an important methylating coenzyme involved in a variety of methylations (e.g., N-methylation of norepinephrine to form epinephrine and O-methylation of catecholamines catalyzed by catechol-*O*-methyltransferases). Adenosylmethionine also participates in the methylation of phosphatidylethanolamine to form phosphatidylcholine, but this pathway is not efficient enough to provide all of the choline required by higher animals; hence, adequate dietary availability of choline is necessary.[2]

Methionine

Choline. Choline is a component of many biomembranes and plasma phospholipids. Dietary sources include eggs, fish, liver, milk, and vegetables. These sources provide choline primarily as the phospholipid lecithin. Lecithin is hydrolyzed to glycerophosphorylcholine by the intestinal mucosa before absorption. The liver liberates choline. Choline can be biosynthesized by humans; consequently, it cannot be considered a true vitamin. Biosynthesis involves methylation of ethanolamine. The methyl groups are provided by methionine or by a reaction involving vitamin B_{12} and folic acid. Therefore, deficiencies can occur only if all methyl donors are excluded from the diet.

Choline

Betaine

The therapeutic uses of choline depend on its physiological functions. Because it is involved in the formation of plasma phospholipids, it is used as a lipotropic agent to alleviate fatty infiltration of the liver, cirrhosis. It has been used, in large doses, in certain central nervous system disorders (e.g., tardive dyskinesia, presenile dementia) because it is a precursor of acetylcholine. Choline also serves as a methyl donor in some reactions after it is converted to betaine.

p-Aminobenzoic Acid, USP. *p*-Aminobenzoic acid (PABA) has been mentioned as a biosynthetic component of folic acid in bacteria, but higher mammalian organisms cannot synthesize folic acid from its precursors. Nevertheless, PABA appears to perform certain metabolic functions in some animals. In the early 1950s, PABA was reported to be an essential factor in the normal growth and life of the chick.

p-Aminobenzoic Acid

Since these original developments in this field, various claims[167] have been made for the chromotrichial value of PABA in rats, mice, chicks, minks, and humans. The problem of nutritional achromotrichia is a complex one that may involve several vitamin or vitamin-like factors and is complicated by the synthesis and absorption from the intestinal tract of several factors produced by bacteria.

PABA is a white, crystalline substance that occurs widely in the plant and animal kingdoms. It occurs both free and combined[168] and has been isolated[169] from yeast, of which it is a natural constituent. It is soluble 1:170 in water and 1:8 in alcohol and freely soluble in alkali.

PABA is thought to play a role in melanin formation and to influence or catalyze tyrosine activity.[170] It inhibits oxidative destruction of epinephrine and stilbestrol, counteracts the graying of fur attributable to hydroquinone in cats and mice, exhibits antisulfanilamide activity, and counteracts the toxic effects of carbarsone and other pentavalent phenylarsonates.[171]

When given either parenterally or in the diet to experimental animals, PABA protects them against otherwise fatal infections of epidemic or murine typhus, Rocky Mountain spotted fever, and tsutsugamushi disease.[172] These diseases have been treated clinically with most encouraging results by maintaining blood levels of 10 to 20 mg/100 mL for Rocky Mountain spotted fever and tsutsugamushi disease. The mode of action of PABA in the treatment of these diseases appears to be rickettsiostatic rather than rickettsicidal, and the immunity mechanisms of the host finally overcome the infection.

PABA appears to function as a coenzyme in the conversion of certain precursors to purines.[173] It has been suggested as an effective sunscreen as a 5% solution in 55 to 75% ethyl alcohol on excessive sunlight-exposed areas of the skin.[174]

The historical significance of the effect of PABA on the antimicrobial action of sulfonamides and sulfones has been reviewed by Anand.[175]

REFERENCES

1. White, A., et al.: Principles of Biochemistry, 6th ed. New York, McGraw-Hill, 1978, pp. 1320, 1333, 1362.
2. American Medical Association: Drug Evaluations, 3rd ed. Littleton, MA, 1977, p. 175.
3. Code of Federal Regulations. Section 101.9. 1977.
4. Funk, C. J.: J. Physiol. 44:50, 1912.
5. Drummond, J. C.: Biochem. J. 14:660, 1920.
6. McCollum, E. V., and Davis, M.: J. Biol. Chem. 19:245, 1914.
7. McCollum, E. V., and Davis, M.: J. Biol. Chem. 21:179, 1915.
8. De Luca, L. M.: Vitam. Horm. 35:1, 1977.
9. Chytil, F., and Ong, D. E.: Vitam. Horm. 36:1, 1978.
10. Wolf, G.: Nutr. Rev. 51:81, 1993.
11. Blomhoff, R.: Nutr. Rev. 53:S13, 1994.
12. Snell, E. E., et al.: J. Am. Chem. Soc. 77:4134, 4136, 1955.
13. Milas, N. A.: Science 103:581, 1946.
14. Arens, J. F., and van Dorp, D. A.: Nature 157:190, 1946.
15. Arens, J. F., and van Dorp, D. A.: Recl. Trav. Chim. 65:338, 1946.
16. Isler, O., et al.: Helv. Chim. Acta 30:1911, 1947.
17. Blomhoff, R., et al.: Physiol. Rev. 71:951, 1991.
18. Blomhoff, R., et al.: Science 250:399, 1990.
19. Wolf, G.: Physiol. Rev. 64:873, 1984.
20. Wolf, G.: Nutr. Rev. 49:1, 1991.
21. Ong, D. E.: Nutr. Rev. 52:S24, 1994.
22. Sheard, N. F., and Walker, W. A.: Nutr. Rev. 46:30, 1988.
23. Carr, F. H., and Price, E. A.: Biochem. J. 20:497, 1926.
24. Ganguly, J.: Biochemistry of Vitamin A. Boca Raton, FL, CRC Press, 1989, p. 1.
25. Goodman, P. S., et al.: J. Biol. Chem. 242:3543, 1967.
26. Goodman, D. S., et al.: Science 149:879, 1965.
27. Glove, J.: Vitam. Horm. (Leipzig) 18:371, 1960.
28. Pett, L. B.: J. Lab. Clin. Med. 25:149, 1939.
29. Hecht, S., and Mandelbaum, J.: JAMA 112:1910, 1939.
30. McLean, F., and Budy, A.: Vitam. Horm. 21:51, 1963.
31. Green, J.: Vitam. Horm. 20:485, 1962.
32. Meyers, D. G., et al.: Arch. Intern. Med. 156:925–935, 1996.
33. Melhus, H., et al.: Ann. Intern. Med. 129:770–778, 1998.
34. Lammer, E. J., et al.: N. Engl. J. Med. 313:837–841, 1985.
35. Rothman, K. J., et al.: N. Engl. J. Med. 333:1369–1373, 1995.
36. Wald, G.: Nature 219:800, 1968.
37. Morton, R. A.: Handb. Sens. Physiol. 7(Pt 1):33, 1972.
38. Kliger, D. S., and Menger, E. L.: Acc. Chem. Res. 8:81, 1975.
39. Hubbel, W. L.: Acc. Chem. Res. 8:85, 1975.
40. Honig, B., et al.: Acc. Chem. Res. 8:92, 1975.
41. Abrahamson, E. W.: Acc. Chem. Res. 8:101, 1975.
42. Williams, T. P.: Acc. Chem. Res. 8:107, 1975.
43. Hecht, S.: Am. Sci. 32:159, 1944.
44. White, A., et al.: Principles of Biochemistry, 6th ed. New York, McGraw-Hill, 1978, pp. 1173–1178.
45. Barry, R. J., Canada, F. J., and Rando, R. R.: J. Biol. Chem. 264: 9231, 1989.
46. Saari, J. C., and Bredberg, L.: Biophys. Acta 716:266, 1982.
47. Wolf, G.: J. Nutr. Biochem. 1:284–289, 1990.
48. DeLuca, L. M.: FASEB J. 5:2924–2933, 1991.
49. Leid, M., and Chambon, P.: Trends Biochem. Sci. 17:427–433, 1992.
50. Gottardi, M. M., Lamph, W. W., Shalinsky, D. R. et al.: Cancer Res. 38:85, 1996.
51. Mangelsdorf, D. J., et al.: Nature 345:224, 1990.
52. Wolf, G.: Nutr. Rev. 51:81, 1993.
53. Dawson, M. I., Elstner, E., Kizaki, M., et al.: Blood 84:446, 1994.
54. Kurie, J. M., Lee, J. S., Griffin, T., et al.: Clin. Cancer Res. 2:287, 1996.
55. Yu, V. C., et al.: Cell 67:1251, 1991.
56. Willett, M. D., et al.: Nutr. Rev. 52:S53, 1994.
57. Ross, A. C., and Ternus, M. E.: J. Am. Diet. Assoc. 93:1285, 1993.
58. Orfanos, C. E., Ehlert, R., and Gollnick, H.: Drugs 34:459, 1987.
59. Klingman, A. M., et al.: J. Am. Acad. Dermatol. 15:836, 1986.
60. Weiss, J. S., et al.: JAMA 259:527, 1986.
61. Product Information: Soritane. Nutley, NJ, Roche Pharmaceuticals, 2001.
62. Miller, W. H., Jakubowski, A., Tong, W. P., et al.: Blood 85:3021, 1995.
63. Asselineau, D., Cavey, M-T., Shrott, B., et al.: J. Invest. Dermatol. 98:128, 1992.
64. Gottardi, M. M., Bischoff, E. D., Shirley, M. A., et al.: Cancer Res. 56:5566, 1996.
65. Hall, R. W.: Inpharma Weekly 965:9, 1994.
66. Chandraratna, R. A. S.: Br. J. Dermatol. 135:18, 1996.
67. AHFS Drug Information 2000. Bethesda, MD, American Society of Health-System Pharmacists, 2000, p. 3275.
68. Mellanby, E.: Lancet 1:407, 1919.
69. Huldschinsky, K.: Dtsch. Med. Wochenschr. 45:712, 1919.
70. Bikle, D. D.: Sci. Med. 2:57–58, 1995.
71. DeLuca, H. D.: Nutr. Today 28:6–11, 1993.
72. Bhattacharyya, M. H., and DeLuca, H. F.: Biochem. Biophys. 160: 58, 1974.
73. Holick, M. F.: J. Invest. Dermatol. 77:51, 1981.
74. Makin, G., Lohnes, D., Byford, V., and Jones, G.: Biochem. J. 262: 173, 1989.
75. Reddy, G. S., and Tserng, K. Y.: Biochemistry 28:1763, 1989.
76. Fraser, D. R.: Lancet 345:104–107, 1995.
77. Marcus, R.: In Hardman, J. G., and Limbird, L. E. (eds.). Goodman and Gilman's The Pharmacological Basis of Therapeutics, 10 ed. New York, McGraw-Hill, 2001, Chap. 62, pp. 1715–1744.
78. Yagci, A., Werner, A., Murer, H., and Bilber, J.: Pflugers Arch. 422: 211, 1992.
79. Suda, T., et al.: Biochemistry 9:1651, 1970.
80. Lowe, K. E., and Norman, A. W.: Nutr. Rev. 50:138–147, 1992.
81. Sjoden, G. O. J., Lindgren, L. U., and DeLuca, H. F.: Bone, 6:231, 1985.
82. Product Information: Hectorol. Bone Care International, Madison, WI, 1999.
83. Takehashi, F., Finch, J. L., Denda, M, et al.: Am. J. Kidney Dis. 30: 105, 1997.
84. Geisman, T. A., and Crout, D. H. G.: Organic Chemistry of Secondary Plant Metabolism. San Francisco, Freeman-Cooper, 1996, p. 292.
85. Stern, M. A., et al.: J. Am. Chem. Soc. 69:869, 1947.
86. Demole, V., et al.: Helv. Chim. Acta 22:65, 1939.
87. Karrer, P., and Bussmann, G.: Helv. Chim. Acta 23:1137, 1940.
88. Weber, F., et al.: Biochem. Biophys. Res. Commun. 14:186, 1964.
89. Bieri, J. G., and Farrell, P. M.: Vitam. Horm. 34:31, 1976.
90. American Medical Association: Drug Evaluations, 3rd ed. Littleton, MA, 1977, pp. 186–187.
91. Williams, R. J.: Nutrition Against Disease. New York, Pitman Publishing, 1971, p. 148.
92. Williams, R. J., and Kalita, D. K.: A Physician's Handbook on Orthomolecular Medicine. New Canaan, CT, Keats Publishing, 1977, p. 64 [for further information].
93. Williams, R. J.: Physician's Handbook of Nutritional Sciences. Springfield, IL, Charles C Thomas, 1978 [general review].
94. Gryglewski, R. J.: Trends Pharmacol. Sci. 1:164, 1980.
95. Geisman, T. A., and Crout, D. H. G.: Organic Chemistry of Secondary Plant Metabolism. San Francisco, Freeman-Cooper, 1969, pp. 291–311.
96. Esmon, C. T., Sadowski, J. A., and Suttie, J. W.: J. Biol. Chem. 250: 4744–4788, 1975.
97. Stenflo, J., et al.: Proc. Natl. Acad. Sci. U. S. A. 71:2730–2733, 1974.
98. Nelsestuen, J. L., Zytkovicz, T. H., and Howard, J. B.: J. Biol. Chem. 249:6347–6350, 1974.
99. Stenflo, J.: Thromb. Hemost. 10:109–121, 1984.
100. Van Hisbergh, V. W. M., et al.: Blood 64:444–451, 1985.

101. Dahlbäck, B., and Stenflo, J.: Proc. Natl. Acad. Sci. U. S. A. 78: 2512–2516, 1981.
102. Suttie, J. W.: FASEB J. 7:445–452, 1993.
103. Sadowski, J. A., et al.: Structure and mechanism of activation of vitamin K antagonists. In Poller, L., and Hirsh, J. (eds.). Oral Anticoagulants. London, Arnold, 1996.
104. Olson, R. E., and Suttie, J. W.: Vitam. Horm. 35:59–108, 1977.
105. Dowd, P., et al.: J. Am. Chem. Soc. 113:7734–7743, 1991.
106. Dowd, P., et al.: J. Am. Chem. Soc. 114:7613–7617, 1992.
107. Sokoll, L. J., and Sadowski, J. A.: Am. J. Clin. Nutr. 63:566–573, 1996.
108. Dowd, P., et al.: Science 269:1684–1691, 1995.
109. Price, P. A., and Baukol, S. A.: J. Biol. Chem. 255:11660–11663, 1980.
110. Schüle, R., et al.: Cell 61:497–504, 1990.
111. Ducy, P., et al.: Nature 382:448–452, 1996.
112. Luo, G., et al.: Nature 386:78–81, 1997.
113. Nakano, T., et al.: J. Biol. Chem.270:5702–5705, 1995.
114. Hauschka, P. V., et al.: Biochem. Biophys. Res. Commun. 71: 1207–1213, 1976.
115. Shanahan, C. M., et al.: J. Clin. Invest 93:2393–2403, 1994.
116. Kulman, J. D.: Proc. Natl. Acad. Sci. U. S. A. 94:9058–9062, 1997.
117. Di Palma, J. R., and Ritchie, D. M.: Annu. Rev. Pharmacol. Toxicol.17:133–148, 1977.
118. Beers, M. H., and Berkow, R. (eds.): The Merck Manual of Diagnosis and Therapy, 17th ed. Whitehouse Station, NJ, Merck Research Laboratories, 1999, pp. 42–45.
119. Dietary Reference Intakes for Vitamin A, Vitamin K, Arsenic, Boron, Chromium, Copper, Iodine, Iron, Manganese, Molybdenum, Nickel, Silicon, Vanadium, and Zinc. Food and Nutrition Board, National Academy of Sciences, Institute of Medicine. Washington, DC, National Academy Press, 2001.
120. Isler, O., and Wiss, O.: Vitam. Horm. 17:35–87, 1959.
121. Kig, T. E., and Strong, F. M.: Science 112:562, 1950.
122. Alhadeff, L., et al.: Nutr. Rev. 42:33–40, 1984.
123. Warburg, O., and Christian, C.: Naturwissenschaften 20:688, 1932.
124. McKenney, J. M., et al.: JAMA 271:672–677, 1994.
125. Gyorgy, P.: Vitam. Horm. 20:600, 1962.
126. Coburn, S. P., et al.: Am. J. Clin. Nutr. 48:291, 1988.
127. Black, A. L., et al.: J. Nutr. 108:670, 1978.
128. Braustein, A. E.: Enzymes 2:115, 1960.
129. Ikawa, K., and Snell, E.: J. Am. Chem. Soc. 76:637, 1954.
130. Rose, D. P.: Vitam. Horm. 36:53, 1978.
131. Schaumburg, H., et al.: N. Engl. J. Med. 309:445–448, 1983.
132. Parry, G. J., and Bredesen, D. E. Neurology 35:1466–1468, 1985.
133. Rickes, E. L., et al.: Science 107:397, 1948.
134. Smith, E. L.: Nature 162:144, 1948.
135. Ellis, B., et al.: J. Pharm. Pharmacol. 1:60, 1949.
136. Herbert, V., and Das, K. C.: Vitam. Horm. 34:1, 1976.
137. Scott, J. M., et al.: Lancet 2:234, 1981.
138. Short, R. M. (ed.): Drug Facts and Comparisons January:25, 2000.
139. Williams, R. J., et al.: J. Am. Chem. Soc. 63:2284, 1941.
140. Williams, R. J., et al.: J. Am. Chem. Soc. 66:267, 1944.
141. Waller, C. W., et al.: J. Am. Chem. Soc. 70:19, 1948.
142. Angier, R. G., et al.: Science 103:667, 1946.
143. Montgomery, J. A.: Drugs for neoplastic disease. In Wolff, M. E. (ed.). Burger's Medicinal Chemistry, 4th ed. New York, John Wiley & Sons, 1979, pp. 602–604.
144. Hunter, R., et al.: Lancet 1(7637):61–63, 1970.
145. Schick, B.: Science 98:325, 1943.
146. Holst, A., and Frolich, T.: J. Hyg. 7:634, 1907.
147. Waugh, W. A., and King, C. C.: Science 75:357, 630, 1932.
148. Waugh, W. A., and King, C. C.: J. Biol. Chem. 97:325, 1932.
149. Svirbely, J. L., and Szent-Gyorgyi, A.: Nature 129:576, 609, 1932.
150. Svirbely, J. L., and Szent-Gyorgyi, A.: Biochem. J. 26:865, 1932.
151. Svirbely, J. L., and Szent-Gyorgyi, A.: 27:279, 1933.
152. Tillmans, J., et al.: Biochem. Z. 250:312, 1932.
153. Szent-Gyorgyi, A.: Biochem. J. 22:1387, 1928.
154. Hirst, E. L., et al.: J. Soc. Chem. Ind. 2:221, 1933.
155. Haworth, W. N., et al.: J. Chem. Soc. 2:1419, 1933.
156. Reichstein, T.: Helv. Chim. Acta 16:1019, 1933.
157. Sato, P., and Udenfriend, S.: Vitam. Horm. 36:33, 1978.
158. Williams, R. J.: Physician's Handbook of Nutritional Science. Springfield, IL, Charles C Thomas, 1978, p. 94.
159. Avery G. S.: Drug Treatment: Principles and Practice of Clinical Pharmacology and Therapeutics. Littleton, MA, Publication Sciences Group, 1976, p. 865.
160. Bram, S., et al.: Nature 284:629, 1980.
161. Manzella, J. P., and Roberts, N. J.: J. Immunol. 123:1940, 1979.
162. Rogers, A. R., and Yacomeni, J. A.: J. Pharm. Pharmacol. 23:2185, 1971.
163. Nelson, E. K., and Keenan, G. L.: Science 77:561, 1933.
164. Anderson, R. J., et al.: J. Biol. Chem. 125:299, 1938.
165. Majerous, P. W., et al.: Science 234:1519, 1986.
166. Nishizuka, Y.: Science 225:1365, 1984.
167. Emerson, G. A.: Proc. Soc. Exp. Biol. Med. 47:448, 1941.
168. Diamond, N. S.: Science 94:420, 1941.
169. Rubbo, S. D., and Gillespie, J. M.: Nature 146:838, 1940.
170. Wisansky, W. A., et al.: J. Am. Chem. Soc. 63:1771, 1941.
171. Sandground, J. H., and Hamilton, C. R.: J. Pharmacol. Exp. Ther. 78: 109, 1943.
172. Yeomans, A.: Am. Prof. Pharm. 13:451, 1947.
173. Shive, W., et al.: J. Am. Chem. Soc. 69:725, 1947.
174. Avery, G. S.: Drug Treatment: Principles and Practice of Clinical Pharmacology and Therapeutics. Littleton, MA, Publication Sciences Group, 1976, p. 345.
175. Anand, N.: Sulfonamides and sulfones. In Wolff, M. E. (ed.). Burger's Medicinal Chemistry, 4th ed, Part 2. New York, John Wiley & Sons, 1979, p. 1.

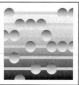

CHAPTER 27

An Introduction to the Medicinal Chemistry of Herbs

JOHN M. BEALE, JR.

According to the World Health Organization, approximately 80% of the world's population uses herbal drugs as part of their normal health care routine.[1] The United States is no exception. In the United States, herbal medicines represent the fastest growing segment of pharmacy trade.[2] Self-medication with herbs cuts across all educational and affluence levels. Senior citizens as well as young, health-conscious persons are using herbs at an incredible rate. The reasons for herbal use are many and certainly cannot be fully enumerated here. Possibly, herbal users desire to assume control over their own health care needs. Perhaps the large, "impersonal" health care system is unpalatable to many, and they turn to herbal medicines as an alternative. Patients may feel alienated by increasingly busy physicians who have less time to spend with them, and they may turn to herbal drugs because they feel that they can gain some control.

Obviously, if people are going to use herbals as part of their health care routine, they must find out about the herbs and what they do. There is no doubt that a definite major factor affecting herbal use is advertising targeted very successfully to specific populations, such as the young professional or the senior citizen. Such advertising is mere pseudoscience, but its flamboyance is a big drawing factor. Herbal ads often convey an attitude that self-medication is safe and effective, and this makes people feel good and as if they do not need the physician who just saw them for 5 minutes. People also tend to believe that natural products are inherently better than synthetic drugs. The natural drugs somehow contain the "vital force" that is going to improve their health. This is actually a belief in the vitalism principle, which Wöhler disproved in 1828.[3] Tyler puts this issue into clear terms: "If it comes in a shrinkwrap, safety-sealed box, or a bottle with a childproof lid, it is not harvested freshly from the earth. It is a manufactured industrial product, no matter how many flowers adorn the wrapper, no matter how many times the label invokes the word 'nature'."[4]

Certainly, the cost of medical care cannot be overlooked when considering the reasons for interest in alternative forms of medicine. Most herbal medicines are far less expensive than prescription drugs. There is danger, however, in self-medicating with herbal drugs. The old adage that "he who tries to diagnose himself has a fool for a physician" becomes very apropos with herbal medicine. When prescription drugs are dispensed, a patient has access to the information that is available from the physician or pharmacist. This is often not the case with herbal medicinals. In the United States, training of health care professionals in the use of herbal

drugs has been nearly nonexistent for years. Hence, herbal users are left to their own devices regarding choice, safety, and quality of the herb chosen.

Until 1882,[5] a number of drugs were monographed and described in *The United States Pharmacopoeia*. Ginseng, for example, was clearly characterized as a drug and could be labeled and described to patients as such. Today, the Food and Drug Administration (FDA) calls ginseng, legally, a "food for beverage use." Outside the United States, it is common to find ginseng recommended for many different medical conditions.[6] At the time of the 1882 *United States Pharmacopoeia* and into the early 1900s, pharmacists were well trained in the use, preparation, and dispensing of herbals and could advise patients on their herbal selection. This is not always the case today.

The convoluted regulatory efforts that began in 1906 and continue today are well described by Tyler.[7] A group of herbs had been grandfathered against the Federal Food, Drug, and Cosmetic Act of 1938 and the Kefauver-Harris amendments of 1962. Most purveyors of herbs assumed that these herbs would continue to be salable with the indications on the label—in other words, marketed as drugs. The FDA declared that all of these grandfathered drugs would be considered misbranded and subject to confiscation if any claims of efficacy were not in accordance with the evaluations of 1 of 17 over-the-counter (OTC) drug evaluation panels that had operated between 1972 and 1990. The net result was that it became possible to sell herbal drugs only if no statements regarding prevention or treatment of a disease state were on the label. The FDA assigned three categories into which herbs were placed. Category I[8] (effective) contains only a select few herbal drugs. These are mostly laxatives such as cascara bark and senna leaf (although as Tyler points out, prune juice is excluded). Category II (unsafe or ineffective) contained 142 herbs, and category III (insufficient evidence to judge) contains 116. As applied to herbs and, in fact, the entire OTC classification, the judgments of the FDA have been harmful and nonscientific.

For the most part, herbal manufacturers decided not to fight the FDA and merely removed the disease- or condition-specific information from the labels and continued to sell the herbs as foods or nutritional supplements. With regard to using herbs as food additives, the FDA has maintained a list of substances "generally recognized as safe" (the GRAS list).[9] The list contains about 250 herbs, primarily relating to their use in beverages and cooking and as food additives. The list, of course, contains no references to herbs as drugs.

In 1990, the Nutrition Labeling and Education Act required consistent, scientifically based labeling on all processed foods. Herbal medicines were still left in limbo. Finally, in 1994, the Dietary Safety Health and Education Act included herbal medicines in the definition of dietary supplements. The act ensures consumers' access to supplements on the market as long as they are safe, and it allows structure and function claims on the label. Despite all of these legislative efforts, herbal drugs have been relegated to the grocery shelf as dietary supplements. They are sold with little or no instruction, and the public has no way of ascertaining purity, standardization, or legitimacy of the use for which the product is sold. Indeed, there is more information on the label of a tube of toothpaste than on a bottle of an herbal drug. Herbal manufacturing companies are making efforts to improve products along these lines, but there is a long way to go. Until testing can be done to prove that herbs are safe and effective, they will probably remain in their present circumstances.

For many years, medicinal chemistry was paired with a science called *pharmacognosy*,[10] a course of study of plants with medicinal uses and analytical techniques for detecting active ingredients. Pharmacognosy was an important science because many of the pharmaceuticals used in the treatment of disease are discovered through the study of ethnobotanical leads and laboratory research. This course of study gave pharmacists the training required to understand, recommend, and counsel on herbs. Today, pharmacognosy is no longer required in most schools, and most practicing pharmacists and physicians have little understanding of herbs.

Medicinal herbs are unlike anything else that appears in the chapters of this book. Although they are unquestionably drugs (a fact that many sellers of herbs will dispute), they are not pure substances. Indeed, most herbal preparations contain many different constituents. Ephedra complex, or *Ma huang*, is a sympathomimetic that contains five or six different β-phenethylamine derivatives. At least one of these, (+)-norpseudoephedrine, is a Schedule IV compound. The alkaloid content[11-13] varies widely in commercial ephedra-containing preparations. In one study, for one single product, lot-to-lot variations in the content of (−)-ephedrine, (+)-pseudoephedrine, and (−)-methylephedrine exceeded 180, 250, and 1,000%, respectively.[11] Total alkaloid content among 20 products ranged from 0.0 to 18.5 mg/dosage unit, and discrepancies were exhibited between the labeled contents and actual measurements.[12] Another study assayed 9 products and found that total alkaloid levels ranged from 0.3 to 56 mg/g of ephedra.[13]

Unlike the situation with ephedra, in many cases we simply have no idea what the components do. The constituents of some herbal drugs seem to work synergistically and cannot be separated without loss of activity of the preparation. Herbal preparations are most often used as crude mixtures and are not standardized or analyzed for the content of the active principle(s). Hence, the chemistry of medicinal herbs cannot be treated in the same way as that of, say, a pure antibiotic or a calcium channel blocker. The medicinal chemistry of the actions, interactions, and side effects of herbal products is complex and difficult to assess clinically and chemically. Frequently, some of the compounds present in a given herb can be identified, but there may be no obvious way to correlate chemical structure with function. Often, assessment of structure–function relationships with herbal products involves a lot of guessing.

WHAT IS AN HERB?

An herb is a substance of plant origin that, according to one's desires, can be used for culinary or medicinal purposes.[14] Obviously, some are more suited to culinary than medicinal uses, but most herbal substances have some identifiable medicinal use. As mentioned in the previous section, a typical herb may contain dozens of different compounds, so it has rarely been advantageous to separate an herb into its component parts. In fact, doing so may completely inactivate the drug. In an herbal mixture, some compounds can reinforce others and vice versa. It is impossible to predict what will happen. In relatively few cases has the active ingredient of an herb been isolated, characterized thoroughly, and tested for activity. We are left with a situation in which herbs are used in crude form as powders, fluidextracts, and teas. The above should not be misconstrued to mean that analysis of herb components is useless. On the contrary, it is essential but just is not done often enough.

HERBAL PURITY AND STANDARDIZATION

In the United States, the issues of herbal purity and adulteration have been neglected for years. Because herbs are not regulated in the United States the same way they are in other countries, the pressure to ensure lot-to-lot standardization and to screen out plant adulterants has been less than optimal. Instances have been reported in the literature[11] in which several bottles of an herb purchased in the same location possessed different concentrations of active ingredient. Ephedra and ginseng are notable examples. Another example is echinacea. This herb is occasionally adulterated with a plant that looks very similar to *Echinacea angustifolia* but has none of the activity of echinacea. Plant parts, insect parts, soil, etc. can all be adulterants. Fortunately, pressure on the herb-producing industry has caused a markedly increased effort to screen and standardize herbs for trade. Possibly, simple high-performance liquid chromatography (HPLC) methods could be used to verify the herb's quality if the time were taken to obtain them. A chromatogram could be supplied to the purchaser to show the purity of the herb. Nevertheless, remember that an herb is a crude material containing multiple pharmacologically active compounds.

AN HERB IS A DRUG

Despite the regulations, an herbal preparation possesses the properties of a drug, albeit a mild one in many cases, and should be treated as such. It is pharmacologically active. It interacts with prescription drugs. It affects the health of the person taking it. Advertisers often tout herbs as "nondrugs" in an attempt to lure consumers. Pharmacists should be cognizant of the truth that herbs are real drugs and that their patients may be self-medicating with them. This practice may affect the outcome of therapy with prescription drugs. For example, suppose a patient is stabilized on Coumadin and starts to take ginkgo. Ginkgo affects platelet-activating factor (PAF)[15] and can effectively cause an overdose effect with Coumadin, and the patient can bleed. Or, suppose a patient taking a monoamine oxidase inhibitor (MAOI) decides to take St. John's wort; the patient may have a toxic reaction.[16] Because pharmacists often do not see what their patients are buying, this is a complex problem.

The herbal drugs available to consumers are far too numerous to discuss in this chapter. This section presents a few of the more commonly used herbs along with their chemistry. Information on other herbs can easily be found in the literature.

TYPES OF HERBS

Echinacea

The medicinal herb that we call *echinacea*, or the purple coneflower, is indigenous to the Great Plains of the United States and, indeed, can be found in much of the Western Hemisphere. The plant gets its name (coneflower) from the narrow florets, which project downward in a conical array from a prominent center toward a substantial stem that bears one flower. Today, the herb is used as an immunostimulant,[17] as a means of lessening the symptoms and duration of a cold or the flu, and sometimes as a wound healer. Recent reports show that echinacea is the best-selling herb in the United States.[3] Folklore[18] tells us that Native Americans used *Echinacea angustifolia* to treat superficial wounds, snakebite, and the common cold. In the latter part of the 19th century, settlers exchanged information about medicines with the Indians and added echinacea to their own "pharmacopoeia." Echinacea even became one of the first patent medicines, sold by a huckster in Missouri at midcentury. In the early 1900s, echinacea was introduced to the European continent, where it occupies a special place in medical therapy. One estimate stated that in Germany alone there are 800 echinacea-containing drugs, including a number of homeopathic preparations.[19]

Three species are identified as echinacea:[20] *Echinacea angustifolia, E. pallida,* and *E. purpura.* All are used for medicinal purposes, and they have similar properties. There are slight differences among the species with regard to the anatomical distribution of active constituents.

CHEMISTRY

There is no doubt that echinacea has immunomodulating properties. The chemistry of the constituents of the plant has been studied extensively, but it is difficult to correlate a major activity with any plant fraction. Indeed, no single component appears to be responsible for the activity of echinacea. Standardization of echinacea preparations has also proved to be a problem. The consumer is presented with three potential preparations sold under the name "echina-

cea"; *E. purpurea, E. angustifolia,* and *E. pallida.* Some medicinal preparations are from the roots (all three species), some from the aerial parts (*E. purpurea),* and some from the whole plant (homeopathic mother tinctures of *E. angustifolia* and *E. pallida*).[20] Another factor that affects the composition of echinacea preparations is the way in which they are extracted. Expressed juices, teas, hydroalcoholic extracts, and tinctures in alcohol are used, as well as solids. It is rarely possible to obtain reproducibility in these preparations.

In 1916, the National Formulary of the United States listed the roots of both *E. angustifolia* and *E. pallida* as official, and the distinction between the two began to be forgotten. In about 1950, *E. purpurea* was introduced as the primary medicinal plant in Europe. Of the three species, *E. pallida* is the most widely cultivated, the tallest, and has the largest flowers. This is considered the official preparation in the United States. *E. purpurea* root preparations are sometimes adulterated with a similar-looking plant called *Parthenium integrifolium.* HPLC analysis can easily detect the adulteration.[21] The above shows how difficult it is to standardize echinacea preparations. Additionally, opinions differ about which plant component is the best for analytical standardization of the drug. Echinacea contains a series of phenylpropanoid glycosides, echinacoside, verbascoside, and 6-*O*-caffeoyl echinacoside.[22, 23] These compounds possess no immunostimulating activity. Some argue that the caffeoyl glycoside echinacoside should be the standard, since it is easy to detect and quantitate; others feel that it makes little sense to standardize the echinacea preparation to a compound that has no medicinal activity.

Echinacoside	R=Glucose (1,6-)	R'=Rhamnose (1,3)-
Verbascoside	R=H	R'=Rhamnose (1,3)-
6-*O*-Caffeoylglycoside	R=6-*O*-caffeoylglucose	R'=Rhamnose (1,3)-

Several fractions of echinacea have been isolated according to polarity and studied for pharmacological activity. The most polar components, the polysaccharides, yielded two immunostimulatory polysaccharides, PS1 and PS2.[24] These stimulate phagocytosis in vivo and in vitro and cause a burst of production of oxygen radicals by macrophages in a dose-dependent way. PS1 is a 4-*O*-methylglucuronoarabinxylan with a molecular weight (MW) of 35,000. PS2 is an acidic arabinorhamnogalactan with an average MW of 45,000. Luettig et al.[25] have shown that different concentrations of polysaccharides from *E. purpurea* could stimulate macrophages to release tumor necrosis factor-α (TNF-α). These constituents also activate B cells and stimulate the production of interleukin-1. Three glycoproteins have also been isolated that exhibit B-cell–stimulating activity and induce the release of interleukin-1, TNF-α, and interferon (IFN) from macrophages, both in vitro and in vivo.[22]

Alcoholic tinctures of the aerial parts and roots of echinacea contain caffeic acid derivatives and lipophilic, polyacetylenic compounds. The roots of *E. angustifolia* and *E. pallida* contain 0.3 to 1.7% echinacoside[26] as the principal conjugate in the plant. *E. angustifolia* contains 1,5-*O*-dicaffeoyl quinic acids (quinic, chlorogenic, and cynarin)[27] in the root tissue, allowing distinction by HPLC. Echinacoside has low bacterial and viral activity but does not stimulate the immune system. The most important set of compounds that seem to be found throughout the tissues of all of the echinacea species are the 2,3-*O*-dicaffeoyl tartaric acids, caftaric acid and chicoric acid.[28] Chicoric acid possesses phagocytic stimulatory activity in vitro and in vivo, while echinacoside lacks this activity. Chicoric acid also inhibits hyaluronidase and protects collagen type III from free radical degradation.

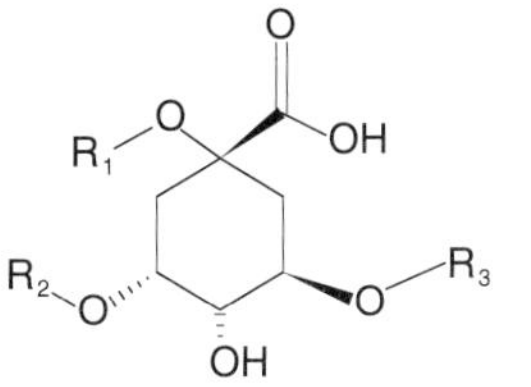

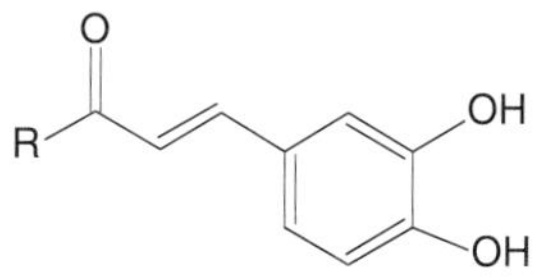

Quinic Acid	R_1=H	R_2=H	R_3=H
Chlorogenic Acid	R_1=H	R_2=R	R_3=H
Cynarin	R_1=R	R_2=R	R_3=H

Shikimate (Quinic Acid) Derivatives

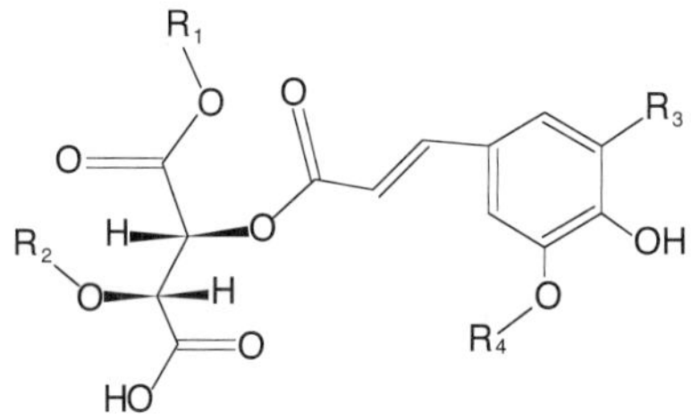

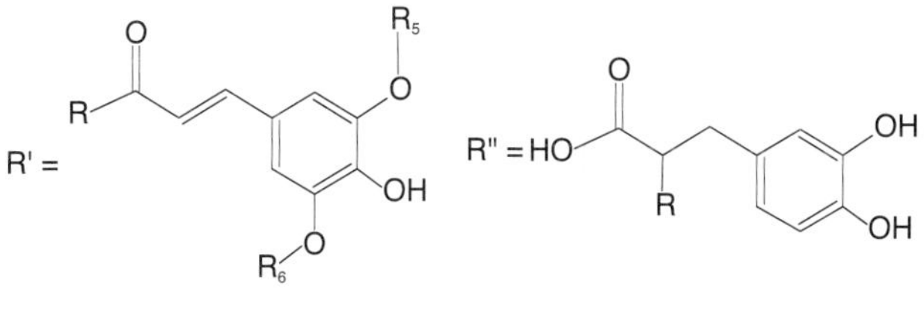

| Caftaric Acid | R_1 = H | R_2 = H | R_3 = OH | R_4 = H | | |
| Chicoric Acid | R_1 = H | R_2 = R' | R_3 = OH | R_4 = H | R_5 = OH | R_6 = H |

The alkamides[29] from the roots and flowers of *E. angustifolia* and *E. purpurea* stimulate phagocytosis in model animal systems. There are a host of these compounds distributed throughout the aerial parts of some *Echinacea* species and the roots of most. One such compound, echinacein,[28] displays sialogogue and insect repellent properties and is believed to be the main immunostimulant in echinacea. The alkamides and ketoalkynes[29, 30] may very well possess activity. One notable effect is the anti-inflammatory effect of a high-molecular-weight arabinogalactan that is about as potent as indomethacin.[25] The lipophilic fractions, the alkamides, stimulate phagocytosis and inhibit 5-lipoxygenase and cyclooxygenase (COX), blocking the inflammatory process.

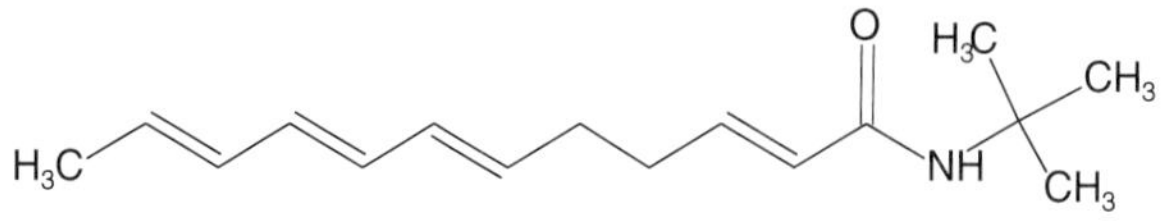

all-*trans*-Echinacein

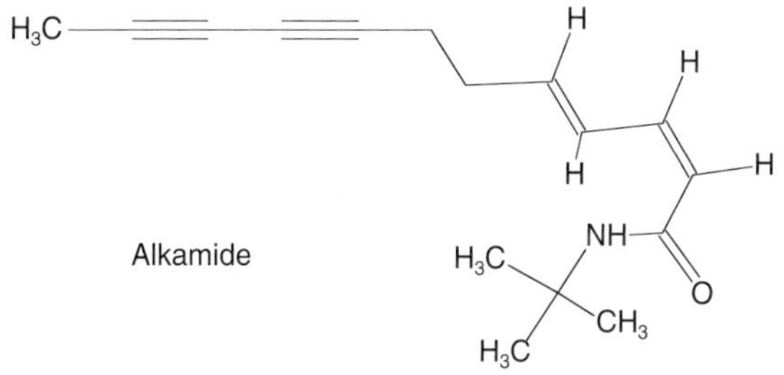

Alkamide

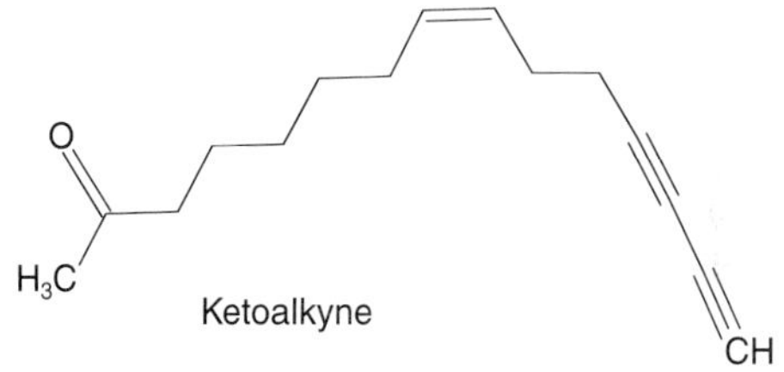

Ketoalkyne

It is clear that echinacea can stimulate components of the innate immune system, but no single component seems to be responsible for the effect. Echinacea, if taken at the onset of symptoms of a cold or flu, will lessen the severity of the disease. It is not recommended that one use echinacea longer than 10 to 14 days, however, and persons under the age of 12 and those who are immunocompromised should never use this herb.

Feverfew

Feverfew, *Tanacetum parthenium* (L.) Schultz Bip,[31] is an herb that was used in antiquity to reduce fever and pain. The literature is replete with anecdotal evidence of the usefulness of the herb, and recent clinical studies have added more support. Feverfew is a member of the aster/daisy family. The plant tissues have a pungent smell and very bitter taste. The medicinal principle of feverfew is concentrated in hairy trichomes on the chrysanthemum-like leaves.[32] The plant displays clusters of daisy-like flowers with yellow centers and radiating white florets. Recent uses of feverfew are for migraine and arthritis, although the indication for arthritis is disputable. The anecdotal evidence that an herb could successfully treat a condition such as migraine headache naturally begged for some scientific proof.

Two prospective clinical studies using dried whole feverfew leaf have been performed[33, 34] to assess the value of the herb in migraine. The two leaf studies on migraine provided good supportive evidence for activity of the herb against migraine. Both studies were double blinded, placebo controlled, and standardized on 0.54 mg parthenolide per capsule. In both studies, the feverfew group demonstrated significant decreases in frequency, severity of attacks, and nausea and vomiting. No adverse effects were observed of the nonsteroidal anti-inflammatory drug (NSAID) type.

MECHANISM OF ACTION

Feverfew inhibits prostaglandin synthesis, but not through an effect on COX.[35] The herb also inhibits the synthesis of thromboxane, again by a COX-independent mechanism. Additionally, feverfew inhibits the synthesis of phospholipase A_2 in platelets,[36, 37] preventing the liberation of arachidonic acid from membrane phospholipids for subsequent conversion to prostaglandins and thromboxane. Feverfew also inhibits the ADP-, collagen-, and thrombin-induced aggregation of platelets, suggesting that the herb has a greater thrombotic effect. In another, similar study, dried leaves of feverfew inhibited prostaglandin and thromboxane synthesis in platelets and inhibited platelet aggregation initiated by ADP and collagen.[38] Surprisingly, this study showed that feverfew inhibited the platelet-release reaction by which intracellular storage granules are released.[39] These storage granules contain serotonin, a positive effector in migraine headache. Some of the more surprising findings for feverfew are that it appears to be a selective inhibitor of inducible COX-2,[40] and it has clear effects on vascular tone in animal models.

The pharmacologically active constituent in feverfew has typically been considered to be parthenolide,[41] an amphiphilic sesquiterpene lactone that is biosynthesized from the germacranolide cation. Parthenolide is present in much greater quantities than any of the other constituents, and its presence does seem to correlate with activity, at least in dried leaves. Parthenolide is an α-methylene lactone,[42] an α,β-unsaturated molecule that can serve as an acceptor in the Michael reaction. In the Michael reaction, a donor nucleophile such as a thiol can attack the acceptor to form a covalent adduct. If parthenolide functions this way, a biological nucleophile such as a thiol on an enzyme could be bound, inactivating that enzyme. The likelihood of this mechanism has been shown by successfully forming adducts with parthenolide itself in vivo.[43, 44] The other components—canin, arteca-

3-β-Hydroxyparthenolide

nin, secotanaparthenolide, and 3-β-hydroxyparthenolide—are present in lower concentrations.[45] Their effects may be important to the activity of feverfew, but this is impossible to judge at present. One study that used an extract of the leaf with known parthenolide content failed to show activity, so questions still remain.

Saint John's Wort

Saint John's wort (*Hypericum perforatum*) is a medicinal herb that has been used since the time of Paracelsus (1493–1541) to treat a variety of psychiatric disorders. Today, the herb remains one of the most important psychotropic drugs in Germany and Western Europe for the treatment of depression, anxiety, and nervousness.[46] The drug has recently become popular among consumers in the United States. The demand for the drug in the United States has been fueled by German studies that reported that St. John's wort was equieffective with fluoxetine in the treatment of depression.

Some interesting circumstances give the herb its name. The plant is a low-growing shrub that grows wild in Europe and Western Asia with yellow flowers that bloom around June 24, the traditional birthdate of St. John. If the flowers are rubbed, a red pigment is released. This red substance has traditionally been associated with the blood of St. John released at his beheading.

The medicinal components of St. John's wort are derived from the flowering tops. A 2001 study in *JAMA*, however, negates about 30 previously published trials and showed that St. John's wort failed to improve major depressive disorder in the first large-scale, multicenter, randomized, placebo-controlled trial in patients diagnosed with major depressive disorder. The herb has a definite mild sedative effect, and in 10 years of controlled clinical trials it has proved effective in the treatment of *mild* depression.

CHEMISTRY[47]

The red components of Saint John's wort are the anthracene derivatives hypericin, present in about 0.15%, and pseudohypericin. Flavonoids present are quercetin, hyperoside, quercitrin, isoquercitrin, and rutin. Two C–C-linked biflavins, amentoflavone and biapigenin, are present, as is the acylphloroglucinol derivative hyperforin. Procyanidin, a chiral flavone dimer, adds to the list of flavones. Some terpenes and *n*-alkanes are present as minor components. The primary active ingredients have traditionally been held to be the hypericins and the flavone/flavonols, especially the hypericins. In fact, the German Commission E Monograph specifies that the herb should be standardized to hypericin content.

Despite the evidence of efficacy, the mechanism of action of St. John's wort remains unclear. Several possibilities have been put forth. Probably the most popular one is the MAOI/

Parthenolide

Canin

Artecanin

Secotanaparthenolide

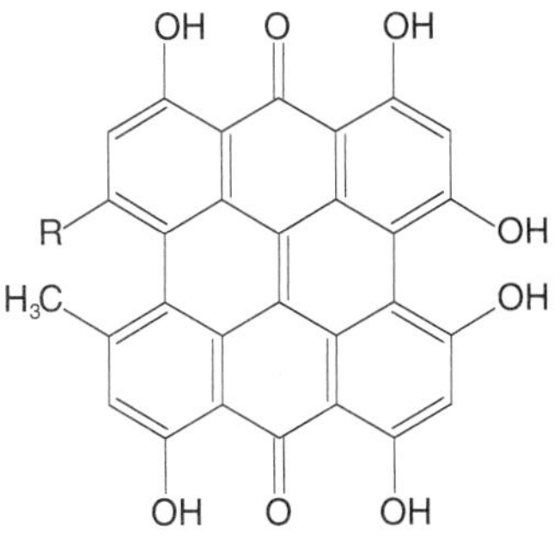

R=CH₃, Hypericin
R=CH₂OH, Pseudohypericin

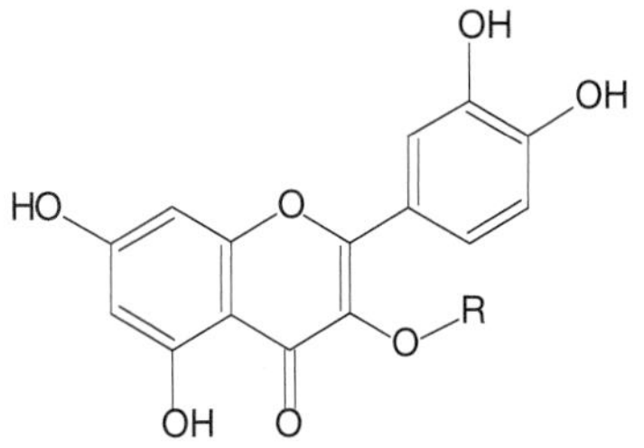

R=H, Quercetin
R=Gal, Hyperoside
R=Rha, Quercitrin
R=Glu, Isoquercitrin
R=Rha-Glu, Rutin

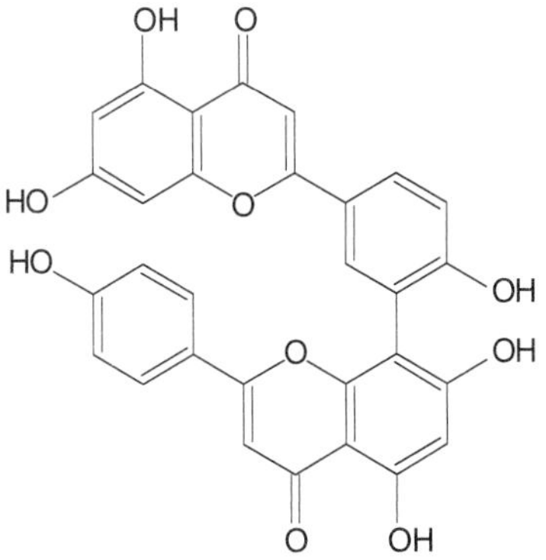

Amentoflavone

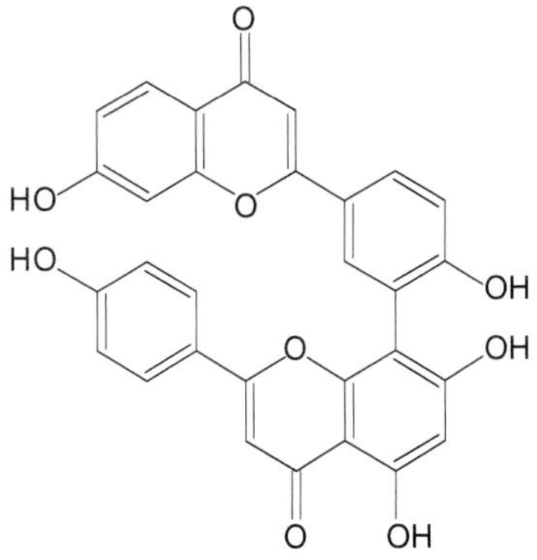

Biapigenin

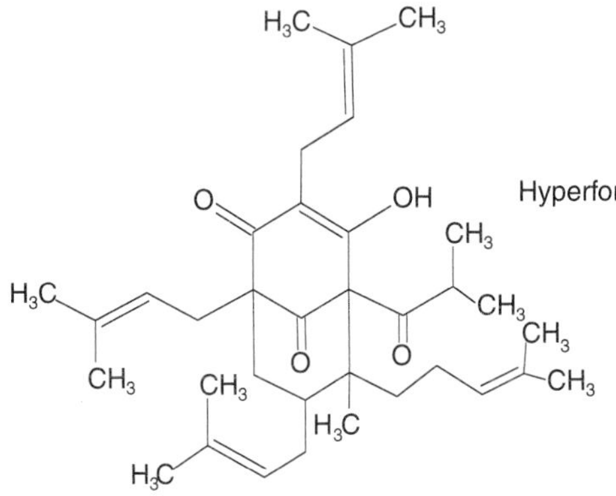

Hyperforin

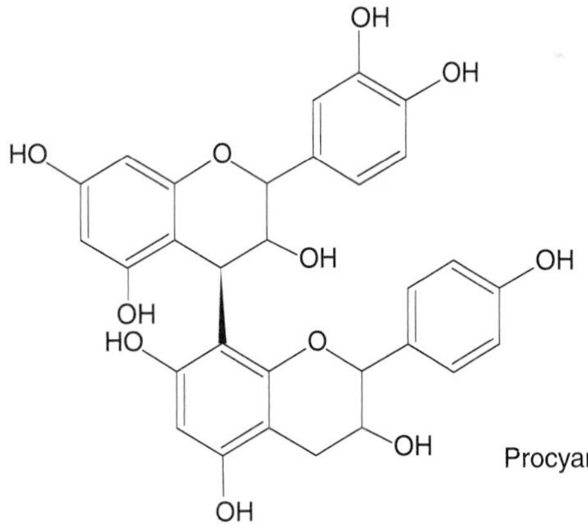

Procyanidine Dimer

COMT hypothesis. According to this hypothesis, St. John's wort increases the levels of catecholamines at the brain synapses by inhibiting their inactivation by oxidative deamination (MAOI) and by catechol functionalization (catechol-*O*-methyltransferase [COMT]).[47] Recent studies have shown that hypericins possess such activities only at pharmacologically excessive concentrations. If true, these effects at normal doses are small and do nothing to alleviate depression. Other hypotheses suggest hormonal effects or effects on the dopaminergic system. Hyperforin has become a candidate for the major antidepressant constituent of St. John's wort,

supposedly inhibiting serotonin reuptake by elevating free intracellular sodium.

St. John's wort also exhibits anti-inflammatory and antibacterial activity. Reports of antiviral activity are unsubstantiated. The main adverse effect with St. John's wort is severe phototoxicity. A sunburn-like condition may occur at normal dosages. St. John's wort should never be taken with MAOIs because of the risk of potentiation of the effects. Selective serotonin reuptake inhibitors (SSRIs) likewise should not be taken with St. John's wort because of the risk of serotonergic syndrome.

Dose (capsules standardized to 0.3% hypericin): 300 mg of standardized extract 3 times daily.

The FDA considers St. John's wort unsafe.

Capsicum (Capsaicin, Chili Pepper, Hot Pepper)

Pepper plants have been used for years as herbal remedies for pain.[48] The therapeutically useful pepper plants are members of the *Solanaceae* family. There are two primary species whose dried fruit is commonly used: *Capsicum frutescens* and *C. annum*. The actual active ingredient, capsaicin, is extracted from an oleoresin that represents up to 1.5% of the plant. Two major components in the oleoresin (among several) are capsaicin and 6,7-dihydrocapsaicin. Volatile oils and vitamins A and C occur in large quantities. The amount of ascorbic acid in the capsaicin oleoresin is reportedly 4 to 6 times that in an orange.[49]

Capsaicin

6,7-Dihydrocapsaicin

Capsaicin is supplied pharmaceutically as a cream, gel, or lotion. The first application of the preparation produces intense pain and irritation at the site of application, but usually no skin reaction occurs. Repeated applications cause desensitization, and eventually analgesic and anti-inflammatory effects occur. Stimulation of afferent nerve tracts causes a heat sensation.

There are several potential explanations for the alleviation of pain by capsaicin. There is believed to be a compound called *substance P* that mediates pain stimuli from the periphery to the spinal cord. One theory is that capsaicin depletes the neuronal supply of substance P so that pain stimuli cannot reach the brain.[50] Additionally, the methoxyphenol portion of the capsaicin molecule may fit the COX receptor site and inhibit the lipoxygenase and cyclooxygenase pathways.[49]

Capsaicin is extremely potent, so topical preparations are compounded in percentage strengths of 0.025 to 0.25%. The preparations deplete substance P most effectively if used 3 to 4 times a day. Capsaicin has been suggested as a remedy for postsurgical pain (postamputation and postmastectomy), postherpetic neuralgia, and a variety of other complex pain situations. Relief of pain may occur as quickly as 3 days or may require up to 28 days.

Patients should be instructed to wash their hands well after applying capsaicin. Contact with mucous membranes and the eyes should be avoided. If contact occurs, one should wash with cool running water.

Capsaicin as the oleoresin is used as a "pepper spray" for self-defense. Spraying into the eyes causes immediate blepharospasm, blindness, and incapacitation for up to 30 minutes.

Garlic

Garlic (*Allium sativum*)[51] is an herbal drug with references to medicinal properties that date back thousands of years. Of all the herbal remedies available to consumers, garlic is probably the most extensively researched.[52] Publications about the effects and benefits of garlic occur with great frequency. Garlic is a bulb. It may be used as such, but it is typically dried, powdered, and compressed into a tablet. Usually, the tablets are enteric coated.

CHEMISTRY

Garlic[53] contains a key component, alliin or *S*-methyl-l-cysteine sulfoxide. Additionally, methiin (methylcysteine sulfoxide), cycloalliin, several γ-L-glutamyl-*S*-alkyl-L-cysteines, and alkyl alkanethiosulfinates are present. The tissues also contain enzymes (alliinase, peroxidase, myrosinase), as well as additional sulfur-containing compounds, ajoene, and other minor components. Garlic itself has the highest sulfur content of all of the *Allium* species. When the garlic clove is crushed, the enzyme alliinase is released, and alliin is converted to allicin. Allicin gives garlic its characteristic odor and is believed to be the pharmacologically active ingredient from the herb. Alliinase will not survive the acidic environment of the stomach, so enteric-coated tablets are used.

Alliin → Allicin

Methiin

Cycloalliin

Ajoene

Garlic is most often studied for its lipid-lowering and antithrombotic[54] effects. A cholesterol-lowering effect is well documented in both animals and humans. Garlic lowers serum cholesterol, triglycerides, and low-density lipoprotein (LDL) while increasing high-density lipoprotein (HDL). Jain reported mean reductions of 6% in total serum cholesterol and 11% in LDL. Methylallyltrisulfide in garlic oil potentially inhibits ADP-induced platelet aggregation, and ajoene inhibits platelet aggregation for short periods.

Compared with the statin drugs, there is a paucity of human research data for garlic. There have been no morbidity and mortality studies for garlic, for instance. All that we can really gather from the literature is that there *may* be an effect on patient lipid profiles, but for every positive response, a negative one can be found. Garlic is certainly not harmful and can be used safely as part of a lipid-reduction program, but this should be done under a physician's supervision.

Chamomile

The herb known as chamomile[55] is derived from the plants *Matricaria chamomilla* (German, Hungarian, or genuine chamomile) and *Anthemis nobilis* (English, Roman, or common chamomile). Plants from the two genera have similar activities. The medicinal components are obtained from the flowering tops. The flowers are dried and used for chamomile teas and extracts. Chamomile has been used medicinally for at least 2,000 years. The Romans used the herb for its medicinal properties, which they knew were antispasmodic and sedative. The herb also has a long history in the treatment of digestive and rheumatic disorders.

The activity of chamomile is found in a light blue essential oil that composes only 0.5% of the flower. The blue color is due to chamazulene, 7-ethyl-1,4-dimethylazulene. This compound is actually a by-product of processing the herb. The major component of the oil is the sesquiterpene $(-)$-α-bisabolol. Also present are apigenin, angelic acid, tiglic acid, the terpene precursors (farnesol, nerolidol, and germacranolide) coumarin, scopoletin-7-glucoside, umbelliferone, and herniarin. Much of the effect of chamomile is due to bisabolol. Bisabolol is a highly active anti-inflammatory agent in a variety of rodent inflammation and arthritis tests. In addition, bisabolol shortens the healing time of burns and ulcers in animal models.

The gastrointestinal (GI) antispasmodic properties of bisabolol and its oxides are well known. In fact, bisabolol is said to be as potent as papaverine in tests of muscle spasticity. Besides bisabolol, the flavone and coumarin components have antispasmodic activities. The blue compound chamazulene possesses both anti-inflammatory and antiallergenic activities, as do the water-soluble components (the flavonoids). Apigenin and luteolin possess anti-inflammatory potencies similar to that of indomethacin. These flavonoids possess acidic phenolic groups, a spacer, and an aromatic moiety that could fit into the COX receptor. None of these effects has been unequivocally documented in humans. The essential oil possesses low water solubility, but teas used over a long period of time provide a cumulative medicinal effect. Typically, 1 teaspoon (3 g) of flower head is boiled in hot water for 15 minutes, 4 times a day.

Apigenin

Luteolin

DRUG INTERACTIONS

Chamomile contains coumarins and may enhance the effect of prescription anticoagulants. The herb is an antispasmodic and slows the motility of the GI tract. This action might decrease the absorption of drugs. Chamomile preparations may be adulterated with chamomile pollen. This may cause allergy, anaphylaxis, and atopic dermatitis.

Ephedra

The varieties of ephedra (*Ephedra sinica, E. nevadensis, E. trifurca, Ma huang*, natural ecstasy, ephedrine, *Herba Ephedrae*) that possess medicinal activity grow in Mongolia or along the Mongolian border region with China. The plant itself, an evergreen with a pine odor, consists of green cane-like structures with small, reddish-brown basal leaves. In the fall, the canes, root, and rhizome are harvested and dried in the sun. The dried material furnishes the active ingredients.

ACTIVITY

Ma huang is a sympathomimetic agent. The active principles are β-phenethylamines.[11-13] These agents can stimulate the release of epinephrine and norepinephrine from nerve endings. Ma huang is a sympathomimetic stimulant in the periphery as well as in the central nervous system (CNS). It has positive inotropic and positive chronotropic effects on the heart; hence, the herb may be dangerous to people with cardiac disease. The amounts of ephedra-type compounds and the relative composition differ so widely that it is difficult to be certain what one is getting in any given preparation. Ma huang's main active ingredient is the β-phenethylamine compound $(-)$-ephedrine. Plants grown in China may contain 0.5 to 2.5% of this compound. Many ephedrine congeners are represented in the plant,[11] and many of these possess considerable pharmacological activity. Some are as follows: $(-)$-ephedrine, $(+)$-pseudoephedrine, norephedrine, norpseudoephedrine, ephedroxane, and pseudoephedroxane.

Chamazulene

$(-)$-α-Bisabolol

$(-)$-Ephedrine

$(+)$-Pseudoephedrine

Norephedrine

Norpseudoephedrine

Ephedroxane

Pseudoephedroxane

Ma huang's principal active ingredient is (−)-ephedrine. This compound is the *erythro*-D(−) isomer with the 2(*S*),3(*R*) configuration. The less potent (+)-pseudoephedrine has the *threo* 2(*S*),3(*S*) structure. Ephedrine acts as a mixed agonist on both α and β receptors.

PHARMACOLOGICAL EFFECTS

Ephedrine's actions occur through mixed stimulation of the α- and β-adrenergic receptors. The drug is a CNS stimulant that increases the strength and rate of cardiac contraction. Additionally, ephedrine decreases gastric motility, causes bronchodilation, and stimulates peripheral vasoconstriction with the predicted increase in blood pressure. The *threo* isomer (+)-pseudoephedrine causes similar effects but is much less potent than (−)-ephedrine. The claims that ephedra causes increased metabolism and "fat burning" are certainly false, and ephedra lacks anorectic effects. Any reports of successful use of ephedra preparations in weight loss probably reflect the stimulant or "energizing" effect and increased physical activity. In the United States, ephedra has been used as a recreational CNS stimulant (natural ecstasy).

E. nevadensis and *E. trifurca* are typically used in teas. The FDA prohibits preparations with more than 8 mg/dose and advises that one should not take an ephedra product more often than every 6 hours and no more than 24 mg/day. Ephedra should not be used for more than 7 days. Dosages over the recommended amount may cause stroke, myocardial infarction, seizures, and death.

Ephedra has been closely linked to methamphetamine production. There are movements in many localities to outlaw the herb. There are many drug interactions with Ma huang. β-Blockers may enhance the sympathetic effect and cause hypertension. MAOIs may interact with ephedra to cause hypertensive crisis. Phenothiazines might block the α effects of ephedra, causing hypotension and tachycardia. Simultaneous use of theophylline may cause GI and CNS effects. In pregnancy, ephedra is absolutely contraindicated (uterine stimulation). Persons with heart disease, hypertension, and diabetes should not take ephedra.

Cranberry

The cranberry plant *(Vaccinium macrocarpon, V. oxycoccus,* and *V. erythrocarpum)* is a trailing evergreen that grows primarily in acidic swamp areas. The whole berries are divested of seeds and skins, and the rest of the fruit is used as a drink or in capsule form. Cranberry juice has been used for many years as a urinary tract disinfectant. In 1923,[56] a report said that the urine of persons who consumed cranberry juice became more acidic. Because an acidic medium hinders the growth of bacteria, it was thought that acidification of the urine inhibited bacterial growth.

An analysis of cranberry juice shows that it contains many different compounds. Citric, malic, benzoic, and quinic acids are present as carboxylic acid components. With pK$_a$s of 3.5 to 5, these compounds should exist in the ionized form in the urine at pH 5.5, thus lowering the pH. We now know that acidification of the urine is not the entire story. In fact, drinking the cocktail does not appreciably acidify the urine. Two other constituents exist in the juice: mannose and a high-molecular-weight polysaccharide.[57–59] With bacteria that use fimbrial adhesins in infecting the urinary tract, mannose binds and inhibits adhesion of the type 1 mannose-sensitive fimbriae, while the high-molecular-weight polysaccharide inhibits binding of the P-type fimbriae. Hence, adhesion of many *Escherichia coli* strains, which cause over half of all urinary tract infections, is inhibited. This inhibition has the effect of blocking infection.

Dosage: Drink between 10 and 16 ounces of juice daily.

Ginkgo biloba

Ginkgo biloba (L.), also known as the maidenhair or Kew tree, has survived essentially unchanged in China for 200 million years.[60] There is a Chinese monograph describing the use of ginkgo leaves dating from 2800 BC. Today, ginkgo is extracted by an extremely complex multistep process that concentrates the active constituents and removes the toxic ginkgolic acid.[61]

The ginkgo extract is a complex mixture of both polar and nonpolar components. The more polar fractions contain flavonol and flavone glycosides. The more nonpolar fractions contain some diterpene lactones, known as ginkgetin, ginkgolic acid, and isoginkgetin, and some interesting caged diterpenes known as ginkgolide A, B, C, J, and M.[62] There is also a 15-carbon sesquiterpene (bilobalide) and other minor components. *Ginkgo biloba* extract is prepared by picking the leaves, drying them, and constituting them into an acetone-water extract that is standardized to contain 24% flavone glycosides and 6% terpenes.[60]

Ginkgolide A

Ginkgolide B

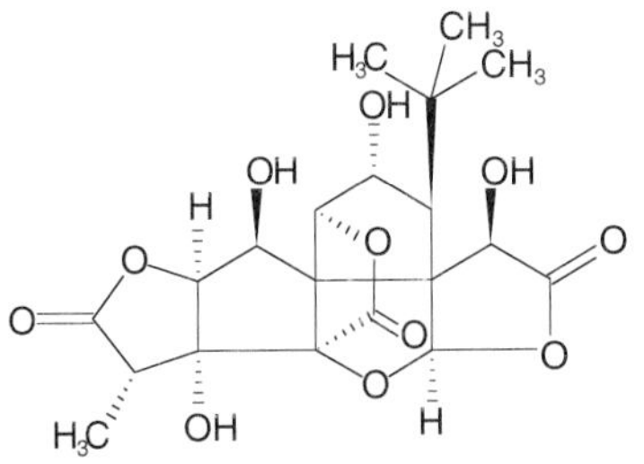

Ginkgolide C

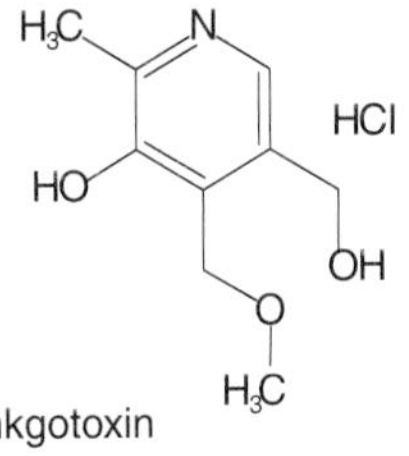

Ginkgotoxin

Ginkgo biloba produces vasodilating effects on both the arterial and venous circulation.[60, 61] The result is increased tissue perfusion (i.e., in the peripheral circulation) and cerebral blood flow. The extract produces arterial vasodilatation (rodent models), dampens arterial spasticity, and decreases capillary permeability, capillary fragility,[60] erythrocyte aggregation, and blood viscosity. There are several possible explanations for these effects. One possibility is that the compounds in *Ginkgo biloba* extract inhibit prostaglandin and thromboxane biosynthesis. It has also been speculated that *Ginkgo biloba* extract has an indirect regulatory effect on catecholamines. Ginkgolide B is reportedly a potent inhibitor of PAF.[15] In any case, the effects are due to a mixture of the constituents, not a single one.

Ginkgo biloba has become popular because of its putative abilities to increase peripheral and cerebral circulation. The herb is called an *adaptogen*,[63] a drug that helps persons handle stress. In the periphery, the herb has been compared to pentoxifylline. If the properties are true, the herb could be used for intermittent claudication. If cerebral blood flow can be increased with *Ginkgo biloba,* the herb might be useful

for disorders of memory that occur with age and Alzheimer's disease. The popular use for the herb is to help people think better under stress and to increase the length of time that someone (e.g., a student) can handle mental stress.

Ginseng

Ginseng is the root of the species *Panax quinquefolius*. This form is commonly known as American, or Western, ginseng. The shape of the root is important to many and may make it highly prized. *Panax* means "all" or "man." Sometimes, the root is shaped like the figure of a human. The doctrine of signatures would say that this root would benefit the whole person. Another species of ginseng, *P. ginseng,* is commonly called Asian, or Korean, ginseng. Chemically, the two species are very similar. Major components are named the *ginsenosides.*[64]

The chemical constituents of ginseng are called *ginsenosides* or *panaxosides.* A total of 12 of these have been isolated but are present in such small quantities that purification is difficult. Sterols, flavonoids, proteins, and vitamins (B_1, B_2, B_{12}, pantothenic acid, niacin, and biotin) are also components with pharmacological activity. The chemistry of ginseng gives a good example of how different compounds in one herb can have opposing pharmacological effects.[65] Ginsenoside Rb-1 acts as a CNS depressant, anticonvulsant, analgesic, and antipsychotic, prevents stress ulcers, and accelerates glycolysis and nuclear RNA synthesis. Ginsenoside Rg-1 stimulates the central nervous system, combats fatigue, is hypertensive, and aggravates stress ulcers. Additionally, ginsenosides Rg and Rg-1 enhance cardiac performance, while Rb depresses that function. Some of the other ginsenosides display antiarrhythmic activity similar to that of the calcium channel blocker verapamil and amiodarone.

Ginseng is popularly believed to enhance concentration, stamina, alertness, and the ability to do work. Longer term use in elderly patients is claimed to enhance "well-being." There are few data from human studies. Clinical studies comparing ginseng to placebo on cognitive function tests showed statistically insignificant improvement. Neverthe-

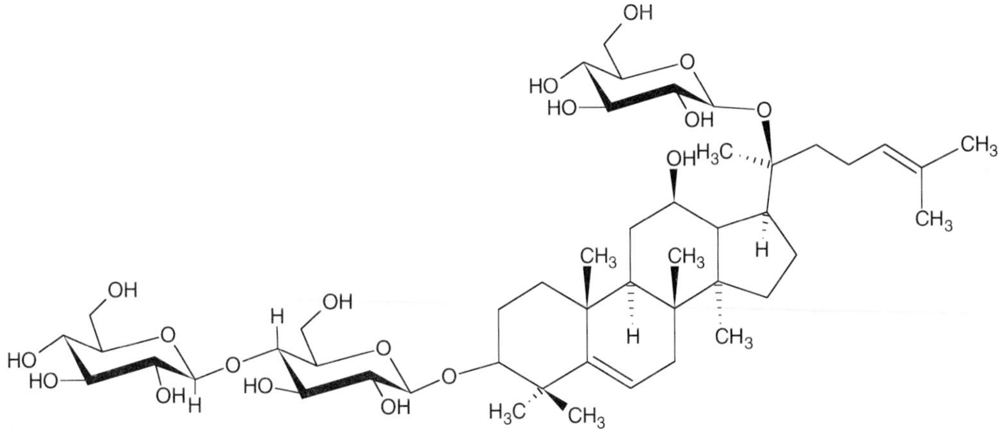

Ginsenoside R_d

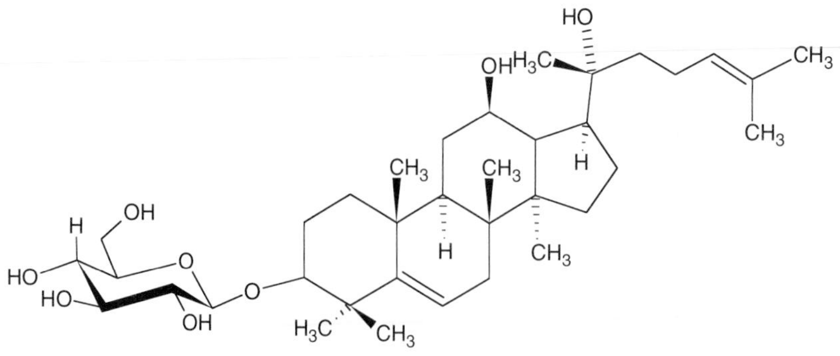

20 (*R*) Ginsenoside

less, ginseng is a popular herbal product recommended by the German Commission E.

Milk Thistle

Milk thistle *(Silybum marianum)* is a member of the Asteraceae, a family that includes daisies, asters, and thistles. The plant has a wide range around the world and is found in the Mediterranean, Europe, North America, South America, and Australia. The seeds of the milk thistle plant have been used for 2,000 years as a hepatoprotectant.[66, 67] This usage can be traced to the writings of Pliny the Elder (AD 23–79) in Rome, who reported that the juice of the plant could be used for "carrying off bile." Culpepper in England reported that milk thistle was useful in "removing obstructions of the liver and spleen and against jaundice."

CHEMISTRY

Milk thistle contains as an active constituent silymarin,[66] which is actually a mixture of three isomeric flavanolignans: silybin (silibinin), silychristin, and silydianin. Silybin is the most active hepatoprotectant and antioxidant compound of the mixture. Also present in the plant are the flavanolignans dehydrosilybin, silyandrin, silybinome, and silyhermin. Other lipid-soluble components are apigenin, silybonol, and linoleic, oleic, myristic, stearic, and palmitic acids.

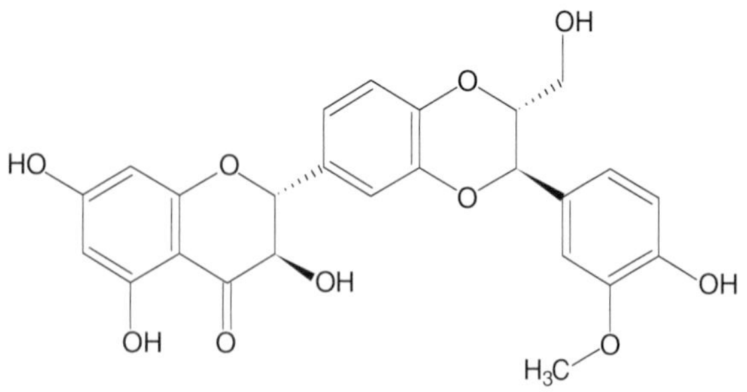

Silymarin

MECHANISM OF ACTION

The silymarin complex is aptly suited for its hepatoprotective actions.[68] Silymarin undergoes enterohepatic cycling, moving from intestine to liver and concentrating in liver cells. Protein synthesis is induced in the liver by silybin, whose steroid structure stimulates both DNA and RNA synthesis. Through these activities, the regenerative capacity of the liver is activated. Silymarin is reported to alter the outer cell membrane structure of liver cells, blocking entrance of toxic substances into the cell. This blockage is so pronounced that it can reduce the death rate from *Amanita phalloides* poisoning. Silymarin's effect can be explained by its antioxidant properties; it scavenges free radicals. By this effect, the level of intracellular glutathione rises, becoming available for other detoxification reactions. Silybin inhibits enzymes like lipoxygenase,[66] blocking peroxidation of fatty acids and membrane lipid damage. Studies also show that silymarin protects the liver from amitriptyline, nortriptyline, carbon tetrachloride, and cisplatin. When treated, patients with alcoholic cirrhosis showed increased liver function as measured by enzymes. In patients with acute viral hepatitis, silymarin shortened treatment time and improved aspartate aminotransferase (AST) and alanine aminotransferase (ALT) levels.

In liver disease, silymarin appears to have an immunomodulatory effect. The activities of superoxide dismutase (SOD) and glutathione peroxidase are increased, which probably accounts for the effect on free radicals. Silymarin, however, has an anti-inflammatory effect on human platelets. Silybin retards release of histamine from human mast cells and inhibits activation of T lymphocytes. The chemical appears capable of reducing the levels of all immunoglobulin classes and enhances the motility of lymphocytes. Milk thistle extract and its components have shown efficacy in treating hepatotoxin poisoning, cirrhosis, and hepatitis. It also plays a role in blood and immunomodulation and in lipids and biliary function. The overall effect is due to the electron-scavenging properties of flavanolignans, the enhanced regenerative capacity of the liver, and the alteration of liver cell membranes that blocks toxin entry.

Valerian

Valerian *(Valeriana officinalis)* is found in temperate regions of North America, Europe, and Asia. The dried rhizome of valerian contains an unpleasant-smelling volatile oil that is attributed to isovaleric acid. Despite the odor, valerian is a safe and effective sleep aid.

CHEMISTRY

Three classes of compounds have been linked to the sedative properties of valerian. The rhizome contains monoterpenes and sesquiterpenes (valerenic acid and its acetoxy derivative), iridoids (valepotrioates), and pyridine alkaloids.[69, 70] At present, it is not possible to state which class of compound is responsible for the sedative activity. Most researchers believe that the valepotrioate is the active component, but some studies have shown that valerenic acid is more potent.

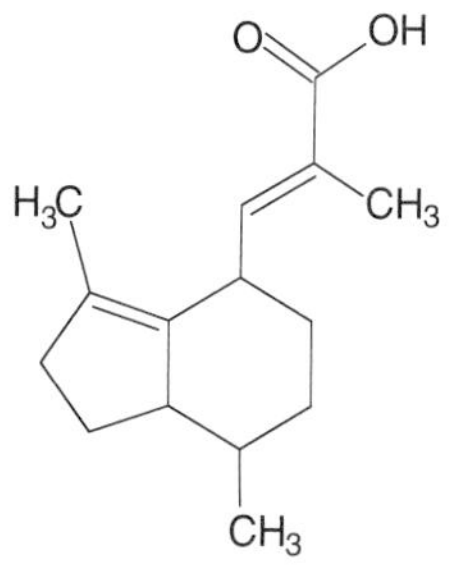

Valerenic Acid

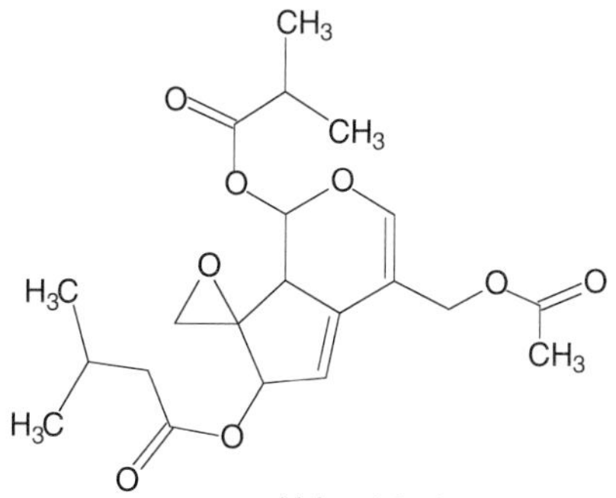

Valepotrioate

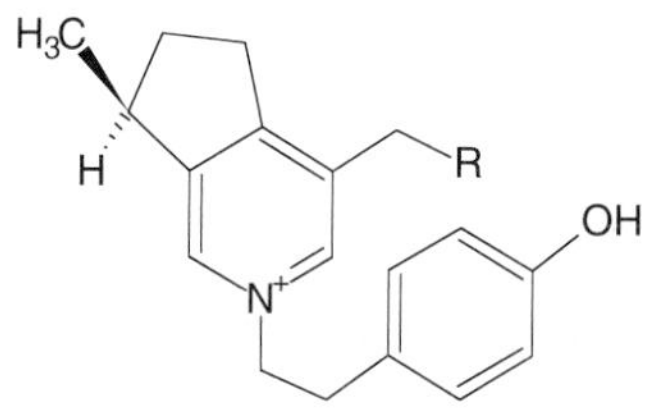

Pyridine Alkaloid

Aqueous and hydroalcoholic extracts of valerian induce the release of [^{3}H] γ-aminobutyric acid (GABA) from synaptosome preparations. The extracts appear to have much the same effects as benzodiazepines, except that valerian does not act on the Na$^+$/K$^+$-ATPase. Valerenic acid inhibits the GABA transaminase. This effect would increase the inhibitory effect of GABA in the CNS.

There is no doubt that valerian is safe and effective as a sleep aid. Used properly, it is one of the more recommendable herbs.

Dose: 400 to 900 mg standardized extract ½ to 1 hour before bedtime.

Pennyroyal

Pennyroyal *(Hedeoma pulegeoides, Mentha pulegium)* is an example of an extremely toxic herb. The plant is a member of the mint family, Labiatae. The dried leaves and flowering tops of the plant contain from 16 to 30% oil, consisting of

the monoterpene pulegone.[71] The oil also contains tannins, α- and β-pinenes, other terpenes, long-chain alcohols, piperitenones, and paraffin.

The toxicity of pennyroyal is believed to be due to the pulegone[71] in the oil. Cytochrome P-450 catalyzes the metabolism of pulegone to yield the toxic metabolite menthofuran. Possibly, some of the other terpenes undergo oxidation to active metabolites as well. Menthofuran, metabolites of other terpenes, and pulegone itself deplete hepatic glutathione, resulting in liver failure. This mechanistic hypothesis is supported by the fact that administration of acetylcysteine reverses the toxicity.

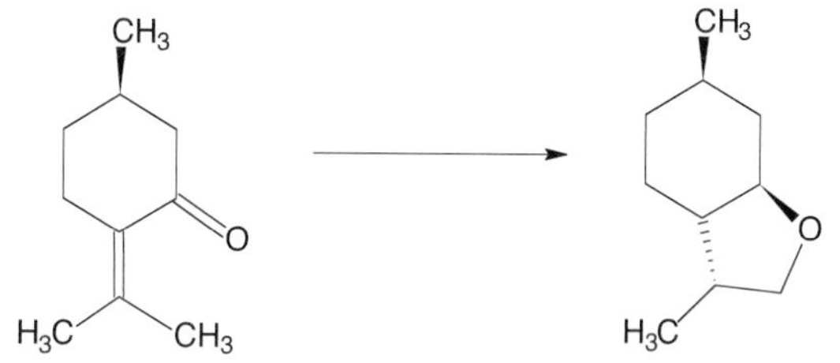

Pulegone   Menthofuran

Pennyroyal has been used as an abortifacient since the time of Pliny the Elder,[72] an insect repellent (the terpenes in the oil have citronellal-like properties), an aid to induce menstruation, and a treatment for the symptoms of premenstrual syndrome. It has also been used as a flea repellent on dogs and cats.

When used as an abortifacient, the drug often causes liver failure and hemorrhage, leading to death. Pennyroyal is sometimes used with black cohosh to accelerate the abortifacient effect. Coma and death have been reported. Pennyroyal is an example of an herb that has no safe uses. It should not be sold.

Herbal Drugs Used in the Treatment of Cancer

Anticancer drugs derived from biological sources are fairly common and are among the most important in the therapeutic armamentarium. Drugs like doxorubicin, mitomycin C, mithramycin, and bleomycin have been around for a long time and have shed much light on the treatment of cancer. Three plant-derived drugs that have found their way through clinical trials deserve mention here. Two of the most famous are vincristine and vinblastine. These are compounds isolated from the periwinkle plant *Catharanthus roseus*. The Vinca alkaloids bind tightly to tubulin in cells and interfere with its normal function in spindle formation. The Vinca alkaloids make the tubulin less stable. The net result is metaphase arrest of cell division. Paclitaxel (Taxol) was originally isolated from the needles or bark of the Pacific yew. Because it occurs in vanishingly small concentration in the plant, a semisynthetic method for its production was developed. Taxol binds to tubulin like the Vinca alkaloids, but it makes the tubulin structure hyperstable so that it cannot function. Again, the net result is metaphase arrest.

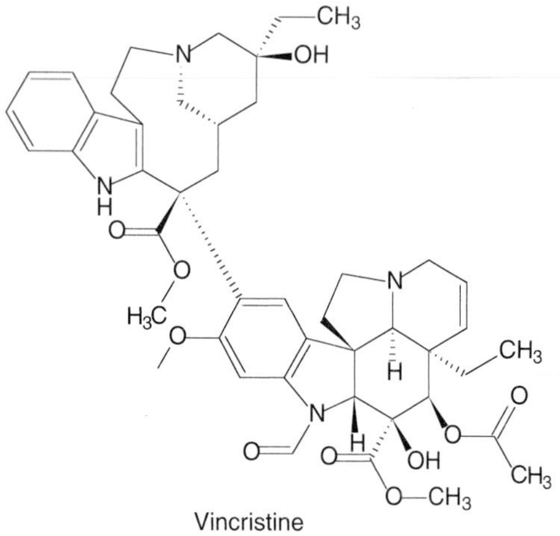

Vincristine

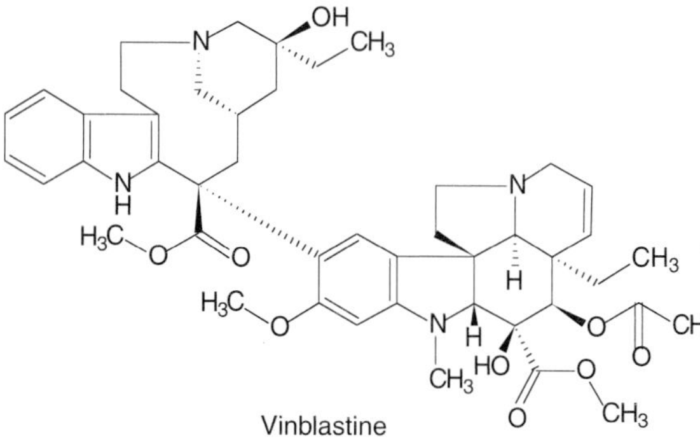

Vinblastine (57)

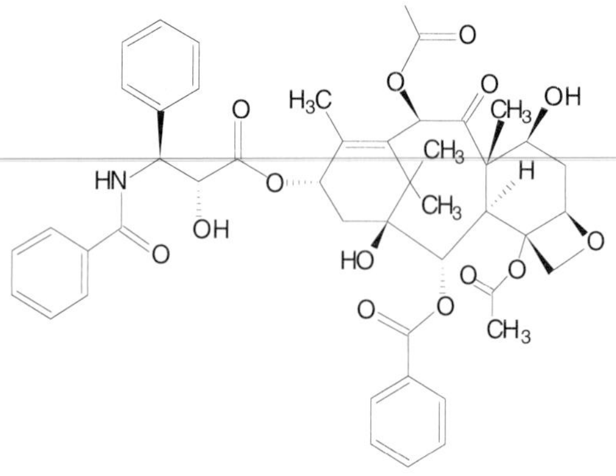

Paclitaxel

Licorice

When we think of licorice, we typically think of the popular candy. Licorice, however, has an important history in herbal medicine. Licorice is a perennial shrub that is indigenous to the Mediterranean and is cultivated in the Middle East, Spain, northern Asia, and the United States. The most common variety used for medicinal purposes is *Glycyrrhiza glabra* var. *typica*. Licorice has been used since Roman times and was described in early Chinese writings.

CHEMISTRY

The root and rhizomes of the licorice plant contain approximately 5 to 9% of a steroidal glycoside called *glycyrrhizin*. In the glycoside form, glycyrrhizin is 150 times sweeter than sugar. Also present are triterpenoids, glucose, mannose, and

sucrose. Concentrated aqueous extracts may contain 10 to 20% glycyrrhizin. When the herb is ingested, the intestinal flora catalyze the conversion of glycyrrhizin into glycyrrhetic acid, the pharmacologically active compound. Glycyrrhizin and glycyrrhetic acid possess mild anti-inflammatory properties. Glycyrrhizin appears to stimulate gastric mucus secretion. This may be the origin of the antiulcer properties of licorice. Glycyrrhizin and glycyrrhetic acid do not act directly as steroids. Instead, they potentiate, rather than mimic, endogenous compounds.

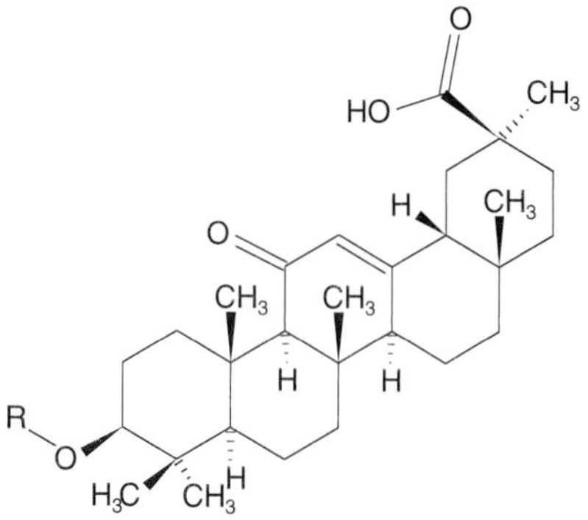

R=Glucuronyl-(1,2)-glucuronate : Glycyrrhizin
R=H : Glycyrrhetic Acid

There is some interesting folklore relating to the use of licorice. During World War II, a Dutch physician[73] noticed that patients with peptic ulcer disease improved dramatically when treated with a paste containing 40% licorice extract. The physician treated many patients in this way, but during the course of his work he noticed that there was a serious side effect from the herbal drug. About 20% of his ulcer patients developed a reversible edema of the face and extremities. Since these original observations, many studies have been conducted with licorice root. The findings have remained the same; licorice is useful for peptic ulcer disease, but potentially serious mineralocorticoid side effects are possible (lethargy, edema, headache, sodium and water retention, excess excretion of potassium, and increased blood pressure).

Licorice exerts its protective effects on the gastric mucosa by inhibiting two enzymes, 15-hydroxyprostaglandin dehydrogenase and Δ^{13}-prostaglandin reductase. Inhibition of these enzymes causes their substrates to increase in concentration, increasing the levels of prostaglandins in the gastric mucosa and causing a cytoprotective effect. The acid also inhibits 11-β-hydroxysteroid dehydrogenase,[74] thus increasing the glucocorticoid concentration in mineralocorticoid-responsive tissues, causing increased sodium retention, potassium excretion, and blood pressure.

In the 1960s, a semisynthetic compound based on glycyrrhetic acid, 4-*O*-succinylglycyrrhetic acid (carbenoxolone), was introduced in Europe. It proved effective against peptic ulcer disease, but it was later shown to be inferior to the H$_2$-receptor antagonists.

Licorice is also an effective demulcent, soothing a sore throat, and is an expectorant and cough suppressant.

Licorice can cause serious adverse reactions. These are mineralocorticoid effects (pseudoprimary aldosteronism), muscle weakness, rhabdomyolysis, and heart failure. Poisoning by licorice is insidious. Long-term high doses are extremely toxic. Licorice can potentiate the digitalis glycosides and cause toxicity. With cardiovascular agents that prolong the QT interval, the effects may be additive.

REFERENCES

1. Strohecker, J.: Alternative Medicine: The Definitive Guide. Puyallup, WA, Future Medicine Publishing, 1994, p. 257.
2. Brevort, P.: HerbalGram 44:33–46, 1998.
3. Solomons, G., and Fryhle, C.: Organic Chemistry, 7th ed. New York, John Wiley & Sons, 2002, pp. 3–4.
4. Tyler, L.: Understanding Alternative Medicine. New York, Haworth Herbal Press, 2000, p. 57.
5. Tyler, V. E.: Herbs of Choice. New York, Pharmaceutical Products Press, 1994, p. 17.
6. Duke, J. A., and Avensu, E. S.: Medicinal Plants of China, vol. 1. Algonac, MI, Reference Publications, 1985, p.122.
7. Tyler, V. E.: Herbs of Choice. New York, Pharmaceutical Products Press, 1994, pp. 17–31.
8. Blumenthal, M.: HerbalGram 23(49):32–33, 1990.
9. Winter, R.: A Consumer's Dictionary of Food Additives. New York, Crown Publishers, 1984.
10. Tyler, V. E., Brady, L. R., and Robbers, J. E.: Pharmacognosy, 7th ed. Philadelphia, Lea & Febiger, 1976.
11. Gurley, B. J., Gardner, S. F., and Hubbard, M. M.: Am. J. Health Syst. Pharm. 57(10):963–969, 2000.
12. Gurley, B. J., Wang, P., and Gardner, S. F.: J. Pharm. Sci. 87(12): 1547–1553, 1988.
13. Betz, J. M., Gay, M. L., Mossaba, M. M., et al.: J. Assoc. Anal. Chem. Int. 80(2):303–315, 1997.
14. Tyler, V. E.: Herbs of Choice. New York, Pharmaceutical Products Press, 1994, p. 1.
15. Koltai, M. et. al.: Drugs 42:9–29, 1991.
16. Suzuki, O., et al.: Planta Med. 50:272–274, 1984.
17. Haas, H.: Arzneipflanzenkunde. Mannheim, B. I. Wissenschafts, Verlag, 1991, pp. 134–135.
18. Moerman, D. E.: Medicinal Plants of Native America. Research Report on Ethnobotany, Contrib. 2, Tech. Rep. no. 19. Ann Arbor, University of Michigan Museum of Anthropology, 1998.
19. Bauer, R.: Echinacea: Biological effects and active principles. In Lawson, L. D., and Bauer, R. (eds.). Phytomedicines of Europe: Chemistry and Biological Activity. American Chemical Society Symposium Series. New York, Oxford University Press, 1998, p. 140.
20. Bauer, R.: Echinacea: Biological effects and active principles. In Lawson, L. D., and Bauer, R. (eds.). Phytomedicines of Europe: Chemistry and Biological Activity. American Chemical Society Symposium Series. New York, Oxford University Press, 1998, p. 141.
21. Bauer, R., Khan, I. A., Lotter, H., et al.: Helv. Chim. Acta 68: 2355–2358, 1985.
22. Egert, D., and Beuscher, N.: Planta Med. 58:426–430, 1988.
23. Bauer, R., Khan, I. A., and Wagner, H.: Planta Med. 54:426–430, 1988.
24. Stimpel, M., Proksch, A., Wagner, H., and Lohmann-Matthes, M.-L.: Infect. Immun. 46:845–849, 1984.
25. Luettig, B., Steinmüller, C., Gifford, G. E., et al.: J. Natl. Cancer Inst. 81:669–675, 1989.
26. Bauer, R., Remiger, P., and Wagner, H.: Dtsch. Apoth. Ztg. 128: 174–180, 1988.
27. Egert, D., and Beuscher, N.: Planta Med. 58:163–165, 1992.
28. Jacobson, M.: J. Org. Chem. 32:1646–1647, 1967.
29. Bauer, R., Remiger, P., and Wagner, H.: Phytochemistry 28:505–508, 1989.
30. Bauer, R.: Echinacea: Biological effects and active principles. In Lawson, L. D., and Bauer, R. (eds.). Phytomedicines of Europe: Chemistry and Biological Activity. American Chemical Society Symposium Series. New York, Oxford University Press, 1998, p. 150.
31. Bauer, R.: Echinacea: Biological effects and active principles. In Lawson, L. D., and Bauer, R. (eds.). Phytomedicines of Europe: Chemistry and Biological Activity. American Chemical Society Symposium Series. New York, Oxford University Press, 1998, pp. 158–159.
32. Blakeman, J. P., and Atkinson, P.: Physiol. Plant Pathol. 15:183–192, 1979.
33. Johnson, E. S., Kadam, N. P., Hylands, D. M., and Hylands, P. J.: Br. Med. J. 291:569–573), 1985.
34. Murphy, J. J., Heptinstall, S., and Mitchell, J. R. A.: Lancet ii:189–192, 1988.
35. Collier, H. O. J., Butt, N. M., McDonald-Gibson, W. J., and Saeed, S. A.: Lancet ii:922–923, 1980.
36. Makheja, A. M., and Bailey, J. M.: Lancet ii:1054, 1981.
37. Makheja, A. M., and Bailey, J. M.: Prostaglandins Leukotrienes Med. 8:653–660, 1982.
38. Thakkar, J. K., Sperelaki, N., Pang, D., and Franson, R. C.: Biochim. Biophys. Acta 750:134–140, 1983.
39. Heptinstall, S., Groenewegen, W. A., Knight, D. W., et al.: In Rose, C. (ed.). Current Problems in Neurology: 4. Advances in Headache Research. Proceedings of the 6th International Migraine Symposium 1987. London, John Libbey & Co. Ltd., 1987, pp. 129–134.
40. Bork, P. M., Lienhard-Schmitz, M. L., Kuhnt, M., et al.: FEBS Lett. 402:85–90, 1997.
41. Bohlmann, F., and Zdero, C.: Phytochemistry 21:2543–2549, 1982.
42. Kupchan, S. M., Fessler, D. C., Eakin, M. A., and Giacobbe, T. J.: Science 168:376–377, 1970.
43. Heptinstall, S., Groenewegen, W. A., Spangenberg, P., and Lösche, W.: Folia Haematol. 115:447–449, 1988.
44. Heptinstall, S., Groenewegen, W. A., Spangenberg, P., and Lösche, W. J.: J. Pharm. Pharmacol. 39:459–465, 1987.
45. Heptinstall, S., Awang, D. V. C., Dawson, B. A., et al.: J. Pharm. Pharmacol. 44:391–395, 1992.
46. German Commission E Monograph, 1999.
47. Reuter, H. D.: Chemistry and biology of *Hypericum perforatum* (St. John's Wort). In Lawson, L. D., and Bauer, R. (eds.). Phytomedicines of Europe: Chemistry and Biological Activity. American Chemical Society Symposium Series. New York, Oxford University Press, 1998, pp. 287–298.
48. Tyler, V. E., Brady, L. R., and Robbers, J. E.: Pharmacognosy, 9th ed. Philadelphia, Lea & Febiger, 1988, pp. 148–150.
49. Fetrow, C. W., and Avila, J. R.: Professional's Handbook of Complementary and Alternative Medicines. Springhouse, PA, Springhouse Corporation, 1999, p. 123.
50. Tyler, V. E.: Herbs of Choice. New York, Pharmaceutical Products Press, 1994, p. 125.
51. Gruenwald, J.: HerbalGram 34:60–65, 1995.
52. Koch, H. P., and Lawson, L. D. Garlic: The Science and Therapeutic Application of *Allium sativum* and Related Species. Baltimore, Williams & Wilkins, 1996, pp. 25–36.
53. Lawson, L. D.: Garlic: A review of its medicinal effects and indicated active compounds. In Lawson, L. D., and Bauer, R. (eds.). Phytomedicines of Europe: Chemistry and Biological Activity. American Chemical Society Symposium Series. New York, Oxford University Press, 1998, pp. 180–186.
54. Koch, H. P., and Lawson, L. D.: Garlic: The Science and Therapeutic Application of *Allium sativum* and Related Species. Baltimore, Williams & Wilkins, 1996, pp. 135–212.
55. Tyler, V. E.: Herbs of Choice. New York, Pharmaceutical Products Press, 1994, pp. 57–58.
56. Blatherwick, N. R., and Long, M. L. J. Biol. Chem. 57:815–818, 1923.
57. Sabota, A. E.: J. Urol. 131:1013–1016, 1984.
58. Soloway, M. S., Smith, R. A.: JAMA 260:1465, 1988.
59. Ofek, I., Goldhar, J., Zafriri, D., et al.: N. Engl. J. Med. 324:1599, 1991.
60. Tyler, V. E.: Herbs of Choice. New York, Pharmaceutical Products Press, 1994, p. 109.
61. Fetrow, C. W., and Avila, J. R.: Professional's Handbook of Complementary and Alternative Medicines. Springhouse, PA, Springhouse Corporation, 1999, p. 278.
62. Hänsel, R., Phytopharmaka, 2nd ed. Berlin, Springer-Verlag, 1991, pp. 59–72.
63. Fetrow, C. W., and Avila, J. R.: Professional's Handbook of Complementary and Alternative Medicines. Springhouse, PA, Springhouse Corporation, 1999, p. 279.
64. Fetrow, C. W., and Avila, J. R.: Professional's Handbook of Complementary and Alternative Medicines. Springhouse, PA, Springhouse Corporation, 1999, p. 282.
65. Tyler, V. E.: Herbs of Choice. New York, Pharmaceutical Products Press, 1994, p. 172.
66. Flora, K.: Am. J. Gastroenterol. 93:139–143, 1998.
67. Salmi, A., and Sarna, S.: Scand. J. Gastroenterol. 174:517–521, 1982.
68. Fetrow, C. W., and Avila, J. R.: Professional's Handbook of Comple-

mentary and Alternative Medicines. Springhouse, PA, Springhouse Corporation, 1999, p. 430.
69. Hänsel, R.: Phytopharmaka, 2nd ed. Berlin, Springer-Verlag, 1991, pp. 252–259.
70. Krieglstein, J., and Grusla, D.: Dtsch. Apoth. Ztg. 128:2041–2046, 1988.
71. Anderson, I. B.: Ann. Intern. Med. 124:726–734, 1996.
72. Fetrow, C. W., and Avila, J. R.: Professional's Handbook of Complementary and Alternative Medicines. Springhouse, PA, Springhouse Corporation, 1999, p. 499.
73. Nieman, C.: Chem. Drug. 177:741–745, 1962.
74. Baker, M. E., and Fanestil, D. D.: Lancet 337:428–429, 1991.

CHAPTER 28

Computational Chemistry and Computer-Assisted Drug Design

J. PHILLIP BOWEN

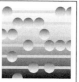

The advent of powerful and inexpensive computers has revolutionized science and medicine. Medicinal chemistry is no exception. Today, drug design methods are widely used in both industrial and academic environments. Through the use of computer graphics, structures of organic molecules can be entered into a computer and manipulated in many ways. Computational chemistry methods are used to calculate molecular properties and generate pharmacophore hypotheses. Once a pharmacophore hypothesis has been developed, structural databases (commercial, corporate, and/or public) of three-dimensional (3D) structures can be searched rapidly for "hits" (i.e., existing compounds that are available with the required functional groups and permissible spatial orientations as defined by the search query). It has become popular to carry out in silico screening of drug–receptor candidate interactions, known as *virtual* high-throughput screening (*v*HTS), for future development. The realistic goal of *v*HTS is to identify potential lead compounds. The drug–receptor fit and predicted physicochemical properties are used to "score" and "rank" compounds according to penalty functions and information filters (molecular weight, number of hydrogen bonds, hydrophobicity, etc.). Although medicinal chemists have always been aware of *a*bsorption, *d*istribution, *m*etabolism, *e*limination, and *t*oxicity (ADMET or ADME/Tox), in recent years, a much more focused approach addresses these issues in the early design stages. This is logical when one considers the compelling statistics associated with clinical evaluations of the safety and efficacy of new drugs. Only approximately 20% of compounds entering clinical trials emerge as marketable drugs. Increased efforts to develop computer-based absorption, distribution, metabolism, and elimination (ADME) models are being pursued aggressively. Many of the *predictive* ADME models use *q*uantitative *s*tructure *a*ctivity *r*elationships (QSAR). In general, understanding what chemical space descriptors are critical for drug-like molecules helps provide insight into the design of chemical libraries for biological evaluation.

With the aid of molecular modeling software, pharmaceutical scientists can modify the structural features of a potential drug candidate in silico and make predictions about its physicochemical properties prior to laboratory synthesis. Crystallographic information about the receptor has allowed scientists to use structure-based drug design approaches with tangible benefits (i.e., marketable drugs). Given the difficulty in preparing organic compounds, one can immediately appreciate the power that computer-based methods offer. Obviously, the computer-generated models must be accurate enough to give scientists a high degree of confidence in them. This means that the computer results must be compared with experimental data. Regardless of the intellectual appeal of *c*omputer-*a*ssisted *d*rug *d*esign (CADD), the methods must be validated for known cases to give confidence in the many situations when the methods will be applied to unknown cases. The inherent differences between a *model* and *reality* should always be appreciated, whether computer simulations are being used for drug design, weather forecasting, or economic prognostication.

The ability to calculate molecular properties, coupled with visualization of molecular structures, has greatly benefited scientists involved in drug discovery. Computer models of drug molecules and drug–receptor interactions are commonly found in the scientific literature. One would be hard-pressed these days to find a journal devoted to drug discovery without one paper showing computer graphics representations of drug molecules. Drug-like molecules can be displayed with molecular surfaces and color-coded according to solvent accessibility, electrostatic potentials, or other properties. With molecular modeling software, it is easy to superimpose two or more molecules. Even pharmaceutical industry marketing campaigns have brightly colored representations of drugs and their molecular surfaces splashed onto magazine ads or swirling across television screens.

In the 1980s, skeptics of the use of computer-based methods for drug discovery often asked the question: what compounds were designed by molecular modeling methods? Few convincing examples could be provided during this period, since CADD had only been in existence for a few years. Furthermore, because it is not uncommon for a drug to take 10 or more years from the design stage to final approval, the fruits of CADD would not be revealed until about a decade later. Unquestionably, many of the major advances in medicinal chemistry have used *rational* drug design but without computers. In some respects, the question regarding CADD success stories is fundamentally flawed, in that no one typically asks how many drugs were designed by a single scientific technique (e.g., nuclear magnetic resonance [NMR] spectroscopy). The NMR analogy was the often-quoted response by computational chemists. In reality, drug discovery is so undeniably complicated that no one single method generally can be credited for the complete design of a drug. An arsenal of methods from diverse scientific areas is brought to bear on drug discovery problems. The scientists involved have to interpret the data. Although molecular modeling methods are just another tool to help scientists make informed decisions on what lead compounds to pursue and what structural features should be modified to enhance biological activity, there is an inherent appeal associated with visualization and predictions. In the final analysis, scientists, not computers, "design" drugs. CADD has two fundamental roles to play in drug research: *lead discovery* and *lead development*.

During the late 20th century, there were many case histories of accurate predictions of in vitro biological activity based on so-called *rational* drug design approaches. In the 1970s, Corwin Hansch demonstrated that simple regression statistics could be used to correlate biological activity indirectly to molecular structure through physical properties such as hydrophobicity (log P), electronic (σ), and steric (E_T) effects (Chapter 2). The seminal contributions of Hansch demonstrated the power of QSAR and helped to usher in the era of computer-based modeling for molecular design. Beginning in the 1980s, there were many reports of computer-based predictions of in vitro biological activity. This is not unreasonable, since there are fewer pharmacodynamic and pharmacokinetic variables to be considered with in vitro testing than with in vivo testing. The use of structure-based design has grown in importance since the early 1980s. Today, there are many examples of drugs on the market or in clinical trials for which computer-based methods, particularly structure-based drug design, have played central roles in their development.

No single chapter can provide all the detailed information necessary to master this specialty, which ranges from quantum physics to 3D database searching. Many of the subtopics discussed have had entire books or series of books devoted to them, and a complete discussion of each topic is simply beyond the scope of this chapter and the purpose of the book. Instead, the goal of this chapter is to provide a brief and accurate overview of a select set of computational chemistry and CADD methods, highlighted with examples when appropriate. In some cases, the concepts are simplified or generalized to make sense of them in a few pages, but this is done without sacrificing accuracy so that the interested reader can continue future studies with a solid foundation in the fundamentals. Finally, computer-based methods do not replace experimental methods. In fact, the purpose of CADD is to aid pharmaceutical scientists in the discovery process, whether through simple visualization or the complex formulation of a pharmacophore model and statistical modeling.

COMPUTER GRAPHICS AND MOLECULAR VISUALIZATION

Ever since chemists have recognized that molecules are made up of atoms, there have been efforts to represent molecular structures accurately. One of the first attempts to develop molecular models can be traced to the early 1800s when John Dalton used wooden spheres drilled with holes to accept metal rod linkers as representations of atoms and chemical bonds, respectively. The original mechanical models are on display at the London Museum of Science.[1, 2]

Prior to computer graphics, the fundamental principles now associated with CADD (or molecular modeling) were used for some landmark discoveries in structural biology. Unquestionably, one of the most widely recognized scientific achievements was the construction of a DNA model proposed by Watson and Crick in 1953.[3] The structure has withstood the test of time, leading to a shared Nobel Prize for Watson and Crick and setting the stage for the age of biotechnology. Initially, crude models were crafted from cardboard. Once a better understanding of the structural requirements of the nucleic acids was developed, more accurate physical models were prepared from metal. Originally, the incorrect tautomeric forms of the heterocyclic bases were used. The incorrect tautomeric forms did not lead to any viable models of DNA, but once Watson and Crick learned that the older literature was in error, they had new nucleic acid models prepared based on the new structural data. With the correct physical models, coupled with their knowledge of the experimental data associated with DNA, they were able to construct the double helical structure[4]—an excellent example of the power of Tinkertoy sets in the right hands.

The modeling principles used by Watson and Crick to arrive at the correct representation of DNA were previously used by Linus Pauling, who correctly predicted that proteins would adopt α-helix or β-sheet conformations.[5] Pauling suggested that solid molecular models would assist in understanding molecular structure, particularly protein structures. Solid models, in which the atomic sizes of the constituent atoms are designed accurately to reflect the relative sizes (the van der Waals radii), were prepared according to International Union of Pure and Applied Chemistry (IUPAC) guidelines. These space-filling molecular models, known as CPK models,[6] became commercially available. They have been used around the world to help understand the molecular shapes of proteins and nucleic acids and their interactions with small drug-like molecules.

Commercially available handheld mechanical models became popular after the impressive structural predictions of the α-helix and β-sheet conformations for proteins, as well as the double helix for DNA. During this time, building on the work of earlier generations, Sir Derek Barton, Ernest Eliel, and others demonstrated the importance of conformational and stereochemical effects for small organic molecules. Medicinal chemists used these models and empirically derived rules to develop hypotheses for drug–receptor interactions. Wooden ball-and-stick models were used by high school and college students to help visualize organic structures. Accurate metal Dreiding and Kendrew models are still useful.[7, 8] These physical models have the advantage that medicinal chemists can hold them, manipulate them, and get a better feel for the structural flexibility. Nevertheless, large macromolecular models usually had to be supported by scaffolding, and they were notoriously troublesome to modify and manipulate. Imagine the difficulties associated with modeling the intercalation of small potential lead structures into DNA. The DNA structure would have to be cranked open mechanically, and the small potential intercalators would have to be inserted and manipulated by hand to get the best fit as determined by visual inspection.

Manipulation of computer models is much superior to the use of traditional physical models (as long as the electricity is flowing). Mathematical models using quantum mechanics or force field methods (see below) better account for the inherent flexibility of molecules than do hard sphere physical models. In addition, it is easy to superimpose one or more molecular models on a computer and to color each structure separately for ease of viewing. Medicinal chemists use the superimposed structures to identify the necessary structural features and the 3D orientation (pharmacophore) responsible for the observed biological activity. The display of the multiple conformations available to a single molecule can provide valuable information about the conformational space available to drug-like molecules. Rather than measuring bond distances with a ruler, as was done years ago with handheld models, it is relatively easy to query a computer-generated molecular display. Because the coordinates for each atom are stored in computer memory, rapid data retrieval is achieved. Moreover, the shape and size of a molecular system can be visualized and quantified, unlike the situation with handheld models, when only visual inspections are possible. Exactly how much energy does it cost to rotate torsion angles from one position to the next? Understanding drug volumes and molecular shapes is critically important when defining the complementary (negative volume image) receptor sites needed to accommodate the drug molecule.

In the 1970s, major advances were made by computer scientists because of increasing computer speeds, which allowed the generation of computer models analogous to the handheld mechanical models. Interestingly, the growth of computer graphics software was driven by the need to have computer-assisted design (CAD) tools for the aircraft manufacturing industry. In the early 1980s, software companies emerged that developed and sold model-building software to the pharmaceutical and agrochemical industries. Today, there are many different software companies that specialize in the interactive manipulations of computer-based molecular images.

High-resolution computer graphics have revolutionized the way drug design is carried out. Once a molecular structure has been entered into a molecular modeling software program, the structure can be viewed from any desired perspective. The dihedral angles can be rotated to generate new conformations, and functional groups can be eliminated or modified almost effortlessly. As indicated above, the molecular features (bond lengths, bond angles, nonbonded distances, etc.) can be calculated readily from the stored 3D coordinates. Significant work by computer scientists has been invested into giving the illusion that flickering computer images are physical 3D objects. With special viewing glasses, 3D computer images can be seen. These are relatively inexpensive and lead to impressive results. The basic idea is that the computer generates two colored images (most commonly green and red) and each structure can only be viewed by one eye. Alternatively, viewing headgear may be worn such that each lens in the glasses is synchronized with the computer monitor to open and shut. To give the illusion of 3D representations, a special optical technique known as depth cueing is used. In this method the brain is tricked into believing that slightly dimmer objects are farther away, while brighter objects are closer. Another approach is to have the molecular structure slowly rock back and forth.

Since the 1970s, the cost of hardware has decreased and the power of computers has increased dramatically. These impressive hardware advances, coupled with advances in software and more efficient algorithms, have made computer-based modeling accessible to anyone. At one time, CADD was the exclusive domain of industry and some specialized academic laboratories. Expensive computer graph-

ics workstations dominated. Today, the power of personal computers makes them an appealing and affordable alternative. Many standard molecular modeling software packages are being ported to run on personal computers, and the cost of computer graphics technology is decreasing because of the demand of the video game market.

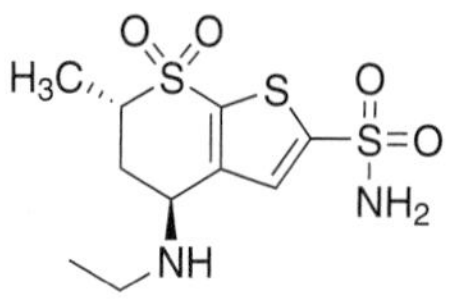

Molecular structures can be represented in many different ways, depending on the properties one decides to highlight. Dorzolamide (Fig. 28-1) is a good example of a drug that involved CADD methods in its development.[9] Figure 28-2 shows a standard representation of dorzolamide from a molecular modeling software package. The atoms can be color-coded in various ways according to the different properties that one might want to highlight. The representation in Figure 28-2 shows the connectivity of the atoms in dorzolamide that one might use during molecular modeling. As noted above, however, it is important to know the size and shape of the molecule. Various representations are possible. One is a CPK solid representation, but insight into the atomic

Figure 28-1 ■ Dorzolamide (Trusopt), the first FDA-approved drug to be designed by structure-based methods, is a carbonic anhydrase inhibitor that is used to lower ocular pressure in glaucoma patients.

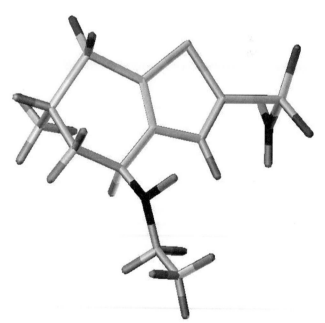

Figure 28-2 ■ A computer-generated representation of dorzolamide (Trusopt). Rather than a ball-and-stick representation, dorzolamide is shown as a tube representation with color-coded atom types. The structure has been energy minimized with the MMFF94 force field in the Sybyl (Tripos, Inc.) molecular modeling software package.

connectivity is difficult with opaque surfaces. Another convenient visualization technique is to have the atoms and bonds displayed simultaneously with the van der Waals surface represented by an even distribution of dots. These dot surfaces are convenient, in that the atomic connectivity is shown along with the appropriate size and shape of the molecular surface. As computer graphics technology has improved, it has become possible to represent the surface as a translucent volume, shown in Figure 28-3, in which the molecular structure appears to be embedded in a clear gelatin material.

Finally, computer graphics images of drug–receptor interactions, whether taken from x-ray crystal data or in silico generated, provide insight into the binding interactions, as shown in Figure 28-4. A full display of all the atomic centers in a protein structure gives too much detail. Most commonly, as shown in Figure 28-4, a ribbon structure traces the backbone of the protein main chain.[10] The Richardson approach is another commonly used display to highlight secondary structural features, in which cylinders denote α helices, arrows denote β sheets, and tubes are used for coils and turns.[11]

Because drug molecules make contact with solvents and receptor sites through surface contacts, it is paramount to have accurate methods to represent molecular surfaces correctly. Algorithms have been developed for such purposes, and they continue to be improved. The most straightforward way to represent a molecular shape is by the so-called van der Waals surface, in which each constituent atom contributes its exposed surface to the overall molecular surface. Each atom is assigned a volume corresponding to its van der Waals radius, and only the union of atomic spheres con-

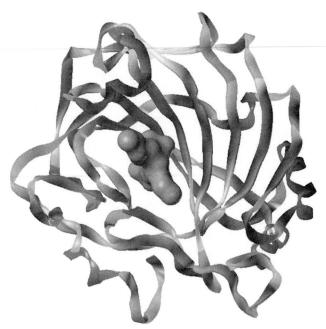

Figure 28–4 ■ A computer-generated representation of a thienothipyran-2-sulfonamide bound to the active site of carbonic anhydrase. Note that the ribbon has been traced through the protein backbone. Proteins are commonly displayed this way.

tributes. These van der Waals surfaces have small crevices and pockets that cannot make contact with solvent molecules. Another surface, known as the solvent-accessible or Connolly surface, can be generated.[12] The algorithm takes the van der Waals surface and rolls a sphere, having the volume of a water molecule with a radius of 1.4 Å, across it. Wherever the sphere makes contact with the original surface, a new surface is created. This expanded surface is a more realistic representation of what water molecules contact. Another similar solvent-accessible surface is known as the Lee and Richards surface.[13] This surface is constructed in an analogous way, with a sphere rolled over the van der Waals surface, but the boundary is taken as a line connecting the center of mass of the sphere from point to point. Also, it is possible to calculate the solvent-excluded surface. The polar and nonpolar surface areas can be used as QSAR descriptors (Chapter 2), and many computer models for solvation use solvent-accessible surface areas (SASA). Commonly, the electrostatic density may be displayed on the surface of a molecular structure, providing an easily recognized color-coded grid that may be used to infer the complementary binding functional groups of the putative receptor.

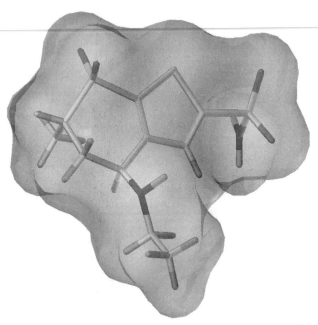

Figure 28–3 ■ Another computer-generated representation of dorzolamide (Trusopt). The structure has been energy minimized with the MMFF94 force field in the Sybyl (Tripos, Inc.) molecular modeling software package and is displayed with a superimposed translucent van der Waals surface. Such representations have the advantages of showing both the atomic connectivity of the molecular structure and its 3D shape and size.

COMPUTATIONAL CHEMISTRY OVERVIEW

Colorful molecular graphics images are based on the foundations of computational chemistry. Computational chemistry methods, which may be defined as the use of theory and computer technology to calculate molecular properties, are widely used in academia and industry to gain insights into complex problems. In many cases, computational chemistry is used to rationalize experiments and to help make sense of the massive amount of data generated. Such practices are important to answer the *why* of chemical and biological phenomena. The greatest potential power of computational chemistry, however, is in the domain of making *predictions* prior to experimental work. Computer experiments are ideally suited to help answer questions that are difficult—and sometimes impossible—to answer by experiments alone. Just what kind of predictions can be made? Energy-based calculations have been used to predict and to understand molecular geometry, chemical conditions, chemical reaction pathways, and transition states, as well as physical, ADME, and biological properties. Usually, computer simulations are less expensive and require less time than carrying out physical experiments.

In general, *computational chemistry* refers to energy-based methods. *CADD* is a more all-encompassing term, including not only energy-based calculations but also QSAR, database searching, and pharmacophore perception methods. Computational chemistry approaches can be divided into two broad categories: quantum mechanics-based and classical mechanics-based. The former covers the areas of semiempirical, ab initio, and density functional theory. The latter refers to force field (molecular mechanics) calculations and molecular dynamics simulations. Each method has its strengths and weaknesses, and it is important to be aware of these. From the practical standpoint of a pharmaceutical scientist, whichever approach gives reliable answers in the shortest time is typically used. The trick, obviously, is knowing when it is appropriate to use one method over another. This understanding comes in time through practice, just as an organic chemist can ''push'' electrons to solve or rationalize complex reaction mechanisms almost instinctively.

The Born-Oppenheimer theorem is a good starting point.[14] The theorem basically states that electrons move in a stationary field of nuclei; and therefore, the electron and nuclear motions can be considered separately. This approximation is valid in most cases of interest to medicinal chemists, since on the time scale of electron motion, the nuclei do not move. The difference in speed is a consequence of the differences in mass of the electron and the particles within the nucleus. It is analogous to speedboats circling a heavy aircraft carrier. On the time scale of the speedboats, during a brief snapshot of time, the aircraft carrier is motionless relative to the lighter craft. These facts, summarized in the Born-Oppenheimer theorem, enable successful use of the various mathematical models used in quantum mechanics and force field-based methods.

Quantum mechanics involves optimizing the electron distributions within molecules. Theoretical physicists first proposed the foundations of quantum mechanics in the 1920s.[15] There were only a few cases where exact solutions existed. More typically, approximate methods had to be used.[16] Although the theory has developed and improved, greater attention began to be placed on computational quantum chemistry in the 1950s when the first commercially available computers were introduced. Once computers became more available to the scientific community, solving problems with computational chemistry became realistic.[17, 18] Force field methods, on the other hand, ignore the electronic distribution and concentrate on the motion of nuclei as if they behaved like a ball-and-spring model, with potential energy functions used to describe the forces holding nuclei together. These methods were shown to be viable in the 1940s.[19–21]

For several reasons, this chapter focuses on force field rather than quantum mechanics methods. First, most medicinal chemistry applications are more amenable to this treatment. Second, most energy-based methods used in molecular modeling software are based on force fields—from conformational searching to scoring functions for drug–receptor fits—and it is critical to have a grasp of the fundamentals. Third, force field methods are conceptually easier to understand, and the mathematics is not as complicated. Finally, for large macromolecular systems with solvation, force field calculations are the only practical way to proceed, given the differences in computer time between classical-based and quantum-based computations.

FORCE FIELD METHODS

Force field methods are not a recent development; in fact, they have a long history. Three independent groups working on different problems reported the first calculations in 1946.[19–21] Of the three papers, the description of biphenyl derivatives examined by Frank H. Westheimer most effectively showed how to solve a problem convincingly.[19] In the early years, the force field or molecular mechanics calculations were known as the *Westheimer method*. Westheimer is considered the father of molecular mechanics. Force field methods were not actively developed until the 1960s and 1970s, as commercial computers were becoming more common. A number of academic research groups began to explore force field calculations as a way to help solve problems of interest. The investigations ranged from small strained organic structures to protein simulations. Most of the current force fields can trace their roots to common sources developed in the 1970s.[22–24]

Force field calculations rest on the fundamental concept that a ball-and-spring model may be used to approximate a molecule.[25, 26] That is, the stable relative positions of the atoms in a molecule are a function of through-bond and through-space interactions, which may be described by relatively simple mathematical relationships. The complexity of the mathematical equations used to describe the ball-and-spring model is a function of the nature, size, and shape of the structures. Moreover, the fundamental equations used in force fields are much less complicated than those found in quantum mechanics. For example, small strained organic molecules require greater detail than less strained systems such as peptides and proteins. Furthermore, it is assumed that the total energy of the molecule is a summation of the individual energy components, as outlined in Equation 28-1. In other words, the total energy (E_{total}) is divided into energy components, which are attributed to bond stretching ($E_{stretching}$), angle bending ($E_{bending}$), nonbonded interactions ($E_{nonbonded}$), torsion interactions ($E_{torsion}$), and coupled energy terms ($E_{cross-terms}$). The cross-terms combine two interrelated motions (bend–stretch, stretch–stretch, torsion–stretch, etc.). The division of the total energy into terms associated with distortions from equilibrium values is the way most chemists and biological scientists tend to think about molecules.

$$E_{total} = \sum_{bonds} E_{stretching} + \sum_{angles} E_{bending}$$
$$+ \sum_{nonbonded} (E_{VDW} + E_{electrostatics})$$
$$+ \sum_{dihedrals} E_{torsion} + \sum E_{cross-terms} \quad \text{(Eq. 28-1)}$$

In the 1600s, Robert Hooke, the scientific rival of the famous Sir Isaac Newton (who among his many scientific contributions invented the calculus, developed a theory of gravitation, and formulated classical mechanics), proposed that if an ideal spring with an attached mass m was compressed or stretched from its equilibrium position by an external force ($\vec{F}_{i \to j}$), the spring would exert a restoring force ($\vec{F}_{j \to i} = -\vec{F}_{i \to j}$) of equal magnitude but in the opposite direction of the distortion. This is an example of Newton's third law: For every action, there is an equal and opposite reaction. For simplicity, it may be assumed that the spring lies along the x axis, where the equilibrium length corresponds to x_0. The position x_0 may be considered the "natural length" of the relaxed spring. Figure 28-5 shows the setup for the classic one-dimensional harmonic oscillator.

Hooke's law for a one-dimensional oscillator oriented along the x axis may be written in mathematical form according to Equation 28-2, where x and x_0 are the distorted and the equilibrium positions, respectively. (Note that in Equation 28-2, $\vec{x}$ is used to symbolize that the displacement is a vector quantity, which alternatively could be represented as $x\hat{i}$, where $\hat{i}$ is a unit vector in the x axis.) If there are no frictional forces present, then the kinetic and potential energies are said to be *conserved*. As shown in Equation 28-3, if we can express the force, $\vec{F}$, as the first derivative of the potential energy, E, with respect to the displacement, then we have a conservative system (i.e., the kinetic and potential energy equal a constant).

$$\vec{F} = -k(\vec{x} - \vec{x}_0) \quad \text{(Eq. 28-2)}$$
$$\frac{dE}{dx} = -\vec{F} \quad \text{(Eq. 28-3)}$$

From elementary physics, the dot product of the force and displacement is defined as the applied work from the surroundings. This external work is the energy required to distort the spring, Equation 28-4. An extension of Newton's third law implies that the spring requires an equal amount of work to be restored, Equation 28-5. Note that work is a scalar quantity. The negative and positive signs assigned to the work reflect whether the surroundings are doing work

on the system (positive) or whether the system is doing work on the surroundings (negative).

According to Hooke's law, the restoring force is proportional to the displacement $-k(\vec{x} - \vec{x}_0)$. Therefore, substitution of Equation 28-2 into Equation 28-5 yields Equation 28-6. Recognizing that the work applied to the system is now the total energy of the system, we generate Equation 28-7.

$$W_{surroundings \to system} = \vec{F}_{external} \bullet d\vec{x} \quad \text{(Eq. 28-4)}$$
$$W_{system \to surroundings} = \vec{F}_{internal} \bullet d\vec{x} = -\vec{F}_{external} \bullet d\vec{x} \quad \text{(Eq. 28-5)}$$
$$W_{system \to surroundings} = -[-k(\vec{x} - \vec{x}_0)] \bullet d\vec{x} \quad \text{(Eq. 28-6)}$$
$$dE_{system} = k(\vec{x} - \vec{x}_0) \bullet d\vec{x} \quad \text{(Eq. 28-7)}$$

Taking the integral of Equation 28-7, where the displacement goes from x_0 to x, with a corresponding energy change E_1 to E_2, gives Equation 28-8.

$$\int_{E_1}^{E_2} dE = k \int_{x_0}^{x} (x - x_0)dx \quad \text{(Eq. 28-8)}$$

Integration of Equation 28-8 yields Equation 28-9, where c is the integration constant.

$$\Delta E = E_2 - E_1 = \frac{1}{2}k(x - x_0)^2 + c \quad \text{(Eq. 28-9)}$$

Equation 28-9 can be simplified by noting that E_2 is the energy corresponding to the distorted spring at position x, whether this is stretching or compression. The energy E_1 can be defined as our zero potential energy when $x = x_0$ relative to any distortion. This means that by our choice of zero potential energy, the integration constant must be zero, $c = 0$, which can clearly be seen if no distortion, $E_2 - E_1 = 0$, occurs. Finally, Equation 28-10 is the generalized one-dimensional potential energy function for stretching and compression of a spring. Note that the ΔE notation has been dropped, since E_1 is defined as the zero energy position. Equation 28-10 is a quadratic function. Figure 28-6 shows the plot of a simple quadratic function with

$$E = -\frac{1}{2}k(x - x_0)^2 \quad \text{(Eq. 28-10)}$$

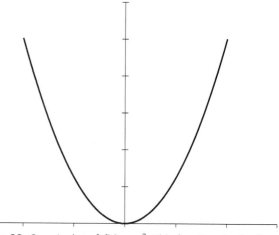

Figure 28–6 ■ A plot of $f(x) = x^2$. This function, in the form of Hooke's law, has been applied successfully in force field calculations to model bond distortions (stretching and compressing).

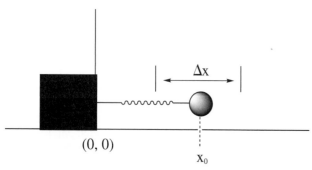

(0, 0)

x_0

Figure 28–5 ■ A simple one-dimensional ball-and-spring (x axis) oscillator serves as a model for bond vibrations.

The distortion of a one-dimensional ball-and-spring model along the x axis can be generalized into the 3D case, where in effect we have replaced x with r and x_0 with r_0. With Equation 28-11, the spring does not depend on being placed along one axis; it may be oriented in any direction. As pointed out above, Equation 28-11 is a quadratic function, used to describe stretching motions in most of the macromolecular force fields (e.g., AMBER[27–30] and CHARMM[31]).

$$E_{stretching} = \frac{1}{2}k_{stretch}\,(r - r_0)^2 \qquad \text{(Eq. 28-11)}$$

The use of a quadratic equation to mimic a chemical bond means that distortion and compression are equivalent in terms of an energy penalty. Think about what the quadratic model suggests: Compression and stretching result in equal increases in energy. This does not make sense physically, since for a diatomic molecule, compression brings the two atoms together, while distortion separates them. It is well known that bond distortion is anharmonic, so immediately we see a flaw in our model, which becomes more obvious in trying to reproduce bond distortions for strained molecules. The energy associated with bond stretching is described by a Morse curve, which is similar to a quadratic function only in the region close to the r_0 (Fig. 28-7). The relatively nondistorted bond lengths, which are characteristic of proteins, fall in the region where the Morse and quadratic functions overlap reasonably well. This is why simple quadratic terms may be acceptable as a first approximation in macromolecular calculations. In fact, given the complexity of nature, it is remarkable that a simple Hooke's law potential energy function works as well as it does.

For small strained organic molecules, more complex equations are usually necessary. Morse curves typically are not used in force field calculations. One approach that takes into account the anharmonicity associated with bond stretching relies on power series approximation. The Morse curve may be expanded into a power series function around the equilibrium position. Such expansions follow a well-known mathematical stratagem embodied in the Taylor series expansion, shown in Equation 28-12, where the expansion occurs about the position a. Complex curves may be approximated by power series. There are many advantages to having a function expressible as $(x - a)^n$, including ease of computation and ease in taking derivatives, which is why a Morse curve is not used directly via force field calculations.

$$f(x) = f(a) + \frac{f(a)}{1!}(x - a)$$
$$+ \frac{f'(a)}{2!}(x - a)^2 + \cdots + \frac{f^{[n]}(a)}{n!}(x - a)^n \quad \text{(Eq. 28-12)}$$

Expanding the Morse curve into a Taylor series using the formula outlined in Equation 28-12 generates Equation 28-13. The first term in the series is a constant, and this may be set equal to zero. The second term in the series may be recognized as the gradient, which stated above without proof and shown in Equation 28-3, is defined as the negative force for conserved systems. At the equilibrium bond length, r_0, the force is equal to zero, which means that the second term is also zero. Therefore, the first two terms in this expansion vanish. The first nonvanishing term in the series is the third term, which is a quadratic term, equivalent to Hooke's law. The fourth and fifth terms correspond to cubic and quartic terms, respectively, in Equation 28-13.

$$E = k_0 + \frac{k_1}{1}(r - r_0) + \frac{k_2}{2}(r - r_0)^2$$
$$+ \frac{k_3}{6}(r - r_0)^3 + \frac{k_4}{24}(r - r_0)^4 + \cdots \quad \text{(Eq. 28-13)}$$

The higher terms can be considered corrections to the quadratic term, which is only a first approximation to bond distortion. New force constants, $k_3^* = k_3/3$ and $k_4^* = k_4/12$, can be defined, giving Equation 28-14. The use of the quadratic function alone is known as the harmonic approximation.

$$E_{stretching} = \frac{k_2}{2}(r - r_0)^2 + \frac{k_3^*}{2}(r - r_0)^3 + \frac{k_4^*}{2}(r - r_0)^4$$
$$\text{(Eq. 28-14)}$$

MMFF94,[32–36] developed by Thomas Halgren at Merck, is currently one of the most widely available force fields. It was developed with medicinal chemistry applications in mind and can be found in various molecular modeling software packages, including Sybyl (Tripos, Inc.),[37] Spartan (Wavefunction, Inc.),[38] PCMODEL (Serena Software),[39] and MacroModel (Schrödinger, Inc.).[40] The force field is robust and can deal with many diverse functional groups found in drug-like molecules, giving accurate answers for small molecules as well as macromolecules. MMFF94 rivals the accuracy of MM3,[41–43] which is known as an excellent small organic molecule force field, as well as those results published for MM4.[44–47] MM3, however, is restricted in its usefulness for medicinal chemistry applications because of limited parameterization. The MM4 force field, a subsequent version of MM3, has modified potential energy functions and an expanded number of cross-terms.[48] These additions should make MM4 more accurate than its predecessor. MM4 will probably suffer from shortcomings similar to those of

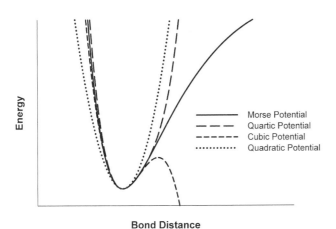

Energy

Bond Distance

—— Morse Potential
– – – Quartic Potential
- - - - Cubic Potential
·········· Quadratic Potential

Figure 28–7 ■ In force field calculations, different levels of approximations are used to reproduce the stretching and compression of chemical bonds. The plot shows a Morse potential energy function superimposed with various power series approximations (quadratic, cubic, and quartic functions). Note that the bottoms of the curves, representing the bond length for most chemical bonds of interest to medicinal chemists, almost overlap exactly. This nearly perfect fit in the bonding region is the reason simple harmonic functions can be used to calculate bond lengths for unstrained molecular structures in the force field method.

MM3, in terms of its ability to calculate diverse drug-like structures, because of the lack of parameters. Interestingly, MM4 has yet to be released publicly, even though it and MMFF94 were reported in 1996, at the same time, in back-to-back publications within the same journal volume. Because MMFF94 is so widely available, it is arguably the standard small molecule force field of choice at this time.

The MM3 and MMFF94 stretching functions may be written as outlined in Equation 28-15, where $\Delta r = r - r_0$, $k_{stretch}$ is the force constant parameter, c_s is a constant used to modify $k_{stretch}$, and 143.9325 is a conversion factor. Note that Equation 28-14 and Equation 28-15 are essentially the same but written in a different form. Equation 28-15 demands that the cubic and quartic force constants be scaled quadratic stretching constants.

$$E_{stretching}^{MMFF94} = 143.9325 \frac{k_{stretch}}{2} (\Delta r)^2 [1 + c_s(\Delta r) + c_s^2(\Delta r)^2]$$

(Eq. 28-15)

Bending strains are treated in an analogous way in force field calculations. Any distortion in bond angles $\theta - \theta_0$ results in a rise in the energy. The increase in energy associated with angle bending may be treated effectively with simple quadratic terms (Eq. 28-16). Equations similar to 28-16 are found in AMBER, CHARMM, and related macromolecular force fields. The use of quadratic terms is just a first approximation applicable to unstrained systems, as seen in the case of bond stretching. Many small molecules require a more complex function. Equation 28-17 is the bending function used in the MMFF94 force field. Again, one can see that the first term is quadratic, while the second term is cubic. The latter may be considered a correction factor.

$$E_{bending} = \frac{1}{2} k_{bend} (\theta - \theta_0)^2 \qquad \text{(Eq. 28-16)}$$

$$E_{bending}^{MMFF94} = 0.043844 \frac{k_{bend}}{2} (\Delta\theta) [1 + c_b(\Delta\theta)^2] \qquad \text{(Eq. 28-17)}$$

To keep C_{sp2}-hybridized centers planar, a special out-of-plane potential energy function is used. This is necessary because force fields are mechanically based and do not treat electrons explicitly. A simple solution regarding out-of-plane bending, found in some force fields, makes use of quadratic potential functions. The idea is simple and effective: Keep the central atom planar. For example and the sake of simplicity, consider formaldehyde. Because by definition three points define a plane, the two hydrogen atoms and oxygen atom (bonded to a carbonyl carbon) form a plane. Without some constraint, the carbonyl carbon will tend to move out of the plane defined by the two hydrogen atoms and the oxygen atom. The projection of the carbonyl carbon onto the plane forms a direct imaginary line, as shown in Figure 28-8. The incorporation of an energy penalty term using a simple quadratic function will achieve the desired purpose of keeping the center atom in the plane. The higher the out-of-plane bending constant, the less puckering will be observed. Equation 28-18 shows the simple form used, where k_{OOP} is the out-of-plane bending constant and $d - d_0$ is the distance from the projection of the atom on the plane to the atom itself.[48]

$$E_{out-of-plane} = \frac{k_{OOP}}{2} (d - d_0)^2 \qquad \text{(Eq. 28-18)}$$

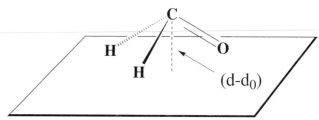

Figure 28–8 ■ To reproduce the out-of-plane bending motions for sp^2-hybridized atoms, a quadratic penalty function is used to constrain the system to be planar. The sp^2-hybridized atom forms a projection onto the plane defined by the three atoms directly bonded to it. For formaldehyde, the two H atoms and the O atom define a plane. The C_{sp2} is constrained to be in the plane by the use of a quadratic function.

Some force fields use an improper torsion angle concept to constrain the central atom of a trigonal planar group. In the case of formaldehyde (Fig. 28-8), the improper torsion angle may be defined as $H-C_{sp2}-O_{sp2}-H$. Note the fact that there is no covalent bond between the oxygen and hydrogen; hence, the name *improper* torsion angle. The use of an improper torsion is an equivalent mathematical method and has the same effect of constraining the central atom to be in the plane as a function of $(\phi - \phi_0)^2$.

Atoms have size and shape. With handheld mechanical models, the size of an atom is invariant regardless of its chemical environment, whereas in reality the van der Waals radii behave as if they were soft spheres rather than hard spheres (i.e., more like marshmallows than wooden balls). One advantage of using computer-based energy calculations is the ability to treat the van der Waals radii more realistically by providing greater flexibility than one can achieve with physical models. Certainly, this approach differs significantly from any hard sphere model. The other important nonbonded energy term arises from electrostatic interactions. Having a good electrostatic model is important, particularly when one considers the significance of electrostatic forces in drug–receptor interactions. Equation 28-19 describes the nonbonded terms.

$$E_{nonbonded} = \varepsilon_{ij} \left[\left(\frac{\sigma_{ij}}{r_{ij}}\right)^{12} - 2\left(\frac{\sigma_{ij}}{r_{ij}}\right)^6 \right] + \frac{1}{4\pi\varepsilon_0\varepsilon} \left(\frac{q_i \cdot q_j}{r_{ij}} \right) \quad \text{(Eq. 28-19)}$$

The first two terms within brackets define the van der Waals repulsions, which vary as $1/r^{12}$, and the London dispersion attractions, which vary as $1/r^6$.[49-51] The constant σ_{ij} is related to the size of the atom pair being considered, r_{ij} is the distance between the atom pairs, and ε_{ij} refers to the depth of the potential energy well. It is based on the Lennard-Jones 6-12 potential. Many force fields use functions of this type to describe steric interactions (Fig. 28-9). Only atoms with a 1,4 nonbonded relationship to one another (i.e., with three chemical bonds separating them) are included in these calculations. The bending and stretching terms include 1,3 nonbonded attractive and repulsion terms implicitly.

Hydrogen bonding may be treated as a special situation requiring a modified Lennard-Jones potential. The nonbonded calculations are the most time consuming, particularly if more complex terms are substituted for the $1/r^{12}$ repulsive part of the Lennard-Jones 6-12 potential, as found in MM3.

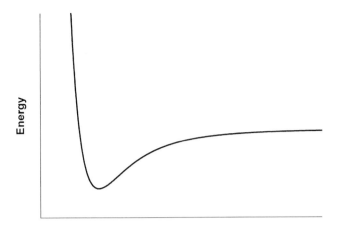

Figure 28–9 ■ When two atoms i and j are separated by infinite distance, there are no interactions between them. As two nonbonded atoms approach one another, two forces have to be considered. Attractive dispersion forces (London forces) result from the interaction of instantaneous dipoles on each atom i and j. As the nonbonded atoms continue to approach one another, a repulsive interaction overwhelms the attractive interaction, and the energy curve rises sharply. The two nonbonded atoms can reach an equilibrium position where repulsive and attractive forces balance. Different mathematical relationships have been used in force field calculations to reproduce the nonbonded steric interactions.

The third term in Equation 28-19 is Coulomb's law, where q_i and q_j are the charges on two nonbonded atoms i and j. The two charged atomic centers are not connected via a chemical bond and do not have a common single atom attached to atoms i and j. In other words, we are talking about 1,4 or greater relationships, as shown in Figure 28-10. The dielectric constant ϵ basically dampens the charge–charge interactions and is a function of the solvent. The greater the

value of the dielectric constant, the less electrostatic interaction exists between the atom pair. In a vacuum, the dielectric constant is 1.0; in water, the dielectric constant is approximately 80.

One of the major limitations of force fields has to do with the assignment of charges to each atomic center. There is no atomic charge operator in quantum mechanics. Atomic charges are determined quantum mechanically by using a population analysis. Consequently, there are many ways charges may be assigned. One popular way is to generate an electrostatic potential from high-level ab initio calculations (discussed below) and then fit the optimal point charge distribution on the atoms via least-squares methods. This approach has been used in AMBER.[30]

As discussed above, most force fields assign point charges to atomic centers and use Coulomb's law. The most notable exception is MM2 and MM3; in both versions, a dipole–dipole scheme for uncharged molecular structures is used.[52] For systems with a net charge, MM3 introduces functions capable of dealing with the additional charge–charge and charge–dipole interactions. Although there should be no difference between the two electrostatic schemes, having dipole–dipole, charge–charge, and charge–dipole terms requires more parameterization time. Improved MM2 and MM3 implementations found in MacroModel have eliminated the dipole–dipole scheme in favor of using point charges and Coulomb's law.

If the stretching, bending, and nonbonded terms were summed over all appropriate pairwise atom contributions within a structure, many important conformational effects in the simplest of hydrocarbons would not be reproduced. For example, Figure 28-11 shows the energy (kcal/mol) versus torsion angle ϕ profile for butane. The energy rises and falls during the rotation around the central C_{sp3}-C_{sp3} bond as a function of the relative positions of the methyl groups. The peaks on the curve correspond to energy maxima, while

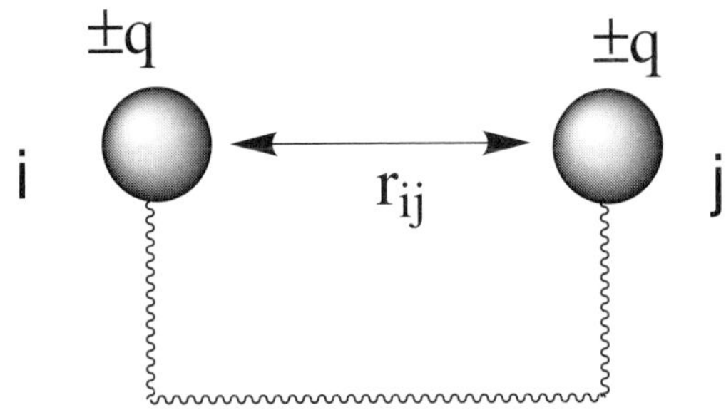

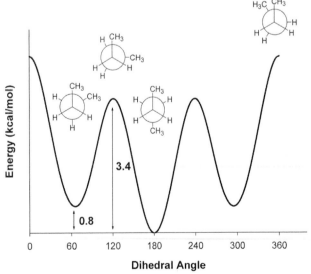

Figure 28–11 ■ Potential energy for butane. The energy (kcal/mol) is plotted on the *y* axis versus the torsion angle C_{sp3}-C_{sp3}-C_{sp3}-C_{sp3}, which is plotted on the *x* axis. There are three minima. The two *gauche* conformers are higher in energy than the *anti* conformer by approximately 0.9 kcal/mol.

Figure 28–10 ■ Two partially charged atoms i and j, not directly connected to each other or connected to a common atom (1,4-interactions or greater), exert an attractive or repulsive electrostatic interaction (depending on the charge) on each other. A Coulomb potential energy function is the most common way used in force field methods to calculate the charge–charge electrostatic energy. Coulomb's law is used in virtually all force fields with the exceptions of the original MM2 and MM3 codes. MM2* and MM3*, improved versions of the original codes, are found in the popular molecular modeling software program MacroModel developed by Clark Still and use charge–charge interaction terms.

the valleys correspond to energy minima. For butane, there are two different types of minima: one is for the *anti* butane conformation, and the other two correspond to the *gauche* butane conformations. The *anti* conformation is the global minimum, meaning it has the absolute lowest energy of the three possible low-energy conformations. The differences in the conformational energies cannot be attributed to steric interactions alone. Structures with more than one rotatable bond have multiple minima available. Knowing the permissible conformations available to drug-like molecules is important for design purposes. It turns out that another nonmechanical effect is needed to reproduce the potential energy curve for butane and other structures.

It has long been known that it requires energy for rotation about single bonds. One of the first conformational effects presented in organic chemistry courses involves the favorable H-C_{sp3}-C_{sp3}-H torsional orientations for ethane. The torsion angles are either *eclipsed* or *staggered*. In 1891, Bischoff proposed that ethane has a preference for a staggered conformation and the rotation in substituted ethanes was restricted.[53–55] The H/H steric interactions alone cannot explain the energy difference. If restricted rotation was considered, Pitzer demonstrated that the calculated and observed entropies for ethane were identical.[56, 57] The *staggered* conformation, where the C_{sp3}-H bonds are not aligned, is preferred because the electron densities in each bond are as far apart as possible. This energetically preferred orientation is reproduced by quantum mechanics calculations, but force field calculations need some equivalent function, since electrons are not treated explicitly but are treated indirectly via classical potential energy functions. For other saturated hydrocarbons, the potential energy terms are just extensions of the fundamental ethane curve with other nonbonded terms superimposed, according to Equation 28-1. In some cases, the energy required to rotate about single bonds is too great, locking structures into chiral conformations (atropisomers). Christie and Kenner first demonstrated restricted rotation in 1922 by resolving 2,2'-dinitrophenyl-6,6'-dicarboxylic acid into optically active isomers.[58]

A solution successfully implemented to reproduce the ethane phenomena, as well as other effects, was accomplished with the introduction of a truncated Fourier series.[59, 60] Although C_{sp3}-C_{sp3}-C_{sp3}-C_{sp3} and H-C_{sp3}-C_{sp3}-H dihedral angles prefer to be staggered, some torsion combinations prefer to be eclipsed.[61] Molecular orbital theory has been used to explain the underlying chemical reasons. Carbonyl oxygens prefer to eclipse the α hydrogens or α carbons of alkyl groups (O_{sp2}=C_{sp2}-C_{sp3}-H or O_{sp2}=C_{sp2}-C_{sp3}-C_{sp3}), and the acyl oxygens of esters prefer to have the O-R groups aligned with the C=O bond (O_{sp2}=C_{sp2}-O_{sp3}-C_{sp3}). These bond alignment effects are reproduced adequately in force field calculations using a three-term truncated Fourier series (Eq. 28-20). Essentially, this torsion function introduces quantum mechanical effects into a classical ball-and-spring system, which transforms our model into a much more powerful tool, with a fraction of the computer costs in terms of CPU cycles compared with using quantum chemical calculations.

$$E_{torsion} = \frac{V_1}{2}(1 - \cos\phi) + \frac{V_2}{2}(1 - \cos2\phi) + \frac{V_3}{2}(1 + \cos3\phi)$$

(Eq. 28-20)

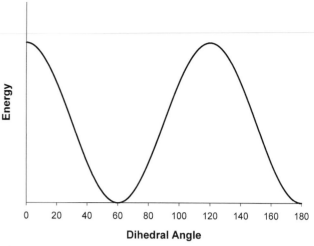

Figure 28–12 ■ A plot of Equation 28-20 with $V_1 = V_2 = 0$, and V_3 is a positive number. Note that this curve has threefold symmetry. The third term in Equation 28-20 is used to reproduce ethane-like torsion profiles about single bonds.

It is illustrative to look at each of the three terms in Equation 28-20 for a full appreciation of how a three-term Fourier series can be used to affect conformational equilibria. Figure 28-12 shows the plot of energy versus dihedral angle rotation with the V_1 and V_2 constants set to zero, and V_3 assigned a positive value. The curve has threefold symmetry. The maxima occur at dihedral angles of 0°, 120°, and 240°; the minima occur at dihedral angles of 60°, 180°, 300°, and 360°. Inspection of Figure 28-12 shows the similarity between it and the ethane torsion curve. Consequently, the third term describes the ethane effect without resorting to any complex calculations.

If the V_1 and V_3 terms are set to zero, plotting the second term shown in Figure 28-13, where V_2 is assigned a positive value in the truncated Fourier series, reveals its physical significance. There are minima at 0°, 180°, and 360° and maxima at 90° and 270°. Therefore, the second term in Equa-

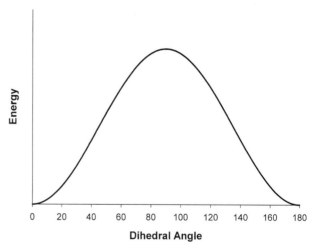

Figure 28–13 ■ A plot of Equation 28-20 with $V_1 = V_3 = 0$, and V_2 is a positive number. Note that this curve has twofold symmetry. The second term in Equation 28-20 is used to reproduce ethylene-like torsion profiles about double bonds.

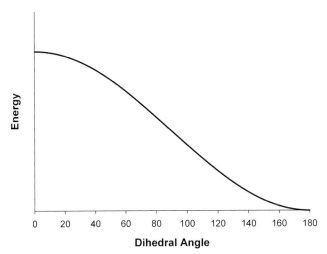

Figure 28–14 ▪ A plot of Equation 28-20 with $V_2 = V_3 = 0$, and V_1 is a positive number. Note that this curve has onefold symmetry. The interpretation is less straightforward than the second and third terms in Equation 28-20. The first term in Equation 28-20 is used to help reproduce torsion curves of the following type, X-C_{sp2}-C_{sp2}-X and X-C_{sp3}-C_{sp3}-X, where X is usually an electronegative element.

tion 28-20 is used to describe the torsional energy profile (arising about $C_{sp2}=C_{sp2}$ double bonds), which has twofold symmetry. The true underlying chemical explanation for the sharp energy rise observed in rotating about carbon–carbon double bonds may be attributed to the breaking of the weak π bond. The π bond is a consequence of the overlap of two adjacent coplanar p-orbitals. Any rotation about the $C_{sp2}=C_{sp2}$ bond shifts the orientation of the p-orbitals, with a reduction in the overlap and a concomitant rise in energy. For example, ethylene, the simplest alkene, prefers a flat conformation with the H-C_{sp2}-C_{sp2}-H dihedral angles at either 0° or 180°. When the H-C_{sp2}-C_{sp2}-H dihedral angle is 90°, the p-orbitals are orthogonal, and there is no overlap. Therefore, the energy is a maximum along the one-dimensional potential energy curve when H-C_{sp2}-C_{sp2}-H is 90°.

The physical significance of the V_1 term is less intuitive. Setting the V_2 and V_3 terms to zero and assigning the V_1 term a positive value yields the curve shown in Figure 28-14. The V_1 term is used primarily as an additional way to increase the repulsive interactions between atoms that have a 1,4 relationship that are not fully accounted for by the nonbonded terms. This situation is commonly found for electron-withdrawing groups X and Y, with torsion combinations X-C_{sp3}-C_{sp3}-Y and X-C_{sp2}-C_{sp2}-Y.

Radom, Hehre, and Pople were the first to give physical interpretations of these torsional terms.[62] For maximum flexibility in developing force fields, it should be noted that the V_1, V_2, and V_3 terms may be either positive or negative. Although the discussion above focuses on carbon–carbon or carbon–hydrogen torsion angles, Equation 28-20 also applies to any other combination i-j-k-l, with any other elements from the periodic table used for i, j, k, and l. Given the number of drugs that have heterocycles, a force field useful for drug design has to address many torsion angle combinations.

Additional energy interaction terms may be added to im-

prove the accuracy of the force field description. Many of these additional terms fall into the category of cross-terms, in which two motions or interactions are connected or correlated. For example, in small molecule force fields one might find stretch–torsion, stretch–bend, bend–bend, torsion–bend, and other interactions. Equation 28-21 shows a stretch–bend function. Some of these cross-terms have been shown to be more important than others. The purpose of cross-terms is to give better geometric results, and they are particularly important in calculating the vibrational spectra.

$$E_{\text{stretch–bend}} = \frac{k_{sb}}{2}[(r - r_0) + (r' - r_0')](\theta - \theta_0) \qquad \text{(Eq. 28-21)}$$

Force field methods are fast and accurate if the potential energy functions and parameters within the potential energy functions have been carefully developed. In addition to calculating molecular geometry, force field calculations are used to determine the energy between conformations.

GEOMETRY OPTIMIZATION

It is important to be able to take a molecular structure in silico and subject it to energy minimization. This is the first step for force field and quantum mechanics calculations and for molecular dynamics simulations. Once a molecular structure finds a stable conformation, the physical and chemical properties can then be calculated. The goal of energy minimization (or geometry optimization) is to take a high-energy state, which is a function of the atomic coordinates, and to reduce the energy by optimizing the geometry. In other words, minimizing the potential energy functions with respect to the coordinates reduces the steric and electrostatic interactions. This is a type of calculus problem familiar to students who have ever had to locate the stationary points of a given equation. Recall that the extrema (maxima and minima) of a mathematical function $f(x)$, with one independent variable x, have first derivatives equal to zero, $f'(x) = 0$. The second derivative $f''(x)$ will be positive if it is a minimum and negative if it is a maximum. Figure 28-15 shows

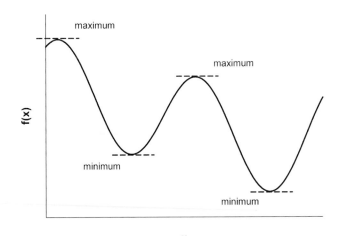

Figure 28–15 ▪ An arbitrary mathematical function with maxima and minima. The first derivative of a function is zero at a maximum or minimum, $f'(x) = 0$. The second derivative is positive ($f''(x) = +$value) if the stationary point is a minimum, or is negative ($f''(x) = -$value) if the stationary point is a maximum.

an example of a function, $f(x)$, with two minima and two maxima.

Typically, a molecular structure is entered into a molecular modeling software package by template fragments or through a sketching mode. It is also possible to download structures from structural databases. Structures built or downloaded do not have an optimum geometry based on the force field potential energy equations; i.e., they are not occupying the lowest energy state in vacuo. Minimization algorithms are written to take a starting structure and minimize the energy, which translates into the structure dropping into the nearest potential energy well on the conformational hyperenergy surface. The more complex the structure, usually the more minima are available in conformational space. Butane, a simple hydrocarbon, is an informative example. It has three minima available. Energy minimization requires a series of iterations because of the nonlinear nature of the force field potential energy functions. The general stratagem is to transform the full nonlinear optimization into a series of local iterative linearizations, and this approach works well. Atoms within a molecular structure are moved in small steps in the direction that results in a decrease in the energy of the system. The size and direction of the steps are determined by the specific method being used, based on Equation 28-3, and illustrated for a one-dimensional case in Figure 28-16.

Geometry optimization may be divided into two broad categories: first-order methods and second-order methods. The former uses first derivatives to determine the step size and direction, while the latter uses both first and second derivatives. First-order methods include *steepest descent* (SD) and *conjugate gradient* (CG). The second-order method discussed below is known as the Newton-Raphson (NR) geometry optimization approach; there are many variations of this method. Again, the concepts of minimizing a function are not new; they were developed years ago. (The "Newton" in Newton-Raphson is Sir Isaac Newton.) The immediate goal of an energy minimization is finding a suitable displacement δ_n, which, as stated above, is opposite to the potential energy gradient. In other words, the atoms are moved in the direction of the forces. The displacement is added to the coordinates at each step and is updated by a quick recalculation of the force field total energy.

SD is the simplest approach.[63–65] The step size in SD δ_n is simply taken as a scaled negative gradient as shown in Equation 28-22, where ∇ (del), a vector operator, is the gradient as defined by Equation 28-23 and λ is a scaling constant. The SD algorithm is inefficient when the potential energy curve is not very steep. So as the minimum is approached, where the slope of the curve is flatter, SD algorithms become inefficient compared with other methods.

$$\delta_n = -\lambda(\nabla_n E_{total}) \qquad \text{(Eq. 28-22)}$$

$$\nabla = \left(\frac{\partial}{\partial x}\hat{i} + \frac{\partial}{\partial y}\hat{j} + \frac{\partial}{\partial z}\hat{k}\right) \qquad \text{(Eq. 28-23)}$$

The CG method, outlined in Equation 28-24, is widely used.[66–67] It gives better convergence than SD algorithms. As the name implies, the previous step size along with the current gradient as determined by the total force field energy is used to determine the next step size. An additional scaling factor c is found to improve results.

$$\vec{r}_{n+1} = \vec{r}_n + c\delta_n \qquad \text{(Eq. 28-24)}$$

The Newton-Raphson method uses information obtained by taking the first and second derivatives of the energy with respect to the coordinates.[22, 63] The combination of both first and second derivatives provides a powerful method to locate minima. This may be a time-consuming process because of the matrix manipulations that must be undertaken for a 3N system, where N is the number of atoms. In Equation 28-25, ∇^2 is the dot product of ∇ multiplied by itself. Note that ∇^2 is a scalar operator.

$$\delta_n = -\frac{1}{\nabla^2 E}(\nabla E) \qquad \text{(Eq. 28-25)}$$

$$\nabla^2 = \nabla \bullet \nabla = \left(\frac{\partial}{\partial x}\hat{i} + \frac{\partial}{\partial y}\hat{j} + \frac{\partial}{\partial z}\hat{k}\right)\left(\frac{\partial}{\partial x}\hat{i} + \frac{\partial}{\partial y}\hat{j} + \frac{\partial}{\partial z}\hat{k}\right)$$
$$= \left(\frac{\partial^2}{\partial x^2} + \frac{\partial^2}{\partial y^2} + \frac{\partial^2}{\partial z^2}\right) \qquad \text{(Eq. 28-26)}$$

None of the geometry optimization methods discussed finds the global minimum.

CONFORMATIONAL SEARCHING

As indicated above, it is important to be able to explore conformational space to determine what arrangements of atoms (conformations) are energetically feasible. Observed physical properties (e.g., heats of formation) are statistical averages of all the conformations available. Most organic molecules have multiple energy minima. In the case of drug design, it may be important to sample the possible number of conformations a drug molecule can adopt. Usually, a drug in the drug–receptor complex adopts a *bioactive conformation* that differs from any of the local minima or the global minimum. From the analysis of many lead and drug pairs, the average drug-like molecule has more degrees of freedom (i.e., is more flexible) than lead-like compounds. Initially, this may seem counterintuitive, since the mission of a drug is to have its functional groups bind to complementary functional groups of the receptor. It turns out that a flexible drug is superior to one with a locked conformation because the exact orientation in a conformationally constrained molecule

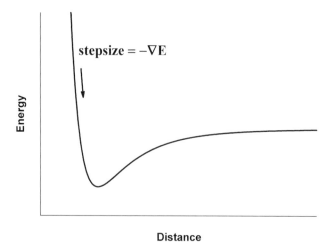

stepsize = $-\nabla$E

Energy

Distance

Figure 28–16 ■ The direction of the step size in an energy minimization is toward the minimum value.

may not be optimal for interactions with the receptor. Moreover, the potential superiority of a flexible drug can be understood when one considers that both receptor and small molecule must mold themselves to form the drug–receptor complex. A flexible drug can contort itself more easily to reach the binding pocket and then adjust itself accordingly to form the necessary interactions. A rigid drug with its functional groups locked into place may be more limited in its ability to get to the target site and, once there, to position itself correctly. Of course, based on the Koshland induced fit hypothesis, it is known that both small molecules and macromolecules adjust themselves to form protein–ligand complexes.

Before conformational searching is discussed in any detail, it is critical to have a common vocabulary. The terms *conformer* and *conformation* can be defined in reference to the butane potential energy curve (Fig. 28-11). There are an infinite number of conformations on the curve, since the distance between any two points on any curve may be as small as desired. *Conformations* refer to both maxima and minima and all positions in between. A *conformer,* on the other hand, refers to the conformation at the bottom of the potential energy well, which is a minimum. Looking at the simple case of butane, it is easily seen that there are three potential energy wells. Every molecular structure has a global minimum, the absolute lowest energy, but there are many minima. For butane, the global minimum corresponds to the *anti* conformer. One speaks of energy minimization, not energy optimization (discussed above), because the potential energy functions are being minimized, not the geometry. *Geometry optimization* is the equivalent term, for the structure is being *optimized* according to the force field equations.

Why is it necessary to explore conformational space? First, as discussed above, energy minimization algorithms are designed to seek the nearest minimum to the starting position. So for butane, if we had an initial input geometry in which the C_{sp3}-C_{sp3}-C_{sp3}-C_{sp3} dihedral angle was 90°, the molecular structure would be energy minimized to the *gauche* conformer. If we started on the other side of the 120° barrier, where the C_{sp3}-C_{sp3}-C_{sp3}-C_{sp3} dihedral angle was 150°, the molecular structure would be energy minimized to the *anti* conformer. Second, some conformations are more important than others. Third, as noted above, many physical problems are a consequence of a statistical average of the conformers present. Fourth, having a conformational search algorithm is a check against having biased structural data. In the case of butane, if only *anti* butane were known, there would be a lot of information missing. The majority of drug-like molecules are structurally more complex than butane, but this hydrocarbon is a straightforward example.

The importance of knowing available conformations for property predictions can be illustrated by looking at substituted cyclohexane. For cyclohexanol, the axial:equatorial ratio is derived by using Boltzmann statistics to calculate the ratio. Equation 28-27 shows the Boltzmann equation, where P_j is the probability of finding one conformation, f_i is a frequency factor indicating the degeneracy of the energy, E_j is the relative energy (kcal/mol), R is the gas constant (0.0199 kcal/mol-K), and T is the temperature (K). For room temperature calculations, the product RT is 0.59 kcal/mol. If one took a single conformation of axial cyclohexanol and compared it with a single conformation of equatorial cyclo-

hexanol, an erroneous answer would result. The right way to do the calculations is to look at all possible axial and equatorial conformations. With cyclohexanol, this is not difficult and can be done by manually altering the orientation of the OH group. For more complex structures, conformational searching routines must be used.

$$P_j = \frac{n_j}{\sum n_i} = \frac{f_i e^{-E_j/RT}}{\sum f_i e^{-E_i/RT}} \qquad \text{(Eq. 28-27)}$$

Table 28-1 shows the three possible axial and equatorial conformations. Substitution in Equation 28-27 generates the calculated ratio of each conformer. Because MMFF94 was parameterized to reproduce the quantum mechanical calculations, it is illustrative to look at the ratio calculated with MMFF94. The Boltzmann-averaged distribution may then be compared with the experimental data as well as the other force field results.

Equation 28-28 outlines the procedures for calculating the denominator in Equation 28-27. Note that in Table 28-1, entries 1 and 2 (as well as 4 and 5) are equivalent in energy, with relative conformational energies of 0.000 kcal/mol and −0.323 kcal/mol, respectively. Consequently, the frequency factor is 2 for both cases. The summation of Equation 28-28 is shown in Equation 28-29 to be 4.057.

$$\sum f_i e^{-E_i/0.593} = (2)e^{\frac{-0.00}{0.593}} + (1)e^{\frac{-0.199}{0.593}}$$
$$+ (2)e^{\frac{-0.323}{0.593}} + (1)e^{\frac{-1.011}{0.593}} \qquad \text{(Eq. 28-28)}$$

$$\sum f_i e^{-E_i/0.593} = 2.00 + 0.715 + 1.160$$
$$+ 0.182 = 4.057 \qquad \text{(Eq. 28-29)}$$

The ratio for each entry in Table 28-1 can be calculated by using Equation 28-27. It is more interesting to look at the summation of the total calculated equatorial versus total axial cyclohexanol conformations, which, on a percentage basis, is calculated by Equations 28-30 and 28-31. MMFF94 results give approximately 67% equatorial and 33% axial. This is in close agreement with the Hartree-Fock (HF) 6-31G(d) quantum mechanical calculations of 66% equatorial and 34% axial, which is in reasonable agreement with experimental data. The calculated percentages with MM3 are 82% equatorial and 18% axial, while the calculated percentages with the Tripos force field yield 46% equatorial and 54% axial. In general, the Tripos force field is qualitative (at best) and does not give particularly good energy values, so one must be cautious when trying to make accurate predictions using force field methods.

$$P_{equatorial} \times 100\% = \left[\frac{\sum\limits_{equatorial} f_i e^{-E_i/RT}}{\sum\limits_{all\ conformers} f_i e^{-E_i/RT}} \right] (100\%)$$

$$= \left[\frac{2.00 + 0.715}{4.057} \right] (100\%) = 66.9\% \quad \text{(Eq. 28-30)}$$

$$P_{axial} \times 100\% = \left[\frac{\sum\limits_{axial} f_i e^{-E_i/RT}}{\sum\limits_{all\ conformers} f_i e^{-E_i/RT}} \right] (100\%)$$

$$= \left[\frac{1.160 + 0.182}{4.057} \right] (100\%) = 33.1\% \quad \text{(Eq. 28-31)}$$

TABLE 28–1   Three Axial and Three Equatorial Conformations of Cyclohexanol With Their Relative Energies Calculated Using Force Field (MMFF94, MM3, Tripos) and Ab Initio Quantum Mechanics (6–31G(d,p) or 6–31G**)

No.	Conformer	MM3	Sybyl	MMFF	HF
1		0.000	0.129	0.000	0.000
2		0.000	0.129	0.000	0.000
3		0.942	0.063	0.199	0.200
4		0.834	0.000	0.323	0.244
5		0.834	0.000	0.323	0.244
6		2.637	0.051	1.011	1.632
	Ratio	81.5:18.5	46.2:53.8	67.0:33.0	66.2:33.8
	$-\Delta G$	0.88	−0.09	0.42	0.40

The goal of conformational searching is to find all possible values of the dihedral angles that could be assigned to each rotatable bond in a molecular structure. Conformational searching may be divided into two general categories: *systematic* and *nonsystematic* searching. As the name implies, systematic searching uses methods that are guaranteed to find all minima within the defined search parameters, while nonsystematic searching uses statistical approaches. Systematic searching includes grid searching, torsion driving, and constrained searching. Nonsystematic searching includes dynamics, stochastic (random), and distance geometry.

Systematic searching has been described as an exhaustive sampling of conformational space,[68, 69] but the success is a function of the number of increments used to explore each rotatable dihedral angle. No conformation will be overlooked (unless the search parameters are not small enough). A simple analogy should make this clear. Imagine walking along a paved highway blindfolded (not recommended) with the goal of discovering all possible potholes. The number of potholes that may be located is a function of the step size and the distance traveled. The longer the gait, the faster one travels down the road, but with a reduced probability of finding all the potholes. Systematic searching generally cannot handle solvents, and the method is only amenable to searching fewer than 10 dihedral angles, because of the exponential explosion of possible conformations that results (see Equation 2-30 in Chapter 2). Large amounts of computer time are expended because small dihedral angle increments are required for each rotatable bond.

In grid searching (GS), each torsion angle is examined, but the structure is not subjected to geometry optimization.

According to Equation 2-30, the number of conformations generated rises exponentially with the number of bonds rotated. Torsion angle driving is GS, while the rest of the structure (with the exception of the torsion being systematically rotated) is energy minimized. Many programs have this feature, and accurate conformational energies are obtained with the minimization.

Nonsystematic searching typically is more suitable for larger molecules, and solvents may be included.[70, 71] In general, more time is necessary to apply statistical analyses for the "completeness" of a search. Although stochastic searches are useful, there is an inherent incompleteness to them. Stochastic searching can use either internal or cartesian coordinates. From a starting low-energy conformation, the cartesian coordinates are randomized with a "kick." If the randomization is not large enough, the structure will return to its starting points. Too large a perturbation generates unrealistic high-energy conformations. The randomized geometry is energy minimized with a force field, and the newly generated structure is compared with the original structure according to the Metropolis algorithm (MA).[72] The current conformation is compared with the newly generated one. If the energy of the newly generated conformation is lower than the energy of the original conformation, the new one is accepted. If the new conformation has a higher energy, there is a statistical chance it may also be retained. In this second case, a Boltzmann factor is calculated (Equation 28-27), which is then compared with a random number between 0 and 1. If the Boltzmann factor is less than the randomly generated number, the conformation is accepted; otherwise, it is rejected.

With all methods, there are strengths and limitations. Conformational searching is no exception. A comparison of the methods was carried out on cycloheptadecane in an effort to find out "what conformations are significantly populated at room temperature or within, say 3 kcal/mol of the global minimum?"[73] The authors reached the following conclusions: *(a)* the effectiveness of the search appears to depend highly on the method used, and *(b)* except for distance geometry, all methods could locate the global minimum; none of the methods found all 262 low-energy conformations in a single search. Because of the importance of conformational searching, newer algorithms have been developed since this benchmark study.

The Confort algorithm, developed in the laboratory of Robert Pearlman, performs a systematic search over all possible combinations of "worthy dihedral angle ranges" rather than searching over all possible combinations of dihedral angles per se. Very fast partial optimizations are carried out for each such combination of dihedral angle ranges. Each of the torsion ranges generated by Confort brackets a single local minimum and is followed by energy minimization. Although still of exponential order, the number of increments used per rotor is typically between 2 and 4, thereby making the Confort algorithm extremely fast and enabling its use for searching rings and ring systems in addition to acyclic substructures.[74]

Methods have been devised that alter the potential energy hyperspace, which have been useful in locating the global minimum. Second-derivative information, discussed above, indicates the curvature of the energy surface, which may be flattened or inflated, depending on whether the surface has a positive curvature (negative second derivative) or negative curvature (positive second derivative), respectively.[75]

Genetic algorithms (GAs) have become popular for many applications in science, including the determination of possible conformations.[76] The widespread use of GAs may be attributed to their robust nature, simplicity, and computational efficiency. One approach to the stochastic sampling of the conformational energy hypersurface uses a GA with a fitness function that attempts to select dihedral angle values leading to low-energy conformers and, possibly, simultaneously attempts to select dihedral angle values corresponding to "diverse" conformations. Although GA-based search results are incomplete, the energies used to "score" various conformations are calculated in an appropriate fashion.[74]

Another stochastic approach involves the "poling" algorithm,[77] which locates minima and artificially increases the conformational energy hyperspace until there are no minima at that location. The name is derived from the analogy of literally placing a pole in the energy well and pulling up the surface around the pole, like raising a circus tent. All methods that involve reshaping the potential energy hypersurface suffer from alterations to the surface being explored. The artificial increase in the conformational energy hypersurface near each low-energy conformation ensures that nearby conformations will not be selected. Although this approach is much faster than GA-based approaches, poling algorithms are often less reliable. They fail to find low-energy conformations because the conformations selected are based on artificially perturbed values of the conformational energy.

MOLECULAR DYNAMICS SIMULATIONS

The molecular configuration is a function of time. Molecular systems are not stationary; molecules vibrate, rotate, and tumble. Force field calculations and the properties predicted by them are based on a stationary model. What is needed is some way to predict what motions the atoms within a molecule will undergo at various temperatures. Molecular dynamics (MD) simulations use classical mechanics—force field methods—to study the atomic and molecular motions to predict macroscopic properties.[78]

MD simulations have the potential to reveal important insights into drug–receptor interactions, but some important assumptions should be reviewed:

1. Molecular systems obey classical mechanics.
2. The forces acting on each atom are equal to the negative gradient of the potential energy.
3. The potential energy may be calculated from force fields.
4. The temperature is proportional to the velocity.
5. The time average is equal to the ensemble average, which is known as the ergodic hypothesis.

In applying classical mechanics to simulate molecular motion, it is necessary to use Newton's laws of motion. The three laws are summarized below:

1. *Law of inertia:* A body stays in motion or at rest unless acted on by outside forces.
2. *Fundamental definition of force:* mass $\times$ acceleration.

$$\vec{F} = m\frac{d^2\vec{r}}{dt^2} = m\vec{a} \qquad \text{(Eq. 28-32)}$$

3. *Law of action–reaction:* For every action, there is an equal and opposite reaction.

$$\vec{F}_{i \to j} = \vec{F}_{j \to i} = -\vec{F}_{i \to j} \qquad \text{(Eq. 28-33)}$$

Using Equation 28-32 as the starting point, the mass m may be eliminated and integrated with respect to time t according to Equation 28-34 to give Equation 28-35, where $\vec{v}$ is the velocity and C is the integration constant. It is a simple matter to determine the integration constant. At the initial time, $t_2 = t_1$, which means that $\vec{a}\Delta t = 0$. Therefore, the integration constant must equal the initial velocity ($C = \vec{v}_0$).

$$\int \frac{d^2\vec{r}}{dt^2}\,dt = \int \vec{a}\,dt \qquad \text{(Eq. 28-34)}$$

$$\frac{d\vec{r}}{dt} = \vec{v} = \vec{a}(t_2 - t_1) + C = \vec{a}\Delta t + \vec{v}_0 \qquad \text{(Eq. 28-35)}$$

Integration of Equation 28-35 provides the distance a particle has traveled from its initial position $\vec{r}$ at time t to its new position $\vec{r}(t + \Delta t)$ at $t + \Delta t$ (Eq. 28-36).

$$\vec{r}(t + \Delta t) = \frac{1}{2}\vec{a}\Delta t^2 + \vec{v}_0 t + \vec{r}(t) \qquad \text{(Eq. 28-36)}$$

Equations 28-35 and 28-36 are known as Newton's equations of motion. MD simulations apply these two equations to all the atoms in a molecular structure. According to the kinetic-molecular theorem, the kinetic energy is proportional to the temperature. This remarkable relationship is shown in Equation 28-37 without derivation, where N is the number of molecules, k is the Boltzmann constant, and T is the absolute temperature. Equation 28-37 connects classical physics to statistical mechanics. The basic idea behind MD simulations is to introduce heat into the system and adjust the velocities to maintain the temperature. The forces on the atoms can be calculated with a force field. Once the forces are known, based on Newton's celebrated second law (Eq. 28-32), the accelerations can be calculated. Using the laws of motion (Eq. 28-35 and 28-36), the velocities and new positions can be calculated. This procedure is repeated for the duration of the simulation.

$$\sum_{i=1}^{n} \frac{1}{2} m_i (\dot{r})^2 = \frac{3}{2} NkT \qquad \text{(Eq. 28-37)}$$

The fundamental steps in a MD simulation may be summarized:

1. Energy minimization
2. Heating
3. Equilibration
4. Production runs
5. Analysis

It is informative to review some of the information regarding MD time steps. It has been learned that the best time step should be 1/10th of the largest frequency in the system. The largest frequency is associated with bond vibrations. The largest frequency ($v_{max} = 10^{14}$ sec^{-1}) involves C-H bonds. Because the largest frequency is inversely proportional to the period of oscillation, the time step Δt is usually 10^{-15} sec or 1 fs. Longer simulation times may be achieved by a factor of 2 or 3 if the C-H bond vibrations are constrained. The SHAKE algorithm was developed whereby constraints are placed on the vibrations of C-H bonds.[79]

When calculating protein structures, one must have a good solvation model. Because water plays a critical role in enzyme reactions and stabilizing proteins, it is important to have effective ways to model water. In the structure-based design of human immunodeficiency virus (HIV) inhibitors, for example, the presence of a single water molecule in the binding cavity was effectively exploited in structure-based drug design. There are essentially two ways to include solvent in MD simulations: *(a)* continuum solvent models and *(b)* explicit solvation models. In principle, the latter should give more accurate protein simulations, but it depends highly on the water model used.

The simplest continuum solvent model simply adjusts the dielectric constant to equal the medium dielectric. An approximation widely used in MD simulations is known as the distance-dependent dielectric constant. In this approach, the dielectric constant is set equal to the distance r_{ij}, as shown in Equation 28-38. The electrostatic energy is now proportional to $1/r^2$ rather than $1/r$. When this was first proposed, the idea was to help reduce CPU time. The rationalization is that the charges on two nonbonded atoms in a macromolecule are separated by the protein, which should reduce the interaction terms. Thus, the interaction energy should fall off faster than $1/r$ because the charges are masked.

$$E_{electrostatic} = \sum_{i<j} \frac{q_i q_j}{4\pi\varepsilon_0 \varepsilon r_{ij}} = \sum_{i<j} \frac{q_i q_j}{4\pi\varepsilon_0 r_{ij}^2} \qquad \text{(Eq. 28-38)}$$

The other approach is to treat the solvent explicitly. There are a number of water models available.[80] Two of the most widely used water solvent models are SPC[81] and TIP3P.[82] In the former, the oxygen atom has a charge of -0.82, and the hydrogens have a charge of 0.41. The H-O-H angle is $109.5°$, and the O-H bond length is 1.0 Å. In the latter, the oxygen atom has a charge of -0.834, and the hydrogens have a charge of 0.417. The H-O-H angle is $104.5°$, and the O-H bond length is 0.957 Å.

To avoid potential water–vacuum interface problems that might arise in a MD simulation, periodic boundary conditions are commonly used.[83] Basically, a protein is surrounded by a rectangular box of water with a defined number of water structures. This water box is then surrounded on each face by another water box. When the MD simulation is being carried out, water near the edges of the central box containing the protein may leave and be replaced with a water coming from the water box on the opposite side. This procedure ensures that the waters inside the central water box remain constant.

The long-range forces found in the nonbonded terms of Equation 28-19 present some unique difficulties for a MD simulation. Calculating these energy terms is CPU intensive. One early solution was to impose 8- to 10-Å cutoffs. Although this saved dramatically on the simulation times, unrealistic protein structures resulted after long runs. There were several potential workarounds, including longer cutoffs and updating these interactions beyond the standard cutoff less frequently.[84] A very attractive approach to circumvent this problem altogether, proposed by Darden, York, and Pedersen, used the particle mesh Ewald (PME) method.[85]

Free energy perturbation (FEP) calculations[86, 87] allow direct $\Delta\Delta G$ comparisons between a drug D that binds to a protein P to form the drug–protein complex D-P and a structural analogue D′ and the same protein P (see Fig. 28-17, which depicts the free energy perturbation cycle). Determining the free energies of binding, ΔG_1 and ΔG_2, experimentally can be difficult and time consuming. Converting D into D′, ΔG_3, and D-P into D′-P, ΔG_4, is experimentally fictitious. Such conversions would amount to alchemy. The conversions can, however, be carried out in silico.

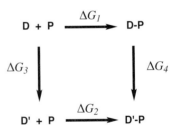

Figure 28-17 ■ Free energy perturbation (FEP) calculations take advantage of a thermodynamic cycle. Here, the *top reaction* shows a drug D combining with a protein P to form the drug–protein complex D-P with a free energy change ΔG_1. The *bottom reaction* shows another drug D′ combining with an identical protein P to form a second drug–protein complex D′-P with a free energy change ΔG_2. Both of these physically observable reactions have a free energy change, ΔG, associated with them. The free energy difference between the two drug–protein reactions is $\Delta\Delta G = \Delta G_2 - \Delta G_1$. According to the first law of thermodynamics (conservation of energy law), the fictitious conversions, ΔG_3 and ΔG_4, must be related to the experimental $\Delta\Delta G$.

In a thermodynamic cycle, Equation 28-39 must hold, as the energy differences depend only on the initial and final states. Subtracting ΔG_3 and ΔG_1 from both sides of Equation 28-39 provides the rearranged Equation 28-40. Recognizing that $\Delta\Delta G = \Delta G_2 - \Delta G_1$, Equation 28-40 can be simplified to give Equation 28-41. This remarkable relationship, taking advantage of the thermodynamic cycle, indicates that the free energy differences based on in silico alchemy must be equivalent to the experimental $\Delta\Delta G$. The method has been used to calculate and compare the binding energies for many different drug–protein complexes. Although the approach is intellectually stimulating, it requires significant computer resources.

$$\Delta G_3 + \Delta G_2 = \Delta G_1 + \Delta G_4 \qquad \text{(Eq. 28-39)}$$

$$\Delta G_2 - \Delta G_1 = \Delta G_4 - \Delta G_3 \qquad \text{(Eq. 28-40)}$$

$$\Delta\Delta G = \Delta G_4 - \Delta G_3 \qquad \text{(Eq. 28-41)}$$

Another application of interest to medicinal chemists involves the thermodynamic perturbation cycle applied to relative property calculations. For example, directly calculating the solvation of a small drug requires extensive simulation times. The drug has to transfer from in vacuo into an aqueous environment. This transfer from the gas phase to the aqueous phase is CPU intensive, given that the solvent has to be reorganized to accommodate the solute. Calculating a second drug analogue will involve a similar process. Making use of a thermodynamic cycle, however, can expedite the process (analogous to the above discussion for the drug–protein binding).

There are two types of motion (harmonic and stochastic) that may be studied by MD simulations. *Harmonic simulations* refer to oscillations near equilibrium (i.e., near the minimum of a potential energy well). *Stochastic* refers to simulations that lead from one local minimum to another local minimum.

From a harmonic oscillator, the frequencies may be calculated according to Equation 28-42, where k is the stretching constant and m is the mass. Extending the concept from a single mass held to a surface by a spring to N particles requires an extension of the Taylor series expansion (Eq. 28-13) to a matrix formulation of partial second derivatives. Each mode has associated its own force constant, frequency, and 3N relative displacements. The normal modes are assigned to the experimental IR or Raman spectrum.

$$\nu = \frac{1}{2\pi}\sqrt{\frac{k}{m}} \qquad \text{(Eq. 28-42)}$$

MD simulations have been applied to generate new conformations.[73, 88] The basic idea is to add enough thermal energy (through high temperatures) and carry out the simulations long enough for the molecular systems to overcome conformational barriers. After the simulations are completed, the trajectory can be reviewed. The temperature of the system can be cooled down to sample potential new conformations. MD simulations are suitable for larger molecules, and solvent may be included. No statistical or geometrical means are used to determine their completeness. In general, MD simulations are not as efficient as stochastic or distance geometry methods.

QUANTUM MECHANICS

One of the great theoretical accomplishments of the 20th century was the development of quantum mechanics.[15] The philosophical interpretations of quantum mechanics may be considered weird from the standpoint of our practical everyday experiences in the macroscopic world. Nevertheless, the applications of quantum mechanics to chemical bonding have changed the way chemists think about molecular structures and have made chemistry a subdiscipline of physics. Many unexplained chemical effects may be understood in the context of molecular orbital (MO) calculations. For example, the anomeric effect seen in carbohydrate chemistry can be rationalized as a combination of MO interactions and electrostatic effects. Although chemists like to follow the example of G. N. Lewis and write simplified molecular structures (Lewis structures), molecules are really nuclei embedded in a sea of electrons. It is remarkable that so many organic structures can be represented, as a first approximation, by localized chemical bonds and lone pairs of electrons. As any student going through a course in organic chemistry can attest, chemical reactivity and physical properties may be explained, in many situations, by extending our simplified bonding concepts to include resonance and electron delocalization. Because most drugs (or organic molecules) and their interactions with macromolecules are responsible for the observed biological effects called "drug action," it is quite reasonable to use theoretical MO methods to understand electron distributions and predict physical properties of drug-like structures. The only way this can be achieved is through the use of quantum chemistry, since force field methods do not explicitly treat electrons.

The history of quantum mechanics, while fascinating, is too lengthy to discuss here, as is a full development of the theory. The goal of this chapter is to present the concepts succinctly for readers who have never taken courses in physical chemistry, where these topics are more fully developed. The emphasis is on following the logical order of concepts, not on the mathematical details, which means some relationships have been simplified. With the fundamentals presented below, it is possible to understand the impact quantum mechanics has, and will continue to have, on medicinal chemistry. The sections that follow contain references to quantum mechanical applications in CADD.

We start with the contributions of Max Planck. At the beginning of the 20th century, physics was in a theoretical crisis. It was believed that Newton's equations and Maxwell's electromagnetic theory could explain all natural phenomena, but the application of these classical mechanics methods to the emission of electromagnetic radiation from perfect "black bodies" did not correlate with experiment. In the theoretical treatments, the radiation was assumed to result from the microscopic oscillators, and the inescapable conclusion of classical mechanics was that a continuous range of energies was available to the oscillator. Planck suggested in 1900 that the energy associated with oscillators was a function of integral values of quanta (Eq. 28-43), where E is the energy of the oscillator, h is Planck's constant (6.626×10^{-34} J-sec), and ν is the frequency. The suggestion worked, but many scientists of that period thought this solution was simply a mathematical trick, because the logical extension meant that energy was available only in discrete quantum values and was not continuous.

$$E = h\nu \qquad \text{(Eq. 28-43)}$$

The quantum idea was used by Einstein to explain the photoelectric effect. When metal surfaces are subjected in vacuo to electromagnetic radiation of specific frequencies, electrons are released. The phenomenon could not be explained by classical mechanics. Einstein used the quantum concept to suggest that electromagnetic radiation was simply a stream of photons where Equation 28-43 correctly defined the energy. Using this quantum idea, Einstein formulated a relationship (Eq. 28-44) between the incident electromagnetic radiation and the expelled electrons. Einstein's work supported the Planck quantum theory. In this equation, Φ is called the work function, which is the minimum energy necessary to eject electrons from the metal surface. Some simple deduction, knowing that the kinetic energy $m\vec{v}^2/2$ cannot be zero, requires that $\Phi = h\nu_0$; therefore, ν_0 is the minimum frequency allowed. (Interestingly, Einstein won the Nobel Prize for his contributions to understanding the photoelectric effect and related matters rather than for his theory of relativity.)

$$h\nu - \Phi = \frac{1}{2} m\vec{v}^2 \qquad \text{(Eq. 28-44)}$$

Because light has particle-like characteristics, de Broglie argued that electrons should therefore exhibit wave-like characteristics. This is odd because it defies our macroscopic experiences. The wave-like character exists for all objects, but only manifests itself—for all practical purposes—with microscopic particles (e.g., electrons). The de Broglie relationship (Eq. 28-45) quantifies the wave-like properties that matter exhibits, where λ is the wavelength, h is Planck's constant, and $m\vec{v}$ is the momentum (mass $\times$ velocity). Clearly, the relationship shows that for tiny masses, the wave property of matter is significant, whereas for large objects, the wave-like character is vanishingly small.

$$\lambda = \frac{h}{m\vec{v}} \qquad \text{(Eq. 28-45)}$$

At this point in 20th century science, it was becoming accepted that matter had both wave-like and particle-like characteristics. Depending on the experimental setup, these seemingly contradictory properties could be observed. If matter has wave-like properties, then there had to exist some generally descriptive wave equation. It was Erwin Schrödinger who recognized that standing waves with imposed boundary conditions yielded sets of integers, which would be consistent with spectroscopic observations.[89–91] He developed the now famous Schrödinger wave equation (Eq. 28-46) for a single particle such as an electron in a 3D box. This equation is a linear (meaning the wave function is raised to a power greater than 1), second-order differential equation (meaning second derivatives are involved), where E is the total energy of the system, U is the potential energy, and $\psi_{el}(x,y,z)$ is the electronic wave function. (Different symbols are used routinely in the literature when discussing wave functions. In this chapter, lower-case psi, ψ, and upper-case psi, Ψ, are used to denote the wave functions for a single particle or a multiparticle system, respectively. Also, lower-case phi, ϕ, is used to represent atomic orbitals,

and lower-case chi, χ, is used for a spin orbital, which is defined below.)

$$\left(\frac{\partial^2}{\partial x^2} + \frac{\partial^2}{\partial y^2} + \frac{\partial^2}{\partial z^2}\right)\psi_{el}(x,y,z) + \frac{8\pi^2 m}{h^2}(E - U)\psi_{el}(x,y,z) = 0$$
$$\text{(Eq. 28-46)}$$

Equation 28-46 can be arranged to give Equation 28-47.

$$\frac{-h^2}{8\pi^2 m}\left(\frac{\partial^2}{\partial x^2} + \frac{\partial^2}{\partial y^2} + \frac{\partial^2}{\partial z^2}\right)\psi_{el}(x,y,z) + U\psi_{el}(x,y,z) = E\psi_{el}(x,y,z)$$
$$\text{(Eq. 28-47)}$$

A more compact (and perhaps less offensive) form of the Schrödinger equation is given by Equation 28-48, where $\hat{H} \equiv -\dfrac{h^2}{8\pi^2 m}\nabla^2 + U(x,y,z)$, ψ_{el} is understood to be a function of the x,y,z coordinates, and ∇^2 was defined earlier in Equation 28-26. (It is not necessary to demand that ψ be a function of cartesian coordinates. The choice of the coordinate system may be dictated by the nature of the problem being solved. In other words, it may be easier to solve a problem within a different reference frame. ψ_{el} may be a function of spherical polar, plane polar, or cylindrical coordinates or of other coordinate systems. For example, solution to the hydrogen atom involves the use of spherical polar coordinates.) $\hat{H}$ is the hamiltonian operator, which is the quantum mechanical equivalent of the classical mechanics formulation $H = T + U$, where T is the kinetic energy and U is the potential energy. Note the similarities between the classical and quantum mechanical formulations of the hamiltonian.

$$\hat{H}\psi_{el} = E\psi_{el} \qquad \text{(Eq. 28-48)}$$

Equation 28-48 is the Schrödinger equation for a single particle. For the application of quantum mechanics to medicinal chemistry, it is necessary to think in terms of electrons moving around nuclei. The Schrödinger equation can be converted into a multiatom problem, given by Equation 28-49. In Equation 28-49, the hamiltonian is

$$\hat{H} \equiv -\frac{h^2}{8\pi^2}\sum_i \frac{1}{m_i}\nabla_i^2 + \sum_i \sum_{j<i} \frac{e_i e_j}{|r_{ij}|}$$

The first term (kinetic energy) is a summation over all the particles in the molecule. The second term (potential energy) uses Coulomb's law to calculate the interaction between every pair of particles in the molecule, where e_i and e_j are the charges on particles i and j. For electrons, the charge is $-e$, while the charge for a nucleus is Ze, where Z is the atomic number. The summation notation $i<j$ for the indices means that one does not doublecount pairwise interaction terms in the summation (e.g., $e_i e_j = e_j e_i$ and should only appear in the potential energy term once). The denominator $|r_{ij}|$ in the second term is the distance between particles i and j. Ψ_{el} is understood to be the electronic wave function for a many-atom system.

$$\hat{H}\Psi_{el} = E\Psi_{el} \qquad \text{(Eq. 28-49)}$$

Originally, Ψ was thought to be a physical wave that was propagated through space. Today, Ψ^2 is more properly interpreted, from the work of Born who first made the proposal, as being proportional to the probability of finding a particle in a small volume element $d\tau$, where $d\tau = dxdydz$. In the more general case, the probability is represented by $\Psi_1^*\Psi$, where Ψ is multiplied by the complex conjugate Ψ^*. The complex conjugate is necessary, in that the wave function may contain imaginary numbers. Because $\Psi^*\Psi d\tau$ represents the probability for a small volume element, it is possible to define Ψ_{el} such that the integral over all space is unity ($\int \Psi_{el}^*\Psi_{el}d\tau = 1$) through the appropriate choice of coefficients. The integral symbol is more complicated than it may appear. It really spans all of coordinate space, so for cartesian coordinates, the range goes from negative to positive infinity for each of the three x, y, and z coordinates. This means that Equation 28-49 is deceptive, since it involves solving a triple integral, $\iiint \Psi_{el}^*(x,y,z)\Psi^*(x,y,z)dxdydz$. To be an "acceptable" Ψ_{el}, there are certain conditions that are required:

1. The wave equation must be well-behaved mathematically.
2. The equation must be a continuous function, which becomes zero at infinity.
3. The wave equation must be single valued.

Equation 28-49 is a complex equation, even in the simplest of examples. It must be applied to every electron in a molecule or molecular system under examination. The Schrödinger equation has exact solutions for only a few simple cases (e.g., a particle in a box, a particle on a ring, the harmonic oscillator, the rigid rotor, the hydrogen atom, the hydrogen molecule ion). Each example listed builds on previous ones but gets more mathematically challenging. Solution of the nonrelativistic Schrödinger equation for the hydrogen atom yields the set of quantum numbers n, l, and m familiar from general chemistry. The spin quantum number s is not one that comes from the Schrödinger treatment. It may be added in an ad hoc fashion, using the magnetic quantum number m as a guide. The fourth quantum number does, however, naturally arise from an alternative mathematical development of quantum mechanics that is formulated by using matrix methods.[92] Later it was shown that both the wave and matrix approaches are equivalent.[93, 94] Exact solutions to drug-like molecules, whether by wave or matrix quantum mechanics, are impossible. Nevertheless, some simplifying assumptions have been developed over the years, beginning in the 1950s when computers made approximate solutions feasible, that result in good electron-based models.

Equation 28-49 may be arranged to give Equation 28-50 by multiplying both sides of the equation by $\int \Psi_{el}^*$ and then solving for the energy of the system E. If the Ψ_{el} function is normalized, meaning it has been scaled such that $\int \Psi_{el}^*\Psi_{el}d;\tau = 1$, the denominator is unity.

$$E = \frac{\int \Psi_{el}^*\hat{H}\Psi_{el}d\tau}{\int \Psi_{el}^*\Psi_{el}d\tau} \qquad \text{(Eq. 28-50)}$$

For a many-electron system, the Hartree-Fock wave function Ψ_{HF}, defined as the product of spin orbitals χ_i as outlined in Equation 28-51, where $A(n)$ is an antisymmetrizer for the electrons, provides good answers.[94] This is the starting point for either semiempirical or ab initio theory. It is necessary to have $A(n)$ to make the wave function antisymmetric, thus obeying the Pauli exclusion principle, which asserts that two electrons cannot be in the same quantum state.

$$\Psi_{HF} = A(n)\chi_1(1)\chi_2(2)\chi_3(3)\cdots\chi_n(n) \qquad \text{(Eq. 28-51)}$$

Another consequence of the Pauli exclusion principle is that the spin orbital is a product of a spatial function ψ and a spin function α or β (Equation 28-52).

$$\chi_i = \begin{cases} \psi_i(x,y,z)\alpha \\ \psi_i(x,y,z)\beta \end{cases} \qquad \text{(Eq. 28-52)}$$

The antisymmetric wave function, shown in Equation 28-51, is a more compact way of writing a Slater determinant (Eq. 28-53). In a Slater determinant, an exchange of any two rows or columns results in the same wave function multiplied by -1. This is another statement of the Pauli exclusion principle. The columns in Equation 28-53 are the single electron wave functions. Equation 28-53, however, is only an approximation, since the electrons are independent of one another and therefore not correlated. This correlation problem reveals itself when calculating the energies and is discussed below.

$$\Psi_{HF} = \frac{1}{\sqrt{N!}} \begin{vmatrix} \chi_1(1) & \chi_2(1) & \cdots & \chi_N(1) \\ \chi_1(2) & \chi_2(2) & \cdots & \chi_N(2) \\ \vdots & \vdots & \vdots & \vdots \\ \chi_1(N) & \chi_2(N) & \cdots & \chi_N(N) \end{vmatrix} \qquad \text{(Eq. 28-53)}$$

Usually, the spatial function ψ is constructed from the summation of one-electron spatial orbitals (atomic orbitals) ϕ, known as the basis set, used to construct a MO. This approach is known as the LCAO method (*l*inear *c*ombination of *a*tomic *o*rbitals).[17, 18] It is an approximation of the accurate many-electron wave function (Eq. 28-54). The atomic orbital contributions are weighted by coefficients c_i. The summation is truncated, so the ψ function is not complete, which has consequences when solving for E.

$$\psi_{MO} = \sum_{i=1}^{n} c_i\phi_i \qquad \text{(Eq. 28-54)}$$

The energy of the system E is a function of ψ. The variational theorem[95] is an important starting point in computational quantum chemistry. It states that the calculated energy of the system is always going to be greater than or equal to the true experimental energy (Eq. 28-55). For the calculated and true energies to be equal, the Ψ function must be exact. Exact wave functions are not possible for molecular structures, since there are an infinite series of atomic orbitals, described above. Therefore, every selection for Ψ will generate a trial wave function, Ψ_{trial}, and the variational theorem demands that the energy will always be higher than the true energy. As Ψ_{trial} approaches the true wave function Ψ, the energy becomes lower and lower, approaching the true experimental energy E.

$$\frac{\int \Psi_{trial}^*\hat{H}\Psi_{trial}d\tau}{\int \Psi_{trial}^*\Psi_{trial}d\tau} \geq E_{true} \qquad \text{(Eq. 28-55)}$$

Solutions to the Schrödinger equation for drug-like molecules may be obtained by making approximations and simplifying assumptions. There are three basic divisions of computational quantum chemistry calculations: *(a)* semiempirical, *(b)* ab initio, and *(c)* density functional theory (DFT).

Early efforts by Pople and coworkers produced a method called CNDO (*c*omplete *n*eglect of *d*ifferential *over*lap).[96–102] In general, the semiempirical approach eliminates integrals that are too complicated to solve analytically. (This is an interesting concept in higher math: if the term is too hard to solve, discard it.) In their place, appropriate factors (constants and equations) are introduced to compensate. Fortunately, the integrals eliminated in the semiempirical approach give relatively small values if solved. Equation 28-56 shows the most complicated type of integrals that are removed in the semiempirical model. They are known as two-electron integrals, where 1 and 2 represent the two electrons, spanning four atomic centers i, j, k, l.

$$\phi_i^*(1)\phi_j(1)\frac{1}{r_{12}}\phi_k^*(2)\phi_l(2) \qquad \text{(Eq. 28-56)}$$

The extensive efforts of Dewar resulted in a series of reasonably accurate semiempirical models: MINDO (*m*odified *i*ntermediate *n*eglect of *d*ifferential *o*verlap).[103, 104] The third version in this series, MINDO/3,[105–109] gave much improved results. The program allowed organic and medicinal chemists to apply electron-based calculations to diverse compounds. The availability of MINDO/3 helped make computational chemistry accessible to experimentalists. The MNDO (*m*oderate *n*eglect of *d*ifferential *o*verlap) model,[110–115] after some modifications of the observed systematic errors, served as the basis for the AM1 (Austin method 1).[116] Stewart took the AM1 model and introduced automated parameterization techniques with a different parameterization philosophy than Dewar. The result was PM3 (parameter method 3).[117]

There are known strengths and weaknesses of each semiempirical method. The AM1 and PM3 models only include s- and p-functions, which limits their usefulness for most elements of the periodic table that require d-orbitals. Many of these elements, however, are not typically found in most drug-like molecules. More recent advances with MNDO/d include the incorporation of d-functions in the NDDO (*n*eglect of *d*iatomic *d*ifferential *o*verlap) model.[118, 119]

Extensive use has been made of semiempirical methods in drug design.[120, 121] Calculations of the highest occupied MO and lowest unoccupied MO (HOMO/LUMO) energies for a series of active and inactive compounds have been used as descriptors for QSAR. AM1, for example, has recently been used to develop a predictive ADME model for P-450 oxidation of drugs, which is discussed below.

The more mathematically rigorous ab initio calculations, as the name implies (''from first principles''), do not use parameters in the same way as the semiempirical models.[95] Unlike semiempirical calculations, no classes of integrals are eliminated. Ab initio methods have, however, a number of approximations. Aside from truncated basis sets, in which the constants have been adjusted to give the optimal basis set, one of the most noteworthy approximations involves the functional form of the wave function ϕ. Solving the Schrödinger equation for the hydrogen atom produces the familiar hydrogenic orbitals, which can be approximated by Slater type (ST) functions. Both are exponential functions having the form $e^{-\alpha u(\bar{r})}$, where ζ is the exponential coefficient and u is a function of the electronic and nuclear positions $\bar{r}$. Solving integrals, which are products of exponential functions, can be CPU intensive. Boys proposed that gaussian type (GT) functions of the form $e^{-\alpha u(\bar{r})}$ could be substituted for ST functions.[122] The theoretical community did not immediately embrace the idea until Pople demonstrated convincingly that a linear combination of GT functions could

mimic ST functions reasonably well. Using three GT functions for every ST function gave rise to a popular basis set known as STO-3G, and many calculations were carried out by using this minimal basis set. STO-3G means three GT functions are used to reproduce every ST function.[123–126]

Pople and coworkers discovered that more extensive combinations of GT functions improved the accuracy of ab initio calculations. The next advance was an attempt to give greater flexibility to the ab initio models. By splitting the GT functions used to describe the valence shell electrons into two separate functions, better agreement between experiment and calculations was achieved. This method is known as split-level basis sets and is more time consuming. For example, 3-21G basis sets quickly replaced STO-3G.[127–129] The symbolism 3-21G means that the inner core or nonvalence electrons are described by three GT functions, and the outer shell or valence electrons are broken into an inner and outer set. The inner set is simulated by two GT functions, while the outer set is simulated by one GT function. Equation 28-57 shows the expansion of the atomic orbitals into GT functions g_i, where a_j represent fixed coefficients.

$$\phi_{(AO)j} = \sum_{i=1}^{n} a_{ij}g_i \qquad \text{(Eq. 28-57)}$$

Additional basis sets may be added to the split-level formulations to achieve greater accuracy. These additional functions are known as polarization functions. For example, 6-31G(d), formerly represented as 6-31G*, has a set of diffuse d-orbitals added to the heavy atoms (nonhydrogen atoms).[130–132] In another example, 6-31G(d,p), formerly known as 6-31G**, has a set of d-orbitals added to each heavy atom, as in 6-31G(d), in addition to a set of three p-orbitals for all the hydrogens.[133] The next level of approximation divides the valence electrons into three sets of GT functions (e.g., 6-311G).[134] An additional set of very diffuse functions can be added to the model to help calculate negatively charged species or hydrogen bonding, denoted by the plus sign in the examples 6-31+G(d,p) and 6-311+G(d,p).[135, 136]

An iterative solution of the Hartree-Fock-Roothaan equations is required for semiempirical and ab initio quantum chemical calculations.[137–139] The approach is also called the *self-consistent field* (SCF) approach. In SCF calculations, each single electron's position in space is optimized in the electric field of all the other electrons. This procedure is repeated until all the electron positions have been optimized, and there is no further significant drop in energy through the adjustment of the electron positions. Hartree-Fock (HF) calculations give good results. The better the basis set, the lower the energy according to the variational theorem. There comes a point of diminishing returns, however, in that the energy approaches a limit known as the Hartree-Fock limit. No further adjustment in the basis set breaks this barrier. The Hartree-Fock limit occurs because the electron motion is correlated, and this is not accounted for in a single Slater determinant. That is, the adjustment of one electron affects the position of the other electrons, and this is not fully taken into account by the SCF approach. To circumvent not taking electron correlation into account, post-SCF calculations must be used in the form of configuration interaction or perturbation methods.

Twsao commonly used post-SCF (or post-Hartree-Fock) methods are used: configuration interaction and perturbation methods.[140–144] In the former, the wave function is a summation of other Hartree-Fock determinants. This is analogous to exciting electrons to higher energy orbitals. In the latter, as the name implies, a perturbation is added to the Hartree-Fock hamilton. Møller-Plesset perturbation theory (MP2, MP3) is not a variational approach, so it is possible to calculate an energy lower than the true value.

There are no quantum mechanical charge operators. Thus, charges are determined on the basis of a population analysis. The electron density $\rho(r)$ is calculated and divided between the atoms of a molecule. The difficulty, however, is in determining how to assign shared electron density between two atoms i and j of different electronegativity. In the Mulliken population analysis,[145] the shared electron density is divided evenly between atoms i and j, regardless of the electronegativity. This, of course, is unrealistic but remains a useful technique. Other electron population analyses have become increasingly popular over the years. As discussed above, fitting charges to electron densities is a way to get more realistic atomic charges. With the electron density distributed throughout a molecular structure, according to an ad hoc population analysis, it is possible to generate dipole moments and color-code the electrostatic potential on molecular surfaces. The electrostatic potential may be useful in developing a pharmacophore and deciding what properties a receptor must have.

Density functional theory (DFT) has been used increasingly over the years.[146] DFT has a radically different approach than that in the preceding discussion on semiempirical and ab initio methods and may be more easily understood. In the DFT formulation, Kohn-Sham equations, electron correlation is built-in.[147] This means that DFT rivals post-SCF calculations for accuracy. Rather than dealing with the multielectron wave function, the electron density is used directly. According to the Kohn-Hohenberg theorem,[148] the energy is minimized when the calculated and true electron densities are equal. DFT calculations rival the accuracy of standard post-Hartree-Fock methods. Of practical importance to medicinal chemists interested in studying drug-like molecular structures with quantum-based energy calculations, there is a significant reduction in the CPU time. Thus, DFT is an attractive alternative. For example, the CPU time required to complete Hartree-Fock calculations, which of course is a function of the number of electrons in the system being examined, is proportional to the number of electrons raised to the fourth power. DFT calculations, however, also a function of the number of electrons in the system, are proportional to the number of electrons raised to the third power.

STRUCTURE-BASED DRUG DESIGN AND PHARMACOPHORE PERCEPTION

The choice of CADD methods that may be applied to drug design depends highly on the availability of the receptor information. If the receptor structure has been characterized by either high-resolution x-ray crystallography or NMR spectroscopy techniques, structure-based drug design methods may be appropriate. (The term *structure-based drug design* refers to the fact that experimental structural data of the macromolecule of the drug–receptor complex is involved in the modeling process explicitly.) The x-ray structures of a receptor and ligand-receptor complex provide information about the binding mode of the ligand. If available, multiple x-ray structures with different ligands provide greater insight into the steric and electrostatic tolerances of the binding cavity. Using sophisticated molecular modeling software, the ligand is modified structurally in silico to achieve a better fit between the complementary binding sites and molecular volumes. The small molecule typically is clipped out of the ligand–receptor complex altogether, and new molecular structures are *docked* into the binding site. It is no coincidence that structure-based modeling began to be applied more frequently in the mid-1980s. The exponential explosion of protein 3D structural information[149] (Fig. 28-18), which was made possible by cloning techniques, made it possible to have macromolecular structural data. The advances in a seemingly unrelated field have helped to usher in the age of structure-based drug design by making proteins available in larger quantities for x-ray studies.

If scant structural information about the receptor is known, which is most commonly the situation confronting medicinal chemists, a more indirect approach is required. This second approach has been characterized as pharmacophore mapping or pharmacophore perception.[150] The critical functional groups and their 3D spatial orientations may be perceived by examining all molecular structures that induce biological activities. A comparison of active versus inactive compounds helps to understand the structural and conformational requirements of a drug candidate. Once a model has been developed, a 3D search query can be submitted to 3D databases. The goal of using a 3D database is to find existing structures that meet the constraints of the query for immediate biological evaluations, thus avoiding synthesis. If the retrieved compounds show activity, they can serve as lead structures for further structural refinements.

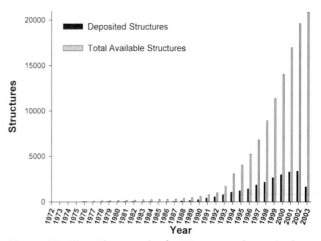

Figure 28–18 ■ The growth of a 3D structural protein database is exponential. The availability of structural information in the Protein Data Bank has helped fuel the growth and success of structure-based drug design. Values are as of May 9, 2003.

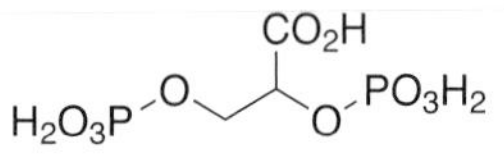

Figure 28–19 ■ Three compounds designed by Beddell and coworkers to mimic the binding of 2,3-diphosphoglycerate (DPG) **(2)** to hemoglobin.

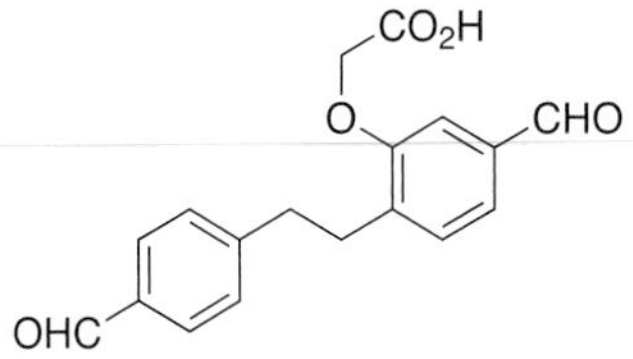

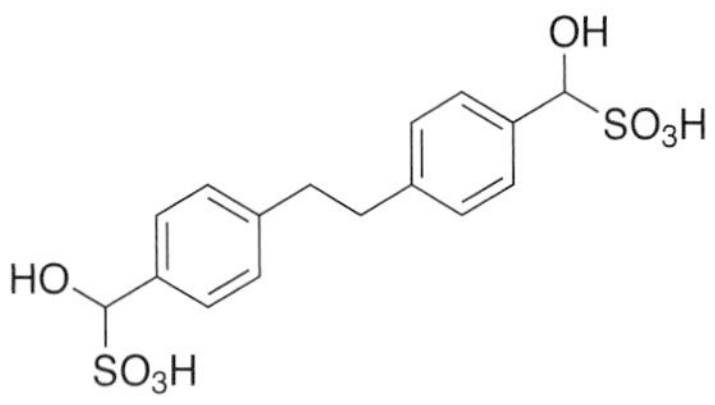

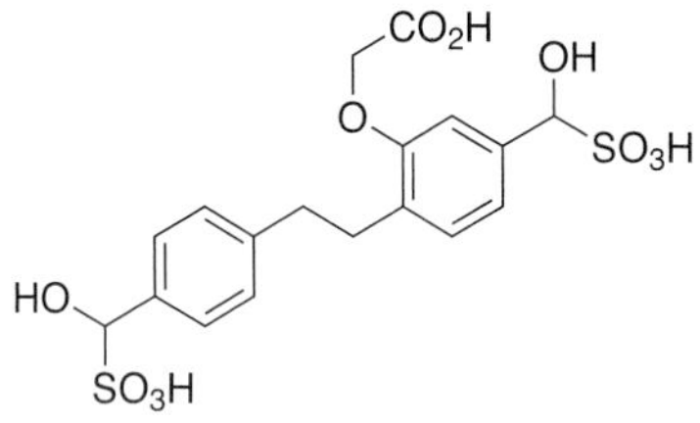

The concepts of structure-based or receptor-based drug design predate the use of computers. Beddell and coworkers are credited in 1976 with successfully predicting compounds that bind to human hemoglobin.[151] Although not strictly a drug–receptor interaction, the approach demonstrated the feasibility of molecular modeling applied to drug design. The goal of their study was to exploit the known binding site of the human deoxyhemoglobin tetramer. The tetramer consists of four single polypeptide chains: two α and two β subunits. The small molecule 2,3-diphosphoglycerate (DPG), **2**, binds with subsequent stabilization of the deoxy conformation (Fig. 28-19). The binding results in the liberation of oxygen, which is readily measured. Wire molecular models of the protein were used to measure bond distances and interacting atoms between the protein and the proposed small molecules. Based on the best fit, predictions were made as to which compounds would bind the best. These early modeling studies suggested that compounds **3–5** would have an affinity for the 2,3-binding site of human hemoglobin. Based on the liberation of oxygen, it was determined that the binding affinities corresponded to **2 ≈ 5 > 4 > 3.**

The often-cited design of the first angiotensin-converting enzyme (ACE) inhibitors by Ondetti and Cushman during this time effectively demonstrated the concept of mechanism-based and structure-based drug design.[152, 153] The Ondetti and Cushman approach resulted in the first marketed ACE inhibitor, captopril, **6** (Fig. 28-20). Many other ACE inhibitors have been designed using computer-based models,

although not by direct structure-based modeling, since to date the structural determination of ACE has not been accomplished. Ondetti and Cushman conceived of captopril based on a related enzyme, carboxypeptidase A, and the earlier reports of succinic acid inhibitors by Wolfenden.[154] Other computer-based methods have been used successfully in ACE inhibitor design. Force field calculations, conformational searching, and analogue design strategies were used by Merck scientists to develop inhibitors. Scientists at Merck have used small molecule structural data (x-ray crystallographic data and NMR solution studies) coupled with conformational methods to design conformationally restricted ACE inhibitors.[155]

Since the 1980s, there have been many success stories using structure-based drug design. One of the first convincing examples of the combined use of an x-ray crystal structure and molecular modeling software was reported in 1982.[156] Again, although this was not a true drug–receptor interaction, the work demonstrated fundamental principles that would be applied later. The x-ray crystallographic coordinates of the L-thyroxine–prealbumin compound have three pairs of symmetry-related cavities (Fig. 28-21). It was noticed that one binding pocket of the symmetric prealbumin

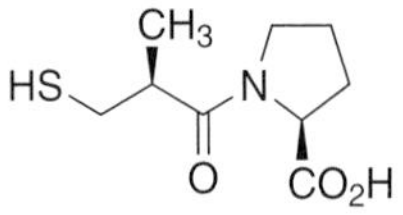

6

Figure 28–20 ■ Captopril was the successful outcome of a rational design approach in which the mechanism of the conversion of angiotensin I to angiotensin II was known. The angiotensin-converting enzyme (ACE) was assumed to have binding cavities similar to the known x-ray structure of carboxypeptidase.

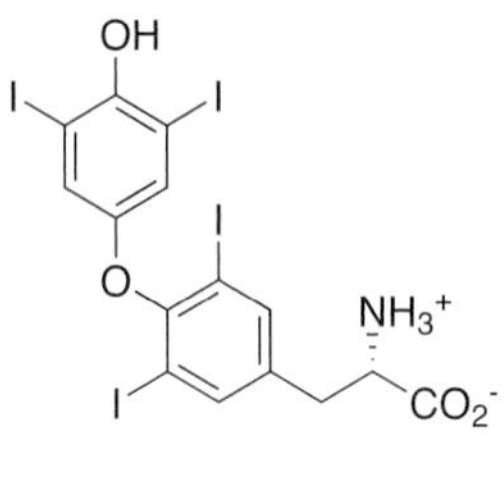

7

Figure 28–21 ■ The molecule L-thyroxine, **7**, binds to prealbumin, a protein found in blood. Based on x-ray data of the L-thyroxine–prealbumin complex, the binding affinity of novel analogues was predicted by using a molecular modeling approach.

dimer was unoccupied by L-thyroxine, **7** (Fig. 28-22). This unoccupied binding pocket had the potential to accommodate a portion of new compound, which presumably would result in greater binding affinity by increasing the contact between the van der Waals surfaces in this hormone–protein complex.

The scientists used a guiding hypothesis that the "tightness of fit" between the computer-generated complementary molecular surfaces of the ligand and prealbumin would correlate to enhanced binding affinities. They modeled the molecular surface interactions with the MS program on an Evans and Sutherland PS2 graphics station. With available modeling software, the UCSF (University of California at San Francisco) scientists stripped L-thyroxine from the binding site and docked various naphthalene-based structures with different substitution patterns, shown in Figure 28-23. The modeling studies were carried out without the aid of force field refinement. After modeling a diverse set of analogues, the scientists concluded that at least three of the four outer binding pockets needed to be filled. Four thyroid hormone analogues (structures **8–11**) were ranked based on visual inspection using their complementarity of fit hypothesis. Structure **8** did not present any bad contacts, while **11** had some obviously bad surface contacts. Structures **9** and **10** appeared to have equally good molecular surface interactions. Once the compounds were ranked (**8** > **9** ≈ **10** > **11**), their binding affinities were determined. The binding data were consistent with the predictions, except structures **9** and **10** were not equivalent. Closer inspection revealed that the phenolic hydroxyl group of **10** had a better surface fit and is in close proximity to Ser-117C and Thr-119C, thus providing additional binding interactions not available to **9**.

Presumably, the additional interactions would have been detected with force field calculations.

In 1985, scientists at Burroughs Wellcome (United States) and the Wellcome Research Laboratories (England) reported some of their CADD efforts for the prediction of dihydrofolate reductase (DHFR) inhibitors.[157] DHFR is an excellent target, since this enzyme pathway is the only known de novo synthetic route to prepare thymine in vivo. Thymine, of course, is one of the four nucleic acids of DNA. For many years DHFR had been a popular drug target for medicinal chemists. Significant drug design activity using the prevailing principles of medicinal chemistry was associated with the development of DHFR inhibitors for antibacterial and antitumor agents. Methotrexate (MTX), **12**, and trimethoprim (TMP), **13**, are good inhibitors of DHFR. Figure 28-24 shows the obvious structural similarities of MTX and folic acid, **14**.

Over the years, literally thousands of inhibitors of DHFR were prepared on the basis of medicinal chemistry intuition preceding the structure-based efforts. A series of 3′-carboxy-alkoxy analogues of TMP were designed based on molecular models of the *Escherichia coli* DHFR–MTX complex. The designed TMP analogues had up to a 55-fold higher enzyme affinity than TMP itself. Kuyper and coworkers noticed that in the *E. coli* DHFR–MTX complex, the α- and γ-carboxyl groups formed ionic interactions with the guanidinium group of Arg-57 and the aminoalkyl side chain of Lys-32, respectively. The observation that there was a possible third ionic interaction with Arg-52 suggested that TMP analogues, with judiciously selected carboxylate groups, could interact with one or more of these complementary residues. The analogue with the carboxylate extended by five methylene units,

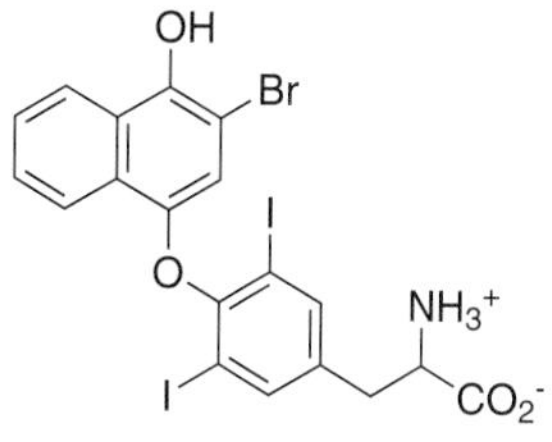

8

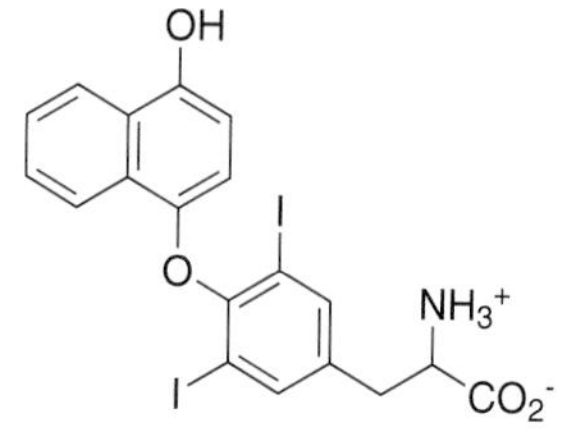

9

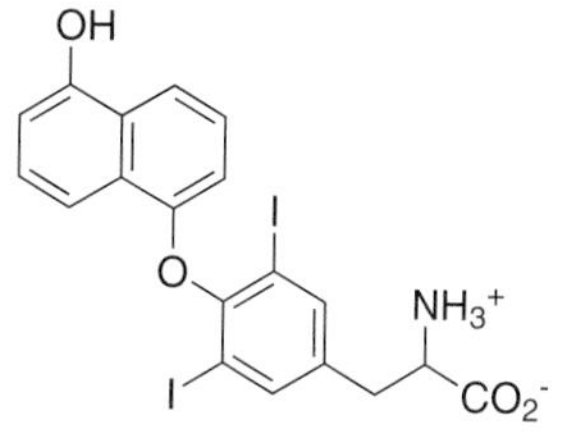

10

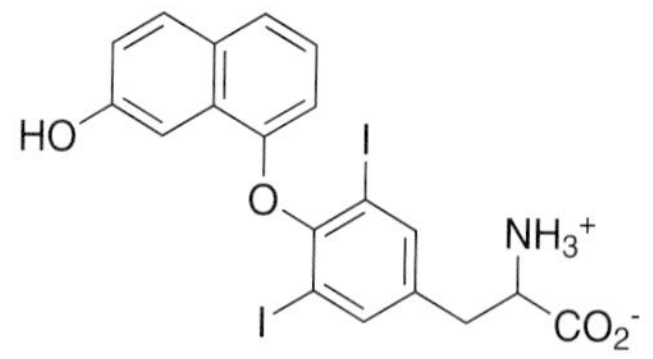

11

Figure 28–23 ▪ Using molecular modeling methods, four L-thyroxine analogues were predicted to have good binding affinity (**8** > **9** ≈ **10** > **11**) to prealbumin.

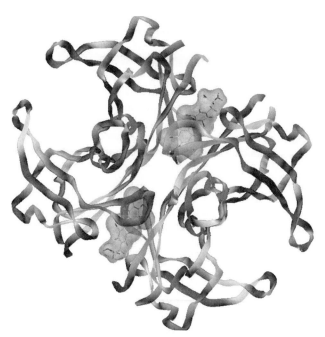

Figure 28–22 ▪ The experimental x-ray crystal structure of prealbumin with bound L-thyroxine. Prealbumin is a tetramer with four identical subunits, A, B, C, and D. The four identical subunits form a channel with two bound L-thyroxine molecules. The binding sites have a C_2 axis of symmetry.

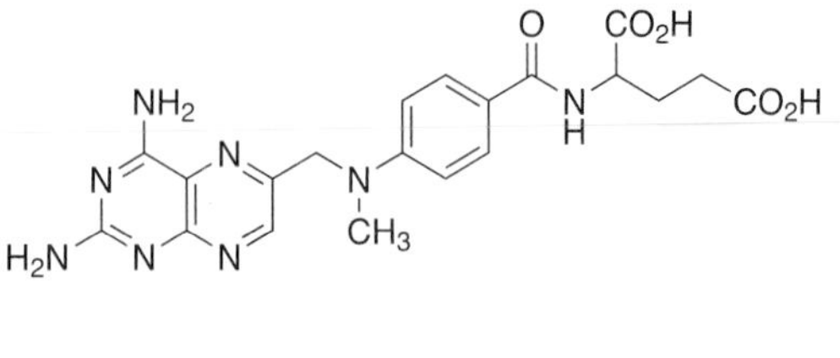

12

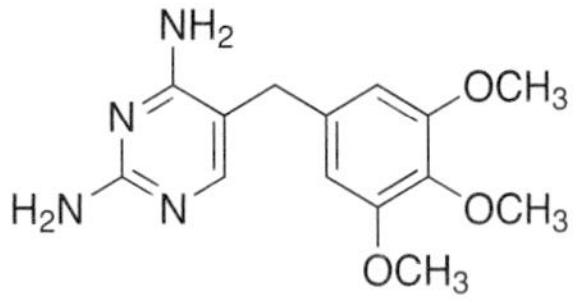

13

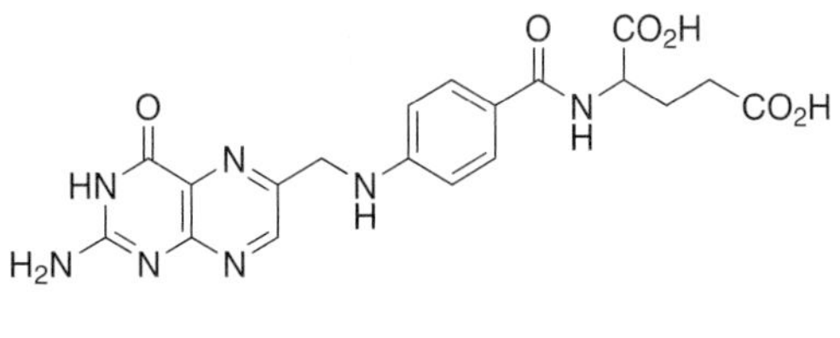

14

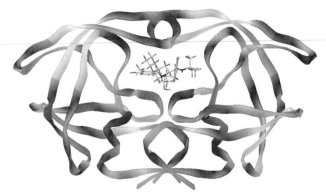

Figure 28–26 ■ Saquinavir (Fortovase, Invirase), **15**, was the first HIV-1 protease inhibitor designed with structure-based CADD methods to receive FDA approval. Here saquinavir is shown inside the binding cavity of HIV-1.

Figure 28–24 ■ Dihydrofolate reductase (DHFR) has been a popular target for drug design. Methotrexate (MTX), **12**, and trimethoprim (TMP), **13**, resemble folic acid, **14**, the natural substrate.

was the HIV protease. The enzyme is one of the proteins coded by the HIV genome, and it is expressed as part of the reproductive cycle of the virus. The x-ray crystal structure for HIV protease has been available for well over a decade now, and it is classified as an aspartyl protease, since there are active aspartate residues present. HIV protease is a symmetric dimer. There are 99 amino acid residues in each monomer. The binding cavity can be seen clearly in Figure 28-26.

In the late 1990s, several HIV-1 protease inhibitors were introduced into the market that were designed using structure-based methods (Fig. 28-27).[158, 159] Hoffmann-La Roche scientists used modeling methods to design saquinavir[160] (Fortovase, Invirase) **15**, which was the first protease inhibitor to be approved. The drug was made available in June 1995 through a compassionate treatment program. Invirase was given Food and Drug Administration (FDA) approval in December 1995, and Fortovase was approved in November 1997. Indinavir[161] (Crixivan), **16**, was developed by Merck scientists and given quick approval in only 42 days in March 1996. In March 1996, Abbott received approval for Ritonavir[162] (Norvir), **17**. The following year, March 1997, Agouron received final approval for Nelfinavir[163] (Viracept), **18**. Each of these drugs, designed using structure-based methods, represents major triumphs of CADD. Agouron originally was a company founded, like Vertex, on the premise that structure-based drug design is an effective approach for drug discovery. Amprenavir (Agenerase), **19**, developed at Vertex, was given FDA approval in April 1999. The ability to collect rapid x-ray crystallographic data allowed scientists at Pharmacia & Upjohn to use structure-

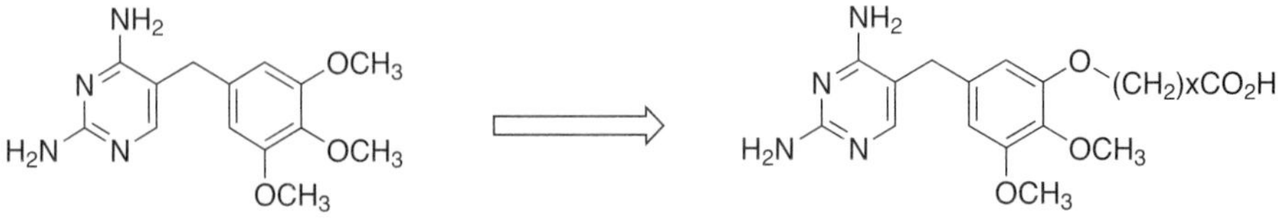

shown in Figure 28-25, was found to have the optimal binding. Much of the experimental binding data were consistent with the molecular modeling studies and the subsequent structural data. Although all the observations could not be explained, this work represents one of the first successful structure-based drug design approaches.

There is a growing body of successful examples using structure-based drug design approaches. Today, many of these have resulted in approved drugs. These methods are applied widely when appropriate experimental data are available. Structure-based drug design is now considered a standard approach to drug design, and the question posed early can be answered with specific examples.

In the 1980s, the target enzyme for inhibitor design was DHFR, as discussed above. In the 1990s, the target enzyme

Figure 28–25 ■ With the aid of x-ray data and molecular modeling, scientists designed trimethoprim (TMP), 13, analogues that had up to 55-fold higher enzyme affinity than the parent inhibitor.

13

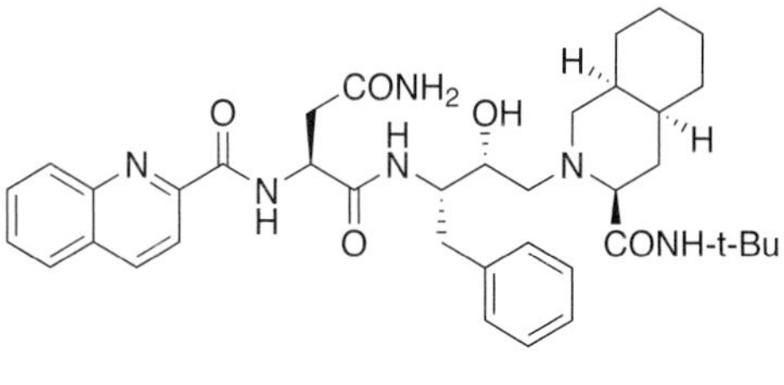

15

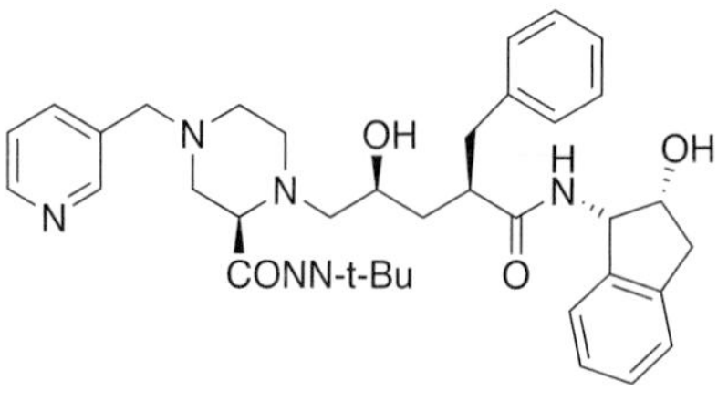

16

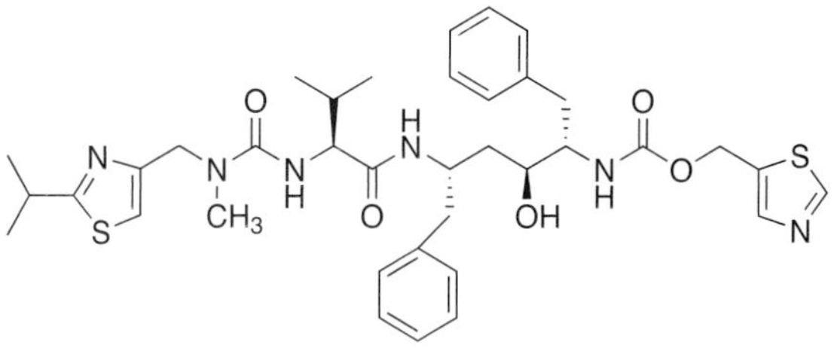

17

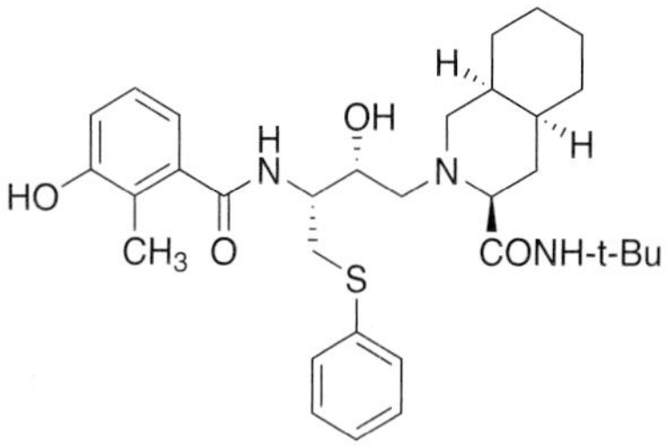

18

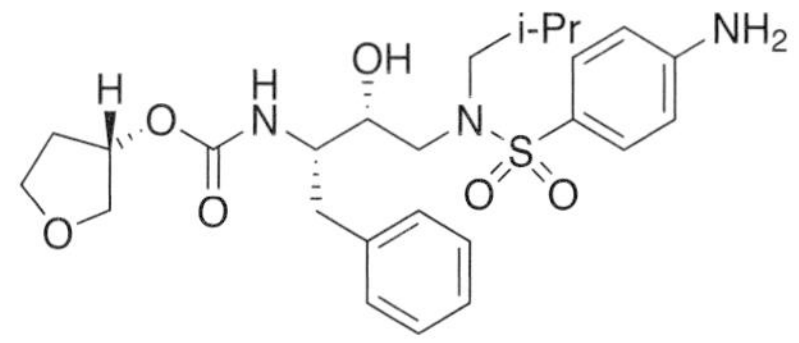

19

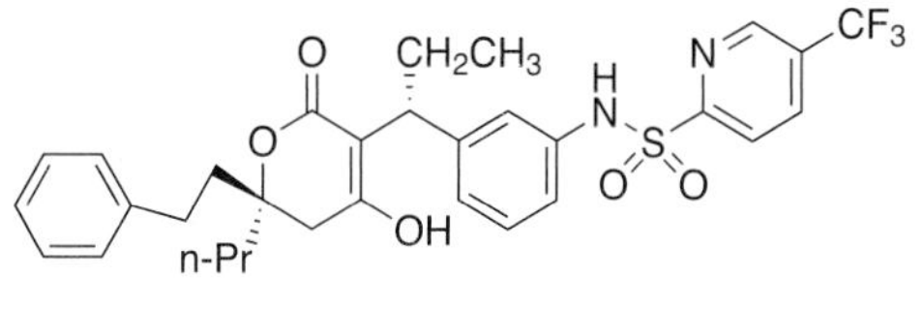

20

Figure 28–27 ■ The six HIV-1 protease inhibitors given FDA approval between 1994 and 1999 were designed by using structure-based drug design methods.

based methods. The resulting compound tipranavir, **20**, is a small nonpeptidic inhibitor that may soon be available.[164]

The first drug designed with structure-based methods to reach the market was dorzolamide[9, 165] (Trusopt), **1**. Ab initio calculations and modeling methods were used to predict substitution patterns. After a decade of research and development at Merck, dorzolamide was given FDA approval in December 1994 and introduced into the market in the sum-

mer of 1995. Dorzolamide is an effective carbonic anhydrase inhibitor used to reduce intraocular pressures that occur in glaucoma patients. It is extremely effective. Inhibition of carbonic anhydrase results in reduced bicarbonate formation in the eye, which has the beneficial effect of lowering sodium ions with the subsequent reduction of fluid secretions. Merck had been working on various lead thienothiopyran-2-sulfonamides by developing models and fitting them into electron density difference maps of carbonic anhydrase. The first carbonic anhydrase inhibitor to lower intraocular pressure in glaucoma patients was MK-927, **21**,[164] which is a close structural analogue of the compound finally approved (Fig. 28-28).

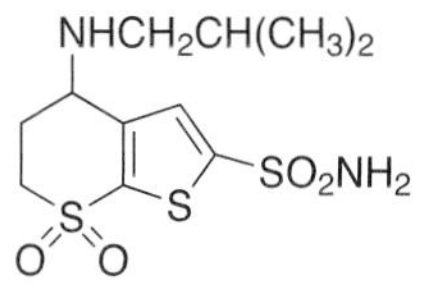

Another successful advance in therapeutics involved a combination of x-ray crystallographic studies and molecular shape analysis (MSA) to produce donepezil[166] (Aricept), **22** (Fig. 28-29). Donepezil is a potent acetylcholinesterase (AChE) inhibitor used in patients with Alzheimer's disease to help stave off the loss of cognitive abilities. Docking simulations of donepezil suggested that the drug does not actually bind to the AChE active site but rather inside the long channel leading to the active site in a tight, narrow region. In addition to the structure-based modeling studies, 3D-QSAR studies were carried out using semiempirical descriptors.

21

Figure 28–28 ■ Dorzolamide (Trusopt), **1**, also a constituent of Cosopt, was the first drug designed with structure-based CADD methods to become commercially available. MK-927, **21,** is a close structural analogue and was the first carbonic anhydrase inhibitor to lower intraocular pressure in glaucoma patients.

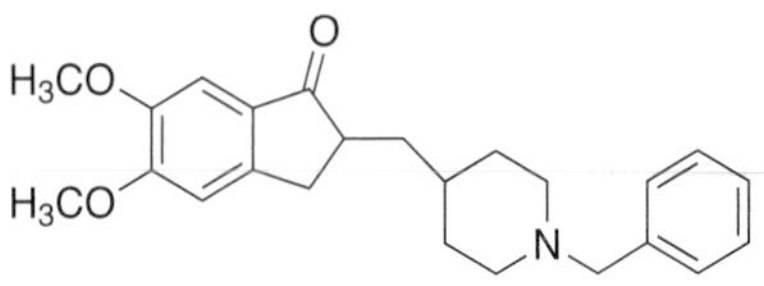

22

Figure 28–29 ■ Donepezil (Aricept), **22**, is a potent acetylcholinesterase (AChE) inhibitor used in the treatment of Alzheimer's disease.

The pharmacophore concept plays a central role in drug design. The pharmacophore, first proposed in the early 1900s by Paul Ehrlich, may be defined as the 3D arrangement of the essential functional groups necessary to cause the biological response. The definition only assumes that it is necessary for a drug to present its properly oriented functional groups to the receptor's complementary amino acid residues. Although the idea may be somewhat simplistic, since it ignores explicit consideration of the molecular structure that correctly orients the functional groups, the idea has withstood the test of time as a first approximation for a model of drug–receptor interactions.

Prior to the explosion of structural data now available to medicinal chemists who may use 3D structures of proteins, typically only indirect information about the nature of the receptor was available. The most common situation faced by medicinal chemists was a series of active and inactive compounds. The fact that there was no structure of the drug bound to its receptor meant that drug design had to follow a procedure of comparing the efficacy of compounds and determining which functional groups were important and which functional groups were not.

The active analogue approach, developed by Garland Marshall, was one of the earliest CADD pharmacophore procedures.[167–169] The approach avoids having to worry excessively about the subtle energy differences between conformations. Systematic conformational searching is applied to a series of biologically active and inactive compounds. The central idea is that there is a limited set of conformations that an active compound (with appropriate functional groups) may adopt. Biological inactivity is assumed, as a first approximation, to result from the competition between small molecules and the receptor for occupation of the same physical space. Usually, the most rigid structure is considered first. Subsequent systematic searches are carried out on the remaining "active" molecular structures. It is possible to add screening filters to eliminate unacceptable conformations; for example, computer-generated structures must be able to adopt conformations similar to those available to the previous molecular structures and not be outside a specified relative energy range. At the conclusion of the process, a volume may be generated representing the union of all available conformations for the biologically active compounds. This "active" volume may be used to glean information about the receptor site. It is possible to generate an "inactive" volume as well, which is the region in 3D space that should not be used to make molecular modifications.

Examination of a series of active and inactive compounds provides important structural information that is used to develop a pharmacophore hypothesis. Once a pharmacophore is developed, it is possible to search 3D structural databases. The first 3D searching software was developed in-house by pharmaceutical firms to mine the corporate 3D databases (ALADDIN,[170] developed at Abbott, and 3DSEARCH,[171] developed at Lederle). The construction of 3D databases was made possible by software such as CONCORD[172] and CORINA[173] that allowed rapid generation of 3D structures from 2D structures. CONCORD has become the standard program used for the creation of 3D structures from 2D input. It is important in 3D searches to account for structural flexibility. There are essentially three ways this may be achieved: *(a)* storing multiple conformations in the database itself; *(b)* developing specialized queries; and *(c)* generating conformations during the search query. The first idea requires that all conformations for every molecular structure be stored in a 3D database. This approach is not practical. Although the second approach is appealing, it requires the scientist to design the query appropriately. The third approach seems to solve the problem, inasmuch as only one (or a few) conformation needs to be stored and adjusted to match the pharmacophore search query. Today, there are several commercial programs available for 3D database and pharmacophore searching.

Goodford proposed that a grid of test points enveloping a molecular structure could be used to calculate favorable interactions (initially with 6–12 nonbonded, electrostatic, and hydrogen-bonding potential energy functions) between it and a target receptor. The program GRID[174] was an interesting innovation. The DOCK[175, 176] program can be considered the first *virtual* high-throughput screening software. The goal was to allow prescreening of compounds that could bind to an active site. A series of molecular structures can be evaluated for their fit into a receptor by use of scoring functions. An early study using α-chymotrypsin ranked several known inhibitors in the top 10 structures, based on the scoring functions used to evaluate the binding potential.[177] Another early academic 3D searching program was CAVEAT.[178]

Predictive pharmacophore models can be generated based on 3D-QSAR analyses. Hansch demonstrated the usefulness of QSAR.[179] In the 1970s, many studies were undertaken to infer biological activity on the basis of physical properties of a molecule. The method remains useful and provides valuable information.[180] Richard Cramer developed a popular program involving a comparative molecular field analysis (CoMFA).[181] The basic idea is to probe a molecular structure for steric and electrostatic interactions directly, and then generate a QSAR equation based on these molecular descriptors, using partial least squares (PLS). The validity of the model can be predicted.

PREDICTIVE ADME

The ultimate goal of CADD is to understand at the molecular level the complex relationships between a disease-causing target (macromolecule) and a drug-like molecule so that reliable predictions can be made to enhance molecular interactions. Other important pharmacokinetic factors are critical, however, for an effective therapeutic medicine. Essentially, potency, solubility, and permeability are the only three physical variables that can be adjusted to enhance the activity of potential oral medications.[182] Lipinski has suggested "poor absorption or permeation is likely when the molecule has more than one of the following properties."

1. More than 5 hydrogen bond donors
2. More than 10 hydrogen bond acceptors
3. Greater than 500 molecular weight
4. Greater than 5 computed log P

Medical professionals must be aware of drug–drug interactions. Because a significant number of drugs are metabolized by the cytochrome P-450 (CYP), it behooves medicinal chemists to consider this oxidative pathway in the design process. Tragic consequences of drug–drug and food–drug interactions have resulted in two FDA-approved drugs, mibefradil (Posicor), **23**, and terfenadine (Seldane), **24**, being removed from the market in recent years. Mibefradil and terfenadine are shown in Figure 28-30. Each drug required P-450 for phase I metabolism.

A more recent predictive model for CYP 3A4 metabolism has been reported.[183] The method relies on PLS, but one of the descriptors is based on AM1-calculated hydrogen abstraction. There are several assumptions: *(a)* CYP 3A4 susceptibility is a function of the electronic environment around the hydrogen that is abstracted. *(b)* Abstraction of the hydrogen atom is the rate-determining step. *(c)* The drug being metabolized tumbles freely in the active site of the enzyme until the most active hydrogen is available. AM1 calculations (using a procedure to account for the fact that unpaired electrons are involved) were carried out on a series of known drugs. The activity, defined as the AM1 H-atom abstraction, is modeled on the presence or absence of chemical descriptors.

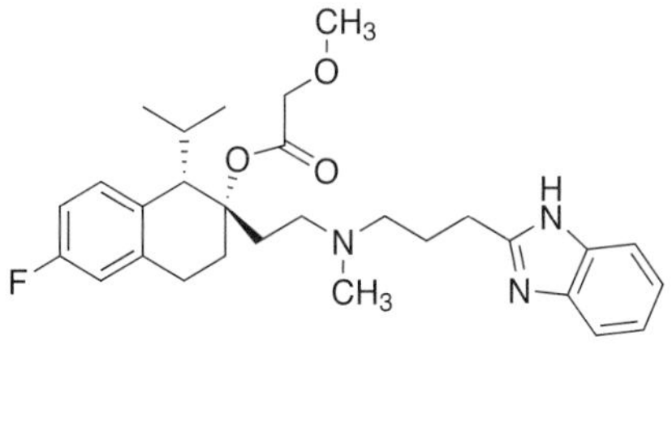

Over the next decade, in silico property and toxicity predictions will increase. As the predictive methods become more reliable and robust, they will be included increasingly in the initial drug design process rather than being an afterthought. There are many other CADD success stories. Although drug discovery is a complex process, in the future, as our understanding of drug action increases, a growing number of therapeutically effective drugs will be designed using computer-based methods.

Acknowledgment

The author acknowledges Tedman Ehlers, who prepared many of the figures for this chapter, and Mark Volmer, who provided valuable manuscript assistance.

REFERENCES

1. Wooden ball-and-stick models attributed to John Dalton, The Science Museum, Exhibition Road, South Kensington, London, England.
2. Bowen, J. P., and Cory, M.: Computer-assisted drug design. In Swarbrick, J., Boylan, J. C. (eds.). Encyclopedia of Pharmaceutical Technology, 2nd ed. New York, Marcel Dekker, 2002, pp. 585–604.
3. Watson, J. D., and Crick, F. H. C.: Nature 171:964, 1953.
4. Watson, J. D.: The Double Helix. New York, New American Library, 1968.
5. Pauling, L., and Corey, R. B.: Proc. Natl. Acad. Sci. U. S. A. 37:205, 729, 1951.
6. Koltun, W.: Biopolymers 3:665, 1965.
7. Dreiding, A. S.: Helv. Chim. Acta 42:1339, 1959.
8. Gordon, A. J.: J. Chem. Educ. 47:30, 1970.
9. Greer, J., Erickson, J. W., Baldwin, J. J., and Varney, M. D.: J. Med. Chem. 37:1035, 1994.
10. Carson, M., and Bugg, C. E.: J. Mol. Graphics 4:121, 1986.
11. Richardson, J. S., and Richardson, D. C.: Trends Biochem. Sci. 14:304, 1989.
12. Connolly, M. L.: Science 221:709, 1983.
13. Lee, B., and Richards, F. M.: J. Mol. Biol. 55:379, 1971.
14. Born, M., and Oppenheimer, R.: Ann. Phys. 84:457, 1927.
15. D'Abro, A.: The Rise of the New Physics: Its Mathematical and Physical Theories. New York, Dover, 1951.
16. Pauling, L., and Wilson, E. B., Jr.: Introduction to Quantum Mechanics, With Applications to Chemistry. New York, McGraw-Hill, 1935.
17. Roberts, J. D.: Notes on Molecular Orbital Calculations. Reading, MA, Benjamin/Cummings, 1961.
18. Streitwieser, A., Jr.: Molecular Orbital Theory for Organic Chemists. New York, John Wiley & Sons, 1961.
19. Westheimer, F. H., and Mayer, J. E.: J. Chem. Phys. 14:733, 1946.
20. Hill, T. L.: J. Chem. Phys. 14:465, 1946.
21. Dostrovsky, I., Hughes, E. D., and Ingold, C. K.: J. Chem. Soc.: 173, 1946.
22. Ermer, O.: Struct. Bonding (Berlin) 27:161, 1976.
23. Altona, C. L., and Faber, D. H.: Top. Curr. Chem. 45:1, 1974.
24. Engler, E. M., Andose, J. D., and Schleyer, P. v. R.: J. Am. Chem. Soc. 95:8005, 1973.
25. Burkert, U., and Allinger, N. L.: Molecular Mechanics. ACS Monograph 177. Washington, DC, American Chemical Society, 1982.
26. Rappe, A. K., and Casewit, C.: Molecular Mechanics Across Chemistry. Sausalito, CA, University Science Books, 1992.
27. Weiner, S. J., Kollman, P. A., Case, D. A., et al.: J. Am. Chem. Soc. 106:765, 1984.
28. Weiner, S. J., Kollman, P. A., Nguyen, D. T., et al.: J. Comput. Chem. 7:230, 1986.
29. Pearlman, D. A., Case, D. A., Caldwell, J. W., et al.: Comput. Phys. Commun. 91:1, 1995.

23

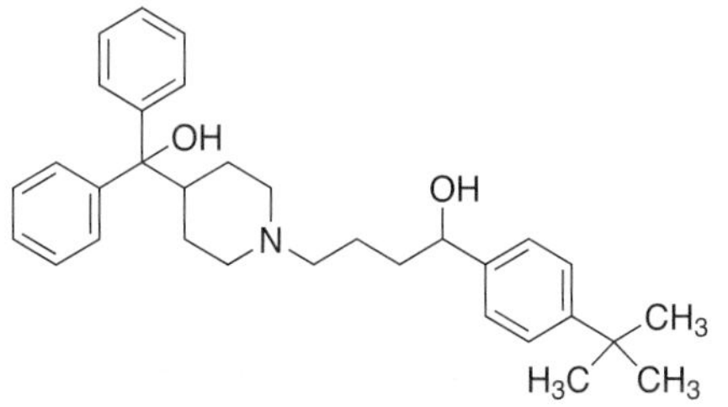

24

Figure 28–30 ■ Predictive ADME is becoming more important in the early stages of drug design. Drug–drug and food–drug interactions have resulted in two FDA-approved drugs, mibefradil (Posicor), **23**, and terfenadine (Seldane), **24**, being removed from the market in recent years.

30. Cornell, W. D., Cieplak, P., Bayly, C. I., et al.: J. Am. Chem. Soc. 117:5179, 1995.
31. Brooks, B. R., Bruccoleri, R. E., Olafson, B. D., et al.: J. Comput. Chem. 4:187, 1983.
32. Halgren, T. A.: J. Comput. Chem. 17:490, 1996.
33. Halgren, T. A.: J. Comput. Chem. 17:5320, 1996.
34. Halgren, T. A.: J. Comput. Chem. 17:553, 1996.
35. Halgren, T. A., and Nachbar, R. B.: J. Comput. Chem. 17:587, 1996.
36. Halgren, T. A.: J. Comput. Chem. 17:616, 1996.
37. Tripos Inc., 1699 South Hanley Rd., Suite 303, St. Louis, MO 63144.
38. Wavefunction, Inc., 18401 Von Karman Ave., Suite 370, Irvine, CA 92715.
39. Serena Software, P.O. Box 3076, Bloomington, IN 47402-3076.
40. Schrödinger, 1500 SW First Ave., Suite 1180, Portland, OR 97201; and 120 West 45th Street, New York, NY 10036.
41. Allinger, N. L. , Yuh, Y. H., and Lii, J.-H.: J. Am. Chem. Soc. 111:8551, 1989.
42. Lii, J.-H., and Allinger, N. L.: J. Am. Chem. Soc. 111:8566, 1989.
43. Lii, J.-H., and Allinger, N. L.: J. Am. Chem. Soc. 111:8576, 1989.
44. Allinger, N. L., Chen, K. S., and Lii, J.-H.: J. Comput. Chem. 17:642, 1996.
45. Nevins, N., Chen, K. S., and Allinger, N. L.: J. Comput. Chem. 17:669, 1996.
46. Nevins, N., Lii, J.-H., and Allinger, N. L.: J. Comput. Chem. 17:695, 1996.
47. Nevins, N., and Allinger, N. L.: J. Comput. Chem. 17:730, 1996.
48. Bowen, J. P., and Liang, G. New vistas in molecular mechanics. In Charifson, P. (ed.). Practical Applications of Computer-Aided Drug Design. New York, Marcel Dekker, 1997, 495–538.
49. London, F.: Z. Phys. 63:245, 1930.
50. Lennard-Jones, J. E.: Proc. R. Soc. London Ser. A 106:463, 1924.
51. Hill, T. L.: J. Chem. Phys. 16:399, 1948.
52. Todebush, P. M., and Bowen, J. P.: Molecular mechanics force field development and applications. In Rami Reddy, R., and Erion, M. D. (eds.). Free Energy Calculations in Rational Drug Design. New York, Kluwer Academic/Plenum Press, 2001.
53. Bischoff, C. A.: Ber. Dtsch. Chem. Ges. 23:620, 1890.
54. Bischoff, C. A.: Ber. Dtsch. Chem. Ges. 24:1074, 1085, 1891.
55. Bischoff, C. A., and Walden, P.: Ber. Dtsch. Chem. Ges. 26:1452, 1893.
56. Kemp, J. D., and Pitzer, K. S.: J. Chem. Phys. 4:749, 1936.
57. Kemp, J. D., and Pitzer, K. S.: J. Am. Chem. Soc., 59:276, 1937.
58. Christie, G. H., and Kenner, J.: J. Chem. Soc. 121:614, 1922.
59. Bartell, L. S.: J. Am. Chem. Soc. 99:3279, 1977.
60. Allinger, N. L., Hindman, D., and Hönig, H.: J. Am. Chem. Soc. 99:3282, 1977.
61. Pitzer, R. M.: Acc. Chem. Res. 16:207, 1983.
62. Radom, L., Hehre, W. J., and Pople, J. A.: J. Am. Chem. Soc. 94:2371, 1972.
63. Jacoby, S. L. S., Kowalik, J. S., and Pizzo, J. T.: Iterative Methods for Nonlinear Optimization Problems. Englewood Cliffs, NJ, Prentice Hall, 1972.
64. Williams, J. E., Stang, P. J., and Schleyer, P. v. R.: Annu. Rev. Phys. Chem. 19:531, 1968.
65. Wiberg, K. B.: J. Am. Chem. Soc. 87:1070, 1965.
66. Fletcher, R., and Reeves, C. M.: Comput. J. 7:149, 1964.
67. Fletcher, R., and Powell, M. J. D.: Comput. J. 6:163, 1963.
68. Dammkoehler, R. A., Karasek, S. F., Berkley Shands, E. F., and Marshall, G. R.: J. Comput. Aided Mol. Des. 3:3, 1989.
69. Motoc, I., Dammkoehler, R. A., Mayer, D., and Labanowski, J.: Quant. Struct. Act. Relat. 5:99, 1986.
70. Ferguson, D., and Raber, D. J.: J. Am. Chem. Soc. 111:4371,1989.
71. Chang, G., Guida, W., and Still, W. C.: J. Am. Chem. Soc. 111:4379, 1989.
72. Metropolis, N., Rosenbluth, A. W., Rosenbluth, M. N., et al.: J. Chem. Phys. 21:1087, 1953.
73. Saunders, M., Houk, K. N., Wu, Y.-D., et al.: J. Am. Chem. Soc. 112:1419, 1990.
74. Personal communication, Robert Pearlman.
75. Kostrowicki, J., and Scheraga, H. A.: J. Phys. Chem. 96:7442, 1992.
76. Judson, R.: Genetic algorithms and their use in chemistry. In Lipkowitz, K., and Boyd, D., (eds.). Reviews in Computational Chemistry, vol 10. New York, VCH, 1997 pp. 1–73.
77. Smellie, A., Teig, S. L., and Textbin, P.: J. Comput. Chem. 16:171, 1995.
78. McCammon, J., Gelin, B., and Karplus, M.: Nature 267:585, 1977.
79. van Gunsteren, W., and Berendsen, H.: Mol. Phys. 34:1311, 1977.
80. Wallquist, A., and Mountain, R. D.: Molecular models of water: Derivation and description. In Lipkowitz, K., and Boyd, D., (eds.). Reviews in Computational Chemistry, vol 13, New York, VCH, 1991, 183–247.
81. Berendsen, H. J. C., Grigera, J. R., and Straatsma, T. P.: J. Phys. Chem. 91:6269, 1987.
82. Jorgensen, W. L., Chandrasekhar, J., Madura, J. D., et al.: J. Chem. Phys. 79:926, 1983.
83. McCammon, J., and Harvey, S.: Dynamics of Proteins and Nucleic Acids. Cambridge, Cambridge University Press, 1987.
84. Berendsen, H., van Gunsteren, W., Zwinderman, H., and Geurtsen, R.: Ann. N. Y. Acad. Sci. 482:269, 1986.
85. Darden, T. A., York, D. M., and Pedersen, L. G.: J. Chem. Phys. 98:10089, 1993.
86. McCammon, J. A.: Science 238:486, 1987.
87. Jorgensen, W. L.: Acc. Chem. Res. 22:184, 1989.
88. Howard, A. E., and Kollman, P. A.: J. Med. Chem. 31:1669, 1988.
89. Schrödinger, E.: Ann. Phys. 79:361, 1926.
90. Schrödinger, E.: Ann. Phys. 80:437, 1926.
91. Schrödinger, E.: Ann. Phys. 81:109, 1926.
92. Heisenberg, W.: Z. Phys. 33:879, 1925.
93. Schrödinger, E.: Ann. Phys. 79:734, 1926.
94. Eckart, C.: Phys. Rev. 28:711, 1926.
95. Hehre, W. J., Radom, L., Schleyer, P., and Pople, J. Ab Initio Molecular Orbital Theory. New York, John Wiley & Sons, 1986.
96. Pople, J. A., and Beveridge, D.: Approximate Molecular Orbital Theory. New York, McGraw-Hill, 1970.
97. Dewar, M. J. S.: The Molecular Orbital Theory of Organic Chemistry. New York, McGraw-Hill, 1969.
98. Murrell, J. N., and Harget, A. J.: Semiempirical Self-Consistent-Field Molecular Orbital Theory of Molecules. London, Wiley-Interscience, 1972.
99. Pople, J. A., Santry, D. P., and Segal, G. A.: J. Chem. Phys. 43:S129, 1965.
100. Pople, J. A., and Segal, G. A.: J. Chem. Phys. 43:3136, 1965.
101. Pople, J. A., and Segal, G. A.: J. Chem. Phys. 44:3289, 1966.
102. Pople, J. A., Beveridge, D. L., and Dobosh, P.A.: J. Chem. Phys. 47:2026, 1967.
103. Dewar, M. J. S., and Thiel, W.: J. Am. Chem. Soc. 99:4899, 1977.
104. Dewar, M. J. S.: J. Mol. Struct. 100:41, 1983.
105. Bingham, R. C., Dewar, M. J. S., and Lo, D. H.: J. Am. Chem. Soc. 97:1285, 1975.
106. Bingham, R. C., Dewar, M. J. S., and Lo, D. H.: J. Am. Chem. Soc. 97:1294, 1975.
107. Bingham, R. C., Dewar, M. J. S., and Lo, D. H.: J. Am. Chem. Soc. 97:1302, 1975.
108. Bingham, R. C., Dewar, M. J. S., and Lo, D. H. J. Am. Chem. Soc. 97:1307, 1975.
109. Dewar, M. J. S., Lo, D. H., and Ramsden, C. A.: J. Am. Chem. Soc. 97:1311, 1975.
110. Dewar, M. J. S., and Thiel, W.: J. Am. Chem. Soc. 99:4907, 1977.
111. Dewar, M. J. S., and McKee, M. L.: J. Am. Chem. Soc. 99:5231, 1977.
112. Dewar, M. J. S., and Rzepa, H. S.: J. Am. Chem. Soc. 100:777, 1978.
113. Davis, L. P., Guidry, R. M., Williams, J. R., et al.: J. Comput. Chem. 2:433, 1981.
114. Dewar, M. J. S., McKee, M. L., and Rzepa, H. S.: J. Am. Chem. Soc. 100:3607, 1978.
115. Dewar, M. J. S., and Healy, E.: J. Comput. Chem. 4:542, 1983.
116. Dewar, M. J. S., Zoebisch, E. G., Healy, E. F., and Stewart, J. J. P.: J. Am. Chem. Soc. 107:3902, 1985.
117. Stewart, J. J. P.: J. Comput. Chem. 10:209, 1989.
118. Theil, W., and Voityuk, A. A.: J. Phys. Chem. 100:616, 1996.
119. Theil, W.: Adv. Chem. Phys. 93:703, 1996.
120. Richards, W. G.: Quantum Pharmacology, 2nd ed. London, Butterworths, 1984.
121. Kier, L. B.: Molecular Orbital Theory in Drug Research. New York, Academic Press, 1971.
122. Boys, S. F.: Proc. R. Soc. London, Ser. A 200:542, 1950.
123. Hehre, W. J., Stewart, R. F., and Pople, J. A.: J. Chem. Phys. 51:2657, 1969.
124. Hehre, W. J., Ditchfield, R., Stewart, R. F, and Pople, J. A.: J. Chem. Phys. 52:2769, 1970.

125. Pietro, W. J., Levi, B. A., Hehre, W. J., and Stewart, R. F.: Inorg. Chem. 19:2225, 1980.
126. Pietro, W. J., Blurock, E. S., Hout, R. F., Jr., et al.: Inorg. Chem. 20: 3650, 1981.
127. Binkley, J. S., Pople, J. A., and Hehre, W. J.: J. Am. Chem. Soc. 102: 939, 1980.
128. Gordon, M. S., Binkley, J. S., Pople, J. A., et al.: J. Am. Chem. Soc. 104:2797, 1982.
129. Dobbs, K. D., and Hehre, W. J.: J. Comput. Chem. 7:359, 1986.
130. Hehre, W. J., Ditchfield, R., and Pople, J. A.: J. Chem. Phys. 56: 2257, 1972.
131. Binkley, J. S., and Pople, J. A.: J. Chem. Phys. 66:879, 1977.
132. Francl, M. M., Pietro, W. J., Hehre, W. J., et al.: J. Chem. Phys. 77: 3654, 1982.
133. Carlsen, N. R.: Chem. Phys. Lett. 51:192, 1977.
134. Krishnan, R., Frisch, M. J., and Pople, J. A.: J. Chem. Phys. 72:4244, 1980.
135. Clark, T., Chandrasekhar, J., , Spitznagel, G. W., and Schleyer, P. v. R.: J. Comput. Chem. 4:294, 1983.
136. Frisch, J. A., Pople, M. J., and Binkley, J. S.: J. Chem. Phys. 80:3265, 1984.
137. Hartree, D. R.: Proc. Cambridge Philos. Soc. 24:105, 1928.
138. Roothaan, C. C. J.: Rev. Mod. Phys. 23:69, 1951.
139. Hall, G. G.: Proc. R. Soc. London, Ser. A 205:541, 1951.
140. Møller, C., and Plesset, M. S.: Phys. Rev. 46:618, 1934.
141. Pople, J. A., Binkley, J. S., and Seeger, R.: Int. J. Quantum Chem. Symp. 10:1, 1976.
142. Pople, J. A., Seeger, R., and Krishnan, R.: Int. J. Quantum Chem. Symp. 11:149, 1977.
143. Krishnan, R., and Pople, J. A.: Int. J. Quantum Chem. 14:91, 1978.
144. Schlegel, H. B.: J. Chem. Phys. 77:3676, 1982.
145. Mulliken, R. S.: J. Chem. Phys. 23:1833, 1955.
146. Parr, R. G., and Yang, W.: Density Functional Theory of Atoms and Molecules. Oxford, Oxford University Press, 1989.
147. Kohn, W., and Sham, L. J.: Phys. Rev. A140:1133, 1965.
148. Hohenberg, P., and Kohn, W.: Phys. Rev. B136:864, 1964.
149. Berman, H. M., Westbrook, J., Feng, Z., et al.: The Protein Data Bank. Nucl. Acids Res. 28:235, 2000.
150. Güner, O. F. (ed.): Pharmacophore Perception, Development, and Use in Drug Design. IUL Biotechnology Series. La Jolla, CA, International University Line, 2000.
151. Beddell, C. R., Goodford, P. J., Norrington, F. E., et al.: Br. J. Pharmacol. 57:201, 1976.
152. Cushman, D. W., Cheung, H. S., Sabo, E. F., and Ondetti, M. A.: Biochemistry 16:5484, 1977.
153. Ondetti, M. A. and Cushman, D. W.: CRC Crit. Rev. Biochem. 16: 381, 1984.
154. Byers, L. D., and Wolfenden, R.: J. Biochem. 247:606, 1972.
155. Thorsett, E. D., Harris, E. E., Aster, S. D., et al.: J. Med. Chem. 29: 251, 1986.

156. Blaney, J. M., Jorgensen, E. C., Connolly, M. L., et al.: J. Med. Chem. 25:785, 1982.
157. Kuyper, L. F., Roth, B., Baccanari, D. P., et al.: J. Med. Chem. 28: 303, 1985.
158. Vacca, J. P., and Condra, J. H.: Drug Discovery Today 2:261, 1997.
159. Kubinyi, H. J.: Receptor Signal Transduction Res. 19:15, 1999.
160. Ghosh, A. K., Thompson, W. J., Fitzgerald, P. M., et al.: J. Med. Chem. 37:2506, 1994.
161. Dorsey, B. D., Levin, R. B., McDaniel, S. L., et al.: J. Med. Chem. 37:3443, 1994.
162. Kempf, D. J., Sham, H. L., Marsh, K. C., et al.: J. Med. Chem. 41: 602, 1998.
163. Kaldor, S. W., Kalish, V. J., Davies, J. F., II, et al.: J. Med. Chem. 40:3979, 1997.
164. Thaisrivongs, S., and Strohbach, J. W.: Biopolymers 51, 51, 1999.
165. Baldwin, J. J., Ponticello, G. S., Anderson, P. S., et al.: J. Med. Chem. 32:2510, 1989.
166. Kawakami, Y., Inoue, A., Kawai, T., et al.: Bioorg. Med. Chem. 4: 1429, 1996.
167. Marshall, G. R., and Motoc, I.: Top. Mol. Pharmacol. 3:115, 1986.
168. Marshall, G. R.: Annu. Rev. Pharmacol. Toxicol. 27:193, 1987.
169. Mayer, D., Motoc, C. B., Motoc, I., and Marshall, G. R.: J. Comput. Aided Mol. Des. 1:3, 1987.
170. Van Drie, J. H., Weininger, D., and Martin, Y. C.: J. Comput. Aided Mol. Des. 3:225, 1989.
171. Sheridan, R. P., Nilakantan, R., Rusinko, A., III, et al.: J. Chem. Inf. Comput. Sci. 29:255, 1989.
172. Pearlman, R.: Chem. Design Automated News 2:1, 1987.
173. Hiller, C., and Gasteiger, J.: Ein Automatisierter Molekülbaukasten. In Gasteiger, J. (ed.). Software-Entwicklung in der Chemie. Berlin, Springer, 1987.
174. Goodford, P. J.: J. Med. Chem. 28:849, 1985.
175. DesJarlais, R. L., Sheridan, R. P., Seibel, G. L., et al.: J. Med. Chem. 31:722, 1988.
176. Kuntz, I. D.: Science 257:1078, 1992.
177. Stewart, K. D., Bentley, J. A., and Cory, M.: Tetrahedron Comput. Methodol. 3:713, 1990.
178. Bartlett, P., Shea, G. T., Telfer, S. J., and Waterman, S.: CAVEAT: A program to facilitate the structure-derived design of biologically active molecules. In Roberts, S. M. (ed.). Molecular Recognition: Chemical and Biological Problems. Cambridge, Royal Society of Chemistry, 1989, pp. 182–196.
179. Hansch, C.: Acc. Chem. Res. 2:232, 1969.
180. Hansch, C., and Leo, A.: Exploring QSAR: Fundamentals and Applications in Chemistry and Biology. Washington, DC, American Chemical Society, 1995.
181. Cramer, R. D., III, Patterson, D. E., and Bunce, J. D.: J. Am. Chem. Soc. 110:5959, 1989.
182. Lipinski, C. A., Lombardo, F., Dominy, B. W., and Feeney, P. J.: Adv. Drug Delivery Rev. 23:3, 1997.
183. Singh, S. B., Shen, L. Q., Walker, M. J., and Sheridan, R. P.: J. Med. Chem. 46:1330, 2003.

APPENDIX

Calculated Log P, Log D, and pK$_a$

The log P, log D at pH 7, and pK$_a$ values are from Chemical Abstracts Service, American Chemical Society, Columbus, OH, 2003, and were calculated by using Advanced Chemistry Development (ACD) Software Solaris V4.67. The pK$_a$ values are for the most acidic HA acid and most weakly acidic BH$^+$ groups. The latter represent the most basic nitrogen. Keep in mind that pK$_a$ values for HA acids that exceed 10 to 11 mean that there will be little, if any, anionic contribution in the pH ranges used in pharmaceutical formulations and in physiological pH ranges. Similarly, for BH$^+$ acids, there will be little, if any, cationic contribution for pK$_a$ values below 2 to 3. Because Chemical Abstracts does not report calculated physicochemical values for ionized compounds including salts and quaternary ammonium compounds, the log P values in this appendix are for the unionized form.

Compound	Log P	Log D at ph 7	pK$_a$ HA	pK$_a$ BH$^+$	Compound	Log P	Log D at ph 7	pK$_a$ HA	pK$_a$ BH$^+$
Abacavir	0.72	0.72		5.08	Amiloride	1.90	1.88	8.58	1.58
Acarbose	−3.03		12.39	5.90	p-Aminobenzoic acid	0.01	−2.12	4.90	2.48
Acebutolol	2.59	0.52	13.78	9.11	Aminoglutethimide	1.41	1.41	11.60	4.41
Acetaminophen	0.34	0.34	9.86		Aminolevulinic acid	−0.93	−3.38	4.00	7.37
Acetazolamide	−0.26	−0.40	7.44		4-Aminosalicylic acid	0.32	−3.02	3.58	2.21
Acetic acid	−0.29	−2.49	4.79		Amiodarone	8.59	6.29		9.37
Acetohexamide	2.24	0.03			Amitriptyline	6.14	3.96		9.24
Acetohydroxamic acid	−1.59	−1.59	9.26		Amlexanox	4.67	1.65	3.95	
Acetylcysteine	−0.15	−3.74	3.25		Amlodipine	3.72	2.00		8.73
Acitretin	5.73	3.52	4.79		Amobarbital	2.10	2.05	7.94	
Acyclovir	−1.76	−1.76	9.18	1.89	Amoxapine	2.59	1.52		8.03
Adapalene	8.04	5.29	4.23		Amoxicillin	0.61	−2.21	2.61	6.93
Adefovir dipivoxil	2.38	2.38		4.63	Amphetamine	1.81	−0.91		9.94
Adenine	−2.12	−2.12		2.95	Amphotericin B	0.18		3.96	8.13
Adenosine	−1.46	−1.46	13.11	3.25	Ampicillin	1.35	−1.54	2.61	6.79
Alanine	−0.68	−3.18	9.62	2.31	Amprenavir	4.20	4.20	11.54	1.76
Alatrofloxacin	0.31	−2.22	0.64	8.12	Amyl nitrite	2.45	2.45		
Albendazole	3.01	2.99	10.46	5.62	Anagrelide	1.13	1.13	11.79	1.48
Albuterol	0.02	−2.15	9.83	9.22	Anastrozole	0.77	0.77		4.78
Alclometasone dipropionate	4.26	4.26	13.73		Anthralin	4.16	3.91	7.16	
Alendronic acid	−3.52	−7.80	0.47	10.56	Apomorphine	2.47	2.34	9.41	6.50
Alfentanil	2.03			7.59	Apraclonidine	0.30	−1.91		9.11
Alitretinoin	6.83	4.62	4.79		Arginine	−1.78	−5.26	2.51	13.64
Allopurinol	−0.48	−0.50	9.20	2.40	Aripiprazole	5.68	5.55		6.50
Almotriptan	1.89	−0.51		9.48	Articaine	2.44	1.41	13.46	7.99
Alosetron	0.96	0.65		6.71	Ascorbic acid	−2.12	−4.96	4.13	
Alprazolam	2.50	2.50		2.39	Asparagine	−1.51	−4.02	2.30	8.34
Alprostadil (prostaglandin E$_1$)	2.25	0.02	4.77		Aspartic acid	−0.67	−4.17	2.28	9.95
					Aspirin	1.19	−2.23	3.48	
Altretamine	2.42	1.90		7.37	Astemizole	5.80	3.62		9.03
Amantadine	2.22	−0.79		10.75	Atazanavir	5.51		11.11	4.81
Amcinonide	3.80	3.80	13.15		Atenolol	0.10	−2.03	13.88	9.17
Amifostine	−1.69	−4.72	1.29	10.16	Atomoxetine	3.84	1.03		10.12
Amikacin	−3.84		12.94	9.52	Atorvastatin	4.22	1.54	4.30	
					Atovaquone	6.18	4.14	4.97	

(*Continued*)

Compound	Log P	Log D at ph 7	pK$_a$ HA	pK$_a$ BH$^+$	Compound	Log P	Log D at ph 7	pK$_a$ HA	pK$_a$ BH$^+$
Atropine	1.53	−1.21		9.98	Calcifediol (25-OH-D$_3$)	7.53	7.53		
Azathioprine	−0.54	−0.54		0.25	Calcipotriene	5.43	5.43	13.98	
Azelaic acid	1.33	−3.01	4.47		Calcitriol (1,25-di (OH)-D$_3$)	6.12	6.12		13.98
Azelastine	3.71	1.60		9.16	Candesartan cilexetil	7.43	4.81	4.22	4.24
Azithromycin	3.33	0.58	13.30	8.59	Capecitabine	0.97	−0.38	5.67	
Aztreonam	−2.07	7.11		2.36	Capsaicin	3.31	3.31	9.91	
Baclofen	1.56	−0.94	4.00	10.32	Captopril	0.27	−2.86	3.82	
Balsalazide	2.70	−2.29	2.97		Carbamazepine	2.67	2.67	13.94	
Beclomethasone dipropionate	4.59	4.59	13.08		Carbenicillin	1.01	−3.99	2.62	
Benazepril	5.50	2.31	3.73	5.02	Carbidopa	−0.19	−2.71	3.40	7.91
Bendroflumethiazide	2.02	2.01	8.63		Carbinoxamine	2.76	1.12	8.65	
Benzocaine	2.49	2.49		2.51	Carboprost	2.49	0.27	4.77	
Benzoic acid	1.90	−0.88	4.20		Carisoprodol	2.15	2.15	12.49	
Benzonatate	0.32	0.32		2.20	Carmustine	1.30	1.30	10.19	
Benzoyl peroxide	3.47	3.47			β- Carotene	15.51	15.51		
Benzphetamine	4.43	2.57		8.88	Carteolol	1.67	−0.42	13.84	9.13
Benzthiazide	2.68	2.67	9.15		Carvedilol	4.23	3.16	13.90	8.03
Benztropine	4.96	2.00		10.54	Cefaclor	0.19	−2.71	1.95	6.80
Bepridil	6.43	4.27	9.21		Cefadroxil	−0.09	−2.89	3.12	6.93
Betamethasone	2.06	2.06	12.14		Cefamandole	1.52	−2.39	2.62	
Betamethasone acetate	2.61	2.61	12.05		Cefdinir	−0.73	−5.13	2.80	3.27
Betamethasone dipropionate	4.23	4.23	12.93		Cefditoren pivoxil	1.23	1.13	7.57	2.89
Betamethasone valerate	3.98	3.97	12.67		Cefixime	−0.51	−5.53	2.10	2.86
Betaxolol	2.69	0.56	13.89	9.17	Cefonicid	0.54	−4.46		
Bexarotene	8.75	6.07	4.30		Cefoperazone	1.43		2.62	
Bicalutamide	4.54	4.54	11.49		Cefotaxime	−0.31	−4.24	2.66	2.90
Bimatoprost	1.98	1.98			Cefoxitin	0.72	−3.19	2.63	
Biperiden	4.52	1.89		9.80	Cefpodoxime proxetil	0.66	0.57	7.61	2.90
Bisoprolol	2.22	0.11	13.86	9.16	Cefprozil	0.15	−2.67	2.92	6.93
Bitolterol	5.25	3.30	13.68	8.97	Ceftibuten	−1.06	−5.08	3.00	5.44
Bosentan	1.15	0.01	5.89		Ceftizoxime	−0.92	−4.70	2.99	2.90
Brimonidine	0.97	−1.34		9.63	Ceftriaxone	−1.76	−5.86	2.57	2.90
Brinzolamide	0.25	−1.06	9.62	8.29	Cefuroxime	−0.54	−4.47	2.59	
Bromocriptine	4.63	4.52	9.61	6.45	Celecoxib	3.01	3.01	9.68	
Brompheniramine	3.57	1.30		9.33	Cephalexin	0.65	−2.22	3.12	6.80
Buclizine	6.24	6.10		6.59	Cephapirin	0.79	−3.05	2.67	4.49
Budesonide	3.24	3.24	12.85		Cephradine	0.98	−1.79	3.12	6.99
Bumetanide	2.78	−0.27	3.18	4.48	Cetirizine	2.97	−0.02	3.27	6.43
Bupivacaine	3.64	2.45		8.17	Cevimeline	1.12	−1.29		9.51
Buprenorphine	3.61	2.40	9.67	8.18	Chloral hydrate	1.68	1.68	10.54	
Bupropion	3.47	3.08		7.16	Chlorambucil	3.70	1.52	4.86	3.66
Buspirone	3.43	3.33		6.43	Chloramphenicol	1.02	1.02	11.03	
Busulfan	−0.52	−0.52			Chlordiazepoxide	2.49	2.49		4.45
Butabarbital	1.56	1.52	7.95		Chlorhexidine	4.54	−0.46		11.73
Butenafine	6.77	5.84		7.87	Chloroprocaine	3.38	1.28		9.13
Butoconazole	6.88	6.69		6.72	Chloroquine	4.69	1.15		10.48
Butorphanol	3.94	2.93	10.26	7.97	Chlorothiazide	−0.18	−0.18	9.17	
Cabergoline	2.39	−0.92	13.06	9.41	Chloroxine	3.75	1.51	2.07	7.20
Caffeine	−0.08	−0.08		1.39	Chlorphenesin carbamate	1.41	1.41	12.99	
					Chlorpheniramine	3.39	1.13		9.33

(Continued)

Compound	Log P	Log D at ph 7	pKa HA	pKa BH+	Compound	Log P	Log D at ph 7	pKa HA	pKa BH+
Chlorpromazine	5.36	3.01		9.43	Dehydrocholic acid	1.77	−0.48	4.74	
Chlorpropamide	2.21	0.28			Delavirdine	−1.23	−3.23	10.10	8.87
Chlorthalidone	−0.74	−0.74	9.57		Demeclocycline	−0.58	−4.34	4.50	9.68
Chlorzoxazone	2.44	2.43	8.92		Desflurane	1.87	1.87		
Cholecalciferol	9.72	9.72			Desipramine	3.97	1.05		10.40
Ciclopirox	2.59	1.76	6.25		Desloratadine	5.26	2.95		9.38
Cidofovir	−3.38	−7.64	1.61	4.54	Desonide	2.72	2.72	12.85	
Cilastatin	2.42	−1.09	2.09	8.83	Desoximetasone	2.40	2.40	12.80	
Cilostazol	3.04	3.04			Dexamethasone	2.06	2.06	12.14	
Cimetidine	0.20	−0.11		6.73	Dexamethasone acetate	2.61	2.61	12.05	
Cinoxacin	−0.53	−4.58		4.31	Dexmedetomidine	3.18	2.85		6.75
Ciprofloxacin	1.31	−1.20	2.74	8.76	Dexrazoxane	−0.37	−0.37	10.74	2.62
Citalopram	2.89	0.41		9.59	Dextromethorphan	4.28	2.22		9.10
Citric acid	−1.72	−7.67	2.93		Diazepam	3.86	3.86		3.40
Cladribine	0.24	0.24	13.75	1.44	Diazoxide	1.07	1.07		
Clarithromycin	3.16	2.00	13.07	8.14	Dibucaine	4.40	1.95	12.90	9.56
Clavulanic acid	1.98	−5.84	2.78		Dichloroacetic acid	0.54	−3.54	1.37	
Clemastine	5.69	2.83		10.23	Dichlorphenamide	0.93	0.92	8.95	
Clindamycin	2.14	0.41	12.87	8.74	Diclofenac	3.28	0.48	4.18	
Clioquinol	4.32	2.35	2.10	7.24	Dicloxacillin	3.02	−0.90	2.60	
Clobetasol propionate	4.18	4.18	12.94		Dicyclomine	6.05	3.87		9.23
Clocortolone pivalate	4.41	4.41	13.10		Didanosine	−0.92	−0.93	8.67	1.98
Clofazimine	7.50	7.43		6.24	Diethylcarbamazine	1.14	1.00		6.57
Clomiphene	8.01	5.58		9.53	Diethylpropion	2.95	1.46		8.48
Clomipramine	5.19	2.80		9.49	Difenoxin	5.73	3.23	3.57	8.91
Clonazepam	3.02	3.02	11.19	1.55	Diflorasone diacetate	2.91	2.91	12.69	
Clonidine	1.41	−0.67		9.16	Diflunisal	4.32	0.54	2.94	
Clotrimazole	5.76	5.71		6.12	Digoxin	1.14	1.14	13.50	
Clozapine	3.48	3.40		6.33	Dihydroergotamine	3.02	1.17	9.64	8.87
Cocaine	3.08	1.14		8.97	Dihydrotachysterol	9.86	9.86		
Codeine	2.04	0.83	13.42	8.29	Dihydroxyacetone	−0.78	−0.78	12.44	
Colchicine	1.03	1.03			Diltiazem	4.53	2.64		8.91
Cortisone	1.24	1.24	12.29		Dimercaprol	0.84	0.83	8.88	
Cromolyn	0.20	−4.80	1.85		Dinoprostone (prostaglandin E_2)	1.88	−0.36	4.76	
Crotamiton	3.10	3.10			Diphenhydramine	3.66	1.92		8.76
Cyclizine	2.42	1.83		7.46	Diphenoxylate	6.57	5.85		7.63
Cyclobenzaprine	6.22	4.06		9.21	Dipivefrin	1.49	−0.49	13.76	9.01
Cyclophosphamide	0.63	0.63		4.09	Dipyridamole	−1.22		13.54	6.37
Cyclopropane	1.69	1.69			Disopyramide	2.86	0.07		10.10
Cycloserine	−1.84	−1.87		5.93	Disulfiram	3.88	3.88		0.86
Cyproheptadine	6.62	4.93		8.70	Dobutamine	2.49	−0.31	9.65	10.37
Cystamine	0.62	−2.53		8.97	Dofetilide	1.56	0.27	9.68	8.28
Cysteamine	0.03	−1.45	7.93	10.47	Dolasetron	2.40	2.10		7.00
Cysteine	0.24	−2.31	2.07	11.05	Donepezil	4.70	2.89		8.82
Cytarabine	−2.30	−2.30	13.48	4.47	DOPA	−0.23	−2.73	2.24	9.30
Dacarbazine	−0.26	−0.26	12.32	4.09	Dopamine	0.12	−2.36	9.41	9.99
Dalfopristin	−0.94	−2.87	13.32	8.95	Dorzolamide	−0.21	−2.02	9.48	8.82
Danazol	4.70	4.70	13.10		Doxapram	3.23	2.67		7.41
Dantrolene	0.95	0.87	7.69		Doxazosin	0.65	0.54		6.47
Dapiprazole	2.44	2.28		6.39	Doxepin	5.08	2.93		9.19
Dapsone	0.94	0.94		1.24	Doxercalciferol	8.15	8.14	13.82	
Daunorubicin	2.39	0.47	7.15	8.64					

(Continued)

Compound	Log P	Log D at ph 7	pK_a HA	pK_a BH⁺	Compound	Log P	Log D at ph 7	pK_a HA	pK_a BH⁺
Doxorubicin	2.29	0.36	7.12	8.64	Felbamate	1.20	1.19	12.99	
Doxycycline	−0.26	−3.83	4.50	9.32	Felodipine	4.92	4.92		3.96
Dronabinol	7.64	7.64	9.81		Fenofibrate	4.80	4.80		
Droperidol	4.10	2.85	11.79	8.23	Fenoldopam	1.72	−0.56	8.51	9.53
Dutasteride	6.85	6.85	13.34		Fenoprofen	3.84	1.06	4.20	
Dyclonine	4.67	2.83		8.86	Fentanyl	3.93	1.90		9.06
Dyphylline	−1.12	−1.12	13.66	0.76	Fexofenadine	5.18	2.68	4.43	9.56
Econazole	5.81	5.64		6.69	Finasteride	3.24	3.24		
Efavirenz	4.90	4.85	7.92		Flavoxate	5.46	4.18		8.27
Eflornithine	0.56	−2.14	1.22	10.45	Flecainide	3.47	0.55	13.63	10.39
Eletriptan	3.27	0.36		10.35	Floxuridine	−1.20	−1.21	8.66	
Emedastine	2.06	−0.98		8.91	Fluconazole	0.31	0.30	11.93	5.23
Enalapril	2.98	−0.12	3.75	5.50	Flucytosine	−2.36	−2.38	8.36	3.68
Enflurane	2.10	2.10			Fludarabine	−2.32	−2.32	13.05	1.73
Entacapone	2.63	1.66	6.07		Fludrocortisone acetate	1.78	1.78	12.04	
Ephedrine	1.05	−1.25	13.96	9.38	Flumazenil	0.87	0.87		1.42
Epinephrine	−0.63	−2.75	9.60	9.16	Flunisolide	2.26	2.26	12.84	
Epirubicin	2.29	0.36	7.12	8.64	Fluocinolone	0.77	0.77	11.43	
Eplerenone	1.05	1.05			Fluocinolone acetonide	2.34	2.34	12.55	
Epoprostenol	2.21	−0.07	4.71		Fluorescein	3.61	3.60	8.56	
Eprosartan	4.96	1.46	3.31	8.73	Fluorexon	2.19	−3.86	1.79	9.24
Ergocalciferol	9.56	9.56			Fluorometholone	2.22	2.21	12.42	
Ergonovine	0.57	0.09		7.30	Fluorouracil	−0.78	−2.29	7.88	
Ergotamine	3.06	2.65	9.62	7.20	Fluoxetine	4.35	1.57	10.05	
Ertapenem	−1.28	−4.81	4.03	7.94	Fluoxymesterone	2.17	2.17	13.43	
Erythromycin	2.83	1.66	13.08	8.14	Fluphenazine	4.84	4.29		7.21
Escitalopram oxalate	2.89	0.41		9.59	Flurandrenolide	1.95	1.95	12.84	
Esmolol	1.91	−0.22	13.88	9.17	Flurazepam	4.71	2.12		9.76
Esomeprazole	1.80	1.80	9.08	4.61	Flurbiprofen	4.11	1.28	4.14	
Estazolam	3.25	3.25		1.67	Flutamide	4.06	4.06	13.12	
Estradiol	4.13	4.13	10.37		Fluticasone propionate	3.92	3.92	12.59	
Estradiol cypionate	7.59	7.59	10.35		Fluvastatin	3.72	1.01	4.28	
Estradiol valerate	6.62	6.62	10.35		Fluvoxamine	3.17	0.86		9.39
Estramustine	5.75	5.75			Folic acid	−2.63	−7.52	3.55	2.11
Ethacrynic acid	3.38	−0.47	2.80		Fomepizole	0.78	0.78		3.21
Ethambutol	−0.05	−2.56		9.60	Formaldehyde	0.35	0.35		
Ethanolamine oleate	7.59	6.82		7.68	Formoterol	1.57	−0.17	8.65	9.09
Ethaverine	5.55	5.43		6.47	Foscarnet	−2.53	−7.64	0.66	
Ethinyl estradiol	4.52	4.52	10.34		Fosfomycin	−2.98	−7.25	1.70	
Ethionamide	7.22	7.22	12.14	4.34	Fosinopril	5.81	2.65	3.78	
Ethosuximide	1.14	1.14		9.70	Fosphenytoin	0.47	−4.61	1.72	
Ethotoin	0.86	0.82	8.00		Frovatriptan	0.84	−2.06		10.34
Ethylene	1.32	1.32			Fumaric acid	−0.01	−4.95	3.15	
Etidronic acid	−3.54	−9.21	0.68		Furazolidone	−0.04	−0.04		3.12
Etodolac	3.31	0.64	4.31		Furosemide	2.92	−0.80	3.04	
Etomidate	3.36	3.36		4.23	Gabapentin	1.19	−1.31	4.72	10.27
Etonogestrel	4.23	4.22		13.02	Galantamine	2.12	1.13	13.98	7.94
Etoposide	1.97	1.96	9.95		Ganciclovir	−2.07	−2.07	9.15	3.05
Exemestane	3.30	3.30			Gatifloxacin	1.59	−0.92		8.82
Ezetimibe	4.39	4.29	9.66		Gemcitabine	−0.68	−0.68	11.65	4.47
Famciclovir	−0.09	−0.09		4.24	Gemfibrozil	4.39	2.14	4.75	
Famotidine	2.18	−3.02	7.61	7.75	Glimepiride	2.94	1.27	5.34	

(Continued)

Compound	Log P	Log D at ph 7	pKa HA	pKa BH+	Compound	Log P	Log D at ph 7	pKa HA	pKa BH+
Glipizide	2.19	0.52	5.34		Inositol	−2.11	−2.11	12.63	
Glutamic acid	−1.44	−4.92	2.17	9.76	Iodoquinol	4.34	2.14	2.21	7.37
Glutamine	−1.60	−4.10	2.27	9.52	Irinotecan	3.81	1.54	11.00	9.33
Glutaraldehyde	−0.34	−0.33			Isocarboxazid	1.03	1.03	11.26	1.23
Glutethimide	2.70	2.70	11.36		Isoetharine	1.13	−1.03	9.26	9.55
Glyburide	3.93	2.28			Isoflurane	2.79	2.79		
Glycerin	−2.32	−2.32	13.52		Isoniazid	−0.89	−0.89	11.27	3.79
Glycine	−1.03	−3.53	2.43	9.64	Isoproterenol	0.25	−1.87	9.60	9.16
Granisetron HCl	1.95	−1.00	12.39	10.50	Isosorbide	−1.75	−1.75		
Griseofulvin	2.36	2.36			Isosorbide dinitrate	0.90	0.90		
Guaifenesin	0.57	0.57	13.38		Isosorbide mononitrate	−0.51	−0.51	13.09	
Guanadrel	−0.08	−3.18		12.76	Isotretinoin	6.83	4.62	4.79	
Guanethidine	1.07	−3.58		13.43	Isoxsuprine	2.58	1.33	9.47	8.24
Guanfacine	1.12	1.12	11.81	3.75	Isradipine	3.68	3.67		3.81
Guanidine	2.57	0.15		9.66	Itraconazole	3.29	3.15		6.39
Halcinonide	3.32	3.32	13.25		Kanamycin	−2.60		12.94	9.52
Halobetasol propionate	3.92	3.92	12.61		Ketamine	2.15	2.01		6.59
Halofantrine	8.86	6.50	13.56	9.43	Ketoconazole	2.88	2.73		6.54
Haloperidol	4.06	2.80	13.90	8.25	Ketoprofen	2.81	0.07	4.23	
Halothane	2.30	2.30			Ketorolac	2.08	−0.44	4.47	
Hexachlorophene	7.20	7.20	6.58		Ketotifen	4.99	3.25		8.75
Histamine	−0.84	−3.68		10.15	Labetalol	2.87	0.99	7.91	9.20
Homatropine	1.57	−1.17	12.10	9.98	Lactulose	−2.41	−2.41	11.67	
Hydrochlorothiazide	−0.07	−0.08	8.95		Lamivudine	−1.02	−1.02	13.83	4.41
Hydrocortisone	1.43	1.43	12.48		Lamotrigine	−0.19	−0.19		3.31
Hydrocortisone acetate	1.98	1.98	12.42		Lanoxin	1.14	1.14	13.50	
Hydrocortisone buteprate	4.12	4.12			Lansoprazole	2.39	2.38	8.48	3.53
					Latanoprost	3.65	3.65		
Hydrocortisone butyrate	2.81	2.80	12.95		Leflunomide	1.95	1.95	11.74	
Hydrocortisone cypionate	4.53	4.53	12.33		Letrozole	1.52	1.52		3.63
Hydrocortisone valerate	3.34	3.34	12.95		Leucovorin	−8.12	−7.91	3.55	5.01
Hydroflumethiazide	0.54	0.54	8.63		Levalbuterol	0.02	−2.15	9.83	9.22
Hydromorphone	−1.23	−0.21	9.61	8.36	Levamisole	0.54	−1.26		8.81
Hydroquinone	0.64	0.64	10.33		Levarterenol	−0.88	−2.19	9.57	8.30
Hydroxyamphetamine	1.07	−1.84	9.82	10.71	Levetiracetam	−0.67	−0.67		
Hydroxychloroquine	3.54	1.08		8.87	Levobetaxolol	2.69	0.56	13.89	9.17
Hydroxyprogesterone caproate	5.74	5.74			Levobunolol	2.86	0.77	13.84	9.13
Hydroxyurea	−1.80	−1.80	10.56		Levobupivacaine	3.64	2.45		8.17
Hydroxyzine	2.31	2.21		6.34	Levocabastine	4.86	2.36	3.56	9.38
Hyoscyamine sulfate	1.53	−1.21		9.98	Levodopa	−0.23	−2.73	2.24	9.30
Ibuprofen	3.72	1.15	4.41		Levofloxacin	1.49	−1.35	2.27	6.81
Ibutilide fumarate	4.17	1.47	9.57	9.47	Levomethadyl acetate	5.45	3.13		9.40
Idarubicin	2.16	0.43	7.79	8.64	Levonorgestrel	3.92	3.92	13.10	
Ifosfamide	0.63	0.63		4.03	Levorphanol	3.63	1.61	10.41	9.01
Imatinib	1.86	1.18	13.28	7.53	Levothyroxine (T₄; L-thyroxine)	5.96	3.16	2.12	8.94
Imipenem	−2.78	−5.28	4.47	10.37	Lidocaine	2.36	0.83		8.53
Imipramine	4.46	2.07		9.49	Lincomycin	0.86	−0.91	12.91	8.78
Imiquimod	2.61	0.57		9.04	Lindane	3.94	3.94		
Indapamide	2.10	2.09	9.35		Linezolid	−0.92	−0.92		3.94
Indinavir	2.29	2.26		5.73	Liothyronine (T₃; triiodothyronine)	5.12	2.59	2.13	8.96
Indomethacin	3.11	0.30	4.17		Lisinopril	1.75	−1.32	2.18	10.51

(Continued)

Compound	Log P	Log D at ph 7	pK_a HA	pK_a BH+	Compound	Log P	Log D at ph 7	pK_a HA	pK_a BH+
Lodoxamide	0.54	−4.46	2.07		Methoxsalen	1.31	1.31		
Lomefloxacin	2.33	−0.17	2.40	8.82	Methoxyflurane	1.66	1.66		
Lomustine	2.76	2.76	10.88		Methsuximide	2.22	2.22		
Loperamide	4.95	3.87	13.89	8.05	Methyclothiazide	1.76	1.76	9.36	
Lopinavir	5.65	5.64	13.89		Methyldopa	0.13	−2.38	2.28	9.30
Loracarbef	−0.95	−3.79	3.24	6.84	Methylergonovine	1.10	0.62		7.30
Loratadine	6.23	6.23		3.80	Methylphenidate	2.55	−0.42		10.55
Lorazepam	2.48	2.48	10.78	0.03	Methylprednisolone	2.18	2.18	12.48	
Losartan	3.50	0.89	4.24	3.10	Methylprednisolone acetate	2.73	2.73	12.42	
Loteprednol	3.69	3.69			Methyltestosterone	4.02	4.02		
Lovastatin	4.07	4.07	13.49		Metipranolol	2.67	0.53	13.91	9.19
Loxapine	2.99	2.91		6.28	Metoclopramide	2.35	−0.15	13.28	9.62
Lysine	−1.04	−4.52	2.48	10.64	Metolazone	3.16	3.16	10.00	
Mafenide	−0.80	−2.38	10.16	8.58	Metoprolol	1.79	−0.34	13.89	9.17
Malathion	2.93	2.93			Metronidazole	−0.02	−0.02		2.58
Mannitol	−4.67	−4.67	13.14		Metyrosine	0.73	−1.77	2.29	9.35
Maprotiline	4.51	1.52		10.63	Mexiletine	2.16	0.58		8.58
Mebendazole	2.43	2.42	10.29	5.02	Miconazole	6.42	6.25		6.67
Mecamylamine	3.06	−0.02		11.35	Midazolam	3.67	3.68		5.65
Mechlorethamine	1.66	1.33		7.06	Midodrine	−0.32	−1.14	13.53	7.75
Meclizine	5.02	4.83		6.73	Mifepristone	4.91	4.90	12.94	5.19
Meclofenamate	5.90	2.57	3.59		Miglitol	−1.40	−1.42	13.71	5.78
Medroxyprogesterone acetate	4.11	4.11			Milrinone	0.41	0.40	8.83	3.36
Medrysone	2.87	2.87			Minocycline	−0.27	−3.81	4.50	9.74
Mefenamic acid	5.33	2.09	3.69		Minoxidil	0.69	0.69		4.35
Mefloquine	2.87	0.05	13.13	10.13	Mirtazapine	2.52	1.38		8.10
Megestrol acetate	3.82	3.82			Misoprostol	2.91	2.91	13.92	
Meloxicam	2.71	0.22	4.50	3.05	Mitomycin	0.44	0.44	13.27	4.89
Melphalan	2.40	−0.11	2.12	9.54	Mitotane	5.39	5.39		
Meperidine	2.81	1.23		8.55	Mitoxantrone	2.62	−0.90	7.08	9.22
Mephentermine	2.29	−0.62		10.38	Modafinil	1.40	1.40		
Mephobarbital	1.85	1.81	7.97		Moexipril	4.47	1.22	3.57	5.38
Mepivacaine	2.04	0.93		8.09	Molindone	1.96	1.73		6.83
Meprobamate	0.70	0.70	13.09		Mometasone furoate	4.73	4.72	13.08	
Mercaptopurine	0.39	0.37	8.46	2.40	Monobenzone	2.96	2.96	10.28	
Meropenem	−3.13	−5.63	4.47	8.00	Monochloroacetic acid	−0.05	−3.95	2.65	
Mesalamine	0.46	−2.19	1.90	5.43	Monoctanoin	2.12	2.12	13.12	
Mesoridazine	3.98	1.45		9.66	Montelukast	7.85		4.76	
Metaproterenol	0.13	−2.02	9.12	9.33	Moricizine	2.67	2.47	10.27	6.77
Metaraminol	0.07	−1.40	9.75	8.47	Morphine	1.27	0.11	9.72	8.14
Metaxalone	2.42	2.42	12.24		Moxifloxacin	1.97	−0.53	2.17	10.77
Metformin	−2.31	−5.41		13.10	Mupirocin	3.44	1.22	4.78	
Methadone	4.20	2.18		9.05	Mycophenolate mofetil	4.10	4.00	9.98	6.39
Methamphetamine	1.94	−0.97		10.38	Nabumetone	2.82	2.82		
Methazolamide	0.13	0.13	0.33		Nadolol	1.29	−0.84	13.91	9.17
Methenamine	2.17	2.16		5.28	Nafcillin	3.52	−0.40	2.61	
Methimazole	−0.02	−0.02	11.64	1.10	Naftifine	5.67	4.64		7.98
Methionine	0.37	−2.13	2.23	9.26	Nalbuphine	1.96	1.53	9.62	7.22
Methocarbamol	0.55	0.54	13.00		Nalidixic acid	0.18	−3.27	1.20	5.95
Methohexital	2.41	2.36	7.92		Nalmefene	2.82	2.16	9.61	7.56
Methotrexate	−0.28		3.54	5.09	Naloxone	1.92	1.77	9.38	6.61

(Continued)

Compound	Log P	Log D at ph 7	pKa HA	pKa BH+	Compound	Log P	Log D at ph 7	pKa HA	pKa BH+
Naltrexone	1.97	1.42	9.39	7.40	Pantoprazole sodium	1.32	1.16	7.36	3.45
Nandrolone decanoate	8.14	8.14			Papaverine	3.42	3.33		6.38
Naphazoline	3.53	0.65		10.27	Paraldehyde	0.31	0.31		
Naproxen	3.00	0.41	4.40		Paricalcitol	5.83	5.83		
Naratriptan	1.81	−0.71	11.52	9.66	Paromomycin	−3.31		12.93	9.52
Natamycin	0.93	−1.59	3.72	8.13	Paroxetine	3.89	1.00		10.32
Nateglinide	4.57	1.26	3.61		Pemirolast	−0.02	−3.12	2.91	
Nedocromil	2.63	−2.37	2.00		Pemoline	0.52	0.52		1.80
Nefazodone	3.50	3.19		6.75	Penbutolol	4.17	2.05	13.90	9.17
Nelfinavir	6.55	5.91	9.58	7.53	Penciclovir	−2.03	−2.03	9.50	3.55
Nevirapine	−0.31	−0.31	10.93	4.74	Penicillamine	0.93	−1.60	2.13	11.54
Niacin	0.82	−2.58	2.17	4.82	Penicillin G	1.67	−2.25	2.62	
Niacinamide	−0.11	−0.11		3.54	Penicillin V	1.88	−2.04	2.62	
Nicardipine	5.22	4.86		7.11	Pentamidine	2.47	−0.65		11.67
Nicotine	0.72	−0.32		8.00	Pentazocine	5.00	3.08	10.36	8.90
Nifedipine	3.05	3.05		3.93	Pentobarbital	2.10	2.04	7.88	
Nilutamide	3.15	3.08	7.73		Pentostatin	−2.82	−3.15	12.88	7.62
Nimodipine	3.94	3.94		4.01	Pentoxifylline	0.37	0.37		1.36
Nisoldipine	4.46	4.46		3.91	Pergolide	3.97	1.44		9.66
Nitazoxanide	0.83	0.83	10.16		Perindopril	3.36	0.27	3.72	5.74
Nitrofurantoin	−0.55	−0.63	7.69	1.20	Permethrin	6.74	6.74		
Nitrofurazone	0.09	0.09	11.15	3.87	Perphenazine	4.49	3.94		7.22
Nitroglycerin	2.22	2.22			Phenazopyridine	2.55	2.55		4.16
Nitrous oxide	−1.28	−1.28			Phendimetrazine	1.62	1.31		7.02
Nizatidine	1.23	0.75		7.31	Phenelzine	1.14	−0.22		8.34
Norelgestromin	4.40	4.40	12.47		Phenindamine	4.41	3.21		8.07
Norethindrone acetate	3.99	3.99	2.75	8.76	Phenobarbital	1.71	1.62	7.63	
Norfloxacin	1.47	−1.03			Phenoxybenzamine	5.18	5.04		6.58
Nortriptyline	5.65	2.86		10.08	Phentermine	2.16	−0.56		9.94
Ofloxacin	1.49	−1.35	2.27	6.81	Phentolamine	3.60	0.70	9.65	10.31
Olanzapine	3.30	3.20		6.37	Phenylacetic acid	1.51	−1.18	4.30	
Olmesartan medoxomil	4.87	2.26	4.23	4.24	Phenylephrine	−0.30	−2.20	9.76	9.22
Olopatadine	4.37	1.86	4.29	9.19	Phenytoin	2.52	2.52	8.33	
Olsalazine	3.94	−1.06	2.70		Physostigmine	1.16	−0.29	12.23	8.44
Omeprazole	1.80	1.80	9.08	4.61	Phytonadione	12.25	12.25		
Ondansetron	2.49	1.84		7.54	Pilocarpine	−0.10	−0.54		7.25
Orlistat	8.95	8.94			Pimecrolimus	5.21	5.21	9.96	
Orphenadrine	4.12	2.41		8.72	Pimozide	6.08	3.74	12.11	9.42
Oseltamivir	1.50	−0.30		8.81	Pindolol	1.97	−0.19	13.94	9.21
Oxacillin	2.05	−1.87	2.61		Pioglitazone	3.16	2.40	6.35	5.56
Oxandrolone	3.33	3.33			Piperacillin	1.88	−2.04	2.62	
Oxaprozin	4.19	1.40	4.19	0.36	Pirbuterol	−1.63	−3.17	7.81	8.82
Oxazepam	2.31	2.31	10.94	1.68	Piroxicam	1.71	−0.78	4.50	3.60
Oxcarbazepine	1.25	1.25	13.73		Plicamycin	1.39		4.54	
Oxiconazole	5.89	5.82		6.19	Podofilox	1.29	1.29	13.42	
Oxybutynin	5.19	3.93	11.94	8.24	Polythiazide	1.55	1.54	9.37	
Oxycodone	1.84	1.19	13.45	7.53	Pramipexole	1.62	−0.77		9.46
Oxymetazoline	4.17	1.20	11.96	10.53	Pramoxine	3.51	2.95		7.42
Oxymetholone	4.22	1.72	4.50		Pravastatin	1.44	−1.24	4.31	
Oxymorphone	1.07	0.46	9.40	7.48	Praziquantel	2.44	2.44		
Oxytetracycline	−1.22	−4.83	4.50	9.26	Prazosin	−1.14	−1.25		6.47
Pamidronic acid	−3.40	−7.80	0.18	8.93	Prednicarbate	3.82	3.82		

(Continued)

Compound	Log P	Log D at ph 7	pK$_a$ HA	pK$_a$ BH$^+$	Compound	Log P	Log D at ph 7	pK$_a$ HA	pK$_a$ BH$^+$
Prednisolone	1.69	1.69	12.47		Ritonavir	5.08	5.08	11.47	3.48
Prednisolone acetate	2.24	2.24	12.41		Rivastigmine	2.14	0.52		8.62
Prednisolone tebutate	4.00	4.00	12.32		Rizatriptan	0.76	−1.64		9.49
Prilocaine	1.74	0.75		7.95	Rofecoxib	1.63	1.63		
Primaquine	2.67	−0.25		10.38	Ropinirole	3.19	0.81		9.47
Primidone	−0.84	−0.84	12.26		Ropivacaine	3.11	1.92		8.17
Probenecid	3.30	0.06	3.69		Rosiglitazone	2.56	1.71	6.34	6.48
Procainamide	1.23	−1.43		9.86	Salicylic acid	2.06	−1.68	3.01	
Procaine	2.91	0.72		9.24	Salmeterol	3.16	0.97	9.82	9.23
Procarbazine	0.77	0.11		7.46	Scopolamine	1.34	0.29		8.01
Prochlorperazine	4.76	3.69		7.82	Secobarbital	2.33	2.27	7.81	
Procyclidine	4.50	1.55		10.48	Selegiline	2.92	2.28		7.53
Progesterone	4.04	4.04			Sertraline	4.77	2.39		9.47
Proguanil	2.46	−0.59		11.30	Sevoflurane	2.48	2.48		
Promethazine	4.69	2.73		8.98	Sibutramine	5.43	2.88		9.68
Propafenone	4.63	2.39	13.82	9.31	Sildenafil	2.28	1.47	9.35	7.74
Proparacaine HCl	3.55	1.40		9.20	Simvastatin	4.41	4.41	13.49	
Propofol	4.16	4.16	11.00		Sirolimus	3.58	3.58	10.40	
Propoxyphene	5.44	3.29		9.19	Sorbitol	−4.67	−4.67	13.14	
Propranolol	3.10	0.99	13.84	9.14	Sotalol	0.32	−1.82	9.55	9.19
Propylthiouracil	1.37	1.24	7.63	0.54	Sparfloxacin	2.87	0.36	2.27	8.88
Protriptyline	5.06	2.08		10.61	Spectinomycin	1.17	−1.00	9.25	8.56
Pseudoephedrine	1.05	−1.25	13.96	9.38	Spironolactone	3.12	3.12		
Pyrantel	1.37	−1.67		10.97	Stanozolol	5.53	5.53		4.08
Pyrazinamide	−0.37	−0.37	13.91		Stavudine	−0.91	−0.91	9.57	
Pyridoxine	−1.90	−2.12	8.37	5.06	Streptozocin	−1.55	−1.55	9.36	
Pyrimethamine	2.87	2.67		6.77	Succinic acid	−0.59	−4.75	4.24	
Pyrithione	−0.05	−2.35	4.70		Sufentanil	3.42	2.16		8.24
Quazepam	3.87	3.87		0.85	Sulconazole	6.03	5.90		6.56
Quetiapine	1.83	1.82		5.34	Sulfacetamide	−0.90	−2.14	5.78	0.93
Quinapril	4.73	1.30	3.29	5.38	Sulfadiazine	−0.12	−0.74	6.50	1.57
Quinidine	−1.55	1.35	13.05	9.13	Sulfadoxine	0.34	−0.56	6.16	3.15
Quinine	3.44	1.35	13.05	9.13	Sulfasalazine	3.18	−0.63	2.88	1.86
Rabeprazole	1.46	1.44	8.50	4.42	Sulfinpyrazone	2.32	−1.01	3.60	
Raloxifene	6.80	5.12	8.98	8.67	Sulfisoxazole	1.01	−1.12	4.83	1.52
Ramipril	3.97	0.85	3.72	5.51	Sulindac	3.56	0.80	4.22	
Ranitidine	1.28	−0.13		8.40	Sumatriptan	0.67	−1.73	11.31	9.49
Remifentanil	2.00	1.87		6.55	Suprofen	2.42	−0.49	4.07	
Repaglinide	4.86	2.10	4.19	5.78	Tacrine	3.32	0.69		9.64
Reserpine	4.37	3.93		7.25	Tacrolimus	3.96	3.96	9.96	
Retinol	6.84	6.84			Tamoxifen	7.88	6.20		8.69
Ribavirin	−2.63	−2.63	12.95	1.00	Tamsulosin	2.24	0.51	10.08	8.74
Riboflavin	−2.02	−4.68	4.32		Tazarotene	6.22	6.21		0.04
Rifabutin	−3.07				Tazobactam	−1.68	−5.68	2.33	0.88
Rifampin	0.49	−1.75	4.92	6.57	Tegaserod	2.19	−0.17		11.21
Rifapentine	1.98				Telmisartan	7.80	4.79	3.83	5.83
Riluzole	2.84	2.75		6.38	Temazepam	3.10	3.10	11.84	1.58
Rimantadine	3.10	0.03		11.17	Temozolomide	−1.32			
Rimexolone	4.21	4.21			Teniposide	3.10	3.10		
Risedronic acid	−2.94	−8.56	0.32	5.09	Tenofovir disoproxil	1.97	1.97		4.67
Risperidone	2.85	1.88		7.91	Terazosin	−0.96	−1.08		6.47
Ritodrine	1.61	−0.48	9.13		Terbinafine	6.49	6.15		7.07

Compound	Log P	Log D at ph 7	pK$_a$ HA	pK$_a$ BH$^+$	Compound	Log P	Log D at ph 7	pK$_a$ HA	pK$_a$ BH$^+$
Terbutaline	0.48	−1.67	9.12	9.33	Triamcinolone hexacetonide	5.08	5.08	13.15	
Terconazole	3.98	3.36		7.46	Triamterene	1.30	1.22		6.30
Testolactone	2.72	2.72			Triazolam	2.67	2.67		2.32
Testosterone	3.47	3.47			Trichlormethiazide	0.57	0.32	7.12	
Testosterone cypionate	6.93	6.93			Trichloroacetic acid	1.67	−2.42	1.10	
Testosterone enanthate	7.03	7.03			Triclosan	5.82	5.75	7.80	
Tetracaine	3.49	2.23		8.24	Trifluoperazine	5.11	4.04		7.82
Tetrahydrozoline	3.31	0.38		10.42	Trifluridine	0.01	−0.69	6.40	
Theophylline	0.05	0.04	8.60	1.05	Trihexyphenidyl	5.06	2.42		9.83
Thiabendazole	2.87	2.86	9.38	3.58	Trimethadione	0.31	0.31		
Thiethylperazine	5.05	3.98		7.82	Trimethobenzamide	2.91	1.25		
Thioguanine	−0.26	−0.40	7.44	3.09	Trimethoprim	0.79	0.28		7.34
Thiopental	3.00	2.93	7.76		Trimetrexate	1.23	−2.03		10.35
Thioridazine	6.13	3.60		9.66	Trimipramine	4.81	2.51		9.37
Thiotepa	0.52				Trioxsalen	3.80	3.80		
Thiothixene	3.89	2.96		7.74	Triprolidine	4.44	2.36		9.12
Threonine	−1.23	−3.73	2.19	9.64	Troleandomycin	3.36	2.46		7.84
Tiagabine	5.65	3.15	3.88	9.44	Tropicamide	1.16	1.14		5.49
Ticarcillin	0.69	−4.31	2.62		Trovafloxacin	1.57	−0.95	0.64	8.43
Ticlopidine	3.53	3.21		7.05	Undecylenic acid	3.99	1.77	4.78	
Tiludronic acid	−0.51	−6.30	0.45		Unoprostone isopropyl ester	4.63	4.63		
Timolol	−4.30	−1.99	13.38	8.86	Urea	−2.11	−2.11		0.10
Tioconazole	5.79	5.61		6.71	Ursodiol	4.66	2.42	4.76	
Tiopronin	−0.33	−3.64	3.62		Valacyclovir	0.40	−0.78	9.17	7.75
Tirofiban	4.14	1.64	3.37	11.23	Valdecoxib	1.44	1.44	9.83	
Tizanidine	0.65	−1.47		9.18	Valganciclovir	−0.36	−1.16	9.13	7.73
Tobramycin	−3.44	−10.01	13.07	9.52	Valproic acid	2.72	0.54	4.82	
Tocainide	0.76	−0.37		8.10	Valrubicin	5.25	4.89	7.11	
α-Tocopherol	11.86	11.86	11.40		Venlafaxine HCl	2.91	0.70		9.26
Tolazamide	1.71	0.47			Verapamil	4.91	2.91		9.03
Tolbutamide	2.34	0.80			Vidarabine	−1.46	−1.46	13.11	3.25
Tolcapone	4.15	1.98	4.78		Vinblastine	4.22	3.45	11.36	7.64
Tolmetin	1.55	−0.98	4.46		Vincristine	2.84	2.10	11.07	7.64
Tolnaftate	5.48	5.48			Vinorelbine	5.42	5.03	11.34	7.09
Tolterodine	5.77	2.80	10.00	10.78	Volsartan	4.38	−0.57	3.69	
Topotecan	0.79	0.55	7.20	2.28	Voriconazole	0.72	0.72	12.00	4.98
Toremifene	7.96	6.32		8.63	Warfarin	3.47	0.98	4.50	
Torsemide	3.17	0.53	3.08	4.80	Xylometazoline	4.91	1.92		10.62
Tramadol	2.51	0.40		9.16	Yohimbine	1.91	0.47		8.44
Trandolapril	4.53	1.41	3.72	5.51	Zafirlukast	6.15	2.65	3.37	
Tranexamic acid	0.32	−2.19	4.77	10.39	Zalcitabine	−1.51	−1.51		4.47
Tranylcypromine	1.21	−0.56		8.78	Zaleplon	1.00	1.00		
Travoprost	4.06	4.06	13.50		Zanamivir	−3.75	−6.25	3.92	11.65
Trazodone	1.66	1.52		6.59	Zileuton	3.74	3.74	9.99	
Treprostinil	4.09	0.47	3.19		Ziprasidone	4.02	2.75	13.34	8.24
Tretinoin	6.83	4.62	4.79		Zoledronic acid	−2.28	−7.04	0.32	6.78
Triacetin	−0.24	−0.24			Zolmitriptan	1.64	−0.78	12.57	9.52
Triamcinolone	1.03	1.03	11.58		Zolpidem	2.61	2.35		6.91
Triamcinolone acetonide	2.60	2.60	12.69		Zonisamide	−0.10	−0.10	9.56	
Triamcinolone diacetate	1.82	1.82	11.21						

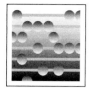

INDEX

Note: Page numbers followed by "f" indicate figures; those followed by "t" indicate tables. Drugs are listed under the generic name.

A

Abbokinase. *See* Urokinase
Abciximab, 190, 634, 860t
Abelcet. *See* Amphotericin B
Ab initio methods, 938
Abortifacients, 795
Absolute ethanol, 220
Acarbose, 672
Accutane. *See* Isotretinoin
ACE. *See* Angiotensin-converting enzyme
Acebutolol, 544–545, 545f
ACE inhibitors
    development of, 940
    prodrug forms of, 646–648, 647f, 647t
Acellular vaccines, 207–208
Acetaminophen, 761t, 762, 822
    arachidonic acid metabolism and, 822
    mechanism of action of, 822
    metabolism of, 96–98, 112, 115, 120
Acetanilid, 760, 761t, 762
Acetazolamide, 603, 604f, 605, 619
Acetohexamide, 668, 669–670
    active metabolites of, 135t
    metabolism of, 82, 103–105
Acetophenone, metabolism of, 103
p-Acetoxyacetanilid, 761t, 762
Acetoxyethyl onium salts, 557t
Acetoxyphenylmercury, 230
2-Acetylaminofluorene (AAF)
    metabolism of, 96
    toxicity of, 115–116
Acetylation, in drug metabolism, 121–124, 123f
    racial/ethnic differences in, 124
Acetylation polymorphism, 122–124
Acetylcholine (ACh), 548
    conformation of, 34–35, 34f, 555–556
    ganglionic stimulation by, 586–588, 587f
    hydrolysis of, 561–563, 561t, 562f, 563t
    muscarinic receptors and, 550, 551, 552, 557–558, 557f, 557t
    neuromuscular junction transmission and, 589
    as neurotransmitter, 548, 550, 551, 552, 557–558, 557f, 557t, 586–588, 587f
    nicotinic effect of, 587–588, 590
    pharmaceutical, 558
    release of, 553f, 554, 683
    storage of, 553f, 554
    structure–activity relationships for, 557–558
    structure of, 550
    synthesis of, 553–554, 553f, 554f
Acetylcholine chloride, 558
Acetylcholine receptor, 549–550, 684–685
Acetylcholinesterase (AChE), 548, 553–554, 553f, 554f, 560–561, 561t
    action of, 561–563, 561t, 562f, 563t
    phosphorylation of, 568, 568f
    reactivation of, 568f, 569
Acetylcholinesterase inhibitors, 563–569, 563t

Acetyl-CoA, 553, 554, 554f
    in drug metabolism, 122
Acetylmethadol, active metabolites of, 135t
N-Acetylprocainamide, metabolism of, 124
Acetylsalicylic acid. *See* Aspirin
Achromycin. *See* Tetracycline
Acid(s), 9–17
    BH$^+$ (ionized), 15–16, 16t
    conjugate, 9
    definition of, 9
    examples of, 10t
    HA (unionized), 15–16, 16t
    ionic form of, 15–16, 15f, 16t
    pH of, calculation of, 13
    pK$_a$ of, 13–14, 14t
    strength of, 11–14
Acid–base balance, 3
Acid–base reactions, 11–13, 12t
    direction of, 13
Acid–conjugate base, 9–11
Aciphex. *See* Rabeprazole sodium
Acitretin, 874
    half-life of, 6
Acivicin, 420
Aclacinomycin A, 416
Aclarubicin, 416
Aclometasone dipropionate, 808f, 812
Aclovate. *See* Aclometasone dipropionate
Acquired immunity, 200, 200t
Acquired immunodeficiency syndrome. *See* Human immunodeficiency virus
Acrivastine, 714–715
Acrodynia, 891
ACTH. *See* Adrenocorticotropic hormone (ACTH)
ACTH-80. *See* Repository corticotropin injection
Acthar. *See* Corticotropin injection
ACTH injection, 842, 842t
Acthrel. *See* Corticorelin
Actidil. *See* Triprolidine hydrochloride
Actimmune. *See* Interferon gamma-1b
Actinomycin C$_1$, 414, 415, 421–422
Actinomycin C$_3$, 415
Actinomycin D, 414, 415
Actinomycins, 300t, 414–415, 421–422
Action potential, 680–681, 683
Activase. *See* Alteplase
Active analogue approach, 944
Activella. *See* Hormone replacement therapy
Active-site–directed irreversible inhibition, 29
Active tubular secretion, 601–602, 602f
Actos. *See* Pioglitazone
Acuretic. *See* Quinapril hydrochloride
Acute phase proteins, 201, 201t
Acyclovir, 377
Acylases, 306
Acylureidopenicillins, 308
Adalat. *See* Nifedipine
Adapalene, 874

Adapin. *See* Doxepin hydrochloride
Adaptive immunity, 200, 200t
Adaptogen, 913
Addiction liability, 732
Addison's disease, 810
Adenohypophysis, 841
Adenosine, as sleep-promoting agent, 488
Adenosine arabinoside, 376, 405, 408
Adenosine deaminase inhibitors, 408
Adenosine monophosphate (AMP), 551, 553
    in smooth muscle relaxation, 623–624, 624f
S-Adenosylmethionine (SAM), in methylation, 125, 126f
Adenylate cyclase, 553
ADMET properties
    definition of, 54, 60
    high-throughput screening for, 54
    Lipinski Rule of Five for, 40, 54
    prediction of, 944–945
    of recombinant drugs, 175
    virtual (in silico) screening for, 55, 919
Adrenal cortex hormones, 803–815. *See also* Glucocorticoid(s); Mineralocorticoid(s)
Adrenaline, 678. *See also* Epinephrine
Adrenergic agents, 524–546
    centrally acting, 652–653
    definition of, 524
    sympatholytics, 524
    sympathomimetics, 524
Adrenergic-blocking agents, 524, 651–652
Adrenergic neurotransmitters, 524–547
    biosynthesis of, 524–525, 524f
    properties of, 524
    receptors for, 527–528
    structure of, 524
    as sympathomimetics, 532
    uptake and metabolism of, 525–527, 526f
Adrenergic receptor antagonists, 539–546
    α, 539–540
    β, 541–546
Adrenergic receptors
    α, 527–528
    β, 528
    heterogeneity of, 169–170, 170t
Adrenergic stimulants, 524
Adrenergic system inhibitors, 649–650
Adrenocorticotropic hormone (ACTH), 805, 841
    biological activities of, 841
    hydrocortisone and, 806
    products, 842–844, 842t
    structure–activity relationships for, 841
Adriamycin. *See* Doxorubicin
Adriamycinol, 416
Advil. *See* Ibuprofen
AeroBid. *See* Flunisolide
Aerosporin. *See* Polymyxin B sulfate
Affinity chromatography, in receptor isolation, 28
Aflatoxin B$_1$, hepatocarcinogenicity of, 76–77